The Royal Marsden Manual of

Clinical Nursing Procedures

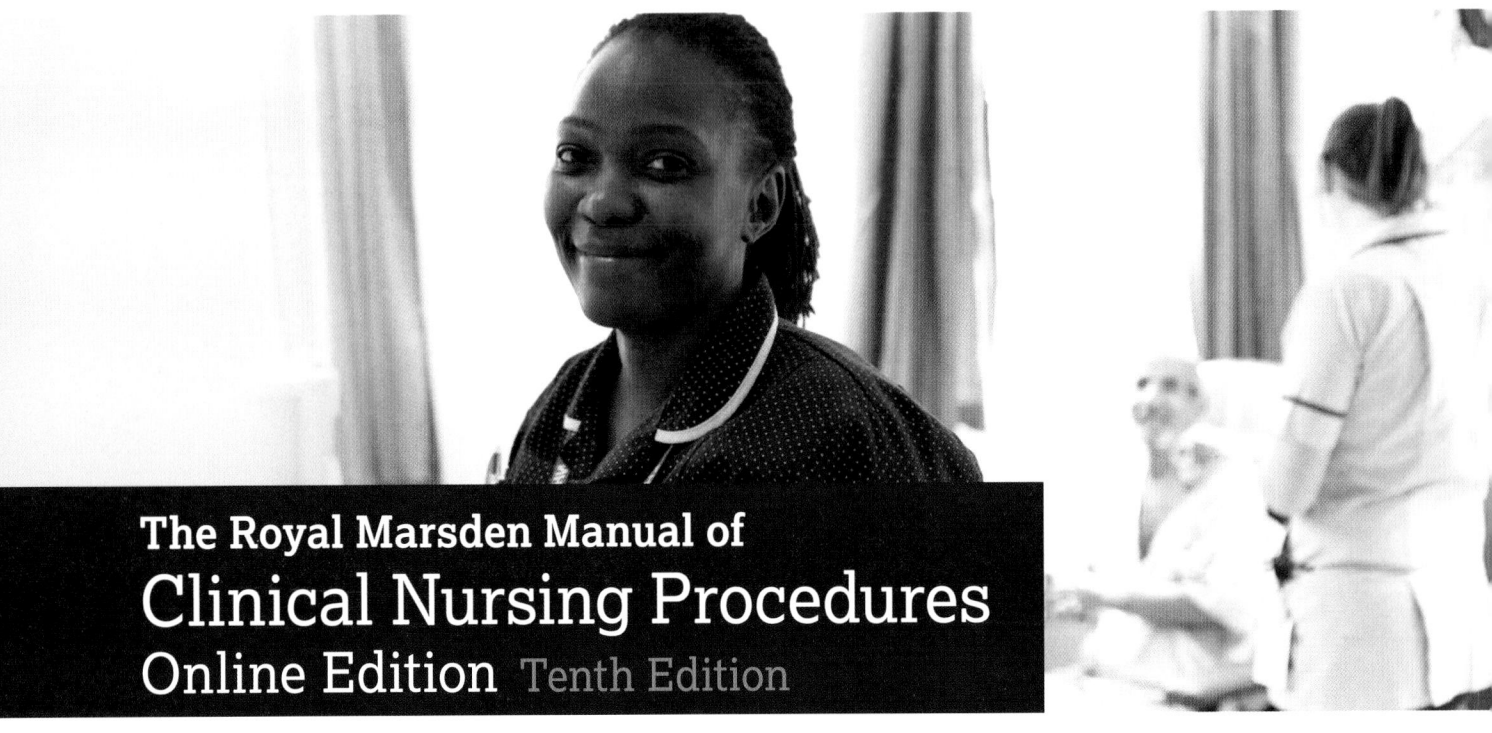

Professional Edition

The Royal Marsden Manual of Clinical Nursing Procedures

Tenth Edition

Edited by

Sara Lister

RN, BSc (Hons), PGDAE, MSc, Dip, MA, MBACP

Head of Pastoral Care and Psychological Support

The Royal Marsden NHS Foundation Trust

Justine Hofland

RN, BSc (Hons), ANP, MSc, PG Dip, ILM Level 5

Divisional Clinical Nurse Director

Cancer Services

The Royal Marsden NHS Foundation Trust

Hayley Grafton

RN, BSc (Hons), CPPD ITU

Chief Nursing Information Officer

The Royal Marsden NHS Foundation Trust

The ROYAL MARSDEN
NHS Foundation Trust

WILEY Blackwell

This edition first published 2020

Edition History
The Royal Marsden NHS Foundation Trust (3e, 1992; 4e, 1996; 5e, 2000; 6e, 2004; 7e, 2008; 8e, 2011; 9e, 2015)

Registered Offices
John Wiley & Sons, Inc., 111 River Street, Hoboken, NJ 07030, USA
John Wiley & Sons Ltd, The Atrium, Southern Gate, Chichester, West Sussex, PO19 8SQ, UK

Editorial Office
9600 Garsington Road, Oxford, OX4 2DQ, UK
For details of our global editorial offices, customer services, and more information about Wiley products visit us at www.wiley.com.

Wiley also publishes its books in a variety of electronic formats and by print-on-demand. Some content that appears in standard print versions of this book may not be available in other formats.

Library of Congress Cataloging-in-Publication Data

Names: Lister, Sara, editor. | Hofland, Justine, editor. | Grafton, Hayley, editor.
Title: The Royal Marsden manual of clinical nursing procedures / edited by Sara Lister, Justine Hofland, Hayley Grafton.
Other titles: Manual of clinical nursing procedures
Description: Tenth edition. | Hoboken, NJ : Wiley-Blackwell, 2020. | Includes bibliographical references and index.
Identifiers: LCCN 2020001579 (print) | LCCN 2020001580 (ebook) | ISBN 9781119510970 (cloth) | ISBN 9781119634386 (paperback) | ISBN 9781119510994 (adobe pdf) | ISBN 9781119511038 (epub)
Subjects: MESH: Nursing Care–methods | Nursing Process | Nursing Theory | Patient Care Planning
Classification: LCC RT41 (print) | LCC RT41 (ebook) | NLM WY 100.1 | DDC 610.73–dc23
LC record available at https://lccn.loc.gov/2020001579
LC ebook record available at https://lccn.loc.gov/2020001580

Cover image: Labor Omnia Vincit Crest is a registered Trademark of The Royal Marsden NHS Foundation Trust
Cover design by Wiley

Set in 9/10pt Lexia by SPi Global, Pondicherry, India

Printed in Singapore
M001033L_000033

Brief table of contents

Detailed table of contents

Foreword to the tenth edition

Being asked to write a foreword for this tenth edition of *The Royal Marsden Manual of Clinical Nursing Procedures* is a great honour. Since it was first published back in 1992, the manual has gained a strong international reputation and is in daily use by nurses across the world, ensuring that their practice is both evidence based and effective. As such, and with the ever-increasing availability of clinical information to all those with vested interests in healthcare, the regular updating of this manual takes on more and more significance.

This manual draws together up-to-date procedures and practices, providing an essential resource of current knowledge against which nurses can critically analyse the judgements they exercise in a variety of clinical settings. Nursing care in 2020 is under constant scrutiny, and nurses are called upon on a daily basis to provide reassurance to patients, their families and loved ones, and the public at large. This *Royal Marsden Manual of Clinical Nursing Procedures* is a real practical help to all engaged in providing nursing care, whether in a ward, over the telephone, in a day-care setting or in the wider community. Users of this tenth edition will discover a new chapter on wellbeing and self-care, as well as additional information on topics such as falls management and antibiotic resistance, to name but two. Keeping up to date also involves embracing new technologies, and as such the manual's online version has been enhanced, further increasing accessibility, and for the first time includes helpful videos of some of the more complex procedures.

The Standards of Proficiency for Registered Nurses, launched by the Nursing and Midwifery Council in January 2019, are an explicit statement to the public of the skills and knowledge they can expect from the nurses who care for them. This manual is an excellent resource for nurses wanting to enhance or update their skills in light of those proficiencies; indeed, each chapter begins with a statement of the proficiencies to which it relates.

Traditionally, one huge strength of this manual has been that it has benefited from contributions from nurses who are both expert and active in clinical practice, and this edition is no exception. There are additional valuable contributions from their healthcare colleagues. This has the double advantage not only of ensuring that the manual reflects the reality of current practice but also ensuring that nurses and other staff at The Royal Marsden NHS Foundation Trust are frequently reviewing the evidence and reflecting upon their care.

Wherever they work across the globe, those involved in nursing are united in their dedication to providing care that is individually and sensitively planned. To provide this care, they need ready access to the most reliable, up-to-date sources of the best available evidence. In commending this tenth edition of *The Royal Marsden Manual of Clinical Nursing Procedures* to you, I have no doubt that it will play a huge part in enabling nurses to perform their core functions. It is fitting that this manual, with its international outlook, should carry the name of the Royal Marsden Hospital, which also enjoys a worldwide reputation for excellence.

A work of this renown and complexity does not come to fruition without a great deal of hard work and I would like to pay a warm tribute to the editors of this tenth edition. Of these, Sara Lister has nurtured the development of the manual since its sixth edition, in 2004; by contrast, Justine Hofland and Hayley Grafton have joined Sara this year as new editors and their input has been considerable. I would also like to pay tribute to all the nurses and allied health professionals at the Royal Marsden Hospital who have worked so diligently to help produce this tenth edition.

Eamonn Sullivan
Chief Nurse
The Royal Marsden NHS Foundation Trust

Preface

It is a privilege to write the preface for this tenth celebratory edition of *The Royal Marsden Manual of Clinical Nursing Procedures*. It is over 30 years since the first edition of the manual was published. The first edition was initially written for the nursing staff of the hospital with the aim of creating a reference that drew together information from diverse sources. The introduction to that first edition stated that intentionally it was 'very different from others [textbooks] that you may have used, because it gives the *why* as well as the *how* for each policy and procedure' (Royal Marsden Hospital 1984). In the foreword, the Chief Nursing Officer, Robert Tiffany, anticipated that 'the work would soon become an essential resource for individuals and organizations alike'. He wasn't wrong – in 2019 it was the best-selling nursing textbook in the UK.

Over the thirty years that the manual has been in use, there have been many expert nurses (and more recently their professional colleagues from other professions) who have given their time to write so that knowledge could be made available to improve care of patients. Over the past 20 years, Dr Lisa Dougherty was 'the manual', and upon her retirement she leaves a legacy with a national and international reputation.

With such a reputation to maintain, the work of updating and revising the manual is not one to be taken lightly. With each new edition come requests for more content and additional procedures alongside – paradoxically – requests to make it a slimmer, easier-to-handle textbook. Core principles guide the decisions that are made about what to include in each new edition:

- The emphasis has always been on the procedures of nursing; the manual is not about the nursing care of an individual with a specific condition.
- The aim is for the manual to be used in practice, so the core of each chapter is the procedures. However, it is not just about *how* to do a procedure but also about understanding the reasons *why*.
- The aim is for the manual to be the 'go-to' reference for clinical areas by drawing together information in one place.
- The rationales underpinning the procedures are drawn from a breadth of sources. As would be expected, these include research findings, national and professional guidelines, and policy, but in addition practice-based evidence is essential. This means that only procedures that are part of nursing care at the Royal Marsden are included to ensure that expertise from practice informs each chapter.

As the first edition of the manual was published in 1984, I was beginning my nursing training at a neighbouring hospital. The focus of nursing, where I trained, was the patient, but alongside that was an increasing awareness that some of the procedures that we carried out were driven by tradition and ritual. There was an appetite for professional research-based practice. *The Royal Marsden Manual* at that time was fulfilling an emerging need.

Over the following years, evidence-based practice came into use more frequently and the scope of practice of nurses broadened, and so too did the structure and content of the manual. In the seventh edition (2008), a system was introduced that made explicit the type of evidence underpinning the steps in a procedure.

The ability to think critically and provide evidence-based care is at the heart of the role of the nurse in the 21st century:

> Registered nurses play a vital role in providing, leading and coordinating care that is compassionate, evidence-based, and person-centred. … The confidence and ability to think critically, apply knowledge and skills, and provide expert, evidence-based, direct nursing care therefore lies at the centre of all registered nursing practice. (NMC 2018a)

In the eighth edition, a new structure was introduced that included more of the background information that might be necessary to fully understand the steps in a procedure, such as anatomy and physiology, explanation of equipment choices, and relevant professional and legislative guidance. Along with this came the first online version, which was available to organizations.

This tenth edition reflects the work that is beginning on preparing nurses for the future, linking content (as appropriate) to *Future Nurse: Standards of Proficiency for Registered Nurses* (NMC 2018b). It also includes expanded content on mental capacity and safeguarding. The 'Legal and professional issues' section has been replaced with 'Clinical governance'. A new chapter on self-care and wellbeing has also been included, reflecting the expectation that nurses 'must be emotionally intelligent and resilient individuals, who are able to manage their own personal health and wellbeing, and know when and how to access support' (NMC 2018b).

I am proud to write the preface to the tenth edition of *The Royal Marsden Manual of Clinical Nursing Procedures*; I am proud that this resource has been invaluable to nurses in the UK and abroad in a variety of clinical settings, as Robert Tiffany hoped it would be; I am proud that nursing has not just talked about ritualized practice but has taken steps to become evidence based, with a critical approach to patient care; I am proud that nurses have read and used the manual, and most importantly have given feedback when what they read wasn't clear or wasn't right. The foreword to the second edition ends by stating that the text wasn't a 'final document'! As the tenth edition goes to print, I would echo that sentiment: the manual is always a work in progress – and even more so with the online edition. Work begins on the next edition as soon as this one goes to print, so please keep telling us what we need to do differently. This is your manual.

Sara Lister
Joint editor of the sixth, seventh, eighth, ninth and tenth editions

References

NMC (Nursing and Midwifery Council) (2018a) *The Code: Professional Standards of Practice and Behaviour for Nurses, Midwives and Nursing Associates.* Available at: https://www.nmc.org.uk/standards/code

NMC (2018b) *Future Nurse: Standards of Proficiency for Registered Nurses.* Available at: https://www.nmc.org.uk/globalassets/sitedocuments/education-standards/future-nurse-proficiencies.pdf

Royal Marsden Hospital (1984) *The Royal Marsden Hospital Manual of Clinical Nursing Policies and Procedures.* London: Harper & Row.

Acknowledgements

Writing a textbook of such breadth and complexity as this is never the task of a few. Over a hundred healthcare professionals who either work for, or are associated with, The Royal Marsden NHS Foundation Trust have contributed to updating the content for this edition. A big thank you to them for the great patience they have shown to the editors every time we went back to them – yet again – with a query. We know how incredibly busy you all are. Among all of those we must thank, we have to make a special mention of the Knowledge Resource Manager, Yi Wen Hon, and her incredible ability to promptly find just the reference we needed. We must also express our gratitude to the medical photographers, Stephen Milward and Denis Underwood.

We acknowledge The Royal Marsden NHS Foundation Trust as an organization. The trust's ongoing commitment to excellence in every aspect of patient care is evident in its continued support of this project, which has now been going for over 30 years.

Our thanks must also go to our publisher, John Wiley & Sons, and specifically to Magenta Styles, who has kept alive the significance of this book for nursing in the UK. She has been very gracious when we have missed deadlines. Thanks also to Alison Nick, our project editor, who has been amazing and who has done so much more than her 'job description', and to Hazel Bird, copy editor, whose intelligent and thoughtful attention to detail has been nothing short of phenomenal.

Finally, as editors, we are very grateful for the support of our families, whether they have provided technical assistance when computers have crashed, read through our drafts to make sure they made sense, or been so understanding when we have 'preferred' to read a manuscript rather than a bedtime story.

Sara Lister
Justine Hofland
Hayley Grafton
Editors

List of contributors

Chapter 1 The context of nursing

Sara Lister RN, BSc (Hons), PGDAE, MSc, Dip, MA, MBACP
Head of Pastoral Care and Psychological Support

Chapter 2 Admissions and assessment

Lorraine Guinan RN, INP, ANP, BSc (Hons), MSc
Advanced Nurse Practitioner, Head and Neck

Victoria Ward RN, INP, ANP, BN (Hons), MSc
Transformation Project Manager

Elizabeth Hendry RN, BN (Hons), PG Dip
Formerly Ward Sister

Emma Masters RN, BSc, MSc
Formerly Advanced Nurse Practitioner, Teenage and Young Adults

Andrew Rayner RN, BSc (Hons), INP, PG Dip
Divisional Clinical Nurse Director, Clinical Services

Emma Thistlethwayte RN, BSc (Hons)
Transplant Clinical Nurse Specialist, Teenage and Young Adult

Manuela Trofor RN, MSc
Matron, Medical Day Unit

Charlotte Weston RN, BSc (Hons), MSc
Formerly Lead Nurse, Teenage and Young Adults

Claire White RN, BSc (Hons)
Acting Matron, Cancer Services

Chapter 3 Discharge care and planning

Caroline Watts RN, BSc (Hons), PG Dip, MSc, INP, ANP
Nurse Lead for Transformation

Emma Collard PG Cert, BSc (Hons), Dip HE
Matron, Palliative Care

Connie Lewis CQSW
Discharge Lead

Chapter 4 Infection prevention and control

Pat Cattini RN, MSc
Lead Nurse and Deputy Director, Infection Prevention and Control

Martin Kiernan RN, ENB 329, MPH
Visiting Clinical Fellow, Richard Wells Research Centre, University of West London, and Director of Clinical Research and Education, GAMA Healthcare

Chapter 5 Communication, psychological wellbeing and safeguarding

Justin Grayer BSc, PG Dip, DClinPsych
Consultant Clinical Psychologist and Lead for Adult Psychological Support Team

Jennie Baxter BSc (Hons), MSc, CPsychol
Counselling Psychologist

Lauren Blackburn BSc
Occupational Therapist

Jill Cooper MBE, MSc, Dip COT
Formerly Head Occupational Therapist

Edwina Curtis BA, BSW
Head of Adult Safeguarding

Lisa Dvorjetz BSc (Hons), DPsych
Counselling Psychologist

Linda Finn RSCN, RHV
Named Nurse

Danielle Gaynor DClinPsych
Family Specialty Clinical Psychologist

Beverley Henderson RN, BSc (Hons), PG Dip
Clinical Nurse Specialist, Psychological Support

Charmaine Jagger BSc (Hons)
Highly Specialist Speech and Language Therapist

Lucy Keating RMN BMedsci
Psychiatric Liaison Team Manager, Central and North West London NHS Foundation Trust

Lauren Leigh-Doyle BSc (Hons)
Highly Specialist Speech and Language Therapist

Sara Lister RN, BSc (Hons), PGDAE, MSc, Dip, MA, MBACP
Head of Pastoral Care and Psychological Support

Raj Mathiah RN, BSc
Clinical Nurse Specialist Liaison, Psychiatry and Adult Psychological Support

Asim Mohammed MBBS, Psych Med, Dip HE
Locum Consultant Psychiatrist, Adult Psychological Support Service

Chapter 6 Elimination

Rebecca Martin MSc, BSc (Hons), RN, INP
Urology Lead Nurse and Advanced Nurse Practitioner

Gemma Allen BSc (Hons), PG Cert, PG Dip
Practice Educator in Critical Care

Katy Hardy BSc (Hons), RN, NIP
Colorectal Clinical Nurse Specialist

Claire McNally RN, BSC (Hons)
Uro-oncology Clinical Nurse Specialist

Jacqueline McPhail RN, PG Cert, Dip M, ENB 338
Stoma Care Clinical Nurse Specialist

Bradley Russell MSc, BSc (Hons), RN, SCP
Urology Surgical Care Practitioner

Laura Theodossy PG Dip
Lecturer Practitioner

Chapter 7 Moving and positioning

Carolyn Moore MCSP
Superintendent Physiotherapist

Jill Cooper MBE, MSc, Dip COT
Head Occupational Therapist

Siobhan Cowan-Dickie MCSP, BSc (Hons), MSc, MCSP
Clinical Specialist Physiotherapist Living with and Beyond Cancer

Lucy Dean BSc (Hons), MCSP
Physiotherapist, Sarcoma Lead

Joanne Jethwa BSc (Hons), MCSP
Specialist Physiotherapist in Neuro-oncology and Complex Rehabilitation

Jessica Whibley BSc (Hons), MCSP
Physiotherapist Respiratory Lead

Leanne Williams BSc (Hons), MSc, MCSP
Clinical Specialist Physiotherapist, Neuro-oncology and Complex Rehabilitation

Chapter 8 Nutrition and fluid balance

Clare Shaw BSc (Hons), PG Dip, PhD
Consultant Dietitian

Laura Askins BSc, PG Dip
Formerly Senior Specialist Dietitian

Grainne Brady BSc (Hons), MRes
Clinical Lead Speech and Language Therapist

Lucy Eldridge BSc (Hons), MSc
Head of Nutrition and Dietetics

Olivia Kate Smith BSc (Hons)
Formerly Senior Specialist Dietitian

Laura Theodossy PG Dip
Lecturer Practitioner

Heather Thexton RN, BSc (Hons)
Senior Staff Nurse, Critical Care Unit

Chapter 9 Patient comfort and supporting personal hygiene

Suzanna Argenio-Haines RN, BA (Hons), Dip
Practice Educator, Clinical Education Team

Helena Aparecida de Rezende RN, PG Cert, MSc
Formerly Practice Educator, Clinical Education Team

Rhiannon Llewelyn, RN, BN (Hons)
Staff Nurse, Critical Care Unit

Chapter 10 Pain assessment and management

Suzanne Chapman RN, BSc (Hons), MSc
Clinical Nurse Specialist, Pain Management

Farzana Carvalho RN, BSc (Hons), MSc
Clinical Nurse Specialist, Pain Management

Caroline Dinen RN, BSc (Hons)
Clinical Nurse Specialist, Pain Management

Chapter 11 Symptom control and care towards the end of life

Anna-Marie Stevens RN, DClinP, MSc, BSc (Hons), Certificate in Oncology
Nurse Consultant, Palliative Care

Anne Doerr BA
Chaplain

Alistair McCulloch MA
Lead Chaplain

Pedro Mendes BSc
Lead Nurse, Interventional Radiology

Jodie Rawlings RN, BN
Formerly Senior Staff Nurse, Critical Care Unit

Laura Theodossy PG Dip
Lecturer Practitioner

Chapter 12 Respiratory care, CPR and blood transfusion

Louise Davison Dip HE, BN
Matron, Acute Oncology Service, Clinical Assessment Unit and Royal Marsden Macmillan Hotline

Wendy McSporran RN, BSc (Hons), PG Dip
Advanced Transfusion Practitioner

Grainne Brady BSc (Hons), MRes
Clinical Lead Speech and Language Therapist

Catherine Forsythe Dip HE, BSc (Hons)
Practice Educator, Critical Care Unit

Olivia Ratcliffe RN, BSc, MSc
Lead Nurse, Sepsis and Acute Kidney Injury

Chapter 13 Diagnostic tests

Andrew Dimech RN, BN, MSc, Dip
Deputy Chief Nurse

Andreia Fernandes RN, BSc, MSc
Clinical Nurse Specialist Gynaecology Oncology

Firza Gronthoud MD, MRCPath
Formerly Consultant Microbiologist

Lilian Li BSc (Hons), MSc, IPres
Lead Antimicrobial Pharmacist

Barbara Witt RN
Nurse Phlebotomist

Chapter 14 Observations

Filipe Carvalho RN, BSc (Hons), PG Dip, MSc, INP
Advanced Nurse Practitioner in Colorectal Surgery

Emma-Claire Breen RN, BSc (Hons)
Senior Staff Nurse and Clinical Practice Facilitator, Critical Care Unit

Zoë Bullock RN, BSc (Hons), PG Dip, PG Cert
Formerly Senior Staff Nurse and Practice Education Facilitator, Critical Care Unit

Sonya Hussein RN, BSc (Hons)
Senior Staff Nurse and Clinical Practice Facilitator, Critical Care Unit

Elodie Malard RN
Sister, Critical Care Unit

Yara Osman De Oliveira RN, BSc (Hons)
Sister, Critical Care Unit

Marie Parsons RN, BSc (Hons), PG Dip
Senior Staff Nurse and Clinical Practice Facilitator, Critical Care Unit

Heather Thexton RN, BSc (Hons)
Senior Staff Nurse, Critical Care Unit

Chapter 15 Medicines optimization: ensuring quality and safety

Lisa Barrott RN, BSc (Hons), MSc
Chemotherapy Nurse Consultant

Emma Foreman MRPharmS, MSc, IPresc, BSc (Hons)
Consultant Pharmacist

Jatinder Harchowal MRPharmS, MSc, BPharm (Hons)
Chief Pharmacist and Clinical Director

Kulpna Daya Reg Pharm Tech, MSc, Dip
Pharmacy Operation Manager and Education & Development Technician

Lisa Dougherty OBE, RN, MSc, DClinP
Formerly editor of *The Royal Marsden Manual of Clinical Nursing Procedures* and Nurse Consultant

Suraya Quadir MRPharmS, MBA, MSc, BPharm (Hons)
Lead Pharmacist, Governance and Education & Training/ Medication Safety Officer

Chapter 16 Perioperative care

Justine Hofland RN, BSc (Hons), ANP, MSc, PG Dip, ILM Level 5
Divisional Clinical Nurse Director, Cancer Services

Hayley Grafton RN, BSc (Hons), CPPD ITU
Chief Nursing Information Officer

Pascale Gruber MBBS, MSc, FRCA, MRCP, FFICM, EDIC
Consultant in Anaesthesia and Intensive Care Medicine, and Clinical Director, Surgery and Inpatients

Tina Kitcher RN, Dip
Practice Educator and Theatre Sister

Lian Lee RN, BSc, MSc, AdvDip OT Nurg
Matron, Theatres and Endoscopy

Chapter 17 Vascular access devices: insertion and management

Gema Munoz-Mozas RN, ONC, BSc (Hons), MSc
Lead Vascular Access Nurse

Lorraine Hyde RN, ONC, BSc (Hons)
Matron/Lead Nurse, Medical Day Unit

Hannah Overland RN, BSc (Hons), MSc
Matron/Lead Nurse, Medical Day Unit

Chapter 18 Wound management

Jenni MacDonald BSc (Hons), RN, BSc TVN, MSc, PGCert
Lead Nurse, Tissue Viability and Harm Free Care

Kumal Rajpaul MSc, BSC (Hons), Dip HE, RN
Assistant Director of Nursing and Patient Experience, Hounslow and Richmond Community NHS Trust

Chapter 19 Self-care and wellbeing

Sara Lister RN, BSc (Hons), PGDAE, MSc, Dip, MA, MBACP
Head of Pastoral Care and Psychological Support

Lorraine Bishop MSc, Dip, Dip MBCT
Formerly Staff Counsellor and Psychotherapist

Lucy Eldridge BSc (Hons), MSc
Dietetic Team Leader

Jayne Ellis RN, BSc (Hons)
Managing Director, EF Training

Tracey Shepherd MSc, MCSP, SRP
Moving and Handling Practitioner, Health Ergonomics Consultancy Ltd

Sara Wright DCR(r), BSc (Hons)
Freelance Moving and Handing Practitioner

Additional contributors

The authors and John Wiley & Sons are hugely grateful to the following staff and students for their help in the development of this edition.

The Nursing and Midwifery Clinical Practice Council at Oxford University Trust were very generous with their time and feedback on the content of the ninth edition of *The Royal Marsden Manual of Clinical Nursing Procedures*. This informed the changes and additions we made for the tenth edition as well as confirming for us what should remain. We would like to extend a large thank-you to them.

We would like to thank the following student nurses and nursing staff who helped to 'test' the revised procedures:

Student nurses (King's College London)

Ade Ajayi
Ciara Doogan
Rebecca Ellis
Jodie Fowler
Terrie Gemal
Rianna Norman
Filipa Santos
Amber Simon

Practice educators (Royal Marsden NHS Foundation Trust)

Sue Argenio-Haines
Catherine Forsythe
Rathai Kanagendram

For the first time, the online version will include videos of some of the procedures. Hayley Grafton led the production of these videos with assistance from the following staff at The Royal Marsden NHS Foundation Trust:

Jackson Young from the Marketing and Communications Team

And the following clinical staff:

Sue Argenio-Haines
Zoë Bullock
Lala Dizon
Catherine Forsythe
Ali Hill
Sara Lister
Jenni Macdonald
Rebecca Martin
Lorraine McHugh, who was a fabulous volunteer patient
Clare McNally
Pedro Medes
Amber Simon (student nurse)

Short Form Film were a great company to work with and we would like to thank them for their flexibility and patience.

Quick reference to the procedure guidelines

For more information on personal protective equipment (specified as the first item in the procedure guideline equipment lists where relevant), see page 87 in Chapter 4: Infection prevention and control.

How to use your manual

Features contained within your manual

The **overview page** gives a summary of the topics covered in each part.

Every chapter begins with a **list of procedures** found within the chapter. Additionally, the *Standards of Proficiency for Registered Nurses* (NMC, 2019) list the knowledge, skills and behaviours that every nurse must have. Each chapter relates to different proficiencies, so the relevant ones are listed in the **being an accountable professional** sections.

Part Two

Supporting patients with human functioning

Chapters

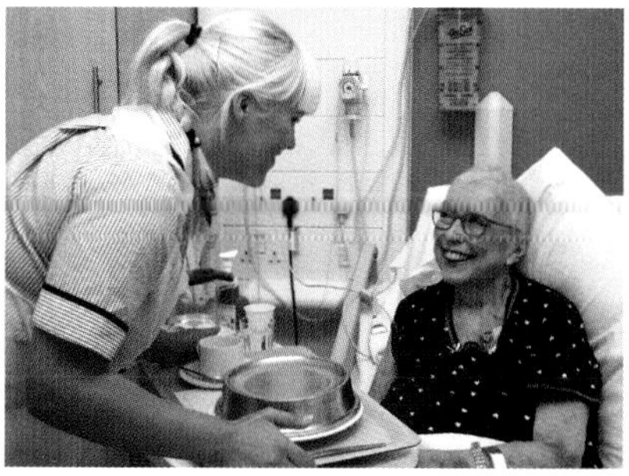

Procedure guidelines

Being an accountable professional

At the point of registration, the nurse will:

1. Use evidence-based, best practice approaches to take a history, observe, recognise and accurately assess people of all ages:
   1.1 mental health and wellbeing status
   1.2 physical health and wellbeing
2. Use evidence-based, best practice approaches to undertake the following procedures:
   2.7 undertake a whole body systems assessment including respiratory, circulatory, neurological, musculoskeletal, cardiovascular and skin status
   2.8 undertake chest auscultation and interpret findings

Future Nurse: Standards of Proficiency for Registered Nurses (NMC 2018)

Your manual is full of **photographs, illustrations and tables**

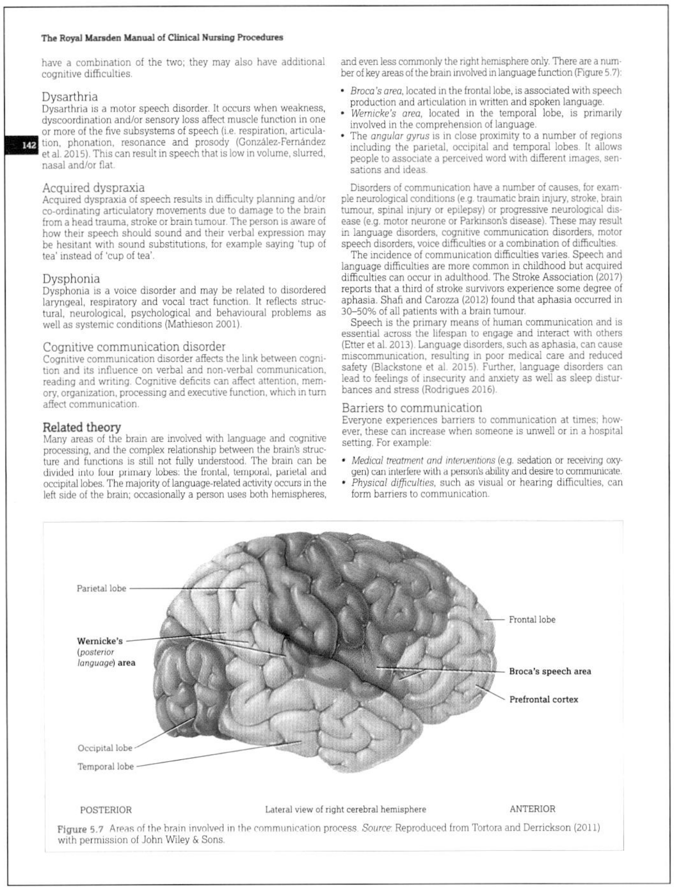

have a combination of the two; they may also have additional cognitive difficulties.

Dysarthria

Dysarthria is a motor speech disorder. It occurs when weakness, dyscoordination and/or sensory loss affect muscle function in one or more of the five subsystems of speech (i.e. respiration, articulation, phonation, resonance and prosody (González-Fernández et al. 2015). This can result in speech that is low in volume, slurred, nasal and/or flat.

Acquired dyspraxia

Acquired dyspraxia of speech results in difficulty planning and/or co-ordinating articulatory movements due to damage to the brain from a head trauma, stroke or brain tumour. The person is aware of how their speech should sound and their verbal expression may be hesitant with sound substitutions, for example saying 'tup of tea' instead of 'cup of tea'.

Dysphonia

Dysphonia is a voice disorder and may be related to disordered laryngeal, respiratory and vocal tract function. It reflects structural, neurological, psychological and behavioural problems as well as systemic conditions (Mathieson 2001).

Cognitive communication disorder

Cognitive communication disorder affects the link between cognition and its influence on verbal and non-verbal communication, reading and writing. Cognitive deficits can affect attention, memory, organization, processing and executive function, which in turn affect communication.

Related theory

Many areas of the brain are involved with language and cognitive processing, and the complex relationship between the brain's structure and functions is still not fully understood. The brain can be divided into four primary lobes: the frontal, temporal, parietal and occipital lobes. The majority of language-related activity occurs in the left side of the brain; occasionally a person uses both hemispheres, and even less commonly the right hemisphere only. There are a number of key areas of the brain involved in language function (Figure 5.7):

- *Broca's area*, located in the frontal lobe, is associated with speech production and articulation in written and spoken language.
- *Wernicke's area*, located in the temporal lobe, is primarily involved in the comprehension of language.
- The *angular gyrus* is in close proximity to a number of regions including the parietal, occipital and temporal lobes. It allows people to associate a perceived word with different images, sensations and ideas.

Disorders of communication have a number of causes, for example neurological conditions (e.g. traumatic brain injury, stroke, brain tumour, spinal injury or epilepsy) or progressive neurological disease (e.g. motor neurone or Parkinson's disease). These may result in language disorders, cognitive communication disorders, motor speech disorders, voice difficulties or a combination of difficulties.

The incidence of communication difficulties varies. Speech and language difficulties are more common in childhood but acquired difficulties can occur in adulthood. The Stroke Association (2017) reports that a third of stroke survivors experience some degree of aphasia. Shafi and Carozza (2012) found that aphasia occurred in 30–50% of all patients with a brain tumour.

Speech is the primary means of human communication and is essential across the lifespan to engage and interact with others (Etter et al. 2013). Language disorders, such as aphasia, can cause miscommunication, resulting in poor medical care and reduced safety (Blackstone et al. 2015). Further, language disorders can lead to feelings of insecurity and anxiety as well as sleep disturbances and stress (Rodrigues 2016).

Barriers to communication

Everyone experiences barriers to communication at times; however, these can increase when someone is unwell or in a hospital setting. For example:

- *Medical treatment and interventions* (e.g. sedation or receiving oxygen) can interfere with a person's ability and desire to communicate.
- *Physical difficulties*, such as visual or hearing difficulties, can form barriers to communication.

Figure 5.7 Areas of the brain involved in the communication process. *Source*: Reproduced from Tortora and Derrickson (2011) with permission of John Wiley & Sons.

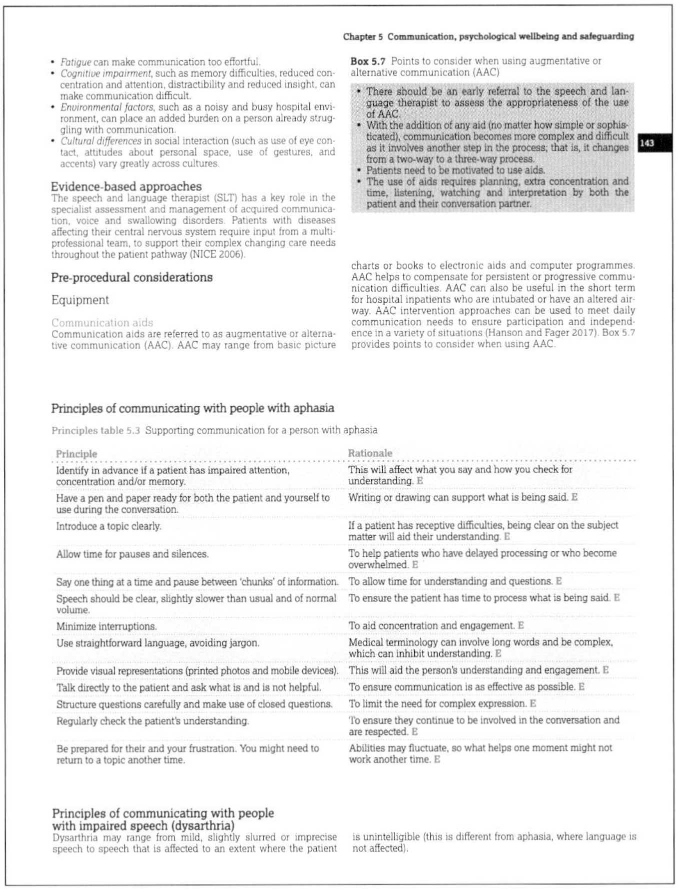

- *Fatigue* can make communication too effortful.
- *Cognitive impairment*, such as memory difficulties, reduced concentration and attention, distractibility and reduced insight, can make communication difficult.
- *Environmental factors*, such as a noisy and busy hospital environment, can place an added burden on a person already struggling with communication.
- *Cultural differences* in social interaction (such as use of eye contact, attitudes about personal space, use of gestures, and accents) vary greatly across cultures.

Evidence-based approaches

The speech and language therapist (SLT) has a key role in the specialist assessment and management of acquired communication, voice and swallowing disorders. Patients with diseases affecting their central nervous system require input from a multiprofessional team, to support their complex changing care needs throughout the patient pathway (NICE 2006).

Pre-procedural considerations

Equipment

Communication aids

Communication aids are referred to as augmentative or alternative communication (AAC). AAC may range from basic picture charts or books to electronic aids and computer programmes. AAC helps to compensate for persistent or progressive communication difficulties. AAC can also be useful in the short term for hospital inpatients who are intubated or have an altered airway. AAC intervention approaches can be used to meet daily communication needs to ensure participation and independence in a variety of situations (Hanson and Fager 2017). Box 5.7 provides points to consider when using AAC.

Box 5.7 Points to consider when using augmentative or alternative communication (AAC)

- There should be an early referral to the speech and language therapist to assess the appropriateness of the use of AAC.
- With the addition of any aid (no matter how simple or sophisticated), communication becomes more complex and difficult as it involves another step in the process; that is, it changes from a two-way to a three-way process.
- Patients need to be motivated to use aids.
- The use of aids requires planning, extra concentration and time, listening, watching and interpretation by both the patient and their conversation partner.

Principles of communicating with people with aphasia

Principles table 5.3 Supporting communication for a person with aphasia

Principle	Rationale
Identify in advance if a patient has impaired attention, concentration and/or memory.	This will affect what you say and how you check for understanding. E
Have a pen and paper ready for both the patient and yourself to use during the conversation.	Writing or drawing can support what is being said. E
Introduce a topic clearly.	If a patient has receptive difficulties, being clear on the subject matter will aid their understanding. E
Allow time for pauses and silences.	To help patients who have delayed processing or who become overwhelmed. E
Say one thing at a time and pause between 'chunks' of information.	To allow time for understanding and questions. E
Speech should be clear, slightly slower than usual and of normal volume.	To ensure the patient has time to process what is being said. E
Minimize interruptions.	To aid concentration and engagement. E
Use straightforward language, avoiding jargon.	Medical terminology can involve long words and be complex, which can inhibit understanding. E
Provide visual representations (printed photos and mobile devices).	This will aid the person's understanding and engagement. E
Talk directly to the patient and ask what is and is not helpful.	To ensure communication is as effective as possible. E
Structure questions carefully and make use of closed questions.	To limit the need for complex expression. E
Regularly check the patient's understanding.	To ensure they continue to be involved in the conversation and are respected. E
Be prepared for their and your frustration. You might need to return to a topic another time.	Abilities may fluctuate, so what helps one moment might not work another time. E

Principles of communicating with people with impaired speech (dysarthria)

Dysarthria may range from mild, slightly slurred or imprecise speech to speech that is affected to an extent where the patient is unintelligible (this is different from aphasia, where language is not affected).

Chapter 1

The context of nursing

Sara Lister

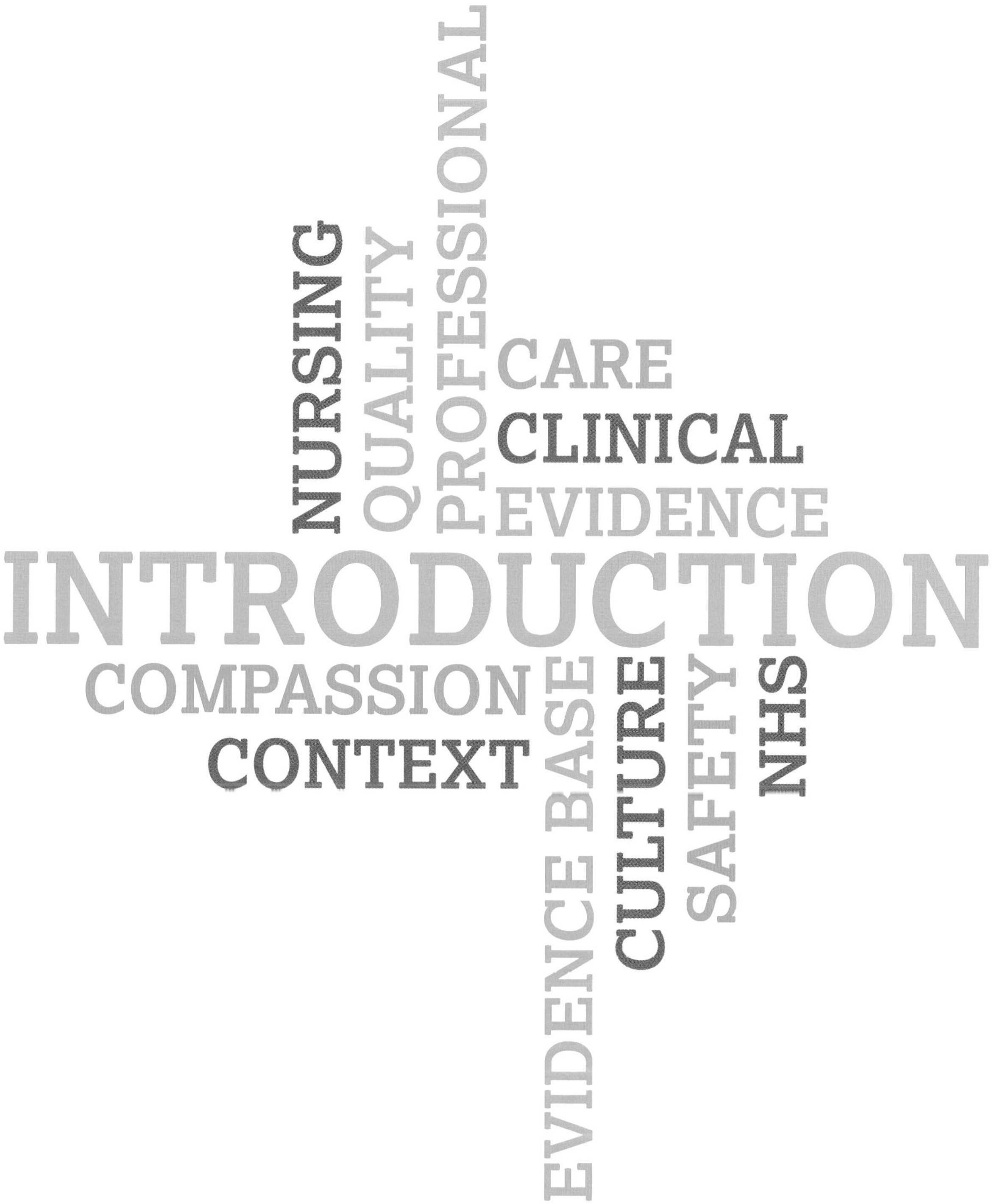

Overview

This introductory chapter presents an overview of the current context of nursing as well as outlining the purpose of the book and providing details of how it is structured. It also includes an explanation of the system used to grade the evidence that supports the clinical procedures.

Background

The first edition of *The Royal Marsden Manual of Clinical Nursing Procedures* was produced in the early 1980s as a core procedure manual for safe nursing practice within The Royal Marsden NHS Hospital, the world's first cancer hospital. Implicit behind that first edition was the drive to ensure that patients received the very best care, including clinical procedures carried out with professional expertise combined with an attitude of respect and compassion. This vision is still at the forefront of nursing in The Royal Marsden today, reflected in two of the themes of The Royal Marsden's *Nursing Strategy 2016–2018* (Royal Marsden NHS Foundation Trust 2015) (Box 1.1).

Context of nursing

It is argued that the role of the nurse is as essential in responding to the healthcare needs of society today as it was over 30 years ago. In the current NHS England *Leading Change, Adding Value: A Framework for Nursing, Midwifery and Care Staff* (NHS England 2016) it is stated that:

> Though the world has changed, our values haven't. As nursing, midwifery and care staff we know that compassionate care delivered with courage, commitment and skill is our highest priority. It is the rock on which our efforts to promote health and well-being, support the vulnerable, care for the sick and look after the dying is built. (NHS England 2016, p.5)

However, in 2020 the context of nursing is different in many ways from that in 1984, when the very first manual was published. In this chapter, two specific influences are identified: political and professional.

Box 1.1 Themes of The Royal Marsden's *Nursing Strategy 2016–2018*

1. Delivering safe, effective and harm-free care
2. Providing a positive experience of care that exceeds expectations

Political context

Nurses are the largest group of employees in the NHS, so the context of nursing in the 21st century is shaped by the situation in the NHS. The aforementioned *Leading Change, Adding Value: A Framework for Nursing, Midwifery and Care Staff* (NHS England 2016) (Figure 1.1) was based on the NHS's *Five Year Forward View* (NHS England 2014), which highlighted the changes taking place in society:

- changes in personal health needs and preferences as we live longer with increasingly complex and more long-term conditions, as well as a need to take increased responsibility for our own wellbeing
- changes in technology and developments in medical research with opportunities arising from these advances that need to be embraced to further enhance treatment and care
- reductions in funding provision because of the global recession that began in 2008.

Unwarranted variation

One of the core principles of the NHS when it was founded 70 years ago was that it should 'meets the needs of everyone' (NHS Liverpool Heart and Chest Hospital 2018, p.1; see also NHS England 2018a). This has continued to guide the development of the NHS; however, as identified in the *Five Year Forward View*

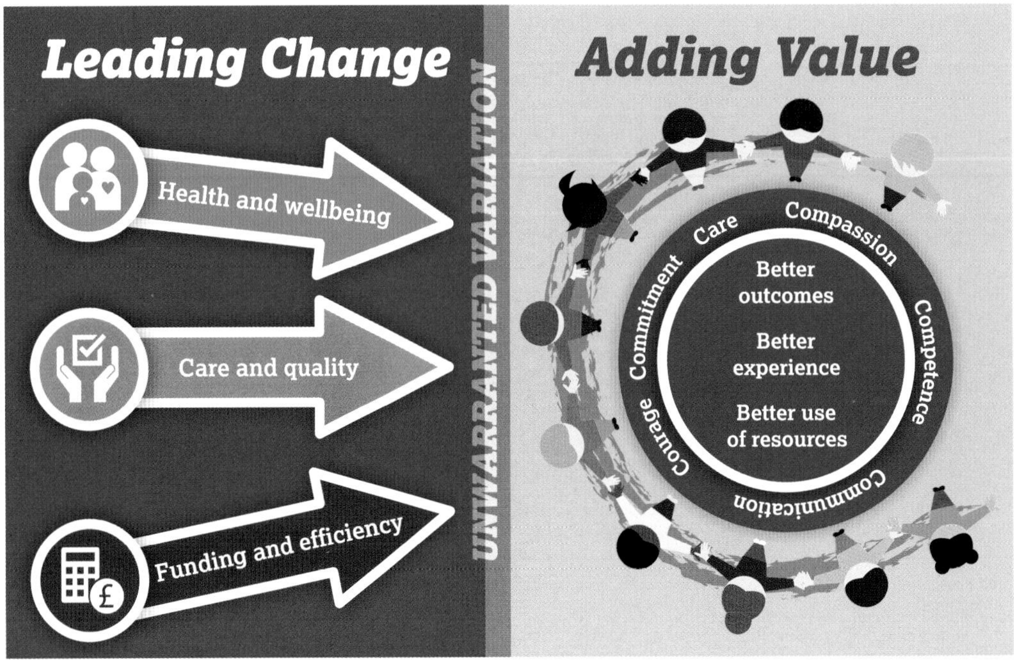

Figure 1.1 *Leading Change, Adding Value: A Framework for Nursing, Midwifery and Care Staff. Source*: Reproduced from NHS England (2016) with permission of the NHS.

Box 1.2 Unwarranted variation: turning intention into action

- Taking a closer look at what we do: for example, benchmarking our procedures against the evidence-based procedures in *The Royal Marsden Manual of Clinical Nursing Procedures*.
- Uncovering activities that we need to change, add or take away.
- Challenging established practice because we understand that service can be delivered in a better way: for example, using the online version of *The Royal Marsden Manual of Clinical Nursing Procedures* to upload and disseminate agreed examples of good practice across an organization.
- Striving for high-value care: for example, reviewing equipment and the medication involved in procedures, or exploring whether procedures are being carried out by the most appropriate member of the team.

Source: Adapted from NHS England (2018b, p.11) with permission of the NHS.

(NHS England 2014), changes in society are contributing to three distinct gaps that, if they are not addressed, will impact the long-term provision of healthcare and increase inequalities:

- *Health and wellbeing*: a focus on prevention is needed or the inequalities in health will continue to grow and the budget for healthcare will need to be spent on avoidable illness and not on the development of new treatments.
- *Care and quality*: health needs will go unmet unless we reshape care, harness technology and address variations in quality and safety (NHS England 2018b, p.8).
- *Funding and efficiency*: without efficiencies, a shortage of resources will hinder care services and progress (NHS England 2018b, p.8).

An implicit part of the role of nursing is therefore to be an integral part of closing these gaps, whether at a strategic, national level or locally at the bedside or in the outpatient department. It is suggested that the impact of these gaps is exaggerated because of 'unwarranted variations', which is 'a term used to describe inequalities that cannot be justified by variations in geography, demography or infrastructure' (NHS England 2018b, p.9). At a local level, nurses can be involved in challenging unwarranted variations in the ways shown in Box 1.2.

NHS Long Term Plan

The NHS Long Term Plan (NHS England 2019) sets out a new service model for the 21st century. This responds to 'concern – about funding, staffing, increasing inequalities and pressures from a growing and ageing population' and optimistically holds 'the possibilities for continuing medical advance and better outcomes of care' (NHS England 2019, p.6).

The plans set out have various implications for nursing. The key chapters of the NHS Long Term Plan with direct relevance to nursing practice in an acute setting are set out in Table 1.1 with reference to the chapters in this manual that might be of specific significance to nurses who are involved in implementing new ways of working.

Professional context

There are many factors influencing the professional context of nursing in 2020. The two highlighted here are patient safety and quality of care, and new roles required to respond to the increasing demand for services.

Patient safety and quality of care

Core to nursing, wherever it takes place, is the commitment to caring for individuals and keeping them safe, so wherever the procedures are used, they are to be carried out within the framework of the Nursing and Midwifery Council's *Code* (NMC 2018a).

One of the original purposes of *The Royal Marsden Manual of Clinical Nursing Procedures* was to promote patient safety through standardized and evidence-based approaches to care. Patient safety is an essential part of nursing care that aims to prevent avoidable errors and patient harm. The Royal College of Nursing (RCN) (2019) highlights four key factors that are important in patient safety:

1. *Developing a culture of safety*: this involves promoting attitudes and behaviours that encourage staff to learn from preventable incidents, which will make it less likely that the incident will happen again. Organizations fostering a proactive approach to patient safety should be open, just and informed, and reporting and learning from error should be the norm (Carthy and Clarke 2009).
2. *Designing for reliability*: this involves making healthcare more reliable – that is, taking a standard approach to patient care, agreeing to ways of working based on research and evidence where it is available, and agreeing at an organizational level to apply that knowledge to practice.
3. *Taking a systemic approach to work*: the system of work – which includes equipment, devices, medication and information systems – makes a considerable difference to quality and safety. Changes to the design of physical things can make a big difference to how well people work. For example, the interfaces of devices, control panels, packaging and lighting levels can improve the speed, accuracy and reliability of a procedure.
4. *Human factors*: this refers to the way teams work together and the culture that influences how they act. The discipline of human factors can be defined as enhancing clinical performance through an understanding of the effects of teamwork, tasks, equipment, workspace, culture, organization of human behaviour and abilities, and application of that knowledge in clinical settings (Clinical Human Factors Group 2019). To paraphrase Ives and Hillier (2015), *nurses* within healthcare are *one of* healthcare's greatest sources of strength and the science of human factors and ergonomics is about providing a system which allows them to work to the very best of their ability *to provide safe, high-quality care for patients.*

Adapted by the RCN, the consultancy Leadership Management and Quality's Human Factors Model (Figure 1.2) illustrates the interaction between the *direct factors* (dexterity (mental or physical), awareness/memory, distraction/concentration and decision – in the orange circle) that impact performance and therefore the patient experience and the *potential factors* (stress, fatigue, safety culture, communication, teamwork, leadership and work environment – in the teal circle), which have the potential to make the situation either better or worse. The *interventions* or *managing* factors (green circle) manage the effect of the potential factors and improve the direct factors (RCN 2019). The interventions or managing factors are many, both at the organizational and the individual levels. The *Royal Marsden Manual of Clinical Nursing Procedures* has a role at the organizational level, providing standardized procedures on which training can be based, and at the individual level, supporting the development of problem prevention and problem solving through the acquisition of knowledge associated with clinical processes.

Professional competency

The development of clinical competency is an integral part of delivering safe care; the Nursing and Midwifery Code states that nurses must:

- have the knowledge and skills for safe and effective practice without direct supervision
- keep their knowledge and skills up to date throughout their working life
- recognize and work within the limits of their competence (NMC 2018a).

Table 1.1 The NHS Long Term Plan (NHS England 2019) and *The Royal Marsden Manual of Clinical Nursing Procedures*

New ways of working identified in the NHS Long Term Plan with direct relevance to nursing practice	Relevant chapter(s) in *The Royal Marsden Manual*	Related content in *The Royal Marsden Manual*
Chapter 1: A New Service Model for the 21st Century		
Personalized health budget and self-care	Chapter 5: Communication, psychological wellbeing and safeguarding	Information giving and decision making.
Same-day emergency care and clinical standards for critical illness	Chapter 12: Respiratory care, CPR and blood transfusion Chapter 13: Diagnostic tests Chapter 17: Vascular access devices: insertion and management	Nursing procedures for emergency care, e.g. CPR.
Improved discharge	Chapter 3: Discharge care and planning	Processes and procedures for arranging discharge with Social Services.
Chapter 3: Further Progress on Care Quality and Outcomes		
Whole chapter	All chapters	The foundation of this textbook is to provide evidence-based procedures and to underpin rationale for the day-to-day procedures used by nurses in the acute setting with the aim of promoting quality care for the best outcome. This is discussed in more detail in the section below.
Chapter 4: NHS Staff Will Get the Backing They Need		
Workforce changes, including increased flexibility and access to professional development to help manage the pressures of working in the NHS	Chapter 19: Self-care and wellbeing	This chapter specifically considers strategies to help nurses cope with the pressures of working in the NHS.
Chapter 5: Upgrading Technology and Digitally Enabling the NHS		
Whole chapter	n/a	This theme is not specifically addressed; however, references are made where appropriate to digital support for procedures, plus the online version of the manual is continually being enhanced.

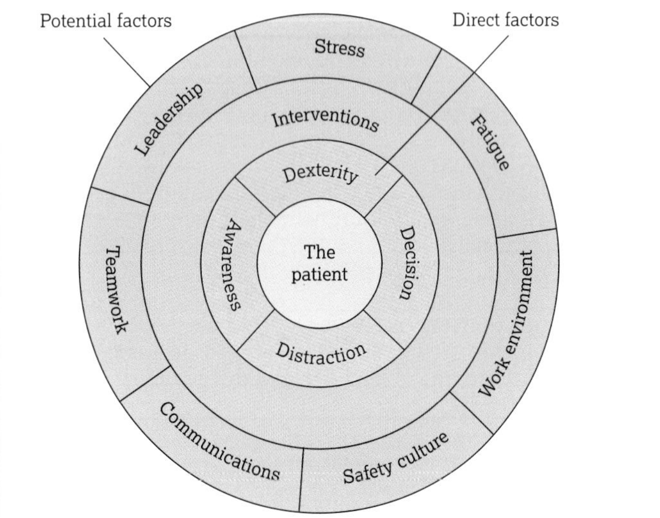

Figure 1.2 The Human Factors Model. *Source*: Adapted from RCN (2019) with permission of the Royal College of Nursing.

The Nursing and Midwifery Council (NMC) 'has a duty to review the standards of proficiency it sets for the professions it registers on a regular basis to ensure that standards remain contemporary and fit for purpose in order to protect the public' (NMC 2018b, p.3). In fulfilling this duty, it published *Future Nurse: Standards of Proficiency for Registered Nurses* (NMC 2018b) (Figure 1.3). This document details the knowledge and skills that all registered nurses must demonstrate when caring for people of all ages and across all care settings, reflecting what the public can expect nurses to know and be able to do in order to deliver safe, compassionate and effective nursing care. These proficiencies have a legal standing, fulfilling Article 5(2) of the Nursing and Midwifery Order 2001, which requires the NMC to establish standards of proficiency necessary for nurses to be admitted to each part of the register and for safe and effective practice under that part of the register (NMC 2018b). The proficiencies are designed to apply across all fields of nursing practice (adult, child, mental health and learning disabilities), 'because registered nurses must be able to meet the person-centred, holistic care needs of the people they encounter in their practice who may be at any stage of life and who may have a range of mental, physical, cognitive or behavioural health challenges' (NMC 2018b, p.60).

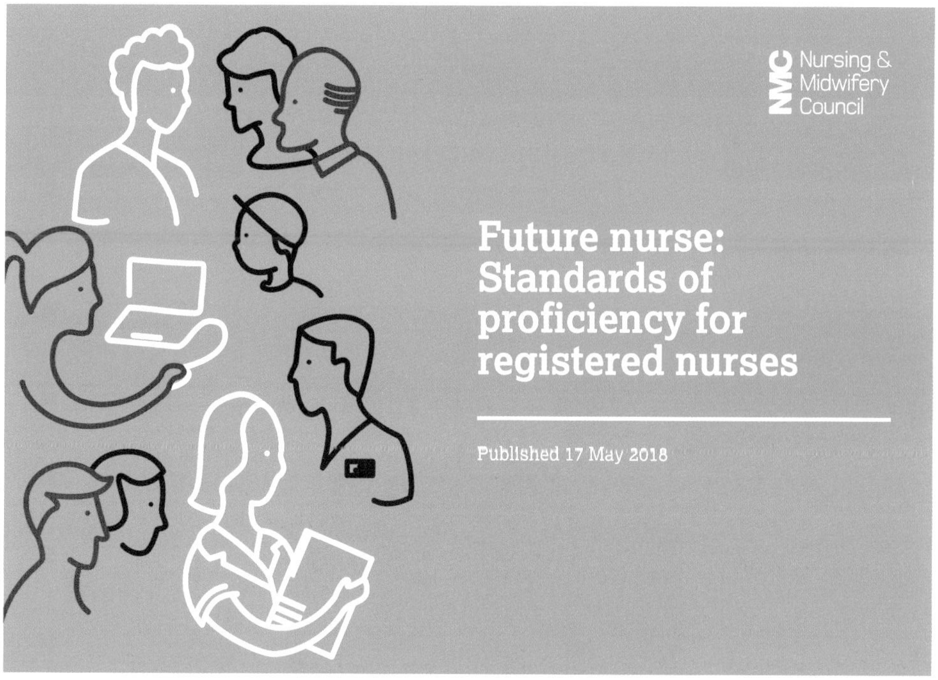

Figure 1.3 *Future Nurse: Standards of Proficiency for Registered Nurses. Source*: Reproduced from NMC (2018b) with permission of the Nursing and Midwifery Council.

Box 1.3 The seven platforms of Standards of Proficiency for Registered Nurses

1 Being an accountable professional
2 Promoting health and preventing ill health
3 Assessing needs and planning care
4 Providing and evaluating care
5 Leading and managing nursing care and working in teams
6 Improving safety and quality of care
7 Co-ordinating care

The proficiencies are grouped around seven platforms (Box 1.3). These reflect what the nursing profession expects a newly registered nurse to know and be capable of doing safely and proficiently at the start of their career (NMC 2018b).

In addition, there are two annexes that describe what registered nurses should be able to demonstrate they can do at the point of registration in order to provide safe nursing care. Annex A specifies the communication and relationship management skills required, and Annex B specifies the nursing procedures that registered nurses must demonstrate that they are able to perform safely (NMC 2018b).

Many of the chapters in this edition of *The Royal Marsden Manual of Clinical Nursing Procedures* map onto the NMC proficiencies in Annex B of the Standards of Proficiency for Registered Nurses (NMC 2018b); these are detailed in the Appendix in this edition of the manual. The manual provides theory and exploration of anatomy and physiology related to nursing procedures, recognizing that competence is not just about knowing how to do something but also about understanding the rationale for doing it and the impact it may have on the patient.

The revision of the standards for nursing also has implications for the education and training of nurses – specifically, ensuring they are prepared for the future roles they will be fulfilling (Figure 1.4).

New roles

The changes in demand for healthcare and the limited resources (particularly staff) available to provide it have prompted government, employers and the profession to consider new roles. These new roles could potentially provide a faster route to solving staffing problems and offer career development opportunities that could also help to improve retention. These include expanding physician associate and advanced nurse practitioner roles and the new nursing associate roles (King's Fund 2018).

Nursing associates

The report *Raising the Bar: Shape of Caring – A Review of the Future Education and Training of Registered Nurses and Care Assistants* (Health Education England 2015), led by Lord Willis, made recommendations for the education of nurses and care assistants. One of the key areas it identified was the skills gap between care assistants and registered nurses (NMC 2018c). The nursing associate role, announced by Ben Gummer, Health Minister, in 2015, was developed to address this gap:

> The new nursing support role is expected to work alongside healthcare support workers and fully qualified nurses to deliver hands on care, ensuring patients continue to get the compassionate care they deserve. Nursing associates will support nurses to spend more time using their specialist training to focus on clinical duties and take more of a lead in decisions about patient care. (Department of Health and Social Care 2015)

The NMC is the regulator for these new roles and has set out standards of knowledge and skills expected of a nursing associate for safe and effective practice (NMC 2018c). The Standards of Proficiency are structured in a similar way to those for registered nurses and are based around six platforms (Box 1.4).

The procedures that it is expected a nursing associate will be able to undertake competently on registration are defined in Annex B of the Standards of Proficiency, which states: 'Nursing associates

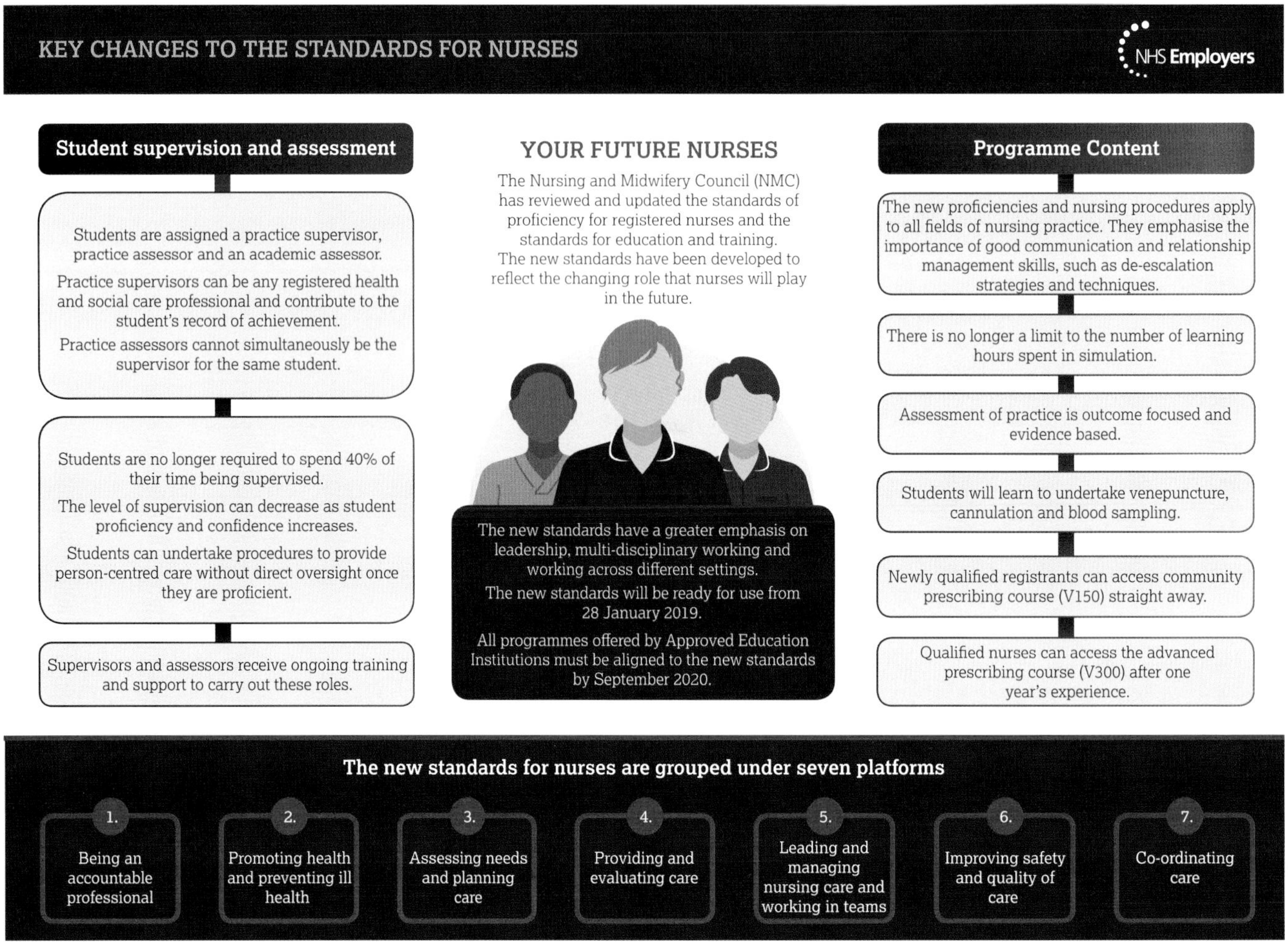
KEY CHANGES TO THE STANDARDS FOR NURSES
NHS Employers
Student supervision and assessment
Students are assigned a practice supervisor, practice assessor and an academic assessor.
Practice supervisors can be any registered health and social care professional and contribute to the student's record of achievement.
Practice assessors cannot simultaneously be the supervisor for the same student.
Students are no longer required to spend 40% of their time being supervised.
The level of supervision can decrease as student proficiency and confidence increases.
Students can undertake procedures to provide person-centred care without direct oversight once they are proficient.
Supervisors and assessors receive ongoing training and support to carry out these roles.
YOUR FUTURE NURSES
The Nursing and Midwifery Council (NMC) has reviewed and updated the standards of proficiency for registered nurses and the standards for education and training.
The new standards have been developed to reflect the changing role that nurses will play in the future.
The new standards have a greater emphasis on leadership, multi-disciplinary working and working across different settings.
The new standards will be ready for use from 28 January 2019.
All programmes offered by Approved Education Institutions must be aligned to the new standards by September 2020.
Programme Content
The new proficiencies and nursing procedures apply to all fields of nursing practice. They emphasise the importance of good communication and relationship management skills, such as de-escalation strategies and techniques.
There is no longer a limit to the number of learning hours spent in simulation.
Assessment of practice is outcome focused and evidence based.
Students will learn to undertake venepuncture, cannulation and blood sampling.
Newly qualified registrants can access community prescribing course (V150) straight away.
Qualified nurses can access the advanced prescribing course (V300) after one year's experience.
The new standards for nurses are grouped under seven platforms
1. Being an accountable professional
2. Promoting health and preventing ill health
3. Assessing needs and planning care
4. Providing and evaluating care
5. Leading and managing nursing care and working in teams
6. Improving safety and quality of care
7. Co-ordinating care

Figure 1.4 Summary of key changes to the standards for nurses. *Source*: Reproduced from NHS Employers (2018) with permission of the NHS.

Box 1.4 Standards of Proficiency for Nursing Associates

- Platform 1: Being an accountable professional
- Platform 2: Promoting health and preventing ill health
- Platform 3: Provide and monitor care
- Platform 4: Working in teams
- Platform 5: Improving safety and quality of care
- Platform 6: Contributing to integrated care

are expected to apply evidence-based best practice across all procedures. The ability to carry out these procedures, safely, effectively, with sensitivity and compassion is crucial to the provision of person-centred care' (NMC 2018c, p.15). It is hoped that this manual will be a resource for nursing associates in helping them to develop the understanding necessary to apply evidence-based practice to all the procedures they undertake. The procedures specified in Annex B of the Standards of Proficiency for Nursing Associates are mapped against the chapters in this manual in the Appendix.

Advanced nurse practitioners

'New solutions are required to deliver healthcare to meet the changing needs of the population. This will need new ways of working, new roles and new behaviours' (NHS England 2017, p.1). Advanced clinical practice roles are seen as an essential part of these solutions (Nuffield Trust 2016). A multi-professional advanced clinical practice framework has been developed to define advanced clinical practice and set out the core capabilities expected across professions and care settings to foster the development of these new roles in a consistent way to ensure safety, quality and effectiveness (NHS England 2017) (see Box 1.5).

Box 1.5 Definition of advanced clinical practice

Advanced clinical practice is defined as follows:

> Clinical practice is delivered by experienced, registered health and care practitioners. It is a level of practice characterized by a high degree of autonomy and complex decision making. This is underpinned by a master's level award or equivalent that encompasses the four pillars of clinical practice, leadership and management, education and research, with demonstration of core capabilities and area specific clinical competence.
>
> Advanced clinical practice embodies the ability to manage clinical care in partnership with individuals, families and carers. It includes the analysis and synthesis of complex problems across a range of settings, enabling innovative solutions to enhance people's experience and improve outcomes. (NHS England 2017, p.7)

Source: NHS England (2017). Reproduced with permission of the NHS.

Developing new roles and taking responsibility for new procedures have obvious risks attached and, although every individual nurse is accountable for their own actions, every healthcare organization has to assume vicarious liability for the care, treatment and procedures that take place. An organization will have expectations of all of its nurses in respect of keeping patients, themselves and the environment safe. There are obvious ethical and moral reasons for this: 'Nurses have a moral obligation to protect those we serve and to provide the best care we have available' (Wilson 2005, p.118). Clinical governance has therefore become an integral part of day-to-day nursing work; for this reason, the clinical governance implications of the areas of practice have been integrated into each chapter of this edition of the manual.

Evidence-based practice

The moral obligation described above extends to the evidence upon which we base our practice. Nursing now exists in a healthcare arena that routinely uses evidence to support decisions, and nurses must justify their rationales for practice. Whereas, historically, nursing and specifically clinical procedures were based on rituals rather than research (Ford and Walsh 1994, Walsh and Ford 1989), over the past 30 years evidence-based practice (EBP) has formed an integral part of practice, education, management, strategy and policy in healthcare. As Draper (2018) states, 'as the global demand for healthcare services increases exponentially, it has never been more important to demonstrate clinical effectiveness to achieve the best outcomes … while ensuring value for money" (p.2480). Research has played a key role in identifying the specific interventions that lead to the best outcomes, or, in other words, identifying the evidence to underpin clinical practice – that is, evidence-based practice.

What is evidence-based practice?

EBP was first described by David Sackett, a pioneer in introducing EBP in UK healthcare, as follows:

> [EBP is] the conscientious, explicit and judicious use of current best evidence in making decisions about the care of the individual patients. The practice of evidence-based medicine [or nursing] means integrating individual clinical expertise with the best available external clinical evidence from systematic research. (Sackett et al. 1996, p.72)

A hierarchy of evidence (Box 1.6) has been developed to provide an indication of the strength of the evidence and therefore, by implication, its usefulness for evidence-based and evidence-informed decision making and clinical practice (Draper 2018, Ingham-Broomfield 2016).

Glover et al. (2006) present for nursing research a hierarchy of evidence as a pyramid (Figure 1.5), with the seventh level or base of the pyramid being ideas, opinions, anecdotes and editorials. Other sources (e.g. Ingham-Broomfield 2016) have created similar pyramids, and it must be noted that the pyramids vary slightly between authors, organizations and professions.

Box 1.6 The traditional hierarchy of evidence

1 Systematic reviews and meta-analyses
2 Randomized controlled trials with definitive results (i.e. confidence intervals that do not overlap the threshold, clinically significant effect)
3 Randomized controlled trials with non-definitive results (i.e. a suggested clinical significant effect but with confidence intervals overlapping)
4 Cohort studies
5 Case-control studies
6 Cross-sectional surveys
7 Case reports

Source: Adapted from Greenhalgh (2014, p.41).

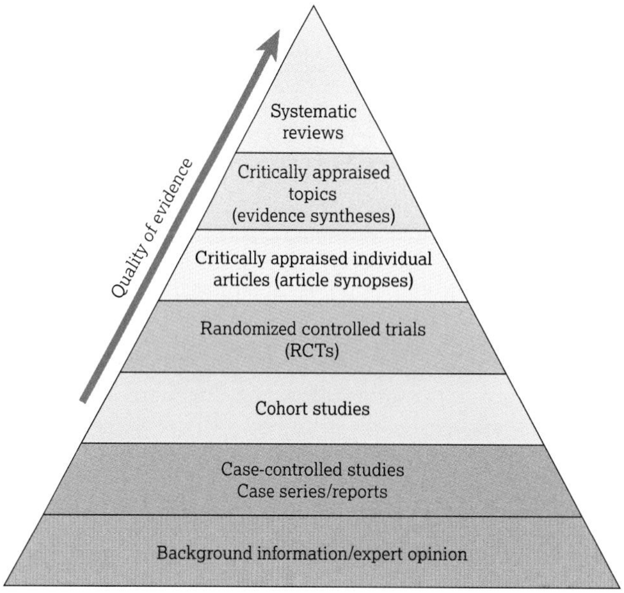

Figure 1.5 Hierarchy of evidence pyramid for nursing. *Source*: Adapted from Glover et al. (2006) with permission of Lei Wang.

These hierarchies assume that the most robust evidence is that derived from systematic reviews and meta analyses of large scale randomized controlled studies (Draper 2018, Greenhalgh 2014, Ingham-Broomfield 2016). However, they provide no means of including qualitative research studies (Greenhalgh 2014) or those seeking to answer questions about patients' experiences or concerns (Del Mar et al. 2013). Draper (2018) therefore proposes that typologies of evidence are a more appropriate way of defining the quality of evidence. Petticrew and Roberts (2003) propose the following features to be used in evaluating evidence: effectiveness, service delivery, salience, safety, acceptability, cost-effectiveness, appropriateness and satisfaction. Glasby et al. (2007) propose a different approach suggesting three different types of evidence: theoretical, empirical and experiential (Box 1.7).

This typology is reflective of the seminal work of Carper (1978), who delineated four different forms of knowing encompassed in clinical expertise in nursing. These are:

- empirical evidence
- aesthetic evidence
- ethical evidence
- personal evidence.

The issue of determining which evidence is acceptable in practice is evident throughout this manual, where clinical expertise

Box 1.7 A typology of evidence to inform practice

- *Theoretical evidence*: ideas, concepts and models used to describe an intervention, and explain how and why it works.
- *Empirical evidence*: information about the actual use of the intervention, its effectiveness and outcomes when it is used.
- *Experiential evidence*: information about people's experiences of the intervention or service.

Source: Adapted from Glasby et al. (2007, p.434).

and guidelines inform the actions and rationales of the procedures. Indeed, these other types of evidence are highly important as long as we can still apply scrutiny to their use.

Porter (2010) describes a wider empirical base upon which nurses make decisions and argues for nurses to take into account and be transparent about other forms of knowledge, such as ethical, personal and aesthetic knowing, echoing Carper (1978). By doing this, and through acknowledging limitations to these less empirical forms of knowledge, nurses can justify their use of them to some extent. Furthermore, in response to Paley's (2006) critique of EBP as a failure to holistically assess a situation, nursing needs to guard against cherry picking (i.e. ensuring that EBP is not brandished ubiquitously and indiscriminately) and know when judicious use of, for example, experiential knowledge (as a form of personal knowing) might be more appropriate.

Evidence-based nursing (EBN) and EBP are differentiated by Scott and McSherry (2009) in that EBN involves additional elements in its implementation. EBN is regarded as an ongoing process by which evidence is integrated into practice and clinical expertise is critically evaluated against patient involvement and optimal care (Scott and McSherry 2009). For nurses to implement EBN, four key requirements are required (Scott and McSherry 2009):

1. to be aware of what EBN means
2. to know what constitutes evidence
3. to understand how EBN differs from evidence-based medicine and EBP
4. to understand the process of engaging with and applying the evidence.

We contextualize our information and decisions to deliver best practice for patients; that is, the ability to use research evidence and clinical expertise, together with the preferences and circumstances of the patient, is essential to arrive at the best possible decision for a specific patient (Guyatt et al. 2004).

Knowledge can be gained that is both *propositional* – that is, from research – and *non-propositional* – that is, implicit knowledge derived from practice (Rycroft-Malone et al. 2004). In more tangible, practical terms, evidence can be drawn from a number of different sources, and this pluralistic approach needs to be set in the context of the complex clinical environment in which nurses work in today's NHS (Pearson et al. 2011, Rycroft-Malone et al. 2004). Rycroft-Malone et al. (2004) proposed that the evidence that informs clinical nursing practice can be considered as arising from four main sources:

1. research
2. clinical experience, expertise and tradition
3. patients, clients and carers
4. the local context and environment (Pearson et al. 2011, Rycroft-Malone et al. 2004).

These four sources have all informed the evidence base that is integral to this manual, which acknowledges that 'in reality practitioners draw on multiple sources of knowledge in the course of their practice and interaction with patients' (Rycroft-Malone et al. 2004, p.88).

Evidence-based practice and *The Royal Marsden Manual of Clinical Nursing Procedures*

The evidence that informs clinical nursing procedures is integral to *The Royal Marsden Manual of Clinical Nursing Procedures*. It is critically discussed in the sections within each chapter on 'related theory' and 'evidence-based approaches'. In these sections, the source of evidence (reflecting the sources described by Rycroft-Malone et al. 2004) is indicated in the rationale that supports the steps in procedures. In previous editions, the level on the research hierarchy was also included, in an attempt to represent the robustness of the evidence. In this edition, that nomenclature has been

Box 1.8 Examples of sources

- Clinical experience and guidelines (Dougherty 2008, **E**)
- Patient (Diamond 1998, **P**)
- Context (NMC 2018a, **C**)
- Research (Stevenson et al. 2017, **R**)

dropped for two reasons: because the hierarchy does not include qualitative studies, some of which are significant in informing nursing practice, and because the hierarchy does not recognize the quality of a study, just the methodological approach.

The following key is used to indicate the sources of evidence:

- Clinical experience (**E**)
  Encompasses expert practical know-how, gained through working with others and reflecting on best practice.
  Example: (Dougherty 2008, **E**). This is drawn from the following article that gives an expert clinical opinion: Dougherty, L. (2008) Obtaining peripheral vascular access. In: Dougherty, L. & Lamb, J. (eds) *Intravenous Therapy in Nursing Practice*, 2nd edn. Oxford: Blackwell.
- Patient (**P**)
  Gained through expert patient feedback and extensive experience of working with patients.
  Example: (Diamond 1998, **P**). This was gained from a personal account of care written by a patient: Diamond, J. (1998) *C: Because Cowards Get Cancer Too*. London: Vermilion.
- Context (**C**)
  Can include audit and performance data, social and professional networks, local and national policy, guidelines from professional bodies (e.g. the RCN) and manufacturers' recommendations.
  Example: (NMC 2018a, **C**). This reference is: NMC (2018a) *The Code: Professional Standards of Practice and Behaviour for Nurses, Midwives and Nursing Associates*. London: Nursing and Midwifery Council.
- Research (**R**)
  Evidence gained through research.
  Example: (Stevenson et al. 2017, **R**). Stevenson, J.C., Emerson, L. & Millings, A. (2017) The relationship between adult attachment orientation and mindfulness: A systematic review and meta-analysis. *Mindfulness*, 8, 1438–1455.

In the text, the source will be represented as shown in Box 1.8. If there is no written evidence to support clinical experience or there are no guidelines to justify undertaking a procedure, the text will be referenced as an '**E**' but will not be preceded by an author's name. Through this process, it is hoped that the reader will be aware of the source of the evidence upon which the care of patients is based and continue to critically evaluate their practice, engaging in research and audit where there are gaps or where best practice is not confirmed.

Structure of the manual

The chapters have been organized into five broad sections that represent – as far as possible – the needs of a patient along their care pathway. The first section, 'Managing the patient journey', presents the generic information that a nurse needs for every patient who enters the acute care environment. The second section, 'Supporting patients with human functioning', relates to the support a patient may require with normal human functions such as elimination, nutrition and respiration, and includes procedures relevant to those areas. The third section, 'Supporting patients through the diagnostic process', relates to all aspects of supporting a patient through the diagnostic process, from simple procedures such as taking a temperature to preparing a patient for complex procedures such as a liver biopsy. The fourth section, 'Supporting patients through treatment', includes procedures related to specific types of treatment or therapies a patient is receiving. An additional final section and chapter has been added focusing on the wellbeing and self-care of the nurse. This has been included for two reasons. Firstly, the new NMC Standards of Proficiency for Registered Nurses state that self-care is a professional responsibility: 'in order to respond to the impact and demands of professional nursing practice, [nurses] must be emotionally intelligent and resilient individuals, who are able to manage their own personal health and wellbeing, and know when and how to access support' (NMC 2018b, p.3). Secondly, there is a common tendency for nurses and other care workers to become 'invisible patients' because their own needs are often ignored or pushed to the bottom of the list (Sheridan 2016). The health and wellbeing of those who care for patients is being recognized as one of the most important aspects of enabling them to care safely (Sign Up to Safety 2019). The final chapter is included to provide accessible strategies that any nurse or care worker can put into practice.

Structure of the chapters

The structure of the chapters is consistent throughout the manual. The core of each chapter is the procedures or guidelines. The other sections provide supporting information so that the procedure can be carried out with understanding of the clinical, technical, physiological, psychological and professional knowledge and evidence from which it has been developed. In each chapter there are the following elements:

- *Overview*: as the chapters are large and have considerable content, each one begins with an overview to guide the reader, informing them of the scope and the constituent sections of the chapter.
- *Definition*: each section begins with a definition of the terms and an explanation of the aspects of care, with any technical or difficult concepts explained.
- *Anatomy and physiology*: if it is necessary to understand the anatomy or physiology of a part of the body to perform a procedure, then the chapter or section includes a discussion of the related anatomy and physiology. If appropriate, this is illustrated with diagrams so the context of the procedure can be fully understood by the reader (e.g. electrical functioning of the heart to explain how electrocardiography works).
- *Related theory*: if it is necessary to understand theoretical principles in order to understand a procedure, then these are included (e.g. theory of communication).
- *Evidence-based approaches*: these sections provide background information and present the research and expert opinion in the relevant area. If appropriate, the indications and contraindications are included, as are any principles of care.
- *Clinical governance*: these sections outline any professional guidance, law or other national policy that may be relevant to the procedures. If relevant, this also includes any professional competences or qualifications required in order to perform the procedures. Any risk management considerations are also included in these sections, including principles of harm-free care.
- *Pre-procedural considerations:* when carrying out any procedure, there are certain actions that may need to be completed, or equipment prepared, or medication given, before the procedure begins. These are made explicit under this heading.
- *Procedure:* each chapter includes the current procedures that are used in the acute hospital setting. They have been drawn from the daily nursing practice at The Royal Marsden NHS Foundation Trust. Only procedures about which the authors have knowledge and expertise are included. Each procedure gives detailed, step-by-step actions, supported by rationales. Where available, the known evidence underpinning these rationales is indicated.
- *Problem solving and resolution*: if relevant, each procedure is followed by a table of potential problems that may be encountered while carrying out the procedure as well as suggestions as to the cause, prevention and any action that may help to resolve the problem.
- *Post-procedural considerations*: care for the patient does not end with the procedure. This section details any documentation the nurse may need to complete, education and information that needs to be given to the patient, and ongoing observations or referrals to other members of the multiprofessional team that may be required.
- *Complications*: any ongoing problems or potential complications associated with the procedure are discussed in a final section. Evidence-based suggestions for resolution are also included.
- *Illustrations*: colour illustrations have been used to demonstrate the steps of some procedures. These will enable the nurse to see in greater detail, for example, the correct position of the hands or the angle of a needle.
- *Websites and references*: many of the chapters have a list of related websites that can be consulted for further information. All of the chapters end with a reference list. Only texts from the past 10 years have been included, unless they are seminal texts.

Finally

This book is intended as a reference and a resource, not as a replacement for practice-based education. None of the procedures in this book should be undertaken without prior instruction and subsequent supervision from an appropriately qualified and experienced professional. We hope that *The Royal Marsden Manual of Clinical Nursing Procedures* will continue to be a resource to help nurses deliver high quality care that maximizes the wellbeing and improves the health outcomes of patients in acute hospital settings.

To paraphrase the quote from *Leading Change, Adding Value* (NHS England 2016, p.5) near the beginning of this chapter, compassionate care delivered with courage, commitment and skill is our highest priority as nurses. This is made more explicit in Commitment 4 of *Leading Change, Adding Value* (NHS England 2016, p.21), which highlights the importance of putting the person at the centre of care (Box 1.9).

It is important to remember that even if a procedure is very familiar to us and we are very confident in carrying it out, it may be new to the patient, so time must be taken to explain it and gain consent, even if this is only verbal consent: 'the views of the person [receiving the treatment] should also be taken into account when choosing which treatment is most likely to be successful for an individual' (NMC 2018a, p.38). The diverse range of technical procedures to which patients may be subjected should act as a

Box 1.9 Commitment 4: We will focus on individuals experiencing high value care

We will ensure that individuals are always supported to influence and direct their own healthcare decisions, so that they are confident that 'no decision is taken about me without me'.

Care planning should involve the development of a personalized plan for each individual who is entering, leaving or transitioning care environments whether within a hospital, in their own home, care home or rehabilitation unit.

We need to encourage people to take more responsibility for their health by focusing on personalized care planning, self-management and behaviour change.

Source: Adapted from NHS England (2016) with permission of the NHS.

reminder not to lose sight of the unique person undergoing such procedures and the importance of individualized patient assessment in achieving this.

When a nurse
Encounters another
What occurs is never a neutral event
A pulse taken
Words exchanged
A touch
A healing moment
Two persons
Are never the same

(Anon. in Dossey et al. 2005)

Nurses have a central role to play in helping patients to manage the demands of the procedures described in this manual. It must not be forgotten that for the patient, the clinical procedure is part of a larger picture, which encompasses an appreciation of their unique experience of the reason they have needed nursing care in the first place.

References

Carper, B. (1978) Fundamental patterns of knowing in nursing. *Advances in Nursing Science*, 1(1), 13–23.

Carthy, J. & Clarke, J. (2009) *The 'How to Guide' for Implementing Human Factors in Healthcare*. Patient Safety First. Available at: https://chfg.org/how-to-guide-to-human-factors-volume-1

Clinical Human Factors Group (2019) *What Are Clinical Human Factors?* Available at: https://chfg.org/what-are-clinical-human-factors

Del Mar, C., Hoffman, T. & Glasziou, P. (2013) Information needs, asking questions, and some basics of research studies. In: Hoffman, T., Bennett, S. & Del Mar, C. (eds) *Evidence Based Practice across the Health Professions*, 2nd edn. Chatswood, Sydney: Churchill Livingstone / Elsevier, pp. 16–37.

Department of Health and Social Care (2015) *Nursing Associate Role Offers New Route into Nursing*. Available at: https://www.gov.uk/government/news/nursing-associate-role-offers-new-route-into-nursing

Diamond, J. (1998) *C: Because Cowards Get Cancer Too*. London: Vermilion.

Dossey, B.M., Keegan, L. & Guzzetta, C.E. (2005) *Holistic Nursing: A Handbook for Practice*, 4th edn. Sudbury, MA: Jones & Bartlett.

Dougherty, L. (2008) Obtaining peripheral vascular access. In: Dougherty, L. & Lamb, J. (eds) *Intravenous Therapy in Nursing Practice*, 2nd edn. Oxford: Blackwell.

Draper, J. (2018) Healthcare education research: The case for rethinking hierarchies of evidence (editorial). *Journal of Advanced Nursing*, 74, 2480–2483.

Ford, P. & Walsh, M. (1994) *New Rituals for Old: Nursing through the Looking Glass*. Oxford: Butterworth-Heinemann.

Glasby, J., Walshe, K. & Harvey, G. (2007) Making evidence fit for purpose in decision-making: A case-study of the hospital discharge of older people. *Evidence & Policy*, 3(3), 425–437.

Glover, J., Izzo, D., Odato, K. & Wang, L. (2006) *EBM Pyramid*. Hanover, NH / New Haven, CT: Dartmouth University / Yale University.

Greenhalgh, T. (2014) *How to Read a Paper: The Basics of Evidence Based Medicine*, 5th edn. London: BMJ Books.

Guyatt, G., Cook, D. & Haynes, B. (2004) Evidence based medicine has come a long way. *BMJ*, 329(7473), 990–991.

Health Education England (2015) *Raising the Bar: Shape of Caring – A Review of the Future Education and Training of Registered Nurses and Care Assistants*. Available at: https://www.hee.nhs.uk/sites/default/files/documents/2348-Shape-of-caring-review-FINAL.pdf

Ingham-Broomfield, R. (2016) A nurses' guide to the hierarchy of research designs and evidence. *Australian Journal of Advanced Nursing*, 33(3), 38–43.

Ives, C. & Hillier, S. (2015) *Human Factors in Healthcare: Common Terms*. Clinical Human Factors Group. Available at: http://s753619566.websitehome.co.uk/wp-content/uploads/2018/06/chfg-human-factors-common-terms.pdf

King's Fund (2018) *Examining the Evidence for New Roles in Health and Social Care*. Available at: https://www.hee.nhs.uk/sites/default/files/documents/Examining%20the%20evidence%20for%20new%20roles%20in%20health%20and%20care.pdf

NHS Employers (2018) *Key Changes to the Standards for Nurses*. Available at: https://www.nhsemployers.org/-/media/Employers/Publications/Workforce-Supply/Key_Changes_to_the_standards_for_nurses.pdf

NHS England (2014) *NHS England: Five Year Forward View*. London: NHS England.

NHS England (2016) *Leading Change, Adding Value: A Framework for Nursing, Midwifery and Care Staff*. Available at: https://www.england.nhs.uk/wp-content/uploads/2016/05/nursing-framework.pdf

NHS England (2017) *Multi-professional Framework for Advanced Clinical Practice in England*. Available at: https://www.hee.nhs.uk/sites/default/files/documents/Multi-professional%20framework%20for%20advanced%20clinical%20practice%20in%20England.pdf

NHS England (2018a) *About the NHS*. Available at: https://www.nhs.uk/using-the-nhs/about-the-nhs/principles-and-values

NHS England (2018b) *Leading Change, Adding Value: A Framework for Nursing, Midwifery and Care Staff – A Learning Tool to Support All Nursing, Midwifery and Care Staff to Identify and Address Unwarranted Variation in Practice*. Available at: https://www.england.nhs.uk/wp-content/uploads/2018/05/lcav-e-learning-tool-v1.pdf

NHS England (2019) *NHS Long Term Plan*. Available at: https://www.longtermplan.nhs.uk/wp-content/uploads/2019/01/nhs-long-term-plan-june-2019.pdf

NHS Liverpool Heart and Chest Hospital (2018) *70 NHS Facts*. Available at: https://www.lhch.nhs.uk/media/5967/nhs70-facts.pdf

NMC (Nursing and Midwifery Council) (2018a) *The Code: Professional Standards of Practice and Behaviour for Nurses, Midwives and Nursing Associates*. Available at: https://www.nmc.org.uk/standards/code

NMC (2018b) *Future Nurse: Standards of Proficiency for Registered Nurses*. Available at: https://www.nmc.org.uk/globalassets/sitedocuments/education-standards/future-nurse-proficiencies.pdf

NMC (2018c) *Standards of Proficiency for Nursing Associates*. Available at: https://www.nmc.org.uk/globalassets/sitedocuments/education-standards/print-friendly-nursing-associates-proficiency-standards.pdf

Nuffield Trust (2016) *Reshaping the Workforce to Deliver the Care Patients Need*. Available at: https://www.nuffieldtrust.org.uk/research/reshaping-the-workforce-to-deliver-the-care-patients-need

Paley, J. (2006) Evidence and expertise. *Nursing Enquiry*, 13(2), 82–93.

Pearson, A., Field, J. & Jordan, Z. (2011) *Evidence-Based Clinical Practice in Nursing and Health Care: Assimilating Research, Experience, and Expertise*. Oxford: Wiley-Blackwell.

Petticrew, M. & Roberts, H. (2003) Evidence, hierarchies and typologies: Horses for courses. *Journal of Epidemiology & Community Health*, 57(7), 527–529.

Porter, S. (2010) Fundamental patterns of knowing in nursing: The challenge of evidence-based practice. *ANS Advances in Nursing Science*, 33(1), 3–14.

RCN (Royal College of Nursing) (2019) *Patient Safety and Human Factors*. Available at: https://www.rcn.org.uk/clinical-topics/patient-safety-and-human-factors

Royal Marsden NHS *Foundation Trust (2015) Nursing Strategy 2016–2018*. Available at: https://shared-d7-royalmarsden-publicne-live.s3.amazonaws.com/files_trust/s3fs-public/nursing-strategy-2016-18.pdf

Rycroft-Malone, J., Seers, K., Titchen, A., et al. (2004) What counts as evidence in evidence-based practice? *Journal of Advanced Nursing*, 47(1), 81–90.

Sackett, D.L., Rosenberg, W.M., Gray, J.A., et al. (1996) Evidence based medicine: What it is and what it isn't. *BMJ*, 312(7023), 71–72.

Scott, K. & McSherry, R. (2009) Evidence-based nursing: Clarifying the concepts for nurses in practice. *Journal of Clinical Nursing*, 18(8), 1085–1095.

Sheridan, C.B. (2016) *The Mindful Nurse: Using the Power of Mindfulness and Compassion to Help You Thrive in Your Work*. Galway: Rivertime Press.

Sign Up to Safety (2019) *Did You Know that Nearly Everyone's Job Affects the Safety of Patients?* Available at: https://www.signuptosafety.org.uk/nearly-everyones-job-affects-safety

Stevenson, J.C., Emerson, L. & Millings, A. (2017) The relationship between adult attachment orientation and mindfulness: A systematic review and meta-analysis. *Mindfulness*, 8, 1438–1455.

Walsh, M. & Ford, P. (1989) *Nursing Rituals, Research and Rational Actions*. Oxford: Heinemann Nursing.

Wilson, C. (2005) Said another way: My definition of nursing. *Nursing Forum*, 40(3), 116–118.

Part One

Managing the patient journey

Chapters

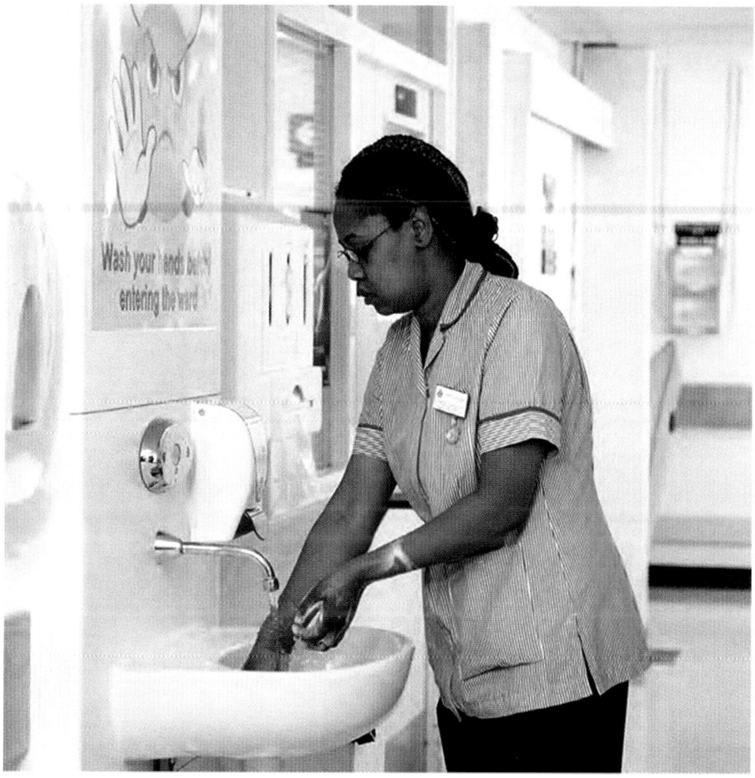

Chapter 2

Admissions and assessment

Lorraine Guinan and Victoria Ward with Elizabeth Hendry, Emma Masters, Andrew Rayner, Emma Thistlethwayte, Manuela Trofor, Charlotte Weston and Claire White

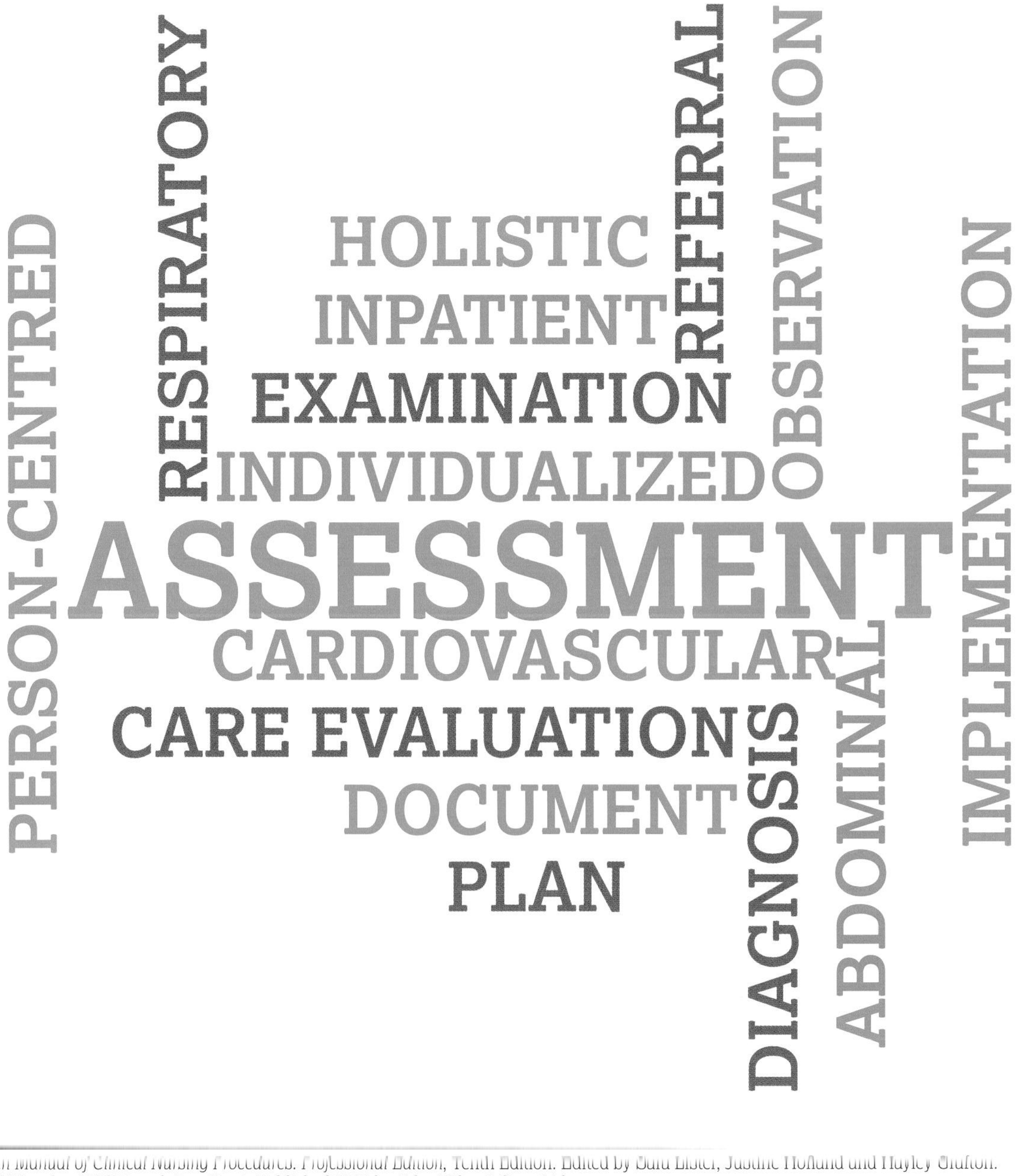
PERSON-CENTRED
RESPIRATORY
HOLISTIC
INPATIENT
REFERRAL
OBSERVATION
EXAMINATION
INDIVIDUALIZED
ASSESSMENT
IMPLEMENTATION
CARDIOVASCULAR
ABDOMINAL
CARE EVALUATION
DIAGNOSIS
DOCUMENT
PLAN

The Royal Marsden Manual of Clinical Nursing Procedures, Professional Edition, Tenth Edition. Edited by Sara Lister, Justine Hofland and Hayley Grafton.

Procedure guidelines

Being an accountable professional

At the point of registration, the nurse will:

1. Use evidence-based, best practice approaches to take a history, observe, recognise and accurately assess people of all ages:
   1.1 mental health and wellbeing status
   1.2 physical health and wellbeing

2. Use evidence-based, best practice approaches to undertake the following procedures:
   2.7 undertake a whole body systems assessment including respiratory, circulatory, neurological, musculoskeletal, cardiovascular and skin status
   2.8 undertake chest auscultation and interpret findings

Future Nurse: Standards of Proficiency for Registered Nurses (NMC 2018)

Overview

This chapter gives an overview of inpatient assessment, the process of care and the importance of observation in the assessment process.

Assessment forms an integral part of patient care and is considered to be the first step in the process of individualized nursing care. It provides information that is critical to the development of a plan of action that enhances personal health status. Early and continued assessments are vital to the success and management of patient care. It is critical that nurses have the ability to assess patients and document their findings in a systematic way.

Advanced nursing practice provides a high quality of care (McLoughlin et al. 2012) and has emerged in response to changing healthcare demands and the need for a flexible approach to care delivery. Key roles within advanced nursing practice include conducting comprehensive health assessments, demonstrating expert skills in diagnosing and treating acute and chronic illness, and making specialist referrals as required. Physical assessment is a core procedure for those undertaking this role and so is incorporated into this chapter.

The patient's age, health and mode of presentation will determine the extent of the physical assessment required (Innes et al. 2018). Observation – coupled with one or more of cardiovascular, respiratory or abdominal examinations – is discussed in this chapter. See Chapter 14: Observations for information on neurological assessment.

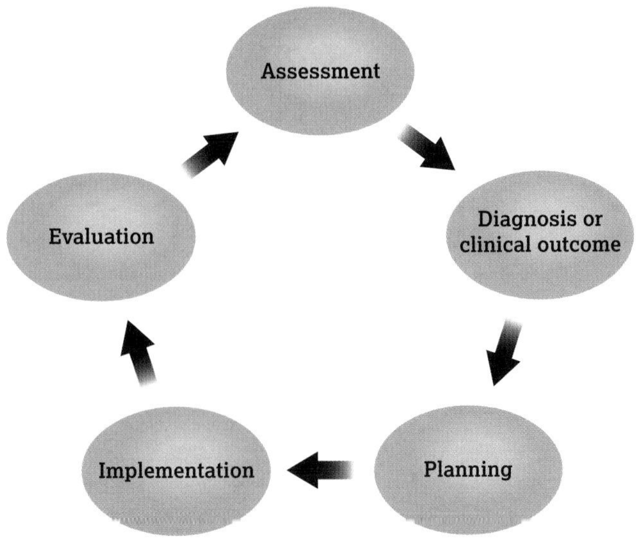

Figure 2.1 Phases of the nursing process. *Source*: Reproduced from Weber and Kelley (2014) with permission of Lippincott Williams & Wilkins.

Inpatient assessment and the process of care

To appropriately care for a patient within the hospital setting or the community, the nurse must assess the patient in order to develop a care plan tailored to the individual (Saxon and Lillyman 2011). The nursing process is an organized, systematic and deliberate approach that aims to improve standards in nursing care (Rush et al. 1996). This process is cyclical, ongoing and generally used in conjunction with various theoretical nursing models or philosophies. The process is both holistic and problem solving; each stage is intimately interconnected with the other stages and is explicable only by reference to the whole – used in partnership with the patient and their family. This process, similar to those used in problem solving and scientific reasoning, incorporates assessment, diagnosis, planning, implementation and evaluation phases, as demonstrated in Figure 2.1 and Table 2.1 (Pratt and Van Wijgerden 2009). Each step of the nursing process depends on the accuracy of the preceding step. This nursing process has evolved over the past decades and is now used by nurses throughout the world as a framework for providing individualized, person-centred care.

Definition

Assessment is the systematic and continuous collection, organization, validation and documentation of information (Berman et al. 2010).

Related theory

Nurses perform assessments on patients to inform professional judgements on what care is required. Assessment takes place from the time a nurse encounters the patient and is ongoing, continuing until discharge from the nurse's care. Nurses use various tools to facilitate the process of assessment (Crouch and Meurier 2005).

A health assessment involves the collection and analysis of data in order to identify the patient's problems. The nursing health assessment incorporates a comprehensive health history and a complete physical examination, both of which are used to evaluate the health status of a person; it is a deliberate and interactive process. The need to solicit information, understand the findings and apply knowledge can initially be daunting to the new nurse. Regardless of who collects the data, a total health assessment is needed when a patient first enters the healthcare system.

Table 2.1 Phases of the nursing process

Phase	Title	Description
1	Assessment	Collecting objective and subjective data
2	Diagnosis	Analysing subjective and objective data to make a professional nursing judgement
3	Planning	Determining outcome criteria and developing a plan
4	Implementation	Carrying out the plan
5	Evaluation	Assessing whether the outcome criteria have been met and revising the plan as necessary

Source: Reproduced from Weber and Kelley (2014) with permission of Lippincott Williams & Wilkins.

The nursing assessment should focus on the patient's response to a health need rather than disease process and pathology (Wilkinson 2007). The process of assessment requires nurses to make accurate and relevant observations and to gather, validate and organize data; this process supports the nurse in making judgements to determine care and treatment needs. The nursing assessment should include physical, psychological, spiritual, social and cultural dimensions; it is vital that these dimensions are explored with the person being assessed.

Effective patient assessment is integral to the safety, continuity and quality of patient care. The main principles of assessment fulfil the nurse's legal and professional obligations in practice (Table 2.2).

Assessment tools

Assessment tools in clinical practice can be used to assess a patient's general needs – for example, via the Supportive Care Needs Survey (Bonevski et al. 2000) – or to assess a specific problem – for example, via the Oral Assessment Guide (Eilers et al. 1988). The choice of tool depends on the clinical setting, although, in general, the aim of using an assessment tool is to link the assessment of clinical variables with the measurement of clinical interventions (Frank-Stromborg and Olsen 2004). To be useful in

Table 2.2 Principles of assessment

1	Assessment is patient focused, being governed by the notion of an individual's actual, potential and perceived needs.
2	It provides baseline information from which to plan the interventions to be used and decide the outcomes of care to be achieved.
3	It facilitates evaluation of the care given and is a dimension of care that influences a patient's outcome and potential survival.
4	It is a dynamic process that starts when problems or symptoms develop and continues throughout the care process, accommodating continual changes in the patient's condition and circumstances.
5	It is an interactive process in which the patient actively participates.
6	Optimal functioning, quality of life and the promotion of independence should be primary concerns.
7	The process includes observation, data collection, clinical judgement and validation of perceptions.
8	Data used for the assessment process are collected from several sources by a variety of methods, depending on the healthcare setting.
9	To be effective, the process must be structured and clearly documented.

Source: Adapted from Alfaro-LeFevre (2014), NMC (2018), Teytelman (2002), White (2003).

clinical practice, an assessment tool must be simple and acceptable to patients, have a clear and interpretable scoring system, and demonstrate reliability and validity (Brown et al. 2001).

The use of patient self-assessment tools appears to facilitate the process of assessment in a number of ways. It enables patients to indicate their subjective experience more easily, gives them an increased sense of participation (Kearney 2001) and prevents them from being distanced from the process by nurses rating their symptoms and concerns (Brown et al. 2001). Many authors have demonstrated the advantages of increasing patient participation in assessment by the use of patient self-assessment questionnaires (Rhodes et al. 2000).

The methods used to facilitate patient assessment are important adjuncts to assessing patients in clinical practice. There is a danger that too much focus can be placed on the framework, system or tool, preventing nurses from thinking about the significance of the information that they are gathering from the patient (Harris et al. 1998). Rather than following assessment structures and prompts rigidly, it is essential that nurses utilize their critical thinking and clinical judgement throughout the process in order to continually develop their skills in eliciting information about patients' concerns and use this to inform care planning (Edwards and Miller 2001).

Structure of assessment

Structuring patient assessment is vital to monitoring the success of care and detecting the emergence of new problems. There are many conceptual frameworks or nursing models, such as Roper's model for assessing activities of daily living (Roper et al. 2000), Orem's self-care model (Orem et al. 2001) and Gordon's functional health patterns framework (Gordon, 1994). There remains, however, much debate about the effectiveness of such models for assessment in practice, with some arguing that individualized care can be compromised by fitting patients into a rigid or complex structure (Kearney 2001, McCrae 2012). Nurses therefore need to take a pragmatic approach and utilize assessment frameworks that are appropriate to their particular area of practice. This is particularly relevant in today's rapidly changing healthcare climate, where nurses are taking on increasingly advanced roles, working across boundaries and setting up new services to meet patients' needs (DH 2006).

The framework of choice at The Royal Marsden NHS Foundation Trust is based on Gordon's functional health patterns framework (Box 2.1; Gordon 1994). This framework facilitates an assessment that focuses on patients' and families' problems and functional status; the framework applies clinical cues to interpret deviations from the patient's usual patterns (Johnson 2000). Gordon's functional health patterns framework is applicable to all levels of care, allowing problem areas to be identified. Information derived from the patient's initial functional health patterns is crucial for interpreting both the patient's and their family's pattern of response to disease and treatment.

Box 2.1 Gordon's functional health patterns

- Health perception and health management
- Nutrition and metabolism
- Elimination
- Activity and exercise
- Sleep and rest
- Cognition and perception
- Self-perception and self-concept
- Coping and stress tolerance
- Roles and relationships
- Sexuality and reproductivity
- Values and beliefs

Source: Adapted from Gordon (1994) with permission of Mosby / Elsevier.

Types of patient assessment

There are several types of assessment, including mini assessment, comprehensive assessment, focused assessment and ongoing assessment (Box 2.2).

Box 2.2 Types of patient assessment

Mini assessment

A snapshot view of the patient based on a quick visual and physical assessment. Consider the patient's ABC (airway, breathing and circulation), then assess mental status, overall appearance, level of consciousness and vital signs before focusing on the patient's main problem.

Comprehensive assessment

An in-depth assessment of the patient's health status, risk factors, and psychological and social aspects of health, along with a physical examination; it usually takes place on admission or transfer to a hospital or healthcare agency. It also considers the patient's health status prior to admission.

Focused assessment

An assessment of a specific condition, problem, identified risk or care need – for example, continence assessment, nutritional assessment, neurological assessment following a head injury, assessment for day care or outpatient consultation for a specific condition.

Ongoing assessment

Continuous assessment of the patient's health status accompanied by monitoring and observation of specific problems identified in a mini, comprehensive or focused assessment.

Source: Ahern and Philpot (2002), Holmes (2003), White (2003).

Evidence-based approaches

Collecting data

Data collection is the process of gathering information about the patient's health needs. Information for assessment is collected by means of:

- interview
- observation
- physical examination.

This information can consist of both objective and subjective data. Objective data are measurable and can be detected by someone other than the patient. Objective data include vital signs, physical signs and symptoms, and laboratory results. Subjective data are based on what the patient perceives. Subjective data may include descriptions of the patient's concerns, their support network, their awareness and knowledge of their abilities/disabilities, their understanding of their illness, and their attitude to and readiness for learning (Wilkinson 2007). While the patient is the primary source of information, data may be elicited from a variety of secondary sources including family, friends, other healthcare professionals and the patient's medical records (Kozier 2012, Walsh et al. 2007).

Assessment is the first and most critical step of the nursing process; it should be systematic and scientific, and should aim to obtain as much accurate and relevant information or data about the patient as possible. Inadequate data or omissions may lead to inaccurate or incorrect judgements.

Assessment interviews

Communication is vital to assessment. It is important to build a good rapport with the patient. The initial assessment interview not only allows the nurse to obtain baseline information about the patient but also facilitates the establishment of a therapeutic relationship (Crumbie 2006). It is vital that the nurse demonstrates interest and respect to the patient from the very start of the interview. Some of the information requested is likely to be of a searching and intimate nature, which may be difficult for the patient to disclose. The nurse should emphasize the confidential nature of the discussion and take steps to reduce anxiety and ensure privacy; the patient may modify their words and behaviour depending on the environment. Taking steps to establish trust and develop the relationship early on will set the scene for effective and accurate information exchange (Silverman et al. 2013).

Interviewing is a skill and an art; it should be both patient centred and clinician centred. The clinician seeks to elicit the full story of the patient's symptoms but must also collect key information in order to complete the assessment and develop a plan. Allowing patients to lead the interview process allows clinicians to understand patients' thoughts, ideas and concerns without adding their own perspective (see Chapter 5: Communication, psychological wellbeing and safeguarding).

In contrast, a clinician-centred or symptom-focused interview is used to elicit specific information in order to identify a disease or problem. Evidence suggests that patients are best served by integrating the two styles as the combination of the two approaches conveys the caring attributes of respect, empathy, humility and sensitivity (Fortin et al. 2012, Haidet and Paterniti 2003). The interview should be open ended, drawing on a range of techniques to cue patients to tell their stories; active listening, guided questioning, non-verbal affirmation, empathetic responses, validation and reassurance are all useful tools (Bickley and Szilagyi 2017).

Observation

Observation is the conscious, deliberate use of the physical senses to gather data from the patient and the environment. For an initial assessment, these observations may include vital signs, physical signs and symptoms, and laboratory results. These are all measurable and objective.

Physical examination

Physical examination is a systematic assessment of all body systems and is concerned with identifying strengths and deficits in the patient's functional abilities. Physical examination elicits both objective and subjective data as it combines elements of both interviewing and observation. It is important to remember that physical examination can be viewed with some anxiety as patients can feel vulnerable, exposed and apprehensive. Good communication (both verbal and non-verbal), together with observational skills, is key, as are ensuring that the environment is appropriate and that all required equipment is readily available.

Principles of an effective nursing assessment

The admitting nurse is responsible for ensuring that an initial assessment is completed when the patient is admitted. The patient's needs, identified following this process, must then be documented in their care plan. Box 2.3 discusses each area of assessment, indicating points for consideration and suggesting questions that it may be helpful to ask the patient as part of the assessment process.

Box 2.3 Points for consideration and suggested questions for use during the assessment process

1 Cognitive and perceptual ability

Communication

The nurse needs to assess the level of sensory functioning with or without aids/support (such as hearing aid(s), speech aid(s), glasses or contact lenses) and the patient's capacity to use and maintain aids/support correctly. Furthermore, it is important during this part of the assessment to assess whether there are or might be any potential language or cultural barriers. Knowing the norm within the patient's culture will facilitate understanding and lessen miscommunication (Galanti 2000).

- How good are the patient's hearing and eyesight?
- Is the patient able to express their views and wishes using appropriate verbal and non-verbal methods of communication in a manner that is understandable by most people?
- Are there any potential language or cultural barriers to communicating with the patient?

Information

During this part of the assessment, the nurse will assess the patient's ability to comprehend the present environment without showing levels of distress. This will help to establish whether there are any barriers to the patient's understanding of their condition and treatment. It may help them to be in a position to give informed consent.

- Is the patient able and ready to understand any information about their forthcoming treatment and care? Are there any barriers to learning?
- Is the patient able to communicate an understanding of their condition, plan of care and potential outcomes/responses?
- Will they be able to give informed consent?

Neurological

It is important to assess the patient's ability to reason logically and decisively, and determine that they are able to communicate in a contextually coherent manner.

- Is the patient alert and orientated to time, place and person?

Pain

To provide optimal patient care, the assessor needs to have appropriate knowledge of the patient's pain and an ability to identify the pain type and location. Assessment of a patient's experience of pain is a crucial component in providing effective pain management. Dimond (2002) asserts that it is unacceptable for patients to experience unmanaged pain or for nurses to have inadequate knowledge about pain. Pain should be measured using an assessment tool that identifies the quantity and/or quality of one or more of the dimensions of the patient's experience of pain.

During the assessment, the nurse should also observe for signs of neuropathic pain, including descriptions such as shooting, burning or stabbing, and descriptions consistent with allodynia (pain associated with gentle touch) (Jensen et al. 2003, Rowbotham and MacIntyre 2003, Schug et al. 2015).

- Is the patient pain free at rest and/or on movement?
- Is the pain a primary complaint or a secondary complaint associated with another condition?
- What is the location of the pain and does it radiate?
- When did it begin and what circumstances are associated with it?
- How intense is the pain, at rest and on movement?
- What makes the pain worse and what helps to relieve it?
- How long does the pain last – for example, continuous, intermittent?
- Ask the patient to describe the character of the pain using quality/sensory descriptors, such as sharp, throbbing or burning.

For further details regarding pain assessment, see Chapter 10: Pain assessment and management.

2 Activity and exercise

Respiratory

Respiratory pattern monitoring addresses the patient's breathing pattern, rate and depth.

- Does the patient have any difficulty breathing?
- Is there any noise when they are breathing, such as wheezing?
- Does breathing cause them pain?
- How deep or shallow is their breathing?
- Is their breathing symmetrical?
- Does the patient have any underlying respiratory problems, such as chronic obstructive pulmonary disease, emphysema, tuberculosis, bronchitis, asthma or any other airway disease?
- If appropriate, discuss smoking cessation.

For further details see Chapter 12: Respiratory care, CPR and blood transfusion.

Cardiovascular

A basic assessment is carried out and vital signs such as pulse (rhythm, rate and intensity) and blood pressure should be noted. Details of cardiac history should be taken for this part of the assessment. Medical conditions and experience of previous surgery should be noted.

- Does the patient take any cardiac medication?
- Do they have a pacemaker?

Physical abilities; personal hygiene, mobility and toileting; independence with activities of daily living

The aim during this part of the nursing assessment is to establish the level of assistance required by the person to tackle activities of daily living such as walking and use of stairs. An awareness of obstacles, level of independent mobility and dangers to personal safety is an important factor and part of the assessment.

- Is the patient able to stand, walk and go to the toilet?
- Is the patient able to move up and down, roll and turn in bed?
- Does the patient need any equipment to be mobile?
- Has the patient good motor power in their arms and legs?
- Does the patient have any history of falling?
- Can the patient take care of their own personal hygiene needs independently or do they need assistance?
- What type of assistance do they need – for example, do they need help with mobility or fine motor movements such as doing up buttons or shaving?

It might be necessary to complete a separate manual handling risk assessment – see Chapter 7: Moving and positioning.

3 Elimination

Gastrointestinal

During this part of the assessment, it is important to determine a baseline with regard to independence.

- Is the patient able to attend to their elimination needs independently and is the patient continent?
- What are the patient's normal bowel habits? Are bowel movements within the patient's own normal pattern and consistency?
- Does the patient have any underlying medical conditions, such as Crohn's disease or irritable bowel syndrome?
- Does the patient have diarrhoea or are they prone to having – or currently having – constipation?
- How does this affect the patient?

For further discussion see Chapter 6: Elimination.

Genitourinary

This part of the assessment is focused on the patient's baseline observations with regard to urinary continence/incontinence. It is also important to note whether there is any penile or vaginal discharge or bleeding.

- Does the patient have a urinary catheter in place? If so, note the type, size and date of insertion. If the patient previously had a urinary catheter, note the date it was removed. Urinalysis results should also be noted here.

(continued)

Box 2.3 Points for consideration and suggested questions for use during the assessment process *(continued)*

- How often does the patient need to urinate (frequency)?
- How immediate is the need to urinate (urgency)?
- Do they wake in the night to urinate (nocturia)?
- Are they able to maintain control over their bladder at all times (incontinence – inability to hold urine)?

For further discussion see Chapter 6: Elimination.

4 Nutrition and oral care

Oral care

As part of the inpatient admission assessment, the nurse should obtain an oral health history that includes oral hygiene beliefs and practices, and current state of oral health. During this assessment it is important to be aware of treatments and medications that affect the oral health of the patient. If deemed appropriate, use an oral assessment tool to perform the initial and ongoing oral assessments.

- Lips – are they pink, moist and intact?
- Gums – are they pink, with no signs of infection or bleeding?
- Teeth – are there dentures, a bridge, crowns or caps?

For details on how to conduct a full oral assessment, see Chapter 9: Patient comfort and supporting personal hygiene.

Hydration

An in-depth assessment of hydration will provide the information needed for nursing interventions aimed at maximizing wellness and identifying problems for treatment. The assessment should ascertain whether the patient has any difficulty drinking. During the assessment, the nurse should observe signs of dehydration – for example, dry mouth, dry skin, thirst or whether the patient shows any signs of an altered mental state.

- Is the patient able to drink adequately? If not, why not?
- How much and what does the patient drink?
- Note the patient's alcohol intake in the format of units per week (see Figure 2.2).
- Also note their caffeine intake, measured in number of cups per day.

Nutrition

A detailed diet history provides insight into a patient's baseline nutritional status. Assessment includes questions regarding chewing or swallowing problems; avoidance of eating related to abdominal pain; changes in appetite, taste or intake; and the use of a special diet or nutritional supplements. A review of past medical history should identify any relevant conditions and highlight increased metabolic needs, altered gastrointestinal function and the patient's capacity to absorb nutrients.

- What is the patient's usual daily food intake?
- Do they have a good appetite?
- Are they able to swallow/chew the food – any dysphagia?
- Is there anything they don't or can't eat?
- Have they experienced any recent weight changes or taste changes?
- Are they able to eat independently?
  (adapted from Arrowsmith 1999, BAPEN and Malnutrition Advisory Group 2000, DH 2005)

For further information, see Chapter 8: Nutrition and fluid balance.

Nausea and vomiting

During this part of the assessment, the nurse should ascertain whether the patient has any history of nausea and/or vomiting. Nausea and vomiting can cause dehydration, electrolyte imbalance and nutritional deficiencies (Marek 2003), and can also affect a patient's psychosocial wellbeing. They may become withdrawn, isolated and unable to perform their usual activities of daily living.

- Does the patient feel nauseous?
- Is the patient vomiting? If so, what are the frequency, volume, content and timing?
- Does nausea precede vomiting?
- Does vomiting relieve nausea?
- When did the symptoms start? Did they coincide with changes in therapy or medication?
- Does anything make the symptoms better?
- Does anything make the symptoms worse?
- What is the effect of any current or past antiemetic therapy, including dose, frequency, duration, effect and route of administration?
- What is the condition of the patient's oral cavity?
  (adapted from Perdue 2005)

For further discussion see Chapter 6: Elimination.

5 Skin

A detailed assessment of a patient's skin is an essential part of the admission and care process. The ASSKING bundle is a tool that can be used to help staff and patients to monitor skin concerns and proactively reduce the risk of developing a pressure ulcer. Documenting each aspect of the ASSKING checklist can help to achieve this (MacDonald and RMH Pressure Ulcer MDT Collaborative 2019).

ASSKING stands for:

A ssessment of risk
S kin inspection and care
S upport surface selection and use
K eep your patient moving
I ncontinence and moisture care
N utrition and hydration management
G iving information

For further information see Chapter 18: Wound management.

6 Controlling body temperature

This assessment is carried out to establish the patient's baseline temperature, determine whether the temperature is within the normal range, and ascertain whether there might be intrinsic or extrinsic factors causing altered body temperature. It is important to note whether any changes in temperature are in response to specific therapies (e.g. antipyretic medication, immunosuppressive therapies, invasive procedures or infection) (Bickley and Szilagyi 2017). White blood count should be recorded to determine whether it is within normal limits (see Chapter 14: Observations).

- Is the patient feeling excessively hot or cold?
- Have they been shivering or sweating excessively?

7 Sleep and rest

This part of the assessment is performed to find out sleep and rest patterns and reasons for variation. The nurse should document the patient's description of their sleep patterns and routines, and the habits they use to achieve a comfortable sleep. The nurse should also include the presence of emotional and/or physical problems that may interfere with sleep.

- Does the patient have enough energy for desired daily activities?
- Do they tire easily?
- Do they have any difficulty falling asleep or staying asleep?
- Do they feel rested after sleep?
- Do they sleep during the day?
- Do they take any aids to help them sleep?
- What are their normal hours for going to bed and waking?

8 Stress and coping

This assessment is focused on the patient's perception of stress and their coping strategies. Support systems should be evaluated and symptoms of stress should be noted. This assessment includes the individual's reserve or capacity to resist challenges to self-integrity, and their modes of handling stress. The effectiveness of a person's coping strategies in terms of stress tolerances may be further evaluated.

- What are the things in the patient's life that are stressful?
- What do they do when they are stressed?
- How do they know they are stressed?
- Is there anything they do to help them cope when life gets stressful?
- Is there anybody they go to for support?

(adapted from Gordon 1994)

9 Roles and relationships

It is important to understand the patient's role in the world and their relationships with others. Assessment in this area includes finding out about the patient's perceptions of the major roles and responsibilities they have in life, and about satisfaction and/or disturbances in their family, work and/or social relationships. An assessment of home life should be undertaken and must include how the patient will cope at home post-discharge, how those at home (e.g. dependants, children and/or animals) will cope while they are in hospital, and whether they have any financial concerns.

- Who is at home?
- Are there any dependants? (Include children, pets and anybody else the patient cares for.)
- What responsibilities does the patient have for the day-to-day running of the home?
- What will happen if they are not there?
- Do they have any concerns about their home while they are in hospital?
- Are there any financial issues related to their hospital stay?
- Will there be any issues related to employment or study while they are in hospital?

10 Perception/concept of self

This assessment concerns body image or self-esteem. Body image is highly personal, abstract and difficult to describe. The rationale for this section is to assess the patient's level of understanding and general perception of self. This includes their attitudes about self, their perception of their abilities (cognitive, affective and physical), their body image, their identity, their general sense of worth and their general emotional pattern. An assessment of body posture and movement, eye contact, voice and speech patterns should also be included.

- How do you describe yourself?
- How do you feel about yourself most of the time?
- Has it changed since your diagnosis?
- Have there been changes in the way you feel about yourself or your body?

11 Sexuality and reproduction

Understanding sexuality as the patient's perceptions of their own body image, family roles and functions, relationships and sexual function can help the assessor to improve assessment and diagnosis of actual or potential alterations in sexual behaviour and activity.

- Are you currently in a relationship?
- Has your condition had an impact on the way you and your partner feel about each other?
- Has your condition had an impact on the physical expression of your feelings?
- Has your treatment or current problem had any effect on your interest in being intimate with your partner?

12 Values and beliefs

This area concerns the patient's religious, spiritual and cultural beliefs. The aim is to assess the patient's needs in this area to provide culturally and spiritually specific care while concurrently providing a forum to explore spiritual strengths that might be used to prevent

(continued)

Box 2.3 Points for consideration and suggested questions for use during the assessment process *(continued)*

problems or cope with difficulties. A patient's experience of their stay in hospital may be influenced by their religious beliefs or other strongly held principles, cultural background or ethnic origin.

- Are there any spiritual or cultural beliefs or practices that are important to you?
- Do you have any specific dietary needs related to your religious, spiritual or cultural beliefs?
- Do you have any specific personal care needs related to your religious, spiritual or cultural beliefs (e.g. washing rituals, dress)?

13 Health perception and management

This assessment concerns any relevant medical conditions, side-effects and complications of treatment. The nurse should document the patient's perceived pattern of health and wellbeing and how their health is managed. Any relevant history of previous health problems, including side-effects of medication, should be noted. Examples of other useful information that should be documented are compliance with medication regimen, use of health promotion activities (such as regular exercise) and whether the patient has annual check-ups.

- What does the patient know about their condition and planned treatment?
- How would they describe their current overall level of fitness?
- What do they do to keep well: exercise, diet, annual check-ups or screening?

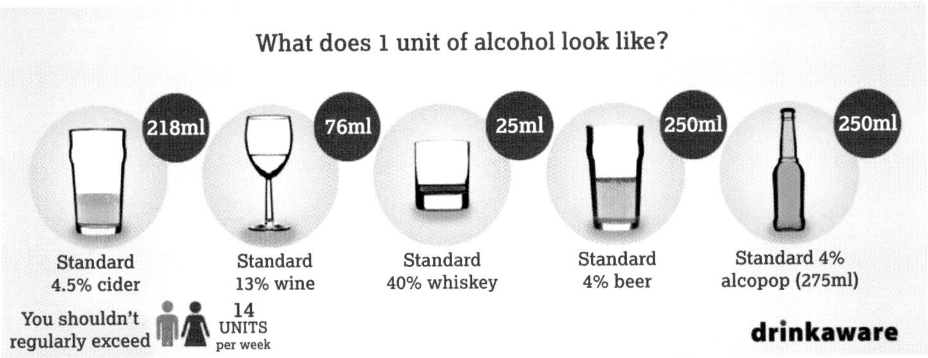

Figure 2.2 Examples of 1 unit of alcohol. *Source*: Drinkaware (2019). Reproduced with permission of Drinkaware.

Post-procedural considerations

Care planning

The purpose of collecting information through the process of assessment is to enable the nurse to make a series of clinical judgements (which are known in some circumstances as nursing diagnoses), and subsequently decisions about the nursing care each individual needs. Nursing diagnoses provide a focus for planning and implementing effective and evidence-based care. This process consists of identifying nursing-sensitive patient outcomes and determining appropriate interventions (Alfaro-LeFevre 2014, Shaw 1998, White 2003). The key steps are:

- To determine the immediate priorities and recognize whether the patient's problems require nursing care or whether a referral should be made to someone else.
- To identify the anticipated outcome for the patient, noting what the patient will be able to do and within what time frame. The use of 'measurable' verbs that describe patient behaviour or what the patient says facilitates the evaluation of patient outcomes (Box 2.4).
- To determine the nursing interventions – that is, what nursing actions will prevent or manage the patient's problems so that the patient's outcomes may be achieved.
- To record the care plan for the patient, which may be written or individualized from a standardized (sometimes called 'core') care plan or a computerized care plan.

Outcomes should be patient focused and realistic, stating how the outcomes or goals are to be achieved and when the outcomes should be evaluated. Outcomes may be short, intermediate or long term, enabling the nurse to identify the patient's health status and progress (stability, improvement or deterioration) over time. Setting realistic outcomes and interventions requires the nurse to distinguish between nursing diagnoses that are life threatening or an immediate risk to the patient's safety, and those that may be dealt with at a later stage.

Box 2.4 Examples of measurable and non-measurable verbs for use in outcome statements

Measurable verbs (use these to be specific)

- state, verbalize, communicate, list, describe, identify
- demonstrate, perform
- will lose, will gain, has an absence of
- walk, stand, sit

Non-measurable verbs (do not use)

- know
- understand
- think
- feel

Source: Reproduced from Alfaro-LeFevre (2014) with permission of Lippincott Williams & Wilkins.

It is important to continue to assess the patient on an ongoing basis while implementing the care planned. Assessing the patient's current status prior to implementing care will enable the nurse to check whether the patient has developed any new problems that require immediate action. During and after any nursing intervention, the nurse should assess and reassess the patient's response to care. The nurse will then be able to determine whether changes to the patient's care plan should be made immediately or at a later stage. If there are any patient care needs that require immediate action – for example, consultation or referral to a doctor – recording the actions taken is essential. Involving the patient and their family or friends will promote the patient's wellbeing and self-care abilities. The use of clinical documentation in the nursing shift report, or 'handover', will help to ensure that the care plans are up to date and relevant (Alfaro-LeFevre 2014, White 2003).

Evaluating care

Effective evaluation of care requires the nurse to critically analyse the patient's health status to determine whether the patient's condition is stable, has deteriorated or has improved. Seeking the patient's and their family's views in the evaluation process will facilitate decision making. By evaluating the patient's outcomes, the nurse is able to decide whether changes need to be made to the care planned. Evaluation of care should take place in a structured manner and on a regular basis by a registered nurse.

Documentation

Nurses have a professional responsibility to ensure that healthcare records provide an accurate account of treatment, care planning and delivery, and are viewed as a tool of communication within the team. There should be clear evidence of the care planned, the decisions made, the care delivered and the information shared (NMC 2018) (Box 2.5). The content and quality of record keeping are a measure of standards of practice relating to the skills and judgement of the nurse (NMC 2018).

Box 2.5 The Royal Marsden NHS Trust's guidelines for nursing documentation (2011) (adopted in line with NMC 2018)

General principles

1 Records should be written legibly in black ink in such a way that they cannot be erased and are readable when photocopied.
2 Entries should be factual, consistent, accurate and not contain jargon, abbreviations or meaningless phrases (e.g. 'observations fine').
3 Each entry must include the date and time (using the 24-hour clock).
4 Each entry must be followed by a signature and the name printed as well as:
- the job role (e.g. staff nurse or clinical nurse specialist);
- if a nurse is a temporary employee (i.e. an agency nurse), the name of the agency.

5 If an error is made, this should be scored out with a single line and the correction written alongside with date, time and initials. Correction fluid should not be used at any time.
6 All assessments and entries made by student nurses must be countersigned by a registered nurse.
7 Healthcare assistants:
- can write on fluid balance and food intake charts;
- must not write on prescription charts, assessment sheets or care plans.

Assessment and care planning

1 The first written assessment and the identification of the patient's immediate needs must begin within 4 hours of admission. This must include any allergies or infection risks of the patient and the contact details of the next of kin.
2 The following must be completed within 24 hours of admission and updated as appropriate:
- nutritional, oral, pressure ulcer and manual handling risk assessments;
- other relevant assessment tools, for example pain and wound assessment.

3 All sections of the nursing admission assessment must be completed at some point during the patient's hospital stay along with the identification of the patient's care needs. If it is not relevant or if it is inappropriate to assess certain functional health patterns (e.g. if the patient is unconscious) then the reasons should be indicated accordingly. The ongoing nursing assessment should identify whether the patient's condition is stable, has deteriorated or has improved.
4 Wherever possible, care plans should be written with the involvement of the patient, in terms that they can understand, and include:
- patient-focused, measurable, realistic and achievable goals;
- nursing interventions reflecting best practice;
- relevant core care plans that are individualized, signed, dated and timed.

5 Update the care plan with altered or additional interventions as appropriate.
6 The nursing documentation must be referred to at shift handover so it needs to be kept up to date.

Principles of assessment

1 Assessment should be a systematic, deliberate and interactive process that underpins every aspect of nursing care (Heaven and Maguire 1996).
2 Assessment should be seen as a continuous process (Cancer Action Team 2007).

Structure of assessment

1 The structure of a patient assessment should take into consideration the speciality and care setting and also the purpose of the assessment.
2 Functional health patterns provide a comprehensive framework for assessment, which can be adapted for use within a variety of clinical specialities and care settings (Gordon 1994).

Methods of assessment

1 Methods of assessment should elicit both subjective and objective assessment data.
2 An assessment interview must be well structured and progress logically in order to facilitate the nurse's thinking and to make the patient feel comfortable in telling their story.
3 Specific assessment tools should be used, where appropriate, to enable nurses to monitor particular aspects of care, such as symptom management (e.g. pain, fatigue), over time. This will help the nurse to evaluate the effectiveness of nursing interventions and it also often provides an opportunity for patients to become more involved in their care (O'Connor and Eggert 1994).

(continued)

Box 2.5 The Royal Marsden NHS Trust's guidelines for nursing documentation (2011) (adopted in line with NMC 2018) *(continued)*

Decision making and nursing diagnosis

1 Nurses should be encouraged to provide a rationale for their clinical judgements and decision making within their clinical practice (NMC 2018).
2 The language of nursing diagnosis is a tool that can be used to make clinical judgements more explicit and enable more consistent communication and documentation of nursing care (Clark 1999, Westbrook 2000).

Planning and implementing care

1 When planning care, it is vital that nurses recognize whether patient problems require nursing care or whether a referral should be made to someone else.
2 When a nursing diagnosis has been made, the anticipated outcome for the patient must be identified in a manner that is specific, achievable and measurable (NMC 2018).
3 Nursing interventions should be determined with the aim of addressing the nursing diagnosis and achieving the desired outcomes (Gordon 1994).

Evaluating care

1 Nursing care should be evaluated using measurable outcomes on a regular basis with interventions adjusted accordingly.
2 Progress towards achieving outcomes should be recorded in a concise and precise manner. Using a method such as charting by exception can facilitate this (Murphy 2003).

Documenting and communicating care

1 The content and quality of record keeping are a measure of standards of practice relating to the skills and judgement of the nurse (NMC 2018).
2 In addition to the written record of care, the important role that the handover plays in the communication and continuation of patient care should be considered, particularly when considering the role of electronic records.

Observation

Definition

Observation is the conscious, deliberate use of the physical senses to gather data from the patient and the environment. Observation occurs whenever the nurse is in contact with the patient. At each patient contact, it is important for the nurse to try to develop a sequence of observations. These might include the following:

1 On approaching the patient, observe for signs of distress, such as pallor, laboured breathing, and behaviours indicating pain or emotional distress.
2 Scan the area for safety hazards, such as any floor spillages.
3 Look at the equipment, such as urinary catheter, intravenous pumps, oxygen and monitors.
4 Notice other people in the area – who is there and how do these people interact with the patient?
5 Observe the patient more closely for physical data such as skin temperature, breath sounds, drainage and dressing odours, condition of drains and dressings, and need for repositioning (Wilkinson 2007).

Accurate measurements of the patient's vital signs provide crucial information about body functions (see Chapter 14: Observations).

Physical assessment

Patient assessment should be systematic; it can be defined as the systematic collection of information concerning the patient's health status with the aim of identifying the patient's current health status, actual and potential health problems, and areas for health improvement (Estes 2013).

Definition

Physical examination is the systematic assessment of all body systems; it is concerned with identifying strengths and deficits in the patient's functional abilities. Physical assessment provides objective data that can be used to validate the subjective data gained when taking the patient's history (Wilkinson 2007).

The patient's history is one of the most important components of a physical assessment; the history guides the nature of the physical assessment that needs to be carried out (Peacock 2004).

The components of a thorough health history are (Bickley and Szilagyi 2017):

- chief complaint
- history of chief complaint
- past medical history
- family history
- social history
- systems review.

The findings of the history will determine which body system to examine and what investigations are required; the nurse will determine whether a focused or comprehensive physical examination is required based on the patient's clinical presentation (Baid 2006).

The aims of the physical examination are:

- to identify potential diagnoses
- to make a diagnosis
- to obtain information on the patient's overall health status
- to enable additional information to be obtained about any symptoms reported by the patient
- to detect changes in the patient's condition
- to evaluate how the patient is responding to interventions
- to establish the patient's fitness for surgery or anaesthetic (Abbott and Ranson 2017; Crouch and Meurier 2005).

During the physical assessment, a systematic approach is taken to build on the patient's history, using the key assessment skills of inspection, palpation, percussion and auscultation (Figure 2.3).

Anatomy and physiology

When examining an area of the body, it is essential to understand the basic anatomy of that area. This will ensure that the appropriate system is examined and that the findings of the examination

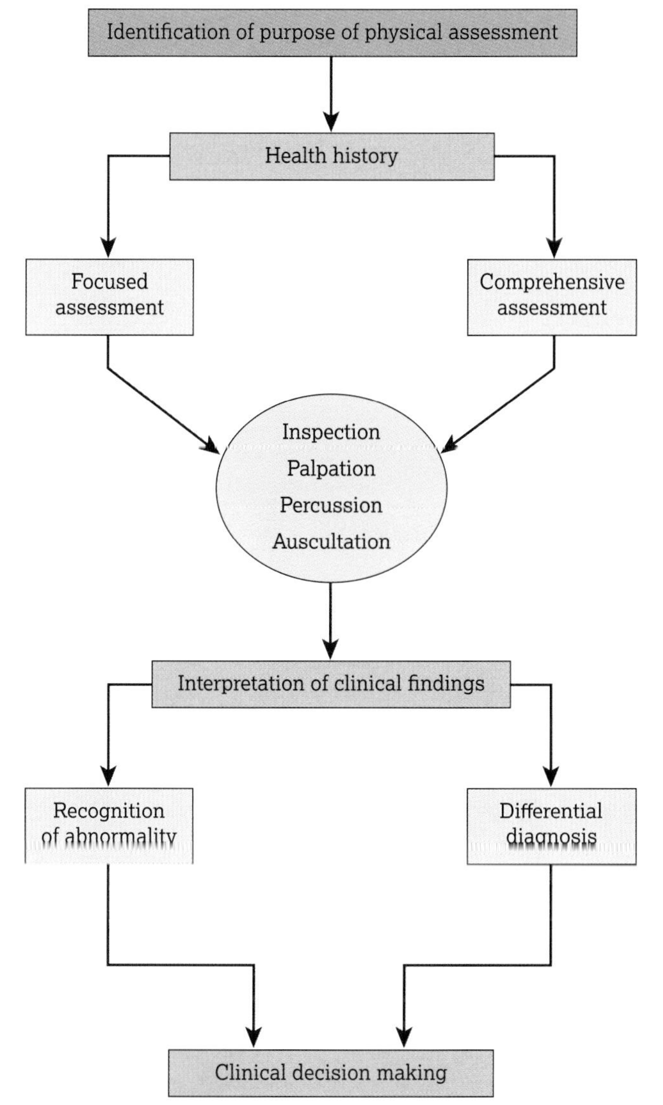

Figure 2.3 Physical assessment framework. *Source*: Reproduced from Baid (2006) with permission of MA Healthcare Limited.

are understood. It will also help in the formation of differential diagnoses and in ensuring that appropriate investigations are ordered.

Related theory

Alongside history taking and investigations, physical assessment is essential to helping a patient from their presenting complaint to diagnosis and treatment. Successful assessment requires critical thinking skills and a good knowledge base to decide which assessments to make, how much information is needed and how to get the information (Wilkinson 2007).

The clinical reasoning model permits the clinician to question and examine an existing problem in order to formulate and critically analyse a comprehensive hypothesis, elaborate strategies, establish a diagnosis and initiate a treatment (Barrows and Pickell 1991). This model represents a step-by-step approach to the clinical decision-making process (Walsh 2006b); it is 'the art of thinking about your thinking while you're thinking so as to make your thinking more clear, precise, accurate, relevant, consistent, and fair' (Paul 1988, pp.2–3).

The systems that this chapter will cover are respiratory, cardiovascular and abdominal. Neurological examination is covered in Chapter 14: Observations.

Evidence-based approaches

Rationale

Before commencing a physical assessment, a detailed health history should be taken. The patient's present complaints, the findings of the history taking, and the nurse's knowledge of anatomy and physiology will determine which body system to examine and what investigations are required (Price et al. 2000). Furthermore, it is also important to consider the patient's entire problem, including from social and psychological perspectives (Barrows and Pickell 1991).

From the history, a list of differential diagnoses will have been generated and the examination should seek to confirm, refute or further establish whether each of the differential diagnoses is a possibility or not. According to Weber and Kelley (2014), the process can be divided into the following steps:

1 Identify abnormal data or the presenting complaint.
2 Cluster the data.
3 Draw interferences and identify the problem.
4 Identify differential diagnoses.
5 Analyse each diagnosis.
6 Confirm or refute each potential diagnosis.
7 Document the conclusion.

Each system-based examination is divided into the following categories:

- inspection (looking)
- palpation (feeling)
- percussion (tapping)
- auscultation (listening).

Inspection

Inspection is simply observing the patient while looking for the presence or absence of physical signs that confirm or refute the differential diagnoses obtained from the history (Dover et al. 2018). A general survey of the patient should include observations of posture, gait, height and weight, posture, mood and alertness (Bickley and Szilagyi 2017).

Prior to taking a history, the nurse should introduce themselves to the patient and define their role. The patient may be particularly worried that the examination will identify a serious problem so it is important to build a rapport and trust. The nurse should provide the patient with their full attention and use appropriate facial expressions. After introducing themselves, the nurse should ask the patient open-ended questions to facilitate conversation (Jarvis 2016). Closed questions can be used to ask for specific information and clarifying questions can be used where appropriate. The nurse must ensure the patient feels confident to share information.

During the interview and the physical examination, the nurse should continue to observe the patient's behaviour, general demeanour and appearance. Having the opportunity to take the patient's history often allows subtle clues about their health to be identified. For example, a patient's voice can provide important clues about neurological and respiratory functions (Baid 2006).

The precise points to consider during inspection are informed to some extent by the history; however, inspection starts as soon as the nurse first sees the patient. This is called the 'global view of the patient', 'general survey' or 'first impression' (Innes et al. 2018). Inspection will then continue throughout the physical examination (Seidel et al. 2011). Typically, the first impression includes looking at the patient as a whole, examining the nails, skin and eyes, and assessing vital signs (Rushforth 2009, Swartz 2014, Tidman 2018). The following should be considered:

- *General appearance*: are they well kept? Are they wearing appropriate clothing?
- *Nutrition*: do they look well nourished?
- *Pain*: do they appear to be in any pain? What is their facial expression?

- *Nausea and vomiting*: are they retching?
- *Posture and gait*: how do they get into the room? Walk? Limp? Wheelchair?
- *Orientation*: are they orientated to time and place? (see Chapter 14: Observations)
- *Consciousness*: what is their level of consciousness? (see Chapter 14: Observations)
- *Symmetry*: are they moving both sides of their body symmetrically?
- *Speech*: is their speech impaired?

Once inspection has been completed, the nurse should move on to the system(s) of concern and examine the area(s) closely.

Palpation

Palpation requires use of the whole hand (including the palm and the full length of the fingers) using touch to feel and assess an area (Bickley and Szilagyi 2017, Rushforth 2009, Swartz 2014).

This includes assessment of:

- texture
- tenderness
- temperature
- contours
- pulse
- lymph nodes
- moisture
- mobility.

The order of palpation is not important unless there is an area of pain or tenderness, in which case always examine that area last. There are two variations of palpation: light palpation and deep palpation:

- *Light palpation* requires a gentle touch, depressing the skin with one hand to a maximum of 2 cm (Rushforth 2009). When lightly palpating, temperature, tenderness, texture, moisture, elasticity, pulsation and any superficial organs or masses should be assessed (see Figure 2.21).
- *Deep palpation* uses the same technique as light palpation but often two hands are used, one on top of the other at a depth of around 4 cm, as illustrated in Figure 2.22. When palpating deeply, internal organs and masses should be assessed. As the nurse palpates, they should watch the patient's face assessing for any discomfort or tenderness (Rushforth 2009).

Percussion

Percussion helps to identify organs, allowing assessment of size and shape. The technique is done by laying the tip and first joint of the middle finger flat on the patient, ensuring that no other part of the finger or hand is touching the patient. The joint is then struck in a quick, fluid movement with the fingertip of the middle finger of the other hand (Bickley and Szilagyi 2017), as illustrated in Figure 2.20. The sound produced by the impact is heard as percussion tones called 'resonance' (Seidel et al. 2011). The percussion technique is the same for all the structures of the body.

The sound produced through percussion can help to identify whether the structures are solid or filled with liquid or air (Table 2.3). It takes experience and practice to be able to hear and identify the different sounds.

Auscultation

Auscultation involves listening to various sounds in the body using a stethoscope (Bickley and Szilagyi 2017, Rushforth 2009). A stethoscope is a medical device and has a bell and a diaphragm (Figure 2.4), which is often used to listen to internal sounds of the human body. The bell should be used to hear low-pitched sounds, for example murmurs; the diaphragm should be used when listening to high-pitched sounds, for example bowel sounds. A good-quality stethoscope will aid diagnosis as more subtle sounds will be heard clearly.

Table 2.3 Different sounds heard on percussion

Sound	Quality	Example of source
Flat	Soft, high-pitched, dull sound	Thigh
Dull	Medium-level, thud-like sound	Liver, spleen
Resonant	Loud, low-pitched, hollow sound	Lung
Hyper-resonant	Very loud, low, booming, hollow sound	No normal organ
Tympanic	Loud, high-pitched, drum-like sound	Gastric air bubble

Source: Adapted from Bickley and Szilagyi (2017), Rushforth (2009).

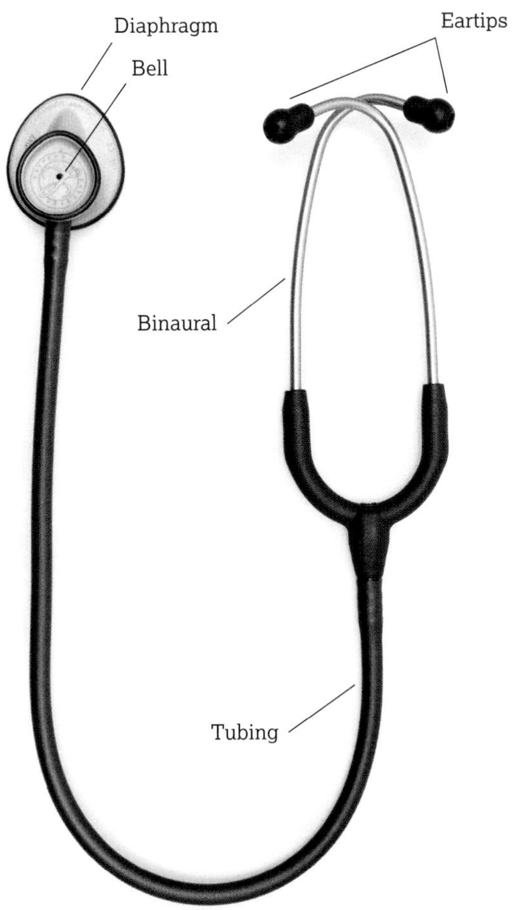

Figure 2.4 Stethoscope.

Clinical governance

As in all aspects of care, nurses must be aware of their ethical and legal responsibilities when assessing patients. Issues of honesty and confidentiality are frequently encountered during assessment (Wilkinson 2007).

Physical assessment is an advanced skill. While nurses may be able to practise skills through reading and work-based learning, many courses are available to help them learn in a structured fashion. It is essential to have a solid understanding of anatomy and physiology, interpretation of findings, and knowledge of appropriate actions to take.

This chapter gives a basic overview of the techniques used when physically assessing patients. In order to perform physical assessment safely, nurses will require further education and supervised clinical experience to ensure competence. The Nursing and Midwifery Council's *Code* (NMC 2018) states that all nurses must be accountable for their actions and omissions and must practise within their sphere of competence at all times.

Consent

The Royal College of Nursing (2017) states that registered nurses must ensure consent is obtained and clearly documented prior to commencing any procedure or treatment. Before gaining consent, information about the procedure should be given to the patient in a clear, honest and jargon-free manner (NMC 2018).

According to Burns et al. (2011), there are three main components of valid consent. To be competent (or to have the capacity) to give consent, the patient must:

- understand the information that has been given
- believe that information
- be able to retain and evaluate the information so as to make a decision.

Pre-procedural considerations

Prior to commencing a patient assessment, the nurse should prepare the physical environment, taking into consideration the patient's privacy and dignity (Smith and Rushton 2015).

Equipment

Prior to the examination, the nurse should ensure the environment is at a suitable temperature and prepare the appropriate equipment. Good preparation of equipment is essential for a competent physical assessment (Crouch and Meurier 2005). The following equipment may be useful as part of a physical examination:

- pen torch
- stethoscope
- examination couch
- tongue depressor
- ruler (must measure in centimetres and be at least 10 cm long).

Patient preparation

During the physical assessment, the use of sheets, blankets and gowns will help to minimally expose the area being examined, maximizing privacy and dignity. Whatever system(s) are being examined, the nurse should organize their steps to minimize the number of times the patient needs to change position (Rushforth 2009). The nurse must consider whether the patient has any needs requiring specific adjustments, whether the patient requires translation and the possibility of a chaperone (Donnelly and Martin 2016).

Respiratory examination

Anatomy

The respiratory system consists of an upper and lower airway (Figure 2.5). The upper airway starts with the nasopharynx and the oropharynx, then continues to the laryngopharynx and the larynx (Rushforth 2009). The lower airway starts at the trachea, which divides into two bronchi; these then divide into lobar bronchi, then secondary bronchi, tertiary bronchi, terminal bronchioles, respiratory bronchioles and alveolar ducts (Rushforth 2009).

The right lung is made up of three lobes: upper, middle and lower. The left lung only has two lobes: upper and lower (Figure 2.6). The lungs are not stationary but expand and contract during inhalation and exhalation (Bickley and Szilagyi 2017). In order for this to happen smoothly, they are covered in two serous membranes: the visceral pleura and the parietal pleura (Bickley and Szilagyi 2017). The space between these two membranes can occasionally become filled with substances such as air, blood and fluid (Rushforth 2009).

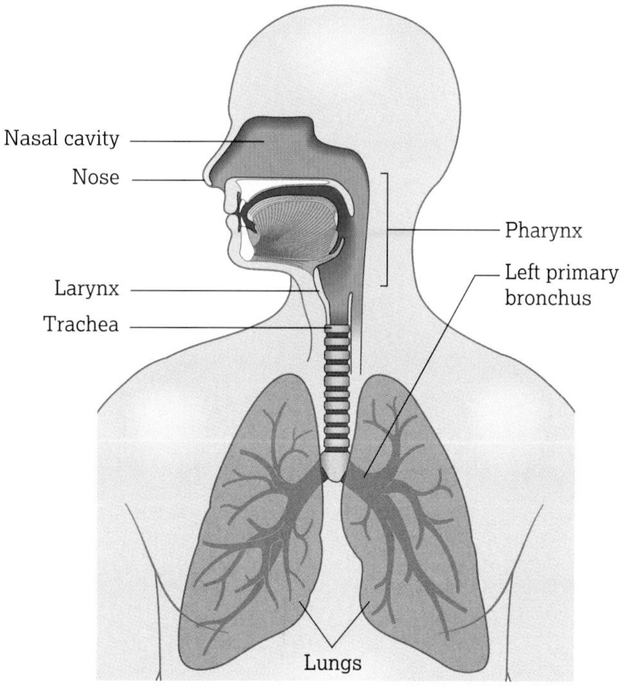

Figure 2.5 Structures of the respiratory system. *Source*: Reproduced from Peate et al. (2014) with permission of John Wiley & Sons, Ltd.

The lungs are within the thorax and are protected by the ribcage which surrounds them; when examining the lungs, it can be helpful to use the thorax as a point of reference when describing the location of findings (Figure 2.7).

Physiology

The respiratory system has two main functions: delivery of oxygen to cells and removal of carbon dioxide, which accumulates as a result of cellular metabolism (Moore 2007). The control of ventilation is either voluntary or involuntary. The former involves regulation of the respiratory muscles (intercostal muscles and diaphragm) via the central nervous system. Involuntary control of the respiratory muscles occurs via the respiratory centre (medulla oblongata and pons) in the brain (Moore 2007). Stimulation of the respiratory centre occurs when carbon dioxide levels in arterial blood become elevated. Detection of raised carbon dioxide levels results in an increase in the rate and depth of breathing to aid carbon dioxide removal. Hence, in normal pathology, the trigger for breathing is carbon dioxide (hypercapnia) and not oxygen levels. It is important to note that in a patient with chronic obstructive pulmonary disease (COPD), the trigger for respiration is hypoxia (low oxygen levels). This is due to chronically elevated carbon dioxide levels. Consequently, patients with COPD are at risk of respiratory arrest if over-oxygenated (Moore 2007).

Related theory

The purpose of the respiratory assessment is to further refine the differential diagnoses identified from the patient history. The respiratory assessment will also assess the adequacy of gas exchange, the delivery of oxygen to the tissues and the removal of carbon dioxide (Moore 2007).

The order of examination for the respiratory system is:

- inspection
- palpation
- percussion
- auscultation.

Both the anterior (front) and the posterior (back) chest must be examined and the same techniques are used for both sides.

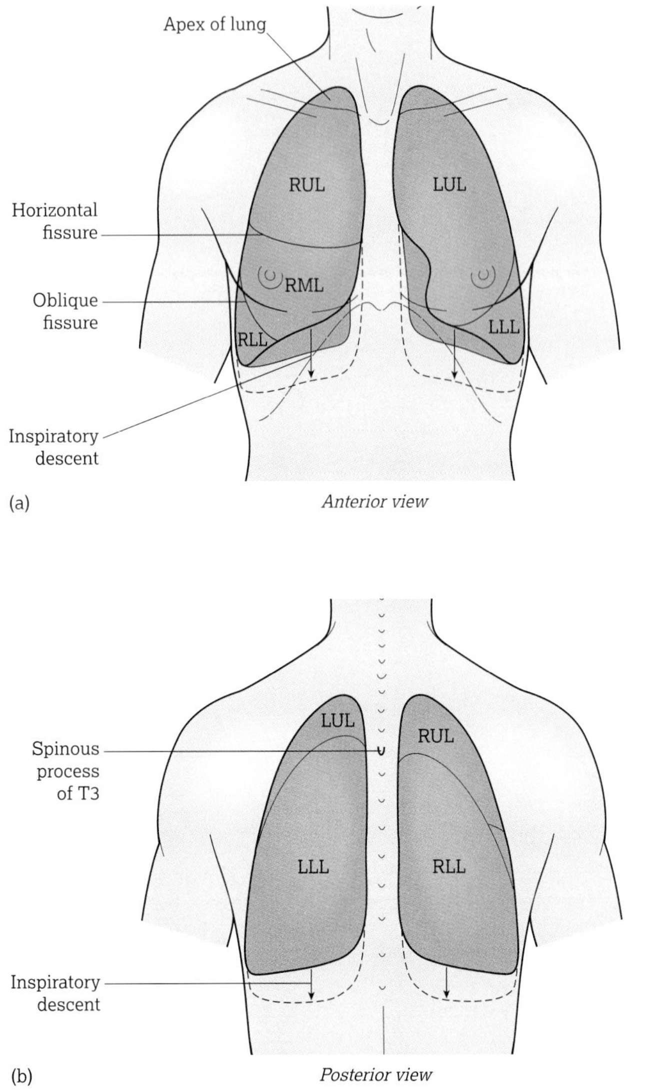

Figure 2.6 Lung, fissures and lobes. RUL, right upper lobe; RML, right middle lobe, RLL, right lower lobe; LUL, left upper lobe; LLL, left lower lobe.

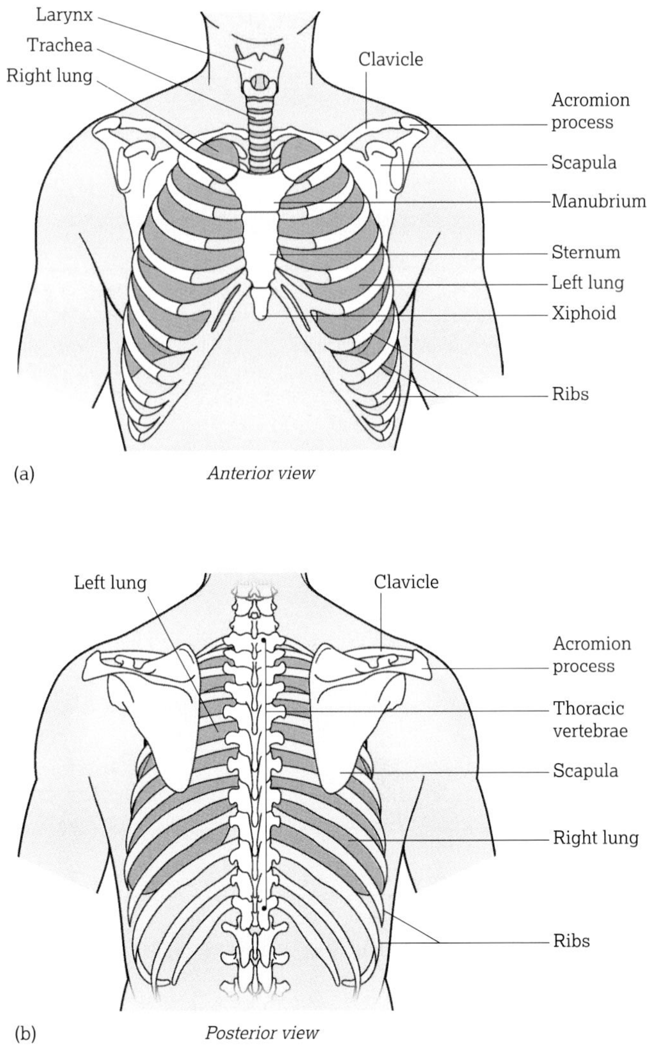

Figure 2.7 Structures of the chest and thorax.

Inspection

Respiratory rate

When inspecting the respiratory rate, consider the rate, rhythm and effort. Signs to look out for include:

- *Rate*: tachypnoea (more than 18 breaths per minute) can be indicative of respiratory distress (acute asthma attack, pain, anxiety). Bradypnoea (less than 10 breaths per minute) can indicate a reduced level of consciousness, opioid overdose or depression of the respiratory centre.
- *Rhythm*: examples of abnormal rhythms include Kussmaul respirations (rapid deep breathing, as seen in states of acidosis such as diabetic ketoacidosis) and Cheyne–Stokes respirations (apnoeic episodes often seen towards the end of life).
- *Effort*: use of accessory muscles (shoulders and sternocleidomastoid muscles), nasal flaring and pursed lip breathing.

Skin colour

When inspecting skin colour, signs to look out for include:

- *Peripheral cyanosis*: this is usually evident in the skin and nail beds and is indicative of poor circulation.
- *Central cyanosis*: this is usually evident in a bluish tinge of the tongue and lips, and is indicative of circulatory or ventilator problems.

Sputum

If the patient has a productive cough, inspection of the sputum can help to ascertain possible causes (Fisher and Potter 2017). The following can be indicative:

- *Purulent, yellow or green*: infection.
- *Mucoid, clear, grey or white*: COPD or asthma.
- *Serous, clear, pink or frothy*: pulmonary oedema.
- *Blood*: malignancy, pulmonary embolus, clotting disorders or infection.

Chest deformities

Some examples of chest deformities are barrel chest, pigeon chest, funnel chest and flail chest (Table 2.4). Also check for the presence of any scars that could be indicative of previous lung surgery, radiotherapy tattoos or previous chest drains (Moore 2007).

Legs

Inspect the legs for any evidence of pulmonary oedema, calf swelling (indicative of a deep vein thrombosis) or erythema nodosum (which can be seen in tuberculosis, sarcoidosis or streptococcal throat infections) (Fisher and Potter 2017).

Table 2.4 Examples of chest deformities

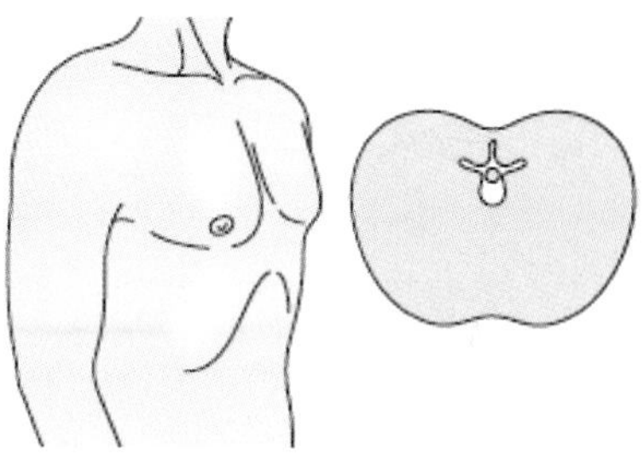	**Normal adult** The thorax in the normal adult is wider than it is deep. Its lateral diameter is larger than its anteroposterior diameter.
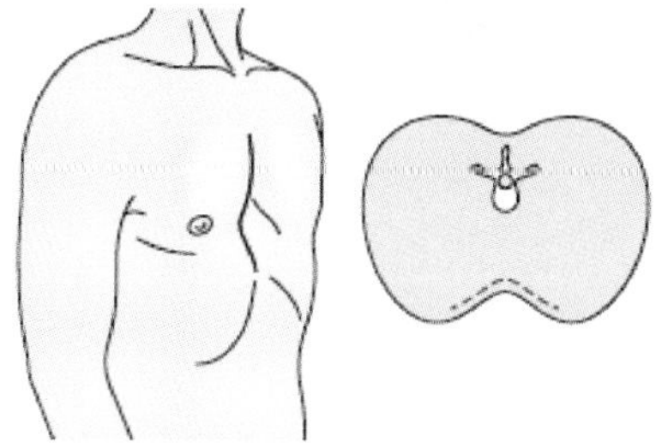	**Funnel chest (pectus excavation)** *Possible cause*: Marfan syndrome Note the depression in the lower portion of the sternum. Compression of the heart and great vessels may cause murmurs.
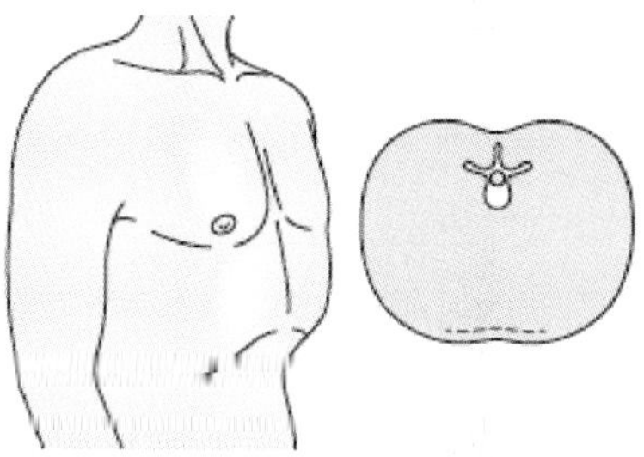	**Barrel chest** *Possible cause*: asthma or chronic obstructive pulmonary disease (COPD) Note the increased anteroposterior diameter. This shape is normal during infancy and often accompanies ageing and COPD.
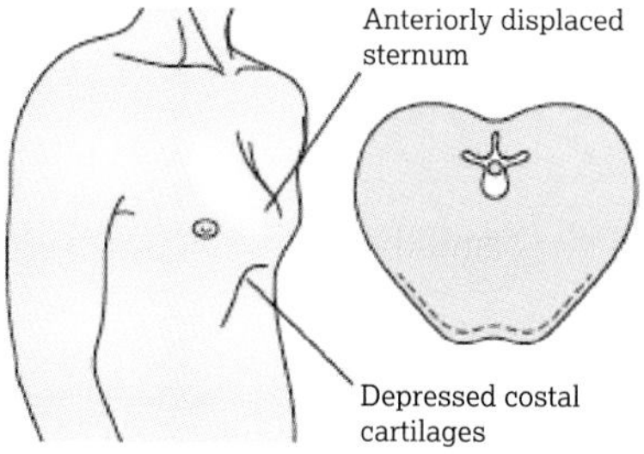	**Pigeon chest (pectus carinatum)** *Possible cause*: severe childhood asthma Note that the sternum is displaced anteriorly, increasing the anteroposterior diameter. The costal cartilages adjacent to the protruding sternum are depressed.
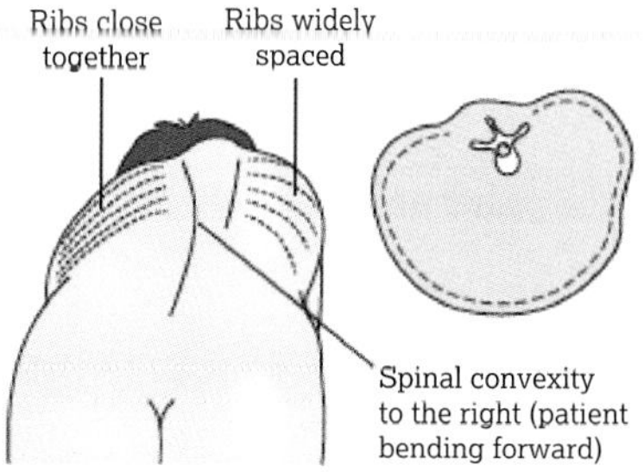	**Thoracic kyphoscoliosis** Note that the abnormal spinal curvatures and vertebral rotation deform the chest. Distortion of the underlying lungs may make interpretation of lung findings very difficult.
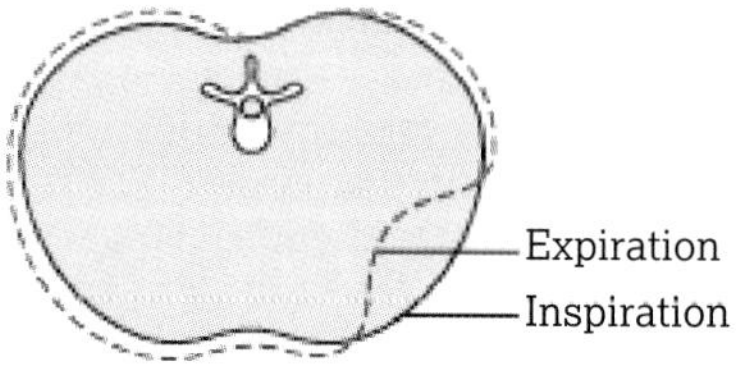	**Traumatic flail chest** Multiple rib fractures may result in paradoxical movements of the thorax. As descent of the diaphragm decreases intrathoracic pressure, on inspiration (breathing in) the injured area caves inward; on expiration (breathing out), it moves outward.

Palpation

Lymph nodes

Part of palpation when examining the respiratory system is to examine the lymph nodes in the neck. Patients often present with a lump or enlarged lymph nodes (lymphadenopathy), which can be an important sign of infection or malignancy (Dover et al. 2018). To do this, stand behind the patient and examine both sides of the neck at the same time. Use your middle and index fingers to softly palpate in circular movements the lymph nodes in the positions illustrated in Figure 2.8.

Chest expansion

To assess for chest expansion and symmetry, adopt the position shown in Figure 2.9 and ask the patient to take a deep breath in. You should be able to see your thumbs move an equal distance apart. Reduced expansion may be indicative of fibrosis, consolidation, effusion or pneumothorax (Fisher and Potter 2017).

Tactile fremitus

Fremitus is the palpable vibration of the patient's voice through the chest wall (Bickley and Szilagyi 2017). See Figures 2.10 and 2.11 for the appropriate locations to feel for fremitus. Compare the two sides of the chest, using the ball or ulnar surface of your hand (Bickley and Szilagyi 2017). The vibrations felt should be symmetrical and will decrease as you work down the chest wall. Fremitus is usually decreased or absent over the precordium. Asymmetry could indicate:

- consolidation
- emphysema
- pneumothorax
- pleural effusion (Rushforth 2009).

Faint or absent fremitus in the upper thorax could indicate:

- obstruction of the bronchial tree
- fluid
- obesity (Rushforth 2009).

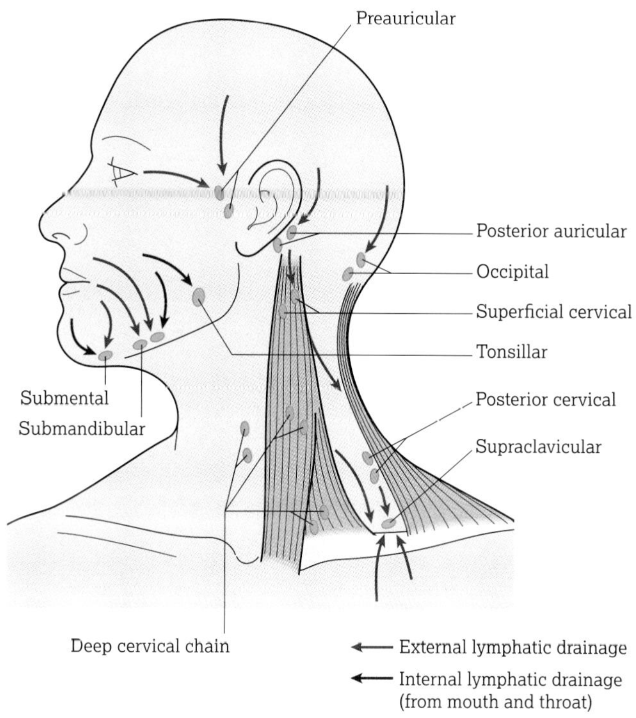

Figure 2.8 The lymph nodes of the head and neck.

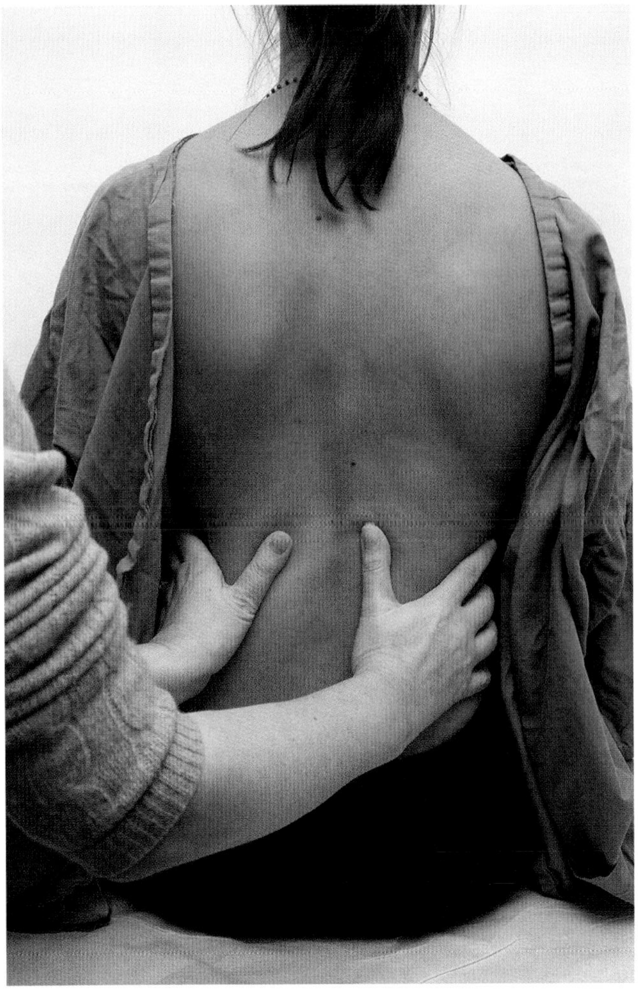

Figure 2.9 Position of hands to assess for chest expansion.

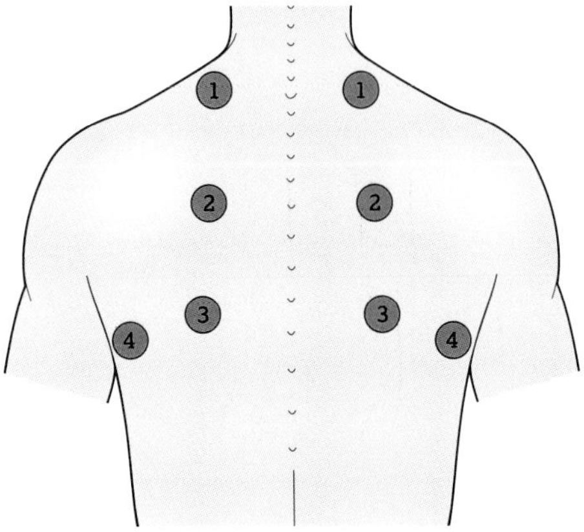

Figure 2.10 Locations for feeling fremitus: back.

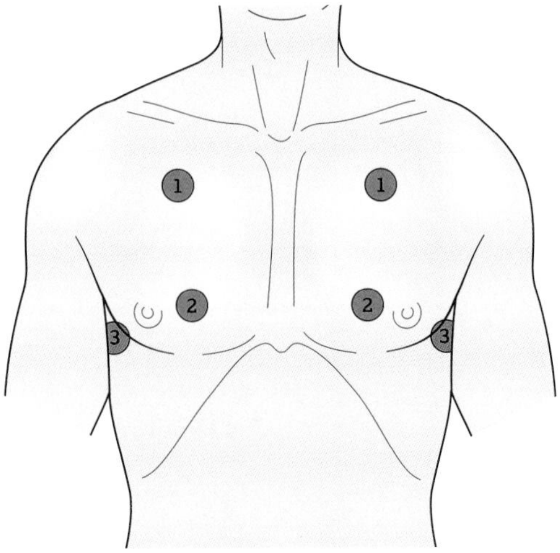

Figure 2.11 Locations for feeling fremitus: front.

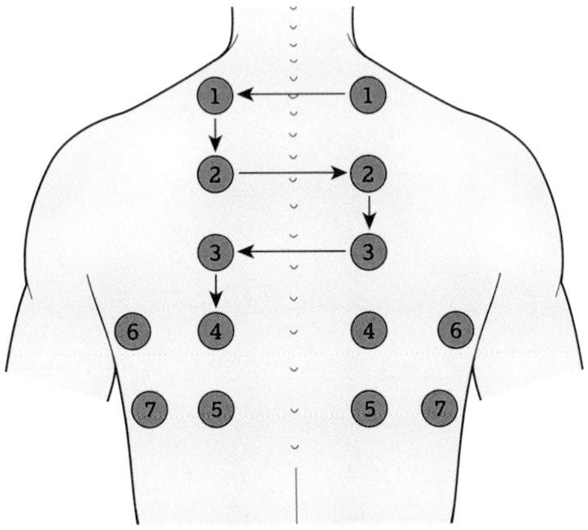

Figure 2.12 Ladder pattern for percussion and auscultation of the chest.

Percussion

When percussing and auscultating, each side of the chest should be compared. To do this, percuss and auscultate in a ladder-like pattern in the positions shown in Figure 2.12.

Resonance is heard over normal aerated lung tissue. There are two main types of percussion notes, which are associated with different lung pathologies. The two notes are dullness and hyper-resonance (Fisher and Potter 2017):

- *Dullness*: heard over solid organ or fluid; can be indicative of a pleural effusion, consolidation or pleural thickening.
- *Hyper-resonance*: heard over hyper-inflated lung tissue or where there is air in the pleural space; can be indicative of a pneumothorax or COPD.

Auscultation

Auscultation should be performed using the bell of the stethoscope (see Figure 2.4) on both the anterior and the posterior chest.

Breath sounds

Normal breath sounds are also known as 'vesicular breath sounds'; they are soft and are louder and longer on breathing in (inspiration) compared with breathing out (expiration) (Talley and O'Connor 2006). Bronchial breaths sound different; they have a hollow quality and are audible throughout expiration (Talley and O'Connor 2006). There is often a short, silent gap between inspiration and expiration (Bickley and Szilagyi 2017).

Adventitious sounds are added sounds on top of breath sounds. See Table 2.5 for examples of adventitious sounds.

Table 2.5 Examples of adventitious sounds

Breath sound	Description	Potential cause
Wheeze	High-pitched, hissing sound	Airway narrowing (bronchospasm or airway swelling), e.g. acute asthma attack
Stridor	High-pitched sound, usually on inspiration	Life threatening: due to laryngeal or tracheal obstruction, e.g. choking or anaphylaxis
Coarse crackles	Low-pitched, bubbling, gurgling sound	Pneumonia, bronchiectasis or fluid overload
Fine crackles	High-pitched, popping sound	Restrictive and obstructive diseases, e.g. pulmonary fibrosis
Rhonchi	Continuous, low-pitched, snoring sound	Problems causing obstruction of the trachea or bronchi, e.g. bronchitis

Vocal resonance can also be assessed as this will give an indication of the lungs' ability to transmit sound. The method of doing this is to ask the patient to say '99' while auscultating over the chest. The patient's voice will become clearer in an area of consolidation while their voice will become muffled if there is a pleural effusion (Fisher and Potter 2017). This can be repeated while asking the patient to whisper '99' (whispering pectoriloquy); increased transmission of sound will be heard over areas of consolidation.

Evidence-based approaches

Rationale

Information obtained from the patient's history, the differential diagnoses identified, and the nurse's knowledge of anatomy and physiology will help to inform when it is appropriate to do a respiratory physical examination. Some examples of presentations that would lead to a respiratory examination are:

- dyspnoea
- cough
- chest pain
- wheezing.

Procedure guideline 2.1 Respiratory examination

Essential equipment

- Personal protective equipment
- Stethoscope
- Examination couch

Action	Rationale
Pre-procedure	
1 Introduce yourself to the patient, explain and discuss the procedure with them, and gain their consent to proceed.	To ensure that the patient feels at ease, understands the procedure and gives their valid consent (NMC 2018, **C**).
2 Gain the patient's verbal consent.	Consent must be gained before any procedure takes place (NMC 2018, **C**).
3 Make sure the patient is warm and comfortable and sitting on the edge of the bed or on a chair.	To ensure that both the anterior (front) and posterior (back) thorax and lungs can be examined (Bickley and Szilagyi 2017, **E**).
4 Expose the patient from head to waist while maintaining privacy and dignity.	To allow a thorough examination (Talley and O'Connor 2006, **E**).
Procedure	
5 Wash and dry hands.	To prevent the spread of infection (NHS England and NHSI 2019, **C**).
General inspection	
6 Take a global view of the patient.	See 'Inspection' above.
7 Look at the patient's skin and nails. Feel the texture, temperature and turgor of the skin.	Abnormalities of the skin and nails can be an indication of a variety of different conditions, for example heart disease, lung disease, cyanosis and/or anaemia (Bickley and Szilagyi 2017, Rushforth 2009). Look for tobacco staining (Innes and Tiernan 2018). **E**
8 Press either side of the patient's finger (first digit) firmly between your finger and thumb for 5 seconds and then let go. Count how many seconds it takes for the colour to return.	To assess capillary refill; this can give an indication of the status of circulation (Paterson and Dover 2018). Normal return is 2 seconds. **E**
9 Ask the patient to hold out their arms with their wrists flexed and their palms facing forwards for 1 minute.	To assess for flapping tremor; a fine tremor can be a side-effect of high-dose beta-agonist bronchodilators. A coarse flapping tremor of the outstretched hands is seen in patients with carbon dioxide retention (Innes and Tiernan 2018, **E**).

(continued)

Procedure guideline 2.1 Respiratory examination *(continued)*

Action	Rationale
10 Look at the patient's eyes.	To assess for any abnormalities, particularly looking for any signs of hypercholesterolaemia (corneal arcus or xanthelasma) or anaemia (conjunctival pallor). Look for any signs of unilateral ptosis or pupillary constriction, which may constitute Horner's syndrome (Innes and Tiernan 2018, **E**).
11 Look at and in the patient's mouth.	The mouth can give a snapshot of the patient's general state of health. Look for signs of malnutrition, infection, central cyanosis and any sores (Bickley and Szilagyi 2017). Look for signs of mouth breathing and upper respiratory tract infection (Innes et al. 2018). **E**
12 Look at and in the patient's nose.	To assess for nasal flare, deviated septum and nasal polyps (Talley and O'Connor 2006, **E**).
13 Listen to the patient's breathing.	To assess for any audible wheeze or stridor (Bickley and Szilagyi 2017, **E**).
14 Look at the patient's neck.	To assess whether accessory muscles are being used and whether the trachea is at the midline (Bickley and Szilagyi 2017, **E**).
15 Check the patient's jugular venous pressure (JVP). To do this, ensure the patient is positioned at 30–45° and ask them to turn their head away from you. Measure the JVP (number of centimetres vertically from the sternal angle to the upper border of pulsation). (For more information, see the section 'Steps for measuring the JVP' below.)	To check for a raised JVP, which can indicate pulmonary hypertension, tension pneumothorax or large pulmonary embolism (Innes and Tiernan 2018, **E**).
16 Palpate the trachea gently with your index finger and thumb.	To ensure it is at the midline with no deviation (Innes and Tiernan 2018, **E**).
17 Palpate the head and neck nodes (see Figure 2.8).	To assess for enlarged nodes; this can be a sign of malignancy or infection (Dover et al. 2018, **E**).
Posterior chest	
18 Inspect the patient's chest.	To assess for any scars, masses, deformities and asymmetry (Bickley and Szilagyi 2017, **E**).
Palpation	
19 Lightly palpate the chest.	To assess for any signs of tenderness, pain or masses (Bickley and Szilagyi 2017, Rushforth 2009, **E**).
20 Place your thumbs at the level of the 10th rib either side of the spine with your fingers fanned out towards the lateral (side) chest. Ask the patient to take a deep breath in (see Figure 2.9).	To assess chest expansion (Bickley and Szilagyi 2017, Rushforth 2009, Talley and O'Connor 2006, **E**).
21 Place the edge of your palm and little finger on the patient's chest at the points seen in Figures 2.10 and 2.11 and ask the patient to say '99'. Assess both sides of the chest together using both hands.	To assess for tactile fremitus (Bickley and Szilagyi 2017, Rushforth 2009, Talley and O'Connor 2006, **E**).
Percussion	
22 Percuss the chest (see Figure 2.12).	To assess for normal resonance in the lungs and identify any abnormalities (Bickley and Szilagyi 2017, **E**).
Auscultation	
23 Auscultate the lungs using the diaphragm of the stethoscope (see Figure 2.12).	To assess for vesicular breath sounds and any adventitious sounds (Bickley and Szilagyi 2017, **E**).
Anterior chest	
24 Inspect the patient's chest.	To assess for any scars, masses, deformities and asymmetry (Bickley and Szilagyi 2017, **E**).
Palpation	
25 Lightly palpate the chest	To assess for any signs of tenderness, pain or masses (Bickley and Szilagyi 2017, Rushforth 2009, **E**).
26 Place your thumbs along each costal margin at about the fifth or sixth rib with your fingers fanned out towards the lateral chest. Ask the patient to take a deep breath in.	To assess chest expansion (Bickley and Szilagyi 2017, Rushforth 2009, Talley and O'Connor 2006, **E**).

27 Place the edge of your palm and little finger on the patient's chest at the points seen in Figure 2.9 and ask the patient to say '99'. Assess both sides of the chest together using both hands.	To assess for tactile fremitus (Bickley and Szilagyi 2017, Rushforth 2009, Talley and O'Connor 2006, **E**).
Percussion	
28 Percuss the chest (see Figure 2.12).	To assess for normal resonance in the lungs and identify any abnormalities (Bickley and Szilagyi 2017, **E**).
Auscultation	
29 Auscultate the lung using the bell of the stethoscope for the apex of the lung (above the clavicle) and the diaphragm of the stethoscope for the rest of the chest (see Figure 2.12).	To assess for vesicular breath sounds and any adventitious sounds (Bickley and Szilagyi 2017, **E**).
Post-procedure	
30 Document fully.	Accurate records should be kept of all discussions and/or assessments made (NMC 2018, **C**).
31 Report any abnormal findings to a senior nurse or to medical staff.	Patients should be cared for as part of a multidisciplinary team and, where appropriate, patient care should be referred to another more experienced practitioner (NMC 2018, **C**).
32 Clean the equipment used and wash hands.	To prevent the spread of infection (NHS England and NHSI 2019, **C**).
33 Explain findings to the patient.	The patient should be told, in a way they can understand, the information they want or need to know about their health (NMC 2018, **C**).
34 Discuss plan of care with the patient.	Where possible, patients should be involved in planning their care (NMC 2018, **C**).
35 Additional bedside investigations: assess vital signs, and inspect sputum and send for microbiology, culture and sensitivity.	This additional information can be used to assess the adequacy of gas exchange (Fisher and Potter 2017, **E**).
36 Order further investigations as needed to include blood, chest X-ray and lung function tests.	This additional information can further refine the differential diagnoses (Fisher and Potter 2017, **E**).

Cardiovascular examination

Anatomy and physiology

The heart is a muscular organ that delivers blood to the pulmonary and systemic systems (Mills et al. 2018) (Figure 2.13). A good understanding of the vascular system of the heart is important.

Related theory

When carrying out a cardiovascular assessment, the order of examination is:

- inspection
- palpation
- auscultation.

Note that percussion is not part of a cardiovascular assessment.

Many symptoms that necessitate a cardiac examination can be life threatening, so first take a moment to assess whether the patient is well enough for a full examination or whether they need immediate treatment in order to be stabilized first (Rushforth 2009).

Inspection

Ideally the patient should be positioned between 30° and 45° and the patient's chest should be exposed to enable a comprehensive assessment. Note that due to the condition of the patient, the patient may be uncomfortable or in pain; in such cases, the assessment should be adjusted to meet the needs of the patient. It can be helpful to visualize the structure of the heart as you undertake inspection.

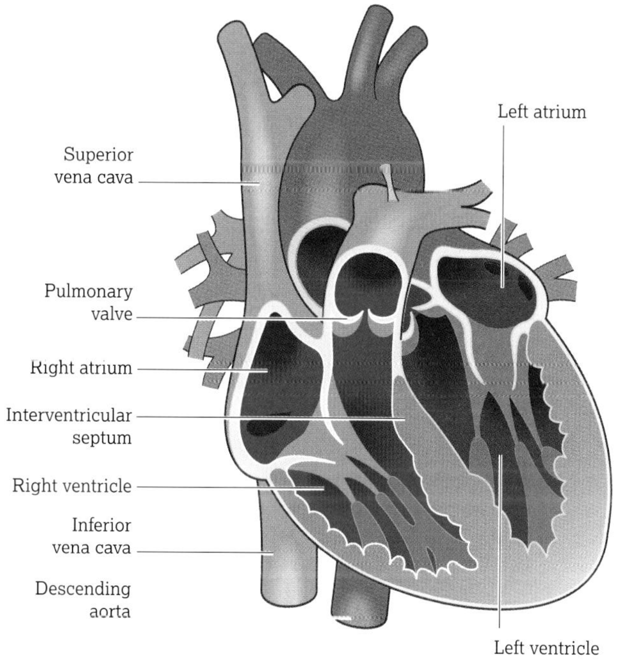

Figure 2.13 Structure of the heart. *Source:* Reproduced from Peate et al. (2014) with permission of John Wiley & Sons, Ltd.

1 Observe the patient for signs of distress, pain or breathlessness.
2 Starting at the hands, assess for cold extremities. Inspect the nails for any unusual changes, such as koilonychia or splinter haemorrhages. Assess capillary refill time (it should be less than 2 seconds). See Procedure guideline 2.2 for further information.
3 Assess skin for turgor, temperature and any rashes or lesions on hands or arms.
4 Observe the patient's face; assess the conjunctiva for signs of anaemia and xanthelasmata around the eyes. Xanthelasmata are fatty deposits that typically present as yellow plaques around the eyes (Nair and Singhal 2018). They can indicate hyperlipidaemia, thyroid dysfunction or diabetes mellitus (Gangopadhyay et al. 1998).
5 Observe for any flushing of the skin on the face. Look at the tongue and mucous membranes for any signs of central cyanosis.
6 Observe the exposed chest for scars, bruising, trauma, surgery or asymmetry (Mills et al. 2018, Powell 2006, Talley and O'Connor 2006).
7 Inspect for heaves or thrills. These are ventricular movements that may be visible over the heart.
8 Inspect the legs and ankles for any sign of peripheral oedema, poor circulation or peripheral vascular disease. Observe for a shiny, hairless appearance of the skin on the legs, and examine the feet and legs for pain, swelling, discoloration, ulceration and temperature (Mills et al. 2018).

Part of cardiovascular inspection is measuring the jugular venous pressure (JVP) (Figure 2.14). JVP reflects the pressure in the right atrium and is a good indicator of cardiac function (Powell 2006). To measure JVP, locating the right internal jugular vein is paramount. The vein runs deep within the sternomastoid muscle so it is not directly visible (Bickley and Szilagyi 2017). Instead, it can be located by looking for its pulsation within the sternomastoid muscle (Bickley and Szilagyi 2017) (Figure 2.14).

Steps for measuring the JVP

1 Make the patient comfortable.
2 Raise the patient's head to an angle of approximately 30° (up to a 45° angle).
3 Turn the patient's head slightly away from the side you are inspecting.
4 Use tangential lighting and examine both sides of the neck. Identify the external jugular vein on each side, then find the internal jugular venous pulsations.

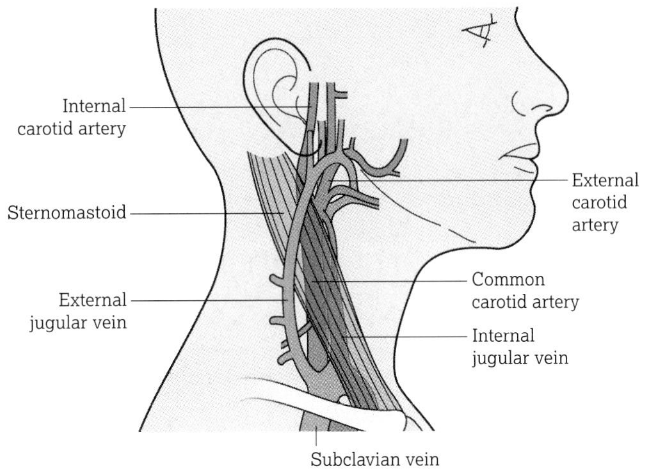

Figure 2.14 Location of the internal jugular veins within the sternomastoid muscles in the neck.

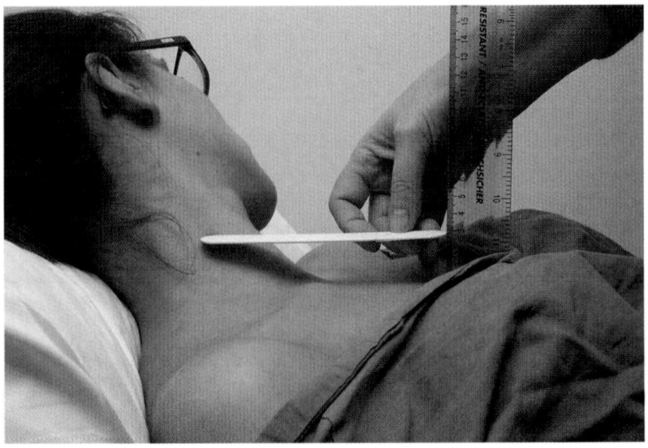

Figure 2.15 Measuring a jugular venous pressure.

5 Focus on the right internal jugular vein. Look for pulsations in the suprasternal notch. Distinguish the pulsations of the internal jugular vein from those of the carotid artery (carotid pulsations are palpable and have a more vigorous thrust with a single outward component; additionally, these pulsations are not eliminated by pressure on the veins at the sternal end of the clavicle, and the height of the pulsations is unchanged by the position of the chest and by inspiration).
6 Identify the highest point of pulsation in the right jugular vein. Extend a long rectangular object or card horizontally from this point and a centimetre ruler vertically from the sternal angle, making an exact right angle (as demonstrated in Figure 2.15). Measure the vertical distance in centimetres above the sternal angle. This is usually less than 3–4 cm (Bickley and Szilagyi 2017).

Palpation

The palpable pulse in an artery reflects the pressure wave generated by the ejection of blood into the circulation from the left ventricle. When taking a pulse assess:

- *Rate*: the number of pulses occurring per minute.
- *Rhythm*: the pattern or regularity of pulses.
- *Volume*: the perceived degree of pulsation.
- *Character*: an impression of the pulse waveform or shape.

The rate and rhythm of the pulse are usually determined at the arterial artery; use the larger pulses (brachial, carotid or femoral) to assess pulse volume and character (Mills et al. 2018).

A weak pulse can be a sign of various conditions, including decreased cardiac output (Rushforth 2009). A bounding pulse can indicate an increased cardiac output, which can be present in hypertension and anaemia (Rushforth 2009). Pulses on each side of the body should be compared simultaneously if possible. There are two exceptions to this: the popliteal pulse and the carotid pulses. The nurse will need to use both hands to assess each popliteal pulse; the carotid pulses should always be palpated separately, as doing both together may make the patient feel faint.

The nurse should feel across the chest for evidence of pain, heaves, thrills and lifts. Lifts and heaves are forceful cardiac contractions that can result in transient movement of the sternum and/or ribs and if present will be felt through the flat of the hand being lifted rhythmically during palpation (Bickley and Szilagyi 2017). They can be a sign of an enlarged ventricle or atrium or sometimes a ventricular aneurysm (Bickley and Szilagyi 2017). Thrills are vibrations that can be felt from light palpation over the chest, usually over the areas of the heart valves, and are the result of a loud heart murmur. They will be felt most clearly using the ball of the hand palpating in the area of the murmur and may feel like a buzzing or vibration (Bickley and Szilagyi 2017).

The nurse should palpate the apical impulse (point of maximum impulse). Start from the fifth intercostal space, inside the mid-clavicular line (Camm and Camm 2016). If the impulse is difficult to find, the patient should be asked to roll slightly onto their left side. Observe the apical impulse for size, amplitude, location, impulse and duration.

Auscultation

When auscultating, the heart sounds should be characterized and identified, as should any added sounds and/or murmurs (Mills et al. 2018). All elements of the cardiac cycle can be heard on auscultation and thus it is important to identify all of them (Camm and Camm 2016). The sound of the beating heart is often described as 'lub dub' and is caused by the closure of valves (Powell 2006). The 'lub', which is also referred to as 'S1', is the sound made when the mitral and tricuspid valves are closing; it is often heard best over the apex. The 'dub' or 'S2' is the sound made when the aortic and pulmonary valves close (Camm and Camm 2016; Powell 2006) and can be heard well across the precordium. There are extra sounds that can sometimes be heard called 'S3' and 'S4'. S3 is occasionally heard immediately after S2 and is caused by the vibration of rapid ventricular filling (Mills et al. 2018). S4 can rarely be heard immediately before S1 and marks atrial contraction. Both of these sounds can indicate a change in ventricular compliance (Bickley and Szilagyi 2017).

Murmurs can be heard in a number of different conditions; they are caused by turbulent blood flow. While murmurs are sometimes harmless, they can indicate valvular heart disease (Bickley and Szilagyi 2017). Heart sounds and murmurs that originate in the four valves radiate widely; see Figure 2.16 for an illustration of the relevant auscultation points.

Assessment of carotid bruits is an important component of cardiovascular assessment. Bruits are often described as 'whooshing' sounds and can indicate atherosclerotic arterial disease (Bickley and Szilagyi 2017).

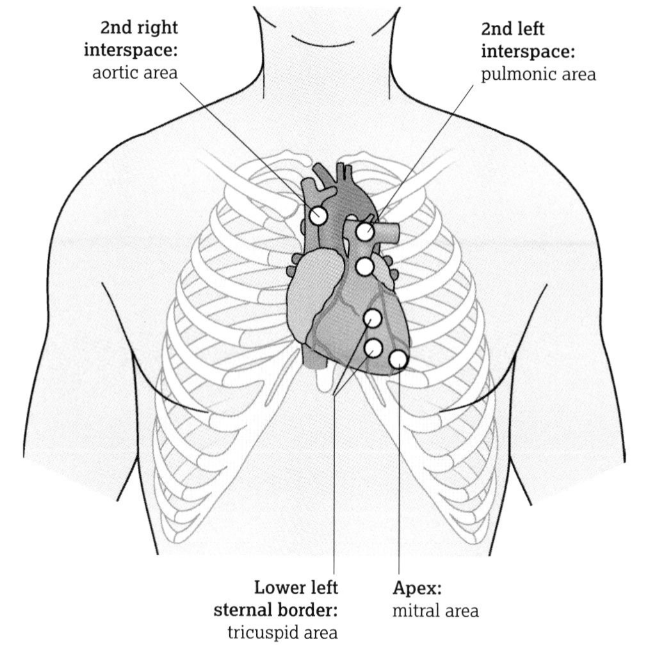

Figure 2.16 Auscultation points and location of the heart valves.

Evidence-based approaches

Rationale

The patient's health history and the nurse's knowledge of anatomy and physiology will help to guide when it is appropriate to do a cardiovascular physical examination. The list of presentations that may lead to a cardiovascular examination is vast; some examples include:

- chest pain
- palpitation
- leg ulcer
- breathlessness
- oedema
- dizziness.

Procedure guideline 2.2 Cardiovascular examination

Essential equipment

- Personal protective equipment
- Stethoscope
- Examination couch
- Pen torch
- Ruler

Action	Rationale
Pre-procedure	
1 Introduce yourself to the patient, explain and discuss the procedure with them, and gain their consent to proceed.	To ensure that the patient feels at ease, understands the procedure and gives their valid consent (NMC 2018, **C**).
2 Gain the patient's verbal consent.	Consent must be gained before any procedure takes place (NMC 2018, **C**).
3 Check that the patient has an empty bladder.	A full bladder will interfere with the examination (Walsh 2006b, **E**).
4 Make sure the patient is warm and comfortable and ideally have them in the supine position, with their head at 30–45° and their arms by their sides.	This is the optimum position from which to assess the jugular venous pressure (JVP) (Talley and O'Connor 2006, **E**).
5 Expose the patient from head to waist while maintaining privacy and dignity. You will also need access to their legs.	To allow a thorough examination (Talley and O'Connor 2006, **E**).

(continued)

Procedure guideline 2.2 Cardiovascular examination *(continued)*

Action	Rationale
Procedure	
6 Wash and dry hands.	To prevent the spread of infection (NHS England and NHSI 2019, **C**).
General inspection	
7 Take a global view of the patient.	See 'Inspection' above.
8 Look at the patient's skin and nails. Feel the texture, temperature and turgor of the skin.	Abnormalities of the skin and nails can be an indication of a variety of different conditions, for example heart disease, endocarditis, hypercholesterolaemia and/or anaemia (Bickley and Szilagyi 2017, Tidman 2018). Also look for tobacco staining. **E**
9 Press the patient's fingernail (on the first digit) firmly between your finger and thumb for 5 seconds and then let go. Count how many seconds it takes for the colour to return to the nail.	To assess the capillary refill; this can give an indication of the status of circulation (Paterson and Dover, 2018). Normal return is 2 seconds. **E**
10 Look at the patient's eyes.	To assess for any abnormalities, particularly looking for any signs of hypercholesterolaemia or anaemia (Talley and O'Connor 2006, **E**).
11 Look at and in the patient's mouth.	The mouth can give a snapshot of the patient's general state of health. Look for signs of malnutrition, infection, central cyanosis and any sores (Innes et al. 2018, **E**).
12 Ask the patient to turn their head to the left, use tangential lighting and locate the highest pulsation point of the internal jugular vein (see Figure 2.15). Place a ruler vertically from the sternal angle, then use a tongue depressor placed horizontally to make a right angle from the pulsation to the ruler. The JVP is measured in centimetres and the measurement is where the tongue depressor meets the ruler.	To assess the JVP (Bickley and Szilagyi 2017, **E**).
13 Inspect the precordium.	To assess for scars, deformities, heaves, lifts and the apical impulse (Bickley and Szilagyi 2017, **E**).
14 Inspect the legs.	To assess for signs of venous disease and ischaemic changes (Mills et al. 2018, **E**).
Palpation	
15 Palpate the pulses.	To assess cardiac output (Rushforth 2009, **E**).
16 Palpate the chest.	To assess for tenderness, heaves, lifts and thrills (Bickley and Szilagyi 2017, Rushforth 2009, **E**).
17 Palpate with the finger tips the fifth intercostal space, inside the mid-clavicular line.	To assess the apical impulse (Bickley and Szilagyi 2017, Rushforth 2009, **E**).
Auscultation	
18 Listen with the bell of the stethoscope to the carotid pulse.	To assess for bruits (Bickley and Szilagyi 2017, **E**).
19 Auscultate at the aortic, pulmonary, tricuspid and mitral valves (see Figure 2.16) with the diaphragm of the stethoscope.	To assess S1 and S2 (Bickley and Szilagyi 2017, Camm and Camm 2016, **E**).
20 Auscultate at the aortic, pulmonary, tricuspid and mitral valves (see Figure 2.16) with the bell of the stethoscope.	To assess for S3, S4 and murmurs (Bickley and Szilagyi 2017, Camm and Camm 2016, **E**).
21 Ask the patient to roll partially onto their left side and listen with the bell of the stethoscope to the apical impulse.	To assess for a mitral murmur (Bickley and Szilagyi 2017, Camm and Camm 2016, **E**).
22 Ask the patient to sit up and lean forward, exhale completely and hold their breath. Listen with the diaphragm of the stethoscope to the apical impulse and along the left sternal border. Make sure to tell the patient to start breathing normally again.	To assess for an aortic murmur and pericardial friction rubs (Bickley and Szilagyi 2017, Camm and Camm 2016, Rushforth 2009, **E**).
23 Ask the patient to sit up and listen to the lung bases with the diaphragm of the stethoscope.	To assess for lung congestion, which can be caused by heart failure (Rushforth 2009, **E**).
Post-procedure	
24 Document fully.	Accurate records should be kept of all discussions and/or assessments made (NMC 2018, **C**).

25 Report any abnormal findings to a senior nurse or to medical staff.	Patients should be cared for as part of a multidisciplinary team and, where appropriate, patient care should be referred to another more experienced practitioner (NMC 2018, **C**).
26 Clean the equipment used and wash hands.	To prevent the spread of infection (NHS England and NHSI 2019, **C**).
27 Explain findings to the patient.	The patient should be told, in a way they can understand, the information they want or need to know about their health (NMC 2018, **C**).
28 Discuss plan of care with the patient.	Where possible, patients should be involved in planning their care (NMC 2018, **C**).

Abdominal examination

Anatomy and physiology

The abdominal cavity houses large parts of the gastrointestinal (GI) system, the renal system and the reproductive system. It is therefore important to have an understanding of the anatomy and physiology of all three systems when examining the abdomen.

The GI system includes the entire GI tract as well as the accessory organs (Figure 2.17). When examining the abdominal area, it is important to be able to visualize which organs are in which quadrant. This will help to form possible differential diagnoses.

The physiology of the GI system is covered in Chapter 6: Elimination and Chapter 8: Nutrition and fluid balance.

Related theory

A full abdominal examination combines the following techniques:

- inspection
- auscultation
- percussion
- palpation.

The assessment of the abdomen starts with inspection, followed by auscultation, then percussion and palpation. Auscultation is performed prior to percussion and palpation to avoid abdomen and small bowel manipulation, which may change findings (Fritz and Becker Weilitz 2016).

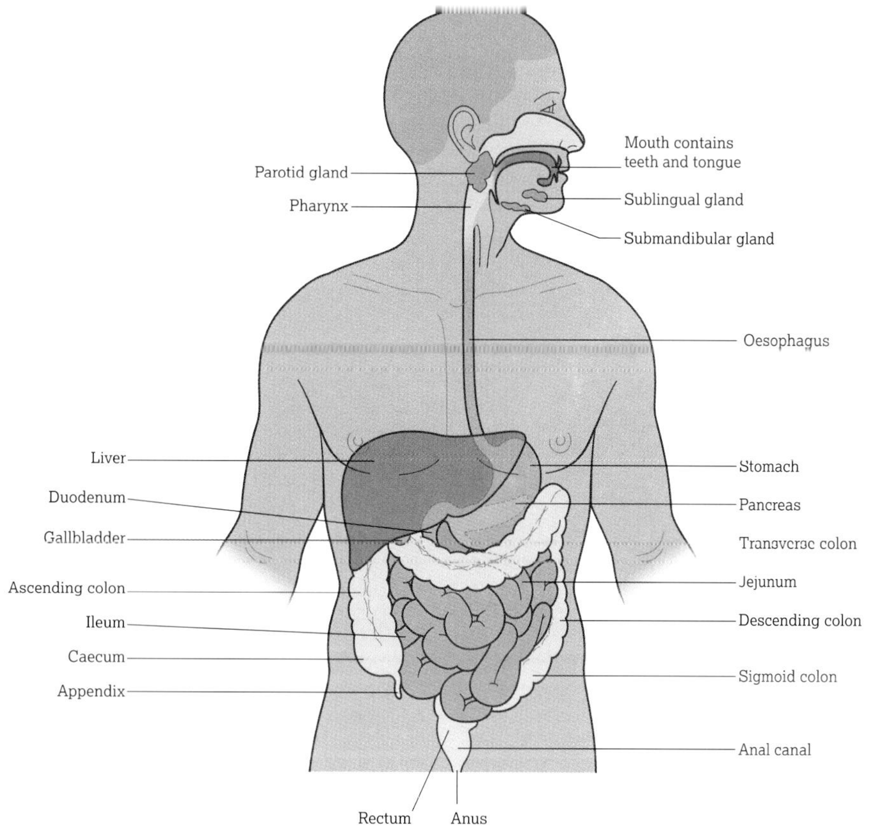

Figure 2.17 Organs of the gastrointestinal system. *Source*: Reproduced from Peate et al. (2014) with permission of John Wiley & Sons, Ltd.

Inspection

Externally, the abdomen should appear flat and symmetrical. The most common causes of abdominal distension are:

- fat in obesity
- flatus in pseudo-obstruction or bowel obstruction
- faeces in subacute obstruction or constipation
- fluid in ascites (accumulation of fluid in the peritoneal cavity)
- tumours (especially ovarian) or distended bladder
- the foetus in pregnancy
- functional bloating (often in irritable bowel syndrome) (Plevris and Parks 2018).

Look at the abdomen for any abnormally prominent veins on the abdominal wall suggestive of portal hypertension or vena cava obstruction. Any abdominal swelling, scars and stomas should also be noted (Plevris and Parks, 2018). The umbilicus position can sometimes help to identify why there is distension.

Auscultation

Bowel sounds should be listened for in all four quadrants of the abdomen (Figure 2.18). Bowel sounds are often described as 'clicks' or 'gurgles' and it should be possible to hear 5–35 clicks in 1 minute. Listening for up to 2 minutes may be required for someone with hypoactive bowel sounds (Fritz and Becker Weilitz 2016). Bowel sounds are often described as active (i.e. normal), absent or hyperactive. Absence of bowel sounds may indicate bowel obstruction and hyperactive bowel sounds may be present if patients are having altered bowel function.

Assessment of bruits is an important component of physical assessment. Bruits are often described as 'whooshing' or harsh intermittent sounds and can indicate atherosclerotic arterial disease (Bickley and Szilagyi 2017). If the bruits are over the renal artery, it can be a sign of renal artery stenosis (Bickley and Szilagyi 2017). See Figure 2.19 for stethoscope positioning.

Percussion

Percussion is used to detect air, fluid, faeces, organs and masses (Walsh 2006a). Predominantly, the abdomen should have a distribution of tympany and dullness – tympany where there is gas in the GI tract and dullness where other organs and faeces lie (Bickley and Szilagyi 2017). Large areas of dullness may indicate organomegaly (enlarged organs), a tumour or ascites (Bickley and Szilagyi 2017). Percussion is also used to locate and measure the size of the liver (Fritz and Becker Weilitz 2016). A normal liver measures 6–12 cm (Talley and O'Connor 2006). See Figure 2.20 for the relevant percussion technique.

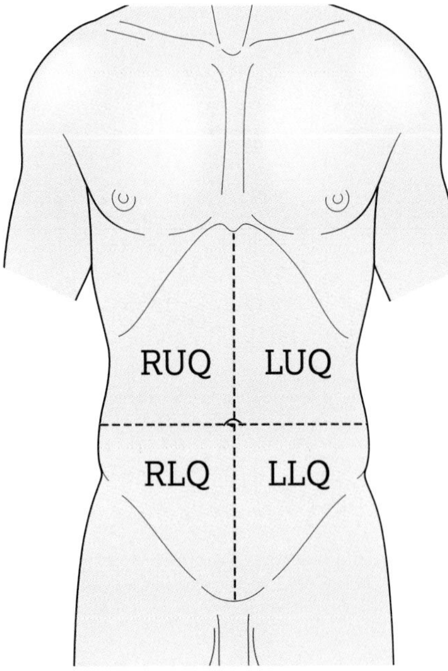

Figure 2.18 The four quadrants of the abdomen. LLQ, left lower quadrant; LUQ, left upper quadrant; RLQ, right lower quadrant; RUQ, right upper quadrant.

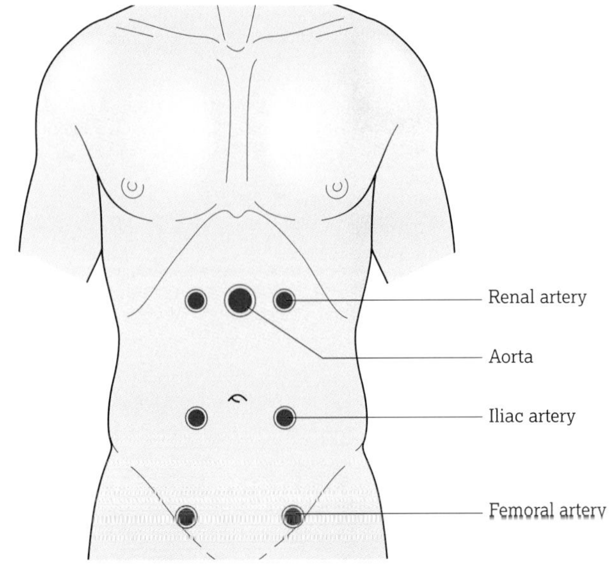

Figure 2.19 Stethoscope positioning for auscultating bruits.

Palpation

Percussion requires indirect tapping of the abdomen to assess the size of the organs and to check for the presence of air or fluid, or air-filled or solid masses (Fritz and Becker Weilitz 2016). If a mass is found, palpation should be used to gather more information about it. Talley and O'Connor (2006) suggest that the following information should be included when describing a mass:

- site
- tenderness
- size
- surface
- edge
- consistency
- mobility
- whether it has a pulse or not.

Likewise, if an organ is found, it should be described. The spleen and kidneys are not normally palpable if they are not enlarged but a normal liver edge can sometimes be felt (Talley and O'Connor 2006). If palpable, it should feel soft, regular and smooth with a well-defined border (Talley and O'Connor 2006). See Figures 2.21 and 2.22 for light and deep palpation techniques to be used during abdominal examination.

Evidence-based approaches

Rationale

The patient's health history and the nurse's knowledge of anatomy and physiology will help to guide when it is appropriate to do an abdominal physical examination. The list of presentations that may lead to an abdominal examination is vast; as discussed in the

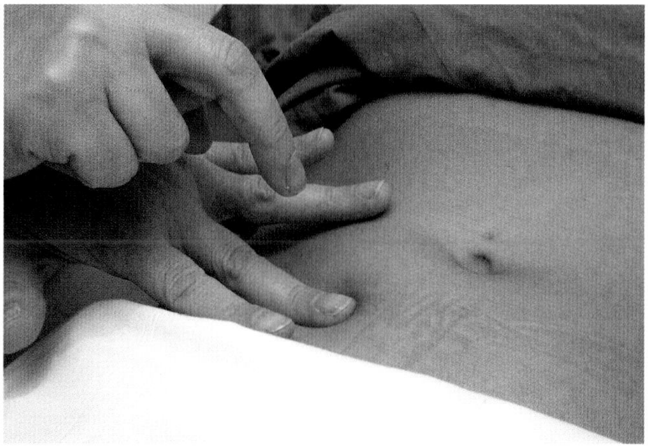

(a)

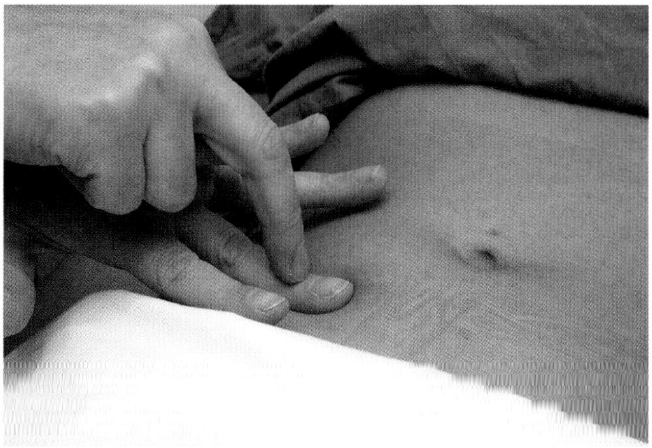

(b)

Figure 2.20 Percussion technique during abdominal examination.

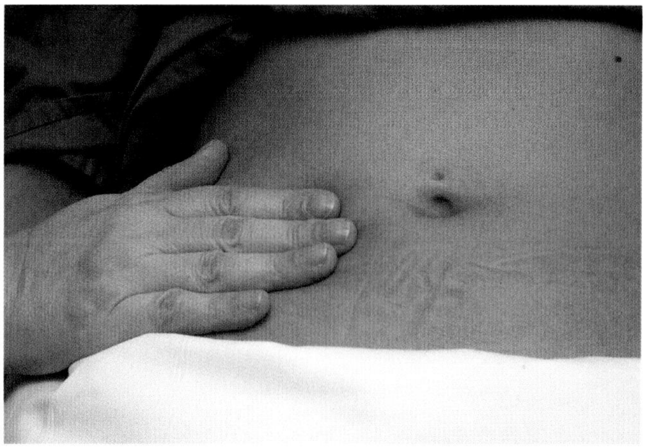

Figure 2.21 Light palpation during abdominal examination.

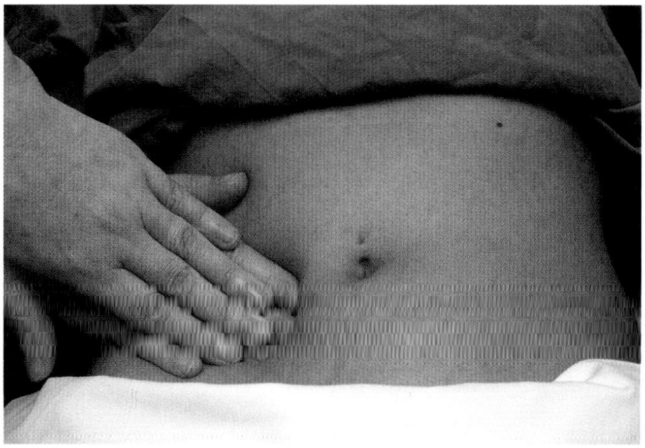

Figure 2.22 Deep palpation during abdominal examination.

anatomy and physiology section, they could involve the GI, renal and/or reproductive systems. Some examples include:

- abdominal pain
- nausea and/or vomiting
- change in bowel habits
- weight change
- jaundice
- bleeding
- dysuria/urgency or frequency
- flank pain
- suprapubic pain

Procedure guideline 2.3 Abdominal examination

Essential equipment

- Personal protective equipment
- Stethoscope
- Examination couch
- Pen torch
- Tongue depressor

Action	Rationale
Pre-procedure	
1 Introduce yourself to the patient, explain and discuss the procedure with them, and gain their consent to proceed.	To ensure that the patient feels at ease, understands the procedure and gives their valid consent (NMC 2018, **C**).
2 Gain the patient's verbal consent.	Consent must be gained before any procedure takes place (NMC 2018, **C**).

(continued)

Procedure guideline 2.3 Abdominal examination *(continued)*

Action	Rationale
3 Check that the patient has an empty bladder.	A full bladder will interfere with the examination (Walsh 2006a, **P**).
4 Make sure the patient is warm and comfortable and ideally have them in the supine position, with their arms by their sides.	If the patient is uncomfortable or cold the abdominal muscles will be tense (Rushforth 2009). The supine position helps to relax the abdominal muscles and is the optimum position for abdominal palpation (Talley and O'Connor 2006). **E**
5 Expose the patient from nipple to pubis, maintaining patient dignity at all times.	To ensure a thorough examination. **E**
Procedure	
6 Wash and dry hands.	To prevent the spread of infection (NHS England and NHSI 2019, **C**).
General inspection	
7 Take a global view of the patient.	See 'Inspection' above.
8 Look at the patient's skin and nails. Feel the texture and turgor of the skin.	Abnormalities of the skin and nails can be an indication of a variety of different conditions, for example bowel disease, malnutrition, liver disease, dehydration and/or anaemia (Bickley and Szilagyi 2017, Dover et al. 2018, Tidman 2018, **E**).
9 Ask the patient to extend their arms, flex their wrists and part their fingers. Ask them to stay in this position for 15 seconds.	To assess for liver flap; this can be a sign of liver and/or renal failure (Talley and O'Connor 2006, **E**).
10 Look at the patient's eyes.	To assess for any abnormalities, particularly looking for any signs of jaundice, hypercholesterolaemia and anaemia (Talley and O'Connor 2006, **E**).
11 Look at the patient's nose.	To assess for signs of telangiectasia, which can indicate liver disease (Bickley and Szilagyi 2017, **E**).
12 Look at and in the patient's mouth	The mouth can give a snapshot of the patient's general state of health. Look for signs of malnutrition, infection and any sores (Innes et al. 2018, **E**).
13 Smell the patient's breath.	To assess for signs of fetor (unpleasant-smelling breath) (Talley and O'Connor, 2006). Sweet-smelling breath can be a sign of ketoacidosis. **E**
14 Ask the patient to shrug their shoulders and lightly palpate, using the finger tips, directly above the clavicle.	To assess for a raised supraclavicular lymph node, which can indicate gastrointestinal malignancy (Talley and O'Connor 2006, **E**).
15 Move to the foot of the bed to inspect the abdomen.	Assessing the abdomen from different angles will help to identify any abnormalities (Walsh 2006a, **E**).
16 Observe the contour of the abdomen and position of the umbilicus.	To assess for asymmetry or distension, peristalsis and/or pulsations (Bickley and Szilagyi 2017, Walsh 2006a, **E**).
17 Move to the side of the bed and observe the contour of the abdomen tangentially.	This will allow any subtle changes in contour to be observed (Cox 2004, **E**).
18 Look at the patient's skin.	To assess for any signs of spider naevi, striae, scars, caput medusa, bruising and rashes (Plevris and Parks 2018, **E**).
Auscultation	
19 Using the diaphragm of the stethoscope, listen in all four quadrants for 1 minute each.	To assess for bowel sounds (Bickley and Szilagyi 2017, **E**). Bowel sounds normally occur every 5–10 seconds but frequency varies (Plevris and Parks 2018, **E**).
20 Using the bell of the stethoscope, listen over the aortic, renal, iliac and femoral arteries (see Figure 2.19).	To assess for bruits (Bickley and Szilagyi 2017, **E**).
Percussion	
21 Percuss in the nine areas of the abdomen.	To listen for a normal distribution of tympany and dullness (see Table 2.3) (Bickley and Szilagyi 2017, **E**).

22 Percuss for liver span. To do this, percuss upwards, starting in the right lower quadrant at the mid-clavicular line. Stop when you hear the dullness of the liver. Next percuss down, starting from the intersection of the nipple line and the mid-clavicular line; stop when the sound changes from the resonant lung to the dull liver. Measure between those two points.	To assess the size and location of the liver (Walsh 2006a, **E**).
23 The above technique can be employed to percuss the spleen, bladder and kidneys.	Not routinely done but may be useful if abnormality, in particular organomegaly, is suspected. **E**
24 Percuss from the midline out to the flanks for dullness. Keep your finger on the site of dullness in the flank, ask the patient to turn onto their opposite side and then percuss again. If the area of dullness is now resonant, shifting dullness is present.	To assess for shifting dullness (Plevris and Parks 2018, **E**).
Palpation	
25 Lightly palpate the abdomen using one hand. Look at the patient's face at all times, to ensure they are not in discomfort.	To assess for tenderness, rebound tenderness, superficial organs and masses (Talley and O'Connor 2006, **E**).
26 Deeply palpate the abdomen.	To assess the organs, identify deeper masses and define masses that have already been discovered (Talley and O'Connor 2006, **E**).
27 Palpate for the liver. To do this, place your left hand in the small of the patient's back and your right in the right lower quadrant pointing towards the upper left quadrant. Ask the patient to take a deep breath and palpate up. If nothing is felt, move up towards the liver and repeat until you reach the ribcage.	To assess for hepatomegaly or gallbladder tenderness (known as Murphy's sign) (Plevris and Parks 2018, **E**).
28 Palpate for the spleen. Ask the patient to tip slightly onto their right side. Start from the umbilicus region and mimic the technique above, moving towards the spleen.	To assess for splenomegaly (Plevris and Parks 2018, **E**).
29 Palpate for the kidneys. Do each kidney separately. For the right side, stand on the right side of the patient, place your left hand just below the 12th rib and lift up. Place your other hand on the right upper quadrant of the abdomen. Ask the patient to take a deep breath. As they do, press your right hand deeply into the abdomen, trying to feel the kidney between your hands. Repeat for the left side, standing on the left of the patient.	To assess for kidney enlargement; if the kidney is normal, it is not usually palpable (Plevris and Parks 2018, **E**).
30 Lightly palpate each costovertebral angle (the area directly overlying the kidneys) for tenderness; if none is felt, place one hand flat over the costovertebral angle and strike the hand firmly with the other fist.	Pain can indicate pyelonephritis (Bickley and Szilagyi 2017, **E**).
Post-procedure	
31 Document fully.	Accurate records should be kept of all discussions and/or assessments made (NMC 2018, **C**).
32 Report any abnormal findings to a senior nurse or to medical staff.	Patients should be cared for as part of a multidisciplinary team and, where appropriate, patient care should be referred to another more experienced practitioner (NMC 2018, **C**).
33 Clean the equipment used and wash hands.	To prevent the spread of infection (NHS England and NHSI 2019, **C**).
34 Explain the findings to the patient.	The patient should be told, in a way they can understand, the information they want or need to know about their health (NMC 2018, **C**).
35 Explain the plan of care to the patient.	Where possible, patients should be involved in planning their care (NMC 2018, **C**).

Post-procedural considerations

Documentation

Nurses should ensure that the following components are documented.

- rationale for examination
- patient's consent to examination
- type of examination performed
- findings from the examination
- plan of care.

As with all record keeping, documentation in relation to physical examinations should be clear, concise, accurate and without jargon or abbreviations (NMC 2018).

Record keeping should include evidence of clinical reasoning in order to identify patients' needs for nursing care. While this becomes more automatic with experience, it should always be possible for a nurse to explain how they arrive at a decision about an individual within their care (Gordon 1994, Putzier and Padrick 1984, Rolfe 1999).

References

Abbott, H. & Ranson, M. (2017) *Clinical Examination Skills for Health Professionals*. Glasgow: M&K Update.

Ahern, J. & Philpot, P. (2002) Assessing acutely ill patients on general wards. *Nursing Standard*, 16, 47–54.

Alfaro-LeFevre, R. (2014) *Applying Nursing Process: The Foundation for Clinical Reasoning*. Philadelphia: Lippincott Williams & Wilkins.

Arrowsmith, H. (1999) A critical evaluation of the use of nutrition screening tools by nurses. *British Journal of Nursing*, 8, 1483–1490.

Baid, H. (2006) The process of conducting a physical assessment: A nursing perspective. *British Journal of Nursing*, 15(13), 710–715.

BAPEN & Malnutrition Advisory Group (2000) *Explanatory Notes for the Screening Tool for Adults at Risk of Malnutrition*. London: British Association for Parenteral and Enteral Nutrition, Malnutrition Advisory Group.

Barrows, H. & Pickell, G. (1991) *Developing Clinical Problem-Solving Skills*. London: Norton Medical Books.

Berman, A., Kozier, B. & Erb, G.L. (2010) *Kozier and Erb's Fundamentals of Nursing*. Frenchs Forest, NSW: Pearson.

Bickley, L.S. & Szilagyi, P.G. (2017) *Bates' Guide to Physical Examination and History Taking*, 12th edn. Philadelphia: Wolters Kluwer.

Bonevski, B., Sanson-Fisher, R., Girgis, A., et al. (2000) Evaluation of an instrument to assess the needs of patients with cancer. *Cancer*, 88, 217–225.

Brown, V., Sitzia, J., Richardson, A., et al. (2001) The development of the Chemotherapy Symptom Assessment Scale (C-SAS): A scale for the routine clinical assessment of the symptom experiences of patients receiving cytotoxic chemotherapy. *International Journal of Nursing Studies*, 38, 497–510.

Burns, E.A., Korn, K., Whyte, J., et al. (2011) *Oxford American Handbook of Clinical Examination and Practical Skills*. New York: Oxford University Press.

Camm, C.F. & Camm, A.J. (eds) (2016) *Clinical Guide to Cardiology*. Oxford: Wiley Blackwell.

Cancer Action Team (2007) *Holistic Common Assessment of Supportive and Palliative Care Needs for Adults with Cancer: Assessment Guidance*. London: Cancer Action Team.

Clark, J. (1999) A language for nursing. *Nursing Standard*, 13, 42–47.

Cox, C.L. (ed) (2004) *Physical Assessment for Nurses*. Oxford: Blackwell.

Crouch, A.T. & Meurier, C. (eds) (2005) *Health Assessment*. Oxford: Blackwell.

Crumbie, A. (2006) Taking a history. In: Walsh, M. (ed) *Nurse Practitioners: Clinical Skills and Professional Issues*, 2nd edn. Edinburgh: Butterworth-Heinemann, pp.14–26.

DH (Department of Health) (2005) *Choosing a Better Diet: A Food and Health Action Plan*. London: Department of Health.

DH (2006) *Modernising Nursing Careers: Setting the Direction*. London: Department of Health.

Dimond, B. (2002) *Legal Aspects of Pain Management*. Dinton, UK: Quay Books.

Donnelly, M. & Martin, D. (2016) History taking and physical assessment in holistic palliative care. *British Journal of Nursing*, 25(22), 1250–1255.

Dover, A.R., Innes, J.A. & Fairhurst, K. (2018) General aspects of examination. In: Innes, J.A., Dover, A.R. & Fairhurst, K. (eds) *Macleod's Clinical Examination*, 14th edn. London: Elsevier, pp.19–36.

Drinkaware (2019) *What Is an Alcoholic Unit?* Available at: https://www.drinkaware.co.uk/alcohol-facts/alcoholic-drinks-units/what-is-an-alcohol-unit

Edwards, M. & Miller, C. (2001) Improving psychosocial assessment in oncology. *Professional Nurse*, 16, 1223–1226.

Eilers, J., Berger, A.M. & Petersen, M.C. (1988) Development, testing, and application of the Oral Assessment Guide. *Oncology Nursing Forum*, 15, 325–330.

Estes, M.E.Z. (2013) *Health Assessment and Physical Examination*, 5th edn. New York: Delmar Cengage Learning.

Fisher, E. & Potter, J. (eds) (2017) *Respiratory Examination*. Available at: www.oxfordmedicaleducation.com/category/clinical-examinations/respiratory-examination

Fortin, M., Stewart, M., Poitras, M.E., et al. (2012) A systematic review of prevalence studies on multimorbidity: Toward a more uniform methodology. *Annals of Family Medicine*, 10(2), 142–151.

Frank-Stromborg, M. & Olsen, S.J. (eds) (2004) *Instruments for Clinical Healthcare Research*. Sudbury, MA: Jones & Bartlett.

Fritz, D. & Becker Weilitz, P. (2016) Abdominal assessment. *Home Healthcare Now*, 34(3), 151–155.

Galanti, G.A. (2000) An introduction to cultural differences. *Western Journal of Medicine*, 172, 335–336.

Gangopadhyay, D.N., Dey S.K., Chandra, M., et al. (1998) Serum lipid profile in xanthelasma. *Indian Journal of Dermatology*, 43, 53–56.

Gordon, M. (1994) *Nursing Diagnosis: Process and Application*. St Louis, MO: Mosby.

Haidet, P. & Paterniti, D.A. (2003). Building a history rather than taking one: A perspective on information sharing during the medical interview. *Archives of Internal Medicine*, 163(10), 1134–1140.

Harris, R., Wilson-Barnett, J., Griffiths, P. & Evans, A. (1998) Patient assessment: Validation of a nursing instrument. *International Journal of Nursing Studies*, 35, 303–313.

Heaven, C.M. & Maguire, P. (1996) Training hospice nurses to elicit patient concerns. *Journal of Advanced Nursing*, 23, 280–286.

Holmes, H.N. (ed) (2003) *Three-Minute Assessment*. Philadelphia: Lippincott Williams & Wilkins.

Innes, J.A., Dover, A.R. & Fairhurst, K. (2018) General aspects of history taking. In: Innes, J.A., Dover, A.R. & Fairhurst, K. (eds) *Macleod's Clinical Examination*, 14th edn. London: Elsevier, pp.9–18.

Innes, J.A & Tiernan, J. (2018) The respiratory system. In: Innes, J.A., Dover, A.R. & Fairhurst, K. (eds) *Macleod's Clinical Examination*, 14th edn. London: Elsevier, pp.75–92.

Jarvis, C. (2016) *Pocket Companion for Physical Examination and Health Assessment*, 7th edn. St Louis, MO: Elsevier.

Jensen, T.S., Wilson, P.R. & Rice, A.S. (2003) *Clinical Pain Management: Chronic Pain*. London: Arnold.

Johnson, T. (2000) Functional health pattern assessment on-line: Lessons learned. *Computers in Nursing*, 18, 248–254.

Kearney, N. (2001) Classifying nursing care to improve patient outcomes: The example of WISECARE. *Nursing Times Research*, 6, 747–756.

Kozier, B. (2012) *Fundamentals of Nursing: Concepts, Process, and Practice*. Harlow, UK: Pearson.

MacDonald, J. & RMH Pressure Ulcer MDT Collaborative (2019) *aSSKINg Bundle Assessment Document NR592*. London: The Royal Marsden NHS Foundation Trust.

Marek, C. (2003). Antiemetic therapy in patients receiving cancer chemotherapy. *Oncology Nursing Forum*, 30, 259–271.

McCrae, N. (2012) Whither nursing models? The value of nursing theory in the context of evidence-based practice and multidisciplinary health care. *Journal of Advanced Nursing*, 68, 222–229.

McLoughlin, A., Shewbridge, A. & Owens, R. (2012) Developing the role of advanced practitioner. *Cancer Nursing Practice*, 11, 14–19.

Mills, N.L., Japp, A.G. & Robson, J. (2018) The cardiovascular system. In: Innes, J.A., Dover, A.R. & Fairhurst, K. (eds) *Macleod's Clinical Examination*, 14th edn. London: Elsevier, pp.39–74.

Moore, T. (2007) Respiratory assessment in adults. *Nursing Standard*, 21(49), 48–56.

Murphy, E.K. (2003) Charting by exception. *AORN Journal*, 78, 821–823.

Nair, P.A. & Singhal, R. (2018) Xanthelasma palpebrarum: A brief review. *Clinical, Cosmetic and Investigational Dermatology*, 11, 1–5.

NHS England and NHSI (NHS Improvement) (2019) *Standard Infection Control Precautions: National Hand Hygiene and Personal Protective Equipment Policy*. Available at: https://improvement.nhs.uk/documents/4957/National_policy_on_hand_hygiene_and_PPE_2.pdf

NMC (Nursing and Midwifery Council) (2018) *The Code: Professional Standards of Practice and Behaviour for Nurses, Midwives and Nursing Associates*. Available at: https://www.nmc.org.uk/standards/code

O'Connor, F.W. & Eggert, L.L. (1994) Psychosocial assessment for treatment planning and evaluation. *Journal of Psychosocial Nursing and Mental Health Services*, 32, 31–42.

Orem, D.E., Taylor, S.G. & Renpenning, K.M. (2001) *Nursing: Concepts of Practice*. St Louis, MO: Mosby.

Paterson, R. & Dover, A.R. (2018) The deteriorating patient. In: Innes, J.A., Dover, A.R. & Fairhurst, K. (eds) *Macleod's Clinical Examination*, 14th edn. London: Elsevier, pp.339–346.

Paul, R. (1988). What, then, is critical thinking? Paper presented at the Eighth Annual and Sixth International Conference on Critical Thinking and Educational Reform, Rohnert Park, CA.

Peacock, S. (2004) Systematic health assessment: A case study. *Practice Nursing*, 15(6), 270–274.

Peate, I., Nair, M. & Wild, K. (2014) *Nursing Practice: Knowledge and Care*. Chichester: Wiley Blackwell.

[illegible] *Nursing Times*, 101, 32–35.

Plevris, J. & Parks, R. (2018) The gastrointestinal system. In: Innes, J.A., Dover, A.R. & Fairhurst, K. (eds) *Macleod's Clinical Examination*, 14th edn. London: Elsevier, pp.93–118.

Powell, A. (2006) The cardiovascular system. In: Walsh, M. (ed) *Nurse Practitioners: Clinical Skills and Professional Issues*, 2nd edn. Edinburgh: Butterworth-Heinemann, pp.98–119.

Pratt, R.J. & Van Wijgerden, J. (2009) Nursing care of patients with tuberculosis In: Schaaf, H.S. & Zumla, A.I. (eds) *Tuberculosis: A Comprehensive Clinical Reference*. London: Elsevier, pp.711–717.

Price, C.I.M., Han, S.W. & Rutherford, I.A. (2000) Advanced nursing practice: An introduction to physical assessment. *British Journal of Nursing*, 9(22), 2292–2296.

Putzier, D.J. & Padrick, K.P. (1984) Nursing diagnosis: A component of nursing process and decision making. *Topics in Clinical Nursing*, 5, 21–29.

Rhodes, V.A., McDaniel, R.W., Homan, S.S., et al. (2000) An instrument to measure symptom experience: Symptom occurrence and symptom distress. *Cancer Nursing*, 23, 49–54.

Rolfe, G. (1999) Insufficient evidence: The problems of evidence-based nursing. *Nurse Education Today*, 19, 433–442.

Roper, N., Logan, W.W. & Tierney, A.J. (2000) *The Roper-Logan-Tierney Model of Nursing: Based on Activities of Living*. New York: Churchill Livingstone.

Rowbotham, D.J. & MacIntyre, P.E. (2003) *Clinical Pain Management: Acute Pain*. London: Arnold.

Royal Collage of Nursing (2017) *Principles of Consent: Guidance for Nursing Staff*. Available at: https://www.rcn.org.uk/professional-development/publications/pub-006047

Rush, S., Fergy, S. & Weels, D. (1996) Professional development: Care planning – Knowledge for practice. *Nursing Times*, 92, 18–23.

Rushforth, H. (2009) *Assessment Made Incredibly Easy!* London: Lippincott Williams & Wilkins.

Saxon, A. & Lillyman, S. (eds) (2011) *Developing Advanced Assessment Skills: Patients with Long-Term Conditions*. Keswick, UK: M&K Publishing.

Schug, S.A., Palmer, G.M., Scott, D.A., et al. (2015) *Acute Pain Management: Scientific Evidence*, 4th edn. Australian and New Zealand College of Anaesthetists and Faculty of Pain Medicine. Available at: http://fpm.anzca.edu.au/documents/apmse4_2015_final

Seidel, H.M., Ball, J.W., Davis, J.E., et al. (2011) *Mosby's Guide to Physical Examination*, 7th edn. New York: Mosby Elsevier.

Shaw, M. (1998) *Charting Made Incredibly Easy*. Springhouse, PA: Springhouse.

Silverman, J., Kurtz, S.M. & Draper, J. (2013) *Skills for Communicating with Patients*. London: Radcliffe.

Smith, J. & Rushton, M. (2015) How to perform respiratory assessment. *Nursing Standard*, 30(7), 34–36.

Swartz, M.H. (2014) *Textbook of Physical Diagnosis: History and Examination*, 7th edn. Philadelphia: Elsevier Saunders.

Talley, N.J. & O'Connor, S. (2006) *Clinical Examination: A Systematic Guide to Physical Diagnosis*. Sydney: Churchill Livingstone Elsevier.

[illegible] *Seminars in Oncology Nursing*, 18, 121–127.

Tidman, M.J. (2018) The skin, hair and nails. In: Innes, J.A., Dover, A.R. & Fairhurst, K. (eds) *Macleod's Clinical Examination*, 14th edn. London: Elsevier, pp.283–293.

Walsh, M. (2006a) Abdominal disorders. In: Walsh, M. (ed) *Nurse Practitioners: Clinical Skills and Professional Issues*, 2nd edn. Edinburgh: Butterworth-Heinemann, pp.139–157.

Walsh, M. (2006b) *Nurse Practitioners: Clinical Skills and Professional Issues*, 2nd edn. Edinburgh: Butterworth-Heinemann.

Walsh, M., Crumbie, A. & Watson, J.E. (2007) *Watson's Clinical Nursing and Related Sciences*. New York: Baillière Tindall / Elsevier.

Weber, J.R. & Kelley, J.H. (2014) *Health Assessment in Nursing*, 5th edn. Philadelphia: Lippincott Williams & Wilkins.

Westbrook, A. (2000) Nursing language. *Nursing Times*, 96, 41.

White, L. (2003) *Documentation and the Nursing Process*. Clifton Park, NY: Thomson / Delmar Learning.

Wilkinson, J.M. (2007) *Nursing Process and Critical Thinking*. Upper Saddle River, NJ: Pearson Prentice Hall.

Chapter 3

Discharge care and planning

Caroline Watts with Emma Collard and Connie Lewis

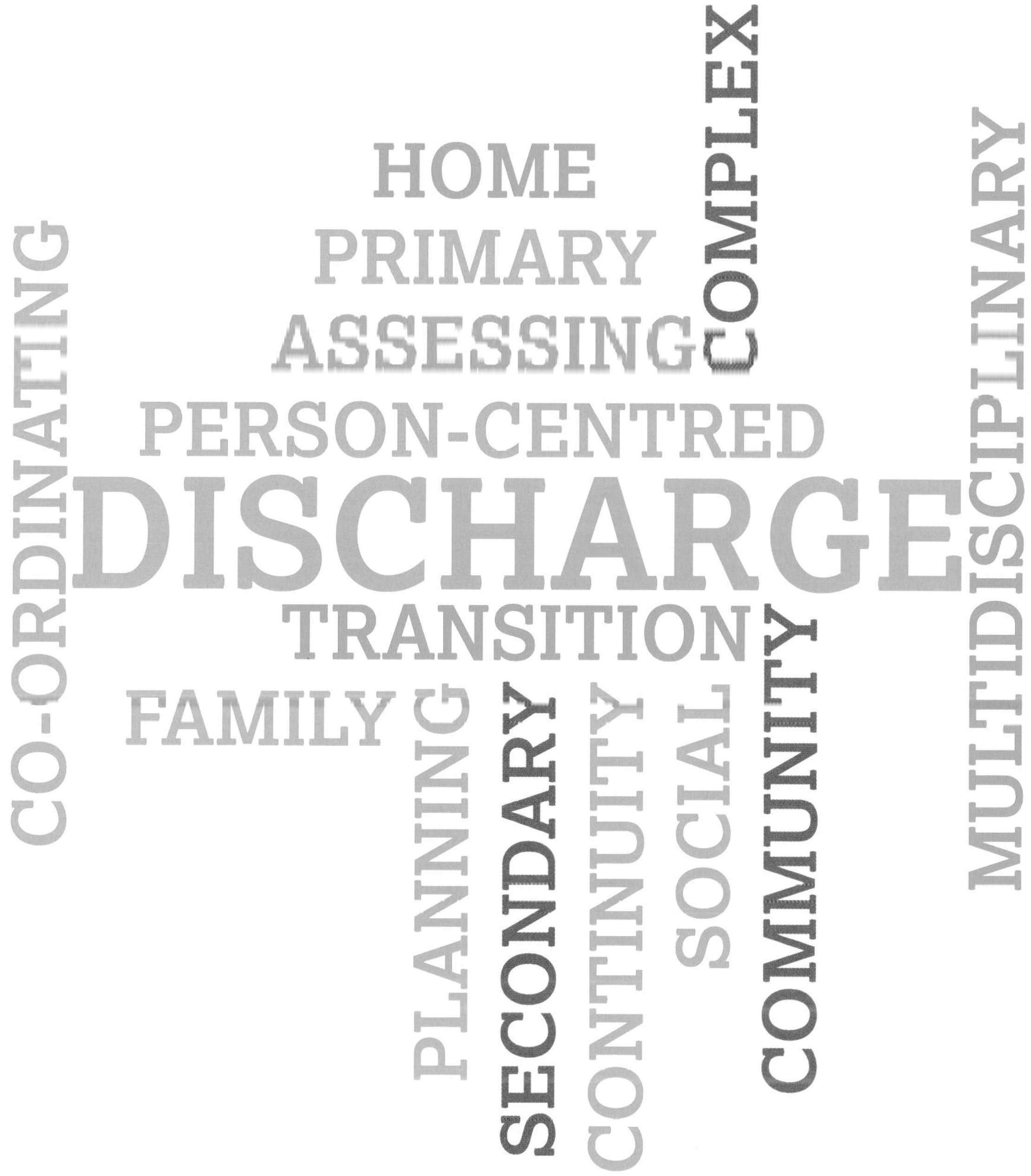

The Royal Marsden Manual of Clinical Nursing Procedures: Professional Edition, Tenth Edition. Edited by Sara Lister, Justine Hofland and Hayley Grafton.

Overview

This chapter addresses the planning and process of discharging patients from hospital. Discharge planning is a routine feature of healthcare systems worldwide and is recognized as the foundation of patients' successful transitions from hospital to home (Pellett 2016). The aim of this multidisciplinary process of assessing, planning and co-ordinating patients' care needs prior to their leaving hospital is to ensure continuity of care with a safe and timely discharge. While discharge planning is a universal priority for all acute inpatient facilities (McNeil 2016), the process and pace of discharge planning have changed beyond all recognition (Lees-Deutsch 2017). The increasing pressure on inpatient beds has meant that despite the clear benefits of reducing the time a patient occupies a hospital bed, 'achieving it has proven difficult' (NHSI 2018, p.3) and effective discharge planning therefore remains one of the major challenges facing the NHS today (Winfield and Burns 2016).

Both internal and external planning processes are included in this chapter. External planning processes are those associated with the interface between primary and secondary care. They include processes related to complex discharges (including for patients with additional needs), discharge to a nursing home and discharge at the end of life.

Discharge care and planning

Definition

Discharge planning is a complex process (Wallace et al. 2017) that is not a discrete event with one model of care but a transitional one with many factors involved (Chenoweth et al. 2015). The process should take into account a patient's physical, psychological, social, cultural, economic and environmental needs. It involves not only patients but also families, friends, informal carers, the hospital multidisciplinary team, and the community health and social services teams.

Related theory

The evidence suggests that a structured discharge plan tailored to the individual is best practice (McNeil 2016). Guidance from the National Institute for Health and Care Excellence (NICE) (2015) emphasizes this person-centred approach by highlighting the importance of information sharing between the patient, their family or carers, and all health and social care practitioners involved to ensure a safe and co-ordinated transition. Patients need to be considered as equal partners in the process where the foundations for decisions are based on what is important to the individual and their needs and preferences (Weiss et al. 2015). This approach also promotes the highest possible level of independence for the patient, their partner and their family by encouraging appropriate self-care activities and participation in the discharge planning process.

The roles of both family members and informal caregivers are crucial in supporting the discharge planning process, as Mabire et al. (2018) indicate. Therefore, providing the patient and their family with information, knowledge and confidence in their care before they leave hospital is an essential component of discharge preparation. Evidence suggests, however, that during a patient's hospitalization, family and carers often receive limited communication and education regarding the care of their loved ones after discharge (Cacchione 2018). This can leave patients unprepared for the transition home; they can feel a sense of abandonment (Wallace et al. 2017) and are rendered more likely to require a readmission. It is therefore vital that nurses and other members of the multidisciplinary team discuss with the patient and their family how they will manage their condition after their discharge and offer appropriate teaching and support to enable self-care. The use of patient information sheets to aid this process has been found to be effective and may help both patients and their families feel more prepared for discharge from hospital (New et al. 2016).

Assessment of patients' individual needs for discharge is of particular importance when considering transfer from an acute care setting. The NICE (2015) guidance indicates that practitioners should work together 'to identify factors that could prevent a safe, timely transfer of care from hospital' (p.12). Assessing risk and the prompt sharing of pertinent concerns regarding a patient's physical, psychological or cognitive ability enables earlier intervention from the multidisciplinary team, thereby helping to ensure patient safety and wellbeing (Lees-Deutsch et al. 2016). Staff should have a clear understanding of their roles and responsibilities and work collaboratively (Elliott and DeAngelis 2017). The NICE (2015) guidance recommends that the multidisciplinary team should be identified as soon as a person is admitted and that there should be regular contact with the community team to provide co-ordinated and planned ongoing support.

To achieve the best continuity of care after discharge, there needs to be effective communication across all disciplines, and with the patient and their family (New et al. 2016, Mabire et al. 2018). This ensures that the patient's wishes are heard and acted upon appropriately (Winfield and Burns 2016).

Co-ordination of discharge care planning should be led by a 'single health or social care practitioner' (NICE 2015, p.10); this nominated person is often a key worker or discharge co-ordinator. A key worker is a single named person who has agreed with the patient to be their first point of contact for support, information and care planning. Discharge co-ordinators are, in general, health or social care professionals who have both hospital and community experience. Their role is to advise, help with planning and assist the co-ordination of the differing care providers that the patient may need when they leave hospital, particularly when their nursing and care needs are complex (Lees 2013).

Clinical governance

Legal, professional and safeguarding issues in discharge planning

There is a requirement in discharge planning for nurses to share information about patients with health and social care providers in the community. Nurses need to ensure they use safe communication procedures so that information is only shared with those who require it. Failing to apply good information governance processes could result in information being shared inappropriately and the breaching of a patient's right to confidentiality. Patients need to be supported and encouraged to make their own decisions; where a patient lacks capacity, the need to share information must be based on a consideration of risk and the person's best interests (this is discussed in more detail in Chapter 5: Communication, psychological wellbeing and safeguarding in the section about the Mental Capacity Act (2005)).

Risk management

Delays in discharge contribute substantially to the financial and capacity pressures facing the NHS, as do readmissions (Winfield and Burns 2016). The total number of NHS hospital beds in England has more than halved in the past 30 years while the number of patients has increased significantly (Ewbank et al. 2017). Anticipating and managing potential delays via proactive planning therefore helps the NHS and other healthcare providers to use their limited resources most effectively, and, more importantly, can improve a patient's quality of life (Alper et al. 2017). Planning care for discharge and involving patients and their families is therefore important in keeping disruption to a minimum to ensure inpatient facilities are maximized and patients move in a seamless fashion back into the community.

Delayed and/or ineffective discharge planning has been shown to have detrimental effects on patients' psychological and physical wellbeing and their illness experience (Lees 2013). Additionally, evidence suggests that inadequate discharge planning in older people leads not only to adverse health outcomes but also to an increased risk of hospital readmission (Chenoweth et al. 2015, Pellett 2016). Older people with dementia or other cognitive impairment are likely to experience an extended length of stay in hospital because of

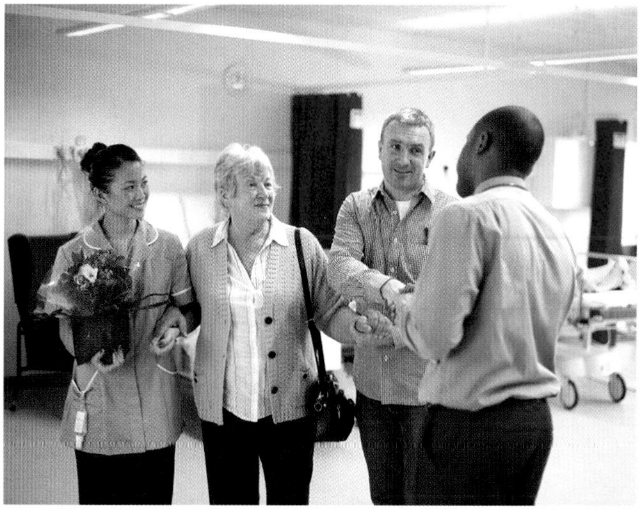

Figure 3.1 A patient leaving hospital. *Source*: Reproduced with permission of Getty Images.

more complex organizational arrangements and an increase in the support needed on discharge (Challis et al. 2014). Elderly patients in acute care do not always get enough opportunity to mobilize and are highly likely to acquire 'deconditioning syndrome', where their bone mass and muscle strength are reduced. Up to 65% of older patients experience this type of decline during hospitalization (British Geriatrics Society 2017). This may result in increased risk of falls, constipation, incontinence, depression, swallowing problems and pneumonia (Arora 2017). Reducing this risk by implementing pro-active planning to ensure timely and safe discharge is therefore paramount; nurses' key role in achieving this is emphasized by The Queen's Nursing Institute (2016), which suggests that nurses are 'at the heart of effective discharge planning' (p.35).

Discharging patients from hospital: internal procedures

Evidence-based approaches

Despite the fact that improved discharge planning has been a consistent recommendation in health policy and research, there is no commonly agreed model for the process of discharge (Waring et al. 2014). The process for discharging patients at ward level should, however, be standard for all simple discharges across the hospital. NHS Improvement (NHSI) (2015) has developed a toolkit on discharge planning and highlighted key elements that are essential for both elective and emergency admissions:

- Specify a date and time of discharge as early as possible within the period of care.
- Identify whether a patient has simple or complex discharge planning needs.
- Identify what the patient's individual discharge needs are and how these will be met.
- Define the specific clinical criteria that a patient must meet for discharge.

NHSI (2015) also says: 'A specific targeted discharge date and time reduces a patient's length of stay, emergency readmissions and pressure on hospital beds' (p.2). Discharge dates in elective care can be planned prior to admission; if patients have attended a pre-assessment appointment, discharge needs should be identified at this point to allow effective planning and to enable clinical staff to notify appropriate services in advance of admission (NICE 2015). Advance planning is not possible in emergency or unscheduled care so in these circumstances robust systems of patient assessment are crucial to gather relevant patient information early (Lees-Deutsch et al. 2016). An estimated date of discharge can then be agreed for everyone to work towards. The date may change depending on clinical and individual patient needs since changes in patients' medical conditions require ongoing reassessment and should be the foundation of decisions about timing (Weiss et al. 2015). The expected date of discharge should therefore be continually reviewed based on the consultant's judgement as to when the patient is likely to have recovered sufficiently to go home. This is best done by establishing the clinical criteria for discharge, which are the functional and physiological parameters that the patient must achieve before discharge (NHSI 2018). These criteria enable everyone to focus on the same factors, which helps in communication and facilitates more effective discharge planning. Due to the rapidly aging population, the increasing number of people living with long-term conditions (such as dementia) and the decreasing number of hospital beds, the pressure to discharge patients quickly is a continuous challenge for the NHS (Ewbank et al. 2017). As a result, there have been many recent reports, recommendations and initiatives to improve discharge planning from statutory and voluntary bodies (e.g. Healthwatch England 2015, NHS England 2016, NICE 2015, QNI 2016, Royal Voluntary Service 2014).

The SAFER Patient Flow Bundle (NHSI 2017a) is a structured approach that uses five elements of best practice to improve discharge planning (Figure 3.2).

The Red to Green approach, which works in tandem with SAFER Patient Flow Bundle, also highlights those days when a patient receives little or no interventions that progresses them towards discharge; these days progress them towards discharge (Figure 3.3). Green days add value to a patient as they receive care that contributes towards them getting home. By using this approach, hospitals can see where there are blockages in their discharge processes and make changes for improvement. For example, a high number of patients may have red days because they are waiting for a scan before discharge. By reviewing the radiology scheduling, the hospital could implement changes to fast-track patients who are awaiting discharge, which could prevent discharge delays.

Nurse-led and criteria-led discharge have both been developed within the past decade as ways to expedite timely discharge for patients. Both require the clinical parameters for a patient's discharge to be clearly defined; once these have been met, discharge can be facilitated by a competent member of staff (Lees-Deutsch and Robinson 2018). For nurse-led discharge to be undertaken, nurses require specific training to ensure competency in the continuing assessment of patients for discharge, whereas criteria-led discharge is an approach that can be used by a range of professionals. Criteria are often developed from clinical guidelines for specific conditions (Cundy et al. 2017) and their use can appropriately inform practitioners about the patient's clinical readiness for discharge. However, effective discharge extends beyond the use of criteria in isolation (Lees-Deutsch and Gaillemin 2018) and nurses must focus on their accountability for delivering holistic care throughout the discharge planning process.

Introducing frameworks and approaches to discharge planning can support the process and improve efficiency, organization and overall satisfaction of patients and staff (Lees-Deutsch and Gaillemin 2018). Such methods help to reduce time lags in the traditional discharge process, thereby reducing length of stay and improving patient safety.

Principles of care

It is essential that nurses are aware of their organization's local discharge procedures, policies and protocols and are able to identify when a patient's discharge needs may be complex; the principles of addressing these are covered below in this chapter.

When planning a patient's discharge from hospital, it is important for nurses to consider that, however well it is structured, discharge can have complex emotional aspects for the patient and

The SAFER Patient Flow Bundle

Introduction

SAFER is a practical tool to reduce delays for patients in adult inpatient wards (excluding maternity).

The SAFER bundle blends five elements of best practice. It's important to implement all five elements together to achieve cumulative benefits. It works particularly well when it is used in conjunction with the '**Red** and Green Days' approach. When followed consistently, length of stay reduces and patient flow and safety improves.

The SAFER patient flow bundle

S - **Senior Review**. All patients will have a senior review before midday by a clinician able to make management and discharge decisions.

A – **All patients** will have an Expected Discharge Date (EDD) and Clinical Criteria for Discharge (CCD), set by assuming ideal recovery and assuming no unnecessary waiting.

F - **Flow** of patients to commence at the earliest opportunity from assessment units to inpatient wards. Wards routinely receiving patients from assessment units will ensure the first patient arrives on the ward by 10 am.

E – **Early discharge**. 33% of patients will be discharged from base inpatient wards before midday.

R – **Review**. A systematic multi-disciplinary team (MDT) review of patients with extended lengths of stay (>7 days – also known as 'stranded patients') with a clear 'home first' mind set.

S - **Senior Review**. All patients should have a senior review before midday:

- Use simple rules to standardise ward and board round processes.
- Minimise variation between individual clinicians and clinical teams to ensure all patients receive an effective daily senior review.
- Daily review undertaken by a senior clinician able to make management and discharge decisions is essential seven days a week.
- Effective ward and board rounds are crucial to decision making and care co-ordination.

Figure 3.2 The SAFER Patient Flow Bundle. *Source*: NHSI (2017a). Reproduced with permission of the NHS.

Red and Green Bed Days

Introduction

'Red and Green Bed Days' are a visual management system to assist in the identification of wasted time in a patient's journey. Applicable to in-patient wards in both acute and community settings, this approach is used to reduce internal and external delays as part of the SAFER patient flow bundle. It is not appropriate for high turnover areas such as Emergency Departments, Assessment Units, Clinical Decision Units/Observation Units, and Short Stay Units where using Red and Green on an hours/minutes basis may be more appropriate.

1	2			3	4			5						6
1	2	3	4	5	6	7	8	9	10	11	12	13	14	15

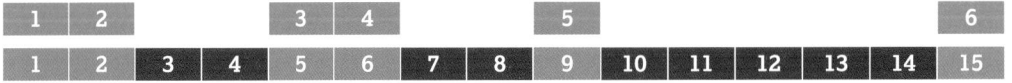

A Red day is when a patient receives little or no value adding acute care. The following questions should be considered:

- Could the care or interventions the patient is receiving today be delivered in a non-acute setting?
- If I saw this patient in out-patients, would their current 'physiological status' require emergency admission?

If the answers are 1. Yes and 2. No, then this is a 'Red bed day'

Examples of what constitutes a Red bed day:

- A planned investigation, clinical assessment, procedure or therapy intervention does not occur.
- The patient is in receipt of care that does not require an acute hospital bed.
- The medical care plan lacks a consultant approved expected date of discharge.
- There are no consultant approved physiological and functional clinical criteria for discharge in the medical care plan.

A RED day is a day of no value for a patient

A Green day is when a patient receives value adding acute care that progresses their progress towards discharge.

A Green day is a day when everything planned or requested gets done.

A Green day is a day when the patient receives care that can only be in an acute hospital bed.

A GREEN day is a day of value for a patient

Figure 3.3 Red and Green Bed Days. *Source*: NHSI (2017b). Reproduced with permission of the NHS.

their family (Teodorczuk 2016). Engaging patients and their carers and families at all stages is therefore an essential part of any discharge planning system as it enables a focus on patients' individual holistic needs. This ultimately ensures not only patients' continued safety but also their general wellbeing (Elliott and DeAngelis 2017).

Pre-procedural considerations

There are certain issues that need to be addressed for all patients, such as transport to enable them to return home and timely prescribing of medications to take home so that they are ready for discharge. NHSI (2015) suggests that checks for all discharge issues should be finalized 48 hours prior to discharge. It is also important to ensure that follow-up arrangements have been made. These may include a clinic appointment or referral to a district nurse for a specific procedure.

Equipment

Patients will frequently require equipment to enable them to return home. Ensuring that all required equipment is available and in working order before discharge facilitates a smooth transition to home (Elliott and DeAngelis 2017). The equipment needs of each patient should be assessed at pre-admission and throughout their stay to ensure nothing is omitted.

Patients may require new additional services at home, such as oxygen, which should be prescribed using the appropriate national Home Oxygen Order Form (HOOF) and the Initial Home Oxygen Risk Mitigation Form (IHORM). In 2017, NHS England changed the process for ordering home oxygen to make it safer as it had been found that patients were not always being asked to sign consent forms when they were started on oxygen (NHS Sunderland Clinical Commissioning Group 2017). The IHORM was therefore introduced to reduce the risk of a serious incident occurring when medicinal oxygen is installed in a home environment. Before a patient is initiated on oxygen, the clinician must ask the patient [illegible] risks and give informed consent.

The HOOF and IHORN forms need to be faxed to the local oxygen supplier but often the task of ordering oxygen is completed by the patient's local clinical commissioning group, which usually has details on its website along with the facility to download forms. It is useful to know how the local procedures work and to ensure consideration is given to the monitoring and reviewing of the patient on oxygen once at home.

Pharmacological support: medication on discharge

Before a patient is discharged, the nurse needs to ensure that the patient and, where appropriate, the carer are competent to self-administer medication at home. Evidence suggests that there are often limited resources in hospitals to ensure patients who are capable of self-care regarding medication maintain their independence (QNI 2016) so supportive measures must be considered. In some areas, tablet dispensers are provided, particularly for those who have difficulty opening containers or who lack competency in remembering which tablets to take when (Figure 3.4). If carers and/or community nurses are involved in giving a patient medication at home, a medicines administration record (MAR chart) should be given on discharge, clearly stating the name of the drug, the dose and frequency, and any special instructions (Figure 3.5). Special considerations are required for medications prescribed for pumps and drivers (e.g. for patients who require end-of-life care or symptom management), and in such circumstances local policies should be referred to.

Non-pharmacological support: nutrition

In some cases, patients may be receiving nutrition via feeding tubes, known as 'enteral feeding'. The common routes for enteral feeding in the community are:

- radiologically inserted gastrostomy (RIG)
- percutaneous endoscopically placed gastrostomy (PEG)
- jejunostomy
- nasogastric (NG).

Dietitians and/or nutrition nurses normally facilitate arrangements for these patients when they are going home. It is important that community teams including nurses and dietitians are contacted in advance of a patient being discharged with supportive feeding *in situ* to ascertain what information and support they need to facilitate the patient's safe and timely discharge home.

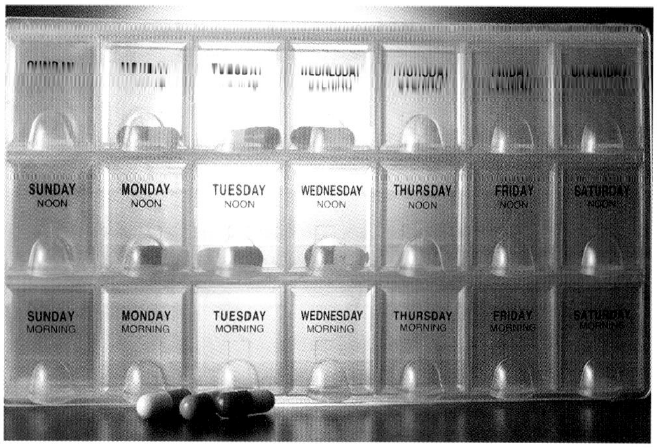

Figure 3.4 An example of a tablet dispenser.

Name	Purpose of medication	Dose	Frequency	Special instructions
Metoclopramide	Anti-sickness	10 mg	Up to 3 times a day	Take if feeling nauseous
Amoxicillin	Antibiotic – to treat infection	500 mg	3 times a day	Do not miss a dose and ensure the course of treatment is completed (take all of the tablets prescribed)

Figure 3.5 A sample medicines administration chart.

Specific patient needs on discharge

It is important to recognize that some patients will have additional needs due to their status or health condition – for example, a continuing disability, learning difficulties, a mental 'illness' or dementia. Patients who live alone or who have limited financial resources also need specific consideration to ensure their needs are met and that they are not vulnerable to further problems once discharged.

There may be practical issues about the transfer home that patients have not considered themselves while in hospital. If, for example, the patient lives alone or is very frail, simple tasks such as shopping may be very difficult. Some trusts have services to provide food packs for elderly patients (QNI 2016) but otherwise arrangements will need to be made prior to discharge to ensure the patient has adequate food provisions. Talking to the patient about what they will need and how they will manage is essential. Carers, family and neighbours should be involved and appropriate local agencies and services considered.

Age UK (www.ageuk.org.uk) provides information and support for older people. Its factsheet on hospital discharge gives useful advice for patients about practical issues to consider when leaving hospital (Box 3.1).

Each year, almost a third of people over the age of 65 fall (NICE 2018). Where patients are frail or at risk of falls, ensuring that they know that a community pendant alarm system or other personal alarm system can be installed may provide them and their family with some reassurance. Information regarding these alarms and local providers is usually held by the local authority (see Chapter 7: Moving and positioning for more information). For many dependent adults, adaptive technologies provide a means to independent living and a decrease in reliance on support from family members or more costly social services.

Accommodation considerations on discharge

On discharge, consideration may need to be given to patient accommodation, such as the suitability of the accommodation and alterations required. The hospital occupational therapy team usually leads on this and makes a domiciliary visit to ensure appropriate aids (e.g. hand rails) are put in place and changes are made to facilitate the safe transition of the patient home. A home visit may also be necessary to ensure the property is habitable – for example, if the patient's property is in a poor state or there are issues in relation to hoarding. This may need to be done by or with social services. Where the patient is a home-owner, however, the housing department may be less likely to intervene, in which case it is up to the patient and their family to address such issues.

It is also possible that prior to admission a patient will have been homeless, or they may become homeless during their hospital stay. The patient may need to be supported to access accommodation through the local authority homelessness team. As part of the process, the patient will need to provide evidence of eligibility for social housing, which will require specific supporting documentation. It is worth noting that all housing assessments are carried out online, which can be difficult for patients who have little or no knowledge of computers, so extra support is needed for such patients to prevent delay in discharge.

Box 3.1 Practical issues for older people when leaving hospital

Attention to practical issues is vital for a safe and smooth discharge:

- Has your carer been given sufficient notice of your discharge date/time?
- Do you have, and are you wearing, suitable clothes for the journey home?
- Is a relative collecting you or is hospital transport required?
- Do you have house keys and money if travelling home alone?
- Will medication be ready on time? This is usually enough fot the next seven days. Has your medication changed since admission? Have changes been explained to you and your carer? Do you know whether some prescribed items are only to be taken in the short term?
- Have you and your carer received training to use new aids or equipment safely and effectively? Will they be there when you get home?
- Do you have a supply of continence products to take home as agreed, know when to expect the next delivery and how to order supplies?
- Is your GP and other community health staff aware of your discharge date and support you need from them? Has a discharge summary with details of any medication changes been forwarded to the practice?
- If returning to your care home, has the manager been informed of the date and likely time of your arrival? Are you to take a copy with you or will staff forward copies of your care plan and medication needs to them promptly?

Source: Age UK (2007). Reproduced with permission of Age UK.

Assessment and recording tools

The use of a discharge checklist or centralized discharge planning record that can be accessed by all hospital staff can aid the process and facilitate rapid transfer of information between teams (Lees 2013, Winfield and Burns 2016). The same checklist can be used for all patients whether they have simple or complex discharge needs, as it minimizes omissions or duplication in discharge actions and ensures a good record of the planning process. An example of a discharge checklist is given in Figure 3.6.

Post-procedural considerations

Every patient leaving hospital should receive a discharge summary that is completed by their clinical team, and a copy should be sent to their GP within 24 hours of the patient being discharged (NHS England 2018). This facilitates improved continuity of care as it is the primary mode of communication between the hospital care team and those who will be providing the aftercare once the patient is at home (Alper et al. 2017). The plan should include an update about the patient's clinical condition and treatment, information about medications and arrangements for follow-up care.

Complications

Delayed discharges

A discharge delay is when a patient remains in hospital beyond the date agreed by the multidisciplinary team and beyond the time when they are medically fit to be discharged. Occasionally the discharge process may not proceed as planned; a discharge may be delayed for a number of reasons and a system should be in place to record this. For every patient who is 'delayed', NHS trusts are required to report the delay to their commissioners. It is the responsibility of the health authorities, in collaboration with local authorities, to monitor and address any issues that result in delays in the transfer of patients from an acute bed to their home or a community bed, such as a care home bed or rehabilitation bed. Trusts closely monitor bed activity and reporting varies from weekly to daily in the winter months.

Discharge against medical advice

Patients may take their own discharge against medical advice and this should be documented accordingly using the hospital's appropriate form (Box 3.2). When patients are assessed as requiring care or equipment but decline these, this does not negate the nurse's duty to ensure a discharge is safe. A discussion should take place with the patient, and their carer if applicable, to assess how they intend to manage without the required care and/or equipment in place. It is crucial that the appropriate community services are made aware of assessed needs that are not being met through patient choice or lack of resources. It is critical that the community teams who will be supporting the patient when they return home are notified: where possible, this should be in writing, enclosing a copy of any form documenting discharge against medical advice.

The ROYAL MARSDEN

NHS Foundation Trust

Discharge checklist

Discharge Criteria		Yes	No	N/A	Comments
1.	**Cognitive and Perceptual Status**				
	Patient is alert and orientated/within patient's 'normal status'	Yes	No		
	Patient/carer demonstrates understanding of treatment and care needs and their concerns have been discussed	Yes	No		
	Patient/carer is aware of warning signs and when to contact hospital	Yes	No		
2.	**Pain**				
	Patient reports pain free/pain is controlled at an acceptable level	Yes	No		
3.	**Respiratory status**				
	O_2 sats above 95% on air; respiratory rate between 12–20 bpm or within patient's normal range if pre-existing respiratory disease	Yes	No		
4.	**Cardiovascular status**				
	Pulse within patient's normal range (rate/rhythm/volume)	Yes	No		
	Blood pressure within patient's normal range	Yes	No		
5.	**Mobility/Activities of Daily Living**				
	Patient's usual level of independence attained or suitable for discharge	Yes	No		
6.	**Elimination**				
	Patient is voiding urine without difficulty and within expected pattern and urine output satisfactory	Yes	No		
	Patient's bowel movements are within patient's expected pattern	Yes	No		
7.	**Nutrition**				
	Patient is eating and drinking	Yes	No	N/A	
	Nutritional supplements supplied and explained to patient	Yes	No	N/A	
	Enteral feeding tube e.g. PEG in situ with no signs of complications	Yes	No	N/A	
8.	**Nausea and Vomiting**				
	Patient reports no nausea or vomiting, or controlled to acceptable level	Yes	No		
9.	**Wound and/or Potential Infection**				
	Temperature between 36.0°C and 37.5°C	Yes	No		
	Surgical wound(s): signs of wound infection absent (no erythema, swelling or discharge)	Yes	No	N/A	
	Surgical wound(s): Patient is aware of type of sutures/clips and arrangements for removal if required	Yes	No	N/A	
	Patient aware of arrangements for wound care/dressing and has been given any dressing required	Yes	No	N/A	

Figure 3.6 Example of a discharge checklist.

(continued)

10.	**Clinically Fit for discharge**				
	Clinical discharge parameters met OR Patient deemed medically fit by clinical team	Yes	No		
	Patient's side effects/complications are managed and the patient's condition is stable for discharge	Yes	No		
	CVADs patent with no signs of complications and/or peripheral cannula removed	Yes	No	N/A	
11.	**Medication**				
	TTOs (including nutritional supps./dressings/CDs and fridge items) given to patient with prescription sheet signed by nurse and patient with copy for GP	Yes	No	N/A	
	Patient/carer demonstrates understanding of purpose of medications and how to administer	Yes	No	N/A	
	If required, patient has medicine administration card to facilitate self-medication at home	Yes	No	N/A	
	Patient has equipment for injections e.g. sharps box if required	Yes	No	N/A	
	Patient has been returned their own medication (including CDs)	Yes	No	N/A	
12.	**Property and Equipment**				
	All required equipment in place/arranged for discharge and patient/carer aware e.g. home oxygen, appliances, nebulisers	Yes	No	N/A	
	Patient has had their property and valuables returned	Yes	No	N/A	
13.	**Information Provision**				
	Patient has been given Discharge summary	Yes	No		
	Patient has been given written information regarding their condition, treatment and/or equipment	Yes	No	N/A	
	Patient knows contact details of Key Worker/RMMH/Ward	Yes	No		
14.	**Follow up and community support**				
	Patient has date and time of next appointment or treatment booked	Yes	No	N/A	
	Referrals made and activated for appropriate community support (e.g. social services, district nurse) if required	Yes	No	N/A	
	Letters/information as required for GP, district nurse, practice nurse given to patient	Yes	No	N/A	
15.	**Transport**				
	Suitable transport agreed and arranged	Yes	No		
16.	**Specific discharge requirements**				
	Specific checklists completed if required e.g. for palliative care patient				

Additional comments

Date:	Signature:	Print name:	Designation:

Figure 3.6 *Continued*

Box 3.2 Example of a form documenting discharge against medical advice

> Name:
>
> Hospital No:
>
> Address:
>
> I wish to discharge myself against medical advice and accept full responsibility for my actions.
>
> Signed:
>
> Date:
>
> Time:
>
> **Statement to be signed by the Doctor**
>
> I have discussed with the patient the medical reasons why he/she should remain in the hospital.
>
> Signed:
>
> **This form should be filed with the patient's medical records**

Readmission following discharge

Premature discharge or discharging the patient to an environment that does not meet their needs may result in them being readmitted to hospital (Alper et al. 2017). Evidence demonstrates that tailored discharge planning can reduce readmission rates and length of stay but that a significant proportion of patients return to hospital within a month due to complications of unplanned care (Teodorczuk 2016). Readmissions are costly and put patients at a higher risk of acquiring infections, of medication errors and of deconditioning, and their impact is therefore negative for both patients' quality of life and the healthcare system (Sheridan et al. 2017). Addressing readmissions by ensuring patients have well-planned and co-ordinated discharge is therefore essential.

The elderly are particularly at risk of readmission following discharge (Lees-Deutsch 2016). Research commissioned by the Royal Voluntary Service (2014) estimated that people aged 75 and older are more than twice as likely as those younger to be readmitted to hospital, if they are not given enough support on discharge. This is particularly true for those who live alone or have long-term healthcare needs. Patients with dementia similarly have higher readmission rates possibly due to the fact that they are less likely to benefit from discharge education, self-care instructions or to report symptoms (Teodorczuk 2016). NICE (2015) guidelines consider referral back to relevant community-based care practitioners and a call or visit from a community-based nurse or GP within 72 hours of discharge to mitigate the possibility of readmission for those at high risk. It is essential that nurses understand the negative impact of readmission in order to ensure timely and safe discharge with maximum continuity of care.

Interface between primary and secondary care: external processes

Related theory

NHS Continuing Healthcare

When a patient with complex and ongoing health or social care needs is ready to be safely discharged from acute care, it is very important that this should happen in a timely manner. It is therefore helpful for nurses to have an understanding of the processes involved in determining the funding for healthcare services and the options available for patients once they have been discharged back into the community.

NHS Continuing Healthcare funding exists to provide a package of ongoing care that is arranged and funded solely by the NHS. It should be awarded only when an individual has been assessed as having a primary health need and it is provided to support the care that people need over an extended period of time as a result of disability, accident or illness, to address both physical and mental health needs (DH 2018). The National Framework for NHS Continuing Healthcare and NHS-Funded Nursing Care (DH 2018) provides guidance and structure on the principles and processes of funding. To be eligible, patients must be assessed by a multidisciplinary team to determine the complexity and intensity of their need and the help they require.

The assessment process for NHS Continuing Healthcare should not be allowed to delay hospital discharge (DH 2018) but it is essential for patients' holistic needs to be placed at the heart of the assessment process as they are frequently facing significant changes in their life and a positive experience of the assessment process is therefore crucial. There is also a legal obligation to inform patients of their right to be assessed for NHS Continuing Healthcare funding, and this can best be done by referring them to an online resource booklet on the Department of Health and Social Care's website (https://www.gov.uk/government/organisations/department-of-health-and-social-care).

Intermediate care and re-ablement services

It is recognized that older inpatients have longer lengths of stay despite proactive discharge planning due to their complex needs (Mabire et al. 2018). This increases the risk of adverse events following their discharge, and initiatives to aid the transition period from hospital to home are therefore important elements in discharge preparation. Following a hospital stay, intermediate-care teams may provide a period of intensive care and/or rehabilitation, which may take place in a care home or in the individual's own home. Intermediate care aims to prevent hospital admissions, support faster recovery from illness or injury, support timely discharge from hospital, and maximize independent living (NICE 2017). Unlike NHS Continuing Healthcare, it is likely to be limited to a maximum of 6 weeks but there are local variations in practice. Intermediate care requires a person-centred approach, involving patients and carers in all aspects of assessment, goal setting and discharge planning.

Re-ablement is a similar service that aims to help people regain their independence following an illness or injury. It is a community-based service that provides assessment and interventions to people in a residential setting such as a care home or a rehabilitation unit. The aim is to optimize individuals' wellbeing by working in partnership with them to enable confidence and independence in activities of daily living and other practical tasks (NICE 2017). Services are delivered by a multidisciplinary team but most commonly by healthcare professionals or care staff if the service is within a care home.

Re-ablement teams are usually made up of the following disciplines:

- social workers
- occupational therapists
- physiotherapists
- rehabilitation support workers
- community nurses.

For patients requiring a long-term package of care, it must be made clear to the patient and/or their family that they will be financially assessed and as a result may be charged for the service. In some local authorities, if the patient is assessed as 'self-funding', social services may only then offer a signposting service to private care providers.

Evidence-based approaches

If a patient does not meet the criteria for NHS Continuing Healthcare, they may still receive assistance with personal care and domestic tasks through social services. This can be through a re-ablement service or a long-term package of care. Where a patient is assessed as requiring care from social services to enable them to return home, the trust should notify the local authority using the Assessment Notification to Social Services from Hospital form and the Discharge Notification form (these forms will be available from the discharge team or social services).

Assessment and recording tools

The local authority will require an Assessment Notification (formerly known as Section 2) no later than 72 hours prior to discharge, but this should be done at the earliest opportunity (see Figure 3.7 for an example). (Again, contact the discharge team or social services for this form.)

The ROYAL MARSDEN
NHS Foundation Trust

ASSESSMENT NOTICE TO LOCAL AUTHORITY

To be completed no later than 2 days before discharge

It is best practice to send this assessment notice as soon as social care requirement is identified

(As required under the Care Act 2014, schedule 3, para (1) (1))

NHS No:		**Hospital No:**			
Part A: Patient Details					
Title:	Given Name: Family Name:	Preferred Name:	DOB:	Sex:	
Address:	House Name/No.: Address Line 1: Address Line 2: City/Town: Postcode: Local Authority:	Patient Email: Patient Land Line No: Patient Mobile No: Other Nos:			
Does the patient live alone?		If No, who do they live with?		Dependants:	
Immigration Status:		Ethnicity:			
Religion:		Other:		First Language: (if not English)	Interpreter needed?

Part B: Carer or Key Contact Details (*may be next of kin, carer, family member, friend, etc - as appropriate*)					
Name:		Tel/Mob:		Relationship to Patient:	
Who is the main carer for the patient?			If other, please specify:		
Part C: General Practitioner Details					
GP Name:		Practice Name:			
GP Address:		Tel:			
Part D: Hospital Details and Patient's Proposed Discharge Date					
Anticipated Discharge Date:		Date of Admission:			
Hospital:	The Royal Marsden Chelsea site Sutton site	Ward Name:		Ward Tel No:	
Lead Clinician		Reason for Admission:		Planned Admission?	

Part E: Patient Consent for Referral/Information Sharing	
What is patient's capacity to give consent to this referral?	
Additional information regarding capacity to consent:	
Has patient consented to this referral?	
Additional Information regarding consent:	
Can Carer or Key Contact be contacted for discussion regarding the patient?	
Part F: Referral Information	
Have you considered whether or not to provide NHS Continuing Health Care (CHC), if so, what was the result of your consideration?	
Reason for referral:	
Accommodation:	
Relevant Medical Information:	
Details of existing support:	
Has the occupational therapy report been completed?	
Part G: Patient's View (*e.g. What support do you think you will need when you leave hospital?*)	
Part H: Carer or Key Contact's View (*e.g. What support do they think the patient/carer will need when they leave hospital?*)	
Part I : Risk Factors	
Are there any safety issues for workers visiting on the ward or at home?	
If yes what are they?	

Part J: Referrer					
Referrer's name:		Job Role:		Fax:	
Date & Time:		Email:		Tel:	

Figure 3.7 Example of a Social Services Assessment Notification form.

How the local authority responds to the Assessment Notification may depend on what local arrangements are in place. Many local authorities have a social worker or social work department within the hospital trust, and this person or team is usually part of the discharge team. Their role is to facilitate the setting up of care packages for discharge. Other authorities may require additional assessments, such as occupational therapy or medical reports, to enable them to set up the care. It is not uncommon for local authorities to request an NHS Continuing Healthcare checklist to be completed as part of the process to assess whether the patient might be entitled to NHS Continuing Healthcare funding.

When the patient has been assessed and is ready for discharge, a Discharge Notification (formerly known as a Section 5) should be sent to the local authority at least 24 hours before the patient leaves hospital (see Figure 3.8 for an example). Nurses need to be aware of the importance of the timeliness of completing this social services documentation and facilitate this being done as soon as possible to avoid discharge delays.

Complications

If the patient becomes unwell or their care needs change significantly prior to discharge, it is the responsibility of the discharge co-ordinator to inform the local authority to put on hold any arranged social services by sending a Withdrawal Notification form (again, contact the discharge team or social services for this form). Once a revised discharge date is confirmed, a new Assessment and Discharge Notification form must be sent to re-establish the services to prevent discharge delay. If a patient is already in receipt of an existing care package and it needs to be re-started without any changes on discharge, Social Services must be informed at least 24 hours prior to discharge to facilitate restarting the existing care package.

The ROYAL MARSDEN
NHS Foundation Trust

DISCHARGE NOTICE TO LOCAL AUTHORITY

To be issued to Social Care at least one day in advance of the confirmed hospital discharge date
It is best practice to send this discharge notice as soon as the discharge date has been agreed

(As required under the Care Act 2014 schedule 3, para 2 (1) (b))

Confirmation of Discharge Date (as agreed by MDT)					
Has Patient been informed of discharge date?			If no, please explain why?		
Has Carer/Key Contact been informed of discharge date?			If no, please explain why?		
NHS No:			**Hospital No:**		
Part A: Patient Details					
Title:	Given Name:	Family Name:	Preferred Name:	DOD:	Sex.
Address:	House Name/No.: Address Line 1: Address Line 2: City/Town: Postcode: London Local Authority:				
Part B: Confirmation of Referring Hospital/Ward Details					
Hospital:	The Royal Marsden	Chelsea Site	Ward Name:		Ward Tel:
Lead Clinician:			Admitted on:		
Diagnosis on Discharge:					
Part C: Confirmation of Health and/ or Social Care Requested for Discharge					
The following health and/or Social Care required will be available on the expected date of discharge:					
Equipment to be provided at home:					
Part D: Notice Status					
Assessment Notice sent to Social Care with admission details confirmed?					
Social Care assessment completed?					
Date Discharge Notice completed					
Has the occupational therapy report been sent to Social Care?					
Part E: Patient Consent for Information Sharing/Referral					
What is patient's capacity to give consent to this referral?					
Additional information regarding capacity to consent:					
Has patient consented to this referral?					
Additional Information regarding consent:					
Can Carer or Key Contact be contacted for discussion regarding the patient?					
Part F: Referrer					
Referrer's name:		Job Role:		Fax:	
Date & Time:		Email:		Tel:	

Figure 3.8 Example of a Social Services Discharge Notification form.

Complex discharges

Definition

For patients requiring specific support on discharge, proactive and systematic planning is essential (Winfield and Burns 2016). A complex discharge may be considered when:

- a large package of care involving various agencies is required
- the patient's needs have changed since admission, with different services requiring co-ordination
- the family and/or carer require intensive input into discharge planning considerations (e.g. psychological interventions)
- the patient is entitled to NHS Continuing Healthcare and requires a package of care on discharge
- the patient requires repatriation
- there is dispute among the family about where the patient should be discharged to or what their care needs are
- the patient is homeless.

Related theory

Patients who have specific social or specialized care needs, who have funding issues or who require a change of residence may have a complex discharge need (Lees-Deutsch et al. 2016) and may require referral to the hospital's discharge team. Hospital trusts may have different titles for staff within the discharge team, but essentially their role is to co-ordinate plans among all involved by liaising with the multidisciplinary team both within the hospital and in the community. In this way they act as 'knowledge brokers' to facilitate sharing and co-ordination (Waring et al. 2014).

If a patient has dementia or a learning disability, the approach to their discharge needs to be carefully planned and tailored to meet their specific additional needs (Poole et al. 2014). If, for example, the patient has been assessed as lacking capacity to make a decision under the Mental Capacity Act (2005) about where they should live, then a 'best interest' decision must be made, ensuring that family and carers are involved. Where the patient is assessed as lacking capacity and has no relatives or friends and so is 'unbefriended' (as defined by the Mental Capacity Act 2005), a referral should be made to a local independent mental capacity advocacy service to ensure the patient gets the required support (Mental Capacity Act 2005). Where there is a concern that a person has a degree of cognitive impairment, it can easily be assumed that they cannot return home or that they need care. These assumptions should be challenged and decisions made on the basis of a needs assessment, which should include a mental capacity assessment. The assessment should evidence that the principles of the Mental Capacity Act (2005) have been applied and that any decisions have been made in the person's best interests. For more detailed information on the principles of capacity and safeguarding, see Chapter 5: Communication, psychological wellbeing and safeguarding.

Evidence-based approaches

NICE (2015) recommend several key principles of care and support that should be considered for more complex patients during the transition from a healthcare facility to home:

- *Person-centred care*: see everyone as an individual, involve families and carers, and identify those at risk.
- *Communication and information sharing*: provide appropriate information in the right format at the right time and ensure discussions take place with all involved.
- *Discharge co-ordinator*: a dedicated individual who works with the multidisciplinary team and involves carers and families in discussions about the care being proposed.
- *Develop a discharge plan*: this should include details about the person's condition, medicines and practicalities of daily living, and should detail which services and sources of support are involved.
- *Plan for care following discharge*: ensure follow-up arrangements are made and communicated effectively.
- *Readmission risk*: ensure those at risk of readmission are referred to appropriate community-based health and social care teams prior to discharge.

For patients who may have additional needs on discharge, it is worth exploring what support services may be available and identifying what services were in place prior to admission. For example, if the person has a learning disability, they may have a learning disability nurse in the community. If so, involving the nurse in the patient's discharge will ensure a safer transition for the patient by enabling access to a professional who has knowledge and expertise in the field of learning disabilities but also in the needs of the patient.

Principles of care

A comprehensive assessment is initially required to ascertain a patient's discharge needs. Joined-up inter-professional care and good carer partnerships can then be established to facilitate safe and seamless transfer of care of the patient from the hospital back to the community (Teodorczuk et al. 2015) (Table 3.1).

Discharge to a nursing home

Related theory

Despite the ageing population and pressure on acute hospital beds, care home admission from hospital is a transition pathway that is poorly understood and little researched (Harrison et al. 2017). Discharging a patient to a care or nursing home requires careful thought as the decision to move into a care home is complex and often difficult and traumatic for individuals and their families (Lord et al. 2016). The impact on a patient and their family or carer may be significant, particularly where the person lives with a partner or family member and the move would be a loss for both of them. A thorough multidisciplinary assessment is essential, taking into account the individual needs of the patient and their family or carer and exploring all the options before deciding on a care or nursing home. Harrison et al. (2017) suggest that it is important in aiding the process to ensure that significant discussions are documented, to include opportunistic conversations that nurses and others have with patients and their families. This ensures decisions and actions are recorded and it also facilitates better continuity of care.

In most cases, the family or carer will look for a care home placement. This can be quite a daunting process and it is worth providing a list of questions and things to look for when assessing a care or nursing home (Table 3.2). Additionally, the local clinical commissioning group will be able to provide the family with a list of registered nursing homes for them to view.

Complications

Nursing and care home placements can be delayed while waiting for funding to be approved or waiting for a suitable bed to become available and it may therefore be necessary to consider an interim placement. It is important that the patient and their carers are aware that there may be time limits on the stay in hospital so they will be required to find a suitable placement within an agreed timescale. Many hospitals have a policy to support staff where patients and their carers are delaying the process of arranging a nursing home placement.

Discharge planning at the end of life

Evidence-based approaches

The National Palliative and End of Life Care Partnership (2015) has set out a framework for end-of-life and palliative care based on key ambitions for the dying person which also relate to carers, families and those important to them. This extends to all aspects of care, including care planning, and is very important when a patient is being discharged for end-of-life care. The condition of a person nearing the end of life may change rapidly, so it is essential that choices are made, decisions are reached and community services are accessed without delay to ensure a timely and smooth transition of care from hospital to home or hospice. Discharging a

Table 3.1 Procedure for the assessment process for complex discharges

1 Nurse conducts a comprehensive assessment on admission	
(a) Identify whether the patient has simple or complex needs.	
(b) Refer to relevant members of the hospital multidisciplinary team.	For example, occupational therapist, physiotherapist, social services or discharge co-ordinator
(c) Liaise with current community services to ascertain current support (if any).	For example, district nurse or community palliative care team.
2 Multidisciplinary team discuss the case at the ward multidisciplinary meeting	
(a) Appoint a discharge co-ordinator.	• To act as discharge planning lead for all social services and NHS Continuing Healthcare referrals. • To act as a point of contact for discharge concerns. • To plan and prepare the family meeting or case conference and to arrange a chairperson and minute-taker for the meeting. • To meet the patient, their carers and their family. • To work in conjunction with multidisciplinary team. • To liaise with the patient's named nurse.
(b) Formulate a discharge plan.	• Formulate a discharge plan based on the patient's assessed needs. • Agree assessments required by the multidisciplinary team. • Agree home visits required (e.g. occupational therapist home visit and functional report).
(c) Set a provisional discharge date.	• Agree a provisional discharge date and time frames. This will only be an approximate date, depending on care needs, equipment, etc. It should be reviewed regularly with the multidisciplinary team. • Discharges should not be arranged for a Friday or a weekend, when skeleton social and care services are in place.
3 Discharge co-ordinator arranges family meeting or case conference	
(a) Invite the patient, their family, their carers and all appropriate healthcare professionals, including community staff where possible.	• Discuss the patient's needs and the services and equipment required, and agree preferred and appropriate place of discharge. • If the patient is not returning to their own neighbourhood, a GP will be required to take the patient on as a temporary resident so this must be arranged. • Agree all relevant Social Services and NHS Continuing Healthcare referrals required. • Discuss any specific and special issues (e.g. infection status, IV therapy, need for syringe driver) to establish an appropriate plan. Notify community services.
4 Ward staff or discharge team make referrals to appropriate community services	
• Refer to community health services.	To include district nurses, community palliative care team, community physiotherapists etc. • Ascertain whether the district nurse is able to undertake any necessary clinical procedures in accordance with their local trust policy (e.g. on care of skin-tunnelled catheters) and make alternative arrangements if not. • Arrange for night sitters via the district nurse if required.
• Refer to Social Services.	The Social Services Assessment Notification (see Figure 3.7 for an example) must be sent at the earliest opportunity and no later than 72 hours prior to discharge.
• Request equipment from community nurse after discussion with patient and family.	For example, hoist, hospital bed, pressure-relieving mattress or cushion, commode or nebulizer. Additionally: • Ascertain the type of accommodation the patient lives in so that the equipment ordered will fit appropriately. • It is important to specify where the patient will be cared for – for example, ground or first floor.
• Request home oxygen if required.	Medical team to complete Home Oxygen Ordering Form (HOOF) and Initial Home Oxygen Risk Mitigation Form (IHORM) for oxygen cylinders and concentrators at home. Fax or email to relevant oxygen supplier.
5 Ward staff or discharge team confirms the discharge date and finalizes the community arrangements	
(a) Confirm *provisional* discharge date.	The provisional date is agreed with the patient and their family and/or informal carer(s). The actual date will then depend on when the following community services can be arranged: • social services package of care • district nurse • re-ablement service • nursing home or residential home placement • hospice bed • rapid response • equipment and home oxygen.

(continued)

Table 3.1 Procedure for the assessment process for complex discharges *(continued)*

(b) Confirm equipment agreed and delivery date.	Ensure the family is informed of the delivery date and knows to contact the ward to confirm receipt of the equipment in the patient's home.
(c) Confirm start date for care and fax or email details.	For example, Social Services, community nurse or community palliative care. • Community care referral forms need to be faxed or emailed to district nurses at least 48 hours prior to discharge. • The Social Services Discharge Notification (see Figure 3.8 for an example) must be sent at least 48 hours prior to discharge. • In some situations, family members are able to bridge the gap before a package of care starts to enable the patient to be discharged sooner. This action should be talked through with the patient and the family to ensure they are able to provide the care needed and that they will not be putting themselves or the patient at risk. • Confirm the agreed discharge date with the patient and their family.
6 Ward staff or discharge team co-ordinates the hospital discharge processes	
(a) Arrange transport and assess need for escort and/or oxygen during transport.	• Assess specific needs for transport – i.e. specify whether the patient needs a walker, chair or stretcher, and/or oxygen or an escort. • Arrange for a do not resuscitate (DNR) form if required for ambulance crew.
(b) Arrange discharge medication.	• Determine whether the patient will self-medicate and requires a self-medication chart or dosette box. • Confirm the name of the person who will provide the prompt or give the medication to the patient at home. • Ensure take-home medication is prescribed and given to the patient or carer with explanations. • Ensure nutrition supplements, dressings and medical appliances are prescribed, ordered and given to the patient or carer with explanations. • If the patient has hospital equipment (e.g. a syringe driver) ensure it is clearly marked for return to the hospital with written instructions for the patient, carer or district nurse.
(c) Make arrangements for suitable access and provision for patient on arrival home.	• Check access issues (e.g. front door keys and steps) and ensure heating has been organized and food will be provided.
(d) Ensure patient has follow-up arrangements made.	• Next inpatient or outpatient appointment.
7 Confirm arrangements 24 hours prior to discharge	
(a) Telephone community services and confirm any special needs of the patient.	For example, infection status update or confirmation of hospital equipment required by patient.
8 After discharge, ward nurse or discharge co-ordinator makes a follow-up phone call to the patient (as agreed)	

patient at the end of life is often complex and multifactorial and requires a multidisciplinary team approach allowing flexibility and responsiveness to the situation. Figure 3.9 shows an example of a checklist that can be used to help structure the process.

Pre-procedural considerations

It is important in the first instance to contact relevant community teams to highlight the need for a rapid response to any referrals being made. Community nursing, the community palliative care team and, where appropriate, the community matron should be notified at the earliest opportunity. A fast-track NHS Continuing Healthcare funding application may need to be submitted to access funding for care provision. This process is used to gain immediate access to funding to allow healthcare professionals to arrange urgent care packages, enabling patients to be cared for and to die in their preferred place, whether it is at home, in a nursing home or in a hospice (Thomas 2017).

Equipment

The patient may also require essential equipment to enable them to return home, such as a profiling bed, commode or hoist. These can often be accessed via the local community nursing team and should be ordered at the first available opportunity. Thomas (2017) found that 25% of discharges were delayed due to problems with the delivery of equipment to patients' homes. Once care and equipment are in place and discharge is proceeding, a medical review should take place and a discharge summary should be written with a copy provided to the patient, their GP, community nurses and the community palliative care team. Telephone contact with all of the above is essential to ensure they are in receipt of all the information they require to take over the care of the patient in the community and to make sure that home visits are requested.

Assessment and recording tools

The introduction of Electronic Palliative Care Co-ordination Systems (EPaCCS) has enabled the recording and sharing of people's care preferences and key details about their care at the end of life. Coordinate My Care (which currently only relates to patients within the London area) allows healthcare professionals to record patients' wishes within an electronic personalized urgent care plan that can be seen by GPs, community teams, emergency and ambulance services; the plan can then guide the care they provide (https://www.coordinatemycare.co.uk). These care plans are accessed repeatedly by the out-of-hours and emergency services, which helps to reduce the number of inappropriate hospital admissions in the last year of life. It is hoped that this type of service will be available nationally in the near future.

Informal carers

Definition

An informal carer can be defined as someone who helps another person, usually a relative or friend, in their day to day life. This is not the same as someone who provides care professionally or through a voluntary organization (NICE 2016).

Table 3.2 Questions and things to look for when assessing a care or nursing home

	Questions
First impressions	• Is the home easy for family and friends to visit, particularly those who have to rely on public transport? • Does the home have its own transport? • Is the main area accessible for people with disabilities, e.g. those with wheelchairs or who are poor sighted or hard of hearing? • Do the staff answer the door promptly? • Do the staff appear friendly and welcoming? • Do there appear to be several members of staff on duty? • Do the residents look well cared for and clean? • Is there an up-to-date registration certificate on display? Note: it is usual to sign a visitors' book on arrival.
The accommodation	• Are the home and the rooms clean and fresh? • Are the rooms single or shared? • Do the rooms have ensuite facilities? • Can you bring your own furniture and personal belongings? • Where are the nearest toilets and are they accessible? • Is there a telephone in the room and/or mobile phone reception? • Is there a Wi-Fi connection? And is there a fee for this? • Are there quiet areas to sit in? • What are the mealtimes? • Is there a choice of meals and diets? • Is there a laundry service on site?
Personal needs	• How often do the hairdresser, dentist, chiropodist, religious support and GP visit? • Does a resident change GP if they move from the local area? • Where are medications stored? • Are there newspapers easily available? • What activities are available to facilitate continuation of hobbies? • Does the home arrange outings? • Are there quiet areas for family and friends to visit? • Can they stay for meals? • Is there an overnight room where they can stay?
Finances and contracts	• What are the fees? • What services do the fees include, e.g. chiropody, hairdresser? • What are the terms and conditions? • Is there a reduction if the patient is admitted to hospital or goes on holiday? • What is the notice period or procedure for terminating a contract? • When is the room available from?
Nursing needs	• How many qualified nursing staff are on duty day and night (in a nursing home)? • How often do qualified nursing staff review a resident (in a nursing home)? • How often does the community nursing team visit and review residents (in a care home)? • What is the daily care routine? • If the patient has very specific nursing needs, how will they be managed? Refer to the list given by the ward staff on the patient's specific healthcare needs. • How often does the community palliative care team visit? • How often is the GP or doctor in the home? • Although a difficult thing to consider, is the home able to support patients to remain in the home for end-of-life care?

Related theory

It is important to recognize that patients do not usually manage their condition in isolation but in the context of their daily lives with people who provide their support network at home, such as family, friends, colleagues and neighbours (Wallace et al. 2017). Engaging and involving both patients and those who support them in an unpaid capacity as equal partners is central to successful discharge planning, and this is clearly recognized in the NICE (2015) guideline on discharge from hospital to the community for adults with identified social care needs.

The hospital discharge process can be a critical time for informal carers, placing an increasing burden of care on them, particularly if they do not feel involved in the discharge process (Harrison et al. 2016). It may be the first time they have been confronted with the reality of their role and the effect it may have on their relationship with the person needing care, their family and their employment. The emotional toll on carers may result in early readmission of the patient and it is therefore vital to involve carers as partners in the discharge planning process.

Carers may have different needs from patients and there may be conflicting opinions about how the patient's care needs can be met. It is not uncommon for patients to report that their informal carer is willing to provide all care whereas the carer is not in agreement with this. Healthcare professionals should allow carers sufficient time and provide appropriate information to enable them to make decisions to promote a successful and seamless transfer from hospital to home (Cacchione 2018). If carers are involved as equal partners throughout the process, they can provide valuable information about the person's needs and circumstances beyond medical conditions or physical needs. This means discharge planning can be more comprehensive and may reduce the likelihood of the person being readmitted to hospital (NICE 2016).

Evidence-based approaches

Under the Care Act (2014), carers are entitled to their own assessment and many support services can be provided, including respite, at no charge. The Act represents the most significant reform of care in many years by putting people and their carers in control

The ROYAL MARSDEN
NHS Foundation Trust

Name: **Hospital No:**

**Patients Being Discharged Home for Complex/urgent Palliative Care-
Checklist for Discharge**

This form should be used to assist with planning an urgent/complex discharge home for a patient with terminal care needs. It should be used in conjunction with the Discharge Policy.

Sign and date to confirm when arranged and equipment given. Document relevant information in the discharge planning section of the nursing documentation. Document if item or care is not applicable.

Appoint a designated discharge lead:

Name: .... Designation: ....Contact No:..........

	Date & Time	Signature & print name
Patient / Family Issues		
Meeting with patient/family to discuss plans for discharge		
Continuing Healthcare funding discussed and information leaflet given.		
Level of care required has been discussed and agreed.		
Role of community services (district nurses and community palliative care team) has been discussed and consent obtained for referral if needed.		
Consent obtained if in area & Coordinate My Care record created or updated. Upload DNaCPR form onto CMC record if this has been discussed with patient & there is a DNaCPR form on EPR.		
Continuing Healthcare application/Fast Track form commenced by Discharge Team & completed by MDT. Fast Track form can be found on the intranet under Discharge support/NHS continuing healthcare & can be accessed on T-drive under each ward/Dept. Contact Discharge team when complete for form to be sent to relevant CCG.		
Communication with District Nurse		
Referral made to District Nurses using the Community Services Referral Form.		
Equipment has been requested (delete as appropriate): - Electric, profiling hospital bed - Pressure relieving mattress - Pressure relieving seat cushion - Commode/urinal/bed pan - Hoist/sling/sliding sheets - Other		
Communication with Community Palliative Care Team		
Referral made to Community Palliative Care Team		
Communication with GP and Community Palliative Care Medical Team-Medical Responsibilities (Hospital medical team to organise -the nurse to confirm when arranged)		
Registrar to discuss patient's condition with GP and request home visit for as soon as possible after discharge.		
Oxygen: HOOF & IHORM (Consent) forms to be completed by the medical team & faxed to relevant company. Please access website below for a list of the oxygen companies & their geographical area. https://www.pcc-cic.org.uk/article/home-oxygen -order-form		
Registrar or Specialist Nurse to discuss with the Community Palliative Care team the patient's needs and proposed plan of care.		

Figure 3.9 Checklist for patients being discharged home for urgent palliative care.

The ROYAL MARSDEN
NHS Foundation Trust

	Date & Time	Signature & print name
Adequate supply of drugs prescribed for discharge (TTOs) including crisis drugs e.g. s/c morphine, midazolam.		
Authorisation for drugs to be administered by community nurses. Please refer to Subcutaneous Drugs policy and complete the discharge checklist for the McKinley T34 syringe pump.		
'Ambulance transfer of palliative care patients' document completed for Ambulance Crew.		

Equipment-		
Has confirmation been received from a family member or the community equipment service provider that the equipment has been delivered to the discharge address?		
Provide an adequate supply of:		
- dressings		
- water/sodium chloride for injection (if going home with end of life care medications for subcutaneous use)		
- sharps bin		
- continence aids		
- supply of needles and syringes		
Transport (confirm by ticking appropriate boxes)	**CHECK OTHER DISCHARGE DOCUMENTATION**	
Escort (family/nurse) Discussed with family that if the patient dies during the journey, the ambulance crew will not attempt resuscitation. Discharge destination in this event has been agreed. DNaCPR form provided?		
Written Information and Documentation		
A discharge summary will need to be completed prior to discharge. The discharge letter must be printed & given to a pharmacist to check the medication list is complete & accurate. Medical summary given to patient or relative.		
Medical discharge summary sent to GP, Community Palliative Care Team and District Nursing Team.		
Prescription sheet of authorisation for drugs to be administered by community nurses. Faxed to District Nurse, GP and Community Palliative Care Team.		
Copies of HOOF & IHORM faxed to GP for information only.		
Patient/carer given list of contact numbers of community services **(including night service)-Discharge information sheet.**		
Medication list, stating reasons for drugs, given and explained to patient/ relative.		
All documentation sent to community services is scanned onto EPR and filed in patient's medical records.		

Signature/print name of designated ward based discharge lead: ....

Date/Time..

File this form in the patient's records on discharge.

Figure 3.9 *Continued*

Box 3.3 Examples of services provided by the voluntary sector in the community

- Personal care – e.g. bathing and dressing
- Practical help at home e.g. gardening and cleaning
- Daily help – e.g. cooking a meal or shopping
- Independent living services – these provide functional support, e.g. transport to enable people to attend hospital appointments, and mobility aids such as wheelchairs
- Short-term support-at-home services – these provide a range of short-term support once a patient has been discharged from hospital to help them regain their confidence, e.g. collecting prescriptions and shopping

of their own support (People First 2018). The aim is to ensure that people and their carers are supported in a practical way by providing information, financial and other support, helping carers to remain at work and to care for themselves. It is particularly important that carers who will be taking on the role for the first time when their family member leaves hospital are made aware of the benefits and support available to them from their local authority, since 'deciding to care or continue caring for someone who is coming out of hospital … can be very difficult' (Carers UK 2018, p.1). Often the first step in raising their awareness might be as simple as letting them know that the role they play with their family member is that of a carer: many people would see themselves as a spouse, child or grandchild rather than a carer.

In addition to understanding that adult carers may be unaware of the support available, it is important to recognize that in some families children take on a caring role, and their needs may go unrecognized. Young carers may struggle with the responsibilities of providing care to parents, and without appropriate support they may feel isolated and distressed (Carers UK 2018). Support for young carers has increased under the Children and Families Act (2014), which aims to ensure that all children and young people are able to access the right support and provision to meet their needs. When a patient is discharged, provided consent is gained from the parents, it is important to inform community health and social care providers that young carers are involved. This will enable young carers to access additional support services so they can continue in their vital role.

The role of voluntary services

Related theory

In many areas, voluntary sector providers have begun to forge ways to deliver efficient, high-quality, patient-centred care. Partnerships between the NHS and the voluntary sector help to facilitate a smooth transition from hospital to the community by providing ongoing support for patients in their own homes (Rivers 2015). When planning discharge for a patient who is elderly or has special needs, it is worth exploring what voluntary services are available locally that could provide support to enable timely discharge and help to prevent a hospital readmission. Examples of services provided by the voluntary sector are shown in Box 3.3, but it is important to consider what is available locally. The provision of practical help, either with personal care or with functional tasks around the home, can give the patient confidence that they will be able to cope and can provide ongoing emotional support once the patient is at home.

References

Age UK (2007) *Factsheet 37: Hospital Discharge.* Available at: https://www.ageuk.org.uk/globalassets/age-uk/documents/factsheets/fs37_hospital_discharge_fcs.pdf

Alper, E., O'Malley, T. & Greenwald, J. (2017) *Hospital Discharge and Readmission.* UpToDate. Available at: https://www.uptodate.com/contents/hospital-discharge-and-readmission

Arora, A. (2017) Time to move: Get up, get dressed, keep moving. *NHS England*, 24 January. Available at: https://www.england.nhs.uk/blog/amit-arora

British Geriatrics Society (2017) *Deconditioning Awareness.* Available at: https://www.bgs.org.uk/resources/deconditioning-awareness

Cacchione, P. (2018) Engaging caregivers during hospitalizations to improve hospital transitions: The CARE Act. *Clinical Nursing Research*, 27(3), 255–257.

Care Act (2014) Available at: www.legislation.gov.uk/ukpga/2014/23/contents/enacted

Carers UK (2018) *Coming Out of Hospital.* Available at: https://www.carersuk.org/images/Factsheets/Coming_out_of_hospital_-_England_April_2019.pdf

Challis, D., Hughes, J., Xie, C. & Jolley, D. (2014) An examination of factors influencing delayed discharge of older people from hospital. *International Journal of Psychiatry*, 29, 160–168.

Chenoweth, L., Kable, A. & Pond, D. (2015) Research in hospital discharge procedures addresses gaps in care continuity in the community, but leaves gaping holes for people with dementia: A review of the literature. *Australasian Journal on Ageing*, 34(1), 9–14.

Children and Families Act (2014) Available at: www.legislation.gov.uk/ukpga/2014/6/contents/enacted

Cundy, T., Sierakowski, K., Manna, A., et al. (2017) Fast-track surgery for uncomplicated appendicitis in children: A matched case control study. *ANZ Journal of Surgery*, 87(4), 271–276.

DH (Department of Health and Social Care) (2018) *National Framework for NHS Continuing Healthcare and NHS Funded Nursing Care.* Available at: https://www.gov.uk/government/publications/national-framework-for-nhs-continuing-healthcare-and-nhs-funded-nursing-care

Elliott, B. & DeAngelis, M. (2017) Improving patient transitions from hospital to home: Practical advice from nurses. *Nursing*, 47(11), 58–62.

Ewbank, L., Thompson, J. & McKenna, H. (2017) *NHS Hospital Bed Numbers: Past, Present and Future.* King's Fund. Available at: https://www.kingsfund.org.uk/publications/nhs-hospital-bed-numbers

Harrison, J.D., Greysen, R.S., Jacolbia, R., et al. (2016) Not ready, not set … discharge: Patient-reported barriers to discharge readiness at an academic medical center. *Journal of Hospital Medicine*, 11(9), 610–614.

Harrison, K., MacArthur, J., Garcia Garrido, A., et al. (2017) Decisions affecting discharge from hospitals directly to care homes. *Nursing Times*, 113(6), 29–32.

Healthwatch England (2015) *Safely Home: What Happens when People Leave Hospitals and Care Settings?* Available at: https://www.healthwatch.co.uk/report/2015-07-21/safely-home-what-happens-when-people-leave-hospital-and-care-settings

Lees, L. (2013) The key principles of effective discharge planning. *Nursing Times*, 109(3), 18–19.

Lees-Deutsch, L. (2016) A framework to discharge frail older people. *Nursing Times*, 112(37/38), 13–15.

Lees-Deutsch, L. (2017) *Principles for Discharge from Acute Medicine Units.* Society for Acute Medicine. Available at: https://www.acutemedicine.org.uk/wp-content/uploads/2010/06/Prinicples-for-dsicharge-from-ACute-Medicine-Units.pdf

Lees-Deutsch, L. & Gaillemin, O. (2018) Dispelling myths around nurse-led and criteria-led discharge. *Nursing Times*, 114(4). Available at: https://www.nursingtimes.net/clinical-archive/patient-safety/dispelling-myths-around-nurse-led-and-criteria-led-discharge/7023726.article

Lees-Deutsch, L. & Robinson, J. (2018) A systematic review of criteria-led patient discharge. *Journal of Nursing Care Quality*, 34(2), 121–126.

Lees-Deutsch, L., Yorke, J. & Caress, A. (2016) Principles for discharging patients from acute care: A scoping review of policy. *British Journal of Nursing*, 25(20), 1135–1143.

Lord, K., Livingston, G., Robertson, S. & Cooper C. (2016) How people with dementia and their families decide about moving to a care home and support their needs: Development of a decision aid, a qualitative study. *BMC Geriatrics*, 16(1), 68.

Mabire, C., Dwyer, A., Garnier, A. & Pellet, J. (2018) Meta-analysis of the effectiveness of nursing discharge planning interventions for older inpatients discharged home. *Journal of Advanced Nursing*, 74, 788–799.

McNeil, A. (2016) Using evidence to structure discharge planning. *Nursing Management (Springhouse)*, 47(5), 22–23.

Mental Capacity Act (2005) Available at: https://www.legislation.gov.uk/ukpga/2005/9/contents

National Palliative and End of Life Care Partnership (2015) *Ambitions for Palliative and End of Life Care: A National Framework for Local Action 2015–2020*. Available at: http://endoflifecareambitions.org.uk/wp-content/uploads/2015/09/Ambitions-for-Palliative-and-End-of-Life-Care.pdf

New, P., McDougall, K.E. & Scroggie, C.P. (2016) Improving discharge planning communication between hospitals and patients. *Internal Medicine Journal*, 46(1), 57–62.

NHS England (2016) *Monthly Delayed Transfers of Care Data, England, March 2016*. Available at: https://www.england.nhs.uk/statistics/wp-content/uploads/sites/2/2016/05/March-16-DTOC-SPN.pdf

NHS England (2018) *NHS Standard Contract 2017/18 and 2018/19 Service Conditions* [January 2018 edition]. Available at: https://www.england.nhs.uk/publication/nhs-standard-contract-201718-and-201819-service-conditions-full-length

NHSI (NHS Improvement) (2015) *Quality, Service Improvement and Redesign Tools: Discharge Planning*. Available at: https://improvement.nhs.uk/documents/2100/discharge-planning.pdf

NHSI (2017a) *SAFER Patient Flow Bundle*. Available at: https://improvement.nhs.uk/resources/safer-patient-flow-bundle-implement

NHSI (2017b) *Red2Green Campaign*. Available at: https://improvement.nhs.uk/improvement-offers/red2green-campaign

NHSI (2018) *Guide to Reducing Long Hospital Stays*. Available at: https://improvement.nhs.uk/documents/2898/Guide_to_reducing_long_hospital_stays_FINAL_v2.pdf

NHS Sunderland Clinical Commissioning Group (2017) *Updated Home Oxygen Order Forms & Consent/ Initial Home Oxygen Mitigation Form IHORM*. Available at: https://www.sunderlandccg.nhs.uk/about-us/prescribing/home-oxygen

NICE (National Institute for Health and Care Excellence) (2015) *Transition between Inpatient Hospital Settings and Community or Care Home Settings for Adults with Social Care Needs* [NICE Guideline NG27]. Available at: https://www.nice.org.uk/guidance/ng27/resources/transition-between-inpatient-hospital-settings-and-community-or-care-home-settings-for-adults-with-social-care-needs-pdf-1837336935877

NICE (2016) *Transition between Inpatient Hospital Settings and Community or Care Home Settings for Adults with Social Care Needs* [NICE Quality Standard QS136]. London: National Institute for Health and Care Excellence.

NICE (2017) *Intermediate Care including Reablement* [NICE Guideline NG74]. London: National Institute for Health and Care Excellence.

NICE (2018) *NICE Impact: Falls and Fragility Fractures*. London: National Institute for Health and Care Excellence.

Pellett, C. (2016) Discharge planning: Best practice in transitions of care. *British Journal of Community Nursing*, 21(11), 542–548.

People First (2018) *Care Act 2014*. Available at: https://www.peoplefirstinfo.org.uk/money-and-legal/care-act-2014

Poole, M., Bond, J., Emmett, C., et al. (2014) Going home? An ethnographic study of assessment capacity and best interests in people with dementia being discharged from hospital. *BMC Geriatrics*, 14(56), 14.

QNI (The Queen's Nursing Institute) (2016) *Discharge Planning: Best Practice in Transitions of Care*. Available at: https://www.qni.org.uk/wp-content/uploads/2016/09/discharge_planning_report_2015.pdf

Rivers, S. (2015) Supporting discharge using a volunteer scheme. *Nursing Times*, 111(23/24). Available at: https://www.nursingtimes.net/roles/older-people-nurses/supporting-discharge-using-a-volunteer-scheme/5085417.article

Royal Voluntary Service (2014) *Going Home Alone: Counting the Cost to Older People and the NHS*. Available at: https://www.royalvoluntaryservice.org.uk/Uploads/Documents/Reports%20and%20Reviews/Going_home_alone.pdf

Sheridan, E., Thompson, C., Pinheiro, T., et al. (2017) Optimizing transitions of care: Hospital to community. *Healthcare Quarterly*, 20(1), 45–49.

Teodorczuk, A. (2016) Understanding safe discharge of patients with dementia from acute hospital. *British Journal of Hospital Medicine*, 77(3), 126–127.

Teodorczuk, A., Mukaetova-Ladinska, E., Corbett, S. & Welfare, M. (2015) Deconstructing dementia and delirium hospital practice: Using cultural historical activity theory to inform education approaches. *Advanced Health Science Theory Practice*, 20, 745–764.

Thomas, C. (2017) Improving hospital discharge for patients at the end of life. *Nursing Times*, 113(11). Available at: https://www.nursingtimes.net/clinical-archive/end-of-life-and-palliative-care/improving-hospital-discharge-for-patients-at-the-end-of-life/7021751.article

Wallace, A., Papke, T., Devissson, E., et al. (2017) Provider opinions and experiences regarding development of a social support assessment to inform hospital discharge: The going home toolkit. *Professional Case Management*, [illegible].

Waring, J., Marshall, R., Bishop, S., et al. (2014) An ethnographic study of knowledge sharing across the boundaries between care processes, services and organisations: The contributions to 'safe' hospital discharge. *Health Services and Delivery Research*, 2(29), 1–160.

Weiss, M., Bobay, K., Bahr, S., et al. (2015) A model for hospital discharge preparation: From case management to care transition. *Journal of Nursing Administration*, 45(12), 606–614.

Winfield, A. & Burns, E. (2016) Let's all get home safely: A commentary on NICE and SCIE guidelines (NG27) transition between inpatient hospital settings and community or care home settings. *Age and Ageing*, 45, 757–760.

Chapter 4

Infection prevention and control

Pat Cattini with Martin Kiernan

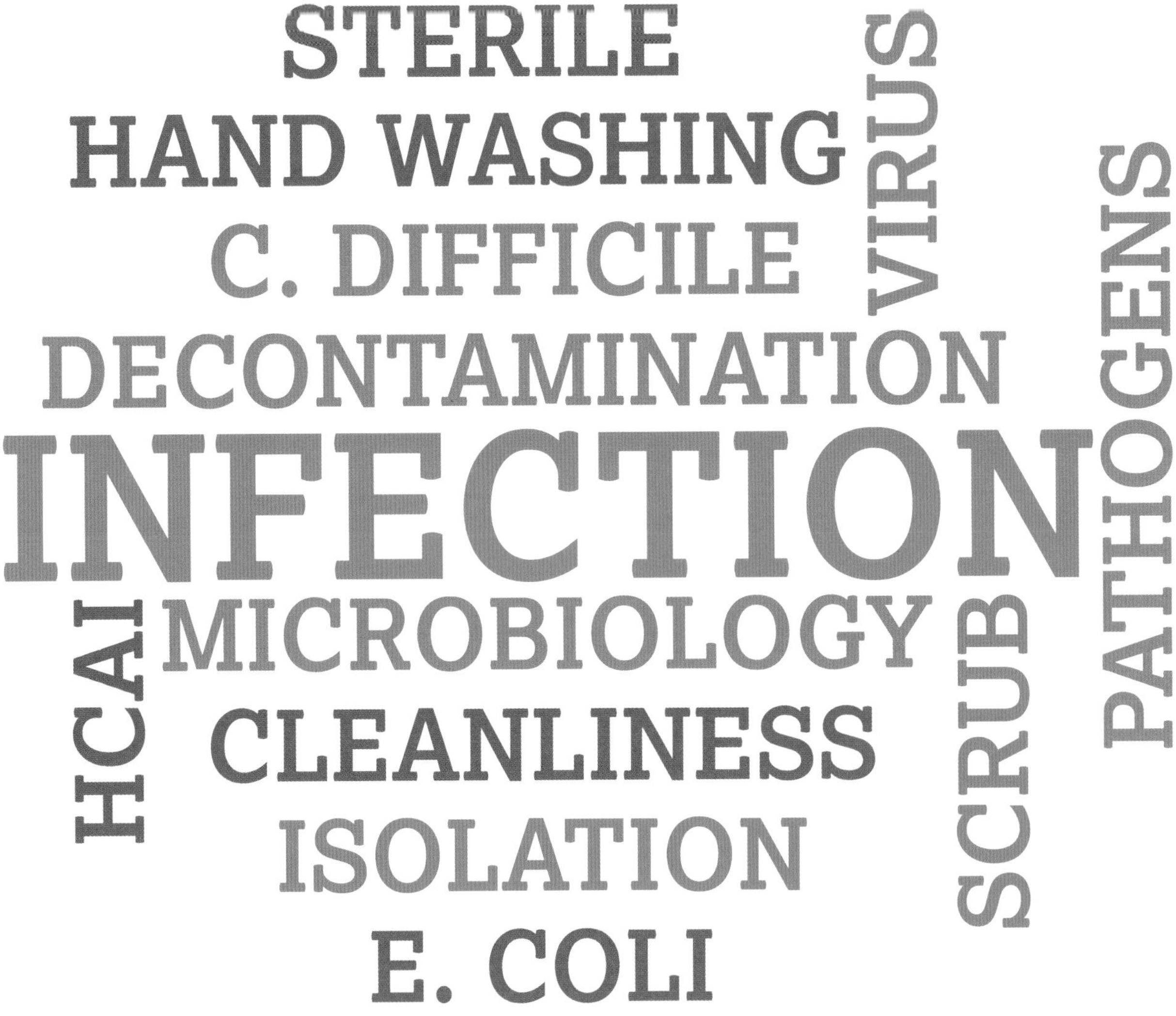

The Royal Marsden Manual of Clinical Nursing Procedures: Professional Edition, Tenth Edition. Edited by Sara Lister, Justine Hofland and Hayley Grafton.

Procedure guidelines

Being an accountable professional

At the point of registration, the nurse will:

9. Use evidence-based, best practice approaches for meeting needs for care and support with the prevention and management of infection, accurately assessing the person's capacity for independence and self-care and initiating appropriate interventions.

Future Nurse: Standards of Proficiency for Registered Nurses (NMC 2018)

Overview

This chapter begins with an explanation of the causes of infection and then focuses on healthcare-associated infections (HCAIs), specifically describing the steps to be taken to minimize the risk of individuals acquiring infections while receiving healthcare. The chapter gives an overview of key principles, terminology and definitions, and describes the standard precautions that must be taken with patients at all times regardless of their known infection status. It also covers additional precautions that may be required because the patient is colonized or infected with micro-organisms that may pose a particular risk to others, or because they are particularly vulnerable to infection themselves. The chapter additionally describes the specific precautions that must be taken during invasive procedures, in particular aseptic technique.

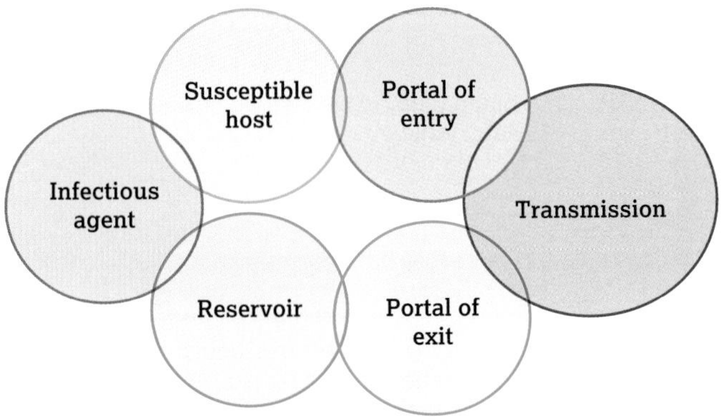

Figure 4.1 The chain of infection: a useful tool for seeing how to prevent transmission.

Infection prevention and control

Definitions

Infection prevention and control

'Infection prevention and control' has been defined as the clinical application of microbiology in practice (RCN 2017); it is a collective term for activities intended to protect people from infection. Such activities may form part of everyday life, such as washing hands after using the toilet or before preparing food. However, the term is most often used in relation to healthcare, with reference in particular to avoiding patients acquiring preventable infections.

Healthcare-associated infection

A healthcare-associated infection (HCAI) is any infection acquired as a result of healthcare contact. It has replaced the term 'hospital-acquired infection' to recognize that not all healthcare is given in a hospital. Such infections are also known as 'nosocomial' infections.

Anatomy and physiology

Pathogens are what cause infection. It is important to understand types of pathogen, how they spread and what kinds of environment are favourable for their growth so that effective infection prevention and control measures can be put in place.

Causes of infection

The term 'infectious agent' is often used to describe anything that may be transmitted from one person to another, or from the environment to a person, and subsequently cause an infection or parasitic infestation.

Distinct types of infectious agent act differently and have different impacts on the infected individual. For example, whether a particular infectious agent will cause an infection in any given circumstance is dependent on many factors, including how *easily* that agent can be transmitted, its *pathogenicity* (its ability to cause disease) and its *virulence* (the severity of the infection produced) (Gillespie and Bamford 2012). The *susceptibility* of the patient to infection is also a significant influence.

To practice effective infection prevention and control, it is helpful to understand the 'chain of infection' (Damani 2011). This is a helpful model to use when considering how infection can be prevented, as it shows how it is possible to break the 'links' in the chain. For an infection to exist, there must be an organism (pathogen) and it must be able to get into a susceptible host, multiply and exit. It may need a place to hide (reservoir) while waiting for the next susceptible host. Figure 4.1 illustrates the chain of infection and Table 4.1 lists the links with examples of how infection can be prevented at each link. The major groups of micro-organisms are described below.

Types and classification of micro-organisms

Historically, the classification of micro-organisms was based on physical characteristics such as their size, shape or ability to retain a particular stain to make them visible under the microscope. Some of these distinctions are still useful, but classification is increasingly based on genetic characteristics, as increasingly sophisticated analysis techniques (such as genomic sequencing) reveal the actual relationships between organisms. This can lead to confusion as new discoveries lead to species being reclassified and renamed. For example, 'methicillin-resistant' *Staphylococcus aureus* is now 'meticillin-resistant' and *Clostridium difficile* is now termed *Clostridioides difficile.*

It should also be noted that there can be a wide variety of characteristics within each species, leading to significant variations in the severity of infection caused by different strains of the same organism. An example of this is Group A *Streptococcus pyogenes*, which is a common cause of sore throat but can also cause skin conditions such as erysipelas, scarlet fever, toxic shock syndrome and necrotizing fasciitis. Another is *Escherichia coli*, which is carried in the gut of all mammals with no ill effects but whose toxin-producing O157:H7 strain can cause serious illness.

In printed text, the names of bacteria are written in italics, with the name of the genus capitalized and the species in lower case, for example *Staphylococcus aureus*. The abbreviation 'spp.' is used to refer to all of the species of a genus, for example *Klebsiella* spp. This section gives an overview of the different types of organism that may be encountered in a healthcare environment as well as the differences between and within the types.

Bacteria

Bacteria are probably the most important group of micro-organisms in terms of infection prevention and control because they are responsible for the majority of opportunistic infections in healthcare. A healthy human being will typically be host to a quadrillion (1000 trillion or 10^{15}) bacteria – around ten times as many organisms as there are cells in the human body – and we need most of these to survive.

The so-called 'human microbiome' is increasingly being recognized as an essential part of human health (Bhalodi et al. 2019, Young 2017) and a variety of conditions – such as Crohn's disease, ulcerative colitis, irritable bowel syndrome, obesity, type 2 diabetes, Parkinson's disease, chronic fatigue syndrome, arthritis and even asthma – may all be related to disturbance of the balance of micro-organisms in the gut, although the question remains as to whether this is a cause or effect (Otter 2014, Tosh and McDonald 2012, Wang et al. 2017). See Table 4.2 for examples of how the human microbiome can be protective.

In normal circumstances, the relationship between bacteria and their host is symbiotic and the organisms are considered to be commensal (i.e. their presence does not cause the host any problems) and mutually beneficial; however, if the host has lowered resistance or a bacteria gains access to a different site, it can become an opportunistic pathogen. For example, *E. coli* from the gut may cause a urinary tract infection (with associated symptoms) if it enters the urethra and ascends the urinary tract.

Table 4.1 Links in the chain of infection

Link	Definition	Example	Examples of breaking the chain
Infectious agent	A potentially pathogenic micro-organism or other agent	• Smallpox • *Staphylococcus aureus* or any other bacteria	• Vaccination – for example, we no longer need to worry about the virus that causes smallpox or how it is transmitted as it does not exist (except in some top-secret laboratories) • Removal of infectious agents through cleaning • Destruction of micro-organisms through sterilization of equipment • Using antibiotics to treat patients with bacterial infections
Reservoir	Any location where micro-organisms hide, exist or reproduce	• Humans • Dust in the healthcare environment • Sink drains	• Cleaning/decontamination of equipment and the environment • Use of handwash basins for hand washing only • Flushing low-use taps and showers • Minimizing the number of people present in high-risk situations such as surgery
Portal of exit	The route by which the infectious agent leaves the reservoir	• Diarrhoea and vomit may carry norovirus • Droplets expelled during coughing or sneezing may contain flu	• Asking a patient with active tuberculosis infection to wear a mask in communal areas of the hospital
Mode of transmission	The way the infectious agent is spread (see definitions section above)	• Contact • Enteric • Droplet • Airborne • Parenteral	• Hands • Diarrhoea • Sneezing • Nebulizer or intubation • Needle stick injury
Portal of entry	The route by which the infectious agent enters a new host	• Organisms introduced into a normally sterile part of the body through use of an invasive device • Intravenous line into the bloodstream • Urinary catheter breaching the bladder • Inhalation of airborne pathogens into the lungs	• Avoiding unnecessary invasive devices • Using strict aseptic technique • Staff members wearing masks when dealing with infectious agents that may be inhaled
Susceptible host	The person that the infectious agent enters has to be susceptible to infection	• The very old and very young are more susceptible • Underlying chronic illnesses	• Ensuring adequate nutrition and personal hygiene • Vaccination – this will often completely prevent or significantly reduce the likelihood of an infection developing

Table 4.2 Examples of how the human microbiome can be protective

Bacteria	Comments
Gut flora including *Bacteroides* spp., *Bifidobacterium* spp., *Enterobacter* spp., *Klebsiella* spp., *Enterococcus* spp. and *Escherichia coli*	Disturbance though antibiotics, surgery or chemotherapy may have far-ranging effects on the human body, including obesity, inflammatory bowel diseases, antibiotic-associated diarrhoea and cancer.
Skin flora including *Staphylococcus epidermidis*, *Staphylococcus aureus*, diphtheroids and *Candida* spp.	A healthy, intact, normal resident skin flora means that pathogenic organisms are less likely to settle on the skin and cause infection.
Vaginal flora including *Lactobacillus* spp. and diphtheroids	Babies born per vagina are more likely to have their skin colonized with the 'right' organisms, which reduces problems with skin and allergies.

Despite the fact that we are surrounded by unquantifiable numbers of bacteria in our world, relatively few are pathogenic to us. There is an important balance to be struck in our home lives; we should not try to disinfect everything we come into contact with, and indeed many things around us are going to be contaminated (money, cash point buttons, our mobile phones and the handles on public transport, to name a few). If we are healthy and have good immunity and intact skin, this will often be of little consequence to us as long as we follow simple precautions such as practising hand hygiene, environmental hygiene (cleaning) and food hygiene.

For a patient receiving interventional healthcare, however, things can be very different and we need to do as much as possible to ensure items introduced into the care environment are free of pathogens. Our increasing understanding of the normal commensal micro-organisms in humans suggests that restoring and maintaining the microbiome may provide a key to preventing colonization and infection, including with multi-drug-resistant organisms (Otter 2014, Tosh and McDonald 2012), which can be 'selected out' when exposed to antibiotics. This means that bacteria that are sensitive to the antibiotics are killed but any resistant ones are left to replicate and become the dominant type. A developing form of treatment is the 'faecal microbiota transplant', or stool transplant, which involves replacing the stool in an affected gut with stool from a healthy donor. This has been shown to be very effective for treatment of intractable *C. difficile* (van Nood et al. 2013) and may be helpful in other conditions.

Sometimes a patient will be 'colonized' with a species of bacteria, which means it is present but not causing them harm. However, if the bacteria are transferred to another patient and gain access to a portal of entry, that person may suffer harm, so there is a need for effective precautions. Whether or not any particular situation will result in an infection depends on a wide range of factors and these are not always predictable. What is certain is that bacterial infections cannot occur when bacteria are not present, hence the importance of measures designed to minimize the risk of transmission.

The presence of an organism in a specimen result does not on its own imply that an infection has occurred. Any laboratory results must always be interpreted in association with an assessment of the patient's condition and symptoms, which will guide the need for treatment.

Morphology

Bacterial cells are much smaller and simpler than human cells; this small size means that bacteria do not have separate structures (such as a nucleus) within their cells. The structure of the cell wall determines another important distinction in medically significant bacteria: whether they are gram positive or gram negative. The 'gram' in these terms refers to Gram staining, named after its Dutch inventor, Hans Christian Gram (1853–1938), who devised the stain in 1884. The structure of the cell wall determines whether or not the bacteria are able to retain a particular stain in the presence of an organic solvent such as acetone. This structure also determines other characteristics of the bacteria, including their susceptibility to particular antibiotics, so knowing whether the cause of a bacterial infection is 'gram positive' or 'gram negative' can help to determine appropriate treatment (Goering et al. 2012). The structures of the two different types of cell wall are shown in Figure 4.2.

Other structures visible outside the cell wall may include pili, which are rigid tubes that help the bacteria attach to host cells (or, in some cases, other bacteria for the exchange of genetic material); flagellae, which are longer, mobile projections that can help bacteria to move around; and capsules, which can provide protection or help the bacteria to adhere to surfaces. These are illustrated in Figure 4.3. The presence or absence of different structures plays a part in determining an organism's pathogenicity – that is, its ability to cause an infection and the severity of that infection (Goering et al. 2012).

A final bacterial structure to consider is the spore. Bacteria reproduce via a process called 'binary fission' – they create a copy of their genetic material and split themselves in two, with each 'daughter' cell being an almost exact copy of the 'parent' (there are mechanisms by which bacteria can transfer genetic material between cells and so acquire characteristics such as antibiotic resistance, but they are beyond the scope of this chapter). Some bacteria, notably the Clostridia, have the capacity, in adverse conditions, to surround a copy of their genetic material with a tough coat called a 'spore'. Once the spore has been formed, the parent cell dies and disintegrates, leaving the spore to survive until conditions are suitable for it to germinate into a normal, 'vegetative'

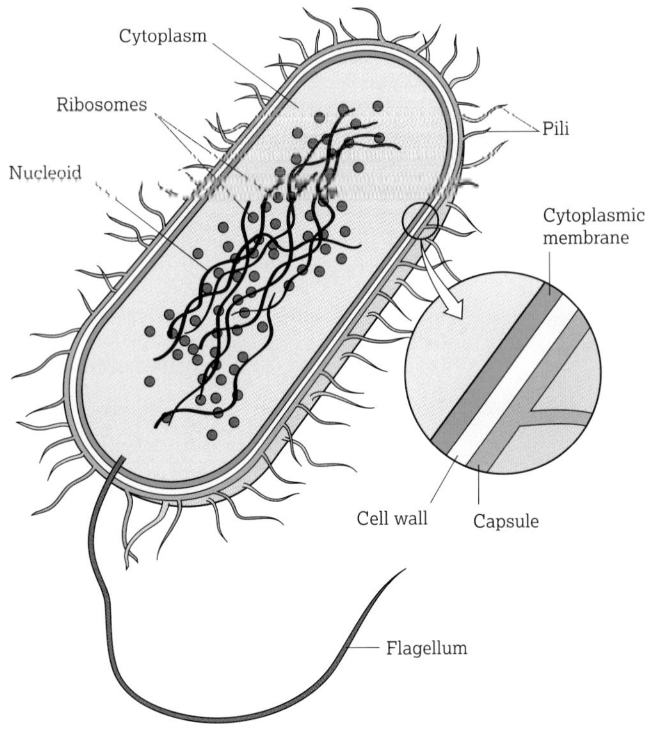

Figure 4.3 Bacterial structures.

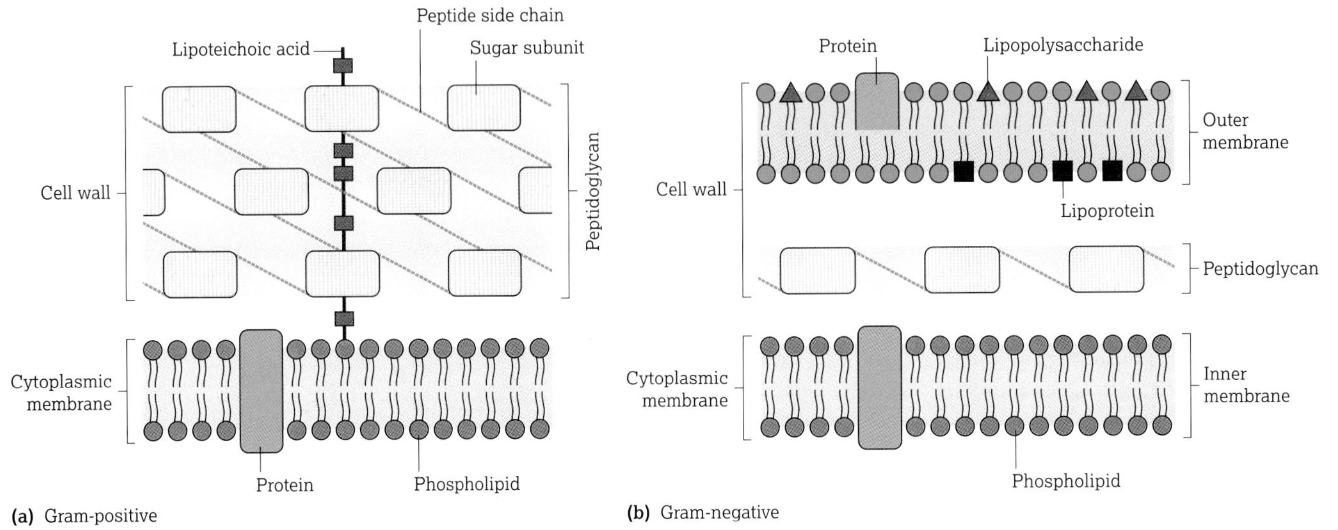

Figure 4.2 (a) Gram-positive and (b) gram-negative bacterial cell walls. *Source*: Adapted from Elliot et al. (2007) with permission of John Wiley & Sons.

Table 4.3 Medically significant bacteria

	Spherical	Rod-shaped
Gram positive	*Staphylococcus aureus* *Streptococcus* spp.	*Clostridioides difficile* *Clostridium tetani* *Bacillus* spp.
Gram negative	*Neisseria meningitidis* *Neisseria gonorrhoeae*	*Escherichia coli* *Pseudomonas aeruginosa* *Klebsiella pneumoniae* *Acinetobacter baumannii* *Salmonella* spp. *Legionella pneumophila*

bacterial cell, which can then reproduce (Goering et al. 2012). Spores are extremely tough and durable. They are not easily destroyed even by boiling or via the alcohol-based handrubs widely used for hand hygiene, hence the need to physically remove them from the hands by washing with soap and water when caring for a patient with *C. difficile* infection. Commonly used disinfectants containing quaternary ammonium compounds (such as benzalkonium chloride) are ineffective against spores.

Some bacteria produce toxins, which are proteins released by the bacteria that can increase the severity of disease. Endotoxins are pieces of the cell wall of gram-negative bacteria; these initiate a strong immune response from the body, which can cause catastrophic damage. For example, endotoxins of *Neisseria meningitidis* cause the breakdown of blood vessels, leading to anoxic tissue and the need for amputation. Antibiotics may kill the bacteria but in doing so flood the body with deadly endotoxins.

Some medically significant bacteria are listed in Table 4.3. A few bacteria do not easily fit into the gram positive/negative dichotomy. The most medically significant of these are the mycobacteria, which have a waxy coat and are responsible for diseases including tuberculosis and leprosy (Goering et al. 2012).

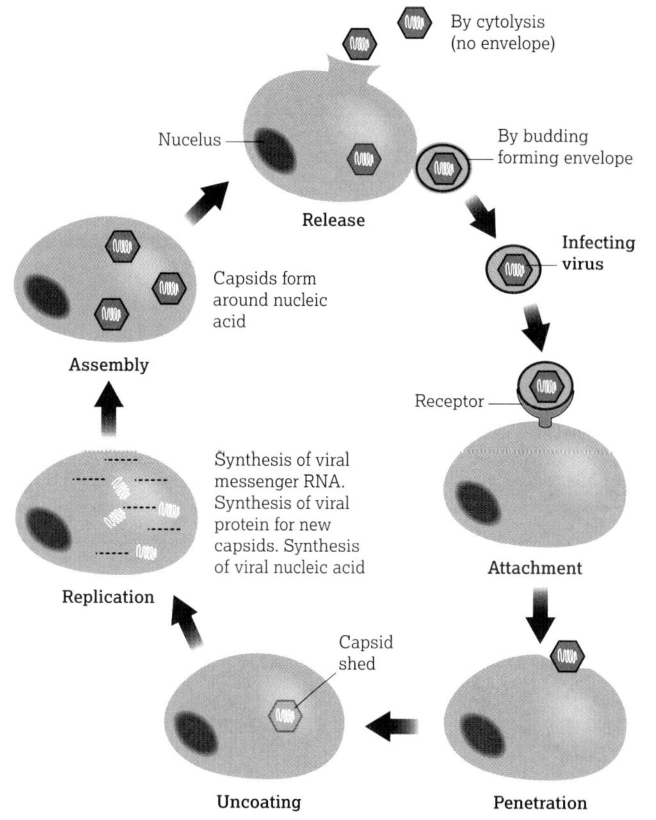

Figure 4.4 The viral life cycle. RNA, ribonucleic acid. *Source:* Adapted from Perry (2007) with permission of John Wiley & Sons.

Culture and sensitivity testing

When a sample arrives in the laboratory, it is put onto agar plates to culture any organisms present. The site of the specimen and clinical information may dictate which tests are deployed and what media are used, which is why it is very important to fill out the microbiology request form with as much detail as possible (for more detail see Chapter 13: Diagnostic tests). The provision of accurate and comprehensive information assists the microbiologist in interpreting the findings in the laboratory and simple information, such as the site of the specimen (if a wound), the type of urine, recent travel and current antibiotic use, can also be helpful.

Different types of agar plate may be used to grow different bacteria. Once the organism has been grown, it can be subjected to further tests to identify it, including a gram stain to see whether it is gram positive or gram negative, examination for the presence of pus cells and sensitivity testing. Sensitivity testing usually involves spreading the organism over an agar plate that contains small antibiotic discs. If the bacteria grow all the way up to the disc, they are resistant to that antibiotic. A 'zone of inhibition' around the disc implies they are sensitive to the antibiotic and that the antibiotic may be used to treat that infection. A faster and more modern technique to identify and speciate microbes involves the use of matrix-assisted laser desorption ionization time-of-flight mass spectrometry (MALDI-TOF MS) (Croxatto et al. 2012).

Modern laboratories use molecular technology to diagnose patients without the need for culture. These techniques include polymerase chain reaction (PCR) and enzyme immuno-assay.

Viruses

Viruses are much smaller, and even simpler, than bacteria. Nobel laureate Peter Medawar is said to have described viruses as 'bad news wrapped in protein' and indeed they are little more than a protein capsule containing some genetic material. They rely on other organisms for their survival and reproduce within a host cell, using the cell's own mechanisms to reproduce, which leads to the death of the host cell (Goering et al. 2012). The life cycle of a virus is illustrated in Figure 4.4. The small size of viruses (e.g. poliovirus is only 30 nanometres across) means that most are smaller than the wavelengths of visible light. They can only be 'seen' with a specialist instrument such as an electron microscope, which will only be available in a very few hospital microbiology laboratories. Diagnosis of viral infections is normally based on the patient's symptoms, with confirmation by laboratory tests designed to detect either the virus itself or antibodies produced by the patient's immune system as a response to infection (Goering et al. 2012). Modern laboratories use PCR to amplify the genes in the sample to make them detectable quickly.

There are viruses that specifically infect humans, other animals or plants, or even bacteria. This is one characteristic that can be used in classifying them. However, the main basis for classification is by the type of genetic material they contain – DNA (deoxyribonucleic acid) or RNA (ribonucleic acid), in either a double or single strand. Other characteristics include the shape of the viral particle and the sort of disease caused by infection (Gillespie and Bamford 2012).

A final point to consider in relation to viral structure and infection prevention and control is the presence or absence of a lipid envelope enclosing the viral particle. Viruses that have a lipid envelope, such as herpes zoster virus (responsible for chickenpox and shingles), are much more susceptible to destruction by alcohol than those without. Norovirus and or rotavirus, which are common causes of viral gastroenteritis (WHO 2009a), are examples of viruses without a lipid envelope. For this reason, alcohol hand sanitizers are not recommended during outbreaks of norovirus in hospitals.

Fungi

Like bacteria, fungi exist in many environments on earth, including occasionally as commensal organisms on human beings. Fungi are familiar to us as mushrooms and toadstools and the yeast that is used in brewing and baking. They also have many uses in the pharmaceutical industry, particularly in the production of antibiotics. Fungi produce spores, both for survival in adverse conditions, as bacteria do, and to provide a mechanism for dispersal in the same way as plants (Goering et al. 2012).

A few varieties of fungi are able to cause opportunistic infections in humans. These are usually found in one of two forms: either as single-celled yeast-like forms, which reproduce in a similar fashion to bacteria (by dividing or budding), or as plant-like filaments called 'hyphae'. A mass of hyphae together forms a 'mycelium'. Some fungi may appear in either form, depending on environmental conditions. Fungal infections are referred to as 'mycoses'. Superficial mycoses, such as ringworm and thrush (*Candida albicans*), usually involve only the skin or mucous membranes and are normally mild, if unpleasant, however, deeper mycoses involving major organs can be life threatening. These occur in patients who have severely impaired immune systems and may be an indicator of such impairment; for example, pneumonia caused by *Pneumocystis jirovecii* (previously *carinii*) is considered a clinical indication of AIDS (acquired immune deficiency syndrome). Superficial infections are generally transmitted by physical contact, whereas deeper infections can result from spores being inhaled. This is why it is important to ensure that patients with impaired immunity are protected from situations where the spores of potentially pathogenic fungi, such as *Aspergillus* spp., are likely to be released, for example during building work (Goering et al. 2012).

Protozoa

Protozoa are single-celled animals, some species of which are medically important parasites of human beings, particularly in tropical and subtropical parts of the world, where diseases such as malaria are a major public health issue. Unlike bacteria, their relationship with humans is almost always parasitic. The life cycles of protozoa can be complex and may involve stages in different hosts.

Medically important protozoa include *Plasmodium* spp., the cause of malaria; *Giardia* spp. and *Cryptosporidium* spp., which can cause gastroenteritis; and *Trichomoniasis* spp., which is a sexually transmitted cause of vaginitis (Gillespie and Bamford 2012).

The most common routes of infection of protozoa are by consuming them in food or water or via an insect vector such as a mosquito (Goering et al. 2012). Cross-infection in the course of healthcare is uncommon but not unknown.

Helminths

'Helminths' is a generic term for parasitic worms. A number of worms from three different groups affect humans: tapeworms (cestodes), roundworms (nematodes) and flukes (trematodes). Transmission generally occurs via ingestion of eggs or larvae, or infected animals or fish, but some are transmitted via an insect vector and some, notably the nematode *Strongyloides* spp., have a larval stage that is capable of penetrating the skin (Gillespie and Bamford 2012).

Helminth infections can affect almost every part of the body, and the effects can be severe. For example, *Ascaris* worms can cause bowel obstruction if there are large numbers present; *Brugia* spp. and *Wuchereria* spp. obstruct the lymphatic system and eventually cause elephantiasis as a result; and infection with *Toxocara* spp. (often after contact with dog faeces) can result in epilepsy or blindness (Goering et al. 2012). However, cross-infection in healthcare is not normally considered a significant risk.

Arthropods

Arthropods (insects) are most significant in infectious disease in terms of their function as vectors of many viral, bacterial, protozoan and helminth-caused diseases. Some flies lay eggs in the skin of mammals, including humans, and the larvae feed and develop in the skin before pupating into the adult form, whereas some, such as lice and mites, are associated with humans for the whole of their life cycle. Such arthropod infestations can be uncomfortable, and there is often significant social stigma attached to them, possibly because the creatures are often visible to the naked eye. The activity of the insects and the presence of their saliva and faeces can result in quite severe skin conditions that are then vulnerable to secondary fungal or bacterial infection (Goering et al. 2012).

Lice

Species of *Pediculus* infest the hair and body of humans, feeding by sucking blood from their host. The adult animal is around 3 mm long and wingless, moving by means of claws. It cannot jump or fly, and dies within 24 hours if away from its host, so cross-infection normally occurs via direct contact or transfer of eggs or adults through sharing personal items (Cummings et al. 2018).

Scabies

Scabies is caused by the mite *Sarcoptes scabiei*, an insect less than 1 mm long that burrows into the top layers of skin. The female mites lay eggs in these burrows and the offspring can spread to other areas of the body. Infestation usually starts around the wrists and in between the fingers because acquisition normally occurs via close contact with an infected individual (e.g. by holding hands). The burrows are visible as a characteristic rash in the areas affected. The skin starts to itch a few weeks after infestation, which is a reaction to the faeces of the mite. A delay in recognition can lead to mass infestation, especially within families or in settings where there is a lot of interpersonal care, such as a nursing home. In immunocompromised hosts and those unable to practise normal levels of personal hygiene, very high levels of infestation can occur, often with thickening of the skin and the formation of thick crusts. This is known as 'Norwegian scabies' and is associated with a much higher risk of cross-infection than the normal presentation.

Scabies is most often associated with long-stay care settings, but there have been outbreaks associated with more acute healthcare facilities (Cassell et al. 2018). Treatment with scabicide must be co-ordinated to ensure untreated hosts do not reinfect those already treated.

Prions

Prions are thought to be the causative agents of a group of diseases called transmissible spongiform encephalopathies (TSEs), the most well known of which are Creutzfeldt–Jakob disease (CJD) and its variant (vCJD) (Table 4.4). These are fatal neurodegenerative diseases with a lengthy incubation period (up to 50 years) and no conventional host response, making them difficult to detect.

TSEs can be naturally occurring, inherited or acquired (Table 4.4). They are characterized by 'plaques' in the brain that are surrounded by holes that give the appearance of a sponge, hence the name.

Table 4.4 Types of transmissible spongiform encephalopathies

Type	Examples
Idiopathic (just happens for no clear reason)	Sporadic (classical) CJD Sporadic fatal insomnia
Inherited (genetic)	Familial CJD Gerstmann–Sträussler–Scheinker syndrome and variants Fatal familial insomnia
Acquired	Derived from humans: • kuru (cannibalism) • iatrogenic CJD (contaminated medical devices or blood products) Derived from bovines: vCJD (diet – meat infected with bovine spongiform encephalopathy)

CJD, Creutzfeldt–Jakob disease; vCJD, variant Creutzfeldt–Jakob disease.

The causative 'organism' is a prion, defined in 1982 by Stanley Prusiner as a proteinaceous infectious particle resistant to procedures that modify nucleic acid.

From an infection control perspective, the key point is that prions contain no genetic material; therefore, it can be argued that they are not alive and so cannot be killed. Control is achieved via recognition of risk and physical removal through cleaning procedures. Prions are not affected by routine decontamination processes such as autoclaving or chemical disinfection. This has led to extensive reviews of decontamination procedures in the UK with increased emphasis on effective washing to remove any residual organic material, and on the tracking of instruments to individual patients to facilitate any look-back exercise. Modern decontamination services are now capable of removing prions from the surface of even complex instruments; however, where risk is identified, single-use instruments are usually recommended, especially for neurological work.

In the 1990s there was a lot of concern about the emergence of vCJD, which was associated with consumption of contaminated beef from cattle who had bovine spongiform encephalopathy (BSE). With intense input from public health initiatives and what was then called the Ministry of Agriculture, Fisheries and Food, beef was made safe again. However, UK citizens born before 1992 are still considered at risk of vCJD due to its long incubation period.

There were also several cases of CJD associated with contaminated medical products, such as human pituitary hormone, dura mater grafts and medical instruments. For this reason, all patients undergoing surgery should be assessed for risk of CJD by asking the following questions:

- Do you have a blood family member who has suffered from CJD?
- Have you ever received hormones derived from a human pituitary gland (e.g. growth hormone)?
- Have you ever had a corneal transplant or a dura mater graft?
- Have you been told that 'you may be at risk of CJD for public health purposes'?

A patient with CJD or vCJD is not infectious to other people under routine circumstances so no special precautions are required other than if dealing with cerebrospinal fluid (CSF). A spillage of CSF should be cleaned up with a strong disinfectant such as 10,000 ppm of chlorine.

Sources of infection

An individual may become infected with organisms already present on their body (endogenous infection) or introduced from elsewhere (exogenous infection). The majority of HCAIs are endogenous, hence the importance of procedures such as effective skin decontamination prior to invasive procedures (NHS England and NHSI 2019).

Indicators and effects of infection

Generally, infection is said to have occurred when infectious agents enter a normally sterile area of the body and cause symptoms as a result. There are obvious exceptions (e.g. the digestive tract is not sterile, being home to trillions of micro-organisms, but many types of infectious gastroenteritis are caused by particular organisms entering this area), but this is a useful working definition. The symptoms of infection are listed below. Not all symptoms will be present in all cases, and it should be noted that many symptoms are caused by the body's response to infection and so may not be present in severely immunocompromised patients (Fishman 2011).

Symptoms of infection

The cardinal signs of inflammation will often be present:

- *Heat*: the site of the infection may feel warm to the touch, and the patient may have a raised temperature.
- *Pain*: at the site of the infection.
- *Swelling*: at the site of the infection.
- *Redness*: at the site of the infection
- *Loss of function*: the affected area may not work properly.

In addition, there may be other signs, such as:

- pus
- raised white cells in blood results
- raised C-reactive protein (CRP) in blood results
- altered blood gases
- feeling of general malaise
- aching joints
- abdominal pain and tenderness
- nausea, diarrhoea and/or vomiting
- oliguria or anuria
- urinary frequency and/or pain on passing urine (strangury)
- confusion (notably in the elderly)
- loin pain.

It is important to look for these clinical signs of infection before making a diagnosis based on the result of a specimen alone.

Related theory

Healthcare-associated infection

An HCAI is acquired while receiving care in a hospital or other healthcare setting and must not have been present prior to that episode of healthcare; 6.6% of people who go into hospital in the UK will develop an HCAI. The figure for Europe is about 4 million people every year, with around 37,000 deaths occurring as a direct result (PHE 2017). The majority of these infections result from the procedures and interventions that patients undergo as treatment, such as insertion of invasive devices, surgery or the administration of antimicrobials that alter natural bacterial flora; all of these ultimately breach the body's natural defences and thereby increase vulnerability to infection. The greater the number of devices and the longer they are *in situ*, the more likely it is that an infection will occur. If the patient is also immunocompromised, the infection risk can be much higher. One report found that patients receiving treatment under oncology or haematology specialities were almost four times as likely to have an HCAI (a similar rate to those in intensive care units) compared to other patients in the same hospital and were twice as likely to be receiving an antibiotic (PHE 2018a).

In addition, bringing many vulnerable people together in a healthcare setting increases the likelihood of exposure to infection and the risk of cross-infection. Patients are often expected to share a room and bathroom facilities with those who may be carrying infection or different normal flora to them. This can lead to cross-infection, for example a patient who has diarrhoea may contaminate a shared toilet, thereby passing the infection to others using the same facilities.

The greater the number of patients that staff are caring for and the greater their workload, the greater the risk of cross-infection between patients. Overcrowding, lack of time and lack of facilities also contribute to non-compliance with best practice (Borg 2003, Eiamsitrakoon et al. 2013, Harbarth et al. 1999, Kampf et al. 2009, WHO 2009a).

Prevalence of healthcare-associated infection

The national Point Prevalence Survey of Healthcare-Associated Infections and Antimicrobial Use in European Acute Care Hospitals (ECDC 2016), conducted by Public Health England and the European Centre for Disease Prevention and Control, identified a prevalence rate of 6.6% (PHE 2017) (Figure 4.5). In acute hospitals, 1 in 15 patients had an HCAI on the day of survey, with the highest prevalence rates in intensive care units (17.6% of patients) followed by surgery (8.5%) and medicine (5.8%).

The most common types of infection were pneumonia and lower respiratory tract infection, urinary tract infections, and surgical site infections. There was very little change from the patterns seen

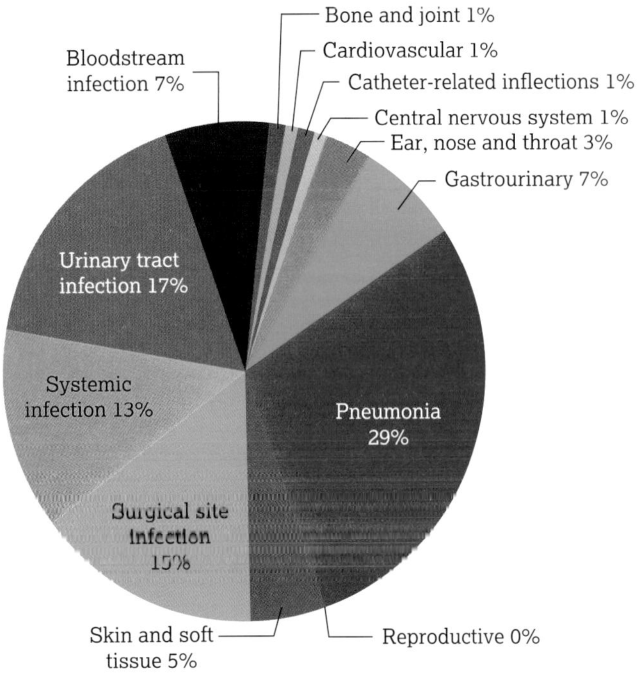

Figure 4.5 Results from the national Point Prevalence Survey in ESPAUR, 2016. Source: Data from *English Surveillance Programme for Antimicrobial Utilisation and Resistance (ESPAUR): Report 2018* (PHE 2018a).

from the previous survey, conducted in 2011 (ECDC 2013). While bacteraemia (bacteria infecting the bloodstream) was less common, it can still have serious consequences for patients. Of the infections identified, gram-negative bacteria species were responsible for 35% of bloodstream HCAIs, which justifies the focus of national prevention strategies in this area.

The most commonly isolated micro-organisms were *E. coli* (18.9%), *S. aureus* (17.6%), *C. difficile* (8.1%), *Pseudomonas aeruginosa* (7.8%), *Klebsiella pneumoniae* (4.9%) and *Enterobacter cloacae* (2.8%). *E. coli* was the most commonly isolated micro-organism in urinary tract infections (50.9%), whereas *S. aureus* was the most commonly isolated micro-organism in pneumonia and lower respiratory tract infections (19.3%), surgical site infections (30.2%) and bloodstream infections (19.2%).

The challenge of antimicrobial resistance

Over the past century, there have been many changes in the types of organism that cause problems in healthcare, largely mirroring advances in medicine. The advent of penicillin and then other antibiotics in the 1940s allowed such advances in medicine and surgery. More complex surgery became possible, such as surgeries requiring implants (joint replacements) or organ transplants, and patients were able to tolerate treatments such as chemotherapy. More and more patients began to survive previously untreatable conditions, largely due to the ability to treat complications such as infection.

With the increasing use of antibiotics, new challenges began to emerge, including *C. difficile* infections (CDI) in the 1970s and epidemic strains of meticillin-resistant *S. aureus* (MRSA) in the 1980s. During the 1990s and early 2000s there was a significant rise in both MRSA and CDI in the UK. Concerted effort engineered by the UK government saw impressive reductions in both these infections (DH 2019); however, the 2000s saw a rise in the prevalence of gram-negative organisms with increasing resistance to antibiotics and an associated increase in untreatable infections. It is fair to argue that increasing antimicrobial resistance is the biggest challenge to healthcare across the world. As stated by the UK Chief Medical Officer Professor Dame Sally Davies, 'We have reached a critical point and must act now on a global scale to slow down antimicrobial resistance' (DH 2014) (see also Box 4.1).

Box 4.1 *Tackling Drug-Resistant Infections Globally: Final Report and Recommendations* (O'Neill 2016)

'The magnitude of the problem is now accepted. We estimate that by 2050, 10 million lives a year are at risk due to the rise of drug-resistant infections if we do not find proactive solutions now to slow down the rise of drug resistance. Antibiotics are a special category of antimicrobial drugs that underpin modern medicine as we know it: if they lose their effectiveness, key medical procedures (such as gut surgery, caesarean sections, joint replacements, and treatments that depress the immune system, such as chemotherapy for cancer) could become too dangerous to perform.'

Nurses, along with other healthcare workers, have a duty to reduce the burden of antimicrobial resistance though effective infection prevention in their everyday work and help to preserve antimicrobials for future generations. An infection prevented means an antibiotic not required.

The term 'antimicrobial stewardship' is widely used to describe efforts to improve and rationalize antimicrobial prescribing. Much of this effort is targeted at doctors, who are the main prescribers of antimicrobials. Examples include the *Start Smart – Then Focus* toolkit (PHE 2015) and *Antimicrobial Stewardship: Systems and Processes for Effective Microbial Medicine Use* (NICE 2015), which exist to improve antimicrobial prescribing and develop a wider understanding of antimicrobial stewardship. 'Start smart' means:

- not starting antimicrobial therapy unless there is clear evidence of infection (ideally supported by appropriate microbiology samples)
- following local antibiotic guidance and taking into account a clear allergy history
- ensuring review dates and rationales for prescribing are all clearly documented.

'Then focus' means:

- reviewing the clinical diagnosis and continuing need for antimicrobials at 48–72 hours
- then clearly documenting a prescribing decision to stop, switch (from intravenous to oral), change (to a narrower-spectrum antibiotic in light of microbiology results), continue (and document the next review date) or use outpatient parenteral antibiotic therapy.

Nurses also have an important role in antimicrobial stewardship even if they are not themselves prescribers. This should include not being afraid to question the use of antimicrobials and encouraging good documentation.

Current infection challenges

In the UK, *E. coli* has increasingly been implicated as a source of bloodstream infection, as can be seen in Figure 4.6. *E. coli* and other gram-negative bloodstream infections caused by organisms such as *Klebsiella* spp. and *P. aeruginosa* are subject to mandatory reporting and reduction targets. A significant proportion of these isolates are showing increasing resistance to antimicrobials, which makes recognition and reduction of risk factors very important in controlling their spread. Such gram-negative infections seem predominantly to originate in the community and are often associated with older age, dehydration and urinary tract problems. Examples include an elderly gentleman with an enlarged prostate that leads to repeated urinary tract infection and an elderly lady becoming dehydrated because she is not drinking due to anxiety about incontinence (PHE 2018b).

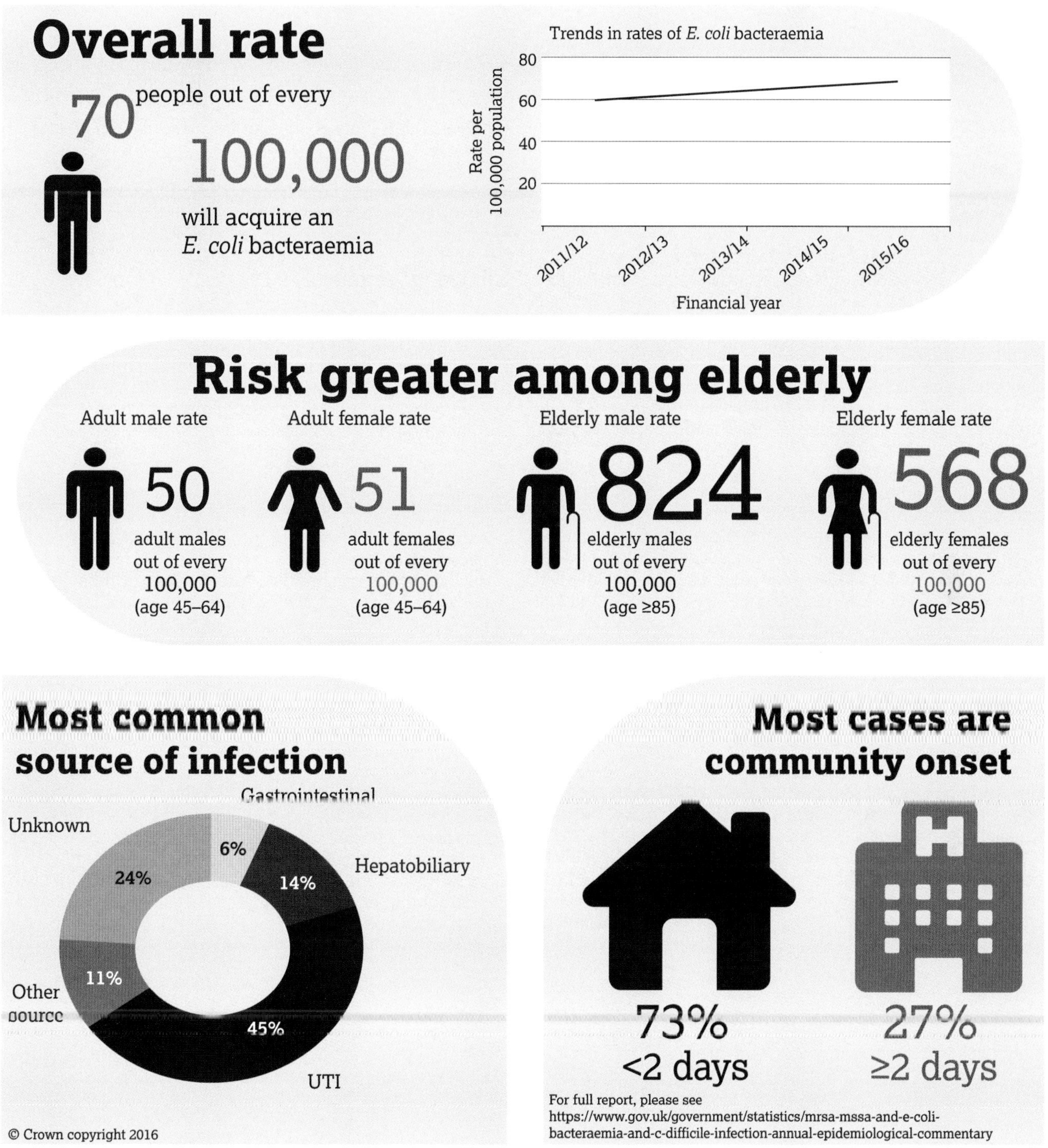

Figure 4.6 *E. coli* bacteraemia rates in England, 2015/2016. *Source*: NHS Improvement (2017). © Crown copyright.

Evidence-based approaches

With good infection prevention and control practice, many HCAIs can be prevented. This has been demonstrated by the significant reductions in MRSA bloodstream infection in English NHS hospitals between 2005 and 2018 (PHE 2018b, 2018c) and the dramatic fall in the number of cases of *C. difficile* infection in England (PHE 2018b, 2018d). These reductions were achieved via the systematic application and monitoring of established practices for the prevention and control of infection, including diligent hand hygiene and correct aseptic technique.

The use of effective infection prevention practices, including hand hygiene, environmental cleaning and care of invasive devices, leads to less cross-transmission, less infection, and less need for antimicrobials and other remedial treatments. It is therefore safer for patients and more cost-effective, and it contributes to reducing the burden of antimicrobial resistance.

Infection prevention and control underpins the clinical practices of all disciplines of healthcare and is fundamental to patient safety. As in other disciplines, robust evidence should underpin and improve practice and be used to ensure patients are receiving optimal care. However, it is not always possible to carry out robust randomized controlled trials (RCTs) to evidence all interventions and in some cases it is very difficult to ascertain which of several interventions implemented concurrently has made a difference. For instance, in early evidence on the importance of hand hygiene, a paper describing a *S. aureus* outbreak in a neonatal unit in the

1960s (Mortimer et al. 1962) demonstrated that babies who were cared for by nurses who were instructed not to wash their hands after coming into contact with a baby who was colonized with *S. aureus* were more likely to acquire the organism than infants cared for by nurses who used the antiseptic hexachlorophene to clean their hands between contact with each baby. This controlled study provided strong evidence that hand washing with an antiseptic agent between patient contact reduces transmission of healthcare-associated pathogens; however, it has never been repeated due to the obvious ethical drawbacks. Hand hygiene must be accepted as good practice on the basis of the results of a multitude of non-RCT studies (Pittet et al. 2000) and experience.

The published studies relating to infection prevention are mostly a mixture of RCTs, cohort studies, case studies, time series intervention analyses, surveillance and feedback, observation and an element of common sense. In many cases, a change may be one of several elements tried at the same time and much of the early evidence was derived from outbreak studies, in which a number of interventions were implemented simultaneously. This 'multimodal' type of study can lead to a situation where it can be difficult to pinpoint which individual measures have made the difference or have been the most beneficial.

One of the most favoured means of presenting best practice is in the form of 'care bundles'. It can even be argued that a set of measures implemented during an outbreak comprises an 'outbreak bundle'. A care bundle is a group of evidence-based interventions that have been put together to be practised consistently with the intention that if all the elements are undertaken together, a particular outcome will occur – or, in the case of infection prevention, will not occur. The bundle normally consists of around five elements, each of which have robust evidence indicating that, if they are implemented reliably, for every patient, on every occasion, they will result in the most benefit of all possible interventions (Rochon et al. 2017).

One of the earliest and most influential bundles was presented in a paper by Pronovost et al. (2006). It described the consistent application of an evidence-based bundle of interventions that demonstrated a sustained reduction in catheter-related bloodstream infection rates across the whole state of Michigan.

In the UK, in 2005 the Department of Health issued Saving Lives, which is a package of 'high impact interventions'. This bundle was put together to reduce infection in key target areas including peripheral vascular devices, central vascular access devices, urinary catheters, surgical wound infection, ventilator-associated pneumonia and nasogastric feeding. The tools were reviewed and reissued by the Infection Prevention Society in 2017. The suite of tools covers:

- prevention of ventilator-associated pneumonia
- prevention of infections associated with peripheral vascular access devices
- prevention of infections associated with central venous access devices
- prevention of surgical site infection
- prevention of infections in chronic wounds
- prevention of urinary-catheter-associated infections
- promotion of stewardship in antimicrobial prescribing.

Clinical governance

Hygiene Code

Infection prevention and control in England is underpinned by the Health and Social Care Act (2008), which has been summarized in a separate code of practice (DH 2015a). Known as the Hygiene Code, this mandates a set of responsibilities to healthcare providers including hospitals, general practitioners, dentists and care homes. This legislation is monitored and enforced by the Care Quality Commission (CQC), which assesses care providers against the requirements of the Code during periodic inspections. Each provider must be registered with the CQC and declare compliance with the 10 criteria of the Hygiene Code. These criteria are summarized in Table 4.5.

All healthcare organizations are required to appoint a senior manager to the role of 'director of infection prevention and control', or DIPC (DH 2003). This person must have the seniority to be able to influence the board of directors to ensure that infection prevention is accorded the highest priority.

All but the smallest healthcare providers should have (or have access to) an infection prevention and control team, who will advise on day-to-day aspects of infection prevention. The team will usually consist of one or more nurses trained in infection prevention along with a consultant microbiologist or infection control doctor and an antimicrobial pharmacist. Some teams will have additional staff working in audit, surveillance, or data collection and analysis. The role of the infection prevention and control team is varied but principally involves providing advice, education and support to healthcare professionals, caregivers and the wider organization to ensure patient and staff safety is maintained and risks are minimized.

Table 4.5 The Hygiene Code

1	Systems to manage and monitor the prevention and control of infection. These systems use risk assessments and consider the susceptibility of service users and any risks that their environment and other users may pose to them.
2	Provide and maintain a clean and appropriate environment in managed premises that facilitates the prevention and control of infections.
3	Ensure appropriate antimicrobial use to optimize patient outcomes and to reduce the risk of adverse events and antimicrobial resistance.
4	Provide suitable accurate information on infections to service users, their visitors and any person concerned with providing further support or nursing/medical care in a timely fashion.
5	Ensure prompt identification of people who have or are at risk of developing an infection so that they receive timely and appropriate treatment to reduce the risk of transmitting infection to other people.
6	Systems to ensure that all care workers (including contractors and volunteers) are aware of and discharge their responsibilities in the process of preventing and controlling infection.
7	Provide or secure adequate isolation facilities.
8	Secure adequate access to laboratory support as appropriate.
9	Have and adhere to policies, designed for the individual's care and provider organizations that will help to prevent and control infections.
10	Providers have a system in place to manage the occupational health needs and obligations of staff in relation to infection.

Source: DH (2015a). © Crown copyright.

Table 4.6 Legislation significant to healthcare infection control policy

Legislation	Coverage
Control of Substances Hazardous to Health (COSHH) (HSE 2002)	Introduced to prevent or reduce healthcare worker exposure to potentially harmful substances. The guidance includes the need to identify hazards, risk assess the potential for harm, if possible remove the harm, and where needed provide measures to reduce the level of harm. This includes the need to provide suitable equipment, training and where necessary health surveillance. The COSHH regulations have forced changes in areas such as endoscopy, where previously harmful chemicals (such as gluteraldehyde) were used with little control. Modern endoscopy units use safer chemicals in special automated processors to significantly reduce the potential for harm to users.
Health Building Note 00-09: Infection Control in the Built Environment (DH 2013c)	Provides guidance on infection prevention measures for new buildings and refurbishments. Includes guidance on finishes, layout and fittings. Should be read in conjunction with other health building notes (HBNs) for specific facilities, such as Health Building Note 04-01 Supplement 1: Isolation Facilities for Infectious Patients in Acute Settings (DH 2013d).
Legionnaires' Disease: The Control of Legionella Bacteria in Water Systems – Approved Code of Practice and Guidance (HSE 2013a)	Sets out the requirements of employers to control legionella, including identifying and assessing sources of risk; preparing a scheme to prevent or control risk; implementing, managing and monitoring precautions; keeping records of precautions; and appointing a responsible manager.
Water Systems: Health Technical Memorandum 04-01 Addendum – *Pseudomonas aeruginosa* – Advice for Augmented Care Units (DH 2013a)	Concerned with controlling or minimizing the risk of morbidity and mortality due to *Pseudomonas aeruginosa* associated with contaminated water outlets. Guidance is provided on assessing the risk to patients, and the document offers remedial actions to take when a water system becomes contaminated with *P. aeruginosa*, including protocols for sampling, testing and monitoring water. It also offers advice on forming a water safety group and developing water safety plans. This guidance came about in response to an outbreak in Belfast where three babies died and several others were infected via water contamination with *P. aeruginosa* (Wise 2012).
Health Technical Memorandum 07-01: Safe Management of Healthcare Waste (DH 2013b)	Sets out the necessary handling of waste to reduce harm to people and the environment.
Food Safety Act (1990)	Sets out regulations for the safe handling and preparation of food

Professional responsibility

In England, nurses must be aware of the measures that are in place in their workplace to ensure compliance with the Hygiene Code. For example, many hospital trusts have a programme of regular visits to clinical areas by senior staff, who carry out inspections against the criteria of the Code as if they were external assessors. This programme ensures that senior staff are familiar with the Code and that everyone is familiar with the inspection process. In addition, nurses may need to carry out activities to promote compliance and provide evidence of assurance, such as audits of hand hygiene performance or compliance with aseptic technique. One such set of audits in place in many hospitals in England is the aforementioned Saving Lives (Infection Prevention Society 2017). Audits are discussed in more detail in the section below on environmental hygiene and the management of waste in the healthcare environment.

Other legal and professional issues

In England, the Health and Safety at Work etc. Act (1974) is the primary piece of legislation relating to the safety of people in the workplace. It applies to all employees and employers, and requires them to do everything that is reasonable and practicable to prevent harm coming to anyone in the workplace. It requires employers to provide training and appropriate protective equipment, and it requires employees to follow the training that they have received, use the protective equipment provided, and report any situations where they believe inadequate precautions are putting anyone's health and safety at serious risk.

The Nursing and Midwifery Council's *Code* (NMC 2018) states that all nurses must work within the limits of their competence. This means, for example, not carrying out aseptic procedures without being competent and confident that this can be done without increasing the risk of introducing infection through lack of knowledge or technique.

In addition to healthcare-specific requirements, items of legislation and regulation have been devised with the objective of reducing the risk of infection; these apply to healthcare as much as they do to any other business or workplace. These include legislation and regulation relating to food hygiene (Food Safety Act 1990), water quality (Water Supply (Water Quality) Regulations 2016), waste management (Waste (England and Wales) Regulations 2011) and other issues that are peripheral to healthcare but must be taken into account when developing policies and procedures for an NHS trust or other healthcare provider. The relevant regulations are summarized in Table 4.6.

Hand hygiene

Definition

Hand hygiene, or hand decontamination as it is also called, is the process used to render the hands physically clean with a reduced microbial load. Hand hygiene may involve the use of soap and water to wash the hands, principally to remove organic soiling, and/or the use of an alcohol-based hand sanitizer, which if applied correctly will remove most micro-organisms (Boyce et al. 2002, Gold and Avva 2018, NHS England and NHSI 2019, Pittet et al. 2000).

Related theory

Hand hygiene is generally accepted as a cornerstone of good infection prevention and so it is essential that wherever care is provided, there are accessible and appropriate facilities for hand hygiene (WHO 2009a). The hands of healthcare workers are a common cause of transmission of micro-organisms between patients and are frequently implicated as the route of transmission in HCAIs (Moolenaar et al. 2000, Mortimer et al. 1962, Pittet et al. 2000, Sax et al. 2007). Transient micro-organisms (bacteria, fungi and viruses) are organisms located on the surface of the skin and beneath the superficial cell of the stratum corneum. The subungual regions of the nails harbour the majority of the micro-organisms found on the hands (AORN 1997, Hedderwick et al. 2000, McNeil et al. 2001). They are acquired from and transfer easily to the animate (patient) and inanimate environments during contact activities. Damaged skin, moisture, false nails and jewellery increase the possibility of colonization with transient micro-organisms (McNeil et al. 2001). Both microbial load and type depend upon the prevalence of micro-organisms in the environment and on the activities being undertaken by healthcare workers. Hands have been found to be contaminated after general ward-based activities including bed making, handling curtains and patients' clothing, and washing materials, and after sluice room activities. Transient micro-organisms, unlike resident bacteria, can easily be removed from the hand surface via effective hand hygiene (Boyce et al. 2002).

There are three main levels of hand hygiene:

1 Hand washing is the process for the physical removal of soil (dirt, blood, body fluids and transient micro-organisms) from the hands (e.g. after using the lavatory or before preparing a meal) using ordinary liquid soap and water. In the clinical setting it should be performed as per the '5 Moments' (discussed below) (Sax et al. 2007, WHO 2009a).
2 Aseptic hand decontamination or hand antisepsis is the destruction of micro-organisms on the hands (e.g. prior to a dressing procedure). If carrying out an aseptic procedure, an antiseptic soap may be used as an alternative to ordinary soap (but it is not essential). This will contain a disinfectant such as chlorhexidine or povidone-iodine. Alternatively, it is very acceptable to wash with ordinary soap and water, dry hands and then apply alcohol-based handrub.
3 Surgical scrub aims to remove dirt and organic matter, kill transient micro-organisms, and reduce the numbers of resident and transient bacteria on the skin prior to surgery. Surgical scrub technique may be carried out using antiseptic soap or approved alcohol-based handrubs. Antiseptic handwash solutions such as chlorhexidine gluconate or povidone-iodine solution should be used with an appropriate technique and for a minimum of 3 minutes as part of surgical preparation. Approved alcohol-based products may be used on physically clean hands for a 90-second scrub.

Taylor (1978) noted that some nurses could wash their hands for a long time but not cover all the surfaces, whereas others could cover all the surfaces within 30 seconds (Figure 4.7). A six-step hand hygiene technique to cover all areas of the skin was first described by Ayliffe et al. (1978) to test the efficacy of different hand disinfectants. The technique has been adopted by the World Health Organization (WHO) (2009a) as standard and is used worldwide; however, more recently some have queryied whether a three-stage technique would be more practical, especially for the use of alcohol-based handrub (Tschudin-Sutter et al. 2017).

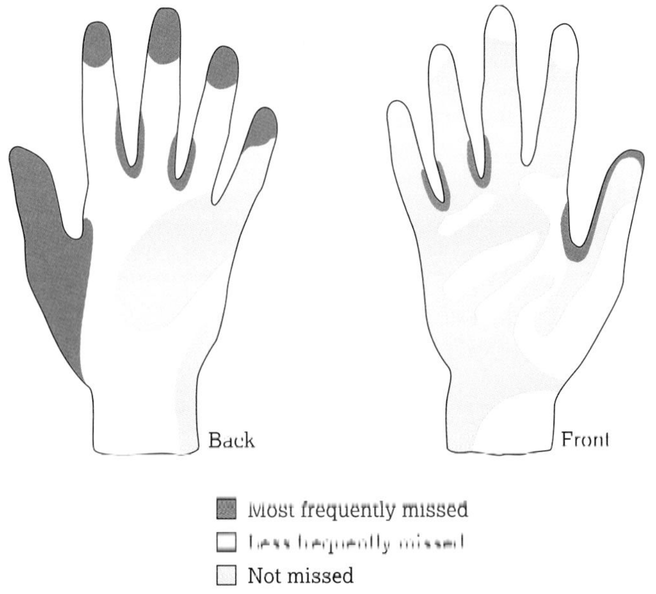

Figure 4.7 Taylor's work in 1978 showed the areas most commonly missed following hand washing – in particular, the thumbs, especially on the dominant hand and in between the fingers. *Source*: Reproduced from Taylor (1978) with permission of EMAP Publishing Ltd.

Evidence-based approaches

The key considerations for hand hygiene are: when should hands be decontaminated, what with and how? The WHO uses the concept of 'My 5 Moments for Hand Hygiene' as a means to focus hand hygiene where it matters – at the point of patient contact (Sax et al. 2007) (Figure 4.8). The WHO describes the 'patient zone' as an imaginary line around the patient. The patient zone is not necessarily a bed or chair; it is wherever the patient is. The WHO then describes the opportunities for hand hygiene within the patient zone. These are:

- *Moment 1*: Entering the patient zone before patient contact.
- *Moment 2*: Carrying out a clean or aseptic procedure.
- *Moment 3*: Handling blood or body fluids.
- *Moment 4*: Leaving the patient zone after patient contact.
- *Moment 5*: After contact with the patient's immediate environment.

Bare below the elbows

In order to facilitate effective hand hygiene it is expected that all healthcare workers should be 'bare below the elbows' when giving patient care (NICE 2017). This involves wearing short-sleeved clothing, not having false nails or nail varnish, and removing all wrist and hand jewellery to allow effective hand hygiene up to and including the wrists (DH 2010a). A plain, smooth metal ring is usually acceptable; however, it should be moveable to ensure decontamination and drying underneath (NHS England and NHSI 2019). There is some debate as to whether it is necessary to be bare below the elbows in a clinical area if not giving care. This may be acceptable in some organizations for non-uniformed staff if they are having no direct patient contact – for example, a ward clerk sat at a desk, or staff visiting other staff in offices on the ward. However, ideally everyone entering a ward should be able to easily decontaminate their hands and this is best facilitated by being bare below the elbows.

Pre-procedural considerations

Equipment

Hand hygiene equipment

Clinical handwash basins

Clinical handwash basins (CHBs) (Figure 4.9) should be available in sufficient numbers such that a healthcare worker does not have to walk too far to decontaminate the hands. In a hospital, a CHB would be expected for roughly every 4–6 beds. While it is important to have an appropriate number of CHBs to allow easy access to hand washing, it should be noted that if they are poorly sited and underutilized they may become a risk for infection. This is because organisms such as *Legionella pneumophilia* can build up in underused pipework – a so-called 'dead leg'. Any water outlet that is not in regular use should be flushed at least twice a week to reduce this risk. Consideration should be given to removal (back to the circulating pipework) of any underused outlets. In some circumstances, point-of-use filters may be employed to ensure water leaving the tap is clean (Garvey et al. 2010, Vonberg et al. 2005).

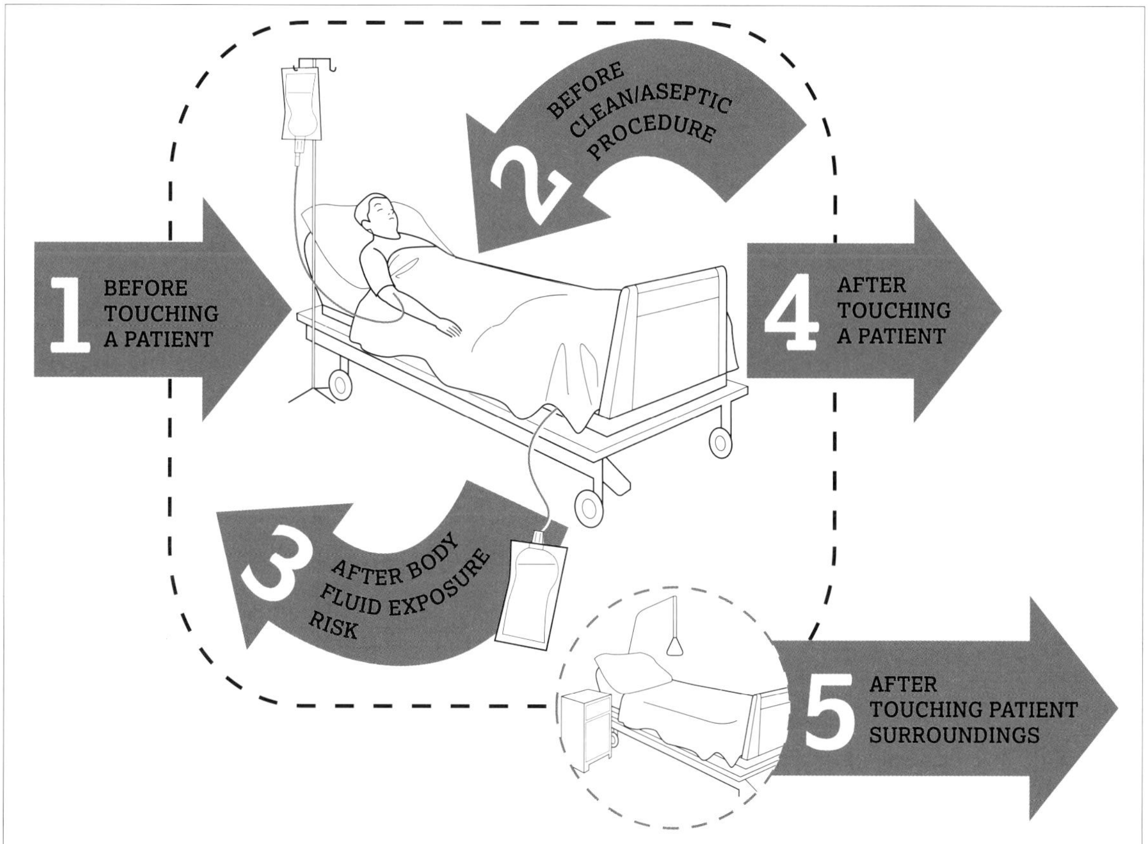

Figure 4.8 'My 5 Moments for Hand Hygiene'. *Source:* Reproduced from Sax et al. (2007) with permission of Elsevier.

CHBs should be used solely by clinical staff for hand hygiene. They should have taps that can be turned on and off without using the hands; that is, they should be non-touch or lever operated (NHS England and NHSI 2019). They should not have plugs (to encourage hand washing under running water) or overflows. Water should be able to drain freely and quickly to discourage growth of microbes from drains (Aranega-Bou et al. 2019, Walker and Moore 2015). CHBs should not be used for the disposal of wash water, intravenous fluids, drugs or beverages as this encourages the growth of harmful organisms such as *Pseudomonas aeruginosa* (Garvey et al. 2018, Kotay et al. 2017, Loveday et al. 2014a). Basins that are also used by patients may require plugs, which will require careful management with some client groups to reduce the risk of flooding. In all cases, the taps should be positioned so that water does not fall directly into the outflow as this may lead to splashes containing organisms from within the drain, which has been implicated in outbreaks of infection (Aranega-Bou et al. 2019, Walker et al. 2014, Wise 2012). Taps should be of a mixer type that allows the temperature to be set before hand washing starts. Access to basins must be unobstructed by any furniture or equipment to ensure that they can easily be accessed whenever required.

Liquid soap dispensers

Liquid soap dispensers should be positioned close to handwash basins and care should be taken to ensure that soap cannot drip onto the floor from the dispenser and cause a slip hazard. Soap should be simple and unscented to minimize the risk of adverse reactions from frequent use. There is no advantage to using soap or detergents containing antimicrobial agents for routine hand washing. Antiseptic preparations may carry a higher risk of adverse reactions. Bar soap should not be used as the wet bar can grow micro-organisms between uses. For surgical scrub or hand antisepsis, the most commonly used preparations contain either chlorhexidine or povidone-iodine; both reduce bacterial counts significantly but chlorhexidine has a residual effect that may reduce rapid regrowth.

Paper towel dispensers

A paper towel dispenser should be fixed to the wall close to each handwash basin. Hand towels should be of adequate quality to ensure that hands are completely dried by the proper use of one or two towels. To conveniently dispose of these towels, a suitable bin with a pedal-operated lid should be positioned close to the basin, but not so that it obstructs access to the basin (WHO 2009a).

Alcohol-based hand sanitizers

Alcohol-based hand sanitizers should be available at the point of care in every clinical area for use immediately before care and between different care activities on the same patient. Dispensers may be attached to the patient's bed or bedside locker, and free-standing pump-top bottles can be used where appropriate, such as on the desk in a room used for outpatient clinics. Dispensers should not be sited close to sinks unless this is unavoidable because of the risk of confusion with soap and the risk of adding organic material to the drains (Kotay et al. 2017). Smaller sized personal-issue bottles are appropriate where there is a risk that alcohol-based handrub may be accidentally or deliberately drunk, such as in paediatric areas or when caring for a patient with alcohol dependency (NPSA 2008).

Pharmacological support

Hand washing is a mechanical process and it is the combination of rubbing and friction to generate a lather that removes dirt, debris and micro-organisms, rather than any 'antiseptic' in the soap. Hands should be washed only with soaps that are designed for hand washing. In a hospital there will usually be one approved brand that meets the European Norms: EN1499 for soap or EN1500

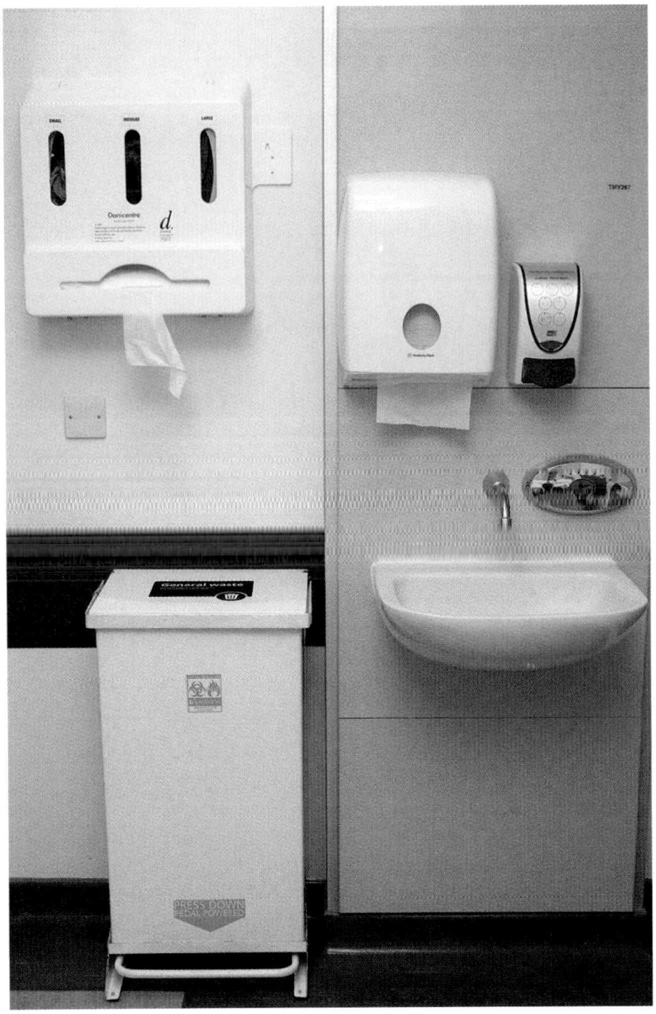

Figure 4.9 Clinical handwash basin.

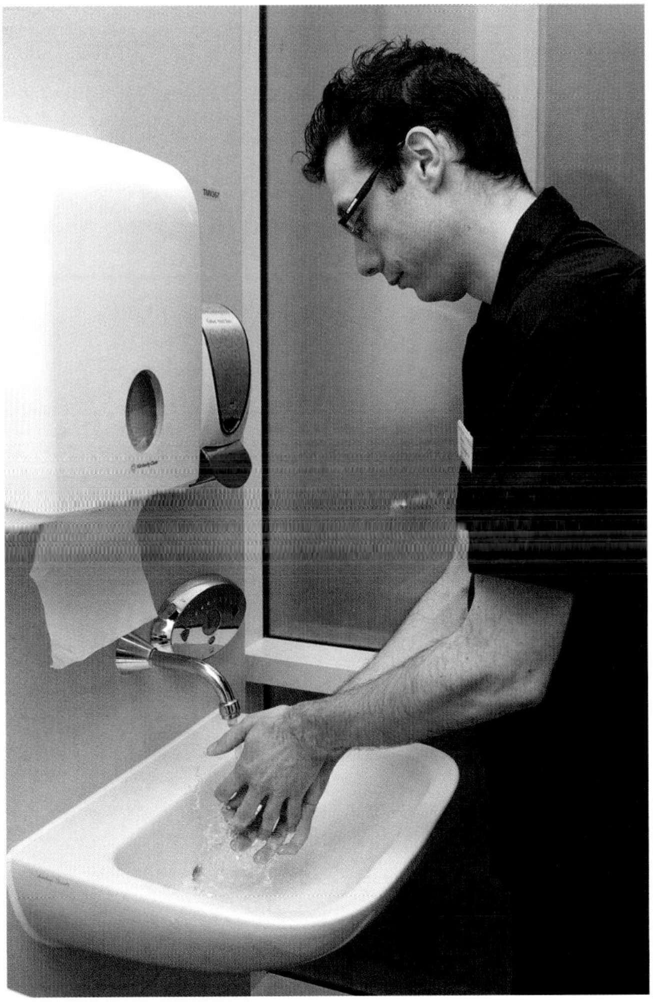

Figure 4.10 Correct position to wash hands.

for surgical hand preparation. The products will usually be unperfumed and hypoallergenic. In a patient's home, a healthcare worker should use any reasonable handwash soap provided.

Detergents

Detergents are surfactants designed to remove organic soiling, including grease, from a surface. They do not specifically kill micro-organisms but may remove them as part of the mechanical action of the process of washing. There are many different types of detergent for use on different surfaces, from washing-up liquid to soap designed for washing hands and keeping skin soft.

Alcohol-based handrub

Alcohol-based handrub may be considered the gold standard for hand hygiene and is recommended for use in most circumstances except if hands are visibly soiled or when caring for patients with vomiting or diarrhoeal illness (Gold and Avva 2018, NHS England and NHSI 2019). This is because alcohol is not effective in the presence of organic soiling, against *C. difficile* spores or against non-enveloped viruses such as norovirus. When compared with soap and water hand washing, alcohol-based handrub is more effective at reducing bacteria on hands, causes less skin irritation, requires less time to use and can be made more easily accessible at the point of care (Boyce et al. 2002, Gold and Avva 2018, Voss and Widmer 1997). Antiseptic handrubs based on non-alcoholic antiseptics are available but evidence suggests that alcohol is the most useful agent in terms of the range and speed of antimicrobial activity (Rotter 2001, WHO 2009a).

Some alcohol-based handrubs may also be used for surgical scrub and there is evidence that they may have greater efficacy than either povidone-iodine or chlorhexidine-based traditional soap products (Kampf and Kramer 2004, NHS England and NHSI 2019, Widmer 2013).

Hand washing

Evidence-based approaches

Hand washing involves three important stages: preparation, washing and rinsing, and drying (NHS England and NHSI 2019).

Hands should always be wet under running tepid water before applying soap. This is to allow the soap to lather when the hands are rubbed together. It is the friction and the lather that removes the dirt and debris and moves the transient organisms to the surface so that they can be effectively rinsed away under the running water. Wetting also reduces the risk of skin irritation. The hands should be rubbed for between 15 and 30 seconds with particular attention paid to the thumbs and the tips of the fingers (Figure 4.10).

It is essential that hands are dried thoroughly after washing; this is because bacteria (especially gram negatives such as *E. coli*) can multiply on a wet surface, leaving hands contaminated. Good-quality paper towels are recommended in hospital settings (NHS England and NHSI 2019). Warm air dryers may be effective but are noisy in clinical areas and there are some concerns that they may increase the number of bacteria in the washroom and lead to them spreading (Best et al. 2018).

Hand care

Hands are used continually by healthcare workers, so it is important that they are maintained in a healthy condition. Dry, excoriated skin is more likely to shed micro-organisms to others and more likely to become contaminated, which may be harmful to the individual. Staff with acute or chronic skin lesions, conditions or reactions, or possible dermatitis, should seek advice from their local occupational health advisor.

Cuts and abrasions must be covered with a water-impermeable dressing prior to clinical contact. It is especially important that staff with skin lesions that cannot be adequately covered seek advice from the occupational health department as it may not be safe for them to work, especially if they are undertaking high-risk aseptic procedures (NICE 2017).

Skin damage and dryness often result from frequent use of harsh soap products, application of soap to dry hands, or inadequate rinsing of soap from the hands. It is essential that correct technique is used to minimize this risk. Alcohol-based sanitizer products may be better for the skin than repeated washing with soap and water, which can remove the skin's natural oils; this is because the alcohol-based products contain emollients, which are rubbed back into the hands as they are decontaminated.

Hand cream may help to prevent dry and chapped skin. This should be supplied from a dispenser or be for personal use, as communal jars may become contaminated and become a source of infection.

Procedure guideline 4.1 Hand washing

Essential equipment

- Handwash basin
- Liquid soap
- Paper towels
- Domestic waste bin

Action	Rationale
Pre-procedure	
1 Remove wristwatch, any rings and/or bracelets and roll up sleeves. *Note*: it is good practice to remove all hand and wrist jewellery and roll up sleeves before entering any clinical area, and the Department of Health has instructed NHS trusts to implement a 'bare below the elbows' dress code.	Jewellery inhibits good hand washing. Dirt and bacteria can remain beneath jewellery after hand washing. Long sleeves prevent washing of wrists and will easily become contaminated and so a route of transmission of micro-organisms (DH 2010b, **C**; WHO 2009a, **C**). Many organizations' dress codes allow staff to wear wedding rings while providing care. Although it can be argued that a smooth ring is less likely to retain dirt and bacteria than one with a stone or engraving, there is no evidence to suggest that wedding rings inhibit hand decontamination any longer than other rings. **E**
2 Cover cuts and abrasions on hands with waterproof dressings.	Cuts and abrasions can become contaminated with bacteria and cannot be easily cleaned. Repeated hand washing can worsen an injury (WHO 2009a, **C**). Breaks in the skin will allow the entry of potential pathogens. **E**
3 Remove nail varnish and artificial nails (most uniform policies and dress codes prohibit these). Nails must also be short and clean.	Long and false nails and imperfections in nail polish harbour dirt and bacteria that are not effectively removed by hand washing (WHO 2009a, **C**).
Procedure	
4 Turn on the taps and where possible direct the water flow away from the plughole. Run the water at a flow rate that prevents splashing.	The plughole and the associated waste are often contaminated with micro-organisms, which could be transferred to the environment or the user if splashing occurs (Aranega-Bou et al. 2019, **R**; Garvey et al. 2016, **C**).
5 Run the water to a comfortable temperature.	Warm water is more pleasant to wash with than cold so hand washing is more likely to be carried out effectively. **E** Water that is too hot could cause scalding (DH 2017, **C**).
6 Wet the surface of the hands and wrists.	Soap applied directly onto dry hands may damage the skin. The water will also quickly mix with the soap to speed up hand washing. **E**
7 Apply liquid soap and water to all surfaces of the hands.	Liquid soap is very effective in removing dirt, organic material and any loosely adherent transient flora. Tablets of soap can become contaminated, potentially transferring micro-organisms from one user to another, but may be used if liquid soap is unavailable (WHO 2009a, **C**). To ensure all surfaces of the hands are cleaned. **E**
8 Rub hands together for a minimum of 10–15 seconds, paying particular attention to between the fingers and the tips of the fingers and thumbs (**Action figure 8**). The areas that are most frequently missed through poor hand hygiene technique are shown in Figure 4.7.	To ensure all surfaces of the hands are cleaned. Areas that are missed can be a source of cross-infection (Fraise and Bradley 2009, **E**).

(continued)

Procedure guideline 4.1 Hand washing *(continued)*

Action	Rationale
9 Rinse soap off hands thoroughly.	Soap residue can lead to irritation and damage to the skin. Damaged skin does not provide a barrier to infection for the healthcare worker and can become colonized with potentially pathogenic bacteria, leading to cross-infection (DH 2017, **C**).
10 Turn off the taps using a wrist or elbow. If the taps are not lever-type, turn them off using a paper hand towel to prevent contact.	To avoid recontaminating hands. **E**
Post-procedure	
11 Dry hands thoroughly with a disposable paper towel from a towel dispenser.	Damp hands encourage the multiplication of bacteria and can become sore (DH 2017, **C**).
12 Dispose of used paper towels in a black bag in a foot-operated waste bin.	Paper towels used to dry the hands are normally non-hazardous and can be disposed of via the domestic waste stream (DH 2013b, **C**). Using a foot-operated waste bin prevents contamination of the hands. **E** Electric hand dryers are generally not recommended for use in clinical areas (Best et al. 2018, **E**)

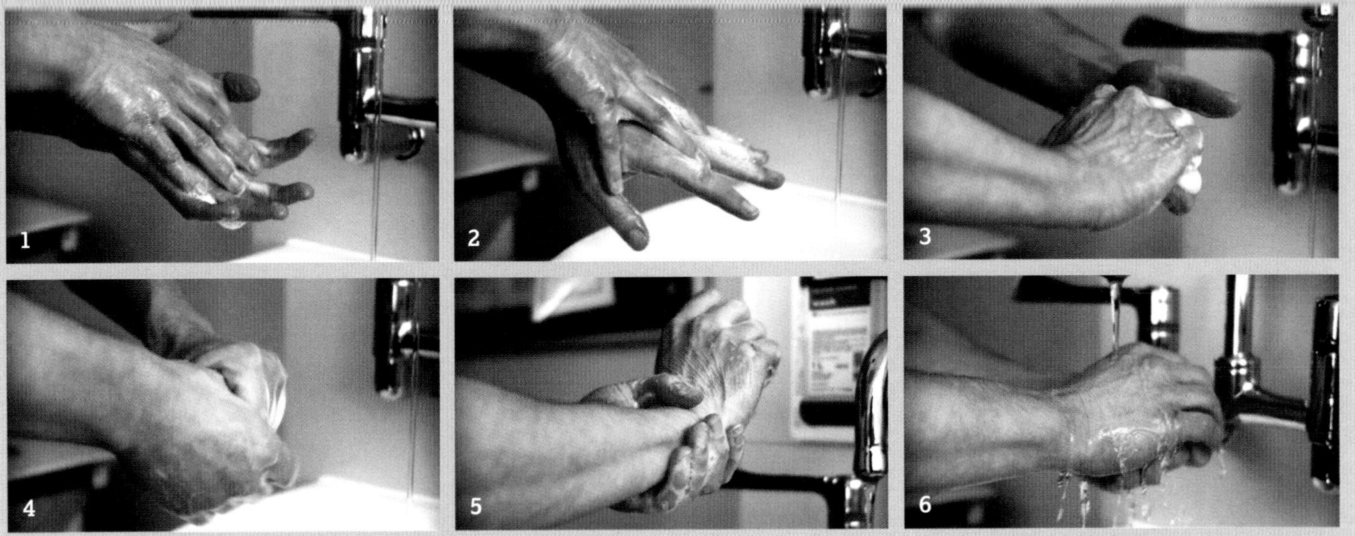

Action Figure 8 (1) Rub hands palm to palm. (2) Rub the back of each hand with the palm of the other hand with fingers interlaced. (3) Rub palm to palm with fingers interlaced. Rub with the backs of the fingers against the opposing palms with fingers interlocked. Rub the tips of the fingers. Rub the tips of the fingers in the opposite palm in a circular motion. (4) Rub each thumb clasped in the opposite hand using a rotational movement. (5) Rub each wrist with the opposite hand. (6) Rinse hands with water.

Use of alcohol-based handrub

Evidence-based approaches

Alcohol-based handrub should be applied in a sufficient quantity to physically clean hands. It should be rubbed into all surfaces until it has evaporated and the hands are dry (NHS England and NHSI 2019).

Procedure guideline 4.2 Hand decontamination using an alcohol-based handrub

Essential equipment

- Alcohol-based handrub

Action	Rationale
Procedure	
1 Dispense the amount of alcohol-based handrub indicated in the manufacturer's instructions into the palm of one hand. If hands are large, a greater amount may be needed to ensure coverage.	Too much handrub will take longer to dry and may consequently cause delays; too little will not decontaminate hands adequately. **E**

2 Rub the alcohol-based handrub into all areas of the hands until the hands are dry, using the illustrated actions in **Action figure 2**.	To ensure all areas of the hands are decontaminated. Alcohol is a rapid-acting disinfectant with the added advantage that it evaporates, leaving the hands dry. This prevents contamination of equipment while facilitating the application of gloves (WHO 2009a, **C**).

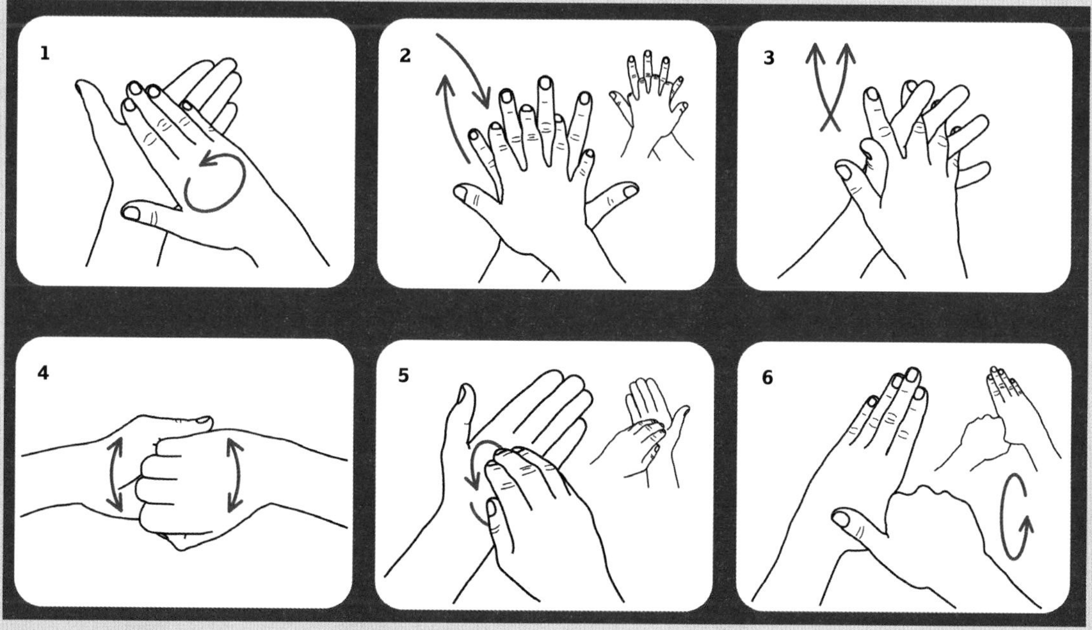

Action Figure 2 Alcohol-based handrub hand hygiene technique for visibly clean hands. After applying a palmful of the product in a cupped hand. (1) rub hands palm to palm. (2) Rub right palm over left dorsum with interlaced fingers and vice versa. (3) Rub palm to palm with fingers interlaced. (4) Rub the backs of the fingers against the opposing palms with fingers interlocked. (5) Rub rotationally, backwards and forwards, with clasped fingers of right hand in left palm and vice versa. (6) Rub rotationally with the left thumb clasped in the right palm and vice versa. *Source*: Reproduced from Stewardson et al. (2014). https://journals.plos.org/plosone/article?id=10.1371/journal.pone.0105866. Licensed under CC BY 4.0.

Surgical hand antisepsis

Evidence-based approaches

Surgical hand antisepsis is the antiseptic surgical scrub or antiseptic handrub performed before donning sterile attire preoperatively. The aim is to reduce the number of resident and transient flora to a minimum and also to inhibit their regrowth for as long as possible, not just on the hands but also on the wrists and forearms (AfPP 2017).

Surgical hand antisepsis can be performed using an approved antiseptic surgical scrub such as chlorhexidine gluconate or povidone-iodine, or an approved alcohol-based handrub. There is evidence that alcohol-based handrub is favourable over soap and water as it has a wide spectrum of activity and better dermal tolerance, and removes the risk of contamination from rinse water (NHS England and NHSI 2019). The practitioner should choose between use of soap and water or alcohol-based handrub as the two procedures should not be combined.

Whichever cleansing agent is used, the hands should be physically clean prior to surgical antisepsis, so any dirt should be removed from the skin or under the nails using ordinary soap and water and a nail pick before entering the theatre (Box 4.2).

Box 4.2 Key steps before starting surgical hand preparation

- Keep nails short and pay attention to them when washing hands – most microbes on hands come from beneath the fingernails.
- Do not wear artificial nails or nail polish.
- Remove all jewellery (rings, watches and bracelets) before entering the operating theatre.
- Wash hands and arms with a non-medicated soap before entering the operating theatre area or if hands are visibly soiled.
- Clean subungual areas with a nail file. Preferably nailbrushes should not be used as they may damage the skin and encourage shedding of cells. If used, nailbrushes must be sterile and single use. Reusable autoclavable nail brushes are available.

Source: Adapted from WHO (2009a).

The principle behind surgical hand antisepsis is to clean the skin thoroughly, moving from the cleanest part (the hands) to the least clean part (the forearm). The procedure should be carried out immediately prior to gowning and gloving for a surgical intervention (AfPP 2017). Each step consists of five strokes rubbing backwards and forwards (AfPP 2017). Hands and forearms should be washed for the length of time recommended by the manufacturer of the alcohol-based handrub or antimicrobial antiseptic solution (WHO 2009a).

Procedure guideline 4.3 Surgical scrub technique using soap and water

Essential equipment

- Surgical scrub sink or handwash basin with sufficient space available under the outlet to allow easy rinsing of hands and forearms
- Antimicrobial antiseptic solution
- Sterile towels
- Domestic waste bin

Optional equipment

- Scrubbing brushes – but note that WHO (2009a) guidelines recommend that scrubbing brushes should only be used for nails and are *not* to be used directly on the skin as they may damage the skin and encourage the shedding of cells (including bacteria)

Action	Rationale
Pre-procedure	
1 Remove any rings, bracelets and wristwatches, and roll up sleeves before entering the operating theatre suite or procedure area. *Note*: most organizations will require staff entering operating theatres to change into 'scrubs'.	To ensure good hand washing as jewellery inhibits this. Dirt and bacteria can remain beneath jewellery after hand washing. Long sleeves prevent washing of wrists and will easily become contaminated ([illegible], **C**; WHO 2009a, **C**).
2 If the skin is damaged with cuts or abrasions, advice should be sought from occupational health as it may not be advisable to proceed with surgical hand antisepsis.	Cuts and abrasions can become contaminated with bacteria and cannot be easily cleaned. Repeated hand washing can worsen an injury. Breaks in the skin will allow the entry of potential pathogens (WHO 2009a, **C**).
3 Remove nail varnish and artificial nails (most uniform policies and dress codes prohibit these). Nails must also be short and clean. Clean beneath the nails using a pick or brush if needed.	Long and false nails and imperfections in nail polish harbour dirt and bacteria that are not effectively removed by hand washing (WHO 2009a, **C**). The area under the nails may harbour dirt and micro-organisms not easily removed by the other stages of the procedure (WHO 2009a, **C**).
Procedure	
4 Turn on the taps and where possible direct the water flow away from the plughole. Run the water at a flow rate that prevents splashing.	Plugholes are often contaminated with micro-organisms, which could be transferred to the environment or the user if splashing occurs (Aranega-Bou et al. 2019, **E**; British Standards Institution 2014, **C**).
5 Run the water until warm.	Warm water is more pleasant to wash with than cold so hand washing is more likely to be carried out effectively. **E** Water that is too hot could cause scalding. **E**
6 Ensuring no part of the sink or taps is touched, wet the surface of the hands, wrists and forearms up to the elbow, working in one direction only from the fingertips to the elbow, keeping the hands higher than the elbows.	Soap applied directly onto dry hands may damage the skin. The water will also quickly mix with the soap to speed up hand washing. **E**
7 Wash the hands again from the hand to the middle of the forearm and then wash from the hand to the wrist area.	As the hand moves up the arm, it may become contaminated. By washing after cleaning to the elbow, this risk of contamination is reduced. **C**
8 Apply appropriate antiseptic soap to all surfaces of the hands in one downwards stroke. Work into the hands palm to palm and then all the areas of the hands and arms just below the elbows as outlined in the following steps.	Liquid soap is very effective at removing dirt, organic material and any loosely adherent transient flora. The bactericidal additive contributes to the reduction in the number of bacteria. Chlorhexidine has a residual effect to prevent regrowth of bacteria for a period after hand decontamination (WHO 2009a, **C**).

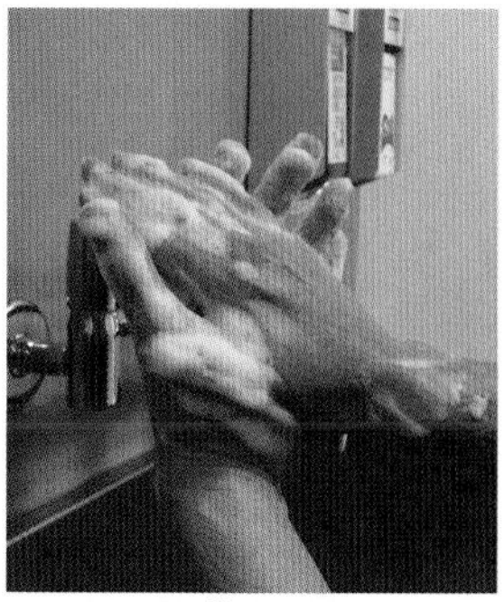

Step 1

Wet hands and forearms. Apply the specified amount of appropriate solution, according to the manufacturer's recommendations, from dispenser (one downward stroke action). Work into hands palm to palm, and then encompass all areas of the hands and arms to just below the elbows as shown in steps 2–9. Perform the same manoeuvres if using alcohol-based handrub but without water and rinsing.

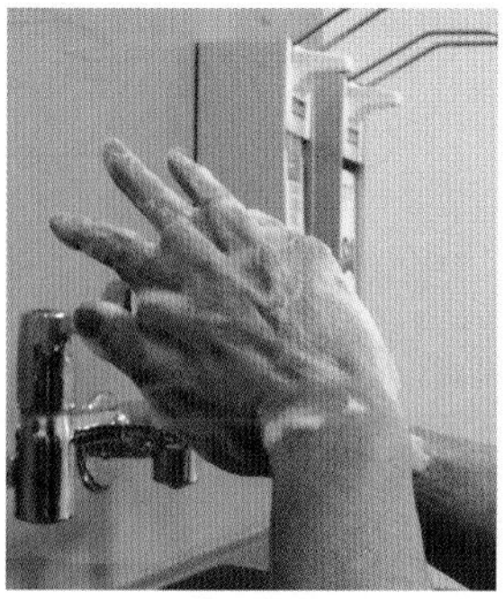

Step 2

Rub with right palm over back of left and vice versa with fingers interlaced.

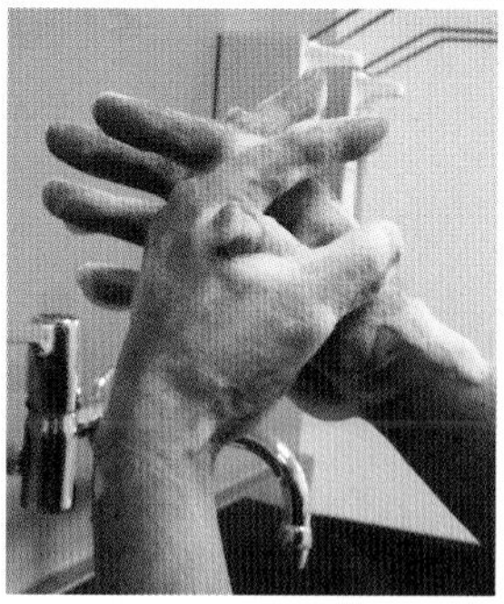

Step 3

Rub palm to palm, fingers interlaced.

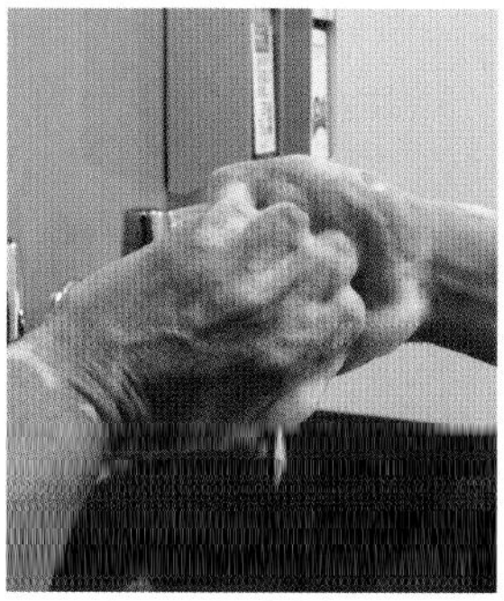

Step 4

Rotational rubbing backwards and forwards with clasped fingers of right hand into left palm and vice versa.

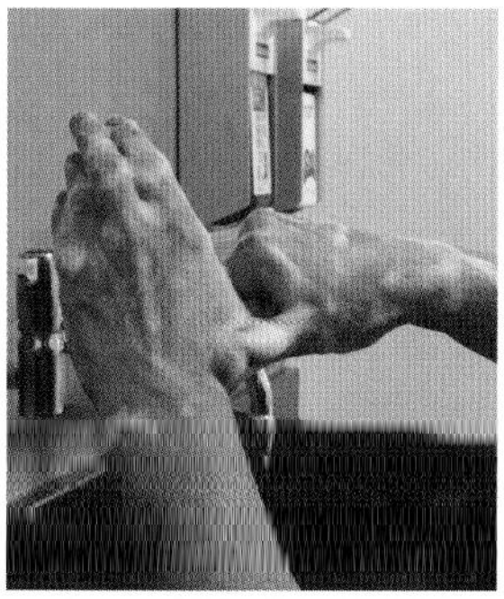

Step 5

Rotational rubbing of right thumb clasped in left hand and vice versa.

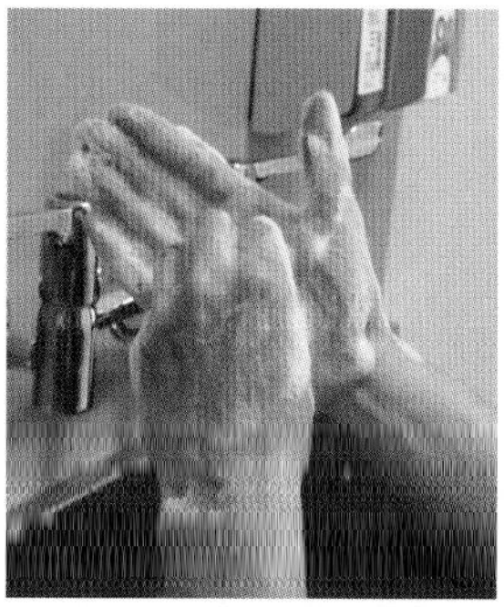

Step 6

Rub finger tips on palms for both hands.

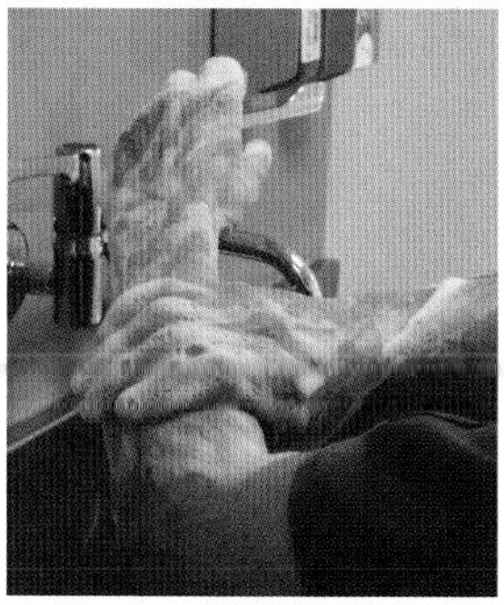

Step 7

Continue with rotating action down opposing arms, working to just below the elbows; do not move back towards the wrist. If using alcohol-based handrub an additional dose may be required here, one for each arm.

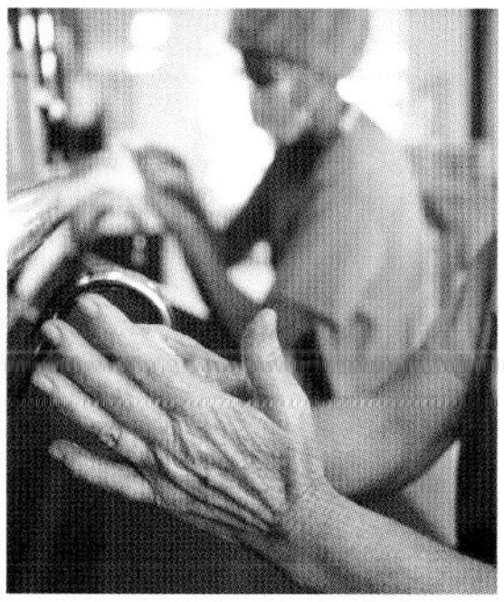

Step 8

Rinse and repeat steps 1–7 keeping hands raised above elbows at all times. **This wash should now only cover two thirds of the forearms to avoid compromising cleanliness of hands.** Local policy may include repeating these steps a third time but to wrists only.

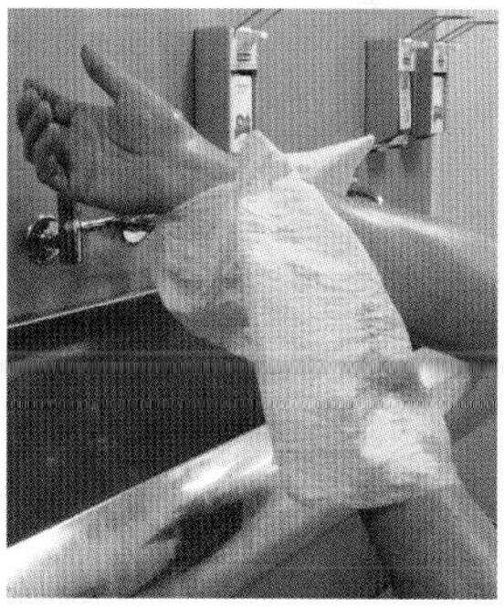

Step 9: ending scrub

If using a solution, rinse hands under running water; clean to dirty area. Turn off tap using elbows if necessary. Open gown pack onto a clean surface and take a hand towel. Hands are dried first by placing the opposite hand behind the towel and blotting the skin, then, using a corkscrew movement, drying from hand to elbow; do not move back down towards wrist. Discard towel. Using a second towel, repeat the process on other hand and forearm before discarding.

If using alcohol-based handrub, allow hands and forearms to dry completely before donning sterile gloves (WHO 2009, 2016).

Action Figure 10 Surgical hand antisepsis. *Source*: Adapted from AfPP (2017) with permission of the Association for Perioperative Practice.

(continued)

Procedure guideline 4.3 Surgical scrub technique using soap and water *(continued)*

Action	Rationale
9 Wash the hands again from the hand to the middle of the forearm and then wash from the hand to the wrist area.	As the hand moves up the arm, it may become contaminated. By washing after cleaning to the elbow, this risk of contamination is reduced. **C**
10 Wash the hands following the steps below: • right palm over back of left and vice versa with fingers interlaced (**Action figure 10**, step two) • rub palm to palm with fingers interlaced (step three) • rotational rubbing backwards and forwards with clasped fingers of right hand into left palm and vice versa (step four) • rotational rubbing of right thumb clasped in left hand and vice versa (step five) • rub finger tips on palms of opposite hands (step six) • continue with rotating action down opposing arms, working to just below the elbows; do not move back to the wrist (step seven). All steps should be carried out thoroughly on both the left and right hands and arms. The scrub procedure should take a minimum of 2–5 minutes, depending on local guidelines (AfPP 2017).	To cover all areas of the skin and prevent bacteria-laden soap and water from contaminating the hands (WHO 2009a, **C**). To prevent recontaminating areas already covered (AfPP 2017, **C**).
11 Rinse hands and arms thoroughly from fingertips to elbows, keeping the hands above the elbows at all times. Avoid passing the hands back and forth through the water.	To avoid recontaminating the hands with water that has been used to clean the arms (WHO 2009a, **C**).
12 At all times take care not to splash water onto clothing.	To avoid contamination. **C**
Post-procedure	
13 Dry hands thoroughly with a sterile paper towel. Hands are dried first by placing the opposite hand behind the towel and blotting the skin, then using a corkscrew movement to dry from hand to elbow (do not move back towards the wrist). Discard the towel and use a second one to repeat the process on the other hand and forearm (**Action figure 10**, step nine).	Damp hands encourage the multiplication of bacteria (DH 2017, **C**). Drying from hands to elbows reduces the risk of contaminating hands with bacteria from parts of the arm that have not been washed. **E**
14 Dispose of used paper towels in a black bag in an open or foot-operated waste bin.	Paper towels used to dry the hands are normally non-hazardous and can be disposed of via the domestic waste stream (DH 2013b, **C**). Using an open or foot-operated waste bin prevents contamination of the hands. **E**

Procedure guideline 4.4 Surgical scrub technique using an alcohol-based handrub

Essential equipment

- An approved alcohol-based handrub, e.g. Desderman or Sterillium

Action	Rationale
Pre-procedure	
1 Remove any rings, bracelets and wristwatches, and roll up sleeves before entering the operating theatre suite or procedure area. *Note*: most organizations will require staff entering operating theatres to change into 'scrubs'.	To ensure good hand washing as jewellery inhibits this. Dirt and bacteria can remain beneath jewellery after hand washing. Long sleeves prevent washing of wrists and will easily become contaminated (NICE 2017, **C**; WHO 2009a, **C**).
2 If the skin is damaged with cuts or abrasions, advice should be sought from occupational health as it may not be advisable to proceed with surgical hand antisepsis.	Cuts and abrasions can become contaminated with bacteria and cannot be easily cleaned. Repeated hand washing can worsen an injury. Breaks in the skin will allow the entry of potential pathogens (WHO 2009a, **C**).
3 Remove nail varnish and artificial nails (most uniform policies and dress codes prohibit these). Nails must also be short and clean. Clean beneath the nails using a pick or brush if needed.	Long and false nails and imperfections in nail polish harbour dirt and bacteria that are not effectively removed by hand washing (WHO 2009a, **C**). The area under the nails may harbour dirt and micro-organisms not easily removed by the other stages of the procedure (WHO 2009a, **C**).

Procedure

4 Before commencing the first scrub of the day, the hands should be washed thoroughly with soap and water and dried with a paper towel (see Procedure guideline 4.1: Hand washing). *Note*: WHO guidelines state that surgical procedures may be carried out one after the other without the need for further hand washing if hands are perfectly clean and dry, provided that the below hand-preparation technique is followed with alcohol-based handrub every time (WHO 2009a).	To ensure all physical dirt and soil is removed as alcohol is inactivated in the presence of dirt. **E**
5 Wet the surface of the hands, wrists and forearms with a generous amount of alcohol-based handrub as advised by the manufacturer.	To ensure the correct amount is used and that skin coverage is appropriate. **E**

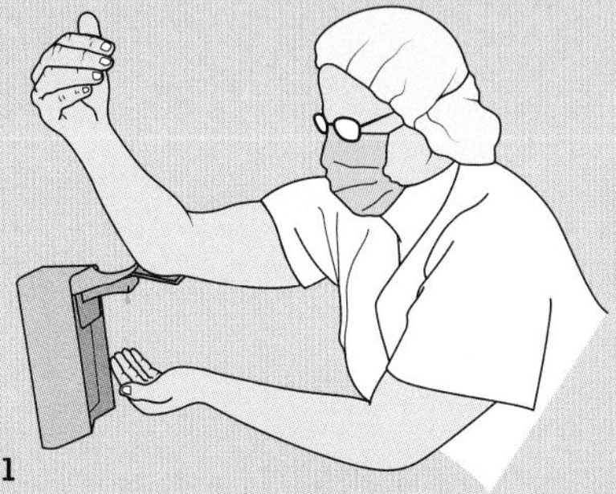

1
Put approximately 5 mL (3 doses) of alcohol-based handrub in the palm of your left hand, using the elbow of your other arm to operate the dispenser.

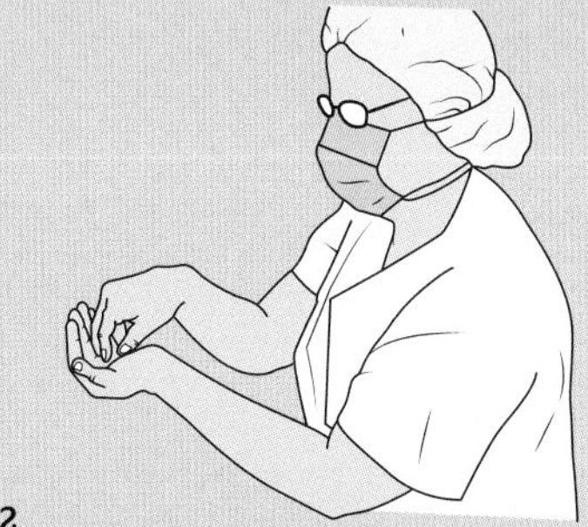

2
Dip the fingertips of your right hand in the handrub to decontaminate under the nails (5 seconds).

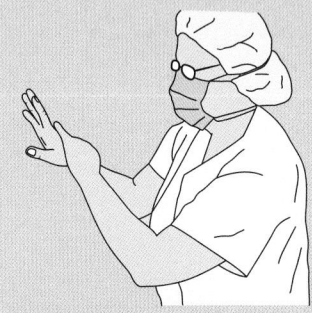

3
Images 3–7: Smear the handrub on the right forearm up to the elbow. Ensure that the whole skin area is covered by using circular movements around the forearm until the handrub has fully evaporated (10–15 seconds).

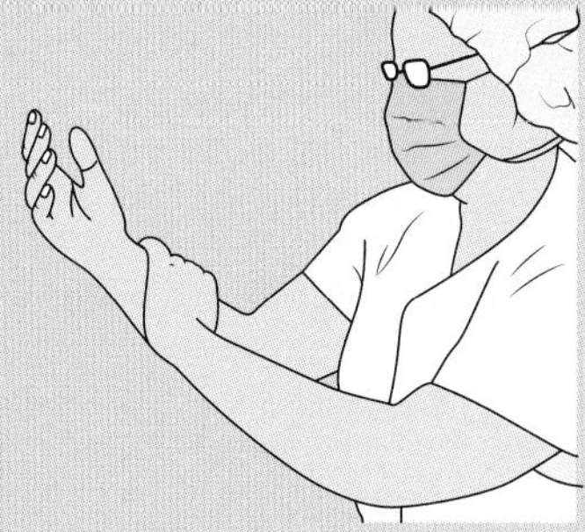

4
See legend for image 3.

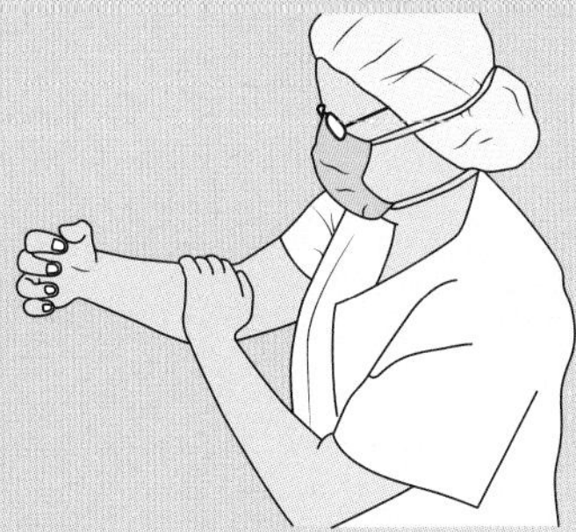

5
See legend for image 3.

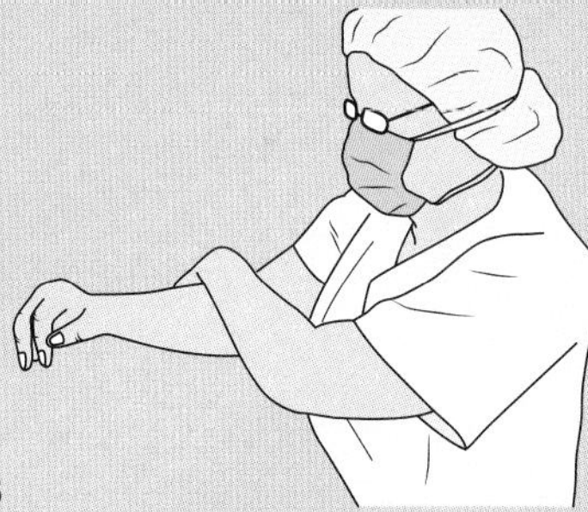

6
See legend for image 3.

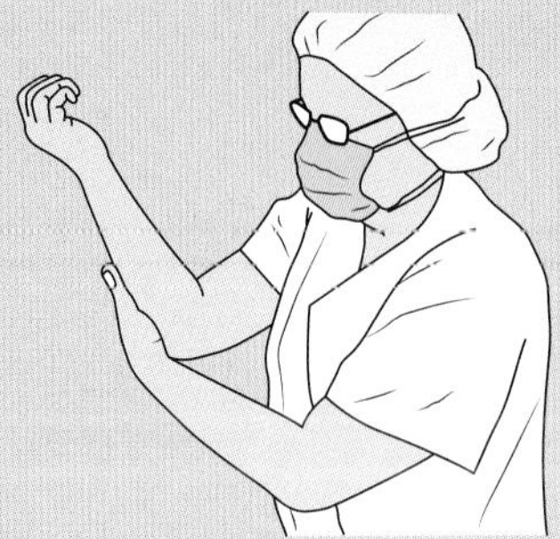

7
See legend for image 3.

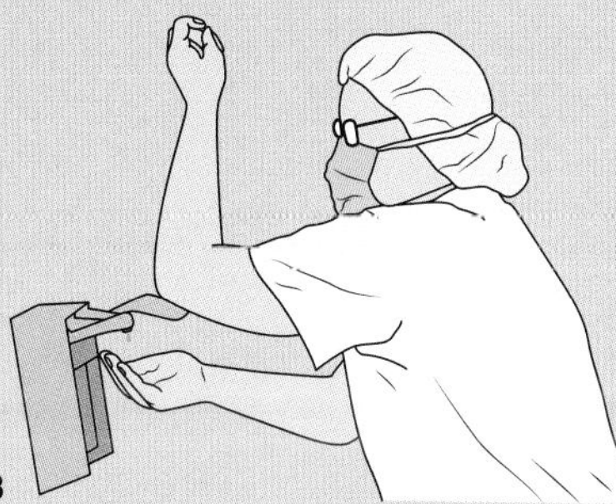

8
Put approximately 5 mL (3 doses) of alcohol-based handrub in the palm of your right hand, using the elbow of your other arm to operate the dispenser.

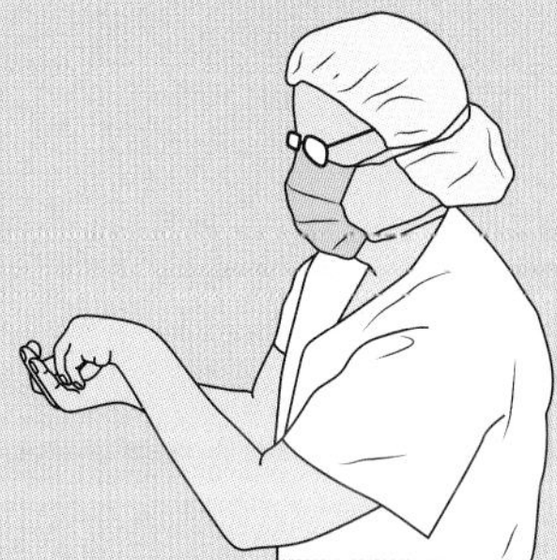

9
Dip the fingertips of your left hand in the handrub to decontaminate under the nails (5 seconds).

Action Figure 6 Surgical hand preparation technique with an alcohol-based handrub formulation. *Source*: WHO (2009a). *Source*: Reproduced from WHO (2009a) with permission of the World Health Organization.

(continued)

Procedure guideline 4.4 Surgical scrub technique using an alcohol-based handrub *(continued)*

Action	Rationale
6 Use steps 1–17 of the surgical hand preparation technique with an alcohol-based rub (**Action figure 6**). The scrub procedure should take between 90 seconds and 3 minutes, depending on the manufacturer's guidelines.	To ensure antimicrobial effectiveness (AfPP 2017, **C**).
7 Apply more alcohol to the hands and work this into the hands and wrists.	As the hand moves up the arm, it may become contaminated. By applying more alcohol after cleaning to the elbow, this risk of contamination is reduced. **C**
8 Allow the alcohol solution to dry on the hands before proceeding to don gown and gloves.	Alcohol needs to be allowed to dry. **E**

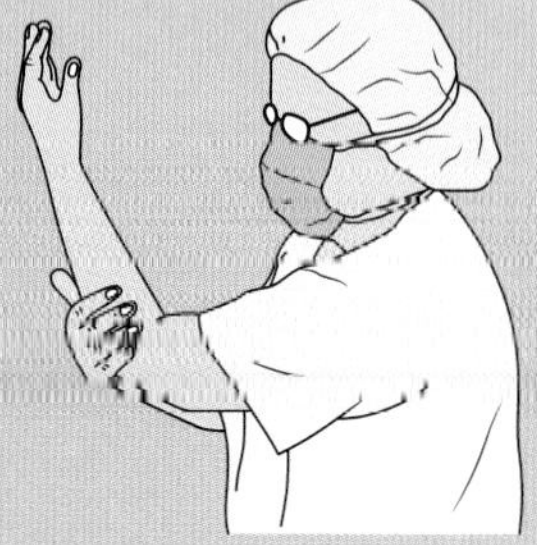

10
Smear the handrub on the left forearm up to the elbow. Ensure that the whole skin area is covered by using circular movements around the forearm until the handrub has fully evaporated (10–15 seconds).

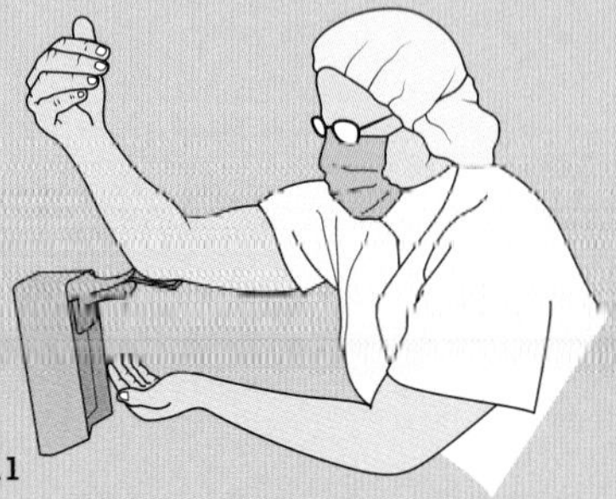

11
Put approximately 5 mL (3 doses) of alcohol-based handrub in the palm of your left hand, using the elbow of your other arm to operate the distributor. Rub both hands at the same time up to the wrists, and ensure that all the steps represented in Images 12–17 are followed (20–30 seconds).

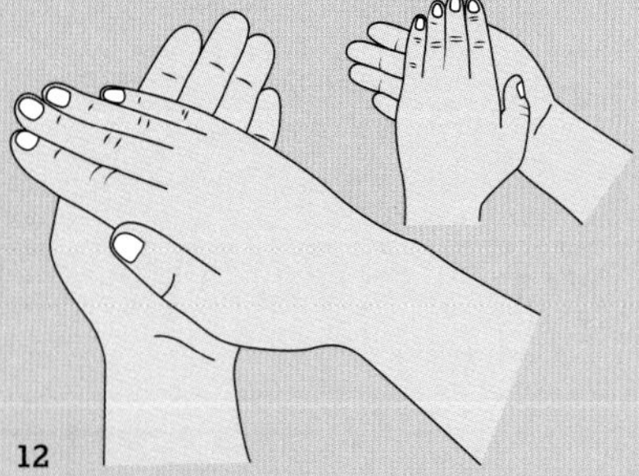

12
Cover the whole surface of the hands up to the wrist with alcohol-based handrub, rubbing palm against palm with a rotating movement.

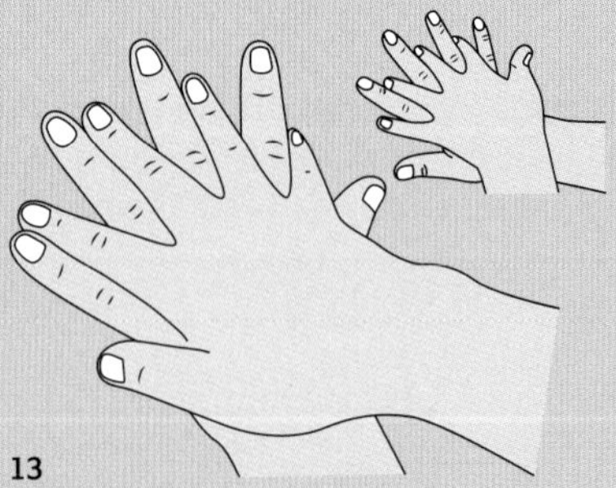

13
Rub the back of the left hand, including the wrist, moving the right palm back and forth, and vice versa.

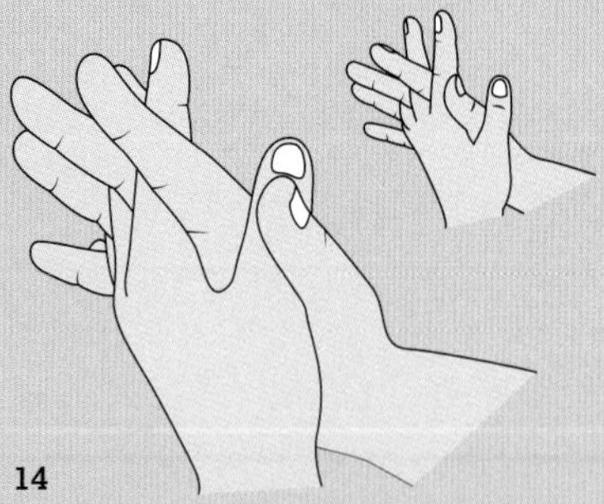

14
Rub palm against palm back and forth with fingers interlinked.

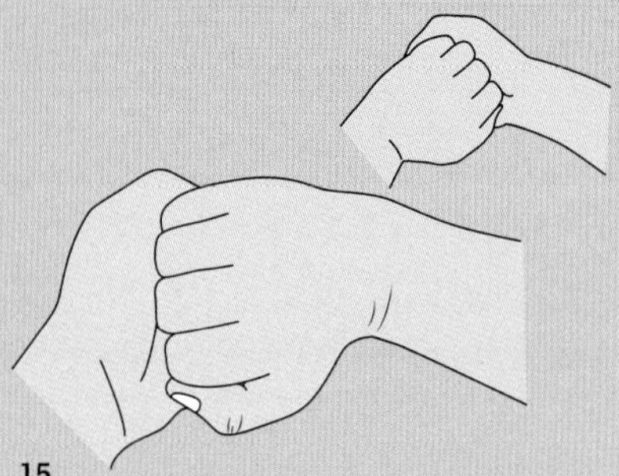

15
Rub the back of the fingers by holding them in the palm of the other hand with a sideways back-and-forth movement.

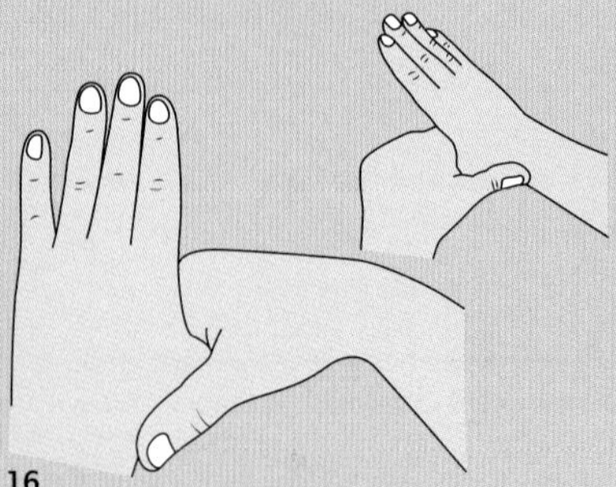

16
Rub the thumb of the left hand by rotating it in the clasped palm of the right hand and vice versa.

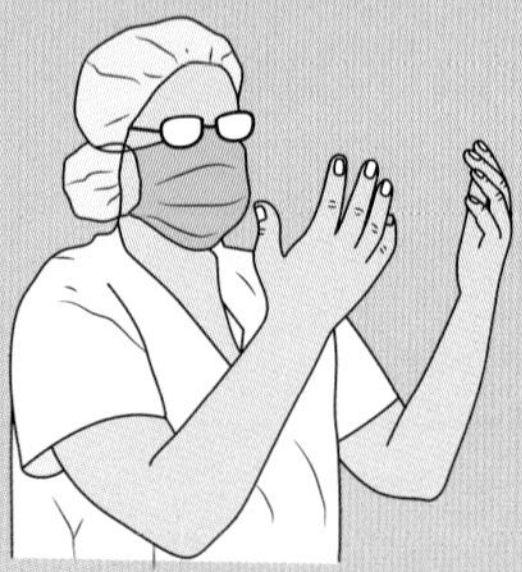

17
When the hands are dry, sterile surgical clothing and gloves can be donned.

Action Figure 6 *Continued*

Personal protective equipment (PPE)

Definition

Personal protective equipment (PPE) is the term for items used to physically protect someone from a potential infection hazard. It can include gloves, aprons, masks, face-shields and gowns.

Related theory

The exact PPE required will depend on the activity being carried out and the organism or risk present. It is a legal requirement in the UK for employers to provide suitable PPE when risks cannot be controlled in other ways, and for employees to use the equipment provided (HSE 2013c).

Basic PPE – that is, non-latex disposable gloves, disposable aprons and eye protection – should be readily available in the clinical area (Loveday et al. 2014a), particularly where regular use is anticipated. For example, it is appropriate to have dispensers for gloves and aprons situated outside isolation rooms. All PPE sold in the UK must comply with the relevant regulations and standards, including being CE marked to demonstrate that it meets these standards (HSE 2013c).

Disposable gloves

Gloves will be necessary in some circumstances but should be worn only when required (Loveday et al. 2014a, RCN 2018, WHO 2009b). Non-sterile disposable gloves are most usefully available packaged in boxes of 100 ambidextrous gloves, in small, medium and large sizes. These boxes should be located close to the point of use, ideally in a fixed dispenser to make removing the gloves from the box as easy as possible. In the past, natural rubber latex was commonly used for these gloves but concerns about latex sensitivity mean that many healthcare organizations have adopted gloves made of alternative materials such as vinyl or nitrile (RCN 2018). All gloves carry a risk of failure, as they may have small holes invisible to the naked eye (Kerr et al. 2004, Korniewicz et al. 2002). The removal process may also contaminate the hands so it is essential that hands are decontaminated after the removal of gloves. Whatever the material, these gloves are single use – they should be used for the task for which they are required and then removed and disposed of. They cannot be cleaned and reused for another task (Loveday et al. 2014a, MHRA 2018).

Disposable aprons

Single-use disposable aprons may be obtained either in a box or linked together on a roll. It is important is to ensure that the product is compatible with the dispensers in use and that it meets the requisite standards (i.e. is CE marked). Aprons are normally made of thin polythene and are available in a range of colours. Different coloured aprons can be used to designate staff doing different tasks or working in different areas to give a visible reminder of the risk of cross-infection. As with disposable gloves, disposable aprons should be used for the task for which they are required and then removed and disposed of (Loveday et al. 2014a, MHRA 2018).

Disposable gowns

Non-sterile long-sleeved gowns are sometimes required to provide greater coverage of uniforms or clothing, for example when caring for a patient with a highly resistant pathogen. The gown should be put on and done up fully to cover the uniform. Like aprons, they should be used for the task for which they are required and then removed carefully and disposed of, with hands decontaminated afterwards.

Sterile gloves

Single-use sterile gloves should be available in any area where their use is anticipated. Sterile gloves are packed as a left-and-right pair and are manufactured in a wide range of full and half sizes (similar to shoe sizes) so as to fit closely and provide the best possible compromise between acting as a barrier and allowing the wearer to work normally. Natural rubber latex is one of the best materials for this; however, if latex gloves are used, care must be taken to ensure alternatives are available for patients and staff with sensitivity to latex (RCN 2018).

Sterile gowns

A sterile, water-repellent gown is required in addition to sterile gloves to provide 'maximal barrier precautions' during surgery and other invasive procedures carrying a high risk of infection, or where infection would have serious consequences to the patient, such as insertion of a central venous catheter.

Face protection

Face protection includes protection for the eyes and/or the mouth and nose and will be required in any situation where the mucous membranes of the face may be exposed to body fluids. This can be from droplets created during aerosol-generating procedures, intubation, surgery with power tools or just close proximity (such as during childbirth). Both single-use and multiple-use options are available. Goggles are normally sufficient for eye protection as long as they are worn in conjunction with a fluid-repellent mask. If greater protection is required, or a mask is not worn for any reason, a face-shield should be used. Face-shields may also be more appropriate for people who wear glasses. Prescription glasses will often not provide sufficient protection and should not be relied upon (DH 1998).

Masks and respirators

When dealing with organisms spread by the airborne or droplet routes, a surgical face-mask or respirator mask will be required. A simple surgical mask will protect the wearer from splashes to the covered area of the face and may impede large droplets. These masks should not be worn for long periods as they can become saturated with water vapour from normal breathing, which will make them permeable.

A respirator mask is a mask that is designed to filter out all but the smallest particles and is usually used to prevent the transmission of respiratory viruses. Masks are available at different grades. Usually the standard FFP3 is accepted in the UK. When using a respirator, a good fit is essential to ensure that there is no leakage around the sides of the mask. Staff who are likely to need to use respirators should be 'fit tested' to ensure that they have the correct size. Fit testing is a formal qualitative test usually performed annually to establish that a particular mask fits a particular face. Fit testing is normally carried out by the occupational health department or infection prevention and control team. Facial hair under the edge of the respirator will prevent a proper seal; staff with beards that prevent a proper seal will not be able to work safely if a respirator is required (HSE 2013d).

Masks and respirators are usually single use; however, reusable respirators are sometimes required where the mask may need to be worn for a long time or for people whose face shape does not allow a good seal with disposable products (DH 2010b). Reusable respirators must be assigned to specific individuals and be cleaned thoroughly every time they are removed.

Removal of personal protective equipment

PPE should be removed in the following sequence to minimize the risks of cross-contamination and self-contamination (Loveday et al. 2014a):

- gloves
- apron
- eye protection (when worn)
- mask/respirator (when worn).

Hands must be decontaminated following the removal of PPE.

Procedure guideline 4.5 Putting on and removing non-sterile gloves

Essential equipment

- Non-sterile gloves

Action	Rationale
Pre-procedure	
1 Decontaminate hands with either soap and water or an alcohol-based handrub before putting on gloves.	Hands must be decontaminated before and after every patient contact or contact with a patient's equipment (NHS England and NHSI 2019, **C**; Wilson 2019, **C**).
Procedure	
2 Remove gloves from the box one at a time (**Action figure 2**). If it is likely that more than two gloves will be required (i.e. if the procedure requires gloves to be changed part-way through), consider removing all the gloves needed before starting the procedure.	To prevent contamination of the finger part of the gloves. **E**
3 Holding the cuff of the glove, pull it into position, taking care not to contaminate the glove from the skin (**Action figure 3**). This is particularly important when the second glove is being put on, as the gloved hand of the first glove can touch the skin of the ungloved second hand if care is not taken.	To prevent cross contamination (WHO 2009b, **C**).
4 During the procedure or when undertaking two procedures with the same patient, it may be necessary to change gloves.	Disposable gloves are single-use items. They cannot be cleaned and reused for the same or another patient (Wilson 2019, **C**).
5 If gloves become damaged during use, they must be replaced.	Damaged gloves are not an effective barrier (WHO 2009b, **C**).
6 Remove the gloves when the procedure is complete, taking care not to contaminate the hands or the environment from the outside of the gloves.	The outside of the glove may be contaminated. **E**
7 Remove the first glove by firmly holding the outside of the glove's wrist and pulling off the glove in such a way as to turn it inside out (**Action figure 7**).	While removing the first glove, the second gloved hand continues to be protected. By turning the glove inside out during removal, any contamination is contained inside the glove. **E**
8 Remove the second glove by slipping the thumb of the ungloved hand inside the wrist of the glove and pulling it off while at the same time turning it inside out (**Action figure 8**).	Putting the thumb inside the glove means they will not be in contact with the potentially contaminated outer surface of the glove. **E**
Post-procedure	
9 Dispose of used gloves immediately in the appropriate bin as per local policy (**Action figure 9**).	Waste that is not contaminated with any infectious material should be disposed of in the 'offensive waste' stream. This is usually a yellow and black 'tiger stripe' bag. If the gloves have been used to deal with any infectious agents thought to pose a particular risk, they should be disposed of as hazardous infectious waste in an orange or yellow bag (DH 2013b, **C**).
10 After removing the gloves, decontaminate hands.	Hands may have become contaminated (NHS England and NHSI 2019, **C**; WHO 2009b, **C**).

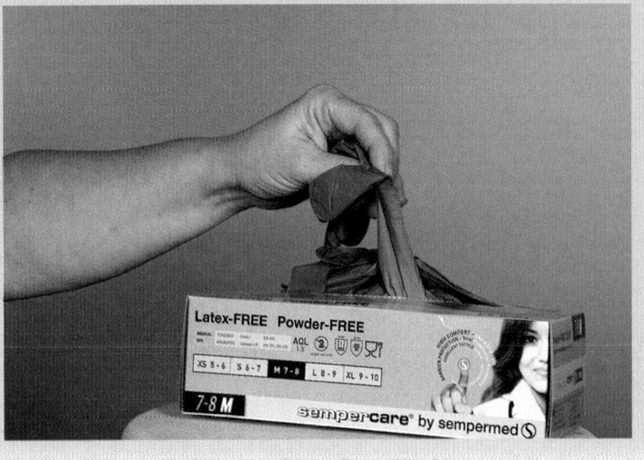

Action Figure 2 Remove gloves from the box.

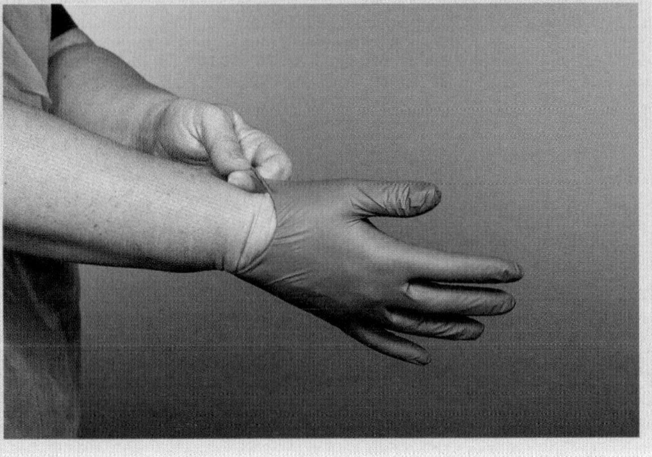

Action Figure 3 Holding the cuff of the glove, pull it into position.

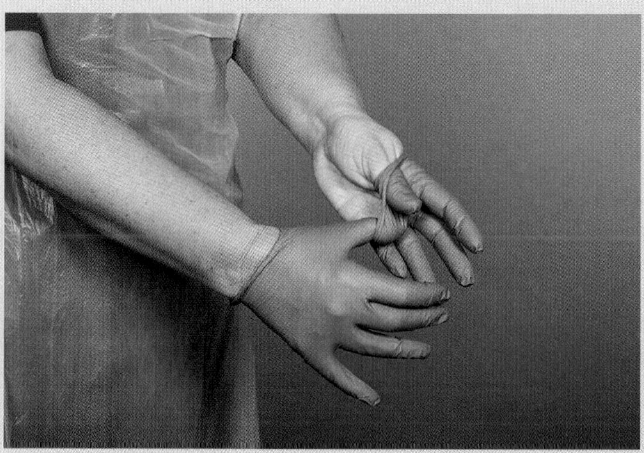

Action Figure 7 Remove the first glove by firmly holding the outside of the glove's wrist, then pull off the glove in such a way as to turn it inside out.

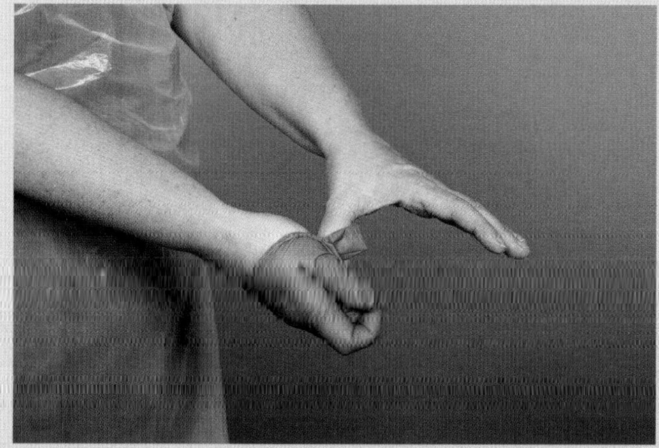

Action Figure 8 Remove the second glove by slipping the thumb of the ungloved hand inside the wrist of the glove and pulling it off while turning it inside out.

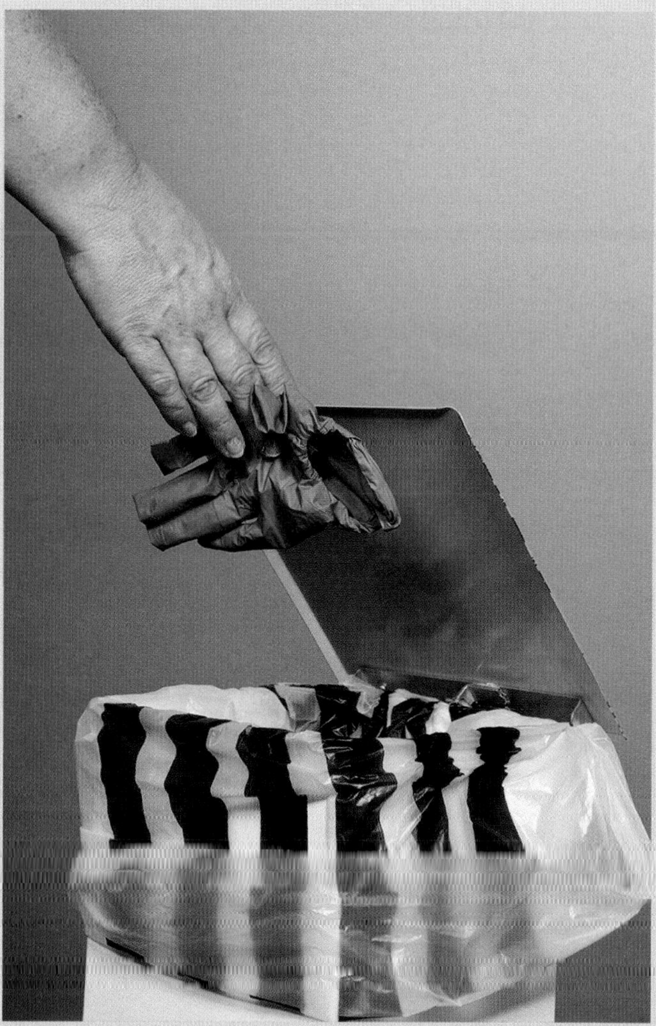

Action Figure 9 Dispose of used gloves in an appropriate clinical waste bag (tiger stripe if non-hazardous and non-infectious).

Procedure guideline 4.6 Applying and removing a disposable apron

Essential equipment
- Disposable apron

Action	Rationale
Pre-procedure	
1 Remove an apron from the dispenser or roll using clean hands and open it out.	To make it easy to put on. **E**
Procedure	
2 Place the neck loop over your head and tie the ties together behind your back, positioning the apron so that as much of the front of your body is protected as possible (**Action figures 2a and 2b**).	To minimize the risk of contamination being transferred between your clothing and the patient, in either direction. **E**
3 If gloves are required, don them as described in Procedure guideline 4.5: Putting on and removing non-sterile gloves. At the end of the procedure, remove gloves first.	The gloves are more likely to be contaminated than the apron and therefore should be removed first to prevent cross-contamination (DH 2010b, **C**).
4 Remove the apron by breaking the ties and neck loop. Then grasp the inside of the apron roll it up (**Action figure 4**).	The inside of the apron should be clean. **E**

(continued)

Procedure guideline 4.6 Applying and removing a disposable apron *(continued)*

Action	Rationale
Post-procedure	
5 Dispose of the used apron immediately in the appropriate bin.	Waste that is not contaminated with any infectious material should be disposed of in the 'offensive waste' stream. This is usually a yellow and black 'tiger stripe' bag. If the apron has been used to deal with any infectious agents thought to pose a particular risk, it should be disposed of as hazardous infectious waste in an orange or yellow bag (DH 2013b, **C**).
6 After removing the apron, decontaminate hands.	Hands may have become contaminated (NHS England and NHSI 2019, **C**).

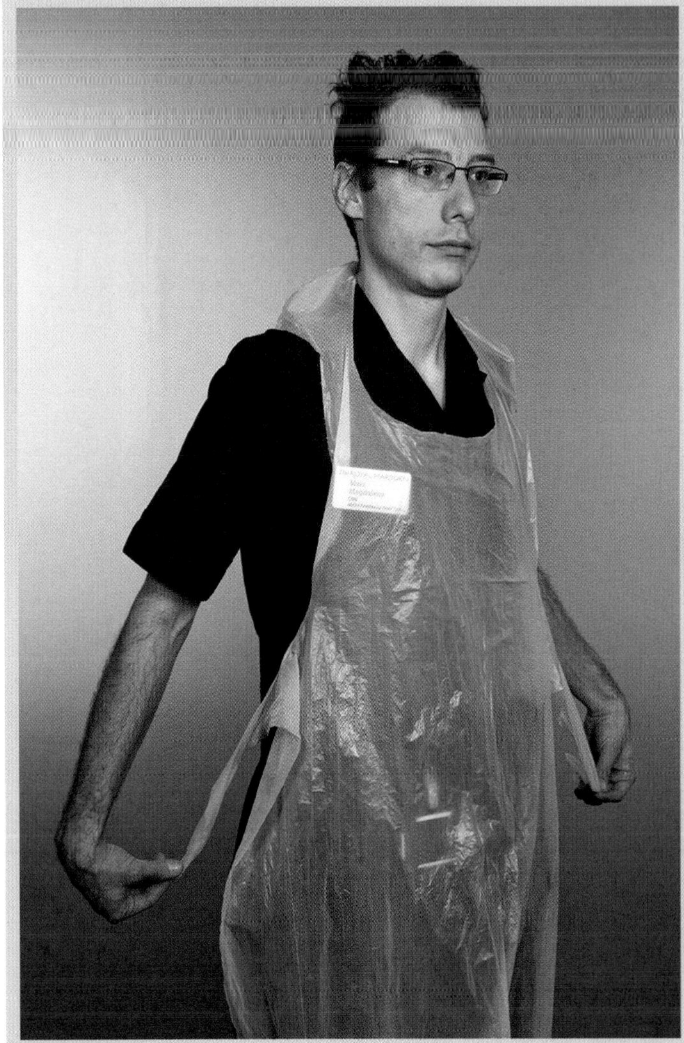

Action Figure 2a Place the neck loop of the apron over your head.

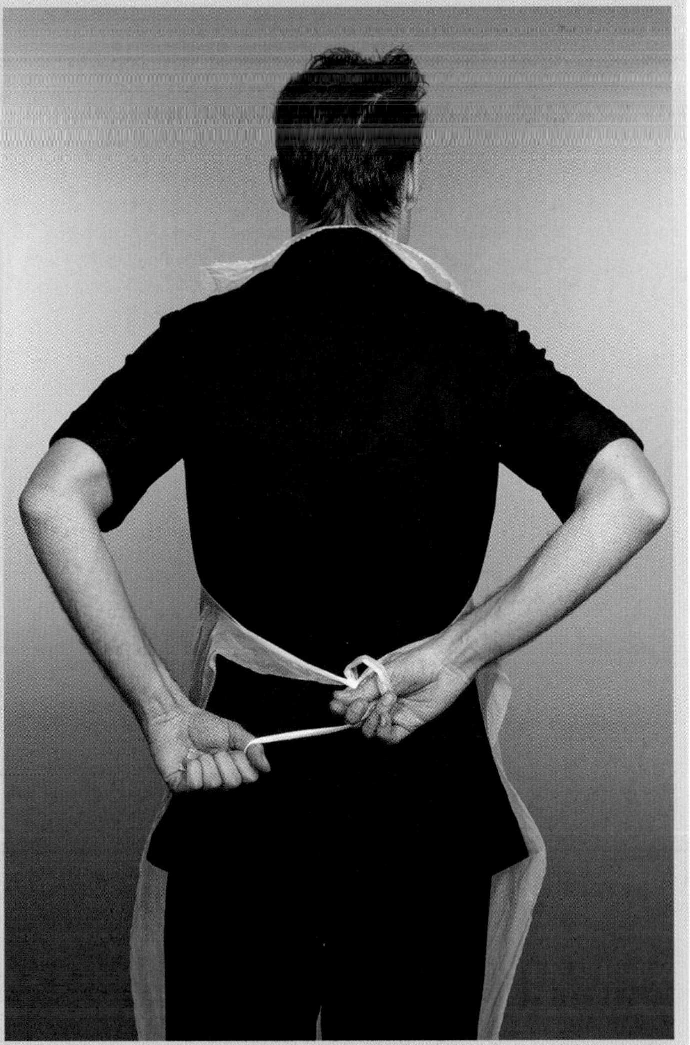

Action Figure 2b Tie the ties together behind your back, positioning the apron so that as much of the front of your body is protected as possible.

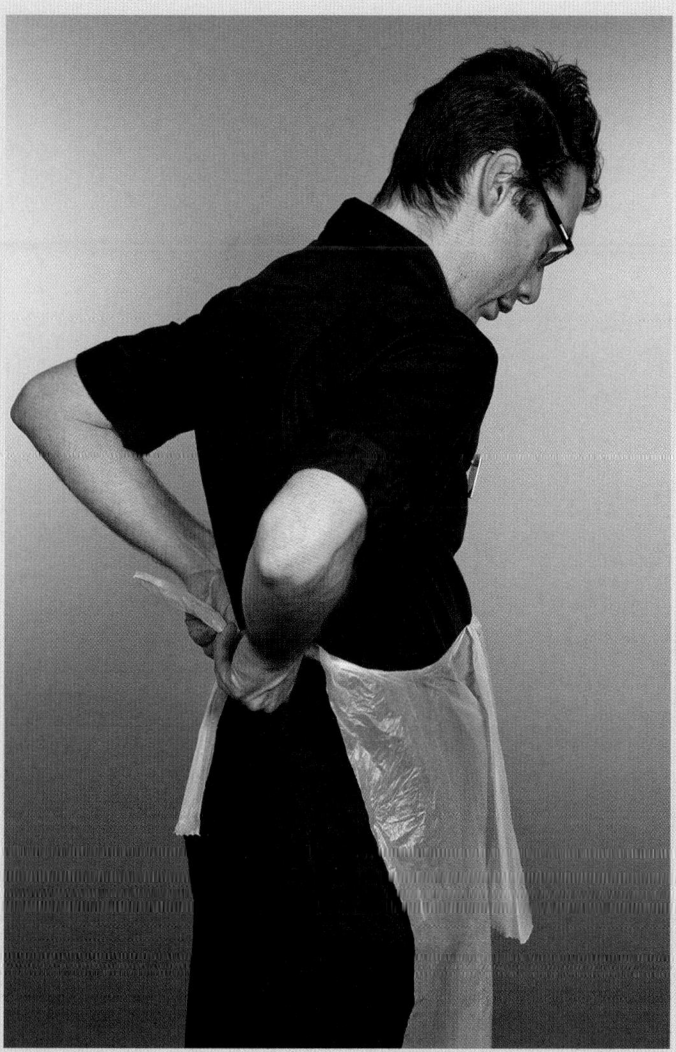

Action Figure 4 Remove the apron by breaking the neck loop and ties.

Procedure guideline 4.7 Putting on and removing a disposable mask or respirator

Essential equipment

- Disposable surgical mask or respirator

Action	Rationale
Pre-procedure	
1 Remove surgical-type masks singly from the box, or remove individually wrapped items from their packaging, with clean hands.	To prevent contamination of the item or others in the box or dispenser. **E**
2 Consider removing glasses, if worn.	Glasses may obstruct the correct positioning of the mask/respirator and may be dislodged or damaged. **E**
Procedure	
3 Place the mask or respirator over your nose, mouth and chin (**Action figure 3**).	To ensure correct positioning. **E**
4 Fit the flexible nose piece over the bridge of your nose if wearing a respirator.	To ensure the best fit. **E**
5 Secure the mask/respirator at the back of your head with ties or fitted elastic straps and adjust to fit (**Action figure 5**).	To ensure the mask or respirator is comfortable to wear and remains in the correct position throughout the procedure. **E**

(continued)

Procedure guideline 4.7 Putting on and removing a disposable mask or respirator *(continued)*

Action	Rationale
6 If wearing a respirator, perform a fit check. First, breathe in – the respirator should collapse or be 'sucked in' to the face. Then breathe out – the respirator should not leak around the edges.	To ensure that there is a good seal around the edge of the respirator so that there is no route for non-filtered air to pass in either direction. Note that this check should be carried out whenever a respirator is worn but is not a substitute for prior fit testing (DH 2010b, **C**).
7 Replace glasses, if previously removed.	To restore normal vision. **E**
8 At the end of the procedure, or after leaving the room in which the mask/respirator is required, remove the mask/respirator by grasping the ties or straps at the back of the head and either break them or pull them forward over the top of the head (**Action figure 8a**). Do not touch the front of the mask/respirator (**Action figure 8b**).	To avoid contaminating the hands with material from the outside of the mask/respirator (DH 2010b, **C**).
Post-procedure	
9 Dispose of used disposable items as hazardous infectious waste, as per local policy.	All waste contaminated with blood, body fluids, excretions, secretions and/or infectious agents thought to pose a particular risk should be disposed of as hazardous infectious waste (DH 2013b, **C**).
10 Clean reusable items according to the manufacturer's instructions, usually with detergent and water or a detergent wipe.	To avoid cross-contamination and ensure the item is suitable for further use (DH 2010b, **C**).

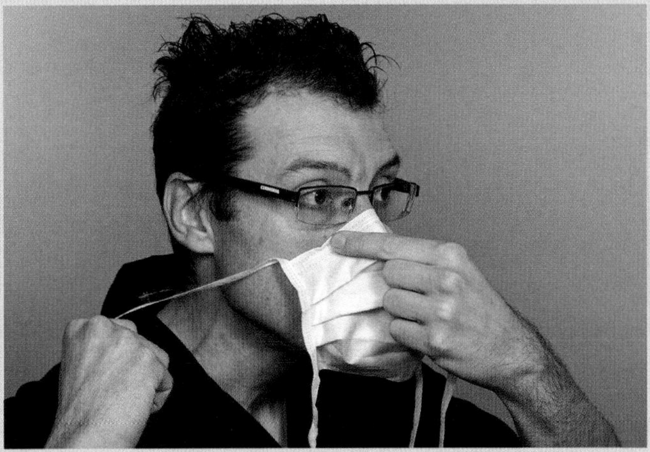

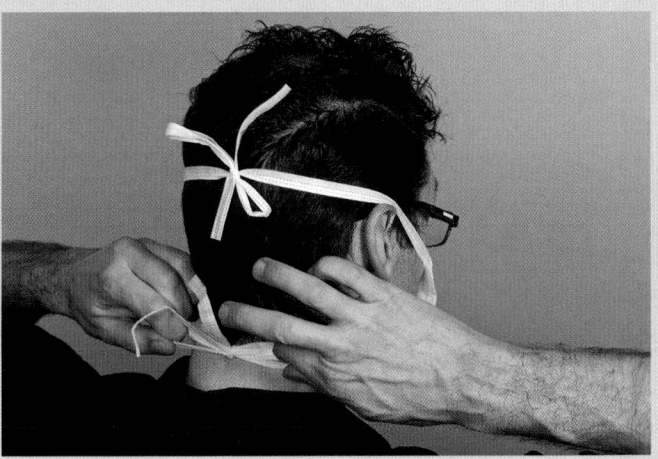

Action Figure 3 Place the mask over your nose, mouth and chin.

Action Figure 5 Secure the mask at the back of your head with ties.

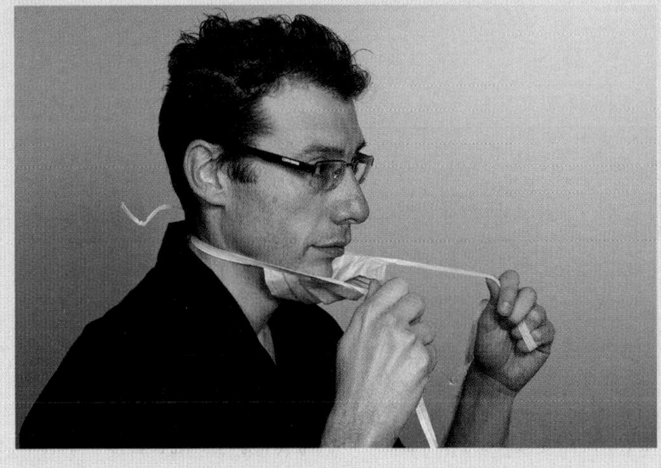

Action Figure 8a After use, remove the mask by untying or breaking the ties and pulling them forward.

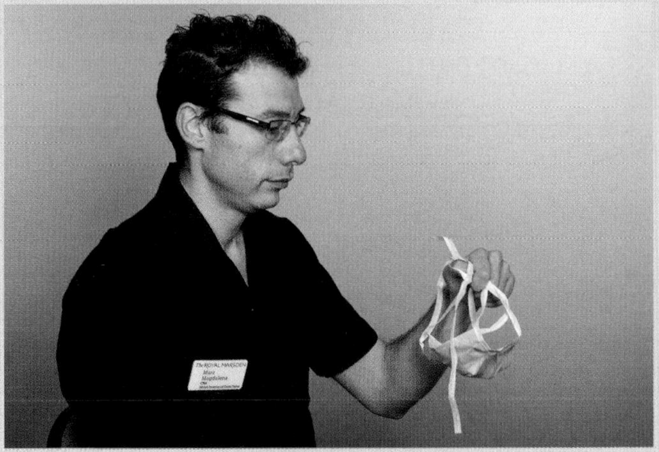

Action Figure 8b Do not touch the front of the mask.

Procedure guideline 4.8 Putting on or removing goggles or a face-shield

The purpose of goggles or a face-shield is to protect the mucous membranes of the eyes, nose and mouth from body fluid droplets generated during aerosol-generating procedures or surgery with power tools.

Essential equipment

- Reusable or disposable goggles or face-shield

Action	Rationale
Pre-procedure	
1 Remove eye protection from any packaging with clean hands.	To prevent cross-contamination. **E**
2 Apply demister solution according to the manufacturer's instructions, if required.	To ensure good visibility throughout the procedure. **E**
Procedure	
3 Position the goggles/face-shield over the eyes and/or face and secure using ear pieces or a headband; adjust to fit (**Action figure 3**).	To ensure the item is comfortable to wear and remains in the correct position throughout the procedure. **E**
4 At the end of the procedure, remove by grasping the ear pieces or headband at the back or side of the head and lifting forward, away from the face. Do not touch the front of the goggles/face-shield.	To avoid contaminating the hands with material from the outside of the eye protection (DH 2010b, **C**).
Post-procedure	
5 Dispose of used disposable items as 'hazardous infectious waste' as per local policy.	All waste contaminated with blood, body fluids, excretions, secretions and/or infectious agents thought to pose a particular risk should be disposed of as hazardous infectious waste (DH 2013b, **C**).
6 Clean reusable items according to the manufacturer's instructions, usually with detergent and water or a detergent wipe.	To avoid cross-contamination and ensure the item is suitable for further use. **E**

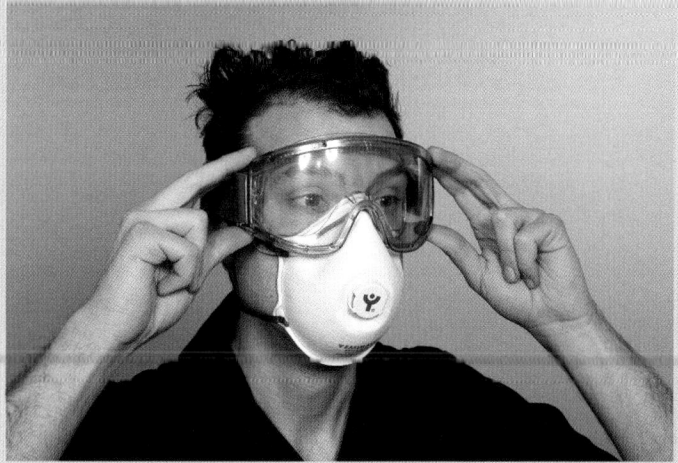

Action Figure 3 Application and removal of protective eye goggles.

Donning theatre attire

Evidence-based approaches

There are two recognized techniques for putting on sterile gloves: a closed and an open method. The open technique may be used on wards for aseptic procedures but is not recommended for use in the operating theatre, where a closed technique should be used.

The open technique is used to create a barrier between the nurse's hands and the patient to prevent the transmission of infectious agents in either direction, and to prevent contamination of a vulnerable area or invasive device. It may be used for aseptic techniques such as inserting a urinary catheter or a sterile wound dressing.

Procedure guideline 4.9 Donning a sterile gown and gloves: closed technique

An assistant is required to open the sterile gloves and tie the back of the gown.

Essential equipment

- Sterile disposable gloves
- Sterile disposable or reusable gown

Action	Rationale
Pre-procedure	
1 Prepare the area where gowning and gloving will take place. Open the gown pack with clean hands. Do not touch the inside of the package.	To ensure that there is adequate room to don gown and gloves and to avoid contaminating either. **E**
2 Wash hands using a surgical scrub technique with either antiseptic handwash or an alcohol-based handrub. Ensure hands are dry.	To both disinfect and physically remove matter and micro-organisms from the hands (WHO 2009a, **C**).
Procedure	
3 Open the inner layer of the gown pack, if present (**Action figures 3a and 3b**).	To allow the gown to be removed. **E**
4 Grasp the gown on its inside surface just below the neck opening (this should be uppermost if the gown pack has been opened correctly) and lift it up, holding it away from the body and any walls or furniture. The gown should fall open with the inside facing towards you (**Action figure 4**).	To open out the gown while keeping its outer surface sterile. **E**
5 Continue to grasp the inside of the gown with one hand. Insert the free hand into the corresponding sleeve of the gown, pulling the gown towards you until your fingers reach, but do not go beyond, the cuff of the sleeve (**Action figure 5**).	To pull on the gown while keeping its outer surface sterile. **E**
6 With the other hand, release the inside surface of the gown and insert that hand into the corresponding sleeve, again until your fingers reach but do not go beyond the cuff of the sleeve The assistant should help to pull the gown on and tie the ties, without touching any part of the gown other than the ties and rear edges (**Action figure 6**).	To pull on the gown while keeping its outer surface sterile. **E**
7 The assistant should open a pair of sterile gloves and present the inner packaging for you to take. Take the package with your hands inside your sleeves, and place it on the sterile area of the open gown package so that the fingers of the gloves point towards you (**Actions figure 7a and 7b**).	To prepare the gloves for donning while keeping them and the gown sterile. **E**
8 Open the inner packaging of the gloves (**Action figure 8a**). The fingers should be towards you, the thumbs uppermost and the cuffs folded over. Keeping your hands within the sleeves of the gown, slide the thumb of your right hand (still inside the sleeve) between the folded-over cuff and the body of the right glove (**Action figure 8b**). Pick up that glove. Grasp the cuff of that glove on the opposite side with the other hand (still inside its sleeve) and unfold it, pulling it over the cuff of the sleeve and the hand inside. Then push your right hand through the cuff of the sleeve into the glove (**Action figures 8c and 8d**). Repeat the process with the left hand (**Action figure 8e**). Adjust the fit once both gloves are on (**Action figure 8f**). Once both hands are inside their respective gloves, there is no risk of contaminating the outside of the gloves or gown with your bare hands. *Note*: never allow the bare hand to touch the gown cuff edge or outside of the glove. Also, the gloves can be put on either hand first; simply exchange 'left' and 'right' in the description if you wish to put on the left-hand glove first.	To don the gloves while keeping their outer surface sterile and ensure that there is no risk of contaminating the outside of the gown. **E**
9 If you need to change a glove because it is damaged or contaminated, pull the sleeve cuff down over your hand as you do so and don the replacement glove using the technique above.	To minimize the risk of contaminating the gown or the sterile field. **E**
10 Dispose of used gloves and disposable gowns as 'hazardous infectious waste', unless instructed otherwise by the infection prevention and control team.	All waste contaminated with blood, body fluids, excretions, secretions and/or infectious agents thought to pose a particular risk should be disposed of as hazardous infectious waste. **C**
11 Once gowned and gloved it is important to maintain sterility, so: • Never drop your hands below the sterile area at which you are working. • Never touch the gown above the level of the axilla or below the sterile area at which you are working. • Never touch an unsterile object. • Never tuck your hands under your armpits.	To avoid contamination of the sterile field. The only part of the gown that is considered sterile is the area at the front between the axilla and the sterile area at which you are working. The armpits are a source of micro-organisms. **C**

Post-procedure

12 At the end of the procedure, remove gown and gloves as a single unit by pulling the gown away from you so as to turn it and the gloves inside out (**Action figures 12a and 12b**).	To avoid cross-contamination of hands. **E**
13 Consign reusable gowns as infected linen according to local arrangements.	To minimize any risk to laundry workers from contaminated items (HSE 2013e, **C**).
14 After removing the gloves and gown, decontaminate hands.	Hands may have become contaminated (NHS England and NHSI 2019, **C**).

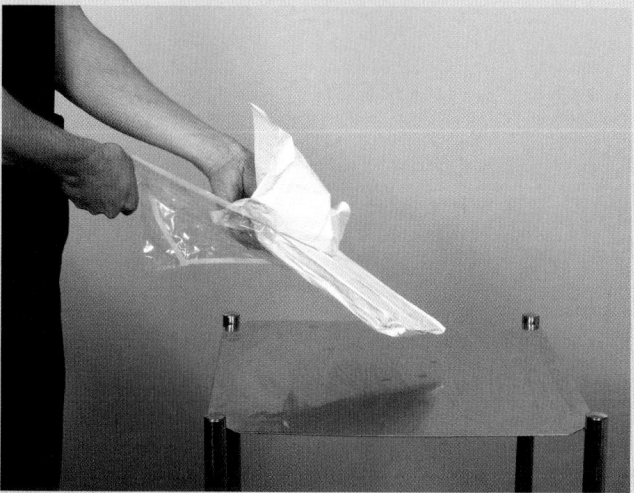

Action Figure 3a Open the gown pack with clean hands onto a clean surface. Do not touch the inner packet until after the surgical scrub.

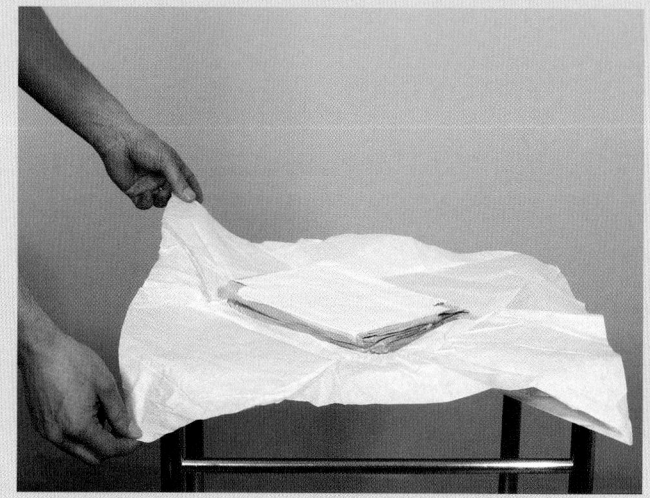

Action Figure 3b Open the inner layer of the pack.

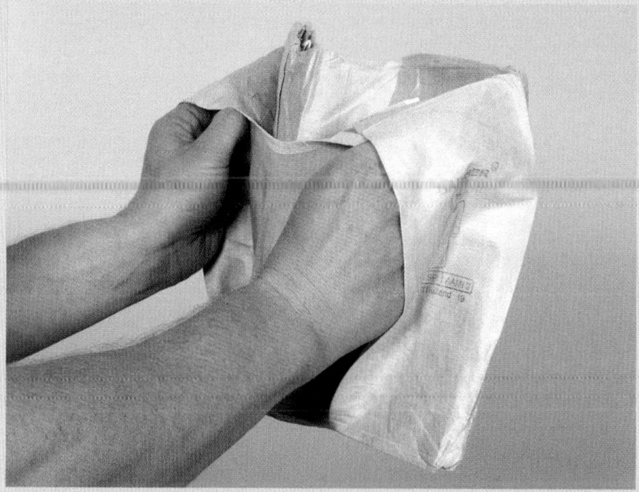

Action Figure 4 Lift up the gown by its inner surface and hold it away from the body.

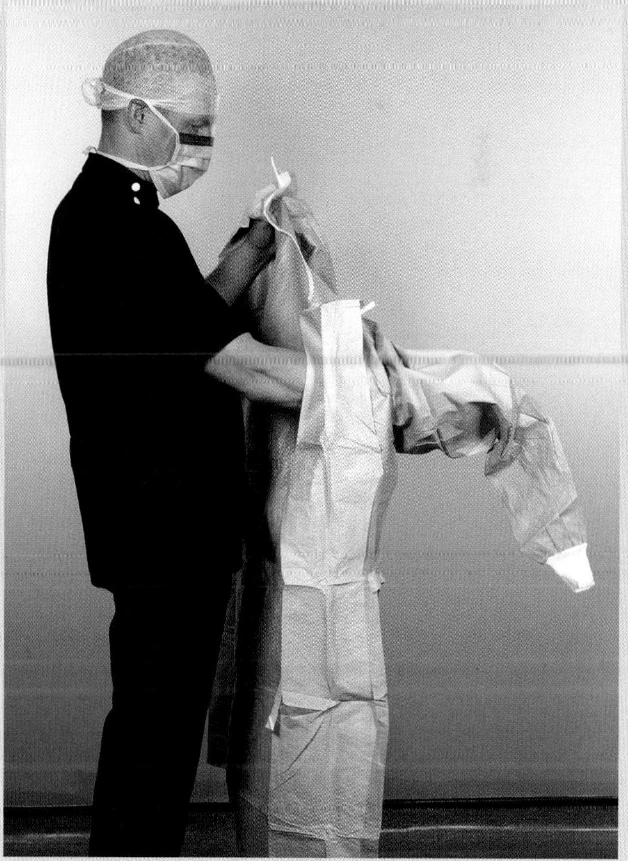

Action Figure 5 Put one hand into the corresponding sleeve and use the other hand to pull the gown towards you. Your hand should not go beyond the cuff.

(continued)

Procedure guideline 4.9 Donning a sterile gown and gloves: closed technique *(continued)*

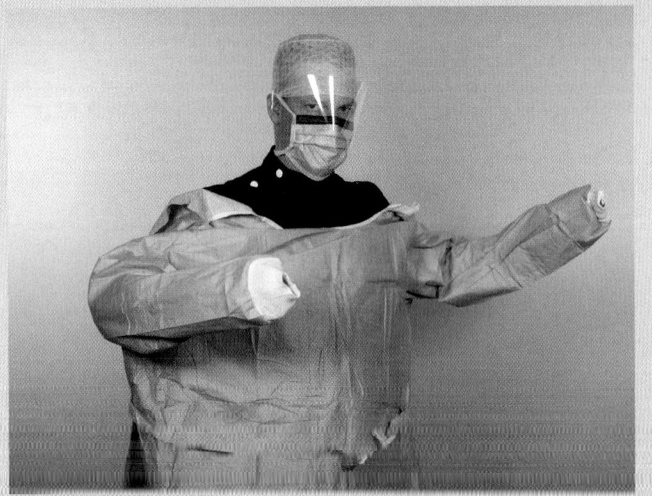

Action Figure 6 Put the other hand into the other sleeve. Again, your hand should not go beyond the cuff.

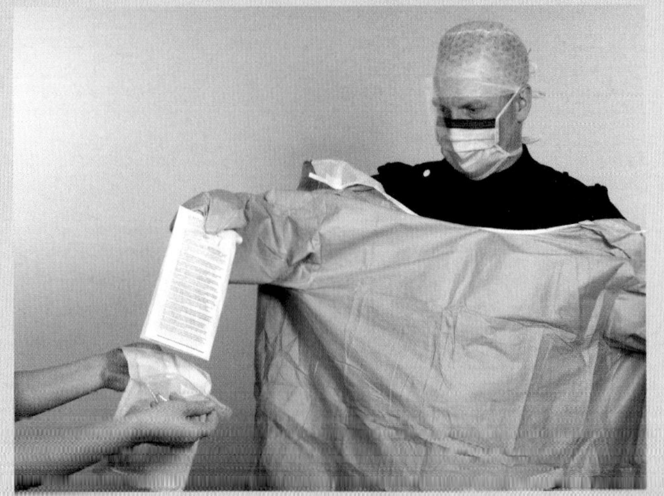

Action Figure 7b Take the gloves, keeping your hands inside your sleeves.

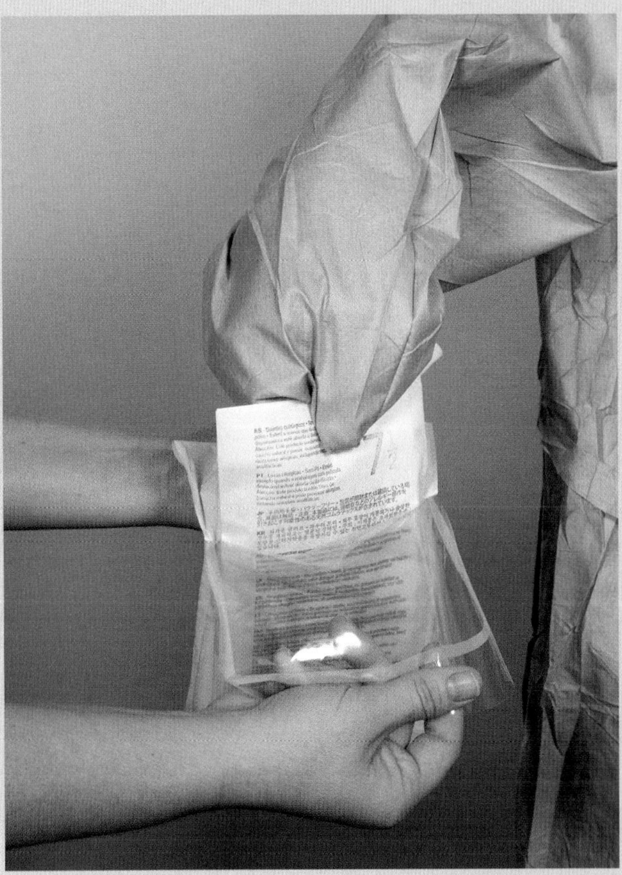

Action Figure 7a The assistant opens a pair of sterile gloves and presents the inner packaging for you to take.

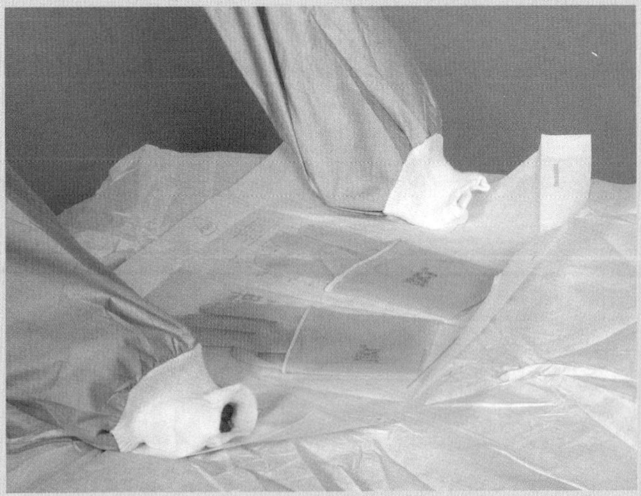

Action Figure 8a Open the inner glove packet onto the sterile open gown package so that the glove fingers point towards you.

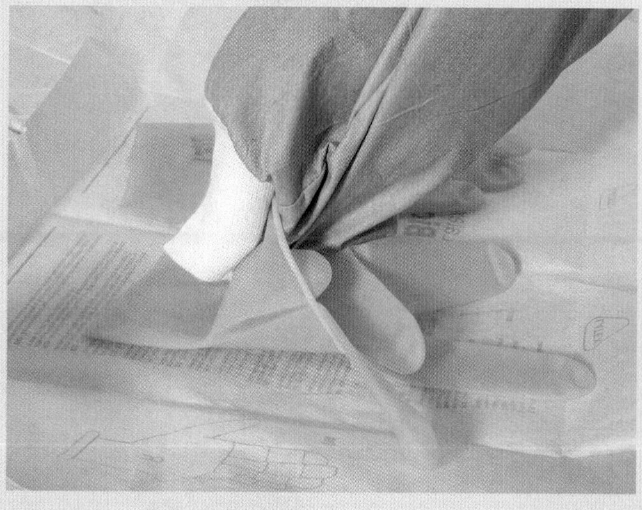

Action Figure 8b Slide the thumb of one hand (still inside the sleeve) under the folded-over cuff of the corresponding glove.

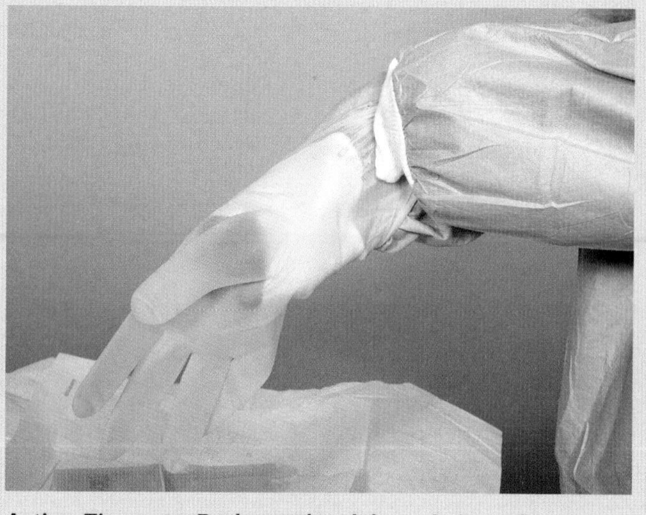

Action Figure 8c Push your hand through the cuff and into the glove.

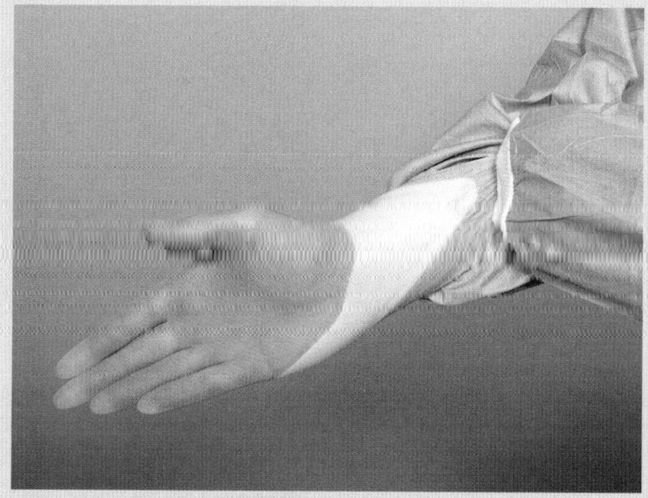

Action Figure 8d Pull the glove into position using the other hand (still inside its sleeve).

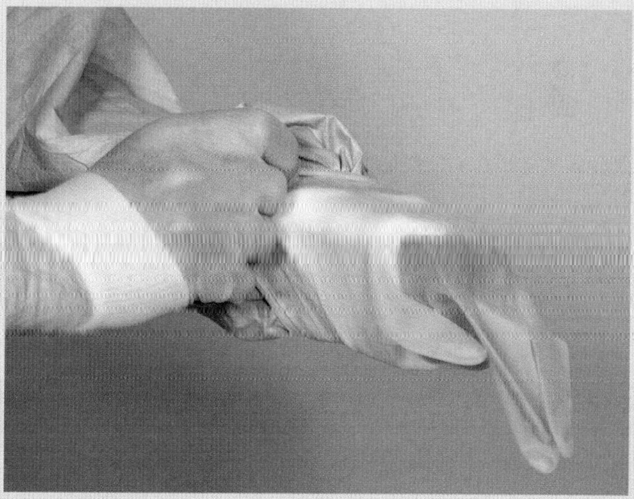

Action Figure 8e Repeat the process with the other glove.

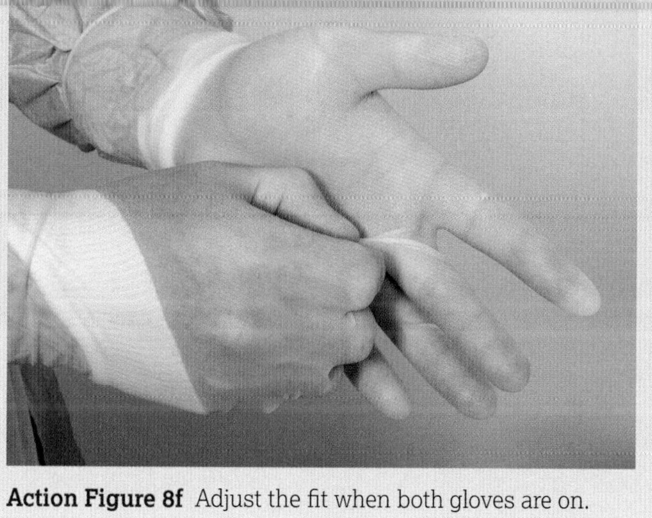

Action Figure 8f Adjust the fit when both gloves are on.

(continued)

Procedure guideline 4.9 Donning a sterile gown and gloves: closed technique *(continued)*

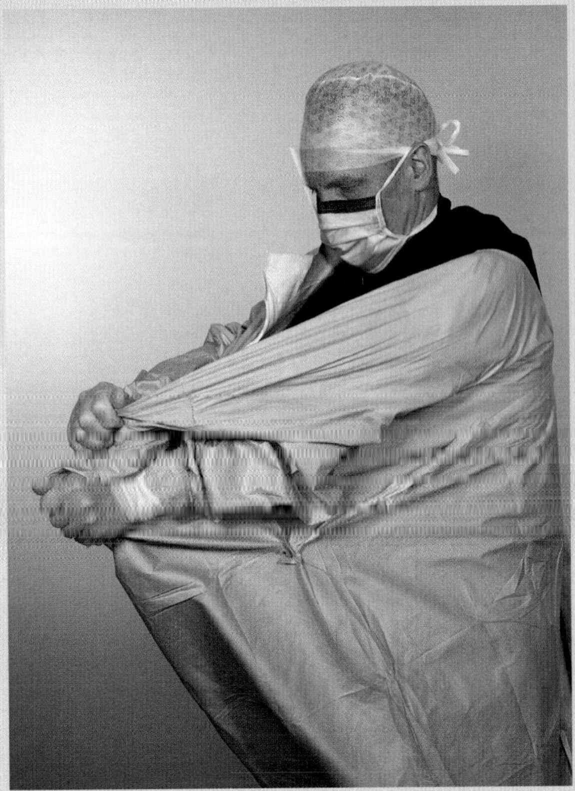

Action Figure 12a At the end of the procedure, remove the gown and gloves as a single unit by pulling the gown away from you.

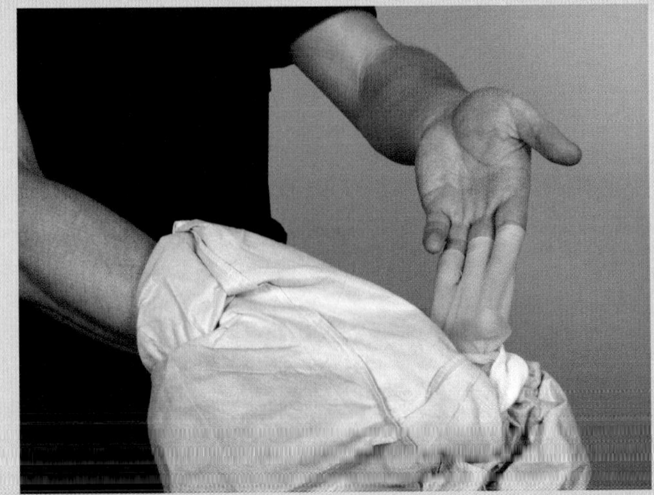

Action Figure 12b Turn the gown and gloves inside out.

Procedure guideline 4.10 Donning sterile gloves: open technique

Essential equipment

- Sterile disposable gloves
- All other equipment required for the procedure for which the gloves are required

Action	Rationale
Pre-procedure	
1 Clean hands using soap and water or an alcohol-based handrub.	Hands must be cleansed before and after every patient contact or contact with a patient's equipment (NHS England and NHSI 2019, **C**).
2 Prepare all the equipment required for the procedure, including setting up the sterile field and tipping sterile items onto it from packets if you do not have an assistant, but do not touch any sterile items before putting on gloves.	To avoid contaminating gloves with non-sterile packets. **E**
Procedure	
3 Open the packet containing the gloves and open out the inside packaging on a clean surface so that the fingers of the gloves are pointed away from you, taking care not to touch the gloves or allow them to come into contact with anything that is non-sterile (**Action figure 3**).	To prevent contamination of the gloves and to place them in the best position for putting them on. **E**
4 Clean hands again using soap and water or an alcohol-based handrub.	Hands must be cleansed before and after every patient contact or contact with patient's a equipment (NHS England and NHSI 2019, **C**).

5 Hold the cuff of the right-hand glove with the left hand, at the uppermost edge where the cuff folds back on itself. Lift this edge away from the opposite edge to create an opening (**Action figure 5a**). Keeping them together, slide the fingers of the hand into the glove, taking care not to contaminate the outside of the glove while keeping hold of the folded edge in the other hand and pulling the glove onto the hand (**Action figure 5b**). Spread the fingers of the right hand slightly to help them enter the fingers of the glove (**Action figure 5c**). *Note*: here and in the next step, the gloves can be put on either hand first; simply exchange 'left' and 'right' in the description if you wish to put on the left-hand glove first.	To prevent contamination of the outside of the glove. **E**
6 Open up the left-hand glove with your right-hand fingertips by sliding them beneath the folded-back cuff. Taking care not to touch the right-hand glove or the outside of the left-hand glove with your left hand, and keeping the fingers together, slide the fingers of your left hand into the left-hand glove (**Action figures 6a and 6b**).	To prevent contamination of the outside of the glove. **E**
7 Again, spread your fingers slightly once inside the body of the glove to help them into the glove fingers. When both gloves are on, adjust the fit by pulling on the body of the gloves to get your fingers to the ends of the glove fingers (**Action figures 7a and 7b**).	To ensure the gloves are comfortable to wear and do not interfere with the procedure. **E**
Post-procedure	
8 Remove the gloves when the procedure is completed, taking care not to contaminate your hands or the environment from the outside of the gloves.	The outside of the gloves is likely to be contaminated. **E**
9 First, remove the first glove by firmly holding the outside of the glove wrist and pulling off the glove in such a way as to turn it inside out.	While removing the first glove, the second gloved hand continues to be protected. By turning the glove inside out during removal, any contamination is contained inside the glove. **E**
10 Then remove the second glove by slipping the fingers of the ungloved hand inside the wrist of the glove and pulling it off while at the same time turning it inside out.	By putting the fingers inside the glove, the fingers will not be in contact with the potentially contaminated outer surface of the glove. **E**
11 Dispose of used gloves as 'hazardous infectious waste', unless instructed otherwise by the infection prevention and control team.	All waste contaminated with blood, body fluids, excretions, secretions and/or infectious agents thought to pose a particular risk should be disposed of as hazardous infectious waste. **E**
12 After removing the gloves, decontaminate your hands.	Hands may have become contaminated (NHS England and NHSI 2019, **C**).

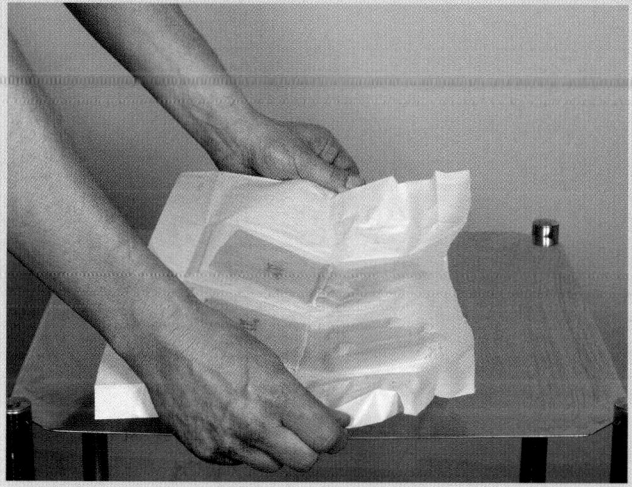

Action Figure 3 Open the packet containing the gloves onto a clean surface and open out the inside packaging so that the fingers of the gloves point away from you.

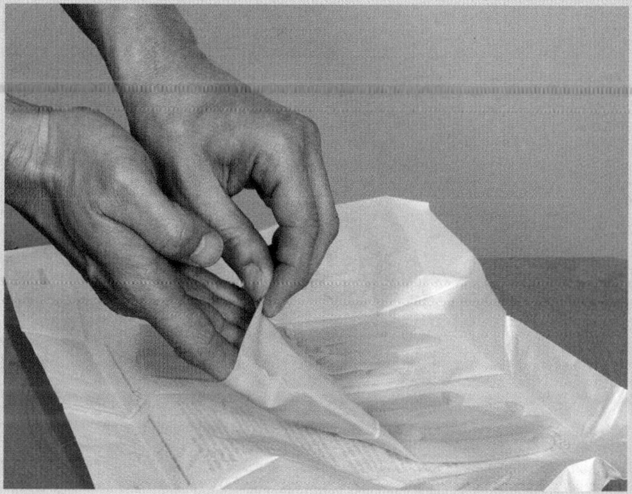

Action Figure 5a Hold the cuff of the first glove with the opposite hand and slide the fingertips of the other hand (the one that the glove is to go on) into the opening.

(continued)

Procedure guideline 4.10 Donning sterile gloves: open technique *(continued)*

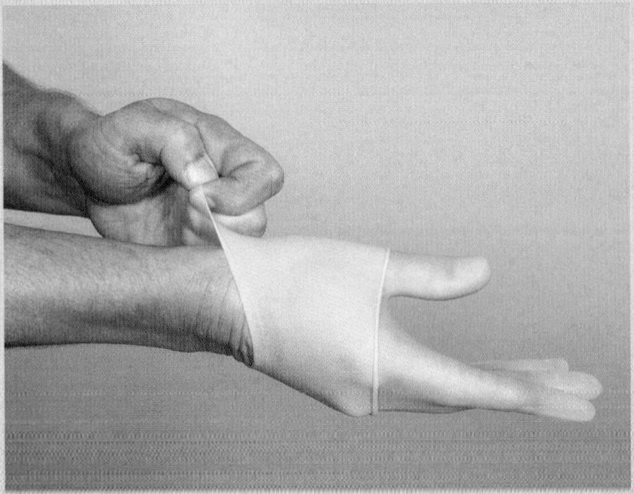

Action Figure 5b Keep hold of the folded edge and pull the glove onto your hand.

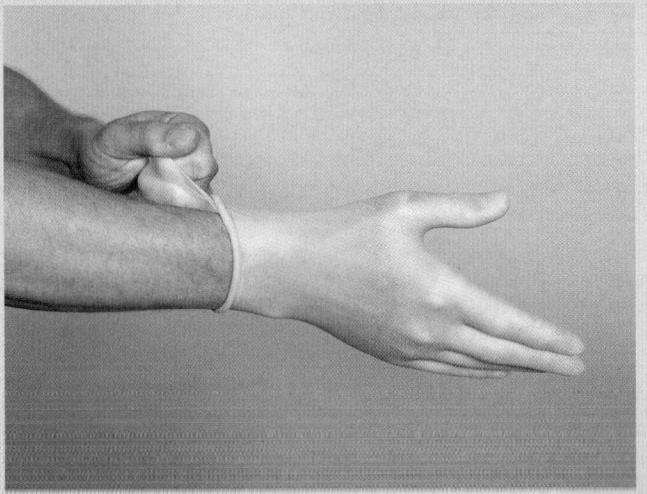

Action Figure 5c Spread your fingers slightly to help them enter the fingers of the glove.

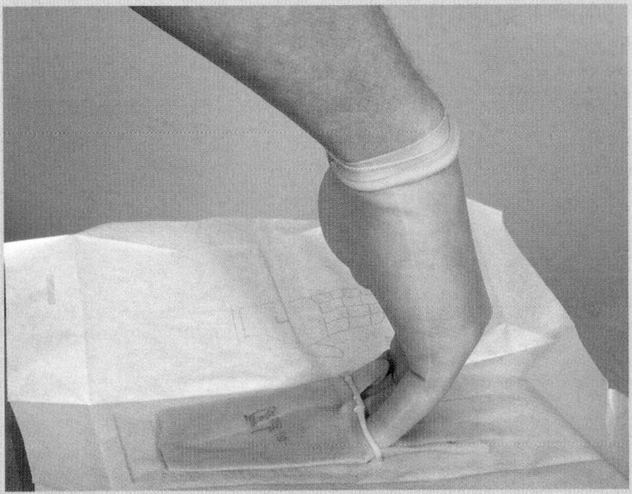

Action Figure 6a Slide the fingertips of your gloved hand beneath the folded cuff of the second glove.

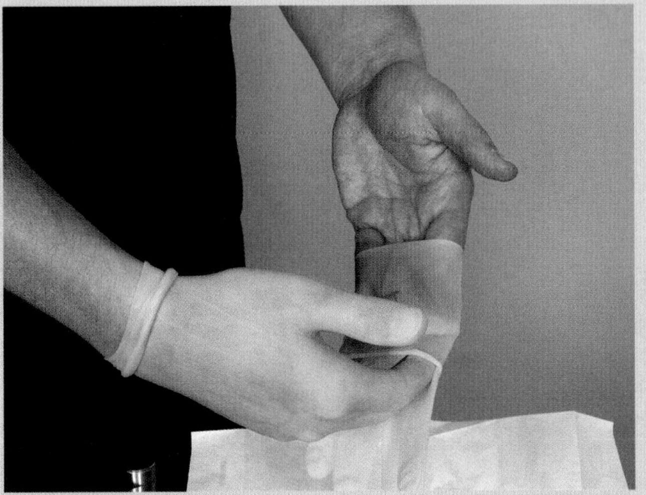

Action Figure 6b Slide the fingertips of your ungloved hand into the opening of the second glove.

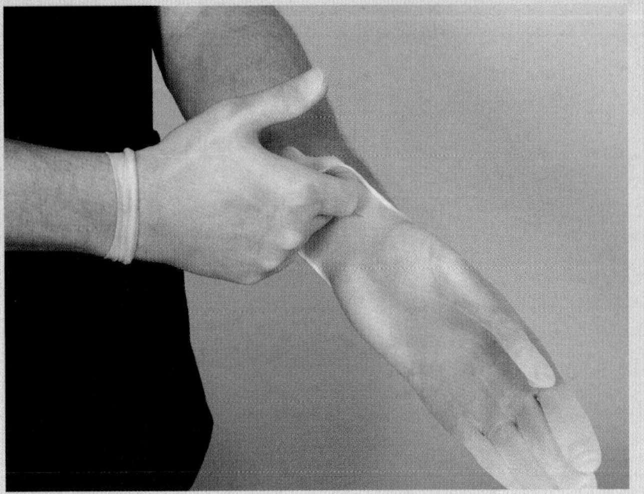

Action Figure 7a Pull the glove onto your hand, again spreading your fingers slightly to help them enter the fingers of the glove.

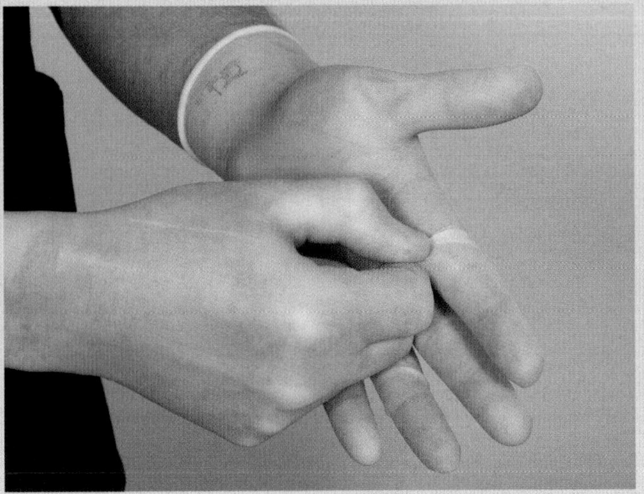

Action Figure 7b When both gloves are on, adjust the fit.

Specific patient-related procedures

Standard precautions

Related theory

The phrase 'standard precautions', or 'standard infection control precautions' (SICPs), is sometimes used to describe the actions that should be taken by all healthcare staff in every care situation to protect patients and others from infection (it is sometimes used interchangeably with 'universal precautions'; however, this term is now considered outdated). Standard precautions include:

- appropriate patient placement to minimize any risk of cross-infection
- hand hygiene at the point of care, as described by the WHO (2009a) in 'My 5 Moments for Hand Hygeine'
- respiratory and cough etiquette
- correct use of PPE for contact with all blood and body fluids
- management of care equipment to ensure it is adequately decontaminated between uses, if not designed for single patient use
- providing care in a suitably clean environment
- safe management of linen, including storage and disposal
- safe management of blood and body fluid spillages
- safe disposal of waste, including care in the use and disposal of sharps
- occupational safety, including prevention and management of inoculation, bite and splash injuries.

Aseptic technique

Definition

Aseptic technique is the practice of carrying out a procedure in such a way as to minimize the risk of introducing contamination into a vulnerable area or an invasive device. The area or device will not necessarily be sterile – wounds, for example, will be colonized with micro-organisms – but the aim is to avoid introducing additional contamination.

Aseptic non-touch technique (ANTT) is the practice of avoiding contamination by not touching key elements, such as the tip of a needle, the seal of an intravenous connector after it has been decontaminated (Figure 4.11), or the inside surface of a sterile dressing where it will be in contact with the wound (Rowley and Clare 2011).

Related theory

As with other infection prevention and control measures, the actions taken to reduce the risk of contamination will depend on the procedure being undertaken and the potential consequences of contamination (Rowley and Clare 2011). Examples of different levels of aseptic technique are given in Table 4.7. It would be difficult to provide a procedure guideline that would apply to the whole range of aseptic procedures; however, the topic is covered in other relevant procedures within this manual, such as those for the insertion of an indwelling urinary catheter (see Chapter 6: Elimination). To provide a context, Procedure guideline 4.11 contains steps for changing a wound dressing but is presented as a guide to aseptic technique in general. Local guidance and training should be sought before carrying out specific procedures.

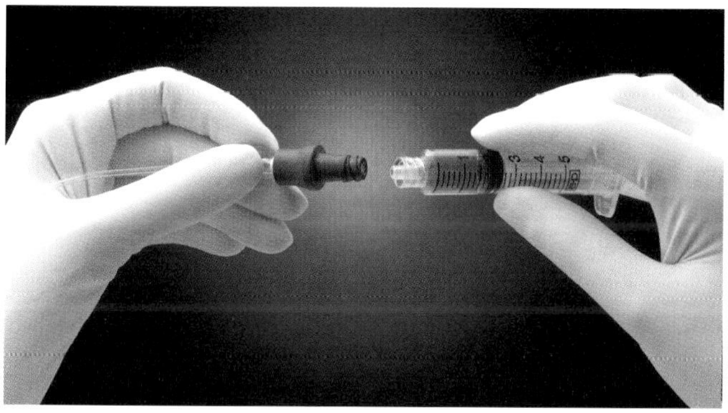

Figure 4.11 Avoiding contamination by avoiding contact with the key elements. *Source*: Reproduced with permission of ICU Medical, Inc.

Table 4.7 Examples of different levels of aseptic procedures

Procedure	Precautions required
Surgery	Carried out in an operating theatre with specialist ventilation by a team whose members wear sterile gowns and gloves
Urinary catheterization	Can be carried out in an open ward by a practitioner wearing an apron and sterile gloves
Peripheral intravenous cannulation	Can be performed in an open ward by a practitioner wearing non-sterile gloves and using an appropriate non-touch technique

Pre-procedural considerations

Equipment

Gloves

Gloves are normally worn for ANTT but they are mainly for the practitioner's, rather than the patient's, protection. Non-sterile gloves are therefore perfectly acceptable.

Sterile dressing pack

This may contain gallipots or an indented plastic tray, low-linting swabs and/or medical foam, disposable forceps, gloves, a sterile field and a disposal bag. There are specific packs available for particular procedures, for example intravenous packs. The usage and availability of these vary between organizations, so reference is generally made to a 'sterile dressing pack'.

Traceabilty system

This is a system for labelling instruments and equipment in such a way that they can be recorded in the patient record, usually as a sticker or a scanned barcode. It allows the opportunity to look back to identify what equipment has been used, where and on whom, in the event of a problem (e.g. with a batch of a product).

Trolley

Dressing trolleys should be cleaned with a detergent wipe prior to each use to remove any dust or soiling. Disinfectant wipes may be used if the trolley is physically clean.

Pharmacological support

Cleansing agents are discussed in more detail in Chapter 18: Wound management.

Specific patient preparation

Education

Wherever possible, patients should be informed about the rationale behind procedures and the steps being taken to reduce the risk of them being exposed to an HCAI during their care. Patients may be offered additional information to help them make informed choices on things that they can do to stay well and prevent infection while they are in hospital or indeed when they are at home. In particular, programmes that encourage patients to ask healthcare workers 'Did you wash your hands?' have been demonstrated to increase healthcare workers' compliance with hand hygiene (McGuckin et al. 2011). They may also empower patients and increase their confidence in the care they are receiving.

Procedure guideline 4.11 Aseptic technique example: changing a wound dressing

Essential equipment (will vary depending on procedure)

- Sterile dressing pack
- Fluids for cleaning and/or irrigation – 0.9% sodium chloride is normally appropriate
- Hypoallergenic tape (if required)
- Appropriate dressing (if required)
- Alcohol-based handrub (hand washing is an acceptable alternative but will take more time and may entail leaving the patient; alcohol-based handrub is the most appropriate method for hand hygiene during a procedure as long as hands are physically clean)
- Any extra equipment that may be needed during the procedure, for example sterile scissors
- Traceability system (sticker or electronic) for any reusable surgical instruments
- Patient record form
- Detergent wipe for cleaning trolley

Action	Rationale
Pre-procedure	
1 Check that all the equipment required for the procedure is available and, where applicable, is sterile (i.e. that packaging is undamaged, intact and dry, and that sterility indicators are present on any sterilized items and have changed colour where applicable).	To ensure that the patient is not disturbed unnecessarily if items are not available and to avoid unnecessary delays during the procedure. **E** To ensure that only sterile products are used (MHRA 2010, **C**).
2 Introduce yourself to the patient, explain and discuss the procedure with them, and gain their consent to proceed.	To ensure that the patient feels at ease, understands the procedure and gives their valid consent (NMC 2018, **C**).
Procedure	
3 Clean hands with an alcohol-based handrub or wash with soap and water and dry with paper towels.	Hands must be cleaned before and after every patient contact and before commencing the preparations for aseptic technique, to prevent cross-infection (NHS England and NHSI 2019, **C**).
4 Clean the trolley with detergent and water or detergent wipes and dry it with a paper towel. Clean from the top surface and work down to the bottom. If disinfection is also required, use disposable wipes saturated with 70% isopropyl alcohol and allow to dry.	Shared pieces of equipment used in the delivery of patient care must be cleaned and decontaminated after each use with products recommended by the manufacturer (Loveday et al. 2014a). **E** To provide a clean working surface (Fraise and Bradley 2009, **E**). Alcohol is an effective and fast-acting disinfectant that will dry quickly (Fraise and Bradley 2009, **E**).
5 Place all the equipment required for the procedure on the bottom shelf of the clean dressing trolley.	To maintain the top shelf as a clean working surface. **E**
6 Take the patient to the treatment room or screen the bed. Ensure that any fans in the area are turned off and windows closed. Position the patient comfortably and so that the area to be dealt with is easily accessible without exposing the patient unduly.	To allow any airborne organisms to settle before the sterile field (and, in this case, the wound) is exposed. To maintain the patient's dignity and comfort. **E**
7 Put on a disposable plastic apron.	To reduce the risk of contaminating clothing and of contaminating the wound or any sterile items via clothing. **E**
8 Take the trolley to the treatment room or patient's bedside, disturbing the curtains as little as possible.	To minimize airborne contamination. **E**
9 Loosen the adhesive or tape on the existing dressing.	To make it easier to remove the dressing. **E**
10 Clean hands with an alcohol-based handrub.	Hands should be cleaned before any aseptic procedure (WHO 2009a, **C**). Using alcohol-based handrub avoids having to leave the patient to go to a sink. **E**
11 Verify that the sterile pack is the correct way up and open the outer cover. Slide the contents, without touching them, onto the top shelf of the trolley.	To minimize contamination of the contents. **E**
12 Open the sterile field using only the corners of the paper.	So that areas of potential contamination are kept to a minimum. **E**
13 Open any other packs, tipping their contents gently onto the centre of the sterile field.	To prepare the equipment and, in the case of a wound dressing, reduce the amount of time that the wound is uncovered. **E**

14 Where appropriate, loosen the old dressing.	To minimize trauma when removing the old dressing. **E**
15 Clean hands with an alcohol-based handrub.	Hands may have become contaminated by handling outer packets or the old dressing (NHS England and NHSI 2019, **C**).
16 Carefully lift the plastic disposal bag from the sterile field by its open end and, holding it by one edge of the open end, place your other hand in the bag. Using it as a sterile 'glove', arrange the contents of the dressing pack and any other sterile items on the sterile field.	To maintain the sterility of the items required for the procedure while arranging them so as to perform the procedure quickly and efficiently. **E**
17 With your hand still enclosed within the disposal bag, remove the old dressing from the wound. Invert the bag so that the dressing is contained within it and stick it to the trolley below the top shelf. This is now the disposal bag for the remainder of the procedure for any waste other than sharps.	To minimize the risk of contamination by containing the dressing in the bag. **E** To ensure that any waste can be disposed of without contaminating the sterile field. **E**
18 Pour any required solutions into gallipots or onto the indented plastic tray.	To minimize the risk of contamination of solutions. **E**
19 Put on gloves, as described in Procedure guideline 4.5: Putting on and removing non-sterile gloves or Procedure guideline 4.10: Donning sterile gloves: open technique. The procedure will dictate whether the gloves should be sterile or non-sterile.	Gloves should be worn whenever any contact with body fluids is anticipated (Loveday et al. 2014a, **C**). Sterile gloves provide greater sensitivity than forceps for procedures that cannot be carried out with a non-touch technique and are less likely to cause trauma to the patient. **E**
20 Carry out the relevant procedure according to local guidelines.	
Post-procedure	
21 Make sure the patient is comfortable.	To minimize the risk of causing the patient distress or discomfort. **E**
22 Dispose of waste, including apron and gloves, in offensive waste bags.	To prevent environmental contamination (DH 2013b, **C**).
23 Draw back the curtains or help the patient back to the bed area and ensure that they are comfortable.	To minimize the risk of causing the patient distress or discomfort. **E**
24 Check that the trolley remains dry and physically clean. If necessary, wash it with liquid detergent and water or detergent wipe and dry thoroughly with a paper towel.	To remove any contamination on the trolley and so minimize the risk of transferring any contamination elsewhere in the ward (Loveday et al. 2014a, **C**).
25 Clean hands with alcohol-based handrub or soap and water.	Hands should be cleaned after any contact with the patient or body fluids (WHO 2009a, **C**).
26 Document the procedure clearly, including details of who carried it out, any devices or dressings used (particularly any left *in situ*), and any deviation from the prescribed procedure. Fix any record labels from the outside packaging of the items used during the procedure on the patient record and add this to the patient's notes.	To provide a record of the procedure and evidence that any items used have undergone an appropriate sterilization process (DH 2007, **C**; NMC 2018, **C**).

Nursing care of patients with suspected or known infection: managing safe care

Related theory

The principle of infection prevention and control is preventing the transmission of infectious agents. However, measures taken to reduce the risk of transmission must be reasonable, practicable and proportionate to the transmission risk. They must not lose sight of the need to provide safe and efficient healthcare and keep services running efficiently for the benefit of all patients. For example, while *S. aureus* can cause severe infections, it is carried by around a third of the population and so isolating every patient who carries it would not be practicable or possible. On the other hand, its antibiotic-resistant version (known as MRSA) can cause equally serious infections and is resistant to common first-line antibiotics that would normally be used to treat these infections. It is carried by far fewer people, and it is therefore reasonable and practical to take additional precautions to prevent its spread in healthcare (Coia et al. 2006).

The management of any individual who is infected or colonized with an organism that may pose a risk to other individuals must be based on a risk assessment that takes into account the following factors (Jones 2010):

- What is the organism responsible for the infection?
- What are the possible routes of transmission and how easily can it be spread?
- How susceptible to infection are any other people being cared for in the same area and what would be the likely consequences if they were to become infected?
- How practical would it be to implement specific infection prevention and control precautions within the relevant area or institution (e.g. bearing in mind the number of single rooms available and staffing levels)?
- What are the individual's other nursing needs?

The infection prevention and control policies of health and social care providers are based on generic risk assessments of their

Box 4.3 Transmission routes

Transmission routes can be divided into the following:
- *Direct contact*: person-to-person spread of infectious agents through physical contact.
- *Indirect contact*: where someone comes into contact with a contaminated object.
- *Enteric*: organisms carried in faeces.
- *Parenteral transmission*: where blood or body fluids containing infectious agents come into contact with mucous membranes or exposed tissue. In healthcare, this can occur through transplantation or infusion (which is why blood and organs for transplantation are screened for blood-borne viruses such as HIV) or through an inoculation injury where blood splashes into the eyes or a used item of sharp equipment penetrates the skin.
- *Faecal–oral transmission*: where an infectious agent present in the faeces of an infected person is subsequently ingested by someone else and enters their gastrointestinal tract. This is the route of most gastrointestinal illness as well as water- and foodborne diseases (salmonella, norovirus and *C. difficile* infections are also spread in this manner).
- *Droplets*: large respiratory particles.
- *Airborne*: smaller airborne particles, usually respiratory.

usual client or patient group and should be adhered to unless there are strong reasons to alter procedures for a particular individual's care. In such circumstances, the advice of the infection prevention and control team (IPCT) should be sought first. Nurses working in organizations without an IPCT should identify the most appropriate source from which to seek advice, preferably before it is needed. The local public health unit will be able to signpost appropriate advice providers.

All patients should have an assessment for infection risk on arrival and where possible beforehand if admission is planned. This assessment may need to be repeated at intervals depending on the changing condition of the patient. Based on this assessment, additional transmission-based precautions may be required for patients known or strongly suspected to be infected or colonized with organisms that pose a significant risk to other patients.

The precautions will vary depending on the route by which the organism can travel from one individual to another, but there will be common elements (Box 4.3).

Evidence-based approaches

Transmission precautions can be grouped as follows.

Contact precautions

Patients known or strongly suspected to be infected or colonized with pathogenic micro-organisms that spread via direct contact with the patient or indirectly from the patient's immediate care environment (including care equipment) should be managed with contact precautions.

Contact precautions normally consist of standard precautions enhanced with isolation of the patient in a single room and use of gloves and apron for any procedure involving contact with the patient or their immediate environment.

Enhanced contact precautions

Enhanced contact precautions are used for patients known or strongly suspected to be infected or colonized with highly resistant organisms. This involves the addition of a long-sleeved gown to the normal contact precautions above.

Enteric precautions

Patients suffering symptoms of diarrhoea or vomiting that do not have an obvious mechanical or non-infectious cause should be cared for using enteric precautions. These should be used from the first instance of diarrhoea or vomiting, regardless of whether a causative organism has been identified, until there is a definitive diagnosis that the symptoms do not have an infectious cause (prompt collection of a stool sample is important). Enteric viruses are highly transmissible and outbreaks occur rapidly if precautions are not speedily implemented.

Enteric precautions consist of prompt isolation of the patient in a single room, ideally with an en suite toilet facility. The door of the room should be closed, and gloves and apron should be used for any procedure involving contact with the patient or their immediate environment (Health Protection Agency 2012).

Droplet precautions

Patients known or strongly suspected to be infected or colonized with pathogenic micro-organisms that are mainly transmitted via droplets of body fluids should be cared for with additional infection control precautions. The infectious agents are most often respiratory secretions expelled during coughing and sneezing but can include droplets from other sources, such as projectile vomiting or explosive diarrhoea.

Droplet precautions consist of isolation of the patient in a single room with the door closed and use of gloves and apron for any procedure involving contact with the patient or their immediate environment. Droplets are heavy and will usually travel no more than a metre from the person before settling on surfaces, so good hand hygiene and frequently touched surface environmental hygiene are essential. The patient should where possible be encouraged to practice good respiratory etiquette. For some infections (high-risk respiratory viruses, e.g. tuberculosis), staff entering the room may be required to wear a mask for close and prolonged contact and during aerosol-generating procedures.

Airborne precautions

Patients known or strongly suspected to be infected or colonized with pathogenic micro-organisms that are transmitted through the airborne route are cared for with airborne precautions. Airborne transmission involves droplets or particles containing infectious agents that are so tiny that the particles can remain suspended in the air for long periods of time. Infections spread via this route include measles and chickenpox.

Airborne precautions consist of isolation of the patient in a single room, if possible with negative pressure ventilation or a positive pressure ventilated lobby, with the door closed. Gloves and apron should be used for any procedure involving contact with the patient or their immediate environment. Staff entering the room should wear a properly fitted respirator (FFP3) mask (Siegel et al. 2007) (Figure 4.12).

Some guidelines merge droplet and airborne precautions in order to provide a single set of instructions for staff caring for

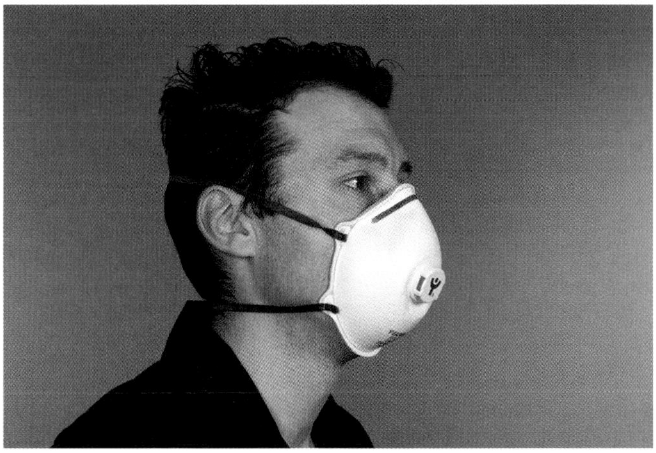

Figure 4.12 A correctly fitted FFP3 mask may be required for aerosol-generating procedures on patients with infections such as tuberculosis or influenza.

patients with any respiratory or airborne infection. A risk assessment should be carried out to determine the most appropriate PPE on a case-by-case basis.

Vector transmission

Many diseases are spread through the action of a vector, most often an insect that travels from one person to another to feed. This route is not currently a concern in healthcare in the UK; however, in some areas of the world, for example where malaria or dengue are endemic, protecting patients from vectors such as mosquitoes is an important element of nursing care. Diseases spread by vector do not generally spread from person to person.

Isolation procedures

Definition

Isolation is the practice of segregating a patient away from others to reduce the risk of spreading infection to others. The type of isolation – source isolation or protective isolation – will depend on the mode of transmission of the pathogen or the risk to the patient.

Source isolation

Definition

Source isolation is used for patients who are infected with, or are colonized by, infectious agents that require additional precautions over and above the standard precautions used with every patient (Siegal et al. 2007) in order to minimize the risk of transmission to other vulnerable persons. The exact precautions needed will depend on the mode of transmission of the organism and are known as 'transmission based precautions'. Patients requiring source isolation are normally cared for in a single room, although during an outbreak it may be necessary for patients affected by the same infection to be nursed in a 'cohort'.

Related theory

A single-occupancy room will physically separate patients who present a risk from others who may be at risk, and will act as a reminder to any staff dealing with patients who present a risk of the need for additional infection control precautions. Single-occupancy rooms used for source isolation should have en suite toilet and bathroom facilities wherever possible, and should contain all items required to meet the patient's nursing needs during the period of isolation (e.g. instruments to assess vital signs). Ideally, these should remain inside the room throughout the period of isolation. However, if this is not possible because insufficient equipment is available on the ward, any items taken from the room must be thoroughly cleaned and disinfected (with locally approved disinfectant) before being used with any other patient (Health Protection Scotland 2017). Conversely, it is important not to have unnecessary equipment in the room that may have to be discarded when the patient leaves.

The air pressure in a source isolation room should be negative or neutral in relation to the air pressure in the rest of the ward (note that some airborne infections will require a negative pressure room) (Siegal et al. 2007). A lobby will provide an additional degree of security and space for donning and removing PPE and performing hand hygiene. Some facilities have lobbies that are ventilated to have positive pressure with respect to both the rest of the ward and the single-occupancy room; this allows the room to be used for both source and protective isolation (DH 2013d).

Where insufficient single rooms are available for source isolation, they should be allocated to those patients who pose the greatest risk to others. As a general rule, patients with highly multiresistant organisms and/or enteric symptoms (such as diarrhoea and vomiting) or serious airborne infections (such as tuberculosis) have the highest priority for single-occupancy rooms (Jeanes et al. 2011). If a patient cannot be isolated, this should be escalated to the site manager and flagged as a risk. While the patient is waiting for an appropriate room, contact precautions will be required in the open ward.

Patients should receive a clear explanation of why they are being isolated and how this is prioritized, or they may be concerned about inconsistency. It is important that the patient's other nursing and medical needs are always taken into account, and infection control precautions may need to be modified accordingly as isolation can have adverse psychological effects (Guilley-Lerondeau et al. 2017).

Evidence-based approaches

Principles of care

Attending to a patient in isolation

Meals

Meals should be served on normal crockery and the patient provided with normal cutlery. Cutlery and crockery should be washed in a dishwasher able to thermally disinfect items – that is, with a final rinse of 80°C for 1 minute or 71°C for 3 minutes. Disposables and uneaten food should be discarded in the appropriate bag. Contaminated crockery is a potential vector for infectious agents, particularly those that cause enteric disease, but thermal disinfection will minimize this risk (Fraise and Bradley 2009).

Urine and faeces

Wherever possible, a toilet should be kept solely for the patient's use. If this is not feasible, the patient should be offered a commode. If there is sufficient stock, the commode should be kept in the patient's room; it should be emptied promptly and cleaned between each use with an appropriate disinfectant. Gloves and apron must be worn by staff when dealing with body fluids. Bedpans and urinals should be covered and taken directly to the sluice for disposal. They should not be emptied before being placed in the bedpan washer or macerator unless the volume of the contents needs to be measured for a fluid balance or stool chart. Weighing scales are recommended for recording volume for fluid balance (1 ml = 1 gram). Gloves and aprons worn in the room should be kept on until the body waste has been disposed of and then removed (gloves first) and discarded as offensive waste.

Spillages

As elsewhere, any spillage must be mopped up immediately to remove the risk of anyone slipping. Blood or body fluids should be cleaned up using a locally approved disinfectant with demonstrable activity against target pathogens, following the manufacturer's instructions and local guidance.

Bathing

Ideally an en suite bathroom or patient specific bathroom should be used. If this is not possible, the patient should use the ward bathroom, which should be thoroughly cleaned after use to minimize the risk of cross-infection to other patients.

Linen

Follow local procedure and place linen in an infected linen bag. This is usually a red water-soluble alginate polythene bag, which must be secured tightly before being put into a red fabric bag. These bags should await the laundry collection in the area designated for this. Placing infected linen into the appropriate bags confines harmful organisms and allows laundry staff to recognize the potential hazard and avoid handling the linen (DH 2013c).

Waste

Hazardous waste bags should be kept in the isolation room for disposal of clinical waste generated in the room. The top of the bag should be sealed and labelled with the name of the ward or department before it is removed from the room.

Cleaning an isolation room

The following principles should be adhered to regarding the cleaning of an isolation room:

- Domestic or environmental services staff must be instructed on the correct procedure to use when cleaning an isolation room; however, they must not be given any confidential patient information.
- They should understand what disinfectants should be used and if necessary how to make them up (dilution) as well as the correct colour coding for cleaning materials. This will reduce the risk of mistakes and ensure that appropriate precautions are maintained (Curran et al. 2019, DH 2017). Cleaning cloths may be reusable microfibre or disposable, depending on the organization's local policy.
- Separate cleaning equipment must be used for isolation rooms. Cross-infection may result from shared cleaning equipment (Wilson 2019).
- Domestic or environmental services staff must wear gloves and plastic aprons while cleaning isolation rooms to minimize the risk of contaminating hands or clothing. Some PPE may also be required for the safe use of some cleaning solutions.
- Isolation rooms should be cleaned last, to reduce the risk of the transmission of contamination to 'clean' areas (NICE 2017).
- Daily cleaning will reduce the number of bacteria in the environment. Organisms, especially gram-negative bacteria, multiply quickly in the presence of moisture and on equipment (Wilson 2019).
- Furniture and fittings should be damp-dusted daily (by nursing or cleaning staff) using a disposable cloth and a detergent or disinfectant solution, as dictated by local protocol. This is to remove dirt and a proportion of any organisms contaminating the environment (Wilson 2019).
- The toilet, shower and bathroom areas must be cleaned at least once a day and, if they become contaminated, using a non-abrasive hypochlorite powder, cream or solution. Non-abrasive powders and creams preserve the integrity of the surfaces.
- Floors must be washed daily with a disinfectant as appropriate. All excess water must be removed and disposed of in a dedicated disposal sink. Floors should have a hard surface: carpeted rooms should not be used in patient care areas.
- Cleaning solutions must be freshly made up each day and the container emptied and cleaned daily after use. This is because disinfectants may lose their effectiveness over time and cleaning solutions can easily become contaminated (Weber et al. 2007).
- After use, the bucket must be cleaned and dried. Contaminated cleaning equipment and solutions will spread bacteria over surfaces being cleaned (Weber et al. 2007).
- Mop heads and reusable cloths should be laundered daily as they become contaminated easily (Wilson 2019). Current methods for decontamination of reusable mops and cloths include ozone or laundry in water above 71°C (minimum 3 minutes). The exact methods will be dictated by local contract arrangements.

Procedure guideline 4.12 Source isolation: preparing an isolation room

Essential equipment

- Personal protective equipment
- Single-occupancy room
- Patient equipment
- Hand hygiene facilities
- Patient information material

Action	Rationale
Pre-procedure	
1 Identify the most suitable room available for source isolation, taking into account the risk to other patients and staff and the patient's other nursing needs.	To ensure the best balance between minimizing the risk of cross-infection and maintaining the safety and comfort of the isolated patient. **E**
Procedure	
2 Remove all non-essential furniture and equipment from the room. The remaining furniture should be easy to clean. Ensure that the room is stocked with any equipment required for patient care and sufficient but not excessive numbers of any disposable items that will be required.	To ensure the availability of everything required for patient care while minimizing the number of items that will require cleaning or disposal at the end of the isolation period and the amount of traffic of people and equipment into and out of the room. **E**
3 Ensure that a bin with a hazardous waste bag is present in the room. This will be used for clinical waste generated in the room. The bag must be sealed before it is removed from the room. Depending on the infection, it may be possible to have a general waste bag as well for non-infected items.	To contain contaminated rubbish within the room and minimize further spread of infection. **E**
4 Place a container for sharps in the room.	To contain contaminated sharps within the infected area (DH 2013b, **C**).
5 Keep the patient's personal property to a minimum. All belongings taken into the room should be washable, cleanable or disposable. Contact the infection prevention and control team for advice as to how best to clean or wash specific items.	The patient's belongings may become contaminated and cannot be taken home unless they are washable or cleanable. **E**
6 Ensure that all personal protective equipment (PPE) required is available outside the room. Wall-mounted dispensers offer the best use of space and ease of use but, if necessary, set up a trolley outside the door or in the ante room for PPE and alcohol-based handrub. Ensure that these arrangements do not cause an obstruction or other hazard.	To have PPE readily available when required. **E**

7 Introduce yourself to the patient, explain the reason for isolation and the precise precautions, and provide relevant patient information material where available. Allow the patient to ask questions and ask for a member of the infection prevention and control team to visit the patient if ward staff cannot answer all questions to the patient's satisfaction. The patient's family and other visitors may require an explanation but *any explanations given must respect patient confidentiality.*	Patients and their visitors may be more compliant if they understand the reasons for isolation, and the patient's anxiety may be reduced if they have as much information as possible about their condition. **E**
8 Fix a suitable notice outside the room where it will be seen by anyone attempting to enter. This should indicate the special precautions required while preserving the patient's confidentiality.	To ensure all staff and visitors are aware of the need for additional infection control precautions. **E**
9 Move the patient into the single-occupancy room.	For effective isolation. **E**
10 Arrange for terminal cleaning of the bed space that the patient has been occupying.	To remove any infectious agents that may pose a risk to the next patient to occupy that bed (NPSA 2009, **C**; Otter et al. 2012, **C**; Passaretti et al. 2013, **R**).
Post-procedure	
11 Assess the patient daily to determine whether source isolation is still required; for example, if enteric precautions have been required, has the patient been without symptoms for 48 hours?	There is often limited availability of isolation rooms (Wigglesworth and Wilcox 2006, **R**) so they must be used as effectively as possible. **E**

Procedure guideline 4.13 Source isolation: entering an isolation room

Essential equipment

- Personal protective equipment as dictated by the precautions required: gloves and apron are the usual minimum; a respirator is required for droplet precautions; eye protection is required if an aerosol-generating procedure is planned
- Any equipment required for any procedure intended to be carried out in the room

Action	Rationale
Pre-procedure	
1 Decontaminate hands and collect all equipment needed.	To avoid entering and leaving the area unnecessarily. **E**
Procedure	
2 Ensure you are 'bare below the elbow' (see Procedure guideline 4.1: Hand washing).	To facilitate hand hygiene and avoid any contamination of long sleeves or cuffs, as this could cause cross-contamination to other patients. **E**
3 Put on a disposable plastic apron.	To protect the front of the uniform or clothing, which is the area most likely to come into contact with the patient. **E**
4 Put on a well-fitting mask or respirator of the appropriate standard if droplet or airborne precautions are required, for example if the patient has: • meningococcal meningitis and has not completed 24 hours of treatment • pandemic influenza • tuberculosis, if carrying out an aerosol-generating procedure or the tuberculosis may be multiresistant.	To reduce the risk of inhaling organisms (DH 2010b, **C**; HSE 2013c, 2013d, **C**).
5 Don eye protection if instructed by the infection prevention and control team (e.g. for pandemic influenza) or if conducting an aerosol-generating procedure (e.g. bronchoscopy or intubation) in a patient requiring airborne or droplet precautions.	To prevent infection via the conjunctiva (DH 2010b, **C**).
6 Clean hands with soap and water or an alcohol-based handrub.	Hands must be cleaned before patient contact (WHO 2009a, **C**).
7 Don disposable gloves if you are intending to deal with blood, excreta or contaminated material, or if providing close personal care where contact precautions are required. Gloves may need to be changed while in the room as per 'My 5 Moments for Hand Hygiene' (WHO 2009a).	To reduce the risk of hand contamination (NHS England and NHSI 2019, **C**).
8 Enter the room, shutting the door behind you.	To reduce the risk of airborne organisms leaving the room (Kao and Yang 2006, **R**). To preserve the patient's privacy and dignity. **E**

Procedure guideline 4.14 Source isolation: leaving an isolation room

Essential equipment

- Hazardous waste bag
- Hand hygiene facilities

Action	Rationale
Procedure	
1 If there is an ante room or lobby, this should be used for removal of personal protective equipment (PPE).	To minimize the amount of waste in the room and provide space for applying and removing PPE.**C**
2 If wearing gloves, remove and discard them in the hazardous waste bag.	To avoid transferring any contamination on the gloves to other areas or items (Loveday et al. 2014a, **C**).
3 Remove apron by holding the inside of the apron and breaking the ties at the neck and waist. Discard it into the hazardous waste bag.	To avoid transferring any contamination on the apron to other areas or items (Loveday et al. 2014a, **C**).
4 Clean hands with soap and water or an alcohol-based handrub. Do not use alcohol based handrub when dealing with faeces.	Hands must be cleaned after contact with the patient or their immediate environment (WHO 2009a, **C**). Alcohol is less effective against *C. difficile* spores and some enteric viruses and in the presence of organic material such as faeces (Fraise and Bradley 2009, **E**).
5 Leave the room, shutting the door behind you.	To reduce the risk of airborne organisms leaving the room (Kao and Yang 2006, **R**). To preserve the patient's privacy and dignity. **E**
6 Clean hands with an alcohol-based handrub on leaving the room.	Hands must be cleaned after contact with the patient or their immediate environment (WHO 2009a, **C**).

Procedure guideline 4.15 Source isolation: transporting infected patients outside a source isolation area

Action	Rationale
Procedure	
1 At the earliest opportunity, inform the department concerned about the procedure and the appropriate infection control precautions required. *Maintain patient confidentiality.*	To allow the department time to make appropriate arrangements. **E**
2 If possible and appropriate, arrange for the patient to have the last appointment of the day. If this is not possible, the patient should be seen quickly and returned to their isolation room.	The department concerned and any intervening areas will be less busy, so reducing the risk of contact with other vulnerable individuals. Also, the additional cleaning required following any procedure will not disrupt subsequent appointments. **E**
3 Inform the portering service of the infection control precautions required.	Explanation will minimize the risk of cross-infection through failure to comply with infection control precautions (Fraise and Bradley 2009, **E**).
4 Introduce yourself to the patient, and explain and discuss the procedure with them.	To ensure that the patient feels at ease and understands the procedure (NMC 2018, **C**).
5 If the patient has an infection requiring droplet or airborne precautions, where the infection may present a risk to people encountered in the other department or in transit, the patient will need to wear a mask or respirator of the appropriate standard. Provide the patient with the mask and explain why it is required and how and when it is to be worn (i.e. while outside their single-occupancy room) and assist them to don it if necessary.	To prevent airborne cross-infection. **E** Providing the patient with relevant information will reduce anxiety. **C**
6 Escort the patient if necessary.	To attend to the patient's nursing needs and to remind others of infection control precautions if required. **E**

Post-procedural considerations

Discharging a patient from isolation

If the patient no longer requires isolation but is still to be a patient on the ward, inform them of this and the reasons why isolation is no longer required before moving them out of the room. Also inform them if there is any reason why they may need to be returned to isolation, for example if diarrhoea returns.

If the patient is to be discharged home or to another health or social care setting, ensure that the discharge documentation includes details of their condition, the infection control precautions taken while they were in hospital, and any precautions or other actions that will need to be taken following discharge. Accurate information on infections must be supplied to any person involved with providing further support or nursing/medical care in a timely fashion (DH 2015a).

Cleaning an isolation room after a patient has been discharged

The following principles should be adhered to regarding the cleaning of an isolation room after a patient has been discharged:

- The room should be stripped. All bed linen and other textiles must be changed and curtains changed (reusable curtains must be laundered and disposable curtains discarded as offensive waste). Dispose of any unused disposable items. Curtains and other fabrics readily become colonized with bacteria (Shek et al. 2018), and paper packets cannot easily be cleaned.
- Impervious surfaces (e.g. locker, bedframe, mattress cover, chairs, floor, blinds and soap dispenser) should be washed with soap and water, or a sporicidal disinfectant if activity against spores is required, and dried. Relatively inaccessible places, for example ceilings, may be omitted, as inaccessible areas are not generally relevant to any infection risk (Wilson 2019). Wiping of surfaces is the most effective way of removing contaminants. Spores from some sources (e.g. *C. difficile*) will persist indefinitely in the environment unless destroyed by an effective disinfectant, and bacteria will thrive more readily in damp conditions.
- The room can be reused as soon as it has been thoroughly cleaned and restocked. Effective cleaning will have removed infectious agents that may pose a risk to the next patient.
- For some high-risk infections, such as *C. difficile* or multi-resistant gram-negative bacteria, it may be helpful to use additional automated room disinfection technology such as hydrogen peroxide vapour or ultraviolet-C light. However, these are not available in all settings; if they are available, they must only be used by specifically trained staff.

Protective isolation

Definition

Protective isolation is the practice of isolating a patient who does not have a competent immune system in order to protect them from potentially harmful organisms. It was formerly known as 'reverse barrier nursing'.

Related theory

Protective isolation is used to minimize the exposure to infectious agents of patients who are particularly at risk of infection. The evidence that protective isolation successfully reduces the incidence of infection is limited (Abad et al. 2010), probably because many infections are endogenous (i.e. caused by the patient's own bacterial flora). Protective isolation is used to reduce the risk of exogenous infection in groups that have greatly impaired immune systems, such as bone marrow transplant patients. Patients who have compromised immune systems often have greatly reduced numbers of a type of white blood cell called a neutrophil; this condition is known as neutropenia and those affected are described as neutropenic. Neutropenia is graded from mild to severe according to how few neutrophils are in the circulation and hence how severe the risk is (Godwin et al. 2018).

Single-occupancy rooms used for protective isolation should have neutral or positive air pressure with respect to the surrounding area.

Evidence-based approaches

Principles of care

The patient should be given information about the importance of good food hygiene in reducing their exposure to potential pathogens. Neutropenic patients should avoid unpasteurized dairy products, raw or runny eggs, pâté and sushi, other potentially hazardous foods such as raw fruit, salads and uncooked vegetables may be eaten as long as good food hygiene is followed. This includes washing raw ingredients, peeling fruit or vegetables, storing foods at correct temperatures and avoiding reheating food.

It is important that the patient and their family understand the importance of good hand hygiene before eating or drinking (as potential pathogens on the hands may be inadvertently consumed) and the need for good food hygiene. Any food brought in for the patient should be in undamaged, sealed tins and packets obtained from well-known, reliable firms and must be within the expiry date, as correctly processed and packaged foods are more likely to be of an acceptable food hygiene standard. Previously served food should not be reheated.

Procedure guideline 4.16 Protective isolation: preparing an isolation room

Essential equipment

- Personal protective equipment
- Single-occupancy room
- Patient equipment
- Hand hygiene facilities
- Patient information material

Action	Rationale
Pre-procedure	
1 Identify the most suitable room available for protective isolation, taking into account the risk to the patient, the patient's other nursing needs and other demands on the available single rooms.	To ensure the best balance between minimizing the risk of infection, maintaining the safety and comfort of the isolated patient, and the need for single rooms for other purposes. **E**

(continued)

Procedure guideline 4.16 Protective isolation: preparing an isolation room *(continued)*

Action	Rationale
Procedure	
2 Remove all non-essential furniture and equipment from the room. The remaining furniture should be easy to clean. Ensure that the room is stocked with any equipment required for patient care and sufficient numbers of any disposable items that will be required.	To ensure the availability of everything required for patient care while minimizing the amount of cleaning required and the amount of traffic of people and equipment into and out of the room. **E**
3 Ensure that all personal protective equipment (PPE) required is available outside the room. Wall-mounted dispensers offer the best use of space and ease of use but, if necessary, set up a trolley outside the door for PPE and an alcohol-based handrub. Ensure that these arrangements do not cause an obstruction or other hazard.	To have PPE readily available when required. **E**
4 Ensure that the room is thoroughly cleaned before the patient is admitted.	Effective cleaning will remove infectious agents that may pose a risk to the patient (NPSA 2009, **C**).
5 Introduce yourself to the patient, explain the reason for isolation and the precise precautions, and provide relevant patient information material where available. Allow the patient to ask questions and ask for a member of the infection prevention and control team to visit the patient if ward staff cannot answer all questions to the patient's satisfaction. The patient's family and other visitors may require an explanation but *any explanations given must respect patient confidentiality.*	Patients and their visitors may be more compliant if they understand the reasons for isolation, and the patient's anxiety may be reduced if they have as much information as possible about their condition. **E**
6 Fix a suitable notice outside the room where it will be seen by anyone attempting to enter the room. This should indicate the special precautions required while preserving the patient's confidentiality.	To ensure all staff and visitors are aware of the need for additional infection control precautions. **E**
7 Move the patient into the single-occupancy room.	To minimize exposure to potentially harmful micro-organisms (Wigglesworth 2003, **E**).
8 Ensure that surfaces and furniture are damp-dusted according to the cleaning schedule using disposable cloths. High-risk areas should usually be cleaned two or three times per day.	Damp-dusting and mopping remove micro-organisms without distributing them into the air. **E** To meet national cleaning standards for a high-risk area. **E**

Procedure guideline 4.17 Protective isolation: entering an isolation room

Essential equipment

- Hand hygiene facilities
- Disposable plastic apron
- Gloves and mask where indicated
- Additional equipment for any procedure to be undertaken

Action	Rationale
Pre-procedure	
1 Collect all equipment needed.	To avoid entering and leaving the room unnecessarily. **E**
Procedure	
2 Ensure you are 'bare below the elbow' (see Procedure guideline 4.1: Hand washing).	To facilitate hand hygiene and to avoid transferring any contamination to the patient from long sleeves or cuffs. **E**
3 Put on a disposable plastic apron.	To provide a barrier over the front of the uniform or clothing, which is the area most likely to come in contact with the patient. **E**
4 Staff who have any coryzal symptoms should not enter the room. If this is unavoidable, they should wear a mask.	To prevent unnecessary exposure of the patient to pathogenic organisms. **E**
5 Clean hands with soap and water or an alcohol-based handrub.	To remove any contamination from the hands that could be transferred to the patient (WHO 2009a, **C**).
6 Close the door after entering.	To reduce the risk of airborne transmission of infection from other areas of the ward and ensure that the ventilation and air filtration systems work as efficiently as possible. **E**

Visitors	
7 Ask the patient to nominate close relatives and friends who may then, after instruction (see steps 1–6 above), visit freely. The patient or their representative should ask other acquaintances and non-essential visitors to avoid visiting during the period of vulnerability.	The risk of infection is likely to increase in proportion to the number of people visiting. Unlimited visiting by close relatives and friends may diminish any sense of isolation in the patient; however, large numbers of visitors may be difficult to screen and educate. **E**
8 Exclude any visitor who has had symptoms of infection or been in contact with a communicable disease in the previous 48 hours.	Individuals may be infectious both before and after developing symptoms of infection (Goering et al. 2012, **E**).
9 Educate all visitors to decontaminate their hands before entering the isolation room.	Hands carry large numbers of potentially pathogenic micro-organisms, but these can be easily removed (WHO 2009a, **C**).
10 Visiting by children, other than very close relatives, should be discouraged.	Children are more likely to have been in contact with infectious diseases but are less likely to be aware of this and are more likely to develop infections because they have less acquired immunity. **E**

Post-procedural considerations

Discharging a neutropenic patient

Patients who have recently been neutropenic should be advised to avoid crowded areas, for example shops, cinemas, pubs and other entertainment venues (Calandra 2000). They should be advised that pets should not be allowed to lick them, and new or other people's pets should be avoided. Pets are known carriers of potential pathogens (Lefebvre et al. 2006).

Certain foods, for example take-away meals, soft cheese and pâté, should continue to be avoided as these foodstuffs are more likely than others to be contaminated with potential pathogens (Gillespie et al. 2005). Salads and fruit should be washed carefully, dried and, if possible, peeled to remove as many pathogens as possible (Moody et al. 2006).

It is vital that the patient and their family know that any signs or symptoms of infection, such as a temperature, should be reported immediately to the patient's GP or to the discharging hospital. Any infection may have serious consequences if not treated promptly.

Environmental hygiene and the management of waste in the healthcare environment

Definition

The term 'environmental hygiene' refers to the standard of cleanliness expected in a clinical area.

Related theory

Providing a clean and safe environment for healthcare is a key priority for the NHS and is a core standard in the Hygiene Code (DH 2015a). The role of cleaning has been recognized as a vital and cost-effective mechanism for ensuring that the risk to patients from HCAIs is reduced to a minimum (Dancer and Kramer 2019, Hall et al. 2016). It is also an important confidence marker for patients and the general public, as a 'dirty' environment is often seen as being synonymous with risk of infection. Many items in the healthcare environment can become contaminated, but the most likely routes for the spread of infection are inadequately decontaminated items of equipment used for diagnosis or treatment. Transmission can be prevented via effective cleaning and decontamination between each use (Curran et al. 2019). Healthcare providers are obliged under the Hygiene Code to provide reasonable standards of cleanliness with an appropriately staffed and resourced cleaning service.

According to the national standards of cleanliness (NPSA 2009), clinical environments are divided into areas of very high, high, significant and low risk, and cleaning standards and frequencies are determined from this categorization. It can be argued that all clinical areas and equipment will carry some risk and items that are used between patients must be subjected to thorough decontamination (Curran et al. 2019). Regular auditing should be undertaken by the organization, and the nurse in a clinical area may be asked to accompany staff on these audits and verify that cleanliness is at a satisfactory standard. The standards are set out in local cleaning specifications (British Standards Institution 2014, NPSA 2009). Some of the key elements a nurse should be looking for include the presence of dust high up or low down on surfaces, and evidence of organic material on surfaces, including residues of blood or body fluids. Particular attention should be paid to the cleanliness of toilets, handwash basins, baths, showers and high-touch surfaces such as door plates and handles, taps, call bells and light switches. Nurses should also consider auditing the cleanliness of clinical equipment that is not usually cleaned by domestic staff; this may include commodes, drip stands, pulse oximeters, blood pressure equipment and pumps (among others). Decontamination of these items is facilitated by availability of effective and properly used decontamination items at the point of use in the same way that local placement of hand hygiene products facilitates hand hygiene (Curran et al. 2019).

It should be noted, though, that decontamination (which includes cleaning) is an important nursing role, as many pieces of equipment (e.g. blood pressure monitors) are used on multiple patients, meaning that decontamination to an appropriate level should take place between each patient use. Nurses have a duty to ensure high standards of hygiene in the care environment. Particularly, they must ensure that equipment that may be used for multiple patients and that has a high risk of contamination (such as commodes) is safe for use by the next vulnerable patient. Nurses should be trained to decontaminate any equipment that they use in line with local policies and the manufacturer's guidance.

Wipes

Wipes (wet wipes) are a modern alternative to traditional cleaning cloths. They are usually impregnated with a detergent and/or a disinfectant, do not require mixing, can be placed at the point of use to facilitate best practice, and when used appropriately can clean and/or disinfect a surface. Wipes, like other cleaning and disinfectant products, are licensed for specific uses such as cleaning/disinfecting skin, hard surfaces or medical devices. A wipe must only be used as instructed by the manufacturer on the designated surface. Note that sometimes the same chemical may be licensed for different uses in different products. Such wipes are not interchangeable and the manufacturer's instructions for use must be respected.

Examples of chemicals that may be found in wipes include quaternary ammonium compounds, chlorine, phenolic, hydrogen peroxide, peracetic acid, chlorhexidine in alcohol, and ethyl or isopropyl alcohol. There are a range of manufacturers that produce wipes. Products chosen for use in healthcare should meet approved standards, should have been tested in appropriate laboratories (accredited or a university laboratory with specific expertise) and be compatible with the surface to which they will be applied.

Indicator tape

An indicator label or tape may be applied to an item after cleaning to indicate that it has been decontaminated after its last use. This system is ideally used for shared equipment (e.g. commodes or drip stands), which may be stored between uses.

Automated room disinfection systems

The environment is a known source of HCAI pathogens, and these may persist on surfaces for weeks or months, in some cases presenting a risk to patients. The use of automated room disinfection systems may be considered to eradicate persistent organisms such as *C. difficile* or high-risk organisms such as multiresistant organisms from the environment. Systems that use hydrogen peroxide or ultraviolet light, although quite expensive, have been employed with very favourable results (Otter et al. 2012, Passaretti et al. 2013).

Procedure guideline 4.18 Cleaning a hard surface without recontamination

Essential equipment

- Personal protective equipment
- Appropriate wipes

Action	Rationale
Pre-procedure	
1 Wash and dry hands.	To reduce the risk of introducing further pathogens into the area to be cleaned. **C**
2 Undertake a risk assessment of the chemical and the environment in which it is to be used. Select appropriate personal protective equipment (PPE) (gloves and apron, and potentially a face-mask) for the task so as to protect the skin and mucous membranes. Also consider adequate ventilation of the area. Follow the manufacturer's instructions.	Some chemicals may be harmful to health if not used correctly. **C**
Procedure	
3 Select an appropriate wipe for the task. 'Appropriate' means that the agents contained within and released by the wipe have been demonstrated to act against the target micro-organism. Take one from the packet and use it, following the principle of one wipe, one direction and one surface. Follow the manufacturer's instructions.	To ensure the product is used effectively. **C**
4 Remove heavy soiling using the wipe.	If an item is physically dirty, some disinfectants (such as chlorine) may be inactivated by soil, impairing their efficacy. **C**
5 Wipe all surfaces, including underneath. Pay specific attention to high touch points, which are surfaces that hands regularly come into contact with. Consider what the item is and how it is used to ensure that it is cleaned correctly.	To ensure that all areas are cleaned appropriately. **C**
6 Wipe items from top to bottom, going from a clean to a dirty area using an S-shaped motion. Overlap the motions slightly, making sure not to go over the same area twice (**Action figure 6**).	To ensure no area is missed and areas are not recontaminated by going back over an area that has previously been decontaminated. **C**
7 Dispose of the wipe between surfaces and if it becomes dry or soiled.	To ensure that micro-organisms are not transferred from a surface to another and to ensure that the efficacy of the wipe is not compromised by the agents becoming used up. **C**
8 Remove any PPE, and wash and dry hands.	To prevent recontamination of surfaces and to render hands clean for the next task. **C**
9 Apply any indicator tape if required by local policy.	So that items in storage can be identified as having been decontaminated after last use and are understood to now be safe to use for the next patient. **C**

Source: Procedure guideline adapted from GAMA Healthcare.

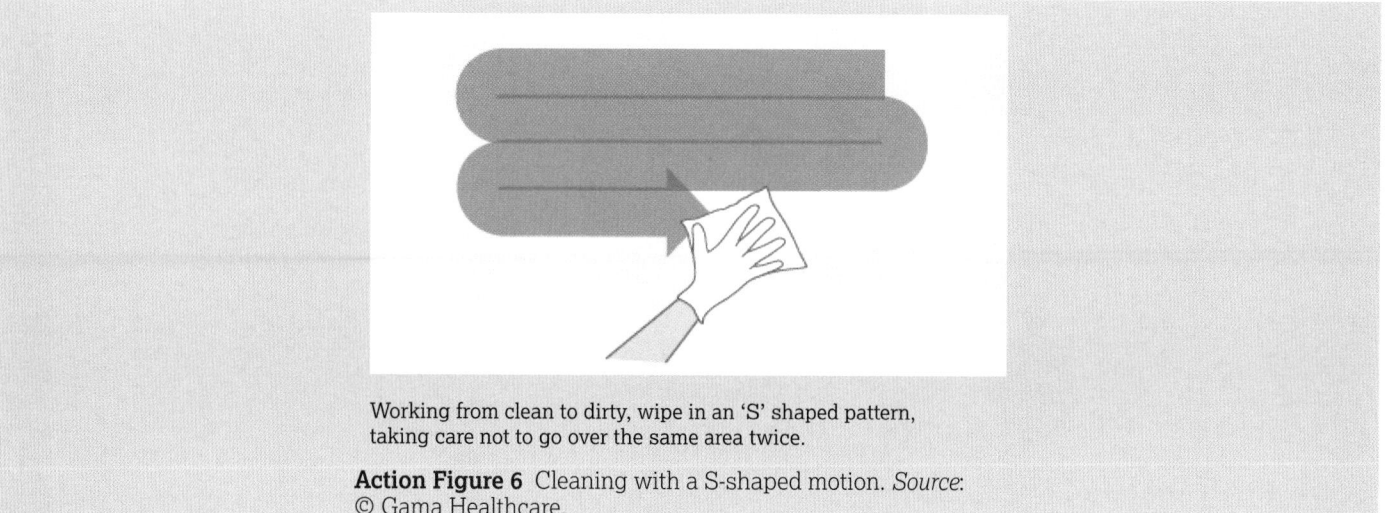

Working from clean to dirty, wipe in an 'S' shaped pattern, taking care not to go over the same area twice.

Action Figure 6 Cleaning with a S-shaped motion. *Source*: © Gama Healthcare.

Waste disposal

Related theory

Waste material produced in the healthcare environment may carry a risk of infection to people who are not directly involved in providing healthcare but who are involved in the transport or disposal of that waste. All waste disposal is subject to regulation and hazardous waste is subject to further controls, depending on the nature of the hazard (DH 2013b). To ensure that everyone involved in waste management is aware of, and protected from, any hazard presented by the waste with which they are dealing, and that the waste is disposed of appropriately, a colour-coding system is used. The colours in general use are shown in Table 4.8.

Table 4.8 Waste colour codes

Colour	Description
Yellow	Waste that requires disposal by incineration Indicative treatment/disposal required is **incineration** in a suitably permitted or licensed facility.
Orange	Waste that may be 'treated' Indicative treatment/disposal required is to be '**rendered safe**' in a suitably permitted or licensed facility, usually alternative treatment plants. However, this waste may also be disposed of by **incineration**.
Purple	Cytotoxic and cytostatic waste Indicative treatment/disposal required is **incineration** in a suitably permitted or licensed facility.
Yellow/black	Offensive/hygiene waste Indicative treatment/disposal required is **landfill** or **municipal incineration/energy from waste** at a suitably permitted or licensed facility.
Red	Anatomical waste for incineration Indicative treatment/disposal required is **incineration** in a suitably permitted facility.
Black	Domestic (municipal) waste Minimum treatment/disposal required is **landfill**, municipal **incineration/energy from waste** or other municipal **waste treatment process** at a suitably permitted or licensed facility. Recyclable components should be removed through segregation. Clear/opaque receptacles may also be used for domestic waste.
Blue	Medicinal waste for incineration Indicative treatment/disposal required is **incineration** in a suitably permitted facility.
White	Amalgam waste For **recovery**.

Source: Adapted from DH (2013b). © Crown copyright

There are several different types of waste containers. They are usually plastic bags or rigid plastic containers of the appropriate colour (Table 4.9). Boxes for disposal of sharps are usually differentiated from rigid boxes for other waste.

Clinical governance

The producer of hazardous waste is legally responsible for that waste, and remains responsible for it until its final disposal by incineration, alternative treatment or landfill (DH 2013b). In order

Table 4.9 Waste containers

Waste type	Waste receptacle	Example description[1]	Waste management requirements[2]	Additional comments
Domestic type waste	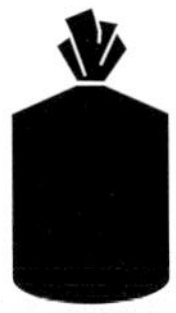 Black bag	Mixed municipal waste	Landfill Municipal incineration Energy from waste Other authorised disposal or recovery	Medical practices must not place any hazardous waste in this waste stream. Recycling options should be considered
Offensive (healthcare)	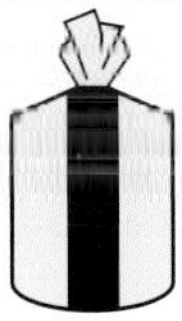	Offensive waste from human/animal healthcare	Landfill Municipal incineration Energy from waste Other authorised disposal or recovery	This is restricted to offensive wastes from healthcare and related activities (including autoclaved wastes from laboratories)
Offensive (municipal)	Yellow and black striped bag	Offensive waste, municipal		This includes municipal hygiene wastes from medical practices
Anatomical waste (chemically preserved)	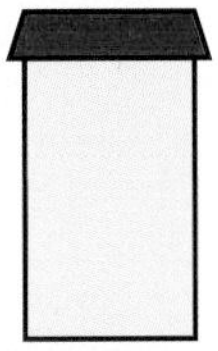	Clinical waste, human/animal anatomical, chemically preserved, for incineration only	Clinical waste incineration	If the waste is not classified as infectious then: • tissue preserved in chemicals remains clinical waste and the transport requirements may be determined by the chemical preservatives, and • where not preserved in chemicals, tissue would not normally be clinical waste
Anatomical waste (not chemically preserved)	Red-lidded, rigid yellow container	Clinical waste, human/animal anatomical, not chemically preserved, for incineration only		
Infectious waste contaminated with chemicals	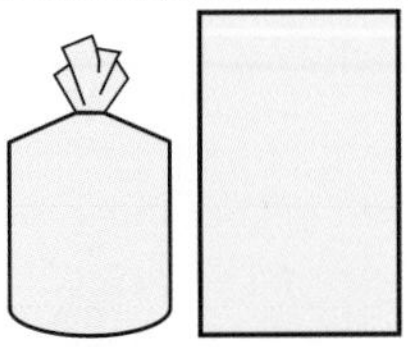	Clinical waste, infectious, containing chemicals from human/animal healthcare, for incineration only	Clinical waste incineration	Waste chemicals must not be placed in this waste stream. It is for infectious materials containing or contaminated with chemicals (eg sample vials and used diagnostic kits)
Infectious waste (not containing chemicals or medicinal contamination)	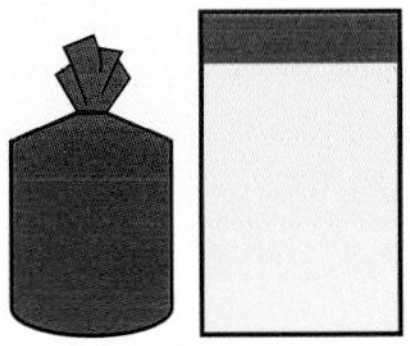 Orange bag or Orange-lidded, rigid yellow container	Clinical waste, infectious, from human/animal healthcare, suitable for alternative treatment	Alternative treatment or clinical waste incineration	This assumes healthcare offensive and domestic wastes are also segregated separately

Table 4.9 Waste containers

Waste type	Waste receptacle	Example description[1]	Waste management requirements[2]	Additional comments
Sharps, non-medicinally contaminated	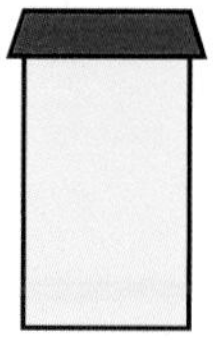 Orange-lidded, yellow sharps box	Clinical waste, sharps, infectious, non-medicinally contaminated, suitable for alternative treatment	Alternative treatment or clinical waste incineration	For producers and disposal sites in England and Wales, sharps that are not contaminated with medicinal products only
		Clinical waste, sharps, infectious, non-medicinally contaminated, from non-healthcare activities suitable for alternative treatment		For producers in Northern Ireland and Scotland whose waste is disposed of in those countries, both sharps that are not contaminated with medicinal products, and fully discharged medicinally contaminated sharps (other than cytotoxic and cytostatic)
Sharps, medicinally contaminated, other than cytotoxic and cytostatic	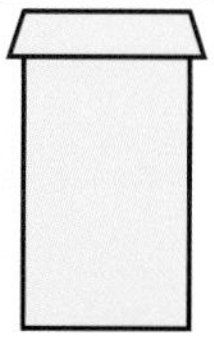	Clinical waste, mixed sharps and pharmaceutical waste (not cytotoxic and cytostatic), infectious, for incineration only	Clinical waste incineration	This may include associated vials, bottles and ampoules of medicine
Sharps, contaminated with cytotoxic and cytostatic medicines	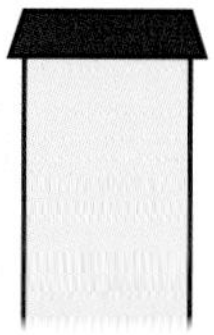 Purple-lidded, yellow sharps box	Clinical waste, mixed sharps and cytotoxic and cytostatic waste, infectious, for incineration only	Clinical waste incineration	This may include associated vials, bottles and ampoules of cytotoxic and cytostatic medicines
Other infectious waste contaminated with cytotoxic and cytostatic medicines	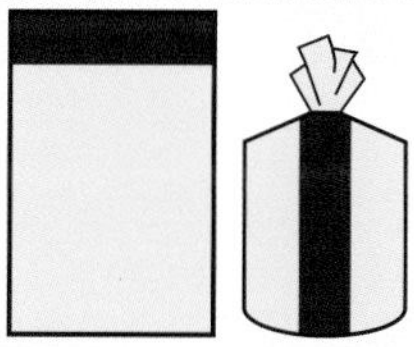 Purple-lidded, rigid yellow container and sack	Clinical waste, cytotoxic and cytostatic waste, infectious, for incineration only		
Cytotoxic and cytostatic medicines (in original packaging)	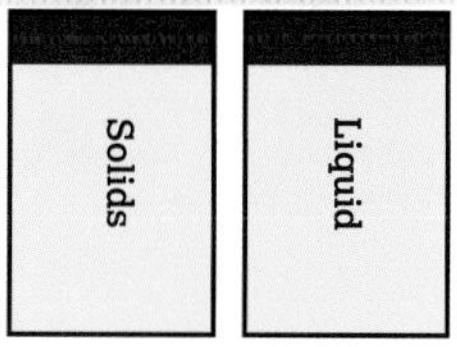 Two purple-lidded, rigid yellow containers (one for solids, one for liquids)	Clinical waste, cytotoxic and cytostatic medicines from animal/human healthcare for incineration only	Clinical waste incineration	
Cytotoxic and cytostatic medicines (not in original packaging)	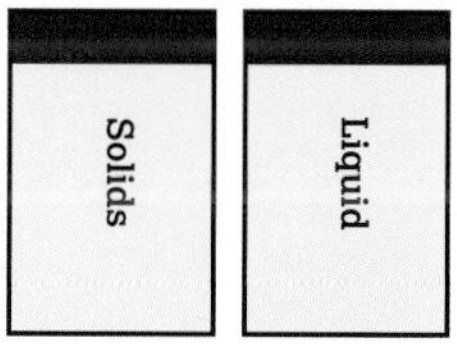 Two purple-lidded, rigid yellow containers (one for solids, one for liquids)			

(continued)

Table 4.9 Waste containers *(continued)*

Waste type	Waste receptacle	Example description[1]	Waste management requirements[2]	Additional comments
Other medicines (in original packaging)	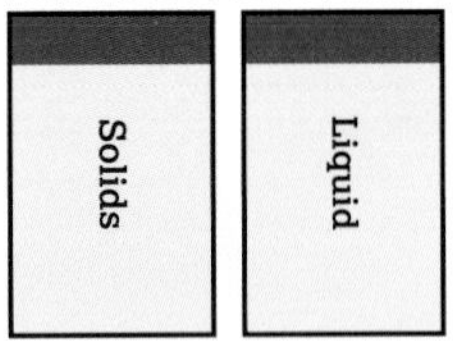 Two blue-lidded, rigid yellow containers (one for solids, one for liquids)	Clinical waste, medicines (not cytotoxic and cytostatic) from animal/human healthcare, for incineration only	Clinical waste incineration	
Other medicines (not in original packaging)	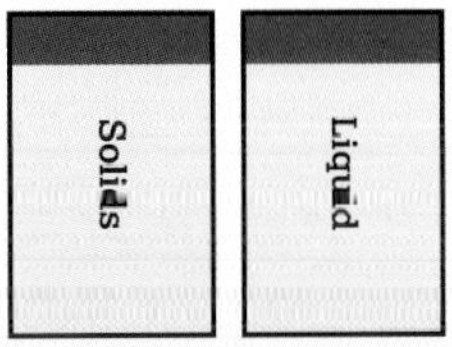 Two blue-lidded, rigid yellow containers (one for solids, one for liquids)			
Dental amalgam	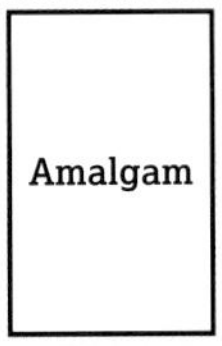 Leak-proof rigid container with Hg suppressant	Dental amalgam and mercury including spent and out-of-date capsules, excess mixed amalgam and contents of amalgam separators	Recovery	Where teeth containing amalgam are present, H9: Infectious (see DH 2013b) may also apply
Photographic (X-ray) wastes	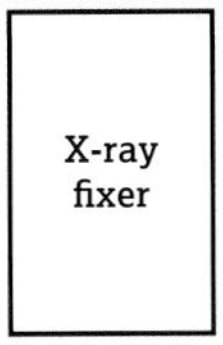	X-ray fixer	Recovery or treatment	
	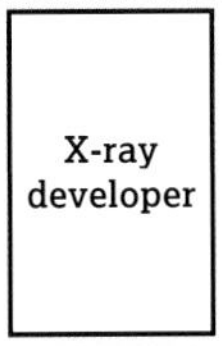	X-ray developer (water based)	Recovery or treatment	
Photographic (X-ray) wastes (contd)	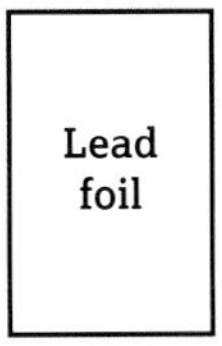	Lead foil	Recovery	
	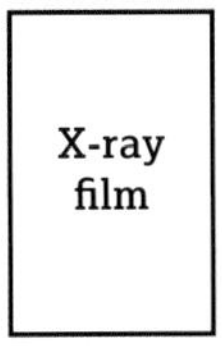	X-ray film containing silver	Recovery	
Gypsum and plaster-cast wastes	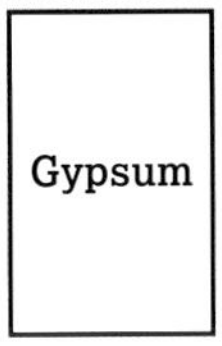	Non-infectious gypsum and plaster waste from healthcare	Gypsum recovery or specialist landfill in separate gypsum cell	See supporting text under 'Gypsum and plaster casts' (see DH 2013b) for advice on the small proportion of this material that may be infectious and clinical waste

Table 4.9 Waste containers

Waste type	Waste receptacle	Example description[1]	Waste management requirements[2]	Additional comments
Radioactive waste	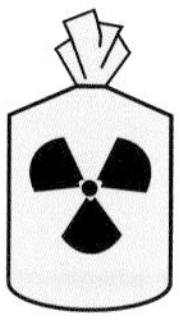	Healthcare waste contaminated with radioactive material	UN number will depend upon isotope. Radioactivity takes precedence for transport class when above the lower threshold	Incineration in hazardous waste incineration facility subject to Radioactive Substances Act (RSA)

Notes:

The information in this table should be used where the assessment framework in 'Healthcare waste definitions and classifications' (see DH 2013b) has identified that it is applicable to the waste in question.

[1] The three entries are generic and will not be appropriate for all cytotoxic and cytostatic medicines. Some waste medicines will have to be classified in accordance with the provisions of ADR (ADR refers to the *Accord européen relatif au transport international desmarchandises dangereuses par route*, or European Agreement Concerning the International Carriage of Dangerous Goods by Road). In most cases a safety data sheet (SDS) for the medicines should show the appropriate transport classification. If this is not available, advice from a dangerous goods safety adviser (DGSA) should be sought.

[2] The waste must be disposed of, or recovered, at a suitably authorised facility.

Source: DH (2013b) *Health Technical Memorandum 07-01: Safe Management of Healthcare Waste.* Department of Health, London. Figure 11. https://www.gov.uk/government/uploads/system/uploads/attachment_data/file/167976/HTM_07-01_Final.pdf

to track waste to its point of origin, for example if it is necessary to identify where waste has been disposed of into the wrong waste stream, healthcare organizations should have a system of identifying waste according to the ward or department where it is produced. This may be through the use of labelling or dedicated waste carts for particular areas. When assembling sharps bins, always complete the label on the outside of the bin, including the date and the initials of the assembler. When sharps bins are closed and disposed of, they should be dated and initialled at each stage (DH 2013b).

Management of soiled linen in the healthcare environment

Related theory

As with waste, soiled linen must be managed so as to minimize any risk to any person coming into contact with it. This is done by clearly identifying any soiled linen that may present a risk through the use of colour coding and limiting any contact with such linen through the use of water-soluble bags to contain the linen so that laundry staff do not have to handle it before it goes into the washer (DH 2013e, 2016).

Linen that may present a risk may be described as foul, infected or infested. The management of all hazardous linen is similar, so the following procedure applies to any linen that:

- is wet with blood or other high-risk body fluids (see the section on prevention and management of inoculation injury below) or faeces
- is from a patient in source isolation for any reason (that is, where enteric, contact or droplet/airborne precautions are in place)
- is from a patient who is infested with lice, fleas, scabies or other ectoparasites.

Note that this procedure can be much more easily carried out by two people working together.

Procedure guideline 4.19 Safe disposal of foul, infected or infested linen

Essential equipment

- Personal protective equipment
- Water-soluble laundry bag
- Red plastic or linen laundry bag in holder
- Orange waste bag

Action	Rationale
Pre-procedure	
1 Assemble all the required equipment.	To avoid having to fetch anything else during the procedure and risk spreading contamination to other areas. **E**
2 Put on disposable gloves and apron.	To minimize contamination of hands or clothing from the soiled linen. **E**
3 Separate the edges of the open end of the water-soluble laundry bag.	To make it easier to put the soiled linen in the bag. **E**

(continued)

Procedure guideline 4.19 Safe disposal of foul, infected or infested linen *(continued)*

Action	Rationale
Procedure	
4 Gather up the foul, infected or infested linen in such a way that any gross contamination (e.g. blood or faeces) is contained within the linen.	To minimize any contamination of the surrounding area. **E**
5 If there are two people, one holds the water-soluble laundry bag open while the other puts the soiled linen into it. If there is one person, hold one edge of the open end of the water-soluble bag in one hand and place the soiled linen in the bag with the other. In either case, take care not to contaminate the outside of the bag.	To remove the need for laundry workers to handle foul, infected or infested linen before it is washed (DH 2013c, **C**).
6 Tie the water-soluble bag closed using the tie provided or by knotting together the edges of the open end.	To keep the soiled laundry inside the bag. **E**
7 Place the full water-soluble bag of soiled linen into the red outer laundry bag without touching the outside of the red bag.	To identify the linen as requiring special treatment. **E**
8 Remove gloves and apron and dispose of them in an orange waste bag.	To avoid transferring contamination to other areas (DH 2013b, **C**).
9 Wash hands and forearms with soap and water. Dry thoroughly with a disposable paper towel.	To avoid transferring contamination to other areas (WHO 2009a, **C**).
10 Close the red outer laundry bag and transfer it to the designated collection area.	To ensure it does not cause an obstruction and is transferred to the laundry at the earliest opportunity. **E**

Prevention and management of inoculation injury

Related theory

Healthcare workers are at risk of acquiring blood-borne infections such as human immunodeficiency virus (HIV), the virus that causes acquired immune deficiency syndrome (AIDS), hepatitis B and hepatitis C. While the risk is small, there were 4830 significant occupational exposures to a blood-borne virus reported among healthcare workers between 2004 and 2013. Of these, half were exposed to hepatitis C, a third to HIV and a tenth to hepatitis B. Of these exposures, 71% involved a percutaneous needle stick injury (the majority were sharps injuries involving a hollow-bore needle) and 65% occurred in wards, theatres or A&E (PHE 2014; Woode Owusu et al. 2014). An understanding of the risk of infection and the preventive measures to be taken is essential in promoting a safer work environment (DH 1998).

Blood-borne viruses are present in the blood and in other high-risk fluids, which should be handled with the same precautions as blood. High-risk fluids include:

- cerebrospinal fluid
- peritoneal fluid
- pleural fluid
- pericardial fluid
- synovial fluid
- amniotic fluid
- semen
- vaginal secretions
- breast milk
- any other body fluid or unfixed tissue or organ containing visible blood (including saliva in dentistry).

Body fluids that do not need to be regarded as high risk, unless they are blood stained, are:

- urine
- faeces
- saliva
- sweat
- vomit.

The most likely route of infection for healthcare workers is through the percutaneous inoculation of infected blood via a sharps injury (often called a needle stick injury) or by blood or other high-risk fluid splashing onto broken skin or a mucous membrane in the mouth, nose or eyes. These incidents are collectively known as 'inoculation injuries'. An EU directive incorporated into UK law requires healthcare organizations to use safe devices and systems of work to minimize the risk of inoculation injury (HSE 2013b). Blood or another high-risk fluid coming into contact with intact skin is not regarded as an inoculation injury. It carries little or no risk due to the impervious nature of intact skin. The guidance in Box 4.4 has been shown to reduce the risk of sharps injuries.

Complications

In the event of an inoculation injury occurring, prompt and appropriate action will reduce the risk of subsequent infection. Relevant actions are described in Box 4.5 and should be taken regardless of what is thought to be known about the status of the patient whose blood has been inoculated. HIV, for example, has a 3-month window following infection during which the patient has sufficient virus in their blood to be infectious but before their immune system is producing sufficient antibodies to be detected by the normal tests for HIV status.

Box 4.4 Actions to reduce the risk of inoculation injury

- Use safety devices as an alternative to sharp items wherever these are available (HSE 2013b).
- Do not resheath used needles.
- Ensure that you are familiar with the local protocols for the use and disposal of sharps (e.g. location of sharps bins) and any other equipment before undertaking any procedure involving the use of a sharp item.
- Do not bend or break needles or disassemble them after use; discard needles and syringes into a sharps bin immediately after use.
- Handle sharps as little as possible.
- Do not pass sharps directly from hand to hand; use a receiver or similar receptacle.
- Discard all used sharps into a sharps container at the point of use; take a sharps container with you to the point of use if necessary. Do not dispose of sharps into anything other than a designated sharps container.
- Do not fill sharps bins above the mark that indicates that it is full.
- Sharps bins that are not full or in current (i.e. immediate) use should be kept out of reach of children and with any temporary closure in place.
- Sharps bins in use should be positioned at a height that enables safe disposal by all members of staff and secured to avoid spillage.
- Wear gloves in any situation where contact with blood is anticipated.
- Avoid wearing open footwear in any situation where blood may be spilt or where sharps are used.
- Always cover any cuts or abrasions, particularly on the hands, with a waterproof dressing while at work. Wear gloves if hands are particularly affected.
- Wear facial protection consisting of a mask and goggles or a face-shield in any situation that may lead to a splash of blood or other high-risk fluid to the face. Do not rely on prescription glasses – they may not provide sufficient protection.
- Clear up any blood spillage promptly and disinfect the area. Use any materials or spillage management packs specifically provided for this purpose in accordance with the manufacturer's instructions.

Source: DH (1998).

Box 4.5 Actions to take in the event of inoculation injury

- Encourage any wound to blood to wash out any foreign material that has been introduced. Do not squeeze the wound, as this may force any virus present into the tissues.
- Wash any wound with soap and water. Wash out splashes to mucous membranes (eyes or mouth) with large amounts of clean water.
- Cover any wound with a waterproof dressing to prevent entry of any other foreign material.
- Ensure the patient is safe then report the injury as quickly as possible to your immediate line manager and occupational health department. This is because post-exposure prophylaxis, which is medication given after any incident thought to carry a high risk of HIV transmission, is more effective the sooner after the incident it is commenced (DH 2015b).
- Follow any instructions given by the occupational health department.
- Co-operate with any action to test yourself or the patient for infection with a blood-borne virus but do not obtain blood or consent for testing from the patient yourself; this should be done by someone not involved in the incident.
- Complete a report of the incident according to local protocols.

Source: DH (1998).

Websites

AMR Local Indicators
https://fingertips.phe.org.uk/profile/amr-local-indicators

Infection Prevention Society
https://www.ips.uk.net

Public Health England
https://www.gov.uk/government/organisations/public-health-england

World Health Organization: Infection Prevention and Control
https://www.who.int/infection-prevention/en

References

Abad, C., Fearday, A. & Safdar, N. (2010) Adverse effects of isolation in hospitalised patients: A systematic review. *Journal of Hospital Infection*, 76(2), 97–102.

AfPP (Association for Perioperative Practice) (2017) *A Guide to Surgical Hand Antisepsis*. Available at: https://www.afpp.org.uk/filegrab/surgical-hand-antisepsis-poster-final.pdf?ref=1908

AORN (Association of Operating Room Nurses) (1997) *Standards, Recommended Practices, and Guidelines*. Denver, CO: Association of Operating Room Nurses.

Aranega-Bou, P., George, R., Verlander, N., et al. (2019) Carbapenem-resistant Enterobacteriaceae dispersal from sinks is linked to drain position and drainage rates in a laboratory model system. *Journal of Hospital Infection*, 102(1), 63–69.

Ayliffe, G.A.J., Babb, J.R. & Quoraishi, A.H. (1978) A test for hygienic hand disinfection. *Journal of Clinical Pathology*, 31, 923–928.

Best, E., Parnell, P., Couturier, J., et al. (2018) Environmental contamination by bacteria in hospital washrooms according to hand-drying method: A multi-centre study. *Journal of Hospital Infection*, 100(4), 469–475.

Bhalodi, A.A., van Engelen, T.S.R., Virk, H.S. & Wiersinga, W.J. (2019) Impact of antimicrobial therapy on the gut microbiome. *Journal of Antimicrobial Chemotherapy*, 74(Suppl. 1), i6–i15.

Borg, M.A. (2003) Bed occupancy and overcrowding as determinant factors in the incidence of MRSA infections within general ward settings. *Journal of Hospital Infection*, 54(4), 316–318.

Boyce, J.M., Pittet, D., Healthcare Infection Control Practices Advisory Committee, & HICPAC/SHEA/APIC/IDSA Hand Hygiene Task Force (2002) Guideline for hand hygiene in health-care settings: Recommendations of the Healthcare Infection Control Practices Advisory Committee and the HICPAC/SHEA/APIC/IDSA Hand Hygiene Task Force. *Morbidity and Mortality Weekly Report*, 51, 1–45.

British Standards Institution (2014) *Specification for the Planning, Application, Measurement and Review of Cleanliness Services in Hospitals* [PAS 5748]. Available at: http://qna.files.parliament.uk/qna-attachments/175888%5Coriginal%5CPAS5748%20Specification%20for%20the%20planning,%20application,%20measurement%20and%20review%20of%20cleanliness%20services%20in%20hospitals.pdf

Calandra, T. (2000) Practical guide to host defence mechanisms and the predominant infections encountered in immunocompromised patients. In: Glauser, M.P. & Pizzo, P.A. (eds) *Management of Infections in Immunocompromised Patients, Part I*. London: W.B. Saunders, pp.3–16.

Cassell, J.A., Middleton, J., Nalabanda, A., et al. (2018) Scabies outbreaks in ten care homes for elderly people: A prospective study of clinical features, epidemiology, and treatment outcomes. *Lancet Infectious Diseases*, 18(8), 894–902.

Coia, J.E., Duckworth, G.J., Edwards, D.I., et al. (2006). Guidelines for the control and prevention of meticillin-resistant *Staphylococcus aureus* (MRSA) in healthcare facilities. *Journal of Hospital Infection*, 63(Suppl. 1), S1–S44.

Croxatto, A., Prod'hom, G. & Greub, G. (2012) Applications of MALDI-TOF mass spectrometry in clinical diagnostic microbiology. *FEMS Microbiology Reviews*, 36(2), 380–407.

Cummings, C., Finlay, J.C. & MacDonald, N.E. (2018) Head lice infestations: A clinical update. *Paediatrics & Child Health*, 23(1), e18–e24.

Curran, E., Wilkinson, M. & Bradley, T. (2019) Chemical disinfectants: Controversies regarding their use in low risk healthcare environments (part 1). *Journal of Infection Prevention*, 20(2), 76–82.

Damani, N.N. (2011) Basic concepts. In: Damani, N.N. (ed) *Manual of Infection Prevention and Control*, 3rd edn. Oxford: Oxford University Press, pp.1–16.

Dancer, S.J. & Kramer, A. (2019) Four steps to clean hospitals: LOOK, PLAN, CLEAN and DRY. *Journal of Hospital Infection*, 103(1), e1–e8.

DH (Department of Health) (1998) *Guidance for Clinical Health Care Workers: Protection against Infection with Blood-Borne Viruses – Recommendations of the Expert Advisory Group on AIDS and the Advisory Group on Hepatitis.* London: Department of Health. Available at: www.dh.gov.uk/en/Publicationsandstatistics/Lettersandcirculars/Healthservicecirculars/DH_4003818

DH (2003) *Winning Ways: Working Together to Reduce Healthcare Associated Infection in England – Report from the Chief Medical Officer.* London: Department of Health.

DH (2007) *Health Technical Memorandum 01-01: Decontamination of Reusable Medical Devices, Part A – Management and Environment.* London: Department of Health.

DH (2010a) *Uniforms and Workwear: Guidance on Uniform and Workwear Policies for NHS Employers.* Available at: https://www.whatdotheyknow.com/request/288156/response/702370/attach/3/uniform%20revised%20guidance%202010.pdf

DH (2010b) *Pandemic (H1N1) 2009 Influenza: A Summary of Guidance for Infection Control in Healthcare Settings.* Available at: https://assets.publishing.service.gov.uk/government/uploads/system/uploads/attachment_data/file/357401/Infection_control_in_healthcare_settings.pdf

DH (2013a) *Water Safety: Health Technical Memorandum 04-01 Addendum –* Pseudomonas aeruginosa *– Advice for Augmented Care Units.* London: Department of Health.

DH (2013b) *Health Technical Memorandum 07-01: Safe Management of Healthcare Waste.* Available at: www.gov.uk/government/uploads/system/uploads/attachment_data/file/167976/HTM_07-01_Final.pdf

DH (2013c) *Health Building Note 00-09: Infection Control in the Built Environment.* Available at: https://assets.publishing.service.gov.uk/government/uploads/system/uploads/attachment_data/file/170705/HBN_00-09_infection_control.pdf

DH (2013d) *Health Building Note 04-01 Supplement 1: Isolation Facilities for Infectious Patients in Acute Settings.* Available at: www.gov.uk/government/uploads/system/uploads/attach-ment_data/file/148503/HBN_04-01_Supp_1_Final.pdf

DH (2013e) *Choice Framework for Local Policy and Procedures 01-04: Decontamination of Linen for Health and Social Care – Guidance for Linen Processors Implementing BS EN 14065.* Available at: https://assets.publishing.service.gov.uk/government/uploads/system/uploads/attachment_data/file/527546/BS_EN14065.pdf

DH (2014) *Prime Minister warns of global threat of antibiotic resistance* [Press Release]. Available at: https://www.gov.uk/government/news/prime-minister-warns-of-global-threat-of-antibiotic-resistance

DH (2015a) *The Health and Social Care Act 2008: Code of Practice on the Prevention and Control of Infections and Related Guidance.* Available at: https://assets.publishing.service.gov.uk/government/uploads/system/uploads/attachment_data/file/449049/Code_of_practice_280715_acc.pdf

DH (2015b) *Updated Guidance on Occupational HIV Post-exposure Prophylaxis (PEP) from the UK Chief Medical Officers' Expert Advisory Group on AIDS (EAGA).* Available at: https://www.gov.uk/government/publications/eaga-guidance-on-hiv-post-exposure-prophylaxis

DH (2016) *Health Technical Memorandum 01-04: Decontamination of Linen for Health and Social Care Management and Provision.* Available at: https://assets.publishing.service.gov.uk/government/uploads/system/uploads/attachment_data/file/527542/Mgmt_and_provision.pdf

DH (2017) *Safe Water in Healthcare Premises* [HTM 04-01]. Available at: https://www.gov.uk/government/publications/hot-and-cold-water-supply-storage-and-distribution-systems-for-healthcare-premises

DH (2019) *MRSA, MSSA and Gram-Negative Bacteraemia and CDI: Annual Report.* Available at: https://www.gov.uk/government/statistics/mrsa-mssa-and-e-coli-bacteraemia-and-c-difficile-infection-annual-epidemiological-commentary

ECDC (European Centre for Disease Prevention and Control) (2013) *Point Prevalence Survey of Healthcare-Associated Infections and Antimicrobial Use in European Acute Care Hospitals 2011–2012.* Available at: https://ecdc.europa.eu/sites/portal/files/media/en/publications/Publications/healthcare-associated-infections-antimicrobial-use-PPS.pdf

ECDC (2016) *Point Prevalence Survey of Healthcare-Associated Infections and Antimicrobial Use in European Acute Care Hospitals.* Available at: https://ecdc.europa.eu/sites/portal/files/media/en/publications/Publications/PPS-HAI-antimicrobial-use-EU-acute-care-hospitals-V5-3.pdf

Eiamsitrakoon, T., Apisarnthanarak, A., Nuallaong, W., et al. (2013) Hand hygiene behavior: Translating behavioral research into infection control practice. *Infection Control & Hospital Epidemiology*, 34(11), 1137–1145.

Elliot, T., Worthington, A., Osman, H. & Gill, M. (2007) *Lecture Notes: Medical Microbiology and Infection*, 4th edn. Oxford: Blackwell.

Fishman, J.A. (2011) Infections in immunocompromised hosts and organ transplant recipients: Essentials. *Liver Transplantation*, 17(Suppl. 3), S34–S37.

Food Safety Act (1990) Available at: www.legislation.gov.uk/ukpga/1990/16/contents

Fraise, A.P. & Bradley, T. (eds) (2009) *Ayliffe's Control of Healthcare-Associated Infection: A Practical Handbook*, 5th edn. London: Hodder Arnold.

Garvey, M.I., Bradley, C.W. & Holden, E. (2018) Waterborne *Pseudomonas aeruginosa* transmission in a hematology unit? *American Journal of Infection Control*, 46(4), 383–386

Garvey, M.I., Bradley, C.W., Tracey, J. & Oppenheim, B. (2016) Continued transmission of *Pseudomonas aeruginosa* from a hand wash basin tap in a critical care unit. *Journal of Hospital Infection*, 94(1), 8–12.

Gillespie, I.A., O'Brien, S.J., Adak, G.K., et al. (2005) Foodborne general outbreaks of *Salmonella enteritidis* phage type 4 infection, England and Wales, 1992–2002: Where are the risks? *Epidemiology & Infection*, 133(5), 795–801.

Gillespie, S. & Bamford, K. (2012) *Medical Microbiology and Infection at a Glance*, 4th edn. Chichester: John Wiley & Sons.

Godwin, J.E., Braden, C.D. & Sachdever, K. (2018) *Neutropenia. Medscape*, 18 September. Available at: http://emedicine.medscape.com/article/204821-overview

Goering, R., Dockrell, H., Zuckermann, M., et al. (2012) *Mims' Medical Microbiology*, 5th edn. London: Saunders.

Gold, N.A. & Avva, U. (2018) *Alcohol sanitizer*. In: *StatPearls*. Available at: https://www.ncbi.nlm.nih.gov/books/NBK513254

Guilley-Lerondeau, B., Bourigault, C., Guille des Buttes, A.C., et al. (2017). Adverse effects of isolation: A prospective matched cohort study including 90 direct interviews of hospitalized patients in a French university hospital. *European Journal of Clinical Microbiology & Infectious Diseases*, 36(1), 75–80.

Hall, L., Farrington, A., Mitchell, B.G., et al. (2016) Researching effective approaches to cleaning in hospitals: Protocol of the REACH study, a multi-site stepped-wedge randomised trial. *Implementation Science*, 11, 44.

Harbarth, S., Sudre, P., Dharan, S., et al. (1999) Outbreak of *Enterobacter cloacae* related to understaffing, overcrowding, and poor hygiene practices. *Infection Control & Hospital Epidemiology*, 20, 598–603.

Health and Safety at Work etc. Act (1974) Available at: www.legislation.gov.uk/ukpga/1974/37

Health and Social Care Act (2008) Available at: www.legislation.gov.uk/ukpga/2008/14/contents

Health Protection Agency (2012) *Guidelines for the Management of Norovirus Outbreaks in Acute and Community Health and Social Care Settings.* London: Health Protection Agency.

Health Protection Scotland (2017) *Roles & Responsibilities for Reusable Patient Care Equipment and Environmental Decontamination.* Available at: https://www.hps.scot.nhs.uk/web-resources-container/roles-responsibilities-for-reusable-patient-care-equipment-and-environmental-decontamination/

Hedderwick, S., McNeil, S., Lyons, M. & Kauffman, C.A. (2000) Pathogenic organisms associated with artificial fingernails worn by healthcare workers. *Infection Control & Hospital Epidemiology*, 21(8), 505–509.

HSE (Health and Safety Executive) (2002) *Control of Substances Hazardous to Health 2002 (COSHH).* Available at: www.hse.gov.uk/nanotechnology/coshh.htm

HSE (2013a) *Legionnaires' Disease: The Control of Legionella Bacteria in Water Systems – Approved Code of Practice and Guidance*, 4th edn (L8). Available at: www.hse.gov.uk/pubns/books/l8.htm

HSE (2013b) *Health and Safety (Sharp Instruments in Healthcare) Regulations 2013.* London: Health and Safety Executive.

HSE (2013c) *Personal Protective Equipment (PPE) at Work: A Brief Guide.* Available at: www.hse.gov.uk/pubns/indg174.htm

HSE (2013d) *Respiratory Protective Equipment at Work: A Practical Guide* [HSG53], 4th edn. Available at: www.hse.gov.uk/pUbns/priced/hsg53.pdf

HSE (2013e) *Laundry Treatments at High and Low Temperatures*. Available at: www.hse.gov.uk/biosafety/blood-borne-viruses/laundry-treatments.htm

Infection Prevention Society (2017) *High Impact Interventions: Care Processes to Prevent Infection*, 4th edn. Infection Prevention Society in association with NHS Improvement. Available at: https://www.ips.uk.net/files/6115/0944/9537/High_Impact_Interventions.pdf

Jeanes, A., Macrae, B. & Ashby, J. (2011) Isolation prioritisation tool: Revision, adaptation and application. *British Journal of Nursing*, 20(9), 540–544.

Jones, D. (2010) How to reduce the negative psychological impact of MRSA isolation on patients. *Nursing Times*, 106(36), 14–16.

Kampf, G., & Kramer, A. (2014) Epidemiologic background of hand hygiene and evaluation of the most important agents for scrubs and rubs. *Clinical Microbiology Review*, 17(4), 863–893.

Kampf, G., Löffler, H. & Gastmeier, P. (2009) Hand hygiene for the prevention of nosocomial infections. *Deutsches Ärzteblatt International*, 106(40), 649–655.

Kao, P.H. & Yang, R.J. (2006) Virus diffusion in isolation rooms. *Journal of Hospital Infection*, 62(3), 338–345.

Kerr, L.N., Chaput, M.P., Cash, L.D., et al. (2004) Assessment of the durability of medical examination gloves. *Journal of Occupational and Environmental Hygiene*, 1(9), 607–612.

Korniewicz, D.M., El-Masri, M., Broyles, J.M., et al. (2002) Performance of latex and nonlatex medical examination gloves during simulated use. *American Journal of Infection Control*, 30(2), 133–138.

Kotay, S., Chai, W., Guilford, W., et al. (2017) Spread from the sink to the patient: In situ study using green fluorescent protein (GFP)-expressing *Escherichia coli* to model bacterial dispersion from hand-washing sink-trap reservoirs. *Applied and Environmental Microbiology*, 83(8), e03327–16.

Lefebvre, S., Waltner-Toews, D., Peregrine, A., et al. (2006) Prevalence of zoonotic agents in dogs visiting hospitalized people in Ontario: Implications for infection control. *Journal of Hospital Infection*, 62(3), 458–466.

Loveday, H.P., Wilson, J.A., Pratt, R.J., et al. (2014a) epic 3: National evidence-based guidelines for preventing healthcare-associated infections in NHS hospitals in England. *Journal of Hospital Infection*, 86(Suppl. 1), S1–S70.

Loveday, H.P., Wilson, J.A., Kerr, K., et al. (2014b) Association between healthcare water systems and *Pseudomonas aeruginosa* infections: A rapid systematic review. *Journal of Hospital Infection*, 86(1), 7–15.

McGuckin, R., Storr, J., Longtin, Y., et al. (2011) Patient empowerment and multimodal hand hygiene promotion: A win-win strategy. *American Journal of Medical Quality*, 26(1), 10–17.

McNeil, S.A., Foster, C.L., Hedderwick, S. & Kauffman, C.A. (2001) Effect of hand cleansing with antimicrobial soap or alcohol-based gel on microbial colonization of artificial fingernails worn by health care workers. *Clinical Infectious Disease*, 32, 367–372.

MHRA (Medicines and Healthcare products Regulatory Agency) (2018) *DB 2006(04) Single-Use Medical Devices: Implications and Consequences of Reuse*. Available at: www.mhra.gov.uk

MHRA (2010) Guidance notes on medical devices which require sterilization. In: *EC Medical Devices Directives: Guidance for Manufacturers on Clinical Investigations to be Carried Out in the UK*. London: MHRA, pp.40–41.

Moody, K., Finlay, J., Mancuso, C., et al. (2006) Feasibility and safety of a pilot randomized trial of infection rate: Neutropenic diet versus standard food safety guidelines. *Journal of Pediatric Hematology/Oncology*, 28(3), 126–133.

Moolenaar, R.L., Crutcher, J.M., San Joaquin, V.H., et al. (2000) A prolonged outbreak of *Pseudomonas aeruginosa* in a neonatal intensive care unit: Did staff fingernails play a role in disease transmission? *Journal of Hospital Epidemiology*, 21(2), 80–84.

Mortimer, E.A., Lipsitz, P.J., Wolinsky, E., et al. (1962) Transmission of staphylococci between newborns. Importance of the hands to personnel. *American Journal of Diseases of Children*, 104, 289–295.

NHS England and NHSI (NHS Improvement) (2019) *Standard Infection Control Precautions: National Hand Hygiene and Personal Protective Equipment Policy*. Available at: https://improvement.nhs.uk/documents/4957/National policy_on_hand_hygiene_and_PPE_2.pdf

NHS Improvement (2017) *Preventing Healthcare Associated Gram-Negative Bloodstream Infections: An Improvement Resource*. London: NHS Improvement.

NICE (National Institute for Health and Care Excellence) (2015) *Antimicrobial Stewardship: Systems and Processes for Effective Antimicrobial Medicine Use* [NG15]. Available at: https://www.nice.org.uk/guidance/NG15/chapter/1-Recommendations#all-antimicrobials

NICE (2017) *Healthcare-Associated Infections: Prevention and Control in Primary and Community Care* [CG139]. Available at: https://www.nice.org.uk/Guidance/CG139

NMC (Nursing and Midwifery Council) (2018) *The Code: Professional Standards of Practice and Behaviour for Nurses, Midwives and Nursing Associates*. Available at: https://www.nmc.org.uk/standards/code

NPSA (National Patient Safety Agency) (2008) *Clean Hands Save Lives (Patient Safety Alert)*. Available at: https://www.nric.org.uk/node/52696

NPSA (2009) *The Revised Healthcare Cleaning Manual*. Available at: https://www.ahcp.co.uk/wp-content/uploads/NRLS-0949-Healthcare-clea-ng-manual-2009-06-v1.pdf

O'Neill, J. (2016) *Tackling Drug-Resistant Infections Globally: Final Report and Recommendations – The Review on Antimicrobial Resistance*. London: Department of Health and Wellcome Trust.

Otter, J. (2014) *Tending the Human Microbiome*. Available at: https://reflectionsipc.com/2014/09/25/tending-the-human-microbiome

Otter, J.A., Yezli, S., Perl, T.M., et al. (2012) The role of 'no-touch' automated room disinfection systems in infection prevention and control. *Journal of Hospital Infections*, 83, 1–13.

Passaretti, C.L., Otter, J.A., Reich, N.G., et al. (2013) An evaluation of environmental decontamination with hydrogen peroxide vapor for reducing the risk of patient acquisition of multidrug-resistant organisms. *Clinical Infectious Diseases*, 56(1), 27–35.

Perry, C. (2007) *Infection Prevention and Control*. Oxford: Blackwell.

PHE (Public Health England) (2014) *Eye of the Needle: United Kingdom Surveillance of Significant Occupational Exposures to Bloodborne Viruses in Healthcare Workers*. Available at: https://assets.publishing.service.gov.uk/government/uploads/system/uploads/attachment_data/file/385300/EoN_2014_-_FINAL_CT_3_sig_occ.pdf

PHE (2015) *Start Smart – Then Focus: Antimicrobial Stewardship Toolkit for English Hospitals*. Available at https://assets.publishing.service.gov.uk/government/uploads/system/uploads/attachment_data/file/417032/Start_Smart_Then_Focus_FINAL.PDF

PHE (2017) *English Surveillance Programme for Antimicrobial Utilisation and Resistance (ESPAUR): Report 2017*. Available at: https://assets.publishing.service.gov.uk/government/uploads/system/uploads/attachment_data/file/656611/ESPAUR_report_2017.pdf

PHE (2018a) *English Surveillance Programme for Antimicrobial Utilisation and Resistance (ESPAUR): Report 2018*. Available at: https://assets.publishing.service.gov.uk/government/uploads/system/uploads/attachment_data/file/759975/ESPAUR_2018_report.pdf

PHE (2018b) *Annual Epidemiological Commentary: Gram-Negative Bacteraemia, MRSA Bacteraemia, MSSA Bacteraemia and C. difficile Infections, Up To and Including Financial Year April 2017 to March 2018*. Available at: https://webarchive.nationalarchives.gov.uk/20190509003205/https://www.gov.uk/government/statistics/mrsa-mssa-and-e-coli-bacteraemia-and-c-difficile-infection-annual-epidemiological-commentary

PHE (2018c) *Staphylococcus aureus (MRSA and MSSA) Bacteraemia: Mandatory Surveillance 2017/18 – Summary of the Mandatory Surveillance Annual Epidemiological Commentary 2017/18*. Available at https://assets.publishing.service.gov.uk/government/uploads/system/uploads/attachment_data/file/724361/S_aureus_summary_2018.pdf

PHE (2018d) *Clostridium difficile Infection: Mandatory Surveillance 2017/18: Summary of the Mandatory Surveillance Annual Epidemiological Commentary 2017/18*. Available at: https://assets.publishing.service.gov.uk/government/uploads/system/uploads/attachment_data/file/724368/CDI_summary_2018.pdf

Pittet, D., Hugonnet, S., Harbarth, S., et al. (2000) Effectiveness of a hospital-wide programme to improve compliance with hand hygiene. *Lancet*, 356, 1307–1312.

Pronovost, P., Needham, D., Berenholtz, S., et al. (2006) An intervention to decrease catheter-related bloodstream infections in the ICU. *New England Journal of Medicine*, 355(26), 2725–2732.

RCN (Royal College of Nursing) (2017) *Infection Prevention and Control*. Available at: https://www.rcn.org.uk/library/subject-guides/infection-prevention-and-control-subject-guide

RCN (2018) *Tools of the Trade: RCN Guidance for Health Care Staff on Glove Use and the Prevention of Contact Dermatitis*. Available at: https://www.rcn.org.uk/professional-development/publications/pdf-006922

Rochon, M., Jarman, J., Gabriel, J., et al. (2017) Multi-centre prospective internal and external evaluation of the Brompton Harefield Infection Score (BHIS). *Journal of Infection Prevention*, 19(2), 74–79.

Rotter, M.L. (2001) Arguments for alcoholic hand disinfection. *Journal of Hospital Infection*, 48, S4–S8.

Rowley, S. & Clare, S. (2011) ANTT: A standard approach to aseptic technique. *Nursing Times*, 107(36), 12–14.

Sax, H., Allegranzi, B., Uçkay, I., et al. (2007) 'My five moments for hand hygiene': A user-centred design approach to understand, train, monitor and report hand hygiene. *Journal of Hospital Infection*, 67(1), 9–21.

Shek, K., Patidar, R., Kohja, Z., et al. (2018). Rate of contamination of hospital privacy curtains in a burns/plastic ward: A longitudinal study. *American Journal of Infection Control*, 46(9), 1019–1021.

Siegel, J.D., Rhinehart, E., Jackson, M., et al. (2007) *Guideline for Isolation Precautions: Preventing Transmission of Infectious Agents in Healthcare Settings*. Centers for Disease Control. Available at: www.cdc.gov/ncidod/dhqp/pdf/isolation2007.pdf

Stewardson, A., Iten, A., Camus, V., et al. (2014) Efficacy of a new educational tool to improve handrubbing technique amongst healthcare workers: A controlled, before-after study. *PLOS ONE*, 9(9), e105866.

Taylor, L. (1978) An evaluation of handwashing techniques: 1. *Nursing Times*, 12 January, 54–55.

Tosh, P.K. & McDonald, L.C. (2012) Infection control in the multidrug-resistant era: Tending the human microbiome. *Clinical Infectious Diseases*, 54, 707–713.

Tschudin-Sutter, S., Rotter, M.L., Frei, R., et al. (2017) Simplifying the WHO 'how to hand rub' technique: Three steps are as effective as six – Results from an experimental randomized crossover trial. *Clinical Microbiology and Infection*, 23(6), 409.e1–409.e4.

van Nood, E., Vrieze, A., Nieuwdorp, M., et al. (2013) Duodenal infusion of donor feces for recurrent *Clostridium difficile*. *New England Journal of Medicine*, 368, 407–415.

Vonberg, R.P., Eckmanns, T., Bruderek, J., et al. (2005) Use of terminal tap water filter systems for prevention of nosocomial legionellosis. *Journal of Hospital Infection*, 60(2), 159–162.

Voss, A. & Widmer, A.F. (1997) No time for handwashing!? Handwashing versus alcoholic rub: Can we afford 100% compliance? *Infection Control & Hospital Epidemiology*, 18(3), 205–208.

Walker, J.T., Jhutty, A., Parks, S., et al. (2014) Investigation of healthcare associated infections associated with *Pseudomonas aeruginosa* biofilm in taps in neonatal units in Northern Ireland. *Journal of Hospital Infection*, 86(1), 16–23.

Walker, J.T. & Moore, G. (2015) *Pseudomonas aeruginosa* in hospital water systems: Biofilms, guidelines, and practicalities. *Journal of Hospital Infection*, 89(4), 324–327.

Wang, B., Yao, M., Lv, L., et al. (2017) The human microbiota in health and disease. *Engineering*, 3(1), 71–82.

Waste (England and Wales) Regulations (2011) Available at: www.legislation.gov.uk/uksi/2011/988/pdfs/uksi_20110988_en.pdf

Water Supply (Water Quality) Regulations (2016) Available at: www.legislation.gov.uk/uksi/2016/614/pdfs/uksi_20160614_en.pdf

Weber, D.J., Rutala, W.A. & Sickbert-Bennett, E.E. (2007). Outbreaks associated with contaminated antiseptics and disinfectants. *Antimicrobial Agents and Chemotherapy*, 51(12), 4217–4224.

WHO (World Health Organization) (2009a) *WHO Guidelines on Hand Hygiene in Health Care: First Global Patient Safety – Challenge Clean Care Is Safer Care*. Available at: http://apps.who.int/iris/bitstream/handle/10665/44102/9789241597906_eng.pdf;jsessionid=67BD4B6DDF1897202C610AD99481BC49?sequence=1

WHO (2009b) *Glove Use Information Leaflet: Outline of the Evidence and Considerations on Medical Glove Use to Prevent Germ Transmission*. Available at: www.who.int/gpsc/5may/Glove_Use_Information_Leaflet.pdf

Widmer, A.F. (2013) Surgical hand hygiene: Scrub or rub? *Journal of Hospital Infection*, 83, S35–S39.

Wigglesworth, N. (2003) The use of protective isolation. *Nursing Times*, 99(7), 26.

Wigglesworth, N. & Wilcox, M.H. (2006) Prospective evaluation of hospital isolation room capacity. *Journal of Hospital Infection*, 63(2), 156–161.

Wilson, J. (2019) *Infection Control in Clinical Practice, updated* 3rd edn. London: Elsevier.

Wise, J. (2012) Three babies die in pseudomonas outbreak at Belfast neonatal unit. *BMJ*, 344, e592.

Woode Owusu, M., Wellington, E., Rice, B., et al. (2014) *Eye of the Needle: United Kingdom Surveillance of Significant Occupational Exposures to Bloodborne Viruses in Healthcare Workers – Data to End 2013*. London: Public Health England.

Young, V. (2017) The role of the microbiome in human health and disease: An introduction for clinicians. *BMJ*, 356, j831.

Part Two

Supporting patients with human functioning

Chapters

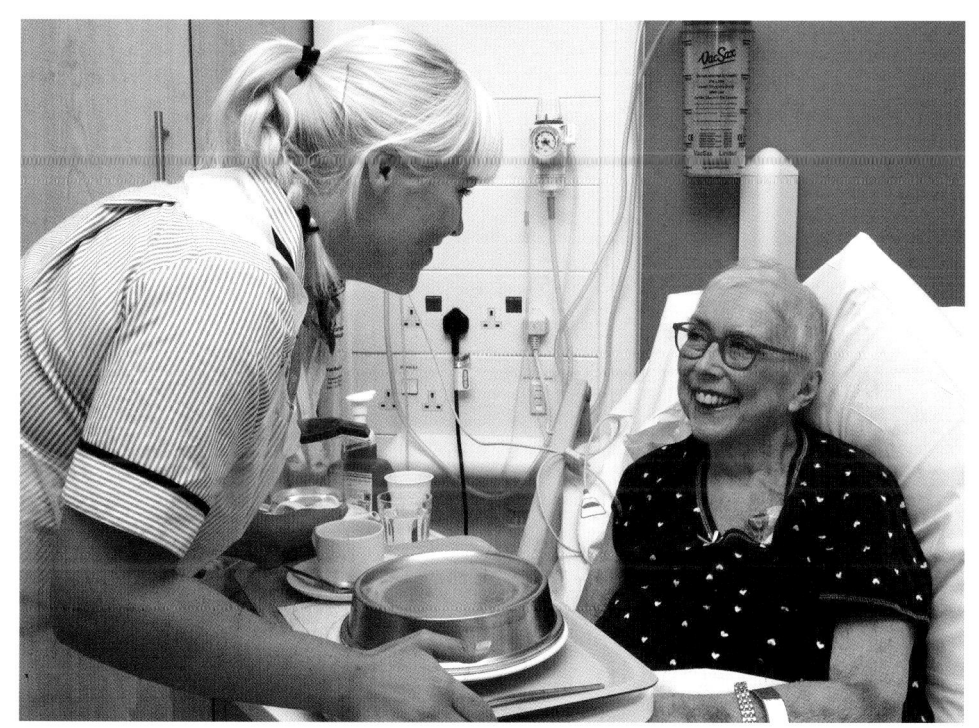

Chapter 5

Communication, psychological wellbeing and safeguarding

Justin Grayer with Jennie Baxter, Lauren Blackburn, Jill Cooper, Edwina Curtis, Lisa Dvorjetz, Linda Finn, Danielle Gaynor, Beverley Henderson, Charmaine Jagger, Lucy Keating, Lauren Leigh-Doyle, Sara Lister, Raj Mathiah and Asim Mohammed

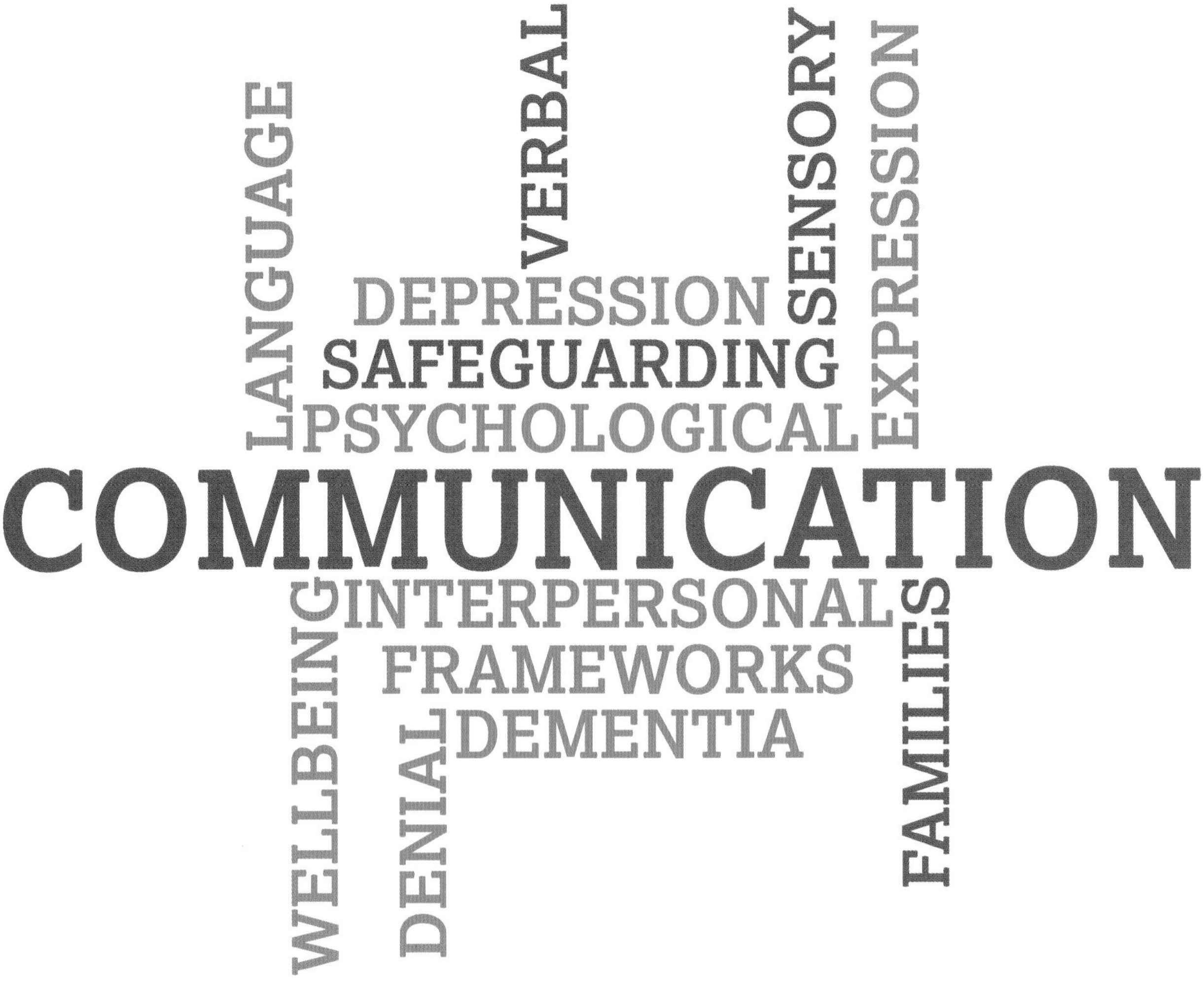

The Royal Marsden Manual of Clinical Nursing Procedures: Professional Edition, Tenth Edition. Edited by Sara Lister, Justine Hofland and Hayley Grafton.

Principles tables

Being an accountable professional

At the point of registration, the nurse will:

1. Use evidence-based, best practice approaches to take a history, observe, recognise and accurately assess people of all ages:
   - **1.1** mental health and wellbeing status
2. Use evidence-based, best practice approaches to undertake the following procedures:
   - **2.11** recognise and respond to signs of all forms of abuse
   - **2.17** recognise and respond to challenging behaviour, providing appropriate safe holding and restraint

Future Nurse: Standards of Proficiency for Registered Nurses (NMC 2018)

Overview

This chapter defines and describes effective communication, factors relating to the psychological wellbeing of patients and those close to them, and issues around safeguarding adults and their families. It discusses interpersonal communication using language comprising verbal and non-verbal expression, and considers the necessary adjustments to communicate with specific populations, such as people with sensory impairment or dementia. The process of offering psychological support to patients and the management of factors that contribute to or compromise psychological wellbeing are considered. There are specific sections on adjustment, denial and collusion, anxiety and panic, depression, anger management and delirium. Finally, ways of working that enhance a patient's safety within and outside healthcare organizations are explored, with relevant legal frameworks outlined.

Communication

Definition

Communication is a universal word with a multitude of definitions. Many definitions describe communication as a transfer of information between a source and a receiver (Kennedy Sheldon 2009): that is, the sending and receiving of verbal and non-verbal messages between two or more people (de Vito 2013). In nursing, this communication is primarily interpersonal: the process by which compassion and support are offered and information, decisions and feelings are shared (McCabe and Timmins 2013). It is also important for nurses to recognize their intrapersonal communication – that is, how they speak and relate to themselves – as this affects their emotions and behaviours and thus their communication with and care of patients (see Chapter 19: Self-care and wellbeing for further information).

Anatomy and physiology

Verbal communication is a complex process that is dependent on intact language, speech and hearing function (González-Fernández et al. 2015). The human voice is produced by exhaled air vibrating the vocal cords in the larynx to set up sound waves in the column of air in the pharynx, nose and mouth. Pitch is controlled by the tension on the vocal cords: the tighter they are, the more they vibrate and the higher the pitch.

Although sound originates from the vibration of the vocal cords, other structures (such as the mouth, pharynx, nasal cavity and paranasal sinuses) convert the sound into recognizable speech (Tortora and Derrickson 2017) (Figure 5.1).

The ear contains receptors for sound waves and the external, or outer, ear is designed to collect sound waves and direct them inward. As the waves strike the tympanic membrane, it vibrates due to the alternate compression and decompression of the air. This vibration is passed on through the malleus, incus and stapes of the middle ear. As the stapes vibrates, it pushes the oval window. The movement of the oval window sets up waves in the perilymph of the cochlea that ultimately lead to the generation of nerve impulses that travel to the auditory area of the cerebral cortex (Tortora and Derrickson 2017) (Figure 5.2).

The glottis consists of a pair of folds of mucous membrane in the larynx (the vocal folds) and the space between them (the rima glottidis).

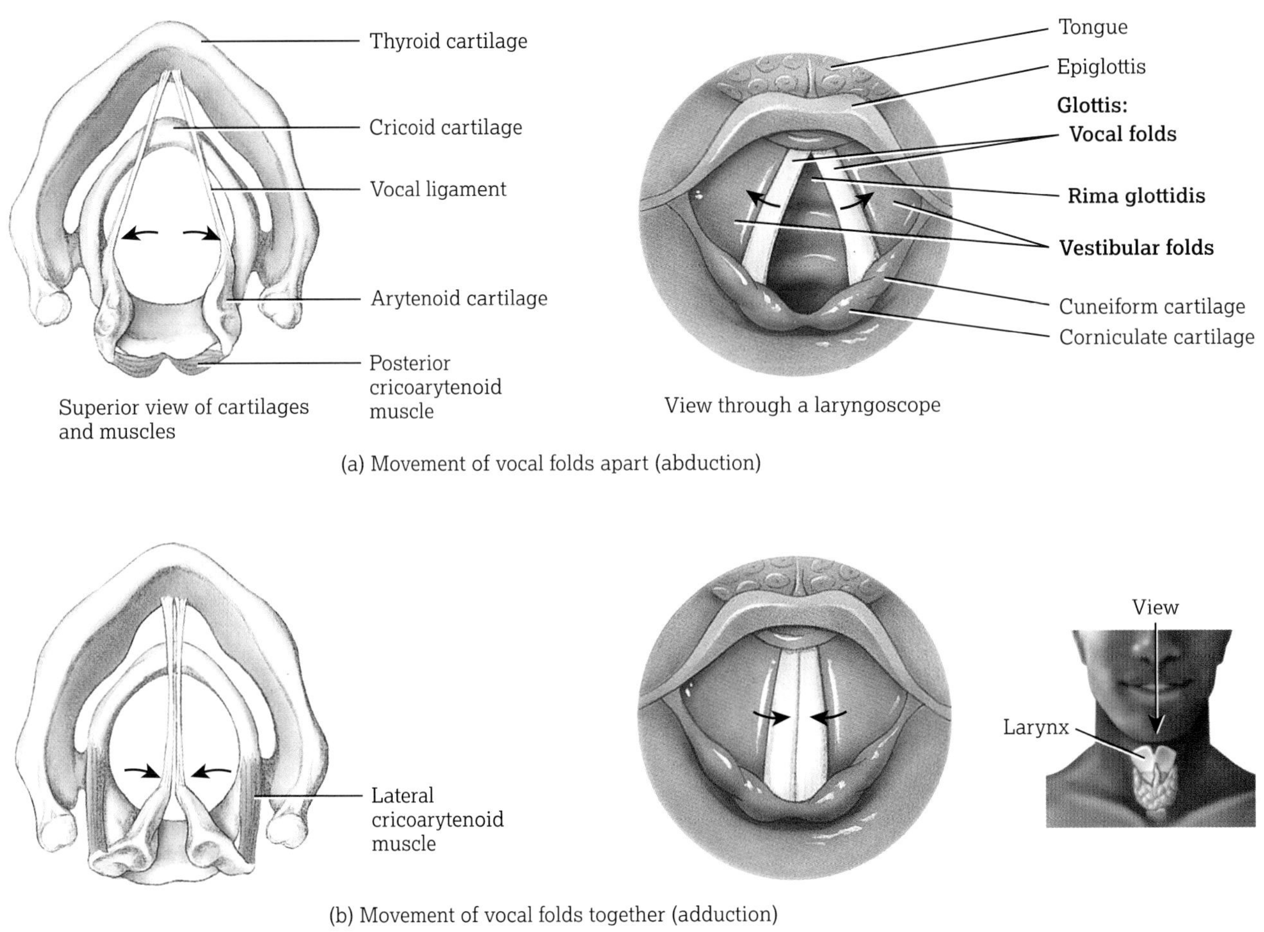

Figure 5.1 Movement of the vocal cords. *Source*: Reproduced from Tortora and Derrickson (2017) with permission of John Wiley & Sons.

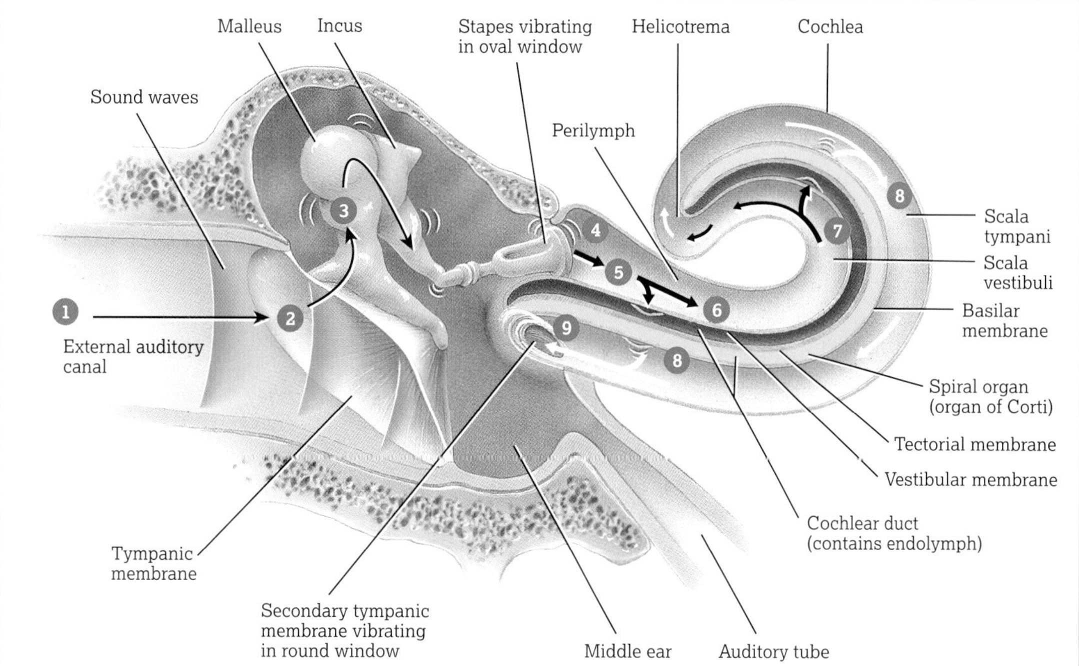

Figure 5.2 Events in the stimulation of auditory receptors in the right ear. *Source*: Reproduced from Tortora and Derrickson (2017) with permission of John Wiley & Sons.

The physiological process of communication is, however, more complex than speech and hearing. The central nervous system (CNS) controls relatively automatic behaviours present from birth and volitional control acquired with development. Voice production includes the volitional acts of speech and singing, but it can also be involuntary in response to pain or fright (Ludlow 2015). Lesions within the CNS can result in speech impairment as there may be paralysis of the muscles of articulation. CNS lesions can be congenital (e.g. in Down syndrome) or acquired following a stroke (Mathieson 2001).

The peripheral nervous system (PNS) controls the laryngeal and palatal muscles; therefore, if the PNS is affected, this can also result in voice and speech impairments. The cerebellum plays an important role in processing motor activity; it regulates the speech, force and timings of movements and if it is damaged bilaterally speech can be affected. Speech may then be described as slurred and unco-ordinated.

Related theory

There are many theories about interpersonal communication. One of the earliest theories is the idea that communication can be represented as a linear process (Miller and Nicholson 1976):

Sender → Message → Receiver

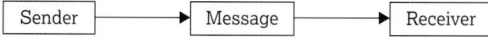

This Linear Model of communication makes certain assumptions, such as the receiver being a willing participant in the process and open to receiving the message, and that all messages will be clear and the sender certain about their purpose (McCabe and Timmins 2013). However, such a model is unidirectional so is more relevant for electronic media and not necessarily representative of the complexity of human communication.

The Transactional Model is more useful, recognizing that human communication is a simultaneous process, so each person involved is a communicator rather than just a sender or receiver (McCabe and Timmins 2013) (Figure 5.3). In addition, the model recognizes that the interpersonal context or environment affects the process significantly, as does the channel of communication (i.e. whether it is visual, aural/vocal, gustatory/taste, olfactory/smell, touch, or kinesic/interpretation of motion). This theory helps nurses to reflect on the multifaceted nature of communicating with patients and so recognize the many factors that can affect an effective process.

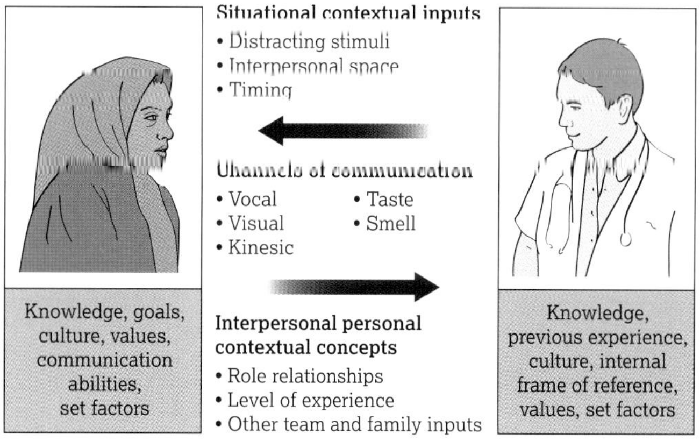

Figure 5.3 Transactional model of communication. *Source*: Adapted from Arnold and Underman Boggs (2011) with permission of Elsevier.

An aim of interpersonal professional communication training is to support and maintain the patient's optimum level of communication while remaining aware of the impact that the disease and its management may have on the patient's ability and/or motivation to speak. It is also important to be aware of the different coping styles and attitudes of the patient and key people in their life, as well as co-morbidities, disease progression, fluctuating cognitive abilities and treatment side-effects. All these factors demand a flexible approach when supporting communication throughout the patient pathway (Dwamena et al. 2012, White 2004).

Non-verbally, people communicate via gestures, body language, posture, facial expression, touch and the items they surround themselves with, such as their personal possessions, which will include their clothing and accessories, means of entertainment (e.g. books and digital media) and photographs in the hospital environment. Communication can be heavily influenced by a multitude of external and internal factors, for example immediate environment, illness, mood, self-esteem, gender, class, status and culture. The influence of these factors needs to be carefully considered in each circumstance.

Evidence-based approaches

Effective communication is widely regarded to be a key determinant of patient satisfaction, adherence and good clinical health outcomes (Boissy et al. 2016). Poor communication is one of the most common causes of complaints in the NHS, and increased 9.7% between 2015–2016 and 2016–2017 (NHS Digital 2017).

Supportive communication is important to create an environment where the individual patient feels heard and understood and can be helped appropriately. In order to deliver personalized patient care, nurses need to consider the patient's feelings, wishes and experiences (Grover et al. 2018). Moreover, communication needs to be flexible and dependent upon cultural, social and environmental factors (Batbaatar et al. 2017).

People with illness want to be approached with a 'caring and humane attitude' that respects their privacy and dignity (Maben and Griffiths 2008, Webster and Bryan 2009). They want to be able to experience a meaningful connection and a sense of 'being known' by the staff they encounter (Thorne et al. 2005, Webster and Bryan 2009). Additionally, patients want their personal values to be respected and to be treated as equals by health professionals. This can be achieved by taking time to communicate, listening and offering emotional support (Smith et al. 2005), and striving for open, clear and honest communication (Heyland et al. 2006, Jenkins et al. 2001). Mazzi et al. (2015) found that when patients were asked to watch recorded medical consultations, they preferred an affective, or emotional, communication style that included empathy, support, interest and active listening skills. However, they cautioned that some patients will not prefer this style and that nurses need to be able to accurately assess how much patients want to share their thoughts and feelings without assuming that they either do or do not wish to.

Communication occurs in a time-pressured environment. Practical and technical tasks demand the nurse's time and tend to be the focus of care over and above the psychological needs of the patient. The task-orientated short communication encounters that emerge do not encourage the disclosure of psychosocial concerns (Silverman et al. 2013). Patients may not expect to discuss psychosocial issues with nurses because of the communication bias towards physical and medical issues (Chant et al. 2004). This can lead to limited communication that prevents effective exploration of psychological issues. Without effective exploration, patients are not sufficiently encouraged to engage with and manage their own care. Additionally, nurses need to be aware of and consider environmental features that may contribute to the nature of the dialogue that takes place (Hargie 2017); for example, a public space may inhibit discussion.

Patient satisfaction is not necessarily related to the acquisition of specific communication skills (Dwamena et al. 2012, Thorne et al. 2005). Nonetheless, listening and appropriate verbal responses that demonstrate empathy remain at the core of effective communication.

Listening

Listening is often assumed to be a simple skill; however, it is a difficult and complex activity. The physical act of hearing is distinct from listening. Hearing can be considered to be passive, but listening requires active processing and attaching meaning to what is heard. It is difficult to answer the question 'How do we listen?' and a procedure on 'how to listen' would not do justice to the sophistication and success of good listeners. However, there are ways of describing the constituent parts of listening that, if followed, would make the person speaking appreciate that they were being listened to.

Active listening involves the assimilation of verbal and non-verbal cues, which are reflected back to the patient using both verbal and non-verbal responses. Problems can emerge when two people interpret the meaning of the same dialogue differently. For example, if the question asked is 'How are you?' and the patient replies 'Getting by', is it assumed that they are doing well and coping or that they are struggling and 'putting on a brave face'? Hopefully, the numerous non-verbal cues will be attended to, in order to decipher what the patient actually means. If the patient sounds upbeat and smiles, it might be concluded that they are coping. However, if there is incongruence between the words 'Getting by' and their delivery – for example, in a low, sad-sounding voice coupled with a simultaneous lowering of the head – it might be thought that they are struggling. Hargie (2017) describes four types of listener (Box 5.1).

Box 5.1 Types of listener

1 *People-orientated listeners.* Their primary concern is for others' feelings and needs. Can be distracted away from the task owing to this focus on psychoemotional perspectives. We seek them out when we need a listening ear. They are good helpers.
2 *Task-orientated listeners.* Are mainly concerned with getting the business done. Do not like discussing what they see as irrelevant information or having to listen to 'long-winded' people or 'whingers'. Can be insensitive to the emotional needs of others.
3 *Content-orientated listeners.* These are analytical people who enjoy dissecting information and carefully scrutinizing it. They often focus on the literal meaning of what has been said. They want to hear all sides and leave no stone unturned, however long the process. Can be slow to make decisions as they are never quite sure if they have garnered all the necessary information. They are good mediators.
4 *Time-orientated listeners.* Their main focus is on getting tasks completed within set time frames. They see time as a valuable commodity, not to be wasted. Are impatient with what they see as prevaricators and can be prone to jumping to conclusions before they have heard all of the information.

Source: Adapted from Hargie (2017) with permission of Routledge.

Non-verbal responses

Non-verbal communication generally indicates information transmitted without speaking. Included in this would be the way a person sits or stands, facial expressions, gestures and posture, whether the person nods or smiles, and the clothes worn; all will have an impact on the total communication taking place (Hargie 2017). Argyle (1988) suggested that only 7% of communication between people is verbal. Hargie (2017) outlines seven non-verbal signs of listening (Box 5.2).

Egan (2018) provides the useful acronym SOLER to summarize the constituent elements of non-verbal communication (Figure 5.4):

Facing the patient	**S**quarely
Maintaining an	**O**pen posture
	Leaning slightly towards the patient to convey interest
Having appropriate	**E**ye contact, not staring nor avoiding (unless culturally appropriate)
Being	**R**elaxed

By being aware of the above factors and making this behaviour part of your normal demeanour, patients will be encouraged to talk more openly, facilitating emotional disclosure.

It can be argued that non-verbal information is more powerful than verbal information, for example in the case of incongruence (discussed above), where the verbal message indicates one meaning and the non-verbal suggests another. There is a tendency to believe the non-verbal message over the verbal in these instances.

	Yes	No
Squarely	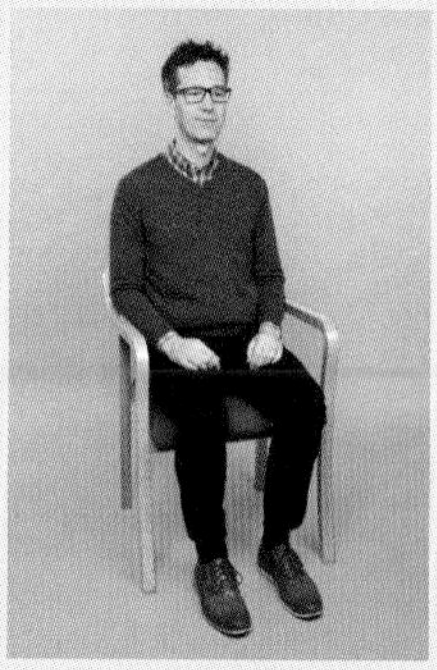	
Open posture	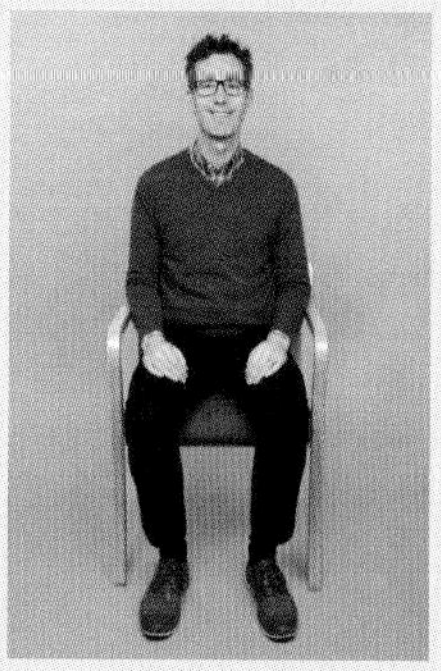	
Leaning slightly towards the patient	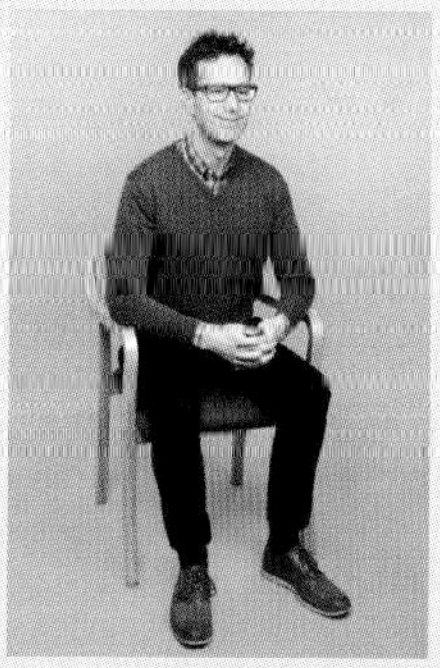	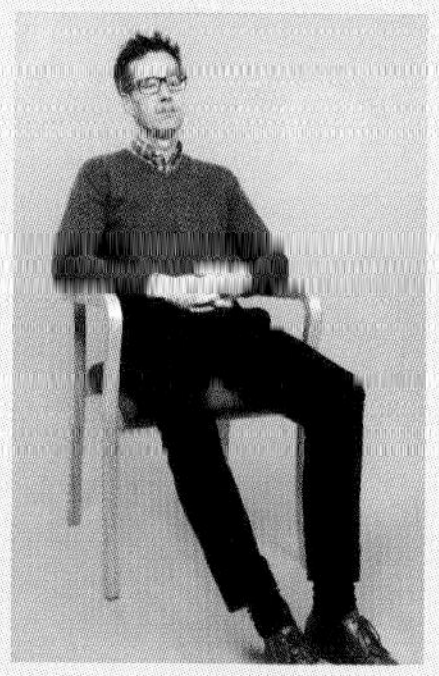
Eye contact		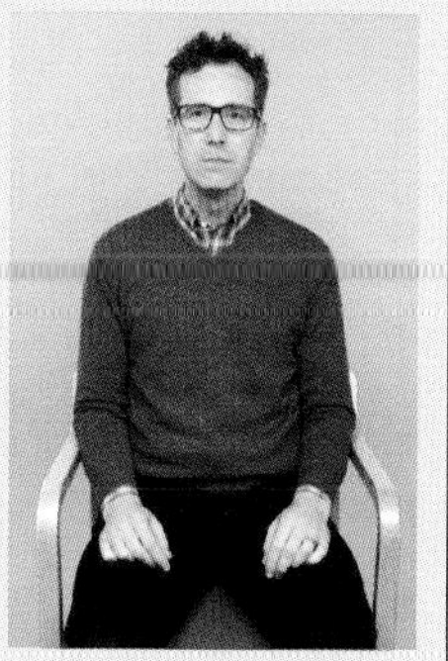
Relaxed		

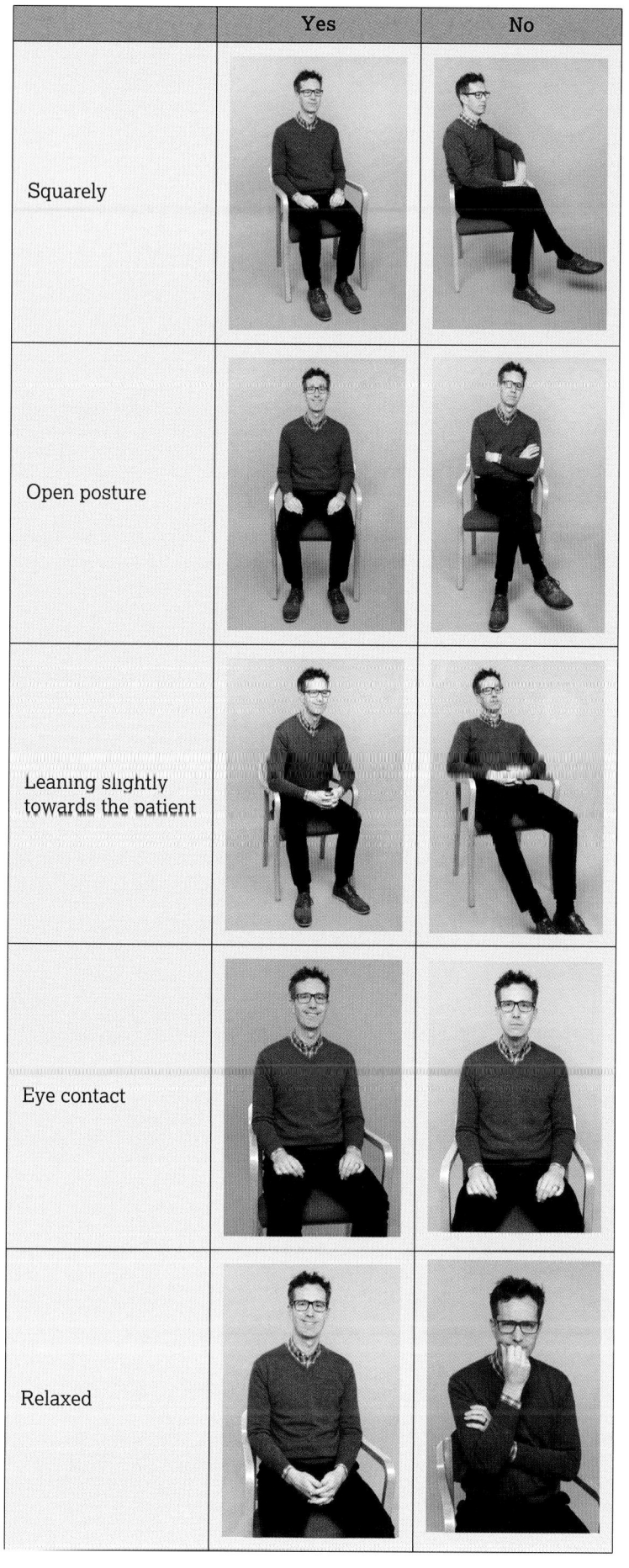

Figure 5.4 Non-verbal communication: SOLER.

Box 5.2 Non-verbal signs of listening

1 *Smiles*: used as indicators of willingness to follow the conversation or pleasure at what is being said.
2 *Direct eye contact*: in Western society, the listener usually looks more at the speaker than vice versa (in other cultures this may not be the case, and direct eye gaze may be viewed as disrespectful or challenging).
3 *Using appropriate paralanguage* to convey enthusiasm for the speaker's thoughts and ideas (e.g. tone of voice, emphasis on certain words, lack of interruption).
4 *Reflecting the facial expressions* of the speaker, in order to show sympathy and empathy with the emotional message being conveyed.
5 *Adopting an attentive posture*, such as a forwards or sideways lean in a chair. Similarly, a sideways tilt of the head (often with the head resting on one hand) is an indicator of listening. What is known as 'sympathetic communication' involves the mirroring of overall posture as well as facial expressions. Indeed, where problems arise in communication, such mirroring usually ceases to occur.
6 *Head nods* to indicate agreement or willingness to listen.
7 *Refraining from distracting mannerisms*, such as doodling with a pen, fidgeting or looking at a watch.

Source: Adapted from Hargie (2017) with permission of Routledge.

This highlights the need to communicate with authenticity. Without this, supportive communication can be severely reduced in its effectiveness.

Non-verbal communication becomes even more important in the case of people whose verbal communication is impaired, for example by dementia, learning disability, stroke or surgery. Hoorn et al. (2016) developed an algorithm to help intensive care nurses identify the best communication aid for intubated patients. Patients need to be supported, ensuring, for example, that they have constant access to pen and paper; communication boards can be used to good effect and it is worth considering the use of information technology and communication software, if available. The experience of losing the ability to speak can be very isolating and frustrating, and preparation of the patient and practice with communication aids are important to maximize the success of communication. It is essential that people with a speech deficit are given more time to communicate their needs, so patience and persistence are essential until interaction and understanding are gained at a satisfactory level. Saying nothing can also be interpreted as a communication with meaning, and so there is always communication, however reluctant or silent the nurse or patient.

Non-verbal behaviour to encourage patients to talk includes nodding or making affirming noises, for example 'hmmm'. This 'affirming' is mostly done naturally, for example at points of eye contact, as specific points are made and during slight pauses in dialogue. It can be especially important to affirm what the patient is saying when they are talking about psychological issues as this will validate that what the patient is saying is an acceptable topic of conversation. Chambers (2003, p.878) suggests that for patients with 'limited verbal expression', nurses have a responsibility to build upon and recognize their non-verbal communication to support the development of a good working relationship with the patient.

Verbal responses

The way words and sentences are spoken makes a considerable difference to communication, so attention needs to be paid to the tone and rate of speech. It is important to sound alert, interested and caring, but not patronizing. In general, speech should be delivered at an even rate, not too fast nor too slow (Hargie 2017). However, when presenting difficult or complex information, particularly when someone is upset, talking more slowly will give the patient additional time, thus reducing the cognitive demand required to understand the information.

Questioning

Questioning is a skill that is used in close collaboration with listening. When specific information is required, for example in a crisis, closed questions are indicated, because they narrow down the number of potential answers (Silverman et al. 2013) and allow the gathering of specific information for a specific purpose. Closed questions, therefore, are ones that are likely to generate a short 'yes' or 'no' answer, for example 'Can you hear me?' or 'Are you in pain?'.

In care situations with significant life-changing implications, a broader assessment of the patient's perspective is required and there is also a need to show compassion and identify any underlying psychosocial issues. Open questions and listening are therefore required. Open questions do the opposite of closed questions; they broaden the number of potential answers (Silverman et al. 2013), giving the agenda and control of the conversation to the patient. For example, instead of asking 'Are you all right?', an open question would be 'How are you today?' or 'What has your experience of treatment been like?'. A question that enquires about a patient's emotional experience indicates that this is also of interest to the nurse – for example, 'How did you feel about that?' or 'What are your main concerns?'.

Open questions cannot be used in isolation as the opportunity for open discussion can easily be blocked by failing to ensure that the rest of the fundamental communication elements are in place. Attention must therefore be paid to providing sufficient time, verbal space (not interrupting) and encouragement (in the form of non-verbal cues, paraphrasing, clarifying and summarizing), so that the patient and/or relative can express their feelings and concerns.

Open questions may not be the most appropriate way of communicating with people who have an acquired communication problem, such as changes to the oral cavity following head and neck surgery, as it may be too difficult or frustrating for them to answer questions at length. However, it is important to provide an opportunity for such patients to express themselves verbally and non-verbally, and a combination of open and closed questions may be appropriate.

Asking one question at a time is important. It is easy to ask more than one question in a sentence, but this can make it unclear where the focus is and lead the patient to answer only one part of the question.

Open questions can also be helpful to respond to cues that the patient may give about their underlying psychological state. Cues can be varied, numerous and difficult to define, but essentially these are either verbal or non-verbal hints of underlying unease or worry. Concerns may be easier to recognize when they are expressed verbally and unambiguously (del Piccolo et al. 2006).

Paraphrasing

This technique involves telling the patient what they have told you using different and often less words that retain the same meaning. For example:

Patient: I need to talk to my partner and parents but whenever they start to talk to me about the future, I just start to get wound up and shut down.
Nurse: You want to talk to your family, but then you get tense and you stop talking …

Reflecting back

Reflecting, sometimes referred to as 'mirroring', includes a reflection of emotion as well as words. When it is used, it needs to be done with thought and authenticity. For example:

Patient: My boss keeps asking me when I am going back to work. I've already had 6 months off, but I feel so tired all the time.
Nurse: It sounds like you are worried that you're not ready to go back to work yet, but you're feeling some pressure from your boss to return.

Box 5.3 Open and closed questions

- Are you feeling like that now? (closed)
- You seem to be down today, am I right? (closed)
- How do you feel about the experience? (closed, although some people may answer it as an open question)
- You say that you've not had enough information: can you tell me what you do know? (open)
- You mention that you are struggling: what kinds of things do you struggle with? (open)
- You say it's been hard getting this far: what has been the hardest thing to cope with? (open)

Clarifying

The aim of this technique is to reduce ambiguity and help the patient to define and explore the central or pivotal aspect of the issues raised. Nurses can be reluctant to explore psychological issues in too much depth for fear that the issues raised will be too emotional and hard to deal with (Perry and Burgess 2002). However, if the principles of good communication are applied and a focus on the patient's agenda is maintained, distressing and difficult situations can be heard and support offered to the patient.

The use of open questions is likely to raise certain issues that would benefit from further exploration. Clarification encourages the expression of detail and context about situations, helping to draw out pertinent matters perhaps not previously considered by either the patient or the nurse. A mixture of open and closed questions can be used in clarification (Box 5.3).

It is sometimes necessary for the nurse to clarify their own position, perhaps acknowledging that they do not know something and cannot answer certain questions. For example, 'I am not in a position to know if the treatment will work.' Sometimes not knowing can be a valuable position, as it prompts an enquiry about the patient's experience rather than making assumptions. The knowledge and experience gained through a nursing career may mean that the experience of the patient or relative is familiar; however, patients and relatives will benefit from the opportunity to share their experience in their own words and to feel 'heard' (Williams and Iruita 2004).

Summarizing

This technique can be used as a way of opening or closing dialogue. An opening can be facilitated by recapping a previous discussion or outlining your understanding of the patient's position. Summarizing can be used to punctuate a longer conversation and highlight specific issues raised. This serves several purposes:

- It informs the patient that they have been listened to and that their situation is understood.
- It allows the patient to correct any mistakes or misconceptions that have arisen.
- It brings the conversation from the specific to the general (which can help to contextualize issues).
- It gives an opportunity for agreement to be reached about what may need to happen.

For example:

> *Nurse*: It sounds like you are tired and are struggling to manage the treatment schedule. It also sounds like you don't have enough information and we could support you more with that …

Summarizing can be a useful opportunity to plan and agree what actions are necessary. However, if summarizing is used in this situation, it is important to avoid getting caught up with planning and solution finding; the patient will gain the greatest benefit from empathetic, attentive listening. Nurses are familiar with 'doing' and correcting problematic situations, and, although interventions can be helpful in psychosocial issues, sometimes it is necessary not to act and to just 'be' with the patient, accepting their experience as it is, however difficult this may be. If it helps you to 'be' with the patient and/or relative, remember that what you are 'doing' is 'being'.

Recognizing when to act and when to sit with distress can be difficult. However, it is important to develop this awareness and to accept that sometimes there are no solutions to difficult situations. The temptation to always correct problems might only serve to negate the patient's experience of being listened to (Connolly et al. 2010). Sometimes all the patient may want in that moment is to be listened to and heard.

Empathy

Sharing time and physical space with other people demands the development of a relationship. In nursing, the relationship with patients is defined by many factors, for example physical and medical care. In clinical roles, it is possible to be emotionally detached and to exist behind a 'professional mask' (Taylor 1998, p.74); however, when working in a supportive role, a shared experience and bond are generated, inclusive of feelings.

Rogers (1975, p.2) seminally described the skill of empathy as 'the ability to experience another person's world as if it were one's own, without losing the "as if" quality'. This means allowing ourselves to step into the patient's shoes and experience some of what they might be experiencing, without allowing ourselves to enter the experience wholly (it is not our experience). Empathy allows for an opportunity to 'taste' and therefore attempt to understand the patient's perspective. Understanding emotions and behaviours in this way encourages an acceptance of them.

Nurses demonstrate empathy when there is a desire to understand the patient as fully as possible and to communicate this understanding back to them (Egan 2018). This means attempting to gain an appreciation of what the patient might be going through, taking into consideration their physical, social and psychological environment. This inferred information can be used to 'connect' with the patient, all the time checking that the interpretation of their experience is accurate. Even if the nurse has experienced similar events, it is important to determine the patient's thoughts and feelings as they can be very different.

Empathy may not always come easily, especially if a patient is angry. Learning the ability to step back from a situation and reflect upon what it is that you, as the nurse, feel and how this relates to what is happening for the patient can be useful in the development and use of empathy.

Maintaining Egan's (2018) 'as if' quality protects nurses from adopting too great an emotional load. Having too much of a sense of loss or sorrow may prevent us from offering effective support, as we are drawn to focus on our own feelings more than is necessary or helpful for ourselves or the patient. Recognizing our own feelings is important to allow us to understand and to 'tolerate another person's pain' (McKenzie 2002, p.34).

Barriers to effective communication

Poor communication with patients can negatively affect decision making and quality of life (Dwamena et al. 2012, Fallowfield et al. 2001, Thorne et al. 2005). The environmental conditions in which nurses work, with competing professional demands and time pressures, can reduce the capacity to form effective relationships with patients (Hemsley et al. 2012, Henderson et al. 2007).

There is a personal, emotional impact when providing a supportive role to patients with psychological issues (Botti et al. 2006, Dunne 2003, Turner et al. 2007) and it is therefore likely that blocking or avoidance of patients' emotional concerns (Box 5.4) relates to emotional self-preservation for the nurse. Young (2012) states that in caring for patients who have dementia, professional caregivers are likely to avoid communication, which can result in further isolation and frustration in the patient, which in turn may lead to angry behaviour.

When communicating and assessing patients' needs, nurses may be anxious about eliciting distress and managing expressed concerns. They may lack confidence in their ability to clarify patients' feelings without 'causing harm to the patient or getting

Box 5.4 Characteristics of blocking behaviours

Blocking can be defined as:

- failing to pick up on cues (ignoring emotional content)
- selectively focusing on the physical and medical aspects of care
- premature or false reassurance, for example telling people not to worry
- inappropriate encouragement or trivializing, for example telling someone they look fine when they have mentioned an altered body image
- passing the buck, for example suggesting it is another professional's responsibility to answer questions or sort out the problem (e.g. doctors or counsellors)
- changing the subject, for example asking about something mundane or about other family members to deflect the conversation away from issues that may make you feel uncomfortable
- jollying along, for example 'You'll feel better when you get home'
- using closed questions (any question that can be answered with a 'yes' or a 'no' is a closed question).

Source: Adapted from Faulkner and Maguire (1994).

into difficulty themselves' (Booth et al. 1996, p.526). As a consequence, nurses can make assumptions, rather than assessing concerns properly (Booth et al. 1996, Kelsey 2005, Schofield et al. 2008). To illustrate this point, Kruijver et al. (2001) demonstrated how nurses verbally focus upon physical issues, which in their study accounted for 60% of communication with patients. Nurses often recognize this bias, with the evidence suggesting that they feel greater competence discussing physical rather than psychological issues; many nurses desire better skills to help them to manage challenging situations (McCaughan and Parahoo 2000).

Intercultural communication and competence require the ability to recognize different cultural identities and meanings. Barriers to intercultural competence are similar to those described above but also include anxiety, stereotyping, non-verbal misinterpretations and language (Roebuck 2017).

Institutions, work environments and the nature of the senior staff within them can influence the nature of communication (Booth et al. 1996, McCabe 2004, Menzies-Lyth 1988, Wilkinson 1991). Approaches to patients who have additional communication needs require consideration and planning. Being supported practically and emotionally by supervisors and/or senior staff can help to decrease blocking behaviours (Booth et al. 1996, Connolly et al. 2010). Clinical supervision can aid the transfer of communication skills into practice (Heaven et al. 2006).

Nurses may improve their own practice by identifying where environmental barriers lie and attempting to mitigate the features of the clinical environment that inhibit psychological care. These barriers to communication may be particularly significant for patients who have cognitive or physical impairment, such as dementia, a learning disability, or a hearing or sight impairment.

Despite the difficulties outlined above, nurses can communicate well when they are supported to provide individual patient-focused care (McCabe 2004).

Clinical governance

There are a number of legal and professional concepts and issues that affect effective communication and psychological support. These include:

- taking professional responsibility for effective communication
- maintaining confidentiality and appropriate disclosure of information about the patient
- gaining informed consent to carry out each procedure and ensuring that the patient is fully cognisant of what it involves, including assessing the patient's mental capacity to engage in care and treatment
- ensuring that issues relating to equality and diversity are taken into account at all times.

Professional responsibility for effective communication

The *Francis Report* (DH 2013b) recommended that there should be an increased focus on a culture of caring, compassion and consideration in nursing. The steps to achieving this were set out in *Compassion in Practice* (DH 2012a), which identified six fundamental values: care, compassion, competence, communication, courage and commitment. These values have been incorporated into *Leading Change, Adding Value: A Framework for Nursing, Midwifery and Care Staff* (NHS England 2016). It is important to note that 'compassionate care delivered with courage, commitment and skill is our highest priority. It is the rock on which our efforts to promote health and wellbeing, support the vulnerable, care for the sick and look after the dying is built' (NHS England 2016, p.6).

Every nurse has a professional responsibility to communicate effectively and compassionately, as explicitly stated in *The Code* (NMC 2018):

- Make the care of people your first concern, treating them as individuals and respecting their dignity.
- You must listen to the people in your care and respond to their concerns and preferences.
- You must make arrangements to meet people's language and communication needs.
- You must share with people, in a way they can understand, the information they want or need to know about their health.
- You must uphold people's rights to be fully involved in their care.

The fifth principle of nursing practice set out by the Royal College of Nursing explicitly describes the role of nurses in the communication process:

> Nurses and nursing staff are at the heart of the communication process: they assess, record and report on treatment and care, handle information sensitively and confidentially, deal with complaints effectively, and are conscientious in reporting the things they are concerned about. (RCN 2019)

Confidentiality

'Information provided in confidence should not be used or disclosed in a form that might identify a patient without his or her consent' (DH 2003, p.7). *The Code* (NMC 2018) states that every nurse must respect a person's right to confidentiality, ensuring that they are informed about how and why information is shared by those who provide their care. In addition, this is a legal obligation and should be part of the terms and conditions of employment of any healthcare professional (DH 2003). However, this does not prevent nurses from communicating with an NHS colleague who is providing direct treatment to their patient – for example, at a multidisciplinary team meeting or on a ward round; the Health and Social Care Act (2012) provides the legal basis for sharing information in this way. Further, if there is a concern that an individual may be at risk of harm, this must be appropriately disclosed following the guidance of the organization in which the nurse works.

Consent

The NHS Constitution states that 'NHS services must reflect the needs and preferences of patients, their families and carers. Patients, with their families and carers where appropriate will be involved and consulted on all decisions about their care and treatment' (DH 2009e, p.4). It also states that a patient has the right to accept or refuse treatment that is offered and not be given any physical examination or treatment unless they have given valid consent.

The Royal College of Nursing's (2017) *Principles of Consent: Guidance for Nursing Staff* outlines the legal and clinical purposes of gaining and documenting consent:

> The legal purpose is to provide those delivering treatment with a defence to a criminal charge of assault or battery or a civil claim for damages for trespass to the person. The clinical purpose comes from the fact that in most cases the co-operation of the person and the person's confidence in the treatment is a major factor in their consenting to the examination, treatment or physical investigation, or the provision of care. (p.5)

The Code (NMC 2018) states that nurses have a responsibility to ensure they gain consent and that they must:

- gain consent before treatment or care starts
- respect and support people's rights to accept or decline treatment or care
- uphold people's rights to be fully involved in decisions about their care
- be aware of the legislation regarding mental capacity
- be able to demonstrate that they have acted in someone's best interests if emergency care has been provided.

For consent to be valid, it must be given voluntarily by a competent person who has been appropriately informed and who has the capacity to consent to the intervention in question (RCN 2017). This will be the patient or someone authorized to give consent on their behalf under a lasting power of attorney, or someone who has the authority to make treatment decisions as a court-appointed deputy (DH 2009d).

The validity of consent does not depend on a signature on a form. Written consent merely serves as evidence of consent. Although completion of a consent form is in most cases not a legal requirement, the use of such forms is good practice where an intervention such as surgery is to be undertaken (DH 2009d).

Obtaining consent is a process and not a one off event (RCN 2017), and consent is not a simple 'yes' or 'no' answer in many situations (RCN 2017). For consent to be valid, the nurse should ensure that the person has understood what examination or treatment is intended, and why (DH 2009d). Legal informed consent is now a requirement in most situations. This means that the person consenting to the procedure, process or treatment must be provided with sufficient information to enable them to make a balanced and informed decision about their care (NMC 2018, RCN 2017).

It is usually the person that is undertaking the procedure that seeks the patient's consent. There may be situations when a nurse has been asked to seek consent on behalf of other staff. Providing the nurse has had training for that specific area, they may seek to obtain that consent (RCN 2017).

Mental capacity

If there is any doubt about a person's capacity to make a decision about consent, the nurse should firstly determine whether or not the person has the capacity to consent to the intervention and secondly establish that they have sufficient information to be able to make an informed decision (DH 2009d). This should be done before the person is asked to sign any form. Documentation is necessary and the nurse should record all discussions relating to consent, details of the assessment of capacity, and the conclusion reached, in the patient's notes (NMC 2018). *The Code* makes explicit the responsibility to be aware of the legislation regarding mental capacity, a factor that can have a significant impact on communication. The Mental Capacity Act (2005) sets out clear guidance and there is an accompanying code of practice to support professionals working with people who may have impairment in their capacity. For more information, see the section on the Mental Capacity Act later in this chapter.

As part of the nursing assessment, the nurse needs to establish whether the person can understand the verbal communication, whether they understand what they are being consented for, and whether they can read, write or communicate their decision in a reliable manner. If they are unable to write, they may be able to make their mark on the form to indicate consent by any reasonable means, for example drawing a line or a squiggle. If consent has been given validly, the lack of a completed form is no bar to treatment, but a form can be important evidence of consent (DH 2009d). If the patient is unable to consent because they do not understand the information, or is unable to communicate their decision, the Mental Capacity Act (2005) allows decisions to be made in the patient's best interest. If the consent is about medical treatment then a best interest decision may be required; whether it is required will depend on the seriousness of the decision (Mental Capacity Act 2005).

A competent adult may refuse to consent to treatment or care, and nurses must respect that decision (NMC 2018). Where a patient declines an intervention, consideration must be given to the patient's capacity; a patient who has capacity is allowed to make what others may consider to be an unwise decision (Mental Capacity Act 2005). When a patient is deemed to have capacity and declines care, this needs to be recorded clearly in their notes.

Equality and diversity

An additional aspect of communication and psychological support from the legal perspective is to ensure that it is as equitable as possible. The Equality Act (2010) reinforces the duty to ensure that everybody has equal access to information and is communicated with equitably, irrespective of disability, sex, gender reassignment, race, age, relationship status, pregnancy and maternity, sexual orientation, religion or faith. This means, for example, that provision is necessary to meet the information needs of blind and partially sighted people (Disability Discrimination Act 1995 (Commencement No. 6) Order 1999, Section 21).

Communication needs are individual and information requirements are culturally sensitive. People may hold different beliefs about why they have developed an illness, for instance thinking that they are being punished for something that they have or have not done (Dein 2006, McEvoy et al. 2009).

Medical language is full of technical vocabulary and jargon that is often difficult to comprehend, even for people who speak English as their first language. The 2011 Census found that in England and Wales 1.6% of respondents did not speak English (in England) or Welsh (in Wales) well or at all and that the vast majority of these respondents lived in London (ONS 2013). Approximately 7.7% of the population reported that English or Welsh was not their main language (this incidence was higher in London and the West Midlands). Furthermore, an increasing number of healthcare staff are trained overseas and speak English as a second language. In nursing conversations where one or more of the people speak English as a second language, there are opportunities for miscommunication, which can result in psychological distress or medical errors (Meuter et al. 2015). Therefore, it is important that nurses use 'short, clear and precise' sentences (Macdonald 2004, p.131) and frequently check the patient's (and family's) understanding.

Patients from minority ethnic backgrounds often take a family member to hospital appointments to assist in the dialogue between them and the medical or nursing practitioner. However, family members may not fully understand what they are being asked to translate, or might misconstrue or misrepresent what is being said (Macmillan Cancer Relief 2002). Most NHS trusts have interpreting services, and there are reputable telephone helplines that can facilitate translation from one language to another. It is good practice that these services be used rather than relying on family or friends of the patient (Macdonald 2004). Guidance for the commissioning of interpreting and translation services is available (NHS England 2018).

Older patients are more likely to have hearing or sight loss (although this should not be assumed) and this needs to be considered alongside the patient's dignity when communicating with them. For example, if a patient is hearing impaired, there may be a temptation to shout, but in a busy clinical environment this might breach the patient's right to confidentiality and to be treated with dignity. Information provided in small print may be inaccessible for a patient with visual difficulties, impacting on their ability to make an informed choice.

Patients with dementia may have additional communication needs, and there is a danger of assuming that because a person has dementia they will not be able to make decisions for themselves. Daniel and Dewing (2012) suggest that this idea needs to be avoided as it fails to meet the requirements of the Mental Capacity Act (2005). The act makes it clear that consent must be decision specific and, as such, each significant decision needs to be assessed. If a patient with dementia has communication issues, it is important to work with them and their family to maximize their ability to be involved in decision making even when the person is assessed as lacking capacity. The Mental Capacity Act 'promotes the autonomy and rights of an individual who lacks decision-making capacity' (Griffith and Tengnah 2008, p.337).

It is estimated that 50–90% of people with learning disabilities experience communication difficulties, such as impaired speech, impaired hearing or sight loss (Jones 2002). It is important to know what tools can be used to support this patient group to communicate their needs while receiving healthcare, bearing in mind that the most important of these tools is the communication skills of the person providing the care (Chambers 2003). Many patients with learning disabilities will have a hospital or My Health passport that will include information on how best to communicate with them. The person with a learning disability may also have a communication book that is full of symbols they can use to communicate their needs.

With any patient who has additional communication needs, it is important to work with the individual and the people who know them well, such as family, carers or other professionals. Family, carers and friends can interpret the non-verbal communication more easily and so can support nurses in providing care; carers should be seen as partners in the caring process. A learning disability liaison nurse role developed in Scotland was found to enhance patient and carer satisfaction, partly through the development and implementation of accessible information (MacArthur et al. 2015).

Competencies

Communication is such an essential aspect of the role of anybody in healthcare that the NHS *Knowledge and Skills Framework* (Agenda for Change Project Team 2004) specifies four levels of skill in communication (Table 5.1). Nurses are expected to be competent as a minimum to Level 3. This is a baseline and much work has been done on developing programmes to advance communication skills further.

The consistency of the success of training interventions has been widely discussed (Chant et al. 2004, Heaven et al. 2006, Schofield et al. 2008). Ongoing development of communication skills should include learning how to negotiate barriers to good communication in the clinical environment, tailoring and individualizing communication approaches for different patients, conflict resolution and negotiation skills (Gysels et al. 2005, Roberts and Snowball 1999, Schofield et al. 2008, Wilkinson 1991).

Courses with a behavioural component of communication training – that is, role-playing situations in the classroom – are preferable as this is indicated to influence effectiveness (Gysels et al. 2005). Skill acquisition and implementation following communication training is more likely when the training is followed up by regular supervision (Eggenberger et al. 2013).

If an issue appears to be beyond the scope of practice of the nurse, it is essential that further advice and help are sought, or that patients are signposted or referred on to specialist psychological practitioners. Self-care and supervision are key factors in maintaining the ability to support other people (see Chapter 19: Self-care and wellbeing).

Pre-procedural considerations

Time

In an acute hospital environment, time is always pressured. This has an impact on communication unless steps are taken to create time for effective, supportive communication to take place. From the patient's perspective, they need to know that they have the nurse's attention for a set period of time. It is therefore essential to be realistic and proactive with the patient to arrange a specific conversation for a prescribed length of time at a prearranged point in the day. It is important to be realistic but also to keep to the arrangement, otherwise there is the potential for the patient to consider that their psychological needs are not important (Towers 2007) or that healthcare providers are unreliable.

Environment

Conversations in a hospital environment can be very difficult, especially if privacy is required. However, there are actions that can be taken to make the environment as conducive as possible to enable supportive communication to take place (Towers 2007) (Box 5.5).

Box 5.5 Making the environment conducive to supportive communication

- Can the patient safely and comfortably move to a more suitable area to talk with more privacy?
- Do they wish to move?
- Is the patient able to sit comfortably?
- Will the patient be too hot or cold?
- Do they wish other people (e.g. members of their family) to be present?
- Clear a space if necessary, respecting the patient's privacy and property.
- If you are in an open area on a ward, draw the curtains (with the patient's permission) to give you some privacy. Obviously, this does not prevent sound transfer and it is worth acknowledging the limitations of privacy.
- Remove distractions – for example, seek the patient's permission to switch off the television if it is on.
- Check whether they prefer sitting on one side or another.
- As far as possible, choose a seat for yourself that is comfortable and on the same level as the patient.
- Position your seat so you can have eye contact with each other easily without having to turn significantly.

Table 5.1 NHS *Knowledge and Skills Framework*: four levels of communication competence

Level 1	Level 2	Level 3	Level 4
Establish and maintain communication with other people on routine and operational matters	Establish and maintain communication with people about routine and daily activities, overcoming any differences in communication between the people involved	Establish and maintain communication with individuals and groups about difficult or complex matters, overcoming any problems in communication	Establish and maintain communication with various individuals and groups on complex, potentially stressful topics in a range of situations

Source: Adapted from Agenda for Change Project Team (2004).

This preliminary work might seem insignificant and time consuming but it underlines the importance of the communication to the patient and demonstrates respect and dignity.

Assessment

Nurses need to make careful assessments of the patient's communication and psychological needs. This will include an assessment of their communication style, skills and ability to relate (see Chapter 2: Admissions and assessment), and will also include observing and enquiring about their current (and past) cognitive state, mood, coping strategies and support networks. Patient needs and presentation are likely to vary at different points in the treatment journey. An ongoing professional relationship between a nurse and a patient can help in the identification of changes in mood and cognitive ability alongside physical health status. Assessment and recording tools may be helpful in supporting discussions with patients as well as noting change over time.

Recording tools

An example of a tool that can be used to facilitate communication about a person's biological, psychological and social situation is the Holistic Needs Assessment (HNA) (Figure 5.5). The HNA includes the Distress Thermometer, which is a validated instrument for measuring distress (Gessler et al. 2008, Mitchell 2007, Ransom et al. 2006). It is similar to a pain analogue scale (0 = no distress, 10 = extreme distress) and is simple to use and understand (Mitchell et al. 2010). The patient marks their distress level for the current moment or for an agreed period preceding the assessment. They are also invited to indicate which practical, family, emotional, spiritual and physical concerns they have and whether they want to discuss these or not. The Distress Thermometer provides a shared language to help patients and staff talk about what is concerning them (Mitchell 2007). A score over 5 would warrant discussion and exploration of whether other support is necessary or desired. It may be that no further referral is necessary and that the structured discussion this tool provides is sufficient in lowering the level of distress (NCCN 2018).

Principles of communication

Communication with a patient that is compassionate and supportive in a clinical environment cannot be described as a simple, linear process; nonetheless, certain principles can increase its effectiveness (see Principles table 5.1: Communication).

RM Partners
West London Cancer Alliance
Hosted by The Royal Marsden NHS Foundation Trust

SELCA
South East London Cancer Alliance

NHS
North Central and East London Cancer Alliance

Pan-London Holistic Needs Assessment

For each item below, please select **yes** or **no** if they have been a concern for you during the last week, including today. Please also select **discuss** if you wish to speak about it with your healthcare professional. Choose not to complete the assessment today by selecting this box. ☐

Date:	
Name:	
Hospital/ NHS number:	

Please **select the number** that best describes the overall level of distress you have been feeling during the last week, including today:

10	☐	Extreme distress
9	☐	
8	☐	
7	☐	
6	☐	
5	☐	
4	☐	
3	☐	
2	☐	
1	☐	
0	☐	No distress

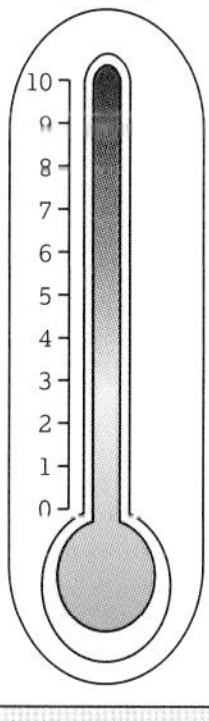

For health professional use	
Date of diagnosis:	
Diagnosis:	
Pathway point:	

Practical concerns	Yes	No	Discuss
Caring responsibilities	☐	☐	☐
Housing or finances	☐	☐	☐
Transport or parking	☐	☐	☐
Work or education	☐	☐	☐
Information needs	☐	☐	☐
Difficulty making plans	☐	☐	☐
Grocery shopping	☐	☐	☐
Preparing food	☐	☐	☐
Bathing or dressing	☐	☐	☐
Laundry/housework	☐	☐	☐
Family concerns			
Relationship with children	☐	☐	☐
Relationship with partner	☐	☐	☐
Relationship with others	☐	☐	☐
Emotional concerns			
Loneliness or isolation	☐	☐	☐
Sadness or depression	☐	☐	☐
Worry, fear or anxiety	☐	☐	☐
Anger, frustration or guilt	☐	☐	☐
Memory or concentration	☐	☐	☐
Hopelessness	☐	☐	☐
Sexual concerns	☐	☐	☐
Spiritual concerns			
Regret about the past	☐	☐	☐
Loss of faith or other spiritual concern	☐	☐	☐
Loss of meaning or purpose in life	☐	☐	☐

Physical concerns	Yes	No	Discuss
High temperature	☐	☐	☐
Wound care	☐	☐	☐
Passing urine	☐	☐	☐
Constipation or diarrhoea	☐	☐	☐
Indigestion	☐	☐	☐
Nausea and/or vomiting	☐	☐	☐
Cough	☐	☐	☐
Changes in weight	☐	☐	☐
Eating or appetite	☐	☐	☐
Changes in taste	☐	☐	☐
Sore or dry mouth	☐	☐	☐
Feeling swollen	☐	☐	☐
Breathlessness	☐	☐	☐
Pain	☐	☐	☐
Dry, itchy or sore skin	☐	☐	☐
Tingling in hands or feet	☐	☐	☐
Hot flushes	☐	☐	☐
Moving around/walking	☐	☐	☐
Fatigue	☐	☐	☐
Sleep problems	☐	☐	☐
Communication	☐	☐	☐
Personal appearance	☐	☐	☐
Other medical condition	☐	☐	☐

Figure 5.5 The London Holistic Needs Assessment tool. *Source*: Reproduced with permission from North Central and East London Cancer Alliance, RM Partners and SEL Cancer Alliance. Adapted with permission from the NCCN Clinical Practice Guidelines in Oncology (NCCN Guidelines®) for Distress Management V.2.2014. © 2014 National Comprehensive Cancer Network, Inc. All rights reserved. The NCCN Guidelines® and illustrations herein may not be reproduced in any form for any purpose without the express written permission of the NCCN. To view the most recent and complete version of the NCCN Guidelines, go online to NCCN.org. NATIONAL COMPREHENSIVE CANCER NETWORK®, NCCN®, NCCN GUIDELINES®, and all other NCCN Content are trademarks owned by the National Comprehensive Cancer Network, Inc.

RM Partners
West London Cancer Alliance
Hosted by The Royal Marsden NHS Foundation Trust

SELCA
South East London Cancer Alliance

NHS
North Central and East London Cancer Alliance

Care Plan

During my holistic needs assessment, these issues were identified and discussed:

Preferred name: **Hospital/NHS number:**

Number	**Issue**	**Summary of discussion**	**Actions required/by (name and date)**
Example	Breathlessness	Possible causes identified Coping strategies discussed Printed information provided	Referral to anxiety management programme; CNS to complete by 24th Dec
1			
2			
3			
4			

Other actions/outcomes e.g. additional information given, health promotion, smoking cessation, 'My actions':

Signed (patient):	Date:
Signed (healthcare professional):	Date:

For healthcare professional use		
Date of diagnosis:	Diagnosis:	Pathway point:

Figure 5.5 *Continued*

Principles table 5.1 Communication

Principle	Rationale
Consider whether the patient is comfortable, needs pain relief or needs to use the toilet before you begin.	Pain, as well as other distractions and discomforts, may limit a patient's ability to reason and concentrate. E
Protect the time. This involves telling other staff that you do not wish to be disturbed for a prescribed period.	Patients may observe how busy nurses are and withhold worries and concerns unless given explicit permission to talk (McCabe 2004, R).
Introduce yourself and your role and check what the patient wishes to be called.	This helps to establish initial rapport (Silverman et al. 2013, C).
Set a realistic time boundary for your conversation at the beginning.	You may only have 10 minutes and therefore you need to articulate the scope of your available time; this will help you to avoid distraction and give your full attention during the time available. Boundaries also help the patient to feel contained. E
Spend a short time developing a rapport and indicating your interest in the patient, for example comment on a picture by the bedside.	Patients want to feel known. P
Be ready to move the conversation on to issues that may be concerning the patient.	Some patients may stay with neutral topics as the central focus of the conversation and withhold disclosure of psychosocial concerns until later in a conversation (Silverman et al. 2013, C).

Principle	Rationale
Suggest the focus of conversation, for example 'I would like to talk about how you have been feeling' or 'I wondered how you have been coping with everything.'	This indicates to the patient that you are interested in their psychological issues. E
Respond and refer to cues. For example, to respond to a cue, you could say: 'I noticed you seemed upset earlier. I have 10 minutes to spare in which we can talk about it if you wish' or 'You seem a little frustrated. Is now a good time to talk about how I can help you with this?'	Patients frequently offer cues – either verbal or non-verbal hints about underlying emotional concerns – and these need to be explored and clarified (Levinson et al. 2000, R; Oguchi et al. 2010, R).
If the patient does not wish to talk, respect this and ask them to let you know if they change their mind and do want to talk (it is still important that you have offered to talk and the patient may well wish to talk at another time).	The patient may not wish to talk at that moment or may prefer to talk to someone else. E
Ask open questions: prefix your question with 'what' or 'how'.	Open questions encourage patients to talk (Hargie 2017, R).
Use closed questions sparingly.	If patients have a complicated issue to discuss, closed questions can help them to be specific and can be used for clarification as well as when closing dialogue (Hargie 2017, R).
Add a psychological focus where you can, for example 'How have you felt about that?'	This will help to elicit information about psychological and emotional issues (Ryan et al. 2005, R).
Listen carefully and feed back your understanding of what is being said at opportune moments.	Listening is a key skill – it is an active process requiring concentration as well as verbal and non-verbal affirmations (Egan 2018, R).
Be empathetic (try to appreciate what the other person may be experiencing and recognize how difficult that may be for them).	Empathy is about creating a human connection with the patient (DH 2012a, C; Egan 2018, R).
Allow for silences.	These can give rise to further expression and allow useful thinking time for yourself and the patient (Silverman et al. 2013, C).
Initially avoid trying to 'fix' people's concerns and the problems that they express. It might be more powerful and important to simply sit, listen and show your understanding.	As an individual is listened to, they may feel comfort, relief and a sense of human connection, which are essential for support (Egan 2018, R).
Ask the patient how they think you may be able to help them.	The patient will know what they need better than you do. E
Avoid blocking (see Box 5.4).	Blocking results in failing to elicit the full range of concerns a patient may have (Back et al. 2005, R).
When you are nearing the end of the time you have agreed to be with the patient, let the patient know; that is, mention that soon you will need to stop your discussion.	The patient can find this easier to accept if you clearly expressed the time you had available in the first place (Towers 2007, R).
Acknowledge that you may not have been able to cover all concerns and summarize what has been discussed, checking with the patient how accurate your understanding is.	The patient can correct any misinterpretations and this can lead to satisfactory agreement about the meeting. It also signifies closure of the meeting (Hargie 2017, R).
If further concerns are raised at this point, make it clear that you cannot support them at the current time. Let the patient know when you or other staff may be available to talk again, or where else they may get further support.	Clarity and honesty are important, as is working within boundaries. Knowing the limits of your time and expertise will help to prevent confusion about where the patient can receive types of support. E
Agree any action points and follow up as necessary. If needs remain unmet, offer support from a clinical nurse specialist or a psychological support service, if available. You must discuss what this means and be realistic with regard to waiting times. Consent from the patient for any further referral is essential (unless you consider the patient to be at risk).	Having made a suitable assessment, you can involve further support if appropriate. E
Document your conversation, having agreed with the patient what is appropriate to share with the rest of the team.	It is essential to document your conversation so that other members of the team are informed and to meet professional requirements (NMC 2018, C).
Reflect upon your own practice.	You may have unintentionally controlled the communication or blocked expression of emotion. Reflection will increase your self-awareness and help to develop your skills. E
Consider the support needs of other people to whom you delegate tasks and your own support needs. If you or others are affected by any discussions you have had, seek discussion with supportive senior members of staff or consider debriefing and/or supervision.	Clinical supervision supports practice, enabling registered nurses to maintain and improve standards of care (NMC 2018, C).

Providing information and making shared decisions

Definition

Providing information and making shared decisions involve giving facts about treatment and care to patients to support them in making choices.

Related theory

Research conducted by the Picker Institute (Ellins and Coulter 2005) shows that 80% of people actively seek information about how to cope with health problems. Information is of prime importance in helping to support people in the decision-making process, particularly when they are vulnerable and feeling anxious. It is important that high-quality, reliable and evidence-based information is accessible to patients, their relatives and carers at the right time, making it an integral part of their care (DH 2008a). This is reiterated in the white paper *Our Health, Our Care, Our Say* (DH 2006), which states that 'everyone with a long-term condition and/or long-term need for support – and their carers – should routinely receive information about their condition' (p.114) and the services available to them. Information prescriptions represent good practice for supporting the information needs of individuals and are often used in, for example, diabetes care (DH 2009b). *High Quality Care for All* (DH 2008b) requires NHS organizations to provide accessible information to patients who have a learning disability.

The term 'giving information' implies that the healthcare professional's agenda is uppermost and can result in a paternalistic model of care (Redsell and Buck 2009). While this approach can at times be justified (e.g. in an emergency situation), wherever possible, it is important to allow patients the opportunity to be a partner in their care and to be involved in a shared decision-making process (DH 2012b). Shared decision making involves engaging the patient in one or more conversations about treatment options (NICE 2012). A nurse's role is to help the patient to choose the option best suited to them; using their clinical expertise and eliciting the patient's wishes, the nurse facilitates conversation(s) in which the patient weighs up the risks and benefits of a decision in the short term and long term (Box 5.6). This can include exploring the patient's understanding of treatment, eliciting their thoughts and feelings about the treatment, exploring what is important to the patient, and helping them to consider whether or not engaging with treatment would be consistent with their values (NICE 2012, Quality Statement 4). Research studies suggest that when professionals engage patients in the shared decision-making process, this improves physical health outcomes (Hack et al. 2006), psychological outcomes (Arora 2003) and quality of life (Street and Voigt 1997) as well as the patient's experience of healthcare (NICE 2016) and their general level of satisfaction (Loh et al. 2007). Further, shared decision making facilitates the informed consent process.

Box 5.6 Questions to ask patients during the shared decision-making process

Information gathering

- What medical procedures or options are available for the patient? What is the patient's understanding of the procedure?
- Do they have all the information they need or do they need additional support or aids in information gathering?
- Do they need communication adjustments (e.g. interpreter or large font)?

The impact of their decision

- What is their understanding of the impact of the treatment or procedure on their physical, psychological and social wellbeing?
- What are their values and how will their decision impact on those values?
- How will their decision impact on their life and those around them?
- What does the patient think and feel about the options? Do they have any concerns, worries or fears? If so, is it possible to clarify any misconceptions that may be contributing towards their worries?

Support from others

- Does the patient have other people to talk to about their decision (if required)?

Consent

- Have they weighed up their options sufficiently to be able to make a fully informed decision to consent to the procedure?

Evidence-based approaches

Shared decision making is essential in complying with national legislation and policy (Health and Social Care Act 2012). NHS England has made shared decision making a policy goal in response to the available evidence base (Churchill 2013). The National Institute for Health and Care Excellence (NICE) guidance also stresses the importance of patients being part of the decision-making process and acknowledges that this can help patients to feel empowered (NICE 2018a).

With any procedure, it is essential that the patient (assuming consciousness and ability to make rational decisions) is psychologically prepared and consented. This requires careful explanation and discussion before a procedure is carried out. Nurses can become so familiar with procedures that they expect them to be considered 'routine' by patients. This can prevent nurses from providing thorough and necessary information and gaining acceptance and co-operation from patients. Nurses therefore need to avoid assuming that repetitive or frequent procedures (e.g. taking a temperature) do not require consent, explanation and potentially discussion.

It is important to consider giving information in small amounts and checking whether the patient understands what has been said after each part has been explained. Keep language simple and clarify common and complex medical terms, for example 'cannula' and 'catheter'.

Check frequently whether the patient wishes you to continue to provide them with the same level of information. It has been shown that getting the level of information wrong (too much or too little) at diagnosis can significantly affect the subsequent level of coping (Fallowfield et al. 2002). If confusion is arising, consider whether you are providing too much detail or using too many medical terms. Be aware of whether the patient is paying attention or appears anxious (e.g. displaying fidgety or non-attentive behaviour). Do not ignore these cues: name them. For example: 'I notice you seem a little anxious while I am describing this' or 'You seem concerned about the procedure – what can I do to help?' This recognition of behaviour will help you to fully explore and support the patient's concerns.

Prior to starting the procedure, establish how the patient can communicate with you while it is being carried out; for example, confirm that they can ask questions, request more analgesia or ask for the procedure to stop (if this is realistic). Giving the patient permission to communicate with the healthcare team facilitates enhanced communication.

Information must be presented accurately and calmly and without 'false reassurance'; for example, do not say that a procedure 'will not hurt' or it 'will not go wrong' when it might. It is better to explain the risks and likely outcome. Explain that working with you and co-operating with instructions are likely to improve the outcome and that every effort will be made to reduce risk and manage any problems efficiently.

Respect a patient's choice to decline treatment; however, you may wish to explore their reasons and explain the potential (realistic) consequences. Carefully document decisions made and discuss them with the multidisciplinary team. If a patient has had a procedure before, do not assume that they are fully aware of the potential experience or risks involved, as there may have been changes to procedures or the patient may have forgotten.

Attention to good communication, honesty, confidence and calmness will help to reassure the patient, thus gaining their compliance and making a good outcome more likely (Maguire and Pitceathly 2002).

Pre-procedural considerations

Written patient information

Patient information in this context refers to information about disease, its treatment, its effects and its side-effects, and the help and support available to people living with a chronic condition, their relatives and carers. When writing information for patients and carers, consideration should be given to information already available on the chosen topic. The purpose of the information may be to:

- address frequently asked questions
- inform about a treatment or service
- reduce anxiety
- give reference material.

Ideas about new patient information should be shared with other members of the team or clinical unit, and patients and carers involved, from the outset. The content of the material should be accurate and evidence based and meet the current Department of Health and Social Care and NHS Litigation Authority requirements.

Within each part of the UK there are significant proportions of adults who lack basic literacy skills (England: 14.9%; Northern Ireland: 17.9%; Scotland: 26.7%; Wales: 12%) (National Literacy Trust 2017). When writing information, everyday language should be used (as if speaking face to face) and jargon should be avoided. However, there is no need to be patronizing or use childish language. The Plain English Campaign (2019) offers a downloadable guide entitled *How to Write in Plain English*.

When producing written information for patients, it may be worth considering accessibility for patients who are non-verbal or have a learning disability. An easy-to-read information resource with pictures, images and few words can support people with learning disabilities to have a greater understanding of information and support their decision making. The Department of Health (2009a) has produced a guide called *Basic Guidelines for People Who Commission Easy Read Information*.

Information should be dated and carry a planned review date. Sources of information should be acknowledged. This gives the reader confidence in the material.

The provision and production of information must take into account diversity in ethnicity, culture, religion, language, gender, age, disability, socioeconomic status and literacy levels, as stated in the Department of Health publication *Better Information, Better Choice, Better Health* (2004).

Information should be ratified according to local trust policy. Where a trust does not produce patient information materials to meet specific patient needs, suitable alternative sources of information should be sought.

Other sources of information

Patients and their families may benefit from information and support available in the wider community, away from the environment of statutory health services. Sources of additional information include:

- *Disease-specific national charities*, for example the National Multiple Sclerosis Society or the British Heart Foundation: these organizations produce written materials in booklet and factsheet format, as well as having websites.
- *'Illness memoirs', internet blogs and digital stories* (e.g. www.patientvoices.org.uk): personal accounts are easily accessible online and through bookstores. It may help patients to hear other people's stories as this can reduce the sense of isolation and powerlessness and promote hope (Chelf et al. 2001). It must be borne in mind that not everyone will benefit from these sources of information.
- *Peer support*: the therapeutic benefits of groups are extensively documented (NICE 2004) and most support charities have a directory of local and national groups available.

Principles of providing information to a patient

The principles of 'facilitative' communication (Wilkinson 1991) are relevant when giving information; this type of conversation is still a dialogue – therefore, patients should be allowed time to contribute to the conversation and be listened to. There are many different theories and models for giving information to patients; the following paragraphs are based on the principles of giving information taken from self-management and person-centred approaches to care.

Giving information implies that there is a message to be shared and someone who is willing and able to receive it. Therefore, a nurse needs to check that these assumptions are correct. It is wise to ensure patients are comfortable and able to absorb information, so attend to analgesia and allow them to visit the toilet beforehand if necessary. It is helpful to outline the purpose of the conversation at the beginning, before any information is shared – this will enable the patient to begin to actively listen, which requires concentration and is tiring. Therefore, make sure that the session is brief and that as much verbal information as possible is supplemented and reinforced with written and visual resources.

Patients should be asked their preferred role in the decision making process before information is given, so that the style of delivery can be tailored to their preferences and wishes (Alexander et al. 2012, Redsell and Buck 2009). In addition, many patients will be well informed about their condition or have existing understanding or knowledge, so it is important to establish and assess patients' existing knowledge and their ability and capacity to learn something new (Price 2013).

Information should be given in 'chunks' or small sections (Smets et al. 2013), pausing after each key point to allow the information to be absorbed and processed, and giving the patient the opportunity to respond, ask questions or make comments.

Giving information is more than a cognitive exercise – it also includes relational, affective aspects (Smets et al. 2013) and therefore the principles of supportive communication apply, especially the need to notice, listen and respond to patients' cues and concerns. During the conversation, remember to use empathetic statements (Egan 2018) and encourage the patient to express their worries and concerns.

Decision support materials have information on the potential outcomes, benefits and risks of treatment options (Health Foundation 2016). They may include DVDs and audio recordings, interactive media and web-based tools. They all present material in a variety of ways to help patients and families better understand the available options and to make informed choices. The most common tools are:

- *patient decision aids* such as those developed by the NHS Right Care Programme for Android phones
- *brief decision aids*: these are used within a consultation and developed from evidence-based guidance
- *option grids*: these are designed to help people compare options during consultations (Figure 5.6).

Many organizations, such as the Alzheimer's Society, Diabetes UK and Macmillan, have also created leaflets for patients explaining different treatment options, their risks and benefits, and what people might experience from choosing certain courses of action.

Herniated Disk in Lower Back: *Treatment Options*

optiongrid

A slipped (herniated) disk is a problem with a cushion (disk) between the bones in your back and causes back or leg pain, or numbness and tingling in your legs.

This decision aid is not for people with back pain from other causes, a herniated disk without symptoms, or symptoms for less than 6 weeks.

Patient questions	Shots in your back (epidural injections)	Surgery (open surgery)	Minimally invasive surgery
What does the treatment involve?	A steroid shot is injected into your back to try to reduce swelling. It takes about an hour. You may need a driver to get home. Discuss costs.	Part of your disk is removed to reduce pressure on the nerves. Surgery takes about 2 hours and you may go home later that day. Discuss costs.	Part of your disk is removed to reduce pressure on the nerves. There is less damage to muscles nearby. Surgery takes about 1 hour and you may go home later that day. Discuss costs.
Will it help my pain?	You may have less pain in 2 weeks or so. Pain will not be less in the long term compared to not having shots.	You may take 2 to 6 weeks to get better. Up to 95 out of 100 people (95%) get better, whether or not they have surgery.	You may take 2 to 8 weeks to get better. Results may be as good as with open surgery.
Might I get surgery later?	About 12 out of 100 people (12%) have surgery by 1 year.	Up to 16 out of 100 people (16%) may have repeat surgery to treat pain that continues or comes back.	From 10 to 45 out of 100 people (10% to 45%) have repeat surgery to treat pain that continues or comes back.
What are the side effects?	Up to 13 out of 100 people (13%) may have worse pain, headache, flushing in the face, or change in voice that lasts for a few hours or days.	Out of 100 people, about: • 30 (30%) have pain at site of surgery for a day or so • 20 (20%) have back or leg pain for up to 3 weeks • 20 (20%) have nausea • 20 (20%) have muscle spasm or cramps	Out of 100 people, about • 30 (30%) have pain running down the leg for up to 3 weeks • 7 (7%) have a burning feeling in the back for up to 2 months
What are the risks?	Up to 3 out of 100 people (3%) may have heavy bleeding or infection.	Out of 100 people, about: • 4 (4%) have nerve damage • 4 (4%) have the disk slip again • 2 (2%) have an infection	Out of 100 people, about: • 7 (7%) have nerve damage • 7 (7%) have the disk slip again • 2 (2%) have an infection
When will I recover?	You can be back to your usual activities the next day.	You can walk by 24 hours, and some return to usual activities by 2 weeks.	You can walk by 24 hours, and some return to usual activities by 2 weeks.

Figure 5.6 Example of an Option Grid™ tool to aid patient decision making. The tool is reviewed regularly and updated based on current evidence. To see the most recent version, visit https://optiongrid.ebsco.com. *Source*: Reproduced from EBSCO Health (2019) with permission of Option Grid.

Principles table 5.2 Giving information about a clinical procedure

Principle	Rationale
Review the changing context of the patient's situation.	People's circumstances and needs change; what may have been relevant before may now be irrelevant. **E**
Prepare for discussion, ensuring you are familiar with the procedure, disease process, medication or other aspect of care to be discussed.	Accurate information giving is an essential part of nursing care. **E**
Ensure patients are well informed.	Informed patients who are part of the shared decision-making process can better manage their health, illness, treatment and medication (Hack et al. 2006, **R**). Informed patients experience anxiety at lower rates (Nordahl et al. 2003, **R**; Scott 2004, **R**). Informed patients have lower levels of pain if they understand the causes of pain and the principles of pain management (Van Oosterwijck et al. 2013, **R**).
If possible, discuss the procedure some time before it is to be carried out for the first time. Provide the patient with leaflets, or audio-visual resources, if available, so they have time to review the information at their own pace.	To give patients the opportunity to digest information in their own time (Lowry 1995, **E**). In certain groups this has been demonstrated to improve clinical outcomes, improve improve satisfaction, increase the chance of meeting the targeted discharge date and lead to quicker return to prior functional status (NICE 2018a, **C**).
Introduce yourself.	To ensure the patient understands who you are and your role and specific aim. To promote patient satisfaction (Delvaux et al. 2004, **R**).
Maintain a warm and approachable demeanour. Do not rush.	To promote understanding and patient satisfaction (Delvaux et al. 2004, **R**).

Principle	Rationale
Consider privacy when giving information.	To promote dignity and preserve confidentiality (NMC 2018, C).
Be honest when giving information.	Patients value honesty from their healthcare professionals – it increases the sense of trust. Honesty is also required by the Health and Social Care Act's (2008) Regulation 20: Duty of Candour. C
Name the procedure and find out what information the patient knows. Clarify and check their understanding of the information.	To promote understanding and patient satisfaction. E
Consider the best way to provide information to the patient and their family.	Anxiety, distressing symptoms, fear and denial can affect a person's ability or willingness to listen and retain information (Kennedy Sheldon 2009, R).
Write down information so that there is a record of the conversation or instructions that can be followed. Keep the written information simple.	People can struggle to remember what they are told; simple language facilitates understanding. C
Avoid using jargon, technical language or abbreviations when giving information to patients. If appropriate, use pictures, for example to explain anatomy. Colours can be used to code information if this would be helpful.	Information that contains words patients understand, supported by images that provide a visual representation of the information, helps patients to concentrate and understand what is being said better. E
Encourage a relative or friend to be present while information is being given.	If someone else hears what is being said, they can more easily support the patient later. E
Divide the information into small sections. Check that the patient has understood before moving on, e.g. ask, 'Do you understand?', 'Is there something you would like to ask at this point?' or 'Would you like to explain to me what I have just shared with you?'	Giving too much information in one session can be overwhelming and prevent a patient from remembering what was said (Smets et al. 2013, R).
Pace the information, regularly checking with the patient that you are progressing at a speed acceptable to them. If you are short of time, give a small part of the information.	Never rush information giving – patients will feel overwhelmed and exhausted. E
Observe the patient closely – read their non-verbal cues and, if necessary, stop.	This helps them to process what they have been told (Smets et al. 2013, R).
Encourage the patient to repeat back to you what you have explained. For example, you could ask the patient to explain what they are going to tell their family when they get home.	This will help you to identify whether they have misunderstood anything you have told them. E
Allow the patient to ask questions.	Listen carefully to the questions the patient asks you – these can indicate where misunderstandings have occurred. E
Monitor the patient's responses and non-verbal cues.	Receiving information is tiring. Be prepared to pause or stop the session and allow the patient time to absorb and process what has been explained. E
Show empathy.	Remember that the information might have an emotional impact on the patient – acknowledge this and be supportive. E
Confirm consent: ensure that the patient is happy for you to proceed. Allow the patient an opportunity to ask further questions or say 'no' to the procedure. (If the patient fully understands what is involved, they may decide that they are not ready to proceed.)	To respect the rights of the individual (NMC 2018, C). To obtain consent correctly (RCN 2017, C).
Start the procedure, reiterating the main issues as you go along and keeping the patient updated on progress.	To maintain open dialogue and address issues and questions as they arise. E
Make it clear when the procedure has finished and what has been achieved. Offer an opportunity for the discussion of implications, disclosing as much information as the patient wishes.	So that the patient is aware and has the information they need and want (Jenkins et al. 2001, R).

Communicating with specific populations

Communicating with people with acquired communication disorders

Definitions

Aphasia or dysphasia

Aphasia or dysphasia (the terms can be used interchangeably) is an acquired communication disorder that impairs a person's ability to process language. It does not affect intelligence but does affect how someone uses language. A neurological condition or acquired brain injury can affect the formulation, expression and/or understanding of language in both written and spoken form (González-Fernández et al. 2015). Aphasia may be temporary or permanent. A patient with receptive aphasia has difficulty understanding spoken or written language. Conversely, expressive aphasia is typically characterized by partial loss of the ability to produce spoken or written language. Someone may have a solely receptive or expressive aphasia but more commonly they will have a combination of the two; they may also have additional cognitive difficulties.

Dysarthria

Dysarthria is a motor speech disorder. It occurs when weakness, dyscoordination and/or sensory loss affect muscle function in one or more of the five subsystems of speech (i.e. respiration, articulation, phonation, resonance and prosody (González-Fernández et al. 2015). This can result in speech that is low in volume, slurred, nasal and/or flat.

Acquired dyspraxia

Acquired dyspraxia of speech results in difficulty planning and/or co-ordinating articulatory movements due to damage to the brain from a head trauma, stroke or brain tumour. The person is aware of how their speech should sound and their verbal expression may be hesitant with sound substitutions, for example saying 'tup of tea' instead of 'cup of tea'

Dysphonia

Dysphonia is a voice disorder and may be related to disordered laryngeal, respiratory and vocal tract function. It reflects structural, neurological, psychological and behavioural problems as well as systemic conditions (Mathieson 2001).

Cognitive communication disorder

Cognitive communication disorder affects the link between cognition and its influence on verbal and non-verbal communication, reading and writing. Cognitive deficits can affect attention, memory, organization, processing and executive function, which in turn affect communication.

Related theory

Many areas of the brain are involved with language and cognitive processing, and the complex relationship between the brain's structure and functions is still not fully understood. The brain can be divided into four primary lobes: the frontal, temporal, parietal and occipital lobes. The majority of language-related activity occurs in the left side of the brain; occasionally a person uses both hemispheres, and even less commonly the right hemisphere only. There are a number of key areas of the brain involved in language function (Figure 5.7):

- *Broca's area*, located in the frontal lobe, is associated with speech production and articulation in written and spoken language.
- *Wernicke's area*, located in the temporal lobe, is primarily involved in the comprehension of language.
- The *angular gyrus* is in close proximity to a number of regions including the parietal, occipital and temporal lobes. It allows people to associate a perceived word with different images, sensations and ideas.

Disorders of communication have a number of causes, for example neurological conditions (e.g. traumatic brain injury, stroke, brain tumour, spinal injury or epilepsy) or progressive neurological disease (e.g. motor neurone or Parkinson's disease). These may result in language disorders, cognitive communication disorders, motor speech disorders, voice difficulties or a combination of difficulties.

The incidence of communication difficulties varies. Speech and language difficulties are more common in childhood but acquired difficulties can occur in adulthood. The Stroke Association (2017) reports that a third of stroke survivors experience some degree of aphasia. [illegible] found that aphasia occurred in 30–50% of all patients with a brain tumour.

Speech is the primary means of human communication and is essential across the lifespan to engage and interact with others (Etter et al. 2013). Language disorders, such as aphasia, can cause miscommunication, resulting in poor medical care and reduced safety (Blackstone et al. 2015). Further, language disorders can lead to feelings of insecurity and anxiety as well as sleep disturbances and stress (Rodrigues 2016).

Barriers to communication

Everyone experiences barriers to communication at times; however, these can increase when someone is unwell or in a hospital setting. For example:

- *Medical treatment and interventions* (e.g. sedation or receiving oxygen) can interfere with a person's ability and desire to communicate.
- *Physical difficulties*, such as visual or hearing difficulties, can form barriers to communication.

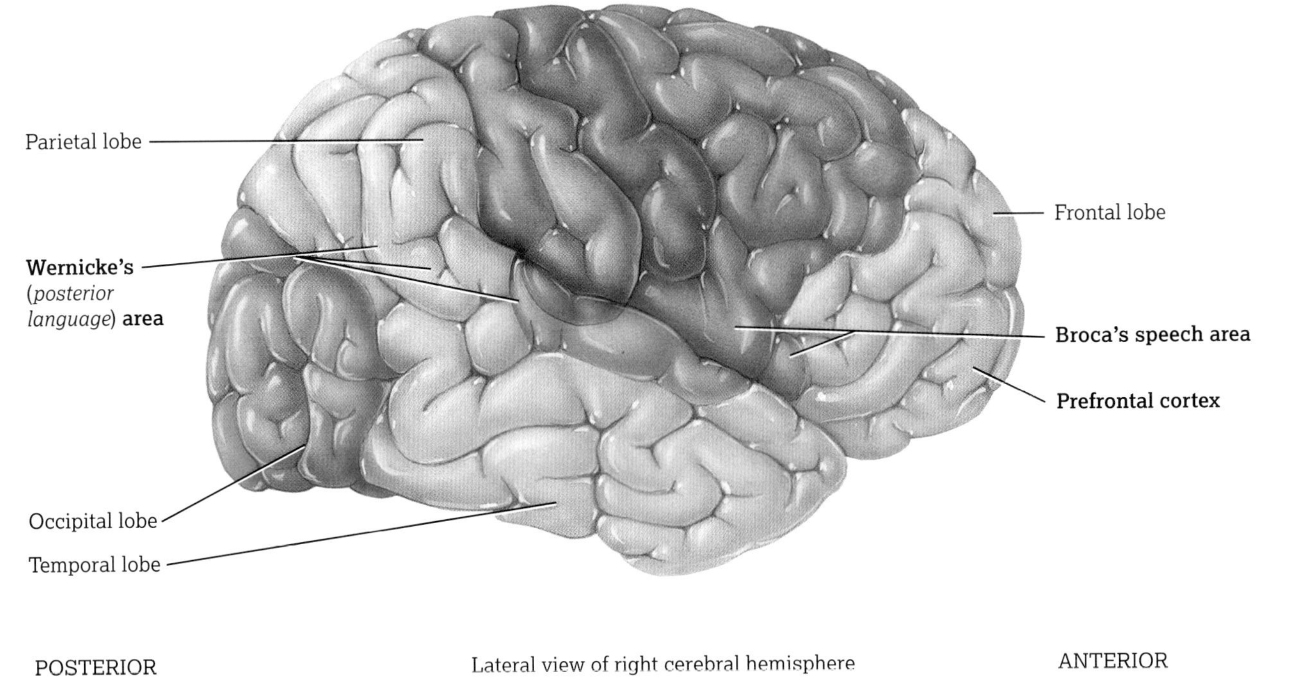

Figure 5.7 Areas of the brain involved in the communication process. *Source*: Reproduced from Tortora and Derrickson (2011) with permission of John Wiley & Sons.

- *Fatigue* can make communication too effortful.
- *Cognitive impairment*, such as memory difficulties, reduced concentration and attention, distractibility and reduced insight, can make communication difficult.
- *Environmental factors*, such as a noisy and busy hospital environment, can place an added burden on a person already struggling with communication.
- *Cultural differences* in social interaction (such as use of eye contact, attitudes about personal space, use of gestures, and accents) vary greatly across cultures.

Evidence-based approaches

The speech and language therapist (SLT) has a key role in the specialist assessment and management of acquired communication, voice and swallowing disorders. Patients with diseases affecting their central nervous system require input from a multiprofessional team, to support their complex changing care needs throughout the patient pathway (NICE 2006).

Pre-procedural considerations

Equipment

Communication aids

Communication aids are referred to as augmentative or alternative communication (AAC). AAC may range from basic picture charts or books to electronic aids and computer programmes. AAC helps to compensate for persistent or progressive communication difficulties. AAC can also be useful in the short term for hospital inpatients who are intubated or have an altered airway. AAC intervention approaches can be used to meet daily communication needs to ensure participation and independence in a variety of situations (Hanson and Fager 2017). Box 5.7 provides points to consider when using AAC.

Box 5.7 Points to consider when using augmentative or alternative communication (AAC)

- There should be an early referral to the speech and language therapist to assess the appropriateness of the use of AAC.
- With the addition of any aid (no matter how simple or sophisticated), communication becomes more complex and difficult as it involves another step in the process; that is, it changes from a two-way to a three-way process.
- Patients need to be motivated to use aids.
- The use of aids requires planning, extra concentration and time, listening, watching and interpretation by both the patient and their conversation partner.

Principles of communicating with people with aphasia

Principles table 5.3 Supporting communication for a person with aphasia

Principle	Rationale
Identify in advance if a patient has impaired attention, concentration and/or memory.	This will affect what you say and how you check for understanding. E
Have a pen and paper ready for both the patient and yourself to use during the conversation.	Writing or drawing can support what is being said. E
Introduce a topic clearly.	If a patient has receptive difficulties, being clear on the subject matter will aid their understanding. E
Allow time for pauses and silences.	To help patients who have delayed processing or who become overwhelmed. E
Say one thing at a time and pause between 'chunks' of information.	To allow time for understanding and questions. E
Speech should be clear, slightly slower than usual and of normal volume.	To ensure the patient has time to process what is being said. E
Minimize interruptions.	To aid concentration and engagement. E
Use straightforward language, avoiding jargon.	Medical terminology can involve long words and be complex, which can inhibit understanding. E
Provide visual representations (printed photos and mobile devices).	This will aid the person's understanding and engagement. E
Talk directly to the patient and ask what is and is not helpful.	To ensure communication is as effective as possible. E
Structure questions carefully and make use of closed questions.	To limit the need for complex expression. E
Regularly check the patient's understanding.	To ensure they continue to be involved in the conversation and are respected. E
Be prepared for their and your frustration. You might need to return to a topic another time.	Abilities may fluctuate, so what helps one moment might not work another time. E

Principles of communicating with people with impaired speech (dysarthria)

Dysarthria may range from mild, slightly slurred or imprecise speech to speech that is affected to an extent where the patient is unintelligible (this is different from aphasia, where language is not affected).

Principles table 5.4 Supporting communication for a person with dysarthria

Principle	Rationale
Find a quiet environment in which to speak.	To reduce distractions and make it easier for the patient to concentrate. **E**
Have a pen and paper to hand, and encourage writing when necessary.	To provide a quick and easy medium of communication during periods of breakdown. **E**
Ask if the patient uses any strategies to help their speech.	Patients may be able to use gesture, writing or drawing to help facilitate their communication. **E**
Encourage a slower rate of speech and regular pauses.	Slowing down rate of speech and ensuring adequate breath support can aid intelligibility for the listener. **E**
Allow more time than usual.	So the person does not feel rushed and pressured, which can reduce intelligibility. **E**
Be encouraging but honest and open if you are having difficulty understanding.	This allows the patient to repeat things or express things in another way that may be more understandable to the listener. **E**

Principles of communicating with people with impaired voice (dysphonia)

The dysphonia may fluctuate from mild voice changes to the patient not being able to give voice at all. All patients with persistent dysphonia may benefit from an early referral to ear, nose and throat specialists followed by a referral to an SLT if appropriate.

Principles table 5.5 Supporting communication for a person with dysphonia

Principle	Rationale
Face-to-face communication is preferable.	The patient will then also be able to use non-verbal communication (such as facial expression) to transmit their messages. **E**
Avoid having to talk where there is background noise.	To reduce the necessity for the individual to strain their voice unnecessarily. **E**
Have pen and paper to hand, and encourage writing when necessary.	To provide another medium of communication during communication breakdown. **E**
Encourage regular sips of water.	To maintain hydration and keep the throat area moist. **E**
Encourage the patient to talk gently and avoid shouting or whispering.	To minimize voice strain. **E**

Principles of communicating with people who are blind or partially sighted

Sight loss varies from mild to complete. For any patient, sight loss is significant, and they will rely more on other senses, especially their hearing. Good communication practice is essential and nurses may need to be the eyes for the patient and relay information they are not aware of – for example, that the patient's visitor has arrived and is waiting. It is important to be open about the visual impairment and identify the person's preferred communication method(s). No single method will suit all people; even the same person might use different methods at different times and under different circumstances.

People who are blind or partially sighted have the same information needs as everyone else and need accessible information in a suitable format, such as large-print documents, Braille or audio. Access to information facilitates informed decisions and promotes independence. The Royal National Institute of Blind People has useful information on its website (RNIB 2019).

Principles table 5.6 Supporting communication for a person who is blind or partially sighted

Principle	Rationale
Gain the attention of the person who is blind by speaking first; when you arrive, introduce yourself and state what your role is as well as where you are in the room. Clearly state when you are leaving the room.	Visual cues are diminished or absent to people who are blind or partially sighted, and they may be disorientated in unfamiliar environments (RNIB 2016, **E**).
Turn down or off any unnecessary background noise; use verbal cues and use names to indicate who is speaking to whom, especially in a group setting.	As visual cues are diminished or absent to a person who is blind, their hearing is particularly important for effective communication (RNIB 2016, **E**).
Ask the person whether they would like help before providing it.	It is polite to check (Stevens 2003, **E**).

Principle	Rationale
Use clear and careful explanations and verbally check that the person you are communicating with understands what you are saying.	A substantial essence of meaning is communicated non-verbally; people who are blind do not receive this information so it may be harder for them to gain full understanding (RNIB 2016, E).
Give clear and precise instructions.	A person who is blind or partially sighted, especially in an unfamiliar environment, needs clarity to be able to follow any instructions (Stevens 2003, E).
Let people know ahead of time about changes to their environment, for example ground surfaces (slopes, slippery floors), whether a door opens towards or away from them, and stairs.	This enables a person to stay safe (Stevens 2003, E).
It is all right to use language such as 'look', 'see' and 'read'.	People who are blind or partially sighted have the same vocabulary (Stevens 2003, E).
Provide information in accessible ways, for example audio (including recordings of appointments), Braille or large print.	To ensure the communication preferences of people who are blind or partially sighted are followed (RNIB 2016, E; Stevens 2003, E).
Ensure glasses are clean and within reach.	Some people who are registered blind do have some sight (RNIB 2016, E).

Principles of communicating with people who are deaf or hard of hearing

As with blindness, the severity of people's hearing impairments vary. If a hearing aid is used, make sure it is fitted and working. Remember that hearing aids amplify everything, including background noise, which can make communication difficult in busy and noisy waiting areas or departments such as A&E. More severe hearing loss will not benefit from an aid and these patients might rely on lip reading and/or signing or writing.

Principles table 5.7 Supporting communication for a person who is deaf or hard of hearing

Principle	Rationale
Find a suitable place to talk – somewhere quiet with no noise or distractions – and close doors when possible.	To reduce noises that may be amplified by hearing aids or be distracting or overwhelming (Ludlow et al. 2018, R).
Ensure that there is good light and that your face can be seen. Use natural facial expressions and gestures and try to keep your hands away from your face.	Facial expressions and body language can help to contextualize information and facilitate understanding (Ludlow et al. 2018, R).
If the person is wearing a hearing aid, ask whether it is on and whether they still need to lip read.	Because at times individuals may turn their hearing aids off because they are not functioning or the interference from background noise is painful. They can then forget to switch the hearing aid on again. E
Ask the person what their preferred mode of communication is.	It is important not to make assumptions about how the person wants to communicate (Burgess 2017, E).
If an interpreter is required, always remember to talk directly to the person you are communicating with, not the interpreter.	This is respectful and confirms that it is them you are addressing. E
Sit or stand on the same level as the person.	This makes it easier for them to see your face and lips (Burgess 2017, E).
Be patient and allow extra time for the consultation or conversation.	It is likely to take longer than normal. E
Make sure you have the listener's attention before you start to speak.	Otherwise they may miss crucial information (Burgess 2017, E).
Contextualize the discussion by giving the topic of conversation first.	Context helps people to understand (Ludlow et al. 2018, R).
Talk clearly but not too slowly, and do not exaggerate your lip movements.	Lip reading is easier when the speaker talks fairly normally (Ludlow et al. 2018, R). Exaggerated mouth movements can distort lip patterns (Burgess 2017, E).
Use plain language; avoid waffling, jargon and unfamiliar abbreviations.	Plain language will be more easily understood. E
Check that the person understands you. Be prepared to repeat or rephrase yourself as many times as necessary.	Many people need to have information repeated to understand it (Ludlow et al. 2018, R).
Depending on the purpose of the consultation, writing down a simple summary of the key points might be helpful.	This will ensure the person has a record of what is said in case they have misunderstood or misheard. E

Communicating with people who are worried or distressed

Related theory

Patients will, naturally, have an emotional response to a serious illness. At its most mild, this will consist of sadness and worry and it is expected that people will adjust to their temporary or permanent health-related circumstances. At its most serious, however, patients experience intense psychological responses such as anxiety states or depression (NICE 2004). This is because illness changes lives, or at least threatens to. Nurses must know how to respond, therefore, to sad and worried patients and their families. The ability to listen fully is perhaps the most frequently used skill or competence of a nurse. Noticing when a patient is worried, listening carefully to their concerns without interrupting, and responding helpfully are components of effective communication with an individual who is distressed. When health workers have such skills, patient outcomes are improved and staff feel more satisfied with their work (Fallowfield and Jenkins 1999, Fellowes et al. 2004, Ong et al. 2000, Razavi et al. 2000, Stewart 1996, Taylor et al. 2005).

Before learning how to listen and respond to patients' worries, it is worth knowing about unhelpful communication habits. For example, health workers often focus on physical and practical concerns but ignore the emotional issues of patients (Booth et al. 1999, Maguire et al. 1996). This is despite the fact that patients often hint at their worries (Uitterhoeve et al. 2010). Health workers may be eager to give advice, reassurance and information before hearing all of a patient's concerns (Booth et al. 1999). Incomplete listening can lead to a rush to fix problems with an inappropriate solution.

Evidence-based approaches

Evidence suggests that nurses and other health workers should listen to all of the concerns of patients who express sadness, nervousness or worry – even those that have no resolution (Booth et al. 1999, Pennebaker 1993). Nurses should enquire about the resources (help) that patients have around them, and patients should be given an opportunity to describe for themselves what would help, before the health worker offers advice, information or reassurance (Booth et al. 1999, Tate 2010). It is also known to be helpful for nurses to use a structure in their own minds to organize their thoughts and questions (Silverman et al. 2013). Patients or their carers will often have disorganized thoughts because their thinking is clouded by emotions. A helpful nurse, on the other hand, needs to be calm, organized and sensitive. The SAGE & THYME model (Connolly et al. 2010) presented below is one way for nurses and other health workers to conduct a structured and evidence-based conversation. The model suggests a sequence of sensitive questions that allow the nurse to hear about strong emotions and remain calm themselves.

Pre-procedural considerations

Patients need privacy to discuss emotions and worries; they also need time. Nurses, therefore, should create suitable conditions for patients to describe their worries. Nurses are often busy because there are many competing demands on their time, yet proper listening requires time and privacy. Nurses create time and privacy to dress a wound. They dress wounds expertly, in a logical and sequential way that has been carefully learned and practised. Listening to the worries of a patient also needs uninterrupted time and a logical sequence. This skill must also be learned and mastered if a nurse is to become an expert listener.

Principles table 5.8 SAGE & THYME

Principle	Rationale
SETTING – think first about the setting. Can you respond to this hint from the patient now or should you return when you and they can protect 10 minutes? Can you create some privacy? Would they like to talk?	Patients notice that nurses are busy and withhold worries unless given an explicit opportunity to describe their concerns (McCabe 2004, **R**). It is important to create a setting or environment within which patients or carers can disclose their concerns (Hase and Douglas 1986, **R**).
ASK – ask the patient what is concerning or worrying them (do not focus on problems that you cannot solve – just listen).	Patients frequently hint about their underlying concerns. These hints need to be noticed and responded to (Oguchi et al. 2010, **R**). Asking specifically about emotions encourages patients to describe psychological and emotional issues (Ryan et al. 2005, **R**). Asking specific questions about psychological concerns is important (Booth et al. 1999, **R**; Maguire et al. 1996, **R**).
GATHER – gather all of the concerns, not just the first few (ask whether there is something else). Repeat back to the patient what you have heard (this proves that you are listening) and make a list of all the concerns (actually write them down).	Listening is an active process, requiring concentration, silences and verbal affirmation that you hear what is being said (Silverman et al. 2013, **R**; Wosket 2006, **R**). It is important to hear all the patient's concerns, to summarize and check that you have understood correctly (Maguire et al. 1996, **R**; Pennebaker 1993, **R**).
EMPATHY – say something that suggests that you are aware of the burden of the patient's worry, such as 'I can see that you have a lot to be worried about at the moment.'	Empathy is about creating a human connection with the patient (Egan 2018, **R**). Empathy shows that you have some sense of how the patient is feeling (Booth et al. 1999, **R**; Maguire and Pitceathly 2002, **R**).
TALK – ask who they have to talk to and what support they have. Make a list of all the people who could help. Ask 'Who do you have that you can talk to about your concerns?'	Patients commonly rely on family and friends for support (Ell 1996, **R**). Good social support is associated with enhanced coping skills of patients (Chou et al. 2012, **R**). Supportive ties may enhance wellbeing by meeting basic human needs for companionship, intimacy and a sense of belonging (Berkman et al. 2000, **R**). It is helpful to know what social support surrounds the patient (Stewart 1996, **R**).
HELP – ask 'How do these people help?'	People's social networks may help them to reinterpret events or problems in a more positive and constructive light (Thoits 1995, **R**). Support from family and friends commonly involves reassurance, comfort and problem solving (Schroevers et al. 2010, **R**).
YOU – ask the patient 'What do you think would help?' or 'What would help?'	It is helpful to use a style of problem solving that seeks the patient's own solutions first (Booth et al. 1999, **R**; Tate 2010, **R**).

Principle	Rationale
ME – ask the patient 'Is there something you would like me to do?'	It is helpful to use a negotiated style of communication that gives the patient control over what, if any, professional help they receive with their concerns or dilemmas (Fallowfield and Jenkins 1999, **R**).
END – summary and strategy. For example, say 'I now know what you are worried about and the support you have. I know what you think would help and what you want me to do. I'll get on with that and come back to you when I can. Is it OK to leave it there for now?'	It is important to summarize and close an interaction (Bradley and Edinberg 1990, **R**). This is respectful to the patient, reinforces for them that they have been listened to, and signals that the interaction has come to an end. **E**

Problem-solving table 5.1 Prevention and resolution (Principles table 5.8)

Problem	Action
Direct requests: patients often have concerns at the same time that they have direct requests or questions. When listening for concerns, it is easy to be distracted by direct requests. The following is an example: 'I keep hearing different things and it makes me feel as though nobody really knows what is happening. That's scary for me. Am I having this scan or not?'	It is tempting to deal only with the direct request (about the scan) and to ignore the other cues and concerns (different messages, nobody knows what is happening, scary). However, the direct request cannot be ignored either. A clear-thinking nurse will notice both the direct question and the other cues and concerns, and will respond accordingly. For example: 'I hear that you are scared, that you feel that nobody knows what is going on, that you are getting different messages and that you want to know about the scan. I promise to find out about the scan; would you prefer me to do that straight away or can I come back to that once we've discussed you feeling scared and that nobody knows what is going on?' In this way, the direct question is addressed but the process of gathering concerns continues. The nurse is back in SAGE because they have 'parked' the request about the scan. Alternatively, they can immediately find out about the scan and then return to the other concerns.
Nobody in the 'T' of THYME: some patients will have nobody to talk to, and no people in their life to help them think through or cope with the difficulties they face. This becomes obvious in the 'T' question in THYME ('Who do you have that you can talk to about your concerns?').	In these circumstances, there is no purpose in asking the 'H' question ('How do these people help?'). Move straight on to the next question, 'What do you think would help?'
Mistaking the 'Y' of THYME: some learners of the SAGE & THYME model misuse the 'You' of THYME by wrongly interpreting this as a challenge to patients: 'What can you do for yourself?'	This is not recommended. It risks the unfair suggestion that the patient is not doing enough for themselves. Nurses should practise hearing themselves asking the correct questions as follows: 'What do *you* think would help?' and 'Is there something else that would help?'. These questions relate to the patient's own ideas about what could be helpful. They are important because it is suggested that nurses should seek the patient's own ideas about what would help before they ask about what they can do to help as this helps patients to retain a sense of control and personal agency in a situation where they often feel out of control. **E**

Psychological wellbeing

Definition

The World Health Organization (WHO) describes 'health' as 'a state of complete physical, mental and social wellbeing and not merely the absence of disease or infirmity' (WHO 1946). Thus, it is important for nurses to be able to address biological, psychological and social factors influencing a patient's health. This is a difficult task when viewed in the context of limited resources. However, a nurse can use their relationship with their patients to offer compassion and curiosity about psychosocial wellbeing alongside technical care. This type of relationship has benefits for staff (e.g. improved job satisfaction) and patients (e.g. increased trust and confidence in healthcare staff), which can save time in the long run (Wiechula et al. 2015).

The WHO's definition of health embraces the biopsychosocial model, rather than a purely biological, or medical, view. This perspective on health has implications for language that are particularly pertinent in the field of psychological wellbeing (Figure 5.8). For example, the phrase 'mental *illness*' implies a biological aetiology such as a disease, whereas 'mental *health* problem' opens up the possibility of a broad range of biopsychosocial factors (e.g. health, thinking styles, loss, unemployment and financial difficulties, and relationships) in the cause and/or maintenance of psychological difficulties. Beliefs about the aetiology of psychological difficulties have significant implications for their treatment (i.e. medication, psychological therapy and/or social interventions).

Related theory

Attachment

The ability to form trusting, secure relationships or 'attachments' across the life course is thought to be influenced by patterns of early childhood relationships. According to attachment theory (Bowlby 1969, 1973, 1980, 1988), a person's attachment style develops from their caregivers' responses to their early physical and emotional needs (e.g. for comfort and security). That is, the way in which a person has experienced care within significant past attachment relationships influences how they experience care in current relationships. Attachment can be thought of as a psychological characteristic whereby these early experiences of care are internalized as working models (Bowlby 1969). Working

Examples: medical diagnostic language	Examples: alternative descriptions
Mental illness	Emotional distress, mental distress, severe mental distress, extreme state, psychological distress.
Disorder	Difficulty (e.g. difficulty with mood or low mood).
Bipolar disorder	Mood swings, severe mood swings, severe changes in mood states, extreme mood state.
Personality disorder	Complex trauma, complex trauma reaction, personality difficulties, relationship or attachment difficulties, complex presentation.
Paranoia	Paranoid thoughts, suspicious thoughts.
Depressive illness, depressive disorder, clinical depression[1] (used in diagnostic sense)	Low mood, misery, depression (contextualized and used in a lay sense)
Anxiety disorder, generalized anxiety disorder	Fear, anxiety, worry, extreme anxiety, feeling threatened.
Obsessive compulsive disorder	Compulsive checking/cleaning, compulsive thoughts/worrying.
Schizophrenia	Hearing voices, having/experiencing visual/auditory/olfactory/tactile hallucinations, having/holding unusual beliefs, beliefs others find unusual, altered state.
X has/suffers from schizophrenia/ bipolar disorder/personality disorder	X has been given a diagnosis of/is in receipt of a diagnosis of schizophrenia/ bipolar disorder/personality disorder.

[1]Depression is an example of a medical term that has entered the everyday vernacular.

Figure 5.8 Terminology in psychological wellbeing. *Source*: Reproduced from BPS (2015) with permission of the British Psychological Society.

models are essentially templates of expectations of self and others, and these templates shape how someone responds in the here and now (Bowlby 1973, 1979). As such, they become particularly evident during times of stress or perceived threat (Mikulincer and Shaver 2008).

Broadly speaking, two types of attachment style are typically described: secure and insecure. Insecure attachments have been further divided into the sub-categories of 'avoidant' or 'ambivalent' following the research of Ainsworth (see Ainsworth and Bell 1970), who collaborated with Bowlby. More recently, a fourth 'disorganized' style of attachment has been described (Main and Solomon 1990).

Where there has been a consistent pattern of availability and responsiveness to needs in early childhood, a secure attachment is likely to form, whereby someone sees themselves as deserving of support and holds a sufficient level of trust in others to deliver the necessary care. Although stressful experiences are still challenging, they do not evoke high levels of anxiety or patterns of avoidance, or they may be shorter lived and the person can reassure themselves during these stressful times. This is because the experience of consistent care that meets our needs is thought to play a significant role in the development of empathy and compassion, including self-compassion (Gilbert 2010).

When early needs for care have not been responded to, or where caregiving has been unpredictable, then an insecure attachment style can develop, either as avoidance or anxiety (Favez et al. 2016). Here, a person may view themselves as unworthy of support, and may view others as untrustworthy, uncaring or unavailable (Harding et al. 2015). For these people, during stressful events the desire or need for care may feel overwhelming. Some individuals may adopt ways of behaving that give some short-term relief from this distress, for example avoiding difficult situations (such as hospital appointments) rather than being present in situations that invoke a sense of vulnerability (Mikulincer and Shaver 2003). Alternatively, some individuals may employ care-seeking behaviours to allay the anxiety that care might stop or be withdrawn, or to elicit reassurance from caregivers where there is little capacity on the part of the individual to soothe themselves or regulate their emotions (Mikulincer and Shaver 2003).

Attachment styles therefore direct the way in which a person can process information, can manage or regulate their emotional states, and can seek or accept help from others. As such, they can exert an influence upon mental health, wellbeing and functioning (Stevenson et al. 2017).

It is important to note that during times of low stress, it may be difficult to identify a person's attachment style. This is because attachment styles most often come to light when we experience stressful life events. In the context of the diagnosis and management of illness, which is arguably a time of stress in which comfort and support are needed, anxious or avoidant attachment styles may become apparent. These can manifest as a patient being easily overwhelmed, having difficulties processing information or adhering to treatment, or experiencing problematic interactions between themselves and their healthcare providers. For example, research among women with breast cancer has highlighted the importance of the nurse–patient relationship, in that a sense of security and trust within the relationship affords the opportunity for fears to be raised and discussed and reassurance sought (Harding et al. 2015). The research found that women's expectations of the nursing staff involved in their care correlated with their attachment styles such that patients with secure attachment styles reported feeling more supported by nurses than patients with anxious or avoidant attachment styles.

It is important for a nurse to hold in mind how a patient's attachment style might influence their perception of care so that the nurse can adapt their own behaviour (as appropriate) to provide patient-centred support. However, Harding et al. (2015) note that an avoidant attachment style can be hard to identify and can be misinterpreted as seemingly unproblematic coping. Some patients who appear able to support themselves ask few questions and do not express emotion in nurse–patient encounters, but they may be doing so because their underlying attachment style incorporates a working model of the self as unworthy of support. Similarly, patients with a working model of others as untrustworthy may express anger or may not attend appointments. These behaviours can be misinterpreted as hostility rather than fear, or as self-sufficient or forgetful (Harding et al. 2015).

Thoughts and emotions, and their function

In Western culture it is common for people to refer to some thoughts and emotions as 'good' or 'positive' and to others as 'bad', 'negative' or 'problematic'. According to some psychotherapists (e.g. Harris 2009), when faced with problems, people tend to use one of two simple problem-solving approaches: fix or avoid. Fixing and avoiding work with 'real-world' problems, such as a flat bike tire: the solutions are to pump up the tyre, repair or change the tire, or avoid riding the bike. Naturally, people apply the fix–avoid approach to their 'problematic' thoughts and emotions, and as this can be successful in the short term they continue with this approach. However, regardless of how hard and creatively people try to fix or avoid thoughts and emotions, at some point they return. This is because thoughts and emotions do not follow the same rules as bike tires; instead, they are more like the weather – that is, they flux and change and are (predominantly) outside human control.

Therefore, it can be helpful for people to enhance their ability to:

- be aware of their thoughts and emotions
- be with those thoughts and emotions (rather than trying to fix or avoid them)
- be self-compassionate about the thoughts and emotions
- be able to refocus on the here and now so that difficult thoughts and emotions do not dominate the mind
- engage with life in a way that is important and meaningful to them.

This approach to coping with our internal, private world is embodied in what are known as third-wave cognitive–behavioural therapies, such as ACT (acceptance and commitment therapy) (Hayes et al. 1999) and compassion-focused therapy (Gilbert 2009). These have had significant success in helping people to cope with physical health problems, for example chronic pain (Dahl and Lundgren 2006).

When someone is diagnosed with a serious illness, it is natural for them to experience a range of challenging thoughts and feelings, and many of these will be uncomfortable, such as worries and fear that their life is going to change or that they will die. Although these emotions can be difficult, they serve a purpose – that is, they help people to understand what is important and orientate their own and other people's behaviour (Ekman 1999) (Box 5.8). Thus, rather than pushing away these difficult thoughts and emotions, it can be helpful for people (including nurses) to pay attention to them.

Box 5.8 Emotions and their function

Emotion	Function of emotion
Anger	Assert, defend self
Disgust	Hide, expel, avoid
Enjoyment	Contact, engage
Fear	Flee, freeze, give up
Sadness	Seek support, withdraw to take care of self
Surprise/ excitement	Attend, explore

Source: Adapted from Ekman (1999).

Families and systems

Traditionally, family networks (or 'systems') are seen as composed of blood relatives and those related by marriage: husbands and wives, children, brothers, sisters, grandparents, aunts, uncles and cousins. In the UK today, however, it is widely accepted that the concept of 'family' extends beyond this traditional view. Same-sex unions are legally recognized. Children may be fostered or adopted, or may live with single parents or step-parents. They may have step-siblings. Migration to, from and within the UK means that biological relatives may scarcely know each other. People may feel far closer to friends or other members of their communities. Moreover, today's families may be composed of people from different cultures, religions, class groups and sexualities (Burnham 1993).

Considering patients within the context of their family systems (Figure 5.9) and wider networks can provide nurses with valuable insight into what is important to the patient, their responses to their circumstances (such as illness), and the challenges arising from these responses. Awareness of the systemic context can provide clues about the strengths that the patient and other members of their system can draw upon to help them face difficulties.

Illness affects the patient *and* their family system. A person's response to the news that they are ill will have an impact upon how others in their system react to the news. Likewise, how family members respond affects the patient and how they behave. For example, a mother's fear about her diagnosis and treatment may frighten her children, and seeing their worry may reinforce her fear (Figure 5.10). On the other hand, the mother's decision to hide her fear may convey that there is nothing to worry about, and she may not receive the care and support she needs.

How people respond to illness often depends upon the various roles they play in relation to other members of their family. For example, one person may inhabit the roles of father, son, brother-in-law, uncle and nephew all at once (Byng-Hall 1995). Each of these roles comes with specific privileges and responsibilities in regard to other members of the system. Simplistically, children are cared for, parents provide care; children obey, parents command. A young parent may occupy both positions, because they are more powerful than and responsible for their children, while remaining the child of their own parents.

Problems can arise when people within the system perceive situations or challenges too differently from each other – for example, when one person perceives a problem when another person does not. For example, a husband may worry about his spouse's 'drinking', which they see as 'just three small glasses of wine with dinner'. Problems can also arise when there is a mismatch in solutions proposed by various members of the system. For example, tensions may arise when a parent cannot bear to lose their terminally ill son, while he can no longer endure the side-effects of his treatment. The son may feel that his parents' preferred solution is

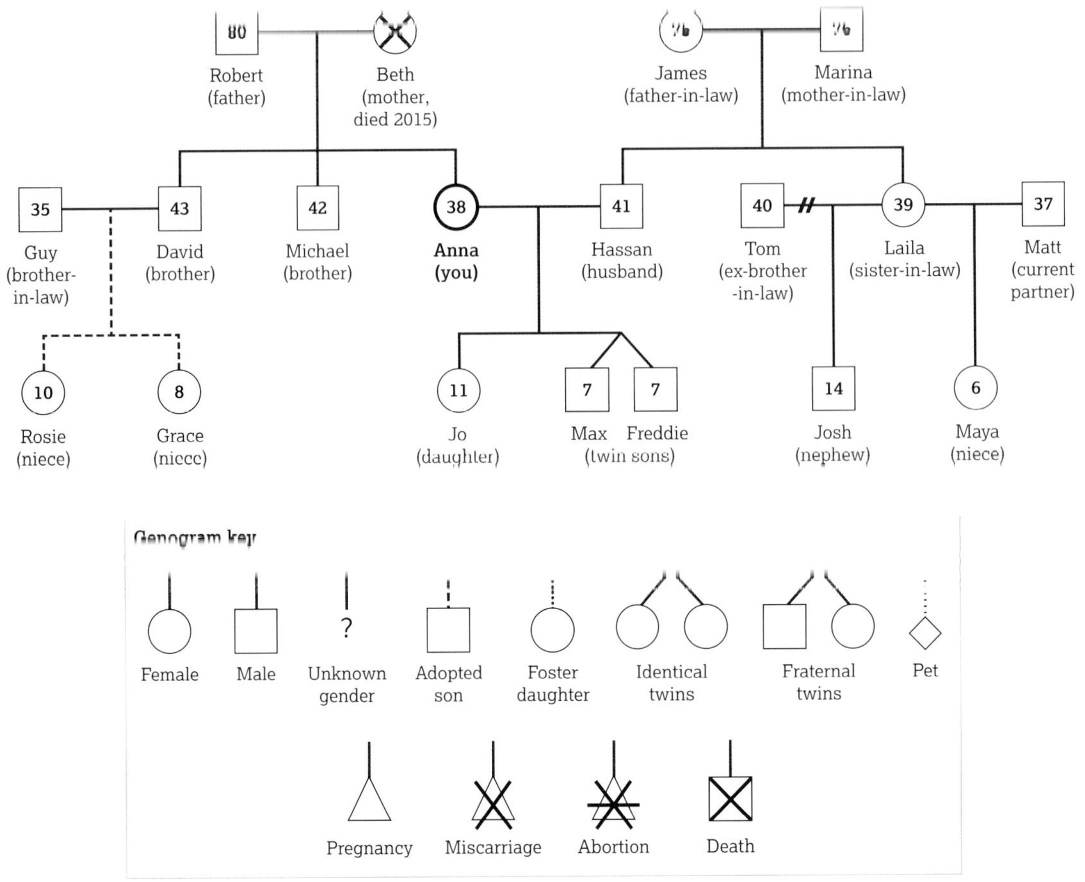

Figure 5.9 Example of a genogram. A genogram is a symbolic representation of who is important in a person's life. In its most basic form, a genogram looks something like this, but it can be adapted to reflect the quality of relationships, health status, cultural heritage or other factors of interest. The key includes additional components that could be used if relevant.

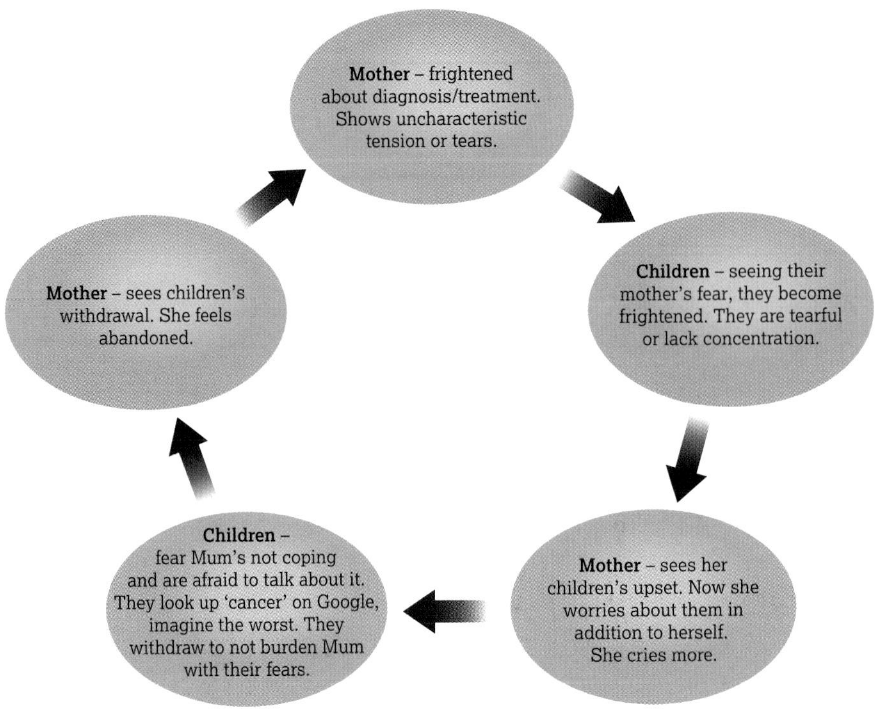

Figure 5.10 Example of a circular interaction within a family.

worse than the original illness, and he may prioritize quality rather than quantity of life. Social roles within people's wider networks (e.g. employee, boss, neighbour, citizen) can also be relevant to a person's response and means of coping with illness. These different roles often come with different priorities; any working parent who has had to leave work early to collect a sick child from school has experienced this.

Moreover, families, like individuals, can be seen to have life cycles (Carter and Goldrick 1999). As a family transitions from one stage to the next, the established roles and expectations that members have of each other change. Power dynamics eventually become reversed. The overlap of social and family systems during a transition can be seen when a parent retires. They lose the social status associated with their professional role and may become increasingly dependent upon their children.

Serious illness can also upset the power balance, and expected order of life cycles, within the family. A previously autonomous person may be forced to adopt the 'sick role' and self-identify as a patient, needing assistance with deeply personal and intimate functions. In receiving care, past as well as current roles may influence a patient's relationship with help (Reder and Fredman 1996), depending upon the beliefs they hold about how to behave within their various roles *in relation* to the others in their multiple systems. This affects how the patient sees themselves in relation to the doctors, nurses and other healthcare professionals involved in their care.

Families are also systems in which attachment relationships (see above) begin and attachment styles develop. While attachment style can be a key factor underpinning a patient's relationship with help, 'family scripts' (Byng-Hall 1995) may also be relevant. For instance, if independence and self-reliance are overvalued within a family's culture, asking for and accepting help can become difficult and suddenly finding oneself in a position of dependence can be extremely uncomfortable. Alternatively, if a family's culture fosters dependence upon a single member, it can be difficult for anyone else to develop belief in their own ability to effectively meet the challenges life presents. Such persons might be at higher risk of becoming overly reliant upon professionals to make decisions for them and manage their care.

Hospitals and multidisciplinary teams as systems

Hospitals, and the treating teams that comprise them, are systems in their own right as well as forming part of the wider network of systems around the patient and their family. As such, it is important to consider interactions not only between patients and individual clinicians but also between the patient and the organization, whether at the level of the team or the whole hospital. Communication and interaction between the individual and the organization will be affected by the roles adopted (such as patient versus professional/expert, or consumer versus service provider) and by the dynamics generated when these roles are assumed.

In the same way that nurses are all members of their own family systems, as workers they are also members of organizational systems. They are affected by the organization's policies, priorities, investment decisions and other aspects. As Reder and Fredman (1996) point out, in addition to being guided by their own personal and family beliefs about receiving and providing assistance and care, nurses must be consistent with professional and service contexts, including statutory obligations as well as ethical ones. Professional contexts come with assumptions regarding roles, duties, responsibilities and rights. At times, these assumptions may clash with those held by patients and their families, as well as those held by colleagues from other professions.

As more teams and services become involved in a patient's care, complexity increases further still. There may be power differences between teams, and the patient's relationships with the various teams may reflect those differences or be impacted by them. Moreover, other systems are commonly involved in complex patient care. These might include education, local authorities and the justice system, all of which can work simultaneously and in conjunction with each other, as illustrated in Figure 5.11.

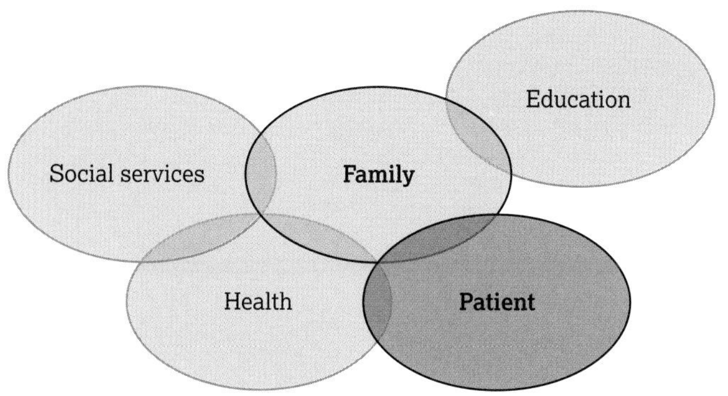

Figure 5.11 Map of overlapping systems.

Adjustment

Definition

The term 'adjustment' refers to the process of adjusting to new and difficult circumstances.

Related theory

As stated above, it is natural to feel frightened or worried when given bad news, especially if this concerns a life-threatening illness. Adjusting to new and difficult circumstances is a process, rather than a one-off event, and is likely to take time.

One useful model of adjustment is Brennan's (2001) Social Cognitive Transition Model. In keeping with ideas from attachment theory, Brennan's model postulates that people hold mental models of the world that influence their assumptions and expectations. When a person's lived experience confirms their expectations and assumptions, their worldview is strengthened. However, when a person's experience disconfirms their worldview, they enter a process of adjustment, whereby new information is assimilated into their working models.

Brennan (2001) posits that there are a number of reasons for the range of psychosocial responses to difficult experiences such as illness:

- People hold different working models about the world (e.g. someone who expects to have a heart attack due to their family history and lifestyle is likely to be less shocked by having one than a person with no family history and a healthy lifestyle).
- The different social groups or contexts (e.g. gender, age, race, sexuality, socioeconomic status) that people belong to influence how an event is perceived (e.g. someone who is financially wealthy may be more confident than someone in poverty that they can access the necessary health and social care to recover from a heart attack).
- People vary in their flexibility around assimilating new information into their mental models (e.g. someone who is able to adjust their view of their parent from 'super-human' to 'human and vulnerable' is more likely to adjust to the parent having had a heart attack).

During this time, the patient is likely to experience some distress as they comprehend the magnitude of their diagnosis or health experience. They may engage (often unconsciously) in emotional regulation strategies such as denial (discussed later in this chapter) or avoidance (behaviour through which a person attempts to escape an unpleasant thought, feeling, sensation or situation). All of these responses may be helpful in the short term but are potentially unhelpful in the longer term as they can block adjustment. Conversely, people may engage in helpful coping strategies, such as problem solving or engaging with appropriate social support.

Adjustment to difficulties can lead to personal development. As people reflect on their lives and the world around them, they can clarify what is important to them, set goals across different domains in their life (e.g. relationships, work or education, leisure and health) and shape their behaviour accordingly.

Adjustment is also a process that takes place in the family of the patient, and how much time it takes varies from family to family. There are a number of factors that can influence the process of family adjustment, including attachment styles within the family, family scripts (the 'story' a family shares that determines how they relate to each other and cope with life, e.g. during illness or celebrations), members' roles and relationships to help, as well as the family's stage within the family life cycle. For example, a young father may fear death all the more because he is aware that his spouse will lose not only a romantic partner but also a co-parent. His children will lose an important source of many kinds of support and guidance. A child may struggle to accept that their father is seriously ill because the loss of a parent is the loss of a significant attachment figure, but it could also change the family structure beyond recognition, if that parent is the sole source of income.

The dilemmas and tensions regarding independence and responsibility that frequently arise between parents and adolescents may be magnified if one or the other develops a serious illness. A child may become a 'young carer', taking on adult responsibilities for their sick parent, or a parent may become overly fearful of letting their child leave home for university.

Circumstances within family members' wider systems also affect adjustment. The cumulative effects of trying to cope with the pressure of school exams while worrying about an ill brother may be beyond the internal resources of a sibling. In the same vein, a supportive work environment can foster resilience by reducing work-related stress.

Principles table 5.9 Adjustment

Principle	Rationale
Allow sufficient time and privacy when giving news that may be perceived as 'bad' and be prepared to provide follow-up support.	Adjusting to new and difficult circumstances is a process rather than a one-off event, and is likely to take time (Brennan 2001, R).
Anticipate that there is a range of possible responses to being diagnosed and treated for a health problem.	A person's response is influenced by their model, or view, of the world and this is informed by family history and social groups (e.g. gender, age, race, sexuality, socioeconomic status) (Brennan 2001, R).
Be prepared to support both the individual and their family to adjust to illness.	Individuals live within the context of systems and these systems need to adjust. The pace and rhythm of family adjustment can depend on the family's developmental stage as well as the roles and responsibilities that are affected by a person being ill (Byng-Hall 1995, R; Carter and Goldrick 1999, R).

Denial and collusion

Definitions

Denial is a complex phenomenon (Vos and de Haes 2010) and can be considered an adaptive mechanism for slowing down and filtering the absorption of traumatic information, 'allowing for avoidance of painful or distressing information' (Goldbeck 1997, p.586).

Collusion is when two or more parties develop a shared, sometimes secret, understanding that may involve withholding information from another person. It can be argued that collusion is consistent with some patients' wishes (Helft 2005) and can be a necessary protection against unbearable facts and feelings (Vos and de Haes 2010, p.227). However, it is important that health professionals resist invitations to collude with patients' or relatives' inaccurate understandings (Macdonald 2004).

Related theory

Diagnosis of any potentially life-threatening illness is experienced in many different ways and can cause strong emotional responses. Patients are likely to feel a degree of distress and experience a wide range of emotions that may be lessened if healthcare professionals are supportive, empathetic, truthful and open with patients about their diagnosis and prognosis.

People may use denial as a way of coping when faced with frightening situations. Denial can be conscious or unconscious and is commonly recognized in cancer settings (Vos and de Haes 2011).

Literature on denial tends to be focused within the cancer field and prevalence rates are difficult to assess. Vos (2008) found that most lung cancer patients displayed some level of denial, which increased over the course of the illness. This was considered to be a normal phenomenon and not a sign of disturbed coping (Vos 2008). Nurses can be unsettled by the presentation of denial as it creates uncertainty about levels of understanding, coping and engagement with treatment. Family members and nurses can collude with patient denial, perhaps as a means of protecting the patient or themselves from facing the full impact and pain of the situation. Nurses need to be aware of the pitfalls of colluding with patient or family denial and consider how they may contribute to it.

As human beings, we live our lives in our own individual, unique ways and also deal with a life-threatening diagnosis in our own way. For some people, focusing on hope and cure is the priority, while for others it is first necessary to prepare themselves and their family for the possibility that their illness may be incurable. Denial is a complex, fluid process, as is living with a life-threatening diagnosis. Patients' understanding of what is happening to them can fluctuate from minute to minute, and denial is not an 'all or nothing' phenomenon (Dein 2005, p.251): a patient may accept their illness in the morning but by evening deny that they have it.

Medical and nursing staff, family members and patients may all be 'in denial' at some point – to protect either themselves or those they care about.

Evidence-based approaches

Assessment of denial

In order to try to understand as fully as possible the emotions that patients are experiencing and the resources they have for coping, a careful assessment of each patient's circumstances is important. Nurses need to establish what information the patient has been given, before assuming that the patient is experiencing denial. They need to be sure that patients have been given adequate, digestible information, if necessary on several occasions.

It is helpful to view denial as a process (Vos and de Haes 2011) and to see its expression as falling somewhere along a continuum. This needs to be acknowledged in the assessment process. Repeated assessments of denial may aid understanding of how various factors might influence denial and how to better understand its dynamic nature.

Principles table 5.10 Supporting a person in denial

Principle	Rationale
Aim to provide honest information to patients with the use of good communication skills, to the depth and detail the patient requests.	This enables patients to have control over the rate at which they absorb and integrate news and information that may have life-threatening implications for them (Maguire 2000, R).
Listening, reflecting and summarizing are useful skills when interacting with individuals in denial.	These techniques will establish a supportive relationship that in the future may provide the patient with the security to acknowledge the gravity of the information they have been given. E
If denial is affecting a treatment regime or decisions for the future, it may need to be gently challenged. This can be done by either questioning any inconsistencies in the patient's story or asking whether at any point they have thought that their illness may be more serious.	These questions may help the patient to get closer to knowledge they may already have about the seriousness of their illness. With the right support, they might be able to face their fears and be more fully involved in decisions about future care and treatment. E
If the patient remains in denial, this should not be challenged any further (Dein 2005).	'Confrontation, if pursued in an insensitive or dismissive way or in the absence of adequate trust and support mechanisms, may increase denial, may reduce treatment compliance, or may even precipitate a complete breakdown in the healthcare professional–patient relationship' (Goldbeck 1997, p.586).
The delivery of bad news and information giving need to be recorded clearly. The degree to which patients will accept the information is variable and needs to be respected and carefully documented.	Good communication can help to prevent patients receiving mixed messages. Clear documentation helps other staff members to understand how the patient is coping. E

Complications

Balancing the reality of the illness with reasonable hope is often difficult for health professionals and caregivers (Kogan et al. 2013, Parker et al. 2010). When working with patients who seem to be in denial, the challenge for healthcare professionals is not so much the confrontation of denial but rather the avoidance of collusion with it (Houldin 2000), as collusion would offer the health professional an opportunity to avoid the distress.

Collusion can leave healthcare professionals, patients and relatives feeling confused. Recognizing collusion, challenging it and discussing concerns with colleagues are important. Working with the multiprofessional team helps to improve communication and ensure a collaborative approach to care. Drawing on the richness of experience of others can help.

Anxiety and panic

Definition

Anxiety is a feeling of fear and apprehension about a real or perceived threat and may cause excessive worry and heightened tension, affecting important areas of normal functioning (NICE 2011a). The source of the feeling may or may not be known (Kennedy Sheldon 2009) and people sometimes refer to it as 'coming out of the blue'. Different people use different words to describe anxiety, for example 'stress', 'nervousness' or 'tension'.

The body has a normal response to fear and stress but, if this response is exaggerated, people might experience a sense of panic. During a panic attack, a number of symptoms can be experienced including palpitations, nausea, trembling, weak legs and dizziness (APA 2013) (Box 5.9). Panic attacks can have a sudden onset and may last 5–20 minutes (MIND 2018). Catastrophic thoughts or images (e.g. having a heart attack, fainting or collapsing) are characteristic of a panic attack and the more frequent and extreme they are the more intense the physiological response becomes (Powell 2009). An indication for many individuals that a panic attack is beginning is a feeling of tightness in the chest or being aware that their breathing is fast. If not managed, this may progress to hyperventilation (Powell 2009).

Box 5.9 Criteria for defining a panic attack according to the *Diagnostic and Statistical Manual of Mental Disorders* (DSM-5)

A panic attack consists of a discrete period of intense fear or discomfort in which four or more of the following symptoms develop abruptly and reach a peak within minutes:

- Palpitations, pounding heart or accelerated heart rate
- Sweating
- Trembling or shaking
- Sensations of shortness of breath or smothering
- Chest pain or discomfort
- Feeling of choking
- Nausea or abdominal distress
- Feeling dizzy, unsteady, light-headed or faint
- Chills or heat sensations
- Paraesthesias (numbness or tingling sensations)
- Derealization (feelings of unreality) or depersonalization (being detached from oneself)
- Fear of losing control or going crazy
- Fear of dying

Source: Adapted from APA (2013) with permission of American Psychiatric Publishing.

Anatomy and physiology

Anxious feelings can result in physical symptoms related to the 'flight or fight' response as the body responds to the threat, real or otherwise (Figure 5.12). The sympathetic nervous system releases adrenaline and other hormones that lead to:

- increase in heart rate and therefore palpitations and raised blood pressure
- faster and shallower breathing (hyperventilation)
- dizziness
- dry mouth and difficulty swallowing
- relaxation of sphincters, leading to an increase in urinary and faecal elimination
- reduction in blood supply to the intestines, leading to feelings of 'butterflies', knotted stomach and nausea
- increase in perspiration as the body seeks to cool down the tense muscles
- musculoskeletal pains (particularly in the back and neck) (Powell and Enright 1990).

These physical symptoms can be perceived as unpleasant by the patient, resulting in further catastrophic worries and an

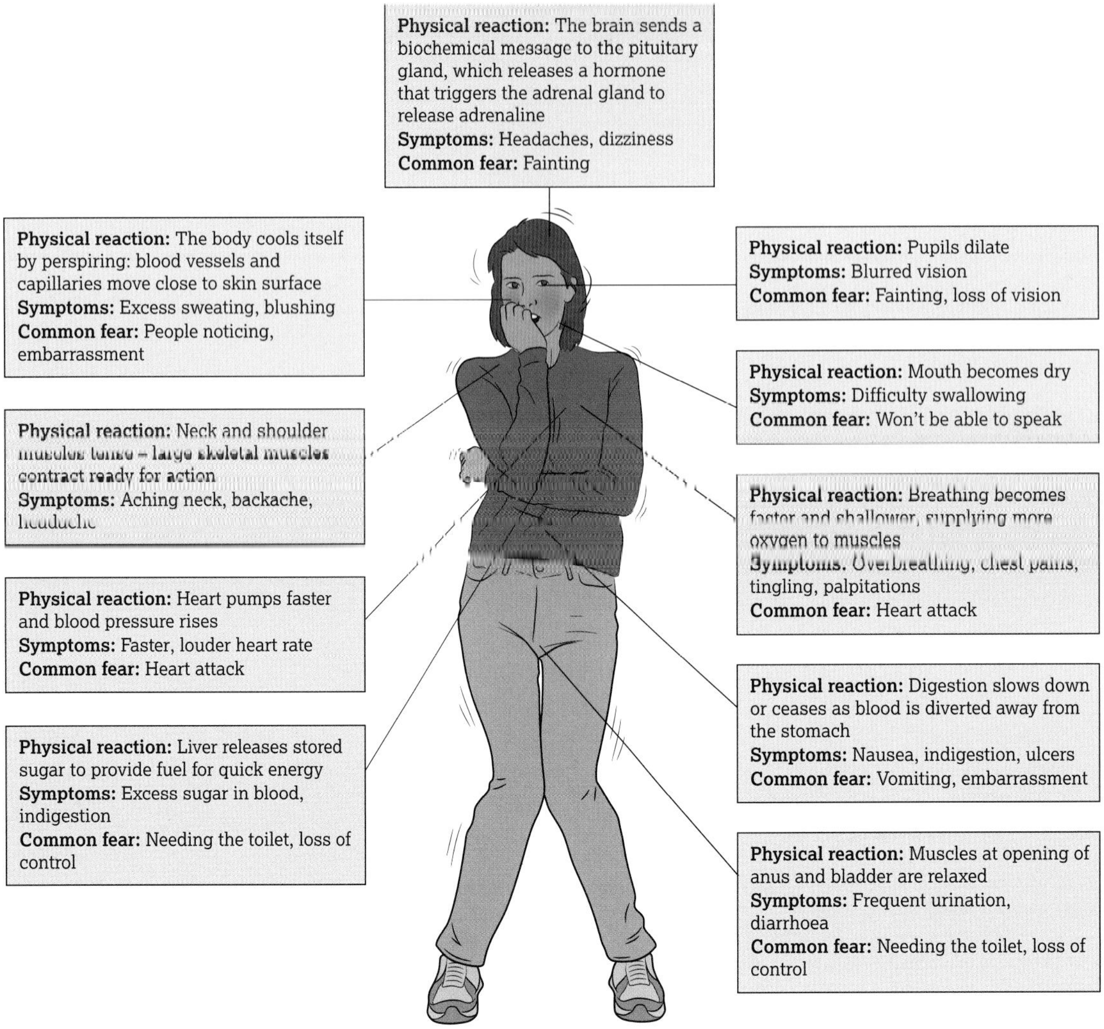

Figure 5.12 The body's arousal system during the fight-or-flight response. *Source*: Adapted from Powell (2009).

escalation in physical symptoms; in this way, a vicious cycle ensues (Figure 5.13). It is useful to note that although people may feel faint and dizzy when they are anxious, increased blood pressure will ensure they do not actually faint. The exception to this is when someone has a needle phobia and blood pressure initially increases and then drops, which can result in fainting (Jenkins 2014). One hypothesis regarding the reason for the reduction in blood pressure in people with a needle phobia is that it is an adaptive mechanism that minimizes any potential loss of blood and therefore enhances a person's chance of survival.

Related theory

Anxiety is a normal and necessary response to threatening events but can become a problem when it is frequent, exaggerated or experienced out of context (Blake and Ledger 2007). There are a number of theories about anxiety, its causes and how to manage it (Powell and Enright 1990); however, all theories consider the role of the situation as well as the patient's thoughts, emotions, physiology and behaviour. To be effective in supporting and communicating with a patient with anxiety, it is necessary to consider the following components of anxiety:

- *Bodily sensations*: as listed above.
- *Thoughts and images*: the ideas, memories, beliefs and mental pictures or images the individual has about what might happen in the feared situation (Powell 2009).
- *Behaviour*: how the individual behaves when faced with the perceived fear, which often involves avoidance or the adoption of behaviours that increase their sense of safety when they cannot avoid the feared situation or activity. For example, a patient may only attend a hospital appointment with a particular friend, while listening to music or with a book to read. While these behaviours can be helpful in the short term, they can present longer-term problems, as they reduce the person's ability to believe that they can cope on their own, and the 'safety behaviour' may not always be possible. That is, the patient's friend may not be able to accompany them, their music device's battery may run out or they may finish their book.

Within the healthcare context, many patients experience anticipatory anxiety, for example worry and anxiety about future appointments, tests and treatments. Patients are frequently required to have tests or treatments that include needles, which are a common fear. McLenon and Rogers' (2018) meta-analysis found that needle fear and phobia were present in the majority of children, 20–50% of adolescents and approximately 20–30% of young adults; they were less prevalent thereafter.

As levels of anxiety increase, a person's awareness and interaction with the environment can decrease, and recall and general function may be impaired (Kennedy Sheldon 2009). Cognitive functions can be affected due to 'emotional hijacking' (Goleman [illegible]). This occurs when the amount of brain activity in the limbic system (the brain's principal emotional system) increases to a level

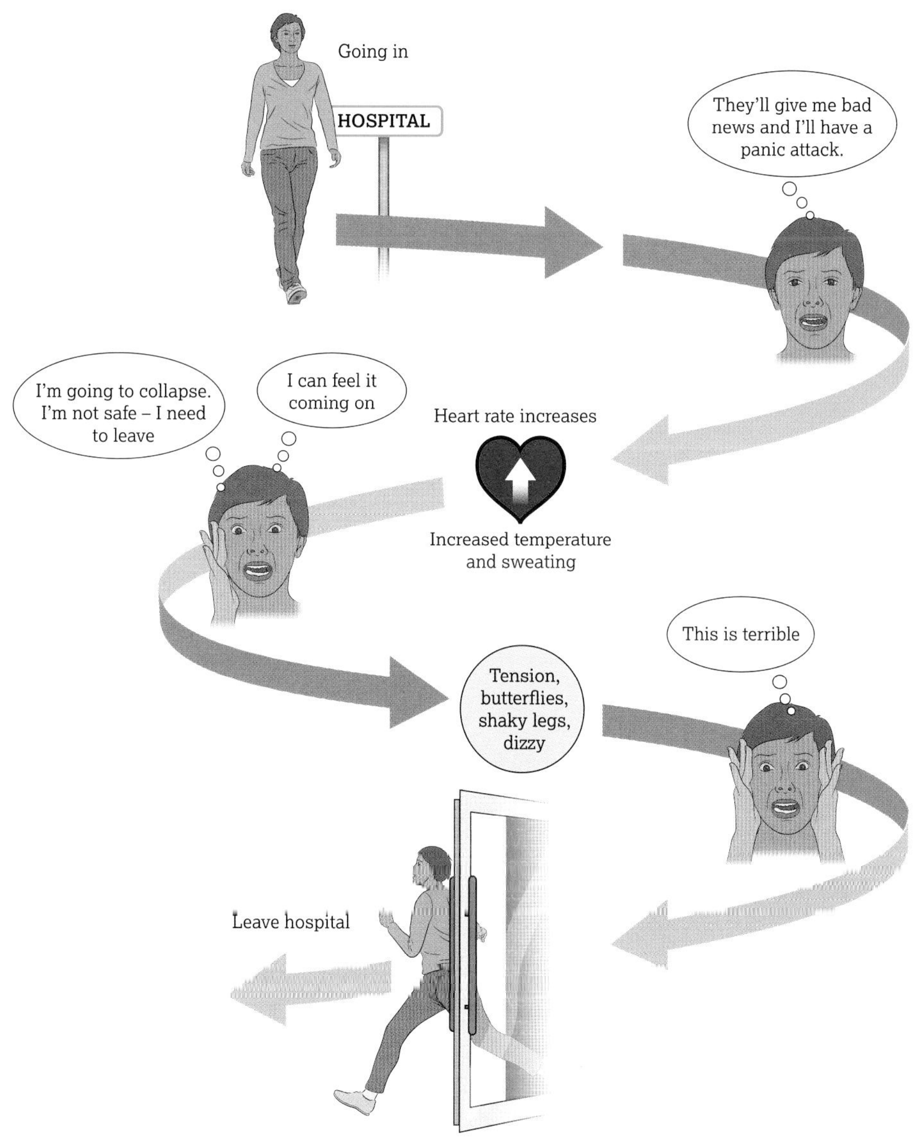

Figure 5.13 Example of an anxious spiral.

where it 'hijacks', or interferes with, the functions of the pre-frontal cortex (where most executive functions are processed, such as thinking, reasoning and attention). Conversely, some anxiety and worry can be helpful when they orientate a person's behaviour towards appropriate problem-solving strategies.

Evidence-based approaches

Managing generalized anxiety is initially about early recognition and helping people to understand the problem. It is recognized that a person's perception of, or behavioural response to, a situation can exacerbate anxiety. Therefore, it is helpful to provide psychoeducation – that is, an explanation or explanatory model for the development and maintenance of the anxiety (Figures 5.12 and 5.13).

Where possible, it is pertinent to allay the source of anxiety. Nurses have more power than patients in the healthcare setting and may be in a position to help change an anxiety-provoking situation. Alternatively, they may be able to support patients in thinking through a difficult situation and helping them to identify what they can do to bring about change. Further, nurses can provide patients with information on how to develop or enhance their problem-solving skills. However, within the healthcare context, many situations or difficulties that provoke anxiety are not changeable or controllable by individuals, so attempting to bring about change can lead to frustration or an experience of failure.

NICE (2011a) promotes a stepped-care approach to managing anxiety, with psychological interventions tried before pharmacotherapy. People can choose between 'individual non-facilitated self-help, individual guided self-help or psycho-educational groups' (NICE 2011a, p.7) and various patient resources are available (see www.ntw.nhs.uk/selfhelp). If these interventions are ineffective, individual high-intensity psychological interventions, such as cognitive–behavioural therapy and relaxation, may be appropriate (Figure 5.14). Third-wave cognitive–behavioural therapies – such as mindfulness-based stress reduction (MBSR), mindfulness-based cognitive therapy (MBCT), acceptance and commitment therapy (ACT), dialectical behavioural therapy (DBT) and compassion focused therapy (CFT) – have a good evidence base for working with anxiety (Gu et al. 2015, Leaviss and Uttley 2015, Swain et al. 2013). NICE guidelines advocate patient preference as a factor in the selection of psychological interventions, and some patients prefer more exploratory therapies such as counselling.

Pre-procedural considerations

During initial nursing consultations or conversations, it is important that nurses ask patients about any history of psychological or mental health difficulties. This will enable the nurse, where possible, to adapt their approach and minimize anxiety triggers.

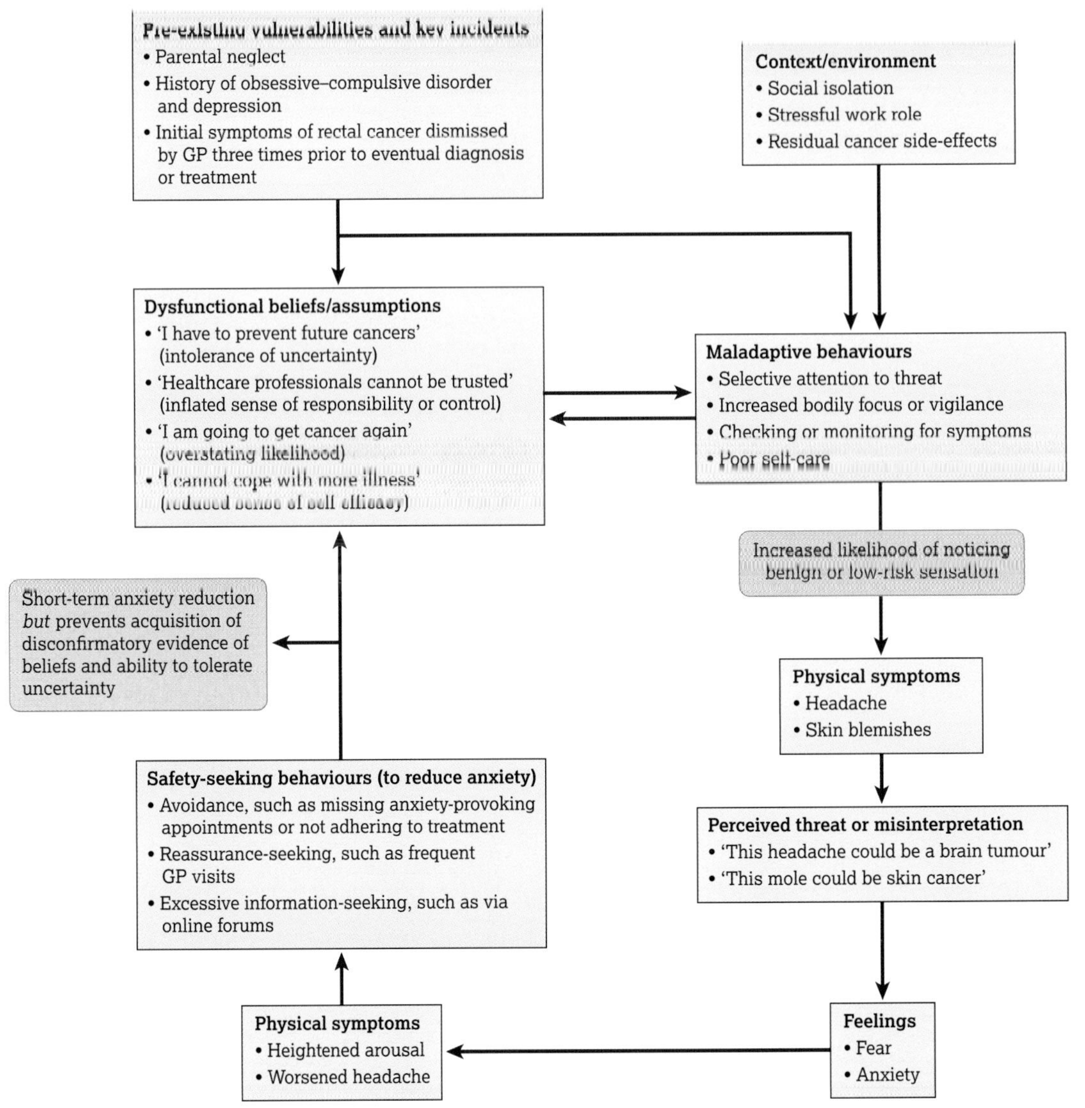

Figure 5.14 Cognitive–behavioural model of anxiety in the context of cancer.

Principles table 5.11 Supporting an anxious person

Principle	Rationale
Be alert to the signs and symptoms of anxiety.	Early recognition and intervention may help to prevent worsening of symptoms. **E**
Encourage the patient to talk about the source of their anxiety if they can. Work openly to explore worries, information requirements and treatment options.	Patients may gain some benefit from expressing their concerns and being heard. **E**
Listen and offer tailored information, but only when the patient has expressed all their concerns. Gentle challenging of misunderstandings about treatment, processes or outcomes may be beneficial if such misunderstandings are the source of the anxiety.	Information about a procedure, particularly an operation, can reduce anxiety and improve outcomes (Nordahl et al. 2003, **R**; Scott 2004, **R**).
If the patient does not know why they are feeling anxious, encourage them to describe what is happening in their body, when it started, what makes it worse and what makes it better.	The patient will feel listened to and less alone, which may increase their sense of security and therefore reduce anxiety. **E**
Ask the patient whether they have had the feelings before. What has helped previously (coping mechanisms) and what do they think may help this time?	This encourages the patient to take control and apply their own coping mechanisms. **E**
Listen to and incorporate individual needs and preferences to promote informed decision making about treatment and care.	If people feel in control, they are likely to feel less worried (NICE 2011a, **C**).

Psychological support

Managing hyperventilation

Managing acute anxiety (including panic attacks) can help to avoid the development of a panic disorder or generalized anxiety disorder. Nurses can support patients to avoid anxiety attacks by taking time to talk through issues. If the anxiety has progressed further and the patient is experiencing the warning signs that they are on the verge of hyperventilation, it is helpful to do the following (adapted from Powell 2009):

- Remind them that the symptoms they are feeling are not harmful even though they are uncomfortable.
- Help them to actively release tension in their upper body by encouraging them to sit up and drop their shoulders in a sideways widening direction. This makes hyperventilation more difficult since the chest and diaphragm muscles are stretched outwards.
- Prompt them to breathe slowly – for example, in to a count of four and out to a count of six. During the in-breath the sympathetic nervous system is activated and during the out-breath the parasympathetic nervous system is activated so it is helpful to have a longer out-breath. The longer, slower out-breath and its activation of the parasympathetic nervous system help to counteract the sympathetic nervous system, which is responsible for the fight-or-flight response, which is activated when a person is anxious and is physiologically responsible for hyperventilation. Slowing down your own breathing can help to model slow breathing to the patient.

Principles table 5.12 Supporting a person having a panic attack

Principle	Rationale
Firstly, exclude any physical reasons for the patient's distress, such as an acute angina episode or asthma attack.	If the symptoms of a panic attack have a physical cause, management needs to be instigated as soon as possible. E
Remain calm and stay with the patient. Ask them about their history of anxiety or panic attacks.	The patient will not be reassured by others reacting with tension or anxiety about the situation. E
Maintain eye contact with the patient.	This helps the patient to be connected to reality and engage with your attempts to support them. Some patients may be reassured by physical touch, but assess each individual for appropriateness. E
Guide the patient to breathe deeply and slowly, demonstrating where necessary.	This gives the patient an activity to concentrate on and may help to normalize any carbon dioxide and oxygen blood imbalance. E

The rebreathing technique

The rebreathing technique involves the patient rebreathing the air they have just breathed out (Box 5.10, Figure 5.15). This air is high in carbon dioxide so has less oxygen. This means that there will be a lower amount of oxygen in the blood, thus activating the parasympathetic nervous system and promoting relaxation (Blake and Ledger 2007).

Further support

After the panic attack, it is important to reflect with the patient about what happened and try to identify any triggers. Explanation and education about physiological responses can help to show the patient the importance of slowing their breathing, which will in turn give them a sense of control.

If the panic attacks continue or if the patient has a history of anxiety, then management could include a referral for psychological support (with consent). Medication may be indicated after assessment (NICE 2011a).

Pharmacological support

Psychological therapies are the first-line treatment for anxiety problems, but pharmacological treatments may be introduced alongside psychological interventions for more severe cases.

Box 5.10 Rebreathing technique: instructions for a patient

1. Make a mask of your hands. Put them over your nose and mouth and keep them there (see Figure 5.15).
2. Breathe in and out through your nose.
3. Breathe in your own exhaled air through your nose.
4. Breathe out hard through your mouth.

This should be done slowly, without holding your breath. Repeat steps 2–4 four or five times but no more. Remain calm and relaxed throughout.

Source: Adapted from Powell (2009) with permission of Speechmark.

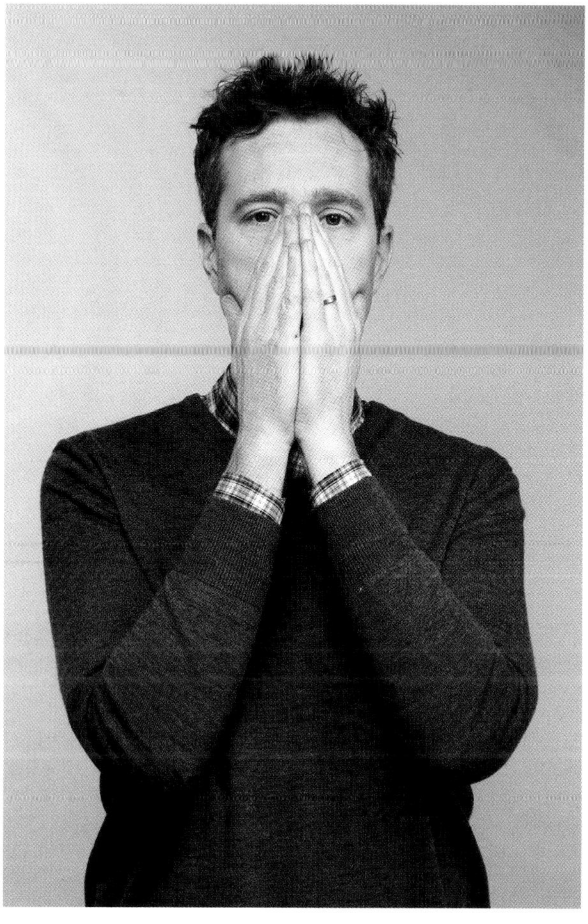

Figure 5.15 Hand position for rebreathing technique.

Anxiety disorders include:

- generalized anxiety disorder (GAD)
- panic disorder
- phobias
- post-traumatic stress disorder (PTSD)
- obsessive compulsive disorder (OCD).

Benzodiazepines are very effective in providing short-term relief from anxiety of all types but are not recommended for long-term use; the Royal College of Psychiatrists recommends that usage does not exceed four weeks, stating that 'around 4 in every 10 people who take them every day for more than 6 weeks will become addicted' (RCPsych 2015a). The most commonly used benzodiazepine for immediate relief is lorazepam (a rapidly acting benzodiazepine with a short half-life). Longer acting benzodiazepines such as diazepam can be used as adjuncts to antidepressants to minimize anxiety, which can occur when starting antidepressant treatment.

Antidepressants are the first-line psychotropic treatment for the following anxiety disorders: GAD, panic disorder and phobias. Among these, selective serotonin reuptake inhibitors (SSRIs) and tricyclic antidepressants are recommended by NICE (2011a). Serotonin–norepinephrine reuptake inhibitors (SNRIs, e.g. venlafaxine) and pregabalin may be considered as alternative initial treatments if SSRIs are judged to be unsuitable.

Other antidepressants, such as trazadone as well as specific anxiolytic drugs such as buspirone, are sometimes effective for treating anxiety. Antipsychotics such as quetiapine and antihistamines such as promethazine may also be used.

Benzodiazepines, antipsychotics and sedating antihistamines are associated with poor long-term outcomes, and pharmacological interventions should consist of either tricyclic or SSRI antidepressant medication (NICE 2011a).

Nurses have an important role in exploring with the patient any concerns they may have about taking an anxiolytic. The patient should be given all the necessary information regarding the optimum time to take the medication and the expected length of time before any therapeutic effect is likely to become apparent.

Box 5.11 Symptoms that indicate a diagnosis of clinical depression

Behavioural

- Irritability
- Socially withdrawn
- Diminished activity
- Changes to sleep pattern
- Changes to eating patterns that are not related to attempts to diet
- Self-harm or suicide attempts

Physical

- Tearfulness
- Exacerbation of pre-existing pains
- Pains secondary to increased muscle tension
- Agitation and restlessness
- Changes in appetite and weight
- Fatigue or loss of energy
- Lack of libido

Cognitive

- Poor concentration
- Reduced attention
- Mental slowing
- Pessimistic thoughts
- Recurring negative thoughts about oneself, past and future
- Rumination
- Suicidal ideation

Emotional

- Guilt
- Worthlessness
- Feeling of being deserving of punishment
- Lowered self-esteem
- Loss of confidence
- Feelings of helplessness and hopelessness
- Reduced enjoyment or interest in most activities

Depression

Definition

Depression is a broad and heterogeneous diagnosis. Central to it is a depressed mood and/or loss of pleasure in most activities (NICE 2009). Depression is often accompanied by symptoms of anxiety and can be short lived (sometimes dependent upon physical symptoms) or chronic.

Related theory

Depression is a common psychological response in patients with a chronic physical illness such as heart disease, diabetes or cancer. When this occurs, it is referred to as 'co-morbid' depression. Co-morbid depression is difficult to detect as symptoms can be similar to the expected side-effects of the illness or treatment, such as fatigue. Psychological screening and outcome measures for depression in physical healthcare settings need to be carefully selected to account for this overlap; the Hospital Anxiety and Depression Scale (Zigmond and Snaith 1983) is an appropriate measure.

Depression can be found in 20% of patients with a chronic physical illness (NICE 2009), which is two to three times higher than the rate in individuals in good physical health. Pitman et al.'s (2018) review of depression in people with cancer reported that it affects up to 20% of adult patients and that 'geographical variations in the diagnosis and treatment … impl[y] under-recognition' (p.1). It is essential, therefore, that patients with a long-term physical illness are regularly assessed for anxiety and depression.

Box 5.11 sets out some of the symptoms of depression (NICE 2009). A normal experience of sadness or low mood is differentiated from what is diagnosed as a depressive episode by the length of time the low mood is experienced and its pervasive and debilitating nature. Low mood that persists for 2 weeks or more, rapid-onset low mood and severe low mood are reasons for concern. The presence of other depressive symptoms contributes to a diagnosis as well as a consideration of how this low mood affects the individual's ability to function. Depression frequently follows a pattern of relapse and remission, and the key aim of intervention is to relieve symptoms (NICE 2009). However, this may or may not include the alleviation of the low mood itself; third-wave cognitive–behavioural therapies aim to support a person with depressed mood to develop psychological flexibility, whereby they can live alongside difficult thoughts and emotions, including depression, and commit themselves to engaging with a meaningful life.

Evidence-based approaches

Approaches to treating depression are influenced by the severity of the condition. Diagnosing depression has improved following the introduction of the 10th edition of the WHO's *International Classification of Diseases* (ICD-10), which lists 10 depressive symptoms (Box 5.12). The level of severity of depression is categorized according to the number and severity of the symptoms a person experiences:

- *mild*: two or three symptoms – the person is distressed but able to continue with most activities
- *moderately depressed*: four or more symptoms – the person is usually having considerable difficulty carrying on with ordinary activities

Box 5.12 The ICD-10's list of 10 depressive symptoms

- Lowering of mood
- Reduction of energy
- Decrease in activity
- Reduction in capacity for enjoyment and interest in life
- Reduction in concentration
- Marked tiredness even after minimum effort
- Sleep disturbance
- Reduced appetite
- Ideas of guilt or worthlessness
- Reduced self-esteem and confidence

Source: Adapted from WHO (2016).

- *severe (without psychotic symptoms)*: an episode of depression in which many symptoms are present; they are obvious and distressing, and loss of self-esteem, feelings of worthlessness and guilt are typically present. Suicidal thoughts may also be present.

Symptoms need to be present for greater than 2 weeks. Core management skills include risk assessment plus the following:

- good communication skills, which will enable the nurse to elicit information from the patient (Brown et al. 2009) and show understanding of the problem
- a sufficient understanding of the signs and symptoms of anxiety and depression and an ability to make a preliminary assessment
- a sufficient understanding of antidepressant medication to enable the nurse to give an explanation of its actions to the patient
- an ability to refer the patient on for further assessment when it is recognized that the issues are beyond the scope of the nurse's experience (this must be done with the patient's consent)
- awareness of the stigma attached to a diagnosis of depression
- sensitivity to diverse cultural, ethnic and religious backgrounds, considering variations in presentations of low mood and its understanding
- awareness of any cognitive impairments or learning disabilities to ensure that specialist therapists are involved (where needed)
- protection of the patient's privacy and dignity.

Use of available psychological support services can assist with the care and treatment of patients as well as providing a supervisory and support framework for staff. Working with psychological support services can enable nurses to develop their assessment skills around anxiety and depression, helping them to identify the appropriate time for referral to a specialist service if required (Towers 2007).

Pre-procedural considerations

Psychological support

Nurses can be involved in assessing depression in patients with physical illness. NICE (2009) guidance sets out a four-step model for managing a patient with depression. The first step (Box 5.13) could be implemented by a nurse in an acute environment.

It is important to assess how the patient's low mood has affected their usual daily activities, such as eating, dressing and sleeping. The nurse can also encourage the patient to engage with activities that would be normal for them as this can provide them with opportunities for connecting, achievement or enjoyment. Some people who are low in mood have thoughts about death and dying – these can be very natural thoughts in the context of a serious physical health problem and do not necessarily imply any risk of harm to self. However, some people do have thoughts about wanting to die or to harm themselves, and it is important that nurses are able to explore these thoughts and feelings with patients (Problem-solving table 5.2). It is important that any conversation about self-harm or suicidality is collaborative and person centred (rather than protocol driven) and aims to understand the social context of these thoughts and feelings with the intention to reduce the causes of the depression where possible (HEE 2018).

Box 5.13 Managing a patient with depression: NICE (2009) guidance, step 1

Key questions

1 During the last month, have you often been bothered by:
- feeling down, depressed or hopeless?
- having little interest or pleasure in doing things?

2 How long have you felt like this for?

If the patient answers 'yes' to question 1 and the timescale is longer than 2 weeks, it is important that a referral is made for further assessment by a healthcare professional with clinical competence in managing depression, such as a psychologist or a registered mental health nurse, so they can determine whether the patient has been bothered by 'feelings of worthlessness, poor concentration or thoughts of death' (NICE 2009, p.9).

Other questions

Further questions should assess for the following:
- other physical health problems that may be significantly affecting the patient's mood, such as uncontrolled pain, sleep disruption, excessive nausea and vomiting, physical limitations on their independence or body image disturbance
- a history of psychological difficulties such as depression
- a consideration of the medication the patient is taking, specifically medication for mental health problems (have they been able to take it and absorb it or have they had any digestive issues?)
- social support for the patient (who else is around to support the person, and are they isolated?).

Source: Adapted from NICE (2009).

Pharmacological support

Antidepressant medication can be both effective and acceptable to patients for the treatment of their depression. There are several classes of antidepressant medication:

- tricyclic antidepressants (TCAs), e.g. amytryptiline
- selective serotonin reuptake inhibitors (SSRIs), e.g. fluoxetine, citalopram and sertraline
- serotonin–norepinephrine reuptake inhibitors (SNRIs), e.g. venlafaxine and duloxetine
- noradrenaline reuptake inhibitors (NARIs), e.g. atomoxetine, reboxetine and bupropion
- monoamine oxidase inhibitors (MAOIs), e.g. phenelzine and moclobomide.

Table 5.2 lists the most commonly prescribed antidepressants.

When a patient is prescribed antidepressants, it is important to consider the presence of other physical health problems, medications the patient is already taking and their side-effect profile, and any history of a good or poor response to antidepressant medication. There is little difference in terms of effectiveness between the types of antidepressant; however, there are clear differences in the side-effects of the different classes and types of antidepressant. SSRIs are safer in overdoses than TCAs, which

Table 5.2 The most commonly prescribed antidepressants

Medication	Trade name	Group
Amitriptyline	Tryptizol	Tricyclic
Clomipramine	Anafranil	Tricyclic
Citalopram	Cipramil	SSRI
Dosulepin	Prothiaden	Tricyclic
Doxepin	Sinequan	Tricyclic
Fluoxetine	Prozac	SSRI
Imipramine	Tofranil	Tricyclic
Lofepramine	Gamanil	Tricyclic
Mirtazapine	Zispin	NaSSA
Moclobemide	Manerix	MAOI
Nortriptyline	Allegron	Tricyclic
Paroxetine	Seroxat	SSRI
Phenelzine	Nardil	MAOI
Reboxetine	Edronax	SNRI
Sertraline	Lustral	SSRI
Tranylcypromine	Parnate	MAOI
Trazodone	Molipaxin	Tricyclic related
Venlafaxine	Efexor	SNRI

MAOI, monoamine oxidase inhibitor; NaSSA, noradrenergic and specific serotonergic antidepressant; SNRI, serotonin-norepinephrine reuptake inhibitor; SSRI, selective serotonin reuptake inhibitor.

can be dangerous. There is an increased risk of gastrointestinal bleeding in the elderly with SSRIs so they should be avoided for patients who are taking non-steroidal anti-inflammatory drugs. Monoamine oxidase inhibitors can affect blood pressure, particularly when certain food types (e.g. cheeses) are eaten. SNRIs are not appropriate for patients with heart conditions as they too increase blood pressure. Citalopram and sertraline (both SSRIs) are associated with fewer interactions and so are more likely to be prescribed if the patient has a long-term chronic condition (NICE 2009).

Due to increased sensitivity to side-effects in the medically ill, treatment may need to be introduced at a lower dose before cautiously increasing it. Dividing the dose may improve tolerance, as may liquid preparations, which can be helpful in low-dose prescribing and for patients who have difficulty swallowing.

Nurses have an important role in exploring with patients any concerns they may have about taking an antidepressant. Patients should be given all the necessary information regarding the optimum time to take the medication, and the expected length of time before any therapeutic effect becomes apparent; this is usually 4 to 6 weeks. Medication should be taken for at least 6 months following remission.

In general, treatment should not be stopped abruptly, and discontinuation of treatment usually requires a gradual reduction of the dose over 4 weeks (NICE 2009). Addiction is unlikely to happen with modern antidepressant treatments, but patients may need to be provided with further information and reassurance that this is the case. Further information on pharmacological interventions can be found in the NICE guidelines on depression (NICE 2009).

Principles table 5.13 Communicating with a person who is depressed

Principle	Rationale
Initiate the conversation and develop rapport. Develop a person-centred communication style.	Good communication is essential to assess and individualize support (NICE 2009, C).
Show understanding, caring and acceptance of behaviours, including tears or anger.	Accepting patients as they are, without attempting to block or contain their emotions, helps them to express their feelings. E
Encourage the patient to identify their own abilities or strategies for coping with the situation.	To promote self-efficacy. E

Problem-solving table 5.2 Prevention and resolution (Principles table 5.13)

Problem	Cause	Prevention	Action
Patient expresses ideas of self-harm or taking their own life; for example, patient says that they sometimes wish they would not wake up in the morning so that they do not have to face their difficulties	Low mood, depression	Assess for risk: this can be as simple as remarking upon the person's low mood and asking them if they have ever thought of hurting themselves. For example: • 'Sometimes when people are low in mood they have thoughts about harming themselves – have you had or do you have thoughts like this?' • 'It sounds like there are times when you struggle and that if you didn't wake up in the morning you wouldn't have to deal with these difficulties, but that you don't actually want to hurt or kill yourself … is that right?' If the patient says that they are actively thinking about harming themselves, you need to explore any plans they have and any intention to act on these plans. For example: • 'Do you have any plans about how you would hurt yourself?' • 'Do you intend to carry out this plan?'	If you have any concerns that the patient is at risk, follow the procedure of your organization. This may include contacting psychiatric liaison services or other psychological support services.

Problem	Cause	Prevention	Action
		Crucially, you will also need to explore what stops the patient from acting (known as 'protective factors') and what changes might cause them to act. For example: • 'What has stopped you from doing this before?' • 'What might happen that would increase the chance of you hurting yourself?' If you consider the patient to be at risk, explain to them that you need to refer them for further support. The patient may be reluctant for you to share this information; however, it is your duty to act in their best interests and reduce the risk of harm. For example: • 'I am concerned for your safety and I would like to speak to my manager about how we can help you to keep yourself safe. Would this be OK with you?' • 'I understand that you are reluctant for me to share this information, however, my priority is to keep you safe and so I do need to speak to my manager. I will let them know what we have discussed and your own ideas about how to look after yourself.'	

Anger, aggression and violence

Definition

Anger is an emotional state experienced as the impulse to behave in order to protect, defend or attack in response to a threat or challenge, and as such can have a legitimate function. Of itself, anger is not classified as an emotional disorder. This emotional state may range in intensity from mild irritation to intense fury and rage, and becomes a problem when it is associated with poor impulse control and related behaviours.

'*Violence and aggression* refer to a range of behaviours or actions that can result in harm, hurt, or injury to another person, regardless of whether the violence or aggression is physically or verbally expressed, physical harm is sustained or the intention is clear' (NICE 2015, p.6).

The phrase 'clinically challenging behaviour' can be used to refer to aggressive, confrontational or threatening behaviour from patients arising from any of the following:

- dementia
- delirium
- brain tumours or metastases
- substance or alcohol use or withdrawal
- other mental health conditions or learning disabilities
- factors such as the receipt of bad news or bereavement
- anxiety, fear or a sense of powerlessness
- adverse reactions to treatment, such as hallucinations (NHS Protect 2013).

Related theory

The Health and Safety Executive (n.d.) reports that violence and aggression form the third most frequently reported group of incidents from the health and social care sector in its RIDDOR incident reporting system. Therefore, nurses will, sadly, be exposed to anger and aggression.

Poor communication is frequently a precursor to anger and aggressive behaviour (Duxbury and Whittington 2005). Aggression and abuse tend to be discussed synonymously in the literature and are reported to occur with some frequency in nursing (McLaughlin et al. 2009). Anger is felt or displayed when someone's annoyance or irritation has increased to a point where they feel or display extreme displeasure. Verbal aggression is the expression of anger via hostile language; this language can cause offence and may result in physical assault. Some people experience verbal abuse as worse than a minor physical assault (Adams and Whittington 1995).

There can be many causes of clinically challenging behaviour, including unmet care needs (such as thirst, pain or the need to eliminate) as well as a lack of meaningful activity, sensory deprivation, sleep deprivation, and impaired ability to communicate or understand a situation. NHS Protect (2013) proposes a framework for explaining challenging behaviour. This includes considering:

- *historical factors* such as substance and alcohol abuse
- *current presentation*: diagnosis and physical factors such as pain
- *triggers or antecedents*, including environmental factors such as other agitated individuals and busy or noisy areas, and situational factors such as inconsistent staff attitude and time of day.

Figure 5.16 presents this framework in more detail.

In some instances, challenging or difficult behaviour can be seen to be related to underlying stress and difficulty in a person's situation. Anger, aggression and violence may have 'biological, psychological, social and environmental roots' (Krug 2002, p.25). People frequently get angry when they feel they are not being heard or when their control of a situation and self-esteem are compromised. Institutional pressures can influence healthcare professionals to act in controlling ways and may contribute to patients' angry responses (Gudjonsson et al. 2004). Patients are often undergoing procedures that threaten them and they may consequently feel vulnerable and react aggressively as a result (NHS Protect 2013). Threats, uncertainty and disempowerment may predispose people to anger, and living with and being treated for a serious condition can be sufficiently threatening and disempowering (NHS Protect 2013). Another source of anger can arise when personal beliefs are contravened via social or religious rules being broken by others. Nurses therefore need to strive to be aware of individual and cultural values and work with them to avoid frustration and upset.

People can become angry when they feel that they have not been communicated with honestly or feel they have been misled about treatments and their outcomes. To prevent people's frustration escalating into anger or worse, health professionals need to ensure that they are communicating openly, honestly and frequently (NHS Protect 2013).

Some patients may appear or sound aggressive when they are not intending to be and nurses must therefore use good judgement to clarify the patient's behaviour in these instances. Nurses also need to be aware of their own boundaries and capabilities when dealing with challenging or abusive situations.

For some people, anger may be the least distressing emotion to feel or display. Sometimes helplessness, sadness and loss are far harder to explore and show to others. Anger therefore can be a way of controlling intimacy and disclosure, but it can escalate to threatening, abusive or violent behaviour.

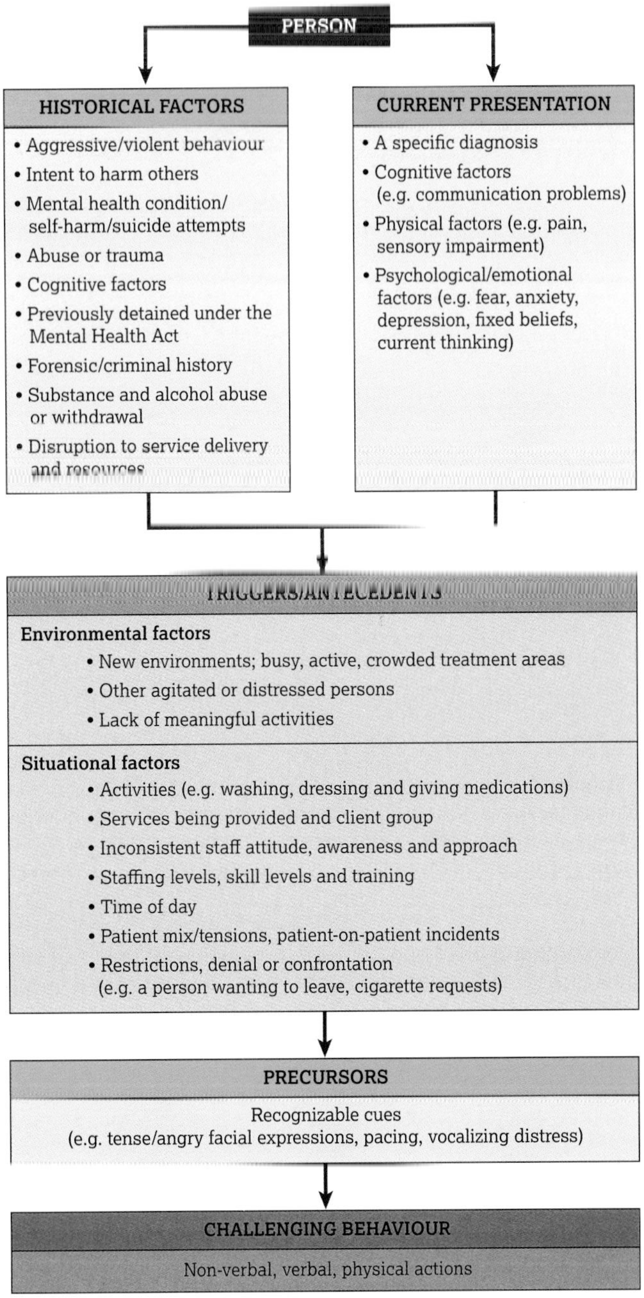

Figure 5.16 Managing and assessing risk behaviours. A framework for explaining challenging behaviour. *Source:* NHS Protect (2013).

Whatever the cause of anger or aggression, people can behave in a number of challenging ways and with varying degrees of resistance to social and hospital rules. People may simply refuse to comply with a request or may behave aggressively, for example by pushing someone aside (without intent to harm) or by deliberately striking out at others. Mental capacity issues should be considered when assessing the causes of aggressive behaviours. However, some patients may feel too depleted by experiences of disease and treatment to express their anger (Bowes et al. 2002).

Evidence-based approaches

Prevention is the most effective method of managing anger – that is, diffusing stressful or difficult interactions before they become a crisis. Understanding why angry or challenging behaviour occurs can be helpful in establishing a comprehensive approach to prevention. The public health model detailed in *Meeting Needs and Reducing Distress* (NHS Protect 2013) focuses on the prevention and management of challenging behaviour that is clinically related. It proposes that the focus should be on *primary prevention* (addressing the root cause before challenging behaviour happens) and then if necessary *secondary prevention* (using de-escalation techniques, empathy and understanding). There should be less emphasis on *tertiary* responses (restrictive interventions including physical intervention and medication).

Clinical governance

Nurses may be inclined to accept aggressive behaviour as part of the job (McLaughlin et al. 2009) due to being encouraged to be caring, compassionate and accepting of others. Despite this, nurses have the right to work without feeling intimidated or threatened and should not tolerate verbal or physical abuse, threats or assault. Personal comments, sarcasm and innuendo are all unacceptable. Any healthcare professional is legally permitted to act in self-defence as long as the response is proportionate to the seriousness of the attack.

Employers have a responsibility to adhere to the Management of Health and Safety at Work Regulations (1999) (see also NHS England 2015, NHS Protect 2013). This involves providing a safe environment for people to work in and one that is free from threats and abuse. With any physical assault, the police should be involved.

Pre-procedural considerations

Assessment

Box 5.14 lists signs indicating that people may be angry. It is necessary to engage people sensitively and carefully to attempt to help them while maintaining a safe environment for all.

Non-physical intervention

It is frequently possible to engage with and manage some of the underlying features of anger and aggression without endangering anyone. People who are behaving aggressively probably do not normally act that way and may apologize when helped.

Talking down or de-escalation of situations where someone is being non-compliant can be achieved with careful assessment of the situation and skilful communication. NICE's (2015) clinical guidelines on managing disturbed and violent behaviour recommend de-escalation, which includes remaining calm when approaching someone and supporting them to be calm and relaxed while offering them choices on how to proceed. It is acknowledged, however, that there is little research indicating the correct procedure to follow (Gaynes et al. 2017). Box 5.15 suggests phrases that might help when talking with an angry person.

Physical intervention

If the challenging or violent behaviour increases and the person or others are considered to be at risk, the situation is considered to be an emergency. If restrictive intervention and then potentially chemical restraint are necessary, it is essential that local policies and procedures are followed. Restrictive intervention is defined as follows:

> Deliberate acts on the part of other person(s) that restrict a patient's movement, liberty and/or freedom to act independently in order to:
> - take immediate control of a dangerous situation where there is a real possibility of harm to the person or others if no action is undertaken, and
> - end or reduce significantly the danger to the patient or others.
>
> (DH 2015, para. 26:36)

Box 5.14 Warning signs that a patient is angry

- Tense, angry facial signs, restlessness and increased volume of speech
- Prolonged eye contact and a refusal to communicate
- Unclear thought process, delusions or hallucinations
- [illegible]

Box 5.15 Phrases and responses that might help when talking with an angry person

Some initial phrases to try include the following:

- 'I can see that you are angry about this.'
- 'I would like to help you try to sort this out. How can I do that?'
- 'I would like to help you and in order for me to do this I need you to stop shouting.'
- 'Please stop [unacceptable behaviour] as it frightens me and other people.'
- 'Can you tell me what is making you so angry so that I might be able to help you sort it out?'
- 'What can I/we do to help you [comply with the rules/ request]?'

Try to agree with the patient where possible (this can be a good way to defuse tensions). For example: 'I can see how that would annoy you … let's see what we can do about it.'

In addition, the following de-escalation approaches may help:

- Where possible, avoid compromising the person's sense of personal space.
- Try to achieve the same level as the person – sit if they sit, stand if they stand.
- Move to a safe place if possible; this means a place where the person will feel secure and that would provide an escape route for you if necessary.
- Explain what you are doing to the person and why you are doing it.
- Try to appear calm and self-controlled; focusing on your breathing may help.
- As far as possible, ensure that non-verbal behaviour is not threatening – for example, avoid sudden movements or crossed arms.
- As far as possible, ask other staff to control other agitating factors in the environment, such as excessive noise or the number of people around.
- It may be necessary for staff to take it in turns to be in the de-escalating role, with one staff member stepping forward to engage with the person and the other stepping back.

Restrictive intervention should only ever be used where de-escalation alone proves insufficient and it should always be used in conjunction with further efforts at de-escalation; it should never be used as a punishment or in a punitive manner (DH 2015, para. 26:36). Key questions to consider in the decision-making process around restraining a patient are detailed in Box 5.16.

Any form of restrictive intervention must follow the principles set out in NICE's guidance *Violence and Aggression: Short-Term Management in Mental Health, Health and Community Settings* (NICE 2015). Specifically, it must:

- be necessary, justifiable and proportionate
- be combined with strategies to de-escalate
- be carried out with the least restrictive interventions possible
- not impact the airway, breathing or circulation
- not include the deliberate application of pain
- be used for the minimum possible amount of time
- not prevent staff from continuing to monitor the physical and medical condition of the patient, including monitoring their vital signs and level of consciousness
- avoid inducing any avoidable physical damage to the individual through
  - holding individual limbs near the joint, not on it
  - protecting vulnerable areas such as the neck, throat, genitals, abdomen and chest
- be formally recorded after the event
- involve the family and patient in reviewing the ongoing care after the event.

Box 5.16 Key questions to consider in the decision-making process around using restraint

- Is there reasonable belief that the person is likely to suffer harm unless proportionate physical intervention is used?
- Are there viable alternatives?
- Is the amount of time or type of physical intervention a proportionate response to the likelihood of and seriousness of the potential harm?
- Is the least possible amount of physical intervention being used for the shortest possible time?
- Could the restraint be justified in a court of law if necessary?

Source: Adapted from NHS Protect (2013).

Pharmacological support

In acute circumstances, if the violent or aggressive behaviour of an inpatient has a clinical cause and is putting them or others at risk, the doctor responsible for their care may consider 'rapid tranquillization' with a benzodiazepine, for example lorazepam. The aim is to render the patient lightly asleep and lying down so that the risks posed to themselves and others by their behaviour are averted. This approach should only be used after careful assessment.

Depending on the degree of disturbed behaviour and taking into account other factors, for example a confusional state, a psychiatrist may prescribe an antipsychotic medication for short-term management, usually haloperidol either orally or as an injection.

Principles table 5.14 Communicating with a person who is angry

Principle	Rationale
Remain calm.	This can help to de-escalate the situation. If the behaviour of others around the agitated person is calm, then distressing and/or provoking them further is minimized. E
Verbally acknowledge the person's distress/anger and suggest that you wish to help.	The person may respond positively and accept help (NHS Protect 2013, C).
Acknowledge issues that may be contributing, for example being kept waiting.	This helps the person feel that their concerns are understood. E
Consider what causes there may be, for example medication or disease (consider diabetes – either hypoglycaemia or hyperglycaemia), medical, circumstantial and so on.	Several factors might be influencing the behaviour. E
Consider safety – try to move to another area (ideally where you can sit down). If others might be intimidated or in danger, move one of the parties away where practical, but do not endanger yourself in the process.	To maintain safety for all (NHS Protect 2013, C).

(continued)

Principles table 5.14 Communicating with a person who is angry *(continued)*

Principle	Rationale
If a person's behaviour is hostile and intimidating, tell them you are finding their behaviour threatening and state clearly that you wish them to stop (see Box 5.15 for suggested phrases).	Some people may not be aware of the impact of their behaviour and will change it when it is pointed out that it is unacceptable (NHS Protect 2013, C).
Assess individual situations and make use of relatives or friends if they are present and can be of assistance in defusing the situation.	Sometimes people will listen more to a person who is close to them. E
Create some physical distance or summon assistance if the patient does not concur and continues to be threatening, abusive or passively non-compliant (e.g. refuses to move).	To maintain safety for all. E
Warn the person that you will contact security staff or the police if necessary – but avoid threatening language. If possible, make a personal or practical appeal.	People need clear information about the consequences of their actions. E
Attempt to talk the individual down; that is, calm them down by remaining calm and professional yourself, keeping your voice at a steady pace and a moderate volume. Try to engage the person in conversation.	Your behaviour will have an impact on theirs (NHS Protect 2013, C).
Avoid personalizing the anger but do not accept unwarranted personal criticism.	If we personalize then we are likely to react in a way that exacerbates the situation, but neither should a nurse accept abuse. E
Suggest walking with the patient to discuss issues but ensure you remain in a public and safe environment.	Changing the environment may help to recontextualize behaviour, and movement can reduce agitation. E
It is important to listen to what the grievance is, treat the person as an individual, preserve their dignity and attempt to help where it is realistic to do so. Avoid passing the buck or blocking in another way.	People need to be heard and understood (NHS Protect 2013, C).
If a patient is no longer abusive or threatening but is struggling to reduce their anger, they may benefit from some further psychological support or medication to help them feel calmer.	The short-term use of some medication may be beneficial. C
In rare and extreme circumstances where patients are violent and do not respond to de-escalation attempts and where the safety of other people is compromised, you must take immediate action by involving security and the police. If the person is an ambulant outpatient, ask them to leave if their behaviour is not acceptable.	To maintain safety for all. E
Physical intervention and tranquillization may be required in some cases. Follow individual hospital security and emergency procedures in these instances.	To maintain the safety of the patient and staff members (NICE 2015, C).
Document the incident according to the hospital incident reporting process.	So such incidents can be investigated. C

Post-procedural considerations

The ideal outcome of an encounter with an angry, aggressive or threatening person is that safety is not compromised and the healthcare professional is able to de-escalate the situation and help the person to express the reason why they are angry. Follow-up support should be offered to help stop the person repeating the same behaviour. However, people should also be made aware of potential sanctions if they are unable to comply, for example withdrawal of treatment and involvement of the police (Box 5.17).

It can be distressing to be exposed to threatening or abusive people and it is good practice to seek a debriefing interview. This can help nurses and the institution reflect upon the experience and put procedures in place to manage such situations. The institution's occupational health or human resources department should have information on how nurses can access support facilities.

Box 5.17 When to call the police

- If all other possible avenues for safely de-escalating or managing the situation have been exhausted or failed, and/or physical or pharmacological intervention is not appropriate
- Where staff, patients or the public remain in imminent or grave danger
- If a crime (such as criminal damage or assault, or bodily harm) has been committed
- If the person is armed with a weapon (a weapon can be defined as an article adapted, made or used with the intention of causing harm)

Delirium

Definition

Delirium is a distressing and underdiagnosed syndrome of acute alteration in mental state. The core clinical features that indicate a diagnosis of delirium are:

- impaired consciousness and attention
- disorientation, impaired recent memory, perceptual distortions and transient delusions
- psychomotor disturbances (hypoactivity or hyperactivity)
- disturbed sleep–wake cycle
- emotional disturbances (various) (WHO 2018).

Delirium can present in three forms:

- *Hypoactive delirium*: a subtype of delirium characterized by becoming withdrawn, quiet and sleepy.
- *Hyperactive delirium*: a subtype of delirium characterized by heightened arousal where people can be restless, agitated or aggressive.
- *Mixed*: with both hypoactive and hyperactive features.

Related theory

In most cases, delirium is caused by a general medical condition, intoxication, or withdrawal of medication or substances that act upon the neurochemical balance of the brain (Ross 1991). Causative factors such as infection, post-anaesthesia and medication (especially analgesics) need to be considered, particularly for sudden onset of delirium in the hospital environment.

The prevalence of delirium in hospital patients is between 20% and 50% (NICE 2010). Certain factors predispose people to delirium or are risk factors for its development:

- other serious illness such as uncontrollable cardiovascular or respiratory conditions, diabetes
- multiple co-morbidities
- older age
- alcohol dependence syndrome
- previous or existing other mental disorder, such as dementia
- hypoalbuminaemia
- infection
- taking medications that affect the mind or behaviour
- uncontrolled pain
- taking high doses of analgesia (Irving et al. 2006).

Being an inpatient in a hospital environment can contribute to the development of delirium. The following factors can increase the risk:

- patient not a UK resident and/or English is not their first language
- changing clinical environment, such as room or ward, on a number of occasions
- absence of any means of gauging the time of day
- absence of family or a close friend
- catheterization.

The greater the number of risk factors present, the greater the likelihood of delirium developing (NICE 2010).

Delirium can develop quickly and fluctuate over the course of a 24-hour period (APA 2013). A patient's behaviour may change to indicate potential delirium before a full set of diagnostic symptoms is observable (Duppils and Wikblad 2004). Environmental cues during the daytime act as stabilizing factors and so at night-time symptoms are typically worse. Delirium can resolve within hours or days, or it can last longer if it co-exists with other problems, such as dementia; it is important to rule out pre-existing neurocognitive disorders when considering treatment responses.

Delirium is associated with considerable morbidity, which can delay recovery and rehabilitation, as well as mortality (Irving et al. 2006, NICE 2010). Recognizing and addressing delirium are important, not only because of the clinical impact but also because of the distress it causes patients, families and staff (Lawlor et al. 2000).

Evidence-based approaches

Nurses play a critical role in the prevention, early detection (Milisen et al. 2005) and management of delirium. Delirium is frequently iatrogenic (i.e. caused by medical intervention) and hence can often be corrected once the causative factor has been identified.

Addressing potential causative factors as part of good nursing and medical care will help to prevent the development of delirium. This means ensuring hydration and nutritional requirements are met and any electrolyte imbalances are monitored and corrected.

Nurses need to be aware that patients over the age of 65 years (especially those having anaesthesia) will be highly prone to developing delirium so they need to be monitored carefully over a period of time to pick up any early signs. The effect of analgesia (especially opiates) also needs to be considered.

The emergence of delirium can also be significant at the end of life and can significantly complicate care provision (Delgado-Guay et al. 2008). Terminal restlessness is a term often used to describe this agitated delirium in end-of-life care, where the causes may require specific management different from that of other types of delirium (Brajtman 2005, White et al. 2007). A progressive shutdown of body organs in the last 2–3 days of life (Lawlor et al. 2000) leads to irresolvable systemic imbalances. The management of delirium in end-of-life care therefore shifts from a focus on reversing the cause to alleviating the symptoms. Nurses should avoid medicating symptoms unless this is in the patient's best interest.

Principles of care

Initial screening for any cognitive issues on admission is important to identify predictive factors and establish a baseline of cognitive functioning. Involving the family can be crucial in an accurate assessment where there are existing changes.

If risk factors are identified, nursing care for an individual with delirium should focus on minimizing hyperarousal from the environment:

- Minimize the frequency of moving the patient from one ward, bed or room to another.
- Ensure that there is cognitive stimulation – for example, make sure the television is working and that the patient is in an environment with other patients.
- Give the patient access to a means of determining the time of day (e.g. a clock or window).
- Ensure the patient has access to hearing aids, glasses, etc.
- Encourage friends, relatives and spiritual advisors (if appropriate) to visit.

In addition, nursing care should include optimizing physical health for the patient to maintain mobility (if appropriate), hydration and nutrition and to prevent constipation and incontinence. This will take place in parallel with the patient's medical management, which should initially focus on attempting to establish potential reversible causes. These include:

- newly started medications
- changes in dosage
- opioid toxicity
- withdrawal from opioids or alcohol
- use of corticosteroids
- metabolic imbalances or organ failure affecting the processing and excretion of drugs
- infections
- hypercalcaemia
- constipation.

Clinical governance

In the case of medium-term to longer-term delirium, another person may make decisions on the patient's behalf as long as this has been agreed as part of a best interest assessment and the principles of the Mental Capacity Act (2005) have been applied. The best interest assessment must include the views of family or informal carers, and the decision maker is generally the lead clinician for the patient (Griffith and Tengnah 2008). However, if the patient has a lasting power of attorney for welfare and this application has been registered with the Office of the Public Guardian, then the relevant person will be able to make decisions on the patient's behalf.

The Mental Capacity Act (2005) sets out principles relating to the protection of liberty when caring for someone with reduced capacity. This must be reliant upon accurate and suitable assessments of capacity and best interests that are well documented and reviewed.

Physical intervention

Wherever possible, nurses must attempt to create an environment where physical intervention will not be necessary. Physical intervention happens very rarely and all feasible steps to avoid it must be explored. Any action taken must be the 'least harmful' intervention in the circumstance. The aim is to balance the patient's right to independence with their and others' safety. However, if physical intervention is necessary to maintain the safety of the patient, then it requires careful ethical and legal consideration.

Physical intervention takes many forms and must be meticulously judged for the potential to benefit or harm an individual. The *Delirium: Diagnosis, Prevention and Management* guidelines (NICE 2010) advise that the use of physical intervention should be a last resort, where the patient is putting themselves or others at risk of harm and all other means of management and deflection have been employed. When physical intervention is employed, this should be for the shortest period possible and use minimum force to ensure the patient is not harmed.

If intervention is required, nurses must explain to the patient why they are doing what they are doing (regardless of the patient's perceived capacity) and act to reduce the negative impact upon the patient's dignity as much as possible.

Documentation

Delirium is under-reported in nursing and medical note taking (Irving et al. 2006). Documentation outlining the onset of behaviours and symptoms is instrumental in assisting the medical team to identify the cause of the problem and its likely solution. The documentation of the assessment and subsequent care must be detailed and accurate.

Pre-procedural considerations

Psychosocial support

It is important, wherever possible, to create an environment conducive to orientation (e.g. a quiet, well-lit environment where normal routines take place). Nurses must help patients to maximize their independence through activity, as mobilization is seen to assist with orientation (Neville 2006). Nursing interventions include creating a well-lit room with familiar objects, limited staff changes (possibly requiring one-to-one nursing care), reduced noise stimulation, and the presence of family or familiar friends.

Pharmacological support

Once diagnosed, symptoms that do not respond to non-pharmacological interventions can be treated with prescribed medication including sedatives, for example haloperidol (NICE 2010). As far as possible, benzodiazepines should be avoided as a side-effect of these can be delirium (BNF 2019). However, they may be used if delirium is caused by alcohol withdrawal.

Use of medication for sedation in the end stages of life needs individual consideration and the family must be involved and communicated with regularly.

It is worth noting that health professionals and family members can mistake the agitation of delirium for symptoms of pain. If opioids are increased as a result, there may be worsening of the delirium (Delgado-Guay et al. 2008).

Principles table 5.15 Communicating with a person with delirium

Principle	Rationale
It is essential to ensure that aids for visual and hearing impairments are functional and being used.	To maximize the patient's ability to communicate normally. E, C
Adjust the environment to promote the patient's orientation, for example install a visible clock or calendar and photographs of family.	To maintain or promote orientation. E, C
Background noise should be kept to a minimum.	Background noise can be very distracting for the patient. E, C
Always introduce yourself to the patient (do not assume they remember you). If possible, limit the number of individuals involved in the person's care.	To promote consistency and reduce the potential for confusion. E
Give simple information in short statements. Use closed questions.	Closed questions are less taxing and only require a 'yes' or 'no' answer. E
Give clear explanations of any procedures or activities carried out with the individual.	To maintain respect and dignity. E, C

Post-procedural considerations

Liaison with the patient's family is important so that they understand what is happening and what they can do to help. It can be distressing to witness or spend time with a delirious family member. The family should therefore be given the opportunity to talk about their concerns and be updated with information about the cause and management. It is good practice to give them written information about delirium, such as the leaflet provided by the Royal College of Psychiatrists (RCPsych 2015b).

Dementia

Definition

Dementia is an umbrella term that describes a degenerative neurological disorder caused by diseases or injury to the brain. Although there are over 200 subtypes, there are four common types of dementia:

- Alzheimer's
- vascular
- Lewy body
- frontotemporal.

Weatherhead and Courtney (2012, p.114) state that 'dementia is not a normal part of the ageing process, but almost all types of dementia are progressive and incurable'.

Related theory

The WHO (2017) estimates that over 50 million people are living with dementia worldwide, and this number is predicted to rise exponentially to 152 million people in 2050. The Alzheimer's Society (2014) estimates that there were 850,000 people living with dementia in the UK in 2015, with a related cost of £26 billion a year.

Although the risk of developing dementia increases as people age, dementia does not exclusively affect older people. Although it is rare, and can be difficult to diagnose, dementia can affect younger people: 40,000 people aged under 65 have a dementia diagnosis in the UK (Alzheimer's Society 2017).

Dementia can be caused by a number of illnesses and manifests as a decline in multiple areas of functioning, most notably a person's ability to think, retain information, reason and communicate (Young Dementia UK 2018). People living with dementia are twice as likely to be hospitalized as people with normal cognitive functioning (Parke et al. 2017). Studies suggest that one-quarter of UK inpatient beds were occupied by people with dementia in 2009 (Alzheimer's Society 2009), and that figure will have risen in the years since then.

Delirium and depression are prevalent in older patients, and it can be difficult to make a differential diagnosis between these presentations and dementia. Due to the differences in the treatments for these conditions, it is essential that healthcare professionals are able to identify key signs and symptoms associated with all three conditions so that appropriate management can be provided (Polson and Croy 2015).

Evidence-based approaches

De Vries (2013) suggests that the 'decline in communication ability for older people with dementia is usually progressive and gradual, with the condition affecting expressive and receptive language abilities' (p.30). It is thought that those in the caring profession avoid communication with people who have dementia and this can have a negative impact on the person's experience and result in behaviour, which can be challenging (Jootun and McGhee 2011). People who have dementia frequently have word-finding difficulties so supporting communication can include finding suitable tools, such as a communication book. The use of non-verbal skills, such as simply allowing the person to point at what they want, can help in the communication process. It is important to engage with people with dementia and, although it may take more time, the results can be rewarding. Excluding or ignoring patients can leave them feeling frustrated and angry, therefore compromising their safety (Tonkins 2011).

The involvement of family and carers is important as they may have a greater understanding of the verbal and non-verbal communication of the person with dementia. However, the involvement of family and carers should not exclude communication between the person with dementia and nurses; the person with dementia should be involved as much as possible in all communication relating to their care. As Jootun and McGhee (2011, p.41) suggest, it is important for nurses to demonstrate sensitivity and encourage the person to communicate in the way they are most able and prefer.

Baillie et al. (2012) suggest that providing personal care to a person with dementia, if done sensitively, can help to develop the relationship between them and the nurse. However, it is important to consider what the person with dementia might be experiencing as their reality may not be the same as the nurse's. For example, the person with dementia may think they are at home and that the nurse is a family member.

There is a higher risk for patients with cognitive impairment (compared to those who do not have cognitive impairment) who are admitted into a hospital to have poorer health outcomes and be discharged into 24-hour care. NICE (2018b) recommends that care plans for patients with dementia should promote and maintain the patient's independence in activities of daily living (such as mobility and personal care) due to the high risk of institutionalization and dependency on others. When writing care plans, the unique needs of people with dementia must be taken into consideration and addressed to ensure person-centred care. Environmental factors, such as signage and a clear, clutter-free bed space, should always be considered to ensure safety and promote independence (RCOT 2015).

Clinical governance

The principles of the Mental Capacity Act (2005) apply to all patients and the first principle of the act, the presumption of capacity, also applies to patients who have dementia. A person's capacity is decision specific and, as such, a person with dementia should have the ability to make decisions as long as they can show that they understand the decision they are making and the risks associated with that decision. If a patient with dementia declines care or treatment, they should be treated as an adult with capacity unless an assessment of capacity has indicated they lack capacity to make the decision. If this is the case, a best interest decision must be made in consultation with the patient's family. Where the person has no family and the decision relates to medical treatment or about where they will be living, a referral must be made to the Independent Mental Capacity Advocate.

For people with dementia who are in hospital or a care setting, consideration needs to be given to the Deprivation of Liberty Safeguards (DoLS). If a patient is unable to consent to being in hospital and there are restrictions on their liberty, they are not free to leave if they wish to, so they may be being deprived of their liberty.

Pre-procedural considerations

Equipment

People who have dementia may only need a nurse's effective communication skills. However, tools such as communication cards or books that allow patients to point to images (e.g. toilet, shower, food and drink) may be very useful.

Assessment

Assessing the pain of a person who has dementia and communication difficulties can be challenging. Using non-verbal pain assessment tools should ensure that the patient's pain is appropriately assessed.

Principles table 5.16 Environmental considerations for the assessment of people with dementia

Principle	Rationale
Ensure that there are recognizable environments and clear signage to identifiable rooms, such as toilets, bathrooms and kitchens.	Visual cues help patients with dementia to navigate their environment, which reduces disorientation and promotes independence (NICE 2018b, C).
Provide orientation cues including a calendar and a working clock with date, time and season.	Orientation cues can help to reduce confusion and agitation and thus be reassuring. It may also help to establish night and day routines to reduce sun-downing (behavioural change in individuals with dementia in the evening). E
Implement effective lighting and a clutter-free environment.	To promote patient safety (RCOT 2015). A clutter-free environment can promote independence by reducing falls risks and distractions. C
Use contrasting colours.	This may improve visual–spatial awareness and orientation (RCOT 2015), although bright colours can also be confusing. C
Install stimulating murals, gardens and therapeutic rooms (which may contain personalized photos as well as rummage and activity boxes; see Figure 5.17).	This can improve stimulation and provide a calm, therapeutic environment (NICE 2018b), as well as a place to talk or reminisce. C

(continued)

Principles table 5.16 Environmental considerations for the assessment of people with dementia *(continued)*

Principle	Rationale
Minimize patient relocation and ensure continuity and stability.	Avoid moving the patient from ward to ward unless medically essential as this will increase disorientation and may lead to deterioration in abilities (NICE 2018b). A side room is preferable, with continuity of care provider where possible. C
Establish a routine at the individual's pace and encourage independence wherever possible.	To maintain the maximum potential for independence for as long as possible to avoid deterioration (NICE 2018b, C).

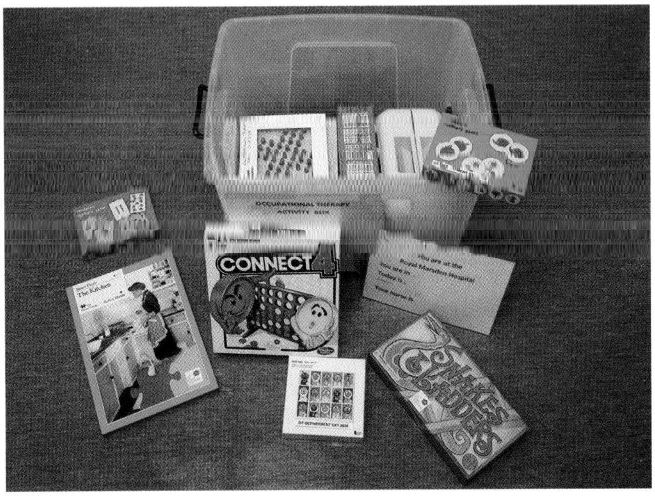

Figure 5.17 Example of an activity box.

Referring on to psychological support services

Evidence-based approaches

Many acute hospitals have in-house psychological support services. It is hoped that the prevalence of psychological services in physical health settings will increase as there is better recognition of the bidirectional relationship between physical and psychological health, and as the 'parity of esteem' principle (Health and Social Care Act 2012) is embedded in NHS services.

There are a range of psychological professionals, such as counsellors, psychologists, psychotherapists (including art, music and psychosexual therapists) and psychiatrists. All of them aim to support people in understanding and improving their psychological, or mental, health. Depending on the type of training they received, professionals will emphasize different aspects of the biopsychosocial model:

- *Psychiatrists* have initial training in medicine and prescribe psychotropic medication, so they tend to focus on the biological factors relating to a person's mental health. Some psychiatrists have completed additional training in psychotherapy and can therefore provide this.

Principles table 5.17 Supporting communication for people with dementia

Principle	Rationale
Be aware of what the patient's communication needs may be.	Knowing the patient's preferred style of communication or communication needs will enhance the patient's and nurse's experience. E
Be aware of the patient's reality, orientating them and if necessary reinforcing this throughout the care intervention.	To give the patient the best possible chance of understanding the context. E
Consider whether the patient has other communication issues.	The patient may have dementia but they may also have a hearing impairment and so they may understand what is being said but not be able to hear what is being asked. E
Consider the environment and its impact on the patient.	The patient may be distracted by the noise of a busy unit. Finding a quieter space may help the communication process. E
Avoid reinforcing a patient's reality when it is not real, and avoid telling them things that are not true.	Telling a patient that a loved one, such as a parent or spouse, has been dead for some years may be very distressing for them but so might telling them they are at home and they will see the person later. It is better to change the subject and orientate the patient to where they are. E
Patients with dementia may need constant reorientation.	Due to anxiety and poor short-term memory, patients with dementia may forget what they have been told very quickly; for instance, when a nurse is assisting with personal care or changing a dressing, the patient may need to be reminded where they are. E
Learn about the patient's past and occupation, e.g. via life story work or memory books.	It is not uncommon for patients with dementia to behave as they did when they were in employment; for instance, a cleaner may want to go around the ward cleaning. These behaviours can give the patient a sense of value but can present risks. If a nurse understands a patient's past, behaviours that are not congruent with their current environment and context can make more sense. E

Principle	Rationale
Be aware of your body language and non-verbal communication; be open and approachable and be on the patient's level.	Patients with dementia may misinterpret non-verbal communication and this can cause them to become distressed or angry. E
Use short, simple sentences and avoid providing too many choices.	Patients with dementia may not recall everything that is being said, so shorter sentences will help. Offering two choices at a time might be better than providing a long list and it can be helpful to refer to pre-existing information about the patient's preferences. E
It is better to use closed questions (such as 'Would you like a cup of tea?) rather than open questions (such as 'What drink would you like?').	Open questions can make it difficult for the person to respond, as they may struggle to remember the words they need. E
If a person with dementia is struggling to find a word, help them find a way around it.	People with dementia can become very frustrated when trying to find a word and may decide to withdraw from the conversation. E
When giving instructions to a patient with dementia, give one instruction at a time.	To help maximize the person's independence. Supporting them to do a task by helping them with the sequencing is enabling. E
Avoid interruption when a person with dementia is speaking.	Interrupting the person while they are speaking may result in them losing track of what they wanted to say and can cause frustration. E

Source: Adapted from Dementia UK (2019), Vasse et al. (2010).

- *Counsellors*, *psychologists* and *psychotherapists* tend to focus on the psychosocial factors that influence a person's mental health.

There are a range of therapy approaches, including:

- non directive and exploratory therapies (e.g. existential, psychodynamic)
- more structured therapies that teach skills and strategies (e.g. cognitive–behavioural therapy, acceptance and commitment therapy, compassion-focused therapy)
- therapies for couples or families (e.g. emotionally focused therapy for couples, systemic therapy).

It can be difficult for nurses, patients and their families to ascertain the differences between types of psychological training and therapy; the links at the end of this chapter may be useful.

Psychological therapists based in acute settings perform a number of functions. In addition to providing direct psychological interventions, psychologists, counsellors and psychotherapists have a consultative role. Thus, they can support teams to think about the psychological impact of contextual issues that may influence a patient or family member's thoughts, emotions, behaviour and choices; this can be particularly helpful when psychological therapy is not appropriate or when a patient does not consent to it. Furthermore, psychological therapists often provide training and supervision to the healthcare workforce as a way of disseminating psychological knowledge and skills. For example, within cancer services, guidelines state that one core member of each multidisciplinary team should be trained to provide Level 2 psychological support with ongoing monthly supervision to supplement this training (NICE 2004).

Similarly to physical health services, NHS mental health services are structured in a stepped-care model (NICE 2011b). In primary care, some GP practices have an in-house psychological therapist; however, most do not. Instead, primary care mental health services are embedded within the Improving Access to Psychological Therapies (IAPT) program, which started in 2008 to help people with anxiety and depression. IAPT has expanded to support people with common physical long-term conditions, including diabetes, respiratory disease, cardiac disease and medically unexplained symptoms. Most IAPT services accept GP and/or self-referrals, and tend to provide a telephone assessment to better understand the person's psychological concerns and needs. Services may include group or individual work via the telephone, online or in person. Waiting times vary from area to area.

As psychological difficulties increase in severity, people will be referred to secondary care services or to specialist tertiary services. Referrals are usually made by a GP and waiting times vary; however, there can be long waits.

It is important to note that as the NHS has reorganized itself over time, some psychological services have come to be provided by third-sector organizations, such as MIND or Relate, and by private companies. If someone is accessing a service via an NHS pathway, it will be free at the point of access regardless of the provider. When young people are affected psychologically, it may be useful to identify counselling services at school, college or university.

Safeguarding, mental capacity and the Mental Health Act

Safeguarding

Definition

The Department of Health and Social Care defines safeguarding as follows:

> Safeguarding means protecting an adult's right to live in safety, free from abuse and neglect. It is about people and organizations working together to prevent and stop both the risks and experience of abuse or neglect, while at the same time making sure that the adult's wellbeing is promoted including, where appropriate, having regard to their views, wishes, feelings and beliefs in deciding on any action. This must recognize that adults sometimes have complex interpersonal relationships and may be ambivalent, unclear or unrealistic about their personal circumstances. (DH 2018, para. 14.7)

Safeguarding duties apply to an 'adult at risk' (which has replaced the term 'vulnerable adult'), who is defined as an adult who 'has needs for care and support; is experiencing, or at risk of, abuse or neglect; and as a result of those care and support needs is unable to protect themselves from either the risk of, or the experience of abuse or neglect' (DH 2018, para. 14.2).

Similarly, safeguarding children and young people consists of action taken to 'protect children from maltreatment; prevent impairment of children's health or development', ensure children grow up 'in circumstances consistent with the provision of safe and effective care' and enable 'all children to have the best outcomes' (DfE 2018, p. 102).

Safeguarding is a key focus for all nurses, healthcare practitioners and organizations. Although this manual is for nurses working in adult contexts, it is imperative that all nurses consider safeguarding in the context of families, as they will work with adults who are in contact with children who require safeguarding.

Related theory

Types of abuse and neglect

The statutory guidance on the Care Act (2014) (DH 2018, paras. 14.17–14.33) describes different forms of abuse and neglect: physical, sexual, psychological, discriminatory, domestic and financial, as well as organizational abuse and modern slavery (Box 5.18). Further adult safeguarding concerns include female genital mutilation, forced marriage, honour-based violence, hate crime, human trafficking, sexual exploitation and mate crime (Box 5.19) (Gov.uk 2018a, 2018b).

Within the child safeguarding arena, there are four identified types of abuse and neglect: physical, psychological, sexual and neglect (DfE 2018) (Box 5.20). The London Child Protection Procedures (London Safeguarding Children Board 2017) provide guidance in relation to safeguarding children in specific circumstances, including children with disabilities and those with fabricated or induced illness (Box 5.21).

Prevalence of abuse and neglect

As abuse usually occurs in secret, it is not possible to accurately state the number of people who are abused in the UK. Abused individuals may not know that they are being abused, or may be too frightened or ashamed to tell others what they are experiencing. Further, 'observers' of abuse may not recognize the signs of abuse and therefore fail to identify and report it.

Box 5.18 Types and indicators of abuse and neglect identified in the Care Act (2014) statutory guidance (DH 2018)

Physical abuse	
Physical abuse includes assault, hitting, slapping, pushing, misuse of medication, restraint and inappropriate physical sanctions.	**Possible indicators** • Black eyes • Unexplained injuries, e.g. fractures, sprains or dislocations • Scalds and/or cigarette burns • Bruises (especially in well-protected areas) • Confusion due to oversedation
Sexual abuse	
Sexual abuse includes rape, indecent exposure, sexual harassment, inappropriate looking or touching, sexual teasing or innuendo, sexual photography, subjection to pornography or witnessing sexual acts, indecent exposure, and sexual assault or sexual acts to which the adult has not consented or was pressured into consenting.	**Possible indicators** • Changes in behaviour (e.g. more withdrawn, depressed, confused, fearful or agitated) • Difficulty in walking or sitting • Torn, bloody or stained underclothes • Pain or itching in the genital area • Bruising or bleeding in the external genitalia or the vaginal or anal areas • Sexually transmitted infections • Sexualized behaviour
Psychological abuse	
Psychological abuse includes emotional abuse, threats of harm or abandonment, deprivation of contact, humiliation, blaming, controlling, intimidation, coercion, harassment, verbal abuse, cyber bullying, isolation, and unreasonable and unjustified withdrawal from services or supportive networks.	**Possible indicators** • Fear • Passivity • Depression • Mental anguish or anxiety • Loss of independence • Behaviour that is out of character • Uncontrolled or unprovoked crying • Unusual weight loss or gain • Disturbed sleep pattern
Neglect and acts of omission	
Neglect and acts of omission include ignoring medical, emotional or physical care needs; failure to provide access to appropriate health, care and support or educational services; and withholding the necessities of life, such as medication, adequate nutrition and heating.	**Possible indicators** • Dehydration and/or malnutrition • Infections • Inadequate clothing • Pressure sores • Unexplained failure to respond to prescribed medication
Self-neglect	
Self-neglect is defined as a wide range of behaviours including neglecting to care for one's personal hygiene, health or surroundings. It includes behaviours such as hoarding.	**Possible indicators** • Poor personal hygiene and/or clothing • Dehydration and/or malnutrition • Untreated or poorly attended medical conditions • Hazardous or unsafe living conditions

Discriminatory abuse

Discriminatory abuse is discrimination on the grounds of protected characteristics (Equality Act 2010), such as race, faith or religion, age, disability, gender reassignment, sexual orientation, relationship status or pregnancy, along with racist, sexist, homophobic or ageist comments or jokes, or comments or jokes based on a person's disability or any other form of harassment, slur or similar treatment. Excluding a person from activities on the basis that they are 'not liked' is also discriminatory abuse.

Possible indicators
- Unable to eat culturally acceptable foods
- Religious observances not encouraged or anticipated
- Isolation due to language or communication barriers
- Public humiliation, such as taunts from strangers

Domestic abuse

Domestic abuse (or domestic violence) is defined as any incident or pattern of incidents of controlling, coercive or threatening behaviour, violence or abuse between individuals aged 16 or over who are or have been intimate partners or family members regardless of gender or sexuality (DH 2013a). It includes psychological, physical, sexual, financial and emotional abuse, and so-called 'honour'-based violence.

Possible indicators
- Changes in behaviour when around partner or family members
- Jealous or possessive partner
- Socially isolated, with many aspects of life controlled by the partner or family member

Financial or material abuse

Financial or material abuse includes theft; fraud; internet scamming; coercion in relation to an adult's financial affairs or arrangements, including in connection with wills, property, inheritance or financial transactions; and the misuse or misappropriation of property, possessions or benefits.

Possible indicators
- A 'disappearing' pension
- Malnutrition
- Inadequate clothing
- Insufficient money to purchase basic necessities
- Inadequate money to pay household bills
- Inadequate heating and/or lighting

Modern slavery

Modern slavery is defined as slavery, servitude and being forced into compulsory labour (Modern Slavery Act 2015). A person commits an offence if:
- they hold another person in slavery or servitude and the circumstances are such that the person knows or ought to know that the other person is held in slavery or servitude, or
- they require another person to perform forced or compulsory labour and the circumstances are such that the other person is being required to perform forced or compulsory labour.

All disclosures of modern slavery must be reported to the National Referral Mechanism by an identified first responder agency.

Possible indicators
- Neglected or abused physical appearance
- Withdrawn
- Isolated – rarely allowed to travel on their own, seem under the control or influence of others, rarely interact with others, or appear unfamiliar with their neighbourhood or where they work
- May have no identification documents, have few personal possessions and always wear the same clothes
- Restricted freedom of movement; may have had their travel documents retained

Organizational abuse

Organizational abuse includes neglect and poor care practice within an institution or specific care setting (e.g. hospital or care home) or in relation to care provided in the person's own home. This may range from one-off incidents to ongoing ill-treatment. It can occur through neglect or poor professional practice as a result of the structure, policies, processes and practices within an organization.

Possible indicators
- Poor standards of cleanliness
- Low staffing levels over a long period of time
- Low staff morale
- High staff turnover
- Lack of knowledge about care guidelines
- Lack of positive communication with adults at risk
- Punitive treatment of adults at risk

Box 5.19 Further safeguarding concerns for adults

Female genital mutilation (FGM)

FGM is any procedure that is designed to alter or injure a girl's (or woman's) genital organs for non-medical reasons. It is sometimes known as 'female circumcision' or 'female genital cutting'. It is mostly carried out on young girls. The Female Genital Mutilation Act (2003) makes it illegal to practise FGM in the UK or to take girls who are British nationals or permanent residents of the UK abroad for FGM whether or not it is lawful in another country (Gov.uk 2018b).

Forced marriage

Forced marriage is when a person faces physical (e.g. threats, physical violence or sexual violence) or psychological pressure to marry. This includes someone being taken overseas with the intention of forcing them to marry (whether or not the forced marriage takes place) and the marriage of someone who lacks the mental capacity to consent to the marriage (whether they are pressured into the marriage or not) (Gov.uk 2018a).

(continued)

Box 5.19 Further safeguarding concerns for adults *(continued)*

Honour-based violence

Honour-based violence is a crime that is committed when families feel that dishonour has been brought on them and they respond with violence. Women are predominantly (but not exclusively) the victims and the violence is often committed with a degree of collusion from family members and/or the community. Some victims contact the police or other organizations; however, some are so isolated and controlled that they are unable to seek help.

Hate crime

Hate crime is any incident that is perceived by the victim, or any other person, to be racist, homophobic, transphobic or due to a person's religion or belief, gender, identity or disability (Law Commission 2019).

Human trafficking

Human trafficking is actively used by serious and organized crime groups in order to make significant amounts of money. Traffickers exploit the social, cultural or financial vulnerability of the victim, or their family, and place large financial and ethical obligations on them. They control almost every aspect of the victim's life with little regard for the victim's welfare and health. Human trafficking is often related to modern slavery and includes trafficking internationally as well as within the UK.

Sexual exploitation

Sexual exploitation involves exploitative situations, contexts and relationships where adults at risk (or a third person or persons) receive 'something' (e.g. accommodation, affection, alcohol, cigarettes, drugs, food, gifts or money) as a result of them performing (and/or allowing another or others to perform on them) sexual activities. An example could be an adult at risk being provided with an incentive (alcohol, drugs or even a place to sleep and 'friendship') in exchange for providing sexual activity with a person or persons. It affects men as well as women. People who are sexually exploited do not always perceive that they are being exploited.

Mate crime

'Mate crime' is when a person pretends to be the friend of another person who has vulnerabilities, such as a learning disability, and then takes advantage of them (Safety Net Project 2019). It may not be an illegal act but still has a negative effect on the individual. Mate crime is often difficult for police to investigate due to its sometimes ambiguous nature, but it should be reported to the police, who will make a decision about whether or not a criminal offence has been committed. Mate crime is carried out by someone the adult knows and often happens in private.

Box 5.20 Types and indicators of child abuse

Physical abuse

Physical abuse may involve hitting, shaking, throwing, poisoning, burning or scalding, drowning, suffocating, or otherwise causing physical harm to a child.

Possible indicators

- Bruising on the head but also on the ear or neck or soft areas (the abdomen, back and buttocks)
- Bruising in non-independently mobile children
- Bruises with dots of blood under the skin
- Bruises in the shape of a hand or object
- Clusters of bruises on the upper arm, outside the thigh or on the body
- Defensive wounds commonly on the forearm, upper arm, or back of the legs, hands or feet
- Burns or scalds with inadequate explanation
- Bite marks
- Fractures to the ribs or the leg bones in babies
- Multiple fractures or breaks at different stages of healing
- Effects of poisoning such as vomiting, drowsiness or seizures
- Respiratory problems from drowning, suffocation or poisoning

Emotional or psychological abuse

Emotional abuse is the persistent emotional maltreatment of a child that causes severe and ongoing effects on the child's emotional development, and may involve:

- conveying to children that they are worthless or unloved, inadequate, or valued only insofar as they meet the needs of another person
- imposing age- or developmentally inappropriate expectations on children (e.g. interactions that are beyond the child's developmental capability, as well as overprotection and limitation of exploration and learning, or preventing the child from participating in normal social interaction)
- causing a child to see or hear the ill-treatment of another (e.g. witnessing domestic abuse)
- serious bullying, causing children frequently to feel frightened or in danger
- exploiting and corrupting children.

Some level of emotional abuse is involved in all types of maltreatment of a child, though it may occur alone.

Possible indicators

Changes in emotions are a normal part of growing up, so it can be difficult to tell whether a child is being emotionally abused. However, signs may be perceptible in a child's actions or emotions.

Babies and *pre-school children* may:

- be overly affectionate towards strangers or people they have not known for very long
- lack confidence or become wary or anxious
- not appear to have a close relationship with their parent (e.g. when being taken to or collected from nursery)
- be aggressive or nasty towards other children and animals.

Older children may:

- use language, act in a way or know about things that would not be expected at their age
- struggle to control strong emotions or have extreme outbursts
- seem isolated from their parents
- lack social skills or have few, if any, friends.

Sexual abuse

Sexual abuse involves forcing or enticing a child or young person to take part in sexual activities (not necessarily involving a high level of violence), whether or not the child is aware of what is happening. The activities may involve physical contact, including assault by penetration (e.g. rape or oral sex) or non-penetrative acts (e.g. masturbation, kissing, rubbing or touching outside clothing). Sexual abuse includes non-contact activities, such as children looking at (including online) or being involved in the production of pornographic materials; children watching sexual activities; encouraging children to behave in sexually inappropriate ways; or grooming a child in preparation for abuse (including via the internet). In addition, sexual abuse includes abuse of children through sexual exploitation.

Possible indicators

Staying away from certain people:
- They might avoid being alone with people, such as family members or friends.
- They could seem frightened of a person or reluctant to socialize with them.

Showing sexual behaviour that is inappropriate for their age:
- A child might become sexually active at a young age.
- They might be promiscuous.
- They could use sexual language or know information that wouldn't be expected.

Physical symptoms:
- anal or vaginal soreness
- an unusual discharge
- sexually transmitted infection (STI)
- pregnancy.

Neglect

Neglect is the persistent failure to meet a child's basic physical and/or psychological needs. It is likely to result in serious impairment of the child's health or development. Neglect may occur during pregnancy as a result of maternal substance misuse, maternal mental ill health or learning difficulties, or a cluster of such issues. Where there is domestic abuse and violence towards a carer, the needs of the child may be neglected. Once a child is born, neglect may involve a parent failing to:
- provide adequate food, clothing and shelter (including exclusion from home or abandonment)
- protect a child from physical and emotional harm or danger
- ensure adequate supervision (including the use of inadequate care-givers)
- ensure access to appropriate medical care or treatment.

It may also include neglect of, or unresponsiveness to, a child's basic emotional, social and educational needs.

Possible indicators

Poor appearance and hygiene. They may:
- be smelly or dirty
- have unwashed clothes
- have inadequate clothing, e.g. not having a winter coat
- seem hungry or turn up to school without having breakfast or lunch money
- have frequent and untreated nappy rash (in infants).

Health and development problems. They may:
- have untreated injuries, medical issues and/or dental issues
- have repeated accidental injuries caused by lack of supervision
- have recurring illnesses or infections
- have not been given appropriate medicines
- have missed medical appointments such as vaccinations
- have poor muscle tone or prominent joints
- have skin sores, rashes, flea bites, scabies or ringworm
- have a thin or swollen tummy
- have anaemia
- have tiredness
- have faltering weight or growth and not reach developmental milestones
- have poor language, communication or social skills.

Housing and family issues. They may:
- live in an unsuitable home environment (e.g. presence of dog faeces or a lack of heating)
- be left alone for a long time.

Source: Adapted from DfE (2018).

Box 5.21 Specific child safeguarding risks

Children with disabilities

Any child with a disability is by definition a 'child in need' under Section 17 of the Children's Act (1989). The available UK evidence on the extent of abuse among disabled children suggests that disabled children are at increased risk of abuse and that the presence of multiple disabilities appears to increase the risks of both abuse and neglect.

Specific risks

Looked-after disabled children are not only vulnerable to the same factors that exist for all children living away from home but are also particularly susceptible to abuse because of their additional dependency on residential and hospital staff for day-to-day physical care needs. Specific risks include:
- force feeding
- unjustified or excessive physical restraint
- rough handling
- extreme behaviour modification, including the deprivation of liquid, medication, food or clothing

(continued)

Box 5.31 Specific child safeguarding risks *(continued)*

	• misuse of medication, sedation or heavy tranquillization • invasive procedures carried out against the child's will • deliberate failure to follow medically recommended regimes • misapplication of programmes or regimes • ill-fitting equipment (e.g. callipers, a sleep board that causes injury or pain, or inappropriate splinting) • undignified intimate care practices that are inappropriate to the child's age or culture.
Fabricated or induced illness	
Fabricated or induced illness is a condition where a child has suffered, or is likely to suffer, significant harm through the deliberate action of their parent and that is attributed by the parent to another cause. There are three main ways of a parent fabricating or inducing illness in a child: • fabrication of signs and symptoms, including fabrication of past medical history • fabrication of signs and symptoms and falsification of hospital charts, records, letters and documents, and specimens of body fluid • induction of illness by a variety of means.	**Possible indicators** • Reported symptoms and signs found on examination are not explained by any 'normal' medical condition • Physical examination and results of investigations do not explain the reported symptoms and signs • New symptoms are reported on resolution of previous ones • Reported symptoms and identified signs are not observed in the absence of the parent • The child's normal daily life activities are being curtailed beyond that which may be expected from any medical disorder from which the child is known to suffer • Treatment for an agreed condition does not produce the expected effects • Repeated presentations to a variety of doctors and with a variety of problems • The child denies parental reports of symptoms • Specific problems (e.g. apnoea, fits, choking or collapse) • Child becomes drawn into the parent's illness • History of unexplained illnesses or deaths, or multiple surgery in parents or siblings of the family • A past history in the parent of child abuse, self-harm or somatizing, or false allegations of physical or sexual assault

Source: Adapted from the London Child Protection Procedures (2017).

Nonetheless, there are a number of sources of data that can be drawn upon to provide a sketch of the level of abuse, for example, government (Figure 5.18), social services and charities such as the NSPCC (Figure 5.19). It is accepted that actual levels of abuse and neglect are higher than the number of reported incidents.

Contextual safeguarding

People are usually abused by someone they know, for example a spouse, parent or other family member, as well as friends, neighbours, professionals and volunteers. This is not to say that strangers cannot be the perpetrators of abuse. Neglect, by definition, can only be carried out by someone who has a personal or professional relationship with the neglected person. Extra-familial threats can arise in educational, work or healthcare establishments; from within peer groups; or from the wider community (including online). Thus, nursing assessments must include an awareness and understanding of the context in which a child or adult exists to enable them to prevent and manage safeguarding risks.

Evidence-based approaches

Rationale

Safeguarding aims to protect people from harm and abuse while concurrently promoting individual (and thereby societal) wellbeing so that everybody can live a healthy life to their fullest potential.

Government safeguarding principles

Government and healthcare guidance includes safeguarding principles that underscore the need for relevant systems to be

Key Facts

394,655 concerns of abuse were raised during 2017–18, an increase of 8.2% on the previous year.

There were 150,070 safeguarding enquiries that started in the year, a decrease of 1,090 (0.7%) on 2016–17.

The number of Section 42 enquiries that commenced during the year fell by 1.1% to 131,860 and involved 107,550 individuals. The number of Other enquiries increased by 1.8% to 18,210 during the same period.

Older people are much more likely to be the subject of a Section 42 safeguarding enquiry; one in every 43 adults aged 85 and above, compared to one in every 862 adults aged 18–64.

The most common type of risk identified in Section 42 enquiries was Neglect and Acts of Omission, which accounted for 32.1% of risks, and most commonly took place in the person's own home (43.5%). In 68.5% of Section 42 enquiries a risk was identified and action was taken.

Figure 5.18 Findings from the *Safeguarding Adults Collection* for 1 April 2017 to 31 March 2018. *Source*: NHS Digital (2018).

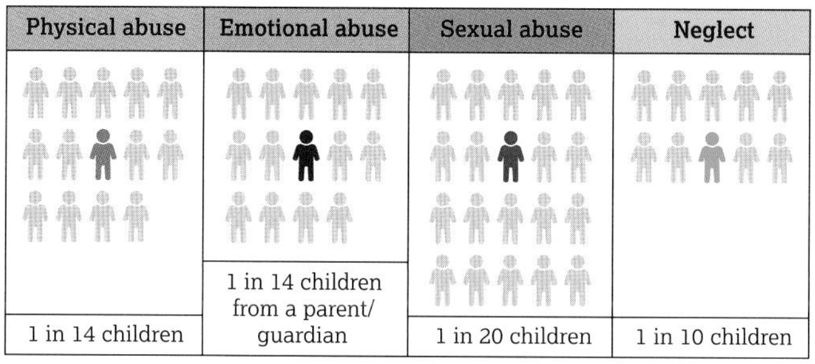
Physical abuse
Emotional abuse
Sexual abuse
Neglect
1 in 14 children
1 in 14 children from a parent/ guardian
1 in 20 children
1 in 10 children

Figure 5.19 Prevalence of child abuse and neglect. *Source*: Bentley et al. (2018).

developed and applied in a robust and appropriate manner. When nurses adhere to the principles outlined below, they can provide an appropriate and personalized approach to safeguarding.

The Care Act (2014) and statutory guidance (DH 2018) define six key principles that underpin all adult safeguarding work. These are the prevention of abuse and neglect, the empowerment and protection of people, the delivery of accountable and proportionate safeguarding responses, and partnership work with other agencies (Table 5.3). These principles are embraced by the nursing profession, which clearly states that safeguarding is a core component of the nursing role:

> You put the interests of people using or needing nursing or midwifery first. You make their care and safety your main concern and make sure that their dignity is preserved and their needs are recognised, assessed and responded to. You make sure that those receiving care are treated with respect, that their rights are upheld and that any discriminatory attitudes and behaviours towards those receiving care are challenged. (NMC 2018, p.6)

The Royal College of Nursing more specifically states that nurses must take both individual and collective responsibility to safeguard others:

> Safeguarding is everyone's responsibility; for services to be effective each professional and organisation should play their full part [and] professionals and organisations must work in partnership to protect children and adults in need. (RCN n.d.)

The concept 'making safeguarding personal' (MSP) (LGA 2018) is an important approach to adult safeguarding that encourages all staff to take personal responsibility for safeguarding patients and their families. This approach was implemented to end a culture of passing safeguarding concerns and responsibilities to others. Thus, MSP encourages staff to see themselves as key to both raising concerns and to implementing appropriate safeguarding responses. Nurses need to have conversations *with* patients that enhance patient involvement, choice and control as well as improving quality of life, wellbeing and safety. MSP frames people as experts in their own lives and supports staff to work alongside them to enable them to reach a better resolution of their circumstances and recovery.

Partnership working

While it is parents and carers who have primary care for their children, local authorities, working with partner organizations and agencies, have specific duties to safeguard and promote the welfare of all children in their area. Local authorities have statutory responsibility for adults in their area. Local authorities can only do their job effectively if there is appropriate partnership work between health, social care and other key support agencies. Co-operation between agencies is important to reduce the risk of cases slipping through the safeguarding system and stopping abuse at an early stage or preventing it from happening in the first place.

In order for organizations, agencies and practitioners to collaborate effectively, it is vital that nurses working with adults, children and families understand the role they should play and the roles of other practitioners (Box 5.22). Nurses should be aware of, and comply with, the published arrangements set out by their local safeguarding partners.

A different form of partnership working is with the families or carers of patients. Families and carers have a wealth of information and knowledge about the person that they care for and support. As well as raising concerns, families and carers are able to support safeguarding enquiries through sharing important information. If a family member or carer speaks up about abuse or neglect, it is

Table 5.3 Safeguarding principles as outlined in the Care and Support Statutory Guidance

Principle	Description	Example
Prevention	Strategies are developed to prevent abuse and neglect that promote resilience and self-determination.	I provide my patients with easily understood information about what abuse is, how to recognize it and what they can do to seek help.
Empowerment	Adults are provided with support, information and encouragement to make their own decisions. This is particularly pertinent in healthcare, as people are often asked to hand over control and power to professionals.	I ensure that my patients are sufficiently informed and consulted about the outcomes they want from the safeguarding process and these directly inform what happens.
Protection	Adults are offered ways to protect themselves, and there is a co-ordinated response to adult safeguarding.	I provide my patients with help and support to report abuse and to take part in the safeguarding process to the extent to which they want and are able.
Proportionate	Safeguarding responses will be the least restrictive possible and appropriate to the risk(s) identified and their context.	I will only get involved as much as is needed and will provide advice and support to my patients consisting of suitable options related to the identified concerns.
Accountable	Accountability and transparency are employed in delivering a safeguarding response.	I ensure that the patient and all those involved in the patient's life understand their roles and responsibilities.
Partnerships	Local solutions are provided through services working together within their communities.	I ensure patient information is appropriately shared in a way that takes into account its personal and sensitive nature and will work with agencies to find the most effective responses to the situation.

Source: Adapted from ADASS (2013, p.13).

Box 5.22 The nurse's safeguarding roles and responsibilities in partnership with colleagues and organizations

Nurse roles and responsibilities

- Nurses must be aware of the signs of abuse and neglect and keep people safe.
- Nurses can escalate their safeguarding concerns by raising these with the patient (unless this might increase the risk of harm), their line manager and their organization's safeguarding team.
- Nurses must clearly and accurately document any signs of abuse and neglect as well as their actions, the actions of others, and the patient's response and wishes.

Safeguarding lead

- All hospitals must have a named safeguarding lead who is responsible for:
  - ensuring the organization has safeguarding policies and procedures in place and has a programme of training
  - consulting with hospital staff so that all employees within the organization can fulfil their own safeguarding responsibilities – it is rare that the safeguarding lead will have direct contact with a patient.
- If a safeguarding allegation is made against a staff member, the safeguarding lead may have direct contact with the patient.
- The safeguarding lead will help staff to escalate safeguarding concerns to a local authority and may continue to liaise with the local authority regarding their response.

Local authority

- Local authority structures vary and not all have safeguarding teams. However, all local authorities have social workers, who will lead the response to a safeguarding enquiry.
- A local authority social worker will screen a safeguarding concern or referral reported on the telephone or by email.
- Nurses can expect to receive a telephone call from the local authority to discuss immediate risks and safety concerns, and to seek clarity or further information (e.g. contextual information such as medical or social factors and needs). The urgency of the return call will depend on the nature of the safeguarding concern.
- Nurses may be invited to attend a case conference. The timing of these varies according to the urgency of the concern reported.
- When a concern is escalated to the local authority, it will contact the person reportedly at risk to better understand the concerns and risks and to identify their preferred outcome of any intervention.
- With respect to a child safeguarding concern, the local authority will normally contact the parents or carers; however, they may not do this if they feel this would increase the level of risk. Additionally, they may approach young people away from home (e.g. at school) to discuss the concerns raised with them away from family members.
- When nurses are advised to liaise with a local authority by their safeguarding lead, nurses need to both share their safeguarding concerns with the relevant local authority and work with it to formulate and implement an appropriate safeguarding response.
- Safeguarding responses may include ongoing monitoring, engaging in multi-agency meetings and taking the lead on a safeguarding intervention (as the nurse may know the patient better than others).

essential that they are listened to and appropriate enquiries are made. Families and carers can identify and mitigate risks as well as advocate for patients. Staff should also be vigilant to recognize the signs of carer stress and potential unintentional neglect; staff must address these directly with carers and discuss key agencies that can provide support.

Section 44 of the Care Act (2014) stipulates that local authorities must conduct a safeguarding adults review (SAR) when an adult in its area with care and support needs has experienced significant harm from, or dies as a result of, abuse or neglect (whether known or suspected) and when there is a concern that partner agencies could have worked more effectively to protect the adult. The purposes of a SAR are to identify lessons to be learned from the case, to apply those lessons to future cases, and to improve how agencies work both independently and together to safeguard adults at risk. Nurses may be asked to contribute to a SAR by providing evidence and/or to participate in learning events following a SAR so that lessons learned can be embedded in health and social care practice.

A thematic review of 27 SARs completed in London identified key lessons (Braye and Preston-Shoot 2017) (Figure 5.20). These included the need to consider risk assessment as a process (rather than a one-off event) that is carried out in a person-centred manner. Thus, nurses need to engage with the person at risk (and others in their system as appropriate) to elicit the history of any concerns and the person's wishes and views about these concerns and needs, bearing in mind that these may differ from the nurse's own view. Moreover, the review identified a need for services to more proficiently assess mental capacity, and, where this is deemed to be lacking, to engage in best interests decision making that incorporates the family's and/or carer's information. Furthermore, the review identified that staff need to report their concerns about services providing substandard care.

The NSPCC (2015) examined a series of safeguarding children reviews and reported a number of consistent errors, including overreliance on parental reporting and a reluctance to challenge parents' views, a failure to flag up missed appointments, uncertainty about how to escalate safeguarding concerns, and inadequate information sharing.

Clinical governance

Confidentiality and information sharing

People have the right to expect that information shared with a nurse will be treated as confidential. However, nurses must make it clear to patients at the beginning of conversations that when they are concerned about the patient's (or another person's) welfare, they have a professional duty to share the information with someone who is in a position to take action, for example a line manager. When a nurse is concerned about safety it is important to discuss with the patient the rationale for sharing information, and how and with whom that information will be shared. Furthermore, the nurse must explain to the patient that they will record their views and wishes about what they want to happen so that these can be taken into account in so far as is possible. There may be times when it is unsafe for a nurse to share their safeguarding concerns with a patient – for example, when the nurse suspects that the patient may feel compelled to tell the alleged perpetrator due to high levels of control and coercion.

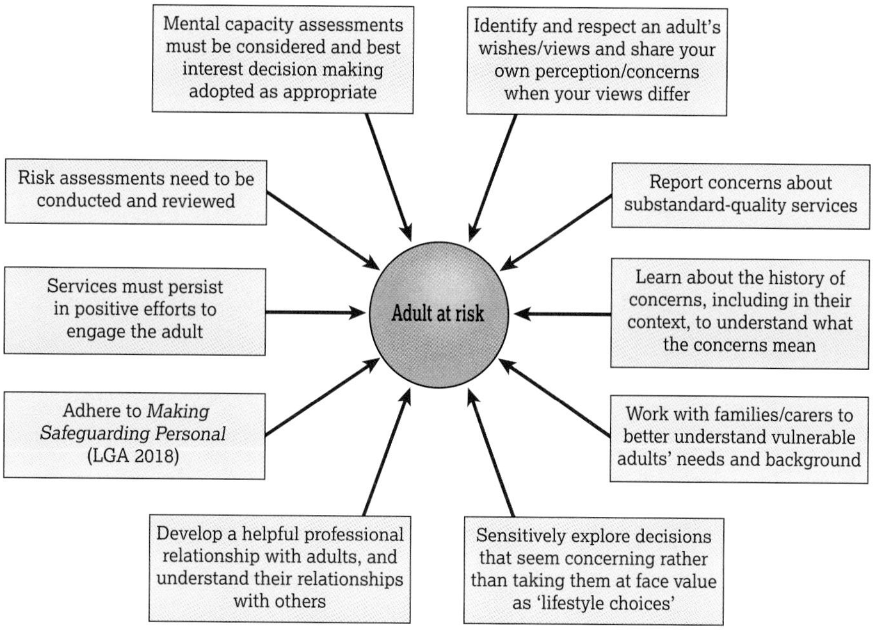

Figure 5.20 Key lessons from safeguarding adults reviews. *Source*: Adapted from Braye and Preston-Shoot (2017).

Sharing the right patient information at the right time with the right professionals is a fundamental part of safeguarding practice. Nurses can be ambivalent about sharing patient information within and between organizations for fear of breaching confidentiality or data protection guidance. However, sharing information in relation to day-to-day safeguarding practice is covered within common-law duty of confidentiality, Crime and Disorder Act (1998), the Human Rights Act (1998), the Care Act (2014) and the General Data Protection Regulation (GDPR) (2018) (Box 5.23). It is important to record on the patient's notes the decision to share, or not, information and the reasons for this decision.

Legal guidance

Some legislation pertinent to safeguarding is only applicable to individual parts of the UK. It is important that nurses familiarize themselves with legislation, guidance and policy that is applicable in the country where they work. Acts of Parliament and guidance that form the legal framework for safeguarding adults are detailed in Box 5.24.

Principles of safeguarding

All nurses will experience times when the behaviour they witness or that has been reported to them raises safeguarding concerns. On

Box 5.23 Myth-busting guide to information sharing for safeguarding purposes

Sharing information enables practitioners and agencies to identify and provide appropriate services that safeguard and promote the welfare of children and adults at risk. Below are common myths that may hinder effective information sharing.

1. Data protection legislation and the Human Rights Act (1998) are barriers to sharing information

No. Legislation does not stop nurses from collecting and sharing patient personal information. Nurses need to balance the common-law duty of confidence and the Human Rights Act (1998) against the effect on individuals or others of not sharing the information. Data protection law provides a framework to make sure that any personal information is shared appropriately.

2. Consent is always needed to share personal information

No. It is good practice to let a patient know the boundaries of confidentiality. For example, at the start of a conversation, let the patient know that if they share information with you that leads you to be concerned about their, or someone else's, safety, then you may need to share that information to keep people safe.

There are circumstances where it is not appropriate to seek consent: because the individual cannot give it, because it is not reasonable to obtain consent or because to gain consent would put a person's safety at risk.

When you do ask for someone's consent to share information that is not related to safety, then they need to provide this consent freely. It is good practice to have written evidence of their consent; however, it is not essential.

3. IT systems are a barrier to effective information sharing

No. IT systems, such as the Child Protection – Information Sharing (CP-IS) project and NHS Spine, can be useful for information sharing. IT systems are most valuable when practitioners use the shared data to make more informed decisions about how to support and safeguard a child or vulnerable adult.

Source: Adapted from DfE (2018, p.18).

Box 5.24 Key Acts of Parliament for safeguarding adults and children

Care Act (2014)

The Care Act (2014) and associated statutory guidance are applicable to England only (DH 2018). They provide a statutory framework and legal footing for safeguarding adults, and give guidance to professionals about how to work in partnership to support, protect and reduce the risk to adults at risk. Under the Care Act (2014), statutory safeguarding adults duties apply to any adult at risk who:

- has care and support needs, and
- is experiencing, or is at risk of, abuse or neglect, and
- is unable to protect themselves from either the risk or the experience of abuse or neglect, because of those needs.

When concerns are identified, professionals must seek the patient's consent and consider their mental capacity. Concerns should only be shared without the patient's consent where there are identified vital or public interests in relation to the concerns raised. These may include significant risk to a vulnerable person or risk to other people.

In other parts of the UK, the following safeguarding legislation applies:

- Northern Ireland: Safeguarding Vulnerable Groups Order (2007)
- Scotland: Adult Support and Protection Act (2007)
- Wales: Social Services and Well-being Act (2014).

Mental Capacity Act (2005)

The Mental Capacity Act (2005) provides a framework for assessing a person's capacity to make decisions about health and social care. The Deprivation of Liberty Safeguards (DoLS) (DH 2009c) are an amendment to the MCA (2005). Both the MCA and the DoLS are discussed in detail later in this section.

Human Rights Act (1998)

The Human Rights Act (1998) affords specific rights to all people living in the UK, such as the right to life, the right to liberty and freedom, and the right to be treated equally (without discrimination).

Equality Act (2010)

The Equality Act (2010) aims to provide people with legal protection from 'discrimination in the workplace and wider society'. The act includes the 'equality duty', which outlines the responsibilities of public sector organizations, including the provision of NHS services. The act defines nine groups of characteristics upon which people cannot be discriminated against: age, disability, gender reassignment, marriage and civil partnership, pregnancy and maternity, race, religion or belief, sex, and sexual orientation.

Counter Terrorism and Security Act (2015)

The Counter Terrorism and Security Act (2015) requires specified authorities to have due regard to the need to prevent people being drawn into terrorism. The government's counter-terrorism strategy CONTEST outlines four key areas, including PREVENT. PREVENT aims to safeguard and support people vulnerable to radicalization so that they do not become terrorists or support terrorism in the pre-criminal space. PREVENT works by identifying vulnerabilities that might make people susceptible to being radicalized and ensures appropriate referral to local channel panels, so that a multi-agency approach can be agreed to support and safeguard vulnerable people (HM Government 2018).

Safeguarding of children

Legislation pertinent to the safeguarding of children includes the Children's Act (1989, 2004), the Children and Social Work Act (2017) and *Working Together to Safeguard Children* (DfE 2018).

these occasions, nurses must adhere to local policies and procedures, which will cover the recognition of abuse and neglect, how to make the individual(s) safe, how to escalate concerns and what to document. Safeguarding concerns may or may not lead to a safeguarding referral (Figure 5.21). It can be helpful for nurses to speak to their manager and their institution's safeguarding team for guidance.

Mental Capacity Act (2005)

Definition

A person is judged to have mental capacity if they can understand and retain information for long enough to consider its meaning and merits and can then communicate their decision to others.

Related theory

In order to protect people who are deemed to lack capacity and to enable them in so far as is possible to be a part of their health-related decision making, the following statutory principles apply:

- Nurses must assume a person has capacity unless it is proved otherwise.
- Nurses must take all practicable steps to help patients to make their own decisions.
- Nurses must not assume incapacity simply because someone makes what the nurse and others consider to be an unwise decision.
- Nurses must act in the best interests of people who are deemed to lack capacity.
- Nurses must carefully consider which actions to take to ensure the least restrictive option is implemented.

Within the environment of a busy hospital, emergencies can be challenging to manage. The nature of the emergency may be such that there is insufficient time to conduct all necessary investigations and to consult with all the relevant people; as a result, there is the potential for capacity to be misjudged. The Mental Capacity Act (2005) states that in these situations, when a nurse or other healthcare professional has acted in the best interests of the patient, they will not be liable for that decision and the following actions. These actions can include restraint if it is judged to be proportionate and necessary to prevent harm (Section 6), and even 'a deprivation of liberty' if this is necessary for 'life sustaining treatment or a vital act' while a court order is sought if need be (Section 4B).

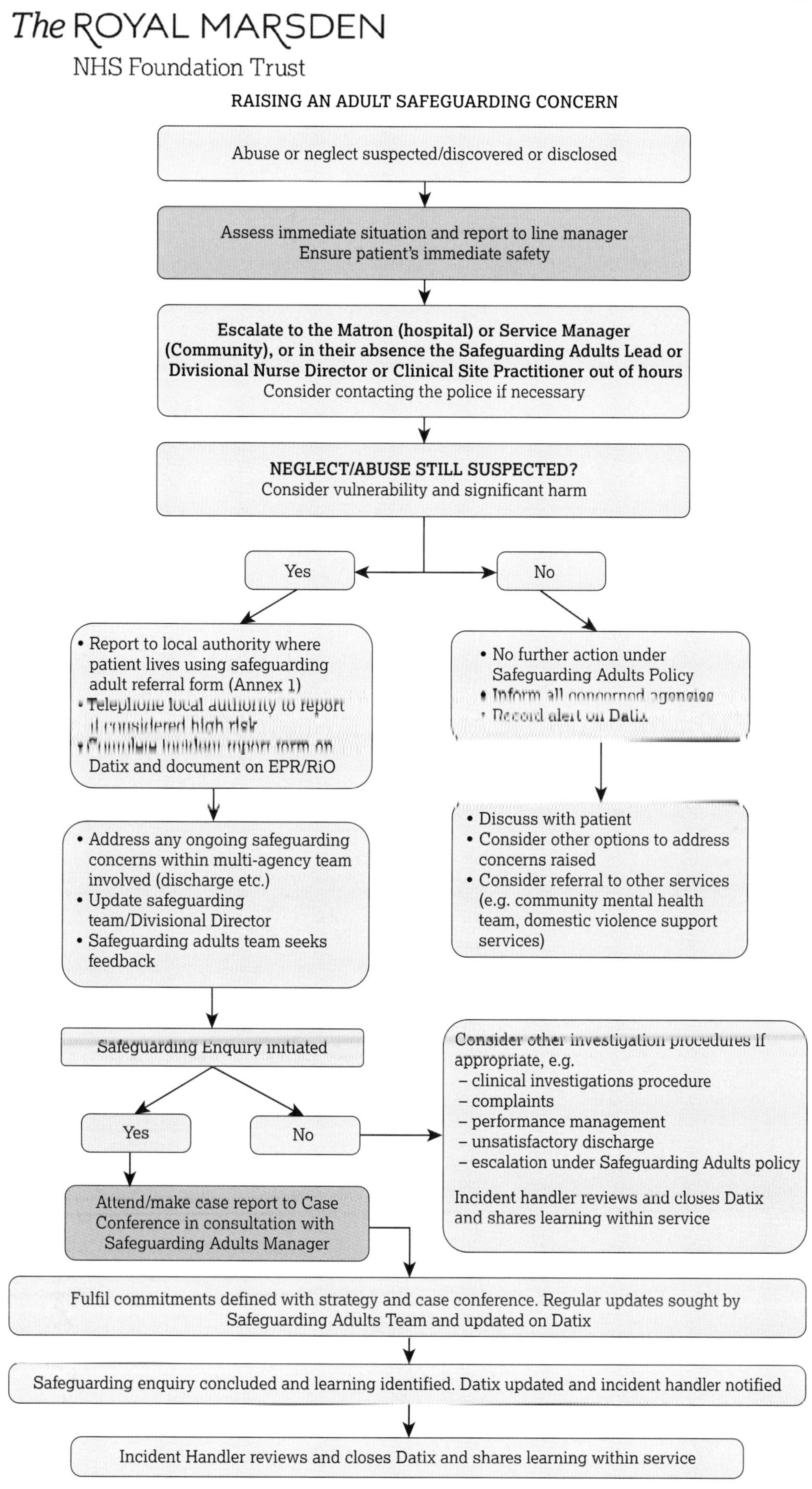

Figure 5.21 Example of a safeguarding protocol. *Source:* Reproduced with permission of the Royal Marsden NHS Foundation Trust.

Principles table 5.18 Responding to safeguarding concerns

Principle	Rationale
Recognition	
Attend safeguarding training so that the signs of abuse and neglect are recognized across biological, psychological and social domains.	Early recognition of people who are at risk of, or experiencing, abuse or neglect is essential for protection (Care Act 2014, C).
Base your assessment of safeguarding concerns within the legal framework and organizational policies and procedures. Ask your manager and safeguarding team for guidance.	The Care Act (2014) provides a legal framework for safeguarding adults. C
Use effective communication skills during safeguarding conversations.	Discussions about safeguarding concerns can be anxiety provoking; thus, nurses need to use their communication skills to establish rapport and carry out a high-quality assessment. E
Engage the patient in a person-centred conversation that enables them to fully express their concerns and needs as well as their wishes and preferences for any outcomes.	You must do everything you can to ensure that the patient is able to engage as fully as possible in the safeguarding processes (LGA 2018, C).
Consider the patient within their social system and the potential risk (or protective) factors in relation to others, for example children or older adults.	The person at risk does not exist in isolation (LGA 2018, C).
Do not ask probing or leading questions that may affect the credibility of the evidence.	The nurse's role is not to investigate the situation but to gain sufficient information to ascertain whether the patient is safe or not, and if or how to escalate the safeguarding concern.
Be open and honest and do not promise to keep a secret.	The nurse's role is to keep people safe, not to keep information (Care Act 2014, C).
Immediate safety	
When the risk of harm is assessed as high, it may be necessary to quickly implement a safety plan.	To take the necessary steps to avoid harm (Care Act 2014, C).
Link with managers and the safeguarding team for guidance on the development of a safety plan.	Nurses are not expected to work in isolation. Use the resources and support systems available to you (ADASS 2015, C).
Interventions need to be proportionate to the risk identified.	It is important that safeguarding responses are the least restrictive possible and appropriate to the risk(s) identified and their context (Care Act 2014, C).
Identify whether there are reasons to act without the patient's consent – for example, where others are at risk, where there is a need to address a service failure that might affect others, or where there are any concerns for children or young people.	Nurses have a duty to protect individuals and the public and do not need consent to share information in these circumstances (Common-law duty of confidentiality, Care Act 2014, Crime and Disorder Act 1998, GDPR 2018, Human Rights Act 1998, C).
If a crime has been committed (e.g. in cases of domestic abuse), the police need to be informed. Note that the police will intervene and they may press charges, but the prosecution may collapse if the person at risk does not want to co-operate with an investigation.	Nurses need to follow the law (Care Act 2014, Female Genital Mutilation Act 2003, C).
Preserve evidence that may be required. This includes securing any patient records and notes to prevent tampering, and considering forensic requirements (e.g. medical examination).	It is important that first responders preserve forensic evidence in situations that may result in criminal or civil charges. E
Escalation	
Consider whether it is safe to tell the person that you have safeguarding concerns.	Some patients may feel compelled by a perpetrator of abuse or neglect to share that a safeguarding concern has been raised and this may put them in increased danger. E
Share information without consent if it is in the vital or public protection interest in order to prevent a crime or protect others from harm (follow your own organization's policy and procedures).	All healthcare professionals have a duty of care to protect the patient and others who may be at risk (Care Act 2014, C).
It is prudent to discuss with appropriate others (e.g. manager, safeguarding team, external organizations) what information has been elicited and your decision-making process.	Local authorities have a statutory responsibility for adults in their area (Care Act 2014, C). A lack of information sharing is repeatedly found in safeguarding children reviews (Braye and Preston-Shoot 2017, R).
Make a clear and concise referral so that the person reading the form understands the key issues.	This makes it easy for the person reading the referral to understand what is happening and to consider how to respond. E
Consider the needs of any other people for whom the patient may have caring responsibilities (e.g. children, older adults).	The person at risk does not exist in isolation (LGA 2018, C).

Principle	Rationale
Consider mental capacity, best interests decision making and deprivation of liberty safeguards.	If a patient has capacity in relation to safeguarding decision making and they, or others, are not at imminent danger and a crime has not been committed, they have the right for their information not to be shared. If the person is deemed to lack capacity, then best interests decisions must be made (Care Act 2014, Mental Capacity Act 2005, C).
If the person is unable to advocate for themselves, ensure that someone else can do this for them, such as the Independent Mental Capacity Advocate.	The Mental Capacity Act makes provision for people to have access to independent advocates to ensure that their interests are met (Mental Capacity Act 2005, C).
Do not delay unnecessarily.	Delays in responsiveness and action may increase a person's danger. E
Concerns about a colleague should be raised internally through your organization's policies on managing allegations against staff or whistleblowing.	Whistleblowers are given protection under the Public Interest Disclosure Act (1998, C).
Documentation	
Make comprehensive, accurate and factual, legible and timely notes in the patient's record; these must include the views and hopes of the adult at risk. Explain the basis of your actions or inaction.	You are accountable for your actions and omissions and must therefore document the rationale behind your decision making (Care Act 2014, C).

Source: Adapted from NHS England North (2017).

Clinical governance

The Mental Capacity Act (2005) and the Mental Capacity Act Code of Practice (2005) apply to people aged 16 years or older in England and Wales. Nurses must have due regard for the legislation and statutory guidance and apply this appropriately in their practice.

Pre-procedural considerations

The Mental Capacity Act (2005) provided the legal framework for the creation of the Independent Mental Capacity Advocate (IMCA). The IMCA helps vulnerable people who lack capacity and are facing important decisions, including serious healthcare treatment decisions, and who have nobody to speak for them. Local IMCA services and organization safeguarding leads can advise when the involvement of the IMCA may be appropriate, for example when a patient who lacks capacity has no appropriate person to speak on their behalf with respect to a serious medical treatment or a change in accommodation.

It is prudent to identify patients who lack capacity, or who are likely to lack capacity in the future, and ascertain whether they have communicated or delegated their decision making in advance. Declarations (some of which are legally binding and some of which are not) can inform best interests decisions and care plans (Box 5.25).

Box 5.25 Processes for communicating or delegating decision making when a person lacks capacity

- A *lasting power of attorney* (LPA) is a person who is legally nominated (and accepts this nomination) by a patient to make decisions on their behalf if they are assessed as lacking capacity. An LPA can be nominated for finances and property, and/or health and welfare (Mental Capacity Act 2005).
- An *advance decision to refuse treatment* (or 'living will') is a legally binding written statement declaring that certain medical treatments in certain situations are to be refused. This information instructs health and social care staff, as well as family, when a person subsequently lacks capacity and is unable to make their own decisions (Mental Capacity Act 2005).
- An *advance statement* is a written statement that outlines a person's wishes and preferences for future health and social care decisions, to help others make decisions on their behalf if they do not have the capacity to make those decisions. An advance statement is not legally binding.

Principles of mental capacity assessment

Assessment of capacity involves a two-stage test (Figure 5.22). Before assessing a person's capacity to make a decision, it is important to be clear about what decision the patient is required to make, so that the capacity decision is specific. Capacity is a fluctuating state and must therefore be assessed each time a decision is made:

- The *first test of capacity* is whether or not a person has an impairment of the mind or brain (e.g. a mental 'illness', dementia or learning disability).
- The *second test of capacity* is whether or not they are able to understand, retain and weigh up information required to make a decision and to then communicate that decision.

If someone is assessed as lacking capacity and is therefore unable to consent to or refuse a medical test or treatment, then nurses and their colleagues need to act in the patient's best interests. This is best achieved by working with the patient, other healthcare staff and, where applicable and appropriate, the patient's carers (Box 5.26).

Post-procedural considerations

Following an assessment of capacity and any best interest decisions, nurses must consider the tasks of confidentiality, communication, record keeping (Box 5.27) and reporting. Nurses must follow local policies and procedures, and seek guidance from their manager as appropriate.

Deprivation of Liberty Safeguards (2009)

Definition

When a person has liberty, they have the freedom to do something. When a person does not have the freedom to act, regardless of whether or not they want to act, they have been deprived of their liberty. The Deprivation of Liberty Safeguards (DoLS) is a set of safeguards designed to protect people from being deprived of their liberty in the context of healthcare (DH 2009c).

Related theory

UK citizens are legally entitled to liberty and freedom, as enshrined in the Human Rights Act (1998). However, some medical treatments deprive a person of their liberty (e.g. sedation and restraint). Some patients may consent to this, having weighed up

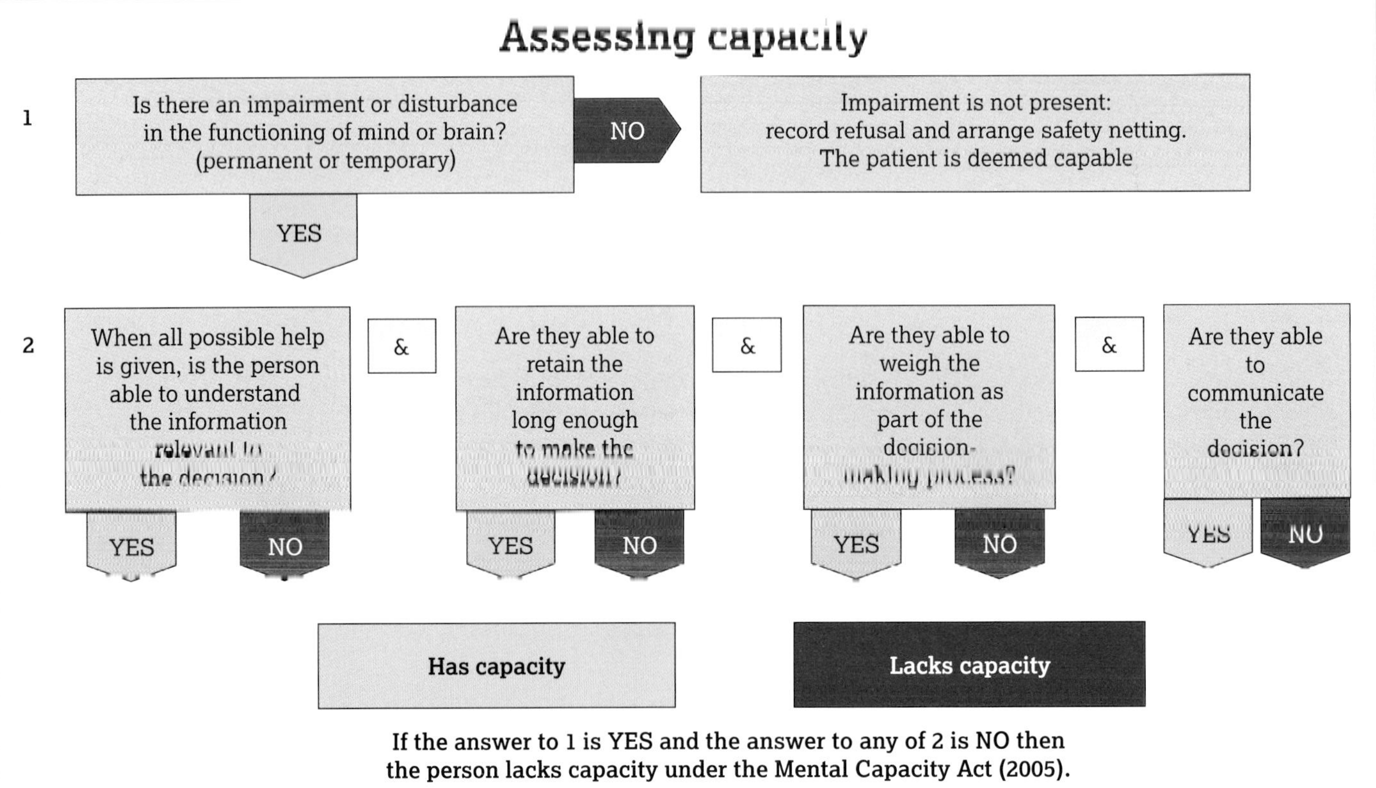

Figure 5.22 Assessing capacity. *Source*: Reproduced from NHS England North (2017) with permission of NHS England.

Box 5.26 Making a best interests decision

When a person is assessed as lacking the capacity to make a specific decision, nurses have a duty of care to support the healthcare team to act in the patient's best interests. To make a best interest decision:

- Do not make assumptions about the person's capacity and what they want based on their age, appearance, condition or diagnosis.
- Consider whether the person will in the future have capacity in relation to the matter in question and continue to assess their capacity.
- Encourage the person to participate as fully as possible in any decision making.
- Consider the person's past and present beliefs, values, wishes and feelings so that decisions made will be respectful of their worldview.
- Consider the views of others who may know the patient well, for example carers, relatives, friends and advocates.
- Consider the pros and cons of any options both in the short term and in the longer term.
- Select the least restrictive option.

Source: Adapted from NHS England North (2017).

the advantages and disadvantages of the treatment. However, when a person does not have the capacity to consent to medical treatment, a best interests decision is made, which may deprive that person of their liberty.

The DoLS (DH 2009c) apply where *all* of the following are true:

- The person lacks capacity to consent to the care or treatment they receive.
- The person is over 18 years of age.
- The person is receiving care in a hospital or a care home setting.
- The care the person receives deprives them of their liberty.
- The person is not detained under the Mental Health Act (1983, 2007) for treatment to which the deprivation relates.

DoLS also apply to people resident in other settings where care is funded by a statutory health body or local authority. In other settings, a deprivation of liberty can be authorized by the Court of Protection.

The test of deprivation of liberty has been revised into an 'acid test' by the Supreme Court as follows:

> The person is under continuous supervision AND control AND is not free to leave. (*P v Cheshire West and Chester Council* 2014)

Every element of this must be satisfied i.e.

- continuous
- supervision
- control
- not free to leave.

The patient might not attempt to leave. However, if they did try to leave and were unable to do so, then they would have been deprived of their liberty if the other elements were met. If a nurse is unsure whether an individual is being deprived of their liberty in a care home, hospital or community setting, they should contact their safeguarding adults lead or the local authority DoLS team for advice.

When a treatment is judged to deprive a non-capacitous patient of their liberty, the treatment provider is expected to speak with family, friends and other professionals who know the patient to maximize the likelihood that the intervention will align with the patient's wishes, be in their best interest, be proportional to the level of risk that the hospital is trying to prevent, and be the least restrictive intervention. In the absence of people who know the patient, the hospital can arrange for an Independent Mental Capacity Advocate (IMCA).

Box 5.27 Record keeping following a capacity assessment and best interests meeting

Documenting the capacity assessment

Before assessing capacity (document details and evidence)
- What decision is to be made?
- Is there an impairment or disturbance in the functioning of the mind or brain (e.g. brain injury, delirium, dementia, learning disability, mental 'illness', or another condition related to a specific disease)? If so, what evidence is there for this impairment or disturbance? Is it temporary or permanent?

Determining capacity (document details and evidence)
- Is the person able to understand the information relating to the decision to be made?
- Is the person able to retain information relating to the decision long enough to make the decision?
- Is the person able to weigh up the information relating to the decision?
- Is the person able to communicate their decision by any means?
- If the answer to any of the above questions is 'no', have all reasonable efforts been made to aid the person's understanding, retention and weighing up of information and to communicate their decision?

Advance statements (document details and evidence)
- Has an advance decision of some kind (e.g. lasting power of attorney, advance statement or advance decision to refuse treatment) been made? If so, what date was this made and what are the details?

Outcome of assessment (document details and evidence)
- What support was provided to the person to maximize their capacity to make the decision required (e.g. additional time to make the decision, simplified materials, involvement of family or carers)?
- Can the decision making be delayed until a time when the person is likely to have regained capacity to make the decision?
- Did the person lack capacity *because of* their impairment or disturbance of the mind or brain (e.g. brain injury, delirium, dementia, learning disability, mental 'illness', or another condition related to a specific disease)?

Documenting the best interests meeting

- Date and location of meeting.
- Who was consulted about the meeting and who was at the meeting? Provide names, roles/relationships (e.g. someone close to the patient, lasting power of attorney, Independent Mental Capacity Advocate, Court of Protection Deputy) and contact details.
- What was the purpose of the meeting?
- Confirm agreement that the person lacked capacity in relation to the decision to be made.
- Confirm that lack of capacity for the decision was permanent, or if it was temporary why the decision making could not wait.
- Is there an advance decision to refuse treatment or an advance statement expressing the patient's views, wishes, values or beliefs? (Include copies of document(s).)
- Name and role of decision maker (include copies of document(s) relating to lasting power of attorney).
- What is the proposed treatment? What are its risks and how might these risks be managed?
- What are the risks of not carrying out the proposed treatment?
- What are the views of the different people in the meeting, including people who know the patient best and the Independent Mental Capacity Advocate (if relevant)? Was there, or could there be, any dispute about the decision made?
- What was the least restrictive option available? Will restraint be used and, if so, are Deprivation of Liberty Safeguards required?
- What were the best interests decision, plan and time frames?
- When was the best interests decision made if it was not made at the meeting?
- The decision maker needs to record their name, designation and contact details.

Source: Adapted with permission of the Royal Marsden NHS Foundation Trust.

When a person has consented to a care plan or treatment prior to losing mental capacity, and the care being delivered is that which the patient consented to, then this may be considered an advance plan. This is applicable to end-of-life care. However, when the care given deviates from the care plan, then a DoLS application must be made.

Clinical governance

The DoLS are an amendment to the Mental Capacity Act (2005) and their aim is to protect patients lacking mental capacity from being deprived of their liberty. In 2018 the UK government published a Mental Capacity (Amendment) Bill, which is yet to be ratified in Parliament; if this becomes law, then the processes outlined in this section will be subject to change. The bill proposes a new scheme called the Liberty Protection Safeguards, which will be applicable to people over 16 years of age staying or living in hospital, a care home, supported living, shared living or private housing. It proposes a simplified best interests decision process with greater emphasis on the patient's wishes and increased checks that the deprivation of liberty is still required.

Pre-procedural considerations

There are times when a person has not, or is unable to, provide consent to treatment and there is no rush for treatment provision – for example, when there is an elective surgical procedure. If the treatment is assessed to deprive the person of their liberty then a DoLS standard application can be made to the local authority where the person usually resides up to 28 days in advance of treatment (Figure 5.23).

However, in medical settings, there are times when there is an urgent need to provide treatment to a person who does not have the capacity to consent to that treatment and it will deprive them of their liberty. In these situations, the hospital submits both an urgent DoLS application and a standard DoLS application to the local authority where the person is usually resident. Urgent applications are authorized by the treatment provider and so treatment can begin before the local authority responds to make an assessment.

The joint social services and Department of Health seven-page DoLS form requires the following information about the patient:

- basic details (name, date of birth, etc.)
- medical history

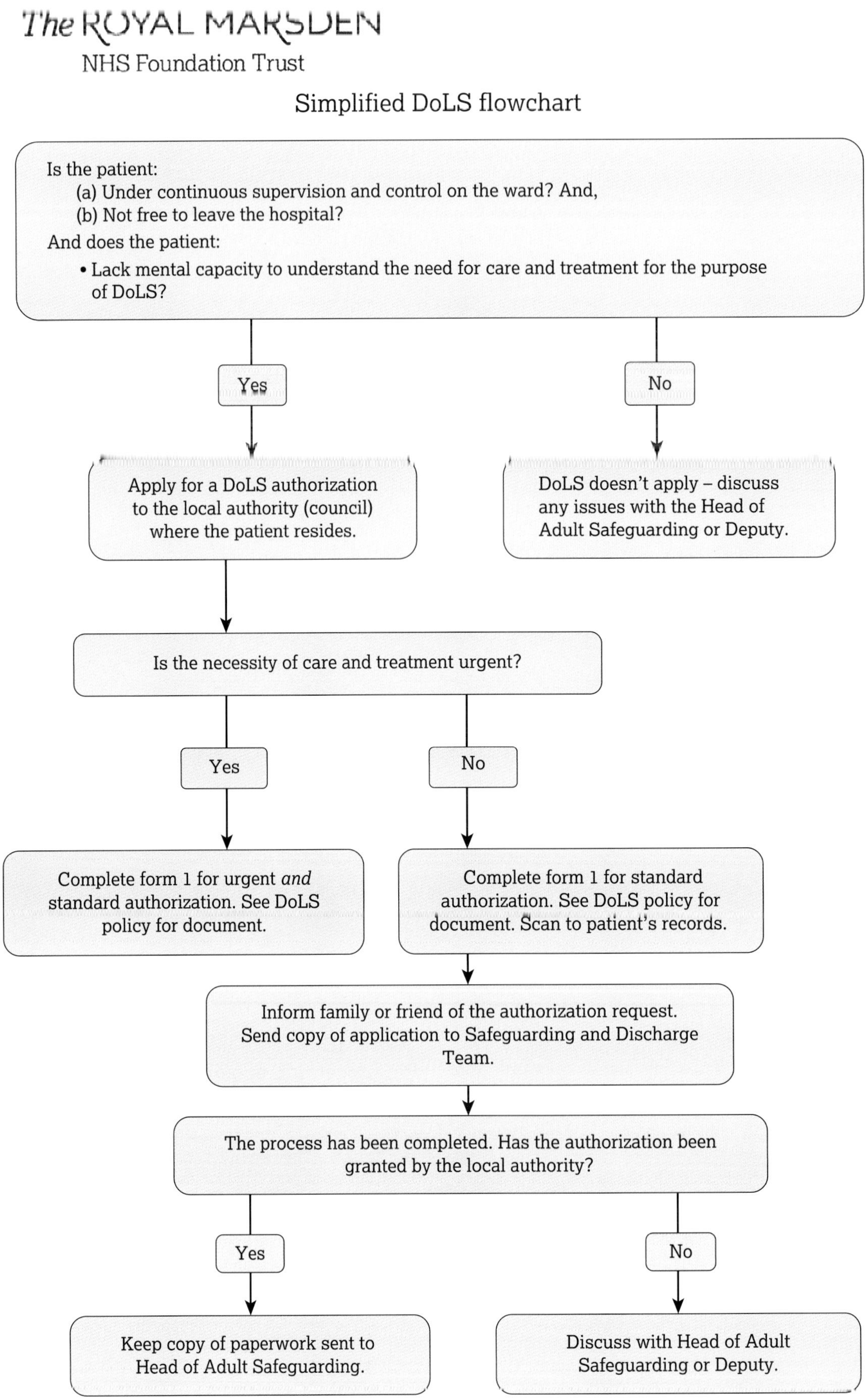
The ROYAL MARSDEN
NHS Foundation Trust
Simplified DoLS flowchart
Is the patient:
(a) Under continuous supervision and control on the ward? And,
(b) Not free to leave the hospital?
And does the patient:
• Lack mental capacity to understand the need for care and treatment for the purpose of DoLS?
Yes
No
Apply for a DoLS authorization to the local authority (council) where the patient resides.
DoLS doesn't apply – discuss any issues with the Head of Adult Safeguarding or Deputy.
Is the necessity of care and treatment urgent?
Yes
No
Complete form 1 for urgent and standard authorization. See DoLS policy for document.
Complete form 1 for standard authorization. See DoLS policy for document. Scan to patient's records.
Inform family or friend of the authorization request. Send copy of application to Safeguarding and Discharge Team.
The process has been completed. Has the authorization been granted by the local authority?
Yes
No
Keep copy of paperwork sent to Head of Adult Safeguarding.
Discuss with Head of Adult Safeguarding or Deputy.

Figure 5.23 Algorithm for assessing whether a Deprivation of Liberty Safeguards (DoLS) application is required. *Source:* Reproduced with permission of The Royal Marsden NHS Foundation Trust.

- communication preferences and requirements
- care requirements
- the rationale for restricting the person's freedom and how this will be done
- information relating to the best interests decision including any known advance statements and any need for an IMCA
- whether the patient is under the care of the Mental Health Act.

Principles relating to deprivation of liberty

When a hospital patient lacks capacity and is deprived of their liberty, the person concerned may, knowingly or unknowingly, attempt to leave the environment in which they have been confined. Sometimes this happens in a state of confusion or anxiety about being in an unfamiliar environment. The nurse's role is to assess and de-escalate the situation. Any intervention to restrain the patient must be proportionate to the risk posed to the patient. For example, a person quietly attempting to leave their room to access a corridor may need a nurse to speak to them or distract them and to guide them back to their room. Any consideration to use medication as a form of restraint should be a last resort with clear considerations of the consequences and a clear justification. All organizations will have their own policies and procedures and it is important that nurses adhere to these and seek guidance from managers and the safeguarding team.

Principles table 5.19 Enacting a deprivation of liberty

Principle	Rationale
Assess the situation and de-escalate it.	Your intervention must be based on clinical judgement; effective communication can help to de-escalate the situation (DH 2009c, C).
Any intervention to restrain the patient must be proportionate to the risk posed; medication as a form of restraint should be a last resort with clear considerations of the consequences and a clear justification.	Deprivation of liberty must be justified and for as short a time as possible (DH 2009c, C).
Follow your organization's policies and procedures; seek guidance from a manager or the safeguarding team.	There are support systems around you to help you do your job (DH 2009c, C).

Post-procedural considerations

Sometimes deprivation of liberty is required to provide care or treatment and protect people from harm. Efforts should be made to prevent deprivations of liberty by making provision to avoid placing restrictions. If a deprivation of liberty cannot be avoided, it should be for no longer than is necessary.

If a nurse is working with someone whom they think has been deprived of their liberty and the appropriate safeguards have not been employed, the nurse should contact their safeguarding adults lead or the local authority DoLS team for advice.

Interface between the Mental Health Act (1983, revised 2007) and the Mental Capacity Act (2005)

Related theory

The purpose of the Mental Health Act (1983) is to provide the statutory framework for the compulsory care and treatment of people with a 'mental disorder' when they are unable or unwilling to consent to that care and treatment, and when it is necessary for that care and treatment to be given to protect them or others from harm. The Mental Health Act is restricted to compulsory treatment for a mental disorder, which it defines as 'any disorder or disability of the mind' (Box 5.28).

The UK government intended to pass a new Mental Health Act to replace the 1983 act. However, opposition to many of its proposals meant that the 2007 act was an amendment to the 1983 act.

The code of practice for the Mental Health Act (DH 2015) provides stronger protection for patients and includes discussion on:

- involving the patient and where appropriate their families and carers in discussions about the patient's care at every stage
- providing personalized care
- minimizing the use of inappropriate blanket restrictions, restrictive interventions and the use of police cells as places of safety.

Box 5.28 Clinically recognized conditions that could fall within the definition of 'mental disorder' under the Mental Health Act (1983)

- Affective disorders, such as depression and bipolar disorder
- Schizophrenia and delusional disorders
- Neurotic, stress-related and somatoform disorders, such as anxiety, phobic disorders, obsessive compulsive disorders, post-traumatic stress disorder and hypochondriacal disorders
- Organic mental disorders such as dementia and delirium (however caused)
- Personality and behavioural changes caused by brain injury or damage (however acquired)
- Personality disorders (see DH 2015, paras. 2.19–2.20 and chapter 21)
- Mental and behavioural disorders caused by psychoactive substance use (see DH 2015, paras 2.9–2.13)
- Eating disorders, non-organic sleep disorders and non-organic sexual disorders
- Learning disabilities (see DH 2015, paras. 2.14–2.18 and chapter 20)
- Autistic spectrum disorders (including Asperger's syndrome) (see DH 2015, paras. 2.14–2.18 and chapter 20)
- Behavioural and emotional disorders of children and young people

Note: this list is not exhaustive.

Evidence-based approaches

Rationale

Indications

The Mental Health Act is only applicable to people with a mental disorder. Its aim is to facilitate assessment and treatment for people with mental disorders who are unable to consent to this (or are unwilling due to a lack of insight). Although it can be invoked to prevent deterioration of mental health, in practice it is generally used where risks to self or others, arising from the mental disorder, have been identified.

Psychiatric disorders associated with substance misuse (e.g. delirium tremens and drug-induced psychoses) are covered by the Mental Health Act. However, alcohol or drug dependence syndrome (addiction) and uncomplicated intoxication are not. Delirium and dementia are both mental disorders in the terms of the Mental Health Act.

Contraindications

The Mental Health Act cannot be used to prevent unwise refusal of medical treatment (or self-discharge from an acute ward) by a person who has no serious mental disorder.

The act is clear that uncomplicated intoxication with drugs or alcohol, or dependence on drugs or alcohol, is not grounds for detention. Intoxicated patients are often incapacitous and can be looked after in the general hospital setting using the Mental Capacity Act until 'sober'. People with substance dependence cannot be detained under the Mental Health Act as a route into treatment for their addiction.

Pre-procedural considerations

When a nurse is concerned that someone with a 'diagnosable mental disorder' is at *imminent* risk of harm to or from themselves and/or others and that the person may need to be confined for their own safety, the nurse should follow local guidance on mental health or psychiatry emergencies. The guidance given here specifically focuses on inpatients.

If an inpatient develops a mental disorder of a nature, severity and riskiness that demands further assessment and treatment, the first step is to seek their consent to all the proposed interventions. This involves inviting their consent to interventions such as special observation by a registered mental health nurse, frequent reviews of mental state, medical investigations to ascertain the cause of the mental disorder, suspension of leave from the hospital and administration of psychotropic medication. If the person lacks the capacity to consent, a decision needs to be made about whether to use the Mental Capacity Act or to invoke the Mental Health Act.

Generally speaking, the Mental Capacity Act is appropriate for the short-term care of medically unwell, acutely confused inpatients. Management should be in the patient's best interests and the least restrictive intervention should be implemented. For all other severe and/or risky 'mental disorders', the Mental Health Act should be used if the person does not or cannot consent.

Principles of using the Mental Health Act

Mental Health Act: Section 2

Section 2 of the Mental Health Act provides for the issuing of a 28-day assessment order. It requires three opinions:

- a psychiatrist with Section 12 approval, i.e. speciality trainees (4–6) or consultant
- the patient's GP or an independent Section 12-approved doctor
- an approved mental health professional (usually a specially trained social worker).

In the acute hospital setting during office hours, this process usually takes several hours. Detention of the person may need to occur more quickly than this to maintain their or other people's safety and to keep the patient on the ward. In these circumstances, Section 5(2) should be invoked.

Mental Health Act: Section 5(2)

Section 5(2) provides the power to immediately, and temporarily, detain a hospital inpatient who has a 'mental disorder' to ensure their (or other people's) immediate safety. A Section 5(2) lasts for up to 72 hours and a person cannot appeal against; it is imperative that once it has been activated, staff trigger the process for a Section 2 assessment to take place.

Any fully registered medical doctor (of any speciality) can act as the 'nominated deputy' of the 'responsible clinician' for the patient's care and complete a Section 5(2) application form. Local guidance should be consulted to identify who can be contacted to implement the Section 5(2). The nominated manager named in local policy should be called upon to support the completion of these forms and the ongoing management of the patient. If a psychiatric liaison service is available, they need to be involved from the outset.

See Mental Health Law Online (2019) for the appropriate forms. These forms can be completed online (see www.mentalhealthlaw.co.uk/Mental_Health_Act_1983_Statutory_Forms), but they must then be printed out and signed.

Post-procedural considerations

Anyone detained under Section 5(2) should be assessed for detention under Section 2 of the Mental Health Act as soon as this can be arranged. Section 5(2) should not be allowed to simply 'run on' until close to its expiry.

Depending on the context and outcome of the Mental Health Act assessment, a nurse may or may not have a role to play following the assessment. At the very least, however, they will need to clearly document what happened and their role in the lead-up to and following the assessment. It will also be important for the hospital treating team to liaise with the mental health provider to ensure ongoing appropriate physical and mental health treatment.

Interface between the Mental Health Act (2007) and Mental Capacity Act (2005)

Related theory

The Mental Health Act (2007) is concerned with the treatment of a person's mental disorder, while the Mental Capacity Act (2005) has a broader scope that includes physical and mental health as well as welfare, finances, property and research participation.

Someone who is deemed to have a mental disorder may or may not have capacity, and someone who does not have capacity may or may not have a diagnosis of a mental disorder. It is entirely possible for someone assessed and detained under the Mental Health Act to have capacity in relation to a treatment decision. Whether an individual patient has or does not have decision-making capacity is not the key determinant of whether the Mental Health Act should be used. If a patient were already detained and subject to the compulsory treatment provisions of the Mental Health Act, the Mental Capacity Act would not be used for the provision of further medical treatment for that mental disorder; thus, best interests principles would not apply in the same way. However, it would still be possible to apply the Mental Capacity Act for other aspects of care if the patient lacked capacity for related decisions. Based on the specific case and needs of a patient with a 'mental disorder', staff must decide which act and subsequent approaches is least restrictive to the individual (Browne Jacobson LLP 2016). Both the Mental Capacity Act and the Mental Health Act provide procedural safeguards to ensure the rights of the person concerned are protected during their detention, and staff need to consider which safeguards will best protect the interest of the patient (Table 5.4).

The interested reader may want to visit www.brownejacobson.com, www.39essex.com or www.no5.com for accessible summaries of the relevant legislation and case law.

Table 5.4 Choosing between the Mental Health Act (1983) and the Mental Capacity Act (2005)

	Mental Health Act (1983)	Mental Capacity Act (2005)
Focus of the act	Relates to a person's status as someone with a 'mental disorder' within the meaning of the act	Relates to a person's (in)capacity to make a particular decision
Scope of the act	A person can be detained solely on the basis of the risk that they pose to themselves or others due to a mental disorder	Requires decisions made or acts done on behalf of the person who lacks capacity to be made or done in their best interests
Decision-making powers	Limited to decisions about care in hospital and medical treatment for a mental disorder	Covers all decision making

Websites

Action for Blind People
www.actionforblindpeople.org.uk

Action on Hearing Loss
www.actiononhearingloss.org.uk

British Association for Counselling and Psychotherapy
www.bacp.co.uk

British Psychological Society
www.bps.org.uk

Compassionate Mind Foundation
www.compassionatemind.co.uk

Dementia UK
www.dementia.org

Depression Alliance
www.depressionalliance.org

Depression UK
www.depressionuk.org

Get Self-Help
www.getselfhelp.co.uk

Mental Health Act
https://www.legislation.gov.uk/ukpga/2007/12/contents

MIND
www.mind.org.uk

Northumberland, Tyne and Wear NHS Foundation Trust: Self Help
www.ntw.nhs.uk/selfhelp

Plain English Campaign
www.plainenglish.co.uk

RNIB: See It Right
www.rnib.org.uk

Royal College of Occupational Therapists
www.rcot.co.uk

Royal College of Speech and Language Therapists
www.rcslt.org

Samaritans
www.samaritans.org

Speakability
www.speakability.org.uk

Stroke Association
www.stroke.org.uk

References

Adams, J. & Whittington, R. (1995) Verbal aggression to psychiatric staff: Traumatic stressor or part of the job? *Psychiatric Care*, 2(5), 171–174.

ADASS (Association of Directors of Adult Social Services) (2015) *London Multi-agency Adult Safeguarding Policy and Procedures*. Available at: http://londonadass.org.uk/wp-content/uploads/2015/02/Pan-London-Updated-August-2016.pdf

Adult Support and Protection (Scotland) Act (2007) Available at: https://www.legislation.gov.uk/asp/2007/10/contents

Agenda for Change Project Team (2004) *The NHS Knowledge and Skills Framework and the Development Review Process*. Available at: www.ksf.scot.nhs.uk/uploads/documents/KSF_Handbook.pdf

Ainsworth, M.D.S. & Bell, S.M. (1970) Attachment, exploration, and separation: Illustrated by the behavior of one-year-olds in a strange situation. *Child Development*, 41, 49–67.

Alexander, S.C., Sullivan, A.M., Back, A.L., et al. (2012) Information giving and receiving in haematological malignancy consultations *Psycho-Oncology*, 21, 297–306.

Alzheimer's Society (2009) *Counting the Cost: Caring for Older People with Dementia on Hospital Wards*. Available at: https://www.alzheimers.org.uk/sites/default/files/2018-05/Counting_the_cost_report.pdf

Alzheimer's Society (2014) *Dementia UK: Update*, 2nd edn. Available at: https://www.alzheimers.org.uk/sites/default/files/migrate/downloads/dementia_uk_update.pdf

Alzheimer's Society (2017) *What is Dementia?* Available at: https://www.alzheimers.org.uk/sites/default/files/pdf/what_is_dementia.pdf

APA (American Psychiatric Association) (2013) *Diagnostic and Statistical Manual of Mental Disorders*, 5th edn. Washington, DC: American Psychiatric Association.

Argyle, M. (1988) *Bodily Communication*, 2nd edn. Abingdon: Routledge.

Arnold, E.C. & Underman Boggs, K. (2011) *Interpersonal Relationships: Professional Communication Skills for Nurses*, 6th edn. St Louis, MO: Saunders.

Arora, N.K. (2003) Interacting with cancer patients: The significance of physicians' communication behavior. *Social Science & Medicine*, 57(5), 791–806.

Back, A.L., Arnold, R.M., Baile, W.F., et al. (2005) Approaching difficult communication tasks in oncology. *CA: A Cancer Journal for Clinicians*, 55(3), 164–177.

Baillie, L., Cox, J. & Merritt, J. (2012) Caring for older people with dementia in hospital: Part one – Challenges. *Nursing Older People*, 24(8), 33–37.

Batbaatar, E., Dorjdagva, J., Luvsannyam, A., et al. (2017) Determinants of patient satisfaction: A systematic review. *Perspectives in Public Health*, 137(2), 89–101.

Bentley, H., Burrows, A., Clarke, L., et al. (2018) *How Safe Are Our Children?* National Society for the Prevention of Cruelty to Children. Available at: https://learning.nspcc.org.uk/media/1067/how-safe-are-our-children-2018.pdf

Berkman, L., Glass, T., Brissette, I. & Seeman, T. (2000) From social integration to health: Durkheim in the new millennium. *Social Science & Medicine*, 51(6), 843–857.

Blackstone, S., Beukelman, D.R. & Yorkston, K.M. (2015) *Patient–Provider Communication: Roles for Speech-Language Pathologists and Other Health Care Professionals*. San Diego: Plural Publishing.

Blake, C. & Ledger, C. (2007) *Insight into Anxiety*. Farnham, UK: CWR.

BNF (British National Formulary) (2019) *British National Formulary*. National Institute for Health and Care Excellence. Available at: https://bnf.nice.org.uk

Boissy, A., Windover, A.K., Bokar, D., et al. (2016) Communication skills training for physicians improves patient satisfaction. *Journal of General Internal Medicine*, 31(7), 755–761.

Booth, K., Maguire, P., Butterworth, T. & Hillier, V.F. (1996) Perceived professional support and the use of blocking behaviours by hospice nurses. *Journal of Advanced Nursing*, 24, 522–527.

Booth, K., Maguire, P. & Hillier, V.F. (1999) Measurement of communication skills in cancer care: Myth or reality? *Journal of Advanced Nursing*, 30(5), 1073–1079.

Botti, M., Endacott, R., Watts, R., et al. (2006) Barriers in providing psychosocial support for patients with cancer. *Cancer Nursing*, 29(4), 309–316.

Bowes, D.E., Tamlyn, D. & Butler, L.J. (2002) Women living with ovarian cancer: Dealing with an early death. *Health Care for Women International*, 23(2), 135–148.

Bowlby, J. (1969) *Attachment and Loss: Volume I – Attachment*. London: Hogarth.

Bowlby, J. (1973) *Attachment and Loss: Volume II – Separation Anxiety and Anger*. New York: Basic Books.

Bowlby, J. (1979) *The Making and Breaking of Affectional Bonds*. London: Tavistock.

Bowlby, J. (1980) *Attachment and Loss: Volume III – Loss: Sadness and Depression*. New York: Basic Books.

Bowlby, J. (1988) *A Secure Base: Clinical Applications of Attachment Theory*. Bristol: Routledge.

BPS (British Psychological Society Division of Clinical Psychology) (2015) *Guidelines on Language in Relation to Functional Psychiatric Diagnosis*. Available at: www.newvisionformentalhealth.com/2018/01/26/guidelines-on-language-in-relation-to-functional-psychiatric-diagnosis/

Bradley, J.C. & Edinberg, M.A. (1990) *Communication in the Nursing Context*, 3rd edn. London: Prentice Hall.

Brajtman, S. (2005) Terminal restlessness: Perspectives of an interdisciplinary palliative care team. *International Journal of Palliative Nursing*, 11, 170, 172–178.
Braye, S. & Preston-Shoot, M. (2017) *Learning from SARs: A Report for the London Safeguarding Adults Board.* Available at: http://londonadass.org.uk/wp-content/uploads/2014/12/London-SARs-Report-Final-Version.pdf
Brennan, J. (2001) Adjustment to cancer: Coping or personal transition? *Psycho-Oncology*, 10, 1–18.
Brown, R.F., Byland, C.L., Kline, N., et al. (2009) Identifying and responding to depression in adult cancer patients. *Cancer Nursing*, 32(3), E1–E7.
Browne Jacobson LLP (2016) *The Interface between the Mental Health Act, the Mental Capacity Act and DoLS.* Available at: https://www.brownejacobson.com/health/training-and-resources/legal-updates/2016/01/the-interface-between-the-mental-health-act-the-mental-capacity-act-and-dols
Burgess, P. (2017) People with hearing loss: Removing the barriers to communication. *British Journal of Healthcare Assistants*, 11(9), 444–450.
Burnham, J. (1993) Systemic supervision: The evolution of reflexivity in the context of the supervisory relationship. *Human Systems*, 4, 349–381.
Byng-Hall, J. (1995) *Rewriting Family Scripts: Improvisation and Systems Change.* New York: Guilford Press.
Care Act (2014) Available at: www.legislation.gov.uk/ukpga/2014/23/contents/enacted
Carter, B. & Goldrick, M. (1999) *The Expanded Family Life Cycle: Individual and Family Perspectives*, 3rd edn. Boston: Allyn & Bacon.
Chambers, S. (2003) Use of non-verbal communication skills to improve nursing care. *British Journal of Nursing*, 12(14), 874–879.
Chant, S., Jenkinson, T., Randle, J. & Russell, G. (2004) Communication skills: Some problems in nurse education and practice. *Journal of Clinical Nursing*, 11, 12–21.
Chelf, J.H., Agre, P., Axelrod, A., et al. (2001) Cancer-related patient education: An overview of the last decade of evaluation and research. *Oncology Nursing Forum*, 28(7), 1139–1147.
Children's Act (1989) Available at: www.legislation.gov.uk/ukpga/1989/41/contents
Children's Act (2004) Available at: www.legislation.gov.uk/ukpga/2004/31/contents
Children and Social Work Act (2017) Available at: www.legislation.gov.uk/ukpga/2017/16/contents
Chou, A.F., Stewart, S.L., Wild, R.C., et al. (2012) Social support and survival in young women with breast carcinoma. *Psycho-Oncology*, 21(2), 125–133.
Churchill, N. (2013) *Ensuring that People Have a Positive Experience of Care.* Available at: https://www.england.nhs.uk/wp-content/uploads/2013/11/pat-expe.pdf
Connolly, M., Perryman, J., McKenna, Y., et al. (2010) SAGE & THYME™: A model for training health and social care professionals in patient-focussed support. *Patient Education and Counseling*, 79(1), 87–93.
Counter Terrorism and Security Act (2015) Available at: https://www.gov.uk/government/collections/counter-terrorism-and-security-bill
Crime and Disorder Act (1998) Available at: www.legislation.gov.uk/ukpga/1998/37/contents
Dahl, J. & Lundgren, T. (2006) *Living Beyond Your Pain: Using Acceptance and Commitment Therapy to Ease Chronic Pain.* Oakland, CA: Harbinger.
Daniel, D. & Dewing, J. (2012) Practising the principles of the Mental Capacity Act. *Nursing & Residential Care*, 14(5), 243–245.
de Vito, J.A. (2013) *Essentials of Human Communication*, 8th edn. London: Pearson.
De Vries, K. (2013) Communicating with older people with dementia. *Nursing Older People*, 25(4), 30–38.
Dein, S. (2005) Working with the patient who is in denial. *European Journal of Palliative Care*, 12(6), 251–253.
Dein, S. (2006) *Culture and Cancer Care: Anthropological Insights in Oncology.* Maidenhead, UK: Open University Press.
del Piccolo, L., Goss, C. & Bergvik, S. (2006) The fourth meeting of the Verona Network on Sequence Analysis: 'Consensus finding on the appropriateness of provider responses to patient cues and concerns'. *Patient Education and Counseling*, 61, 473–475.
Delgado-Guay, M.O., Yennurajalingam, S. & Bruera, E. (2008) Delirium with severe symptom expression related to hypercalcemia in a patient with advanced cancer: An interdisciplinary approach to treatment. *Journal of Pain and Symptom Management*, 36(4), 442–449.
Delvaux, N., Razavi, D., Marchal, S., et al. (2004) Effects of a 105 hours psychological training program on attitudes, communication skills and occupational stress in oncology: A randomised study. *British Journal of Cancer*, 90, 106–114.
Dementia UK (2019) *Tips for Better Communication.* Available at: https://www.dementiauk.org/understanding-dementia/advice-and-information/dementia-first-steps/tips-for-better-communication-2
DfE (Department for Education) (2018) *Working Together to Safeguard Children: A Guide to Inter-agency Working to Safeguard and Promote the Welfare of Children.* Available at: https://assets.publishing.service.gov.uk/government/uploads/system/uploads/attachment_data/file/779401/Working_Together_to_Safeguard-Children.pdf
DH (Department of Health) (2003) *Confidentiality: NHS Code of Practice.* Leeds: Department of Health.
DH (2004) *Better Information, Better Choice, Better Health.* London: Department of Health.
DH (2006) *Our Health, Our Care, Our Say: A New Direction for Community Services.* London: Department of Health.
DH (2008a) *Information Accreditation Scheme.* Available at: http://webarchive.nationalarchives.gov.uk/+/dh.gov.uk/en/Healthcare/PatientChoice/BetterInformationChoicesHealth/Informationstandard/index.htm
DH (2008b) *High Quality Care for All.* London: Department of Health.
DH (2009a) *Basic Guidelines for People Who Commission Easy Read Information.* London: Department of Health.
DH (2009b) *Information Prescriptions.* London: Department of Health.
DH (2009c) *Mental Capacity Act 2005: Deprivation of Liberty Safeguards – Deprivation of Liberty Safeguards (DoLS) Resources for Health and Care Professionals.* Available at: https://www.gov.uk/government/collections/dh-mental-capacity-act-2005-deprivation-of-liberty-safeguards
DH (2009d) *Reference Guide to Consent to Examination or Treatment.* Available at: https://assets.publishing.service.gov.uk/government/uploads/system/uploads/attachment_data/file/138296/dh_103653__1_.pdf
DH (2009e) *NHS Constitution: Interactive Version.* Available at: https://www.nhs.uk/NHSEngland/aboutnhs/Documents/NHS_Constitution_interactive_9Mar09.pdf
DH (2012a) *Compassion in Practice Nursing, Midwifery and Care Staff: Our Vision and Strategy.* Leeds: Department of Health.
DH (2012b) *The Handbook to the NHS Constitution.* Leeds: Department of Health.
DH (2013a) *Guidance for Health Professionals on Domestic Violence.* Available at: https://www.gov.uk/government/publications/guidance-for-health-professionals-on-domestic-violence
DH (2013b) *Report of the Mid-Staffordshire NHS Foundation Trust Public Inquiry.* London: House of Commons.
DH (2015) *Mental Health Act 1983: Code of Practice.* Available at: https://www.gov.uk/government/news/new-mental-health-act-code-of-practice
DH (2018) *Statutory Guidance: Care and Support Statutory Guidance.* Available at: https://www.gov.uk/government/publications/care-act-statutory-guidance/care-and-support-statutory-guidance#safeguarding-1
Disability Discrimination Act 1995 (Commencement No. 6) Order (1999) Available at: www.legislation.gov.uk/uksi/1999/1190/contents/made
Dunne, K. (2003) The personal cost of caring: Guest editorial. *International Journal of Palliative Nursing*, 9(6), 232.
Duppils, G.S. & Wikblad, K. (2004) Delirium: Behavioural changes before and during the prodromal phase. *Journal of Clinical Nursing*, 13(5), 609–616.
Duxbury, J. & Whittington, R. (2005) Causes and management of patient aggression and violence: Staff and patient perspectives. *Journal of Advanced Nursing*, 50(5), 469–478.
Dwamena, F., Holmes-Rovner, M., Gaulden, C.M., et al. (2012) Interventions for providers to promote a patient-centred approach in clinical consultations. *Cochrane Database of Systematic Reviews*, 12, CD003267.
EBSCO Health (2019) *Option Grid™ Decision Aids: Herniated Disk in Lower Back – Treatment Options.* Ipswich, MA: EBSCO Health.
Egan, G. (2018) *The Skilled Helper: A Client-Centred Approach*, 2nd edn. Andover, UK: Cengage Learning.

Eggenberger, E., Heimerl, K. & Bennett, M.I. (2013) Communication skills training in dementia care: A systematic review of effectiveness, training content, and didactic methods in different care settings. *International Psychogeriatrics*, 25(3), 345–358.

Ekman, P. (1999) Basic emotions. In: Dalgleish, T. & Power, M. (eds) *Handbook of Cognition and Emotion*. Oxford: John Wiley & Sons, pp.45–60.

Ell, K. (1996) Social networks, social support and coping with serious illness: The family connection. *Social Science & Medicine*, 42(2), 173–183.

Ellins, J. & Coulter, A. (2005) *How Engaged Are People in Their Healthcare? Findings of a National Telephone Survey*. Oxford: Picker Institute.

Equality Act (2010) Available at: www.equalities.gov.uk/equality_act_2010.aspx

Etter, N.M., Stemple, J.C & Howell, D.M. (2013) Defining the lived experience of older adults with voice disorders. *Journal of Voice*, 27(1), 61–67.

Fallowfield, L. & Jenkins, V. (1999) Effective communication skills are the key to good cancer care. *European Journal of Cancer*, 35(11), 1592–1597.

Fallowfield, L., Jenkins, V.A. & Beveridge, H.A. (2002) Truth may hurt but deceit hurts more: Communication in palliative care. *Palliative Medicine*, 16, 297–303.

Fallowfield, L., Ratcliffe, D., Jenkins, V. & Saul, J. (2001) Psychiatric morbidity and its recognition by doctors in patients with cancer. *British Journal of Cancer*, 84, 1011–1015.

Faulkner, A. & Maguire, P. (1994) *Talking to Cancer Patients and Their Relatives*. Oxford: Oxford University Press.

Favez, N., Notari, S.C., Charvoz, L., et al. (2016). Distress and body image disturbances in women with breast cancer in the immediate postsurgical period: The influence of attachment insecurity. *Journal of Health Psychology*, 21(12), 2994–3003.

Fellowes, D., Wilkinson, S. & Moore, P. (2004) Communication skills training for health care professionals working with cancer patients, their families and/or carers. *Cochrane Database of Systematic Reviews*, 2, CD003751.

Female Genital Mutilation Act (2003) Available at: www.legislation.gov.uk/ukpga/2003/31/contents

Gaynes, B.N., Brown, C.L., Lux, L.J., et al. (2017) Preventing and de-escalating aggressive behavior among adult psychiatric patients: A systematic review of the evidence. *Psychiatric Services*, 68(8), 819–831.

GDPR (General Data Protection Regulation) (2018) Available at: https://gdpr-info.eu

Gessler, S., Low, J., Daniells, E., et al. (2008) Screening for distress in cancer patients: Is the Distress Thermometer a valid measure in the UK and does it measure change over time? A prospective validation study. *Psycho-Oncology*, 17(6), 538–547.

Gilbert, P. (2009) Introducing compassion-focused therapy. *Advances in Psychiatric Treatment*, 15, 199–208.

Gilbert, P. (2010) *The Compassionate Mind*. London: Constable & Robinson.

Goldbeck, R. (1997) Denial in physical illness. *Journal of Psychosomatic Research*, 43(6), 575–593.

Goleman, D. (2005) *Emotional Intelligence: Why It Can Matter More than IQ*. New York: Bantam Books.

González-Fernández, M., Brodsky, M.B. & Palmer, J.B. (2015) Poststroke communication disorders and dysphagia. *Physical Medicine and Rehabilitation Clinics of North America*, 26(4), 657–670.

Gov.uk (2018a) *Forced Marriage*. Available at: https://www.gov.uk/stop-forced-marriage

Gov.uk (2018b) *Multi-agency Statutory Guidance on Female Genital Mutilation*. Available at: https://www.gov.uk/government/publications/multi-agency-statutory-guidance-on-female-genital-mutilation

Griffith, R. & Tengnah, C. (2008) Mental Capacity Act: Determining best interests. *British Journal of Community Nursing*, 13, 335–340.

Grover, C., Mackasey, E., Cook, E., et al. (2018) Patient-reported care domains that enhance the experience of 'being known' in an ambulatory cancer care centre. *Canadian Oncology Nursing Journal*, 28(3), 166–171.

Gu, J., Strauss, C., Bond, R. & Cavanagh, K. (2015). How do mindfulness-based cognitive therapy and mindfulness-based stress reduction improve mental health and wellbeing? A systematic review and meta-analysis of mediation studies. *Clinical Psychology Review*, 37, 1–12.

Gudjonsson, G.H., Rabe-Hesketh, S. & Szmukler, G. (2004) Management of psychiatric in-patient violence: Patient ethnicity and use of medication, restraint and seclusion. *British Journal of Psychiatry*, 184, 258–262.

Gysels, M., Richardson, R. & Higginson, I.J. (2005) Communication training for health professionals who care for patients with cancer: A systematic review of effectiveness. *Journal of Supportive Care in Cancer*, 13(6), 356–366.

Hack, T.F., Degner, L.F., Watson, P. & Sinha, L. (2006) Do patients benefit from participating in medical decision making? Longitudinal follow-up of women with breast cancer. *Psycho-Oncology*, 15, 9–19.

Hanson, E.K. & Fager, S.K. (2017) Communication supports for people with motor speech disorders. *Topics in Language Disorders*, 37(4), 375–388.

Harding, R., Beesley, H., Holcombe, C., et al. (2015). Are patient–nurse relationships in breast cancer linked to attachment style? *Journal of Advanced Nursing*, 71(10), 2305–2314.

Hargie, O. (2017) *Skilled Interpersonal Communication: Research, Theory and Practice*, 6th edn. Abingdon, UK: Routledge.

Harris, R. (2009). *ACT Made Simple: An Easy-to-Read Primer on Acceptance and Commitment Therapy*. Oakland, CA: New Harbinger.

Hase, S. & Douglas, A.J. (1986) *Human Dynamics and Nursing: Psychological Care in Nursing Practice*. Melbourne: Churchill Livingstone.

Hayes, S.C., Strosahl, K.D. & Wilson, K.G. (1999) *Acceptance and Commitment Therapy: An Experiential Approach to Behaviour Change*. New York: Guilford Press.

Health Foundation (2016) *Person-Centred Care Resource Centre*. Available at: https://www.health.org.uk/what-we-do/supporting-health-care-improvement/analysis-publications-and-resources-on-quality-improvement/person-centred-care-resource-centre

Health and Social Care Act (2008) Available at: https://www.legislation.gov.uk/ukpga/2008/14/contents

Health and Social Care Act (2012) Available at: www.legislation.gov.uk/ukpga/2012/7/contents/enacted

Heaven, C., Clegg, J. & Maguire, P. (2006) Transfer of communication skills training from workshop to workplace: The impact of clinical supervision. *Patient Education and Counseling*, 60, 313–325.

HEE (Health Education England) (2018) *Self-Harm and Suicide Prevention Competence Framework*. National Collaborating Centre for Mental Health University College London and Health Education England. Available at: https://www.ucl.ac.uk/pals/research/clinical-educational-and-health-psychology/research-groups/core/competence-frameworks/self

Helft, P.R. (2005) Necessary collusion: Prognostic communication with advanced cancer patients. *Journal of Clinical Oncology*, 23(13), 3146–3150.

Hemsley, B., Balandin, S. & Worrall, L. (2012) Nursing the patient with complex communication needs: Time as a barrier and a facilitator to successful communication in hospital. *Journal of Advanced Nursing*, 68(1), 116–126.

Henderson, A., van Eps, M.A., Pearson, K., et al. (2007) 'Caring for' behaviours that indicate to patients that nurses 'care about' them. *Journal of Advanced Nursing*, 60(2), 146.

Heyland, D.K., Dodek, P., Rocker, G., et al. (2006) What matters most in end-of-life care: Perceptions of seriously ill patients and their family members. *Canadian Medical Association Journal*, 174(5), 627–633.

HM Government (2018) *CONTEST: The United Kingdom's Strategy for Countering Terrorism*. Available at: https://assets.publishing.service.gov.uk/government/uploads/system/uploads/attachment_data/file/716907/140618_CCS207_CCS0218929798-1_CONTEST 3.0 WEB.pdf

Hoorn, S., Elbers, P.W., Girbes, A.R. & Tuinman, P.R. (2016) Communicating with conscious and mechanically ventilated critically ill patients: A systematic review. *Critical Care*, 20(1), 333.

Houldin, A. (2000) *Patients with Cancer: Understanding the Psychological Pain*. Philadelphia: Lippincott Williams & Wilkins.

HSE (Health and Safety Executive) (n.d.) *Violence in Health and Social Care*. Available at: www.hse.gov.uk/healthservices/violence/index.htm#know

Human Rights Act (1998). Available at: https://www.legislation.gov.uk/ukpga/1998/42/contents

Irving, K., Fick, D. & Foreman, M. (2006) Practice development – delirium. Delirium: A new appraisal of an old problem. *International Journal of Older People Nursing*, 1(2), 106–112.

Jenkins, K. (2014) II. Needle phobia: A psychological perspective. *BJA*, 113(1), 4–6.

Jenkins, V., Fallowfield, L. & Saul, J. (2001) Information needs of patients with cancer: Results from a large study in UK cancer centres. *British Journal of Cancer*, 84, 48–51.

Jones, J. (2002) *Factsheet: Communication*. Worcester: British Institute of Learning Disabilities.

Jootun, D. & McGhee, D. (2011) Effective communication with people who have dementia. *Nursing Standard*, 25, 40–46.

Kelsey, S. (2005) Improving nurse communication skills with the cancer patient. *Cancer Nursing Practice*, 4(2), 27–31.

Kennedy Sheldon, L. (2009) *Communication for Nurses*. Sudbury, MA: Jones & Bartlett.

Kogan, N.R., Dumas, M. & Cohen, S.R. (2013) The extra burdens patients in denial impose on their family caregivers. *Palliative & Supportive Care*, 11(2), 91–99.

Krug, E.G. (2002) *World Report on Violence and Health*. Geneva: World Health Organization.

Kruijver, I.P., Kerkstra, A., Bensing, J.M. & van de Weil, H.B. (2001) Communication skills of nurses during interactions with simulated cancer patients. *Journal of Advanced Nursing*, 34(6), 772–779.

Law Commission (2019) *Hate Crime*. Available at: https://www.lawcom.gov.uk/project/hate-crime

Lawlor, P.G., Gagnon, B., Mancini, I.L., et al. (2000) Occurrence, causes, and outcome of delirium in patients with advanced cancer: A prospective study. *Archives of Internal Medicine*, 160(6), 786–794.

Leaviss, J. & Uttley, L. (2015) Psychotherapeutic benefits of compassion focused therapy: An early systematic review. *Psychological Medicine*, 45, 927–945

Levinson, W., Gorawara Bhat, R. & Lamb, J. (2000) A study of patient clues and physician responses in primary care and surgical settings. *JAMA*, 284(8), 1021–1027.

LGA (Local Government Association) (2018) *Making Safeguarding Personal: Outcomes Framework*. Available at: https://www.local.gov.uk/sites/default/files/documents/msp-outcomes-framework-final-report-may-2018.pdf

Loh, A., Simon, D., Wills, C.E., et al. (2007) The effects of a shared decision-making intervention in primary care of depression: A cluster-randomized controlled trial. *Patient Education and Counseling*, 67(3), 324–332.

London Safeguarding Children Board (2017) *London Child Protection Procedures and Practice Guidance*. Available at: www.londoncp.co.uk

Lowry, M. (1995) Knowledge that reduces anxiety: Creating patient information leaflets. *Professional Nurse*, 10(5), 318–320.

Ludlow, C.L. (2015) Central nervous system control of voice and swallowing. *Journal of Clinical Neurophysiology*, 32(4), 294–303.

Ludlow, K., Mumford, V., Makeham, M., et al. (2018) The effects of hearing loss on person-centred care in residential aged care: A narrative review. *Geriatric Nursing*, 39(3), 269–302.

Maben, J. & Griffiths, P. (2008) *Nurses in Society: Starting the Debate*. London: King's College.

MacArthur, J., Brown, M., McKechanie, A., et al. (2015) Making reasonable and achievable adjustments: The contributions of learning disability liaison nurses in 'getting it right' for people with learning disabilities receiving general hospitals care. *Journal of Advanced Nursing*, 71(7), 1552–1563.

Macdonald, E. (2004) *Difficult Conversations in Medicine*. Oxford: Oxford University Press.

Macmillan Cancer Relief (2002) *Macmillan Black and Minority Ethnic Toolkit: Effective Communication with African-Caribbean and African Men Affected by Prostate Cancer*. London: Macmillan Cancer Relief.

Maguire, P. (2000) *Communication Skills for Doctors*. London: Arnold.

Maguire, P., Booth, K., Elliott, C. & Jones, B. (1996) Helping health professionals involved in cancer care acquire key interviewing skills: The impact of workshops. *European Journal of Cancer*, 32(9), 1486–1489.

Maguire, P. & Pitceathly, C. (2002) Key communication skills and how to acquire them. *BMJ*, 325, 697–700.

Main, M., & Solomon, J. (1990) Procedures for identifying infants as disorganized/disoriented during the Ainsworth Strange Situation. In: Greenberg, M.T., Cicchetti, D. & Cummings, E.M. (eds) *Attachment in the Preschool Years: Theory, Research, and Intervention*. Chicago: University of Chicago Press, pp.121–160.

Management of Health and Safety at Work Regulations (1999) Available at: www.legislation.gov.uk/uksi/1999/3242/contents/made

Mathieson, L. (2001) *The Voice and Its Disorders*, 6th edn. London: Whurr.

Mazzi, M.A., Rimondini, M., Deveugele, M., et al. (2015) What do people appreciate in physicians' communication? An international study with focus groups using videotaped medical consultations. *Health Expectations*, 18(5), 1215–1226.

McCabe, C. (2004) Nurse–patient communication: An exploration of patients' experiences. *Journal of Clinical Nursing*, 13, 41–49

McCabe, C. & Timmins, F. (2013) *Communication Skills for Nursing Practice*, 2nd edn. Basingstoke: Palgrave Macmillan.

McCaughan, E. & Parahoo, K. (2000) Medical and surgical nurses' perceptions of their level of competence and educational needs in caring for patients with cancer. *Journal of Clinical Nursing*, 9, 420–428.

McEvoy, M., Santos, M.T., Marzan, M., et al. (2009) Teaching medical students how to use interpreters: A three year experience. *Medical Education Online*, 14(1), 4507.

McKenzie, R. (2002) The importance of philosophical congruence for therapeutic use of self in practice. In: Freshwater, D. (ed) *Therapeutic Nursing: Improving Patient Care through Self-Awareness and Reflection*. London: Sage, pp.22–38.

McLaughlin, S., Gorley, L. & Moseley, L. (2009) The prevalence of verbal aggression against nurses. *British Journal of Nursing*, 18(12), 25.

McLenon, J. & Rogers, M.A.M. (2018) The fear of needles: A systematic review and meta-analysis. *Journal of Advanced Nursing*, 75(1), 30–42.

Mental Capacity Act (2005) Available at: https://www.legislation.gov.uk/ukpga/2005/9/contents

Mental Capacity Act Code of Practice (2005) Available at: https://www.gov.uk/government/publications/mental-capacity-act-code-of-practice

Mental Health Act (1983) Available at: https://www.legislation.gov.uk/ukpga/1983/20/contents

Mental Health Act (2007) Available at: https://www.legislation.gov.uk/ukpga/2007/12/contents

Mental Health Law Online (2019) *Mental Health Act 1983 Statutory Forms*. Available at: www.mentalhealthlaw.co.uk/Mental_Health_Act_1983_Statutory_Forms

Menzies-Lyth, I. (1988) *Containing Anxiety in Institutions: Selected Essays*. London: Free Association Books.

Meuter, R.F.I., Gallois, C., Segalowitz, N.S., et al. (2015) Overcoming language barriers in healthcare: A protocol for investigating safe and effective communication when patients or clinicians use a second language. *BMC Health Services Research*, 15, 371.

Mikulincer, M. & Shaver, P.R. (2003) The attachment behavioral system in adulthood: Activation, psychodynamics, and interpersonal processes. *Advances in Experimental Social Psychology*, 35, 53–152.

Mikulincer, M., & Shaver, P.R. (2008) Adult attachment and affect regulation. In: Cassidy, J. & Shaver, P.R. (eds) *Handbook of Attachment: Theory, Research, and Clinical Applications*. New York: Guilford Press, pp.503–531.

Milisen, K., Lemiengre, J., Braes, T. & Foreman, M.D. (2005) Multicomponent intervention strategies for managing delirium in hospitalized older people: Systematic review. *Journal of Advanced Nursing*, 52(1), 79–90.

Miller, G.R. & Nicholson, H.E. (1976) *Communication Inquiry: A Perspective on a Process*. Reading, MA: Addison-Wesley.

MIND (2018) *Anxiety and Panic Attacks*. Available at: https://www.mind.org.uk/information-support/types-of-mental-health-problems/anxiety-and-panic-attacks/panic-attacks/#.W8ry13tKjZ4

Mitchell, A.J. (2007) Pooled results from analysis of the accuracy of Distress Thermometer and other ultra short methods of detecting cancer related mood disorders. *Journal of Clinical Oncology*, 25, 4670–4681.

Mitchell, A.J., Baker-Glenn, E.A., Park, B., et al. (2010) Can the Distress Thermometer be improved by additional mood domains? Part II: What is the optimal combination of emotion thermometers? *Psycho-Oncology*, 19(2), 134–140.

Modern Slavery Act (2015) Available at: www.legislation.gov.uk/ukpga/2015/30/contents/enacted

National Literacy Trust (2017) *What is Literacy?* Available at: https://literacytrust.org.uk/information/what-is-literacy

NCCN (National Comprehensive Cancer Network) (2018) *Distress Management: Clinical Practice Guidelines in Oncology*. Available at: https://oncolife.com.ua/doc/nccn/Distress_Management.pdf

Neville, S. (2006) Practice development – delirium. Delirium and older people: Repositioning nursing care. *International Journal of Older People Nursing*, 1(2), 113–120.

NHS Digital (2017) *Data on Written Complaints in the NHS 2016–2017*. Available at: https://files.digital.nhs.uk/pdf/l/a/data_on_written_complaints_in_the_nhs_2016-17_report.pdf

NHS Digital (2018) *Safeguarding Adults Collection (SAC) Annual Report, England (April 2017–March 2018)*. Available at: https://digital.nhs.uk/

data-and-information/publications/statistical/safeguarding-adults/annual-report-2017-18-england

NHS England (2015) *Health and Safety Policy: Policy & Corporate Procedures.* Available at: https://www.england.nhs.uk/wp-content/uploads/2017/04/pol-1002-health-safety-policy.pdf

NHS England (2016) *Leading Change, Adding Value: A Framework for Nursing, Midwifery and Care Staff.* Available at: https://www.england.nhs.uk/wp-content/uploads/2016/05/nursing-framework.pdf

NHS England (2018) *Guidance for Commissioners: Interpreting and Translation Services in Primary Care.* Available at: https://www.england.nhs.uk/publication/guidance-for-commissioners-interpreting-and-translation-services-in-primary-care

NHS England North (2017) *Safeguarding Adults.* Available at: https://www.england.nhs.uk/wp-content/uploads/2017/02/adult-pocket-guide.pdf

NHS Protect (2013) *Meeting Needs and Reducing Distress: Guidance on the Prevention and Management of Clinically Related Challenging Behaviour in NHS Settings.* Available at: https://learn.canvas.net/courses/510/files/299314/download?verifier=7cbESZckm38jnVADwLQPSn1rlFAqtQOTHUN2varz&wrap=1

NICE (National Institute for Health and Care Excellence) (2004) *Improving Supportive and Palliative Care for Adults with Cancer: The Manual.* London: National Institute for Health and Care Excellence.

NICE (2006) *Guidance on Cancer Services: Improving Outcomes for People with Tumours of the Brain and Central Nervous System.* London: National Institute for Health and Care Excellence.

NICE (2009) *Depression in Adults with a Chronic Physical Health Problem: Recognition and Management* [CG91]. Available at: https://www.nice.org.uk/guidance/cg91/chapter/1-Guidance

NICE (2010) *Delirium: Diagnosis, Prevention and Management* [CG103]. London: National Institute for Health and Care Excellence.

NICE (2011a) *Generalised Anxiety Disorder and Panic Disorder (with or without Agoraphobia) in Adults: Management in Primary, Secondary and Community Care* [CG113]. London: National Institute for Health and Care Excellence.

NICE (2011b) *Common Mental Health Problems: Identification and Pathways to Care* [CG123]. Available at: https://www.nice.org.uk/guidance/cg123/chapter/1-guidance

NICE (2012) *Patient Experience in Adult NHS Services* [QS15]. Available at: https://www.nice.org.uk/guidance/qs15

NICE (2015) *Violence and Aggression: Short-Term Management in Mental Health, Health and Community Settings* [NG10]. Available at: https://www.nice.org.uk/guidance/ng10/resources/violence-and-aggression-shortterm-management-in-mental-health-health-and-community-settings-pdf-1837264712389

NICE (2016) *Patient Experience in Adult NHS Service* [CG138]. Available at: https://www.nice.org.uk/guidance/cg138

NICE (2018a) *Shared Decision Making.* Available at: https://www.nice.org.uk/about/what-we-do/our-programmes/nice-guidance/nice-guidelines/shared-decision-making

NICE (2018b) *Dementia: Assessment, Management and Support for People Living with Dementia and Their Carers.* Available at: https://www.nice.org.uk/guidance/ng97/resources/dementia-assessment-management-and-support-for-people-living-with-dementia-and-their-carers-pdf-1837760199109

NMC (Nursing and Midwifery Council) (2018) *The Code: Professional Standards of Practice and Behaviour for Nurses, Midwives and Nursing Associates.* Available at: https://www.nmc.org.uk/standards/code

Nordahl, G., Olofsson, N., Asplund, K. & Sjoling, M. (2003) The impact of pre-operative information on state anxiety, postoperative pain and satisfaction with pain management. *Patient Education and Counseling*, 51(2), 169–176.

NSPCC (National Society for the Prevention of Cruelty to Children) (2015) *Health: Learning from Case Reviews – Overview of Risk Factors and Learning for Improved Practice for all Professionals Working in the Health Sector.* Available at: https://learning.nspcc.org.uk/media/1340/learning-from-case-reviews_health.pdf

Oguchi, M., Jansen, J., Butow, P., et al. (2010) Measuring the impact of nurse cue-response behaviour on cancer patients' emotional cues. *Patient Education and Counseling*, 82(2), 163–168.

Ong, L.M., Visser, M.R., Lammes, F.B. & de Haes, J.C. (2000) Doctor–patient communication and cancer patients' quality of life and satisfaction. *Patient Education and Counseling*, 41(2), 145–156.

ONS (Office for National Statistics) (2013). *Language in England and Wales: 2011.* Available at: https://www.ons.gov.uk/peoplepopulationandcommunity/culturalidentity/language/articles/languageinenglandandwales/2013-03-04

P v Cheshire West and Chester Council [2014] UKSC 19. Available at: https://www.supremecourt.uk/cases/docs/uksc-2012-0068-judgment.pdf

Parke, B., Boltz, M., Hunter, K., et al. (2017) A scoping literature review of dementia-friendly hospital design. Gerontologist, 57(4), e62–e74.

Parker, P.A., Ross, A.C., Polansky, M.N., et al. (2010) Communicating with cancer patients: What areas do physician assistants find most challenging? *Journal of Cancer Education*, 25(4), 524–529.

Pennebaker, J.W. (1993) Putting stress into words: Health, linguistic, and therapeutic implications. *Behaviour Research and Therapy*, 31(6), 539–548.

Perry, K.N. & Burgess, M. (2002) *Communication in Cancer Care.* Oxford: Blackwell.

Pitman, A., Suleman, A., Hyde, N. & Hodgkiss, A. (2018) Depression and anxiety in patients with cancer. *BMJ*, 361, k1415.

Plain English Campaign (2019) *How to Write in Plain English.* Available at: www.plainenglish.co.uk/how-to-write-in-plain-english.html

Polson, J. & Croy, S. (2015) Differentiating dementia, delirium and depression. *Nursing Times*, 113(16), 18–19.

Powell, T. (2009) *The Mental Health Handbook*, 3rd edn. Milton Keynes: Speechmark.

Powell, T. & Enright, S. (1990) *Anxiety and Stress Management.* London: Routledge.

Price, B. (2013) Six steps to teaching cancer patients. *Cancer Nursing Practice*, 12(6), 25–33.

Public Interest Disclosure Act (1998) Available at: www.legislation.gov.uk/ukpga/1998/23/contents

Ransom, S., Jacobsen, P.B. & Booth-Jones, M. (2006) Validation of the Distress Thermometer with bone marrow transplant patients. *Psycho-Oncology*, 15(7), 604–612.

Razavi, D., Delvaux, N., Marchal, S., et al. (2000) Testing health care professionals' communication skills: The usefulness of highly emotional standardized role-playing sessions with simulators. *Psycho-Oncology*, 9(4), 293–302.

RCN (Royal College of Nursing) (n.d.) *Safeguarding.* Available at: https://www.rcn.org.uk/clinical-topics/safeguarding

RCN (2017) *Principles of Consent: Guidance for Nursing Staff.* Available at: https://www.rcn.org.uk/-/media/royal-college-of-nursing/documents/publications/2017/june/pub-006047.pdf

RCN (2019) *Principles of Nursing Practice.* Available at: https://www.rcn.org.uk/professional-development/principles-of-nursing-practice

RCOT (Royal College of Occupational Therapists) (2015) *Occupational Therapy and the Prevention and Management of Falls in Adults.* Available at: https://www.rcot.co.uk/practice-resources/rcot-practice-guidelines/falls

RCPsych (Royal College of Psychiatrists) (2015a) *Benzodiazepines.* Available at: https://www.rcpsych.ac.uk/mental-health/treatments-and-wellbeing/benzodiazepines

RCPsych (2015b) *Delirium.* Available at: https://www.rcpsych.ac.uk/mental-health/problems-disorders/delirium

Reder, P. & Fredman, G. (1996) Relationship to help: Interacting beliefs about the treatment process. *Clinical Child Psychology and Psychiatry*, 1, 457–467.

Redsell, S.A. & Buck, J. (2009) Health-related decision making: The use of information giving models in different care settings. *Quality in Primary Care*, 17(6), 377–379.

RNIB (Royal National Institute of Blind People) (2016) *Ten Tips to Help You Communicate with a Person with Sight Loss.* Available at: https://www.rnib.org.uk/nb-online/top-tips-communication

RNIB (2019) *Top Tips for Healthcare Professionals.* Available at: https://www.rnib.org.uk/top-tips-healthcare-professionals

Roberts, D. & Snowball, J. (1999) Psychosocial care in oncology nursing: A study of social knowledge. *Journal of Clinical Nursing*, 8, 39–47.

Rodrigues, A. (2016) *Exploring the Relationships among Attachment, Emotion Regulation, Differentiation of Self, Negative Problem Orientation, Self Esteem, Worry, and Generalized Anxiety* [doctoral dissertation]. Department of Applied Psychology and Human Development, University of Toronto.

Roebuck, T. (2017) *Rethinking Communication in Health and Social Care.* London: Palgrave.

Rogers, C.R. (1975) Empathic: An unappreciated way of being. *Counseling Psychologist*, 5, 2–10.

Ross, C.A. (1991) CNS arousal systems: Possible role in delirium. *International Psychogeriatrics*, 3(2), 353–371.
Ryan, H., Schofield, P., Cockburn, J., et al. (2005) How to recognize and manage psychological distress in cancer patients. *European Journal of Cancer Care*, 14(1), 7–15.
Safeguarding Vulnerable Groups (Northern Ireland) Order (2007) Available at: https://www.legislation.gov.uk/nisi/2007/1351/contents
Safety Net Project (2019) *Safety Net*. Available at: https://arcuk.org.uk/safetynet
Schofield, P.E., Butow, P.N., Thompson, J.F. & Tattersall, M.H. (2008) Physician communication. *Journal of Clinical Oncology*, 26(2), 297–302.
Schroevers, M.J., Helgeson, V.S., Sanderman, R., et al. (2010) Type of social support matters for prediction of posttraumatic growth among cancer survivors. *Psycho-Oncology*, 19(1), 46–53.
Scott, A. (2004) Managing anxiety in ICU patients: The role of pre-operative information provision. *Nursing in Critical Care*, 9(2), 72–79.
Shafi, N. & Carozza, L. (2012) Treating cancer-related aphasia. *ASHA Leader*, 17(9). DOI: 10.1044/leader.FTR3.17092012.np.
Silverman, J.D., Kurtz, S.M. & Draper, J. (2013) *Skills for Communicating with Patients*, 3rd edn. London: Radcliffe.
Smets, E.M., Hillen, M.A., Douma, K.F., et al. (2013) Does being informed and feeling informed affect patients' trust in their radiation oncologist? *Patient Education and Counseling*, 90(3), 330–337.
Smith, C., Dickens, C. & Edwards, S. (2005) Provision of information for cancer patients: An appraisal and review. *European Journal of Cancer Care*, 14, 282–288.
Social Services and Well-being (Wales) Act (2014) Available at: https://www.legislation.gov.uk/anaw/2014/4/contents
Stevens, S. (2003) Assisting the blind and visually impaired: Guidelines for eye health workers and other helpers. *Community Eye Health*, 16(45), 7–9.
Stevenson, J.C., Emerson, L. & Millings, A. (2017) The relationship between adult attachment orientation and mindfulness: A systematic review and meta-analysis. *Mindfulness*, 8, 1438–1455.
Stewart, M.A. (1996) Effective physician-patient communication and health outcomes: A review. *Canadian Medical Association Journal*, 152, 1423–1433.
Street, R.L. Jr. & Voigt, B. (1997) Patient participation in deciding breast cancer treatment and subsequent quality of life. *Medical Decision Making*, 17(3), 298–306.
Stroke Association (2017) *State of the Nation: Stroke Statistics*. Available at: https://www.stroke.org.uk/sites/default/files/state_of_the_nation_2017_final_1.pdf
Swain, J., Hancock, K., Hainsworth, C. & Bowman, J. (2013) Acceptance and commitment therapy in the treatment of anxiety: A systematic review. *Clinical Psychology Review*, 33, 964–978.
Tate, P. (2010) *The Doctor's Communication Handbook*. London: Radcliffe Medical Press.
Taylor, B. (1998) Ordinariness in nursing as therapy. In: McMahon, R. & Pearson, A. (eds) *Nursing as Therapy*. Cheltenham: Stanley Thornes, pp.64–75.
Taylor, C., Graham, J., Potts, H., et al. (2005) Changes in mental health of UK hospital consultants since the mid-1990s. *Lancet*, 366(9487), 742–744.
Thoits, P.A. (1995) Stress, coping, and social support processes: Where are we? What next? *Journal of Health and Social Behavior*, 35, 53–79.
Thorne, S.E., Kuo, M., Armstrong, E.-A., et al. (2005) 'Being known': Patients' perspectives of the dynamics of human connection in cancer care. *Psycho-Oncology*, 14(10), 887–898.
Tonkins, S. (2011) Dementia care. *Nursing Standard*, 25(50), 59.
Tortora, G.J. & Derrickson, B.H. (2011) *Principles of Anatomy & Physiology*, 13th edn. Hoboken, NJ: John Wiley & Sons.
Tortora, G.J. & Derrickson, B.H. (2017) *Principles of Anatomy & Physiology*, 15th edn. Hoboken, NJ: John Wiley & Sons.
Towers, R. (2007) Providing psychological support for patients with cancer. *Nursing Standard*, 28(12), 50–58.
Turner, J., Clavarino, A., Yates, P., et al. (2007) Oncology nurses' perceptions of their supportive care for patients with advanced cancer: Challenges and educational needs. *Psycho-Oncology*, 16, 149–157.
Uitterhoeve, R.J., Bensing, J.M., Grol, R.P., et al. (2010) The effect of communication skills training on patient outcomes in cancer care: A systematic review of the literature. *European Journal of Cancer Care*, 19(4), 442–457.
Van Oosterwijck, J., Meeus, M., Paul, L., et al. (2013) Pain physiology education improves health status and endogenous pain inhibition in fibromyalgia: A double-blind randomized controlled trial. *Clinical Journal of Pain*, 29(10), 873–882.
Vasse, E., Vernooij-Dassen, M., Spijker, A., et al. (2010) A systematic review of communication strategies for people with dementia in residential and nursing homes. *International Psychogeriatrics*, 22(2), 189–200.
Vos, M.S. (2008) Denial in lung cancer patients: A longitudinal study. *Psycho-Oncology*, 17, 1163–1171.
Vos, M.S. & de Haes, H.J. (2010) Complex rather than vague. *Lung Cancer*, 70(2), 227–228.
Vos, M.S. & de Haes, H.J. (2011) Denial indeed is a process. *Lung Cancer*, 72(1), 138.
Weatherhead, I. & Courtney, C. (2012) Assessing the signs of dementia. *Practice Nursing*, 23(3), 114–118.
Webster, C. & Bryan, K. (2009) Older people's views of dignity and how it can be promoted in a hospital environment. *Journal of Clinical Nursing*, 18(12), 1784–1792.
White, C., McCann, M. & Jackson, N. (2007) First do no harm … terminal restlessness or drug-induced delirium. *Journal of Palliative Medicine*, 10, 345–351.
White, H. (2004) Acquired communication and swallowing difficulties in patients with primary brain tumours. In: Booth, S. & Bruera, E. (eds) *Palliative Care Consultations Primary and Metastatic Brain Tumours*. Oxford: Oxford University Press, pp.117–134.
WHO (World Health Organization) (1946) *Constitution of WHO: Principles*. Available at: https://www.who.int/about/mission/en/
WHO (2016) *ICD-10 Version: 2016*. Available at: https://icd.who.int/browse10/2016/en
WHO (2017) *Dementia*. Available at: https://www.who.int/en/news-room/fact-sheets/detail/dementia
WHO (2018) *ICD-11: The 11th Revision of the International Classification of Diseases*. Geneva: World Health Organization.
Wiechula, R., Conroy, T., Kitson, A.L., et al. (2015) Umbrella review of the evidence: What factors influence the caring relationship between a nurse and patient? *Journal of Advanced Nursing*, 72(4), 723–734.
Wilkinson, S. (1991) Factors which influence how nurses communicate with cancer patients. *Journal of Advanced Nursing*, 16, 677–688.
Williams, A.M & Iruita, V.F. (2004) Therapeutic and non-therapeutic interpersonal interactions: The patient's perspective. *Journal of Clinical Nursing*, 13(7), 806–815.
Wosket, V. (2006) *Egan's Skilled Helper Model: Developments and Applications in Counselling*. London: Routledge.
Young, T. (2012) Devising a dementia toolkit for effective communication. *Nursing & Residential Care*, 14(3), 149–151.
Young Dementia UK (2018) *Young Onset Dementia Facts and Figures*. Available at: https://www.youngdementiauk.org/young-onset-dementia-facts-figures
Zigmond, A.S. & Snaith, R.P. (1983) The Hospital Anxiety and Depression Scale. *Acta Psychiatrica Scandinavica*, 67(6), 361–370.

Chapter 6

Elimination

Rebecca Martin with Gemma Allen, Katy Hardy, Claire McNally, Jacqueline McPhail, Bradley Russell and Laura Theodossy

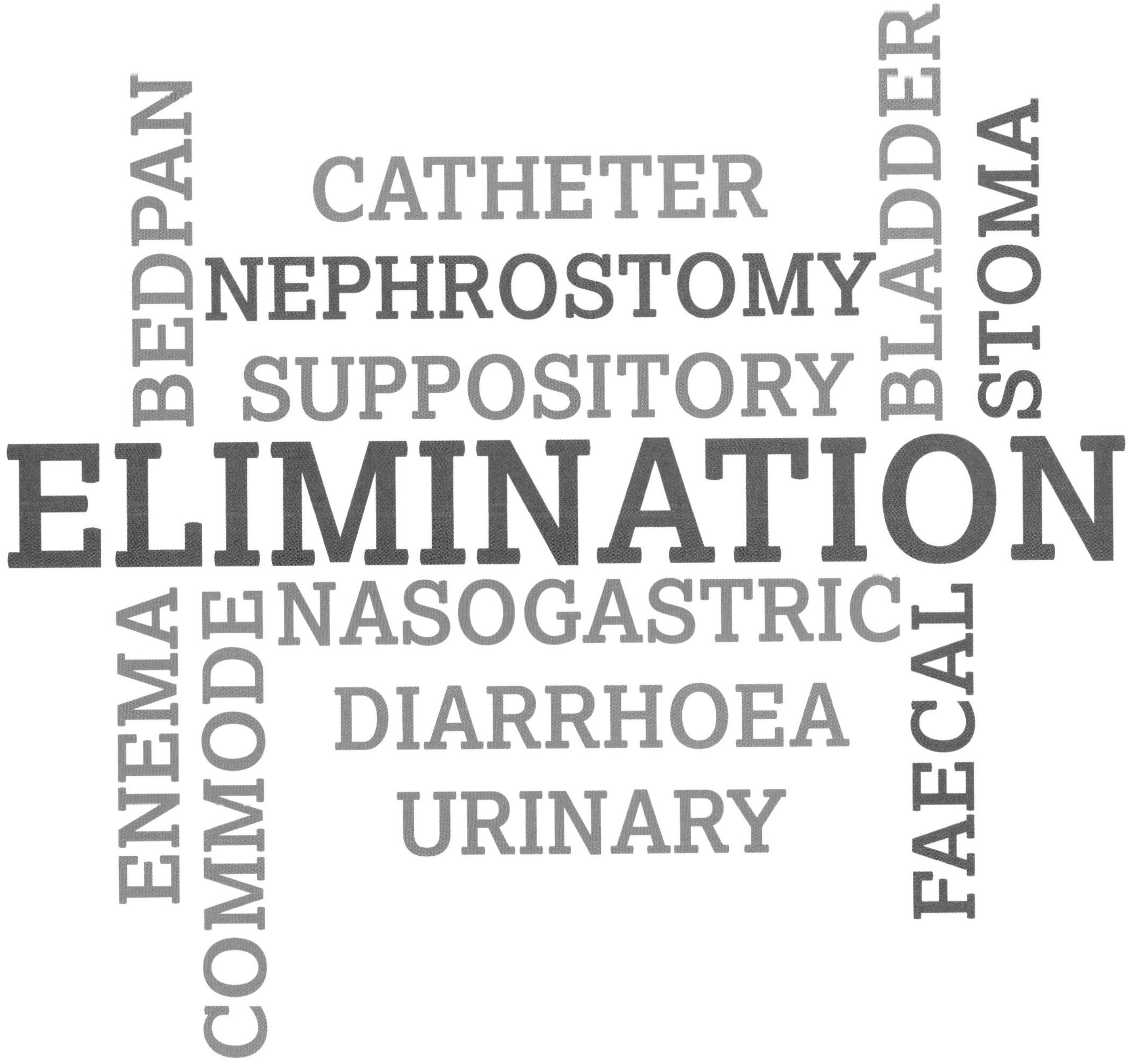

Procedure guidelines

Being an accountable professional

At the point of registration, the nurse will:

6. Use evidence-based, best practice approaches for meeting needs for care and support with bladder and bowel health, accurately assessing the person's capacity for independence and self-care and initiating appropriate interventions

Future Nurse: Standards of Proficiency for Registered Nurses (NMC 2018)

Overview

This chapter provides an overview of elimination and is divided into four main sections. The first reviews normal elimination. The second section examines altered urinary elimination, including penile sheaths, urinary catheterization, urinary diversions and bladder irrigation. The third section considers altered faecal elimination, including diarrhoea, constipation, enemas, suppositories, digital rectal examination and digital removal of faeces. The final section provides an overview of stoma care, both urinary and faecal.

Normal elimination

Urinary elimination

Definition

Urinary elimination is the excretion of urine from the body (Patton 2018). Urine is made by the kidneys and is the liquid by-product of metabolism; it contains, among other products, urea, uric acid and creatinine (Marieb and Hoehn 2015).

Anatomy and physiology

The urinary tract (see Figure 6.1) consists of the two kidneys, the two ureters, the bladder and the urethra. The urinary system produces, stores and eliminates urine. The kidneys are responsible for excreting wastes such as urea and ammonium and for the reabsorption of glucose and amino acids. They are involved in the production of hormones including calcitrol, renin and erythropoietin. The kidneys also have homeostatic functions, including the regulation of blood volume and electrolytes, acid-base balance and blood pressure (Tortora and Derrickson 2017).

Each kidney excretes urine into a ureter, which arises from the renal pelvis on the medial aspect of each kidney. In adults, the ureters are approximately 25–30 cm long and 2–4 mm in diameter (Tortora and Derrickson 2017). The ureters are muscular tubes that propel urine from the kidneys to the urinary bladder. They enter through the back of the bladder, running within the wall of the bladder for a few centimetres. Ureterovesical valves prevent the backflow of urine from the bladder to the kidneys.

The bladder sits on the pelvic floor and is a hollow, muscular, distensible organ that stores urine until it is convenient to expel it. Urine enters the bladder via the ureters and exits via the urethra. As the bladder fills, stretch receptors in the muscular wall signal the parasympathetic nervous system to contract the bladder, initiating the conscious desire to expel urine. In order for urine to be expelled, both the automatically controlled internal sphincter and the voluntarily controlled external sphincter must be opened.

Urine leaves the bladder via the urethra. In females this lies in front of the anterior wall of the vagina and is approximately 3.8 cm long. In males it passes through the prostate and penis and is approximately 20 cm long (Tortora and Derrickson 2017).

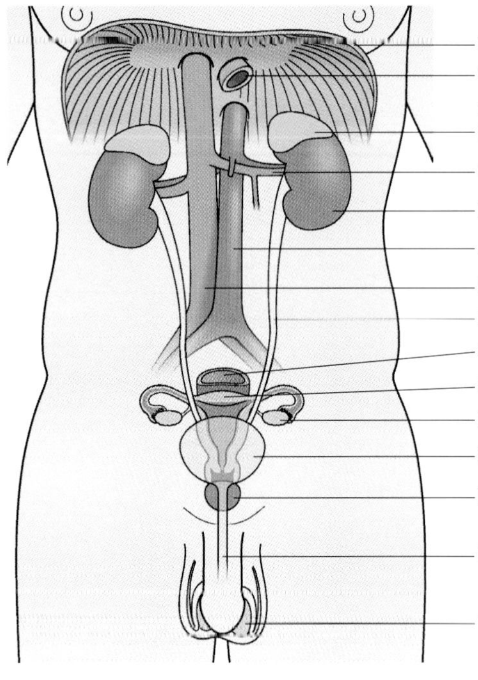

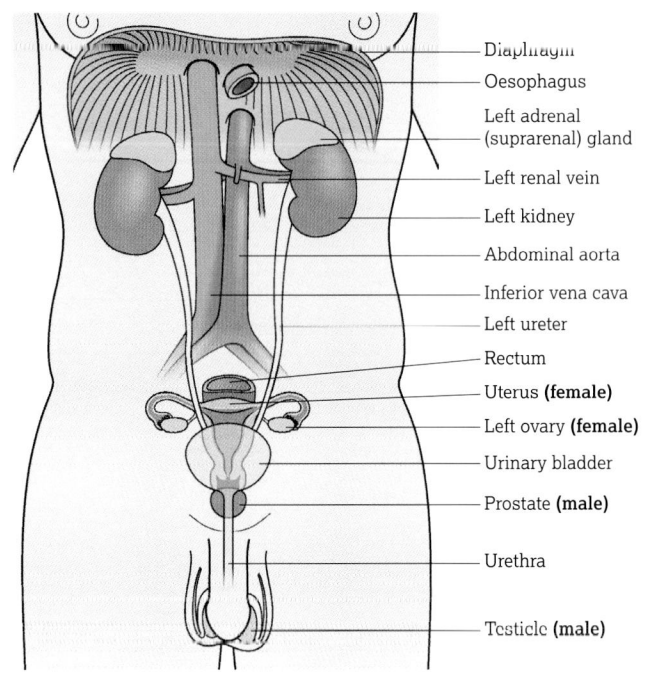

Figure 6.1 The (a) male and (b) female genitourinary tracts.

Faecal elimination

Definition

Faecal elimination is the expulsion of the residues of digestion (faeces) from the digestive tract (Patton 2018). The act of expelling faeces is called defaecation.

Anatomy and physiology

This section considers the normal structure and function of the bowel, which includes the small and large intestines (Figure 6.2). The small intestine begins at the pyloric sphincter of the stomach; it then coils through the abdomen and opens into the large intestine at the ileocaecal junction. It is approximately 6 m in length and is divided into three segments: the duodenum (25 cm), jejunum (2.5 m) and ileum (3.5 m) (Patton 2018). The mucosal surface of the small intestine is covered with finger-like processes called villi, which increase the surface area available for absorption and digestion. A number of digestive enzymes are secreted by the small intestine (Tortora and Derrickson 2017).

Movement through the small bowel is divided into two types – segmentation and peristalsis – and is controlled by the autonomic nervous system. Segmentation refers to the localized, concentric contraction of the intestine, aided by constant lengthening and shortening of the villi; this results in mixing the intestinal contents and bringing particles of food into contact with the mucosa for absorption. Once the majority of a meal has been absorbed through this process, intestinal content is then pushed along the small intestine by repeated peristaltic wave like actions. Intestinal content usually remains in the small bowel for 3–5 hours (Tortora and Derrickson 2017).

The total volume of fluid, including ingested liquids and gastrointestinal secretions, that enters the small intestine daily is about 9.3 L. The small intestine is responsible for absorbing around 90% of the nutrients, electrolytes and water by diffusion, facilitated diffusion, osmosis and active transport (Tortora and Derrickson 2017). Water is able to move across the intestinal mucosa in both directions but is influenced by the absorption of nutrients and electrolytes. As various electrolytes and nutrients are actively transported out of the lumen, they create a concentration gradient, promoting water absorption, via osmosis, in order to maintain an osmotic balance between intestinal fluid and blood. This ultimately leads to only about 1 L of effluent passing through into the colon (Patton 2018, Tortora and Derrickson 2017).

From the ileocaecal sphincter to the anus, the colon is approximately 1.5–1.8 m in length and 4–6 cm in diameter. Its main function is to eliminate the waste products of digestion by the propulsion of faeces towards the anus. In addition, it produces mucus to lubricate the faecal mass, thus aiding its expulsion. Other functions include the absorption of fluid and electrolytes (including sodium and potassium), the storage of faeces and the synthesis of vitamins B and K by bacterial flora (Patton 2018, Tortora and Derrickson 2017).

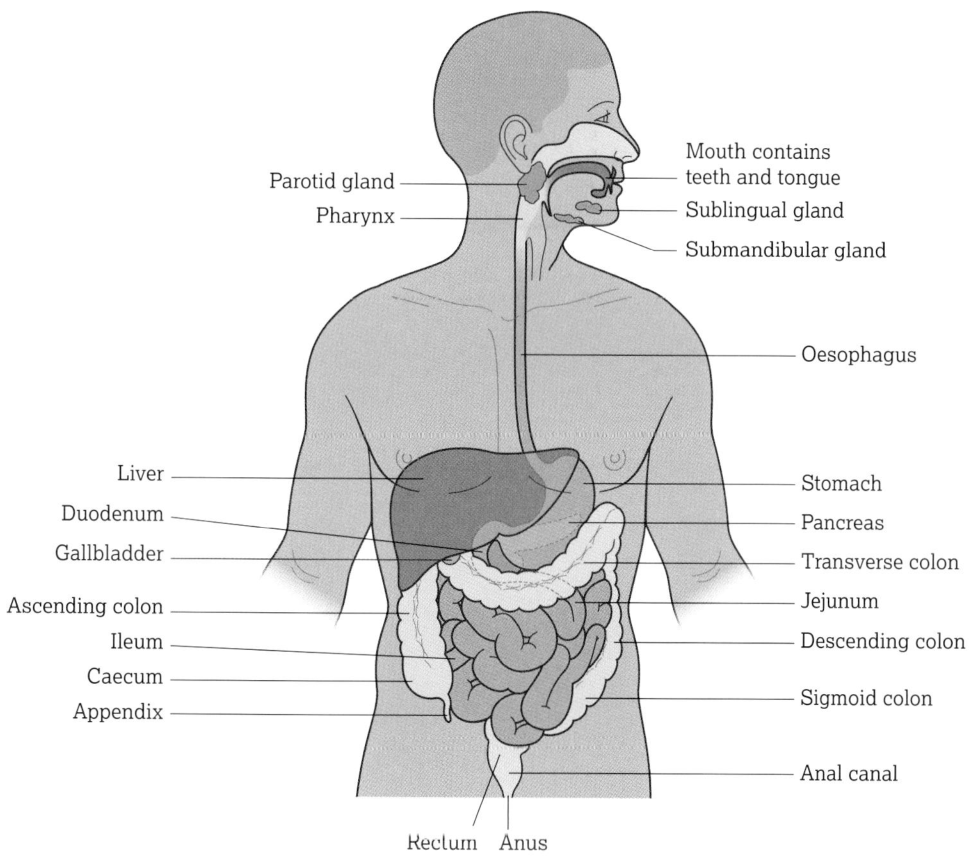

Figure 6.2 The gastrointestinal tract. *Source:* Reproduced from Peate et al. (2014) with permission of John Wiley & Sons, Ltd.

Faeces consist of the unabsorbed end-products of digestion: bile pigments, cellulose, bacteria, epithelial cells, mucus and some inorganic material. They are normally semi-solid in consistency and contain about 70% water (Tortora and Derrickson 2017). The colon absorbs about 2 L of water in 24 hours, so if faeces are not expelled they will gradually become hard (due to dehydration) and more difficult to expel. If there is insufficient roughage (fibre) in the faeces, colonic stasis occurs, which leads to continued water absorption and further hardening of the faeces. Faeces will, therefore, vary in consistency, as illustrated in the Bristol Stool Chart (Figure 6.3).

The movement of faeces through the colon towards the anus occurs via mass peristalsis, a gastrocolic reflex initiated by the presence of food in the stomach. Mass peristalsis begins at the middle of the transverse colon and quickly drives the colonic contents into the rectum. This mass peristaltic movement generally occurs three to five times a day (Perdue 2005). In response to this stimulus, faeces move into the rectum (Tortora and Derrickson 2017). This rectal distension triggers the desire to defaecate, also known as the 'call to stool'.

Assisting the patient with elimination

Evidence-based approaches

Principles of care

Elimination can be a sensitive issue and providing effective care and management for problems associated with it can sometimes be problematic. The difficulties associated with this can be minimized if the nurse seeks to respect the patient's dignity when carrying out procedures such as assisting them with using a bedpan or a commode.

Clinical governance

The privacy and dignity of the patient must be respected at all times (NMC 2018). It is essential that the procedure is explained clearly to the patient to ensure consent is obtained and patient co-operation is agreed. A moving and handling assessment is vital in order to establish whether additional equipment, such as a hoist, is required.

Pre-procedural considerations

Equipment

Before commencing the procedure, ensure that appropriate equipment and staff are available for safe moving and handling of the patient and, depending on the patient's mobility, that either a bedpan or commode is available for immediate use (Figures 6.4 and 6.5).

Pharmacological support

Incontinence-associated dermatitis (IAD) is a term used for the breakdown of the natural skin barrier that happens when the skin becomes macerated as a consequence of faecal and/or urinary incontinence (Yates 2018) and has been clearly differentiated from other forms of skin damage, such as pressure ulcers or skin tears (Gray et al. 2012). It can affect the perineum, buttocks, groin folds, labia majora (in women) or scrotum (in men) (Beeckman et al. 2015). Current nursing practice includes the use of a wide range of skin moisturizers and barrier creams with varying evidence of their efficacy and effectiveness (Gray et al. 2012). Callaghan et al. (2018) suggest that barrier creams can be effective in promoting skin integrity when selected appropriately. A review suggests that the use of barrier creams with a pH near to that of normal skin can be useful in the prevention of skin problems (Beeckman et al. 2009, Geraghty 2011).

Procedure guideline 6.1 Slipper bedpan use: assisting a patient

Essential equipment

- Personal protective equipment
- Manual handling equipment as appropriate
- Slipper bedpan and paper cover
- Additional nurse or healthcare assistant if required to assist with manual handling
- Toilet paper
- Washbowl, warm water, disposable wipes and a towel

Action	Rationale
Pre-procedure	
1 Carry out an appropriate manual handling assessment prior to commencing procedure and establish whether an additional nurse or equipment such as a hoist is necessary.	To maintain a safe environment. **E**
2 Introduce yourself to the patient, explain and discuss the procedure with them, and gain their consent to proceed.	To ensure that the patient feels at ease, understands the procedure and gives their valid consent (NMC 2018, **C**).
Procedure	
3 Take the equipment to the bedside. Wash hands and put on gloves and apron.	To ensure the procedure is as clean as possible and minimize the risk of spreading infection (NHS England and NHSI 2019, **C**).
4 Close the door or draw the curtains around the patient's bed area.	To maintain privacy and dignity and avoid any unnecessary embarrassment for the patient (NMC 2018, **C**).
5 Remove the bedclothes and, providing there are no contraindications (e.g. if patient is on flat bedrest), assist the patient into an upright sitting position.	An upright, 'crouch-like' posture is considered anatomically correct for defaecation. Poor posture adopted while using a bedpan has been shown to cause extreme straining during defaecation. Patients should therefore be supported with pillows in order to achieve an upright position on the bedpan (Woodward 2012, **E**).
6 Ask the patient to raise their hips and buttocks, and insert the bedpan beneath the patient's pelvis, ensuring that the wide end of the bedpan is between the legs and the narrow end is beneath the buttocks.	A slipper bedpan provides more comfort for a patient who is unable to sit upright on a conventional bedpan (Nicol 2008, **E**).
7 Offer the patient the use of pillows and encourage them to lean forward slightly if possible.	To provide support and optimize positioning for defaecation (Woodward 2012, **E**).
8 Once the patient is on the bedpan, encourage them to move their legs slightly apart and check to ensure that their positioning is correct.	To avoid any spillage onto the bedclothes and reduce the risk of contamination and cross-infection. **E**
9 Cover the patient's legs with a sheet.	To maintain privacy and dignity (NMC 2018, **C**).
10 Ensure that toilet paper and a call bell are within the patient's reach and leave the patient, but remain nearby.	To maintain privacy and dignity (NMC 2018, **C**).
11 When the patient has finished using the bedpan, remove it, replace the paper cover and bring washing equipment to the bedside. Assist the patient to clean the perianal area. Apply a small amount of barrier cream to the perineal and/or buttock area if appropriate.	Talcum powder should not be used. Barrier creams should be applied sparingly and gently layered on in the direction of the hair growth rather than rubbed into the skin (Le Lievre 2002, **E**).
12 Offer a bowl of water or moistened wipes for the patient to clean their hands.	For infection prevention and control, and for the patient's comfort (Fraise and Bradley 2009, **E**).
13 Ensure the bedclothes are clean, straighten the sheets and the rearrange pillows, and assist the patient into a comfortable position. Ensure the call bell is within reach of the patient.	For the patient's comfort. **P**
14 Take the bedpan to the dirty utility (sluice) room and, where necessary, measure urine output and note characteristics and amount of faeces using the Bristol Stool Chart (Figure 6.3).	To monitor and evaluate the patient's elimination patterns. **E**
Post-procedure	
15 Dispose of the contents safely and place the bedpan in the washer or disposal unit.	For infection prevention and control (Fraise and Bradley 2009, **E**).
16 Remove disposable apron and gloves. Wash hands using soap and water and/or alcohol-based handrub.	For infection prevention and control (NHS England and NHSI 2019, **C**).
17 Record any urine output and/or bowel action in the patient's documentation.	To maintain accurate documentation (NMC 2018, **C**).

Procedure guideline 6.2 Commode use: assisting a patient

Essential equipment

- Personal protective equipment
- Manual handling equipment as appropriate
- A clean commode with conventional bedpan inserted below seat
- Additional nurse or healthcare assistant if required
- Toilet paper
- Washbowl, warm water, disposable wipes and a towel

Action	Rationale
Pre-procedure	
1 Carry out an appropriate manual handling assessment prior to commencing procedure and ensure that patient's weight does not exceed the maximum recommended for the commode (see manufacturer's guidelines).	To maintain a safe environment. **E**
2 Introduce yourself to the patient, explain and discuss the procedure with them, and gain their consent to proceed.	To ensure that the patient feels at ease, understands the procedure and gives their valid consent (NMC 2018, **C**).
3 Wash hands and/or use an alcohol-based handrub, and put on gloves and an apron. Take the equipment to the bedside.	For infection prevention and control (NHS England and NHSI 2019, **C**).
Procedure	
4 Close the door or draw the curtains around the patient's bed area.	To maintain privacy and dignity and avoid any unnecessary embarrassment for the patient (NMC 2018 **C**).
5 Remove the commode cover and ensure the brakes are on. Assist the patient out of the bed/chair and onto the commode.	To ensure the patient can safely position themselves on the commode. **E**
6 Once they are seated, ensure the patient's feet are positioned directly below their knees and flat on the floor or footplates of commode. The use of a small footstool and/or pillows may help to achieve a comfortable position.	An upright, crouching posture is considered anatomically correct for defaecation. Pillows and a footstool can provide support and optimize positioning for defaecation (Woodward 2012, **E**)
7 Cover the patient's knees with a towel or sheet.	To maintain privacy and dignity (NMC 2018, **C**).
8 Ensure that toilet paper and a call bell are within the patient's reach and leave the patient, but remain nearby.	To maintain privacy and dignity (NMC 2018, **C**) and to prevent falls.
9 When the patient has finished using the commode, bring washing equipment to the bedside. Assist the patient to clean the perianal area using toilet paper and, where necessary, warm water or wipes. Apply a small amount of barrier cream to the perineal and/or buttock area if appropriate.	Talcum powder should not be used, and barrier creams should be applied sparingly and gently layered on in the direction of the hair growth rather than rubbed into the skin (Le Lievre 2002, **E**).
10 Offer a bowl of water for the patient to wash their hands.	For infection control and patient dignity (Fraise and Bradley 2009, **E**).
11 Assist the patient to stand and walk to the bed/chair, ensuring that they are comfortably positioned. Ensure the call bell is within reach of the patient.	For the patient's comfort. **P**
Post-procedure	
12 Replace the cover on the commode and return it to the dirty utility (sluice) room.	To reduce any risk of contamination or cross-infection (Fraise and Bradley 2009, **E**) and to avoid patient embarrassment (NMC 2018, **C**).
13 Remove the pan from underneath the commode and, where necessary, measure urine output and note characteristics and amount of faeces using the Bristol Stool Chart (see Figure 6.3).	To monitor and evaluate the patient's elimination patterns. **E**
14 Dispose of the contents safely and place the pan in the washer or disposal unit.	For infection prevention and control (Fraise and Bradley 2009, **E**).
15 Clean the commode using chlorine wipes or chlorine cleaning solution according to local guidelines.	For infection prevention and control (Fraise and Bradley 2009, **E**).
16 Remove disposable apron and gloves. Wash hands using bactericidal soap and water.	For infection control (NHS England and NHSI 2019, **C**).
17 Record any urine output and/or bowel action in patient's documentation.	To maintain accurate documentation (NMC 2018, **C**).

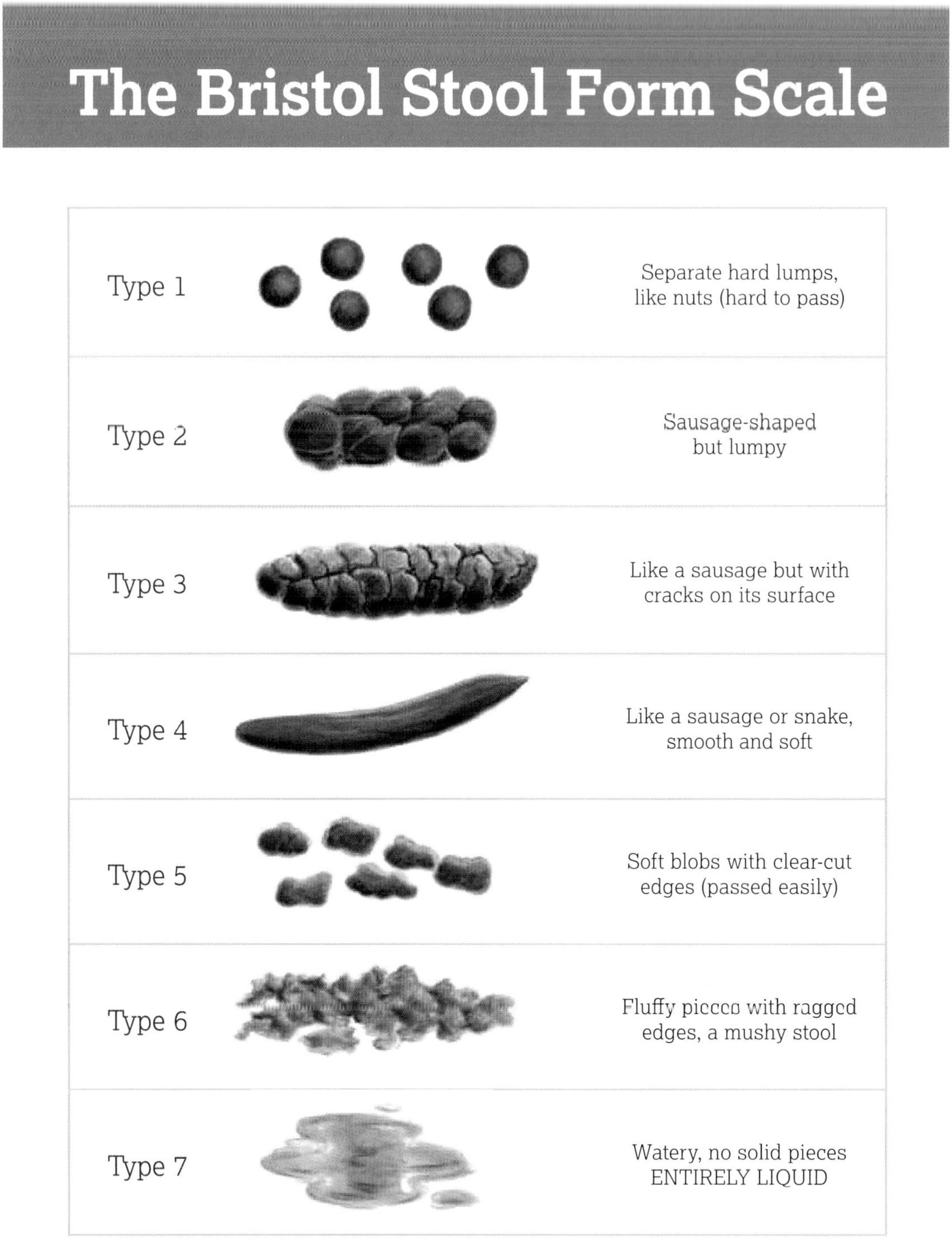
The Bristol Stool Form Scale
Type 1
Separate hard lumps, like nuts (hard to pass)
Type 2
Sausage-shaped but lumpy
Type 3
Like a sausage but with cracks on its surface
Type 4
Like a sausage or snake, smooth and soft
Type 5
Soft blobs with clear-cut edges (passed easily)
Type 6
Fluffy pieces with ragged edges, a mushy stool
Type 7
Watery, no solid pieces ENTIRELY LIQUID

Figure 6.3 Bristol Stool Chart. *Source*: Courtesy of Dr. K.W. Heaton, Reader in Medicine at the University of Bristol. Reproduced with permission of Norgine Pharmaceuticals Ltd.

Altered urinary elimination

This section first examines urinary incontinence and then reviews different approaches to its management. Surgical interventions and supportive care for altered urinary elimination are considered, including insertion of nephrostomy tubes and urinary diversions.

Urinary incontinence

Related theory

Urinary incontinence affects both men and women throughout the world. Roughly 11–34% of men over the age of 65 suffer with urinary incontinence (Clemens et al. 2018), and it is thought that 12–53% of women of all ages suffer from urinary incontinence

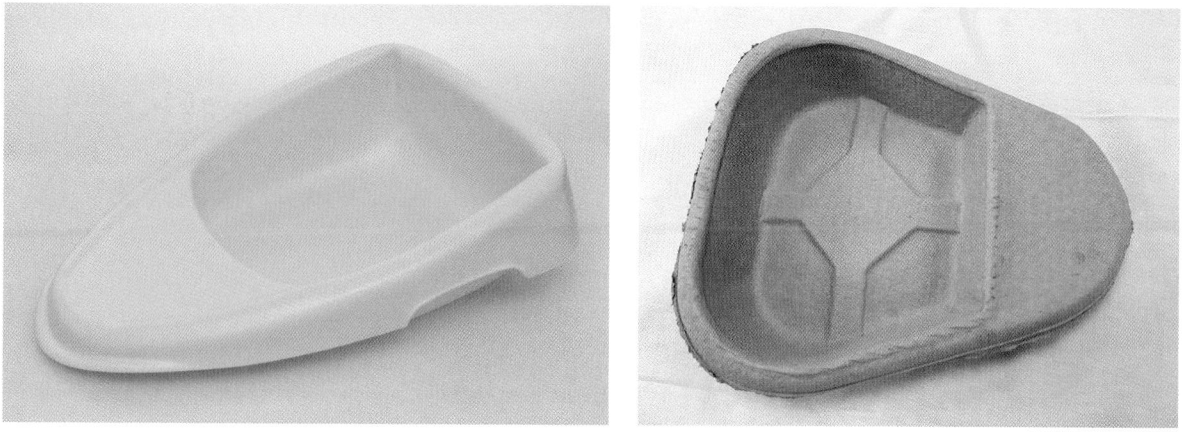

(a) (b)

Figure 6.4 Slipper bed pans: (a) reusable, (b) disposable.

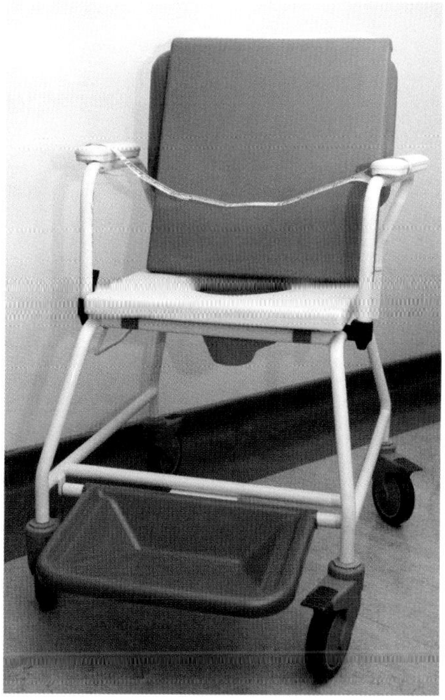

Figure 6.5 Commode.

(Serati and Ghezzi 2016). Urinary incontinence can be defined in many ways. Throughout this section you will find evidence-based approaches to managing urinary incontinence.

Urinary incontinence has many impacts on the lives of those who suffer from it and should be fully assessed to find the cause, which will signpost the suitable management approach. Urinary incontinence can have a negative effect on sleep, psychological and emotional wellbeing, relationships, working life and social life, and overall quality of life can be altered with any form of urinary incontinence (Abrams et al. 2014). Studies have shown that people affected by urinary incontinence feel ashamed, embarrassed and anxious around their condition (Nazarko 2018b).

Risk factors include the following:

- age (Devore et al. 2012)
- neurological conditions (multiple sclerosis, motor neurone disease or spinal cord injury) (Nethercliffe 2012)
- surgical procedures (e.g. hysterectomy, pelvic surgery) (Stothers and Friedman 2011)
- diabetes (Stothers and Friedman 2011)
- higher body mass index (Devore et al. 2012)
- physical trauma (e.g. childbirth) (Nethercliffe 2012)
- menopause (Legendre et al. 2013)
- cystitis and urinary tract infections (UTIs) (Mody and Juthani-Mehta 2014)
- enlargement of the prostate, known as benign prostatic hyperplasia
- prostate surgery (Macaulay et al. 2015)
- prostate cancer (Macaulay et al. 2015).

Penile sheaths

Evidence-based approaches

Rationale

Penile sheaths are external devices made from soft and flexible latex or silicone tubing. They are applied over the penis to direct urine into any standard urinary drainage bag, from where it can be conveniently emptied (see Figure 6.6) (Kyle 2011a). They can be used by men to manage urinary incontinence.

Penile sheaths (also known as condom catheters or male external catheters, or by the trade name Conveen) are only to be considered once other methods of promoting continence have failed,

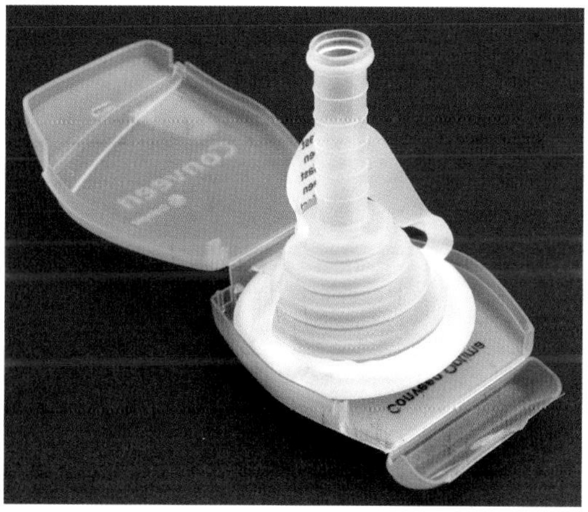

Figure 6.6 Penile sheath: standard design.

as the promotion of continence and treatment of incontinence should be the primary concern of the multidisciplinary team (Smart 2014). Penile sheaths should be considered as a preferable alternative to other methods of continence control, such as pads, which can quickly become sodden and cause skin problems, and catheters, which have several potential complications (discussed further below) (Smart 2014).

Indications

Penile sheaths (Figure 6.6) may be used to relieve incontinence when no other means is practicable or when all other methods have failed. Penile sheaths are also used to avoid or prevent catheter-associated UTIs (Gray et al. 2016). Penile sheaths are associated with many common problems, which are identified by Smart (2014); these include difficulties relating to fitting, leaking, kinking, falling off, allergies and UTIs.

Contraindications

Penile sheaths are contraindicated for men with very small or retracted penises, sensitive skin and allergies to specific materials such as latex (Nazarko 2018b).

Pre-procedural considerations

Equipment

Silicone types are now preferred due to concerns about latex allergies; additionally, the use of silicone enables the wearer or carer to assess and monitor the condition of the skin of the penis (Nazarko 2018b; Smart 2014).

Sizing and fitting

Modern sheaths come in a variety of sizes and the correct size can be determined by measuring the girth of the penile shaft. The penis should be measured in the flaccid state (Nazarko 2018b). Most devices come with a manufacturer's sheath sizing guide with different diameters cut into it, so that the correct size can be easily determined. Sheaths are available in a variety of different sizes, which generally increase in increments of 5–10 mm and in either standard or short lengths (Macaulay et al. 2015).

The main methods of fixation in current use follow two different approaches. First, the sheaths can be self-adhesive, so that the sheath itself has a section along its length with adhesive on the internal aspect that sticks to the penile shaft as it is applied. The second method is a double-sided strip of hypoallergenic or foam material applied in a spiral around the penis (which increases the surface area of the sheath adhered to the penis) and then the sheath is applied over the top.

Additionally, newer devices have been developed that move away from the condom catheter-based system and employ a unique hydrocolloid 'petal' design that adheres only to a small area of the glans penis, around the meatus, ensuring a comfortable and secure fit; these are ideal for men with a retracted penis (Nazarko 2018b).

Sheath material

As mentioned, silicone sheaths are advantageous as they are transparent, allowing the patient's skin to be observed. A silicone sheath also allows the skin to breathe, thus avoiding moisture build-up and preventing skin damage (Kyle 2011a).

Procedure guideline 6.3 Penile sheath application

Essential equipment

- Personal protective equipment
- Bowl of warm water, soap and clean, dry wipes
- Scissors or a disposable razor
- Drainage bag and stand or holder
- Selection of appropriate-sized penile sheaths
- Leg strap
- Catheter leg bag
- Trolley

Action	Rationale
Pre-procedure	
1 Introduce yourself to the patient, explain and discuss the procedure with them, and gain their consent to proceed.	To ensure that the patient feels at ease, understands the procedure and gives their valid consent (NMC 2018, **C**).
2 Screen the bed.	To ensure the patient's privacy (NMC 2018, **C**). To allow dust and airborne organisms to settle before the field is exposed (Fraise and Bradley 2009, **E**).
3 Take the trolley to the patient's bedside, disturbing the screens as little as possible.	To minimize airborne contamination (Fraise and Bradley 2009, **E**).
4 Wash hands using bactericidal soap and water or alcohol-based handrub.	To reduce the risk of infection (NHS England and NHSI 2019, **C**).
5 Put on personal protective equipment.	To reduce the risk of cross-infection (NHS England and NHSI 2019, **C**).
6 Assist the patient into a comfortable position. The patient can lie on the bed in the supine position or sit on the edge of the bed.	To ensure the appropriate area is easily accessible. **E**
Procedure	
7 Assist the patient to remove his underwear. Use a sheet or disposable towels to cover his thighs.	To maintain privacy and dignity (NMC 2018, **C**).

8 Position a disposable pad under the patient's buttocks and thighs.	To ensure urine does not leak onto the bedclothes. **E**
9 Clean hands with an alcohol-based handrub.	Hands may have become contaminated by handling the patient, bedding and pads (NHS England and NHSI 2019, **C**).
10 Put on non-sterile gloves.	To reduce the risk of cross-infection (NHS England and NHSI 2019, **C**).
11 With one hand, retract the foreskin (if necessary) and with the other hand clean the penis with soap and water. Dry completely and reduce or reposition the foreskin.	To remove old adhesive and ensure the sheath sticks to the skin. **E** To prevent retraction and constriction of the foreskin behind the glans penis (paraphimosis), which may occur if this is not performed (Nazarko, 2018b, **E**).
12 Using scissors, trim any excess pubic hair from around the base of the penis.	To prevent the sheath from painfully pulling pubic hair when applied. (Woodward 2015, **E**).
13 Apply the sheath following the manufacturer's guidelines, ensuring that there is a space between the glans penis and the sheath. Squeeze the sheath gently around the penile shaft.	To prevent the sheath from rubbing the glans penis and causing discomfort and potential skin irritation, and to ensure the sheath has adhered to the penis (Nazarko, 2018b, **E**).
14 Connect the catheter bag and ensure the tubing is not kinked.	To facilitate drainage of the urine into the catheter bag. **E**
15 Remove gloves and apron. Dispose of all waste and equipment in a clinical waste bag and seal the bag as per local policy.	For infection control (NHS England and NHSI 2019, **C**).
Post-procedure	
16 Provide any assistance the patient may need to dress, encouraging loose clothing where possible. Draw back the curtains once the patient is dressed.	To maintain the patient's dignity (NMC 2018, **C**) and to avoid any unnecessary kinking of the sheath or its tubing. **E**
17 Record information in the relevant documents; this should include: • reasons for applying penile sheath • date and time of application • sheath type • sheath length and size • sheath manufacturer • any problems negotiated during the procedure • a review date to assess the need for reapplication.	To provide a point of reference or comparison in the event of later queries (NMC 2018, **C**).

203

Problem-solving table 6.1 Prevention and resolution (Procedure guideline 6.3)

Problem	Cause	Prevention	Action
Leaking or backflow of urine under the sheath	Penile sheath is the wrong size or incorrectly applied	Measure penile shaft using the sizing tool.	Re-measure the penile shaft, select the correct size and apply using guidance above.
Twisting or kinking of sheath	Lack of care taken when applying; drainage tube unsecured	Assess patient mobility before application and select suitable type and method of securing the drainage bag.	Secure drainage bag to leg or stand.
Difficulty fitting sheath to patient with a retracted penis	Anatomy of the patient	It may be that a penile sheath is not the most appropriate device.	Observe the penile length when the patient is sitting. If the length of the penis is less than 5 cm when sitting, use a hydrocolloid petal-design sheath.

Urinary catheterization

Evidence-based approaches

Rationale

Urinary catheterization is the insertion of a specially designed tube into the bladder using an aseptic technique for any of the indications listed below. It is an invasive procedure and should not be undertaken without full consideration of the benefits and risks. The presence of a catheter can be a traumatic experience for patients and have huge implications for body image, mobility, pain and discomfort (Chapple et al. 2014; Fowler et al. 2014). Indwelling catheters are the primary source of UTIs within acute care (Nicolle 2014). It is essential that they are only used if clinically necessary, and they should not stay in place longer than required (Murphy et al. 2014).

Indications

Urinary catheterization may be carried out for the following reasons (EAUN 2012, RCN 2019):

- acute and chronic urinary retention
- to maintain a continuous outflow of urine for patients with voiding difficulties as a result of neurological disorders that effect urination
- for patients who require prolonged immobilization (e.g. resulting from traumatic spinal injuries)
- for urological investigations and for accurate measurements of urinary output, such as in critically ill and perioperative patients
- in perioperative use for some surgical procedures, especially those involving urological surgery on contiguous structures of the genitourinary tract
- to assist in healing of open sacral or perineal wounds in incontinent patients
- to facilitate continence and maintain skin integrity (in cases of failure of conservative treatment methods)
- for bladder irrigation or lavage
- for the instillation of medications such as chemotherapy
- to ensure comfort for end-of-life care when indicated
- for management of intractable incontinence.

When to remove a catheter

The HOUDINI protocol (Table 6.1) is a nurse-led patient safety tool that outlines clear criteria designed to guide nurses on when continued catheterization is indicated; patients who fall outside these criteria should have their catheter removed (Adams et al. 2012). The tool is designed to reduce the risk of catheter-associated urinary tract infections (CAUTIs) by reducing unnecessary duration of catheterization (Roser et al. 2012). However, if in any doubt, seek advice from the medical team first.

CAUTI is considered one of the most prevalent hospital-acquired infections (Tatham et al. 2015). Reducing CAUTIs is the focus of many safety improvement programmes across the UK and championed by NHS Improvement as part of the reducing gram-negative blood stream infections initiative. For further information on CAUTIs refer to the 'Catheter-associated complications' section below.

Clinical governance

Competencies

Nurses performing female and/or male urinary catheterization must have demonstrated the appropriate level of competency to carry out these procedures. They must be sure these procedures are within their scope of professional practice (NMC 2018, RCN 2019). Each organization will have its own arrangements for assessing individual competency.

Pre-procedural considerations

Patients should be risk assessed individually (RCN 2019) with regard to the ideal time to insert or change their catheter. This should be done in line with the manufacturer's guidance (EAUN 2012). The HOUDINI protocol (Table 6.1) can assist with identifying when catheters can be removed rather than changed. Always ensure the correct type of indwelling catheter is selected for the intended purpose (Table 6.2). To improve consistency of catheter care, the Royal College of Nursing (RCN) (2019) advocates the use of a catheter diary or passport; this will also help to ascertain any pattern of catheter blockages so that changes can be planned accordingly.

Prior to opening any equipment, check the allergy status of the patient to ensure they are not allergic to any of the contents (e.g. equipment containing latex, chlorhexadine or lidocaine).

Table 6.1 The HOUDINI protocol

H	Haematuria
O	Obstruction, urinary
U	Urological surgery
D	Decubitus ulcers
I	Input/output measurements (in critical illness/ haemodynamic instability)
N	Neurogenic bladder dysfunction/chronic indwelling catheter
I	Immobilization due to physical constraints

Source: Adapted from Adams et al. (2012).

Table 6.2 Types of catheter

Catheter type	Materials	Uses
Balloon (Foley) two-way catheter: two channels, one for urine drainage and a second, smaller channel for balloon inflation	Latex, PTFE-coated latex, silicone elastomer coated, 100% silicone, hydrogel coated	Most commonly used for patients who require bladder drainage (short, medium or long term).
Balloon (Foley) three-way irrigation catheter: three channels, one for drainage, one for irrigation fluid and one for balloon inflation	Latex, PTFE-coated latex, silicone, plastic	To provide continuous irrigation (e.g. after transuretheral resection of the bladder/prostate). The potential for infection is reduced by minimizing the need to break the closed drainage system (Madeo and Roodhouse, 2009).
Non-balloon, straight catheter (e.g. Nelaton or Scotts), or intermittent catheter (one channel only)	PVC and other plastics	To empty the bladder or continent urinary reservoir intermittently; to instil solutions into the bladder.

PTFE, polytetrafluoroethylene; PVC, polyvinyl chloride.

Equipment

Catheter selection

A wide range of urinary catheters are available, made from a variety of materials and with various design features. Careful assessment of the most appropriate material, size and balloon capacity will ensure that the catheter selected is as effective as possible for the intended purpose, that complications are minimized, and that patient comfort and quality of life are promoted (EAUN 2012). Types of catheter are listed in Table 6.2 and illustrated in Figure 6.7, together with their suggested uses. Catheters should be used in line with the manufacturer's recommendations, in order to avoid product liability.

Balloon size

In 1932, Dr Fredrick Foley designed a catheter with an inflatable balloon to keep it positioned inside the bladder. This is commonly known as a 'Foley catheter'. Balloon sizes vary from 2.5 mL for children to 30 mL for adult bladder irrigation. A 5–10 mL balloon is recommended for adults and a 3–5 mL balloon for children for most indications.

With a Foley catheter, care should be taken to inflate the balloon according to the manufacturer's guidelines. Under- or overinflation can cause occlusion of draining eyelets, leading to possible irritation to the bladder wall and subsequent bladder spasms and/or spontaneous catheter loss (EAUN 2012).

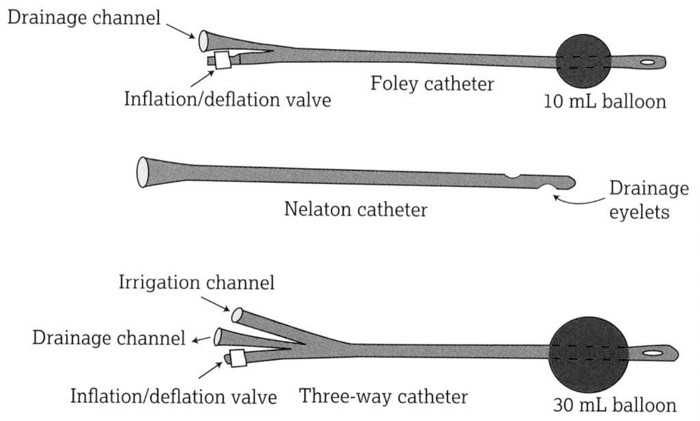

Figure 6.7 Types of catheter.

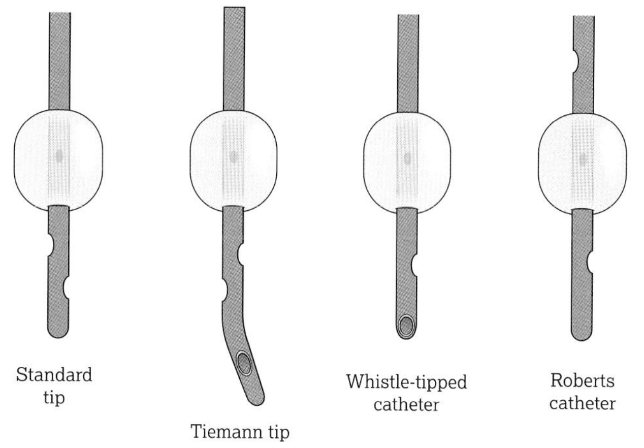

Figure 6.8 Catheter tips.

Sterile water should be used to inflate the balloons of all types of catheter. Inflation of silicone catheters with water can sometimes lead to water loss from the catheter balloon over time, although this has been found to be minimal (Huang et al. 2009). This may increase the risk of inadvertent catheter loss; silicone catheters should be used with caution where catheters are used to protect an anastomosis (EAUN 2012).

Catheter size

Urethral catheters are measured in charrières (ch). The charrière is the outer circumference of the catheter in millimetres and is equivalent to three times the diameter. Thus, a 12 ch catheter has a diameter of 4 mm. The bigger the catheter, the more the urethra is dilated. 12 ch is normally suitable for men and women (Nazarko 2012). The urethra is approximately 6 mm in diameter, which is equivalent to a size 16 ch catheter. This is useful to know as it has implications for patient comfort.

Potential side-effects of large-gauge catheters include:

- pain and discomfort
- pressure ulcers, which may lead to stricture formation
- blockage of paraurethral ducts
- abscess formation (Dellimore et al. 2013)
- bypassing – urethral leakage.

The most important guiding principle is to choose the smallest size of catheter necessary to maintain adequate drainage (Yates 2017). If the urine to be drained is likely to be clear, a 12 ch catheter should be considered. Larger-gauge catheters may be necessary if debris or clots are present in the urine as the diameter of the catheter directly correlates to the size of the drainage channel and also the eyelets (EAUN 2012).

Catheter length

There are three lengths of catheter currently available:

- female length: 23–26 cm (*not for use in males*)
- paediatric: 30 cm
- standard length: 40–44 cm.

The shorter female-length catheter is often more discreet and less likely to cause trauma or infections because movement in and out of the urethra is reduced. Infection may also be caused by a longer catheter looping or kinking (Mangnall 2014, Yates 2017). In obese women or those in wheelchairs, however, the inflation valve of the shorter catheter may cause soreness by rubbing against the inside of the thigh, and the catheter is more likely to pull on the bladder neck; therefore, the standard-length catheter should be used (Simpson 2017).

The male urethra is approximately 15–20 cm long and the female urethra is approximately 3–5 cm long. Conditions such as benign prostatic hyperplasia in a male may extend the distance into the bladder further.

It is vital to stress that female catheters must not be used for male catheterization. A National Patient Safety Agency alert (NPSA 2009b) was issued in 2009 after a series of incidents relating to the shorter female catheters being inserted into males. Female catheters are often too short to reach the bladder of a male patient; therefore, their use in males can cause severe trauma to the urethra as the balloon may be inflated inside the urethra. This can cause haematuria, penile swelling, retention and impaired renal function. For this reason, many organizations stock only male-length catheters to avoid serious incidents.

Catheter tip design

Several different types of catheter tip are available in addition to the standard round tip (Figure 6.8). Each tip is designed to overcome a particular problem:

- The *Tiemann-tip* or *coude tip catheter* has a curved tip with one to three drainage eyes to allow greater drainage. This catheter is designed to negotiate the membranous and prostatic urethra in patients with prostatic hypertrophy. It is recommended that these catheters are only inserted by a urology specialist.
- The *whistle-tip catheter* has a lateral eye in the tip and eyes above the balloon to provide a large drainage area. This design is intended to facilitate drainage of debris, for example blood clots.
- The *Roberts catheter* has one eye above the balloon and another below it to facilitate the drainage of residual urine.
- Several new and novel tip designs are available for Nelaton catheters for intermittent catheterization. Some were developed for patients with a tortuous urethra; examples include the IQ-Cath and the SpeediCath Flex.

Catheter material

A wide variety of materials are used to make catheters. The key criterion in selecting the appropriate material is the length of time the catheter is expected to remain in place. Three broad timescales have been identified:

- short term (1–7 days), e.g. polyvinyl chloride and intermittent catheters
- short to medium term (up to 28 days), e.g. polytetrafluoroethylene catheters
- medium to long term (6–12 weeks), e.g. hydrogel, all-silicone and silastic catheters.

The principal catheter materials are as follows

Polyvinyl chloride

Catheters made from polyvinyl chloride (PVC) or plastic are quite rigid. They have a wide lumen, which allows a rapid flow rate, but their rigidity may cause some patients discomfort. They are mainly used for intermittent catheterization or post-operatively. They are recommended for short-term use (Gilbert 2018).

Latex

Latex is a purified form of rubber and is the softest of the catheter materials. It has a smooth surface, with a tendency to allow crust formation. It has been shown to cause urethral irritation; therefore, latex catheters are now usually coated with silicone elastomer or Teflon (as below).

Hypersensitivity to latex is well documented within the literature. Therefore, care must be taken to check allergy status and select an alternative, where indicated, to avoid anaphylaxis (Feneley et al. 2015).

Teflon and silicone elastomer coatings

A Teflon (polytetrafluoroethylene, or PTFE) or silicone elastomer coating is applied to latex catheters to render the latex inert and reduce urethral irritation (Bell 2010). Teflon is recommended for short-term use and silicone-elastomer-coated catheters are used for long-term catheterization.

All-silicone

Silicone is an inert material that is less likely than other materials to cause urethral irritation. Silicone catheters are not coated and therefore have a wider lumen. The lumen of these catheters, in cross-section, is crescent- or D-shaped, which may induce formation of encrustation. Silicone permits gas diffusion; therefore, balloons may lose water and cause the spontaneous loss of the catheter. For this reason, they should be used with caution in patients having urological surgery. These catheters may be more uncomfortable than the latex-cored types as they are more rigid. All-silicone catheters are suitable for patients with latex allergies. Silicone catheters are suitable for long-term use (Singha et al. 2017).

Hydrogel coatings

Hydrophilic coated catheters provide improved patient comfort as the polymer coating is well tolerated by the urethral mucosa. They are composed of an inner core of latex encapsulated in a hydrophilic polymer coating and are commonly used for long-term catheterization. Hydrogel-coated catheters become smoother when rehydrated, reducing friction with the urethra. They are reported to be resistant to bacterial colonization; however, there is conflicting data surrounding this issue, and the lower level of colonization could be attributed to the different properties of catheter material or the type of hydrogel coating (Siddiq and Darouiche 2012).

Conformable catheter

Conformable catheters are designed to conform to the shape of the female urethra and allow partial filling of the bladder. The natural movement of the urethra against the collapsible catheter is intended to prevent obstructions. They are made of latex and have a silicone elastomer coating. Conformable catheters are approximately 3 cm longer than conventional catheters for women.

Other materials

Research into new types of catheter materials is ongoing, particularly examining materials that resist the formation of biofilms (bacterial colonies that develop and adhere to the catheter surface and drainage bag) and consequently reduce the incidence of UTIs (Hook et al. 2012, Loveday et al. 2014, Mandakhalikar et al. 2016).

Current preventive strategies include coating catheter surfaces with antibiotic drugs or silver toxins to create a hostile environment for bacteria. A Cochrane review examining the available evidence concluded that these coatings are often not effective in reducing infection rates, with any benefit likely to be small (Lam et al. 2014). Such catheters were found to be more likely to cause patient discomfort and were more expensive to purchase, adding overall cost and inefficiency to patient treatment (Singha et al. 2017).

Drainage bags

A wide variety of drainage systems are available. When selecting a system, consideration should be given to the reasons for catheterization, the intended duration, the patient's wishes and infection control issues.

To reduce the number of possible entry sites for pathogens into the urinary system, a closed catheter drainage system should be adopted. This is an aseptic system in which the path from the catheter tip to the drainage bag remains as one system. However, this path must be broken to allow emptying and changing of drainage bag (EAUN 2012).

Urine drainage bags should only be changed according to clinical need – that is, when the catheter is changed or if the bag is leaking, or at times dictated by the manufacturer's instructions, for example every 5–7 days (Loveday et al. 2014). Urine drainage bags positioned above the level of the bladder and full bags cause urine to reflux, which is associated with infection. Therefore, bags should always be positioned below the level of the bladder (dependent drainage) to maintain an unobstructed flow, and they should be emptied appropriately. Urine drainage bags should be hung on suitable stands to avoid contact with the floor. When emptying drainage bags, separate clean containers should be used for each patient and care should be taken to avoid contact between the drainage tap and the container (Loveday et al. 2014).

Urine drainage bags are available in a wide selection of sizes ranging from large 2 L bags, which are most commonly used in non-ambulatory patients and overnight, to 350–750 mL leg bags (Figures 6.9 and 6.10). There are also large drainage bags that incorporate urine-measuring devices (urometers), which are used when very close monitoring of urine output is required (Figure 6.11).

There are a number of different styles of drainage bags in addition to the standard leg worn bags. They allow patients greater mobility and can be worn under the patient's own clothes and therefore are much more discreet, helping to preserve the patient's privacy and dignity. Shapes vary from oblong to oval, and some have cloth backing for greater comfort when in contact with the skin. Others are ridged to encourage an even distribution of urine through the bag, resulting in better conformity to the leg. The length of the inlet tube also varies (direct, short, long or adjustable length), as does the intended position on the leg (thigh, knee or lower leg) (Yates 2017). The patient should be asked to identify the most comfortable position for the bag (Yates 2017). The majority of drainage bags are fitted with an anti-reflux valve to prevent the backflow of urine into the bladder. Several different tap designs exist and selection should be based on the patient's manual dexterity. Most leg bags allow for larger 1–2 L bags to be connected via the outlet tap, to increase capacity for night-time use.

A variety of supports are available for use with these bags, including sporran waist belts, leg holsters, knickers/pants and leg straps.

Leg straps

The use of thigh straps (e.g. the Simpla G-Strap) and other fixation devices (e.g. the Bard StatLock™ Foley stabilization device

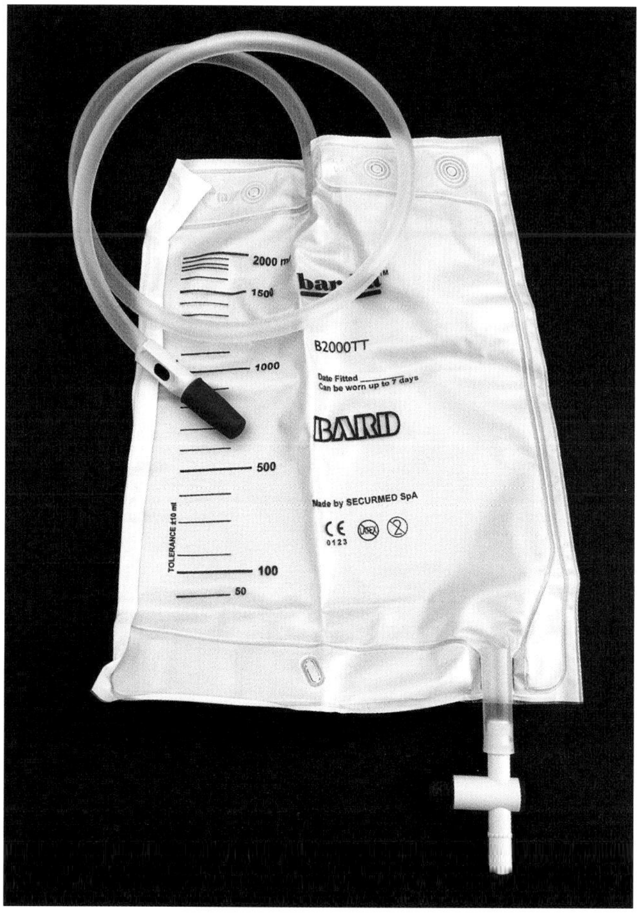

Figure 6.9 Urinary catheter bag: large.

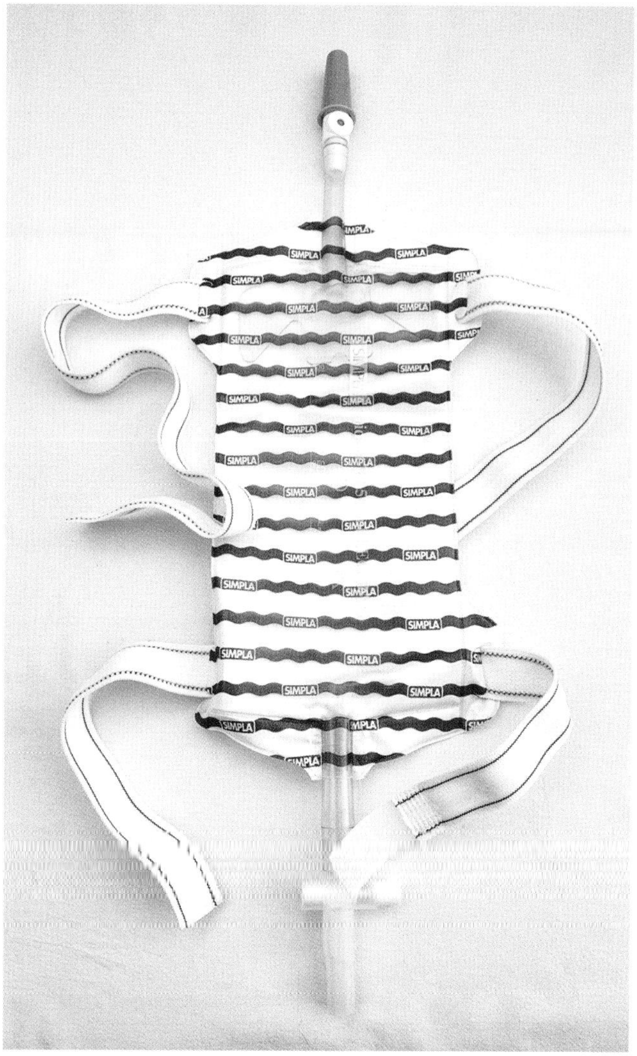

Figure 6.10 Urinary catheter leg bag.

(Figure 6.12), the Loc-Strap™ or the Clinimed CliniFix) helps to immobilize the catheter and thus reduce the trauma potential to the bladder neck and urethra (Eastwood 2009). It is recommended that all catheter users secure their catheter in this way. Guidance from the RCN (2012a) and NHS Scotland (NHSQIS 2004) reiterates the importance of catheter tetherage to promote patient comfort and to limit the potential complications of catheter migration and subsequent need for recatheterization. The application of these devices is not without potential complications; for example, restriction of the circulation to the limb with a thigh strap may give rise to deep vein thrombosis, while tension and traction to the urethra can cause trauma and necrosis, especially in men (Yates 2018). For this reason, the thigh fixation device should be fitted by an appropriately trained individual.

Catheter valves

Catheter valves, which eliminate the need for drainage bags, are also available. The valve allows the bladder to be emptied intermittently and is particularly appropriate for patients who require long-term catheterization and do not require a drainage bag.

Catheter valves are only suitable for patients who have good cognitive function, sufficient manual dexterity to manipulate the valve and an adequate bladder capacity (Woodward 2013). It is important that catheter valves are released at regular intervals to ensure that the bladder does not become over-distended. These valves must not be used on patients following surgical procedures to the prostate or bladder, as continuous drainage of the bladder is required and free drainage is the preferred method. As catheter valves preclude free drainage, they are not appropriate for patients with uncontrolled detrusor overactivity, ureteric reflux or renal impairment. Catheter valves are designed to fit with linked systems so it is possible for patients to connect them to a drainage bag. This may be necessary when access to toilets may be limited, for example overnight or on long journeys.

Catheter valves are recommended to remain *in situ* for 5–7 days, which corresponds with most manufacturers' recommendations (Woodward 2013).

Pharmacological support

The use of anaesthetic lubricating gels is well recognized for male catheterization, but there is some uncertainty about the benefits in female catheterization. Loveday et al. (2014) recommend the use of a lubricant to minimize urethral discomfort and trauma during catheterization. In male patients the anaesthetic lubricating gel is typically instilled directly into the urethra; this can then be milked along the length of the urethra or a gentle clamp applied to the tip of the penis. Onset of anaesthetic action is typically achieved within 5 minutes (Ahluwalia et al. 2018, Losco et al. 2011). Evidence suggests that increasing numbers of individuals are experiencing hypersensitivity reactions to the antiseptic ingredient chlorhexidine, which is in many catheterization gels; therefore, allergy status must be checked before use and the gel should be

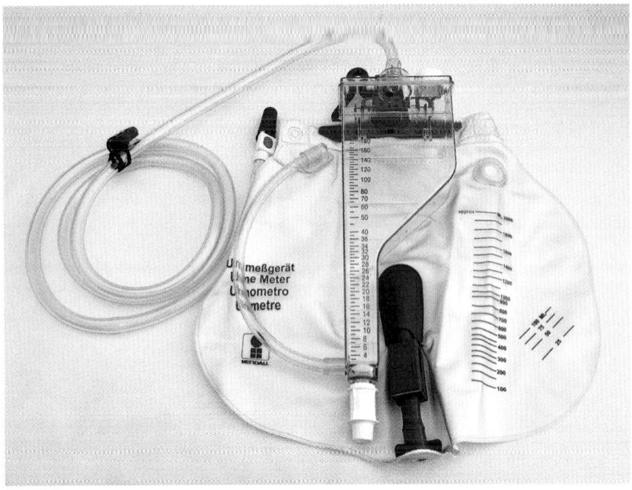

Figure 6.11 Urinary catheter bag with urometer.

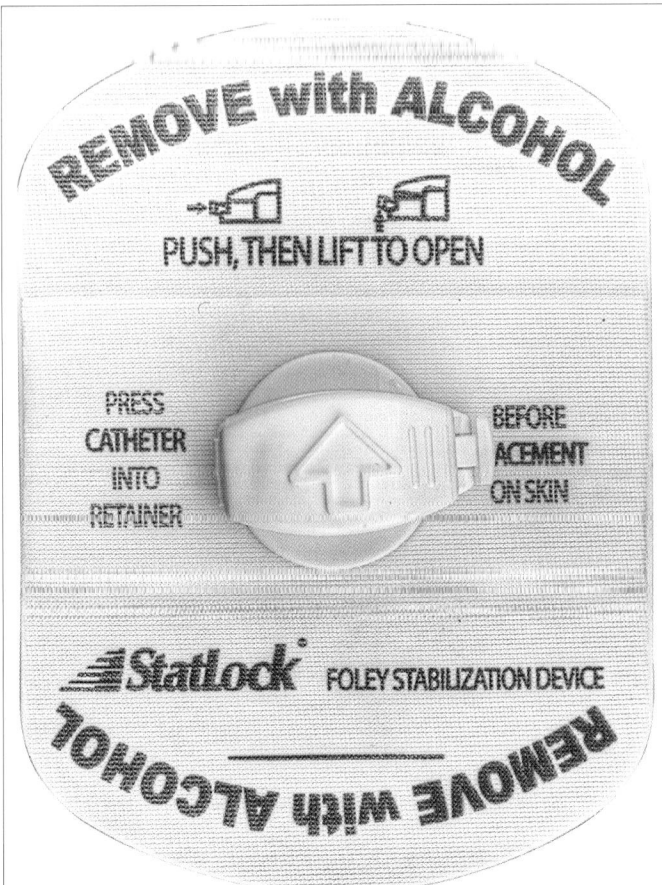

Figure 6.12 Bard StatLock™ Foley stabilization device. *Source*: Reproduced with permission of C.R. Bard, Inc.

used with caution (Williams 2017). In female patients, anaesthetic lubricating gel is applied to the meatus and slowly instilled into the urethra (EAUN 2012). This process also maintains mild ureteral dilation, thereby assisting with the insertion of the catheter (EAUN 2012, Williams 2017).

Routine use of antiseptic lubricants for catheter insertion is not necessary (EAUN 2012). This said, anaesthetic lubricant gel without chlorhexidine is widely available in the UK and should be considered for routine catheterization. Furthermore, Loveday et al. (2014) and Wilson (2016) found limited evidence to support the routine use of antiseptic or antimicrobial agents for meatal cleaning prior to insertion to minimize CAUTI. Loveday et al. (2014) recommend cleansing the meatus with normal sterile saline, whereas NICE (2017) recommends checking local guidelines.

Procedure guideline 6.4 Urinary catheterization: male

Essential equipment

- Personal protective equipment
- Sterile pack containing gallipots, receiver, gauze swabs, disposable towels and forceps
- Disposable pad
- 0.9% sodium chloride or chlorhexidine 0.1% solution
- Leg strap for tethering
- Sterile gloves
- Sterile water
- Selection of appropriate catheters
- Syringe (if required to obtain a urine sample)
- Anaesthetic lubricating gel
- Universal specimen container (if a sample is required)
- Drainage bag and stand or holder
- Clean towel or similar cover

Action	Rationale
Pre-procedure	
1 Introduce yourself to the patient, explain and discuss the procedure with them, and gain their consent to proceed. Offer a chaperone.	To ensure that the patient feels at ease, understands the procedure and gives their valid consent (NMC 2018, **C**; RCN 2019, **C**).

2 Screen the bed.	To ensure the patient's privacy. To allow dust and airborne organisms to settle before the sterile field is exposed (Fraise and Bradley 2009, **E**).
3 Prepare the trolley, placing all equipment required on the bottom shelf. (See also 'Catheter selection' under 'Equipment' above.)	The top shelf acts as a clean working surface. **E**
4 Take the trolley to the patient's bedside, disturbing the screens as little as possible.	To minimize airborne contamination (Fraise and Bradley 2009, **E**).
5 Assist the patient to get into the supine position with the legs extended on the bed.	To ensure the necessary area is easily accessible. **E**
6 Remove the underpants or trousers and use a towel to cover the patient's thighs and genital area.	To maintain the patient's dignity and comfort (NMC 2018, **C**).
7 Wash hands using bactericidal soap and water or alcohol-based handrub and apply personal protective equipment.	To reduce the risk of infection (NHS England and NHSI 2019, **C**). To reduce the risk of cross-infection from micro-organisms on the uniform (Fraise and Bradley 2009, **E**).
Procedure	
8 Open the outer cover of the catheterization pack and slide the pack onto the top shelf of the trolley.	To prepare the equipment. **E**
9 Using an aseptic technique, open the sterile catheter pack. Pour 0.9% sodium chloride or 0.1% chlorhexidine solution into a gallipot. Open the outer packaging of an appropriately selected catheter onto the sterile field.	To reduce the risk of introducing infection into the bladder (NICE 2017, **C**; RCN 2019, **C**).
10 Remove the cover from the patient's genital area, maintaining the patient's privacy, and position a disposable pad under the patient's buttocks and thighs.	To ensure urine does not leak onto the bedclothes. **E**
11 Clean hands with an alcohol-based handrub.	Hands may have become contaminated by handling the outer packs (NHS England and NHSI 2019, **C**).
12 Put on sterile gloves.	To reduce the risk of cross-infection (NICE 2017, **C**)
13 On the sterile field, place the catheter into the sterile receiver with drainage bag attached.	To ensure a closed system, minimizing the infection risk (EAUN 2012, **C**).
14 Place a sterile towel across the patient's thighs.	To create a sterile field. **E**
15 With your non-dominant hand, wrap a sterile gauze swab around the penis. Use this to retract the foreskin, if necessary, and clean around the glans penis with swabs soaked with 0.9% sodium chloride or 0.1% chlorhexidine solution held between forceps, being careful not to touch the penis or gauze with your hand.	To reduce the risk of introducing infection to the urinary tract during catheterization (Loveday et al. 2014, **R**).
16 Confirm patient's allergy status first. If no allergies to products exist, then insert the nozzle of the local anaesthetic or lubricating gel into the urethra. Squeeze the gel into the urethra and withdraw the nozzle, being sure not to touch the penis with your dominant hand. Wait 2 to 5 minutes (as per manufacturer's instructions).	Adequate lubrication helps to prevent urethral trauma. Use of a local anaesthetic minimizes the discomfort experienced by the patient (Ghaffary et al. 2013, **E**). To allow the anaesthetic gel to take effect (Ahluwalia et al. 2018, **E**).
17 With your non-dominant hand, hold the penis firmly behind the glans, raising it until it is almost totally extended (maintain this hold until the catheter is inserted and urine flows).	This manoeuvre straightens the penile urethra and prevents damage to the penoscrotal junction. Maintaining a grasp of the penis prevents contamination and retraction (EAUN 2012, **C**).
18 With your free hand, place the receiver containing the catheter between the patient's legs. Take the catheter with your dominant hand and advance the catheter into the urethra.	
19 If resistance is felt at the external sphincter, increase the traction on the penis slightly and apply steady, gentle pressure on the catheter. Ask the patient to cough gently or wiggle his toes (to distract the patient).	Some resistance may be due to spasm of the external sphincter. Gentle coughing helps to relax the external sphincter (Yates 2017, **E**).
20 When the urine begins to flow, advance the catheter up to the bifurcation (hilt). If urine is not flowing, gently compress the lower abdomen with your hand to place pressure on bladder.	Advancing the catheter ensures that it is correctly positioned in the bladder. This helps to ensure the balloon is in the bladder and not in the urethra (EAUN 2012, **C**).
21 Gently inflate the balloon according to the manufacturer's instructions, having ensured that the catheter is draining properly beforehand.	Inadvertent inflation of the balloon in the urethra causes pain and urethral trauma (Davis et al. 2016, **R**).

(continued)

Procedure guideline 6.4 Urinary catheterization: male (continued)

Action	Rationale
22 Withdraw the catheter slightly so that the balloon is sitting at the bladder neck.	To ensure that the balloon is inflated and the catheter is secure. **E**
23 Secure the catheter using a specially designed support, for example the Simpla G-Strap or the Bard StatLock™ Foley stabilization device (see Figure 6.12). Ensure that the catheter does not become taut when the patient is mobilizing or when the penis becomes erect. Ensure that the catheter lumen is not occluded by the fixation device.	To maintain patient comfort and to reduce the risk of urethral and bladder neck trauma. Care must be taken when applying securing devices to ensure these do not interfere with drainage of the catheter by being applied too tightly. Leg straps must not impair circulation (Yates 2018, **E**).
24 Ensure that the glans penis is clean and dry and then extend the foreskin (if patient is not circumcised).	Retraction and constriction of the foreskin behind the glans penis (paraphimosis) may occur if this is not done (EAUN 2012, **C**).
Post-procedure	
25 Assist the patient to replace his underwear and clothing, feeding the catheter down the leg. Ensure that the area is dry.	To ensure clothing does not occlude drainage. **E** If the area is left wet or moist, secondary infection and skin irritation may occur (Voegeli 2013, **E**).
26 Measure the amount of urine.	To be aware of the bladder capacity of patients who have presented with urinary retention. To monitor renal function and fluid balance if clinically indicated. It is not necessary to measure the amount of urine if the patient is having the urinary catheter changed routinely (EAUN 2012, **C**).
27 If required, take a urine specimen for urinalysis or laboratory examination.	For further information, see Procedure guideline 14.7: Urinalysis: reagent strip and Chapter 13: Diagnostic tests.
28 Dispose of equipment (including apron and gloves) in a clinical waste bag as per local policy.	To reduce the risk of infection (NHS England and NHSI 2019, **C**).
29 Draw back the screen.	
30 Wash hands thoroughly with soap and water.	To reduce the risk of infection (NHS England and NHSI 2019, **C**).
31 Record information in relevant documents; this should include: • reasons for catheterization • date and time of catheterization • catheter type, length and size • amount of water instilled into the balloon • batch number • manufacturer • any problems negotiated during the procedure • review date to assess the need for continued catheterization or date of change of catheter.	To ensure accurate documentation and to provide a point of reference or comparison in the event of later queries (NMC 2018, **C**).

Procedure guideline 6.5 Urinary catheterization: female

Essential equipment

- Personal protective equipment
- Sterile catheterization pack containing gallipots, receiver, gauze swabs, disposable towels and forceps
- Leg strap for tethering
- 0.9% sodium chloride or 0.1% chlorhexidine solution
- Two syringes
- Drainage bag and stand or holder
- Clean towel or similar cover
- Disposable pad
- Sterile gloves
- Selection of appropriate catheters
- Sterile anaesthetic lubricating gel
- Universal specimen container (if a sample is required)
- Light source

Action	Rationale
Pre-procedure	
1 Introduce yourself to the patient, explain and discuss the procedure with them, and gain their consent to proceed. Offer a chaperone.	To ensure that the patient feels at ease, understands the procedure and gives their valid consent (NMC 2018, **C**; RCN 2019, **C**).

2 Screen the bed.	To ensure the patient's privacy. To allow dust and airborne organisms to settle before the sterile field is exposed (Fraise and Bradley 2009, **E**).
3 Prepare the trolley, placing all equipment (**Action figure 3**) required on the bottom shelf. (See also 'Catheter selection' under 'Equipment' above.)	The top shelf acts as a clean working surface. **E**
4 Take the trolley to the patient's bedside, disturbing the screens as little as possible.	To minimize airborne contamination (Fraise and Bradley 2009, **C**).
5 Remove the patient's underwear. Assist the patient to get into the supine position with knees bent, hips flexed and feet resting about 60 cm apart (**Action figure 5**).	To enable the genital area to be seen. **E**
6 Place a towel over the patient's thighs and genital area.	To maintain the patient's dignity and comfort (NMC 2018, **C**).
7 Ensure that a good light source is available.	To enable the genital area to be seen clearly. **E**
8 Wash hands using bactericidal soap and water or alcohol-based handrub. Apply personal protective equipment.	To reduce the risk of cross-infection (NHS England and NHSI 2019, **C**).
Procedure	
9 Open the outer cover of the catheterization pack and slide the pack onto the top shelf of the trolley.	To prepare the equipment. **E**
10 Using an aseptic technique, open the sterile pack. Open the selected catheter and place it on the sterile field.	To reduce the risk of introducing infection into the urinary tract. **E**
11 Remove the towel, maintaining the patient's privacy, and position a disposable pad under the patient's buttocks.	To ensure urine does not leak onto the bedclothes. **E**
12 Clean hands with alcohol-based handrub.	Hands may have become contaminated by handling of outer packs (Fraise and Bradley 2009, **C**).
13 Put on sterile gloves.	To reduce the risk of cross-infection (NICE 2017, **C**).
14 On the sterile field, place the catheter into the sterile receiver.	To ensure a closed system, minimizing infection risk (EAUN 2012, **C**).
15 Place sterile towels under the patient's buttocks.	To create a sterile field. **E**
16 Using gauze swabs, separate the labia minora so that the urethral meatus is seen. Your non-dominant hand should be used to maintain labial separation until the catheter is inserted and urine is flowing (**Action figure 16**).	This manoeuvre provides better access to the urethral orifice and helps to prevent labial contamination of the catheter. **E**
17 Clean around the urethral orifice with swabs soaked with 0.9% sodium chloride or 0.1% chlorhexidine solution held between forceps using single downward strokes, being careful not to touch the surrounding skin (**Action figure 16**).	To clean the urethra orifice and thereby reduce the risk of CAUTI (Loveday et al. 2014, **R**).
18 Apply anaesthetic lubrication to the meatus and then insert the nozzle of the syringe into the urethra and instil gel into the urethra, being careful not to touch the surrounding skin (**Action figure 18**).	Adequate lubrication helps to prevent urethral trauma. Use of a local anaesthetic minimizes the patient's discomfort (Ghaffary et al. 2013, **E**).
19 Place the catheter, in the sterile receiver, between the patient's legs and attach the drainage bag.	To ensure a closed system, minimizing infection risk (EAUN 2012, **C**).
20 Using your dominant hand, introduce the tip of the catheter into the urethral orifice in an upward and backward direction. If the meatus is difficult to identify, this may be due to vaginal atrophy (see Problem-solving table 6.2). Advance the catheter until urine is draining and up to the bifurcation (hilt) (**Action figure 20**).	The direction of insertion and the length of the catheter inserted should relate to the anatomical structure of the area. **E**
21 If there is no urine present, check that the catheter has not accidentally been inserted into the vagina. If the urethral meatus is clearly visible, consider removing the catheter and re-attempting the procedure with a second sterile catheter. If the meatus is not clearly visible, see Problem-solving table 6.2.	This prevents repeated misplacement of the catheter. **E**
22 Inflate the balloon according to the manufacturer's instructions, having ensured that the catheter is draining adequately (**Action figure 22**).	Inadvertent inflation of the balloon within the urethra is painful and causes urethral trauma (Ghaffary et al. 2013, **E**).
23 Withdraw the catheter slightly so that the balloon is sitting at the bladder neck.	To ensure that the balloon is inflated and the catheter is secure. **E**

(continued)

Procedure guideline 6.5 Urinary catheterization: female *(continued)*

Action	Rationale
24 Support the catheter using a specially designed support, for example the Simpla G-Strap or the Bard StatLock™ Foley stabilization device. Ensure that the catheter does not become taut when the patient is mobilizing. Ensure that the catheter lumen is not occluded by the fixation device.	To maintain patient comfort and to reduce the risk of urethral and bladder neck trauma. Care must be taken when applying securing devices to ensure these do not interfere with the drainage of the catheter by being applied too tightly. Leg straps must not impair circulation (Yates 2018, **E**).
Post-procedure	
25 Assist the patient to replace her underwear and clothing, feeding the catheter down the leg. Replace the bedcovers and ensure that the area is dry.	So that the catheter it is not occluded by clothing or tight underwear and is aided to drain by gravity. **E** If the area is left wet or moist, secondary infection and skin irritation may occur (Voegeli 2013, **E**).
26 Measure the amount of urine.	To be aware of bladder capacity for patients who have presented with urinary retention. To monitor renal function and fluid balance if clinically indicated. It is not necessary to measure the amount of urine if the patient is having a routine catheter change (EAUN 2012, **C**).
27 If required, take a urine specimen for laboratory examination.	For further information, see Procedure guideline 14.7: Urinalysis: reagent strip and Chapter 13: Diagnostic tests.
28 Dispose of equipment (including apron and gloves) in a clinical waste bag as per local policy.	To reduce the risk of infection (NHS England and NHSI 2019, **C**).
29 Draw back the screen.	
30 Wash hands thoroughly with soap and water.	To reduce the risk of infection (NHS England and NHSI 2019, **C**).
31 Record information in relevant documents; this should include: • reasons for catheterization • date and time of catheterization • catheter type, length and size • amount of water instilled into the balloon • batch number and manufacturer • any problems negotiated during the procedure • a review date to assess the need for continued catheterization or date of change of catheter.	To ensure accurate documentation and provide a point of reference or comparison in the event of later queries (NMC 2018, **C**).

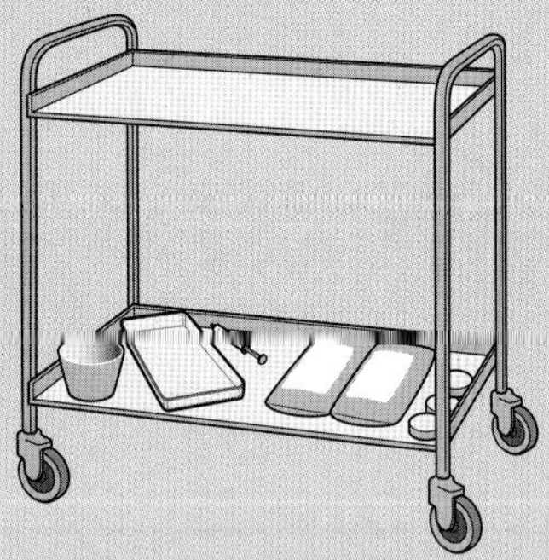

Action Figure 3 Prepare the trolley, placing all required equipment on the bottom shelf. *Source*: Adapted from Yates (2017) with permission of EMAP Publishing Limited.

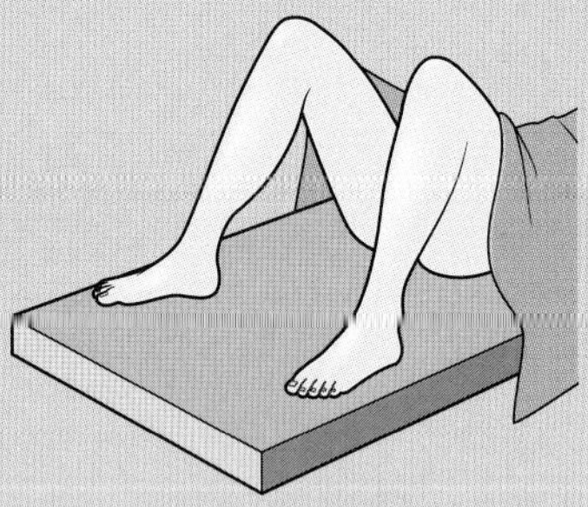

Action Figure 5 Assist the patient into the supine position with knees bent, hips flexed and feet resting about 60 cm apart. *Source*: Adapted from Yates (2017) with permission of EMAP Publishing Limited.

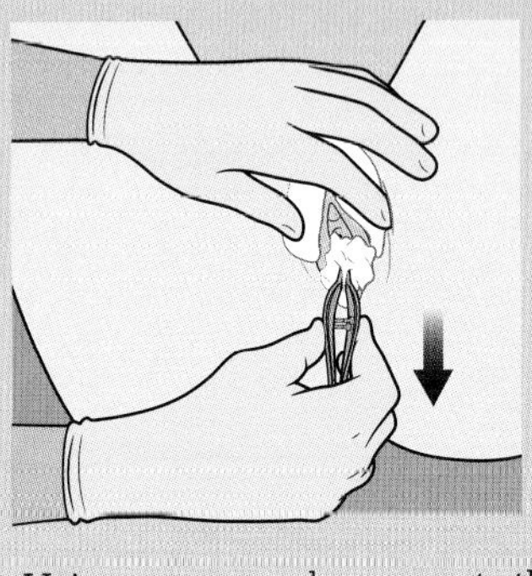

Action Figure 16 Using gauze swabs, separate the labia minora, and with the other hand clean the meatus with gauze swabs soaked in 0.9% sodium chloride, using single downward strokes. *Source*: Adapted from Yates (2017) with permission of EMAP Publishing Limited.

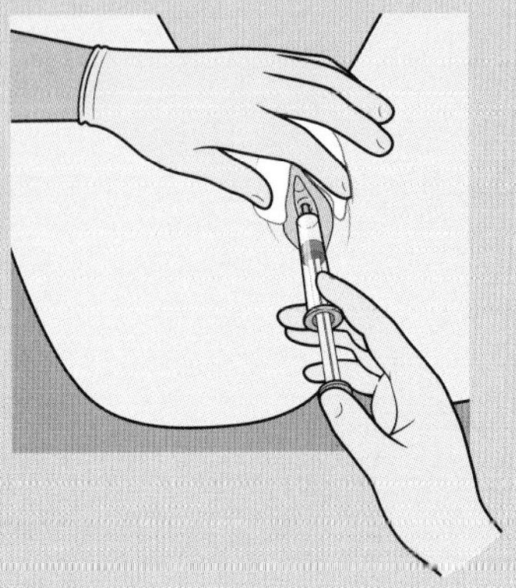

Action Figure 18 Apply anaesthetic lubrication to the meatus and then insert the nozzle of the syringe into the urethra and instil gel into the urethra. *Source*: Adapted from Yates (2017) with permission of EMAP Publishing Limited.

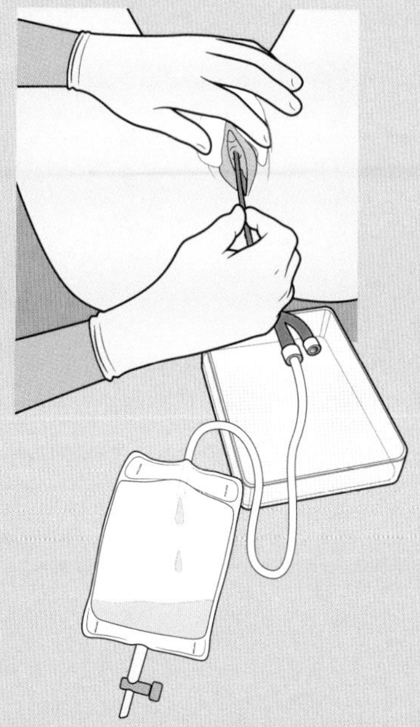

Action Figure 20 Advance the catheter until urine is draining and up to the bifurcation (hilt). *Source*: Adapted from Yates (2017) with permission of EMAP Publishing Limited.

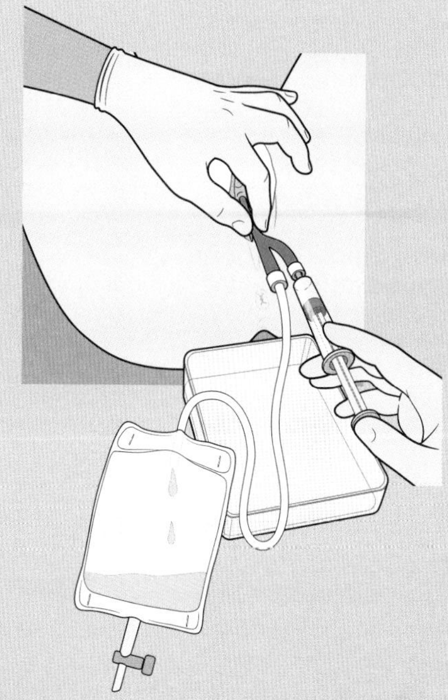

Action Figure 22 Inflate the balloon according to the manufacturer's instructions, having ensured that the catheter is draining adequately. *Source*: Adapted from Yates (2017) with permission of EMAP Publishing Limited.

Suprapubic catheterization

Evidence-based approaches

Rationale

Suprapubic catheterization is the insertion of a catheter through the anterior abdominal wall into the dome of the bladder (Figure 6.13). The procedure is performed under general or local anaesthesia, using a percutaneous system (Robinson 2008). In 2009, a National Patient Safety Agency alert stated that the insertion of a suprapubic catheter should only be undertaken by experienced urology staff using ultrasound imaging, due to the risk of injury to the bowel (NPSA 2009a).

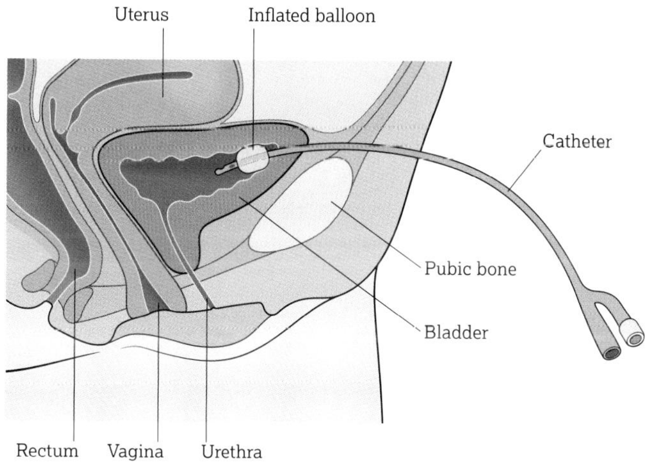

Figure 6.13 Suprapubic catheter. *Source*: Reproduced with permission of Shutterstock.com.

Indications

Indications for the use of suprapubic catheters over indwelling catheters include the following:

- post-operative drainage of urine after lower urinary tract or bowel surgery
- management of neuropathic bladders
- long-term conditions, for example multiple sclerosis or spinal cord injuries
- people with long-term catheters – to minimize the risk of urethral infections or urethral damage (NPSA 2009a).

However, there are a number of risks and disadvantages associated with suprapubic catheterization (BAUS 2017):

- bowel perforation or haemorrhage at the time of insertion
- infection, swelling, encrustation or granulation at the insertion site
- pain, discomfort or irritation for some patients
- bladder stone formation and possible long-term risk of squamous cell carcinoma
- urethral leakage and discharge from the insertion site is not uncommon.

Contraindications

Contraindications to suprapubic catheterization include the following (adapted from EAUN 2012 in RCN 2019):

- known or possible bladder carcinoma
- lower abdominal surgery
- clotting disorder
- ascites
- any prosthetic devices (e.g. hernia mesh).

Related theory

Evidence-based research on the use of suprapubic catheters is limited (EAUN 2012). However, it is believed that there are advantages to their use when compared to urethral catheterization, such as greater patient comfort (especially for those who are chair bound) and greater ease of access to the entry site for cleaning and for catheter and drainage bag changing. The risk of patients developing infections from micro-organisms commonly found in the bowel is reduced, as are the risks of urethral trauma, necrosis and catheter-induced urethritis. Clamping the suprapubic catheter allows urethral voiding to occur, and the clamp can be released if voiding is incomplete. Patient satisfaction is increased as, for some, their level of independence is increased and sexual intercourse can occur with fewer impediments (EAUN 2012).

Post-procedural considerations

Care of a suprapubic catheter is the same as that for a urethral catheter. Immediately following insertion of a suprapubic catheter, aseptic technique should be employed to clean the insertion site (Robinson 2008). Keyhole dressings around the insertion site may be required if secretions soil clothing, but they are not essential. Once the insertion site has healed (7–10 days), the site and catheter can be cleaned during bathing using soap, water and a clean cloth (Rigby 2009).

Changing a suprapubic catheter

Changes of a suprapubic catheter should be completed by staff who are appropriately trained and competent with regard to the technique and potential complications. It should be undertaken at the intervals recommended by the catheter manufacturer (EAUN 2012). The first change should take place no sooner than between 6–12 weeks.

The loss of the catheter tract can occur during a catheter change, usually as a result of the replacement catheter not being advanced into the bladder adequately so that the retaining balloon is inflated in the catheter tract, potentially causing trauma (RCN 2019). Partially filling the bladder with sterile saline or water before changing the catheter can be helpful in some cases (Sweeny 2017). Immediate access to a urology unit should be available in the event of a failed catheter change. It is advised that the first change takes place in a hospital for this reason; after this the tract should be well established. The second reason for the first change to take place in hospital is the very rare risk of a late presentation of bowel perforation at first catheter change.

Procedure guideline 6.6 Changing a suprapubic catheter

Essential equipment

- Personal protective equipment
- Sterile pack containing gallipots, receiver, gauze swabs, disposable towels and forceps
- Disposable pad
- 0.9% sodium chloride or 0.1% chlorhexidine solution
- Leg strap for tethering
- Sterile gloves × 2
- Sterile water
- Selection of appropriate catheters
- Two syringes (the second if required to obtain a urine sample)
- Sterile anaesthetic lubricating gel
- Universal specimen container (if a sample is required)
- Drainage bag and stand or holder
- Clean towel or similar

Action	Rationale
Pre-procedure	
1 Introduce yourself to the patient, explain and discuss the procedure with them, and gain their consent to proceed. Offer a chaperone.	To ensure that the patient feels at ease, understands the procedure and gives their valid consent (NMC 2018, **C**).
2 Screen the bed.	To ensure the patient's privacy. To allow dust and airborne organisms to settle before the sterile field is exposed (Fraise and Bradley 2009, **E**).
3 Prepare the trolley, placing all equipment required on the bottom shelf.	The top shelf acts as a clean working surface. **E**
4 Take the trolley to the patient's bedside, disturbing the screens as little as possible.	To minimize airborne contamination (Fraise and Bradley 2009, **E**).
5 Assist the patient to get into the supine position with the legs extended on the bed.	To ensure the appropriate area is easily accessible. **E**
6 Remove any necessary clothing and use a towel to cover the patient's thighs and genital area.	To maintain the patient's dignity and comfort (NMC 2018, **C**).
7 Wash hands using soap and water or alcohol-based handrub.	To reduce the risk of infection (NHS England and NHSI 2019 **R**).
8 Put on a disposable plastic apron.	To reduce the risk of cross-infection from micro-organisms on the uniform (Fraise and Bradley 2009, **E**).
Procedure	
9 Open the outer cover of the catheterization pack and slide the pack onto the top shelf of the trolley.	To prepare the equipment. **E**
10 Using an aseptic technique, open the sterile catheter pack. Pour 0.9% sodium chloride into a gallipot. Open the outer packaging of an appropriately selected catheter onto the sterile field.	To reduce the risk of introducing infection into the bladder (NICE 2017, **C**).
11 Remove the bedclothes from the patient's abdomen, exposing the catheter exit site.	To ensure urine does not leak onto the bedclothes. **E**

12 Clean hands with an alcohol-based handrub.	Hands may have become contaminated by handling the outer packs (Fraise and Bradley 2009, **C**).
13 Put on sterile gloves.	To reduce the risk of cross-infection (NICE 2017, **C**).
14 On the sterile field, place the catheter into the sterile receiver with the drainage bag attached.	To ensure a closed system, minimizing the infection risk (EAUN 2012, **C**).
15 Place a sterile towel across the patient's thighs.	To create a sterile field. **E**
16 Observe the current suprapubic site for the lie of the catheter, angle of insertion and length of catheter exposed outside the body as this will aid insertion of the new catheter.	To assist with reinsertion of the suprapubic catheter (EAUN 2012, **C**).
17 Clean around the insertion site with 0.9% sodium chloride or 0.1% chlorhexidine solution, holding the indwelling catheter using a gauze swab.	To reduce the risk of introducing infection (Mangnall 2014, **E**).
18 Put on new sterile gloves and place a new sterile drape over the change site.	To minimize infection risk with sterile gloves during insertion of the new catheter and maintain a sterile field (EAUN 2012, **C**).
19 Deflate the balloon and remove the existing catheter. Cover the change site with sterile gauze.	A two-person approach can be adopted at this stage with one person remaining 'aseptic' to insert the new catheter (EAUN 2012, **C**).
20 Instill 5–10 mL of water-soluble lubricant or anaesthetic gel into the suprapubic tract.	Adequate lubricant reduces trauma to the tissues, helping to glide the catheter along the existing tract (EAUN 2012, **C**).
21 Advance the catheter into the tract 3 cm deeper than it was prior to removal. If no urine drains, press gently on the patient's lower abdomen to elicit urine drainage.	Further advancement can inadvertently pass the catheter into the proximal urethra, leading to tissue damage on balloon inflation. **E**
22 Inflate the catheter balloon, after ensuring that urine is draining, then gently withdraw the catheter.	To ensure the balloon is inflated and maintains adequate urine drainage. **E**
23 Support the catheter using a specially designed support, for example the Simpla G-Strap or the Bard StatLock™ Foley stabilization device. Ensure that the catheter does not become taut when the patient is mobilizing. Ensure that the catheter lumen is not occluded by the fixation device.	To maintain patient comfort and to reduce the risk of urethral and bladder neck trauma. Care must be taken when applying securing devices to ensure these do not interfere with drainage of the catheter by being applied to tightly. Leg straps must not impair circulation (Yates 2018, **E**).
Post-procedure	
24 Assist the patient into a comfortable position and feed the catheter bag along the patient's leg. Ensure that drainage is aided by gravity. Replace the bedcovers and make sure the area is dry.	If the area is left wet or moist, secondary infection and skin irritation may occur (Voegeli, 2013, **E**).
25 Measure the amount of urine drained.	To be aware of bladder capacity for patients who have presented with urinary retention. To monitor renal function and fluid balance if clinically indicated. It is not necessary to measure the amount of urine if the patient is having a routine suprapubic catheter change (EAUN 2012, **C**).
26 If required, take a urine specimen for laboratory examination.	For further information, see Chapter 13: Diagnostic tests.
27 Dispose of equipment (including apron and gloves) in a clinical waste bag as per local policy.	To ensure correct and safe disposal of clinical waste (DEFRA 2005, **C**).
28 Draw back the screen.	
29 Wash hands thoroughly with soap and water.	To reduce the risk of infection (Fraise and Bradley 2009, **E**).
30 Record information in relevant documents; this should include: • reasons for catheterization • date and time of catheterization • catheter type, length and size • amount of water instilled into the balloon • batch number and manufacturer • any problems negotiated during the procedure • a review date to assess the need for continued catheterization or date of change of catheter.	To provide a point of reference or comparison in the event of later queries (NMC 2018, **C**).

Intermittent catheterization

Some patients need a catheter long term to empty their bladder. This is often managed by teaching them clean intermittent self catheterization (CISC). This involves passing a catheter into their bladder to drain urine and then removing it immediately when the bladder is empty (Logan 2012).

Patients who may need to do this include those who are unable to empty their bladder effectively (with a residue of 150 mL or more). This could be due to a number of factors including urethral or meatal strictures or prostatic issues such as benign prostatic hypertrophy or prostate cancer (Logan 2012).

Intermittent self-catheterization can also be used short term for the management of post-operative voiding – for example, following surgery for stress incontinence or pelvic-surgery-related neuropathy (Rantell 2012).

Evidence-based approaches

Rationale

Indications

This procedure may be required by patients who have undergone continent reconstruction surgery to manage post-operative incontinence. Patients with a Mitrofanoff reconstruction will need to perform this procedure to facilitate bladder emptying through their abdominal tract, for life. Additionally, many patients with an orthotopic neobladder reconstruction will have to perform this procedure on a regular basis to either facilitate neobladder emptying or drain residual urine.

Patients suitable for intermittent self-catheterization include those:

- with a bladder capable of storing urine without leakage between catheterizations
- who can comprehend the technique
- with sufficient dexterity and mobility to position themselves for the procedure and manipulate the catheter
- who are highly committed to carrying out the procedure (Nazarko 2012).

Contraindications

Contraindications for intermittent self-catheterization include the following:

- insuffient bladder control (bladder not capable of storing urine without leakage between catheterizations)
- insufficient dexterity and/or mobility
- patient resistance.

Related theory

CISC is not a new technique, although it has become noticeably more popular in recent years. The procedure involves the episodic introduction of a catheter into the bladder to remove urine. After this, the catheter is removed, leaving the patient catheter free between catheterizations. In hospital, this should be a sterile procedure because of the risk of hospital-acquired infection. However, in the patient's home a clean technique may be used (Stafford 2017). Catheterization should be carried out as often as necessary to stop the bladder becoming over-distended and to prevent incontinence (Naish 2003). How frequent this is will depend on the individual.

The advantages of intermittent catheterization over indwelling urethral catheterizations include improved quality of life, as patients are free from bulky pads or indwelling catheters, greater patient satisfaction and greater freedom to express sexuality. In addition, urinary tract complications are minimized and normal bladder function is maintained (Wilson 2016).

There are challenges to intermittent catheterization. Patients need to have an understanding of their anatomy, an understanding of what is causing their voiding problems and an understanding of how intermittent catheterization works (Logan 2012, RCN 2019).

There can be physical and psychological barriers to intermittent catheterization:

- Physical barriers include poor eyesight, reduced mobility and reduced dexterity.
- Psychological barriers include anxiety about intermittent catheterization, fear of pain or discomfort, concern regarding sexual function, lack of understanding and cultural concerns (Wilson 2016).

Nurses can help allay some of these anxieties through teaching and encouragement. Continued nursing support can be offered in the community (Nazarko 2012).

Pre-procedural considerations

Equipment

Nelaton catheters are generally used to carry out intermittent self-catheterizations (see Figure 6.7). These catheters are available in standard, female and paediatric lengths and in charrière sizes 6–24; as they are not left in the bladder, they do not have a balloon. They are normally manufactured from plastic but there is also a non-PVC, chlorine-free catheter available. Many Nelaton catheters are coated with a water-activated lubricant; others are packaged with a lubricant gel that coats the catheter as it slides out of the packaging (these catheters are for single use only). Some Nelaton catheters are also available with an integral drainage bag, which is useful when toilet facilities are unavailable or the environment is not conducive to performing a clean procedure safely or comfortably.

Procedure guideline 6.7 Urinary catheterization: intermittent self-catheterization patient guidance: male

Essential equipment

- Personal protective equipment
- Appropriately sized catheter (if carrying out this procedure in hospital, a new catheter must be used every time)
- Lubricating gel if using a non-coated catheter

Optional equipment

- Suitable container (clean jug or receiver) if required
- Mirror if required

Action	Rationale
Pre-procedure	
1 Wash hands using soap and water or an alcohol-based handrub.	To prevent infection (NHS England and NHSI 2019, **C**).
2 Stand in front of a toilet, or (if easier) in front of a low bench with a suitable container, such as a jug or bottle. Standing in front of a mirror is helpful for patients with a large abdomen.	To catch urine. **E** For ease of observation. **E**
Procedure	
3 Clean the glans penis with water or 0.9% sodium chloride. If the foreskin covers the penis, it will need to be held back during the procedure.	To reduce the risk of infection (Loveday et al. 2014, **R**).
4 Wash hands using soap and water and alcohol-based handrub.	To prevent infection (NHS England and NHSI 2019, **C**).

5 Open the catheter packaging or container. If using an uncoated catheter, a water-soluble lubricating gel may be applied to the surface of the catheter. If using a coated catheter, presoak it in water to activate the slippery coating.	To prepare the catheter and to ease insertion. **E**
6 Hold the penis, with the non-dominant hand, upwards towards the stomach.	To straighten the penile urethra and prevent trauma to the penoscrotal junction. **E**
7 Hold the catheter with the dominant hand, being careful not to touch the part of the catheter entering the body, and gently insert it into the opening of the urethra. Advance the catheter into the bladder.	To reduce the risk of introducing an infection (Fraise and Bradley 2009, **E**).
8 There will be a change of feeling as the catheter passes through the prostate gland and into the bladder. It may be a little sore on the first few occasions only. If there is any resistance, do not continue. Withdraw the catheter and contact a nurse or doctor.	The prostate gland surrounds the urethra just below the neck of the bladder and consists of much firmer tissue. This can enlarge and cause an obstruction, especially in older men (Tortora and Derrickson 2017, **C**).
9 Drain the urine into the toilet or a suitable container. When the urine stops flowing, slowly remove the catheter, halting if more urine starts to flow.	To ensure that the bladder is completely emptied. **E**
10 Before removing the catheter from the urethra, put a finger over the funnel end of the catheter and then remove the catheter from the urethra.	To trap urine in the catheter and prevent spillage onto clothing or the floor. **E**
11 Hold the catheter over the toilet or a suitable container and remove finger from the funnel end to release the trapped urine.	To prevent urine spillage. **E**
Post-procedure	
12 Dispose of the catheter in a suitable receptacle.	To prevent environmental contamination. **E**
13 Wash hands with soap and water or alcohol-based handrub.	To reduce the risk of infection (NHS England and NHSI 2019, **C**).

Procedure guideline 6.8 Urinary catheterization: intermittent self-catheterization patient guidance: female

Essential equipment

- Personal protective equipment
- Appropriately sized catheter (if carrying out this procedure in hospital, a new catheter must be used every time)
- Mirror
- Lubricating gel if using uncoated catheter
- Suitable container (clean jug or receiver)

Action	Rationale
Pre-procedure	
1 Wash hands using soap and water or an alcohol-based handrub.	To reduce the risk of cross-infection (NHS England and NHSI 2019, **C**).
2 Take up a comfortable position, depending on mobility (e.g. sitting on toilet or standing with one foot placed on toilet seat).	To facilitate insertion of intermittent catheter. **E**
Procedure	
3 Wash genitalia from front to back, with soap and water or 0.9% normal saline solution, then dry.	To reduce the risk of introducing infection (Loveday et al. 2014, **R**).
4 Wash hands using soap and water and alcohol-based handrub.	To reduce risk of cross-infection (NHS England and NHSI 2019, **C**).
5 Open catheter packaging or container. If using an uncoated catheter, a water-soluble lubricating gel may be applied to the surface of the catheter. If using a coated catheter, presoak it in water to activate the slippery coating.	To prepare the catheter and to ease insertion. **E**
6 Find the urethral opening above the vagina. A mirror can be used to help identify it. Gently insert the catheter into the urethra, taking care not to touch the part of the catheter entering the body.	To reduce the risk of introducing infection (Loveday et al. 2014, **R**).
7 Drain the urine into the toilet or a suitable container. When the urine stops flowing, slowly remove the catheter, halting if more urine starts to flow.	To ensure that the bladder is completely emptied. **E**
8 Before removing the catheter from the urethra, put a finger over the funnel end of the catheter and then remove the catheter from the urethra.	To trap urine in the catheter and prevent spillage onto clothing or the floor. **E**
9 Hold the catheter over the toilet or a suitable container and remove finger from the funnel end to release the trapped urine.	To prevent urine spillage. **E**
Post-procedure	
10 Dispose of the catheter in a suitable receptacle.	To prevent environmental contamination. **E**
11 Wash hands with soap and water.	To reduce the risk of infection (NHS England and NHSI 2019, **C**).

Problem-solving table 6.2 Prevention and resolution (Procedure guidelines 6.4, 6.5, 6.6, 6.7 and 6.8)

Problem	Cause	Prevention	Action
Urethral mucosal trauma	Incorrect size of catheter, procedure not carried out correctly or skilfully, or movement of the catheter in the urethra	Select an appropriate size of catheter (smallest diameter for type of drainage required). Ensure adequate training is received before carrying out the procedure.	Reinsert the catheter using the correct size of catheter. Check the catheter support and apply or reapply as necessary.
	Inadequate lubrication of the catheter	Ensure adequate lubrication.	Add additional lubrication as required.
	Trauma to the urethral tissue due to rapid insertion of the catheter	Ensure the catheter is inserted slowly and gently.	It may be necessary to remove the catheter and wait for the urethral mucosa to heal.
Patient has a vasovagal attack	This is caused by the vagal nerve being stimulated so that the heart slows down, leading to syncope (fainting)	Difficult to predict or prevent; however, ensure the person performing the procedure is prepared and trained in the actions to take following a vasovagal attack.	Patient should lie down in the recovery position (see Figure 12.9) and their doctor should be informed.
Male			
Paraphimosis	Failure to extend the foreskin after catheterization	Ensure adequate training is received before carrying out the procedure.	Refer to a relevant medical colleague to review and attempt to extend the foreskin. The foreskin must not be left in a retracted position.
Female			
No drainage of urine	Incorrect identification of the external urinary meatus	Ensure there is sufficient light to observe the area. Review the female anatomy prior to the procedure.	Check that the catheter has been sited correctly. If the catheter has been wrongly inserted in the vagina, leave it in position to act as a guide, reidentify the urethra and perform the catheterization. Remove the inappropriately sited catheter.
Difficulty in visualizing the urethral orifice	Vaginal atrophy and retraction of the urethral orifice into anterior vaginal wall		The index finger of one hand (for nurses carrying out the procedure in hospital, this will be the 'dirty' hand) may be inserted in the vagina and the urethral orifice can be palpated on the anterior wall of the vagina. The index finger is then positioned just behind the urethral orifice. This then acts as a guide so that the catheter can be correctly positioned (Robinson 2007).

Procedure guideline 6.9 Urinary catheter bag: emptying

Essential equipment

- Personal protective equipment
- Alcohol wipe
- Container (jug or urine bottle)
- Paper towel to cover the jug

Action	Rationale
Pre-procedure	
1 Introduce yourself to the patient, explain and discuss the procedure with them, and gain their consent to proceed.	To ensure that the patient feels at ease, understands the procedure and gives their valid consent (NMC 2018, **C**).
2 Wash hands using soap and water or alcohol-based handrub, and put on disposable gloves.	To reduce risk of cross-infection (NHS England and NHSI 2019, **C**).
Procedure	
3 Open the catheter valve. Allow the urine to drain into the jug or urine bottle.	To empty the drainage bag and accurately measure the volume of the contents. **E**
4 Close the outlet valve and clean it with an alcohol wipe.	To reduce the risk of cross-infection (Fraise and Bradley 2009, **E**).
5 Note and record the amount of urine if this is required for fluid balance records.	To ensure accurate fluid balance monitoring. **E**
6 Cover the jug or urine bottle and dispose of the contents in the sluice or down the toilet.	To reduce the risk of environmental contamination (DEFRA 2005, **C**).
Post-procedure	
7 Wash hands with soap and water or an alcohol-based handrub.	To reduce the risk of infection (NHS England and NHSI 2019, **C**).

Procedure guideline 6.10 Urinary catheter removal

Essential equipment

- Personal protective equipment
- Dressing pack containing sterile towels, gallipots, and swabs or non-linting gauze
- Syringe, alcohol wipe, clamp and a specimen container (if a specimen is requested)
- Syringe for deflating the balloon

Action	Rationale
Pre-procedure	
1 Catheters can be removed at any time. However, it is sensible to remove them early in the morning.	So that any retention problems can be dealt with during the day, thus avoiding delays in recatheterization if required. **E**
2 Introduce yourself to the patient, explain and discuss the procedure with them, and gain their consent to proceed. Inform them of potential post-catheter symptoms, such as urgency, frequency and discomfort, which are often caused by irritation of the urethra by the catheter.	To ensure that the patient feels at ease, understands the procedure and gives their valid consent (NMC 2018, **C**). So that the patient knows what to expect and can plan their daily activity. **E**
3 Wash hands using soap and water and/or an alcohol-based handrub, and put on personal protective equipment.	To reduce the risk of cross-infection (NHS England and NHSI 2019, **C**).
Procedure	
4 If a specimen is required, clamp below the sampling port until sufficient urine collects. Swab the port with an alcohol wipe and take a catheter specimen of urine using the needle-free sampling port.	To obtain an adequate urine sample and to assess whether post-catheter antibiotic therapy is needed (Fraise and Bradley 2009, **E**).
5 Wearing gloves, use saline-soaked gauze to clean the meatus and catheter, always swabbing away from the urethral opening. *Note*: in females, wipe from front to back.	To reduce the risk of infection (Fraise and Bradley 2009, **E**). To help reduce the risk of bacteria from the vagina and perineum contaminating the urethra. **E**
6 Release the leg support.	For easier removal of the catheter. **E**
7 Having checked the volume of water in the balloon (see patient documentation), use a syringe to deflate the balloon.	To confirm how much water is in the balloon. To ensure the balloon is completely deflated before removing the catheter. **E**

(continued)

Procedure guideline 6.10 Urinary catheter removal (continued)

Action	Rationale
8 Ask the patient to breathe in and then out; as the patient exhales, gently (but firmly with continuous traction) remove the catheter. *Note*: male patients should be warned of discomfort as the deflated balloon passes through the prostate gland.	To relax the pelvic floor muscles. **E** It is advisable to extend the penis as per the process for insertion to aid removal. **E**
Post-procedure	
9 *Males*: clean the meatus and make the patient comfortable. *Females*: clean the area from front to back and make the patient comfortable.	To maintain patient comfort and dignity and reduce the risk of cross-contamination. **E**
10 Advise the patient to exercise and to drink 2–3 L of fluid per day.	To prevent urinary tract infections. **E**
11 Dispose of equipment (including apron and gloves) in a clinical waste bag.	To ensure correct and safe disposal of clinical waste (DEFRA 2005, **C**).
12 Wash hands thoroughly with soap and water and/or an alcohol-based handrub.	To reduce the risk of infection (NHS England and NHSI 2019, **C**).
13 Record information in relevant documents; this should include: • date and time of catheter removal • any samples taken and why • any problems associated with the catheter removal • follow-up instructions for care after catheter removal.	To provide a point of reference or comparison in the event of later queries. To ensure the patient has a follow-up plan clearly documented (NMC 2018, **C**).

Catheter-associated complications

A number of complications can arise from having a urinary catheter. UTIs are one of the most common and are discussed in detail below. Other complications are outlined in Table 6.3.

Infections

UTI is the most common healthcare-associated infection and accounts for up to 36% of all such infections, and CAUTI accounts for up to 80% of UTIs (Parker et al. 2017). Several key areas have been identified as having a direct link with the development of a UTI:

- The risk of developing a catheter-associated infection increases with the length of time that a catheter is *in situ* (Bernard et al. 2012). Therefore, assessing the need for catheterization and monitoring the length of time the catheter is *in situ* are essential (EAUN 2012).
- It is important to select the most appropriate type of catheter and drainage system.
- It is important to ensure that aseptic conditions are used during insertion and that a closed drainage system is maintained.
- It is important to ensure timely and appropriate catheter removal as per the HOUDINI protocol (Adams et al. 2012) (see Table 6.1).
- The person performing the procedure and those undertaking the aftercare (i.e. patients, relatives and health professionals) should be appropriately trained and competent.
- Patient education is essential in preventing catheter-associated infections. Adequate information and teaching for patients may help to reduce infection by helping patients to take care of their catheters with good hygiene (RCN 2019).

The maintenance of a closed drainage system is central to reducing the risk of catheter-associated infection. It is thought that micro-organisms reach the bladder by two possible routes: from the urine in the drainage bag and via the space between the catheter and the urethral mucosa (Ostaszkiewicz and Paterson 2012). To reduce the risk of infection, it is important to keep manipulation of the closed system to a minimum; this includes unnecessary emptying, changing the drainage bags or taking samples (Ostaszkiewicz and Paterson 2012). There is now an integral catheter and drainage bag available to reduce the number of potential disconnection sites and minimize the infection risk. Before handling catheter drainage systems, hands must be decontaminated and a pair of clean non-sterile gloves should be worn (Loveday et al. 2014). All urine samples should only be obtained via the specially designed sampling ports using an aseptic technique.

An important aspect of management for patients in whom a clear pattern of catheter history can be established is the scheduling of catheter changes prior to likely blockages (Wilde et al. 2016). In patients in whom no clear pattern emerges, or for whom frequent catheter changes are traumatic, acidic bladder washouts can be beneficial in reducing catheter encrustations (Wilson 2012). The administration of catheter maintenance solutions to eliminate catheter encrustation can also be timed to coincide with catheter bag changes (every 5–7 days) so that the catheter system is not opened more than necessary (Peate and Gill 2015).

A UTI may be introduced during catheterization because of an inadequate aseptic technique, inadequate urethral cleaning or contamination of the catheter tip. It may also be introduced via the drainage system because of faulty handling of equipment, breaking the closed system or raising the drainage bag above bladder level, causing urine reflux.

If a UTI is suspected, a catheter specimen of urine must be sent for analysis. The patient should be encouraged to have a fluid intake of 2–3 L per day. Medical staff should be informed if the problem persists so that antibiotics can be prescribed; however, all healthcare practitioners have a responsibility to adhere to the *Antimicrobial Stewardship* guidelines, which cover the effective use of antimicrobials and are aimed at reducing resistance (NICE 2015b). Implementing good catheter care techniques helps to reduce UTI rates.

Meatal cleansing

EAUN (2012) found no reduction in bacteriuria between routine bathing or showering when compared to antiseptic or antimicrobial solutions for meatal cleansing. However, Fasugba et al. (2017) found that using 0.1% chlorhexidine solution (as opposed to 0.9% sodium chloride) for meatal cleansing before urethral catheterization led to a reduced rate of CAUTI. Further

Table 6.3 Complications of catheterization

Problem	Cause	Suggested action
Inability to tolerate an indwelling catheter	Urethral mucosal irritation	Nurse may need to remove the catheter and seek an alternative means of urine drainage.
	Previous trauma (e.g. sexual abuse)	Explain the need for and the functioning of the catheter and consider referral to psychological support for assessment and possible therapy.
	Unstable bladder Radiation cystitis	Pharmacological support may assist with catheter tolerance. If patient remains intolerant to indwelling catheter, refer to urology.
Inadequate drainage of urine	Incorrect placement of a catheter	Resite the catheter.
	Kinked drainage tubing	Inspect the system and straighten any kinks.
	Blocked tubing, e.g. from pus, urates, phosphates or blood clots	If a three-way catheter, such as a Foley, is in place, irrigate it. If a two-way Foley catheter is in use, milk the tubing in an attempt to dislodge the debris, then attempt a gentle bladder washout. Failing this, the catheter will need to be replaced; a three-way catheter should be used if the obstruction is being caused by clots and associated haematuria.
Fistula formation	Pressure on the penoscrotal angle	Ensure the catheter is correctly secured.
Penile pain on erection	Not allowing enough length of catheter to accommodate penile erection	Ensure that an adequate length is available to accommodate penile erection.
Formation of crusts around the urethral meatus	Increased urethral secretions collect at the meatus and form crusts, due to irritation of the urothelium by the catheter (Fillingham and Douglas 2004)	Regular meatal cleansing using recommended technique.
Leakage of urine around the catheter	Incorrect catheter size	Replace with the correct size, usually 2 ch smaller.
	Incorrect balloon size	Select a catheter with a 10 mL balloon.
		Use a Roberts tipped catheter.
	Bladder hyperirritability	Consider pharmacological support such as anticholinergic drugs (MacDiarmid 2008).
Inability to deflate the balloon	Valve expansion or displacement	Check the non-return valve on the inflation/deflation channel. If jammed, use a syringe and needle to aspirate the inflation channel above the valve.
	Channel obstruction	Obstruction by a foreign body can sometimes be relieved by the introduction of a guidewire through the inflation channel (only under advice from urology).
		Inject 3.5 mL of 0.9% sodium chloride into the inflation arm (only under advice from urology).
		Alternatively, the balloon can be punctured suprapubically using a needle under ultrasound visualization.
		Following catheter removal, the balloon should be inspected to ensure it has not disintegrated, leaving fragments in the bladder.
		Note: the steps above should only be attempted by or under the direction of a urologist. The patient may require cystoscopy following balloon deflation to remove any balloon fragments and to wash the bladder out.
Dysuria	Inflammation of the urethral mucosa	Encourage a fluid intake of 2–3 L per day. Advise the patient that dysuria is common but will usually be resolved once micturition has occurred at least three times. Inform medical staff if the problem persists.

studies support the view that vigorous meatal cleaning is unnecessary and may compromise the integrity of the skin, thus increasing the risk of infection (Leaver 2007, Panknin and Althaus 2001). Therefore, it is recommended that routine daily personal hygiene with soap and water (NICE 2017) is all that is needed to maintain meatal hygiene (Loveday et al. 2014, Pomfret 2004). Nursing intervention is necessary if there is a poor standard of hygiene or a risk of contamination (Gilbert 2006); removal of a smegma ring, where the catheter meets the meatus, is important to prevent ascending infections and meatal trauma (Wilson 2005). It is imperative that the individual perfoming meatal cleansing returns the foreskin to the natural position in uncircumcised men.

Bladder irrigation

Definition

Bladder irrigation is the continuous washing out of the bladder, whereas bladder lavage or bladder washout is the intermittent washing out of the bladder. Bladder irrigation is usually carried out with 0.9% normal saline (BAUN 2012) via a three-way catheter (Peate and Gill 2015).

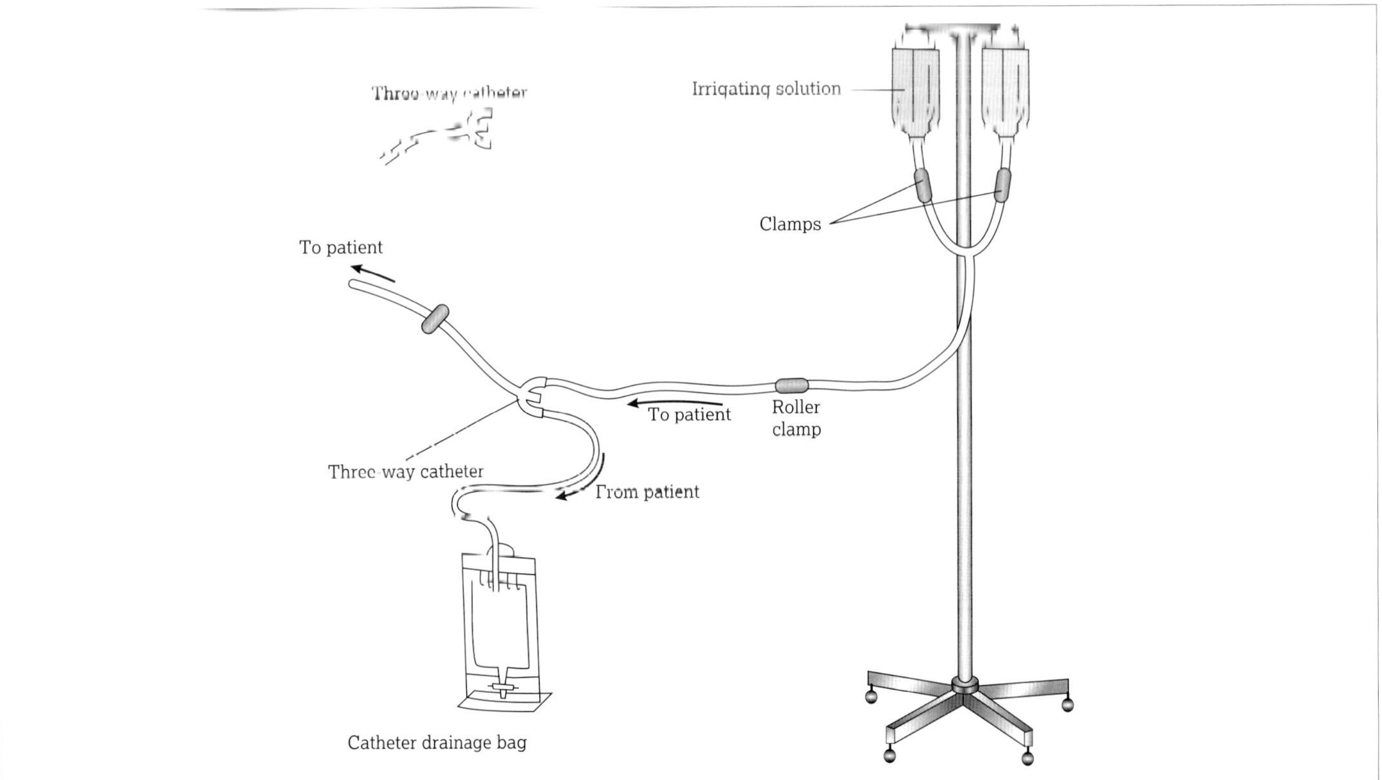

Figure 6.14 Closed urinary drainage system with provision for intermittent or continuous irrigation.

Evidence-based approaches

Rationale

Indications

Bladder irrigation is performed to prevent the formation and retention of blood clots, for example following prostatic surgery, such as transurethral resection of bladder tumour (TURBT) or transurethral resection of prostate (TURP). Other indications include irrigation for the delivery of pharmacological agents, irrigation for candida cystitis, prevention of haematuria following chemotherapy or surgical procedures (Abt et al. 2013).

Principles of care

There are a number of risks associated with bladder irrigation (including introducing infection) and the procedure should not be undertaken lightly (Siddiq and Darouiche 2012). Prior to taking a decision to use bladder maintenance solutions, patients should be assessed. The guiding principle for effective catheter management always involves addressing the individual needs of the patient (Wilde et al. 2016). Assessment of all aspects of catheter care and irrigation should be undertaken, including:

- patient activity and mobility (catheter positioning, catheter kinking)
- diet and fluid intake
- standards of patient hygiene
- patient's and/or carer's ability to care for the catheter (EAUN 2012).

Pre-procedural considerations

Equipment

A three-way urinary catheter must be used for irrigation in order that fluid may simultaneously be run into, and drained out from, the bladder (Davis et al. 2016). A large-gauge catheter (16–24 ch) is often used to accommodate any clots or debris that may be present. This catheter is commonly passed in theatre, for example after transurethral resections (Bijalwan et al. 2017). Occasionally, if a patient is admitted with a heavily contaminated bladder (e.g. by blood clots or pus), bladder irrigation may be started on the ward. If the patient has a two-way catheter, this must be replaced with a three-way type (Peate and Gill 2015).

It is recommended that a three-way catheter is passed if frequent intravesical instillations of drugs or antiseptic solutions are prescribed and the risk of catheter obstruction is not considered to be very great. In such cases, the most important factor is minimizing the risk of introducing infection and maintaining a closed urinary drainage system, which the three-way catheter allows (Figure 6.14).

Pharmacological support

The agent most commonly recommended for irrigation is 0.9% sodium chloride (RCN 2019), which should be used in every case unless an alternative solution is prescribed. 0.9% sodium chloride is isotonic so it does not affect the body's fluid or electrolyte levels, enabling large volumes of the solution to be used as necessary (Clarebrough et al. 2018). In particular, 2 L bags and bottles of 0.9% sodium chloride are available for irrigation purposes. It has been proposed that sterile water should never be used to irrigate the bladder as it can be readily absorbed via osmosis (Gupta et al. 2010). However, a study has demonstrated that sterile water is a safe irrigating fluid for TURP (Bijalwan et al. 2017). Other irrigation fluids include 3.23% and 6% citric acid used in catheter care or maintenance to dissolve or remove encrustations and crystallization in the bladder (RCN 2019).

Although not a common complication, absorption of irrigation fluid can occur during bladder irrigation. This can produce a potentially critical situation, as absorption may lead to electrolyte imbalance and circulatory overload. Absorption is most likely to occur in theatre when glycine irrigation fluid, devoid of sodium or potassium, is forced under pressure into the prostatic veins (Hermanns et al. 2013). 0.9% sodium chloride cannot be used during surgery as it contains electrolytes, which interfere with diathermy (Forristal and Maxfield 2004). However, the risk of absorption remains while irrigation continues post-operatively. For this reason, it is important that fluid balance is monitored carefully during irrigation (Hahn 2015).

Procedure guideline 6.11 Commencing bladder irrigation

Essential equipment

- Personal protective equipment
- Sterile dressing pack and sterile gloves
- Chlorhexidine antiseptic solution or wipe
- Clamp
- Disposable irrigation set
- Infusion stand
- Sterile jug
- Absorbent sheet
- Trolley
- Sterile irrigation fluid

Action	Rationale
Pre-procedure	
1 Introduce yourself to the patient, explain and discuss the procedure with them, and gain their consent to proceed.	To ensure that the patient feels at ease, understands the procedure and gives their valid consent (NMC 2018, **C**).
2 Screen the bed. Ensure that the patient is in a comfortable position, allowing the nurse access to the catheter.	For the patient's privacy and to reduce the risk of cross-infection (Fraise and Bradley 2009, **E**).
3 Wash hands with soap and water and/or alcohol-based handrub and apply personal protective equipment.	To decontaminate hands and reduce the risk of cross-infection (NHS England and NHSI 2019, **C**).
Procedure	
4 Perform the procedure using an aseptic technique.	To minimize the risk of infection (Loveday et al. 2014, **R**).
5 Open the outer wrappings of the sterile dressing pack and place it on the top shelf of the trolley.	To prepare the equipment. **E**
6 Insert the end of the irrigation giving set into the fluid bag and hang the bag on the infusion stand. Allow the fluid to run through the tubing so that air is expelled.	To prime the irrigation set so that it is ready for use. Air is expelled in order to prevent discomfort from air in the patient's bladder. **E**
7 Clamp the catheter and place an absorbent sheet under the catheter junction.	To prevent leakage of urine through the irrigation arm when the spigot is removed. **E**
8 Clean hands with an alcohol based handrub. Put on clean gloves.	Handling the packets may have contaminated hands; to minimize the risk of cross-infection (NHS England and NHSI 2019, **C**).
9 Place a sterile paper towel under the irrigation inlet of the catheter and remove the spigot.	To create a sterile field and to prepare the catheter for connection to the irrigation set (Clarebrough et al. 2018, **E**).
10 Discard the spigot and gloves. Clean hands with an alcohol-based handrub.	To prevent reuse and reduce the risk of cross-infection (NHS England and NHSI 2019, **C**).
11 Put on sterile gloves. Clean around the end of the irrigation arm with sterile low-linting gauze and an antiseptic solution or wipe.	To remove surface organisms from the gloves and the catheter and to reduce the risk of introducing infection into the catheter (Loveday et al. 2014, **R**).
12 Attach the irrigation giving set to the irrigation arm of the catheter. Keep the clamp of the irrigation giving set closed.	To prevent over-distension of the bladder, which can occur if fluid is run into the bladder before the drainage tube has been unclamped (Clarebrough et al. 2018, **E**).
13 Release the clamp on the catheter tube and allow any accumulated urine to drain into the catheter bag. Empty the urine from the catheter bag into a sterile jug.	Urine drainage should be measured before commencing irrigation so that the fluid balance may be accurately monitored (Clarebrough et al. 2018, **E**).
14 Discard the gloves.	These will be contaminated, having handled the cathether bag (NHS England and NHSI 2019, **C**).
15 Set irrigation at the required rate (see Box 6.1), titrated to the colour of the urine output, and ensure that fluid is draining into the catheter bag.	To check that the drainage system is patent and to prevent fluid accumulating in the bladder. **E**
Post-procedure	
16 Make the patient comfortable, remove unnecessary equipment and clean the trolley.	To reduce the risk of cross-infection (Fraise and Bradley 2009, **E**).
17 Remove gloves and apron and dispose according to local policy. Wash hands or use an alcohol-based handrub.	To reduce the risk of cross-infection (NHS England and NHSI 2019, **C**).
18 Check blood results 8–12 hours after irrigation has been commenced.	To ensure absorption has not occurred. **E**
19 Record information in relevant documents; this should include: • reason for irrigation • date and time irrigation commenced • volume, colour and characteristics of urine output.	To provide a point of reference or comparison in the event of later queries (NMC 2018, **C**).
20 Ensure an accurate fluid balance is commenced and maintained throughout irrigation (Figure 6.15 provides an example of a bladder irrigation chart).	To monitor irrigation and to ensure fluid irrigated is also being drained. This will also enable monitoring for any absorption. **E**

Problem-solving table 6.2 Prevention and resolution (Procedure guideline 6.11)

Problem	Cause	Prevention	Action
Fluid retained in the bladder when the catheter is in position	Fault in drainage apparatus, e.g. kinked tubing blocking catheter	Empty the drainage bag every 2–4 hours, depending on how fast the fluid is running.	Straighten the tubing. 'Milk' the tubing. Wash out the bladder with 0.9% sodium chloride using an aseptic technique.
	Overfull drainage bag		Empty the drainage bag.
	Catheter clamped off		Unclamp the catheter.
Distended abdomen related to an overfull bladder during the irrigation procedure	Irrigation fluid is infused at too rapid a rate	Monitor fluid drainage rate every 15 minutes.	Slow down the infusion rate.
	Fault in drainage apparatus		Check the patency of the drainage apparatus.
Leakage of fluid from around the catheter	Catheter slipping out of the bladder	Use appropriate size of catheter.	Insert the catheter further in. Decompress the balloon fully to assess the amount of water necessary. Refill the balloon until it remains *in situ*, taking care not to overfill beyond a safe level (see manufacturer's instructions).
	Catheter too large or unsuitable for the patient's anatomy		If leakage is profuse or catheter is uncomfortable for the patient, replace it with one of a smaller size.
Patient experiences pain during the lavage or irrigation procedure	Volume of fluid in the bladder is too great for comfort	Titrate slowly and assess pain level frequently.	Reduce the fluid volume or rate.
	Solution is painful to raw areas in the bladder		Inform the doctor. Administer analgesia as prescribed.
Retention of fluid with or without distended abdomen, with or without pain	Perforated bladder		Stop irrigation. Maintain in recovery position. Call for urgent medical assistance. Monitor vital signs. Monitor patient for pain or a tense abdomen.

Box 6.1 Care of patients undergoing bladder irrigation

- Adjust the rate of infusion according to the degree of haematuria. This will be greatest in the first 12 hours following surgery (average fluid input is 6–9 L during the first 12 hours, falling to 3–6 L during the next 12 hours). The aim is to obtain a drainage fluid that is rosé in colour. Check the bags of irrigation fluid regularly and renew as required. The overall aim is to remove blood from the bladder before it clots and to minimize the risk of catheter obstruction and clot retention (Scholtes 2002).
- Check the volume in the drainage bag frequently when the infusion is in progress, and empty bags before they reach their capacity (e.g. half-hourly or hourly, or more frequently as required). This will ensure that fluid is draining from the bladder and that blockages are detected as soon as possible; it will also prevent over-distension of the bladder and patient discomfort.
- Annotate the fluid balance chart accurately. The fluid balance of all patients having bladder irrigation must be closely monitored so that urine output is known and any related problems, such as renal dysfunction, may be detected quickly and easily.

Post-procedural considerations

Documentation: bladder irrigation recording chart

A bladder irrigation recording chart (see Figure 6.15) is designed to provide an accurate record of the patient's urinary output during the period of irrigation. Record the time (column A) and the fluid volume in each bag of irrigating solution (column B) as it is put up.

When the irrigating fluid has all run from the first bag into the bladder, record the original volume in the bag in column C. Record the corresponding time in column A. Do not attempt to estimate the fluid volume run-in while a bag is in progress as this will be inaccurate. If, however, a bag is discontinued, the volume run-in can be calculated by measuring the volume left in the bag and deducting this from the original volume. This should be recorded in column C (Clarebrough et al. 2018).

The catheter bag should be emptied as often as is necessary; the volume should be recorded in column D and the corresponding time in column A. The catheter bag must also be emptied whenever the bag of irrigating fluid is empty, with the volume recorded in column D.

When each bag of fluid has run through, add up the total volume drained by the catheter in column D, and write this in red. Subtract from this the total volume run-in (column C) to find the urine output (D – C = E). Write this in column E. Draw a line across the page to indicate that this calculation is complete and continue underneath for the next bag.

Nephrostomy tubes and ureteric stents

Related theory

A nephrostomy tube is a pigtail drain inserted under fluoroscopic, ultrasonographic or CT (computed tomography) guidance, with a local anaesthetic, usually by an interventional radiologist. The procedure involves the passing of a needle and guidewire, followed by a pigtail drain, through the skin, subcutaneous tissue, muscle layers and renal parenchyma into the renal pelvis (McDougal et al. 2015). The drain is attached to a drainage bag (Figure 6.16) and the system is secured to the skin with a suture and in many cases a drain fixation dressing.

Patient name:			**Hospital no:**		
(A) Date and time	**(B) Volume put up**	**(C) Volume run in**	**(D) Total volume out**	**(E) Urine**	**(F) Urine running total**
10/7/20					
10.00	2000				
10.30			700		
11.10			850		
11.40		2000	600		
			2150	150	150
11.45	2000				
12.30			500		
13.15			700		
14.20		2000	800		
			2100	400	550
14.25	2000				
15.30			850		
17.00	Irrigation stopped	1200	800		
			1650	450	1000

Figure 6.15 Example bladder irrigation chart.

The percutaneous nephrostomy diverts urine away from the ureter and bladder into an externalized drainage bag (Hohenfellner and Santucci 2010). The nephrostomy can be unilateral, with a tube and drainage bag on one side and the other kidney continuing to drain through the ureter into the bladder. Alternatively, bilateral tubes may be inserted, with a tube and drainage bag on each side and with minimal urine draining through the ureters into the bladder.

In most cases a nephrostomy is temporary and will be removed when the obstruction has resolved, when the obstruction can be bypassed with an internalized ureteric stent or when the therapeutic intervention has been completed. Rarely, a nephrostomy is a permanent or semi-permanent solution; this is the case when bypassing the obstruction is not possible or when it is inadvisable.

Externalized ureteric stents are used following the formation of an ileal conduit or a continent urinary diversion. Stents are inserted into each kidney, and these then drain into the urostomy pouch or are externalized cutaneously or rectally and drain directly into a bag. These maintain the patency of the ureters following surgery and ensure that the kidneys are able to drain; they also act to protect the anastomosis (Geng et al. 2009). Urine drains both through and around the ureteric stent. In the context of urinary diversion, stents usually remain in situ for 7–14 days depending on patient factors such as previous radiotherapy.

Evidence-based approaches

Rationale

The decision to perform a percutaneous nephrostomy is taken by the patient's medical and/or surgical team in discussion with the radiologist.

Indications

Indications for a nephrostomy include:

- relief of urinary obstruction (the most common reason for insertion, characterized by any of the following: imaging demonstrating obstruction nephropathy, rising creatinine, acute renal failure, loin pain, nausea and vomiting, fever or urosepsis)

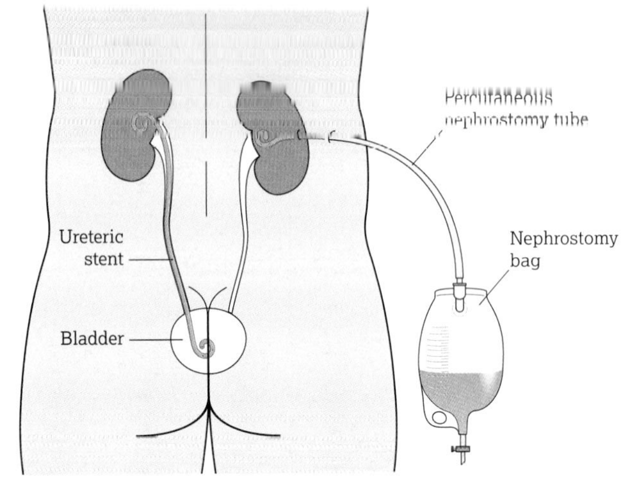

Figure 6.16 Nephrostomy bag.

- urinary diversion (e.g. following a ureteral injury, ureteral fissure or fistula, or haemorrhagic cystitis) (Geng et al. 2009)
- access for therapeutic interventions (e.g. stone removal, antegrade stent insertion, removal of a foreign body such as a broken ureteric stent, delivery of medications or ureteral biopsy)
- diagnostic testing (e.g. antegrade pyelography or a ureteral perfusion test) (Dagli and Ramchandani 2011).

Contraindications

Alternatives to the nephrostomy are retrograde stent insertion (stent insertion from below) or ureteroscopy (investigation into the patency of the ureter); the medical and/or surgical team will be guided by the urologist when making this decision. In general, a retrograde approach is preferred as it has a lower associated morbidity rate. When a retrograde approach is possible for the patient, a nephrostomy is contraindicated.

Other contraindications include:

- coagulation conditions that increase the tendency to bleed
- anticoagulant use (Patel et al. 2012).

Principles of care

The principles of care for a patient with a nephrostomy tube are similar to those for a patient with an indwelling catheter. Accurate measurement of urine output from each of the indwelling tubes is required and should be recorded separately (usually marked 'left', 'right' or 'urethral') and with a total output also recorded.

Good wound site care is essential to avoid exit site infection. Flushing of the nephrostomy should be avoided where possible to avoid introducing infection and potentially causing pyelonephritis. Where flushing of the nephrostomy tube is required, this should be performed by appropriately trained staff with 5 mL of 0.9% sodium chloride using an aseptic technique; see Procedure guideline 6.13: Nephrostomy tube: flushing technique.

With ureteric stents, the output should be recorded and the stents checked to ensure that both are draining; when they are draining into an ileal conduit bag, total urine output should be measured only. If drainage is compromised, this may be due to occlusion or it may be due to dehydration (Geng et al. 2009). The stent should be flushed to assess for patency. If there is no improvement in urine output, the urological surgical team should be informed immediately.

Anticipated patient outcomes

Whether the nephrostomy is short or long term, it is anticipated that the patient will have an uneventful episode of care. The nephrostomy tube will continue to drain urine without occlusion, the patient will remain free from infection and their fluid balance will be maintained (Hsu et al. 2016).

Clinical governance

The nurse looking after the patient must have an understanding of the principles, anatomy and indications for a nephrostomy tube. All staff managing a patient with a nephrostomy tube should be appropriately trained and working within their scope of practice (NMC 2018). If formal competencies are required at the place of employment, these must be met prior to managing the patient's care.

Removal of the nephrostomy tube should be performed by a trained member of staff and under the instruction of the medical and/or surgical team (see Procedure guideline 6.14: Nephrostomy tube: removal of locking pigtail drainage system). If there is a stent *in situ*, the nephrostomy tube should be removed under radiological guidance to avoid misplacement of the ureteric stent.

Following formation of the ileal conduit or continent urinary diversion, ureteric stents should be removed by a trained nurse or member of the surgical team as guided by the consultant surgeon.

Pre-procedural considerations

For a long term nephrostomy, the patient and/or carer should be taught to change both the drain site dressing and the drainage bag on a regular basis. If self-care and independence are not possible, the patient should be referred to the community nursing team.

The recommended dressing is one that supports the nephrostomy tube to prevent accidental tugging and also secures the tube to the patient's skin. There are several drain-specific types available, including the Drain-Guard, Drain-Fix and OPSITE Post-Op Visible drain dressings. When selecting the dressing, it is important to consider the comfort factor for the patient as the exit site is directly on the patient's back and therefore can present discomfort when lying down or sitting against a chair. When such dressings are unavailable or unobtainable, many teams choose to dress the nephrostomy with a simple gauze-and-tape method. If the gauze-and-tape method is used, it is essential to make sure the nephrostomy tube is sutured in position.

To perform the dressing change or drainage bag change, the patient will need to be sitting upright on a stool, couch or a bed with their back facing towards you. The dressing change and drain removal are best performed from behind, so preparing the patient well and good communication are essential (NMC 2018). If the patient is unable to sit upright, then positioning the patient on their side in a bed is an alternative with the patient's back facing towards you.

Post-procedural considerations and complications

After initial nephrostomy insertion, if the kidney has been obstructed, the patient may enter a phase of diuresis. This is characterized by high-volume outputs from the nephrostomy tube (polyuria). Close monitoring of the patient's fluid balance and vital signs is required. The patient's fluid intake (intravenous or oral) should closely match the output. A closely monitored and adjusted fluid balance will prevent deterioration in the patient's condition associated with rapid fluid loss (Hsu et al. 2016, Jairath et al. 2017).

The patient is at risk of pyelonephritis (inflammation of the kidney, usually due to infection) from the foreign body puncturing the kidney (Hsu et al. 2016). The patient should be monitored for signs of infection or sepsis, such as loin pain, elevated temperature, fever or chills, purulent urine output or deterioration in their vital signs. A urine specimen should be taken when infection is suspected. In such cases, medical advice should be sought and the patient treated accordingly. Ensuring the drain site remains clean and dry is essential to prevent infection, and flushing of the nephrostomy tube should only be done when patency of the tube is compromised. Drainage bags should be changed every 5–7 days. Ensure good hand hygiene when handling the drain and exit site and when emptying the drainage bag. Nephrostomy tubes should be routinely changed every 3 months.

The nephrostomy bag should be emptied when it becomes three-quarters full (see Procedure guideline 6.9: Urinary catheter bag:

emptying). Where appropriate, the patient or carer should be taught how to do this. Note that many hospital-supplied nephrostomy drainage bags are not widely available in the community setting and are also not comfortable as body-worn products. An example of a comfortable body-worn system is shown in Figure 6.17.

All patients being discharged out of hospital with a nephrostomy should be referred to the community nursing team for support and assistance when required. They must also be discharged with information on when and how to obtain clinical supplies such as dressings and bags. The patient must also have a written follow-up plan of review and/or a planned date for their tube to be changed. Some manufacturers produce a 'nephrostomy passport', which is a very useful patient-held tool for recording and monitoring this information.

Procedure guideline 6.12 Nephrostomy tube: weekly dressing and bag change and sample collection

Essential equipment

- Personal protective equipment
- 0.9% sodium chloride
- Drainage bag with security straps
- Dressing pack with gauze
- Drain fixation dressing (e.g. Drain-Fix, Drain-Guard or OPSITE Post-Op Visible drain dressing) or if sutured in position can use a simple gauze-and-tape dressing
- Blunt disposable clamps
- Alcohol (chlorhexidine) wipe
- Adhesive remover
- Micropore tape or similar
- A sample container (if required)

Action	Rationale
Pre-procedure	
1 Introduce yourself to the patient, explain and discuss the procedure with them, and gain their consent to proceed.	To ensure that the patient feels at ease, understands the procedure and gives their valid consent (NMC 2018, **C**).
2 Screen the bed.	To ensure patient privacy. To allow dust and airborne organisms to settle before the field is exposed to contamination (Fraise and Bradley 2009, **E**).
3 Wash hands using soap and water or alcohol-based handrub. Put on a disposable plastic apron.	To reduce the risk of cross-infection from micro-organisms on uniform/clothing (NHS England and NHSI 2019, **C**).
4 Prepare the trolley, placing all equipment required on the bottom shelf.	The top shelf acts as a clean working surface. **E**
5 Take the trolley to the patient's bedside, disturbing the screens as little as possible.	To minimize airborne contamination (Fraise and Bradley 2009, **E**).
6 Assist the patient onto the edge of the bed/trolley, sitting in an upright position with their back exposed. Or, if the patient is unable to sit up, assist them to lie on their side with their back towards you.	To enable access to the nephrostomy site. **E**
Procedure	
7 Decontaminate hands using an alcohol-based handrub.	To minimize the risk of cross infection and contamination (NHS England and NHSI 2019, **C**).
8 Keeping the drain secure with one hand, carefully remove the existing drain fixation dressing and inspect the incision site. Check the suture remains intact (if present).	To assess skin for signs of infection, inflammation and overgranulation. The suture should remain intact to ensure the drain remains secure. **E**
9 Pour a small amount of adhesive remover onto a gauze square. Keeping the drain secure with one hand, use the adhesive remover to remove any dressing residue from the drain tubing (check the manufacturer's guidance to ensure the adhesive remover is safe for use on a drain).	Removing the sticky residue from the tubing minimizes the risk of infection. **E**
10 Clean hands with soap and water and/or an alcohol-based handrub.	Hands may have become contaminated by handling the outer packs and the old dressing (NHS England and NHSI 2019, **C**).
11 Put on non-sterile gloves.	To reduce the risk of cross-infection (NHS England and NHSI 2019, **C**).
12 Clean the drain site with 0.9% sodium chloride, working from the drain outwards. Gently remove any encrustation. Allow the site to dry.	This is performed at least weekly to reduce the number of micro-organisms present; to remove exudate, blood and wound debris from around the site and the device, which may be a medium for bacterial growth; and also to prevent overgranulation (NICE 2017, **C**).

(continued)

Procedure guideline 6.12 Nephrostomy tube: weekly dressing and bag change and sample collection *(continued)*

Action	Rationale
13 When the site is dry, apply a sterile drain fixation dressing according the manufacturer's guidelines (e.g. Drain-Fix or OPSITE Post-Op Visible drain dressing). 'Window frame' the edges of the dressing to prevent it rucking up by using surgical tape on each edge of the dressing.	To improve the security of the nephrostomy drain and enable patient mobility. **E**
14 Clean hands with soap and water and/or an alcohol-based handrub.	Hands may have become contaminated by handling the outer packs and the old dressing (NHS England and NHSI 2019, **C**).
15 Gently clamp the nephrostomy tube using blunt disposable clamps.	To prevent leakage of urine. **E**
16 Disconnect the drainage bag, and connector if attached, from the nephrostomy tube.	This is performed every 5–7 days or according to the manufacturer's guidelines. **E**
17 Clean the connector hub with alcohol-impregnated chlorhexidine wipe. *Note*: if a sample is required, it could be obtained at this point by unclamping the drainage tube and allowing drainage of the urine into a sample tube.	To minimize the risk of infection. **E**
18 Apply a new sterile drainage bag, and connector if required, to the nephrostomy tube, being careful not to touch the hubs and unclamp the drain. Urine should begin to flow.	To enable clean passage of urine and to minimize contamination from bacteria within the drainage bag. **E**
19 Secure the bag to the patient with a leg strap or waist strap according to patient preference. Be careful to ensure that the tube is not taut nor pulling at the exit site.	To enable independent mobility and maintain patient dignity. **E** To maintain tube security and to maintain dependent drainage. **E**
Post-procedure	
20 Dispose of waste in a clinical waste bag and seal the bag before moving the trolley.	To ensure correct and safe disposal of contaminated waste (DEFRA 2005, **C**).
21 Cover the patient and then draw back the curtains.	To maintain the patient's dignity (NMC 2018, **C**).
22 Record information in relevant documents; this should include: • date and time of procedure • procedure(s) performed • dressing and bag type used • condition of skin • any problems or concerns during the procedure • any swabs or samples taken during the procedure (e.g. exit site swab or urine sample) • any referrals made following the procedure • a review date for next dressing and/or bag change.	To provide a point of reference or comparison in the event of later queries (NMC 2018, **C**).
23 If the patient is being discharged home, refer them to the community nurse and provide clear guidelines for equipment provision and plan for review and/or change of nephrostomy.	To ensure continuity of care. **E**
24 If a sample was obtained, clearly label the specimen at the patient's bedside and place it with a request form.	To ensure correct patient's details are added to the form and the laboratory is aware of the sample type and what to test for. **E**

Problem-solving table 6.4 Prevention and resolution (Procedure guideline 6.12)

Problem	Cause	Prevention	Action
Wound site infection	Foreign body puncturing the skin	Maintain good exit site care. Change dressing and check site at least every 7 days. Ensure good hand hygiene.	Monitor patient for signs of infection, e.g. purulent discharge, exit site erythema, pain/itching, pyrexia. Send swab for MC&S (microscopy, culture and sensitivity) when indicated. Seek medical advice. Treat patient according to medical advice.
Nephrostomy tube falls out	Locking mechanism on drain has failed Retaining suture has become loose Drain fixation dressing has fallen off	Ensure that all the elements securing the nephrostomy are well situated. Check the locking mechanism on the drain is in the 'lock' or 'drain' position. Check the retaining suture is intact during weekly dressing changes. Be careful to correctly apply and secure the drain fixation dressing.	Seek urgent medical assistance. Nephrostomy tube will need to be replaced by a physician.

Problem	Cause	Prevention	Action
Nephrostomy tube stops draining	No urine output	Monitor urine output and vital signs.	Check the patient's vital signs and seek urgent medical assistance if the patient is unwell. Ensure there are no kinks in the tube that have occluded flow of urine and straighten tube. The tube may be blocked with debris, flush tube with 5 mL NaCl 0.9% using aseptic technique to unblock as per Procedure guideline 6.13: Nephrostomy tube: flushing technique.
	Blocked tube Kinked tube	Escalate concerns to the medical team. Carefully secure the drain and tubing to prevent kinking.	Ensure there are no kinks in the tube that have occluded the flow of urine and straighten the tube. The tube may be blocked with debris; flush the tube with 5 mL 0.9% sodium chloride using an aseptic technique to unblock as per Procedure guideline 6.13: Nephrostomy tube: flushing technique.

Procedure guideline 6.13 Nephrostomy tube: flushing technique

Essential equipment

- Personal protective equipment
- 0.9% sodium chloride
- 10 mL Luer-Lok or Luer tip syringe
- Sterile gloves
- Dressing pack with sterile sheet and gauze
- Blunt disposable clamps
- Alcohol (chlorhexidine) wipe
- Sterile nephrostomy drainage bag

Action	Rationale
Pre-procedure	
1 Introduce yourself to the patient, explain and discuss the procedure with them, and gain their consent to proceed.	To ensure that the patient feels at ease, understands the procedure and gives their valid consent (NMC 2018, **C**).
2 Screen the bed.	To ensure patient privacy. To allow dust and airborne organisms to settle before the field is exposed (Fraise and Bradley 2009, **E**).
3 Wash hands using soap and water and alcohol-based handrub, and apply personal protective equipment.	To reduce the risk of infection from micro-organisms on uniform/clothing (NHS England and NHSI 2019, **C**).
4 Prepare the trolley, placing all equipment required on the bottom shelf.	The top shelf acts as a clean working surface. **E**
5 Take the trolley to the patient's bedside, disturbing the screens as little as possible.	To minimize airborne contamination (Fraise and Bradley 2009, **E**).
6 Assist the patient onto the edge of the bed/trolley sitting in an upright position with their back exposed, or lying on their side with their back exposed.	To enable access to the nephrostomy site. **E**
Procedure	
7 Prepare the dressing pack on the top shelf of the trolley.	To ensure the sterile field is ready for the procedure. **E**
8 Clean hands with soap and water and an alcohol-based handrub.	Hands may have become contaminated by handling the outer packs (NHS England and NHSI 2019, **C**).
9 Clamp the nephrostomy tube.	To temporarily cease drainage. **E**
10 With a clean gloved hand, disconnect the drainage bag and discard.	To allow access to the nephrostomy tube. **E**
11 Put on non-sterile gloves.	To reduce the risk of cross-infection (NHS England and NHSI 2019, **C**).
12 Clean the connector hub with alcohol-impregnated chlorhexidine wipe.	To minimize the risk of infection (Loveday et al. 2014, **R**).
13 Attach a sterile syringe containing 5 mL 0.9% sodium chloride to the nephrostomy tube.	To prepare to flush. **E**

(continued)

Procedure guideline 6.13 Nephrostomy tube: flushing technique *(continued)*

Action	Rationale
14 Unclamp the nephrostomy tube. With gentle pressure, flush the 0.9% sodium chloride into the nephrostomy tube and gently aspirate. Clamp the nephrostomy tube.	To remove potential occlusions from the drainage channel (Radecka and Magnusson 2004, **E**). To temporarily cease drainage. **E**
15 Apply a new sterile drainage bag, and connector if required, to the nephrostomy tube, being careful not to touch the hubs. Unclamp the drain. Urine should begin to flow.	To enable clean passage of urine and to minimize contamination from bacteria within the drainage bag. **E**
16 Apply a leg strap or waist strap according to patient preference to secure the bag to the patient. Be careful to ensure that the tube is not taut nor pulling at the exit site.	To enable independent mobility and maintain patient dignity. To maintain tube security. To maintain dependent drainage. **E**
Post-procedure	
17 Dispose of waste in a clinical waste bag and seal the bag before moving the trolley.	To ensure correct and safe disposal of contaminated waste (DEFRA 2005, **C**).
18 Draw back the curtains once the patient has been covered.	To maintain the patient's dignity (NMC 2018, **C**).
19 Record information in relevant documents; this should include: • date and time of procedure • procedure(s) performed • dressing and bag type used • condition of skin • any problems or concerns during the procedure • any swabs or samples taken during the procedure (e.g. exit site swab or urine sample) • any referrals made following the procedure • a review date for next dressing and/or bag change.	To provide a point of reference or comparison in the event of later queries (NMC 2018, **C**).
20 If the patient is being discharged home, refer them to the community nurse and provide clear guidelines for equipment provision and plan for review and/or change of nephrostomy.	To ensure continuity of care. **E**

Procedure guideline 6.14 Nephrostomy tube: removal of locking pigtail drainage system

Essential equipment

- Personal protective equipment
- Sterile dressing pack containing gallipots or an indented plastic tray, low-linting swabs and/or medical foam, disposable forceps, gloves, sterile field and disposable bag
- Scissors or stitch cutter (refer to patient notes for directions if dressing is in place)
- Key or alternative device to unlock the pigtail drain
- Sterile absorbent dressing to place over drainage site
- 0.9% sodium chloride solution

Action	Rationale
Pre-procedure	
1 Introduce yourself to the patient, explain and discuss the procedure with them, and gain their consent to proceed. Another member of staff may be needed to reassure the patient during the procedure.	To ensure that the patient feels at ease, understands the procedure and gives their valid consent (NMC 2018, **C**).
2 Check the patient's medical notes to confirm which nephrostomy tube is to be removed. Once confirmed, establish the number and site(s) of sutures (both internal and external).	To ensure only documented drains are removed. To ensure all non-absorbable sutures are removed prior to attempting removal of the drain. **E**
3 Offer the patient analgesia as prescribed.	To promote the patient's comfort (NMC 2018, **C**).
4 If the patient has a ureteric stent *in situ*, removal of the nephrostomy should be done under X-ray or ultrasound guidance.	To ensure that the ureteric stent does not become misplaced during removal. **E**

Procedure	
5 Perform all steps of the procedure (below) using aseptic technique. Clean the drain site using 0.9% sodium chloride.	To reduce the risk of infection (Loveday et al. 2014, **R**).
6 If the drain is sutured in place, hold the knot of the suture with metal forceps and gently lift upwards.	To facilitate removal. **E** Plastic forceps tend to slip against nylon sutures. To allow space for the scissors or stitch cutter to be placed underneath. **E**
7 Cut the shortest end of the suture as close to the skin as possible and remove the suture.	To minimize cross-infection by allowing the suture to be liberated from the drain without drawing the exposed part through tissue (Pudner 2010, **E**).
8 Disconnect the drainage bag from the stopcock. Using the 'key' or alternative items that fit in the slot of the stopcock, rotate the stopcock counter-clockwise exactly 180° to the 'unlocked' position. *Note*: the retention stopcock is turned 180° to the locked position after insertion; this *must* be unlocked prior to removal; you must rotate the stopcock counter-clockwise 180° to unlock it	To unlock and release the pigtail. This straightens the tip of the nephrostomy tube, allowing for removal of the drain. Always follow the manufacturer's guidelines. **E**
9 Warn the patient of the pulling sensation they will experience and reassure them throughout.	To promote comfort and co-operation. Another member of staff may be needed to reassure the patient during the procedure. **E**
10 Loosening up of the drain should be done if possible, especially for a drain that has been in for some time. This can be done by gently rotating the drain to loosen it from the embedded tissue.	To minimize pain and reduce trauma. **E** Drains that have been left in for an extended period will sometimes be more difficult to remove due to tissue growing around the tubing (Walker 2007, **E**).
11 With one gloved hand, place a finger on each side of the drain exit site, exerting gentle pressure to stabilize the skin around the drain. Using the other gloved hand, take a firm grasp of the drain as close to the skin as possible and gently pull to start removing it. Steady, gentle traction should be used to remove the drain rather than sudden, jerky movements. If there is resistance, ensure that the other gloved hand is still exerting gentle pressure around the drain exit site.	Using a firm grasp for the shortest possible length of time minimizes patient discomfort. This is especially important for supple drains such as those made from silicone or rubber, which can stretch for some distance, then suddenly break free, causing undue pain to the patient (Walker 2007, **E**).
12 Once removed, the drain should be inspected to ensure that it is intact. The end of the drain should be clean cut and not jagged.	This clean appearance ensures that the whole drain has been removed. **E** If you have any doubt that the drain is intact, the surgeons should be contacted to inspect the drain before disposal. In rare cases an X-ray may be used to confirm complete removal (Cox and Friess 2017, **R**).
13 Cover the drain site with a sterile dressing and tape securely.	To prevent infection entering the drain site. **E**
14 If the site is inflamed or there is a request for the tip to be sent to microbiology, cut it off cleanly, using sterile scissors, and send it in a sterile pot. Also send a wound swab of the exit site.	To recognize and treat suspected infection (Fraise and Bradley 2009, **E**; Walker 2007, **E**).
Post-procedure	
15 Dispose of the used drainage system in a clinical waste bag.	To ensure correct and safe disposal of contaminated waste (DEFRA 2005, **C**).
16 Observe the drain site for signs of haematoma, urinoma or infection.	To identify any complications early. **E**
17 Record information in relevant documents; this should include: • date and time of procedure • procedure(s) performed • any problems or concerns during the procedure • any swabs or samples taken during the procedure (e.g. exit site swab or urine sample) • any referrals made following the procedure.	To provide a point of reference or comparison in the event of later queries (NMC 2018, **C**).

Procedure guideline 6.15 Flushing externalized ureteric stents

Essential equipment

- Personal protective equipment
- 0.9% sodium chloride
- 10 mL Luer-Lok or Luer tip syringe
- Sterile gloves
- Dressing pack with sterile sheet and gauze
- Blunt disposable needle or Bander stent adapter
- Alcohol (chlorhexidine) wipe
- Sterile nephrostomy drainage bag

Action	Rationale
Pre-procedure	
1 Introduce yourself to the patient, explain and discuss the procedure with them, and gain their consent to proceed.	To ensure that the patient feels at ease, understands the procedure and gives their valid consent (NMC 2018, **C**).
2 Screen the bed.	To ensure patient privacy (NMC 2018, **E**). To allow dust and airborne organisms to settle before the field is exposed (Fraise and Bradley 2009, **E**).
3 Wash hands using bactericidal soap and water and alcohol-based handrub, and apply personal protective equipment.	To reduce the risk of infection (NHS England and NHSI 2019, **C**).
4 Prepare the trolley, placing all equipment required on the bottom shelf.	The top shelf acts as a clean working surface. **E**
5 Take the trolley to the patient's bedside, disturbing the screens as little as possible.	To minimize airborne contamination (Fraise and Bradley 2009, **E**).
6 Assist the patient into the supine position and expose the ureteric stent.	To enable access to the externalized ureteric stent. **E**
Procedure	
7 Prepare the dressing pack on the top shelf of the trolley.	To ensure the sterile field is ready for the procedure. **E**
8 Clean hands with soap and water and/or an alcohol-based handrub.	Hands may have become contaminated by handling the outer packs (NHS England and NHSI 2019, **C**).
9 With a clean gloved hand, disconnect the drainage bag and discard.	To allow access to the stent. **E**
10 Put on non-sterile gloves.	To reduce the risk of cross-infection (NHS England and NHSI 2019, **C**).
11 Clean the stent and connect the Bander stent adaptor if not adapted or insert a blunt needle into the end of the stent.	To minimize the risk of infection (Loveday et al. 2014, **R**) and to enable instillation of the flush.
12 Attach a sterile syringe containing 5 mL 0.9% sodium chloride to the stent connector or blunt needle.	To prepare to flush. **E**
13 With gentle pressure, flush the liquid into the stent and gently aspirate.	To remove potential occlusions from the drainage channel (Radecka and Magnusson 2004, **R**).
14 Apply a new sterile drainage bag, and connector if required, to the stent, being careful not to touch the hubs. Urine should begin to flow.	To enable clean passage of urine and to minimize contamination from bacteria within the drainage bag. **E**
Post-procedure	
15 Dispose of waste in a clinical waste bag and seal the bag before moving the trolley.	To ensure correct and safe disposal of contaminated waste (DEFRA 2005, **C**).
16 Cover the patient and then draw back the curtains.	To maintain the patient's dignity (NMC 2018, **C**).
17 Record information in relevant documents; this should include: • date and time of procedure • procedure(s) performed • dressing and bag type used • condition of skin • any problems or concerns during the procedure • any swabs or samples taken during the procedure (e.g. exit site swab or urine sample) • any referrals made following the procedure • a review date for next dressing and/or bag change.	To provide a point of reference or comparison in the event of later queries (NMC 2018 **C**).
18 If the patient is being discharged home, refer them to the community nurse and provide clear guidelines for equipment provision and plan for review and/or change of nephrostomy.	To ensure continuity of care. **E**

Procedure guideline 6.16 Removal of externalized ureteric stents

Essential equipment

- Personal protective equipment
- Sterile dressing pack containing gallipots or an indented plastic tray, low-linting swabs and/or medical foam, disposable forceps, gloves, a sterile field and a disposable bag
- Scissors or stitch cutter
- 0.9% sodium chloride solution
- Replacement stoma bag (if ileal conduit)

Action	Rationale
Pre-procedure	
1 Check with surgical team whether prophylactic antibiotics are required prior to removal.	To prevent infection secondary to a colonized stent (Abbott et al. 2016, **E**).
2 Introduce yourself to the patient, explain and discuss the procedure with them, and gain their consent to proceed. Another member of staff may be needed to reassure the patient during the procedure.	To ensure that the patient feels at ease, understands the procedure and gives their valid consent (NMC 2018, **C**; Walker 2007, **C**).
3 Check the patient's medical notes to confirm which ureteric stent is to be removed. Once confirmed, establish the number and site(s) of sutures (both internal and external).	To ensure only documented stents are removed. To ensure all non-absorbable sutures are removed prior to attempting removal of the stent. **E**
4 Offer the patient analgesia as per chart.	To promote comfort (NMC 2018, **C**).
5 Empty the ileal conduit bag and remove. Or empty drainage bags.	To prepare for stent removal. **E**
Procedure	
6 Perform all steps of the procedure (below) using aseptic technique. Clean the site using 0.9% sodium chloride.	To reduce the risk of infection (Fraise and Bradley 2009, **E**).
7 If the stent is sutured in place, hold the knot of the suture with metal forceps and gently lift upwards.	To facilitate removal. **E** Plastic forceps tend to slip against nylon sutures. To allow space for the scissors or stitch cutter to be placed underneath. **E**
8 Cut the shortest end of the suture as close to the skin as possible and remove the suture.	To minimize cross-infection by allowing the suture to be liberated from the drain without drawing the exposed part through tissue (Pudner 2010, **E**).
9 Warn the patient of the pulling sensation they will experience and reassure them throughout.	To promote patient comfort and co-operation (Walker 2007, **E**). Another member of staff may be needed to reassure the patient during the procedure.
10 Loosening up of the stent should be done if possible, especially for a stent that has been in for some time. This can be done by gently rotating the drain to loosen it from the embedded tissue.	To minimize pain and reduce trauma. **E** Drains that have been left in for an extended period will sometimes be more difficult to remove due to tissue growing around the tubing (Walker 2007, **E**).
11 With one gloved hand, place a finger on each side of the stent exit site, exerting gentle pressure to stabilize the skin around the stent. Using the other hand, take a firm grasp of the stent as close to the skin as possible and gently pull downwards to start removing it. Steady, gentle traction should be used to remove the stent rather than sudden, jerky movements. If there is resistance, ensure that the other gloved hand is still exerting gentle pressure around the exit site.	Using a firm grasp for the shortest possible length of time minimizes patient discomfort (Walker 2007, **E**). The stent should be removed easily; if there is resistance then discontinue the procedure and contact the surgical team. **E**
12 Once removed, the stent should be inspected to ensure that it is intact. The end of the stent should be clean cut and not jagged.	This clean appearance ensures that the whole stent has been removed. **E** If you have any doubt that the stent is intact, the surgeons should be contacted to inspect the stent before disposal.
13 If there is a request for the tip to be sent to microbiology, cut it off cleanly, using sterile scissors, and send it in a sterile pot. Also send a wound swab of the exit site.	To recognize and treat suspected infection (Fraise and Bradley 2009, **E**; Walker 2007, **E**).
Post-procedure	
14 Dispose of the used drainage system in a clinical waste bag.	To ensure correct and safe disposal of contaminated waste. **E**
15 Replace the patient's stoma bag if an ileal conduit (refer to stoma care section later in this chapter).	To ensure the stoma is covered and to avoid urine leakage. **E**
16 Record information in relevant documents; this should include: • date and time of procedure • procedure(s) performed • any problems or concerns during the procedure • any swabs or samples taken during the procedure (e.g. exit site swab or urine sample) • any referrals made following the procedure.	To provide a point of reference or comparison in the event of later queries (NMC 2018, **C**).

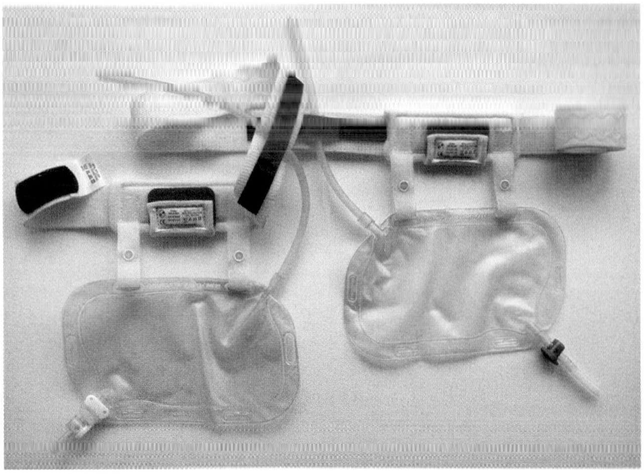

Figure 6.17 Body-worn nephrostomy drainage bag and belt system. *Source*: Reproduced with permission of ManFred Sauer.

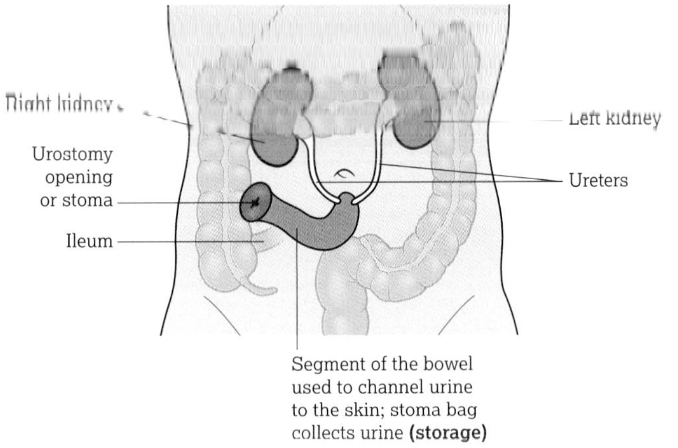

Figure 6.18 Ileal conduit.

Surgical urinary diversions

Definition

A urinary diversion is a surgically created system for removing urine from the body when either the bladder or the urethra is non-existent or no longer viable.

Evidence-based approaches

Rationale

Muscle-invasive bladder cancer is the most common condition for which urinary diversions are performed in adults. Other conditions that may lead to urinary diversion include:

- pelvic cancers, for example gynaecological cancers or sarcoma
- congenital abnormalities, for example bladder extrophy
- neuropathic bladder, a condition where the nerve impulses do not reach the bladder as a result of an underlying disease or injury, for example myelomeningocele
- trauma
- irreparable fistula
- interstitial cystitis
- radiation fibrosis
- intractable incontinence (Geng et al. 2009).

There are two main types: incontinent and continent diversions. Incontinent diversions take the form of an ileal conduit or urostomy, where the urine is stored in a body-worn pouch. Continent urinary diversions differ in that a system is created to collect and store urine, known as a neobladder, before it is removed from the body. Examples of continent urinary diversions include continent cutaneous, orthotopic neobladder and rectal diversion (such as Mainz II) (Geng et al. 2010, Spencer et al. 2018).

The main aim in the selection of a urinary diversion is to provide patients with a diversion that gives the lowest potential for complications and the best quality of life and, for those patients with cancer, the best cancer control (Lee et al. 2014, Spencer et al. 2018).

Indications

A urinary diversion is formed to:

- eliminate urine from the body if the lower urinary tract is defective or absent (as in cystectomy)
- preserve the upper urinary tract
- avoid metabolic disturbance
- store the urine either internally or externally until convenient to empty.

Continent diversions:

- store an adequate volume of urine at low pressure
- offer patients a choice of urinary diversion
- improve or maintain the individual's body image and their psychological and social wellbeing by removing the necessity of wearing external devices, for example a urostomy pouch or incontinence pads (Geng et al. 2010).

Incontinent diversions

An ileal conduit is the most common form of urostomy; the colon (colonic conduit) may also be used. The word 'urostomy' comes from the Greek *uros*, meaning urine, and *stoma*, meaning mouth or opening (Nazarko 2008).

A section of bowel is isolated, along with its mesentery vessels, and the remaining ends of the bowel are anastomosed to restore continuity. The isolated section is mobilized, the proximal end is closed and the ureters, once resected from the bladder, are implanted at this end. The distal end is brought out onto the surface of the abdominal wall and everted to form a spout (Figure 6.18). Urine from a urostomy will contain mucus from the bowel used in its construction (Geng et al. 2009).

A cutaneous ureterostomy is another form of incontinent diversion where the ureters are brought out onto the abdominal wall together (one stoma) or separately (two stomas). This may be a permanent or temporary procedure, and it may be used for patients with poor renal function and when less extensive abdominal surgery is indicated. Stomas formed in this way are often small and flush to the abdomen. They are prone to stenosis and it is often difficult to maintain a leak-proof appliance, and they often require permanent stent placement to maintain patency (Rodriguez et al. 2011).

Continent diversions

All continent diversions consist of three components:

- A reservoir to store urine, which may be the bladder itself, an augmented bladder or one made completely of de-tublarized ileum or colon.
- A continence mechanism to retain urine in the reservoir, which may be an existing valve or sphincter, such as the ileocaecal valve, urethral sphincter or anal sphincter. A valve may also be constructed using the same tissue used to construct the reservoir, such as a flutter valve created by the intussusception of a segment of bowel or a flap valve created by tunnelling a narrow tube between muscle and mucosal layers of the reservoir (Geng et al. 2010).
- A channel or tunnel to let the urine out, which may be formed by using other tube- or tunnel-like structures such as the appendix, ureter, urethra or fallopian tube. Alternatively, a segment of ileum or colon can be used (Geng et al. 2010).

Table 6.4 Long- and short-term risk factors of urinary diversion

	Ileal conduit	Continent cutaneous	Rectal bladder	Orthotopic bladder
Failure to catheterize		✓		
Recurrent infection		✓	✓	✓
Hyperchloraemia		✓	✓	✓
Stones		✓	✓	✓
Pouch rupture		✓	✓	✓
Incontinence			✓	✓
Inability to empty pouch				✓
Anastomotic stricture				✓
Urine malodour			✓	
Risk of colorectal neoplasm			✓	

There are three main types of continent diversion: continent cutaneous diversion, rectal bladder and orthotopic neobladder. There are many considerations long and short term that should be factored into decision making (see Table 6.4).

Continent cutaneous diversion

There are a number of different types of continent cutaneous diversion; they differ in construction, using different structures to form the reservoir and the tunnel, and different techniques to create the continence mechanism. The outcomes for patients and the nursing care involved are essentially similar in most cases. The most commonly performed procedure of this type is arguably the Mitrofanoff procedure, which uses the appendix to form the conduit from skin to pouch (Figure 6.19a).

In this type of diversion, urine drains into the urinary reservoir (which is constructed from bowel or bladder) through the ureters. One end of the tissue used to construct the channel is buried in a submuscular tunnel in the neobladder, forming an obstructing flap valve. The other end is brought to the surface of the abdominal wall to form a continent stoma. As the bladder fills with urine, more pressure is put on the valve, causing it to become even more obstructed. A catheter is passed into the stoma along the channel, through the valve and into the bladder when the patient wants to empty their bladder (Geng et al. 2010). Patients can self-catheterize into the continent urinary stoma every 4–6 hours to empty the urine reservoir (Figure 6.19b; see also Procedure guideline 6.17: Continent urinary diversion stoma: self-catheterization).

Rectal bladder

As with continent cutaneous diversions, there are a number of different surgical techniques that can be used to create a continent rectal bladder; the most commonly used is the sigma rectum pouch known as the Mainz II (Figure 6.20). There are good reported outcomes for continence rates with this technique (Afak et al. 2009). The technique uses a section of de-tubularized sigmoid to create a pouch that empties rectally, creating a mix of urine and faeces. Continence is tested pre-operatively using the 'porridge test', in which up to 500 mL of loose-consistency porridge is instilled into the rectum and retention is measured in time (Woodhouse 2015). Patients who fail this test are considered unable to hold sufficiently for this type of urinary diversion.

Patients must be counselled about the ongoing risk of hyperchloraemia due to reabsorption of urine from the pouch and also the long-term risk of neoplasm. There is also the risk of

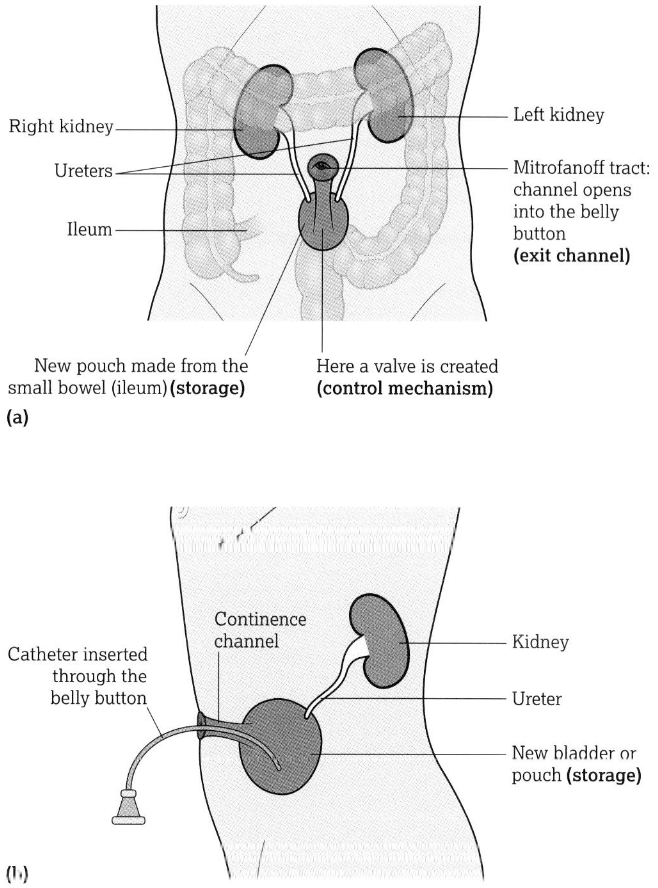

Figure 6.19 A Mitrofanoff urinary diversion. (a) Front view. (b) Side view with a catheter *in situ*.

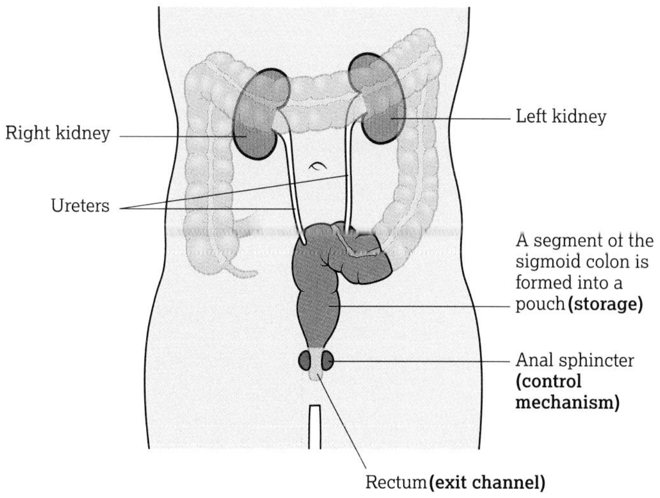

Figure 6.20 A Mainz II urinary diversion.

incontinence, which may occur immediately or over time. Those with this type of diversion require lifelong careful monitoring.

Orthotopic neobladder

This type of diversion is suitable only for those who have disease suitable for the retention of their native urethra and a functional sphincter. A neobladder is created using a section of de-tubularized sigmoid and attached to the patient's native urethra (Figure 6.21). The patient will then void per urethra. As the neobladder does not

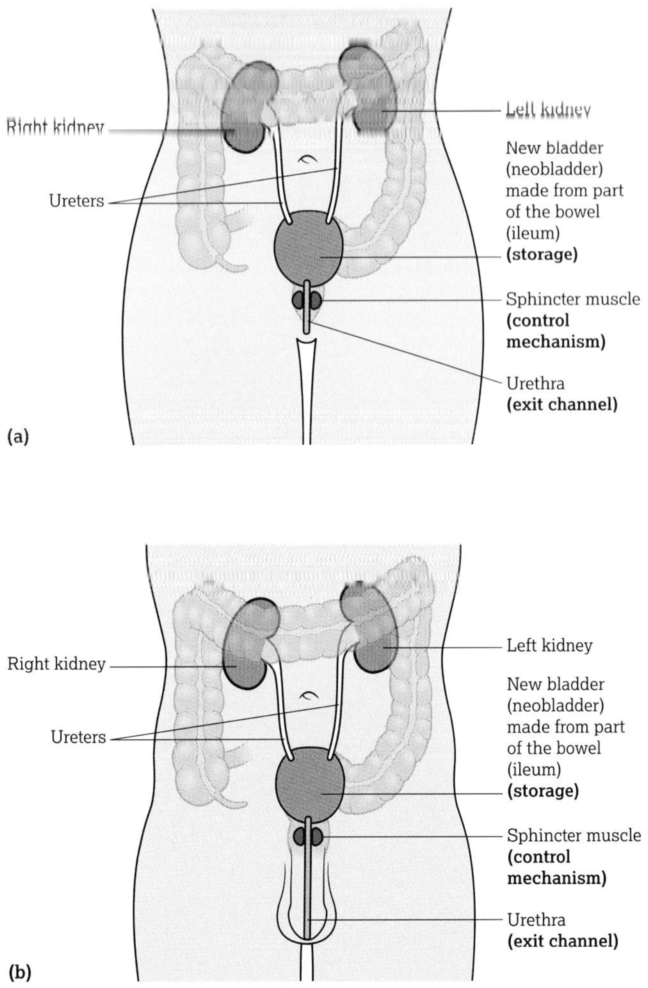

Figure 6.21 (a) Female orthotopic neobladder. (b) Male orthotopic neobladder.

[illegible] bladder, the patient is required to perform a Valsalva manoeuvre (which involves forcing expiration against a closed airway by closing the mouth and pinching the nose while trying to forcefully expire) to generate pressure to void and/or perform intermittent self-catheterization (see Procedure guideline 6.17: Continent urinary diversion stoma: self-catheterization).

Principles of care

Patient-reported outcomes relating to physical functioning and quality of life are often higher in patients with continent diversions (Philip et al. 2009, Singh et al. 2013). However, the decision making around urinary diversions (particularly for the continent types of diversion) needs to be carried out carefully based on many patient and disease factors (Spencer et al. 2018). Patients' general levels of health, their co-morbidities, and their renal and hepatic function are all taken into consideration when deciding on the type of urinary diversion. Intestinal disease (such as inflammatory bowel disease or diverticulitis), stress incontinence, bladder cancer involving the bladder neck or prostatic urethra, concurrent prostate cancer and previous pelvic radiotherapy are contraindications for continent diversion (Hautmann et al. 2006, Kwan et al. 2010).

Patients undergoing continent diversions must be motivated towards self-care, and those needing to self-catheterize must be dextrous enough to manipulate Nelaton or intermittent catheters (Geng et al. 2010). Good anal sphincter control is essential for those undergoing a rectal bladder; this is tested pre-operatively using a 'porridge test' (Woodhouse 2015).

Encouraging patients' independence in living with a urinary diversion is a key aim of care. Practical help, advice and support are employed in encouraging patients to continue with all necessary activities of daily living.

It is important to note that surgery for all urinary diversions, and particularly those involving cystectomy, will have an impact on the patient's sexual function. Frequently, sexual function and libido are affected in males and females. The nurse should take time to counsel the patient and their partner on this outcome of surgery. See also the section 'Sex and the ostomate' below.

Procedure guideline 6.17 Continent urinary diversion stoma: self-catheterization

Essential equipment

- Personal protective equipment
- Catheter for catheterization, with the size depending upon the size of the stoma (usually 14 ch)
- Tissues
- Clean jug or bowl
- Gauze

Action	Rationale
Pre-procedure	
1 Introduce yourself to the patient, explain and discuss the procedure with them, and gain their consent to proceed.	To ensure that the patient feels at ease, understands the procedure and gives their valid consent (NMC 2018, **C**).
2 Collect all equipment necessary for the procedure.	To ensure all the equipment required is easily available. **E**
3 Take the equipment to the toilet, a bathroom or a screened bed area. Ensure there is a good light and a full-length mirror.	To ensure the patient's privacy. To ensure the patient can see the stoma clearly. **E**
4 The equipment should be arranged on a clean surface and within easy reach. The nurse remains in the room with the patient.	To reduce the risk of contamination by surface bacteria. So that the equipment is easily available. **E**
5 The patient needs to remove any inhibiting clothing.	To ensure the patient can examine the stoma. **E**
6 The patient should wash their hands with soap and water and dry them.	To ensure the hands are clean (NHS England and NHSI 2019, **C**).

Procedure	
7 The patient should look at the stoma, if necessary with the aid of a mirror.	To look for mucus and swelling around the stoma (Leaver 2016, **E**).
8 The patient should wipe away any mucus with a tissue soaked in warm water and gently pat dry.	To ensure the opening of the stoma is clear and mucus does not block the catheter during insertion into the stoma. **E**
9 A lubricated catheter should be used; there are many types available. Selection should be based on patient choice or specialist advice.	To allow the catheter to enter the urinary reservoir without causing internal trauma. **E**
10 The patient should ensure the drainage end of the catheter is in a receiver, such as a jug, bowl or toilet.	To ensure the urine goes into the receiver and not onto the patient. **E**
11 The patient can either use a mirror to guide the tube into the opening of the stoma or feel the opening with two fingers slightly apart with the stoma between.	To act as a guide to pass the catheter into the continent urinary stoma. **E**
12 The patient should insert the catheter gently into the stoma, following the pathway inside (usually towards the middle of the abdomen) until urine starts to flow, then insert the tube a further 4–6 cm to reduce the risk of contamination.	The direction of insertion and the diameter of the catheter inserted will depend on the type, size and shape of the continent urinary stoma. **E** To negotiate the continence device. **E**
13 When all the urine has stopped flowing, the patient should advance the catheter to ensure the bladder is completely empty. If urine starts flowing again, they should wait until it stops before removing the catheter any further.	To ensure complete emptying of the urinary reservoir. Moving the tube may dislodge any debris or mucus blocking the tube and allow the urine to flow (Leaver 2016, **E**).
14 The patient should remove the tube, cover the end of the catheter with a finger just before it is removed from the tunnel, and then hold the catheter over the receptacle before removing the finger.	To trap urine in the catheter and stop it leaking onto the patient (Leaver 2016, **E**). To allow complete drainage of the tube. **E**
Post-procedure	
15 The patient should dispose of the catheter in a clinical waste bag.	To ensure correct and safe disposal of contaminated waste (DEFRA 2005, **C**).
16 If required (usually not), the patient should cover the stoma with a non-adherent dressing and secure with skin-protective tape.	To prevent mucus staining the patient's clothing. **E**
17 The patient should wash their hands with soap and water, and then dry them.	To remove any urine on the hands. **E**
18 The patient can then dress, collect the equipment and dispose of any soiled dressings.	To prevent cross-infection (Fraise and Bradley 2009, **E**).

Altered faecal elimination

This section focuses on altered faecal elimination, including diarrhoea and constipation, and considers a range of pharmacological and non-pharmacological strategies that can be used to manage these conditions.

Diarrhoea

Definition

The term 'diarrhoea' originates from the Greek for 'to flow through' (Bell 2004) and can be characterized according to its onset and duration (acute or chronic) or by type (e.g. secretory, osmotic or malabsorptive). Diarrhoea can also be defined in terms of stool frequency, consistency, volume or weight (Metcalf 2007). The World Health Organization defines diarrhoea as the passage of three or more loose stools per day, or more frequently than is normal for the individual (WHO 2018).

Related theory

Diarrhoea is a serious global public health problem, in particularly in low- and middle-income countries due to poor sanitation. There are almost 1.7 billion cases of diarrhoeal disease each year, with approximately 600,000 children each year dying as a result (WHO 2018). The disease pathogens are most commonly transmitted via the faecal–oral route (Ejemot-Nwadiaro et al. 2015). Diarrhoea should be classified according to time (acute or chronic) and the characteristics of the stools (see the Bristol Stool Chart in Figure 6.3) (Baldi et al. 2009).

Acute diarrhoea

Acute diarrhoea is very common, is usually self-limiting, generally lasts less than 2 weeks and often requires no investigation or treatment (Carlson et al. 2016). Causes of acute diarrhoea include:

- dietary indiscretion (eating too much fruit, or alcohol misuse)
- allergy to food constituents
- infective:
  - travel associated
  - viral
  - bacterial (usually associated with food)
  - antibiotic related.

One of the most common causes of acute diarrhoea in the adult population worldwide is viral gastroenteritis resulting from norovirus. Its low infectious dose, its resistance to extreme temperatures and to many household cleaning products, and its viral shedding (before and after symptoms are apparent) have resulted in this virus being prolific during the colder months and becoming widely known as the winter vomiting bug (Krenzer 2012).

Chronic diarrhoea

Chronic diarrhoea generally lasts longer than 3–4 weeks and may have more complex origins. Chronic causes can be divided as follows (Arasaradnam et al. 2018):

- *colonic*: colonic neoplasia, ulcerative colitis and Crohn's disease, microscopic colitis
- *small bowel*: small bowel bacterial overgrowth, coeliac disease, Crohn's disease, Whipple's disease, bile acid malabsorption, disaccharidase deficiency, mesenteric ischaemia, radiation enteritis, lymphoma, giardiasis
- *pancreatic*: chronic pancreatitis, pancreatic carcinoma, pancreatic insufficiency, cystic fibrosis
- *endocrine*: hyperthyroidism, diabetes, hypoparathyroidism, Addison's disease, hormone-secreting tumours
- *other causes*: laxative misuse, drugs, alcohol, autonomic neuropathy, small bowel resection or intestinal fistulas, radiation enteritis.

Pre-procedural considerations

Assessment

The cause of diarrhoea needs to be identified before effective treatment can be instigated. This may include clinical investigations such as stool cultures for bacterial, fungal and viral pathogens or a more formal medical evaluation of the gastrointestinal tract (Bossi et al. 2018).

Ongoing nursing assessment is essential to ensure individualized management and care. Nurses need to be aware of contributing factors and be sensitive to patients' beliefs and values in order to provide holistic care. A comprehensive assessment is therefore essential and should include the all the aspects outlined in Box 6.2.

All episodes of acute diarrhoea must be considered potentially infectious until proven otherwise. The immediate management should comply with local infection control guidelines on precautions and decontamination (RCN 2013); these will often include wearing gloves, aprons and gowns; disposing of all excreta immediately; and, ideally, nursing the patient in a side room with access to their own toilet. Advice should always be sought from the infection control team. At this stage, nursing care should also include educating patients about careful hand washing.

Diarrhoea can have profound physiological and psychosocial consequences for a patient. Severe or extended episodes of diarrhoea may result in dehydration, electrolyte imbalance and malnutrition. Patients not only have to cope with increased frequency of bowel movement but also may have abdominal pain, cramping, proctitis, and anal or perianal skin breakdown. Food aversions may develop or patients may stop eating altogether as they anticipate subsequent diarrhoea following intake. Consequently, this may lead to weight loss and malnutrition. Fatigue, sleep disturbances, and feelings of isolation and depression are all common consequences for those experiencing diarrhoea. The impact of severe diarrhoea should not be underestimated; it is highly debilitating and may cause patients on long-term therapy to be non-compliant (Bossi et al. 2018).

Once the cause of diarrhoea has been established, management should be focused on resolving the cause and providing physical and psychological support for the patient. Most cases of chronic diarrhoea will resolve once the underlying condition is treated, for example drug therapy for Crohn's disease or dietary management for coeliac disease. Episodes of acute diarrhoea, usually caused by bacteria or viruses, generally resolve spontaneously and rarely require professional input (Caramia et al. 2015).

Pharmacological support

The treatment for diarrhoea depends on the cause.

Antimotility drugs

Antimotility drugs such as loperamide or codeine phosphate may be useful in some cases, for example in blind loop syndrome and radiation enteritis. These drugs reduce gastrointestinal motility in order to relieve the symptoms of abdominal cramps and reduce the frequency of diarrhoea (Kaufman 2015). It is important to rule out any infective agent as the cause of diarrhoea before using any of these drugs, as the drugs may make the situation worse by slowing the clearance of the infective agent.

Antibiotics

Empirical antibiotic treatment can eradicate the normal bowel flora, which can increase the risk of potentially fatal infections and multidrug resistance organisms (Caramia et al. 2015). Therefore, treatment with antibiotics is recommended only in patients who are very symptomatic and show signs of systemic involvement. When dealing with antibiotic-associated diarrhoea, most patients will notice a cessation of their symptoms with discontinuation of the antibiotic therapy. If diarrhoea persists, it is important to

Box 6.2 Assessment of a patient experiencing diarrhoea

Assessment should cover:

- History of onset, frequency and duration of diarrhoea: patient's perception of diarrhoea is often related to stool consistency (Arasaradnam et al. 2018).
- Consistency, colour and form of stool, including the presence of blood, fat and mucus. Stools can be graded using a scale such as the Bristol Stool Chart (see Figure 6.3), where diarrhoea would be classified as above type 5 (Arasaradnam et al. 2018).
- Associated symptoms: pain, nausea, vomiting, fatigue, weight loss or fever.
- Physical examination: check for gaping anus, rectal prolapse and prolapsed haemorrhoids (Nazarko 2007).
- Recent lifestyle changes, emotional disturbances or travel abroad.
- Fluid intake and dietary history, including any cause-and-effect relationships between food consumption and bowel action.
- Regular medication, including antibiotics, laxatives, oral hypoglycaemics, appetite suppressants, antidepressants, statins, digoxin or chemotherapy (Nazarko 2007).
- Effectiveness of antidiarrhoeal medication (dose and frequency).
- Significant past medical history: bowel resection, pancreatitis or pelvic radiotherapy.
- Hydration status: evaluation of mucous membranes and skin turgor.
- Perianal or peristomal skin integrity: enzymes present in faecal fluid can cause rapid breakdown of the skin (Beeckman et al. 2015).
- Stool cultures for bacterial, fungal and viral pathogens: to check for infective diarrhoea (Kelly et al. 2018). Treatment may not be commenced until results are available except if the patient has been infected by *Clostridioides difficile* in the past.
- Blood tests: full blood count, urea and electrolytes, liver function tests, vitamin B_{12}, folate, calcium, ferritin, erythrocyte sedimentation rate (ESR) and C-reactive protein.
- Patient's preferences and own coping strategies including non-pharmacological interventions and their effectiveness (Arasaradnam et al. 2018).

exclude pseudomembranous colitis by performing a sigmoidoscopy and sending a stool for cytotoxin analysis.

Over recent years there has been increasing evidence supporting the use of probiotics in cases of diarrhoea associated with antibiotics (Agamennone et al. 2018). Researchers believe that probiotics restore the microbial balance in the intestinal tract previously destroyed by the inciting antibiotics (Agamennone et al. 2018). There are a variety of probiotic products available and their effectiveness appears to be related to the strain of bacteria causing the diarrhoea (Łukasik and Szajewska 2018).

Fluid replacement

The prevention and/or correction of dehydration is the first step in managing an episode of diarrhoea. Adults normally require 1.5–2 L of fluid in 24 hours. A patient who has diarrhoea will require an additional 200 mL for each loose stool. Dehydration can be corrected by using intravenous fluids and electrolytes or by using oral rehydration solutions. The extent of dehydration dictates whether a patient can be managed at home or will need to be admitted to hospital. Nursing care should also include monitoring signs or symptoms of electrolyte imbalance, such as muscle weakness and cramps, hypokalaemia, tachycardia and hypernatraemia (NICE 2018).

Non-pharmacological support

Maintaining dignity

Preserving the patient's privacy and dignity is essential during episodes of diarrhoea. The nurse has an important role in minimizing the patient's distress by adjusting language and using terms that are appropriate to the individual to reduce embarrassment and by listening to the patient's preferences for care (Ostaszkiewicz et al. 2018). Additionally, the use of deodorizers and air fresheners to remove the smell caused by offensive diarrhoea contributes to the person's dignity.

Skin care

It is important that the patient has easy access to clean toilet and washing facilities and that requests for assistance are answered promptly. Skin care is also essential to prevent bacteria present in faecal matter from destroying the skin's cellular defences and causing skin damage. This is particularly important with diarrhoea since it has high levels of faecal enzymes, which come into contact with the perianal skin (Gray et al. 2012). The anal area should be gently cleaned with warm water immediately after every episode of diarrhoea. Frequent washing of the skin can alter the pH and remove protective oils from the skin. Products aimed at maintaining healthy perianal skin should be used to protect patients with diarrhoea (RCN 2013). Soap should be avoided, unless it is an emollient, to avoid excessive drying of the skin. Gentle patting of the skin is preferred for drying to avoid friction damage. The use of incontinence pads should be carefully considered in a person with severe episodes of diarrhoea. This particular material does not absorb fluid stools, protect the skin from damage or contain smells.

Diet

A diet rich in fibre can cause diarrhoea. In such cases, individuals should be advised to reduce their intake of foods including cereals, fruit and vegetables and space them out over the day (RCN 2013). Chilli and other spices can irritate the bowel and should be avoided. Sorbitol (artificial sweetener), beer, stout and high doses of vitamins and minerals should also be avoided.

Faecal incontinence

Definition

Faecal incontinence is a clinical symptom usually associated with diarrhoea. As mentioned above, diarrhoea is defined as the passage of three or more loose or liquid stools per day (or more frequent passage than is normal for the individual) (Barrie 2018).

Box 6.3 Faecal incontinence: high-risk groups

- Frail older people
- People with loose stools or diarrhoea from any cause
- Women following childbirth (especially following third- or fourth-degree obstetric injury)
- People with neurological or spinal disease or injury (e.g. spina bifida, stroke, multiple sclerosis, spinal cord injury)
- People with severe cognitive impairment
- People with urinary incontinence
- People with pelvic organ prolapse and/or rectal prolapse
- People who have had colonic resection or anal surgery
- People who have undergone pelvic radiotherapy
- People with perianal soreness, itching or pain
- People with learning disabilities

Source: NICE (2007). Reproduced with permission of NICE.

Related theory

Faecal incontinence is a sign or a symptom, not a diagnosis. Therefore, it is important to diagnose the cause or causes for each individual. For many people, faecal incontinence is the result of a complex interplay of contributing factors, many of which can co-exist (NICE 2007). Healthcare professionals must be mindful that faecal incontinence is a socially stigmatizing condition and therefore professionals must sensitively enquire about symptoms in patients reporting (or who are reported to have) faecal incontinence, particularly within high risk groups (Box 6.3).

Factors that cause or contribute to the development of faecal incontinence are (Hayden and Weiss 2011):

- obstetric trauma
- anal surgery or pelvic radiation
- neurological diseases
- congenital conditions
- accidental or iatrogenic trauma
- colorectal disease
- diarrhoea, laxative abuse or faecal impaction.

Healthcare professionals should explain to patients that a combination of initial management interventions is likely to be needed. These will be based on the patient assessment and should consider the patient's personal preferences. This will form the basis of the patient's care plan. Initial management strategies may include a medication review; stool sampling and infection treatment; assessment of diet, bowel habit and toilet access; and discussions that focus on skin care advice, continence products, and the offer of emotional and psychological support. Specialist management may be required for those patients who still experience faecal incontinence after initial management options have been exhausted (NICE 2007).

Faecal collection devices (Figure 6.22) consist of a tube that is inserted into the rectum and held *in situ* by a water-filled balloon (similar to that of the Foley catheter). Fluid stools then drain into a drainage bag. It is imperative that such devices are fitted by appropriately trained, competent healthcare professionals and that both local policies and the manufacturer's instructions are followed to ensure this equipment is used in an appropriate and safe manner (Ritzema 2017) (see Procedure guideline 6.18: Insertion of a faecal management system). When used correctly, they can be very beneficial.

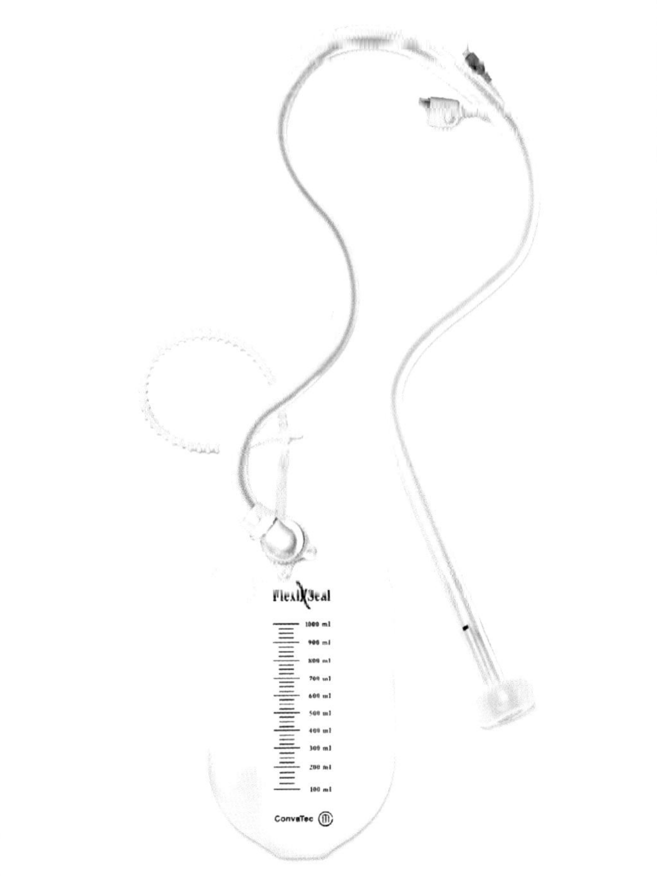

Figure 6.22 Flexi-Seal Faecal Management System. *Source*: Reproduced with permission of ConvaTec Ltd.

Rationale

Indications

Faecal management systems are indicated for patients who are passing liquid or semi liquid stools, usually in association with one or more of the following criteria:

- patient unable to mobilize to toilet or commode (i.e. bed-bound)
- patient has surgical considerations (i.e. to protect surgical sites or skin grafts)
- patient has skin excoriation associated with or exacerbated by faecal incontinence, or is at risk of developing this (Kowal-Vern et al. 2009)
- patient would benefit from help to reduce the spread of infectious diarrhoea by diverting it away from the patient's skin and keeping it contained in the closed system (Kowal-Vern et al. 2009).

Contraindications

Contraindications to the use of faecal management systems include the following:

- solid or formed stool
- suspected or confirmed rectal mucosa impairment
- recent large bowel surgery
- rectal surgery within the past year
- sensitivity or allergy to any of the materials used in the device
- rectal or anal injury
- bowel obstruction
- faecal impaction
- anal tumour
- severe haemorrhoids
- spinal cord injury
- antithrombotic treatment
- thrombocytopenia (ConvaTec 2012).

Procedure guideline 6.18 Insertion of a faecal management system

Essential equipment

- Personal protective equipment
- Faecal management device kit
- Sterile water or saline
- Lubricant

Action	Rationale
Pre-procedure	
1 Introduce yourself to the patient, explain and discuss the procedure with them, and gain their consent to proceed.	To ensure that the patient feels at ease, understands the procedure and gives their valid consent (NMC 2018, **C**).
2 Position the patient lying on their left side (if the patient is unable to tolerate this, position the patient so that access to the rectum is possible). Maintain privacy and dignity throughout.	This position offers the easiest access to the rectum. **E**
3 Undertake a digital examination.	To evaluate suitability for the insertion of the device (ConvaTec 2012, **C**). The rectum should be empty.
4 Remove any residual air from the balloon by attaching the syringe to the inflation port and withdrawing the plunger.	To ensure the balloon is fully deflated prior to insertion. **E**
5 Fill the empty syringe with sterile water or saline. Do not overfill. Follow the manufacturer's guidelines.	To prepare to fill the balloon. **E**
Procedure	
6 Unfold the length of the flexiseal tubing (catheter) and lay it flat on the bed, extending the collection bag towards the foot of the bed.	This is the correct positioning of the tubing and bag to optimize drainage. **E**

7 Insert a lubricated gloved index finger into the retention balloon cuff finger pocket and coat the balloon end of the catheter with lubricant.	To minimize patient discomfort and aid insertion (ConvaTec 2012, **C**).
8 Gently insert the balloon through the anal sphincter until it is well beyond the external orifice and well inside the rectal vault.	This is the correct position for the device (ConvaTec 2012, **C**).
9 Inflate the balloon to the correct volume according to the manufacturer's instructions. Never inflate the balloon with more water than instructed.	Inflating the balloon too much may cause damage to the integrity of the device or damage to the surrounding tissues (ConvaTec 2012, **C**).
10 Remove the syringe from the inflation port and gently pull back on the catheter.	To check the catheter is securely positioned within the rectum. **E**
11 Take note of the position indicator line relative to the patient's anus.	Observing changes in the location of the indicator line can determine movement of the retention balloon in the patient's rectum. This may indicate the need for the balloon or the device to be repositioned (ConvaTec 2012, **C**).
12 Position the length of the catheter along the patient's leg. Make sure to avoid pressure, kinks and obstructions.	To optimize drainage. **E**
13 Hang the collection bag by the strap on the bedside, positioning the bag at a lower level than the patient.	To ensure unobstructed flow. **E**
Post-procedure	
14 Observe the device for obstruction from kinks, solid faecal particles or external pressure. Repeat regularly according to local policy.	To ensure appropriate use of the device and unobstructed flow. **E**
15 Observe the anus for signs of leakage or pressure-related damage.	To ensure the flexiseal is working correctly and that it is not causing any pressure damage. **E**

Problem-solving table 6.5 Prevention and resolution (Procedure guideline 6.18)

Problem	Cause	Prevention	Action
Lack of stool flow	External obstruction, e.g. pressure from equipment or body part or kink in tubing	Ensure the tubing is positioned without kinks or obstruction.	Conduct a complete check of the catheter's patency and ensure it is free of any external obstruction and is positioned lower than the patient. Reposition the patient. Strip the drainage tube by using thumb and forefinger to manually move the contents along the length of the tube.
	Blockage		Flush the drainage tube according to the manufacturer's instructions.
	Stools too solid to pass through tubing	Ensure the stool is liquid or semi-liquid.	If the stools are too solid, discontinue use of the device.
Leakage	Patient position Blockage Deflation of balloon	Ensure correct positioning of the patient and tubing.	Reposition the patient.
Rectal bleeding	Pressure necrosis or ulceration of rectal or anal mucosa	Use the correct technique for insertion and filling the balloon. Undertake regular monitoring.	Notify a senior clinician.

Constipation

Definition

Constipation results when there is a delayed movement of intestinal content through the bowel. It has been described as persistently difficult, infrequent or incomplete defaecation, which may or may not be accompanied by hard, dry stools (Konradsen et al. 2017). Constipation is a subjective disorder, being perceived differently by different people owing to the wide variety of bowel habits among healthy people (Woodward 2012). Consequently, there is a lack of consensus among both healthcare professionals and the general public as to what actually constitutes constipation (Kyle 2011b, Perdue 2005).

Anatomy and physiology

The rectum is very sensitive to rises in pressure, even of 2–3 mmHg, and distension will cause a perianal sensation with a subsequent desire to defaecate. A co-ordinated reflex empties the bowel from the mid-transverse colon to the anus. During this phase, the diaphragm, abdominal muscles and levator ani muscles contract and the glottis closes. Waves of peristalsis

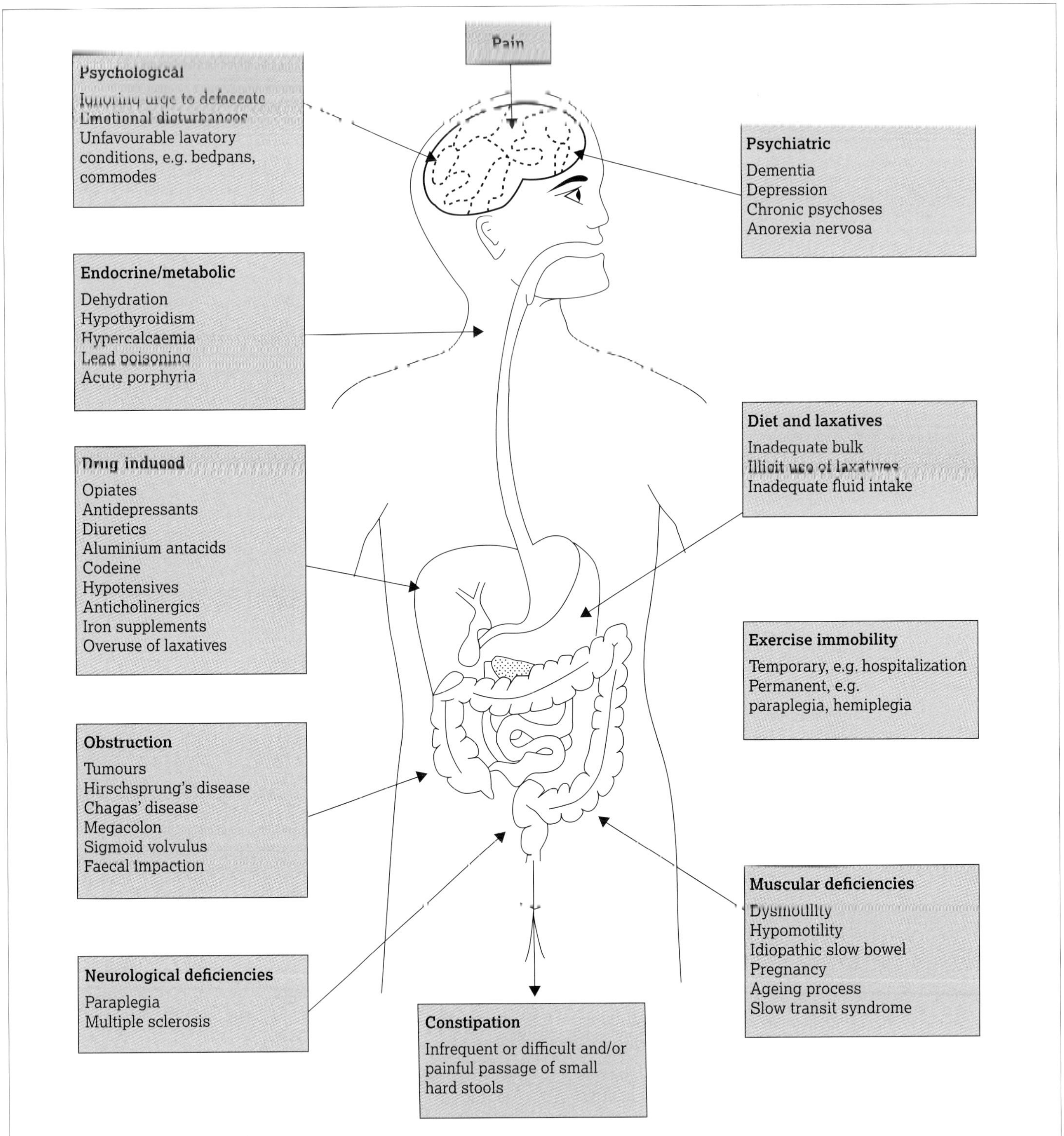

Figure 6.23 Classification of constipation.

occur in the distal colon and the anal sphincter relaxes, allowing the evacuation of faeces (Tortora and Derrickson 2017). The stimulus to defaecate varies in individuals according to habit, and, if a decision is made to delay defaecation, the stimulus disappears and a process of retroperistalsis occurs whereby the faeces move back into the sigmoid colon (Naish and Court 2018). If these natural reflexes are inhibited on a regular basis, they are eventually suppressed and reflex defaecation is inhibited, resulting in such individuals becoming severely constipated.

Related theory

It has been estimated that up to 27% of a given population experience constipation (Dutcher et al. 2018), with an average prevalence of 20% across the general population (Roque and Bouras 2015). Constipation occurs when there is either a failure of colonic propulsion (slow colonic transit) or a failure to evacuate the rectum (rectal outlet delay), or a combination of these problems (Woodward 2012).

The management of constipation depends on the cause. There are numerous possible causes, with many patients being affected by more than one causative factor (Figure 6.23). While constipation in itself is not life threatening, it can lead to bowel perforation, aspiration of vomit or faecal impaction, any of which can be life threatening (Nazarko 2018a). Particularly, constipation can be associated with abdominal pain or cramps, feelings of general malaise or fatigue, and feelings of bloatedness. Nausea, anorexia, headaches, confusion, restlessness, retention of urine, faecal incontinence and halitosis may also be present in some cases (Fritz and Pitlick 2012, Kyle 2011b).

The effective treatment of constipation relies on the cause being identified by thorough assessment, to prevent polypharmacy, which can exacerbate the problem (Wald and Talley 2017). Constipation can be categorized as primary, secondary or functional (RCN 2012b). Primary constipation has no pathological cause (RCN 2012b). Factors that lead to the development of primary, or idiopathic, constipation are extrinsic (or lifestyle related) and include:

- an inadequate diet (low fibre)
- poor fluid intake
- a lifestyle change
- ignoring the urge to defaecate.

Secondary constipation is attributed to another disorder; whether this be metabolic, neurological or psychological, there is an identifiable cause of the constipation (RCN 2012b). Examples of disease processes that may result in secondary constipation include anal fissures, colonic tumours, irritable bowel syndrome and conditions such as Parkinson's disease. Constipation may also result as a side-effect of certain medications, such as opioid analgesics (RCN 2012b, Woodward 2012).

Functional constipation can result from pelvic floor dysfunction or inadequate relaxation of these muscles during defaecation (dyssynergic defaecation) and/or inadequate propulsive forces. Treatment of these will depend on the cause and resulting symptoms. Patients who have not responded to the usual constipation treatments should go on to have their functional ability tested (Skadoon et al. 2017).

Bowel obstruction and ileus

Bowel obstruction occurs when the passage of contents through the bowel lumen is inhibited, either by mechanical (anatomical) or non-mechanical causes. The alternative term 'ileus' is sometimes used to describe the failure of passage of intestinal contents in the absence of any mechanical obstruction (Morton and Fontaine 2017).

Intestinal obstructions are caused by a physical narrowing or internal blockage of the gut lumen, extrinsic compression of the bowel, or a disruption or failure in motility. In cancer patients, malignant bowel obstruction can be either partial or complete, with acute or gradual onset of symptoms (Franke et al. 2017). Obstruction can occur at a single site or, in the case of disseminated intra-abdominal disease, such as intra-abdominal carcinomatosis, in multiple sites (Franke et al. 2017).

Intestinal obstruction is a potentially devastating complication for patients, with a vast number of possible clinical causes, and is a condition that can rapidly progress to cause life-threatening problems (Franke et al. 2017). Intestinal obstruction precipitates a cascade of pathophysiological events that lead to complex and unpleasant symptoms. Thoughtful nursing assessment and evaluation, and meticulous symptom control, can make an important contribution to improving the experience of a patient with bowel obstruction. Management of bowel obstruction may be conservative or surgical and the location of the obstruction, patient prognosis and goal of treatment should be considered when formulating a management plan (Obita et al. 2016). Conservative management usually involves placement of a nasogastric tube (see Procedure guideline 6.19: Insertion of a nasogastric drainage tube), keeping the patient nil by mouth, and managing fluid and medication requirements via intravenous or subcutaneous routes (Ozturk et al. 2018).

Evidence-based approaches

Rationale

Taking a detailed history from the patient is pivotal in establishing the appropriate treatment plan. It is therefore of vital importance that nurses adopt a proactive preventive approach to the assessment and management of constipation. Kyle and colleagues (Kyle 2011b, Kyle et al. 2005) have developed, refined and tested a constipation risk assessment tool, now known as the Norgine Risk Assessment Tool (NRAT). This assesses a range of risk factors that appear consistently within the relevant literature on the development of constipation, including:

- nutritional intake and recent changes in diet
- fluid intake
- immobility and lack of exercise
- medication, for example analgesics, antacids, iron supplements or tricyclic antidepressants
- toileting facilities, for example having to use shared toilet facilities, commodes or bedpans
- medical conditions, for example inflammatory bowel disease, irritable bowel syndrome, colorectal cancer, diabetes, or neurological conditions such as multiple sclerosis or muscular dystrophy.

In addition to the identification of these risks and contributing factors, it is important to take a careful history of a patient's bowel habits, taking particular note of the following:

- Any changes in the patient's usual bowel activity. How long have these changes been present and have they occurred before?
- Frequency of bowel action.
- Volume, consistency and colour of the stool. Stools can be graded using a scale such as the Bristol Stool Chart (see Figure 6.3), where constipation would be classified as type 1 or type 2 (Longstreth et al. 2006).
- Presence of mucus, blood, undigested food or offensive odour.
- Presence of pain or discomfort on defaecation.
- Use of oral or rectal medication to stimulate defaecation and its effectiveness.

A digital rectal examination can also be performed, providing the nurse has received sufficient training or instruction to perform it competently. This procedure can be used to assess the contents of the rectum and anal sphincter tone and to identify conditions that may cause discomfort such as haemorrhoids, anal fissures or rectal prolapse (Kyle 2011c, RCN 2012b). See Procedure guideline 6.23: Digital rectal examination for further information.

Additional investigations or referral to specialist services may be indicated if there are any 'red flag' symptoms (see Box 6.4), if treatment is unsuccessful, faecal incontinence is present, or if there is ongoing pain or bleeding on defaecation (Bardsley 2017).

Over recent years, international criteria (known as the Rome Criteria) have been developed and revised (Simren et al. 2017) that can help to more accurately and consistently define constipation. According to the Rome IV Criteria, an individual who is diagnosed with constipation should report having at least two of the following symptoms within the past 3 months where those symptoms began at least 6 months prior to diagnosis (Simren et al. 2017):

- straining for at least 25% of the time
- lumpy or hard stool for at least 25% of the time
- a sensation of incomplete evacuation for at least 25% of the time
- a sensation of anorectal obstruction or blockage for at least 25% of the time
- manual manoeuvres used to facilitate defaecation at least 25% of the time (e.g. manual evacuation)
- less than three bowel movements a week
- loose stools rarely present without the use of laxatives.

Box 6.4 Red flag symptoms that may need referral to a specialist

Refer adults using a 'suspected cancer pathway referral (for an appointment within 2 weeks) for colorectal cancer if:

- they are aged 40 or over with unexplained weight loss and abdominal pain *or*
- they are aged 50 or over with unexplained rectal bleeding *or*
- they are aged 60 or over with
  - iron-deficiency anaemia *or*
  - changes in their bowel habit *or*
- tests show occult blood in their faeces.

Consider a suspected cancer pathway referral (for an appointment within 2 weeks) for colorectal cancer in adults aged under 50 with rectal bleeding *and* any of the following unexplained symptoms or findings:

- abdominal pain
- changes in bowel habit
- weight loss
- iron-deficiency anaemia.

Source: Adapted from NICE (2015a).

The myth that daily bowel evacuation is essential to health has persisted through the centuries. This has resulted in laxative abuse becoming one of the most common types of drug misuse in the Western world. The annual cost to the NHS of prescribing medications to treat constipation is in the region of £101 million (Coloplast 2017).

Given that there is a wide normal range, it is important to establish the patient's usual bowel habit and the changes that may have occurred. Many people attempt to manage constipation by themselves with over-the-counter remedies before seeking advice despite the impact that it has on their quality of life (Harris et al. 2017). Generally, the patient will complain that they either have diarrhoea or are constipated. These should be seen as symptoms of some underlying disease or malfunction and managed accordingly. The nurse's priority is to effectively assess the nature and cause of the problem, to help find appropriate solutions, and to inform and support the patient. This requires sensitive communication skills to dispel embarrassment and ensure a shared understanding of the meanings of the terms used by the patient (RCN 2013).

Pre-procedural considerations

Pharmacological support

Laxatives

Laxatives work through direct stimulation of the bowel, by softening faecal matter or a combination of both (Candy et al. 2015). A laxative with a mild or gentle effect is also known as an aperient and one with a strong effect is referred to as a cathartic or purgative. Purgatives should be used only in exceptional circumstances – that is, where all other interventions have failed or when they are prescribed for a specific purpose. The aim of laxative treatment is to achieve comfortable rather than frequent defaecation and, wherever possible, the most natural means of bowel evacuation should be employed, with preference given to the use of oral laxatives where appropriate (NICE 2017). The many different laxatives available may be grouped into types according to the action they have (Table 6.5).

Table 6.5 Classification of laxatives

Type of laxative	How it works	Name of drug	Notes
Bulk forming	These drugs act by holding onto water so the stool remains large and soft and thereby encourages the gut to move.	Fybogel Normacol	This is to be avoided if the patient's bowel activity is not normal or their fluid intake is limited.
Stimulant	These drugs cause water and electrolytes to accumulate in the bowel and stimulate the bowel to move.	Senna tablet/liquid Bisacodyl tablet/ suppositories	This group of drugs is to be avoided if the bowel is not moving very well as these drugs can cause abdominal cramps.
Mixed stimulant and softener	Two-in-one preparations.	Co-danthramer liquid or capsules	This drug may cause the urine to change colour. It is a mild stimulant.
Softener	These drugs attract and retain water in the bowel.	Milpar (liquid paraffin and magnesium hydroxide) Docusate Arachis oil enema	If the patient is allergic to nuts, they must tell the nurse or doctor as an arachis oil enema should be avoided.
Osmotic	These drugs act in the bowel by increasing the stimulation of fluid secretion and movement in the bowel.	Lactulose Movicol Laxido Phosphate enema Microlax enema	Can cause bloating, excess wind and abdominal discomfort.
5-HT4 (5-hydroxy-tryptamine receptor 4) receptor agonists (prokinetic agents)	These drugs enhance gut motility by mimicking the effects of serotonin on the gut wall.	Prucalopride	This is not a laxative. It causes an increase in gut motility, resulting in an increase in bowel movements.
Peripheral opioid receptor antagonists	These drugs bind to peripheral opioid receptors and so reverse opioid-induced constipation.	Methylnaltrexone bromide	This is a subcutaneous injection that is only given in advanced stages of illness, in consultation with a specialist palliative care team, where oral laxatives can no longer be taken by mouth.

Bulk-forming laxatives

Bulk-forming agents work by increasing the amount of fibre and therefore water retained in the colon, increasing faecal mass and stimulating peristalsis (Woodward 2012). Ispaghula husk (e.g. manufactured under the brand names Isogel and Regulan) and sterculia (e.g. brand name Normacol) both trap water in the intestine by the formation of a highly viscous gel that softens faeces, increases weight and reduces transit time. These agents need plenty of fluid in order to work (2–3 L per day), as faecal impaction can occur if there is not sufficient fluid intake (Schuster et al. 2015). They also take a few days to exert their effect (Woodward 2012) so are not suitable to relieve acute constipation. Furthermore, bulk-forming laxatives are contraindicated in some patients, including those who have bowel obstruction, faecal impaction, acute abdominal pain and or reduced muscle tone, or those who have had recent bowel surgery.

Increasing the bulk may produce side-effects including flatulence and bloating (Woodward 2012). It may also worsen impaction, lead to increased colonic faecal loading or even intestinal obstruction, and in some cases increase the risk of faecal incontinence. Other potentially harmful effects include causing malabsorption of minerals, calcium, iron and fat-soluble vitamins, and reducing the bioavailability of some drugs.

Stool softeners

Stool-softening preparations, such as docusate sodium and glycerol (glycerine) suppositories, act by lowering the surface tension of faeces, which allows water to penetrate and soften the stool (BNF 2019). Liquid paraffin acts as a lubricant as well as a stool softener by coating the faeces and allowing easier passage. However, its use should be avoided as there are a number of problems associated with this preparation. It interferes with the absorption of fat-soluble vitamins and can also cause skin irritation and changes to the bowel mucosa, while accidental inhalation of droplets of liquid paraffin may result in lipoid pneumonia (BNF 2019).

Osmotic laxatives

Osmotic laxatives, such as lactulose or macrogols (polyethylene glycol), increase the amount of water within the large bowel either through osmosis or by retaining the water they are administered with (BNF 2019). Lactulose is a semi-synthetic disaccharide that draws water into the bowel through osmosis, resulting in a looser stool. However, it can be metabolized by colonic bacteria, which not only reduces the osmotic effect but also produces gas, which can result in abdominal cramps and flatulence, thereby causing discomfort as well as delaying the osmotic effect by as much as 3 days (BNF 2019, Woodward 2012). By contrast, polyethylene glycol is an inert polymer that is iso-osmotic and binds to water molecules, so it acts by retaining the water it is diluted with when administered (BNF 2019, Woodward 2012). Both lactulose and polyethylene glycol are commonly used in the treatment of constipation. A Cochrane review in 2010 recommended that polyethylene glycol is used in preference to lactulose (Lee-Robichaud et al. 2010) as it results in more frequent bowel motions, softer stools and a reduced need for additional laxative products.

Magnesium and phosphate preparations also exert an osmotic effect on the gut. They have a rapid effect, so fluid intake is important as patients may experience diarrhoea and dehydration. These preparations should be avoided in elderly patients and those with renal or hepatic impairment (BNF 2019). These products are often used as bowel cleansers prior to interventional procedures.

Stimulant laxatives

Laxatives including bisacodyl, dantron and senna stimulate the nerve plexi in the gut wall, increasing peristalsis and promoting the secretion of water and electrolytes in the small and large bowel to improve stool consistency (Rogers 2012, Woodward 2012). Stimulant laxatives can cause abdominal cramping, particularly if the stool is hard, and so a stool softener or osmotic laxative may be recommended for use in combination with this group of drugs (BNF 2019, Connolly and Larkin 2012). Other adverse effects with high doses of stimulant laxatives include electrolyte disturbances in frail older people and loose stools (Rogers 2012, Woodward 2012).

Preparations containing dantron (such as co-danthramer) are restricted to certain groups of patients, such as the terminally ill, as some studies on rodents have indicated a potential carcinogenic risk (BNF 2019). Dantron preparations should be avoided in incontinent patients, especially those with limited mobility, as prolonged skin contact may cause irritation and excoriation (BNF 2019).

5-HT4 receptor agonists (prokinetic agents)

5-HT4 (5-hydroxytryptamine receptor 4) receptor agonists are not laxatives but enhance gut motility by mimicking the effects of serotonin on the gut wall. Serotonin is usually released when the gut mucosa is stimulated following a meal and its attachment to 5-HT4 receptors triggers a co-ordinated contraction and relaxation of the gut's smooth muscle known as the peristaltic wave. Prokinetic agents, such as prucalopride, mimic this action, thereby increasing peristalsis and increasing stool frequency (Rogers 2012, Woodward 2012).

Peripheral opioid receptor antagonists

Methylnaltrexone bromide is a parenteral preparation that is usually administered by subcutaneous injection. It is a peripherally acting selective antagonist of opioid binding to the mu-receptors, thus reversing peripherally mediated opioid-induced constipation. As this preparation does not cross the blood–brain barrier, it does not interfere with the centrally mediated analgesic effects of opioids (Rauck et al. 2017). The indications for use are opioid induced constipation in patients with advanced illness receiving palliative care and who are unable to take oral laxatives. It is necessary to exclude bowel obstruction prior to their use and they should be used under the advice of a palliative care team (Connolly and Larkin 2012).

Non-pharmacological support

Diet

Dietary manipulation may help to resolve mild constipation, although it is much more likely to help prevent constipation from recurring. Increasing dietary fibre increases stool bulk, which in turn improves peristalsis and stool transit time (Rogers 2012). The current recommended daily intake of dietary fibre for an adult is 30 g (British Nutrition Foundation 2018).

There are two types of fibre: insoluble fibre is contained in foods such as wholegrain bread, brown rice, fruit and vegetables, and soluble fibre is contained in foods such as oats, pulses, beans and lentils. It is recommended that fibre should be taken from a variety of both soluble and insoluble foods and eaten at times spread throughout the day (British Nutrition Foundation 2018). Care should be taken to increase dietary fibre intake gradually as bloating and abdominal discomfort can result from a sudden increase, particularly in older people and those with slow-transit constipation (Rogers 2012).

Dietary changes need to be made in combination with other lifestyle changes. There is little evidence to support the benefit of increasing fluid intake for constipation, but there is arguably a benefit in encouraging people to drink the recommended daily fluid intake of at least 2 L (Fritz and Pitlick 2012, Rogers 2012). There is a need for further studies to examine the role of dietary manipulation in the management of constipation, particularly concerning the functions of dietary fibre and fluid intake.

Positioning

Patients should be advised not to ignore the urge to defaecate and to allow sufficient time for defaecation. It is important that the correct posture for defaecation is adopted: crouching or a 'crouch-like' posture is considered anatomically correct (Denby 2006, Woodward 2012) and the use of a footstool by the toilet may enable patients to adopt a better defaecation posture (NICE 2014, RCN 2012b, Woodward 2012) (Figure 6.24). The use of a bedpan should always be avoided if possible as the poor posture adopted while using one can cause extreme straining during defaecation.

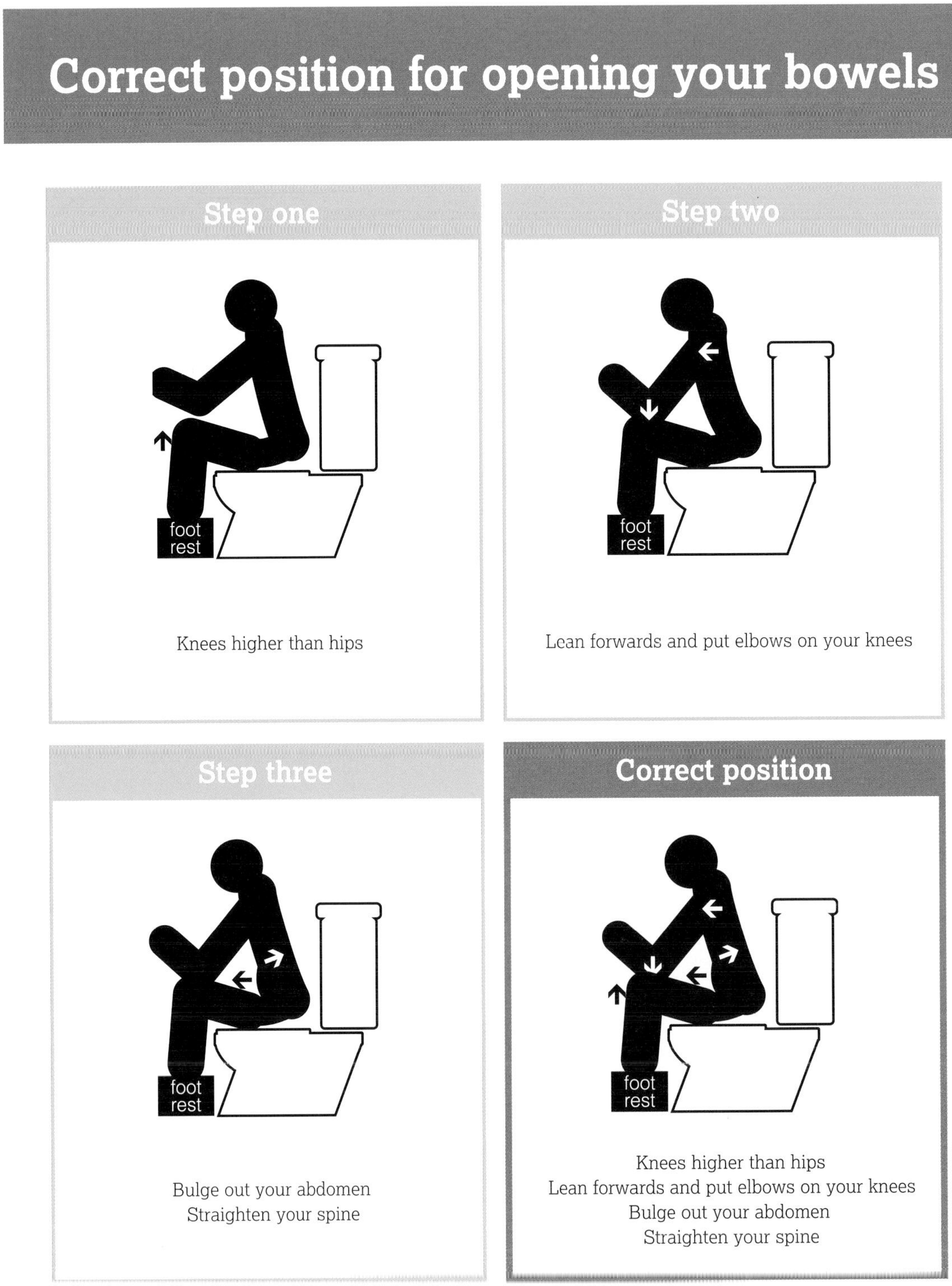
Correct position for opening your bowels
Step one
foot rest
Knees higher than hips
Step two
foot rest
Lean forwards and put elbows on your knees
Step three
foot rest
Bulge out your abdomen
Straighten your spine
Correct position
foot rest
Knees higher than hips
Lean forwards and put elbows on your knees
Bulge out your abdomen
Straighten your spine

Figure 6.24 Correct positioning for opening your bowels. *Source*: Reproduced with permission of Norgine Pharmaceuticals Ltd.

Exercise

Constipation is known to be associated with immobility (Krogh et al. 2017) and increasing physical activity is one of the primary management techniques offered to patients (Emly and Marriott 2017). This is because colonic transit time is reduced as physical activity stimulates bowel motility in healthy individuals (Krogh et al. 2017). Patients with chronic idiopathic constipation may benefit from an exercise programme consisting of 30–60 minutes of physical activity per day (De Schryver et al. 2005).

Other treatments

Biofeedback is a behaviour modification technique that encourages bracing of the abdominal wall and relaxation of the pelvic floor muscles to achieve effective defaecation. It is reported to be effective in a significant number of cases but further blinded research is required to test its efficacy more fully (Thakur et al. 2018).

Rectal irrigation is increasingly being offered as a treatment for both chronic constipation (particularly where biofeedback has not worked) and faecal incontinence. It involves instilling lukewarm water into the rectum using a rectal catheter with the aim of ensuring the rectum, sigmoid and descending colon are emptied of faeces (Rogers 2012, Woodward 2012).

Overall, lifestyle changes and laxatives (see Table 6.5) are the most commonly used treatments for constipation. In general, laxatives should be used as a short-term measure to help relieve an episode of constipation as long-term use can perpetuate constipation and create dependence. The development of newer aperients has broadened the treatment options, particularly for those patients with chronic constipation that has not responded to lifestyle modification or traditional laxatives.

Insertion of a nasogastric drainage tube

For some patients it may be appropriate to insert a nasogastric drainage tube in order to conservatively treat a bowel obstruction and associated nausea and vomiting for which antiemetics are unsuccessful (Walsh et al. 2017).

Anticipated patient outcomes

The patient has a nasogastric drainage tube inserted comfortably and safely. The position is checked and it is confirmed that the tube is placed in the stomach.

Evidence-based approaches

Rationale

Contraindications

Prior to performing this procedure, the patient's medical and nursing notes should be consulted to check for potential complications. For example, anatomical alterations due to surgery, such as a flap repair, or the presence of a cancerous tumour can prevent a clear passage for the nasogastric tube, resulting in pain and discomfort for the patient and further complications. Patients who have recurrent retching or vomiting, who have swallowing dysfunction or are comatose have a high risk of placement error or migration of the tube so care must be taken when placing a nasogastric tube under these circumstances (NPSA 2011). Any patient with coagulation derangements should have these corrected prior to insertion (Curtis 2013). The nurse should clearly document the assessment of the patient, the risks and the patient's consent.

Clinical governance

Those passing the nasogastric tube should have achieved competencies set by the local trust and be clear that the purpose of inserting the tube is for drainage of gastric contents only.

Pre-procedural considerations

Equipment

A wide-bore nasogastric drainage tube must be used for this procedure. This should not be confused with a fine-bore nasogastric tube, which is used for the sole purpose of enteral feeding (see Procedure guideline 8.10: Nasogastric intubation with tubes using an internal guidewire or stylet).

Specific patient preparation

The planned procedure should be discussed with the patient so they are aware of the rationale for the insertion of a nasogastric tube. The decision to insert a nasogastric tube must be made by at least two healthcare professionals, including the senior doctor responsible for the patient's care. Verbal consent for the procedure must be obtained from the patient. Coagulation should be checked prior to insertion to assess the risk of bleeding.

Procedure guideline 6.19 Insertion of a nasogastric drainage tube

Essential equipment

- Personal protective equipment
- Clean tray
- Receiver
- Nasogastric tube
- Drainage bag
- Tape
- Lubricating jelly
- Gauze squares
- 50 mL syringe

Action	Rationale
Pre-procedure	
1 Introduce yourself to the patient, explain and discuss the procedure with them, and gain their consent to proceed.	To ensure that the patient feels at ease, understands the procedure and gives their valid consent (NMC 2018, **C**).
2 Arrange a signal by which the patient can communicate if they want the nurse to stop, for example by raising their hand.	To maintain communication and minimize discomfort and trauma to the patient during the procedure. **E**

(continued)

Procedure guideline 8.11 Insertion of a nasogastric drainage tube (continued)

Action	Rationale
3 Assist the patient to sit in a semi-upright position in the bed or chair. Place a pillow behind their head for support. *Note*: the head should be in a neutral position (not tilted backwards or forwards).	To maintain a suitable position during the procedure to help with the correct insertion of the tube (Fan et al. 2016, **R**).
4 Wash hands with soap and water or an alcohol-based handrub, and assemble the equipment required. Apply personal protective equipment.	To ensure the procedure is as clean as possible (NHS England and NHSI 2019, **C**).
5 Select the appropriate distance mark on the tube by performing a NEX measurement. To do this, using the tube, measure the distance from the patient's nose to their earlobe plus the distance from the earlobe to the bottom of the xiphisternum (see Action figure 5 in Procedure guideline 8.10: Nasogastric intubation with tubes using an internal guidewire or stylet).	To identify the approximate length of tube that needs to be inserted to ensure it is in the correct position. **E**
Procedure	
6 Check the nostrils are patent by asking the patient to sniff with one nostril closed. Repeat with the other nostril.	To avoid any blockages or anatomical abnormalities. **E**
7 Lubricate about 15–20 cm of the tube with a thin coat of lubricating jelly that has been placed on a gauze swab.	To make insertion of the tube easier. **E**
8 Ensure the receiver is placed beneath the end of the tube.	To prevent spillage and reduce the risk of infection (Fraise and Bradley 2009, **E**).
9 Insert the proximal end of the tube into the clearer nostril and slide it backwards and inwards along the floor of the nose to the nasopharynx. If an obstruction is felt, withdraw the tube and try again in a slightly different direction or use the other nostril.	To avoid unnecessary trauma to the nose and nasopharynx. **E**
10 As the tube passes down into the nasopharynx, ask the patient to start swallowing. Offer sips of water (if they are able to take oral fluids).	To help ensure that the tube passes easily into the oesophagus. **E**
11 Advance the tube through the pharynx as the patient swallows until the predetermined mark (NEX measurement) has been reached. If the patient shows signs of distress, for example gasping or cyanosis, remove the tube immediately.	Reaching the NEX measurement on the tube indicates that it should have advanced far enough down the oesophagus to be correctly positioned in the stomach. If there are signs of respiratory distress, this may indicate that the tube is incorrectly positioned in the bronchus. **E**
12 Secure the tube to the nostril with adherent dressing tape or an adhesive nasogastric stabilization/securing device. An adhesive patch (if available) will secure the tube to the cheek.	To ensure the tube remains in the correct position. **E**
13 Use the syringe to gently aspirate any stomach contents and then attach the tube to a drainage bag.	Aspiration and/or drainage of stomach contents or bile will indicate that the tube is in the correct position in the stomach. **E**
14 Assist the patient to find a comfortable position.	To ensure comfort following the procedure. **E**
Post-procedure	
15 Use the pH below to check the position of the nasogastric drainage tube. To carry out the test, aspirate 0.5–1 mL of stomach contents and test its pH on indicator strips (NPSA 2011). Nothing should be instilled into the nasogastric tube until placement has been confirmed.	To ensure correct placement into the stomach. **E** A pH level of between 1 and 5.5 reflects the acidity of the stomach, so aspirate with this level is unlikely to be pulmonary (Metheny and Meert 2004, **R**; NPSA 2011, **C**). If a pH of 6 or above is obtained, then a second person should retest the sample or a chest X-ray should be ordered.
16 Remove gloves and apron and dispose of all equipment safely. Wash hands using soap and water or an alcohol-based handrub.	For infection prevention and control (NHS England and NHSI 2019, **C**).
17 Record the procedure, NEX measurement, length of visible portion of the tube from tip of nose, and tip position in the patient's notes.	To maintain accurate documentation (NMC 2018, **C**).
18 Assess the skin integrity of the nostril in which the tube is placed every 2–4 hours and carefully reposition as required.	To maintain skin integrity and relieve pressure from the plastic tubing. **E**
19 Reassess tube length and pH if there is any suspicion that the tube may have moved or migrated.	To ensure the tube remains in the stomach. **E**

Procedure guideline 6.20 Removal of a nasogastric drainage tube

Essential equipment

- Personal protective equipment
- Contaminated waste disposal bag
- Bowl of warm water and wipes

Action	Rationale
Pre-procedure	
1 Introduce yourself to the patient, explain and discuss the procedure with them, and gain their consent to proceed.	To ensure that the patient feels at ease, understands the procedure and gives their valid consent (NMC 2018, **C**).
2 Assist the patient to sit in a semi-upright position in the bed or chair. Support the patient's head with pillows.	To allow for easy removal of the tube. **E**
3 Wash hands with soap and water or an alcohol-based handrub, and assemble the equipment required. Apply personal protective equipment.	Hands must be cleansed before patient contact to minimize the risk of cross-infection (NHS England and NHSI 2019, **C**).
Procedure	
4 Remove any tape securing the nasogastric tube to the nose.	To assist in the removal of the nasogastric tube. **E**
5 Using a steady and constant motion, gently pull the tube until it has been completely removed.	To remove the nasogastric tube. **E**
6 Place the used nasogastric tube directly into the contaminated waste bag, as per local policy.	For infection prevention and control (Fraise and Bradley 2009, **E**).
7 Using warm water and wipes, clean the nose and face to remove any traces of tape.	To ensure patient comfort and dignity. **E**
8 Assist the patient to find a comfortable position.	To ensure comfort following the procedure. **E**
Post-procedure	
9 Remove gloves and apron and dispose of all equipment safely. Decontaminate hands.	For infection prevention and control (NHS England and NHSI 2019, **C**).
10 Document the removal of the nasogastric tube in the patient's care plan and notes.	To ensure adequate records and to enable continued care of the patient (NMC 2018, **C**).

Enema administration

Definition

An enema is the administration of a substance in liquid form into the rectum, either to aid bowel evacuation or to administer medication (Peate 2015a) (Figure 6.25). Enemas may also be administered into a colostomy by an appropriately trained nurse (Peate 2015a).

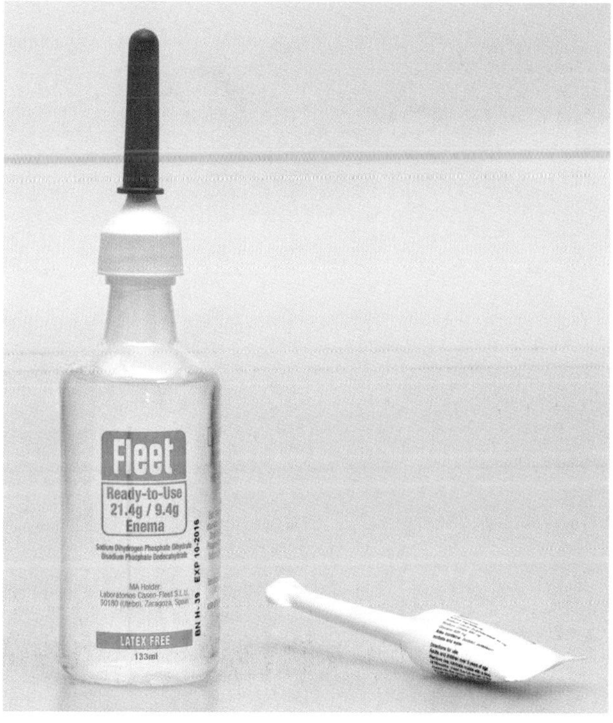

Figure 6.25 Examples of enemas.

Evidence-based approaches

Rationale

Indications

Enemas may be prescribed for the following reasons:

- to clean the lower bowel before surgery, X-ray examination of the bowel using contrast medium or endoscopy examination
- to treat severe constipation when other methods have failed
- to introduce medication into the bowel
- to soothe and treat irritated bowel mucosa
- to decrease body temperature (due to contact with the proximal vascular system)
- to stop local haemorrhage
- to reduce hyperkalaemia (calcium resonium)
- to reduce portal systemic encephalopathy (phosphate enema).

Contraindications

Enemas are contraindicated under the following circumstances (BNF 2019):

- in paralytic ileus
- in colonic obstruction

- where the administration of tap water or soap and water enemas may cause circulatory overload, water intoxication, mucosal damage and necrosis, hyperkalaemia and/or cardiac arrhythmias
- where the administration of large amounts of fluid high into the colon may cause perforation and haemorrhage
- following gastrointestinal or gynaecological surgery, where suture lines may be ruptured (unless medical consent has been given)
- where the patient is frail
- where the patient has proctitis.
- where the patient has inflammatory or ulcerative conditions of the large colon (for microenemas and hypertonic saline enemas).

Clinical governance

Enema administration must be performed by a practitioner with the appropriate knowledge and skills and where it is within their scope of professional practice to carry out this procedure.

Pre-procedural considerations

All types of enema need to be prescribed and checked against the prescription before administration. It is essential that the implications and procedure are fully explained to the patient so as to relieve anxiety and embarrassment.

Evacuant enemas

An evacuant enema is a solution introduced into the rectum or lower colon with the intention of it being expelled, along with faecal matter and flatus, within a few minutes. The osmotic activity increases the water content of the stool so that rectal distension follows and induces defaecation by stimulating rectal motility.

The following solutions are often used:

- Phosphate enemas with standard or long rectal tube in single-dose disposable packs. Although these are often used for bowel clearance before X-ray examination and surgery, there is little evidence to support their use due to the associated risks and contraindications. Wickham (2017) highlights the risk of phosphate absorption resulting from pooling of the enema due to lack of evacuation and also the risk of rectal injury caused by the enema tip. Studies have found that if evacuation does not occur, patients may suffer from hypovolaemic shock, renal failure and oliguria. When using this type of enema, it is vital that good fluid intake is encouraged and maintained.
- Dioctyl sodium sulphosuccinate 0.1% and sorbitol 25% in single-dose disposable packs are used to soften impacted faeces.
- Sodium citrate 450 mg, sodium alkylsulphoacetate 45 mg and ascorbic acid 5 mg are used in single-dose disposable packs.

Retention enemas

A retention enema is a solution introduced into the rectum or lower colon with the intention of it being retained for a specified period of time. Two types of retention enema have been most commonly used: arachis oil enemas (which are contraindicated in patients with nut allergies) and prednisolone enemas. These work by penetrating faeces, increasing the bulk and softness of stools. They are classified as stool softeners, but there is little evidence to support the use of this group of laxatives in the treatment of constipation (Woodward 2012).

Procedure guideline 6.21 Enema administration

Essential equipment

- Personal protective equipment
- Disposable incontinence pad
- Rectal tube and funnel (if not using a commercially prepared pack)
- Solution required, or a commercially prepared enema
- Gauze squares
- Commode or bedpan (if required)
- Lubricating gel
- New stoma appliance (if inserting into a colostomy)

Action	Rationale
Pre-procedure	
1 Introduce yourself to the patient, explain and discuss the procedure with them, and gain their consent to proceed.	To ensure that the patient feels at ease, understands the procedure and gives their valid consent (NMC 2018, **C**).
2 Wash hands with soap and water or use an alcohol-based handrub.	For infection prevention and control (NHS England and NHSI 2019, **C**).
3 Draw curtains around the patient or close the door.	For privacy, to avoid unnecessary embarrassment and to promote dignified care (NMC 2018, **C**).
4 Allow the patient to empty their bladder first if necessary.	A full bladder may cause discomfort during the procedure (Peate 2015a, **E**).
5 Ensure that a bedpan, commode or toilet is readily available.	In case the patient feels the need to expel the enema before the procedure is completed. **P**
Procedure	
6 Warm the enema to room temperature by immersing it in a jug of hot water.	Heat is an effective stimulant of the nerve plexi in the intestinal mucosa. An enema at room temperature or just above will not damage the intestinal mucosa. The temperature of the environment, the rate of fluid administration and the length of the tubing will all have an effect on the temperature of the fluid in the rectum (Peate 2015a, **E**).
7 Assist the patient to lie on their left side with knees well flexed, the upper knee higher up the bed than the lower one, and with the buttocks near the edge of the bed. See Problem-solving table 6.6 if the patient is unable to lie on their left.	This allows easy passage into the rectum by following the natural anatomy of the colon. In this position, gravity will aid the flow of the solution into the colon. Flexing the knees ensures a more comfortable passage of the enema nozzle or rectal tube (Peate 2015a, **E**).
8 Place a disposable incontinence pad beneath the patient's hips and buttocks.	To reduce potential infection caused by soiled linen. To avoid embarrassing the patient if the fluid is ejected prematurely following administration. **P**

9	Decontaminate hands with soap and water or an alcohol-based handrub and put on disposable gloves.	For infection prevention and control (NHS England and NHSI 2019, **C**).
10	Place some lubricating gel on a gauze square and lubricate the nozzle of the enema or the rectal tube.	This prevents trauma to the anal and rectal mucosa, which reduces surface friction (Peate 2015a, **E**).
11	Expel excessive air from the enema and introduce the nozzle or tube slowly into the anal canal while separating the buttocks. (A small amount of air may be introduced if bowel evacuation is desired.)	The introduction of air into the colon causes distension of its walls, resulting in unnecessary discomfort for the patient. The slow introduction of the lubricated tube will minimize spasming of the intestinal wall (evacuation will be more effectively induced due to the increased peristalsis). **E**
12	Slowly introduce the tube or nozzle to a depth of 10–12.5 cm.	This will bypass the anal canal (2–3 cm in length) and ensure that the tube or nozzle is in the rectum. **E**
13	If a retention enema is used, introduce the fluid slowly and leave the patient in bed with the foot of the bed elevated by 45° for as long as prescribed. Ask the patient to retain the fluid for the prescribed time. Now skip to step 20.	To avoid increasing peristalsis. The slower the rate at which the fluid is introduced, the less pressure is exerted on the intestinal wall. Elevating the foot of the bed aids retention of the enema by the force of gravity. **C**
14	If an evacuant enema is used, introduce the fluid slowly by rolling the pack from the bottom to the top to prevent backflow, until the pack is empty or the solution is completely finished.	The faster the rate of flow of the fluid, the greater the pressure on the rectal walls. Distension and irritation of the bowel wall will produce strong peristalsis that is sufficient to empty the lower bowel (Peate 2015a, **E**).
15	If using a funnel and rectal tube, adjust the height of the funnel according to the rate of flow desired.	The forces of gravity will cause the solution to flow from the funnel into the rectum. The greater the elevation of the funnel, the faster the flow of fluid. **E**
16	Clamp the tubing before all the fluid has run in.	To avoid air entering the rectum and causing further discomfort. **E**
17	Slowly withdraw the tube or nozzle.	To avoid reflex emptying of the rectum. **E**
18	Dry the patient's perineal area using gauze squares.	To promote patient comfort and avoid excoriation. **P**
19	Ask the patient to retain the enema for 10–15 minutes before evacuating the bowel.	To enhance the evacuant effect. **P**
20	Ensure that the patient has access to the nurse call system; is near to a bedpan, commode or toilet; and has adequate toilet paper.	To enhance patient comfort and safety. To minimize the patient's embarrassment. **P**
Post-procedure		
21	Remove and dispose of equipment, gloves and apron. Decontaminate hands using soap and water or an alcohol-based handrub.	For infection prevention and control (NHS England and NHSI 2019, **C**).
22	Record in the appropriate documents that the enema has been given, the effect on the patient and the result (colour, consistency, content and amount of faeces produced), using the Bristol Stool Chart (see Figure 6.3).	To monitor the patient's bowel function (Peate 2015a, **C**).
23	Observe the patient for any adverse reactions.	To monitor the patient for complications (Peate 2015a, **C**).

Suppositories

Definition

A suppository is a solid or semi-solid bullet-shaped pellet that is prepared by mixing a medication with a wax-like substance that melts once inserted into the rectum (Peate 2015b).

Related theory

Enema and suppository administration is possible via a stoma; however, the medications are unlicensed for this use and therefore local policy for this practice should be adhered to.

Evidence-based approaches

Rationale

Indications

The use of suppositories is indicated in the following circumstances:

- to empty the bowel prior to certain types of surgery and some investigations
- to empty the bowel to relieve acute constipation or when other treatments for constipation have failed
- to empty the bowel before endoscopic examination
- to administer medication
- to soothe and treat haemorrhoids or anal pruritus.

Contraindications

The use of suppositories is contraindicated when one or more of the following pertain:

- chronic constipation, which would require repetitive use
- paralytic ileus
- colonic obstruction
- malignancy of the perianal region
- low platelet count
- following gastrointestinal or gynaecological operations, unless on the specific instructions of the doctor.

Methods of administration of suppositories

The use of suppositories dates back to about 460 BCE. Hippocrates recommended the use of cylindrical suppositories of honey smeared with ox gall (Hurst et al. 1969). The torpedo-shaped suppositories commonly used today came into being in 1893, when it was recommended that they were inserted apex (pointed end) first (Moppett 2000).

This practice was questioned by Abd-el-Maeboud et al. (1991), who suggested that suppositories should be inserted blunt end first. The rationale for this is based on anorectal physiology; if a suppository is inserted apex first, the circular base distends the anus and the lower edge of the anal sphincter fails to close tightly. The normal squeezing motion (reverse vermicular contraction) of the anal sphincter therefore fails to drive the suppository into the rectum. These factors can lead to anal irritation and rejection of the suppository (Moppett 2000, Pegram et al. 2008). The research study by Abd-el-Maeboud et al. (1991) was very small and remains the only research evidence supporting this practice. Following this, Bradshaw and Price (2006) performed a further search of the literature and no further evidence was available. This remains the case. A distinction can be made between suppositories administered for constipation, requiring a local effect, and those given to achieve a systemic effect.

In the management of constipation, a suppository placed against the bowel wall, rather than within faecal matter, enables body heat to soften the suppository. This requires an accurate insertion technique, which may be better achieved by inserting the suppository apex first (Kyle 2009). However, Kyle (2009) suggests that patients may find it more acceptable to self-administer suppositories blunt end first as the sucking action means there is no need to insert the finger into the anal canal. Suppositories for systemic use are best absorbed by the lower rectum. Here, venous drainage avoids the portal circulation moving to the inferior vena cava quickly, resulting in a more rapid therapeutic effect (Kyle 2009). There is a need for further research in this area but until such work is carried out, expert opinion such as that of Kyle (2009) and manufacturers' guidelines should steer practice (Peate 2015b).

Pre-procedural considerations

Pharmacological support

There are several different types of suppository available. Retention suppositories are designed to deliver drug therapy, for example analgesia, antibiotics and non-steroidal anti-inflammatory drugs (NSAID). Those designed to stimulate bowel evacuation include glycerine, bisacodyl and sodium bicarbonate. Lubricant suppositories, for example glycerine, should be inserted directly into the faeces and allowed to dissolve. They have a mild irritant action on the rectum and also act as faecal softeners (BNF 2019). However, stimulant types, such as bisacodyl, must come into contact with the mucous membrane of the rectum if they are to be effective as they release carbon dioxide, causing rectal distension and thus evacuation.

Procedure guideline 6.22 Suppository administration

Essential equipment

- Personal protective equipment
- Disposable incontinence pad
- Gauze squares or tissues
- Lubricating gel
- One or more suppositories as required (check prescription before administering any suppository)
- Bedpan or commode (if required)
- New stoma pouch (if inserting into a colostomy)

Action	Rationale
Pre-procedure	
1 Introduce yourself to the patient, explain and discuss the procedure with them, and gain their consent to proceed. If administering a medicated suppository, it is best to do so after the patient has emptied their bowels.	To ensure that the patient feels at ease, understands the procedure and gives their valid consent (NMC 2018, **C**). To ensure that the active ingredients are not prevented from being absorbed by the rectal mucosa and that the suppository is not expelled before its active ingredients have been released (Moppett 2000, **E**).
2 Wash hands and/or use an alcohol-based handrub, and apply personal protective equipment	To ensure the procedure is as clean as possible and for infection control (NHS England and NHSI 2019, **C**).
3 Draw the curtains around the patient or close the door.	To ensure privacy and dignity for the patient (NMC 2018, **C**).
4 Ensure that a bedpan, commode or toilet is readily available.	In case of premature ejection of the suppository or rapid bowel evacuation following its administration. **P**
Procedure	
5 Assist the patient to lie on their left side with the knees flexed, the upper knee higher up the bed than the lower one, with the buttocks near the edge of the bed.	This allows ease of passage of the suppository into the rectum by following the natural anatomy of the colon (Peate 2015b). Flexing the knees will reduce discomfort as the suppository is passed through the anal sphincter (Peate 2015b, **E**).
6 Place a disposable incontinence pad beneath the patient's hips and buttocks.	To avoid unnecessary soiling of linen, leading to potential infection and embarrassment to the patient if the suppository is ejected prematurely or there is rapid bowel evacuation following its administration. **E**
7 Wash hands with soap and water or use an alcohol-based handrub and put on apron and gloves.	For infection prevention and control (NHS England and NHSI 2019, **C**).
8 Place some lubricating jelly on a gauze square and lubricate the blunt end of the suppository if it is being used to obtain systemic action. Separate the patient's buttocks and insert the suppository blunt end first, advancing it for about 2–4 cm. Repeat this procedure if additional suppositories are to be inserted.	Lubrication reduces surface friction and thus eases insertion of the suppository and avoids anal mucosal trauma. The suppository is more readily retained if inserted blunt end first (Abd-el-Maeboud et al. 1991, **R**). The anal canal is approximately 2–3 cm long. Inserting the suppository beyond this point ensures that it will be retained (Abd-el-Maeboud et al. 1991, **R**; Pegram et al. 2008, **E**).

9 Once the suppository has been inserted, clean any excess lubricating jelly from the patient's perineal and perianal areas using gauze squares.	To ensure the patient's comfort and avoid anal excoriation (Peate 2015b, **E**).
10 Ask the patient to retain the suppository for 20 minutes or until they are no longer able to do so. If a medicated suppository is given, remind the patient that its aim is not to stimulate evacuation and that the patient should retain the suppository for at least 20 minutes or as long as possible. Inform the patient that there may be some discharge as the medication melts in the rectum.	This will allow the suppository to melt and release the active ingredients (Peate 2015b, **E**).
Post-procedure	
11 Remove and dispose of equipment, gloves and apron. Wash hands with soap and water or use an alcohol-based handrub.	For infection prevention and control (NHS England and NHSI 2019, **C**).
12 Record that the suppository has been given, the effect on the patient and the result (amount, colour, consistency and content, using the Bristol Stool Chart; see Figure 6.3), if appropriate, in the relevant documents.	To monitor the patient's bowel function (Peate 2015b, **C**) and to maintain accurate records (NMC 2018, **C**).
13 Observe the patient for any adverse reactions.	To monitor for any complications (Peate 2015b, **E**).

Problem-solving table 6.6 Prevention and resolution (Procedure guidelines 6.21 and 6.22)

Problem	Cause	Prevention	Action
Patient unable to lie on their left side	Multiple possible causes (e.g. pain, surgical site, disability)	Control pain.	Lie the patient on their right side to perform the procedure. However, consider the usual anatomy of the bowel; gently advance the enema or suppository and stop if any resistance is felt.
Unable to insert the nozzle of the enema pack or the rectal tube into the anal canal	Tube not adequately lubricated; patient in an incorrect position	Ensure the patient is relaxed and in the correct position.	Apply more lubricating jelly. Ask the patient to draw their knees up further towards their chest. Ensure the patient is relaxed before inserting the nozzle or rectal tube.
	Patient unable to relax anal sphincter; patient apprehensive and embarrassed about the situation	Ensure the patient is relaxed and in the correct position.	Ask the patient to take deep breaths and 'bear down' as if defaecating.
Unable to advance the tube or nozzle into the anal canal	Spasm of the canal walls	Ask the patient to take slow, deep breaths to help them relax.	Wait until the spasm has passed before inserting the tube or nozzle more slowly, thus minimizing spasm. Ensure adequate privacy and give frequent explanations to the patient about the procedure.
Unable to advance the tube or nozzle into the rectum	Blockage by faeces		Withdraw the tubing slightly and allow a little solution to flow, and then insert the tube further.
	Blockage by tumour		If resistance is still met, stop the procedure and inform a doctor.
Patient complains of cramping or the desire to evacuate the enema before the end of the procedure	Distension and irritation of the intestinal wall produces strong peristalsis sufficient to empty the lower bowel	Encourage the patient to retain the enema.	Stop instilling the enema fluid and wait with the patient until the discomfort has subsided.
Patient unable to open their bowels after an evacuant enema	Reduced neuromuscular response in the bowel wall		Inform the doctor that the enema was unsuccessful and reassure the patient.

Digital rectal examination

Definition

A digital rectal examination (DRE) is an invasive procedure that can be carried out as part of a nursing assessment by a registered nurse who can demonstrate competence to an appropriate level in accordance with *The Code* (NMC 2018). The procedure involves the nurse inserting a lubricated gloved finger into the rectum.

Evidence-based approaches

Rationale

Indications

This examination can be performed in the following circumstances:

- to establish whether faecal matter is present in the rectum and, if so, to assess the amount and consistency

- to ascertain anal tone and the ability to initiate a voluntary contraction and to what degree
- to teach pelvic floor exercises
- to assess anal pathology for the presence of foreign objects
- prior to administering rectal medication to establish the state of the rectum
- to establish the effects of rectal medication
- to administer suppositories or an enema prior to endoscopy
- to determine the need for digital removal of faeces (DRF) or digital rectal stimulation and to evaluate for bowel emptiness
- to assess the need for rectal medication and to evaluate its efficacy in certain circumstances, for example in patients who have diminished anal and/or rectal sensation
- to trigger defaecation by digitally stimulating the rectoanal reflex (Peate 2015b)
- to establish anal and rectal sensation (RCN 2012b).

Clinical governance

As DRE is an invasive and intimate procedure, it is important that consent is obtained from the patient prior to it being performed (Kyle 2011c, Steggall 2008). A DRE should form part of the bowel assessment, rather than being a stand-alone procedure (Kyle 2011c), and can be undertaken by registered nurses who demonstrate competency in this procedure, possessing the knowledge, skills and abilities required for lawful, safe and effective practice (RCN 2012b).

As nursing roles develop, nurse specialists and nurse practitioners are increasingly involved in areas of care that necessitate undertaking DRE as part of a physical assessment or procedure. Such instances may include:

- the assessment of prostate size, characterization, mobility and anatomical limits
- during procedures such as the placement of a rectal probe or sensor prior to urodynamic studies or the placement of catheters used in the treatment of constipation or anismus
- prior to using transanal irrigation
- during the placement of an endoscope prior to colonoscopy or sigmoidoscopy (RCN 2012b).

Pre-procedural considerations

Specific patient preparation

Before carrying out a DRE, the perineal and perianal area should be checked for signs of rectal prolapse, haemorrhoids, anal skin tags, fissures or lesions, foreign bodies, scarring, infestations or a gaping anus. The condition of the skin should be noted, as should the type and amount of any discharge or leakage. If any of these abnormalities are seen, a DRE should not be carried out until advice is taken from a specialist nurse or medical practitioner (RCN 2012b, Steggall 2008).

Precautions

Special care should be taken in performing DRE in patients whose disease processes or treatments in particular affect the anus or bowel mucosa. These conditions include (RCN 2012b):

- active inflammation of the bowel, for example ulcerative colitis
- recent radiotherapy to the pelvic area
- rectal and/or anal pain
- rectal surgery or trauma to the anal and/or rectal area in the past 6 weeks
- obvious rectal bleeding – consider possible causes for this
- spinal cord injury at or above the sixth thoracic vertebra, because of the risk of autonomic dysreflexia
- known allergies, for example latex
- a known history of abuse
- tissue fragility related to age, radiation or malnourishment.

Procedure guideline 6.23 Digital rectal examination

Essential equipment

- Personal protective equipment
- Disposable incontinence pad
- Lubricating gel
- Gauze squares or tissues
- Bedpan or commode (if required)

Action	Rationale
Pre-procedure	
1 Introduce yourself to the patient, explain and discuss the procedure with them, and gain their consent to proceed.	To ensure that the patient feels at ease, understands the procedure and gives their valid consent (NMC 2018, **C**).
2 Ensure privacy.	To avoid unnecessary embarrassment to the patient and to promote dignity and privacy (NMC 2018, **C**).
3 Ensure that a bedpan, commode or toilet is readily available.	DRE can stimulate the need for a bowel movement (Weisner and Bell 2004, **E**).
Procedure	
4 Assist the patient to lie in the left lateral position with knees flexed, the upper knee higher up the bed than the lower knee, with the buttocks towards the edge of the bed.	This allows ease of digital examination into the rectum by following the natural anatomy of the colon (RCN 2012b, **C**). Flexing the knees reduces discomfort as the examining finger passes the anal sphincter (Kyle et al. 2005, **E**).
5 Place a disposable incontinence pad beneath the patient's hips and buttocks.	To reduce potential infection caused by soiled linen. To avoid embarrassing the patient if faecal staining occurs during or after the procedure. **E**
6 Wash hands with soap and water or an alcohol-based handrub and put on disposable gloves.	For infection prevention and control (NHS England and NHSI 2019, **C**).

7 Observe the anal area prior to the insertion of the finger into the anus for evidence of skin soreness, excoriation, swelling, haemorrhoids, rectal prolapse or infestation.	May indicate incontinence or pruritus. Swelling may be indicative of mass or abscess. Abnormalities such as bleeding, discharge or prolapse should be reported to medical staff before any examination is undertaken (RCN 2012b, **C**).
8 Palpate the perianal area starting at 12 o'clock, moving clockwise to 6 o'clock and then moving from 12 o'clock anticlockwise to 6 o'clock.	To assess for any irregularities, swelling, indurations, tenderness or abscesses in the perianal area (RCN 2012b, **C**).
9 Place some lubricating gel on a gauze square and gloved index finger. Inform the patient you are about to proceed.	To minimize discomfort as lubrication reduces friction and to ease insertion of the finger into the anus and rectum. Lubrication also helps to minimize anal mucosal trauma from digitization (Peate 2016, **E**). Informing the patient assists with co-operation during the procedure (NMC 2018, **C**).
10 Prior to insertion, encourage the patient to breathe out or talk, and/or place gloved index finger on the anus for a few seconds prior to insertion.	To prevent spasm of the anal sphincter on insertion (RCN 2012b, **C**). Gently placing a finger on the anus initiates the anal reflex, causing the anus to contract and then relax (RCN 2012b, **C**).
11 On insertion of the finger, assess for anal sphincter control; resistance should be felt.	Digital insertion with resistance indicates good internal sphincter tone; poor resistance may indicate the opposite (RCN 2012b, **C**).
12 With finger inserted in the anus, swoop clockwise then anticlockwise, noting any irregularities.	Palpating around 360° enables the nurse to establish whether there is any swelling or tenderness within the rectum (RCN 2012b, **C**; Steggall 2008, **E**).
13 Digital examination may allow the nurse to feel faecal matter within the rectum; note the consistency of any faecal matter.	May establish a loaded rectum and indicate constipation and the need for rectal medication (RCN 2012b, **C**).
14 Carefully remove the finger and change gloves.	To enable the cleaning of the patient. **E**
15 Clean the anal area after the procedure.	To prevent irritation and soreness occurring. To preserve the patient's dignity and personal hygiene. **P**
Post-procedure	
16 Remove gloves and apron and dispose of equipment in an appropriate clinical waste bin. Wash hands with soap and water or an alcohol-based handrub.	For infection prevention and control (NHS England and NHSI 2019, **C**).
17 Assist the patient into a comfortable position and offer a bedpan, commode or toilet facilities as appropriate.	To promote the patient's comfort. **P**
18 Document the findings and report them to the appropriate members of the multidisciplinary team.	To ensure continuity of care and ensure appropriate corrective action may be initiated (NMC 2018, **C**; RCN 2012b, **C**).

Digital removal of faeces

Definition

Digital removal of faeces (DRF) is an invasive procedure involving the removal of faeces from the rectum using a gloved finger. This should only be performed when necessary and after individual assessment (RCN 2012b).

Related theory

Managing bowel problems such as constipation and prolonged bowel evacuation in patients following spinal cord injury requires a multimodality approach. This includes dietary fibre, digital stimulation, enemas, suppositories, stool softeners and abdominal massage (Peate 2016).

Autonomic dysreflexia (AD) is unique to patients with spinal cord injury at the sixth thoracic vertebra or above. It is an abnormal response from the autonomic nervous system to a painful (noxious) stimulus below the level of the spinal cord injury (RCN 2012b). The signs and symptoms of AD are headache, flushing, sweating, nasal obstruction, blotchiness above the lesion and hypertension, the most significant being the rapid onset of a servere headache. Distended bowel caused by constipation or impaction can lead to AD and therefore it is important that an effective programme of bowel management is established and followed (Eldahan and Rabchevsky 2018). Acute AD may occur in response to digital intervention. It is therefore important that all healthcare professionals who carry out digital interventions on individuals with spinal cord injury are aware of the signs and symptoms; should any occur, the intervention must be stopped immediately (RCN 2012b).

Evidence-based approaches

Rationale

Advances in orally and rectally administered medicines as well as surgical treatments have reduced the need for DRF to be performed; however, for certain groups of patients, such as those with spinal injuries, spina bifida or multiple sclerosis, this procedure may be the only suitable bowel-emptying technique, forming a long-standing, integral part of their bowel routine (RCN 2012b).

DRF can be distressing, painful and dangerous. In particular, stimulation of the vagus nerve in the rectal wall can slow the patient's heart, and there is a risk of bowel perforation and bleeding (Peate 2016).

Indications

Indications for assisted evacuation of bowels (DRF or digital stimulation) include:

- faecal impaction/loading
- incomplete defaecation
- inability to defaecate
- failure or unsuitability of other bowel-emptying techniques
- neurogenic bowel dysfunction
- spinal cord injury (RCN 2012b).

Patients are at risk of rectal trauma if these procedures are not performed with care or knowledge. The nurse should be aware of any conditions that may contraindicate performance of these procedures (see 'Precautions' in the section on digital rectal examination above).

Clinical governance

DRF should be performed by registered nurses who demonstrate competency in this procedure, possessing the knowledge, skills and abilities required for lawful, safe and effective practice (RCN 2012b). In addition, they should ensure that their employer has defined policies and procedures for undertaking this role (RCN 2012b). If appropriate, the patient and their personal carer may wish for the carer to maintain the established programme of bowel management once the patient has left hospital (Peate 2016).

Pre-procedural considerations

Specific patient preparations

If this procedure is used as an acute intervention, the patient's pulse rate should be recorded before and during the process. Patients with a spinal cord injury should also have their blood pressure measured before, during and after the procedure. A baseline blood pressure measurement should be available for comparison (RCN 2012b). Every time the procedure is performed, the consistency of the stool should be noted before continuing. If the stool is hard and dry, lubricant suppositories should be inserted and left for 30 minutes before commencing. If the stool is too soft to remove effectively, consider delaying the procedure for 24 hours to allow further water reabsorption to occur.

During the procedure, the nurse should observe the patient for signs of:

- distress, pain or discomfort
- bleeding
- autonomic dysreflexia: hypertension, bradycardia, headache, flushing above the level of the spinal injury, sweating, pallor below the level of the spinal injury or nasal congestion (RCN 2012b)
- collapse (RCN 2012b).

Procedure guideline 6.34 Digital removal of faeces

Essential equipment

- Personal protective equipment
- Disposable incontinence pad
- Receiver and clinical waste bag
- Specimen pot (if required)
- Bedpan or commode (if appropriate)
- Tissues or topical swabs
- Lubricating gel

Action	Rationale
Pre-procedure	
1 Introduce yourself to the patient, explain and discuss the procedure with them, and gain their consent to proceed.	To ensure that the patient feels at ease, understands the procedure and gives their valid consent (NMC 2018, **C**).
2 Draw a curtain around the patient or close the door.	To ensure privacy and to avoid unnecessary embarrassment to the patient (NMC 2018, **C**).
3 In spinal cord injury, patients who are at risk of autonomic dysreflexia (AD) should have a blood pressure reading taken prior to the procedure. A baseline blood pressure reading should be available for comparison. For such patients where this procedure is routine and tolerance is well established, this is not required.	In spinal cord injury, stimulus below the level of injury may result in symptoms of AD including headache and hypertension (Peate 2016, **C**; RCN 2012b, **C**).
Procedure	
4 Assist the patient to lie in the left lateral position with knees flexed, the upper knee higher up the bed than the lower knee, with the buttocks towards the edge of the bed.	This allows ease of digital insertion into the rectum, by following the natural anatomy of the colon (RCN 2012b, **C**). Flexing the knees reduces discomfort as the finger passes the anal sphincter (Peate 2016, **C**).
5 Place a disposable incontinence pad beneath the patient's hips and buttocks.	To reduce potential infection caused by soiled linen. To avoid embarrassing the patient if faecal staining occurs during or after the procedure. **E**
6 Wash hands with bactericidal soap and water or an alcohol-based handrub and put on disposable apron and gloves.	For infection prevention and control (NHS England and NHSI 2019, **C**).
7 Place some lubricating gel on a gauze square and gloved index finger.	To minimize discomfort as lubrication reduces friction and to ease insertion of the finger into the anus and rectum. Lubrication also helps to minimize anal mucosal trauma (Peate 2016, **E**).
8 Inform the patient you are about to proceed.	To assist with patient co-operation with the procedure (NMC 2018, **C**).
9 In spinal cord injury patients, observe for signs of AD throughout the procedure	In spinal cord injury, stimulus below the level of the injury may result in symptoms of AD, including hypertension (Peate 2016, **E**; RCN 2012b, **C**).
10 Observe the anal area prior to the insertion of the finger into the anus for evidence of skin soreness, excoriation, swelling, haemorrhoids or rectal prolapse.	May indicate incontinence or pruritus. Swelling may be indicative of mass or abscess. Abnormalities such as bleeding, discharge or prolapse should be reported to medical staff before any examination is undertaken (RCN 2012b, **C**).

11 Proceed to insert finger into the anus and rectum. Proceed with caution in those patients with spinal cord injury.	The majority of spinal cord injury patients will not experience any pain (Peate 2016, **C**).
12 If the stool is type 1 (see Figure 6.3), remove one lump at a time until no more faecal matter is felt.	To relieve patient discomfort (Peate 2016, **C**).
13 If a solid faecal mass is felt, split it and remove small pieces until no more faecal matter is felt. Avoid using a hooked finger to remove faeces.	To relieve patient discomfort (Peate 2016, **C**). Use of a hooked finger may cause damage to the rectal mucosa and anal sphincter (RCN 2012b, **C**).
14 If faecal mass is too hard to break up or more than 4 cm across, stop the procedure and discuss with the multidisciplinary team.	To avoid unnecessary pain and damage to the anal sphincter. The patient may require the procedure to be carried out under anaesthetic (Peate 2016, **C**).
15 As faeces are removed, they should be placed in an appropriate receiver.	To assist in appropriate disposal and reduce the risk of contamination and cross-infection. **E**
16 Encourage patients who receive this procedure on a regular basis to have a period of rest or, if appropriate, to assist using the Valsalva manoeuvre.	Patient and nurse education is required to use this technique safely. Therefore, further guidance should be sought before introducing this manoeuvre as it may lead to complications such as haemorrhoids (Peate 2016, **C**).
17 Change gloves, then wash and dry the patient's anal area and buttocks.	To ensure the patient feels comfortable and clean. **P**
Post-procedure	
18 Remove gloves and apron and dispose of equipment in an appropriate clinical waste bin. Wash hands.	For prevention and control of infection (NHS England and NHSI 2019, **C**).
19 Assist the patient into a comfortable position.	To promote comfort. **P**
20 In spinal cord injury patients, take a blood pressure reading.	In spinal cord injury, stimulus below the level of the injury may result in symptoms of AD, including hypertension (Peate 2016, **C**).
21 Document the findings and report them to the appropriate members of the multidisciplinary team.	To ensure continuity of care and enable appropriate actions to be initiated (NMC 2018, **C**; RCN 2012b, **C**).

Stoma care

Definition

A stoma is an opening, either natural or surgically created, which connects a portion of the body cavity to the outside environment. The names of surgical procedures in which stomas are created end in the suffix -ostomy and begin with the prefix denoting the organ or area being operated on (Zulkowski et al. 2014).

Related theory

It is believed that in the UK around 25,000 new stoma operations take place each year; in 2017 there were approximately 11,000 new colostomies, 9000 new ileostomies and 1660 new ileal conduits created (BAUS 2018). The most common underlying conditions resulting in the need for stoma surgery are:

- colorectal cancer
- bladder cancer
- ulcerative colitis
- Crohn's disease.

Other causes of stoma surgery include:

- pelvic cancer, for example gynaecological cancer
- trauma
- neurological damage
- congenital disorders
- diverticular disease
- familial polyposis colitis
- intractable incontinence
- fistula
- radiation bowel disease
- bowel perforation (Burch 2015).

Types of stoma

Colostomy

A colostomy may be formed from any section of the large bowel. Its position along the colon will dictate the output and consistency of the faeces. Therefore, an understanding of the relevant anatomy and physiology is essential to fully care for stoma patients.

The most common site for a colostomy is on the sigmoid colon. This will produce a semi-solid or formed stool and is generally positioned in the left iliac fossa and is flush to the skin (Boyles and Hunt 2016). Stomas formed higher up along the colon will produce a slightly more liquid stool. A colostomy tends to be active on average two or three times per day, but this can vary between individuals.

Colostomies can either be permanent or temporary (Figure 6.26). Permanent (end) (Figure 6.27) colostomies are often formed following removal of rectal cancers, as in abdominoperineal resections of the rectum, whereas temporary (loop) colostomies (Figure 6.28) may be formed to divert the faecal output, to allow healing of a surgical join (anastomosis) or repair, or to relieve an obstruction or bowel injury (Rostas 2012). Temporary stomas have increased in prevalence over the years and now there are more temporary ileostomies and colostomies than permanent ones (Lim et al. 2013).

As is evident from Figures 6.27 and 6.28, end and loop colostomies are very different in appearance. An end colostomy tends to be flush to the skin and sutured to the abdominal wall and consists of an end-section of bowel, whereas a loop colostomy is larger. During the perioperative period, a loop colostomy is supported by a stoma bridge or rod (see Figure 6.28). This is placed under the section of bowel and generally left in place for approximately 5 days following surgery and then removed (Whiteley et al. 2016).

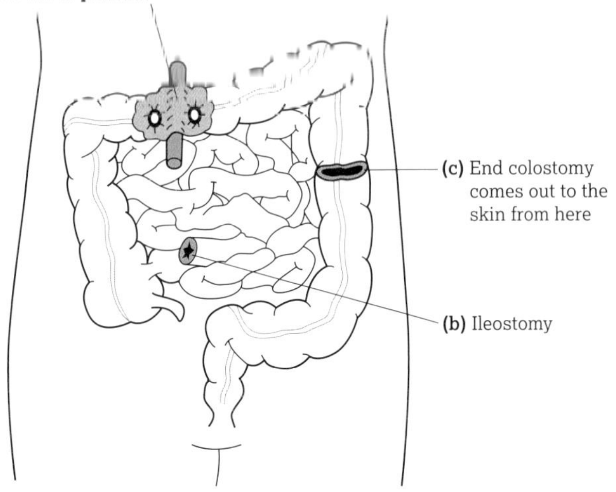

Figure 6.26 (a) Transverse (loop) colostomy, (b) ileostomy and (c) end colostomy.

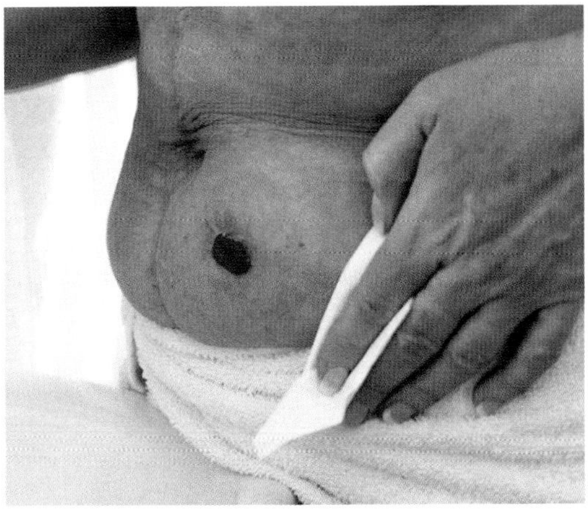

Figure 6.27 End colostomy.

Ileostomy

Ileostomies are formed when a section of ileum is brought out onto the abdominal wall. This is generally positioned at the terminal end of the ileum on the right iliac fossa, but it can be anywhere along the ileum (Black 2015b). Consequently, the output tends to be a looser, more liquid stool, as waste is eliminated before the water is absorbed from the large bowel (colon). Due to the more alkaline, abrasive nature of the stool at this stage, a spout is formed with this type of stoma. The ileum is everted to form a spout, which allows the effluent to drain into an appliance without coming into contact with the peristomal skin (Figure 6.29). This prevents skin breakdown and allows for better management (Burch 2011b). The average output from an ileostomy is 200–600 mL per day.

Ileostomies can also be either permanent (end) (Figure 6.29) or temporary (loop). Permanent ileostomies are often formed following total colectomies (removal of the entire colon). Loop ileostomies are increasingly common and are often formed to allow healing of a surgical join (anastomosis) or an ileoanal pouch (Black 2015a). These are sometimes held in place by a stoma bridge or rod. See Procedure guideline 6.28: Stoma bridge or rod removal for more information on bridge and rod care and removal.

Urostomy or ileal conduit

An ileal conduit is the most common form of urostomy; the colon (colonic conduit) may also be used. Urostomy comes from the Greek words *uros*, meaning urine, and *stoma*, meaning mouth or opening (Nazarko 2008).

A section of bowel is isolated, along with its mesentery vessels, and the remaining ends of the bowel are anastomosed to restore continuity. The isolated section is mobilized, the proximal end is closed and the ureters, once resected from the bladder, are implanted at this end. The distal end is brought out onto the surface of the abdominal wall and everted to form a spout (Figure 6.29), as in an ileostomy (Leach 2015). Urine from a urostomy will contain mucus from the bowel used in its construction (Geng et al. 2009, Leach 2015).

Some patients who are obese may have a Turnbull's loop ileal conduit formed. The distal and proximal ends of the loop can expel urine. There is an improved blood supply to the distal portion of the conduit by delivering mesenteric blood supply to this area. Selected obese patients and those in which the tension to the distal end of the stoma may contribute to ischaemia and stomal stenosis are given this type of ileal conduit. These patients may have a stoma rod in addition to ureteric stents *in situ*.

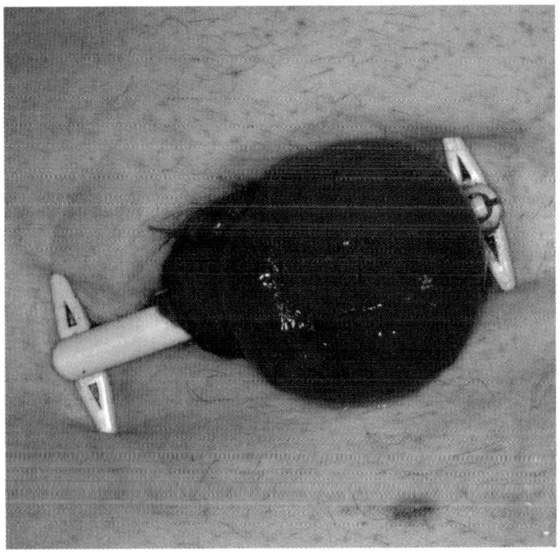

Figure 6.28 Loop colostomy with bridge *in situ*.

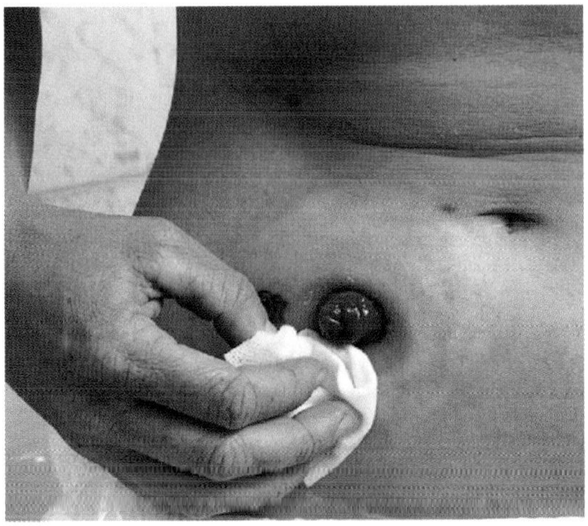

Figure 6.29 End ileostomy illustrating the 'spout'. *Source*: Reproduced with permission of Dansac Ltd.

Stents are removed following advice from the urological surgeon. This can be done after 7 days; however, the timing of removal is dependent on whether the patient has undergone previous radiotherapy, or has one kidney or other underlying renal issues, in which case the amount of time the stents are *in situ* may be longer. The stoma bridge is removed after approximately 5 days.

Ureteric stents protect the anastomosis at the ureteroileal junction by allowing healing, and preventing strictures and leakage (Leach 2015). They also ensure the kidneys can drain urine freely and prevent upper urinary tract obstruction caused by compression due to post-operative oedema. The stents need to be monitored; although they facilitate the flow of urine, they may become obstructed due to bleeding, calculi or sediment (for example). Obstruction can result in hydronephrosis and kidney damage. The stent is a foreign body in the urinary tract and can increase the risk of a urinary tract infection. A two-piece bag system aids stoma management immediately post-operatively, while the stents are *in situ*, and allows the healthcare professional to check the stents. The stents should be checked daily for drainage. If they are not draining, the urology team should be informed as they may need to be flushed (refer to Procedure guideline 6.15: Flushing externalized ureteric stents) (Leach 2015). The patient should have adaptors for the stents from the time of surgery to assist with flushing.

Carter double-barrelled wet colostomy

The Carter double-barrelled wet colostomy – commonly known as a Carter stoma or DBWC – is a specialist technique offered to patients having a total pelvic exenteration in some institutions. The procedure involves performing bipolar colostomy, with the section and sutured closure of the distal end of the colon at about 10–15 cm distal to the stoma, and implantation of ureters into the formed colon conduit. After the intervention, a urine reservoir, which is formed distal to the stoma, empties out freely without faecal contact (Pavlov et al. 2013) (Figure 6.30). The main advantage to the patient is managing just one stoma. A specialist bag is required to manage the mixed output (Figure 6.31).

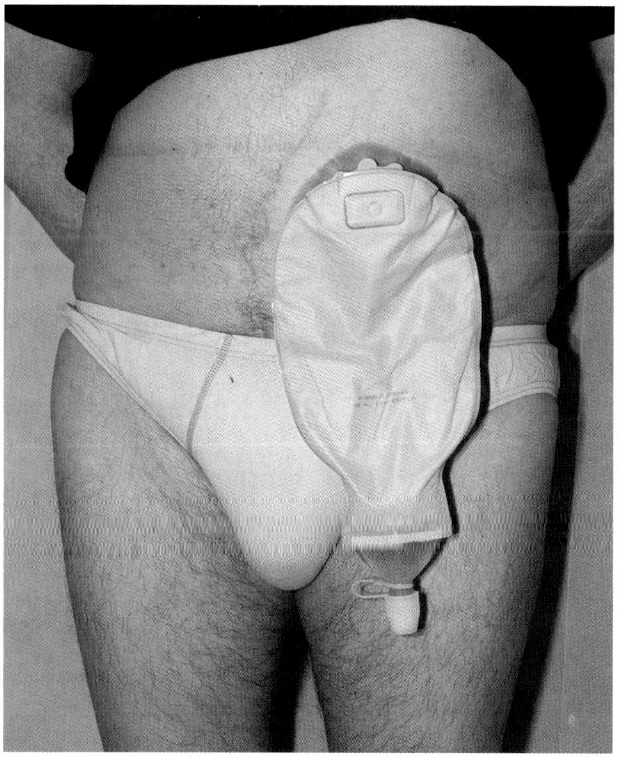

Figure 6.31 A patient wearing a specialist stoma product for the Carter stoma.

Evidence-based approaches

Stoma care has developed greatly over the years. Although an evidence base does exist, it mainly centres on clinical practice and experience (Davenport and Hayles 2018). There is a paucity of high-quality evidence (McPhail 2018). A limited number of randomized controlled trials of ostomy equipment (Berg and Seidler 2005, Colwell et al. 2018, Kelly et al. 2000, Moller Kruse and Storling 2015, Walker et al. 2016) provide information on evidence-based practice.

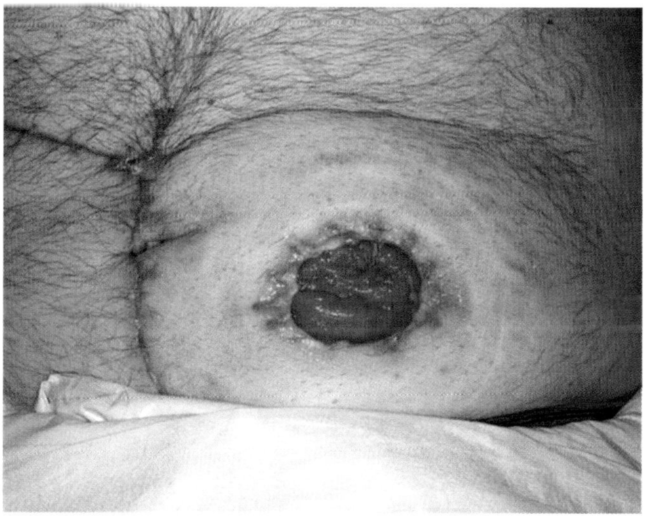

Figure 6.30 A newly formed Carter double-barrelled wet colostomy.

Stoma care is very individual and requires full holistic patient assessment. The primary aim is to promote patient independence by providing care and advice on managing the stoma, thereby allowing the patient, commonly known as the ostomate, to continue with all the necessary activities of daily living.

Rationale

Indications

Stoma care is essential:

- to collect faeces and/or urine in an appropriate appliance
- to achieve and maintain patient comfort and security
- to support psychological adaptation and independence.

Clinical governance

Stoma care is primarily based on experience. It is a fundamental area of nursing practice that all registered nurses should have the competence to undertake. It has been recognized that many of the core nursing skills in stoma care are being carried out by healthcare assistants and carers (Black 2011b, 2011c). Therefore, there is an increasing demand for education in this area. Due to the increasing demand for good, effective stoma care, many courses and conferences now exist to improve patient care and enhance professional knowledge and skills. The Association of Stoma Care Nurses (ASCN) UK has issued national clinical guidelines (ASCN 2016) recommending that pre-operative counselling and stoma siting should be undertaken by a clinical nurse specialist with appropriate stoma care qualifications. Each organization will have local arrangements for who should perform this function based on the local governance structure, but it is clear that training and competency assessment are essential.

Pre-procedural considerations

Equipment

The appliances that are now available vary in style, colour, skin barrier types and efficiency. Patients need to learn the principles of stoma care while they are inpatients, and sometimes before, to ensure they are able to manage independently with the stoma on discharge.

The aim of good stoma care is to empower patients to return to their normality. One of the ways in which this can be facilitated is to provide patients with a safe, reliable appliance. This means that there should be no fear of leakage or odour and the appliance should be comfortable, unobtrusive, easy to handle and disposable. The ostomate should be allowed a choice from the management systems available. It is also important to identify and manage problems with the stoma or peristomal skin at an early stage.

When choosing the appropriate management system for a new ostomate, factors that need to be considered include:

- type of stoma
- type of effluent
- allergies
- condition of the skin
- cognitive ability
- manual dexterity
- lifestyle
- condition of peristomal skin
- siting of stoma
- abdominal topography
- patient preference (Black 2015b).

Appliances

Stoma appliances (Figure 6.32) are made from an odour-proof plastic film. They adhere to the peristomal skin using an adhesive hydrocolloid base or flange (Williams 2011). Appliances may be opaque or clear and often have a soft backing to absorb perspiration. They usually have a built-in integral filter containing charcoal to neutralize any odour. The type of appliance used will depend on the type of stoma and the expected effluent. Refer to Figure 6.33 and Table 6.6 to assist with appliance selection.

Choosing the right size

It is important that the flange of the appliance fits snugly around the stoma (Black 2011a). The appliance must not rub on the stoma. Stoma appliances usually come with measuring guides to allow for choice of size. During the initial weeks following surgery, the oedematous stoma will gradually reduce in size and the appliance needs to be adapted accordingly, so a cut-to-fit pouch is used (Black 2011a). After this time a pre-cut pouch can be ordered.

Fear of malodour

As mentioned, colostomy and ileostomy appliances usually have a built-in integral filter containing charcoal to deodorize any odour when flatus is released. Therefore, smell should only be noticeable when emptying or changing an appliance, unless the pouch is not adhering correctly. There are also various deodorizers (which may be put into the pouch) and sprays (which can be sprayed into the air just before changing or emptying the pouch) (NHSBSA 2018a). The individual should be reassured that any problems with odour or leakage will be investigated and that in most circumstances the problem will be solved with alternative appliances and accessories, or modification of their technique.

Types of pouch

Drainable pouches

Drainable pouches are used when the effluent is fluid or semi-formed, in the case of an ileostomy or transverse colostomy (Figure 6.32c). These pouches have specially designed filters, which are less likely than other non-drainable pouches to become blocked or leak faecal fluid. They need to be emptied regularly and the outlet rinsed carefully and then the integral closure should be sealed; rarely, a clip may be used. They may be left on for up to 3 days depending on the skin barrier and the patient's preference.

Closed pouches

Closed pouches are mainly used when formed stool is expected, for example in the case of a sigmoid colostomy (Figure 6.32a). They have a flatus filter and need to be changed once or twice a day depending on output.

Urostomy pouches

Urostomy pouches have a drainage tap for urine and should be emptied regularly (Figure 6.32b). They can be attached to a large

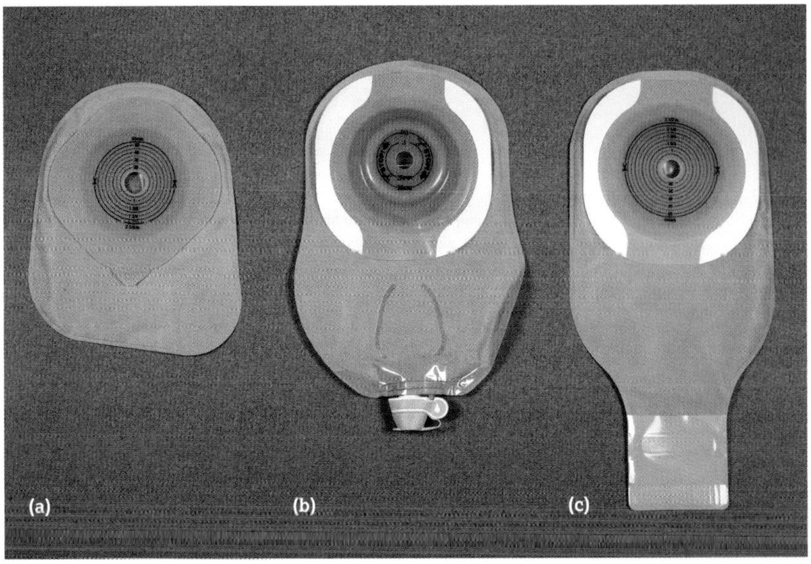

Figure 6.32 Examples of stoma pouches. (a) Closed pouch. (b) Urostomy pouch. (c) Drainable pouch.

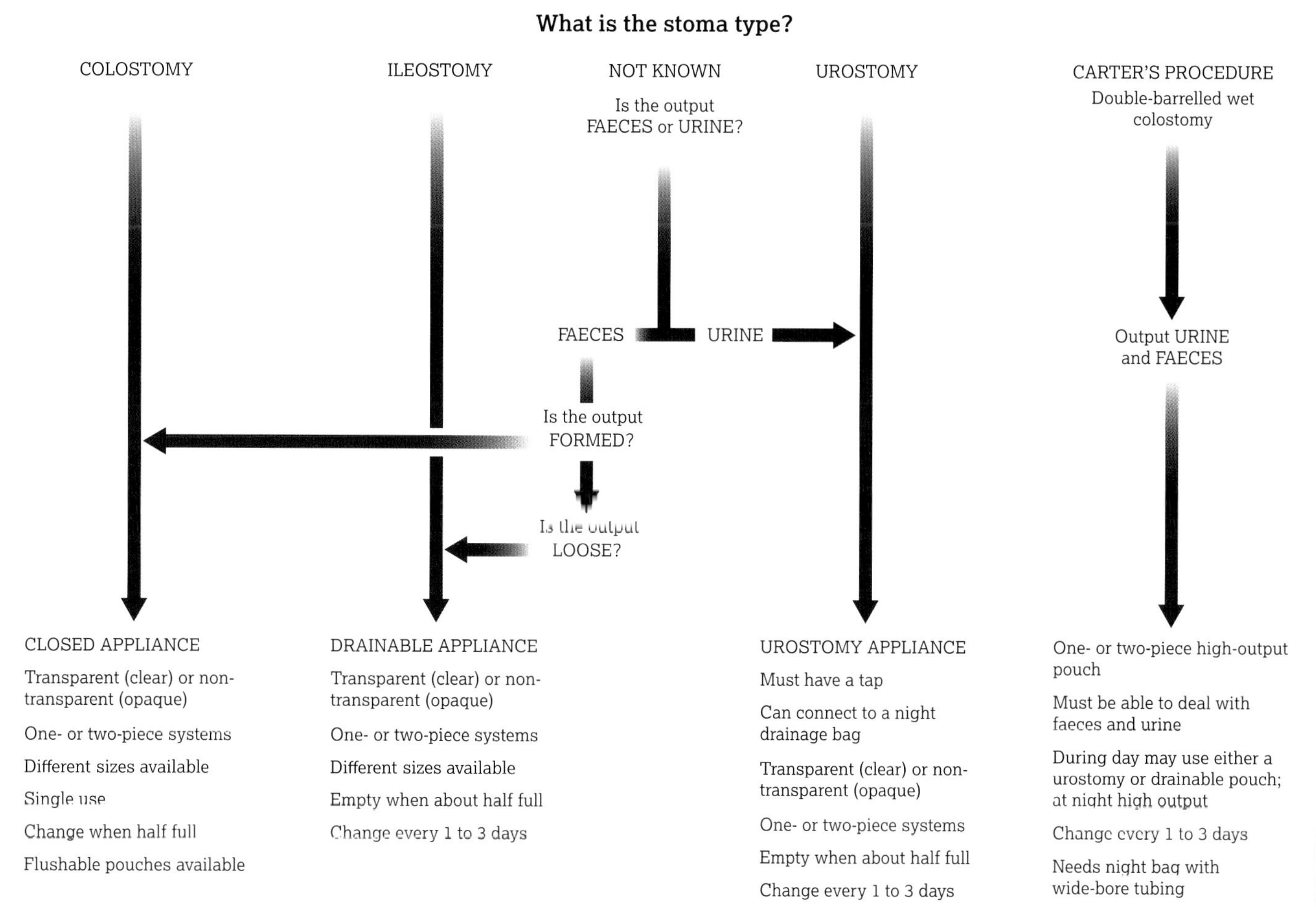

Figure 6.33 Flow chart for choosing appliances: International Ostomy Forum Group (2006) *Observation Index*. *Source*: Reproduced with permission of Dansac Ltd.

bag and tubing for night drainage. These pouches can remain on for up to 3 days, depending on the skin barrier and the patient's preference.

One- or two-piece systems

All types of pouch (closed, drainable or with a tap) fall into one of two broad categories: one-piece or two-piece systems (Burch 2011b). The prescription cost analysis data for 2017 (NHSBSA 2017) indicates that the majority of individuals with a stoma in the UK use a one-piece system. It also indicated that that this time there were 65,000 ileostomy patients, 43,000 colostomy patients and 12,000 people with a urostomy in the UK, giving a total population of people with a stoma of 120,000.

- *One-piece system*: this comprises a pouch that is already attached to an adhesive skin barrier. The barrier is removed completely when the pouch is changed. Compared to a two-piece system, this is an easier system for an ostomate with dexterity problems, such as arthritis or peripheral neuropathy, to handle.
- *Two-piece system*: this comprises a skin barrier onto which a pouch is clipped or stuck. It can be used with sore and sensitive skin because when the pouch is removed, the skin barrier is left intact and so the skin is left undisturbed.

Plug system

Patients with colostomies may be able to stop the effluent by inserting a plug into the stoma lumen. This plug swells in the moist environment and behaves as a seal so that faeces can be passed at a more convenient time (Burch 2011a, Durnal et al. 2011).

Solutions for skin and stoma cleaning

Warm water is sufficient for skin and stoma cleaning. All adhesive remover spray must be washed off as this may interfere with the pouch's adhesion. In addition, wet wipes are not recommended as they too can leave a residue on the skin and prevent the skin barrier from adhering. Detergents, disinfectants and antiseptics cause dryness and irritation and should not be used. The stoma is not a wound or a lesion and should be regarded as a resited urethra or anus.

See Table 6.7 for a summary of products used in managing problems associated with a stoma.

Deodorants

Aerosols

Aerosols are used to absorb or mask odour. One or two puffs are discharged into the air before emptying or removing the appliance. See the section on deodorants in the *Drug Tariff* (NHSBSA 2018a).

Drops

Drops are used to deodorize bag contents. Before fitting a pouch or after emptying and cleaning a drainable pouch, squeeze drops into the colostomy or drainable bag, not the urostomy bag.

Pre-procedural assessment and care

Pre-procedural care can be divided into two sections: physical and psychological.

Table 6.6 A summary of products used for problems associated with stoma (the examples shown are not the only products, it is recommended to review full availability on the latest edition of the *Drug Tariff*: NHSBSA 2019)

Accessory	Product example	Use	Precautions
Protective films	Skin protective barrier films in spray or wipe form (NHSBSA 2018c)	To prevent irritation and give protection	If contains alcohol, avoid use on broken skin
Protective wafers	Skin barrier in wafer form (NHSBSA 2018c)	To cover and protect skin	Allergies (rare)
Seals/washers/ barrier rings	See section in *Drug Tariff* (NHSBSA 2018d)	To provide skin protection around the stoma. Useful to fill gaps and dips in skin	Allergies (rare)
Caulking pastes	Stomahesive paste Adapt paste	To fill gaps and dips in skin and provide a smoother surface for applying the pouch, or to protect an area of dehiscence	If contains alcohol, avoid use on broken skin Should not be used as a solution to an ill-fitting pouch
Protective pastes	Orabase paste	To protect excoriated, painful peristomal skin	
Powders	Ostomy powders: see section in *Drug Tariff* (NHSBSA 2018c)	To dry any wet, moist areas to aid adhesion of the skin barrier	Can sometimes affect adherence Need to ensure that excess is removed
Adhesive preparations	See section in *Drug Tariff* (NHSBSA 2018d)	To improve adherence of the product	Should not be used as a solution to an ill-fitting pouch
Adhesive removers	Hollister Adapt Medical Adhesive Remover For more examples see *Drug Tariff* (NHSBSA 2018b)	To aid removal of the pouch if the patient is experiencing pain when the pouch is removed	Some contain alcohol and should not be used on broken skin Must not be used near naked flame (risk of burns)
Flange extenders (Black 2016)	Brava Elastic Tape Dansac X-tra Strips flange extenders	To improve patient security; useful for patients with parastomal hernias	Should not be used as a solution to an ill-fitting pouch or if the pouch is leaking
Thickening agents	Gel-X capsules, Ostosorb gel	To help solidify loose stoma output	If output is loose, cause should be investigated
Convex devices	Adapt Convex Ring	To prevent ostomy output from leaking under the pouch; particularly useful for retracted stomas	Bruising and ulceration may result if used incorrectly
Aerosol deodorants	LiMone FreshAire (NHSBSA 2018a)	To mask and absorb odour	Must not be used near a naked flame (risk of burns)
Drops	Nodor S Drops	To deodorize the bag contents	

Physical pre-procedural care

Physical care consists of surgical preparation, which can be in the form of bowel preparation, where patients are required to take laxatives to cleanse their bowel prior to surgery. This arguably improves surgical visibility and prevents contamination. This depends on the surgeon's preference and needs to be checked with the patient's surgical team on admission.

Many hospitals now carry out enhanced recovery programmes for colorectal patients. These involve intensive preparation preoperatively, where selected patients are required to take nutritional drinks and are given a pre-operative stoma pack to practice with a stoma model and pouches to develop their skills in changing a stoma bag. This improves recovery and management and consequently reduces the length of hospital stays.

Stoma siting is one of the most important elements of preoperative care (Leyk et al. 2018); the site of the stoma can have a huge impact on post-operative quality of life. Appropriate siting of a stoma minimizes future difficulties such as the stoma interfering with clothes, or skin problems caused by leakage of the appliance (Cronin 2012). Stoma siting should be carried out by a nurse who has been deemed competent to do so. For patients undergoing total pelvic exenteration leading to two stomas, care should be taken with the siting of both stomas (Hardy and McPhail 2018).

The use of accessory items should be limited to those that are key in assisting with skin health, skin barrier adhesion or leakage prevention. They should be suitable for the patient's condition (Black 2015b).

Patient assessment is necessary, taking into account:

- physical restrictions and disabilities
- psychological status
- visual impairment
- manual dexterity
- lifestyle
- occupation
- hobbies, leisure activities and sporting activities.

All these factors need to be carefully considered and discussed with the patient while siting the stoma. Patient involvement is important as it allows the patient control and enhances their ability to cope with a newly formed stoma.

Procedure guideline 6.25 Stoma siting

Essential equipment

- Personal protective equipment
- Stoma appliance
- Permanent marker pen
- Adhesive tape
- Clear dressing (check allergy status)
- Bed, trolley or couch to enable the patient to lie flat
- Chair to enable the patient to sit down

Action	Rationale
Pre-procedure	
1 Introduce yourself to the patient, explain and discuss the procedure with them, and gain their consent to proceed. Ensure they are aware that any mark made on their body is for guidance purposes only.	To ensure that the patient feels at ease, understands the procedure and gives their valid consent (NMC 2018, **C**). To familiarize the patient with the procedure. **E**
2 Draw curtains around the patient or close the door to ensure privacy.	To avoid unnecessary embarrassment and to promote dignified care (NMC 2018, **C**).
3 Wash hands thoroughly using soap and water or an alcohol-based handrub.	To prevent the spread of infection by contaminated hands (NHS England and NHSI 2019, **C**).
Procedure	
4 Ensure the patient is in a supine position with one pillow under their head. Ask the patient to lift their clothing to expose the abdomen.	In order to locate the rectus muscle and observe the characteristics and contours of the abdomen. **E**
5 Locate the rectus muscle. The muscle can be identified by asking the patient to raise their head. The muscle may also be palpated and easily felt when the patient coughs.	Placing the stoma in the rectus muscle reduces the risk of peristomal herniation and prolapse (Leyk et al. 2018, **E**).
6 Identify a flat area of skin on the abdomen, as this facilitates safe adhesion of the appliance. Avoid siting on bony prominences, skinfolds, the waistline or belt areas.	Avoiding skin creases, especially in the region of the groin or umbilicus, will help to prevent urine or faecal matter tracking along the skin creases, causing leaks. This also helps the patient to visualize the stoma more easily. Restrictive clothing, such as belts, over the site may lead to unnecessary pressure and leaks or trauma to the stoma. **E**
7 Imagine a line running from the umbilicus to the top of the pelvic bone on the appropriate side. Place a piece of tape on the midpoint of this line or at the closest point to it on a flat piece of skin. Mark the tape with an 'X'.	This initial marking is used to assess the suitability of the site when the patient is sitting, walking, bending and moving (Leyk et al. 2018, **E**).
8 Allow the patient to sit up and move around as much as possible to reassess the positioning. Encourage the patient to carry out movements or activities that are associated with their occupation or hobbies. Ensure the patient can see the site.	This will help to determine the most appropriate site for the patient. **E**
9 Secure an appliance to the temporary site and encourage the patient to spend some time wearing the appliance. Where possible, ensure the position allows the patient to view the stoma site and appliance sufficiently.	Correct positioning will enable self-care of the stoma and post-operative rehabilitation (Leyk et al. 2018, **E**).
10 Once both the nurse and the patient are satisfied with the site, use a permanent marker pen to indicate the site. Cover this mark with a film dressing.	To ensure the stoma site remains clearly marked until the time of surgery (Leyk et al. 2018, **E**).
Post-procedure	
11 Wash hands thoroughly using soap and water or an alcohol-based handrub.	To prevent the spread of infection by contaminated hands (NHS England and NHSI 2019, **C**).
12 Document your actions and report them to the appropriate members of the multidisciplinary team.	To ensure continuity of care and maintain accurate records (NMC 2018, **C**).

Psychological pre-procedural care

Psychological preparation of individuals facing stoma surgery should begin as soon as surgery is considered, preferably by using the skills of a trained stoma care nurse. It is important that the information and discussions are tailored to the individual's needs, taking into account their level of anxiety and distress (Di Gesaro 2016).

It is important that patients meet all members of the multidisciplinary team who are involved in their care and that they fully understand the need for the stoma surgery. This needs to be explained in order to obtain informed consent. It is beneficial if the patient is met in pre-assessment or at home prior to surgery to discuss the implications of stoma care and the patient's own role in rehabilitation. At this point it is also helpful to provide the patient with written information, audio visual information (if available), access to self-help support groups, and access to peer support including the chance to speak or meet with an experienced ostomate.

Stoma counselling is ideally carried out by the specialist stoma care nurse involved in the patient's care, but all nurses involved in the care of patients undergoing a stoma should be aware of the impact of having a stoma on:

- body image
- family relationships
- sexual relationships
- depression and anger
- fears and concerns.

It is often beneficial to provide patients with some patient information or literature to take home. This gives them an opportunity to digest the information and write down any questions that they have. There are many different aids available, such as information booklets, samples of various products, diagrams, audio-visual information, stoma pre-operative packs and websites. These help to reinforce and clarify the verbal information given to the patient.

Specific patient preparation

Education

Patients undergoing stoma formation have to make major physical and psychological adjustments following surgery. If the surgery is elective, patient education should begin in the pre-operative period (Cronin 2012, Wallace 2016). Adequate pre- and post-operative support is mandatory to maintain quality of life for stoma patients (Metcalf 2017). Individual holistic patient assessment is key as it is important to identify appropriate teaching strategies for each patient. One of the most important ways in which a nurse can support the patient is to teach them stoma care, ensuring independence before discharge (ASCN 2016, Burch 2011a). It is important that the patient is able to independently change their stoma bag, recognize problems, and obtain support and supplies once they have been discharged home. Providing patients with adequate information and input helps to promote patient decision making by allowing them control (ASCN 2016, Black 2011a).

All healthcare professionals are required to wear disposable gloves and an apron when changing an appliance, and this practice should be explained to patients so that they do not feel it is just because they have a stoma that these precautions are being taken (Cronin 2012).

Procedure guideline 6.26 Stoma bag change

This procedure may also be applied when teaching a patient how to care for their stoma.

Essential equipment

- Personal protective equipment
- Dry wipes
- New appliance
- Measuring device or template
- Scissors
- Disposal bags for used appliances and wipes
- Adhesive remover spray
- Other relevant accessories, for example protective film, and seals and washers
- Bowl of warm water
- Gauze
- Jug or receiver for contents of appliance
- Protection for bed or patient's clothing

Action	Rationale
Pre-procedure	
1 Introduce yourself to the patient, explain and discuss the procedure with them, and gain their consent to proceed.	To ensure that the patient feels at ease, understands the procedure and gives their valid consent (NMC 2018, **C**).
2 Ensure that the patient is in a suitable and comfortable position where they will be able to watch the procedure, if well enough. A mirror may be used to aid visualization.	To allow good access to the stoma for cleaning and for secure application of the stoma bag. The patient will become familiar with the stoma and will also learn about the care of the stoma by observing the nurse. **E**
3 Use a small protective pad to protect the patient's clothing from drips if the effluent is fluid.	To avoid the necessity of changing clothing or bedclothes and to avoid demoralization of the patient as a result of soiling. **E**
4 Wash hands with soap and water and/or an alcohol-based handrub. Apply personal protective equipment: non-sterile gloves and a plastic apron.	To reduce the risk of cross-infection (NHS England and NHSI 2019, **C**).
Procedure	
5 If the bag is of the drainable type, empty the contents into a jug before removing the bag.	For ease of handling the appliance and prevention of spillage. **E**
6 Remove the appliance slowly using an adhesive remover. Peel the adhesive off the skin with one hand while exerting gentle pressure on the skin with the other.	To reduce trauma to the skin (Burch 2011b, **C**).
7 Fold the appliance in two to ensure there is no spillage and place it in a disposal bag.	To ensure safe disposal according to environmental policy (DEFRA 2005, **C**).
8 Remove excess faeces or mucus from the stoma with a piece of gauze soaked in tap water.	So that the stoma and surrounding skin are clearly visible. **E**

9 Examine the skin and stoma for soreness, ulceration and other unusual phenomena. If the skin is unblemished and the stoma is a healthy red colour, proceed. Report any abnormalities to the stoma care nurse or surgical team.	To identify complications or to treat existing problems. **E**
10 Wash the peristomal skin and stoma gently with gauze soaked in warm water until they are clean.	To promote cleanliness and prevent skin excoriation. **E**
11 Dry the peristomal skin gently but thoroughly.	Because the appliance will only attach securely to dry skin. **E**
12 Measure the stoma and cut appliance, leaving 3 mm clearance. Apply a clean appliance.	The appliance should provide skin protection. The aperture should be cut just a little larger than the stoma so that effluent cannot cause skin damage, but it should not touch the stoma (Kirkwood 2006, **C**).
Post-procedure	
13 Dispose of soiled tissues, the used appliance, gloves and apron as per local policy.	To ensure safe disposal. **E**
14 Wash hands thoroughly using soap and water or an alcohol-based handrub.	To prevent the spread of infection by contaminated hands (NHS England and NHSI 2019, **C**).

Procedure guideline 6.27 Obtaining a clean-catch urine sample from an ileal conduit

Essential equipment

- Personal protective equipment
- Dry wipes
- New appliance
- Measuring device or template
- Scissors
- Disposal bags for used appliances and wipes
- Adhesive remover spray
- Other relevant accessories, for example protective film, and seals and washers
- Bowl of warm water
- Jug or receiver for contents of appliance
- Protection for bed or patient's clothing
- Sample pot

Action	Rationale
Pre-procedure	
1 Introduce yourself to the patient, explain and discuss the procedure with them, and gain their consent to proceed.	To ensure that the patient feels at ease, understands the procedure and gives their valid consent (NMC 2018, **C**).
2 Ensure that the patient is in a suitable and comfortable position where they will be able to watch the procedure, if well enough. A mirror may be used to aid visualization.	To allow good access to the stoma for cleaning and for secure application of the stoma bag. The patient will become familiar with the stoma and will also learn about the care of the stoma by observing the nurse. **E**
3 Use a small protective pad to protect the patient's clothing from drips if the effluent is fluid.	To avoid the necessity of changing clothing or bedclothes and to avoid demoralization of the patient as a result of soiling. **E**
4 Wash hands with soap and water and/or an alcohol-based handrub. Apply personal protective equipment: non-sterile gloves and a plastic apron.	To reduce the risk of cross-infection (NHS England and NHSI 2019, **C**).
Procedure	
5 Empty the contents of the pouch into a jug before removing the bag.	For ease of handling the appliance and prevention of spillage. **E**
6 Remove the appliance slowly using an adhesive remover. Peel the adhesive off the skin with one hand while exerting gentle pressure on the skin with the other.	To reduce trauma to the skin (Burch 2011b, **C**).
7 Fold the appliance in two to ensure there is no spillage and place it in a disposal bag.	To ensure safe disposal according to environmental policy (DEFRA 2005, **C**).
8 Examine the skin and stoma for soreness, ulceration and other unusual phenomena. If the skin is unblemished and the stoma is a healthy red colour, proceed. Report any abnormalities to the stoma care nurse or surgical team.	To identify complications or to treat existing problems. **E**
9 Wash the peristomal skin and stoma gently with gauze soaked in warm water until they are clean.	To promote cleanliness and prevent skin excoriation. **E**
10 Take the sample pot and place it below the ileal conduit to allow urine to drip directly into the pot.	To obtain urine from the conduit for sampling. **E**

(continued)

Procedure guideline 6.27 Obtaining a clean catch urine sample from an ileal conduit *(continued)*

Action	Rationale
11 Dry the peristomal skin gently but thoroughly.	The appliance will only attach securely to dry skin. E
12 Measure the stoma and cut appliance, leaving 3 mm clearance. Apply a clean appliance.	The appliance should provide skin protection. The aperture should be cut just a little larger than the stoma so that effluent cannot cause skin damage (Kirkwood 2006, **C**).
Post-procedure	
13 Dispose of soiled tissues, the used appliance, gloves and apron as per local policy	To ensure safe disposal. **E**
14 Wash hands thoroughly using soap and water or an alcohol-based handrub.	To prevent the spread of infection by contaminated hands (NHS England and NHSI 2019, **C**).
15 At the patient's bedside, clearly label the sample pot and place it inside the request form.	To ensure the correct patient's details are entered. **E**

Procedure guideline 6.28 Stoma bridge or rod removal

Essential equipment

- Personal protective equipment
- Dry wipes
- New appliances
- Disposal bags for used appliances and wipes
- Adhesive remover spray
- Relevant accessories, for example belt and washers
- Bowl of warm water
- Jug for contents of appliance
- Gauze
- Protection for bed or patient's clothing

Action	Rationale
Pre-procedure	
1 Introduce yourself to the patient, explain and discuss the procedure with them, and gain their consent to proceed.	To ensure that the patient feels at ease, understands the procedure and gives their valid consent (NMC 2018, **C**).
2 Ensure the patient is in a suitable and comfortable position.	To allow good access to the stoma for cleaning and for secure application of the stoma bag. **E**
3 Wash hands with soap and water and/or an alcohol-based handrub. Apply personal protective equipment.	To reduce the risk of cross-infection (NHS England and NHSI 2019, **C**).
4 If the bag is of the drainable type, empty the contents into a jug before removing the bag.	For ease of handling the appliance and prevention of spillage. **E**
Procedure	
5 Remove the appliance. Gently peel the adhesive off the skin using an adhesive remover spray.	To reduce trauma to the skin (Burch 2011a, 2011b, **C**).
6 Remove excess faeces or mucus from the stoma and bridge with a piece of gauze soaked in tap water.	So that the stoma and surrounding skin are clearly visible. **E**
7 If using the **Convatec bridge**, slide the bridge gently to one side to ensure the mobile wing of the bridge is away from the stoma. Turn this wing so that it becomes flush with the bridge. Gently slide the bridge through the stoma loop.	To prepare the bridge for removal. **E**
8 If using the **Coloplast bridge**, slide the bridge gently to one side to ensure that the end that folds back off the bridge is away from the stoma. Fold back the end of the bridge. Gently slide the bridge through the stoma loop (see **Action figure 8**).	To prepare the bridge for removal. **E**
9 Examine the skin and stoma for soreness, ulceration and other unusual phenomena. If the skin is unblemished and the stoma is a healthy red colour, proceed. Also note if the stoma retracts once the bridge is removed.	To prevent complications or treat existing problems. **E**
10 Wash the skin and stoma gently with gauze soaked in warm water until they are clean.	To promote cleanliness and prevent skin excoriation. **E**

11	Dry the skin gently but thoroughly.	The appliance will only attach securely to dry skin. **E**
12	If the skin is red and/or broken, apply barrier film and notify the stoma care nurse. If the stoma is not a healthy red colour, inform the medical and/or stoma care nurse.	To promote skin healing. **E**
13	Apply a clean appliance.	To contain effluent from the stoma. **E**
Post-procedure		
14	Dispose of soiled wipes, the bridge, the used appliance, gloves and apron.	To prevent environmental contamination. **E**
15	Wash hands with soap and water or an alcohol-based handrub.	To reduce the risk of cross-infection (NHS England and NHSI 2019, **C**).

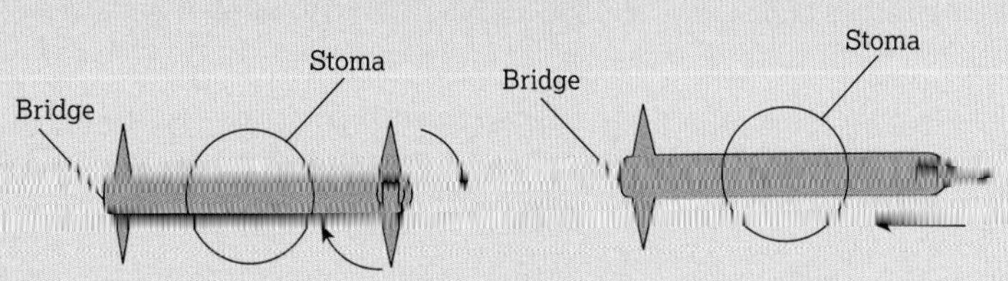

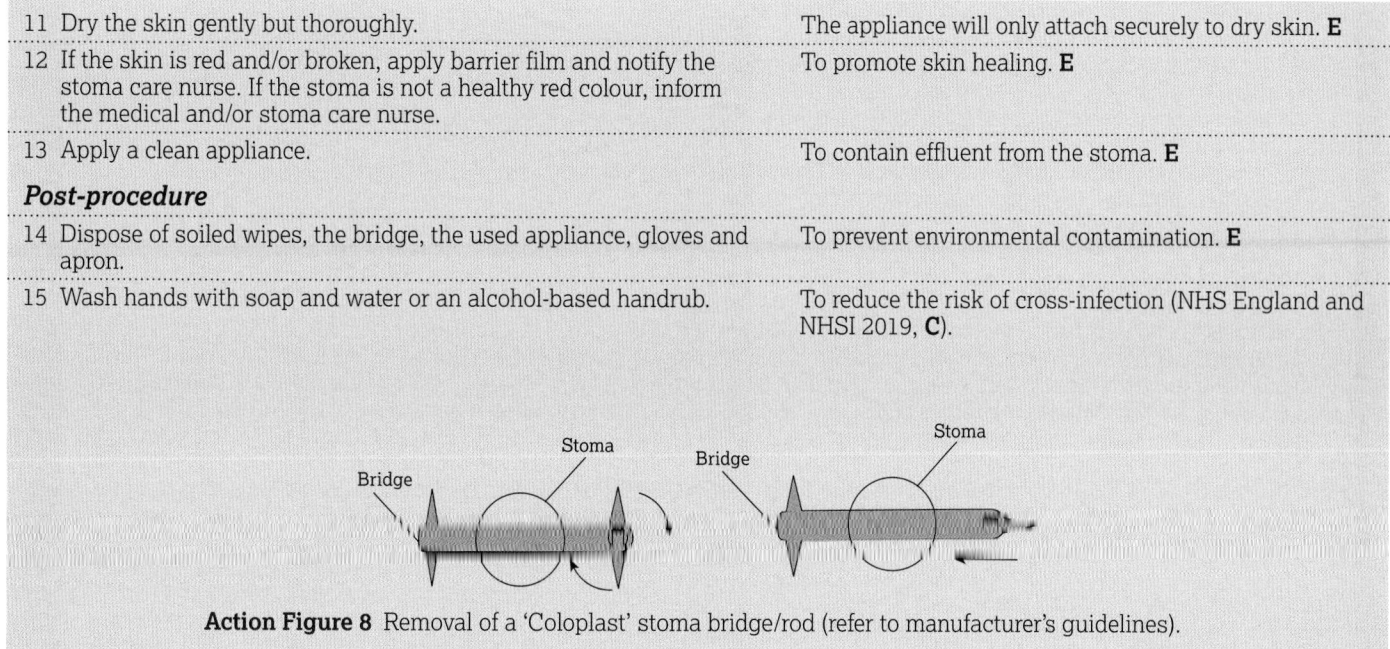

Action Figure 8 Removal of a 'Coloplast' stoma bridge/rod (refer to manufacturer's guidelines).

Post-procedural considerations

Initial and ongoing care

Post-operative stoma care

In theatre, an appropriately sized transparent drainable appliance should be applied. This should be left on for approximately 2 days. For the first 48 hours post-operatively, the stoma should be observed for signs of ischaemia or necrosis, and stoma colour (a pink and healthy appearance indicates a good blood supply), size and output should be noted, as should the presence of any devices, such as ureteric stents or a bridge with a loop stoma (Boyles and Hunt 2016).

Table 6.7 recommends the most appropriate bag type to use on each type of stoma and the expected output. The drainable appliance should always be emptied frequently and gas should be filtered out of the pouch via the filter; however, if gas builds up, allow it to be emptied from the pouch to prevent ballooning. The appliance should not be allowed to get more than half full with effluent. If the appliance becomes too full, leaks may occur and the weight from the effluent or the pressure from gas may cause the appliance to fall off. A leak-proof, odour-resistant, well-fitted appliance does much to promote patient confidence at this time (Black 2015b).

The first time a bowel stoma acts, the type, appearance, quantity and consistency of the matter passed should be recorded; this includes any flatus that may be passed (Black 2011a).

Immediately post-operatively, patients should not be expected to perform their own stoma care. However, if appropriate, teaching begun pre-operatively can be put into practice within the first 24–48 hours following surgery. During appliance changes, observations should be made of the following:

- *Stoma*: colour, size and general appearance: oedematous, flush with abdomen or retracted.
- *Peristomal skin*: presence of any erythema, broken areas, rashes, pain or itchiness.
- *Stoma/skin margin (mucocutaneous margin)*: sutures intact, tension on sutures and separation of stoma edge from skin (mucocutaneous separation).

Any abnormalities should be reported to the stoma care nurse and medical staff (Black 2011b). Viewing the stoma may be difficult for the patient, who may be very aware of other people's reactions to it. The patient's reaction to their stoma should be observed and recorded.

Table 6.7 Decision tool to use when selecting an appropriate bag or pouch

Type of stoma	Expected post-operative output	Recommended bag to be used	Expected stoma output on discharge	Recommended bag to be used on discharge
Colostomy	Haemoserous fluid Flatus Liquid or loose stool	Clear drainable bag	Soft formed stool: bowel action one to three times a day	Closed opaque bag with viewing option
Ileostomy	Haemoserous fluid Liquid or loose stool Flatus	Clear drainable bag	Loose stool: approximately >600 mL per day	Opaque drainable bag with viewing option
Urostomy	Urine and mucus	Two-piece clear urostomy bag with tap	Urine: 0.5 mL/kg/h	Clear or opaque urostomy bag with tap, plus a urostomy night bag
Double-barrelled wet colostomy	Urine, mucus and faecal output	Two-piece system with a high-output pouch, or a urostomy pouch	First few days urine only, then soft stool with the urine	One- or two-piece beige pouch with viewing option, plus a high-output night bag

Source: Adapted from Adams et al. (2012).

Colostomy function

Typically in the first few days, a sigmoid colostomy will produce haemoserous fluid and flatus. By day 5 there should be some faecal fluid and then by day 7–14 some semi-formed stool. A closed appliance can be used once the output has thickened up. Rarely, a stoma may be formed in the transverse colon, usually as a result of an emergency procedure (Cronin 2012), and in such cases only a small amount of water will be reabsorbed from the faecal matter, so the stool will be less formed. Therefore, a drainable pouch will be required.

Patients with a sigmoid colostomy (ostomates) should generally be advised to have a balanced and mixed diet. To avoid constipation, ostomates are advised to take adequate oral fluids and fibre in the form of five portions of fruit and vegetables per day (Burch 2011c). If either constipation or loose stool is a problem, then dietary intake should be reviewed. Ostomates may find that their colostomy is usually active at particular times of the day, but ultimately the only means of gaining control with a sigmoid colostomy is by using a plug system or by regular irrigation. Stoma care nurses will need to assess patients for their suitability for using either a plug system or irrigation. The patient's consultant must approve of irrigation for the patient.

Ileostomy function

Typically, for the first few days, the stoma will produce haemoserous fluid and flatus. By days 5–10 there will be brown faecal matter. The fluid output after surgery can be as much as 1500 mL every 24 hours but this should gradually reduce to 500–850 mL every 24 hours as the bowel settles down (Black 2016). It is important that fluid balance recordings are made and serum electrolytes are measured as patients are at risk of sodium, potassium and/or magnesium depletion (Goodey and Colman 2016). Sometimes the output from a stoma remains high (>1000 mL every 24 hours), which may be due to the amount of small bowel removed during surgery or an underlying bowel condition; these patients require careful management. Patients who continue to have a high output from their stoma may need to be managed by specialist teams that include gastroenterologists, dietitians and stoma care nurses in order to provide ongoing support (Slater 2012).

The effluent from an ileostomy takes on a porridge-like consistency when a normal intake of food is established (Burch 2011c). A drainable appliance is therefore used. The effluent contains enzymes, which will excoriate the skin (Burch 2011b); therefore, if the pouch leaks, it must be changed promptly to prevent skin breakdown. The effluent cannot be controlled but may vary throughout the day. Patients with ileostomies often find that the output is thicker first thing in the morning and after meals, or the output is looser with reduced dietary intake (Burch 2011c). Output can vary between watery, loose and soft stool depending on the time of day and what the patient has eaten. Sometimes medication that reduces peristaltic action, for example codeine or loperamide, may be used to control excessive watery output. If using loperamide, this should be taken half an hour to an hour before food in order to achieve an optimal effect.

Urostomy or ileal conduit function

Urine will dribble from the stoma every 20–30 seconds and it will start to drain immediately. Normal output is 1500–2000 mL every 24 hours but it may be less after periods of reduced fluid intake, for example at night. Urinary stents (fine-bore catheters) may be in place, from the ureters past the anastomosis and out of the stoma. They are placed to maintain patency and protect the suturing until primary healing is completed (Geng et al. 2009, Leach 2015). Stents usually remain *in situ* for 7–14 days depending on the surgeon and patient factors such as condition of the stoma, previous radiotherapy and renal function.

Body image

Stoma formation creates many issues for patients and many struggle with body image. Studies suggest that this is often overlooked (Wallace 2016). The circumstances in which the stoma is formed will influence psychological recovery (Di Gesaro 2016). Communication is key and it is important to allow the patient and their family to discuss their concerns and anxieties. Therefore, stoma care nurses play a vital role in supporting the patient and their family. It is important to promote patient independence and acceptance.

Diet

Initially, all patients will start with sips of water, then move on to free fluids, and then to a light diet. In the absence of nausea and vomiting, they can proceed with building up their dietary intake. Colostomists and urostomists should be encouraged to eat a wide variety of foods and drink 1.5–2 L of fluids each day. People's digestive systems react in individual ways to different foods and so it is important that patients try a wide range of foods on several occasions and that none should be specifically avoided (Burch 2011c). Patients can then make decisions about different foods based on their own experiences. Explanations should be given of how the gut functions, how it has been changed since surgery and the effects certain foodstuffs may cause.

However, patients with an ileostomy should use caution with foods that will increase output as these may cause a high-output stoma. A person with an ileostomy should also be aware of what to do if the output is watery for longer than 24 hours (Goodey and Colman 2016). The normal output from an ileostomy should be toothpaste-like or porridge-like in consistency and the patient should empty the pouch approximately six to eight times a day (approximately 600–800 mL in 24 hours) (Cronin 2013). If the patient has watery stool for over 12 hours, they should consider increasing the amount of starch in their diet, such as white bread, white pasta, white rice, noodles and potatoes. They should avoid fibre, and in particular they should reduce their intake of fruit (including fruit juice) and green leafy vegetables. In addition, they can stagger eating and drinking so that they are not doing both at the same time, spacing them at least half an hour apart (Goodey and Colman 2016).

The patient should have been prescribed some medication to reduce diarrhoea, such as loperamide. They should take this in accordance with instructions from their prescriber. Loperamide needs to be taken half an hour before each meal to slow the bowel down (Goodey and Colman 2016).

If a person with an ileostomy has had a watery output for more than 24 hours or consistently has a watery output, they should contact their stoma care nurse or doctor. They must be aware of the symptoms of dehydration, such as headaches, dizziness, thirst, reduced and darker-coloured urine, cramps and tingling in the hands (Goodey and Colman 2016). Patients may be at risk of acute kidney injury if the dehydration continues. In particular, their electrolytes (sodium, potassium and magnesium) are likely to be outside normal parameters.

An ileostomy patient can help to rehydrate themselves by making up a rehydration solution (Box 6.5) and drink a litre of this during the course of 24 hours. They should reduce their intake of tea and coffee and not take any fizzy drinks (Goodey and Colman 2016).

Box 6.5 An example of an oral rehydration solution: St Mark's rehydration solution

- 6 level teaspoons (5 mL spoonfuls) or 20 g of glucose powder
- Half a teaspoon (2.5 mL) or 2.5 g of sodium bicarbonate
- 1 level teaspoon (5 mL spoonful) or 3.5 g of salt
- 1 L of tap water

The patient may add squash or cordial to flavour the solution.

Source: Cronin (2013), Goodey and Colman (2016).

Patients with colostomy or ileostomy formation do not have the same control as with an anal sphincter, so passage of wind cannot be controlled. High-fibre foods such as beans and pulses produce wind as they are broken down in the gut; hence, individuals who eat large quantities of these foodstuffs may be troubled by wind. There are several non-food causes of wind, such as chewing gum, eating irregularly and drinking fizzy drinks, and these should be considered before blaming a particular food. Eating yoghurt or drinking buttermilk may help to reduce wind for these patients. Green vegetables, pulses and spicy food are examples of foods that may cause colostomy and ileostomy output to increase or become watery. Boiled rice, smooth peanut butter, apple sauce and bananas are some of the foods that may help to thicken stoma output (Black 2000, Burch 2011c).

Some foods, for example tomato skin and pips, may be seen unaltered in the output from an ileostomy. Celery, dried fruit, nuts, fibrous fruit (such as mango) and potato skins are some of the foods that can temporarily block ileostomies (Burch 2011c). The blockage is usually related to the amount eaten and the offending food can be tried at another time in small quantities, ensuring it is chewed well and not eaten in a hurry.

There are no dietary restrictions with a urostomy, although bowel activity may be temporarily affected if a portion of the ileum has been used for the stoma. It must be stressed, however, that an adequate fluid intake must be maintained to minimize the risk of urinary tract infection due to a shortened urinary tract. The recommended fluid intake for all individuals is 1.5–2 L per day (Burch 2011c). Fluid intake should be increased in hot weather and at times when there is an increase in sweating, for example with exercise or fever. Patients should be made aware of certain foods that may cause a change to the usual character of the urine. For example, beetroot, radishes, spinach and some food dyes may discolour urine; some drugs may also have this effect, for example metronidazole and nitrofurantoin. Similarly, following consumption of asparagus or fish, urine may develop a strong odour.

Fear of malodour

This is a common fear for patients with bowel stomas, often based on hearsay or experience with other ostomates in hospital or the community. Appliances are odour free when fitted correctly. Flatus may be released via charcoal filters, and deodorizers are available. The individual must be reassured, however, that any problems that occur post-operatively will be investigated, with a good possibility of their being solved by such means as the use of alternative appliances (Black 2016).

Sex and the ostomate

The possibility of sexual impairment for both men and women after stoma surgery depends on the nature of the operation and the ensuing damage to the nerves and tissues involved. The psychological impact of the surgery and its effect on the individual's body image must also be taken into consideration. Surgery that results in physical sexual disability will have psychological repercussions, while some sexual difficulties may be of psychological origin (Humphreys 2017, Reese et al. 2014, Williams 2012). Impairment may be permanent or temporary. In the latter case, resolution of the difficulty may take anywhere up to 2 years. Pre- and post-operative counselling should be offered for both patient and partner.

All patients may experience loss of libido and sexual desire. Females having cystectomy for cancer will in most cases require anterior exenteration and vaginal reconstruction. This includes removal of the urethra and a vaginal reconstruction, which affects both vaginal length and blood supply to the vagina and clitoris. Consequent sexual dysfunction occurs and patients must be counselled accordingly in the pre-operative period (Zippe et al. 2004). In males, ejaculatory disturbances occur following cystectomy so men facing this surgery should be offered sperm banking prior to surgery. Erectile dysfunction is a common complication of all pelvic surgery and there are a number of treatment options available. These include oral medications, such as phosphodiesterase type 5 inhibitors (PD5 inhibitors), sublingual apomorphine, intraurethral and intracavernosal injections, vacuum devices and penile implants (Broholm et al. 2014, Geng et al. 2010, NHSBSA 2018e, Park et al. 2015). Patients with persistent erectile dysfunction should be referred for penile rehabilitation.

Female sexual dysfunction after colorectal and pelvic surgery is common (Bregendahl et al. 2015, Burch 2016). Typically, a loss of libido and satisfaction occurs. Female patients may experience dyspareunia; this may be due to narrowing or shortening of the vagina, a reduction in the volume of vaginal secretions or changes in genital sensations (Reese et al. 2014). The use of a lubricant, adopting different positions during penetrative intercourse or encouraging greater relaxation by extending foreplay may help to resolve painful intercourse (Humphreys 2017).

Planning for discharge

Discharge planning for a patient with a stoma should commence once the patient is admitted. It is important to set a provisional discharge date and set realistic goals with the patient. Prior to discharge, ideally the patient should have returned to their prior level of independence, be eating a normal diet and be competent in stoma care. Family or close friends are likely to require support and information so that they are in a position to help the ostomate and this should be provided as much as possible before discharge. If family or close friends are involved during all stages of stoma surgery, and patients are well informed, patients are better able to adapt to life with a stoma (ASCN 2016, Cronin 2012).

Acceptance of the stoma is a gradual process and, on discharge from hospital, patients may only be beginning to adapt to life with a stoma. Indeed, in a survey of 100 patients following stoma formation, 56% felt that support was needed for the first 6 months, indicating the ongoing need for professional advice and support for a substantial amount of time after stoma surgery (Wallace 2016). Continuity of care for these patients is crucial. Effective communication and collaboration between healthcare professionals are key to psychological adaptation and successful rehabilitation (Borwell 2009, Di Gesaro 2016). See Figure 6.34 for an example of a discharge checklist.

Follow-up support

Patients should be discharged home with:

- 2 weeks of stoma supplies
- contact details of the community stoma care nurse
- prescription details of the products being used
- information on the delivery company, if relevant (ASCN 2016).

Patients should be discharged with enough stoma products to last until a prescription is obtained from their GP. Written reminders should also be provided on how to care for the stoma, how to obtain supplies of appliances and any other information that may be required. Patients should have the details of non-medical stoma clinics, details about the relevant agencies and information about voluntary associations. Arrangements should also be made for a home visit from the stoma care nurse and/or the community nurse (Davenport 2014). Figure 6.34 provides an example of a discharge checklist. Patients should then have annual reviews to ensure that the product remains suitable for them (Black 2015b, Davenport 2014).

Obtaining supplies

All NHS patients with a permanent stoma or cancer are entitled to free prescriptions for their stoma care products, and should complete the relevant forms for exemption from payment. Appliances can then be obtained from the local chemist or free home delivery services.

The ROYAL MARSDEN
NHS Foundation Trust

Stoma Care Discharge Letter

Please write details or affix label

Name: Address:	GP: Address:
Post code Telephone No:	Post code Telephone No:
Date of Birth:	Next of Kin:

Diagnosis:	
Previous Medical History :	
Operation:	
Date of Operation:	
Type of Stoma:	
Admission Date:	Discharge Date:

Appliance Details: *Please include; Manufacturer, Product name, Order code and quantity given/ordered (details can be found on the product box or on the appliance itself)*
Delivery Arrangements:
Additional Information: *(i.e. is patient self caring; sutures in-situ; peristomal skin condition; current bowel action, any significant information relating to stoma care capabilities)*

Community Stoma Care Nurse:		Telephone No: Fax No:
Form Completed By: *(Please print)*	Signature:	
Ward:	Telephone No:	Date:
Stoma Care Nurse :	Telephone No:	

Figure 6.34 An example of a stoma discharge checklist. *Source*: Reproduced with permission of The Royal Marsden.

Complications

As a healthcare professional providing support and care to stoma patients, it is important to be able to distinguish normal from abnormal. The observational index (Figure 6.35) provides a reference guide to use when observing, recording and reporting the condition of a stoma. If any of the complications are noted, it is important to ensure that the medical team and/or stoma care nurse is informed. Advice on how to manage these problems should be obtained from a specialist stoma care nurse. Early recognition of problems and complications can prevent more serious complications later.

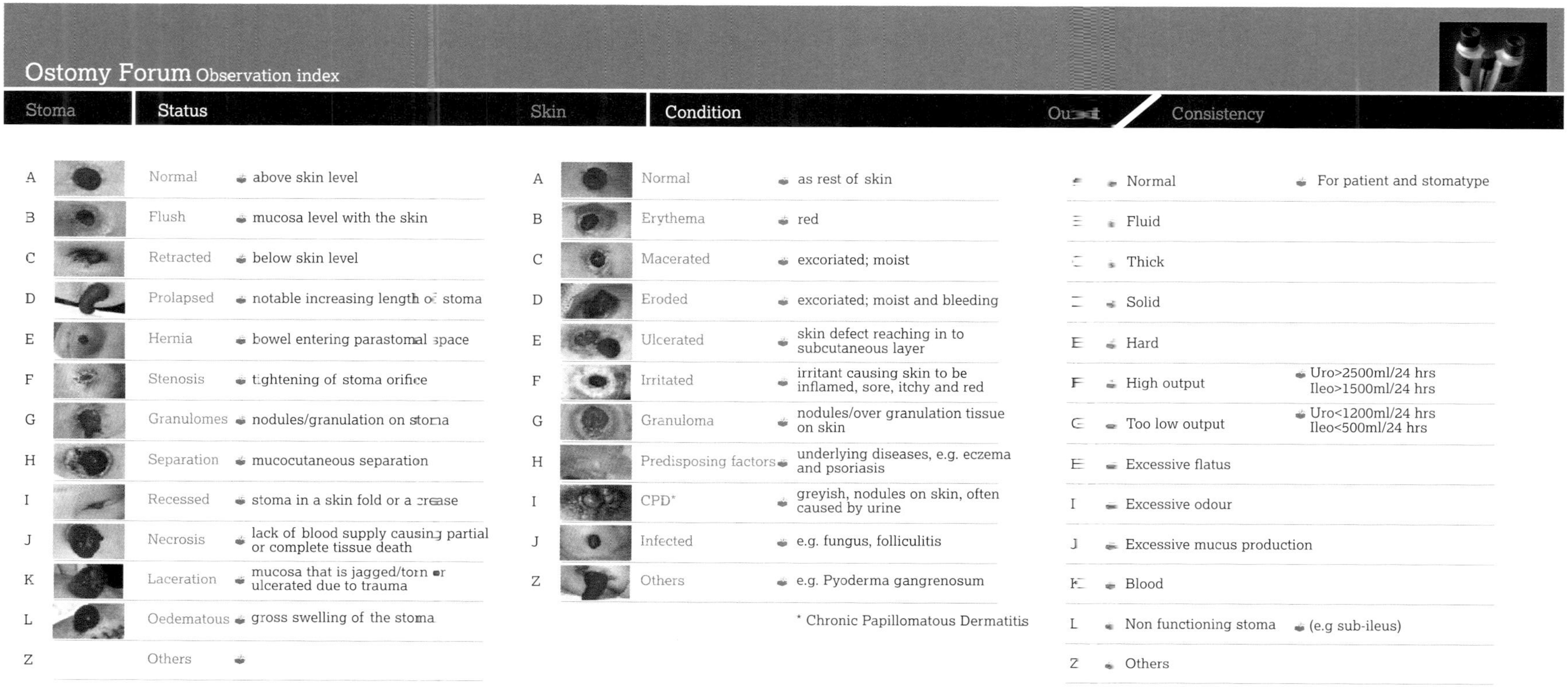

Ostomy Forum Observation index
Stoma
Status
Skin
Condition
Consistency
A Normal above skin level
B Flush mucosa level with the skin
C Retracted below skin level
D Prolapsed notable increasing length of stoma
E Hernia bowel entering parastomal space
F Stenosis tightening of stoma orifice
G Granulomes nodules/granulation on stoma
H Separation mucocutaneous separation
I Recessed stoma in a skin fold or a crease
J Necrosis lack of blood supply causing partial or complete tissue death
K Laceration mucosa that is jagged/torn or ulcerated due to trauma
L Oedematous gross swelling of the stoma
Z Others
A Normal as rest of skin
B Erythema red
C Macerated excoriated; moist
D Eroded excoriated; moist and bleeding
E Ulcerated skin defect reaching in to subcutaneous layer
F Irritated irritant causing skin to be inflamed, sore, itchy and red
G Granuloma nodules/over granulation tissue on skin
H Predisposing factors underlying diseases, e.g. eczema and psoriasis
I CPD* greyish, nodules on skin, often caused by urine
J Infected e.g. fungus, folliculitis
Z Others e.g. Pyoderma gangrenosum
* Chronic Papillomatous Dermatitis
Normal For patient and stomatype
Fluid
Thick
Solid
Hard
F High output Uro>2500ml/24 hrs Ileo>1500ml/24 hrs
Too low output Uro<1200ml/24 hrs Ileo<500ml/24 hrs
Excessive flatus
I Excessive odour
J Excessive mucus production
Blood
L Non functioning stoma (e.g sub-ileus)
Z Others

Figure 6.35 Ostomy observational index. *Source*: Reproduced with permission of Dansac Ltd.

Websites

Colostomy UK
www.colostomyuk.org

Ileostomy & Internal Pouch Association
www.iasupport.org

MedicAlert
www.medicalert.org.uk

Sexual Advice Association
https://sexualadviceassociation.co.uk

Urostomy Association
www.uagbi.org

References

Abbott, J.E., Han, A., MacDonald, M., et al. (2016) Are antibiotics necessary during routine cystoscopic stent removal? *Translational Andrology and Urology*, 5(5), 784–788.

Abd-el-Maeboud, K.H., el-Naggar, T., el-Hawi, E.M., et al. (1991) Rectal suppository: Commonsense and mode of insertion. *Lancet*, 338(8770), 798–800.

Abrams, P., Smith, A.P. & Cotterill, N. (2014) The impact of urinary incontinence on health-related quality of life (HRQoL) in a real-world population of women ages 45–60 years: Results from a survey in France, Germany, the UK and the USA. *BJU International*, 115, 143–152.

Abt, D., Bywater, M., Engeler, D.S. & Schmid, H. (2013) Therapeutic options for intractable hematuria in advanced bladder cancer. *International Journal of Urology*, 20(7), 651–660.

Adams, D., Bucior, H., Day, G. & Rimmer, J.A. (2012) HOUDINI: Make that urinary catheter disappear – nurse-led protocol. *Journal of Infection Prevention*, 13(2), 44–46.

Afak, Y.S., Wasir, B.S., Hamid, A., et al. (2009) Comparative study of various forms of urinary diversion after radical cystectomy in muscle invasive carcinoma urinary bladder. *International Journal of Health Sciences*, 3(1), 3–11.

Agamennone, V., Krul, C.A.M., Rijkers, G. & Kort, R. (2018) A practical guide for probiotics applied to the case of antibiotic-associated diarrhea in the Netherlands. *BMC Gastroenterology*, 18(1), 1–12.

Ahluwalia, A., Rossiter, D. & Menezes, P. (2018) Urinary catheterisation: Indications, techniques and managing failure. *InnovAIT*, 11(1), 29–34.

Arasaradnam, R.P., Brown, S., Forbes, A., et al. (2018) Guidelines for the investigation of chronic diarrhoea in adults: British Society of Gastroenterology, 3rd edition. *Gut*, 67, 1380–1399.

ASCN (Association of Stoma Care Nurses UK) (2016) *ASCN Stoma Care National Clinical Guidelines*. Available at: http://ascnuk.com/wp-content/uploads/2016/03/ASCN-Clinical-Guidelines-Final-25-April-compressed-11-10-38.pdf

Baldi, F., Bianco, M.A., Nardone, G., et al. (2009) Focus on acute diarrhoeal disease. *World Journal of Gastroenterology*, 15(27), 3341–3348.

Bardsley, A. (2017) Assessment and treatment options for patients with constipation. *British Journal of Nursing*, 26(6), 312–318.

Barrie, M. (2018) Nursing management of patients with faecal incontinence. *Nursing Standard*, 33(2), 69–74.

BAUS (British Association of Urological Surgeons) (2017) *Having a Permanent Suprapubic Catheter (in men)*. Patient information leaflet. Available at: https://www.baus.org.uk/_userfiles/pages/files/Patients/Leaflets/Suprapubic%20care%20male.pdf

BAUS (2018) *Analyses of Radical Cystectomies Performed Between Jan 1st and December 31st 2017*. Available at: https://www.baus.org.uk/_userfiles/pages/files/Publications/Audit/FinalAnalysisCystectomy2017.pdf

Beeckman, D., Campbell, J., Campbell, K., et al. (2015) Incontinence-associated dermatitis: Moving prevention forward. *Wounds International*. Available at: https://www.woundsinternational.com/resources/details/incontinence-associated-dermatitis-moving-prevention-forward

Beeckman, D., Schoonhoven, L., Verhaeghe, S., et al. (2009) Prevention and treatment of incontinence-associated dermatitis: Literature review. *Journal of Advanced Nursing*, 65(6), 1141–1154.

Bell, M.A. (2010) Severe indwelling urinary catheter-associated urethral erosion in four elderly men. *Ostomy Wound Management*, 56(12), 36–39.

Bell, S. (2004) Investigations and management of chronic diarrhoea in adults. In: Norton, C. & Chelvanayagam, S. (eds) *Bowel Continence Nursing*. Beaconsfield, UK: Beaconsfield Publishers, pp.92–102.

Berg, K. & Seidler, H. (2005) Randomised crossover comparison of adhesively coupled colostomy pouching systems. *Ostomy Wound Management*, 51(3), 30–34.

Bernard, M.S., Hunter, K.F. & Moore, K.N. (2012) A review of strategies to decrease the duration of indwelling urethral catheters and potentially reduce the incidence of catheter-associated urinary tract infections. *Urologic Nursing*, 32(1), 29–37.

Bijalwan, P., Pooleri, G.K. & Thomas, A. (2017) Comparison of sterile water irrigation versus intravesical mitomycin C in preventing recurrence of nonmuscle invasive bladder cancer after transurethral resection. *Indian Journal of Urology*, 33(2), 144–148.

Black, P. (2000) Practical stoma care. *Nursing Standard*, 14(41), 47–53, quiz 54–45.

Black, P. (2011a) Choosing the correct stoma appliance. *Journal of Community Nursing*, 25(6), 44–49.

Black, P. (2011b) The role of the carer and patient in stoma care. *Nursing & Residential Care*, 13(9), 432–436.

Black, P. (2011c) Stoma care: Training in an era of health service setbacks. *British Journal of Healthcare Assistants*, 5(4), 191–193.

Black, P. (2015a) Accessories in stoma care. *Nursing & Residential Care*, 17(2), 68–70.

Black, P. (2015b) Selecting appropriate appliances and accessories for ileostomates. *Gastrointestinal Nursing*, 13(7), 42–50.

Black, P. (2016) The use of flange extenders to support patient care. *British Journal of Nursing Stoma Supplement*, 25(5), S12.

BNF (British National Formulary) (2019) *British National Formulary*. National Institute for Health and Care Excellence. Available at: https://bnf.nice.org.uk

Borwell, B. (2009) Continuity of care for the stoma patient: Psychological considerations. *British Journal of Community Nursing*, 14(8), 326, 328, 330–331.

Bossi, P., Antonuzzo, A., Cherny, N.I., et al. (2018) Diarrhoea in adult cancer patients: ESMO clinical practice guidelines. *Annals of Oncology*, 29(Suppl. 4), iv126–iv142.

Boyles, A. & Hunt, S. (2016) Care and management for a stoma: Maintaining peristomal skin health. *British Journal of Nursing*, 25(17), S14–S21.

Bradshaw, A. & Price, L. (2006) Rectal suppository insertion: The reliability of the evidence as a basis for nursing practice. *Journal of Community Nursing*, 16(1), 98–103.

Bregendahl, S., Emmertsen, K.J., Lindegaard, J.C. & Laurberg, S. (2015) Urinary and sexual dysfunction in women after resection with and without preoperative radiotherapy for rectal cancer: A population-based cross-sectional study. *Colorectal Disease*, 17(1), 26–37.

British Nutrition Foundation (2018) *Dietary Fibre*. Available at: https://www.nutrition.org.uk/healthyliving/basics/fibre.html

Broholm, P., Pommergaard, H.C. & Gogenur, I. (2014) Possible benefits of robot-assisted rectal cancer surgery regarding urological and sexual dysfunction: A systematic review and meta-analysis. *Colorectal Disease*, 17(5), 375–381.

Burch, J. (2011a) Resuming a normal life: Holistic care of the person with an ostomy. *British Journal of Community Nursing*, 16(8), 366–373.

Burch, J. (2011b) Peristomal skin care and the use of accessories to promote skin health. *British Journal of Nursing*, 20(7), S4, S6, S8–S10.

Burch, J. (2011c) Providing information and advice on diet to stoma patients. *British Journal of Community Nursing*, 16(10), 479–480, 482, 484.

Burch, J. (2015) Troubleshooting stomas in the community setting. *Journal of Community Nursing*, 29(5), 93–96.

Burch, J. (2016) Intimacy for patients with a stoma. *British Journal of Nursing*, 25(17), S26.

Callaghan, R., Hunt, S., Mohamud, L. & Small, B. (2018) Case study series: Medi Derma-S Total Barrier Cream for the management and prevention of mild incontinence-associated dermatitis. *Wounds UK*, 14(1), 76–82.

Candy, B., Jones, L., Larkin, P.J., et al. (2015) Laxatives for the management of constipation in people receiving palliative care. *Cochrane Database of Systematic Reviews*. Available at: https://www.cochranelibrary.com/cdsr/doi/10.1002/14651858.CD003448.pub4/full

Caramia, G., Silvi, S., Verdenelli, M.C. & Coman, M.M. (2015) Treatment of acute diarrhea: Past and now. *International Journal of Enteric Pathology*, 3(4), 8–19.

Carlson, A.A., Rose, T.N. & Gelinas, A. (2016) The rundown: Management of acute and chronic diarrhoea. *Drug Topics*, 160(6), 55–63.

Chapple, A., Prinjha, S. & Salisbury, H. (2014) How users of indwelling urinary catheters talk about sex and sexuality: A qualitative study. *British Journal of General Practice*, 64(623), e364–e371.

Clarebrough, E., McGrath, S., Christidis, D. & Lawrentschuk, N. (2018) CATCH 22: A manual bladder washout protocol to improve care for clot retention. *World Journal of Urology*, 36(12), 2043–2050.

Clemens, J.Q., O'Leary, M.P. & Givens, J. (2018) Urinary incontinence in men. *UpToDate*. Available at: www.uptodate.com/contents/urinary-incontinence-in-men

Coloplast (2017) *The Cost of Constipation*. Available at: https://www.coloplast.co.uk/Global/UK/Continence/Cost_of_Constipation_Report_FINAL.pdf

Colwell, J.C., Pittman, J., Raizman, R. & Salvadalena, G. (2018) A randomised controlled trial determining variances in ostomy skin conditions and the economic impact (ADVOCATE Trial). *Journal of Wound, Ostomy and Continence Nursing*, 45(1), 37–42.

Connolly, M. & Larkin, P. (2012) Managing constipation: A focus on care and treatment in the palliative setting. *British Journal of Community Nursing*, 17(2), 60, 62–64, 66–67.

ConvaTec (2012) *Guidelines for the Management of Fecal Incontinence with Flexi-Seal® Signal® Fecal Management System (FMS)*. ConvaTec. Available at: https://www.convatec.co.uk/continence-critical-care/faecal-incontinence/product-range/flexi-seal-fms

Cox, J.S. & Friess, D. (2017) Retained surgical drains in orthopedics: Two case reports and a review of the literature. *Case Reports in Orthopedics*, 2017(2), 1–3.

Cronin, E. (2012) What the patient needs to know before stoma siting: An overview. *British Journal of Nursing*, 21(22), 1304, 1306–1308.

Cronin, E. (2013) Dietary advice for patients with a stoma. *Gastrointestinal Nursing*, 11(3), 14–24.

Curtis, K. (2013) Caring for adult patients who require nasogastric feeding tubes. *Nursing Standard*, 27(38), 47–56.

Dagli, M. & Ramchandani, P. (2011) Percutaneous nephrostomy: Technical aspects and indications. *Seminars in Interventional Radiology*, 28(4), 424–437.

Davenport, R. (2014) A proven pathway for stoma care: The value of stoma care services. *British Journal of Nursing*, 23(22), 1174–1180.

Davenport, R. & Hayles, K. (2018) Clinical evidence: Does it exist in stoma care practice? Do we need it? Association of Stoma Care Nurses poster presentation P6, 9–11 September, Birmingham, UK.

Davis, N.F., Quinlan, M.R., Bhatt, N.R., et al. (2016) Incidence, cost, complications and clinical outcomes of iatrogenic urethral catheterisation injuries: A prospective multi-institutional study. *Journal of Urology*, 196, 1473–1477.

De Schryver, A.M., Keulemans, Y.C., Peters, H.P., et al. (2005) Effects of regular physical activity on defecation pattern in middle-aged patients complaining of chronic constipation. *Scandinavian Journal of Gastroenterology*, 40(4), 422–429.

DEFRA (Department for Environment, Food and Rural Affairs) (2005) *Hazardous Waste Regulations: List of Wastes Regulations 2005*. London: Department for Environment, Food and Rural Affairs.

Dellimore, K.H., Helyer, A.R. & Franklin, S.E. (2013) A scoping review of important urinary catheter induced complications. *Journal of Materials Science: Materials in Medicine*, 24, 1825–1835.

Denby, N. (2006) The role of diet and lifestyle changes in the management of constipation. *British Journal of Community Nursing*, 20(9), 20–24.

Devore, E.E., Townsend, M.K., Resnick, N.M., et al. (2012) The epidemiology of urinary incontinence in women with type 2 diabetes. *Journal of Urology*, 188(5), 1816–1821.

Di Gesaro, A. (2016) The psychological aspects of having a stoma: A literature review. *Gastrointestinal Nursing*, 14(2), 38–44.

Durnal, A.M., Maxwell, T.R., Kiran, R.P. & Kommala, D. (2011) International study of a continence device with 12 hour wear times. *British Journal of Nursing*, 20(16), S4–S11.

Dutcher, G., Flood, D., Curry, M.A., et al. (2018) Improving documentation of pain and constipation management within the cancer center of a large public healthcare network. *Journal of Clinical Oncology*, 36(15 Suppl.), 6596–6596.

Eastwood, L. (2009) Safe and secure: Improving practice in the UK. *Journal of Community Nursing*, 23(5), 30–32.

EAUN (European Association of Urology Nurses) (2012) *Evidence-based guidelines for best practice in urological health care, catheterisation: Indwelling catheters in adults – Uretheral and suprapubic*. Available at: https://nurses.uroweb.org/guideline/catheterisation-indwelling-catheters-in-adults-urethral-and-suprapubic

Ejemot-Nwadiaro, R.I., Ehiri, J.E., Arikpo, D., et al. (2015) Hand washing promotion for preventing diarrhoea. *Cochrane Database of Systematic Reviews*. Available at: http://cochranelibrary-wiley.com/doi/10.1002/14651858.CD004265.pub3/full

Eldahan, K.C. & Rabchevsky, A.G. (2018) Autonomic dysreflexia after spinal cord injury: Systemic pathophysiology and methods of management. *Autonomic Neuroscience*, 209, 59–70.

Emly, M. & Marriott, A. (2017) Revisiting constipation management in the community. *British Journal of Community Nursing*, 22(4), 168–172.

Fan, L., Liu, Q. & Gui, L. (2016) Efficacy of non-swallow nasogastric tube intubation: A randomised controlled trial. *Journal of Clinical Nursing*, 25(21–22), 3326–3332.

Fasugba, O., Koerner, J., Mitchell, B.G., et al. (2017) Systematic review and meta-analysis of the effectiveness of antiseptic agents for meatal cleaning in the prevention of catheter-associated urinary tract infections. *Journal of Hospital Infections*, 95(3), 233–242.

Feneley, R.C.L., Hopley, I.B. & Wells, N.T. (2015) Urinary catheters: History, current status, adverse events and research agenda. *Journal of Medical Engineering & Terminology*, 39(8), 459–470.

Fillingham, S. & Douglas, J. (eds) (2004) *Urological Nursing*, 3rd edn. Edinburgh: Baillière Tindall.

Forristal, H. & Maxfield, J. (2004) Prostatic problems. In: Fillingham, S. & Douglas, J. (eds) *Urological Nursing*, 3rd edn. Edinburgh: Baillière Tindall, pp 161–184.

Fowler, S., Godfrey, H., Fader, M., et al. (2014) Living with a long-term, indwelling urinary catheter: Catheter users' experience. *Journal of Wound, Ostomy and Continence Nursing*, 41(6), 597–603.

Fraise, A. P. & Bradley, T. (2009) *Aycliffe's Control of Healthcare-Associated Infections: A Practical Handbook*, 5th edn. London: Hodder Arnold.

Franke, A.J., Iqbal, A., Starr, J.S., et al. (2017) Management of malignant bowel obstruction associated with GI cancers. *Journal of Oncology Practice*, 13(7), 426–434.

Fritz, D. & Pitlick, M. (2012) Evidence about the prevention and management of constipation: Implications for comfort part 1. *Home Healthcare Nurse*, 30(9), 533–540, quiz 540–532.

Geng, V., Corbussen-Boekhorst, H., Fillingham, S., et al. (2009) *Good Practice in Health Care: Incontinent Urostomy*. Arnhem: European Association of Urology Nurses.

Geng, V., Eelen, P., Fillingham, S., et al. (2010) *Good Practice in Health Care: Continent Urinary Diversion*. Arnhem: European Association of Urology Nurses.

Geraghty, J. (2011) Introducing a new skin-care regimen for the incontinent patient. *British Journal of Nursing*, 20(7), 409–415.

Ghaffary, C., Yohannes, A., Villanueva, C. & Leslie, S.W. (2013) A practical approach to difficult urinary catheterizations. *Current Urology Reports*, 14, 565–579.

Gilbert, B. (2018) Ins and outs of urinary catheters. *Royal Australian College of General Practitioners*, 47(3), 132–136.

Gilbert, R. (2006) Taking a midstream specimen of urine. *Nursing Times*, 102(18), 22–23.

Goodey, A. & Colman, S. (2016) Safe management of ileostomates with high output stomas. *British Journal of Nursing*, 25(22), S4–S9.

Gray, M., Beeckman, D., Bliss, D.Z., et al. (2012) Incontinence-associated dermatitis: A comprehensive review and update. *Journal of Wound, Ostomy and Continence Nursing*, 39(1), 61–74.

Gray, M., Skinner, C. & Kaler, W. (2016) External collection devices as an alternative to the indwelling urinary catheter: Evidence-based review and expert clinical panel deliberations. *Journal of Wound, Ostomy and Continence Nursing*, 43(3), 301–307.

Gupta, K., Rastogi, B., Jain, M., et al. (2010) Electrolyte changes: An indirect method to assess irrigation fluid absorption complication during transurethral resection of prostate. A prospective study. *Saudi Journal of Anaesthesia*, 4(2), 142–146.

Hahn, R.G. (2015) Fluid absorption and the ethanol monitoring method. *Acta Anaesthesiologica Scandinavica*, 59(9), 1081–1093.

Hardy, K. & McPhail, J. (2018) Pre-operative preparation of patients undergoing total pelvic exenteration (TPE). Association of Stoma Care Nurses oral presentation O22, 9–11 September, Birmingham, UK.

Harris, L.A., Horn, J., Kissous-Hunt, M., et al. (2017) The Better Understanding and Recognition of the Disconnects, Experiences, and Needs of Patients with Chronic Idiopathic Constipation (BURDEN-CIC) study: Results of an online questionnaire. *Advances in Therapy*, 34(12), 2661–2673.

Hautmann, R.E., Volkmer, B.G., Schumacher, M.C., et al. (2006) Long-term results of standard procedures in urology: The ileal neobladder. *World Journal of Urology*, 24(3), 305–314.

Hayden, D.M. & Weiss, E.G. (2011) Fecal incontinence: Etiology, evaluation and treatment. *Clinics in Colon and Rectal Surgery*, 24(1), 64–70.

Hermanns, T., Funkhauses, C.D., Hafermehl, L.J., et al. (2013) Prospective evaluation of irrigation fluid absorption during pure transurethral bipolar plasma vaporisation of the prostate using expired-breath ethanol measurements. *BJU International*, 112(5), 647–654.

Hohenfellner, M. & Santucci, R.A. (2010) *Emergencies in Urology*. New York: Springer.

Hook, A.L., Chang, C.-Y., Yang, J., et al. (2012) Combinatorial discovery of polymers resistant to bacterial attachment. *Nature Biotechnology*, 30(9), 868–887.

Hsu, L., Li, H., Pucheril, D., et al. (2016) Use of percutaneous nephrostomy and ureteral stenting in management of ureteral obstruction. *World Journal of Nephrology*, 5(2), 172–181.

Huang, J.G., Ooi, J., Lawrentschuk, N., et al. (2009) Urinary catheter balloons should only be filled with water: Testing the myth. *British Journal of Urology International*, 104(11), 1693–1695.

Humphreys, N. (2017) Sexual health and sexuality in people with a stoma: A literature review. *Gastrointestinal Nursing*, 15(10), 18–26.

Hurst, A.F., Hunt, T. & British Society of Gastroenterology (1969) *Selected Writings of Sir Arthur Hurst (1879–1944)*. London: British Society of Gastroenterology.

International Ostomy Forum Group (2006) Flow chart for choosing appliances. *ObservationIndex*. Dansac Ltd.

Jairath, A., Ganpule, A. & Desai, M. (2017) Percutaneous nephrostomy step by step. *Minimally Invasive Surgery*, 1, 180–185.

Kaufman, S. (2015) Short bowel syndrome. In: Wyllie, R., Hyams, J.S. & Kay, M. (eds) *Pediatric Gastrointestinal and Liver Disease*, 5th edn. Philadelphia: Elsevier, pp.405–417.

Kelly, A.W., Nelson, M.L., Heppel, J., et al. (2000) Disposable plastic liners for colostomy appliance: A controlled trial and follow up survey of convenience, satisfaction and costs. *Journal of Wound, Ostomy and Continence Nursing*, 27(5), 272–278.

Kelly, L., Jenkins, H. & Whyte, L. (2018) Symposium: Gastroenterology – Pathophysiology of diarrhoea. *Paediatrics & Child Health*, 28(11), 520–526.

Kirkwood, L. (2006) Postoperative stoma care and the selection of appliances. *Journal of Community Nursing*, 20(3), 12–18.

Konradsen, H., Rasmussen, M.L.T., Noiesen, E. & Trosborg, I. (2017) Effect of home care nursing on patients discharged from hospital with self-reported signs of constipation. *Gastroenterology Nursing*, 40(6), 463–468.

Kowal-Vern, A., Poulakidas, S., Barnett, B., et al. (2009) Fecal contaminant in bedridden patients: Economic impact of 2 commercial bowel catheter systems. *American Journal of Critical Care*, 18(3 Suppl.), S2–S14.

Krenzer, M.E. (2012) Viral gastroenteritis in the adult population: The GI peril. *Critical Care Nursing Clinics of North America*, 24(4), 541–553.

Krogh, K., Chiarioni, G. & Whitehead, W. (2017) Management of chronic constipation in adults. *United European Gastroenterology Journal*, 5(4), 465–472.

Kwan, M.L., Leo, M.C., Danforth, K.N., et al. (2019) Factors that influence selection of urinary diversion among bladder cancer patients in 3 community-based integrated health care systems. *Urology*, 125, 222–229.

Kyle, G. (2009) Practice questions: Solving your clinical dilemmas. *Nursing Times*, 105(2). Available at: https://www.nursingtimes.net/practice-questions-solving-your-clinical-dilemmas/1963570.article

Kyle, G. (2011a) The use of urinary sheaths in male incontinence. *British Journal of Nursing*, 20(6), 338.

Kyle, G. (2011b) Risk assessment and management tools for constipation. *British Journal of Community Nursing*, 16(5), 224, 226–230.

Kyle, G. (2011c) Digital rectal examination. *Nursing Times*, 107(12), 18–19.

Kyle, G., Prynn, P., Oliver, H., et al. (2005) The Eton Scale: A tool for risk assessment for constipation. *Nursing Times*, 101(18), 50–51.

Lam, T.B.L., Omar, M.I., Fisher, E., et al. (2014) Types of indwelling urethral catheters for short-term catheterisation in hospitalised adults. *Cochrane Database of Systematic Reviews*. DOI: 10.1002/14651858.CD004013.pub4.

Le Lievre, S. (2002) An overview of skin care and faecal incontinence. *Nursing Times*, 98(4), 58–59.

Leach, D. (2015) Ureteric stent removal post cystectomy. *British Journal of Nursing*, 24(22), S20–S26.

Leaver, R.B. (2007) The evidence for urethral meatal cleansing. *Nursing Standard*, 21(41), 39–42.

Leaver, R.B. (2016) Managing the aftercare of patients with a Mitrofanoff pouch. *Journal of Community Nursing*, 30(1), 40–46.

Lee, R.K., Abol-Enein, H., Artibani, W., et al. (2014) Urinary diversion after radical cystectomy for bladder cancer: Options, patient selection, and outcomes. *British Journal of Urology*, 113(1), 11–23.

Lee-Robichaud, H., Thomas, K., Morgan, J., et al. (2010) Lactulose versus polyethylene glycol for chronic constipation. *Cochrane Database of Systematic Reviews*. Available at: http://onlinelibrary.wiley.com/doi/10.1002/14651858.CD007570.pub2/pdf.

Legendre, G., Ringer, V., Fauconnier, A. & Fritel, X. (2013) Menopause, hormone treatment and urinary incontinence at midlife. *Maturitas*, 74(1), 26–30.

Leyk, M., Stevens, P., Stelton, S., et al. (2018) Revisiting the history of stoma siting and its impact on modern day practice. *WCET Journal*, 38(1), 22–29.

Lim, S.W., Kim, H.J., Kim, C.H., et al. (2013) Risk factors for permanent stoma after low anterior resection for rectal cancer. *Langenbeck's Archives of Surgery*, 398(2), 259–264.

Logan, K. (2012) An overview of male intermittent self-catheterisation. *British Journal of Nursing*, 21(18), S18–S22.

Longstreth, G.F., Thompson, W.G., Chey, W.D., et al. (2006) Functional bowel disorders. *Gastroenterology*, 130(5), 1480–1491.

Losco, G., Antoniou, S. & Mark, S. (2011) Male flexible cystoscopy: Does waiting after insertion of topical anaesthetic lubricant improve patient comfort? *British Journal of Urology*, 108(Suppl. 2), 42–44.

Loveday, H.P., Wilson, J.A., Pratt, R.J., et al. (2014) Epic3: National evidence-based guidelines for preventing healthcare associated infections in NHS hospitals in England. *Journal of Hospital Infection*, 86(Suppl. 1), S1–S70.

Łukasik, J. & Szajewska, H. (2018) Effect of a multispecies probiotic on reducing the incidence of antibiotic-associated diarrhoea in children: A protocol for a randomised controlled trial. *BMJ Open*, 8(5), e021214.

Macaulay, M., Broadbridge, J., Gage, H., et al. (2015) A trial of devices for urinary incontinence after treatment for prostate cancer. *BJU International*, 116(3), 432–442.

MacDiarmid, S. (2008) Maximizing the treatment of overactive bladder in the elderly. *Reviews in Urology*, 10(1), 6–13.

Madeo, M. & Roodhouse, A.J. (2009) Reducing the risks associated with urinary catheters. *Nursing Standard*, 23(29), 47–55, quiz 56.

Mandakhalikar, K.D., Rongyuan R.C. & Tambyah, P.A. (2016) New technologies for prevention of catheter associated urinary tract infection. *Current Treatment Options in Infectious Diseases*, 8(1), 24–41.

Mangnall, J. (2014) Urinary catheterisation: Reducing the risk of infection. *Nursing & Residential Care*, 16(6), 310–318.

Marieb, E. & Hoehn, K. (2015) *Human Anatomy & Physiology, Global Edition*, 9th edn. Cambridge: Pearson.

McDougal, W.S., Wein, A., Kavoussi, L., et al. (2015) *Campbell-Walsh Urology*, 11th edn. Philadelphia: Elsevier.

McPhail, J. (2018) Literature search for randomised controlled trials of ostomy skin barriers within the last 10 years; to support evidence based practice with high level evidence. Association of Stoma Care Nurses poster presentation P3, 9–11 September, Birmingham, UK.

Metcalf, C. (2007) Chronic diarrhoea: Investigation, treatment and nursing care. *Nursing Standard*, 21(21), 48–56, quiz 58.

Metcalf, C. (2017) Evaluating nursing standards in a stoma care service: Results of an internal audit. *Gastrointestinal Nursing*, 15(4), 35–41.

Metheny, N.A. & Meert, K.L. (2004) Monitoring feeding tube placement. *Nutrition in Clinical Practice*, 19(5), 487–495.

Mody, L. & Juthani-Mehta, M. (2014) Urinary tract infections in older women: A clinical review. *JAMA*, 311, 844–854.

Moller Kruse, T. & Storling, Z.M. (2015) Considering the benefits of a new stoma appliance: A clinical trial. *British Journal of Nursing*, 24(22), S12–S18.

Moppett, S. (2000) Which way is up for a suppository? *Nursing Times*, 96(19), 12–13.

Morton, P.G. & Fontaine, D.K. (eds) (2017) *Critical Care Nursing: A Holistic Approach*, 11th edn. Philadelphia: Lippincott Williams & Wilkins.

Murphy, C., Fader, M. & Prieto, J. (2014) Interventions to minimise the initial use of indwelling urinary catheters in acute care: A systematic review. *International Journal of Nursing Studies*, 51(1), 4–13.

Naish, J. & Court, D.S. (2018) *Medical Sciences*, 3rd edn. Amsterdam: Elsevier.

Naish, W. (2003) Intermittent self-catheterisation for managing urinary problems. *Nursing Times*. Available at: https://www.nursingtimes.net/intermittent-self-catheterisation-for-managing-urinary-problems/200048.article

Nazarko, L. (2007) Managing diarrhoea in the home to prevent admission. *British Journal of Community Nursing*, 12(11), 508–512.

Nazarko, L. (2008) Caring for a patient with a urostomy in a community setting. *British Journal of Community Nursing*, 13(8), 354–361.

Nazarko, L. (2012) Intermittent self-catheterisation: Past, present and future. *British Journal of Community Nursing*, 17(9), 408–412.

Nazarko, L. (2018a) The healthcare assistant and bowel care. *British Journal of Healthcare Assistants*, 12(4), 162–168.

Nazarko, L. (2018b). Male urinary incontinence management: Penile sheaths. *British Journal of Community Nursing*, 23(23), 110–116.

Nethercliffe, J.M. (2012) Urinary incontinence. In: Dawson, C. & Nethercliffe, J. (eds) *ABC of Urology*, 3rd edn. Chichester: Wiley Blackwell, pp.14–18.

NHS England and NHSI (NHS Improvement) (2019) *Standard Infection Control Precautions: National Hand Hygiene and Personal Protective Equipment Policy*. Available at: https://improvement.nhs.uk/documents/4957/National_policy_on_hand_hygiene_and_PPE_2.pdf

NHSBSA (National Health Service Business Service Authority) (2017) *Prescription cost analysis for January to December 2017*. Available at: https://www.nhsbsa.nhs.uk/prescription-data/dispensing-data/prescription-cost-analysis-pca-data.

NHSBSA (2018a) Deodorants. *Drug Tariff*, June, pp.637–638.

NHSBSA (2018b) Skin fillers and protectives. *Drug Tariff*, June, pp.705–709.

NHSBSA (2018c) Skin protectors. *Drug Tariff*, June, pp.710–714.

NHSBSA (2018d) Adhesives. *Drug Tariff*, June, p.549.

NHSBSA (2018e) Vacuum pumps and constrictor rings for erectile dysfunction. *Drug Tariff*, November, pp.510–513.

NHSBSA (2019) *Drug Tariff* [continually updated]. Available at: https://www.nhsbsa.nhs.uk/pharmacies-gp-practices-and-appliance-contractors/drug-tariff

NHSQIS (NHS Quality Improvement Scotland) (2004) *Urinary Catheterisation and Catheter Care: Best Practice Statement*. Available at: www.healthcareimprovementscotland.org/his/idoc.ashx?docid=feaef66c-08e3-4168-ae5c-85eba638ae8b&version=-1

NICE (National Institute for Health and Care Excellence) (2007) *Faecal Incontinence: The Management of Faecal Incontinence in Adults* [CG49]. Available at: www.nice.org.uk/guidance/cG49

NICE (2014) *Faecal Incontinence in Adults* [QS54]. Available at: https://www.nice.org.uk/guidance/qs54

NICE (2015a) *Suspected Cancer: Recognition and Referral* [NG12]. Available at: http://tinyurl.com/px4ykkv

NICE (2015b) *Antimicrobial Stewardship: Systems and Processes for Effective Antimicrobial Medicine Use* [NG15]. Available at: https://www.nice.org.uk/guidance/ng15

NICE (2017) *Healthcare-Associated Infections: Prevention and Control in Primary and Community Care* [CG139]. Available at: https://www.nice.org.uk/guidance/cg139/chapter/1-Guidance#long-term-urinary-catheters

NICE (2018) *Diarrhoea: Adult's Assessment Clinical Knowledge Summary*. London National Institute for Health and Care Excellence. Available at: https://cks.nice.org.uk/diarrhoea-adults-assessment#!scenarioRecommendation:1

Nicol, M. (2008) *Essential Nursing Skills*, 3rd edn. London: Mosby Elsevier.

Nicolle, L.E. (2014) Catheter associated urinary tract infection. *Antimicrobial Resistance & Infection Control*, 3(1), 23.

NMC (Nursing and Midwifery Council) (2018) *The Code: Professional Standards of Practice and Behaviour for Nurses, Midwives and Nursing Associates*. Available at: https://www.nmc.org.uk/standards/code

NPSA (National Patient Safety Agency) (2009a) *Minimising Risks of Suprapublic Catheter Insertion (Adults Only): Rapid Response Report* [NPSA/2009/RRR005]. London: National Patient Safety Agency.

NPSA (2009b) *Female Urinary Catheters: Rapid Response Report* [NPSA/2009/RRR02]. London: National Patient Safety Agency.

NPSA (2011) *Reducing the Harm Caused by Misplaced Nasogastric Feeding Tubes in Adults, Children and Infants: Patient Safety Alert* [NPSA/2011/PSA002]. London: National Patient Safety Agency.

Obita, G.P., Boland, E.G., Currow, D.C., et al. (2016) Somatostatin analogues compared to placebo and other pharmacological agents in the management of symptoms of inoperable malignant bowel obstruction: A systematic review. *Journal of Pain and Symptom Management*, 52(6), 901–919.

Ostaszkiewicz, J. & Paterson, J. (2012) Nurses' advice regarding sterile or clean urinary drainage bags for individuals with a long-term indwelling urinary catheter. *Journal of Wound, Ostomy and Continence Nursing*, 39(1), 77–83.

Ostaszkiewicz, J., Tomlinson, E. & Hutchinson, A.M. (2018) 'Dignity': A central construct in nursing home staff understandings of quality continence care. *Journal of Clinical Nursing*, 27(11–12), 2425–2437.

Ozturk, E., van Iersel, M., Stommel, M.M., et al. (2018) Small bowel obstruction in the elderly: A plea for comprehensive acute geriatric care. *World Journal of Emergency Surgery*, 13(1), 48.

Pankhin, H.T. & Althaus, P. (2001) Guidelines for preventing infections associated with the insertion and maintenance of short-term indwelling urethral catheters in acute care. *Journal of Hospital Infection*, 49(2), 146–147.

Park, S.Y., Choi, G.S., Park, J.S., et al. (2015) Efficacy and safety of udenafil for the treatment of erectile dysfunction after total mesorectal excision of rectal cancer: A randomized, double-blind, placebo-controlled trial. *Surgery*, 157(1), 64–71.

Parker, V., Giles, M., Graham, L., et al. (2017) Avoiding inappropriate urinary catheter use and catheter-associated urinary tract infection (CAUTI): A pre-post control intervention study. *BMC Health Services Research*, 17(1), 314.

Patel, I.J., Davidson, J.C., Nikolic, B., et al. (2012) Consensus guidelines for periprocedural management of coagulation status and hemostasis risk in percutaneous image-guided interventions. *Journal of Vascular and Interventional Radiology*, 23(6), 727–736.

Patton, K.T. (2018) *Anatomy & Physiology*, 10th edn. St Louis: Elsevier

Pavlov, M.J., Ceranic, M.S., Nale, D.P., et al. (2013) Double-barreled wet colostomy versus ileal conduit and terminal colostomy for urinary and fecal diversion: A single institution experience. *Scandinavian Journal of Surgery*, 103, 189–194.

Peate, I. (2015a) How to administer an enema. *Nursing Standard*, 30(14), 34–36.

Peate, I. (2015b) How to administer suppositories. *Nursing Standard*, 30(1), 34–36.

Peate, I. (2016) How to perform digital removal of faeces. *Nursing Standard*, 30(40), 36.

Peate, I. & Gill, M. (2015) Closed and open catheter irrigation by a skilled and competent healthcare worker. *British Journal of Healthcare Assistants*, 9(2), 71–76.

Peate, I., Nair, M., & Wild, K. (2014) *Nursing Practice: Knowledge and Care*. Chichester: Wiley Blackwell.

Pegram, A., Bloomfield, J. & Jones, A. (2008) Safe use of rectal suppositories and enemas with adult patients. *Nursing Standard*, 22(38), 39–41.

Perdue, C. (2005) Managing constipation in advanced cancer care. *Nursing Times*, 101(21), 36–40.

Philip, J., Manikandan, R., Venugopal, S., et al. (2009) Orthotopic neobladder versus ileal conduit urinary diversion after cystectomy: A quality-oflite based comparison. *Annals of The Royal College of Surgeons of England*, 91(7), 565–569.

[illegible] (2004) Urinary catheters and associated UTIs. *Journal of Community Nursing*, 18(9), 15–19.

[illegible] Tindall.

Radecka, E. & Magnusson, A. (2004) Complications associated with percutaneous nephrostomies: A retrospective study. *Acta Radiologica*, 45(2), 184–188.

Rantell, A. (2012) Intermittent self-catheterisation in women. *Nursing Standard*, 26(42), 61–68.

Rauck, R., Slatkin, N.E., Stambler, N., et al. (2017) Randomized, double-blind trial of oral methylnaltrexone for the treatment of opioid-induced constipation in patients with chronic noncancer pain. *Pain Practice*, 17(6), 820–828.

RCN (Royal College of Nursing) (2012a) *Catheter Care: RCN Guidance for Nurses.* London: Royal College of Nursing.

RCN (2012b) *Management of Lower Bowel Dysfunction, Including DRE and DRF: RCN Guidance for Nurses.* London: Royal College of Nursing.

RCN (2013) *The Management of Diarrhoea in Adults.* London: Royal College of Nursing.

RCN (2019) *Catheter Care: RCN Guidance for Health Care Professionals.* London: Royal College of Nursing.

Reese, J.B., Finan, P.H., Haythornthwaite, J.A., et al. (2014) Gastrointestinal ostomies and sexual outcomes: A comparison of colorectal cancer patients by ostomy status. *Support Care Cancer*, 22, 461–468.

Rigby, D. (2009) An overview of suprapubic catheter care in community practice. *British Journal of Community Nursing*, 14(7), 278–284.

Ritzema, J. (2017). Bowel management systems in critical care: A service evaluation. *Nursing Standard*, 31(22), 42–49.

Robinson, J. (2007) Female urethral catheterization. *Nursing Standard*, 22(8), 48–56.

Robinson, J. (2008) Insertion, care and management of suprapubic catheters. *Nursing Standard*, 23(8), 49–56.

Rodriguez, A., Lockhart, A., King, J., et al. (2011) Cutaneous ureterostomy technique for adults and effects of ureteral stenting: An alternative to the ileal conduit. *Journal of Urology*, 186(5), 1939–1943.

Rogers, J. (2012) How to manage chronic constipation in adults. *Nursing Times*, 108(41), 12–18.

Roque, M.V. & Bouras, E.P. (2015) Epidemiology and management of chronic constipation in elderly patients. *Clinical Interventions in Aging*, 10, 919.

Roser, L., Altpeter, T., Anderson, D., et al. (2012). A nurse driven Foley catheter removal protocol proves clinically effective to reduce the incidents of catheter related urinary tract infections. *American Journal of Infection Control*, 40(5), e92–e93.

Rostas, J. (2012) Preventing stoma-related complications: Techniques for optimal stoma creation. *Seminars in Colon & Rectal Surgery*, 23, 2–9.

Scholtes, S. (2002) Management of clot retention following urological surgery. *Nursing Times*, 98(28), 48–50.

Schuster, B.G., Kosar, L. & Kamrul, R. (2015) Constipation in older adults: Stepwise approach to keep things moving. *Canadian Family Physician*, 61(2), 152–158.

Serati, M. & Ghezzi, F. (2016). The epidemiology of urinary incontinence: A case still open. *Annals of Translational Medicine*, 4(6), 123.

Siddiq, D.M. & Darouiche, R.O. (2012) New strategies to prevent catheter-associated urinary tract infections. *Nature Reviews Urology*, 9, 305–314.

Simpson, P. (2017) Long-term urethral catheterization: Guidelines for community nurses. *British Journal of Nursing*, 26(9), S22–S26.

Simren, M., Palsson, O.S. & Whitehead, W.E. (2017) Update on Rome IV criteria for colorectal disorders: Implications for clinical practice. *Current Gastroenterology Reports*, 19(4), 15.

Singh, V., Yadav, R., Sinha, R.J. & Gupta, D.K. (2013) Prospective comparison of quality-of-life outcomes between ileal conduit urinary diversion and orthotopic neobladder reconstruction after radical cystectomy: A statistical model. *British Journal of Urology International*, 113(5), 726–732.

Singha, P., Locklin, J. & Handa, H. (2017) A review of the recent advances in antimicrobial coatings for urinary catheters. *Acta Biomaterialia*, 50, 20–40.

Skardoon, G.R., Khera, A.J., Emmanuel, A.V. & Burgell, R.E. (2017) Review article: Dyssynergic defaecation and biofeedback therapy in the pathophysiology and management of functional constipation. *Alimentary Pharmacology & Therapeutics*, 46, 410–423.

Slater, R. (2012) Managing high output stomas. *British Journal of Nursing*, 21(22), 1309–1311.

Smart, C. (2014). Male incontinence. Using the urinary sheath. *Nursing & Residential Care*, 16(10), 568–572.

Spencer, E.S., Lyons, M.D. & Pruthi, R.S. (2018) Patient selection and counseling for urinary diversion. *Urologic Clinics of North America*, 45(1), 1–9.

Stafford, T. (2017) Intermittent self-catheterisation today. *British Journal of Community Nursing*, 22(5), 214–217.

Steggall, M.J. (2008) Digital rectal examination. *Nursing Standard*, 22(47), 46–48.

Stothers, L. & Friedman, B. (2011) Risk factors for the development of stress urinary incontinence in women. *Current Urology Reports*, 12(5), 363–369.

Sweeny, A. (2017) Suprapubic catheter change methods: A crossover comparison cohort trial. *Journal of Wound, Ostomy and Continence Nursing*, 44(4), 368–373.

Tatham, M., Macfarlane, G., MacRae, M., et al. (2015) Development and implementation of a catheter associated urinary tract infection (CAUTI) 'toolkit'. *BMJ Quality Improvement Reports*, 4(1), u205441.w3668.

Thakur, E.R., Shapiro, J., Chan, J., et al. (2018) A systematic review of the effectiveness of psychological treatments for IBS in gastroenterology settings: Promising but in need of further study. *Digestive Diseases and Sciences*, 63(9), 2189–2201.

Tortora, G.J. & Derrickson, B.H. (2017) *Principles of Anatomy & Physiology*, 15th edn. Hoboken, NJ: John Wiley & Sons.

Voegeli, D. (2013) Moisture-associated skin-damage: An overview for community nurses. *British Journal of Nursing*, 18(1), 6–12.

Wald, A. & Talley, N.J. (2017) Management of chronic constipation in adults. *UpToDate*. Available at: https://www.uptodate.com/contents/management-of-chronic-constipation-in-adults

Wallace, A. (2016) The key factors that affect psychological adaption to a stoma: Literature review. *Gastrointestinal Nursing*, 14(6), 39–47.

Walker, H., Hopkins, G., Waller, M. & Storling, Z.M. (2016) Raising the bar: New flexible convex ostomy appliance – A randomised controlled trial. *WCET Journal*, 36(1 Suppl.), S6–S11.

Walker, J. (2007) Patient preparation for safe removal of surgical drains. *Nursing Standard*, 21(49), 39–41.

Walsh, D., Davis, M., Ripamonti, M., et al. (2017) 2016 updated MASCC/ESMO consensus recommendations: Management of nausea and vomiting in advanced cancer. *Support Cancer Care*, 25, 333–340.

Weisner, P. & Bell, S. (2004) Bowel dysfunction: Assessment and management in the neurological patient. In: Norton, C. & Chelvanayagam, S. (eds) *Bowel Continence Nursing*. Beaconsfield: Beaconsfield Publishers, pp.181–203.

Whiteley, I., Russell, M., Nassar, N. & Gladman, M.A. (2016) Outcomes of support rod usage in loop stoma formation. *International Journal Colorectal Disease*, 31, 1189–1195.

WHO (World Health Organization) (2018) *Health Topics: Diarrhoea*. Available at: www.who.int/topics/diarrhoea/en

Wickham, R.J. (2017) Managing constipation in adults with cancer. *Journal of the Advanced Practitioner in Oncology*, 8(2), 149.

Wilde, M.H., McMahon, J.M., Crean, H.F. & Brasch, J. (2016) Exploring relationships of urinary tract infection and blockage in people with long-term indwelling urinary catheters. *Journal of Clinical Nursing*, 26, 2558–2571.

Williams, C. (2017) Making a choice of catheterisation gel and the role of chlorhexidine. *British Journal of Community Nursing*, 22(7), 346–351.

Williams, J. (2011) Stoma appliances: It's all about the bag! *British Journal of Nursing*, 20(9), 534.

Williams, J. (2012) Stoma care: Intimacy and body image issues. *Practice Nursing*, 23(2), 91–93.

Wilson, L.A. (2005) Urinalysis. *Nursing Standard*, 19(35), 51–54.

Wilson, M. (2012) Addressing the problems of long-term urethral catheterization: Part 2. *British Journal of Nursing*, 21(1), 16, 18–20, 22.

Wilson, M. (2016) Urinary catheterisation in the community: Exploring challenges and solutions. *British Journal of Community Nursing*, 21(10), [illegible].

Woodhouse, C.R.J. (2015) *Adolescent Urology and Long Term Outcomes*. Oxford: John Wiley & Sons.
Woodward, S. (2012) Assessment and management of constipation in older people. *Nursing Older People*, 24(5), 21–26.
Woodward, S. (2013) Catheter valves: A welcome alternative to leg bags. *British Journal of Nursing*, 22(11), 650, 652–654.
Woodward, S. (2015) Selecting and fitting a penile sheath. *British Journal of Nursing*, 24(5), 290–292.
Yates, A. (2017) Urinary catheters 3: Catheter drainage and support systems. *Nursing Times*, 113(3), 41–43.
Yates, A. (2018) Catheter securing and fixation devices: Their role in preventing complications. *British Journal of Nursing*, 27(6), 290–294.
Zippe, C., Raina, R., Shah, A., et al. (2004) Female sexual dysfunction after radical cystectomy: A new outcome measure. *Urology*, 63(6), 1153–1157.
Zulkowski, K., Ayello, E.A. & Stelton, S. (eds) (2014) *WCET International Ostomy Guideline*. Perth: World Council of Enterostomal Therapists.

Chapter 7

Moving and positioning

Carolyn Moore with Jill Cooper, Siobhan Cowan-Dickie, Lucy Dean, Joanne Jethwa, Jessica Whibley and Leanne Williams

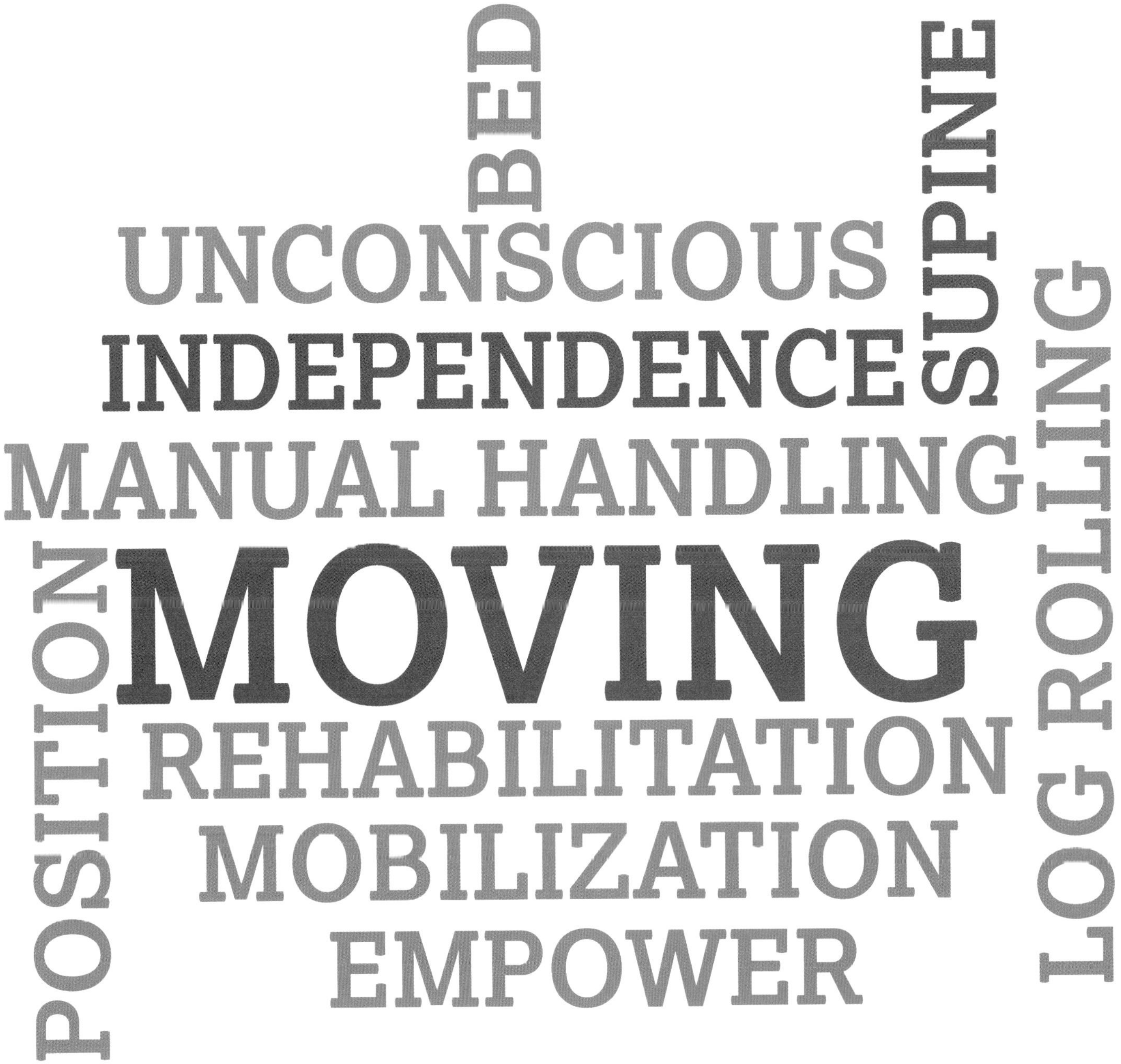
BED
SUPINE
UNCONSCIOUS
INDEPENDENCE
MANUAL HANDLING
LOG ROLLING
POSITION
MOVING
REHABILITATION
MOBILIZATION
EMPOWER

The Royal Marsden Manual of Clinical Nursing Procedures: Professional Edition, Tenth Edition. Edited by Sara Lister, Justine Hofland and Hayley Grafton.

Procedure guidelines

Being an accountable professional

At the point of registration, the nurse will:

7. Use evidence-based, best practice approaches for meeting needs for care and support with mobility and safety, accurately assessing the person's capacity for independence and self-care and initiating appropriate interventions

Future Nurse: Standards of Proficiency for Registered Nurses (NMC 2018)

Overview

This chapter provides guidance on moving and positioning patients, acknowledging the need to be clinically effective and, where possible, evidence based. It is important to emphasize that moving and positioning is just one aspect of rehabilitation, where the overall goal is to enable independence. Wherever possible, the aim should be to empower and enable the patient to actively move as much as possible. This chapter relates to moving and positioning of adults and does not specifically cover positioning of children or neonates.

The main objectives of the chapter are to:

- outline the general considerations regarding moving and positioning
- provide guidance on the principles of moving and positioning, whether the patient is in bed, sitting or preparing to mobilize
- consider optimal moving and positioning, including modifications for patients with different clinical needs.

The chapter includes the following:

- general principles of moving and handling
- moving and positioning unconscious patients and patients with an artificial airway
- considerations and modifications for patients with different respiratory requirements
- moving and handling for patients with neurological problems, including spinal cord compressions and those with raised intracranial pressure
- moving and handling considerations for upper and lower limb amputees.

The general principles of moving and positioning are discussed first followed by considerations of positioning for patients with specific clinical needs.

Moving and positioning: general principles

Definition

'To move' is to 'go in a specified direction or manner' or 'change position' (Oxford Dictionaries 2019a) and 'to position' is described as 'a particular way in which someone or something is placed or arranged' (Oxford Dictionaries 2019b). In medical terms, 'position' relates to body position or posture. Moving and positioning lie within the broader context of manual handling.

Anatomy and physiology

The human body is a complex structure that relies on the musculoskeletal system to provide support and to assist in movement. The musculoskeletal system is an integrated system consisting of bones, muscles and joints.

While bones provide the structural framework for protecting vital organs and enabling stability, skeletal muscles maintain body alignment and create movement (Tortora and Derrickson 2017). In order for the skeletal muscles to provide these functions, they often cross at one or more joints and attach to the articulating bones that form the joint so that when a muscle contracts, movement of a joint can occur in one direction. Muscles tend to work in synergy with each other (rather than in isolation) not just to create but also to control the movement. However, muscles will waste if not used and can also become shortened if not stretched regularly.

Joints are supported not just by the muscles but also by ligaments, which are strong connective tissue structures attached to either side of the joint. Ligaments can also become shortened if they are left in one position repeatedly or over a long period of time, which can then lead to problems maintaining full joint movement.

Evidence-based approaches

Rationale

Moving and positioning are important aspects of patient care because together they have a major impact on patients' rehabilitation and wellbeing, affecting them physically and psychologically. Optimum positioning is a good starting point to maximize the benefit of other interventions, such as bed exercises and breathing exercises; it can also assist rest and mobility, thereby facilitating recovery and enhancing function. However, although it is important, it must not be seen in isolation and is just one aspect of patient management where the overall goal is to optimize independence.

It is essential to frequently evaluate the effect that moving and positioning is having on the individual to ensure that the intervention is helping to achieve the desired result or goal. Consider whether the moving and positioning procedure is being clinically effective and, where possible, is evidence based.

There are several points to consider with regard to the clinical effectiveness of moving and positioning:

- Is the timing right for moving the patient? For example, is the pain relief adequate?
- Is it being carried out in the correct way? This relates to manual handling with regard to preventing trauma to both the patient and the practitioner. Manual handling causes over a third of all workplace injuries. These include work-related musculoskeletal disorders (MSDs) such as pain and injuries to arms, legs and joints, and repetitive strain injuries of various sorts (HSE 2018). Approved patient handling techniques are essential for safe practice.
- Is the required position taking into account all the pertinent needs of the patient? This emphasizes the need to consider the patient in a holistic manner and take into account any co-morbidities as well as the primary issue that is being addressed.
- Is it achieving the desired outcome or preventing a detrimental result?

Indications

Patients should always be encouraged to move themselves. Assistance in moving and positioning is indicated for patients who have difficulty moving or require periods of rest when normal function is impaired. The severity of an illness may leave no choice except bedrest, but rest alone is rarely beneficial.

Contraindications

There are no general contraindications for moving and positioning; however, some clinical conditions may require special considerations, preparation and specialist assistance.

Principles of care

The main principles underpinning all interventions regarding patient positioning and mobilization focus on the short- and long-term goals of rehabilitation and management for each specific patient. It is imperative that a thorough assessment is carried out prior to any intervention in order to plan appropriate goals of treatment. Wherever possible, goal setting should be a joint patient and healthcare professional discussion. It may be necessary to compromise on one principle, depending on the overall goal. For example, for the palliative patient, after discussing the patient's goals it may be that the primary aim of any intervention is to facilitate comfort at the cost of reducing function. Regular reassessment is necessary to allow for modification of plans to reflect changes in status. Communication and involvement of the multidisciplinary team will assist rehabilitation interventions as treatment can be incorporated during positional changes. This potentially allows an opportunity for multiprofessional working and allows many individuals to act with a common purpose and with co-ordinated activity (Health Foundation 2016).

Benefits of optimal positioning and mobilizing

Encouraging a normal routine and the provision of supported self-management can only be beneficial to patients. Encouraging patients to sit out of bed for meals, get dressed and mobilize (as able) reduces the risk of:

- pressure ulcers
- falls
- deep vein thrombosis
- chest infections
- increased length of stay in hospital.

Facilitating mobility supports harm-free care, with significant benefits to clinical outcomes and the costs of patient care (Chief Allied Health Professions Officer's Team 2017). For many, wearing pyjamas reinforces being sick and can prevent recovery. Studies show that three in five immobile, older patients in hospital had no medical reason that required bedrest and doubling the amount of walking while in hospital reduces the length of stay (NHS England 2018). The #EndPJparalysis initiative is global social movement embraced by nurses, therapists and medical professionals to get patients up, dressed and moving. Having patients in their day clothes while in hospital, rather than in pyjamas (PJs) or gowns, enhances dignity and autonomy and, in many instances, shortens their length of stay. For patients over the age of 80, a week in bed can lead to 10 years of muscle ageing and 1.5 kg of muscle loss, and may lead to increased dependency and demotivation. Getting patients up and moving has been shown to reduce falls, improve patient experiences and reduce length of stay by up to 1.5 days (NHS England 2018).

Effects of bedrest and decreased mobility

Patients with acute medical conditions and decreased mobility are at risk of developing secondary complications (Ye et al. 2017). Bedridden patients are prone to dehydration, progressive cardiac deconditioning and postural hypotension. They show reduced lung function and increased susceptibility to respiratory tract infections. Prolonged bedrest often leads to venous stasis and blood vessel damage, which, together with increased blood coagulability, predisposes bedridden patients to deep vein thrombosis and potentially pulmonary embolism (Ye et al. 2017).

Therefore, patients should be encouraged and/or assisted to mobilize or change position, at frequent intervals. All healthcare professionals should see facilitating mobility as part of their role. For example, nurses and healthcare support staff are perfectly placed to initiate rehabilitation and to identify those whose mobility is deteriorating during their inpatient stay. Early referrals to therapy services ensure that patients regain their independence in the shortest possible time. Starting rehabilitation early can improve physical and non-physical functioning and prevent future problems. The needs of a person in intensive or critical care can change very quickly; therefore, goals should be continually reviewed and updated within the rehabilitation programme.

Prolonged immobility is harmful, with rapid reductions in muscle mass, bone mineral density and impairment in other body systems evident within the first week of bedrest, which is further exacerbated in individuals with critical illness (Parry and Puthucheary 2015). Research has shown that many patients who survive critical illness (and therefore prolonged immobility) suffer long-term effects (NICE 2017b).

Patients should be encouraged to maintain muscle strength and length. Active ankle movements (Figure 7.1) are to be encouraged to assist the circulation.

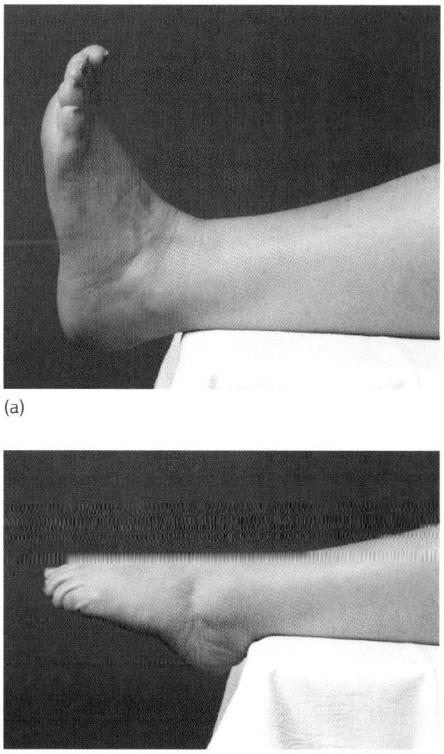

(a) (b)

Figure 7.1 (a) Ankle in dorsiflexion (DF). (b) Ankle in plantarflexion (PF).

Risk assessment

There is an absolute requirement to assess the risks arising from moving and handling patients (CSP 2014). Local policy on risk assessment and documentation should be referred to and local manual handling training adhered to. Once the risk of not moving the patient is deemed to be greater than moving the patient, consider the following (TILE):

T *Task/operation*: achieving the desired position or movement.
I *Individual*: this refers to the handler(s). In patient handling, this relates to the skills, competence and physical capabilities of the handlers. It is also important to consider health status, height, gender, pregnancy status, age and disability.
L *Load*: in the case of patient handling, the load is the patient. The aim of rehabilitation is, where possible, to encourage patients to move for themselves or contribute towards this goal. This may mean that additional equipment is needed. For assistance and guidance, liaise with the physiotherapist and/or occupational therapist.
E *Environment*: before positioning or moving the patient, think about the space, placement of equipment and removal of any hazards.

Other factors, for example any intravenous infusions or monitoring attached to the patient, must also be considered when undertaking a risk assessment. The key points to consider are summarized in Box 7.1.

Where there is any doubt about patients with complex needs, seek advice from the physiotherapist or the occupational therapist. Once a risk assessment has been carried out, this needs to be recorded prior to proceeding with any manual handling intervention (CSP 2014).

Consent must be obtained before any intervention is started. Consent is the voluntary and continuing permission of the patient to receive a particular treatment based on an adequate knowledge of the purpose, nature and likely risks of the treatment, including the likelihood of its success and any alternatives to it. Valid consent must be obtained before commencing an examination, starting treatment or physical investigation, or providing care (RCN 2017).

Clinical governance

For recommendations and further information on safe manual handling, refer to professional guidance (CSP 2014), government and local trust policy (HSE 2018), and the local manual handling

Box 7.1 Risk assessment

1 Assess the patient holistically.
2 Consider realistic clinical goals and functional outcomes in discussion with the patient and ascertain the level at which the patient will be able to participate in the task.
3 Consider whether the proposed intervention involves hazardous manual handling and reduce the hazard by:
   a adapting the technique
   b introducing equipment as needed following assessment
   c seeking advice/assistance from appropriately skilled colleagues.
4 Risk assessment should be an ongoing process and be constantly updated.
5 After the procedure, document the risk assessment, being sure to include the date, the number of staff involved and the equipment needed to perform the task. Also document any changes in the patient's condition, such as skin redness. It is important to also document the intended duration for which the patient should be maintained in this new position.

Source: Adapted from CSP (2014). Reproduced with permission of The Chartered Society of Physiotherapy.

advisor or physiotherapist. This is particularly relevant when dealing with complex, high-risk situations.

Pre-procedural considerations

Before positioning or moving the patient, carry out a comprehensive assessment. Consider the following factors.

Pressure and skin care

All clinical staff should be aware of the risk factors for developing pressure damage. These include:

- significantly limited mobility (e.g. in people with a spinal cord injury)
- significant loss of sensation
- a previous or current pressure ulcer
- nutritional deficiency
- incontinence
- significant cognitive impairment.

Direct pressure and friction during movement of patients are two of the most common causes of injury to the skin that can lead to pressure damage. Also consider shearing forces, which may occur when patients are at risk of sliding down in the bed or chair. Consider using a validated scale to support clinical judgement. Any patient with pressure damage or a pressure ulcer or who is thought to be at risk should be positioned with the use of pressure-relieving equipment such as a specialist mattress and cushion. Additional use of pillows and/or towels may be required depending on individual assessment.

Using a tool such as the ASSKING bundle can manage and prevent pressure damage. ASSKING is a five-step approach to preventing and treating pressure ulcers (NHS Improvement 2018):

- **A**ssess risk.
- **S**urface: consider the pressure exerted by the bed or chair. Provide specialist equipment where needed.
- **S**kin inspection: early inspection means early detection. Show patients and carers what to look for.
- **K**eep your patients moving.
- **I**ncontinence/moisture: your patients need to be clean and dry.
- **N**utrition/hydration: help patients have the right diet and plenty of fluids.
- **G**ive information.

See Chapter 18: Wound management for further information.

Wounds

Consider the location of wounds and injuries when selecting a comfortable position. Ideally positions should avoid pressure on or stretching of any wounds, and consideration should be given to the timing of dressing changes, which ideally should be done prior to positioning to avoid disturbing the patient twice. Specific surgical needs may also be apparent that will require a patient to remain in certain positions, posing further complications to the moving and positioning of the patient.

Sensation

Take extra care in positioning patients with decreased sensation as numbness and paraesthesia (abnormal skin sensation) may result in skin damage as the patient is unaware of pressure or chafing. These patients may not be aware of the need to adjust their position or alert nursing staff to discomfort so it is very important to reposition them frequently and check their skin regularly for areas of redness or breakdown.

Oedema/swelling

Where possible, swollen limbs should not be left dependent but be supported on pillows or a footstool, as elevation will help to maximize venous return and minimize further swelling. Oedema may result in pain, fragile skin or loss of joint movement.

Pain

It is important to ensure the patient has optimal pain relief before they move. Pain is often a barrier to early mobilization in intensive care settings and after surgery (Dubb et al. 2016, Jønsson et al. 2018). It is important to allow adequate time for any pain medication to take effect.

Weakness

The patient's ability to maintain the position should be considered. Additional support may be required in the form of pillows or towels to maintain the desired posture.

Limitations of joint and soft tissue range (contractures)

Changes in the soft tissue and joint range benefit from being identified early as some will respond to physiotherapy. Soft tissue changes and contractures can occur through disuse although the pathology is poorly understood (Wong et al. 2015). As a result, restrictions in joint range may mean that positions need to be modified or are inappropriate altogether.

If there is the potential for any joint or soft tissue restriction then it is necessary to liaise with the physiotherapist or occupational therapist regarding any specific exercises or positions necessary for the patient to avoid developing contractures, as this may affect position choice or involve incorporating appropriate splinting to maintain muscle length.

Fracture or suspected fracture

Patients with unstable fractures or suspected fractures should not be moved and the area should be well supported. A change of position could result in pain, fracture displacement and associated complications. Patients with osteoporosis or metastatic bone disease with unexplained bony pain should be treated as having a suspected fracture until this is ruled out.

Osteoporosis refers to a reduction in the quantity and quality of bone due to loss of both bone mineral and protein content. Risk factors for osteoporosis increase with age and include being female, Caucasian or postmenopausal; having a low body mass index (BMI), a positive family history of osteoporosis or a sedentary lifestyle; and having Coeliac or Crohn's disease (NHS 2016).

Altered tone

Muscle tone can be defined as the degree of resistance to a passive movement. The degree of resistance is determined to be less than normal (hypotonic), normal or more than normal (hypertonic). The last of these three may be referred to as spasticity (Latish and Zatsiorsky 2015).

Tone can be altered by positioning with either positive or negative consequences. Further information on moving and handling patients either with neurological impairment or who are unconscious is outlined later in this chapter.

Spinal stability

It is important to establish spinal stability before positioning or moving a patient. Failure to do so could lead to further complications such as paralysis. The specifics of moving and positioning a patient with spinal cord compression are discussed later in this chapter.

Medical devices associated with treatment

Care should be taken to avoid pulling on or causing an occlusion if the patient has a catheter, intravenous infusion, venous access device or drain. Pulling on devices may cause pain and/or injury. Prior to any moving or positioning procedure, it is important to ensure that any electrical pumps have been disconnected and sets are untangled and flowing freely. Once the moving or positioning procedure has been completed, a check must be made to ensure all devices are reconnected.

Medical status and cardiovascular instability

Patients who are medically unstable may become increasingly so during movement. Orthostatic tolerance (postural hypotension) deteriorates rapidly with immobility. Bedrest lessens carotid–cardiac baroreceptor reflex responsiveness, contributing to postural hypotension and tachycardia and, as a result, a reduction in stroke volume and cardiac output (Vollman 2012); therefore, patients who are acutely unwell should be monitored carefully during and after any change of position or when mobilizing. Post-operative patients may have a drop in blood pressure when sat up in the early post-operative period. It is advisable to sit a post-operative patient on the edge of the bed for a few minutes before transferring them into a chair to ensure blood pressure is maintained in a seated posture and the patient is not at risk of fainting.

Fatigue

Fatigue can be a distressing symptom, so advice and help should be given to the patient about how to pace their everyday activities. Therefore, prioritizing activities may help to avoid engaging in tasks that are unnecessary or of little value (de Raaf et al. 2012). Graded exercise programmes can be beneficial in managing fatigue (White et al. 2011).

Cognitive state

It is important to explain to the patient the reasons for moving and positioning, and to do so in a manner appropriate to their level of understanding. Step-by-step explanations and clear instructions should be given to enable them to participate in the movement. It is known that impaired cognition (the mental process involved in gaining knowledge and comprehension) and depression are intrinsic risk factors for falls in older people (NICE 2013).

Privacy and dignity

Shutting the door and/or the curtains prior to moving the patient will help to maintain privacy and dignity, and will ensure that the environment is as private as possible (CSP 2014). It may be appropriate to ask visitors to wait outside. The process of uncovering the patient may make them feel vulnerable and/or distressed, so keep them covered as much as is practically possible during the procedure. Catheter bags and drains should be hung as discreetly as possible under the patient's bed or chair.

Explanation and instructions for the patient

Before changing a patient's position, it is important to fully inform them of the planned change in position so they are able to consent and to participate with the manoeuvre and reduce the need for assistance. Explaining the potential complications associated with immobility may also help to motivate the patient.

Documentation and liaison with multidisciplinary team

There may be instructions or indications regarding moving and positioning the patient in their health records. If there is uncertainty, advice should be sought from the medical team or physiotherapists involved in the patient's care. It is also important to consider the result of the manual handling risk assessment and recommendations from the physiotherapy staff for any special precautions that need to be taken into account prior to moving and positioning.

Prevention of falls

Based on data submitted to the National Reporting and Learning System (NHS Improvement 2017), around 250,000 falls were reported in 2015/16 across acute, mental health and community hospital settings. During this period, 77% of all reported inpatient falls happened to patients over the age of 65 despite that group representing only 40% of total admissions across these three hospital settings combined (NHS Improvement 2017). The human costs of falling include distress, pain, injury, loss of confidence, loss of independence and mortality. Falling also affects the family members and carers of people who fall. Falls are estimated to cost the NHS more than £2.3 billion per year (NICE 2013). Therefore, falling has an impact on quality of life, health and healthcare costs (NICE 2013).

Definition

A fall is an event that results in a person coming to rest unintentionally on the ground, the floor or other lower level (CSP 2014).

Related theory

Falls among inpatients are the most frequently reported safety incident in NHS hospitals. Between 30% and 50% of falls result in physical injury, and fractures occur in 1–3% of falls. No fall is harmless, with psychological sequelae leading to lost confidence, delays in functional recovery and prolonged hospitalization (Morris and O'Riordan 2017).

Evidence-based approaches

Falls from the bed account for 30% of falls and this must be considered when positioning a patient in bed (Richardson and Carter 2015). Preventing falls in older people has been well described in national guidance and all prevention programmes should include particular reference to the care of older people (Age UK 2013). The causes of falls are complex and elderly hospital patients are particularly likely to be vulnerable to falling due to medical conditions including delirium; cardiac, neurological or musculoskeletal conditions; side-effects from medication; or problems with their balance, strength, mobility and/or eyesight. Problems such as reduced or poor memory can lead to disorientation and therefore create a greater risk of falls when someone is out of their normal environment and on a hospital ward. Continence problems can mean patients are vulnerable to falling while making urgent journeys to the toilet. However, patient safety has to be balanced with independence, rehabilitation, privacy and dignity. A patient who is not allowed to walk alone will very quickly become a patient who is unable to walk alone. Specialist exercise programmes include STEEP (the Staying Steady Exercise and Education Programme), which consists of advice and an exercise session run over a 7-week period (NICE 2017a). The prevention of falls requires a systematic multiprofessional approach in order to nurture a culture of vigilant safety consciousness by all staff (Morris and O'Riordan 2017). Individual needs and the various environmental factors associated with different settings – for example, home, care home or hospital – will need to be assessed regularly.

Increasing patient awareness by advising and educating on reducing the risk of falls should be encouraged. The use of booklets such as *Falls Prevention in Hospital: A Guide for Patients, Their Families and Carers* (Royal College of Physicians 2017) clearly outlines ways to reduce the risk factors. It is the responsibility of all staff to report any environmental hazards within their working areas and to ensure that spillages are removed and appropriate signage is used to warn people of hazards.

Risk factors

It is important to consider the risk of falls when undertaking a manual handling risk assessment on patient admission. The patient's risk of falls should be reconsidered at weekly intervals,

Table 7.1 Falls: risk factors

Intrinsic risk factors	Extrinsic risk factors	Behavioural risk factors
• [illegible] • Impaired balance and gait, or restricted mobility • Medical history of Parkinson's disease, stroke, arthritis or cardiac abnormalities • Fear of falling • Medication, including polypharmacy and psychotropic medication • Dizziness • Postural hypotension • Syncope • Reduced muscle strength • Foot problems • Incontinence • Cognitive impairment • Impaired vision • Low mood • Pain	• [illegible] • Clutter and tripping hazards, for example rugs and trailing wires • Floor coverings • Poor lighting, glare and shadows • Lack of appropriate adaptations such as grab rails and stair rails • Low furniture • No access to telephone or alarm call system • Poor heating • Thresholds and doors • Difficult access to property, bins, garden and uneven ground • Inappropriate walking aids • Pets	• Limited physical activity or exercise • Poor nutrition or fluid intake • Alcohol intake • Carrying, reaching and bending • Risk-taking behaviours such as climbing on chairs, use of ladders • Inappropriate footwear

or if the patient experiences a fall or their condition changes significantly. Risk factors can be broadly divided into intrinsic and extrinsic risks (Table 7.1).

Once the risk has been assessed, any identified risk factors need to be addressed and managed. In order to reduce the risk, it is important to investigate every fall that does occur and understand the circumstances surrounding it. A useful way of analysing falls is to categorize them and to map areas on the ward or areas in the hospital where more than one patient has fallen. Common themes can then be identified and strategies can be implemented to reduce the risk.

Positioning a patient: in bed

Evidence-based approaches

Rationale

Effective positioning of a patient in bed is essential, not only to ensure their comfort but also to prevent injury, such as pressure, muscle or joint damage.

Indications

Positioning in bed is indicated for any patient who is unable to reposition themselves independently.

Contraindications

There are no absolute contraindications; however, some patients will have specific conditions to take into account prior to undertaking this procedure and some of these are considered in the following sections.

Equipment

Whenever safe and possible, patients should always be encouraged to take the initiative to be as independent as possible in positioning themselves and changing their position in bed. If they do require assistance, sliding sheets should be used to assist patients to roll or change position in bed. Due to the slippery surface of the sliding sheet fabric, friction is reduced and patients can be moved or relocated with very minimal effort or discomfort (Ruszala and Alexander 2015).

Procedure guideline 7.1 Positioning a patient: supine

Essential equipment

- Personal protective equipment
- Sliding sheets
- Pillows
- Clean linen (if required)

Action	Rationale
Pre-procedure	
1 Introduce yourself to the patient, explain and discuss the procedure with them, and gain their consent to proceed.	To ensure that the patient feels at ease, understands the procedure and gives their valid consent (NMC 2018, **C**).
2 Wash hands thoroughly with soap and water or use an alcohol-based handrub.	To reduce the risk of contamination and cross-infection (NHS England and NHSI 2019, **C**; WHO 2012, **C**).
Procedure	
3 Ensure the bed is at the optimum height for the handlers. If two handlers are required, try to match the handlers' heights as far as possible.	To minimize the risk of injury to practitioners (Treadwell 2013, **E**).
4 *Either*: Place one pillow squarely under the patient's head.	To support the head in a neutral position and to compensate for the natural lordosis (anatomical concavity) of the cervical spine (Fragala 2015, **E**). To increase patient support and comfort (Fragala 2015, **E**).

Or: Use two pillows in a 'butterfly' position so that two layers of pillow support the head with one layer of pillow under each shoulder.	This may be necessary for a patient with pain, breathlessness (see the section 'Moving and positioning a patient with respiratory compromise' below) or an existing kyphosis (anatomical convexity of the spine) (Fragala 2015, **E**).
Or: Use a folded towel under the patient's head if this provides natural spinal alignment.	To prevent excessive neck flexion (Fragala 2015, **E**).
5 Ensure the patient lies centrally in the bed.	To ensure spinal and limb alignment. To reduce the risk of falls by ensuring the patient is not too close to the edge of the bed. To prevent peripheral nerve injury (Bouyer-Ferullo 2013, **E**).
6 Place pillows and/or towels under individual limbs to provide maximum support for a patient with painful, weak or oedematous limbs.	To ensure patient comfort (Bouyer-Ferullo 2013, **E**).
7 Ensure the patient's feet are fully supported by the mattress. For taller patients, use a bed extension if required.	To ensure patient comfort (Bouyer-Ferullo 2013, **E**).
8 Place a pillow at the end of the bed to support the ankles at 90° of flexion if the patient has weakness or is immobile around the ankle.	To ensure patient comfort (Fragala 2015, **E**). To prevent loss of ankle movement (Bouyer-Ferullo 2013, **E**).
Post-procedure	
9 Document the details of the procedure.	To fulfil the legal requirements of the professional body and employing institution (NMC 2018, **C**).

Positioning a patient: sitting up in bed

Evidence-based approaches

Rationale

Indications

Patients should be encouraged to sit up in bed (Figure 7.2) regularly if their medical condition prevents them from sitting out in a chair. If the patient is unable to participate fully in the procedure, manual handling equipment should be used to help achieve the desired position. Attention should also be given to the sitting posture. Poor posture is one of the most common causes of low back pain, which is frequently brought on by sitting for a long time in a poor position (Perry 2013).

Contraindications

After a lumbar puncture, patients should lie flat to prevent dural headache in accordance with local policy.

Spinal instability

Refer to the section 'Moving and positioning a patient with actual or suspected spinal cord compression or spinal cord injury' below and see Procedure guideline 7.13: Log rolling a patient with suspected or confirmed cervical spinal instability (above T6).

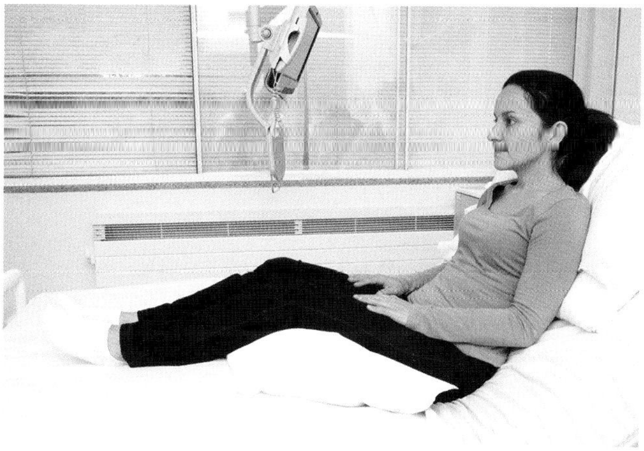

Figure 7.2 Sitting up in bed.

Procedure guideline 7.2 Positioning a patient: sitting up in bed

Essential equipment

- Personal protective equipment
- Pillows
- Other manual handling equipment (as required and as advised by local policy)

Action	Rationale
Pre-procedure	
1 Introduce yourself to the patient, explain and discuss the procedure with them, and gain their consent to proceed.	To ensure that the patient feels at ease, understands the procedure and gives their valid consent (NMC 2018, **C**).
2 Wash hands thoroughly with soap and water or use an alcohol-based handrub.	To reduce the risk of contamination and cross-infection (NHS England and NHSI 2019, **C**; WHO 2012, **C**).

(continued)

Procedure guideline 7.2 Positioning a patient: sitting up in bed *(continued)*

Action	Rationale
Procedure	
3 Ensure the bed is at the optimum height for the handlers. If two handlers are required, try to match the handlers' heights as far as possible.	To minimize the risk of injury to the practitioners (Treadwell 2013, **E**).
4 Ask the patient to sit up in the centre of the bed. The angle at which the patient sits may be influenced by pain, fatigue, abdominal distension or level of confusion/agitation.	To reduce the risk of falls by ensuring the patient is not too close to the edge of the bed (Richardson and Carter 2015, **E**). To encourage haemodynamic stability (Heravi et al. 2015, **E**). To enable effective breathing patterns, maximizing basal expansion (Katz et al. 2018, **R**). To assist in functional activities such as eating and drinking (Szczygieł et al. 2017, **E**).
5 Ask the patient to position their hips in line with the hinge of the automatic mattress elevator or backrest of the bed.	To ensure good postural alignment – that is, flexing at the hip when sitting up in bed (McInnes et al. 2014, **E**). To prevent strain on the spine. (Szczygieł et al. 2017, **E**).
6 Place a pillow under the patient's knees or use the electrical control of the bed to slightly bend the patient's knees (Figure 7.2). Extra care should be taken if the patient has a femoral line.	To reduce strain on the lumbar spine (Szczygieł et al. 2017, **E**). To maintain the position (McInnes et al. 2014, **E**)
7 Place a pillow under individual or both upper limbs for patients with a chest drain, upper limb weakness, trunk weakness, or surgery involving the shoulder(s), upper limb, breast(s) or thorax. Also do this for fungating wounds involving the axilla, breast(s) or shoulder(s); for upper limb or truncal lymphoedema; and for fractures involving ribs or upper limbs.	To provide upper limb support (McInnes et al. 2014, **E**). To maintain trunk alignment (McInnes et al. 2014, **E**). To encourage basal expansion (Katz et al. 2018, **R**).
Post-procedure	
8 Document the details of the procedure.	To fulfil the legal requirements of the professional body and employing institution (NMC 2018, **C**).

Positioning a patient: side-lying

Evidence-based approaches

Rationale

Indications

This can be a useful position for patients with:

- compromised venous return, for example due to pelvic or abdominal mass, or pregnancy
- global motor weakness
- risk of developing pressure sores
- unilateral pelvic or lower limb pain
- altered tone (see the 'Moving and positioning a patient with neurological impairment' section)
- fatigue
- chest infection, for gravity-assisted drainage of secretions
- lung pathology (see the section 'Moving and positioning a patient with respiratory compromise' below)
- abdominal distension (e.g. ascites) or bulky disease, to optimize lung volume (see the section 'Moving and positioning a patient with respiratory compromise' below).

Contraindications

This procedure is contraindicated in patients with suspected or actual spinal fracture or instability. Refer to the section 'Moving and positioning a patient with actual or suspected spinal cord compression or spinal cord injury' below.

Procedure guideline 7.3 Positioning a patient: side-lying

Essential equipment

- Personal protective equipment
- Pillows
- Manual handling equipment (e.g. sliding sheets or a hoist) may be required following risk assessment, depending on local policy

Action	Rationale
Pre-procedure	
1 Introduce yourself to the patient, explain and discuss the procedure with them, and gain their consent to proceed.	To ensure that the patient feels at ease, understands the procedure and gives their valid consent (NMC 2018, **C**).
2 Wash hands thoroughly with soap and water or use an alcohol-based handrub.	To reduce the risk of contamination and cross-infection (NHS England and NHSI 2019, **C**; WHO 2012, **C**).

Procedure

3 Ensure the bed is at the optimum height for the handlers. If two handlers are required, try to match the handlers' heights as far as possible.	To minimize the risk of injury to the practitioners (Treadwell 2013, **E**).
4 Place one or two pillows in a 'butterfly' position under the patient's head, ensuring the airway remains patent. Extra care should be taken for those patients with an artificial airway, central lines, or recent head or neck surgery.	To support the head in the midline position (Yoshikawa et al. 2015, **E**). To support the shoulder contours (Yoshikawa et al. 2015, **E**).
5 Ask or assist the patient to semi-flex the lowermost leg at the hip and the knee and roll onto their side. Extra care should be taken with the degree of flexion for those patients who have hip or knee pain or loss of movement, fracture involving the femur or pelvis, leg oedema, femoral lines or other venous access devices. Ensure the patient is lying centrally in the bed.	To support the patient in a stable position and prevent rolling (Yoshikawa et al. 2015, **E**). To reduce the risk of falls by ensuring the patient is not too close to the edge of the bed (Richardson and Carter 2015, **E**).
6 *Either:* Ask or assist the patient to semi-flex the uppermost leg at the hip and knee. Use a pillow for support under the leg placed on the bed. *Or:* Place a pillow between the patient's knees.	To prevent lumbar spine rotation (Yoshikawa et al. 2015, **E**). To support the pelvic girdle (Yoshikawa et al. 2015, **E**). To aid pressure care. **E**
7 Place the underneath arm in front with scapula protracted (**Action figure 7**) – that is, pushed forward (this would not be appropriate for patients with shoulder pathology). Extra care should be taken with patients with low tone in the affected arm, swollen arms or access lines in that arm.	To promote patient comfort. **E** To promote shoulder alignment. **E** To provide additional support and comfort. **E**

Post-procedure

8 Document the details of the procedure.	To fulfil the legal requirements of the professional body and employing institution (NMC 2018, **C**).

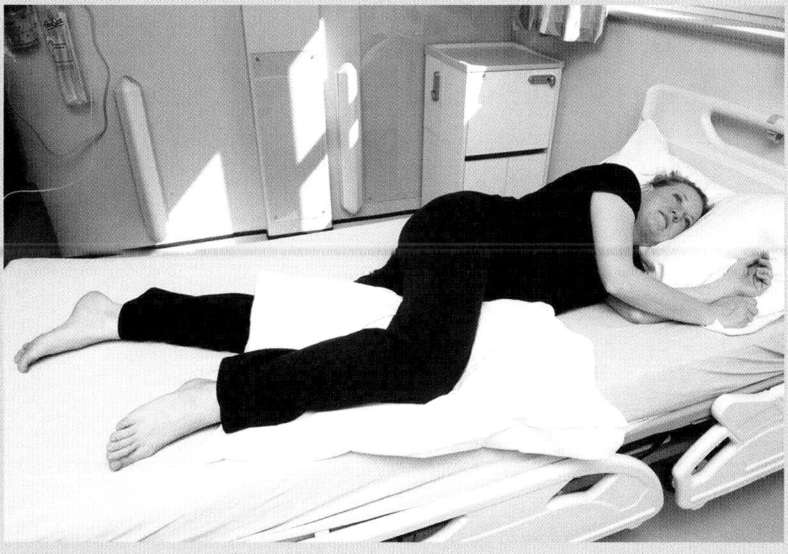

Action Figure 7 Side-lying position.

Procedure guideline 7.4 Positioning a patient: lying down to sitting up

Essential equipment

- Personal protective equipment
- Manual handling equipment (e.g. sliding sheet) or 2 people may be required following risk assessment, depending on local policy

Action	Rationale
Pre-procedure	
1 Introduce yourself to the patient, explain and discuss the procedure with them, and gain their consent to proceed.	To ensure that the patient feels at ease, understands the procedure and gives their valid consent (NMC 2018, **C**).
2 Wash hands thoroughly or use an alcohol-based handrub.	To reduce the risk of contamination and cross-infection (NHS England and NHSI 2019, **C**).
Procedure	
3 Ensure the bed is at the optimum height for the handlers. If two handlers are required, try to match the handlers' heights as far as possible.	To minimize the risk of injury to the practitioners (Treadwell 2013, **E**).
4 Ask the patient to bend both knees and turn their head towards the direction they are moving. Ask the patient to reach towards the side of the bed with the uppermost arm and roll onto their side. Abdominal wounds should be supported by the patient's hands. Extra care should be taken with patients who have joint pathology, oedema, ascites or positional vertigo (dizziness or giddiness).	To assist the patient to roll using their bodyweight. **E**
5 Ask the patient to bend their knees and lower their feet over the edge of the bed (**Action figure 5a**). Ask the patient to push through the underneath elbow and the upper arm on the bed to push up into a sitting position (**Action figure 5b**). As the patient sits up, monitor changes in pain or dizziness, which could indicate postural hypotension or vertigo. Be aware that a patient with neurological symptoms or weakness may not have safe sitting balance and may be at risk of falling. Refer to Procedure guideline 7.10: Positioning the neurological patient with tonal problems in bed.	To help to lever the patient into a sitting position using the weight of their legs. **E**
6 Assist the patient to achieve an upright sitting position with appropriate alignment of the body parts.	To ensure a safe sitting position. **E**
Post-procedure	
7 Once the patient is on the edge of the bed, safely supported as required, continue to mobilize or transfer them to a wheelchair, commode or chair using local mobilizing policy.	To ensure safe transfers. **E**
8 Document the details of the procedure.	To fulfil the legal requirements of the professional body and employing institution (NMC 2018, **C**).

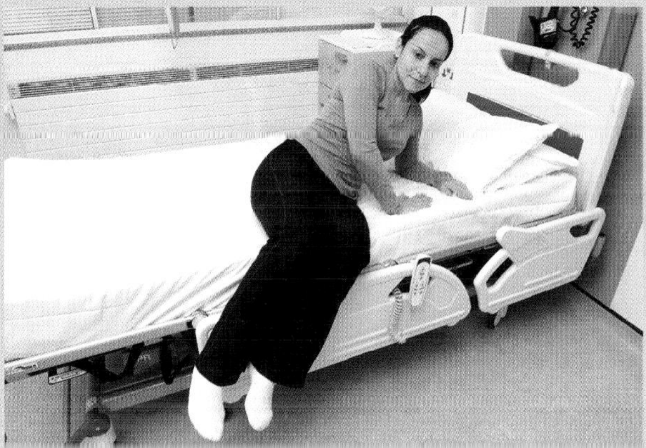

Action Figure 5a Lying to sitting

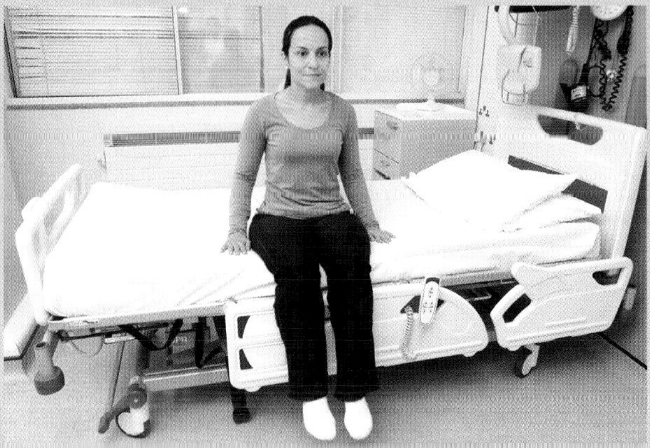

Action Figure 5b Sitting on the edge of the bed (from side-lying).

Moving a patient from sitting to standing

Evidence-based approaches

Rationale

Indications

The patient should be encouraged to take the initiative to stand up safely from the edge of the bed by pushing down on the mattress with both hands, leaning forwards by flexing from the hips, and standing in a controlled and safe manner. Once the patient feels safe in their standing balance, they can start to walk safely and independently. This will improve their confidence in mobilizing safely, encourage good lung capacity, promote improved strength in their posture and quadriceps, and promote balance.

Contraindications

If the patient does not feel safe or feels dizzy or unsteady, they should sit back down gently and in a controlled manner by placing their hands back to feel for the mattress, feeling the bed behind the back of their legs and lowering themselves back to sitting. The patient should be assessed, and observations and vital signs should be recorded to ensure there are no concerns regarding these.

If the patient has attachments (e.g. catheter, intravenous drip or feeding tubes) in place, they will require the assistance and supervision of at least one person to ensure they do not trip over or dislodge these.

A physiotherapy referral may be appropriate.

Procedure guideline 7.5 Moving a patient from sitting to standing: assisting the patient

Essential equipment

- Personal protective equipment
- Walking aid (if required)
- Suitable non-slip, well-fitting, supportive and flat footwear (if not available then bare feet are preferable to socks or stockings, which may slip)

Action	Rationale
Pre-procedure	
1 Introduce yourself to the patient, explain and discuss the procedure with them, and gain their consent to proceed.	To ensure that the patient feels at ease, understands the procedure and gives their valid consent (NMC 2018, **C**).
2 Wash hands thoroughly with soap and water or use an alcohol-based handrub.	To reduce the risk of contamination and cross-infection (NHS England and NHSI 2019, **C**; WHO 2012 **E**).
3 Ask or assist the patient to put on their shoes.	To reduce the risk of falls (Treadwell 2013, **E**).
4 Ensure walking aids are positioned and ready to use.	To reduce the risk of falls (Treadwell 2013, **E**).
5 Disconnect any unnecessary lines and attachments, or ensure they have plenty of slack.	To reduce the risk of falls (Treadwell 2013, **E**).
Procedure	
6 Ask the patient to lean forwards and 'shuffle' (by transferring their weight from side to side) and bring their bottom closer to the front of the chair or edge of the bed.	To bring the patient's weight over their feet. **E**
7 Ask the patient to move their feet back so they are slightly tucked under the chair or bed with their feet hip-width apart.	To provide a stable base prior to moving. **E**
8 Instruct the patient to lean forwards from their trunk (**Action figure 8**).	To help initiate movement. **E** To facilitate a normal pattern of movement. **E**
9 Instruct the patient to push through their hands on the arms of the chair or surface of the bed as they stand. Encourage a forward and upward motion while extending their hips and knees (**Action figure 9**).	To minimize energy expenditure and maximize safety. **E**
10 Once the patient is standing, provide aids as required and ask the patient to stand still for a moment to ensure balance is achieved before they attempt to walk.	To ensure safe, static standing and reduce the risk of falling. **E**
Post-procedure	
11 Document the details of the procedure.	To fulfil the legal requirements of the professional body and employing institution (NMC 2018, **C**). To communicate ability and assessment to other healthcare professionals. **E**

(continued)

Procedure guideline 7.5 Moving a patient from sitting to standing: assisting the patient (continued)

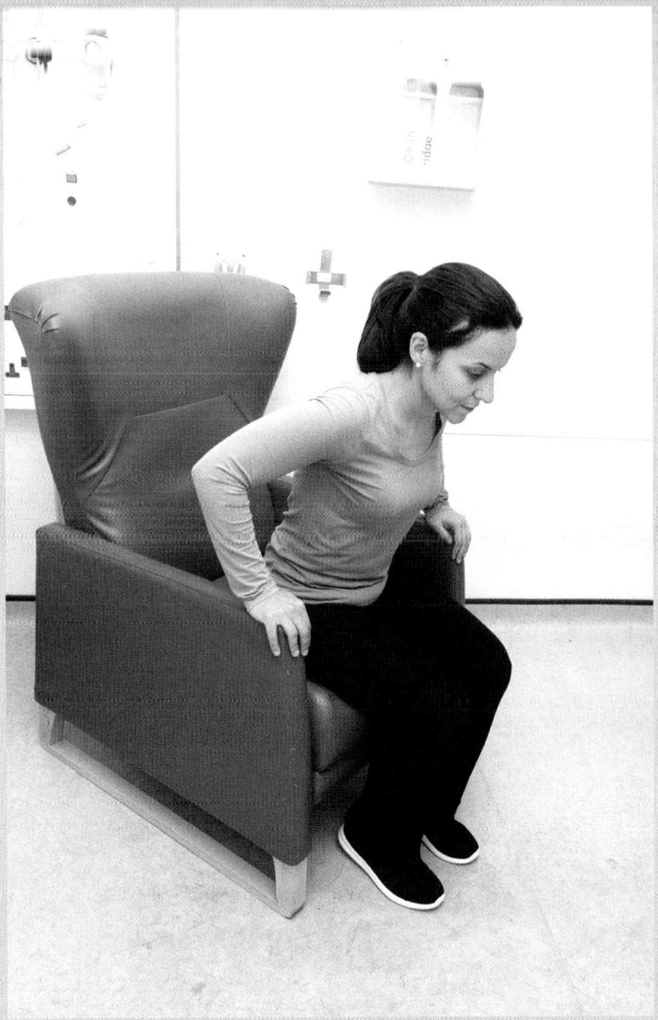

Action Figure 8 Preparing to stand from sitting.

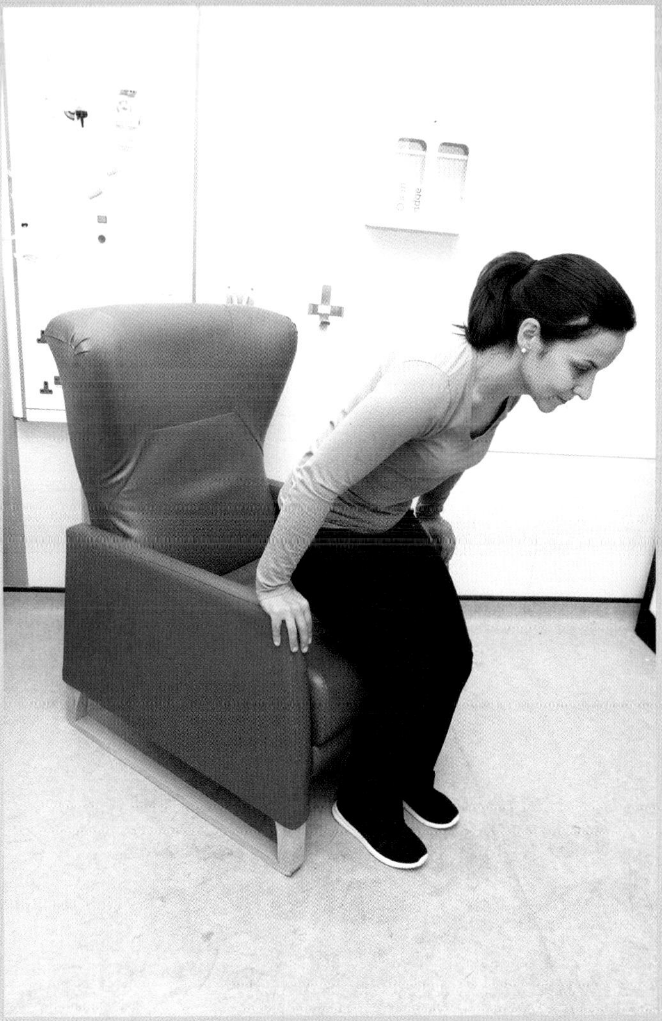

Action Figure 9 Sitting to standing from a chair.

Positioning a patient: in a chair or wheelchair

Evidence-based approaches

Rationale

Indications

The patient should sit out in a chair or wheelchair whenever possible to prevent chest infections, normalize blood pressure, allow the bodyweight to be distributed evenly over both hips and thighs, and increase their sitting tolerance and stamina. It will also encourage the patient to socialize and participate in their surroundings rather than being confined to bed, which will have an important impact on their psychological wellbeing (McDaniel and Browning 2014, Szczygieł et al. 2017).

If the patient is assessed and identified as being at risk of pressure ulcers, they will require a pressure-relieving cushion to distribute their weight evenly, prevent skin breakdown, and encourage sitting tolerance and improved posture. There are various types available and they are usually assessed for and provided by the occupational therapist, depending on the specific needs and requirements of the patient (NPUAP, EPUAP and PPPIA 2014).

Contraindications

The patient must be monitored regularly to ensure there is no risk of pressure ulcers developing. It is recommended that bony prominences and vulnerable areas of skin are monitored and recorded on a body chart or photographed to keep an accurate record (NPUAP, EPUAP and PPPIA 2014).

Procedure guideline 7.6 Positioning a patient: in a chair or wheelchair

Essential equipment

- Personal protective equipment
- Upright chair with arms that provide support from the elbow to wrist – if using a wheelchair, make certain that the chair has been measured by an occupational therapist to ensure correct fit and position of the footrests
- Manual handling equipment (e.g. a hoist) may be required following risk assessment, depending on local policy
- Pillows or a rolled-up towel
- Footstool if the patient has lower limb oedema
- Pressure cushion

Action	Rationale
Pre-procedure	
1 Introduce yourself to the patient, explain and discuss the procedure with them, and gain their consent to proceed.	To ensure that the patient feels at ease, understands the procedure and gives their valid consent (NMC 2018, **C**).
2 Wash hands thoroughly or use an alcohol-based handrub.	To reduce the risk of contamination and cross-infection (NHS England and NHSI 2019, **C**; WHO 2012 **C**).
Procedure	
3 Place a pressure-relieving cushion in the chair and ask the patient to sit well back in the chair. They should have a maximum of a 90° angle at their hips and knee joints. The patient may not be able to achieve this position if they have hip, back or any other pain, or abdominal distension. It may be necessary to refer the patient to an occupational therapist for assessment of the potential need to raise the height of the chair, provide a specialized cushion or provide other seating if a comfortable or safe position cannot be achieved.	Patients with reduced mobility are at greater risk of pressure skin damage (NPUAP, EPUAP and PPPIA 2014, **C**). To provide a stable base of support for balance and reduce the risk of falls. **E** To ensure good body alignment. **E** To achieve a safe sitting position. **E**
4 Place a pillow or rolled-up towel in the small of the patient's back according to what is comfortable for the patient.	To allow the patient's back to be supported in a good position. **E**
5 Ensure the patient's feet are resting on the floor or a supportive surface. Use pillows or a rolled-up towel to provide support under the feet if necessary. Make sure the patient's feet are supported on the footrests if using a wheelchair.	To provide postural alignment and support the lumbar spine. **E**
6 If the patient has lower leg oedema, use a footstool, ensuring the whole leg and foot are supported and avoiding hyperextension (defined as excessive extension of a limb or joint) at the knees.	To improve venous drainage (Doughty and Sparks 2016, **E**).
Post-procedure	
7 Document the details of the procedure.	To fulfil the legal requirements of the professional body and employing institution (NMC 2018, **C**).

Walking

Definition

Walking is defined as 'to move at a regular pace by lifting and setting down each foot in turn, never having both feet off the ground at once' (Oxford Dictionaries 2019c).

Related theory

There are a variety of different walking aids designed to improve balance and safety, thus reducing the risk of falls. These should be assessed for by the physiotherapist, who will provide equipment as appropriate.

It is assumed that, if possible, the patient will take equal amounts of bodyweight through both legs, defined as being fully weight bearing (FWB). If the patient has to be non-weight bearing (NWB) or partially weight bearing (PWB), this will be due to bone or joint pathology – for example, fracture, joint instability, inflammation or infection.

If a patient has any difficulty walking, appears unsafe or is at risk of falling for any reason, refer them for a physiotherapy assessment. The physiotherapist will assess and issue the patient with an appropriate walking aid and provide appropriate advice.

Evidence-based approaches

Rationale

Indications

Patients should be encouraged to walk as soon as is safe and appropriate for their condition. This will promote their safety and independence, ensuring they return to their previous routine as soon as possible.

Contraindications

Certain surgical procedures or injuries may restrict a patient's ability to walk, or walking may be detrimental to their recovery for a period of time. Effective weight bearing and therefore walking may also be affected by pain, weakness and sensory changes, and may be contraindicated, especially without assistance or rehabilitation.

Procedure guideline 7.7 Assisting a patient to walk

Essential equipment

- Personal protective equipment
- Walking aid if required (if previously issued by physiotherapist)
- Suitable non-slip, well-fitting, supportive and flat footwear (if not available then bare feet are preferable to socks or stockings, which may slip)

Action	Rationale
Pre-procedure	
1 Introduce yourself to the patient, explain and discuss the procedure with them, and gain their consent to proceed.	To ensure that the patient feels at ease, understands the procedure and gives their valid consent (NMC 2018, **C**).
2 Wash hands thoroughly with soap and water or use an alcohol-based handrub.	To reduce the risk of contamination and cross-infection (NHS England and NHSI 2019, **C**; WHO 2012 **C**).
3 Ask or assist the patient to put on footwear, and provide walking aids.	To maximize safety and promote independence. **E**
4 Where possible, disconnect any attachments or devices (e.g. drainage bags, catheters or intravenous infusions). Ensure others are safely secured.	To prevent harm and to ensure attachments are not displaced. **E**
Procedure	
5 Stand next to and slightly behind the patient. Assistance is mostly given with a palm-to-palm hold, with the other hand under the patient's forearm. The nurse should not allow the patient to lean too heavily on them or grasp their thumb as this restricts them letting go in the event of a fall.	To give appropriate support. **E** To increase the patient's confidence. **E**
6 Observe changes in pain or breathlessness as the patient walks.	To assess patient safety and reduce the risk of falls (Ruszala and Alexander 2015, **E**).
7 Give verbal supervision and/or cueing as required to achieve safe walking.	To provide encouragement. **E** To ensure patient safety. **E**
Post-procedure	
8 Document the details of the procedure.	To fulfil the legal requirements of the professional body and employing institution (NMC 2018, **C**).

Problem-solving table 7.1 Prevention and resolution (Procedure guidelines 7.1, 7.2, 7.3, 7.4, 7.5, 7.6 and 7.7)

Problem	Cause	Prevention	Action
Increase in pain	Change in posture and position of joints and soft tissues. Patients who are symptom-controlled at rest may suffer incidental pain when moving.	Pre-procedural symptom control. Ongoing assessment of symptoms and adjustment of medication.	Assist the patient to move slowly and offer support and reassurance where needed.
Increase in nausea	Change in posture and position of joints and soft tissues. Patients who are symptom-controlled at rest may suffer incidental nausea when moving.	Pre-procedural symptom control. Ongoing assessment of symptoms and adjustment of medication.	Assist the patient to move slowly and offer support and reassurance where needed.
Change in clinical condition	Change in position may cause a drop in blood pressure or cause cardiovascular instability.	Monitor carefully.	Always have two people present if the patient is at risk of cardiovascular instability. Be prepared to return to the original position.
Bowel or bladder elimination	Change in position may stimulate bladder and bowels.	Have a commode nearby, or the ability to get the patient to the toilet should they need it. If the patient is incontinent, put pads and pants on the patient before moving.	It may be necessary to allow the patient to pass urine or open their bowels before continuing to move or position them.

Problem	Cause	Prevention	Action
Increase in loss of fluid, e.g. from a wound	Change in position may cause breakdown of primary healing or increase in muscular activity, which may increase fluid loss.	Give support to wounds during movement where possible. Seek advice from surgical teams prior to mobilizing.	Stop and alert the medical team for assessment.
Loss of consciousness, fainting	Change in position may cause a decrease in blood pressure.	Allow adequate time for the patient to adjust to a more upright position. Sit the patient up in bed and then sit them over the edge of the bed and allow time for positional adjustment in blood pressure before they attempt to stand.	Call for help and follow the emergency procedure. Refer to local procedure for managing a falling patient.
Fall	Multifactorial.	Risk assessment and planning.	Call for help and follow the emergency procedure. Refer to local procedure for managing a falling patient.
Poor adherence to or toleration of sitting position	Discomfort, reduced tolerance or cognitive issues	Use pillows and/or towels to ensure the patient is well supported and comfortable. A timed goal often helps with patient compliance. Start with a short time, for example 30 minutes, and build up the time slowly. Always tell the patient how long they are aiming to sit out for and make sure the call bell is within reach.	Combine sitting out with a mealtime as this can help the patient to eat more easily and also help to distract the patient from the length of time they have to sit out.
Inability to maintain the position	Patients who are weak and/or fatigued may be at risk of slipping or falling.	Careful positioning of towels and pillows may be needed to maintain a central, safe posture in the chair.	Observe the patient regularly.

Moving and positioning an unconscious patient

Definition

Consciousness is a state of awareness of self, environment and one's response to that environment. Being fully conscious means that the individual appropriately responds to external stimuli. An altered level of consciousness represents a decrease in this full state of awareness and response to environmental stimuli (Blume et al. 2015).

Anatomy and physiology

Unconsciousness is a physiological state in which the patient is unresponsive to sensory stimuli and lacks awareness of self and the environment (Wislowska et al. 2014). There are many central nervous system conditions that can result in a patient being in an unconscious state. In addition, an unconscious state can be medically induced, such as during general anaesthesia. The depth and duration of unconsciousness span a broad spectrum of presentations from fainting, with a momentary loss of consciousness, to prolonged coma lasting several weeks, months or even years. The physiological changes that occur in unconscious patients will depend on the cause of unconsciousness, the length of immobility while unconscious and the quality of care. Drugs (e.g. some muscle relaxants used in intensive care) can contribute to muscle weakness, raised intraocular and intracranial pressure, electrolyte imbalances and reduced airway tone (Murray et al. 2016). Unconsciousness can lead to problematic changes for patients that have implications for nursing interventions, including moving and positioning.

Evidence-based approaches

Principles of care

The general principles of care already mentioned in this chapter are relevant to the care of unconscious patients. However, there are some additional principles that should be considered.

Sedation

In critically ill patients, sedation is often an integral part of management. While the patient is sedated, the nurse must incorporate a rehabilitation framework to maintain intact function, prevent complications and disabilities, and restore lost function to the maximum extent possible. It may be appropriate to gain assistance from therapists to achieve this and assist in the rehabilitation process.

Titration of sedation to achieve patient comfort and compliance with interventions (e.g. mechanical ventilation) is essential. Daily sedation breaks are useful in order to assess whether the level of sedation is appropriate, with an aim of using the minimal amount to achieve patient comfort. Some studies have suggested that using this strategy results in a reduction of ventilator days and length of stay (Jackson et al. 2010). However, a Cochrane review by Burry et al. (2014) did not find conclusive support for this concept. Daily sedation holds remain common practice throughout intensive care practice (Richards-Belle et al. 2016).

Communication

There is evidence that unconscious patients are aware of what is happening to them and can hear conversations around them (Boyle 2018). It is therefore important to tell patients what is going to happen (e.g. that they are going to be moved) and explain the procedure just as it would be explained to a conscious patient.

Immobility

The human body is designed for physical activity and movement. Therefore, any lack of movement, regardless of reason, can result in multisystem deconditioning as well as anatomical and physiological changes. Guidance from a physiotherapist for passive exercises early in the period of unconsciousness may help in the prevention of further complications, for example joint stiffness and loss of joint movement. There is, however, no evidence to justify the inclusion of regular passive movements within the standard management of a patient's care. Intervention should be specific to the patient's presentation.

Despite sedation and critical illness, patients may be able to participate in some active movements and it has been shown that it is safe and appropriate for them to do so (Hodgson et al. 2014). Therefore, it is also important to assist the patient to complete early mobilization and functional movements, such as sitting over the edge of the bed, sitting in a chair and mobilizing. Guidance and intervention from physiotherapists and occupational therapists is essential to assist in the patient's rehabilitation and restore normal movement, and thus to minimize the effects and complications of prolonged immobility and bedrest (Denehy et al. 2017).

Effects of immobility of muscle

There are two major effects of muscle immobility:

- *Decreased muscle strength*: the degree of loss varies between muscle groups and according to the degree of immobility (Jolley et al. 2016, Puthucheary et al. 2010). The anti-gravitational muscles of the legs lose strength twice as quickly as the arm muscles and their recovery takes longer.
- *Muscle atrophy (loss of muscle mass)*: when a muscle is relaxed, it atrophies about twice as rapidly as when it is in a stretched position (Hickey and Powers 2011). Critical illness accelerates the rate of muscle wasting (weakness and atrophy) (Parry and Puthucheary 2015).

Respiratory function

Due to the immobility of the unconscious patient, there is an increased threat of them developing respiratory complications such as atelectasis, pneumonia, aspiration and airway obstruction. Respiratory assessment should be carried out prior to moving the patient and changing their position in order to provide a baseline that can be referred to following the procedure. The assessment should include checking the patency of the airway; monitoring the rate, pattern and work of breathing; testing peripheral oxygen saturations using a pulse oximeter; and measuring blood gases to assess adequacy of gaseous exchange (Hodgson et al. 2014).

Patients may require mechanical ventilation for the following reasons:

- inability to ventilate adequately, for example post-anaesthesia, due to inspiratory muscle weakness, or in cases of respiratory failure due to respiratory disease
- inability to protect their own airway or presenting with upper airway obstruction
- ability to breathe adequately but may be inadvisable depending on diagnosis, for example with an acute head injury for neuro-protection.

Mechanical ventilation may be required for days, weeks or even months (Damuth et al. 2015). It is worth remembering that mechanically ventilated patients often cannot express any sort of preference for certain body positions. If the patient is intubated with an endotracheal tube, they are at increased risk of developing nosocomial infections (Kalil et al. 2016, Wang et al. 2016), so it is important that lung volumes and respiratory mechanics are continuously monitored in these patients. Consequently, early mobilization is of great benefit for this patient group. Referral to the physiotherapy team is vital to instigate early intervention and rehabilitation to minimize respiratory complications (Parry and Puthucheary 2015).

Cardiovascular function

Immobility can cause changes in cardiovascular function, for example increased cardiac workload, decreased cardiac output, decreased blood pressure and decreased circulating volume (Koo and Fan 2013). Immobility causes a reduction in patients' maximum oxygen uptake (VO_2 max) which is the body's ability to extract and utilize oxygen for work. This affects the body's reserve capacity and therefore the ability to perform exercise and everyday functional movements (Koo and Fan 2013). In addition, the positioning of the unconscious patient will cause central fluid shift, from the legs to the thorax and head, so the head of the unconscious patient with raised intracranial pressure may need to be elevated to at least 30° (Jeon et al. 2014).

Circulatory function

The risk of deep vein thrombosis and pulmonary embolism is increased in the unconscious patient. This is due to several factors, including blood pooling in the legs, hypercoagulability and prolonged pressure from immobility in bed (Adam et al. 2017).

Moving and positioning a patient with an artificial airway

Definition

Patients who are unable to maintain their own safe airway, whether unconscious or not, will require an artificial airway to support their respiratory system; the choice of airway will depend on individual need and presentation.

The different airways include:

- nasal
- endotracheal
- tracheostomy (see Figures 7.3 and 7.4).

For more detailed information regarding these and other specific care issues and including anatomy and physiology, see Chapter 12: Respiratory care, CPR and blood transfusion.

Evidence-based approaches

Principles of care

Maintaining a patent artificial airway

When moving a patient with an artificial airway, it is important to maintain neutral head and neck alignment within the movement plane. It is sensible to have one member of staff in sole charge of

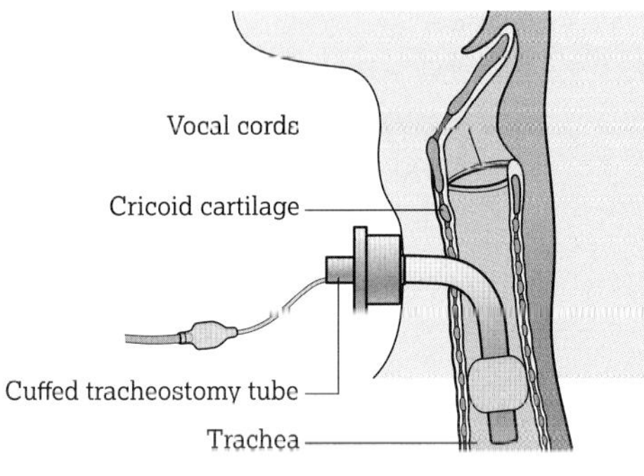

Figure 7.3 A tracheostomy tube *in situ*. *Source*: Reproduced from Munir and Clarke (2013). © 2013 Nazia Munir and Ray Clarke. Published 2013 by Blackwell Publishing Ltd.

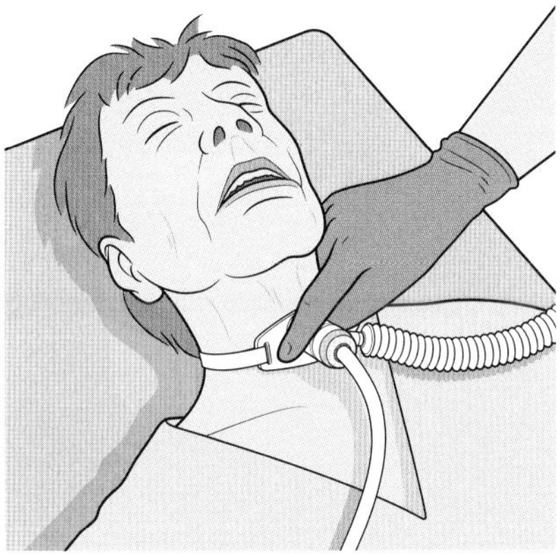

Figure 7.4 A patient with an artificial airway.

looking after the patient's artificial airway to avoid risks of trauma, dislodgement and occlusion and, if the patient is ventilated, prolonged disconnection from the ventilatory and oxygen source. Changing position will also alter the neck musculature so it is important to ensure the tracheostomy tapes are tied securely before and after moving the patient.

With newly formed tracheostomies, there is an increased risk of dislodgement 7–10 days following the procedure as the surrounding fascia and muscle need to repair to form the tract (McGrath 2014, NCEPOD 2014). During this time, it is important to have the following equipment by the patient's bedside and to display signage regarding the type of artificial airway and the emergency tracheostomy care algorithm (McGrath et al. 2012) (see Figure 12.34):

- tracheal dilators
- two spare tracheostomy tubes, one a size smaller than the one *in situ*
- tracheostomy tapes
- spare inner cannula
- inner tube cleaners, oxygen supply and tracheostomy mask
- humidification
- suction equipment
- bag-valve mask
- lubricant
- stitch cutter.

These are essential in case the patient's airway is compromised (for guidance on how to use this equipment, see Chapter 12: Respiratory care, CPR and blood transfusion).

Emergency situations

The three most significant life-threatening emergency situations with a tracheostomy tube are blockage, displacement and haemorrhage. If any of these occur while moving the patient, stop and call for assistance immediately.

Staff should not be moving a patient with a tracheostomy, particularly a new tracheostomy, unless they are experienced in managing these emergency situations or working alongside someone who is (NCEPOD 2014).

Clinical governance

Consent

If an individual is unconscious, an understanding of the Mental Capacity Act (2005) is essential.

Pre-procedural considerations

It is important to ensure regular positional changes, as with any patient unable to move themselves, to help prevent pressure damage and reduce the complications of prolonged bedrest (NHS Improvement 2018). Ideally, the patient should be moved every 2 hours and positioned alternating between side-lying and supine.

Equipment

Artificial airway

When the patient has an artificial airway, such as a tracheostomy or endotracheal tube, ensure that the appropriate equipment is at the bedside and that the airway tapes are tightly secured (NCEPOD 2014).

Procedure guideline 7.8 Positioning an unconscious patient or a patient with an artificial airway in supine

Essential equipment

- Personal protective equipment
- Manual handling equipment (e.g. sliding sheets) may be required following risk assessment, depending on local policy
- Pillows
- Towels
- Splints
- Bed extension for tall patients
- At least three members of staff to move the patient, including one dedicated staff member to be responsible for the airway (refer to local trust policy)
- Appropriate emergency airway equipment at the bedside in line with local trust policy

Action	Rationale
Pre-procedure	
1 Introduce yourself to the patient and explain the procedure. If the patient is alert, discuss the procedure with them and gain their consent to proceed.	To ensure that the patient feels at ease, understands the procedure and gives their valid consent, even if they are unconscious (NMC 2018, **C**).
2 Wash hands thoroughly with soap and water or use an alcohol-based handrub.	To reduce the risk of contamination and cross-infection (NHS England and NHSI 2019, **C**; WHO 2012, **C**).

(continued)

Procedure guideline 7.8 Positioning an unconscious patient or a patient with an artificial airway in supine *(continued)*

Action	Rationale
3 Ensure the bed is at the optimum height for the handlers. If two handlers are required, try to match the handlers' heights as far as possible.	To minimize the risk of injury to the practitioners (Aslam et al. 2015, **C**).
4 Document the patient's vital signs prior to moving.	This is important as it will provide a baseline for any changes that may occur during the moving or positioning procedure. **E**
Procedure	
5 Ensure one person is in charge of the artificial airway, ensuring it remains in place and supporting the tubing throughout the movement and repositioning.	To reduce the risk of artificial airway displacement or dislodgement when moving (NCEPOD 2014, **E**).
6 *Head*: maintain proper alignment of the head and neck; support them with a pillow or towel roll.	To help maintain a patent airway. **P**
7 Elevate the head of the bed by 30°.	To reduce the risk of nosocomial pneumonia (McGrath 2014, Morris et al. 2011, Wang et al. 2016). This facilitates the drainage of secretions from the oropharynx, minimizes the risk of aspiration, assists the maintenance of adequate cerebral perfusion pressure and promotes an effective breathing pattern (Jeon et al. 2014, **E**).
8 *Body*: position in alignment with spine (use towels and pillows).	To maintain correct alignment of the body and minimize complications. **E**
9 *Upper limbs:* support arms on pillows. *Lower limbs:* place a pillow between the knees; use pillows or splints (if prescribed by the physiotherapist) to flex the ankles parallel to the feet (**Action figure 9**); align the hips with the head.	To provide joint protection. **E** To prevent skin breakdown, foot-drop and internal rotation of the upper leg (Hickey and Powers 2011, **E**).
10 Refer to physiotherapists or occupational therapists to review limb movement and provide appropriate intervention to prevent the loss of movement.	To ensure the patient is assessed by a physiotherapist and an appropriate care plan is put in place. **E**
Post-procedure	
11 Monitor the patient's respiratory and cardiovascular observations.	To ensure the patient has not become unstable. **E**
12 Monitor the colour, temperature and pulses of the limbs.	To help preserve musculoskeletal function and prevent deep vein thrombosis (Hickey and Powers 2011, **E**).

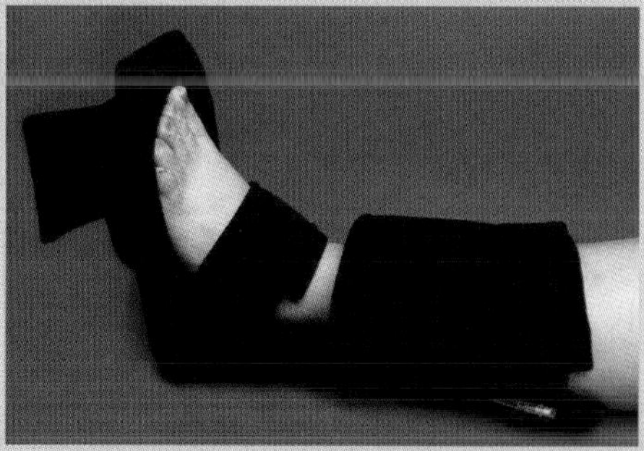

Action Figure 9 Foot resting in a splint.

Procedure guideline 7.9 Positioning an unconscious patient or a patient with an artificial airway in side-lying

Essential equipment

- Personal protective equipment
- Manual handling equipment (e.g. sliding sheets) may be required following risk assessment, depending on local policy
- Pillows
- Towels
- Splints
- Bed extension for tall patients
- At least three members of staff to move the patient, including one dedicated staff member to be responsible for the airway (refer to local trust policy)
- Appropriate emergency airway equipment at the bedside in line with local trust policy

Action	Rationale
Pre-procedure	
1 Introduce yourself to the patient and explain the procedure. If the patient is alert, discuss the procedure with them and gain their consent to proceed.	To ensure that the patient feels at ease, understands the procedure and gives their valid consent, even if they are unconscious (NMC 2018, **C**).
2 Wash hands thoroughly with soap and water or use an alcohol-based handrub.	To reduce the risk of contamination and cross-infection (NHS England and NHSI 2019, **C**; WHO 2012, **C**).
3 Ensure the bed is at the optimum height for the handlers. If two handlers are required, try to match the handlers' heights as far as possible.	To minimize the risk of injury to the practitioners (Aslam et al. 2015, **C**).
Procedure	
4 Place one or two pillows under the patient's head, ensuring the airway remains patent. Extra care should be taken for those patients with an artificial airway, central lines or recent head/neck injury or surgery.	To support the head in the midline position. **E**
5 Semi-flex the lowermost leg at the hip and the knee. Extra care should be taken with the degree of flexion for those patients who have hip or knee pain, loss of movement (including fractures), leg oedema, femoral lines or other venous access devices.	To support the patient in a stable position. **E**
6 Ask or assist the patient to semi-flex the uppermost leg at the hip and knee. Place one pillow under the patient's back and one pillow under the patient's bottom.	To prevent lumbar spine rotation. **E** To support the pelvic girdle. **E** To increase the comfort for the patient resting in side-lying. **E**
7 Place a pillow between the patient's knees.	To aid pressure care. **E**
8 Place the underneath arm in front with scapula protracted (this may not be appropriate for patients with shoulder pathology). Extra care should be taken with patients with low tone in the affected arm, swollen arms or lines in that arm.	To promote patient comfort. **E** To promote shoulder alignment. **E** To provide additional support and comfort. **E**
9 Place a pillow under the uppermost arm with the elbow resting in a flexed position (**Action figure 9**).	To support the arm and shoulder, particularly if the patient has low muscle tone and subluxation (Ada et al. 2005, **E**). To promote patient comfort. **E** To reduce upper limb swelling. **E**
Post-procedure	
10 Monitor the patient's respiratory and cardiovascular observations.	To ensure the patient has not become unstable. **E**
11 Monitor the colour, temperature and pulses of the limbs.	To help preserve musculoskeletal function and prevent deep vein thrombosis (Hickey and Powers 2011, **E**).

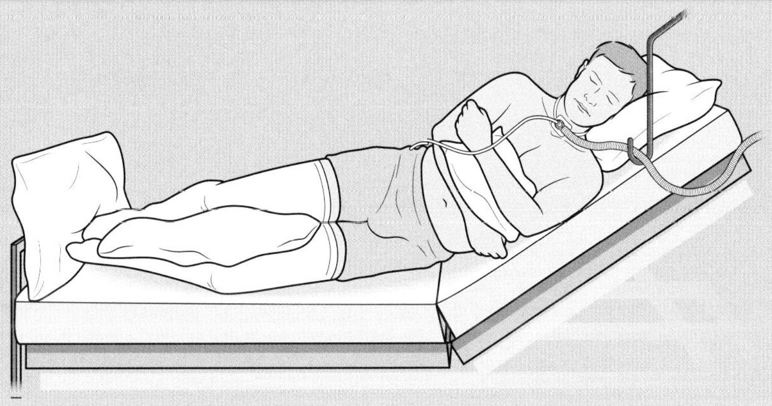

Action Figure 9 Positioning an unconscious patient or a patient with a tracheostomy in side-lying.

Problem-solving table 7.2 Prevention and resolution (Procedure guidelines 7.8 and 7.9)

Problem	Cause	Prevention	Action
Change in medical condition	With any change in position, transient changes in vital signs also occur.	Any changes in respiratory or cardiovascular status should be closely monitored with any positional change or intervention (Hodgson et al. 2014).	If oxygen saturation (SpO_2) drops and does not return to its usual value within 5 minutes, or heart rate increases or decreases by over 10 beats per minute and does not settle, the patient should be returned gently to the previous position (Hodgson et al. 2014). Inform the medical team about the change in the patient's condition and increase the frequency of observation.
Intensive-care-acquired muscle weakness	Muscle atrophy can start to develop within hours of a patient being mechanically ventilated (Hodgson and Tipping 2016, Paratz et al. 2016).	Ensure upon changing the patient's position that all limbs are in appropriate positions and not overstretched.	Once the patient has been repositioned, ensure the limbs are well supported and use resting splints to maintain muscle length.
Risk of excess pressure on body parts	Body parts, such as ears, positioned without due care and attention.	If the patient is in side-lying, ensure the ear is not twisted under the head (NICE 2014).	Check all bony prominences and pressure areas regularly. Move the patient's head to shift the ear to a more comfortable position.
Loss of artificial airway patency (e.g. blocked, displaced or dislodged)	Change of position of neck or of airway.	Ensure the endotracheal or tracheostomy tube is secure. This will involve checking the position of the tube, the cuff pressure, and the endotracheal or tracheostomy ties, as movement will alter the soft tissue distribution, which will affect all of these (McGrath 2014). Monitor vital signs closely to ensure the values return to normal within 5 minutes of position change. Ensure there are enough persons present to assist with the movement. Ensure one person is in sole charge of the airway when moving. Ensure there is visible signage at the patient's beside about the type of altered airway and the appropriate emergency algorithm (McGrath 2014, NCEPOD 2014)	Call for assistance immediately. Refer to Chapter 12: Respiratory care, CPR and blood transfusion for more specific guidance on emergency management of the airway.

Post-procedural considerations

The general principles of care mentioned earlier in the this chapter are relevant to this section. Close monitoring of the patient after a position change will ensure any change in observations is noted and acted on appropriately.

Documentation

Details of the patient's position should be documented, as should the length of time they spend in that position. Any incidents or changes in condition during the procedure should be clearly reported and documented.

Moving and positioning a patient with respiratory compromise

Definition

The causes of respiratory compromise may be multifactorial and should be established before undertaking positioning interventions. Compromise may be due to medical intervention (e.g. side-effects of medication) or to metabolic, surgical or primary respiratory pathologies. The general principles provided at the beginning of this chapter regarding the principles of moving and positioning are applicable to these patients, but in particular observation is required regarding their response to the intervention.

Anatomy and physiology

Both the skeletal and the muscular structures that make up the thoracic cage and surround the lungs play vital roles in respiration (see Chapter 12: Respiratory care, CPR and blood transfusion). Compromise of one or more of these (e.g. abdominal muscle dysfunction due to abdominal surgery, ascites or deconditioning) may lead to an alteration in normal respiratory function and the inability to generate an effective cough (Schellekens et al. 2016).

Evidence-based approaches

Principles of care

The main aim of positioning a patient with respiratory symptoms is to:

- maximize ventilation/perfusion (V/Q) matching
- minimize the work of breathing
- maximize the drainage of secretions.

Positioning may enhance medical management by using the effects of gravity to help achieve the aims listed above. This may reduce the need for more invasive intervention (Pathmanathan et al. 2015), such as mechanical ventilation. Therefore, the most advantageous positioning should be integrated into the overall 24-hour plan.

Positioning a patient to maximize ventilation/perfusion matching

Anatomy and physiology

For optimal gaseous exchange to take place, it is necessary that the air and the blood are in the same area of lung at the same time. Matching of these is expressed as a ratio of alveolar ventilation to perfusion (V/Q). A degree of mismatch can occur due to either adequate ventilation to an underperfused area (dead space) or inadequate ventilation to a well-perfused area (shunt) (West 2012).

The function of the lungs is to exchange oxygen and carbon dioxide between the blood and atmosphere. Oxygen from the atmosphere comes into close contact with blood via the alveolar capillary membrane. Here, it diffuses across into the blood and is carried around the body. The amount of oxygen that reaches the blood depends on the rate and depth of the breath, the compliance of the chest and any airway obstruction (Lumb and Nunn 2010).

In a self-ventilating individual in the upright position, ventilation will be preferential in the dependent regions (lowest part in relation to gravity) as:

- the apex of the lung is more inflated and therefore has less potential to expand
- the bases of the lung are compressed by the weight of the lungs and the blood vessels and therefore have more potential to inflate.

Perfusion to the alveoli is approximately equal to that to the systemic circulation; however, as the pressure is far less, the distribution is gravity dependent. The variability in the distribution of perfusion throughout the lungs is far greater than that of ventilation (West 2012).

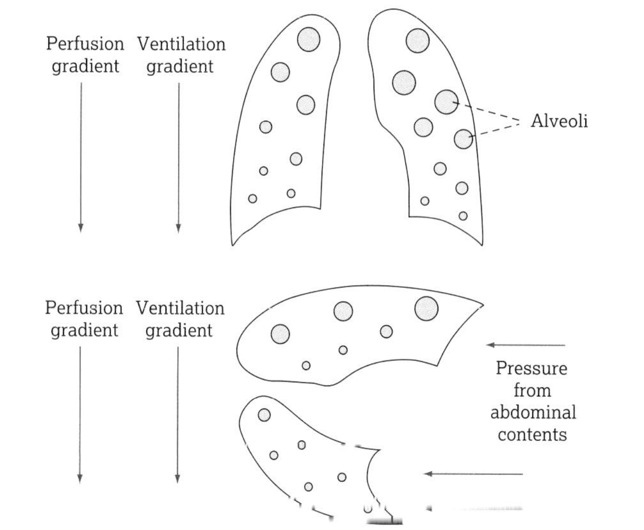

Figure 7.5 The effect of gravity on the distribution of ventilation and perfusion in the lung in the upright and lateral positions. *Source*: Reproduced from Hough (2001) with permission of Oxford University Press.

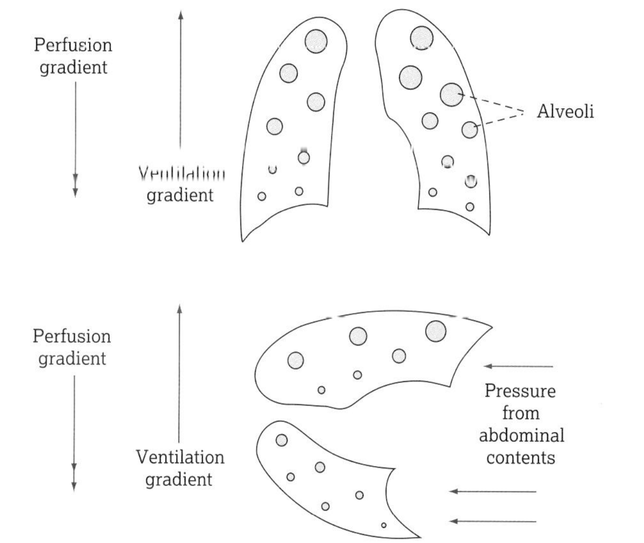

Figure 7.6 The effect of controlled mandatory ventilation on ventilation and perfusion gradients. In contrast to spontaneous respiration, the perfusion gradient increases downwards and the ventilation gradient is reversed. *Source*: Reproduced from Hough (2001) with permission of Oxford University Press.

Evidence-based approaches

Principles of care

In a self-ventilating upright position, V/Q is not exactly matched even in a healthy lung but is regarded as optimal in the bases (Figure 7.5) because this where is the greatest perfusion and ventilation occur. Similarly, in a side-lying position, the effect of gravity alters the distribution of perfusion and ventilation so that the dependent area of lung – that is, the lowermost lung – has the best V/Q ratio (West 2012).

In a patient receiving mechanical ventilation, especially in a mandatory mode (where the ventilator rather than the patient initiates and terminates the breath), the distribution of ventilation and perfusion will alter (Figure 7.6). As ventilation is driven by a positive pressure (rather than the negative pressure involved in self-ventilation), air will take the path of least resistance. Ventilation will therefore be optimal in the apex of the lungs in the upright position or the non-dependent/uppermost lung in side-lying. This can be altered further in the presence of lung pathology. Perfusion will remain preferentially delivered to the bases (in the upright position) or the dependent/lowermost lung (in the side-lying position) and have a higher gradient (variability from apex to bases) than in self-ventilating patients as the positive pressure displaces blood from the areas of highest ventilation. These two situations mean that the V/Q ratio of those receiving mechanical ventilation can have a higher degree of mismatch than in self-ventilating patients. Strategies such as positive end-expiratory pressure (PEEP) and a higher rate of oxygen delivery will help to overcome this (West 2012).

The prone position may be used in intensive care when patients are mechanically ventilated to improve oxygenation in severe respiratory failure or to manage acute respiratory distress syndrome (ARDS) (Guerin et al. 2013).

Positioning a patient to minimize the work of breathing

Anatomy and physiology

At rest, inspiration is an active process whereas expiration is passive. The main muscle involved in inspiration is the diaphragm (Figure 7.7). The diaphragm contracts, thereby increasing the volume of the thoracic cavity. Additionally, the external intercostal muscles work by pulling the sternum and ribcage upwards and outwards, in a process likened to a pump and bucket handle (Figure 7.8).

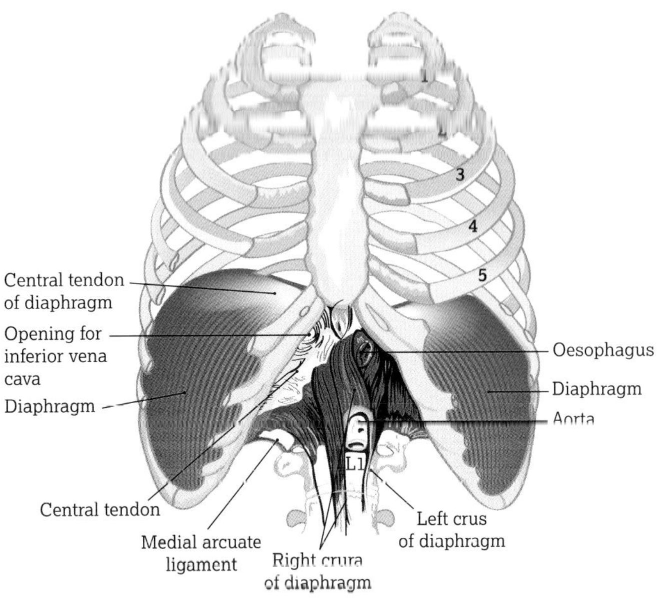

Figure 7.7 The diaphragm as seen from the front. Note the openings in the vertebral portion for the inferior vena cava, oesophagus and aorta.

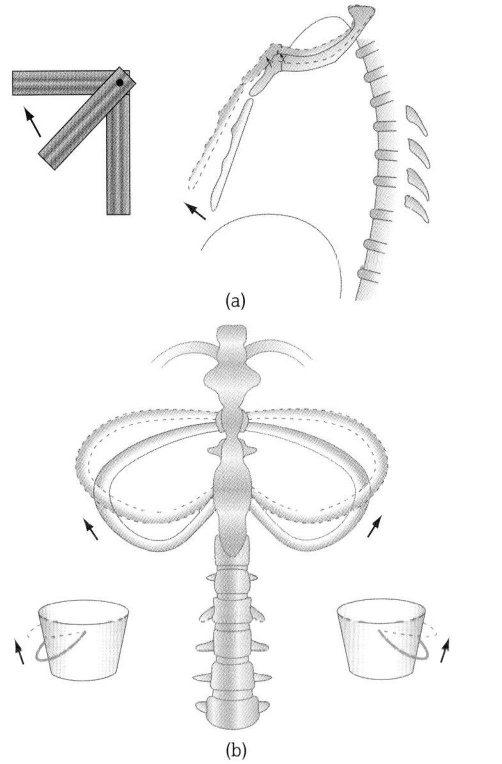

Figure 7.8 Movement of the chest wall on inspiration. (a) The upper ribs move upwards and forwards, increasing the anteroposterior dimension of the thoracic cavity. As a result, the sternum also rises forwards. (b) The lower ribs move like bucket handles, increasing the lateral dimension of the thorax. *Source*: Aggarwal and Hunter (2007). Reproduced with permission of BMJ Publishing Group Ltd.

When increased ventilation is required (e.g. with exercise or in disease), the accessory muscles (the scalenes and sternocleidomastoid) assist with this process (Tortora and Derrickson 2017).

If ventilation is increased for a prolonged period of time, as in respiratory disease, the diaphragm's activity reduces and the accessory muscles take on a higher proportion of the work. This can be observed in a patient who adopts a posture with raised shoulders.

Although expiration should be passive in normal conditions, the internal intercostals and muscles of the abdominal wall (the transversus abdominis, the rectus abdominis, and the internal and external obliques) are used in times of active expiration to push the diaphragm upwards, reducing the volume of the thoracic cavity and forcefully expelling air. This can be observed clinically when the abdominal wall visibly contracts and pulls in the lower part of the ribcage during expiration (Tortora and Derrickson 2017).

Evidence-based approaches

Principles of care

Many people suffering with long-term breathlessness adopt positions that will best facilitate their inspiratory muscles (Bott et al. 2009). The aim of any position is to restore a normal rate and depth of breathing in order to achieve efficient but adequate ventilation (Box 7.2).

Pre-procedural considerations

The general procedural considerations mentioned earlier in this chapter are all relevant to this section. However, there are also some other general principles that need to be considered for these patients.

Pharmacological support

Administering nebulizers

If prescribed, administering nebulizers approximately 15 minutes prior to moving a patient will help to dilate the airways, making breathing more efficient and ensuring better oxygen delivery to the blood (Boe et al. 2001).

Oxygen requirements

Repositioning can cause a temporary fall in oxygen saturation or a raised respiratory rate. If the fall is greater than 4% or recovery time is protracted, supplemental oxygen delivery may be required for several minutes before, during and after moving. Consideration should be given to patients who have chronic obstructive pulmonary disease or who are chronic carbon dioxide retainers as supplementary oxygen will cause a negative impact on their respiratory function by reducing their respiratory drive (Kent et al. 2011).

Non-pharmacological support

Pacing

It may be necessary to allow the patient time to rest during the process of getting into a new position to limit the exertion and therefore decrease the respiratory demand.

Environment

A breathless patient may be anxious about carrying out a task that could exacerbate their breathlessness. By reducing additional stressors such as noise and a cluttered environment, this can be minimized.

Positioning a patient to maximize the drainage of secretions

Anatomy and physiology

The trachea branches into two bronchi, one to each lung (Figure 7.10). Each main bronchus then divides into lobar and then segmental bronchi (upper, middle and lower on the right; upper and lower on the left), each one branching into two or more segmental bronchi with smaller and smaller diameters, until they reach the bronchioles and finally the alveoli (Tortora and Derrickson 2017).

Box 7.2 Positioning to minimize the work of breathing

There are certain resting positions that can help to reduce the work of breathing, as shown in Figure 7.9.

- High side-lying (Figure 7.9a)
- Forward lean sitting (Figure 7.9b)
- Relaxed sitting (Figure 7.9c)
- Forward lean standing (Figure 7.9d)
- Relaxed standing (Figure 7.9e)

These positions serve to:

- support the body, reducing the overall use of postural muscles and oxygen requirements
- improve lung volumes
- optimize the functional positions of the respiratory (thoracic and abdominal) muscles (De Troyer and Boriek 2011).

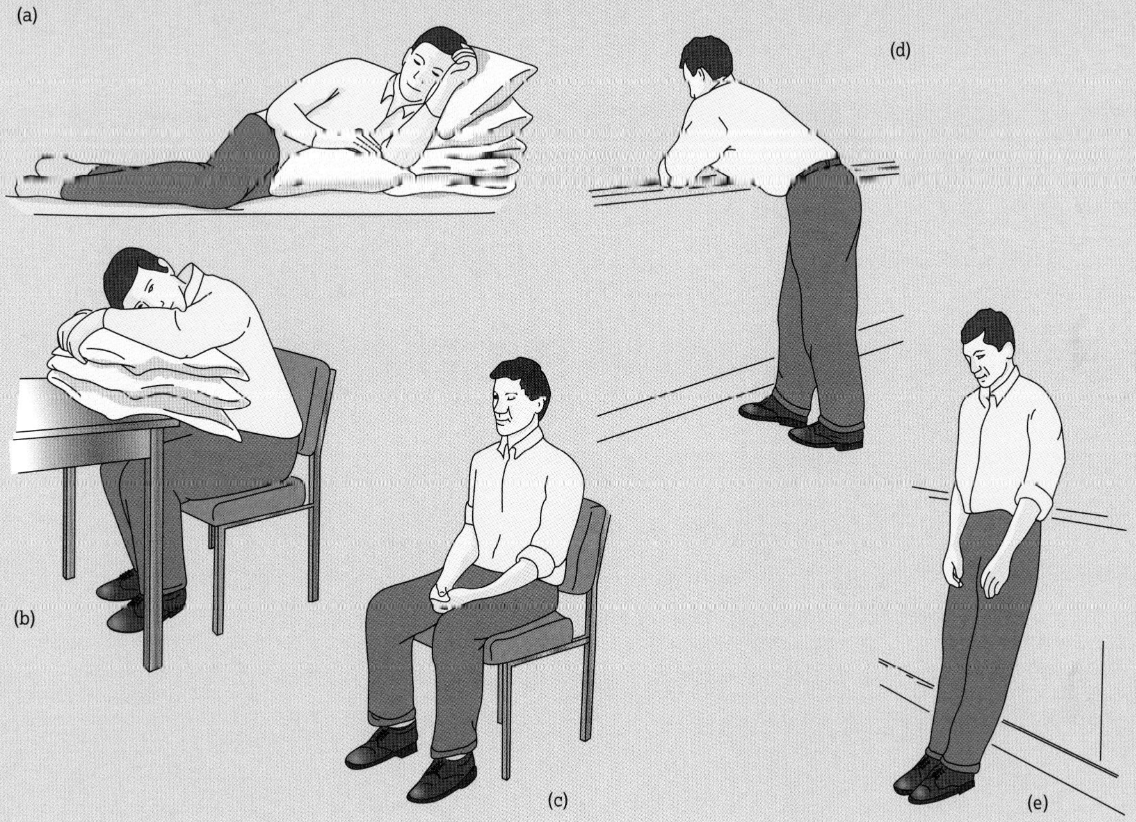

Figure 7.9 Positions to reduce the work of breathing.

The walls of the airways are lined with epithelium, which contains cilia. The cilia constantly beat in a co-ordinated movement, propelling the mucus layer towards the pharynx. The mucus layer traps any dust particles or foreign objects, which can then be transported along the 'mucociliary escalator', which is an important part of the lungs' defence mechanism (Figure 7.11). An increased volume of mucus is produced in response to airway irritation and in some disease states (Tortora and Derrickson 2017).

A reduced ability to effectively remove this mucus can lead to an increased bacterial load and therefore may compromise respiratory functioning by causing airway obstruction. This can lead to segmental atelectasis or lobar collapse, and long term it can lead to chronic inflammation and airway destruction (Lumb and Nunn 2010).

Pre-procedural considerations

Pharmacological support

Administering nebulizers

Drugs such as mucolytic agents or bronchodilators can be prescribed and administered via a nebulizer. These drugs can assist with secretion clearance and be used prior to patients being placed in positions intended to optimize the drainage of secretions (Rubin 2014, Strickland et al. 2015).

Non-pharmacological support

Humidification

Drainage of secretions will be optimized if the patient and therefore the mucus layer and cilia are well hydrated. This can be ensured via adequate humidification.

Moving and positioning a patient with neurological impairment

The general principles of positioning discussed earlier in this chapter can be applied for this group of patients. However, the variation and complexity of presentation with these patients means a uniform approach to overall management cannot be adopted. Therefore, this section looks at some of the variations in presentation of this patient group and suggests principles to be considered when positioning these patients. It covers recommendations for

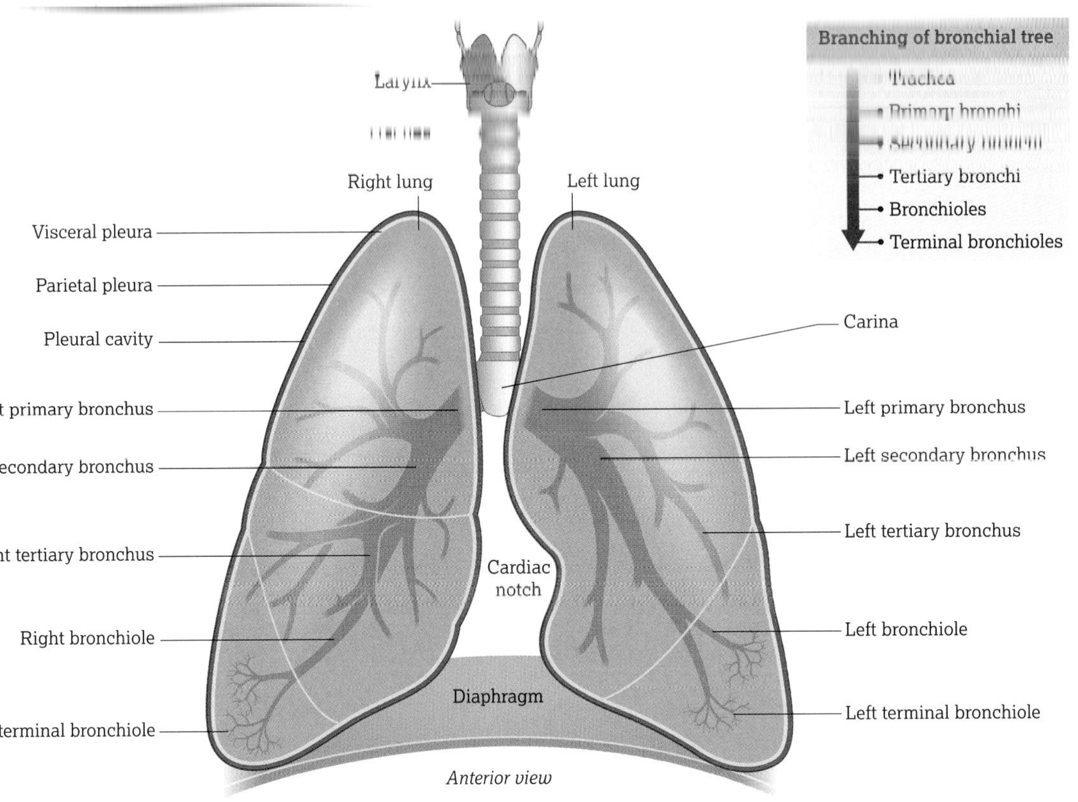

Figure 7.10 The bronchial tree. *Source*: Reproduced from Peate et al. (2014) with permission of John Wiley & Sons, Ltd.

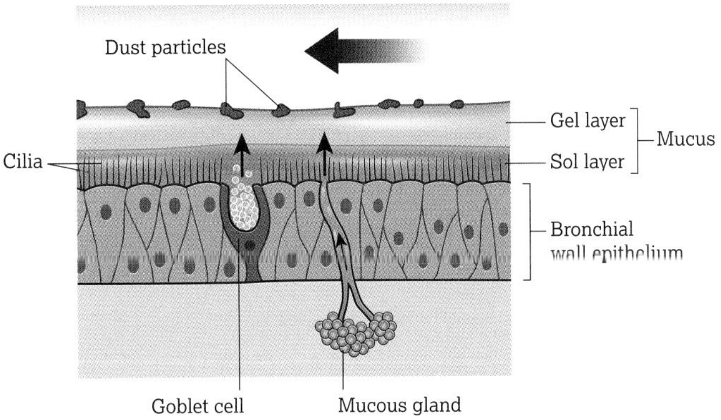

Figure 7.11 The mucociliary escalator. *Source*: Reproduced from DeTurk and Cahalin (2010) with permission of The McGraw Companies.

assisting patients presenting with neurological symptoms arising from changes to their central nervous system and/or peripheral nervous system, either as a consequence of their disease or as a consequence of their treatment.

Definition

Neurological impairment occurs through disease or illness, which can cause damage to patients' central, peripheral and autonomic nervous systems, affecting the relay of messages along nerve pathways and preventing normal motor and sensory function. This in turn affects a person's functional ability.

Anatomy and physiology

The nervous system is divided into the central nervous system (CNS), which comprises the brain and spinal cord, and the peripheral nervous system (PNS), which comprises all the nerves outside the brain and spine, including the spinal and cranial nerves. The PNS is further divided into the autonomic nervous system (ANS) and the somatic nervous system (SNS) (Lundy-Ekman 2018a). This is illustrated in Figure 7.12.

The central nervous system

The brain consists of four lobes (frontal, temporal, parietal and occipital), the brainstem and the cerebellum. Each area has specific functions, as detailed in Figure 7.13.

The brain connects to the spinal cord via the brainstem and relays messages between the brain and the body via the PNS. The spinal cord exits the skull through an opening called the foramen magnum and travels down the spinal column through a channel at the back of each spinal bone (vertebrae) called the spinal canal. The vertebrae are numbered according to their location. The cervical spine has 7 vertebrae (C1–C7 from top to bottom), the thoracic spine has 12 vertebrae (T1–T12) and the lumbar spine has 5 vertebrae (L1–L5). The spinal cord (and therefore the CNS) stops at around L1 or L2 and forms the cauda equina, which is part of the PNS (Figure 7.14) (Lundy-Ekman 2018b).

The peripheral nervous system

Between each vertebrae, a nerve branches off the spinal cord and exits to the body. These are called the spinal nerves and are numbered accordingly (Figure 7.14).

The PNS is divided into the autonomic nervous system (ANS) and the somatic nervous system (SNS) (Figure 7.12). The SNS controls moving and feeling within the body. Efferent or motor nerves carry messages from the brain to the body to cause movement. Afferent or sensory nerves carry sensory information from the body back to the brain to provide feedback. The ANS regulates structures not under conscious control, such as blood pressure, gut motility, sweating and body temperature (Lundy-Ekman 2018b).

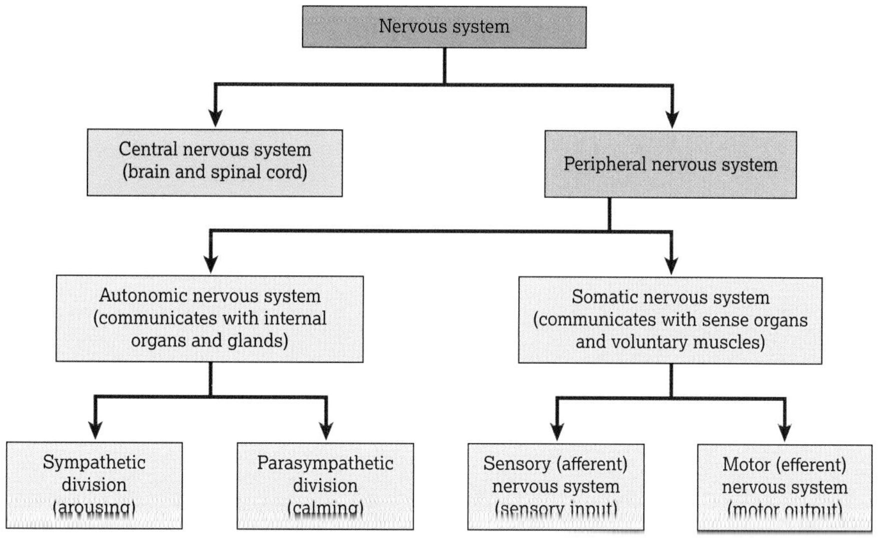

Figure 7.12 Divisions of the nervous system. *Source*: Reproduced from PsychLogic (2017) with permission of CC.

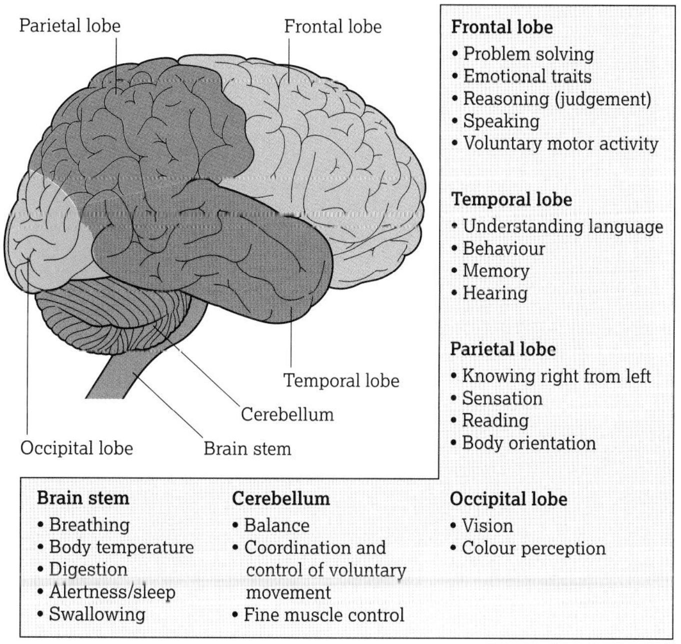

Figure 7.13 The lobes of the brain and their functions.

Illness, disease and side-effects of treatment can affect any or all of these parts of the nervous system, which will have implications for moving, positioning and patient management.

Normal movement

Normal movement is dependent on a neuromuscular system that can receive, integrate and respond appropriately to multiple intrinsic and extrinsic stimuli. Key components include:

- *Muscle tone*: this is the amount of activity in a muscle. Postural muscle tone is continuous partial contraction of the postural muscles to keep the body upright against gravity (Vander et al. 2016a, 2016b).
- *Muscle reflexes*: these are involuntary and nearly instantaneous muscle contractions in response to a stimulus (Vander et al. 2016a, 2016b).
- *Biomechanical properties of muscle*: resting muscle is soft and can be easily stretched. To move a joint, a muscle must contract and shorten (Vander et al. 2016a, 2016b).
- *Reciprocal innervation of muscles*: when a muscle contracts, its opposite muscle relaxes to an equal extent, allowing smooth movement. For example, when the biceps contracts to bend the elbow, the triceps relaxes (Vander et al. 2016a, 2016b).
- *Sensory-motor feedback and feed-forward mechanisms*: the brain gathers information from the body about movement that has happened and sends messages to the muscles to correct the movement or adjust for changes (Duff et al. 2012).
- *Balance reactions*: the brain uses the feedback and feed-forward mechanisms described above to make adjustments to the ankle, hip and trunk muscles to maintain balance and prevent falling (Vander et al. 2016a, 2016b).

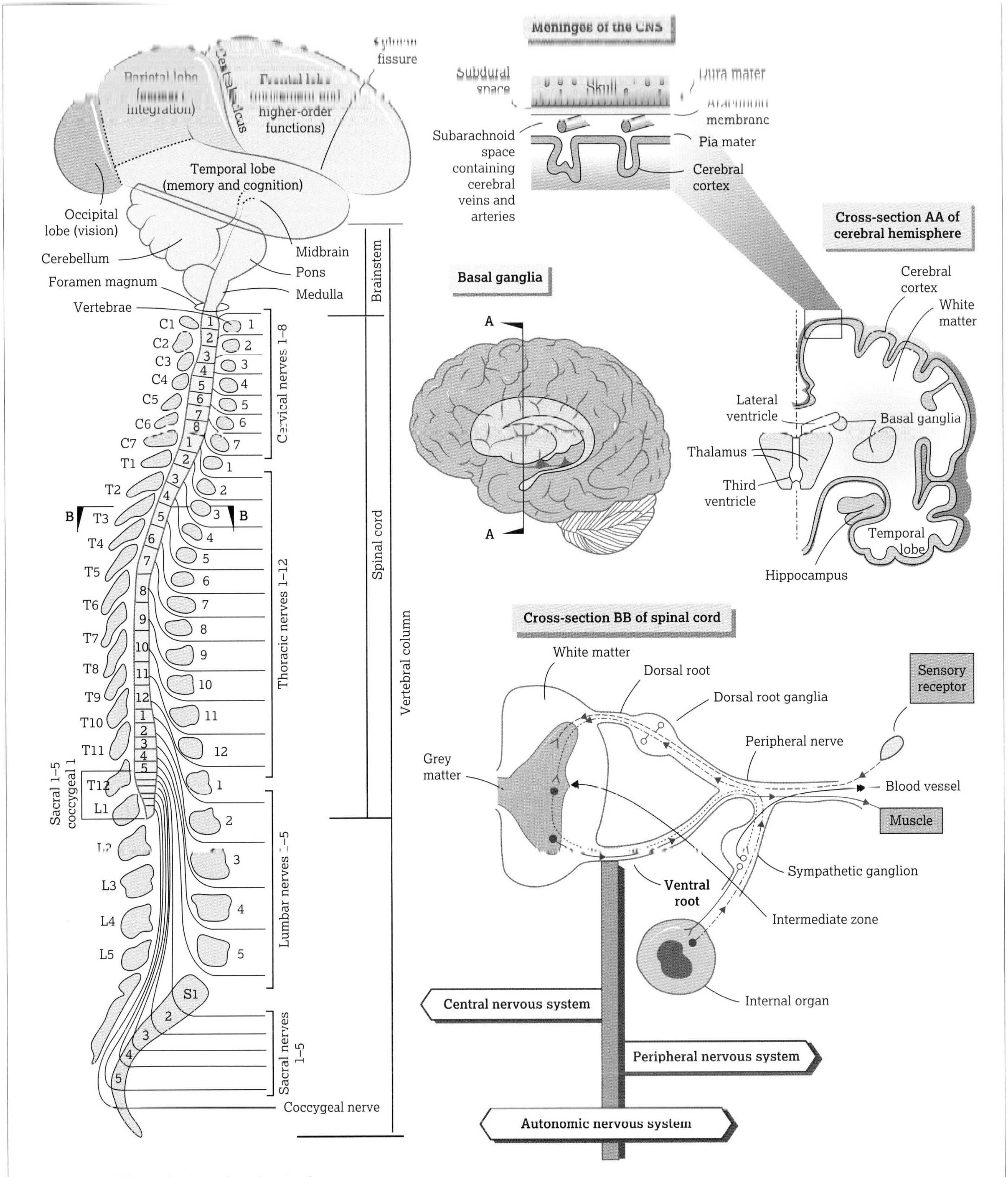

Figure 7.14 The spinal cord and spinal nerves.

When any of these components are altered (e.g. if there is damage to or disease of the CNS or PNS; Box 7.3), abnormal movement patterns will exist, and these will affect the patient's functional ability. Positioning and active movement are key strategies in managing the influence of these changes.

Related theory

Consequences of neurological damage

Disease or damage to the CNS or PNS can lead to temporary or permanent complex physical, cognitive, psychological and

Box 7.3 Possible causes of neurological deficit

- Acquired brain injury, such as cerebral palsy (CP), traumatic brain injury (TBI), infection or stroke
- Brain tumour
- Congenital conditions such as spina bifida
- Progressive neurological disorders such as Parkinson's disease (PD) or multiple sclerosis (MS)
- Peripheral motor or sensory neuropathy, such as diabetic neuropathy
- Neuromuscular diseases such as motor neurone disease (MND)
- Spinal cord injury (SCI) or compression

Source: Adapted from Lindsay et al. (2010).

psychosocial problems, including the inability to move independently (Box 7.4).

If a person with a neurological presentation has problems moving, they are deprived of the physical benefits of movement and are at risk of developing secondary complications such as those described in Table 7.2. These changes can occur in as little as one week. They also present a challenge to health professionals assisting these patients' mobility. Effective management of patients with neurological impairment requires holistic assessment and multidisciplinary management.

Altered muscle tone

A person with neurological damage often suffers from changes in their muscle tone. A decrease in muscle tone is known as low tone or flaccidity, whereas an increase in muscle tone is known as high tone, which may be spasticity or rigidity (Lundy-Ekman 2018d).

Low tone

A patient with low tone will find it hard to move their affected limbs and may even have difficulty sitting up against gravity. They may have little or no activity in the muscles that lift the foot, meaning that they cannot clear their foot when walking. This is known as foot-drop, and it can cause inefficiencies in walking, or even falls if the patient catches their toes and trips.

Because the integrity of the shoulder joint is reliant on muscle tone, patients with low tone in the arm will often present with a shoulder glenohumeral joint subluxation. In this case the humeral head is pulled downwards and forwards in relation to the glenoid fossa because the weight of the flaccid arm is unopposed by the shoulder joint muscles. This causes a palpable gap between the humeral head and the acromion. A shoulder subluxation (Figure 7.15) and hemiparetic shoulder pain can occur with many neurological conditions, but they are particularly prevalent in the stroke population (Ada et al. 2005, Harpreet et al. 2014). This can be very painful if not managed well and will ultimately affect the patient's functional outcomes. The use of an orthopaedic splint or shoulder subluxation brace may provide support and comfort for the patient (Table 7.3).

High tone

Increased tone is a state of muscle overactivity. This is sometimes referred to as spasticity, although this is just one cause of high tone. Spasticity is caused by overactive stretch reflexes in the muscle. High tone may also be caused by an overactive flexor withdrawal reflex or by rigidity, the latter of which is a type of overactivity seen in Parkinson's disease where a muscle is stiff throughout movement.

Spasticity, the most commonly seen presentation of high tone, can occur in any muscle, but common patterns do exist (see Table 7.2). It can vary relative to the time of day, environmental factors, activity and time since onset. Spasticity is made worse with effort, pain, infection and fatigue, to name a few factors. It causes involuntary muscle movements, pain, stiffness and tightness, and ultimately affects a person's functional ability. Spasticity and its consequences can have a negative effect on a person's quality of life, so optimum management of this troublesome symptom is paramount (Bhimani and Anderson 2014, Pandey and Berman 2018).

Box 7.4 Neurological symptoms that can affect a person's capacity to move independently

- Muscle weakness or paralysis:
  - affecting single muscles or joint movements – such as weak ankle muscles
  - affecting one limb
  - affecting one side of the body – known as hemiparesis (weakness) or hemiplegia (paralysis)
  - affecting both legs and trunk, depending on the level of damage – known as paraplegia
  - affecting all four limbs and trunk – known as quadriplegia or tetraplegia
- Altered muscle tone – spasticity, flaccidity or rigidity
- Difficulties with co-ordination, such as ataxia
- Nerve pain
- Sensory impairment – numbness, pins and needles, hypersensitivity or proprioceptive loss
- Balance impairments
- Visual problems
- Autonomic dysfunction, such as blood pressure changes
- Seizure activity
- Changes to bladder or bowel function
- Confusion
- Altered mood
- Perceptual changes – difficulty with the interpretation of sensation into meaning
- Cognitive changes – difficulties with concentration, understanding, comprehension, memory, planning, problem solving, safety awareness and memory
- Behavioural changes
- Speech and language difficulties:
  - dysarthria – difficulty forming words due to changes in control of the mouth muscles
  - expressive dysphasia – difficulty finding words
  - receptive dysphasia – difficulty understanding words

Source: Adapted from Lundy-Ekman (2018c) with permission of Elsevier.

Table 7.9 Common postural problems seen in patients with neurological impairment

Presentation	Posture	Complications
Low-tone patients	• Extended neck and protracted chin • Protracted and depressed shoulder with glenohumeral subluxation • Flexed thoracic spine • Flattened lumbar spine • Pelvis tilted backwards (posterior pelvic tilt) • Feet fall into plantar flexion	• Difficult sitting or standing up against gravity • May fall or slump forward or to the side when sitting • Heavy arm when standing or walking may affect balance • Foot-drop affects walking • At risk of shoulder joint subluxation
Spasticity of the upper limb (commonly seen in CP, TBI or stroke)	• Adduction and internal rotation of the shoulder • Flexion of the elbow and wrist • Pronation of the forearm • Flexion of the fingers and adduction of the thumb	• Difficulty accessing under the arm when washing and dressing • Difficulty holding and manipulating objects • Joint and muscle pain
Spasticity of the lower limb	*Flexor patterns commonly seen in CP, MS or TBI:* • Hip adduction and flexion • Knee flexion • Ankle plantar flexion and/or inversion *Extensor patterns commonly seen after TBI:* • Knee extension or flexion • Ankle plantarflexion and eversion • Great toe extension	• Difficulty maintaining hygiene • Difficulty dressing • Difficulty toileting • Difficulty positioning in bed and seating • Difficulty standing, transferring and walking

CP, cerebral palsy; MS, multiple sclerosis; TBI, traumatic brain injury.
Source: Adapted from Pandey and Berman (2018).

Certain medications can be used to manage spasticity in appropriate patients. There are a variety of pharmacological options for managing tone, and it is important to be aware of these when treating patients with high tone. The most commonly used are (Chang et al. 2013):

- *Oral baclofen*: this is the first-line antispasmodic. It is centrally acting and can cause drowsiness, so may not be appropriate for all patients.
- *Diazepam*: a benzodiazepine that has benefits for managing tone overnight, allowing more comfortable sleep. As it tends to act on flexor reflexes, it is better suited to managing spinal spasticity than cerebral spasticity.
- *Botulinum toxin injection*: a locally acting, long-lasting treatment for focal spasticity.

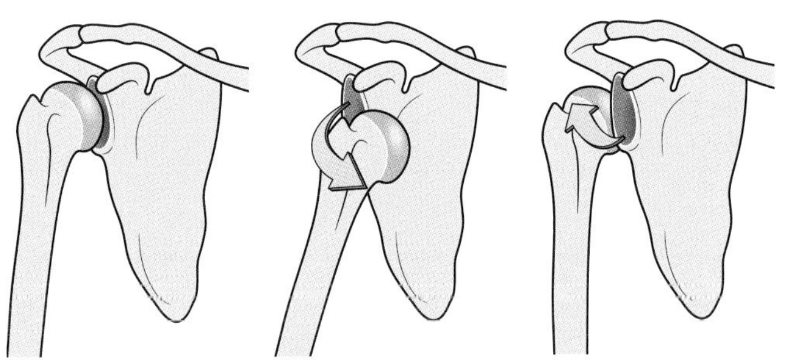

Figure 7.15 Shoulder subluxation.

Posture

Posture and postural control will be affected in patients with neurological impairment. 'Posture' describes the biomechanical alignment of the joints and orientation of the body to the environment (Duff et al. 2012), while 'postural control' describes the body's ability to balance and move against gravity. If a patient is unable to maintain a good postural alignment or actively change their own posture, it becomes important for those caring for them to ensure good positioning and regular movement to reduce complications such as pain and soft tissue shortening. Therefore, additional considerations should be applied for neurological patients with tonal issues, and these should always be discussed with the physiotherapist (Preston and Edmans 2016).

Evidence-based approaches

The general principles of moving and positioning patients mentioned earlier in this chapter are all relevant to this section and can be applied when assisting those with complex neurological impairment. Patients with neurological impairment may be able to participate in the usual transfer techniques but the risk assessment will consider several additional factors. This section identifies considerations for staff in their decision making. Where there is any doubt when moving patients with complex needs, guidance should be sought from a physiotherapist or occupational therapist.

For those with acute and long-standing neurological issues, the principles of moving and positioning can be applied at any time along the patient's treatment trajectory from rehabilitation to deteriorating function to palliative management.

Consequences of incorrect positioning and handling

There are various potential consequences of incorrect positioning and handling (Lundy-Ekman 2018d):

- Shoulder joint subluxation (Figure 7.15) in patients with low tone if their shoulder joint is not correctly supported.
- Traumatic shoulder injury if there is inappropriate handling of a patient during transfers, especially in low-tone patients.
- Pain from being in sustained postures and positions.
- Exacerbation of spasticity due to pain.
- Muscle shortening from sustained positioning. This most commonly occurs in the ankles where the feet fall or pull into plantarflexion (pointed toes) and stay in that position for extended periods, especially when a patient is not standing and stretching

Table 7.3 Shoulder subluxation supports

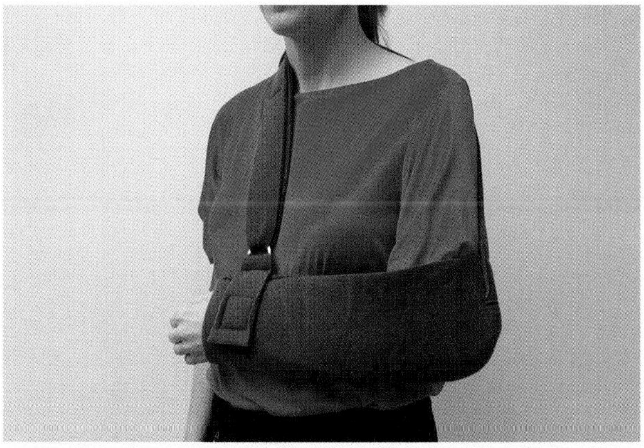	An orthopaedic sling can provide enough support to a flaccid arm in the early stages of rehabilitation to prevent complications.
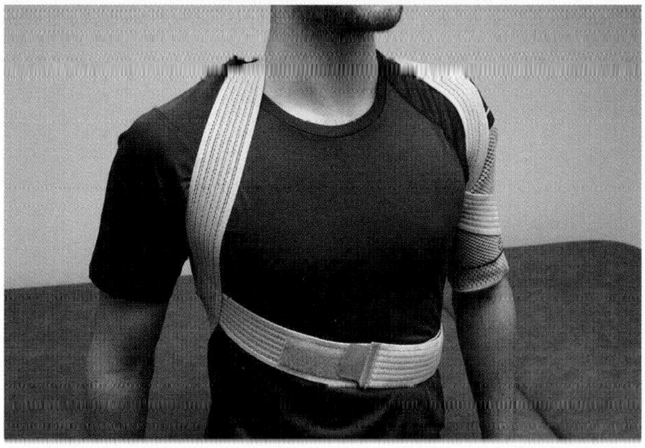	Specially designed subluxation braces are appropriate for some patients.

the posterior ankle muscles. This can become permanent if it is prolonged and is known as contracture. Contracture is most evident in people with high tone, because it is difficult to stretch their muscles in the normal way.

Patients with neurological deficits may vary in their presentation on a daily basis. The additional considerations for positioning and moving patients with neurological impairment are listed in Box 7.5.

Positioning a neurological patient with tonal problems in bed

Pre-procedural considerations

Equipment

Splints and orthoses

An orthosis or splint is an external device designed to apply, distribute or remove forces to or from the body in a controlled manner in order to control body motion and prevent alteration in the shape of body tissues. The aim is to compensate for weak or absent muscle function or to resist unopposed activity of a high tone muscle (Charlton 2009).

They may be used to:

- enable a high-tone muscle to be stretched to improve or maintain joint range of movement, with the aim of enabling participation in personal care, positioning, transferring and feeding, and reducing the risk of pressure ulcer development
- help the patient to gain better joint alignment for proximal and truncal activity
- enable more balanced and efficient walking
- maintain and assist function (ACPIN and College of Occupational Therapy 2015, Ada et al. 2005, Shumway-Cook and Woollacott 2012).

Box 7.5 Considerations for moving patients with neurological impairment

- Variations in tone, for example flaccidity or spasm
- Cognitive problems including attention deficit
- Behavioural problems
- Communication problems
- Variable patient ability, for example 'on/off' periods for patients with Parkinson's disease and patients with changing presentations, for example multiple sclerosis and degenerative conditions
- Sensory and proprioceptive problems, including reduced midline awareness
- Pain and/or altered sensitivity
- Decreased balance and co-ordination
- Visual disturbance
- Varying ability over 24 hours, for example fatigue at the end of the day or at night
- Effects of medication
- Varying capability of the patient according to the experience and/or skill mix of handler(s)
- Post-surgery: presence of tracheotomy, chest and other drains
- Traumatic and non-traumatic spinal injury: risk of spinal instability
- Importance of maintaining privacy and dignity

Source: Adapted from CSP (2014) with permission of The Chartered Society of Physiotherapy.

Table 7.4 Examples of commonly used resting splints

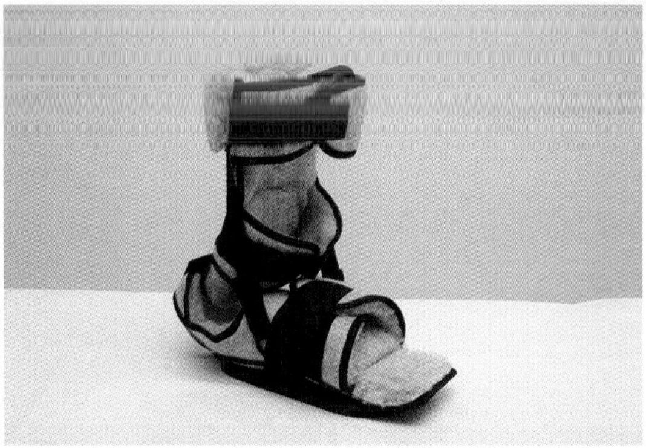	A resting ankle splint – used to maintain ankle range of movement in patients who are resting in bed for prolonged periods.
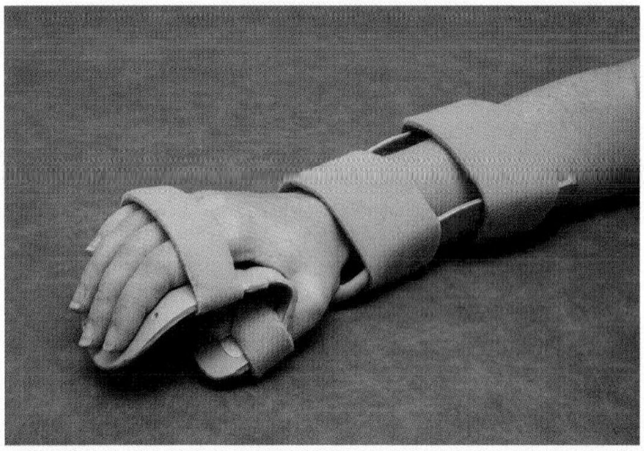	Resting splints to maintain wrist and finger position.
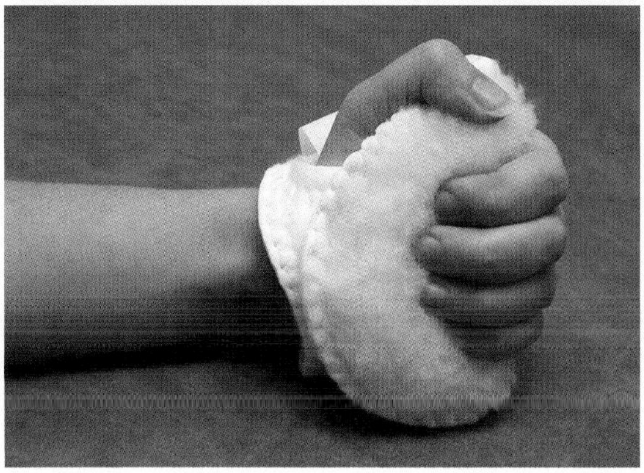	Palm protector – used where spasticity pulls the hand into a fist, risking the integrity of the skin of the palm, but where contractures in finger flexors mean fingers cannot be stretched out.

As with all therapeutic interventions, splints and orthoses (see examples in Table 7.4) should only be used after detailed assessment and based on sound clinical reasoning. If a splint or an orthosis is required, then this will normally be provided and fitted by a physiotherapist, occupational therapist or orthotist. They will also give instructions on how to use it.

Positioning aids

When patients do not have normal postural control, we often need to use equipment to help support or prevent certain postures. This can consist of simple things such as pillows and towels, or specialist postural management equipment such as wedges and T-rolls (Preston and Edmans 2016) (Figure 7.16).

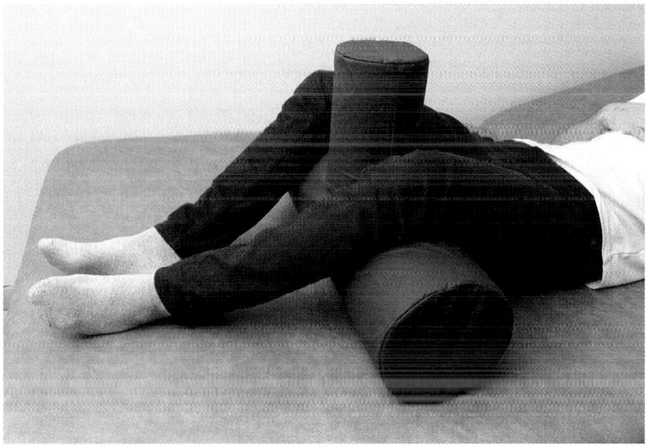

Figure 7.16 T-roll.

Procedure guideline 7.10 Positioning a neurological patient with tonal problems in bed

Essential equipment

- Personal protective equipment
- Pillows or towels for support when positioning

Optional equipment

- Any resting splints recommended or provided by the patient's physiotherapist or occupational therapist

Medicinal products

- Analgesia as required
- Antispasmodics as required

Action	Rationale
Pre-procedure	
1 Introduce yourself to the patient, explain and discuss the procedure with them, and gain their consent to proceed.	To ensure that the patient feels at ease, understands the procedure and gives their valid consent (NMC 2018, **C**).
2 Wash hands thoroughly with soap and water or use an alcohol-based handrub.	To reduce the risk of contamination and cross-infection (NHS England and NHSI 2019, **C**; WHO 2012, **C**).
3 Ensure the bed is at the optimum height for the handlers. If two handlers are required, try to match the handlers' heights as far as possible.	To minimize the risk of injury to the practitioners (CSP 2014, **C**).
Procedure	
4 Follow the basic advice for positioning the patient in the supine position (Procedure guideline 7.1: Positioning a patient: supine), side-lying (Procedure guideline 7.3: Positioning a patient: side-lying) or sitting up in bed (Procedure guideline 7.2: Positioning a patient: sitting up in bed).	To ensure patient comfort. **E** To allow pressure relief. **E** As a part of the patient's rehabilitation programme. **E**
5 *Positioning the patient in supine*: consider and apply possible modifications for positioning in supine (**Action figure 5**): • Place a pillow under a hemiplegic arm to support and align the shoulder. • Place additional pillows, wedges or T-rolls under the knees to support hemiparetic legs or maintain the position of high-tone legs. • Apply resting splints to hands and feet if provided (see Table 7.4). It is important to ensure any splint is fitted correctly, to only apply it for the recommended time and to check the integrity of the skin when removing the splint. • If the patient does not have resting splints, consider placing a folded pillow or rolled towel to support the feet in the neutral (plantargrade) position.	To promote alignment of body segments for patients with high or low tone resulting in asymmetrical posture (Preston and Edmans 2016, **R**). To control pelvic and spinal alignment. **E** To optimize patient comfort. **E** To maintain joint and soft tissue range (Duff et al. 2012, **E**).
6 *Positioning the patient in side-lying*: consider and apply possible modifications as specified below for side-lying (**Action figure 6**): • Ensure that the top hip is either directly on top of the lower hip or slightly in front of it (this prevents the patient rolling back). • Place a pillow between the legs. • Place folded pillows behind the back. • Ensure that the lower arm is not under the trunk. It is important to take care when checking this, particularly when moving a low-tone shoulder. • If the patient is lying on their unaffected side (i.e. the hemiplegic arm is uppermost), place their affected arm on pillow(s) and apply a resting splint for the hand or forearm if required.	To support the patient's affected shoulder and upper limb due to a risk of trauma, pain, or muscle and soft tissue shortening (Ada et al. 2005, **R**). To reduce the influence of asymmetrical posturing of the head and trunk in patients with high or low tone. **E** To maintain soft tissue and joint range (Duff et al. 2012, **E**).
7 *Positioning the patient sitting in bed*: consider and apply possible modifications as specified below for sitting in bed (**Action figure 7**): • If possible, raise the knee break of the bed to prevent the patient slipping down the bed. If this is not an option, consider placing pillows under the knees. • Place folded pillows, blocks or rolled towels under the affected elbow to support a low-tone or subluxed shoulder, or apply a shoulder brace.	To promote alignment of body segments for patients with high or low tone when sitting (Preston and Edmans 2016, **R**). To maintain soft tissue and joint range and minimize pain (Duff et al. 2012, **E**).

(continued)

Procedure guideline 7.10 Positioning a neurological patient with tonal problems in bed (*continued*)

Action	Rationale
• Place rolled towels or wedges between the arm and the body in high-tone arms to maintain range. • Place wedges, rolled towels or pillows along the trunk if support is required to prevent the patient leaning or falling laterally. • Place rolled towels or wedges under the head pillow to help maintain the head position.	
Post-procedure	
8 Reassess and record neurological symptoms. In the event of any worsening pain or neurological symptoms, arrange for a reassessment by the medical team.	To ensure clinical status is maintained (MASCIP 2015, **C**).

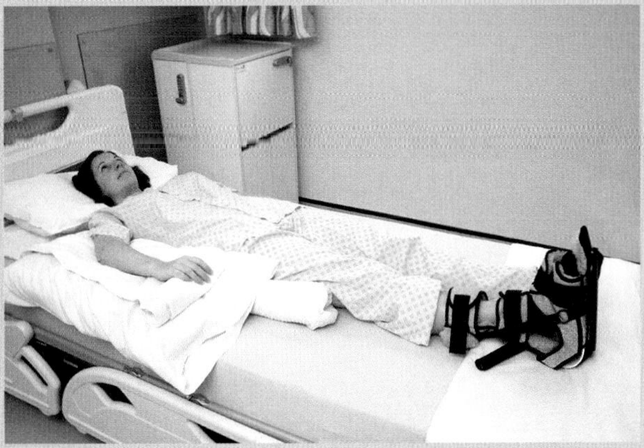

Action Figure 5 Positioning a patient with tonal problems in bed: supine.

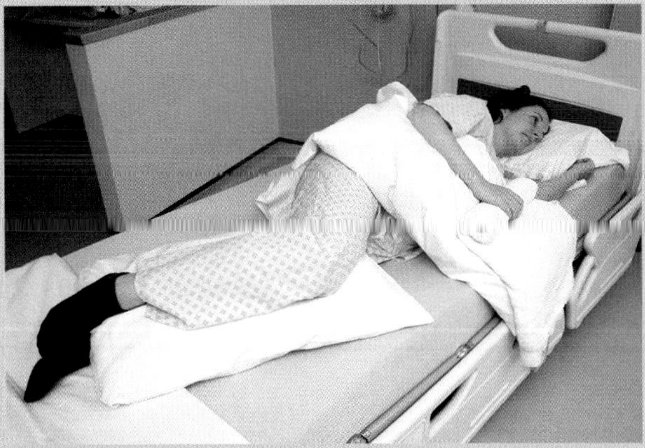

Action Figure 6 Positioning a patient with tonal problems in bed: side-lying.

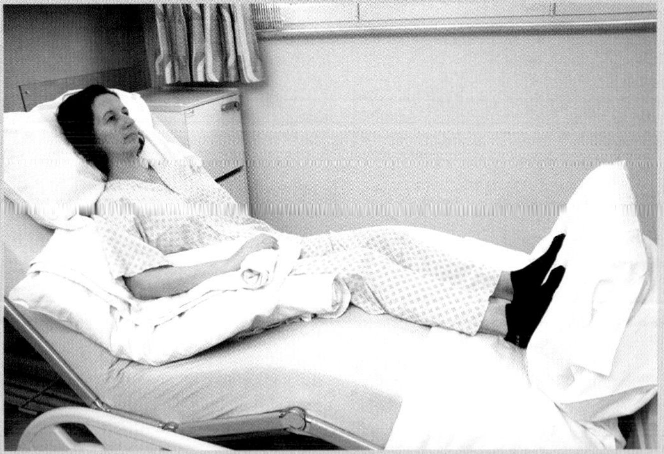

Action Figure 7 Positioning a patient with tonal problems in bed: sitting in bed.

Positioning a neurological patient with tonal problems in a chair

Pre-procedural considerations

Equipment

When people with shoulder subluxation and weak trunk muscles sit, gravity can exacerbate the subluxation and challenge the weak trunk muscles. It is therefore important to support the trunk and shoulders to optimize the patient's position and reduce the risk of joint damage (Ada et al. 2005).

Seating

Appropriate seating is advocated as an adjunct to management for effective postural support (Crawford and Stinson 2015, Preston and Edmans, 2016). Occupational therapists and physiotherapists will consider this for the management of patients with complex needs and provide appropriate seating if required.

Initially, patients may require chairs with plenty of support that can tilted backwards to reduce the challenges gravity presents. As they gain more control, they may be able to sit in a standard chair or wheelchair (see Table 7.5).

Table 7.5 Types of wheelchair

Type of chair	Purpose and advantages
Attendant-propelled wheelchair 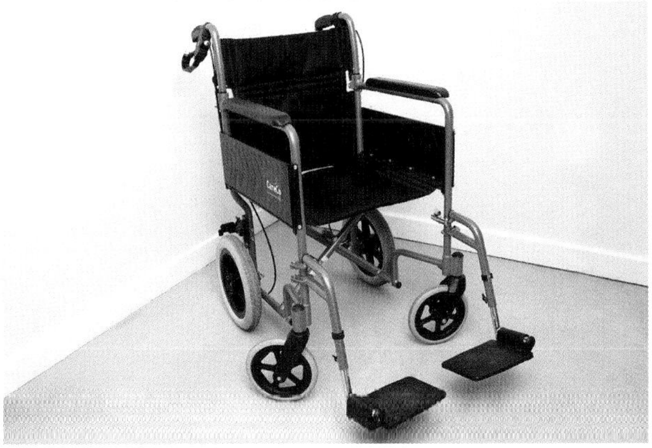	• Used for patients with good sitting balance but who are unable to propel themselves, whether due to arm weakness, fatigue or cognitive impairment.
Self-propelled wheelchair 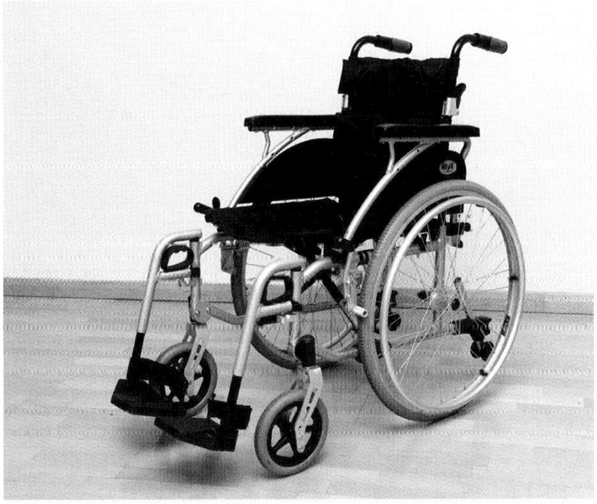	• Used for patients with good sitting balance who can use their upper limbs to propel themselves. • Promotes independence.
Tilt-in-space wheelchair 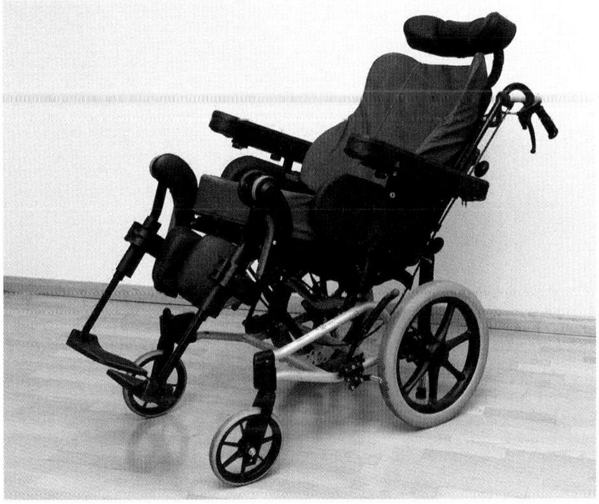	• Used for patients who have limited postural control or sitting endurance. • These chairs usually have two modes of adjustment: the backrest can tilt back, or the whole chair can tilt backwards on its axis. • These are available in attendant- and self-propelling options.

(continued)

Table 7.5 Types of wheelchair (*continued*)

Type of chair	Purpose and advantages
Powered wheelchair 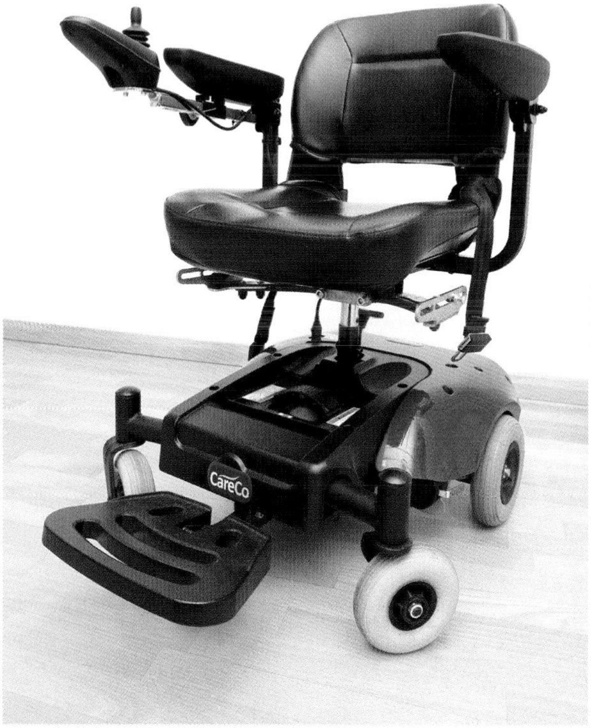	• Options are available with varying levels of support depending on a patient's postural control. • Allows independent movement for those patients who are unable to self-propel. • Patients must not have any cognitive impairment that would affect their safety when driving a powered chair.

Procedure guideline 7.11 Positioning a neurological patient with tonal problems in a chair

Essential equipment

- Personal protective equipment
- Appropriate chair or wheelchair
- Appropriate positioning aids (e.g. pillows and towels)
- Appropriate splints and/or supports

Action	Rationale
Pre-procedure	
1 Introduce yourself to the patient, explain and discuss the procedure with them, and gain their consent to proceed.	To ensure that the patient feels at ease, understands the procedure and gives their valid consent (NMC 2018, **C**).
2 Always use the chair recommended by the treating therapist.	To ensure the chair adequately meets the needs of the patient. **E**
3 Using local moving and handling guidelines, move the patient into the chair. Once the patient is in the chair, use the following steps to ensure correct positioning.	To ensure correct local procedures are followed for safe moving and handling. **E**
Procedure	
4 Ensure that the pelvis is neither rotated (so that one leg is further forward) nor tilted (so that one hip is lower than the other).	To maximize sitting stability to increase function and energy levels (Crawford and Stinson 2015, **E**).
5 Place any leg, lateral trunk or head supports as recommended (e.g. rolled towels between the knees to maintain hip alignment) (**Action figure 5**).	To maintain correct position and alignment, **E**.
6 Protect low-tone shoulders with shoulder supports or pillows as recommended.	To avoid any further problems associated with low tone (Crawford and Stinson 2015, **E**).

7 Ensure the patient's feet are well positioned on the footplates.	For the patient's comfort and to maintain pelvis alignment (Crawford and Stinson 2015, **E**).
8 Apply and tilt or recline to the chair as recommended.	To ensure the patient's comfort. **E**
Post-procedure	
9 Closely monitor the skin condition of patients requiring the use of an external splint to maintain joint position and range.	To monitor skin integrity and pressure care. **E**

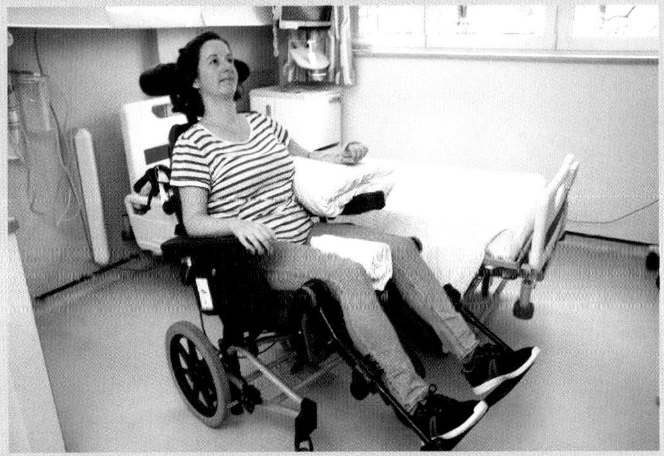

Action Figure 5 Positioning a patient with tonal problems in a chair.

Post-procedural considerations

For patients requiring the use of an external splint to maintain joint position and range, skin condition must be closely monitored at regular intervals for marking to avoid pressure areas. If there are any concerns about the fit, the use of the splint should be discontinued and the issue should be reported to the providing therapist as soon as possible.

Moving and positioning a patient with actual or suspected spinal cord compression or spinal cord injury

Definition

Spinal cord compression (SCC) or spinal cord injury (SCI) is when there is damage to the spinal cord either from trauma or non-traumatic causes, leading to functional impairment.

Anatomy and physiology

The spinal cord extends from the base of the brain to the pelvis within the vertebral canal, protected by the surrounding vertebrae (Figure 7.17). The spinal cord is part of the central nervous system, which carries messages along the spinal tracts between the brain and the spinal nerves (Lundy-Ekman 2018b).

The spinal nerves branch out from the spinal cord at each vertebral level to communicate with specific areas of the body to control sensory, motor and autonomic functions (see the section 'Moving and positioning a patient with neurological impairment' above for further detail). Each spinal nerve innervates a specific group of muscles or an area of skin. A myotome is the group of muscles that a single spinal nerve innervates. A dermatome is an area of skin supplied by a single spinal nerve (Figure 7.18) (Lundy-Ekman 2018b).

Related theory

The spinal canal is a rigid, contained cavity. Therefore, any expanding disease process will eventually cause spinal cord and/or nerve root compression. This results in impaired function or loss of function, causing reduced movement or sensation. The spinal cord does not have to be severed in order for a loss of functioning to occur (Lindsay et al. 2010).

Following damage to the spinal cord, 'spinal shock' may occur. This is the temporary suspension of spinal cord activity or loss of reflexes caused by oedema at and below the level of the injury. A complex series of physiological and biochemical reactions occur due to resulting oedema and vascular damage. Circulation of blood and oxygen is disrupted, and ischaemic tissue necrosis follows with immediate cessation of conductivity within the spinal cord neurones. Following 2–6 weeks there will be a return of reflex activity, often resulting in spasticity (Bonner and Smith 2013).

The causes of SCC and SCI are characterized as 'traumatic' or 'non-traumatic'.

Traumatic spinal cord injury

It is estimated that 1000–1200 people sustain traumatic SCI in the UK each year (RNOH 2016). Traumatic injuries are caused by an impact that fractures, dislocates or compresses one or more of the vertebrae. Common causes of trauma include falls, road traffic collisions, sporting injuries, gunshots and stabbing.

Non-traumatic spinal cord injury

Non-traumatic spinal cord injuries form a heterogeneous group of diseases, with the leading causes being tumours and degenerative

Problem-solving table 7.3 Prevention and resolution (Procedure guidelines 7.10 and 7.11)

Problem	Cause	Prevention	Action
Abnormally high tone or spasms, leading to difficulty positioning the patient's arms or legs in bed or in a chair	• Inadequate pain control • Inadequate anti-spasticity medication • Poor postural alignment • Bladder and bowel dysfunction • Noxious stimuli such as ill-fitting splint, ingrowing toenail or infection (UCLH 2012)	• Ensure pain control • Ensure bowel management • Ensure effective catheter drainage • Ensure adequate anti-spasticity medication (UCLH 2012)	• Assess for painful stimuli, infection, constipation and catheter drainage, which may increase tone in patients with CNS disease • Use leg flexion position on electric bed controls and/or position a small folded pillow or rolled towel under the patient's knees • Avoid contact of the patient's feet against the end of the bed as this can stimulate increased tone in legs • Liaise with physiotherapist • Consider a medical review
Pain	• High tone • Injury • Neuropathic pain • Ill-fitting splint • Pressure area • Sustained or poorly aligned posture	• Ensure adequate pain relief • Ensure correct management of tone (as above) • Ensure good alignment and regular position changes (ACPIN 2015) • Check fit of splint	• Liaise with physiotherapist • Consider a medical review
Unable to fit splint	• Swelling • Increased tone (ACPIN 2015)	• Encourage ankle circle exercises • Manage tonal changes (as above)	• Refer to therapists for consideration of compression garments
Splint marking the skin or causing pain	• Splint not fitting properly • Splint not applied correctly • Splint left in place for too long (ACPIN 2015)	• Follow therapist's instructions regarding fitting, positioning and length of time the splint remains *in situ* (ACPIN 2015)	• Remove splint and discontinue use until reviewed • Liaise with treating therapist
Inattention or neglect: patient may be unaware of the affected side of their body or environment	• Sensory/motor inattention • Neglect	• Draw patient's awareness to their neglected side	• Ensure affected limbs are supported by pillows, or folded or rolled towel, as required • Liaise with OT, who will recommend strategies to draw attention to the neglected side
Reduced conscious level: changes in the patient's consciousness affecting their ability to participate in positioning and/or sitting	• Symptom of neurological condition • Side-effect of certain medications • Changes in neurological status	• Consider timing of sedating medications as far as possible • Increase arousal levels with activity	• Liaise with medical team
Cognitive impairment impacting on the ability of the patient to sit in a chair safely	• Symptom of neurological condition or pre-existing cognitive disorder • Acute illness • Side-effect of treatment or medication	• Determine any reversible causes	• Liaise with OT to discuss management strategies to allow safe seating • Consider one-to-one support
Communication difficulties	• Language barrier • Dysphasia • Dysarthria	• Use interpreter services or family to overcome language barrier	• Liaise with a speech and language therapist to establish communication strategies for dysphasia and dysarthria
Fatigue	• Symptom of neurological condition • Acute illness • Side-effect of treatment or medication (Abd-Elfattah et al. 2015)	• Limit time sitting in bed or chair • Allow rest periods • Ensure adequate nutrition and hydration	• Liaise with OT for fatigue-management strategies

CNS, central nervous system; OT, occupational therapist.

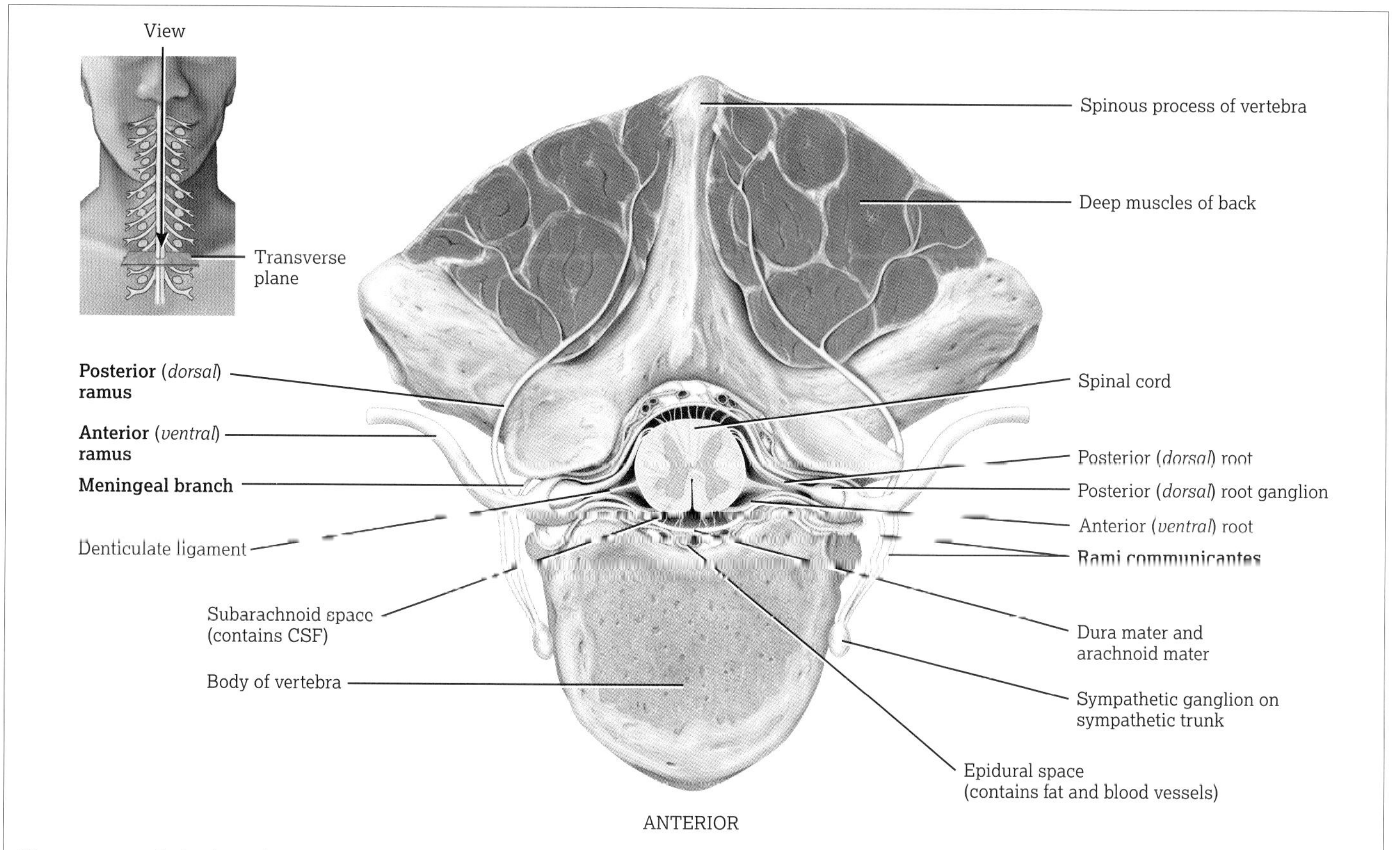

Figure 7.17 Spinal cord cross section. *Source*: Reproduced with permission of Pearson

diseases of the spinal column. Due to the heterogeneity of causes, it is difficult to know the numbers of non-traumatic SCI cases within the UK. They can be split into the following types:

- *Vascular*: involves damage to the blood vessels or supply. This can include haemorrhage, hypotension or embolism (SIA 2015).
- *Inflammatory and infections*: involves conditions such as tuberculosis, abscess, transverse myelitis and autoimmune disorders (SIA 2015).
- *Degenerative conditions*: involves degeneration of the vertebrae surrounding the spinal cord leading to compression. Includes osteoarthritis, osteoporosis and degenerative disc disease (SIA 2015).
- *Neoplastic*: either from a primary spinal tumour or from metastatic disease. Around 5% of all cancers can lead to SCC (SIA 2015).
  - *Primary tumours*: classified into two broad categories: intradural intramedullary tumours and intradural extramedullary tumours. Intramedullary tumours are composed predominantly of gliomas (astrocytomas and ependymomas). Extramedullary tumours are either peripheral nerve sheath tumours or meningiomas) (Louis et al. 2016).
  - *Metastatic spinal cord compression (MSCC)*: an oncological emergency caused by direct pressure and/or induction of vertebral collapse or instability by metastatic spread, leading to a risk of (or actual) neurological disability (GAIN 2014).

Classification

SCC and SCI are classified in general terms as being neurologically 'complete' or 'incomplete' based upon the sacral sparing definition. Sacral sparing refers to the presence of sensory and motor function in the most caudal sacral segments (i.e. preservation of light touch and/or pin prick at S4–S5 dermatome and voluntary anal sphincter contraction) (Kirshblum et al. 2011).

- *Complete spinal cord injury*: when the cord 'loses all descending neuronal control below the level of the lesion' (Lundy-Ekman 2018d, p.373). There is the absence of sacral sparing.
- *Incomplete spinal cord injury*: when 'the function of some ascending and/or descending fibres is preserved within the spinal cord' (Lundy-Ekman 2018d, p.373). There is the presence of sacral sparing.

On initial presentation, imaging will confirm both the presence of SCI and whether the spine is 'stable' or 'unstable':

- *Stable spine*: this is where spinal alignment is intact, with no further risk of progression of neurological symptoms as the spine is still able to maintain and distribute weight appropriately.
- *Unstable spine*: this is where the spinal fractures or lesions pose a risk of potential irreversible neurological symptoms due to movement of the fracture site.

Clinical presentation

The clinical presentations of SCI and SCC are dependent on the location within the spinal cord or cauda equina and the degree and duration of compression. In SCC, early diagnosis is crucial in order to at best prevent and otherwise minimize irreversible neurological damage.

Common symptoms of SCI include:

- back pain and/or radicular pain
- nerve root symptoms resulting in pain or loss of sensation within a dermatome
- respiratory compromise
- limb weakness
- sensory loss
- bladder and/or bowel dysfunction
- sexual dysfunction.

The level and extent of the injury will determine the functional impairment. Lesions within the thoracic and lumbar region may lead to paraplegia, and cervical or upper thoracic lesions may lead to quadriplegia/tetraplegia (Table 7.6) (Kirshblum et al. 2011).

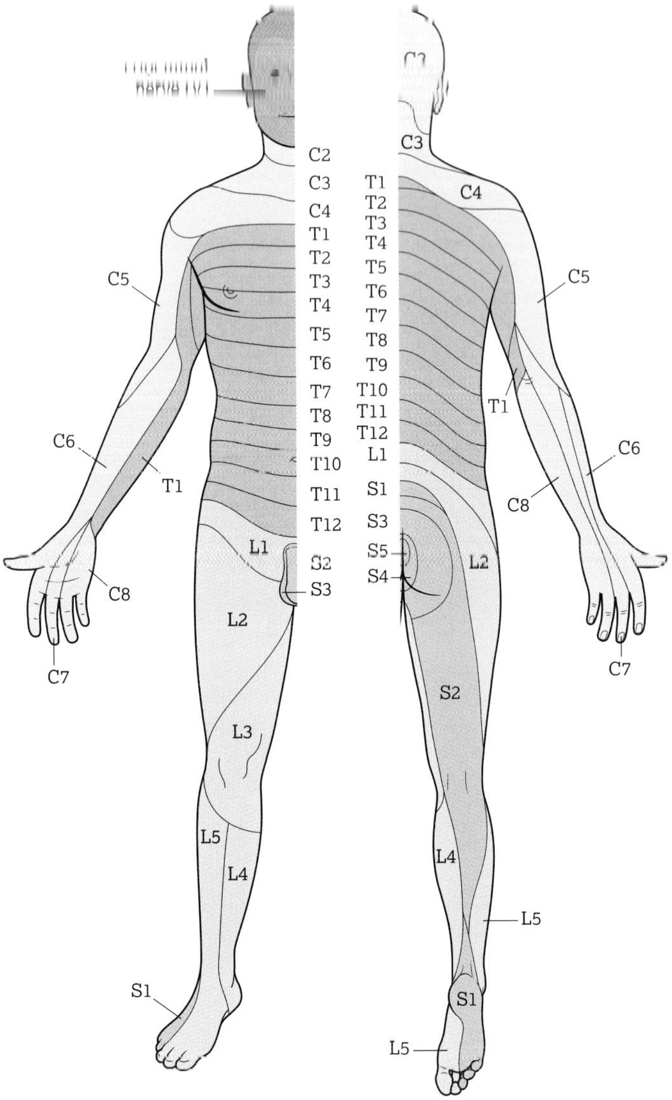

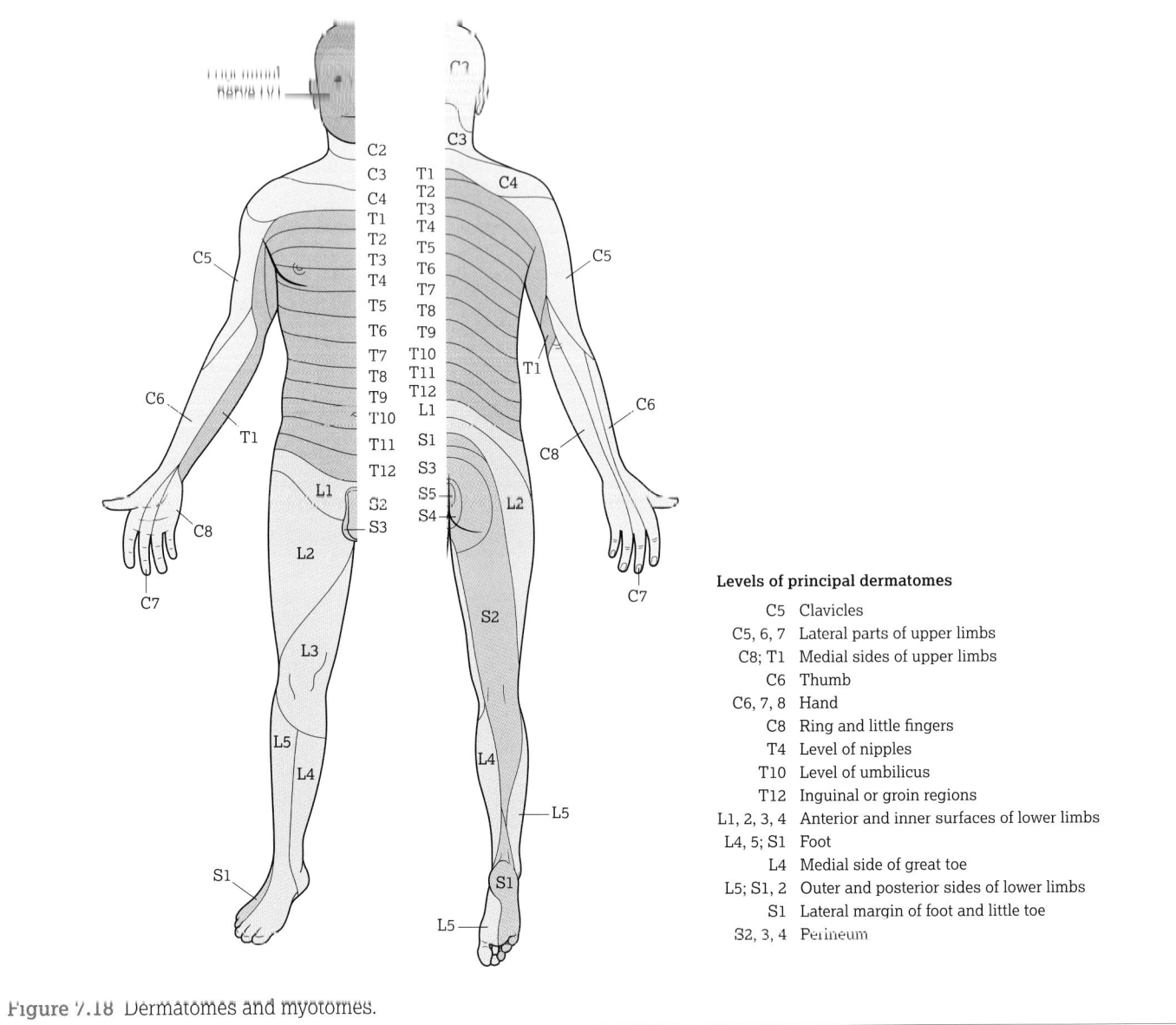

Levels of principal dermatomes

C5	Clavicles
C5, 6, 7	Lateral parts of upper limbs
C8; T1	Medial sides of upper limbs
C6	Thumb
C6, 7, 8	Hand
C8	Ring and little fingers
T4	Level of nipples
T10	Level of umbilicus
T12	Inguinal or groin regions
L1, 2, 3, 4	Anterior and inner surfaces of lower limbs
L4, 5; S1	Foot
L4	Medial side of great toe
L5; S1, 2	Outer and posterior sides of lower limbs
S1	Lateral margin of foot and little toe
S2, 3, 4	Perineum

Figure 7.18 Dermatomes and myotomes.

It is important to consider respiratory function in patients with lesions of T12 and above due to the involvement of respiratory muscles. Patients with significant respiratory muscle involvement will require assistance with coughing and considerations of positioning to prevent respiratory compromise. Refer to the physiotherapist to assist with respiratory management (Bonner and Smith 2013).

If patients are assessed to have reduced bowel function, they will require a bowel management regime to prevent complications such as constipation, faecal incontinence and autonomic dysreflexia (see the 'Complications' section below).

Evidence-based approaches

Principles of care

Stable spine

The general principles of positioning mentioned earlier in this chapter are all relevant to this group of patients. However, patients need to be assessed for adequate pain control prior to moving and positioning, and care should be taken to avoid excessive rotation of the spine when turning.

Mobilization requires a graduated and carefully monitored approach, and sitting must be trialled with regular review of neurology and observations (CRGSCI 2016). Clinical vigilance should be exercised with moving and positioning patients with an SCC. Such interventions should be ceased if there is worsening of pain or neurological symptoms. Medical advice should be sought regarding spinal stability.

Unstable spine

For patients with an unstable spine or severe mechanical pain suggestive of spinal instability, specific instructions for moving must be followed until bony and neurological stability is radiologically confirmed and discussed with appropriate medical teams. This is to ensure spinal alignment and reduce the risk of further spinal damage and potential loss of function. If a thoracolumbar injury is suspected, do not flex the hip more than 45° (CRGSCI 2016).

This patient group will require particular considerations to enable safe practice without compromising their clinical condition. These may include (CRGSCI 2016):

- lateral surface transfer (e.g. bed to trolley) using a spinal board or scoop stretcher

Table 7.6 Levels of spinal injury with resulting function loss.

Site of spine	Level	Affected area of body
Cervical	C4 (tetraplegia)	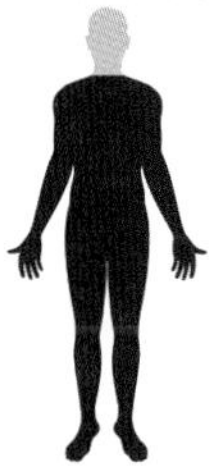
Cervical	C6 (tetraplegia)	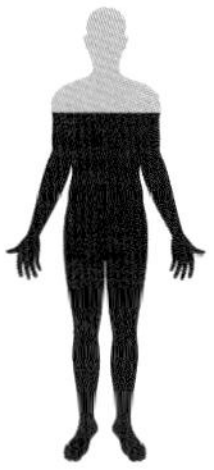
Thoracic	T6 (paraplegia)	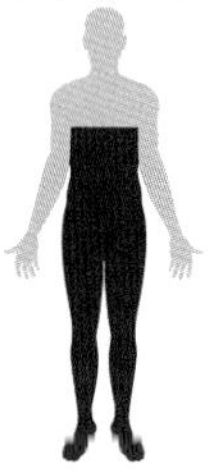
Lumbar	L1 (paraplegia)	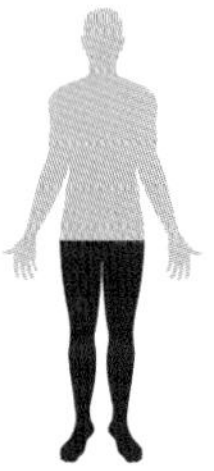

- manual support of the patient's head and neck for any flat surface transfer of patients with lesions above T6 (this ensures appropriate spinal alignment and patient comfort)
- log rolling for personal and pressure care for patients with unstable SCI.

When moving and turning patients with confirmed or suspected spinal instability who are being nursed flat, log rolling must be used. This is a technique used to maintain neutral spinal alignment. It is an essential method to enable continence and pressure area care.

Repositioning frequency will be determined by the individual's skin integrity, continence needs and degree of spinal instability (GAIN 2014). Patients should only be moved by adequate numbers of staff who have been fully trained in moving patients with SCC or SCI. Differing methods are recommended depending on the level of the lesion or injury:

- *Cervical and high thoracic lesions (T6 and above)*: log roll with five people (MASCIP 2015; see also Procedure guideline 7.13: Log rolling a patient with suspected or confirmed cervical spinal instability (above T6)).
- *Thoracolumbar lesions (T7 and below)*: log roll with four people (MASCIP 2015; see also Procedure guideline 7.14: Log rolling a patient with suspected or confirmed thoracolumbar spinal instability (T7 and below)).

Early and accurate diagnosis and, if appropriate, treatment are necessary to optimize neurological functioning. Timely referral to rehabilitation services (such as physiotherapists and occupational therapists) is imperative for assessment and appropriate intervention, and thorough discharge planning is required to enable a smooth transition back into the community (GAIN 2014).

Active rehabilitation may be postponed until the medical team has confirmed that the patient's spine is stable. However, there is a significant role for members of the rehabilitation team in the management of these patients in terms of:

- assessing motor and sensory function
- minimizing further complications, such as chest infections, which may arise as a result of prolonged bedrest and respiratory muscle weakness
- effective, co-ordinated discharge planning – the positioning and moving needs of these patients are often complex and so discharge planning may be lengthy and multifaceted, with the patient requiring ongoing support and rehabilitation in the community to optimize their functional independence (GAIN 2014).

Patients with neurological symptoms will require a physiotherapist to ensure correct manual handing is carried out, especially the first time a patient is moved out of bed. Patients may be able to assist with moving, positioning and transfers depending on:

- spinal stability
- pain
- level of lesion
- muscle power
- sensory impairment
- exercise tolerance
- patient confidence.

Pre-procedural considerations

Equipment

Cervical collar or spinal brace

Where there is a risk of spinal instability due to vertebral injury or collapse, patients may require external spinal support. This may be in the form of a spinal brace or collar. A properly fitted hard collar must be used when there is suspicion of spinal instability in the cervical spine (MASCIP 2015). If there is suspected spinal instability in the thoracolumbar region then a spinal brace may be prescribed (GAIN 2014). Depending on local policy, these are available from surgical appliances or orthotics suppliers, or some physiotherapy departments. The manufacturer's product details and care instructions will be provided with the equipment. Staff should be guided by medical advice and local policy on the application of a collar or brace. It is essential that correct fitting and application of the collar or brace is adhered to, so as to ensure spinal stability and prevention of damage to pressure areas.

Moving and handling aids

Patients with stable injuries may be able to assist with transfers using transfer boards, standing aids, mobility aids, frames, crutches or sticks. If they are unable to assist, there is a variety of moving and handling aids, for example lateral patient transfer boards, hoists and standing hoists, which maintain the safety of both the patient and the carer.

Assessment and recording tools

The focus of an initial neurological assessment is to establish the level of cord injury and act as a baseline against which future improvements or declines may be compared (Harrison 2007).

Standard assessments, including pain, motor and sensory, should be used as a baseline and updated with any change in a patient's presentation. It is vital that anal tone and sensation are assessed in all patients to establish the extent of damage to the spinal cord and whether bowel management strategies are required.

Assessments will depend on local policy and may include:

- the American Spinal Injury Association's International Standards for Neurological Classification of Spinal Cord Injury (ASIA 2015)
- a pain assessment tool, for example a visual analogue scale (Dijkers 2010)
- a bladder and bowel management assessment (MASCIP 2012)
- a pressure ulcer assessment (see Chapter 18: Wound management).

Pain management: pharmacological and non pharmacological

As already discussed, spinal and radicular pain can be an indicator of MSCC in the first instance but, in relation to moving and handling, it can also be suggestive of changes in neurology. Implementation of a pain assessment chart can enable continuity of care, allowing accurate assessment and evaluation of all pharmacological interventions (i.e. non-steroidal anti-inflammatory drugs, opiates, bisphosphonates and epidural) and non-pharmacological interventions (i.e. relaxation and therapeutic management). Chapter 10: Pain assessment and management provides more specific information.

Procedure guideline 7.12 Application of a two-piece cervical collar

See also the manufacturer's instructions

Essential equipment

- Personal protective equipment
- Collar

Action	Rationale
Pre-procedure	
1 Introduce yourself to the patient, explain and discuss the procedure with them, and gain their consent to proceed.	To ensure that the patient feels at ease, understands the procedure and gives their valid consent (NMC 2018, **C**).
2 Wash hands thoroughly with soap and water or use an alcohol-based handrub.	To reduce the risk of contamination and cross-infection (NHS England and NHSI 2019, **R**; WHO 2012, **C**).
3 Ensure the bed is at the optimum height for the handlers. If two handlers are required, try to match the handlers' heights as far as possible.	To minimize the risk of injury to the practitioners (Smith et al. 2011, **C**).
4 Ensure that there are sufficient personnel available to assist with the procedure.	Because one staff member is needed to maintain spinal alignment and one or two are needed to apply the collar (MASCIP 2015, **C**).
Procedure	
5 Measure the neck using a sizing guide (provided by the manufacturer) and then select the most appropriate size collar.	To ensure correct sizing for spinal stability and comfort, and to minimize skin damage. **E**
6 The lead practitioner stabilizes the patient's neck, supporting the patient's head without obstructing the ears so that the patient can hear explanations. The first assistant gently feeds the back piece of the collar into position, pressing it into the mattress (**Action figure 6**).	To immobilize the patient's head. **E** To ensure spinal alignment is monitored throughout the procedure (MASCIP 2015, **C**). To minimize movement of the spine and to ensure correct positioning of collar. **E**
7 The front piece is then brought into position by the assistant, who scoops the collar up and under the chin (**Action figure 7**).	Scooping enables best fit and comfort of collar. **E**
8 The collar is secured with Velcro fastenings (**Action figure 8**).	To ensure it remains securely in place. **E**
Post-procedure	
9 Check the comfort and fit with the patient.	For patient comfort. **E**
10 Remove the collar daily to check the skin and pressure areas and for hygiene purposes.	To maintain skin integrity. **E**
11 Reassess and record neurological symptoms. In the event of any worsening pain or neurological symptoms, arrange for a reassessment by the medical team.	To ensure clinical status is maintained (MASCIP 2015, **C**).

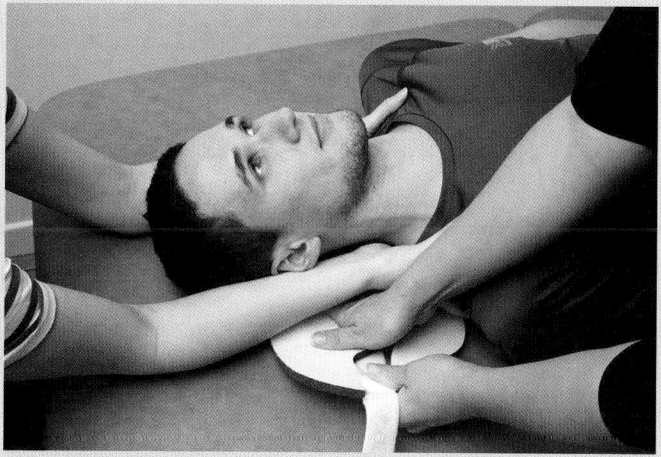

Action Figure 6 Neck stabilization throughout the application of the neck collar.

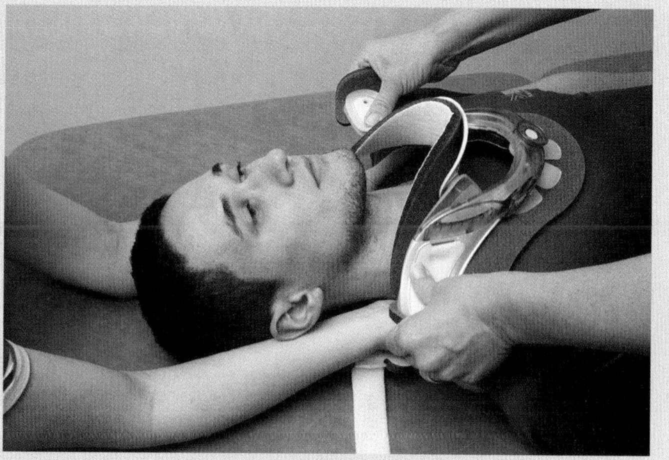

Action Figure 7 Application of the collar around the patient's neck while maintaining neck stabilization.

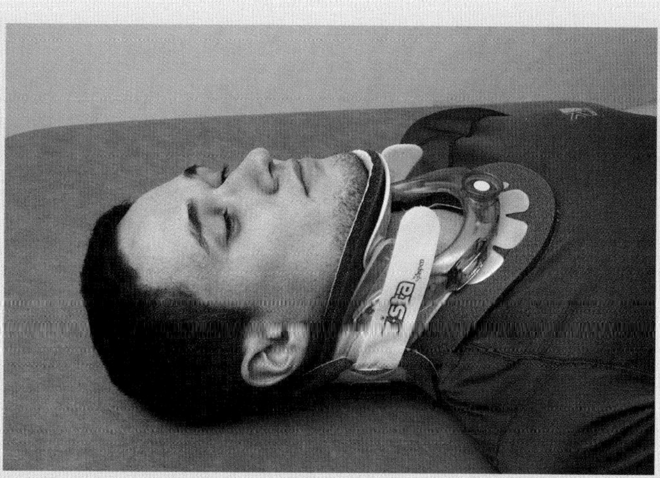

Action Figure 8 Securing the collar.

Procedure guideline 7.13 Log rolling a patient with suspected or confirmed cervical spinal instability (above T6)

Essential equipment

- Personal protective equipment
- Collar (if required)

Optional equipment

- Slipper pan
- Clean sheets
- Hygiene equipment

Action	Rationale
Pre-procedure	
1 Introduce yourself to the patient, explain and discuss the procedure with them, and gain their consent to proceed.	To ensure that the patient feels at ease, understands the procedure and gives their valid consent (NMC 2018, **C**).
2 Wash hands thoroughly with soap and water or use an alcohol-based handrub.	To reduce the risk of contamination and cross-infection (NHS England and NHSI 2019, **C**; WHO 2012, **C**).
3 Ensure the bed is at the optimum height for the handlers. If two handlers are required, try to match the handlers' heights as far as possible.	To minimize the risk of injury to the practitioners (Smith et al. 2011, **C**).

(continued)

Procedure guideline 7.13 Log rolling a patient with suspected or confirmed cervical spinal instability (above T6) *(continued)*

Action	Rationale
4 Ensure there are sufficient personnel available to assist with the procedure (minimum of five for patients with cervical spinal instability).	Because four staff are needed to maintain spinal alignment and one is needed to perform the personal and pressure care check during the procedure (MASCIP 2015, **C**).
Procedure	
5 Assess the patient's motor and sensory function using neurological observations (see Procedure guideline 14.9: Neurological observations and assessment).	To provide a baseline to compare against after the procedure (MASCIP 2015, **C**).
6 The lead practitioner stabilizes the patient's neck, supporting the patient's head (**Action figure 6**).	To stabilize the cervical spine to prevent any further injury (MASCIP 2015, **C**). To co-ordinate and lead the log roll. **E** To take responsibility for providing instructions (MASCIP 2015, **C**).
7 Ideally, the lead practitioner's hands should offer support for the entire cervical curve from the base of the skull to C7.	To immobilize the patient's head. **E** To ensure spinal alignment is monitored throughout the procedure (MASCIP 2015, **C**).
8 The second practitioner stands at the thorax and positions their hands over the patient's furthest shoulder and hip.	To ensure the lower spine remains aligned (MASCIP 2015, **C**).
9 The third practitioner stands at the hip area (on the same side as the second practitioner) and places one hand on the patient's furthest hip and the other underneath the furthest thigh.	To prevent movement at the thoracolumbar site (MASCIP 2015, **C**).
10 The fourth practitioner stands at the patient's lower leg (on the same side as the second and third practitioners) and places their hands under the knee and ankle of the furthest leg.	To ensure the lower spine remains aligned (MASCIP 2015, **C**).
11 Ensure there is a fifth person standing on the opposite side of the bed from practitioners two, three and four.	To position the equipment or take care of hygiene needs. **E** To assess the skin condition of the upper back and occiput (MASCIP 2015, **C**).
12 The lead practitioner (holding the head) provides clear instructions to the team to ensure the roll is well co-ordinated and alignment is maintained – for example, 'We will move on "roll". Ready, steady, roll.' The patient's upper leg should be maintained in alignment throughout (**Action figure 12**).	To ensure all practitioners are aware of when to move, so this is done in a co-ordinated manner (MASCIP 2015, **C**).
13 Those performing the manoeuvre should roll the patient in co-ordination with each other, maintaining the patient's spinal alignment throughout the procedure.	To maintain spinal stability and reduce the risk of further injury or damage (MASCIP 2015, **C**).
14 Each practitioner remains in place while the necessary care or intervention is performed.	To maintain spinal alignment throughout the procedure (MASCIP 2015, **C**).
15 The person holding the head then provides clear instructions to return the patient to supine. The patient's position and alignment should be checked.	To complete the move. **E**
Post-procedure	
16 Reassess and record the patient's motor and sensory function (refer to Procedure guideline 14.9: Neurological observations and assessment).	To ensure clinical status is maintained (MASCIP 2015, **C**).

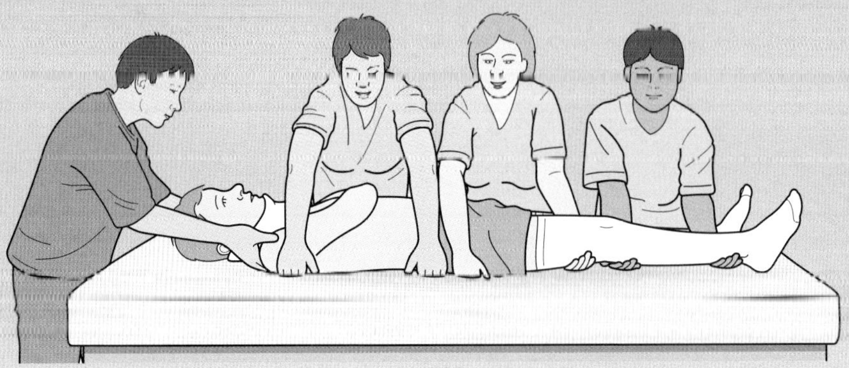

Action Figure 6 The practitioners position themselves as described in the steps above. Source: Illustrations © Louisa E. Hunt and SIA. Reproduced from the Spinal Injuries Association (www.spinal.co.uk) with permission.

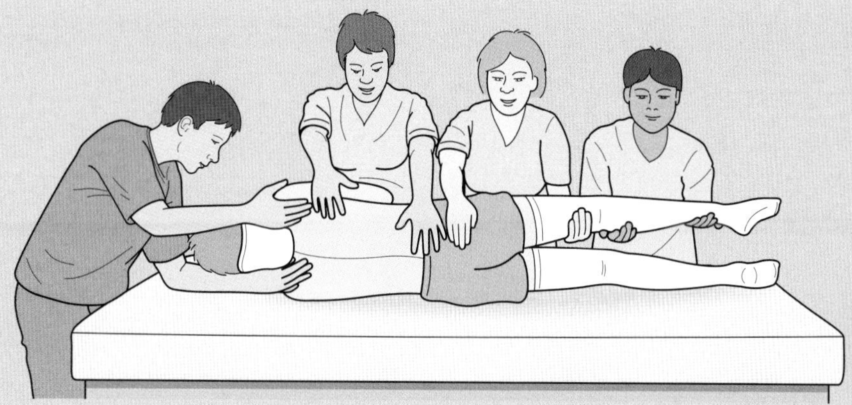

Action Figure 12 The roll is co-ordinated by the lead practitioner, with the patient's upper leg maintained in alignment throughout. *Source*: Illustrations © Louise E. Hunt and SIA. Reproduced from the Spinal Injuries Association (www.spinal.co.uk) with permission.

Procedure guideline 7.14 Log rolling a patient with suspected or confirmed thoracolumbar spinal instability (T7 and below)

Equipment

- Personal protective equipment
- Slipper pan
- Clean sheets
- Hygiene equipment
- Spinal brace (if requested by medical team)

Action	Rationale
Pre-procedure	
1 Introduce yourself to the patient, explain and discuss the procedure with them, and gain their consent to proceed.	To ensure that the patient feels at ease, understands the procedure and gives their valid consent (NMC 2018, **C**; RCN 2017, **C**).
2 Wash hands thoroughly with soap and water or use an alcohol-based handrub.	To reduce the risk of contamination and cross-infection (NHS England and NHSI 2019, **C**; WHO 2012, **C**).
3 Ensure the bed is at the optimum height for the handlers. If two handlers are required, try to match the handlers' heights as far as possible.	To minimize the risk of injury to the practitioner (Smith et al. 2011, **C**).
4 Ensure there are sufficient personnel available to assist with the procedure (a minimum of four for patients with thoracolumbar spinal instability).	Because three staff are needed to maintain spinal alignment and one is needed to perform the personal and pressure care check during the procedure (MASCIP 2015, **C**).
Procedure	
5 Assess the patient's motor and sensory function using neurological observations (Procedure guideline 14.9: Neurological observations and assessment).	For assessment before and after the log roll (MASCIP 2015, **C**).
6 The lead practitioner stands at the patient's thorax and positions their hands over the patient's furthest shoulder and top of hip (**Action figure 6**).	To co-ordinate and lead the log roll. **E** To take responsibility for providing instructions and ensuring all other practitioners are ready before commencing the manoeuvre (MASCIP 2015, **C**). To ensure the lower spine remains aligned (MASCIP 2015, **C**).
7 The second practitioner stands at the hip area (on the same side as the first practitioner) and places one hand on the patient's furthest hip next to the lead practitioner's hand and the other underneath the furthest thigh.	To prevent movement at the thoracolumbar site (MASCIP 2015, **C**).

(continued)

Procedure guideline 7.14 Log rolling a patient with suspected or confirmed thoracolumbar spinal instability (T7 and below) *(continued)*

Action	Rationale
8 The third practitioner stands at the patient's lower leg (on the same side as the first and second practitioners) and places their hands under the knee and ankle of the furthest leg.	To ensure the lower spine remains aligned (MASCIP 2015, **C**).
9 Ensure there is a fourth person standing on the opposite side of the bed.	To position the equipment or take care of hygiene needs (MASCIP 2015, **C**). To assess pressure areas (MASCIP 2015, **C**).
10 The lead practitioner provides clear instructions to the team to ensure the roll is well co-ordinated and alignment is maintained – for example, 'We will move on "roll". Ready, steady, roll.' The patient's upper leg should be maintained in alignment throughout (**Action figure 10**).	To ensure a co-ordinated approach to the move. **E** To ensure spinal alignment (MASCIP 2015, **C**).
11 Each practitioner remains in place while the necessary care or intervention is performed.	To maintain spinal alignment throughout the procedure (MASCIP 2015, **C**).
12 The person holding the head then provides clear instructions to return to supine, in a co-ordinated manner, maintaining alignment. Patient's position, and alignment should be checked.	To complete the move. **E**
Post-procedure	
13 Reassess and record neurological observations (see Procedure guideline 14.9: Neurological observations and assessment). In the event of a worsening of pain or neurological symptoms, ask the medical team to reassess the patient.	To ensure clinical status is maintained (NICE 2016, **C**)

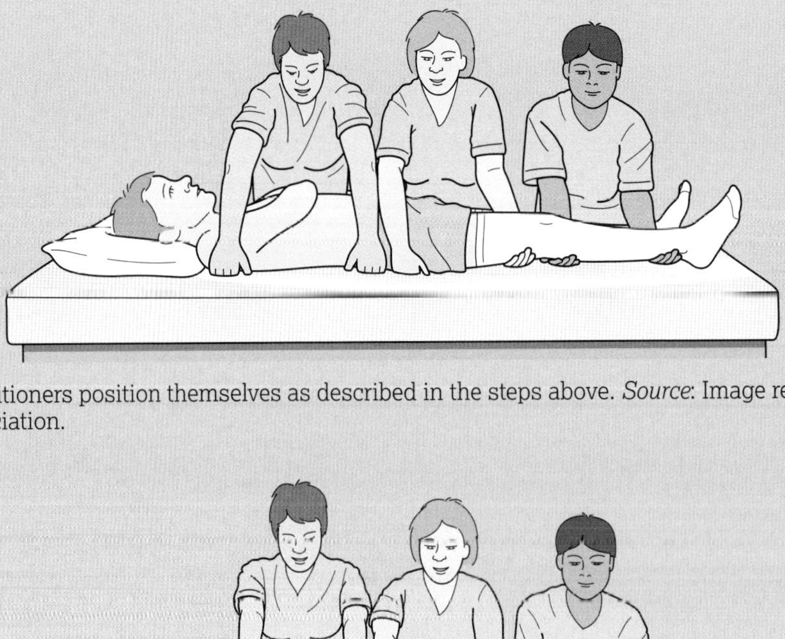

Action Figure 6 The practitioners position themselves as described in the steps above. *Source*: Image reproduced with permission of the Spinal Injuries Association.

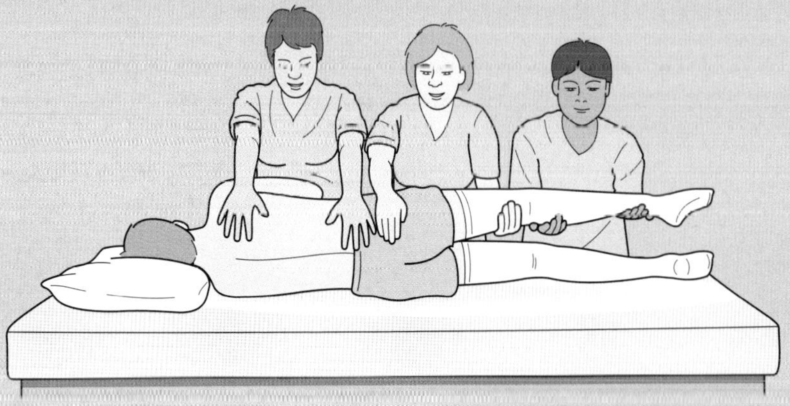

Action Figure 10 The roll is co-ordinated by the lead practitioner, with the patient's upper leg maintained in alignment throughout. *Source*: Image reproduced with permission of the Spinal Injuries Association.

Procedure guideline 7.15 Early mobilization of a patient with spinal considerations

Essential equipment

- Personal protective equipment
- Collar or spinal brace for patients with an unstable spine

Action	Rationale
Pre-procedure	
1 Introduce yourself to the patient, explain and discuss the procedure with them, and gain their consent to proceed.	To ensure that the patient feels at ease, understands the procedure and gives their valid consent (NMC 2018, **C**).
2 Wash hands thoroughly with soap and water or use an alcohol-based handrub.	To reduce the risk of contamination and cross-infection (WHO 2012, **C**; NHS England and NHSI 2019, **C**).
3 Ensure the bed is at the optimum height for the handlers. If two handlers are required, try to match the handlers' heights as far as possible.	To minimize the risk of injury to the practitioners (Smith et al. 2011, **C**).
4 Ensure there are sufficient staff available to assist with the procedure.	To ensure the safety of the patient and the people assisting. **E**
Procedure	
5 Assess motor and sensory function using neurological observations (see Procedure guideline 14.9 Neurological observations and assessment).	To assess and evaluate clinical symptoms (MASCIP 2015, **C**).
6 Discuss mobilization concerns or restrictions with medical staff.	To ensure there are no contraindications or added risks. **E**
7 Ensure a collar or brace is *in situ* for patients with an unstable spine (following Procedure guideline 7.12: Application of a two-piece cervical collar).	To ensure safety and stability (MASCIP 2015, **C**).
8 Assist the patient to move from supine to sitting (following Procedure guideline 7.4: Positioning a patient: lying down to sitting up).	
9 Perform regular close monitoring of blood pressure and neurological symptoms (for details see Chapter 14: Observations).	To assess and evaluate clinical symptoms (GAIN 2014, **C**).
10 On confirmation of stable symptoms, assist the patient to sit over the edge of the bed unsupported (following Procedure guideline 7.4: Positioning a patient: lying down to sitting up).	To ensure safe handling (CSP 2014, **C**).
11 Closely monitor any changes in symptoms.	To assess and evaluate clinical symptoms (GAIN 2014, **C**).
12 On confirmation of stable symptoms, proceed to the standard principles of mobilization (following Procedure guideline 7.5: Moving a patient from sitting to standing: assisting the patient) and using the general principles for moving patients with neurological impairment.	To ensure safe handling (CSP 2014, **C**).
Post-procedure	
13 Reassess the patient.	To ensure there have been no changes to their neurological status or condition. **E**
14 Document the procedure and its outcome in the patient's notes.	To ensure effective communication between healthcare professionals and effective documentation of care completed (NMC 2018, **C**).

Post-procedural considerations

Ongoing care

Reassessment by the medical team will be necessary in the event of an increase in pain or neurological symptoms.

Documentation

Any changes in neurological presentation and/or function must be documented both prior to and following any procedure.

Potential complications and problem solving

There are a number of potential long-term complications that may occur during or after moving and positioning SCI patients; these may be due to the initial injury, the subsequent effects of changes in bowel and bladder functions, and the paralysis (i.e. the complete loss of motor function) associated with their disease or injury. In addition, bedrest contributes to long-term complications.

Problem-solving table 7.4 Prevention and resolution (Procedures guidelines 7.13, 7.14 and 7.15)

Problem	Cause	Prevention	Action
Autonomic dysreflexia: a mass reflex due to excessive activity of the sympathetic nervous system by noxious stimuli below the level of the lesion. It is a potential complication for all patients with complete lesions above T6. Symptoms: • bradycardia • hypertension • pounding headache • flushing, sweating or blotchy appearance of skin above the level of the lesion.	• Overstretching of bladder or rectum (urinary obstruction being the most common cause) • Ingrowing toenail or other painful stimulus • Fracture below level of lesion • Pressure sore, burn, scald or sunburn • Urinary tract infection or bladder spasm • Visceral pain or trauma	• Closely monitor urinary drainage • Bowel management regime • Early recognition that an individual with SCI above T6 often has a normal systolic blood pressure in the 90–110 mmHg range; blood pressure of 20 to 40 mmHg above baseline may be a sign of autonomic dysreflexia	• *This is a medical emergency* as it could induce a myocardial infarct or a cerebrovascular accident • Sit the patient up • Loosen or remove tight clothing • Monitor blood pressure every 2–5 minutes • The patient's bladder and bowel should be checked as these are the most common causes • If the blood pressure is >150 mmHg, start pharmacological management (10 mg nifedipine sublingual or GTN spray: 1–2 sprays); repeat every 20–30 minutes if needed (RNOH 2018)
Orthostatic hypotension: low blood pressure when moving from lying to upright position.	• Loss of sympathetic vasoconstriction • Loss of muscle-pumping action for blood return	• Antiembolic stockings • Careful assessment and monitoring during early mobilization and upright position changes	• Medical review: use of medication prior to mobilization • Trial of abdominal binder (Lundy-Ekman 2018d)
Pain: increased pain on movement to the extent that it is perceived by the patient as severe or does not reverse with rest.	• Potential extension of spinal cord compression	• Ensure patients with unstable spine are moved correctly	• Nurse patient flat • Reassess spinal stability prior to further movement (GAIN 2014)
Impaired respiratory function: reduced respiratory function in a patient with lesions of T12 and above, especially T6 and above (GAIN 2014).	Respiratory function following SCI is determined by the level and extent of injury. Alterations of respiratory function following SCI include: • reduction in lung capacity • impaired ability to cough • altered breathing pattern • imbalance in ANS following SCI above the level of T6, with relative bronchoconstriction (airway narrowing) and increased secretion production • chronic secondary changes including reduction in lung and chest wall compliance.	• Routine assessment of respiratory function (e.g. vital capacity) (GAIN 2014) • Consideration of prophylactic management including manual cough assistance and use of a cough assist machine (contact physiotherapist) • Education to promote long-term self-management (RNOH 2018)	• If patient's respiratory function decreases, contact medical team urgently
Reduced skin integrity: risk to skin integrity and the development of pressure sores.	• Reduced mobility • Poor circulation • Altered sensation • Friction and shearing damage (GAIN 2014)	• Use of correct manual handling equipment • Regular positional changes • Regular assessment of the skin and pressure areas • Consider nutritional status	• Contact local tissue viability service

ANS, autonomic nervous system; GTN, glyceryl trinitrate; SCI, spinal cord injury.

Moving and positioning a patient with raised intracranial pressure

Definition
Intracranial pressure (ICP) is the pressure exerted within the cranial cavity. Normal pressure is 5–15 mmHg (Hawthorne and Piper 2014).

Anatomy and physiology
Injury or disease within the brain can lead to raised ICP. As the skull is a rigid structure and its contents – the brain, blood and cerebrospinal fluid (CSF) – are non-compressible, any increase in one of these or an expanding mass results in an increase in ICP (Lindsay et al. 2010). As the volume increases, the pressure rises exponentially to a critical level (Figure 7.19).

Causes of raised ICP include:

- expanding mass: tumour, haematoma or abscess
- hydrocephalus (excess CSF)
- cerebral oedema (Lindsay et al. 2010).

Related theory

Clinical presentation
Clinical features of raised ICP include:

- headache
- vomiting
- pupillary dysfunction
- reduction in level of consciousness.

As the pressure rises, the risk of brain shift and eventual brain herniation increases, potentially leading to death. Early identification and management of raised ICP is critical to minimize complications and ICP's catastrophic results (Lindsay et al. 2010).

Medical management
Patients with raised ICP are likely to be monitored closely using an ICP bolt within the critical care setting. Depending on the cause of the raised ICP, management may include:

- management of cerebral blood flow or maintenance of cerebral perfusion pressure
- sedation or paralysing agents
- CSF drainage (e.g. extraventricular drainage)
- surgery – excision of haematoma or tumour and decompressive craniectomy (Denehy and Main 2016).

Evidence-based approaches

Rationale
Positioning and moving patients with uncontrollable or raised ICP should be limited to essential tasks only, as such interventions can lead to further increases in ICP. Monitoring the effects on ICP of positioning and interventions, including how quickly any increase in ICP returns to baseline, is essential. If it takes a significant amount of time for ICP to return to baseline, then the medical team should be informed for further management.

Indications
Patients with raised ICP should be moved only for essential care, including:

- pressure area relief
- respiratory management
- cleaning and hygiene.

Contraindications
When handling patients with ICP:

- Consider the risks versus the benefits to the patient before moving and handling.
- Keep in mind that persistently raised ICP that does not settle quickly could be detrimental to the patient.

Pre-procedural considerations
Considerations of positioning patients with raised ICP within the critical care setting include:

- maintaining the head of the bed up at 30° to facilitate venous drainage, which will aid in reducing ICP
- keeping the head and neck in the neutral position to improve cerebral venous drainage and reduce ICP

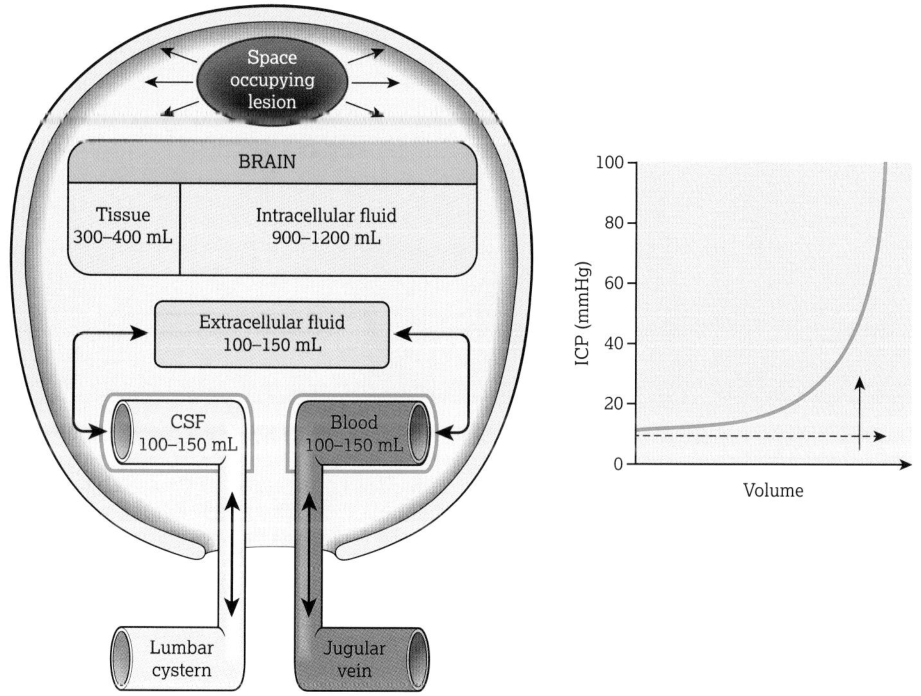

Figure 7.19 Causes of raised intracranial pressures. CSF, cerebrospinal fluid; ICP, intracranial pressure.

- avoiding compression of internal and external jugular veins from a tight cervical collar ([illegible] and [illegible] 2016).

Once ICP has stabilized and is within normal limits (5–15 mmHg), moving and positioning patients should be guided by the general principles of moving and positioning patients with neurological impairment (discussed earlier in this chapter).

Moving and positioning a patient with an amputation

Definition

Amputation refers to the loss of part of a limb or an entire limb. The different types and levels of amputation are shown in Figure 7.20. Vascular disease is the most common cause of amputation in contemporary healthcare but it can also be the result of trauma or congenital deficiency, and may be performed in the management of some malignancies, such as extremity sarcoma (Richardson 2010, Virani et al. 2015).

Related theory

The level of the amputation and the surgical technique can affect an individual's body image as well as their functional ability and suitability for prosthesis fitting (British Society of Rehabilitation Medicine 2018, Devinuwara et al. 2018).

Evidence-based approaches

Rationale

Patients will have reduced mobility in the immediate post-operative phase and a multidisciplinary approach to care and rehabilitation is essential in achieving the best outcomes (Smith et al. 2016).

Frequent changes of position should be encouraged to prevent skin breakdown and contractures ([illegible] 2017). Early physiotherapy intervention is important to teach bed mobility as well as exercises to help prevent contractures, strengthen muscles and assist early mobilization.

Indications

Any patient who has had an upper or lower limb amputation. Moving and positioning a patient with an amputation may be required to:

- minimize pain and maximize comfort
- decrease oedema
- prevent pressure area damage
- promote wound healing.

Contraindications

There are no absolute contraindications, but specialist techniques and/or adaptations may be required as described in the following procedure guidelines.

Principles of care

The main goals of moving and positioning with regard to amputee management are to:

- prevent problems arising as a consequence of reduced mobility
- prevent compromise to the remaining, contralateral limb in lower limb amputees
- help to control residual limb oedema in order to assist wound healing
- help to decrease phantom (sensation in the part of the extremity that has been amputated) and residual limb pain
- prevent contractures and maintain joint range of movement and muscle strength in order to maximize function and rehabilitation potential (particularly if the patient's goal is prosthetic rehabilitation)
- assist the restoration of functional independence as soon as possible.

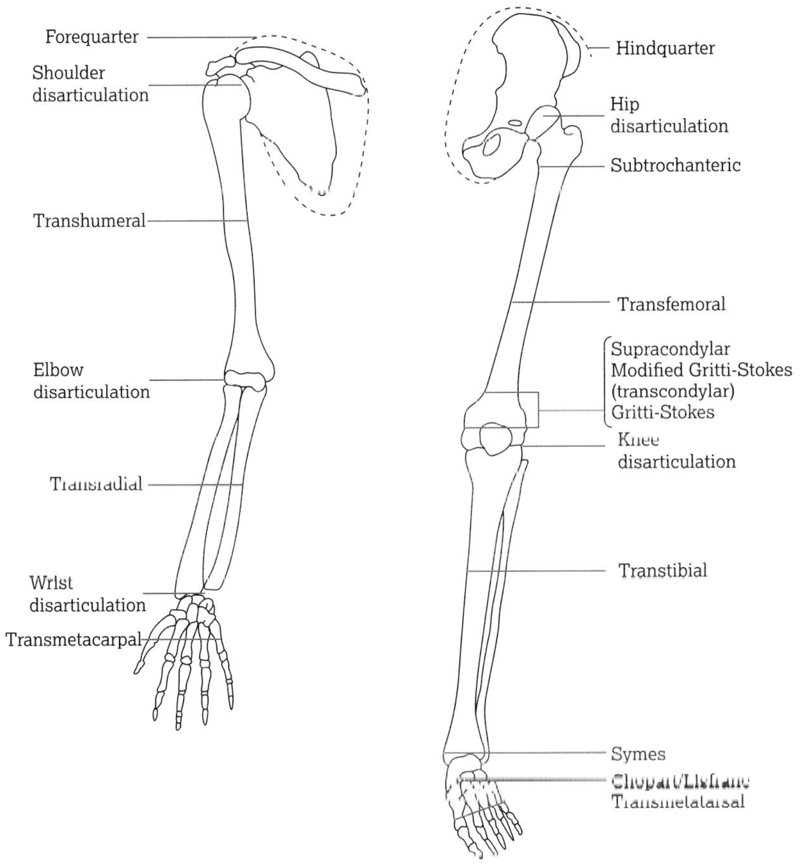

Figure 7.20 Levels of amputation in the upper and lower limbs.

When assisting an amputee, it is important to consider the following points:

- Any level of amputation, either of an upper or lower limb, will alter the patient's centre of gravity, potentially resulting in decreased balance. This, in turn, will increase the risk of falls in this patient group.
- Body symmetry and posture will be altered, which can affect balance and may lead to poor postural habits that will hinder recovery and function.

The British Association of Chartered Physiotherapists in Amputee Rehabilitation (Smith et al. 2016) recommends a comprehensive assessment by key professionals to establish rehabilitation goals. This assessment should be carried out as soon as possible following the decision to amputate and there will need to be regular reviews. Nurses play a vital role at all stages providing technical and physical care, including wound care and assisting with personal hygiene (Schreiber 2017).

Where possible, care relating to positioning should commence during the pre-operative stage. Patients should be encouraged to keep as mobile and independent as possible within their pain limits to reduce the effects of deconditioning. In the presence of pre-operative pain, patients are frequently less able to mobilize and, as a result, may adopt positions of comfort that can lead to contractures. These positions are often maintained after amputation due to comfort and habit but are also due to changes in muscle balance (Devinuwara et al. 2018, Ghazali et al. 2018). For example, transfemoral (above-knee) amputees may adopt a flexed and abducted position of their residual limb due to an alteration in muscle balance and pain, but this can lead to contractures over time if not corrected. Contractures can profoundly affect the potential for prosthetic rehabilitation and overall function, so optimization of pain control and early correct positioning are paramount (Devinuwara et al. 2018, Virani et al. 2015).

The general principles of care mentioned earlier in this chapter are all relevant to these patients. However, particular attention should be given to any possible balance issues for both upper limb and lower limb amputees. In the post-operative phase, lower limb amputees should mobilize using the wheelchair provided for them unless the physiotherapist or occupational therapist has advised otherwise (Smith et al. 2016). This is because standing for long periods or hopping can:

- negatively influence residual limb oedema and wound healing
- increase the risk of falls and subsequently impede wound healing
- overtire a patient, particularly elderly patients and those who are physically deconditioned prior to the amputation
- encourage patients to adopt poor gait patterns due to excessive weight bearing on the remaining limb, leading to difficulty with prosthetic rehabilitation.

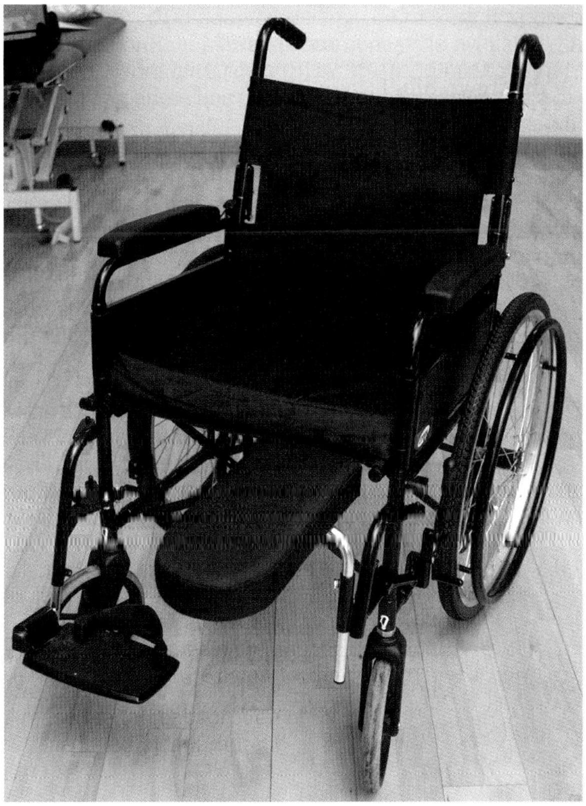

Figure 7.21 Wheelchair with amputee stump support. *Source*: Reproduced from Musculoskeletal Key (n.d.).

Pre-procedural considerations

Equipment

Wheelchair and pressure relief

Patients who have undergone lower limb amputation should be provided with an appropriate wheelchair including anti-tippers (to prevent the wheelchair from tipping over) and a suitable pressure-relieving cushion (Smith et al. 2016).

Residual limb support board

Residual limb support boards are required for below-knee (transtibial) amputees when sitting out in a wheelchair to ensure that the limb is fully supported and help to prevent knee flexion contractures (Figure 7.21). Dependent positioning or dangling of the residual limb is not advisable during the early post-operative phase due to the risk of increased oedema (Virani et al. 2015).

Procedure guideline 7.16 Positioning a patient with an amputation

Essential equipment

- Personal protective equipment
- Residual limb support board (for below-knee amputees sitting out in a wheelchair)
- Pillows
- Hoists and appropriate amputee and rehabilitation slings or sliding sheets may be required if the patient presents as a manual handling risk

Action	Rationale
Pre-procedure	
1 Introduce yourself to the patient, explain and discuss the procedure with them, and gain their consent to proceed.	To ensure that the patient feels at ease, understands the procedure and gives their valid consent (NMC 2018, **C**).

(continued)

Procedure guideline 7.18 Positioning a patient with an amputation (continued)

Action	Rationale
2 Wash hands thoroughly with soap and water or use an alcohol-based handrub.	To reduce the risk of contamination and cross-infection (NHS England and NHSI 2019, C; WHO 2017, C).
3 Assess the patient's pain and provide prescribed analgesia if required.	Pain levels should be considered and adequately controlled prior to moving and positioning (Smith et al. 2016, **C**).
4 Ensure the bed is at the optimum height for the patient and handlers. If two handlers are required, try to match the handlers' heights as far as possible.	To minimize the risk of injury to the practitioners and patient (Aslam et al. 2015, **R**).
Procedure	
Upper limb amputee	
5 Ensure the patient is maintaining full range of motion of all remaining joints of the upper limb by encouraging active movements of the limb.	To prevent contractures in case of possible prosthetic rehabilitation and functional use (Virani et al. 2015, **R**).
Transfemoral amputee (above knee)	
6 Maintain hip in a neutral position. • *In bed*: ensure the patient is periodically lying supine *or* consider prone-lying or side-lying with the hip in a neutral position. • *In a chair*: ensure that the patient does not place a towel or pillow under the residual limb.	To maintain hip extension and reduce the risk of developing a hip flexion contracture (Ghazali et al. 2018, **R**).
Transtibial amputee (below knee)	
7 Maintain knee extension. • *In bed*: do not place a towel or pillow under the knee unless it is supporting the whole of the residual limb; that is, do not encourage the knee to be maintained in a flexed position. • *In a chair*: use a residual limb board on the wheelchair if one has been issued. If the patient is sitting out in a chair then support the stump with a footstool and pillows.	To prevent knee flexion contracture (Ghazali et al. 2018, **R**). To aid oedema management in the residual limb and promote healing (Smith et al. 2016, **C**). To improve patient comfort and protect the residual limb (Bouch et al. 2012, **C**).
Post-procedure	
8 Document the procedure and its outcome in the patient's notes.	To ensure effective communication between healthcare professionals and effective documentation of care completed (NMC 2018, **C**).

Problem-solving table 7.5 Prevention and resolution (Procedure guideline 7.18)

Problem	Cause	Prevention	Action
Painful residual limb following transfer or change of position	• Fear of movement • Pressure on distal end of residual limb over wound • Residual limb dependent, leading to increased oedema and reduced blood flow • Unsupported residual limb	• Reassure patient • Ensure that the residual limb is well supported following the change of position • Ensure adequate analgesia prior to movement and support residual limb wherever possible during the procedure	• Explain the procedure to the patient prior to moving their position • Ensure that there is no pressure over the wound site following the procedure • Offer prescribed analgesia
Wound breakdown	• Unsupported residual limb during movement • Infection • Vascular insufficiency	• Ensure that the residual limb is well supported during and following the change of position	• Ensure that there is no pressure over the wound site following the procedure • Seek medical review

Post-procedural considerations

Mobilization following amputation

The same principles apply as are outlined earlier in this chapter. The main considerations following both upper and lower limb amputation are balance and pain issues. If a lower limb amputee has a prosthesis, ensure that this is correctly applied and fitted prior to standing and mobilizing the patient.

Complications

Limb contracture

This can occur due to:

- immobility
- alteration in muscle balance around the joints
- pain
- habit.

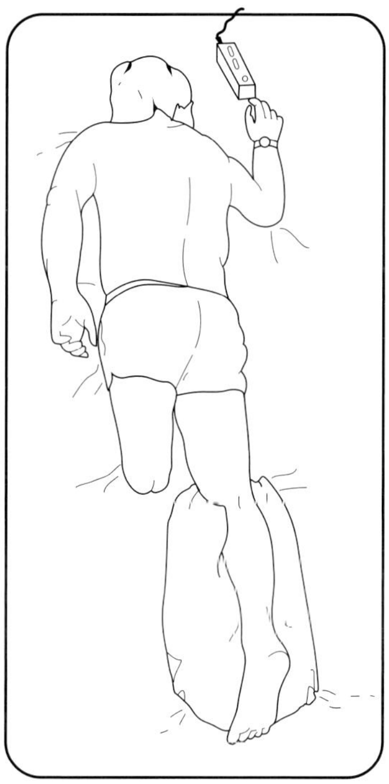

Points to remember

1. To roll prone, the amputee must turn towards the unaffected side, the nurse ensuring that the residual limb is lowered gently.
2. Initially the amputee lies prone for about 10 minutes.
3. The amputee should then build up to lying prone for 30 minutes three times a day.

Figure 7.22 The correct position for prone lying. *Source*: Reproduced from Engstrom and van de Ven (1999) with permission of Elsevier.

In order to help prevent limb contracture, the patient will require adequate analgesia to control their pain. It is also important to help patients increase their awareness of the positions they adopt, particularly those that may lead to limb contracture. The physiotherapist may recommend that the patient adopts certain positions for periods during the day to help prevent contractures, such as prone-lying for lower limb amputees (Figure 7.22).

Ongoing phantom limb pain

This can be a persistent problem and will need referral to the pain team for appropriate management.

Wound infection or delayed healing

Review by medical team and tissue viability team for appropriate management.

Websites

Age UK
www.ageuk.org.uk

American Spinal Injury Association
www.asia-spinalinjury.org

British Society of Rehabilitation Medicine
www.bsrm.org.uk

Chartered Society of Physiotherapy
www.csp.org.uk

Council for Allied Health Professions Research
https://cahpr.csp.org.uk

European Pressure Ulcer Advisory Panel
www.epuap.org

Health Foundation: Patient Safety Resource Centre
https://patientsafety.health.org.uk

Multidisciplinary Association for Spinal Cord Injury Professionals
www.mascip.co.uk

NHS England and NHS Improvement
www.england.nhs.uk

Royal National Orthopaedic Hospital
www.rnoh.nhs.uk

References

Abd-Elfattah, H., Abdelazeim, F. & Elshennawy, S. (2015) Physical and cognitive consequences of fatigue: A review. *Journal of Advanced Research*, 6(3), 351–358.

ACPIN (Association of Chartered Physiotherapist in Neurology) & College of Occupational Therapy (2015) *Splinting for the Prevention and Correction of Contractures in Adults with Neurological Dysfunction*. Available at: https://www.rcot.co.uk/file/926/download?token=ZyFUmQMR

Ada, L., Foongchomcheay, A. & Canning, C.G. (2005) *Supportive devices for preventing and treating subluxation of the shoulder after stroke. Cochrane*

Database of Systematic Reviews. Available at: https://www.cochranelibrary.com/cdsr/doi/10.1002/14651858.CD00[illegible].pub3/full

Adam, S., Osborne, S. & Welch, J. (2017) *Critical Care Nursing: Science and Practice*, 3rd edn. Oxford: Oxford University Press.

Age UK (2013) *Staying Steady Guide*. Available at: www.ageuk.org.uk/Documents/EN-GB/Information-guides/AgeUKIG14_staying_steady_inf.pdf?dtrk=true

Aggarwal, R. & Hunter, A. (2007) How exactly does the chest wall work? *Student BMJ*, 334, 070252.

ASIA (American Spinal Injury Association) (2015) *Impairment Scale*. Available at: www.asia-spinalinjury.org/wp-content/uploads/2016/02/International_Stds_Diagram_Worksheet.pdf

Aslam, I., Davis, S.A., Feldman, S.R. & Martin, W.E. (2015) A review of patient lifting interventions to reduce health care worker injuries. *Workplace Health & Safety*, 63(6), 267–276.

Bhimani, R. & Anderson, L. (2014) Clinical understanding of spasticity: Implications for practice. *Rehabilitation Research and Practice*, 2014, 1–10.

Blume, C., del Giudice, R., Wislowska, M., et al. (2015) Across the consciousness continuum: From unresponsive wakefulness to sleep. *Frontiers in Human Neuroscience*, 10(9), 105.

Boe, J., Dennis J.H., O'Driscoll, B.R., et al. (2001) European Respiratory Society guidelines on the use of nebulizers: Guidelines prepared by a European Respiratory Society Task Force. *European Respiratory Journal*, 18(1), 228–242.

Bonner, S. & Smith, C. (2013) Initial management of acute spinal cord injury. *Continuing Education in Anaesthesia, Critical Care & Pain*, 13(6), 224–231.

Bott, J., Blumenthal, S., Buxton, M., et al. (2009) Guidelines for the physiotherapy management of the adult, medical, spontaneously breathing patient. *Thorax*, 64 (Suppl. 1), i1–i51.

Bouch, E., Burns, K., Geer, E., et al. (2012) *Guidance for the Multi-Disciplinary Team on the Management of Post-operative Residuum Oedema in Lower Limb Amputees*. London: British Association of Chartered Physiotherapists in Amputee Rehabilitation.

Bouyer-Ferullo, S. (2013) Preventing perioperative peripheral nerve injuries. *AORN Journal*, 97(1), 111–121.

Boyle, B. (2018) I can't move or speak but I can hear and feel. *BMJ*, 363, k4036.

British Society of Rehabilitation Medicine (2018) *Amputee and Prosthetic Rehabilitation: Standards and Guidelines*, 3rd edn. London: British Society of Rehabilitation Medicine.

Burry, L., Rose, L., McCullagh, I.J., et al. (2014) *Daily sedation interruption versus no daily sedation interruption for critically ill adult patients requiring invasive mechanical ventilation. Cochrane Database of Systematic Reviews*. Available at: https://www.cochranelibrary.com/cdsr/doi/10.1002/14651858.CD009176.pub2/full

Chang, E., Ghosh, N., Yanni, D., et al. (2013) A review of spasticity treatments: Pharmacology and interventional approaches. *Critical Reviews in Physical and Rehabilitation Medicine*, 25(1/2), 11–22.

Charlton, P.T. (2009) Orthotic management. In: Lennon, S. & Stokes, M. (eds) *Pocketbook of Neurological Physiotherapy*. Edinburgh: Churchill Livingstone, pp.261–272.

Chief Allied Health Professions Officer's Team (2017) *AHPs in Action: Using Allied Health Professionals to Transform Health and Wellbeing, Case Study 4 – Eat, Drink, Move! – Supporting People to Keep Well During Hospital Admission*. Available at: www.england.nhs.uk/wp-content/uploads/2017/01/ahp-action-transform-hlth.pdf

Crawford, S. & Stinson, M. (2015) Management of 24 hour body positioning. In: Söderback, I. (ed) *International Handbook of Occupational Therapy*, 2nd edn. Cham: Springer, pp.189–203.

CRGSCI (Clinical Reference Group for Spinal Cord Injury) (2016) *The Initial Management of Adults with Spinal Cord Injuries: Advice for Major Trauma Networks*. Available at: www.rnoh.nhs.uk/sites/default/files/advice_for_acute_centres_on_acute_sci_in_adults.pdf

CSP (Chartered Society of Physiotherapy) (2014) *Guidance in Manual Handling for Chartered Physiotherapists*, 4th edn. London: Chartered Society of Physiotherapy.

Damuth, E., Mitchell, J.A., Bartock, J.L., et al. (2015) Long-term survival of critically ill patients treated with prolonged mechanical ventilation: A systematic review and meta-analysis. *Lancet Respiratory Medicine*, 3(7), 544–553.

de Raaf, P.J., de Klerk, C., Timman, R., et al. (2012) Differences in fatigue experiences among patients with advanced cancer, cancer survivors and the general population. *Journal of Pain and Symptom Management*, 44(6), 823–830.

De Troyer, A. & Boriek, A.M. (2011) Mechanics of the respiratory muscles. *Comprehensive Physiology*, 1(3), 1273–1300.

Denehy, L. & Main, E. (2016) Cardiorespiratory management of special populations. In: Main, E. & Denenhy, L. (eds) *Cardiorespiratory Physiotherapy*, 5th edn. Edinburgh: Elsevier, pp.658–660.

Denehy, L., Lanphere, J. & Needham, D. (2017) Ten reasons why ICU patients should be mobilised early. *Intensive Care Medicine*, 43(10), 86–90.

DeTurk, W. & Cahalin, L. (2010) *Cardiovascular and Pulmonary Physical Therapy: An Evidence Based Approach*, 2nd edn. New York: McGraw-Hill Professional.

Devinuwara, K., Dworak-Kula, A. & O'Connor, R. (2018) Rehabilitation and prosthetics post-amputation. *Orthopaedics and Trauma*, 32(4), 234–240.

Dijkers, M. (2010) Comparing quantification of pain severity by verbal rating and numerical rating scales. *Journal of Spinal Cord Medicine*, 33(3), 232–242.

Doughty, D.B. & Sparks, B. (2016) Wound-healing physiology and factors that affect the repair process. In: Bryant, R.A. & Nix, D.P. (eds) *Acute & Chronic Wounds: Current Management Concepts*, 5th edn. St Louis, MO: Elsevier, pp.63–81.

Dubb, R., Nydahl, P., Hermes, C., et al. (2016) Barriers and strategies for early mobilization for patients in intensive care units. *Annals of the American Thoracic Society*, 13(5), 724–730.

Duff, S.V., Shumway-Cook, A. & Woollacott, M.H. (2012) Clinical management of the patient with reach, grasp and manipulation disorders. In: Shumway-Cook, A. & Woollacott, M.H. (eds) *Motor Control: Translating Research into Clinical Practice*, 4th edn. Philadelphia: Lippincott Williams & Wilkins, pp.552–594.

Engstrom, B. & van de Ven, C. (1999) *Therapy for Amputees*, 3rd edn. Edinburgh: Churchill Livingstone.

Fragala, G. (2015) Bed care for patients in palliative settings: Considering risks to caregivers and bed surfaces. *International Journal of Palliative Nursing*, 21(2), 66–70.

GAIN (Guidelines and Audit Implementation Network) (2014) *Guidelines for the Rehabilitation of Patients with Metastatic Spinal Cord Compression*. Available at: www.rqia.org.uk/RQIA/files/cb/cba33182-deab-46ae-acd1-d27279d9847c.pdf

Ghazali, M., Razak, N.A.A., Osman, N.A.A. & Gholizadeh, H. (2018) Awareness, potential factors and post-amputation care of stump flexion contractures among transtibial amputees. *Turkish Journal of Physical Medicine and Rehabilitation*, 64(3), 268–276.

Guerin, C., Reignier, J., Richard, J., et al. (2013) Prone positioning in severe acute respiratory distress syndrome. *New England Journal of Medicine*, 368(23), 2159–2168.

Harpreet, K., Singh, S., Jeyaraj, D. & Kaur, S. (2014) Prevalence of post stroke shoulder subluxation and pain. *Indian Journal of Physiotherapy & Occupational Therapy*, 18(1), 5–8.

Harrison, P. (2007) *The First 48 Hours: Managing Spinal Cord Injury*. Milton Keynes: Spinal Injury Association.

Hawthorn, C. & Piper, I. (2014) Monitoring of intracranial pressure in patients with traumatic brain injury. *Frontiers in Neurology*, 5(121). DOI: 10.3389/fneur.2014.00121.

Health Foundation (2016) *Teamwork and Communication*. Available at: https://patientsafety.health.org.uk/area-of-care/safety-management/teamwork-and-communication

Heravi, Y., Amin, M., Mohsen, Y. & Simin, J. (2015) Effect of change in patient's bed angles on pain after coronary angiography according to vital signals. *Journal of Research in Medical Sciences*, 20(10), 937–943.

Hickey, J.V. & Powers, M.B. (2011) Management of patients with a depressed state of consciousness. In: Hickey, J.V. (ed) *The Clinical Practice of Neurological and Neurosurgical Nursing*, 6th edn. Philadelphia: Wolters Kluwer/Lippincott Williams & Wilkins Health, pp.336–351.

Hodgson, C.L., Stiller, K., Needham, D.M., et al. (2014) Expert consensus and recommendations on safety criteria for active mobilization of mechanically ventilated critically ill adults. *Critical Care*, 18(6), 58.

Hodgson, C.L. & Tipping, C.J. (2016) Physiotherapy management of intensive care unit-acquired weakness. *Journal of Physiotherapy*, 63, 4–10.
Hough, A. (2001) *Physiotherapy in Respiratory Care: An Evidence-Based Approach to Respiratory and Cardiac Management*, 3rd edn. Cheltenham: Nelson Thornes.
HSE (Health and Safety Executive) (2018) *The Health and Safety Toolbox: How to Control Risks at Work*. Available at: www.hse.gov.uk/toolbox/manual.htm
Jackson, D.L., Proudfoot, C.W., Cann, K.F. & Walsh, T. (2010). A systematic review of the impact of sedation practice in the ICU on resource use, costs and patient safety. *Critical Care Journal*, 14(2), R59.
Jeon, S., Koh, Y., Choi, A., et al. (2014) Critical care for patients with massive ischemic stroke. *Stroke*, 16(3), 146–160.
Jolley, S., Bunnell, A. & Hough, C. (2016) ICU-acquired weakness. *Chest*, 150(5), 1129–1140.
Jønsson, L., Ingelsrud, L., Tengberg, L., et al. (2018) Physical performance following acute high-risk abdominal surgery: A prospective cohort study. *Canadian Journal of Surgery*, 61(1), 42–49.
Kalil, A.C., Metersky, M.L., Klompas, M., et al. (2016). Management of adults with hospital-acquired and ventilator-associated pneumonia: Clinical practice guidelines by the Infectious Diseases Society of America and the American Thoracic Society. *Clinical Infectious Diseases*, 63(5), e61–e111.
Katz, S., Arish, N., Rokach, A., et al. (2018) The effect of body position on pulmonary function: Systematic review. *BMC Pulmonary Medicine*, 18, 159.
Kent, B.D., Mitchell, P.D. & McNicholas, W.T. (2011) Hypoxemia in patients with COPD: Cause, effects, and disease progression. *International Journal of Chronic Obstructive Pulmonary Disease*, 6, 199–208.
Kirshblum, S., Burns, S. & Waring, W. (2011) International standards for neurological classification of spinal cord injury. *Journal of Spinal Cord Medicine*, 34(6), 535–546.
Koo, K.Y. & Fan, E. (2013) ICU-acquired weakness and early rehabilitation in the critically ill. *Journal of Science Communication*, 20(5), 223–231.
Latish, M. & Zatsiorsky, V. (2015) *Biomechanics and Motor Control: Defining Central Concepts*. London: Elsevier.
Lindsay, K.W., Bone, I., Fuller, G., et al. (2010) *Neurology and Neurosurgery Illustrated*, 5th edn. Edinburgh: Churchill Livingstone.
Louis, D.N., Perry, A., Reifenberger, G., et al. (2016) The 2016 World Health Organization classification of tumors of the central nervous system: A summary. *Acta Neuropathologica*, 131, 803–820.
Lumb, A.B. & Nunn, J.F. (2010) *Nunn's Applied Respiratory Physiology*, 7th edn. London: Elsevier.
Lundy-Ekman, L. (2018a) Introduction to neuroscience. In: *Neuroscience: Fundamentals for Rehabilitation*, 5th edn. St Louis, MO: Saunders Elsevier, pp.1–3.
Lundy-Ekman, L. (2018b) Neuro-anatomy. In: *Neuroscience: Fundamentals for Rehabilitation*, 5th edn. St Louis, MO: Saunders Elsevier, pp.4–43.
Lundy-Ekman, L. (2018c) Motor systems: Motor neurons and spinal motor function. In: *Neuroscience: Fundamentals for Rehabilitation*, 5th edn. St Louis, MO: Saunders Elsevier, pp.241–257.
Lundy-Ekman, L. (2018d) Spinal region. In: *Neuroscience: Fundamentals for Rehabilitation*, 5th edn. St Louis, MO: Saunders Elsevier, pp.351–384.
MASCIP (Multidisciplinary Association of Spinal Cord Injury Professionals) (2012) *Guidelines for Management of Neurogenic Bowel Dysfunction in Individuals with Central Neurological Conditions*. Available at: www.rnoh.nhs.uk/sites/default/files/sia-mascip-bowelguidenew2012.pdf
MASCIP (2015) *Moving and Handling Patients with Actual or Suspected Spinal Cord Injuries (SCI)*. Available at: www.mascip.co.uk/wp-content/uploads/2015/02/MASCIP-SIA-Guidelines-for-MH-Trainers.pdf
McDaniel, J.C. & Browning, K.K. (2014) Smoking, chronic wound healing, and implications for evidence-based practice. *Journal of Wound, Ostomy and Continence Nursing*, 41(5), 415–423.
McGrath, B. (2014). *Comprehensive Tracheostomy Care: The National Tracheostomy Safety Project Manual*. Chichester: Wiley Blackwell.
McGrath, B.A., Bates, L., Atkinson, D. & Moore, J.A. (2012) Multidisciplinary guidelines for the management of tracheostomy and laryngectomy airway emergencies. *Anaesthesia*, 67(9), 1025–1041.
McInnes, E., Chaboyer, W., Murray, E., et al. (2014) The role of patients in pressure injury prevention: A survey of acute care patients. *BMC Nursing*, 13(1), 41.
Mental Capacity Act (2005) Available at: https://www.legislation.gov.uk/ukpga/2005/9/contents
Morris, A.C., Hay, A.W., Swann, D.G., et al. (2011) Reducing ventilator associated pneumonia in intensive care: Impact of implementing a care bundle. *Critical Care Medicine*, 39(10), 2218–2224.
Morris, R. & O'Riordan, S. (2017) Prevention of falls in hospital. *Clinical Medicine*, 17(4), 360–362.
Munir, N. & Clarke, R. (2013) *Ear, Nose and Throat at a Glance*. Chichester: Wiley Blackwell.
Murray, M.J., DeBlock, H., Erstad, B., et al (2016) Clinical practice guidelines for sustained neuromuscular blockade in the adult critically ill patient. *Critical Care Medicine*, 44(11), 2079–2103.
Musculoskeletal Key (n.d.) *Amputees*. Available at: https://musculoskeletalkey.com/amputees
NCEPOD (National Confidential Enquiry into Patient Outcome and Death) (2014) *Tracheostomy Care: On the Right Trach?* Available at: https://www.ncepod.org.uk/2014tc.html
NHS (2016) *Overview: Osteoporosis*. Available at: https://www.nhs.uk/conditions/osteoporosis
NHS England (2018) *70 Days to End Pyjama Paralysis*. Available at: www.england.nhs.uk/2018/03/70-days-to-end-pyjama-paralysis
NHS England and NHSI (NHS Improvement) (2019) *Standard Infection Control Precautions: National Hand Hygiene and Personal Protective Equipment Policy*. Available at: https://improvement.nhs.uk/documents/4957/National_policy_on_hand_hygiene_and_PPE_2.pdf
NHS Improvement (2017) *The Incidence and Costs of Inpatient Falls in Hospitals: Summary*. Available at: https://improvement.nhs.uk/documents/1473/Falls_summary_July2017.pdf
NHS Improvement (2018) *Pressure Ulcer Core Curriculum*. Available at: https://improvement.nhs.uk/documents/2921/Pressure_ulcer_core_curriculum_2.pdf
NICE (National Institute for Health and Care Excellence) (2013) *Falls: Assessment and Prevention of Falls in Older People* [CG161]. Available at: www.nice.org.uk/nicemedia/live/14181/64088/64088.pdf
NICE (2014) *Pressure Ulcers: Prevention and Management* [CG179]. Available at: www.nice.org.uk/guidance/cg179/chapter/1-Recommendations
NICE (2016) *Spinal Injury: Assessment and Initial Management* [NG41]. Available at: https://www.nice.org.uk/guidance/ng41/chapter/recommendations
NICE (2017a) *Falls Prevention Exercise and Education Programme*. Available at: www.nice.org.uk/sharedlearning/falls-prevention-exercise-and-education-programme
NICE (2017b) *Rehabilitation after Critical Illness Quality Standard* [QS15]. Available at: https://www.nice.org.uk/guidance/qs158/chapter/Quality-statement-1-Rehabilitation-goals
NMC (Nursing and Midwifery Council) (2018) *The Code: Professional Standards of Practice and Behaviour for Nurses, Midwives and Nursing Associates*. Available at: https://www.nmc.org.uk/standards/code
NPUAP (National Pressure Ulcer Advisory Panel), EPUAP (European Pressure Ulcer Advisory Panel) & PPPIA (Pan Pacific Pressure Injury Alliance) (2014) *Prevention and Treatment of Pressure Ulcers: Quick Reference Guide*. Available at: www.internationalguideline.com/guideline
Oxford Dictionaries (2019a) *Move*. Available at: https://en.oxforddictionaries.com/definition/move
Oxford Dictionaries (2019b) *Position*. Available at: https://en.oxforddictionaries.com/definition/position
Oxford Dictionaries (2019c) *Walk*. Available at: https://en.oxforddictionaries.com/definition/walk
Pandey, K. & Berman, S. (2018). *Spasticity clinical presentation. Medscape*. Available at: https://emedicine.medscape.com/article/2207448-clinical
Paratz, J., Ntoumenopoulos, G., Jones, A. & Fitzgerald, C. (2016) Adult intensive care. In: Main, E. & Denehy, L. (eds) *Cardiorespiratory Physiotherapy: Adults and Paediatrics*, 5th edn. Elsevier, pp.415–454.
Parry, S. & Puthucheary, Z. (2015) The impact of extended bed rest on the musculoskeletal system in the critical care environment. *Extreme Physiology and Medicine*, 4(16). DOI: 10.1186/s13728-015-0036-7.
Pathmanathan, N., Beaumont, N. & Gratrix, A. (2015) Respiratory physiotherapy in the critical care unit. *Continuing Education in Anaesthesia, Critical Care & Pain*, 15(1), 20–25.
Peate, I., Nair, M. & Wild, K. (2014) *Nursing Practice: Knowledge and Care*. Chichester: Wiley Blackwell.
Perry, M. (2013) Low back pain: Tackling a common problem. *Practice Nursing*, 24(7), 356–358.

Preston, J. & Edmans, J. (2016) Using technology to support participation. In: *Occupational Therapy and Neurological Conditions*. Chichester: Wiley Blackwell, pp.150–170.
PsychLogic (2017) *Biological Psychology*. Simply Psychology. Available at: https://www.simplypsychology.org/a-level-biological.html
Puthucheary, Z., Harridge, S. & Hart, N. (2010) Skeletal muscle dysfunction in critical care: Wasting, weakness, and rehabilitation strategies. *Critical Care Medicine*, 38(10), s676–s682.
RCN (Royal College of Nursing) (2017) *Principles of Consent: Guidance for Nursing Staff*. Available at: www.rcn.org.uk/professional-development/publications/pub-006047
Richards-Belle, A., Canter, R., Power, S., et al. (2016) National survey and point prevalence study of sedation practice in UK critical care. *Critical Care*, 20, 355.
Richardson, A. & Carter, R. (2015) Falls in critical care: A local review to identify incidence and risk. *Nursing in Critical Care*, 22(5), 270–275.
Richardson, C. (2010) Phantom limb pain: Prevalence, mechanisms and associated factors. In: Murray, C. (ed) *Amputation, Prosthesis Use, and Phantom Limb Pain: An Interdisciplinary Perspective*. New York: Springer, pp.137–156.
RNOH (Royal National Orthopaedic Hospital) (2016) *Aetiology of Spinal Cord Injury: Traumatic vs Non-traumatic*. Available at: www.rnoh.nhs.uk/sites/default/files/traumatic_vs_non-traumatic.pdf
RNOH (2018) *Respiratory Complications*. Available at: www.rnoh.nhs.uk/our-services/spinal-cord-injury-centre/medical-management-advice/respiratory-complications
Royal College of Physicians (2017) *Falls Prevention in Hospital: A Guide for Patients, Their Families and Carers*. Available at: www.rcplondon.ac.uk/projects/outputs/falls-prevention-hospital-guide-patients-their-families-and-carers
Rubin, B.K. (2014) Secretion properties, clearance, and therapy in airway disease. *Translational Respiratory Medicine*, 2(6). DOI: 10.1186/2213-0802-2-6.
Ruszala, S. & Alexander, P. (2015) *Moving & Handling in the Community and Residential Care*. Towcester, UK: National Back Exchange.
Schellekens, W.M., van Hees, H.W.H., Doorduin, J., et al. (2016) Strategies to optimize respiratory muscle function in ICU patients. *Critical Care*, 20(1), 103.
Schreiber, M. (2017) Lower limb amputation: Postoperative nursing care and considerations. *MEDSURG Nursing*, 26(4), 274–277.
Shumway-Cook, A. & Woollacott, M.H. (eds) (2012) *Motor Control: Translating Research into Clinical Practice*, 4th edn. Philadelphia: Lippincott Williams & Wilkins.
SIA (Spinal Injuries Association) (2015) *Non-trauma Spinal Cord Injury*. Available at: www.spinal.co.uk/wp-content/uploads/2015/07/Non-Trauma-SCIs-Aug-2014.pdf
Smith, J., National Back Exchange & BackCare (2011) *The Guide to the Handling of People: A Systems Approach*, 6th edn. Teddington, UK: BackCare.
Smith, S., Pursey, H., Jones, A., et al. (2016) *Clinical Guidelines for the Pre and Post Operative Physiotherapy Management of Adults with Lower Limb Amputations*, 2nd edn. London: British Association of Chartered Physiotherapists in Amputee Rehabilitation.
Strickland, S.L., Rubin, B.K., Haas, C.F., et al. (2015) Clinical practice guideline: Effectiveness of pharmacologic airway clearance therapies in hospitalized patients. *Respiratory Care*, 60(7), 1071–1077.
Szczygiel, E., Zielonka, K., Mętel, S. & Golec, J. (2017) Musculo-skeletal and pulmonary effects of sitting position: A systematic review. *Annals of Agricultural and Environmental Medicine*, 24(1), 8–12.
Tortora, G.J. & Derrickson, B.H. (2017) *Principles of Anatomy & Physiology*, 15th edn. Hoboken, NJ: John Wiley & Sons.
Treadwell, L. (2013) Safe manual handling practices in the UK and USA: More than just a training exercise. *International Journal of Therapy and Rehabilitation*, 20(7), 326–327.
UCLH (University College London Hospitals) (2012) *Managing Spasticity*. Available at: www.ucl.ac.uk/cnr/docs/nhnninfo/Spasticity_information_for_patients
Vander, A., Sherman, J. & Luciano, D. (2016a) Muscle. In: *Vander's Human Physiology: The Mechanisms of Body Functions*. Boston: McGraw-Hill, pp.256–281.
Vander, A., Sherman, J. & Luciano, D. (2016b) Control of body movement. In: *Vander's Human Physiology: The Mechanisms of Body Functions*. Boston: McGraw-Hill, pp.298–316.
Virani, A., Werunga, J., Ewashen, C. & Green, T. (2015) Caring for patients with limb amputation. *Nursing Standard*, 30(6), 51–58.
Vollman, K. (2012) Hemodynamic instability: Is it really a barrier to turning critically ill patients? *Critical Care Nurse*, 32(1), 70–75.
Wang, L., Li, X., Yang, Z., et al. (2016) *Semi-recumbent position versus supine position for the prevention of ventilator-associated pneumonia in adults requiring mechanical ventilation (review). Cochrane Database of Systematic Reviews*. Available at: www.cochranelibrary.com/cdsr/doi/10.1002/14651858.CD009946.pub2/full
West, J.B. (2012) *Respiratory Physiology: The Essentials*, 9th edn. Philadelphia: Lippincott Williams & Wilkins.
White, P., Goldsmith, K., Johnson, A., et al. (2011) Comparison of adaptive pacing therapy, cognitive behaviour therapy, graded exercise therapy, and specialist medical care for chronic fatigue syndrome (PACE): A randomised trial. *Lancet*, 377(9768), 823–836.
WHO (World Health Organization) (2012) WHO highlights importance of good hand hygiene for patient safety. *Central European Journal of Public Health*, 20(2), 155.
Wislowska, M., del Giudice, R. & Schabus, M. (2014) Searching for neuronal correlates of consciousness: What do we learn from coma and disorders of consciousness. *Functional Neurology Rehabilitation and Ergonomics*, 4(2/3), 135–147.
Wong, K., Trudel, G. & Laneuville, O. (2015) Noninflammatory joint contractures arising from immobility: Animal models to future treatments. *BioMed Research International*, 2015, 1–6.
Ye, F., Stalvey, C., Khuddus, M., et al. (2017) A systematic review of mobility/immobility in thromboembolism risk assessment models for hospitalized patients. *Journal of Thrombosis and Thrombolysis*, 44(1), 94–103.
Yoshikawa, Y., Maeshige, N., Sugimoto, M., et al. (2015) Positioning bedridden patients to reduce interface pressures over the sacrum and greater trochanter. *Journal of Wound Care*, 24(7), 319–325.

Chapter 8

Nutrition and fluid balance

Clare Shaw with Laura Askins, Grainne Brady, Lucy Eldridge, Olivia Kate Smith, Laura Theodossy and Heather Thexton

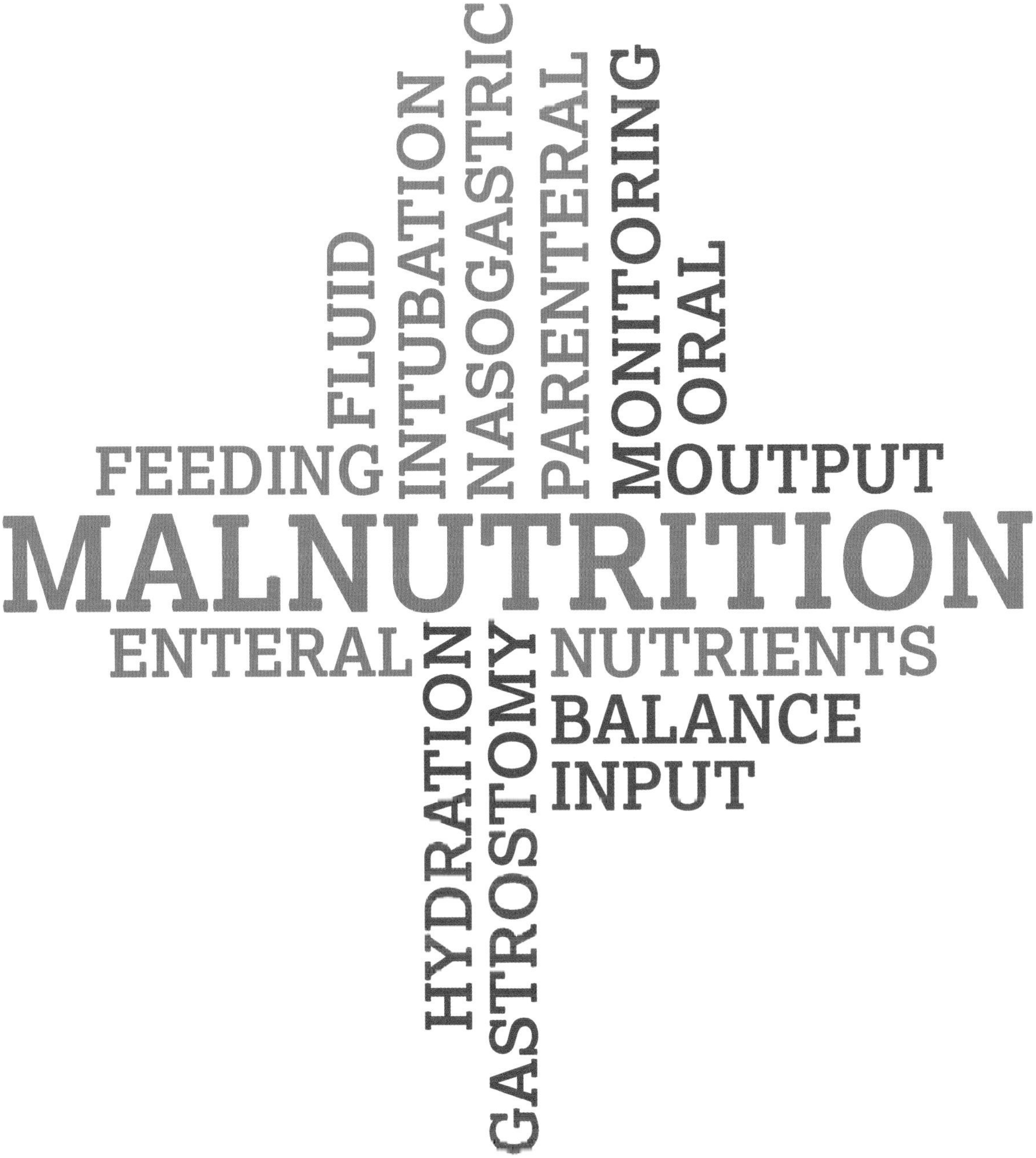

The Royal Marsden Manual of Clinical Nursing Procedures: Professional Edition, Tenth Edition. Edited by Sara Lister, Justine Hofland and Hayley Grafton.

Procedure guidelines

Being an accountable professional

At the point of registration, the nurse will:

2 Use evidence-based, best practice approaches to undertake the following procedures:
  2.6 accurately measure weight and height, calculate body mass index and recognise healthy ranges and clinically significant low/high readings

5. Use evidence-based, best practice approaches for meeting needs for care and support with nutrition and hydration, accurately assessing the person's capacity for independence and self care and initiating appropriate interventions

Future Nurse: Standards of Proficiency for Registered Nurses (NMC 2018)

Overview

Good nutrition, the supply of optimal nutrients and fluid to meet requirements, is an essential component of health, with poor nutrition contributing to ill health and prolonged recovery from illness or disease. It is therefore crucial that the nutritional status of all patients is assessed and considered during the whole of the patient's care. This chapter addresses how fluid and nutrition can influence body composition, how to identify patients who are dehydrated and/or malnourished or at risk of malnutrition and, most importantly, how the patient's nutritional needs can be met.

The provision of food and fluids to patients is an integral part of basic care. In normal circumstances, adequate nutritional intake enables the body to maintain homeostasis of body composition and function but in disease states this balance can be altered. The majority of patients will achieve adequate nutrition through the oral route of diet and fluids; however, for some, additional artificial nutritional support will be required to maintain optimal body composition and function. This chapter describes how the patient's needs can be assessed and met through oral, enteral and parenteral routes of fluid and nutrition.

Fluid balance

Definition

In the human homeostatic state, fluid intake should equal output, thereby maintaining optimal hydration (Marieb and Hoehn 2018). In nursing practice, 'fluid balance' refers to the procedure of measuring fluid input and output to determine whether they are balanced.

Anatomy and physiology

Body composition

The human body is made up of approximately 60% water but this varies with age, gender and percentage of fatty tissue. The higher percentage of fat in women's bodies means a lower water content (approximately 50%), while a higher muscle mass contains a higher water content (Marieb and Hoehn 2018, Tortora and Derrickson 2017). Bodily water/fluid is essential to life and vital for:

- controlling body temperature
- the delivery of nutrients and gases to cells
- the removal of waste
- acid-base balance
- the maintenance of cellular shape (Baumberger-Henry 2008).

Total body water is distributed between two main compartments: intracellular fluid (ICF, within the cell) and extracellular fluid (ECF, outside the cell) (Table 8.1). ECF is further divided into the intravascular space, within the blood vessels (known as plasma); the interstitial space, which surrounds the cells; and the transcellular space. The transcellular space contains specialized fluids, such as cerebrospinal fluid, that are not readily exchanged with other compartments and so are rarely considered in fluid balance or management (Rhoda et al. 2011).

Body fluid is a composition of water and a variety of dissolved solutes known as electrolytes or non-electrolytes (Marieb and Hoehn 2018) (Figure 8.1). Non-electrolytes (such as glucose, lipids, creatinine and urea) are molecules that do not dissociate in solution and have no electrical charge. Electrolytes (such as potassium, sodium, chloride, magnesium and bicarbonate) all dissociate in solution into charged ions that conduct electricity. Concentration of these solutes varies depending on the compartment in which they are contained; for example, ECF has a high sodium content (135–145 mmol/L) and is relatively low in potassium (3.5–4.5 mmol/L) and ICF is the reverse: high in potassium but lower in sodium. The movement and distribution of fluid and solutes between compartments are controlled by the semi-permeable phospholipid cellular membranes (Figure 8.2) that separate them (Tortora and Derrickson 2017).

Transport and movement of water and solutes

Water can readily and passively pass across the cell semi-permeable membrane and does so by osmosis (Table 8.2) in response to changing solute concentrations (Tortora and Derrickson 2017). The amount of solute in solution determines the osmolarity – the higher the solute concentration, the higher the osmolarity; this is also referred to as the osmotic pressure (or pull). Electrolytes move across the membrane via the protein channels, some by diffusion (Table 8.2) and some via a passive mode of transport where solutes move towards an area of low solute concentration. Sodium and potassium are exceptions to this rule, as they are required to move against the concentration gradient in order to preserve higher intravascular sodium concentrations. Energy is used to pump sodium out of the cell via the protein channels and pump potassium back into the cell; this is known as the sodium/potassium pump (Figure 8.3).

The movement of water and solutes out of the intravascular space and into the interstitial space is dependent on opposing osmotic and hydrostatic pressures (Tortora and Derrickson 2017). Hydrostatic pressure is caused by the pumping action of the heart and the diameter (resistance) of the vessels and capillaries; this forces water and molecules that are small enough to pass through the membrane out of the vessel and into the interstitial fluid. Within the vascular system, only the capillaries have semi-permeable membranes and this is where 'filtration' occurs. At the arteriole end of the capillary, the hydrostatic pressure exceeds the osmotic pressure, which results in solutes moving out of the plasma and into the interstitial space. At the venous end, hydrostatic pressure is reduced and the osmotic pressure within the vessel (plasma) is higher so water is pulled back into the vessel and circulating volume (Tortora and Derrickson 2017). The osmotic pressure within the vessels is provided by plasma proteins that are too large to pass through the membrane even under pressure. Conditions such as sepsis or a systemic inflammatory response can cause the membranes to become permeable to plasma proteins; osmotic pressure is then reduced, resulting in an excess of water moving into the interstitial space, which in turn leads to oedema. Pulmonary oedema is caused by this mechanism in the lungs.

Table 8.1 Body fluid compartments

			Volume (L)	Distribution
Total body water, made up of:			40	60% of bodyweight
	Intracellular fluid (ICF)		25	40% of bodyweight
	Extracellular fluid (ECF), made up of:		15	20% of bodyweight
		Interstitial fluid (IF)	12	80% of ECF
		Plasma	3	20% of ECF

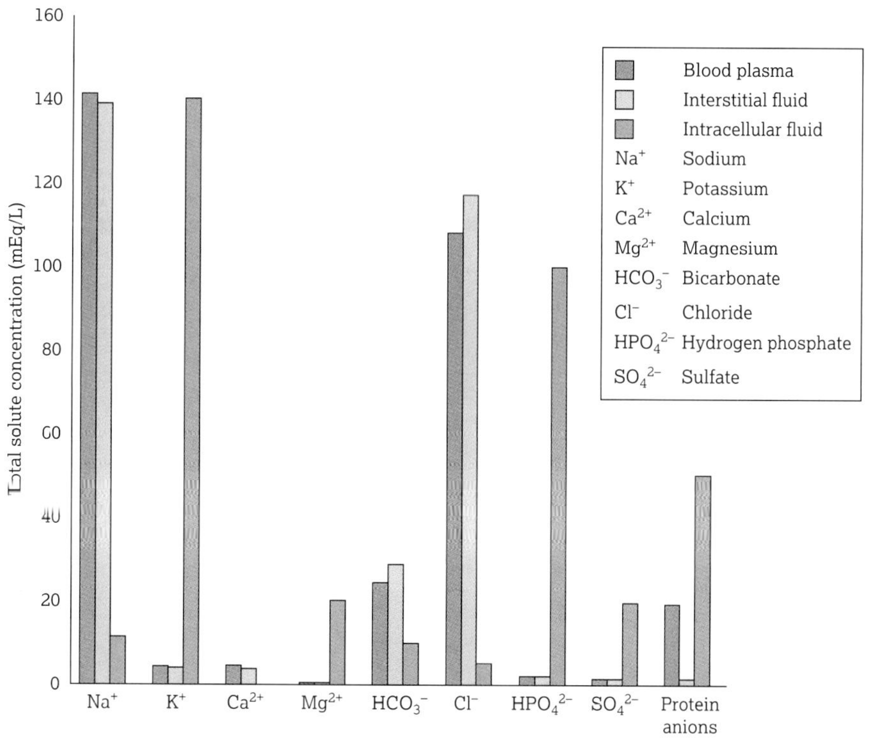

Figure 8.1 Electrolyte composition of blood plasma, interstitial fluid and intracellular fluid. *Source*: Reproduced with permission of Pearson.

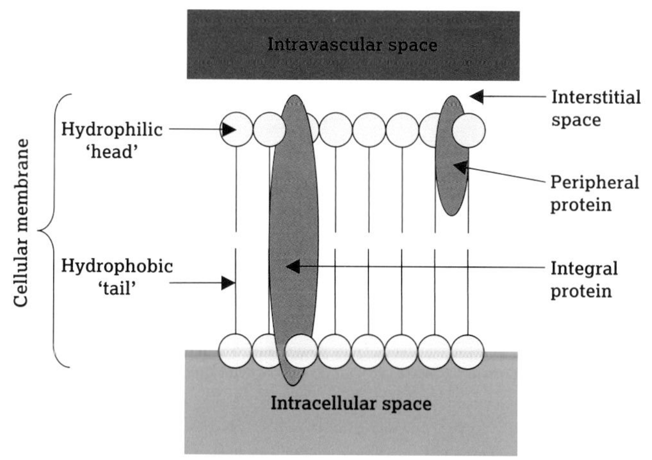

Figure 8.2 Cellular membrane.

Osmolarity and fluid balance

Sodium is the most influential electrolyte in fluid balance and is the primary cation (positively charged ion) of the ECF. The concentration of sodium in the ECF has the most profound effect on its osmolarity and therefore water balance (Rhoda et al. 2011). If ECF osmolarity increases (e.g. with increased intake of sodium, reduced fluid intake or increased fluid loss), even very slightly (by 1–2%), osmoreceptors in the hypothalamus detect and trigger the thirst response (Figure 8.4), which in turn encourages oral fluid intake in an attempt to restore the balance.

Hormonal mechanisms and the kidneys are highly influential in fluid and electrolyte balance and again are also triggered in response to changing osmolarity and/or plasma volumes. Antidiuretic hormone (ADH) is released from the posterior pituitary gland in response to osmoreceptor (in the hypothalamus) stimulation (Figure 8.5) (Tortora and Derrickson 2017). ADH then acts on the tubules and collecting ducts of the kidneys, inhibiting water excretion and encouraging water reabsorption. If plasma osmolarity falls (indicating water excess), these mechanisms are suppressed by a negative feedback loop and the osmoreceptors are no longer stimulated. This in turn inhibits ADH release; the renal tubules no longer conserve water and thirst is reduced, leading to a reduction of oral intake and restoration of balance. ADH is also released in the renin–angiotensin–aldosterone system (Figure 8.6) response to a reduction in blood pressure (detected by baroreceptors in blood vessels).

Aldosterone is a mineralocorticoid secreted by the adrenal cortex in response to increased osmolarity and/or decreased blood pressure (part of the renin–angiotensin–aldosterone system; Figure 8.6). It acts on the renal tubules, initiating the active transport of sodium (and hence water) from the tubules and collecting ducts back into the plasma and circulating volume (Tortora and Derrickson 2017).

These homeostatic mechanisms are very effective in maintaining fluid and electrolyte balance in health and act to compensate for fluid imbalances to ensure effective cellular function. However, these compensatory mechanisms are not sustainable and will eventually fail if ill health or imbalance persists. For example, in continued haemorrhage, the body will compensate by conserving water and constricting blood vessels in an attempt to increase blood pressure and volume. Failure to replace lost fluids, improve volume and thereby increase perfusion eventually leads to cellular and organ dysfunction, which in turn leads to organ failure and possibly death (Goldstein 2014).

Dehydration is a particular concern in ill health as often fluid intake is reduced by poor appetite, being nil by mouth or experiencing nausea, and often coincides with an increased output due to, for example, vomiting, diarrhoea, haemorrhage, drain output or fever. The elderly are at particular risk of dehydration as the effectiveness of the thirst response diminishes with age (Bak and Tsiami 2016, Welch 2010). When the osmolarity of the ECF

Table 8.2 Molecular transport modes

Transport mode	Description	Diagram
Osmosis	Movement of water from an area of low solute concentration to an area of high solute concentration.	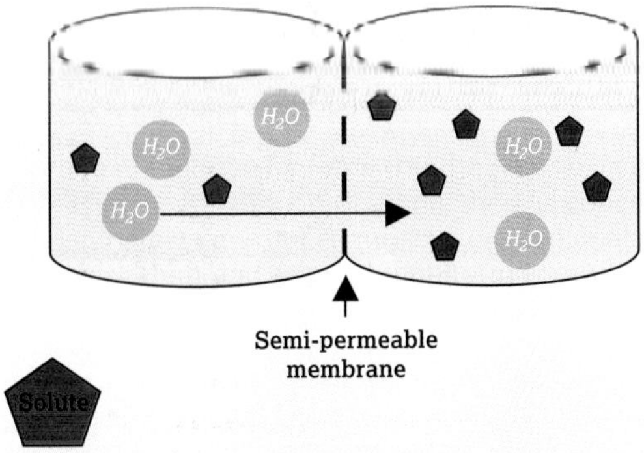
Diffusion	Movement of solutes from an area of high concentration to an area of low concentration.	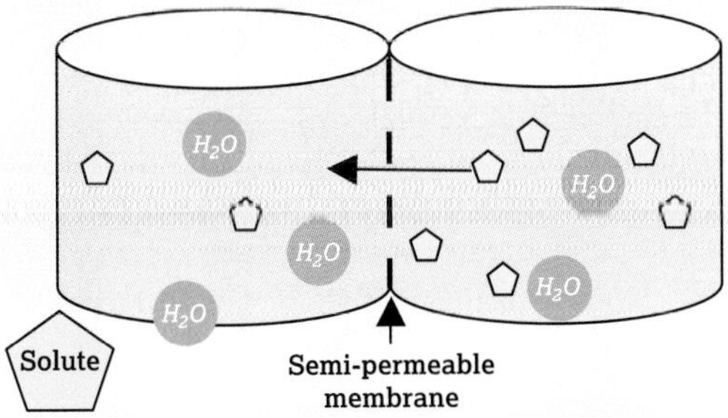
Facilitated diffusion	Movement of solutes from an area of high concentration to an area of low concentration, facilitated by a carrier molecule (e.g. glucose only enters the cell carried by insulin).	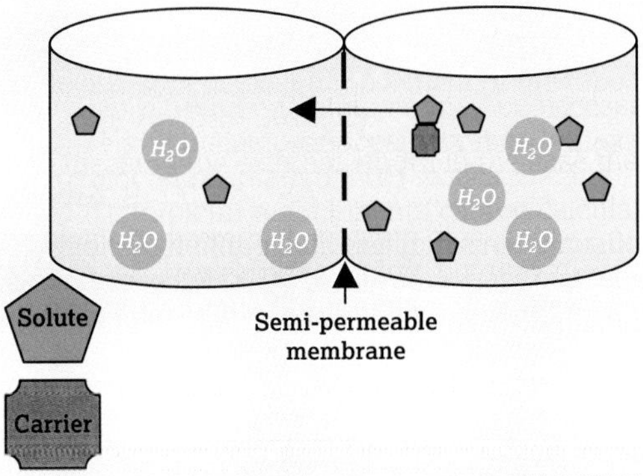
Active transport	Movement of solutes against the concentration gradient from an area of low concentration to an area of high concentration. This mode of transport requires energy synthesized within the cell (i.e. the sodium/potassium pump).	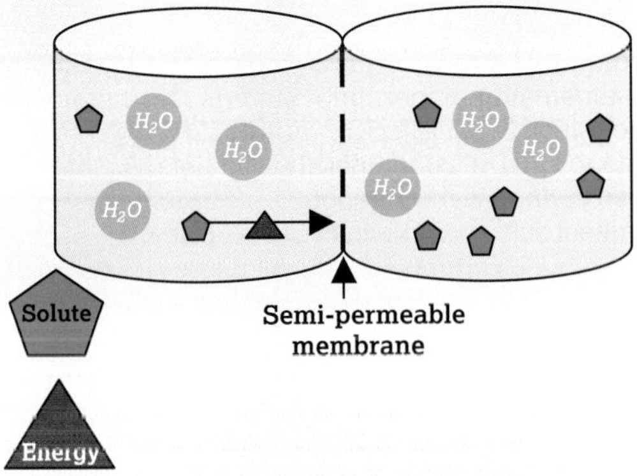

increases, it encourages water out of the cell and into the ECF, which eventually leads to cellular dehydration, impaired metabolism, disturbed cellular shape and impaired cellular function (Tortora and Derrickson 2017).

If the osmolarity of the ECF falls, water moves into the cell; if this continues, it will lead to water toxicity, causing cells to expand and eventually burst. Care should therefore be taken when administering intravenous fluids (Powell-Tuck et al. 2011, Rhoda et al. 2011), as fluids that are of lower osmolarity than ECF (hypotonic) will cause a shift of water into the cells. Conversely, hypertonic solutions will cause a shift of fluid from the cells, causing cellular dehydration. Maintenance fluids are usually isotonic (have the same osmolarity as ECF) (Gross et al. 2017, Rhoda et al. 2011).

Evidence-based approaches

Fluid and electrolyte balance monitoring and management are integral and vital to nursing care (Davies et al. 2015, Jevon and Ewens 2012). The fluid balance chart serves as a non-invasive tool for monitoring fluid status and guides the prescription and administration of intravenous fluids (Davies et al. 2015).

Fluid balance charting allows healthcare professionals to carefully monitor a patient's fluid input and output and calculate their

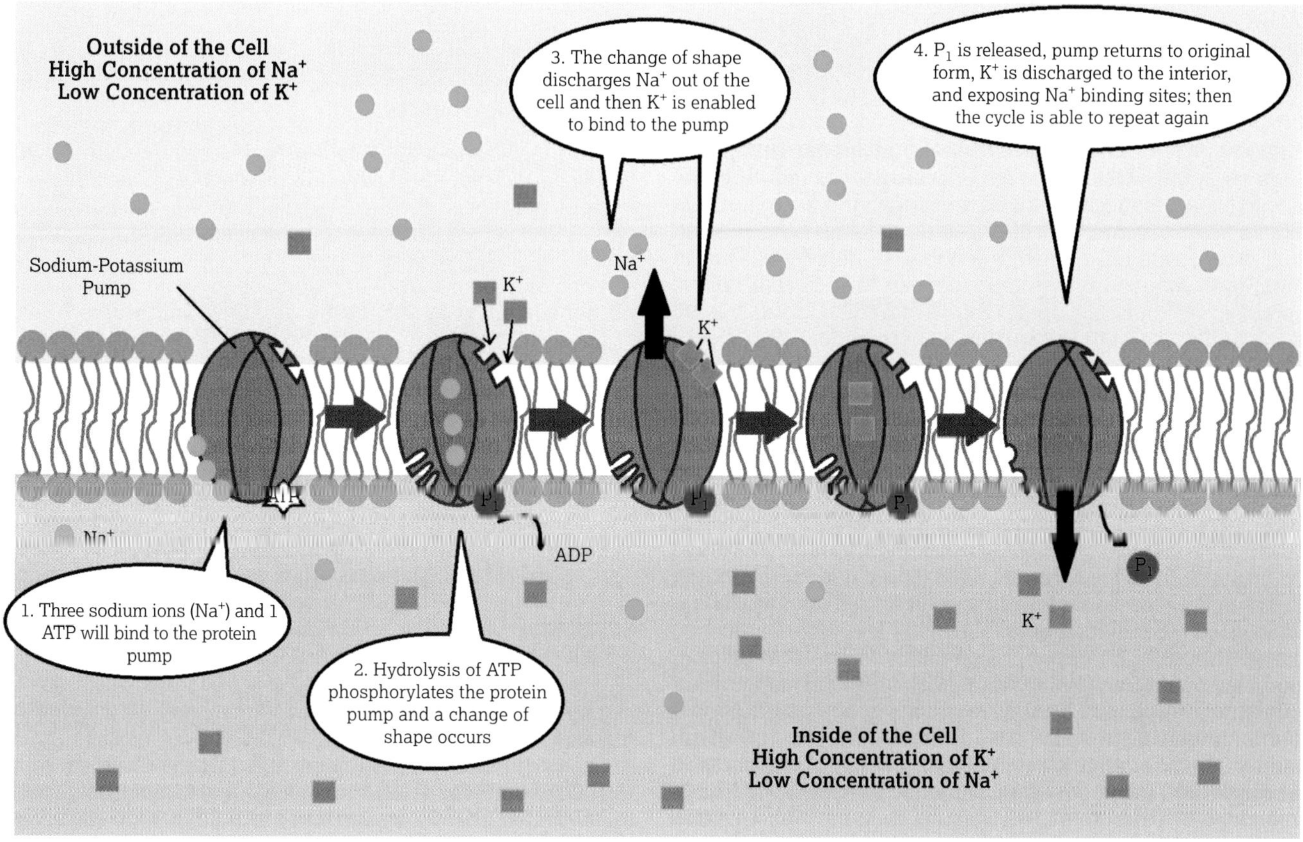

Figure 8.3 Active transport: sodium/potassium pump. *Source*: Clod94, CC BY-SA 4.0, https://creativecommons.org/licenses/by-sa/4.0.

fluid balance. This is usually measured over a 24-hour period (Jevon and Ewens 2012, Pinnington et al. 2016). A positive fluid balance indicates that the input has exceeded the output, and a negative fluid balance indicates the reverse – that is, that the output has exceeded the input. Although a fluid balance chart is a good indication of fluid balance, it is not an exact measurement, for several reasons. Some losses are insensible, such as those from perspiration, respiratory secretions and immeasurable bowel losses. The calculation of fluid balance also relies heavily on the accurate measuring, charting and calculating of input, output and overall balance. For such measurements to be taken accurately, additional interventions (such as catheterization) may be required. The benefit of accurate fluid balance measurement in critically or acutely unwell patients must be considered to outweigh the risks associated with such interventions (NICE 2017b). Table 8.3 identifies routes and sources of fluid intake and output.

Although a very useful tool, fluid balance charting should not be used in isolation. When considering fluid and electrolyte balance, physical assessment and monitoring electrolyte levels in the plasma should be integral to the observation and care of a patient with actual or potential fluid and electrolyte imbalances (NICE 2017b).

Nursing assessment is discussed in detail in Chapter 2: Admissions and assessment, and the assessment of a patient's fluid status should be an integral part of any admission. There should also be subsequent daily assessments, particularly if the patient is critically ill, if a fluid deficit has been identified, if the patient requires continuous intravenous fluid replacement or if the patient is at risk of acute kidney injury. See Table 8.4 for details of what should be included in a fluid status assessment.

A simple way to assess whether a patient will be responsive to fluid replacement is to perform a passive leg raise (Figure 8.7). Raising the legs to 45° while simultaneously lowering the patient from a semi-recumbent position to supine can cause a fluid shift from the legs to the central vascular system, which mimics a fluid bolus (Pickett et al. 2017). This can increase blood pressure and indicate whether the patient is likely to respond to fluid resuscitation (Cooke et al. 2018, Monnet et al. 2016, Pickett et al. 2017). However, the existing evidence on the use of the passive leg raise focuses on critically ill patients and evaluating the response using invasive cardiac output monitoring (such as LiDCO) to assess change in stroke volume. Assessing changes in systolic blood pressure has been suggested (Pickett et al. 2017); however, the lack of quality evidence to support the accuracy of this method means its routine use in practice is not recommended.

Haemodynamic monitoring methods in critical care (such as LiDCO, PiCCO or oesophageal Dopplar) can help to assess fluid status and efficacy of fluid challenges through the analysis of stroke volume as well as cardiac output, central venous pressure and mean arterial pressure (Cecconi et al. 2014, Michard 2016, Polderman and Varon 2015). Changes in cardiac output should be assessed 1 minute after a fluid challenge (Aya et al. 2016).

Throughout the literature, it is recognized that fluid balance monitoring is often poorly performed by nurses. Many authors identify barriers to accurate monitoring of fluid status and suggest that nurses must have a good understanding of the concepts involved in fluid balance in order to recognize and anticipate imbalances (Alexander and Allen 2011, Davies et al. 2015, Nazli et al. 2016, NICE 2017b, Pinnington et al. 2016, Shepherd 2011). They suggest the use of a fluid management policy to guide both nursing and medical staff and to standardize practice. NICE (2017b) offers guidance on the management of adult patients in hospital receiving intravenous fluids; it suggests that history taking, full clinical assessment, review of current medications, fluid balance charts and laboratory investigations are all required in order to fully assess the need for intravenous fluid and/or electrolyte administration.

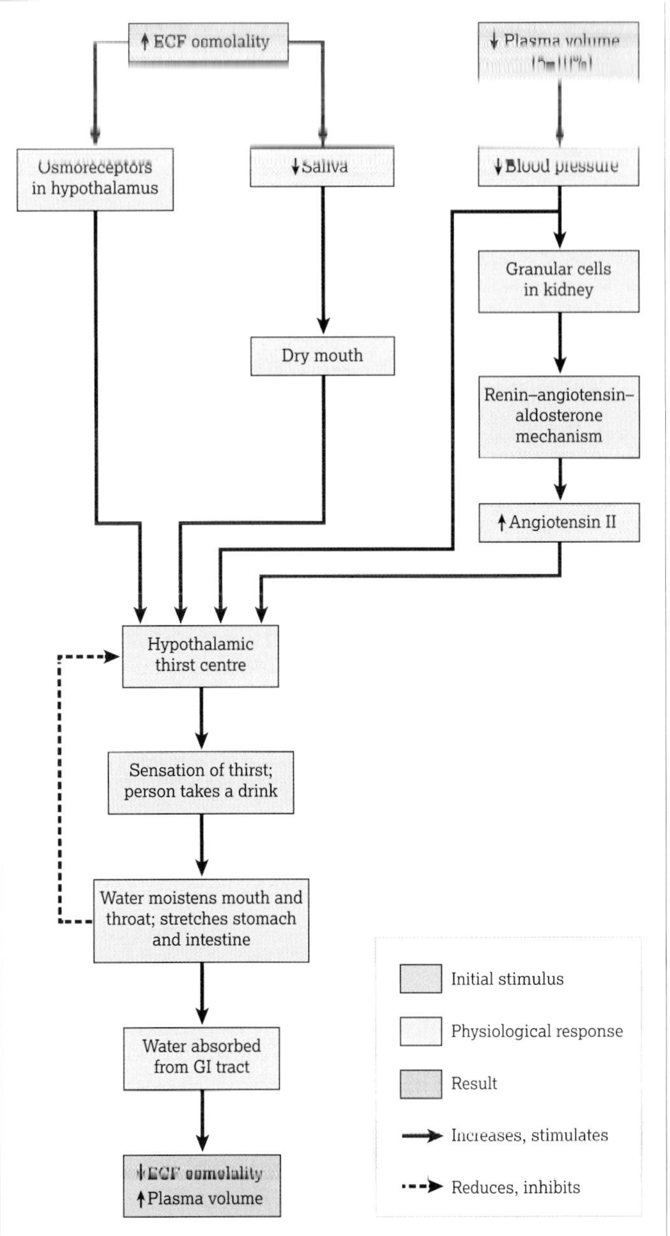

Figure 8.4 Thirst response.

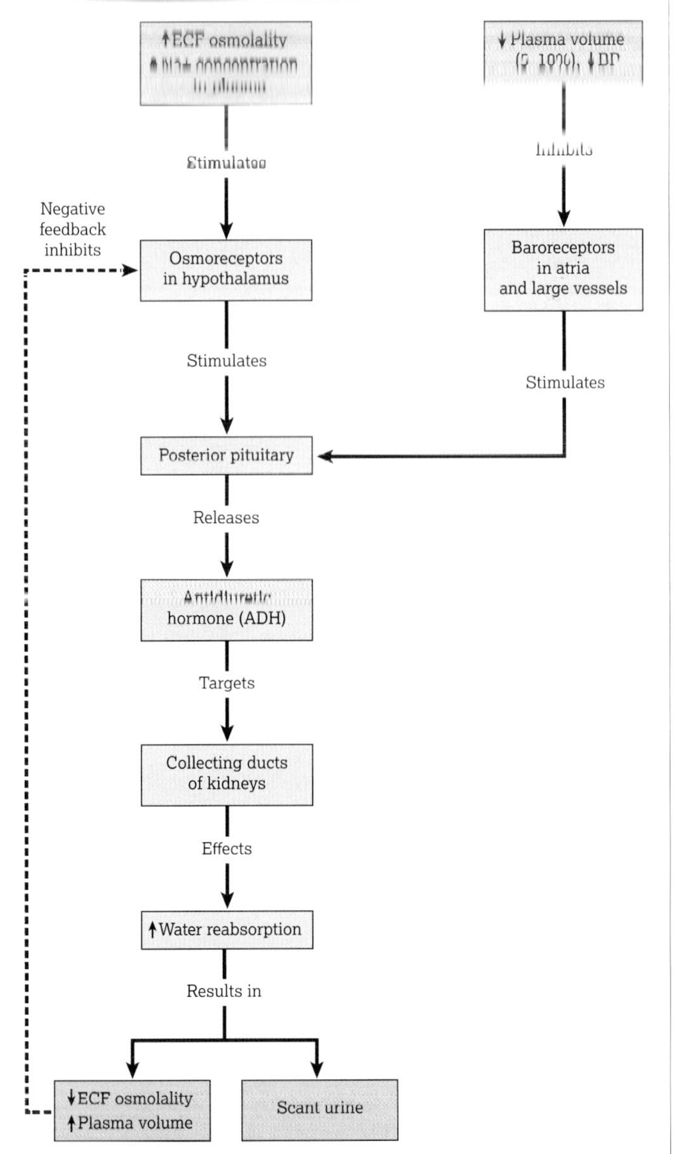

Figure 8.5 Mechanisms and consequences of antidiuretic hormone (ADH) release.

Understanding of the physiological mechanisms and potential implications will ensure fluid balance charting is carried out with knowledge and thought. Nazli et al. (2016) suggest that it is vital for staff involved in patient care to understand why fluid balance recording is important in maintaining patient safety. NICE (2017b) guidance on intravenous fluid therapy in adults has highlighted detrimental effects of fluid overload, such as pulmonary oedema, cardiac failure, cerebral oedema, impaired bowel function, delayed wound healing and tissue breakdown (Cooke et al. 2018, Gross et al. 2017), and therefore the importance of accurate fluid balance monitoring. Recommendations include the need for improved accuracy and the need for medical staff to review these charts regularly, particularly prior to prescribing any intravenous fluids. Nazli et al. (2016) highlight the implications of incorrect fluid balance calculations (by nurses and doctors), which may lead to under- or overprescribing of intravenous fluids and ultimately affect patient outcome. Inaccurate fluid balance monitoring can accumulate over the length of a patient's stay due to underestimation of fluid gains and losses. Measuring patients' weights on a daily basis, where able, can be a reliable method of assessing fluid overload (Alexander and Allen 2011, Davies et al. 2015, NICE 2017b). The organization Kidney Disease: Improving Global Outcomes (KDIGO 2012) uses urine output to classify the stage of acute kidney injury, emphasizing the need for accurate fluid output monitoring for any patient at risk of acute kidney injury (see the section on acute kidney injury below).

NICE (2017b) recommends that all patients receiving intravenous fluids should have at least a daily assessment of their fluid status and that clinicians should be mindful of the electrolyte content of the intravenous fluids they prescribe. Over-administration of normal saline 0.9% can lead to hyperchloraemia and metabolic acidosis, which are linked to increased mortality. This can be avoided by using a buffered salt solution such as compound sodium lactate (also called Hartmann's solution) (Finfer et al. 2010, Gross et al. 2017). Recent studies have compared saline and buffered salt solutions in relation to adverse renal events (Self et al. 2018, Semler et al. 2018). No difference was found in mortality rates, but buffered solutions were found to be less harmful to patients with poor renal function.

With regard to fluid resuscitation, the current recommended practice is to attempt to restore normovolaemia with crystalloids (Resuscitation Council 2015, Rhodes et al. 2017) but avoid dextrose as this can rapidly dilute plasma sodium and lead to the redistribution of fluid from the intravascular space and because it may cause hyperglycaemia. Albumin administration is suggested

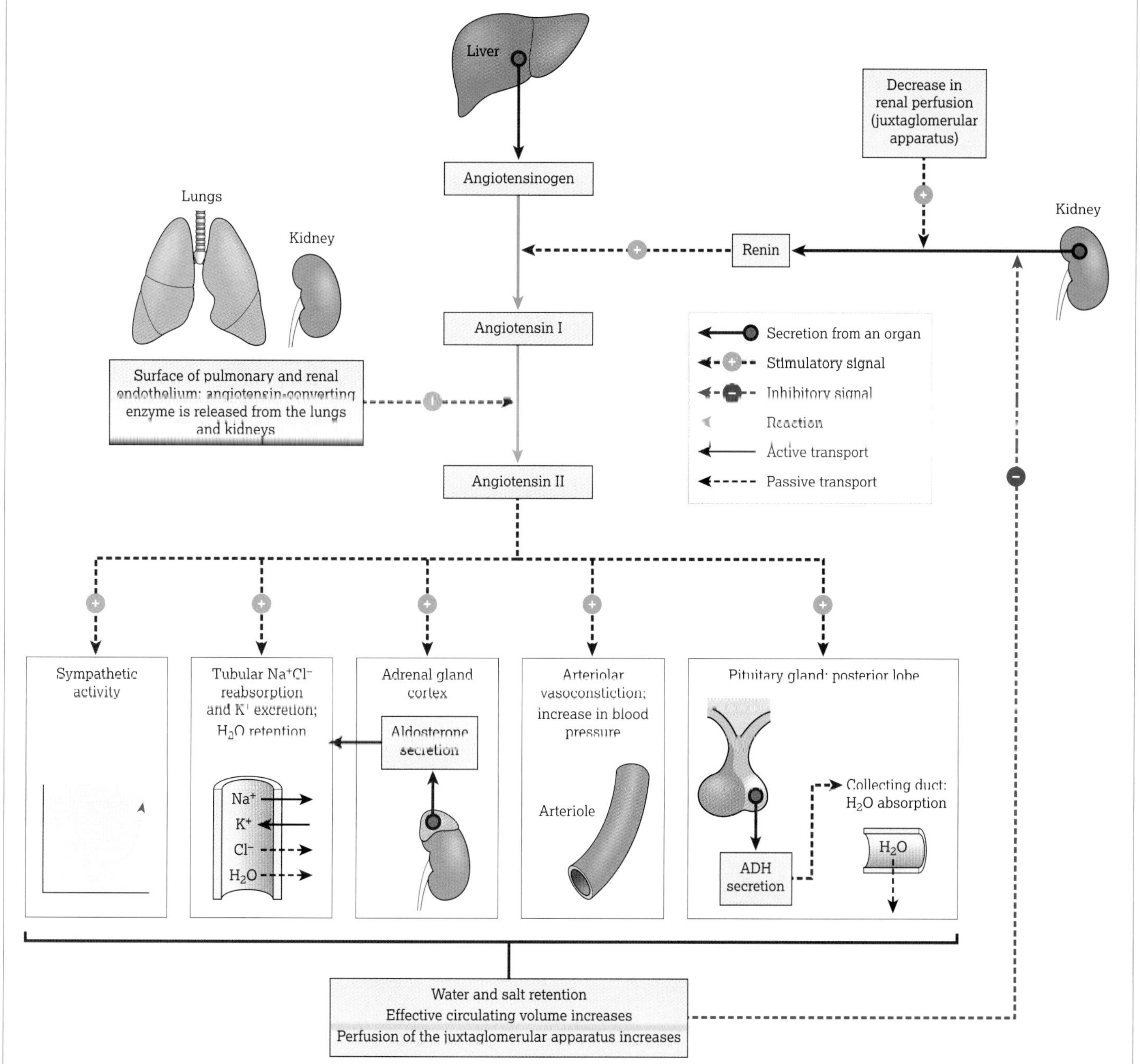

Figure 8.6 The renin–angiotensin–aldosterone system. *Source*: Reproduced with permission of Soupvector – Own work, CC BY-SA 4.0 https://commons.wikimedia.org/w/index.php?curid=66583851.

as a supplement to crystalloids in sepsis (NICE 2017b, Rhodes et al. 2017) but is contraindicated in traumatic brain injury (Gross et al. 2017). The Resuscitation Council (UK) (2015) and NICE (2017c) suggest a bolus of 500 mL of warmed crystalloid solution (e.g. Hartmann's solution or 0.9% sodium chloride) over less than 15 minutes if the patient is hypotensive. Use smaller volumes (e.g. 250 mL) for patients with known cardiac failure or trauma and use closer monitoring (listen to the chest for crackles after each bolus). Rhodes et al. (2017) recommend 30 mL/kg within the first 3 hours for sepsis-induced hypoperfusion.

A wide variation in practice can be evident across trusts and even individual departments. NICE (2017b) offers clear, standardized guidance with regard to intravenous fluid administration for adult patients in hospital (excluding patients with diabetes, severe liver or renal disease, pregnant women and patients under the age of 16 years). A summary and useful form of this guidance can be found in the section on algorithms for intravenous fluid therapy in adults in NICE (2017b). See also Figure 8.8.

Synthetic colloid fluids containing hydroxyethyl starch have previously been utilized in fluid replacement. However, the relative benefits and risks of these have come under scrutiny and it was decided by the European Medicines Agency (2013) that production and use of these be suspended. If a colloid is deemed to be necessary, NICE (2017c) recommends human albumin 4.5% for use *only* in patients with sepsis and shock.

Rationale

Indications

Any patient who has shown signs or symptoms of a fluid imbalance, who has undergone surgery or acute illness that has led to critical care admission, or who is at significant risk of acute

Table 8.3 Fluid intake and output

Intake	Output
Oral	**Urine output**
Food and drinks *Normally 2000 mL per day**	*Normally approx. 1500 mL per day*
Parenteral/intravenous	**Faeces**
Maintenance fluids, intravenous infusion, intermittent drugs, flushes	*Normally approx. 100 mL per day*
Additional to or replaces oral intake	**Perspiration**
	Normally approx. 200 mL per day
Enteral	**Gastric secretions**
Nasal gastric/nasal jejunostomy, percutaneous gastric jejunostomy feed, flushes	Vomit, nasal gastric/ gastrostomy drainage
Additional to or replaces oral intake	*Additional to normal output*
	Wounds and drains
	Additional to normal output
	Insensible losses
	Perspiration, respiratory secretions
	Additional to normal output

* NICE (2017b) recommends a total intake of 30–35 mL/kg; however, this guidance should take into account the patient's clinical condition and careful consideration of their fluid needs at the time.
Source: Adapted from Sheppard and Wright (2006) with permission of Elsevier.

kidney injury should have their fluid intake and output monitored and fluid balance calculated on an hourly basis (Davies [illegible] multidisciplinary care; however, it is usually the responsibility of the bedside nurse, healthcare worker or nursing associate to ensure this is done accurately.

Clinical governance

The Code (NMC 2018) clearly states that unambiguous and accurate records must be kept; this includes fluid balance charts (Figure 8.9). Nurses should have an understanding of the mechanisms of fluid balance and identify potential imbalances and the problems associated with them.

Pre-procedural considerations

In order to monitor fluid balance, both input and output must be accurately measured. Below are procedural guidelines for measuring input and output. If the patient is awake, able to take oral fluids and mobile, they must be educated about the fact that their fluid balance is being monitored and each drink must be recorded, as should each episode of passing urine, bowel motion, vomiting and so on. It is helpful to provide a cup with markings showing volume.

It is important to note that patients may have other means of urine output, for example an ileal conduit, ureteric stents, suprapubic catheterization or a neobladder. The same concepts can be used to measure the output in such cases, by attaching an urometer to the catheter or urostomy bag.

Post-procedural considerations

Every hour, the findings of fluid input/output monitoring should be recorded; any deficit or change in fluid balance should be reported. Any imbalance noted will require action and a management plan. The nurse recording the fluid balance should have an appreciation of the importance of fluid imbalance management and should notify the appropriate person of any imbalance.

Table 8.4 Assessment of fluid status

		Indications	
Assessment and symptoms	**Usual findings**	**Fluid deficit**	**Fluid overload**
History (to establish any condition, medication or lifestyle that may contribute to or predispose the patient to a fluid imbalance)	Differs for each patient	For example, chronic or acute diarrhoea, medication such as diuretics, poor oral fluid intake, presence of gastrointestinal stoma	Ingestion of too much water/fluid, renal failure/dysfunction
Thirst (ask the patient)	Occasional; resolved by taking an oral drink	Unusually thirsty	No thirst, normal
Mucosa and conjunctiva (inspect)	Usually moist and pink	Dry and whitened mucosa, dry conjunctiva and 'sunken' eyeballs	Moist, pink and glistening
Clinical signs			
Heart rate	Usual resting rate of 60–100 bpm	Raised	Normal or raised
Peripheral pulse character	Radial pulse is felt just under the skin at the wrist, using light palpation with two or three fingers	Thready, difficult to palpate	Bounding, easy to palpate
Blood pressure	Patient's own normal should be used as a guide	Blood pressure will fall if blood volume falls beyond compensatory mechanisms; patient may experience postural hypotension	Rise in blood pressure, or may remain normal
Central venous pressure	3–10 mmHg	Low	Raised

Table 8.4 Assessment of fluid status *(continued)*

Assessment and symptoms	Usual findings	Indications: Fluid deficit	Indications: Fluid overload
Respiratory rate	12–20 breaths/min	High, to meet increased oxygen demands of compensatory mechanisms	High, if overload present
Capillary refill	Usually 2–3 seconds	Slower	Faster
Urine output	0.5–1 mL/kg	Low	Increase, if good renal function
Lung sounds (auscultation)	Vesicular breath sounds, 'rustling' heard mainly on inspiration	Normal	Additional sounds (crackles) may indicate fluid overload
Skin turgor	Following a gentle pinch, the fold of skin should return to normal	Skin will take much longer to 'bounce' back to normal; unreliable in the elderly, who may have lost some elasticity of their skin	May be normal; however, may be oedematous, in which case skin will remain dented/pinched
Serum electrolyte levels*			
Sodium	135–145 mmol/L	Raised	Lowered
Potassium	3.5–5 mmol/L	May be lowered if cause of fluid deficit is gastrointestinal losses	Normal
Urea	2.5–6.4 mmol/L	Increased** Increased renal reabsorption of urea mediated by antidiuretic hormone	Normal
Creatinine	Male: 63–116 μmol/L Female: 51–98 μmol/L	Normal, but eventually rises with prolonged poor renal perfusion	Normal, unless cause of overload is renal dysfunction
Other			
Serum osmolarity	275–295 mOsmol/kg	Increased	Decreased
Urine osmolarity	50–1400 mOsmol/kg	Increased	Decreased
Daily weight	A person's daily weight should be fairly stable; large losses or gains in weight may indicate fluid imbalance	Reduced each day	Increased each day
Temperature	36.5–37.5°C	May be elevated and this may also contribute to the fluid deficit (increased insensible losses by sweating)	Normal

*This is a basic examination of serum electrolytes in fluid balance. There are several conditions and treatments that may affect these so they should not be used in isolation to assess or treat fluid imbalance.
**Although note that there is a decrease in urea in central diabetes insipidus.
Source: Adapted from Adam et al. (2017), Levi (2005), NICE (2018).

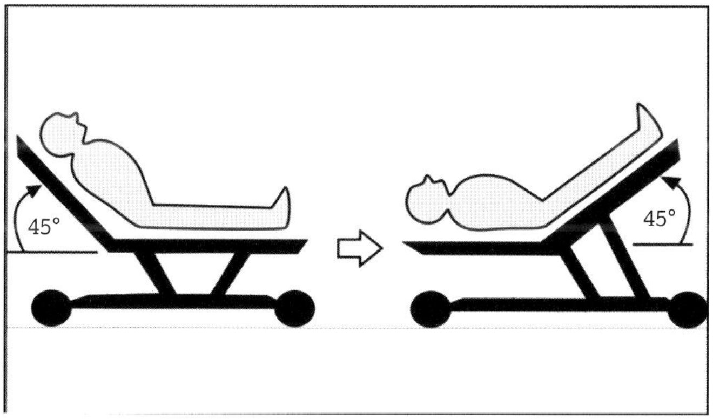

Figure 8.7 Passive leg raise.

Complications

Correct fluid balance monitoring is essential in the successful management of actual or potential fluid balance disturbances (Jevon and Ewens 2012). Over- or underestimation of a patient's fluid status could lead to incorrect management, resulting in fluid overload (hypervolaemia), dehydration (hypovolaemia) (Davies et al. 2015, Pinnington et al. 2016) and/or electrolyte disturbances, all of which will ultimately lead to organ dysfunction.

Fluid overload (hypervolaemia)

Underestimating fluid balance may lead to continued or increased administration of intravenous fluids, which if monitored incorrectly could result in circulatory overload. Excess intravenous fluid administration is not the only cause of circulatory overload, which can also result from acute renal failure, heart failure or excessive sodium intake (Rhoda et al. 2011).

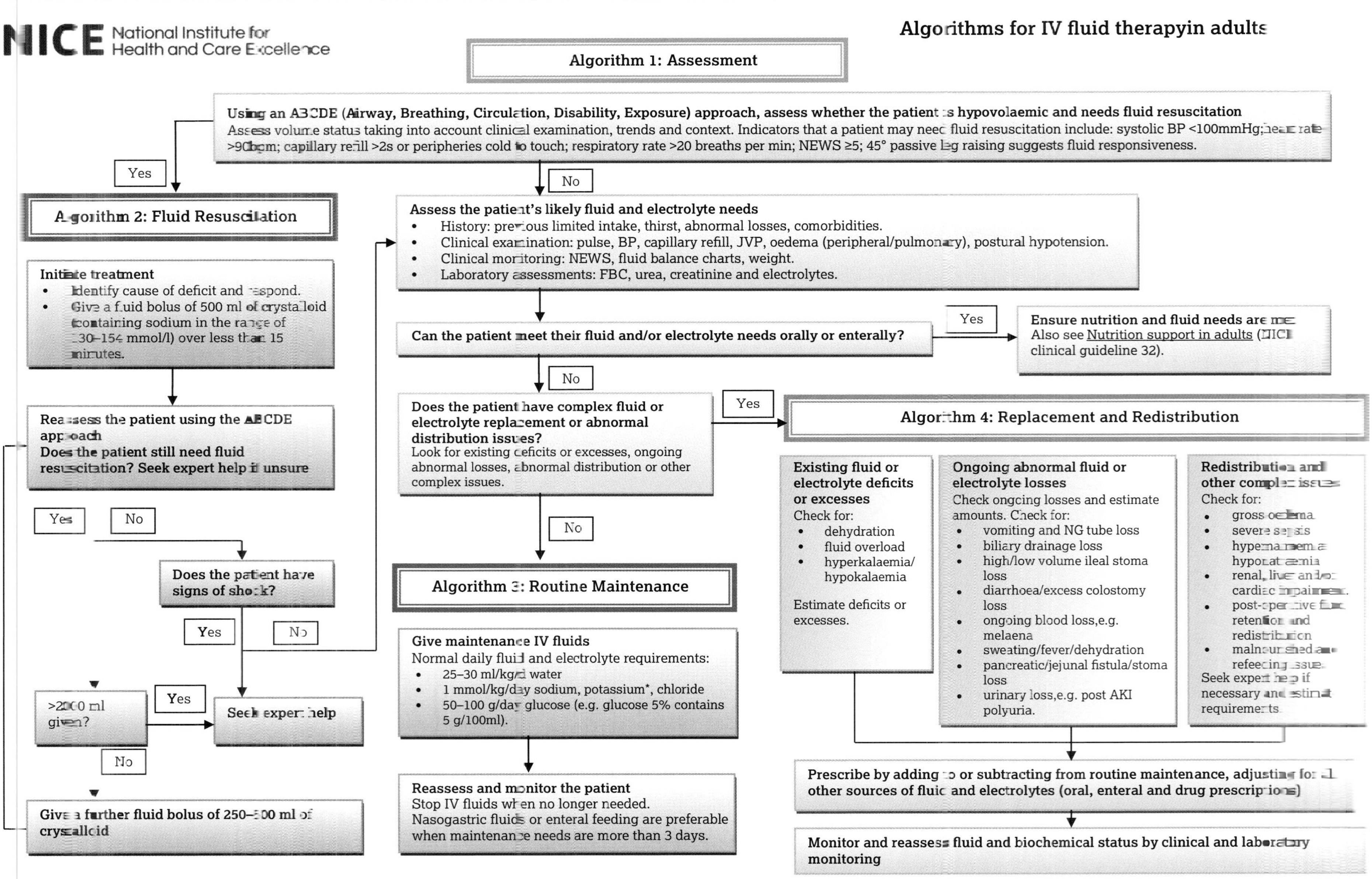
NICE National Institute for Health and Care Excellence
Algorithms for IV fluid therapy in adults
Algorithm 1: Assessment
Using an ABCDE (Airway, Breathing, Circulation, Disability, Exposure) approach, assess whether the patient is hypovolaemic and needs fluid resuscitation
Assess volume status taking into account clinical examination, trends and context. Indicators that a patient may need fluid resuscitation include: systolic BP <100mmHg; heart rate >90bpm; capillary refill >2s or peripheries cold to touch; respiratory rate >20 breaths per min; NEWS ≥5; 45° passive leg raising suggests fluid responsiveness.
Yes
No
Algorithm 2: Fluid Resuscitation
Initiate treatment
• Identify cause of deficit and respond.
• Give a fluid bolus of 500 ml of crystalloid containing sodium in the range of 130–154 mmol/l) over less than 15 minutes.
Reassess the patient using the ABCDE approach
Does the patient still need fluid resuscitation? Seek expert help if unsure
Yes
No
Does the patient have signs of shock?
Yes
No
>2000 ml given?
Yes
No
Seek expert help
Give a further fluid bolus of 250–500 ml of crystalloid
Assess the patient's likely fluid and electrolyte needs
• History: previous limited intake, thirst, abnormal losses, comorbidities.
• Clinical examination: pulse, BP, capillary refill, JVP, oedema (peripheral/pulmonary), postural hypotension.
• Clinical monitoring: NEWS, fluid balance charts, weight.
• Laboratory assessments: FBC, urea, creatinine and electrolytes.
Can the patient meet their fluid and/or electrolyte needs orally or enterally?
Yes
Ensure nutrition and fluid needs are met
Also see Nutrition support in adults (NICE clinical guideline 32).
No
Does the patient have complex fluid or electrolyte replacement or abnormal distribution issues?
Look for existing deficits or excesses, ongoing abnormal losses, abnormal distribution or other complex issues.
Yes
No
Algorithm 3: Routine Maintenance
Give maintenance IV fluids
Normal daily fluid and electrolyte requirements:
• 25–30 ml/kg/d water
• 1 mmol/kg/day sodium, potassium*, chloride
• 50–100 g/day glucose (e.g. glucose 5% contains 5 g/100ml).
Reassess and monitor the patient
Stop IV fluids when no longer needed.
Nasogastric fluids or enteral feeding are preferable when maintenance needs are more than 3 days.
Algorithm 4: Replacement and Redistribution
Existing fluid or electrolyte deficits or excesses
Check for:
• dehydration
• fluid overload
• hyperkalaemia/hypokalaemia
Estimate deficits or excesses.
Ongoing abnormal fluid or electrolyte losses
Check ongoing losses and estimate amounts. Check for:
• vomiting and NG tube loss
• biliary drainage loss
• high/low volume ileal stoma loss
• diarrhoea/excess colostomy loss
• ongoing blood loss,e.g. melaena
• sweating/fever/dehydration
• pancreatic/jejunal fistula/stoma loss
• urinary loss,e.g. post AKI polyuria.
Redistribution and other complex issues
Check for:
• gross oedema
• severe sepsis
• hypernatraemia/hyponatraemia
• renal, liver and/or cardiac impairment
• post-operative fluid retention and redistribution
• malnourished and refeeding issues
Seek expert help if necessary and estimate requirements.
Prescribe by adding to or subtracting from routine maintenance, adjusting for all other sources of fluid and electrolytes (oral, enteral and drug prescriptions)
Monitor and reassess fluid and biochemical status by clinical and laboratory monitoring

*Weight-based potassium prescriptions should be rounded to the nearest common fluids available (for example, a 67 kg person should have fluids containing 20 mmol and 40 mmol of potassium in a 24-hour period).
Potassium should not be added to intravenous fluid bags as this is dangerous.

'Intravenous fluid therapy in adults in hospital', NICE clinical guideline 174 (December 2013. Last update December 2016)

Figure 8 Algorithm for intravenous fluid therapy in adults. *Source:* NICE (2017b). Reproduced with permission of NICE.

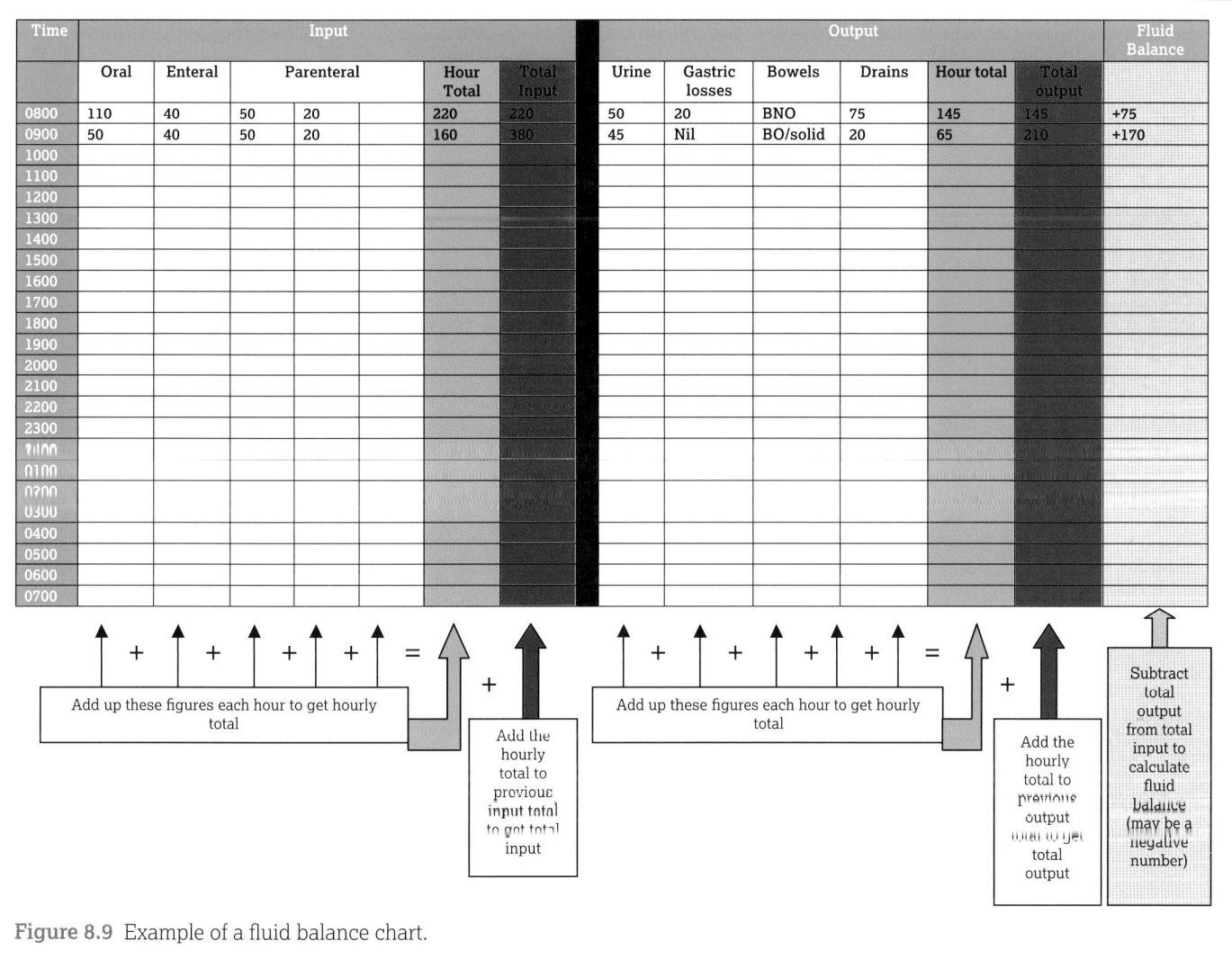

Time	Input							Output						Fluid Balance
	Oral	Enteral	Parenteral			Hour Total	Total Input	Urine	Gastric losses	Bowels	Drains	Hour total	Total output	
0800	110	40	50	20		220	220	50	20	BNO	75	145	145	+75
0900	50	40	50	20		160	380	45	Nil	BO/solid	20	65	210	+170
1000														
1100														
1200														
1300														
1400														
1500														
1600														
1700														
1800														
1900														
2000														
2100														
2200														
2300														
0000														
0100														
0200														
0300														
0400														
0500														
0600														
0700														

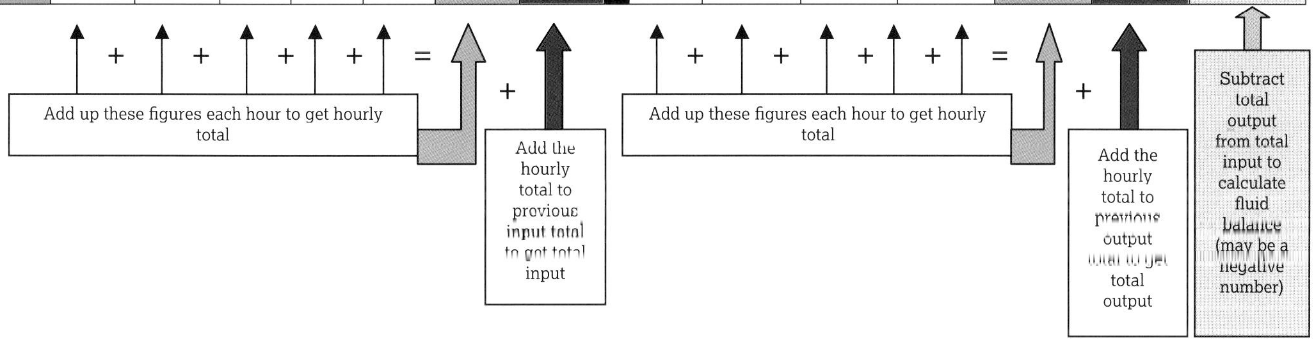

Add up these figures each hour to get hourly total
Add the hourly total to previous input total to get total input
Add up these figures each hour to get hourly total
Add the hourly total to previous output total to get total output
Subtract total output from total input to calculate fluid balance (may be a negative number)

Figure 8.9 Example of a fluid balance chart.

Procedure guideline 8.1 Fluid input: measurement

Essential equipment

- Personal protective equipment
- Fluid balance chart
- Appropriate pumps for fluid or feeding
- Cup with markings

Action	Rationale
Pre-procedure	
1 Introduce yourself to the patient, and explain and discuss the procedure with them. Educate the patient about the fact that their fluid input is being monitored and ask them to communicate any oral intake. Additionally, obtain their consent to continue this monitoring. It can be helpful to provide a cup with millilitre markings or a diagram with estimated volumes.	To ensure the patient is aware of the need to record any oral intake so this can be noted accurately (Baraz et al. 2009, **R**; Georgiades 2016, **E**). To ensure that the patient feels at ease, understands the procedure and gives their valid consent (NMC 2018, **C**).
2 Obtain a fluid balance chart and complete the patient's details and the date commenced, or add the necessary document to the appropriate electronic documentation system.	To ensure the chart is labelled with the details of the correct patient, allowing accurate documentation (Powell-Tuck et al. 2011, **C**).
3 Ensure pumps are available for continuous intravenous fluids and nasogastric/jejunostomy feeds.	To enable accurate hourly recording of intake (Reid et al. 2004, **E**).

(continued)

Procedure guideline 8.1 Fluid input: measurement *(continued)*

Action	Rationale
Procedure	
4 Measure oral fluid intake hourly, noting it on the fluid balance chart (see Figure 8.9).	To obtain an accurate real-time fluid balance status (Davies et al. 2015, **R**; Sumnall 2007, **E**).
5 Note any enteral or parenteral intake.	To obtain an accurate real-time fluid balance status and ensure all possible inputs are considered (Davies et al. 2015, **R**; Smith and Roberts 2011, **E**).
6 Add together the values for oral, enteral and parenteral intake for the hour.	To assess hourly fluid intake (Davies et al. 2015, **R**; Scales and Pilsworth 2008, **E**).
7 Add this value to the cumulative total for intake (see Figure 8.9).	To assess total intake and enable calculation of the fluid balance (Scales and Pilsworth 2008, **E**).
Post-procedure	
8 Once output totals have been calculated (see Procedure guidelines 8.2–8.7), subtract output from input.	To calculate fluid balance (Powell-Tuck et al. 2011, **C**).
9 Document this on the chart.	To ensure accurate documentation (NMC 2018, **C**).

Procedure guideline 8.2 Fluid output: monitoring/measuring output if the patient is catheterized

Essential equipment

- Personal protective equipment
- Urometer
- Fluid balance chart

Action	Rationale
Pre-procedure	
1 Introduce yourself to the patient, explain and discuss the procedure with them, and gain their consent to proceed.	To ensure that the patient feels at ease, understands the procedure and gives their valid consent (NMC 2018, **C**).
2 Determine the relevant sources of fluid output (see Table 8.3) and note them on the fluid balance chart.	To ensure all possibilities have been considered and to ensure accurate (as far as possible) output determination (Scales and Pilsworth 2008, **E**).
3 Wash hands thoroughly and/or use an alcohol-based handrub and apply personal protective equipment necessary for handling body fluids.	To appropriately decontaminate hands and avoid cross-contamination (NHS England and NHSI 2019, **C**).
Procedure	
4 Explain to the patient that it is necessary to monitor their urine output and that you will be doing so every hour.	To ensure that the patient is not alarmed by frequent observation and that they are kept informed about their current care (Bryant 2007, **E**).
5 Attach a urometer to the catheter using an aseptic technique (see Procedure guideline 4.11: Aseptic technique example: changing a wound dressing).	To allow accurate assessment of hourly urine output. **E** To prevent cross-infection (Loveday et al. 2014, **R**).
6 Each hour, on the hour, note the volume of urine in the urometer, recording this on the fluid balance chart.	To determine urine output and to keep accurate records of this, enabling the assessment of fluid balance (Scales and Pilsworth 2008, **E**).
7 Empty the urometer into the collection bag (until the bag is three-quarters full; this will then need emptying).	To ensure the urometer is empty for the next hour's determination and that there is no backflow of urine. **E**
8 Add recorded urine output to the other values for output, giving an hourly total.	To allow for fluid balance determination. **E**
Post-procedure	
9 Once all output has been determined and noted on the chart, calculate the total hourly output and then subtract the total output from the total input.	To calculate hourly fluid balance. **E**
10 Document all values on the chart and record any other actions relating to your findings in the patient's notes.	To ensure accurate documentation (NMC 2018, **C**).

Procedure guideline 8.3 Fluid output: monitoring/measuring output if the patient is not catheterized

Essential equipment

- Personal protective equipment
- Measuring jugs (with volume indicators)
- Bedpan, urinary bottles or commode
- Scales

Action	Rationale
Pre-procedure	
1 Introduce yourself to the patient, explain and discuss the procedure with them, and gain their consent to proceed.	To ensure that the patient feels at ease, understands the procedure and gives their valid consent (NMC 2018, **C**).
2 Determine the relevant sources of fluid output (see Table 8.3) and note them on the fluid balance chart.	To ensure all possibilities have been considered to ensure accurate (as far as possible) output determination (McGloin 2015, **E**; Scales and Pilsworth 2008, **E**).
Procedure	
3 Explain to the patient that it is necessary to measure their urine output.	To ensure that the patient knows that any urine they pass needs to be measured in order to record output and to obtain their co-operation in ensuring accuracy of measurement (Georgiades 2016, **E**).
4 Provide the patient with bedpans or a commode, even if able to mobilize to the bathroom; ask them to place the bedpan over the toilet bowl; ask them to inform you of each episode.	To ensure the urine is kept for measuring and not disposed of (Georgiades 2016, **E**).
5 Use personal protective equipment required for body fluids when handling used bottles or bedpans.	To prevent cross-infection (NHS England and NHSI 2019, **C**).
6 Place bedpan or bottle onto the scales, subtracting the appropriate value to compensate for the weight of the item.	To obtain the amount of urine in grams, which equates to the same in millilitres. **E**
7 If no scales are available, use a jug with volume markings; pour the urine into a jug (using standard precautions), noting the level of urine.	To measure urine volume. **E**
8 Once noted, dispose of urine appropriately.	To prevent contamination and/or cross-infection (Loveday et al. 2014, **R**).
9 Record the value on the fluid balance chart, adding this to the rest of the output values for the hour.	To determine fluid output for the hour (McGloin 2015, **E**).
Post-procedure	
10 Once all output has been determined and noted on the chart, calculate the total hourly output and then subtract the total output from the total input.	To calculate hourly fluid balance. **E**
11 Document all values on the chart and record any other actions relating to your findings in the patient's notes.	To ensure accurate documentation (NMC 2018, **C**).

Procedure guideline 8.4 Fluid output: monitoring/measuring output from drains

Essential equipment

- Personal protective equipment
- Measuring jugs (with volume indicators)
- Tape and/or pen

Action	Rationale
Pre-procedure	
1 Introduce yourself to the patient, explain and discuss the procedure with them, and gain their consent to proceed.	To ensure that the patient feels at ease, understands the procedure and gives their valid consent (NMC 2018, **C**).
2 Determine the relevant sources of fluid output (see Table 8.3) and note them on the fluid balance chart.	To ensure all possibilities have been considered to ensure accurate (as far as possible) output determination (McGloin 2015, **E**).
3 Wash hands and/or use an alcohol-based handrub and apply personal protective equipment necessary for handling body fluids.	To appropriately decontaminate hands and prevent cross-contamination (NHS England and NHSI 2019, **C**).

(continued)

Procedure guideline 8.4 Fluid output: monitoring/measuring output from drains *(continued)*

Action	Rationale
Procedure	
4 Explain to the patient that the output from the drains will be monitored hourly.	To inform the patient about their current care and to ensure they are not alarmed by the frequent observations (Liaw and Goh 2018, **R**).
5 If the drain is drainable, empty the contents into a jug, noting the volume.	To determine the volume of the fluid drained. **E**
6 If it is not possible to drain the fluid out of the bag, use some tape (stuck along the length of the bottle) and/or a suitable pen and mark the level the fluid reaches each hour. Date and time each marking.	To determine drainage each hour. To ensure consistency in reading and to communicate to other members of the multidisciplinary team regarding drainage (Sumnall 2007, **E**).
7 Note volume/drainage on fluid balance chart.	To determine drainage each hour (McGloin 2015, **E**).
8 Add this figure to the rest of the output values for the hour.	To accurately determine total fluid lost each hour (McGloin 2015, **E**).
Post-procedure	
9 Once all output has been determined and noted on the chart, calculate the total hourly output and then subtract the total output from the total input.	To calculate hourly fluid balance (Davies et al. 2015, **R**).
10 Document all values on the chart and record any other actions relating to your findings in the patient's notes.	To ensure accurate documentation (NMC 2018, **C**).

Procedure guideline 8.5 Fluid output: monitoring/measuring output from gastric outlets, nasogastric tubes or gastrostomy

Essential equipment

- Personal protective equipment
- Urometer
- Measuring jugs (with volume indicators)
- Bile drainage bag/gastrostomy drainage bag

Action	Rationale
Pre-procedure	
1 Introduce yourself to the patient, explain and discuss the procedure with them, and gain their consent to proceed.	To ensure that the patient feels at ease, understands the procedure and gives their valid consent (NMC 2018, **C**).
2 Determine the relevant sources of fluid output (see Table 8.3) and note them on the fluid balance chart.	To ensure all possibilities have been considered to ensure accurate (as far as possible) output determination (McGloin 2015, **E**).
3 Wash hands and/or use an alcohol-based handrub and apply personal protective equipment necessary for handling body fluids.	To appropriately decontaminate hands and prevent cross-contamination (NHS England and NHSI 2019, **C**).
Procedure	
4 Explain to the patient that it is necessary to monitor drainage every hour.	To inform the patient of their current care and interventions (Liaw and Goh 2018, **R**).
5 Ensure the gastric outlet device has a drainage bag attached.	To collect any output for measurement. **E**
6 If instructed, leave the bag open to drain (this may differ depending on the patient's condition).	To enable drainage. **E**
7 Drain contents into marked jug every hour (if quantity allows), using standard precautions.	To determine volume. **E**
8 Attach a urometer if output is high.	To ensure accurate reading and for ease of measuring. **E**
9 Note volume on fluid balance chart, adding this value to the rest of the output values for that hour.	To enable determination of fluid balance (McGloin 2015, **E**; Sumnall 2007, **E**).
Post-procedure	
10 Once all output has been determined and noted on the chart, calculate the total hourly output and then subtract the total output from the total input.	To calculate hourly fluid balance (McGloin 2015, **E**)
11 Document all values on the chart and record any other actions relating to your findings in the patient's notes.	To ensure accurate documentation (NMC 2018, **C**)

Procedure guideline 8.6 Fluid output: monitoring/measuring output from bowels

Essential equipment

- Personal protective equipment
- Measuring jugs (with volume indicators)
- Scales
- Bedpan or commode
- Flexi-Seal rectal tube (if required)

Action	Rationale
Pre-procedure	
1 Introduce yourself to the patient, explain and discuss the procedure with them, and gain their consent to proceed.	To ensure that the patient feels at ease, understands the procedure and gives their valid consent (NMC 2018, **C**).
2 Determine the relevant sources of fluid output (see Table 8.3) and note them on the fluid balance chart.	To ensure all possibilities have been considered to ensure accurate (as far as possible) output determination (McGloin 2015, **E**).
3 Wash hands and/or use an alcohol-based handrub and apply personal protective equipment necessary for handling body fluids.	To appropriately decontaminate hands and prevent cross-contamination (NHS England and NHSI 2019, **C**).
Procedure	
4 Explain to the patient that it is necessary to monitor the volume of fluid excreted, including that from the bowel, particularly if the stool is loose/watery.	To keep the patient informed about their current care and observations, to ensure co-operation in monitoring fluid output (Liaw and Goh 2018, **R**).
5 Provide the patient with bedpans or commodate, even if able to mobilize to the bathroom; ask them to place the bedpan over the toilet bowl; ask them to inform you of each episode.	To enable inspection and measurement of fluid lost via the bowel. **E**
6 If the stool is loose enough, this can be transferred into a jug and the volume measured. Alternatively, weigh the bedpan as per local policy.	To quantify fluid output from stool (Scales and Pilsworth 2008, **E**).
7 If the stool is formed and it is not possible to accurately quantify, still note on fluid balance chart that bowels were opened.	To take into account any insensible losses (Shepherd 2011, **E**).
8 A rectal tube may be suitable in some patients; refer to local policy regarding the use of rectal tubes. Note any output on the fluid balance chart.	To ensure correct use of tube and to quantify any fluid losses from the bowel. **E**
9 Add losses to the previous losses for the hour.	To calculate hourly fluid output (Shepherd 2011, **E**).
Post-procedure	
10 Once all output has been determined and noted on the chart, calculate the total hourly output and then subtract the total output from the total input.	To calculate hourly fluid balance (Shepherd 2011, **E**).
11 Document all values on the chart and record any other actions relating to your findings in the patient's notes.	To ensure accurate documentation (NMC 2018, **C**).

Procedure guideline 8.7 Fluid output: monitoring/measuring output from stoma sites

Essential equipment

- Personal protective equipment
- Measuring jugs (with volume indicators)

Action	Rationale
Pre-procedure	
1 Introduce yourself to the patient, explain and discuss the procedure with them, and gain their consent to proceed.	To ensure that the patient feels at ease, understands the procedure and gives their valid consent (NMC 2018, **C**).
2 Determine the relevant sources of fluid output (see Table 8.3) and note them on the fluid balance chart.	To ensure all possibilities have been considered to ensure accurate (as far as possible) output determination (McGloin 2015, **E**).
3 Wash hands and/or use an alcohol-based handrub and apply personal protective equipment necessary for handling body fluids.	To appropriately decontaminate hands and prevent cross-contamination (NHS England and NHSI 2019, **C**).

(continued)

Procedure guideline 8.7 Fluid output: monitoring/measuring output from stoma sites *(continued)*

Action	Rationale
Procedure	
4 Explain to the patient that you are monitoring hourly output.	To ensure the patient understands why their stoma is being checked hourly. To ensure they are up to date with current care (Liaw and Goh 2018, **R**).
5 Check that the stoma bag is drainable; if not, change it (see Procedure guideline 6.26: Stoma bag change).	To ensure ease of draining the bag's contents and to reduce the number of times the adhesive flange is removed, in order to protect the skin. **E**
6 Using protective equipment such as incontinence pads, empty the contents of the stoma bag into the measuring jug, noting the volume.	To determine output from the stoma for 1 hour. **E**
7 Dispose of contents using protective equipment, adhering to local policy.	To ensure correct disposal of contents and prevent cross-infection (Loveday et al. 2014, **R**).
8 Note the volume of the stool on the chart; add this to any other losses for the hour.	To ensure correct documentation of output and allow calculation of fluid balance (NICE 2017b, **C**).
9 Add the hourly total (all outputs) to the cumulative output (see Figure 8.9).	To enable fluid balance determination (Shepherd 2011, **E**).
Post-procedure	
10 Once all output has been determined and noted on the chart, calculate the total hourly output and then subtract the total output from the total input.	To calculate hourly fluid balance. **E**
11 Document all values on the chart and record any other actions relating to your findings in the patient's notes.	To ensure accurate documentation (NMC 2018, **C**).

Problem-solving table 8.1 Prevention and resolution (Procedure guidelines 8.1, 8.2, 8.3, 8.4, 8.5, 8.6 and 8.7)

Problem	Cause	Prevention	Action
Non-compliance or lack of co-operation from patients	Usually misunderstanding or lack of education regarding the importance of monitoring fluid balance	Effective patient education and teaching.	Determine effective teaching methods. Considering individual needs, for example poor hearing or illiteracy. Re-educate the patient, using appropriate means.
Inability to record input due to lack of pumps to regulate intravenous fluids or enteral feeds	Not available, unable to use or inappropriate	Request more equipment from appropriate sources, or request training.	Calculate drip rates on free-flowing fluids to ensure correct hourly input calculated.
Insensible losses	Inability to measure some losses	Not applicable.	Note on chart if perspiration is excessive, if patient is pyrexial, or if bowels were opened and immeasurable, to highlight possible inaccuracy in fluid balance.
Leaking drains	Inevitable with some drains	Inevitable with some drains; however, the surrounding opening may require further suturing. Request a surgical review if necessary.	Use stoma bag or wound drainage bag to collect drainage, to enable measurement.
Incorrect fluid balance calculation	Incorrect fluid input determination, incorrect fluid output determination or incorrect calculation	Appropriate teaching and education for nurses performing these procedures; check competence. Encourage use of a calculator if needed.	Ensure nurses are educated appropriately and that they access information and education if they are unsure of a procedure or technique.

In health, homeostatic mechanisms exist to compensate and redistribute excess fluids; however, in ill health, these mechanisms are often inadequate, leading to increasing circulatory volumes. As the volume within the circulatory system rises, so does the hydrostatic pressure, which, when excessive, results in leaking of fluid from the vessels into the surrounding tissues. This is evident as oedema, initially apparent in the ankles and legs (Figure 8.10) or buttocks and sacrum if the patient is in bed. This can progress to generalized oedema, where even the tissues surrounding the eyes become puffy and swollen. A bounding pulse

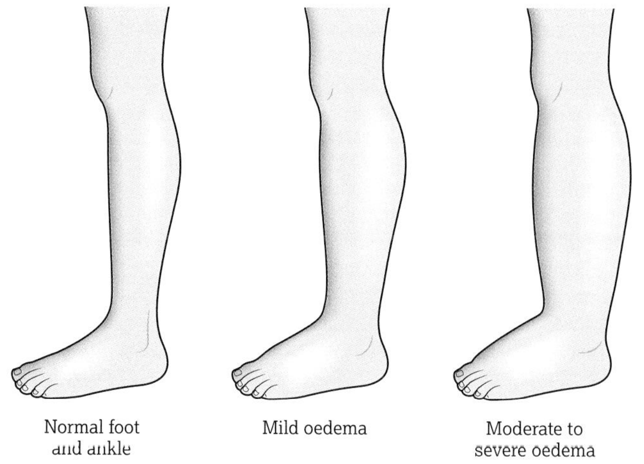

Figure 8.10 Foot and ankle oedema.

and an increased blood pressure are also signs of fluid overload, as are an increased cardiac output and raised central venous pressure (Gross et al. 2017).

One of the most dangerous symptoms of fluid overload is pulmonary oedema, which occurs when rising hydrostatic pressure within the vessels leads to congestion within the pulmonary circulation, causing fluid to leak into the lungs and pulmonary tissues (Chioncel et al. 2015). This presents with respiratory symptoms, including shortness of breath, increased respiratory rate, a cough (Tidy 2018) (often associated with pink, frothy sputum), and finally reduced oxygen saturations due to inadequate gaseous exchange at the alveolar level (Tidy 2018). Left untreated, this can be fatal as the lungs fail to provide essential cells and organs with oxygen; this eventually leads to organ dysfunction and then failure.

Cardiac dysfunction can result from fluid overload, not only from the reduced availability of oxygen to the cardiac cells due to the pulmonary oedema, but also from the increase in volume, which causes the cardiac muscle to stretch, leading to cell damage and inability to contract effectively (Tidy 2018).

Treatment of hypervolaemia involves restricting fluid intake, monitoring electrolytes and using diuretics in an attempt to offload some of the excess fluid (Thomsen et al. 2012). Vasodilators may also be considered to reduce the pressure in the vessels in patients with congestive heart failure. If these mechanisms fail, it may be necessary to use renal replacement therapy to drive the fluid out of the circulation.

In some cases, fluid overload is part of the disease process. However, with effective monitoring, fluid balance recording and assessment, it may be possible to avoid the devastating complications.

Dehydration (hypovolaemia)

Dehydration implies a negative fluid balance: when the fluid output exceeds the fluid intake (Jevon 2010). Overestimation of the fluid balance may lead to inadequate replacement of lost fluids. Dehydration can, however, be caused by a loss of fluids to 'third spaces' such as ascites or lost due to a reduction in colloid osmotic pressure (hypoalbuminaemia) (Frost 2015) – losses that are not easy to account for. Fluid balance charts should therefore always be used in association with physical assessment of the patient, weight measurement and laboratory results.

There are three categories of dehydration (Mentes and Kang 2013) – isotonic, hypertonic and hypotonic – each related to the type of fluid and solutes lost. Isotonic describes the loss of both water and sodium from the ECF; hypertonic is excessive loss of water only, which leads to a rise in ECF sodium, causing a shift in fluid from the intracellular space to the extracellular. Hypotonic dehydration results from excessive sodium loss, particularly with the overuse of diuretics or in the case of high-output ileostomies (Chan et al. 2018, Welch 2010).

Table 8.5 Kidney Disease: Improving Global Outcomes (KDIGO) staging classification

Stage	Serum creatinine	Urine output
Stage 1	1.5–1.9 × baseline	<0.5 mL/kg/hr 6–12 hrs
Stage 2	2.0–2.9 × baseline	<0.5 mL/kg/hr for >12 hrs
Stage 3	3.0 × baseline	<0.3 mL/kg/hr for >24 hrs

Source: KDIGO (2012).

Dehydration can ultimately cause a reduction in circulating volume (Tortora and Derrickson 2017). As with any change in a homeostatic state, in health the body has the ability to compensate but in ill health these mechanisms are often inadequate. Untreated dehydration will quickly lead to a drop in blood pressure and a rise in heart rate (to compensate for the fall in blood pressure). A fall in blood pressure will initially lead to inadequate renal perfusion, causing a rise in metabolites, acidosis, acute kidney injury and cerebral ischaemia. If this is untreated, other organs will suffer from poor perfusion, possibly resulting in ischaemia, organ dysfunction and eventually organ failure (Adam et al. 2017).

Additional signs and symptoms of dehydration are thirst, weight loss, decreased urine output, dry skin and mucous membranes, fatigue and increased body temperature (Rhoda et al. 2011).

Treatment of dehydration includes the replacement of lost fluid and electrolytes but caution must be exercised. If the dehydration is mild, slower fluid replacement is advised, in order to prevent further complications in shifts in electrolytes. However, if hypovolaemia exists with the signs and symptoms of circulatory shock, low blood pressure and organ dysfunction, aggressive fluid replacement is advised (Jevon 2010, NICE 2017b). By restoring circulatory volume with fluid administration or resuscitation, renal perfusion can be improved and acute kidney injury may be prevented (Perner et al. 2017).

Acute kidney injury

Acute kidney injury (which can be due to a multitude of causes) is a common feature in the acutely or critically unwell patient and will require even more careful approaches to monitoring and maintenance of fluid balance (Goldstein 2014). The National Confidential Enquiry into Patient Outcome and Death (NCEPOD 2009) reviewed the care delivered to patients with acute kidney injury and found that 50% received suboptimal care. NICE responded to these findings by producing guidance for the prevention, detection and management of acute kidney injury (NICE 2013). The relevant recommendations from this guidance include the need for reliable monitoring of urine output and early recognition of oliguria. The KDIGO (2012) grading system also reinforces the need for accurate and reliable fluid balance monitoring, particularly monitoring urine output (Table 8.5). All assessments, investigations and results require the healthcare professional undertaking them to have an appreciation and understanding of the implications of the findings so they can act accordingly.

Nutritional status

Definition

Nutritional status refers to the state of a person's health as determined by their dietary intake and body composition. Nutritional support refers to any method of giving nutrients that encourages an optimal nutritional status. It includes modifying the types of foods eaten, dietary supplementation, enteral tube feeding and parenteral nutrition (NCCAC 2006).

Anatomy and physiology

The normal process of ingestion of food or fluids occurs via the oral cavity, which opens into the gastrointestinal tract. Swallowing is a complex activity with voluntary and reflexive components. It is usually described as having four stages and requires intact and ority and sensorimotor functioning of the cranial nerves (Bass 1997, Butler and Leslie 2012, Logemann 1998). It starts with the oral preparatory stage, which is influenced by the sight and smell of food. Food or liquid is placed in the mouth and the lips are closed. With chewing and mixing with saliva, the food forms a cohesive mass (bolus) that is held on the centre of the tongue. The second (oral) stage of the swallow is initiated as food is moved through the oral cavity towards the pharynx. These swallowing stages are voluntary.

The third stage of swallowing is pharyngeal and is involuntary (Figure 8.11); this occurs as the food bolus crosses the mandible/tongue base as the palate closes, sealing entry to the nasal cavity and reducing the risk of nasal regurgitation. Movement of the tongue base and posterior pharyngeal wall squeezes the bolus down the pharynx. Involuntary movements of the larynx (voice box), vocal cords and epiglottis protect the airway and open the cricopharyngeus. In the fourth stage, the bolus travels from the cricopharyngeus to the gastro-oesophageal junction and peristaltic action then transfers the bolus down the oesophagus (Atkinson and McHanwell 2002, Butler and Leslie 2012).

The gastrointestinal tract is the site where food is ingested, digested and absorbed, thus enabling nutrients to be used by the body for growth and maintenance of body functions. Food ingested is moved along the gastrointestinal tract by peristaltic waves through the oesophagus, stomach, small intestine and large intestine. The passage of food and fluid through the gastrointestinal tract is dependent on the autonomic nervous system, gut hormones (such as gastrin and cholecystokinin), the function of exocrine glands (such as the parotid, pancreas and liver), and psychological aspects (such as anxiety). Sphincters situated between the stomach and duodenum, the ileocaecal valves and the anal sphincter also regulate the rate of passage of food and fluids through the tract (Barrett 2014).

Before food can be absorbed, it must be digested and broken down into molecules that can be transported across the intestinal epithelium, which lines the gastrointestinal tract. This process is dependent on digestive enzymes (secreted by the pancreas and lining of the intestinal tract) that act on specific nutrients. Bile, from the liver, is required to emulsify fat, thus enabling it to be broken down by digestive enzymes. The absorption of nutrients is dependent on an active, or energy dependent, transport across

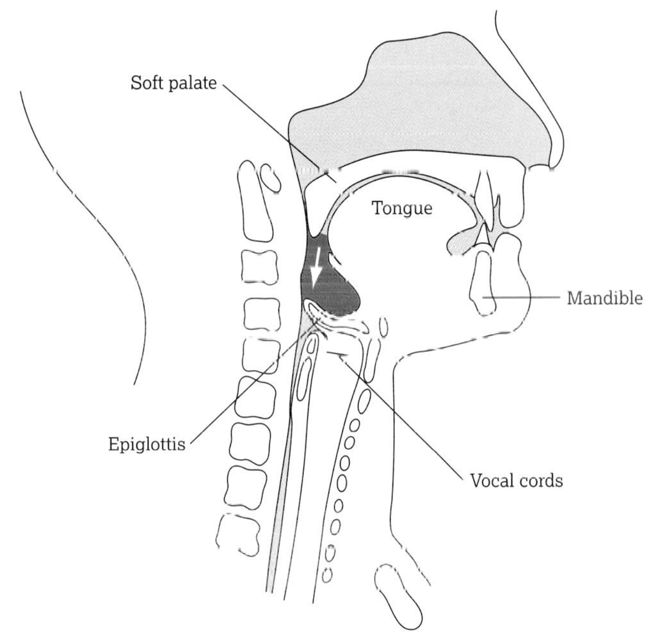

Figure 8.11 The pharyngeal stage of swallowing.

the intestinal epithelium lining the digestive tract. Villi (finger-like projections) increase the surface area of the small intestine to aid absorption.

Most nutrients are absorbed from the small intestine, although some require specific sites within the gastrointestinal tract: for example, vitamin B_{12} is absorbed in the terminal ileum. Mucosa shed into the lumen of the intestine is broken down and absorbed along with fluid and electrolytes secreted into the lumen during the process of digestion. The volumes of fluid secreted into the gut are large and may amount to 8–9 L per day when combined with an oral intake of 1.5–2 L daily. The majority of fluid is reabsorbed in the small intestine with the remainder being absorbed in the large intestine. Bacteria in the large intestine metabolize non-starch polysaccharides (dietary fibre), increasing faecal bulk and producing short-chain fatty acids, which are absorbed and metabolized for energy (Fuller et al. 2016).

Related theory

Bodyweight is the most widely used measure of nutritional status in clinical practice. However, while weight provides a simple, readily obtainable and usually fairly precise measure, it remains a one-dimensional metric and as such has limitations. In contrast, an understanding of anatomy and physiology and in particular the changes that can occur in body composition, in addition to frank weight gain or loss, provides valuable clinical insight (Thibault et al. 2012). In the so-called 'two-compartment' model of body composition, bodyweight is described in terms of, firstly, fat-free mass, that is bones, muscles and organs, which includes the hepatic carbohydrate energy store glycogen, and secondly, fat mass or adipose tissue (Thibault et al. 2012). In health, water constitutes up to 60% of total bodyweight. It is distributed throughout the fat-free and fat compartments with approximately two-thirds present as intracellular and one-third as extracellular fluid. Thus, a healthy 70 kg male comprises 42 kg of water, which amounts to 60% of total bodyweight. This is made up of 28 L of intracellular fluid and 14 L of extracellular fluid (Santanasto et al. 2017).

Body composition and nutritional status are closely linked and are dependent on a number of factors, including age, sex, metabolic requirements, dietary intake and the presence of disease. Depletion of lean body mass occurs in both critical illness and injury; it negatively affects physical functioning and immune function, and can be associated with increased mortality and length of hospital stay (Carlsson et al. 2013, Jensen et al. 2012, Shachar et al. 2016). Generalized loss of skeletal muscle mass and strength with a risk of adverse outcomes (such as physical disability, poor quality of life and death) is called sarcopenia. Sarcopenia plays a major role in the increased frailty and functional impairment that come with age (van den Berg et al. 2019). Shifts in body water compartments are readily observed in conditions such as ascites and oedema (Jaffee et al. 2018, Schol et al. 2016). Both of these conditions result from abnormally increased extracellular water and, despite a gain in total bodyweight, are indicative of worsening outcome.

The physiological characteristics of the different body compartments can be exploited by various assessment tools and techniques, such as bioimpedance analysis (BIA) or measurement of cross-sectional areas of muscle from computed tomography (CT) scanning, to determine changes indicative of nutritional risk (Santanasto et al. 2017). Such changes are masked if weight alone is used as the sole measurement.

Evidence-based approaches

Rationale

Nutritional support, to maintain or replete body composition, should be considered for anybody unable to maintain their nutritional status by taking their usual diet (NCCAC 2006). Supports include the following:

- Patients unable to eat their usual diet (e.g. because of anorexia, mucositis, taste changes or dysphagia) should be given advice on modifying their diet.

- Patients unable to meet their nutritional requirements, despite dietary modifications, should be offered oral nutritional supplements.
- Patients unable to take sufficient food and dietary supplements to meet their nutritional requirements should be considered for an enteral tube feed.
- Patients unable to eat at all should have an enteral tube feed. Reasons for complete inability to eat are outlined in Box 8.1.
- Parenteral nutrition may be indicated in patients with a non-functioning or inaccessible gastrointestinal tract who are likely to be 'nil by mouth' for 5 days or longer. Reasons for a non-functioning or inaccessible gastrointestinal tract include the conditions outlined in Box 8.2.

Enteral nutrition should always be the first option when considering nutritional support.

Patients in any group may have an increased requirement for nutrients due to an increased metabolic rate, as found in those with burns, major sepsis, trauma or cancer cachexia (Arends et al. 2017, Gandy 2014, Todorovic and Mafrici 2019). Patients should have their nutritional requirements estimated prior to the start of nutritional support and should be monitored regularly.

Methods of assessing nutritional status

Before the initiation of nutritional support, the patient must be assessed. The purpose of assessment is to identify whether a patient is undernourished, determine why this may have occurred, and provide baseline data for planning and evaluating nutritional support (NCCAC 2006, Robertson 2018). It is helpful to use more than one method of assessing nutritional status. For example, a dietary history may be used to assess the adequacy of a person's diet but does not reflect actual nutritional status, whereas percentage weight loss does give an indication of nutritional status. However, percentage weight loss taken in isolation gives no idea of either dietary intake or the likelihood of improvement or deterioration in nutritional status (NCCAC 2006).

A holistic assessment of a patient can be carried out with the use of the appropriate performance status or frailty questionnaire. These include the ECOG (Eastern Cooperative Oncology Group) scale (ECOG-ACRIN Cancer Research Group 2019), the Karnofsky Performance Scale (Mor et al. 1984) and the PRISMA-7 Questionnaire (Guidelines and Protocols Advisory Committee 2017). More differentiated tools may be used to monitor daily activities or to quantify physical performance, such as the Five-Times Sit-to-Stand Test and the Timed 'Up & Go' Test, and hand dynamometers can be used to assess muscle function (Makizako et al. 2017).

Box 8.1 Reasons for complete inability to eat

- Carcinoma of the head and neck area or oesophagus
- Surgery to the head or oesophagus
- Radiotherapy treatment to the head or neck
- Fistulae of the oral cavity or oesophagus
- Dysphagia due to cerebrovascular accident (CVA)
- Head injury
- Persistent vegetative state (PVS)

Box 8.2 Reasons for a non-functioning or inaccessible gastrointestinal tract

- Bowel obstruction
- Short bowel syndrome
- Gut toxicity following bone marrow transplantation or chemotherapy
- Uncontrolled vomiting and enterocutaneous fistulae

Bodyweight and weight loss

Body mass index (BMI), or comparison of a patient's weight with a chart of ideal bodyweight, gives a measure of whether the patient has a normal weight, is overweight or is underweight. It may be calculated from weight and height using the following equation:

$$BMI = \frac{Weight\ (\text{kg})}{Height\ (\text{m})^2}$$

Tables are available to allow the rapid and easy calculation of BMI (BAPEN 2018a). These comparisons, however, are not good indicators of whether the patient is at risk nutritionally, as an apparently normal weight can mask severe muscle wasting.

Of greater use is the comparison of current weight with the patient's usual weight. Percentage weight loss is a useful measure of the risk of malnutrition:

$$Percentage\ weight\ loss = \frac{Usual\ weight - Actual\ weight}{Usual\ weight} \times 100$$

A patient would be identified as malnourished if they had any of the following:

- BMI less than 18.5 kg/m^2
- Unintentional weight loss greater than 10% within the past 3–6 months
- BMI less than 20 kg/m^2 and unintentional weight loss greater than 5% within the past 3–6 months (NCCAC 2006).

Unwell children should have their weight and height measured frequently. It may be useful to measure them on a daily basis (Shaw and McCarthy 2014). These measurements must be plotted onto centile charts. A single weight or height cannot be interpreted as there is much variation of growth within each age group. It is a matter of concern if a child's weight begins to fall across the centiles or if the weight plateaus.

Obesity and oedema may make interpretation of bodyweight difficult; both may mask loss of lean body mass and potential malnutrition (Cederholm et al. 2017).

Accurate weighing scales are necessary for measurement of bodyweight. Patients who are unable to stand may require sitting scales or hoist scales.

It is often not appropriate to weigh palliative care patients, who may experience inevitable weight loss as disease progresses. Psychologically, it may be difficult for patients to see that they are continuing to lose weight (Shaw 2011). Measures of nutritional status, such as clinical examination and current food intake, may still be used in addition to measures of bodyweight.

Skinfold thickness and bioelectrical impedance

Skinfold thickness measurements can be used to assess stores of body fat. They are rarely used in routine nutritional assessment due to the insensitivity of the technique and the variation between measurements made by different observers. They are more appropriate for long-term assessments or research purposes and the technique should only be used by practitioners who are practised in using skinfold thickness callipers because of the potential for intra-investigator variation in results (Durnin and Womersley 1974).

Bioelectrical impedance analysis (BIA) is a convenient body composition assessment tool that is non-invasive, provides rapid results and requires minimal operator training (Cederholm et al. 2017). BIA estimates body composition indirectly. A low-voltage current is passed through the body, and tissue resistance and reactance is measured. Empirical equations are then used to estimate body composition (Raeder et al. 2018). This technique works well in healthy individuals, as the validation equations in the individual devices are based on the body composition of healthy individuals. It may be of limited use in some hospital patients with abnormal hydration status (e.g. severe dehydration or ascites) and it is also less reliable at the extremes of the BMI ranges (Gonzalez and Heymsfield 2017, Leahy et al. 2012).

Clinical examination

Observation of the patient may reveal signs and symptoms indicative of nutritional depletion:

- *Physical appearance*: emaciated or wasted appearance; loose dentures, teeth, clothing or jewellery.
- *Oedema*: will affect weight and may mask the appearance of muscle wastage. It may also indicate plasma protein deficiency and is often a reflection of the patient's overall condition rather than a measure of nutritional status.
- *Mobility*: weakness and impaired movement may result from loss of muscle mass.
- *Mood*: apathy, lethargy and poor concentration can be features of undernutrition.
- *Pressure sores and poor wound healing*: may reflect impaired immune function as a consequence of undernutrition and vitamin deficiencies (Gandy 2014).

Specific nutritional deficiencies may be identifiable in some patients. For example, thiamine deficiency characterized by dementia is associated with high alcohol consumption. Rickets is seen in children with vitamin D deficiency.

A more structured approach can be taken by using an assessment tool such as Subjective Global Assessment (SGA) or patient-generated SGA (PG-SGA) (Bauer et al. 2002). This involves a systematic evaluation of muscle and fat sites around the body and assessment for oedema in the ankles or sacral area in immobile patients. Such an assessment can be used to determine whether the patient is malnourished and can be repeated to assess changes in nutritional status.

Dietary intake

Nutrient intake can be assessed via a diet history (Gandy 2014). A 24-hour recall may be used to assess recent nutrient intake and a food chart may be used to monitor current dietary intake. A diet history may also be used to provide information on food frequency, food habits, preferences, meal pattern, portion sizes, the presence of any eating difficulties and changes in food intake (Robertson 2018). A food chart on which all food and fluid taken is recorded is a useful method of monitoring nutritional intake, especially in the hospital setting or when dietary recall is not reliable (Gandy 2014).

Biochemical investigations

Biochemical tests carried out on blood may give information on the patient's nutritional status. The most commonly used are as follows:

- *Plasma proteins*: changes in plasma albumin may arise due to physical stress, changes in circulating volume, changes in hepatic and renal function, shock conditions or septicaemia. Plasma albumin and changes in plasma albumin are not direct reflections of nutritional intake and nutritional status as it has been shown that they may remain unchanged despite changes in body composition (NCCAC 2006). In addition, albumin has a long half-life of 21 days, so it cannot reflect recent changes in nutritional intake. It may be useful to review serum albumin concentrations in conjunction with C-reactive protein (CRP), which is an acute-phase protein produced by the body in response to injury or trauma. CRP greater than 10 mg/L and serum albumin less than 30 g/L suggest 'illness' (Arends et al. 2017). Prealbumin and retinol binding protein levels are more sensitive measures of nutrition support, reflecting recent changes in dietary intake rather than nutritional status. However, they may be expensive to measure and are not measured routinely in hospital.
- *Haemoglobin*: this is often below haematological reference values in malnourished patients (men 135–175 g/L; women: 115–155 g/L). This can be due to a number of reasons, such as loss of blood from circulation, increased destruction of red blood cells, or reduced production of erythrocytes and haemoglobin, for example due to dietary deficiency of iron or folate.
- *Serum vitamin and mineral levels*: clinical examination of the patient may suggest a vitamin or mineral deficiency. For example, gingivitis may be due to a deficiency of vitamin C. Goitre is associated with iodine deficiency, and muscle weakness and cramps may be caused by magnesium deficiency (Gandy 2014). Serum vitamin and mineral levels are rarely measured routinely; however, they should be monitored in people receiving long-term artificial nutritional support or where there is concern about vitamin and mineral status, for example in cases of malabsorption. Long-term vitamin and mineral monitoring should be carried out in accordance with NICE guidelines (NCCAC 2006).
- *Immunological competence*: total lymphocyte count may reflect nutritional status although levels may also be depleted with malignancy, chemotherapy, zinc deficiency, age and non-specific stress (Gandy 2014).

If a patient is considered to be malnourished by one or more of the above methods of assessment then referral to a dietician should be made immediately (NCCAC 2006).

Methods of calculating nutritional requirements

The body requires protein, energy, fluid and micronutrients (such as vitamins, minerals and trace elements) to function optimally. Nutritional requirements should be estimated for patients requiring any form of nutritional support to ensure that these needs are met.

Resting energy requirements may be estimated using figures per kilogram of bodyweight or fat-free mass, depending on body mass index and disease state. Total energy requirements can be estimated by taking into account activity level (Todorovic and Mafrici 2019) (Table 8.6). Careful adjustments may be necessary in cases of low bodyweight, oedema or obesity, in order to avoid overfeeding.

Fluid and nitrogen (i.e. protein) requirements can be calculated in a similar way. If additional nitrogen is being given in situations where losses have increased (e.g. due to trauma, gastrointestinal losses or major sepsis), then it is important to ensure that energy balance is met to assist in promoting a nitrogen balance.

Vitamin and mineral requirements can be calculated as detailed in *Dietary Reference Values for Food Energy and Nutrients for the United Kingdom* (COMA and DH 1991). However, these requirements apply to groups of healthy people and are not necessarily appropriate for those who are ill. A patient deficient in a vitamin or mineral may benefit from additional supplements to improve their condition. Macronutrient and micronutrient requirements for children are also listed in the COMA and DH (1991). Calculations are usually done using the reference nutrient intake (RNI). For children, the actual bodyweight, not the expected bodyweight, is used when calculating requirements. This is to avoid excessive feeding.

Table 8.6 Guidelines for estimation of a patient's daily energy and protein requirements

Factor	Amount per kilogram of bodyweight
Energy (kcal)	25–30
Energy (kJ)	105–126
Protein (g)	1–1.5
Fluid (mL)	35 (18–60 years)
	30 (>60 years)
	Plus consider an additional 2–2.5 mL per °C in temperatures above 37 °C

Note: these guidelines will not always be appropriate for patients who are severely ill or who are outside the body mass index range of 18.5–30 kg/m^2 (Gandy 2014).
Source: Data from Arends et al. (2017) and Todorovic and Mafrici (2019). Reproduced with permission of PENG – Parenteral and Enteral Nutrition Group (www.peng.uk.com) of the British Dietetic Association (www.bda.uk.com).

Methods of measuring the height and weight of an adult patient

Accurately measuring the height and weight of a patient is an essential part of nutrition screening. Accurate measurements of bodyweight may also be required for estimating body surface area and calculating drug dosages, such as for anaesthesia and chemotherapy. All patients should have their height and weight measured on admission to hospital, and weight should be measured at regular intervals during their hospital stay according to local policy and individual clinical need.

When height cannot be measured, it may be estimated using ulna length, which has been shown to have a moderate correlation with height (Madden et al. 2008). See also the section on pre-procedural considerations below.

Clinical governance

Discrepancies in recording patient bodyweight, as well as using inaccurate or inappropriate weighing equipment, can have a negative impact on patient care (Clarkson 2012). This can increase the risk of errors in diagnosis, interventions, treatment and/or medication dosage. Weight should be recorded in patients' medical notes at the time the measurement is taken.

Pre-procedural considerations

Check that the patient is able to stand or sit on the appropriate scales. The patient should remove outdoor clothing and shoes before being weighed and having their height measured.

When obtaining a height measurement, check that the patient is able to stand upright while the measurement is taken. For patients who are unable to stand, height may be determined by measuring ulna length and using conversion tables (see Figure 8.12). If neither height nor weight can be measured or obtained, BMI can be estimated using the mid-upper arm circumference (MUAC) (BAPEN 2018a, Benítez Brito et al. 2016). It may not be possible to weigh patients who cannot be moved or are unable to sit or stand. Alternative methods to obtain weight should be explored, for example bed scales (which can be placed under the wheels of the bed), scales as an integral part of a bed or a patient hoist with a weighing facility

Equipment

Scales

Scales (either sitting or standing) must be calibrated and positioned on a level surface. If electronic or battery scales are used then they must be connected to the mains or have appropriate working batteries prior to the patient getting on the scales.

Stadiometer

These are devices for measuring height and may be mounted on weighing scales or wall mounted.

Tape measure

This is required if estimating height from ulna length or MUAC or for measurement of waist circumference. The tape measure should use centimetres, and it must be disposable or made of plastic that can be cleaned with a detergent wipe between patient uses.

Assessment tools

Identification of patients who are malnourished or at risk of malnutrition is an important first step in nutritional care. There are a number of screening tools available that consider different aspects of nutritional status. National screening initiatives have demonstrated that 25% of patients admitted to hospital were found to be at risk of malnutrition – 18% high risk and 7% medium risk (BAPEN 2012a). Particular diagnoses, such as cancer, increase the risk of malnutrition.

All patients who are identified as at risk of malnutrition should undergo a nutritional assessment. Subjective Global Assessment (SGA) and patient-generated SGA (PG-SGA) are comprehensive assessment tools that necessitate more time and expertise to carry out than most screening tests and therefore are more likely to be used by those with specialist skills, for example dietitians. The Malnutrition Universal Screening Tool (MUST) (BAPEN 2018a) is an example of a screening tool that is based on the patient's BMI, weight loss and illness score; it is less time consuming and easier to use. Other tools may be specific to the patient's age or diagnosis; for example, the Mini Nutrition Assessment (MNA) is used in the elderly and the Royal Marsden Nutrition Screening Tool is used for patients with cancer (Kondrup et al. 2003, Shaw et al. 2015). The most important feature of using any screening tool is that patients identified as having a nutritional deficit or concern, or as requiring intervention have a nutritional care plan initiated and are referred to a dietitian for further advice if appropriate.

Measurement of waist circumference

Table 8.7 shows the waist circumference measurements for men and women at which there is an increased relative risk of heart disease, type 2 diabetes and cancer. In some populations, waist circumference may be a better indicator of risk than BMI, e.g. in persons of Asian descent. In very obese patients (those with a BMI above 35 kg/m^2), waist circumference adds little to the predictive power of disease risk (National Obesity Forum 2016).

Table 8.7 Waist circumference measurements

	Increased risk	Substantially increased risk
Men	≥94 cm	≥102 cm
Women	≥80 cm	≥88 cm

Height (m)	Men (<65 years)	1.94	1.93	1.91	1.89	1.87	1.85	1.84	1.82	1.80	1.78	1.76	1.75	1.73	1.71
	Men (≥65 years)	1.87	1.86	1.84	1.82	1.81	1.79	1.78	1.76	1.75	1.73	1.71	1.70	1.68	1.67
	Ulna length (cm)	32.0	31.5	31.0	30.5	30.0	29.5	29.0	28.5	28.0	27.5	27.0	26.5	26.0	25.5
Height (m)	Women (<65 years)	1.84	1.83	1.81	1.80	1.79	1.77	1.76	1.75	1.73	1.72	1.70	1.69	1.68	1.66
	Women (≥65 years)	1.84	1.83	1.81	1.79	1.78	1.76	1.75	1.73	1.71	1.70	1.68	1.66	1.65	1.63
Height (m)	Men (<65 years)	1.69	1.67	1.66	1.64	1.62	1.60	1.58	1.57	1.55	1.53	1.51	1.49	1.48	1.46
	Men (≥65 years)	1.65	1.63	1.62	1.60	1.59	1.57	1.56	1.54	1.52	1.51	1.49	1.48	1.46	1.45
	Ulna length (cm)	25.0	24.5	24.0	23.5	23.0	22.5	22.0	21.5	21.0	20.5	20.0	19.5	19.0	18.5
Height (m)	Women (<65 years)	1.65	1.63	1.62	1.61	1.59	1.58	1.56	1.55	1.54	1.52	1.51	1.50	1.48	1.47
	Women (≥65 years)	1.61	1.60	1.58	1.56	1.55	1.53	1.52	1.50	1.48	1.47	1.45	1.44	1.42	1.40

Figure 8.12 Conversion chart for estimating height from ulna length. *Source*: Reproduced from BAPEN (2018b) with permission.

Procedure guideline 8.8 Measuring the weight and height of a patient

Essential equipment

- Personal protective equipment
- Scales
- Stadiometer (preferably fixed to the wall)
- Tape measure

Action	Rationale
Pre-procedure	
1 Introduce yourself to the patient, explain and discuss the procedure with them, and gain their consent to proceed.	To ensure that the patient feels at ease, understands the procedure and gives their valid consent (NMC 2018, **C**).
2 Position the scales for easy access and apply the brakes (if appropriate).	To ensure that the patient can get on and off the scales easily and to avoid accidents should the scales move. **E**
3 Ask the patient to remove their shoes and outdoor garments. The patient should be wearing light indoor clothes only (**Action figure 3**).	Outdoor clothes and shoes will add additional weight and/or height and make it difficult to obtain accurate measurements. **E**
Procedure	
Measuring weight	
4 Ensure that the scales record zero, then ask the patient to stand on the scales (or sit if using sitting scales). Ask the patient to remain still and check that the patient is not supporting any weight on any object (e.g. the wall or a stick) and that neither of their feet is on the floor.	To record an accurate weight (NMC 2018, **C**).
5 Note the reading on the scale and record it immediately. Check with the patient that the weight reflects their expected weight and that the weight is similar to previous weights recorded. This may require conversion of weight from kilograms to stones and pounds or vice versa.	To check that the weight is correct. If the weight is not as expected then the patient should be reweighed. **E**
Measuring height	
6 Ask the patient to stand straight with heels together. If the stadiometer is wall mounted, the heels should touch the heel plate or the wall. With a freestanding device, the person's back should be toward the measuring rod.	To ensure that the patient is standing upright. If the person does not have their back against the measuring rod then the measuring arm may not reach the head. **E**

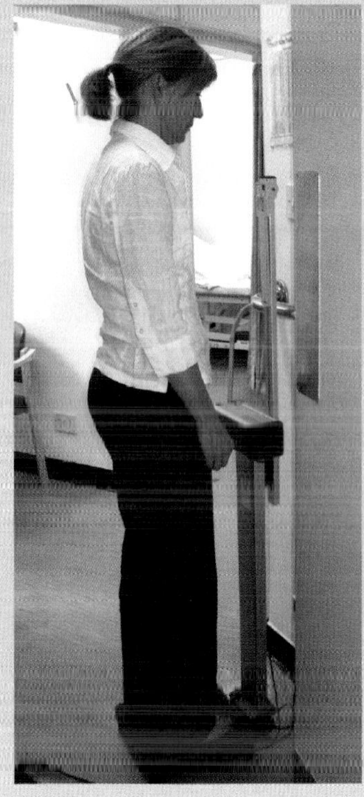

Action Figure 3 Weigh the patient.

7 The patient should look straight ahead and with the bottom of the nose and the bottom of the ear in a parallel plane. The patient should be asked to stretch to reach maximal height.	To ensure an accurate height is measured. **E**
8 Record the height to the nearest millimetre.	To record an accurate measurement of the patient's height (NMC 2018, **C**).
Estimating height using ulna length (only use this method if not possible to measure height in the usual way; Silva and Figueira 2017)	
9 To estimate the height of a patient from ulna length, ask the patient to remove any long-sleeved jacket, shirt or top.	To be able to access the patient's left arm (if possible) for measurement purposes. **E**
10 Measure between the point of the elbow (olecranon process) and the midpoint of the prominent bone of the wrist (styloid process), on the left side if possible (**Action figure 10**).	To obtain a measurement of the length of the ulna. The measurement is taken on the left arm as this is usually the non-dominant arm. **E**
11 Estimate the patient's height to the nearest centimetre, using a conversion table (see Figure 8.12).	To estimate the patient's height (BAPEN 2018a, **C**).
Estimating BMI from mid-upper arm circumference (MUAC)	
12 To estimate BMI from the MUAC, ask the patient to remove any long-sleeved jacket, shirt or top.	To be able to access their left arm (if possible) for measurement purposes (BAPEN 2018a, **C**).
13 Measure the distance between the top of the shoulder (acromion) and the point of the elbow (olecranon process), on the left side if possible (**Action figure 13a**). Identify the midpoint between the two points and mark the arm (**Action figure 13b**).	To obtain the mid-point of the upper arm. The measurement is taken on the left arm as this is usually the non-dominant arm. **E**
14 Ask the patient to let the arm hang loosely by their side and, with a tape measure, measure the circumference of the arm at the midpoint (**Action figure 14**).	To obtain an accurate measurement of the MUAC. **E**
15 Document the measurement.	To record an accurate measurement of the MUAC (BAPEN 2018a, **C**).
16 Estimate the patient's BMI: • If MUAC is <23.5 cm, BMI is likely to be <20 kg/m^2 • If MUAC is >32.0 cm, BMI is likely to be >30 kg/m^2 (BAPEN 2018b)	To estimate the patient's BMI (BAPEN 2018b, **C**).

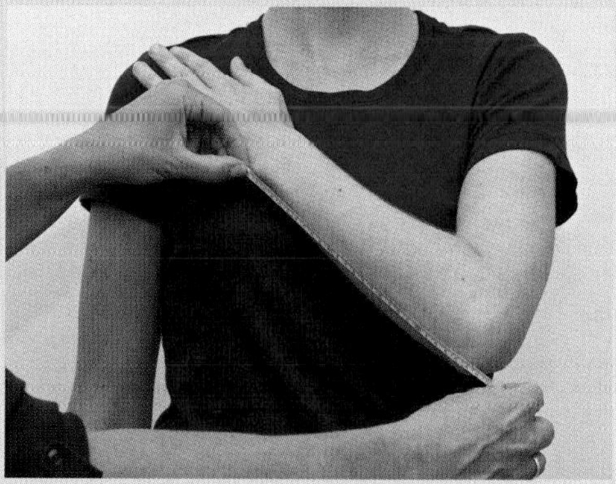

Action Figure 10 Measure between the point of the elbow (olecranon process) and the midpoint of the prominent bone of the wrist (styloid process).

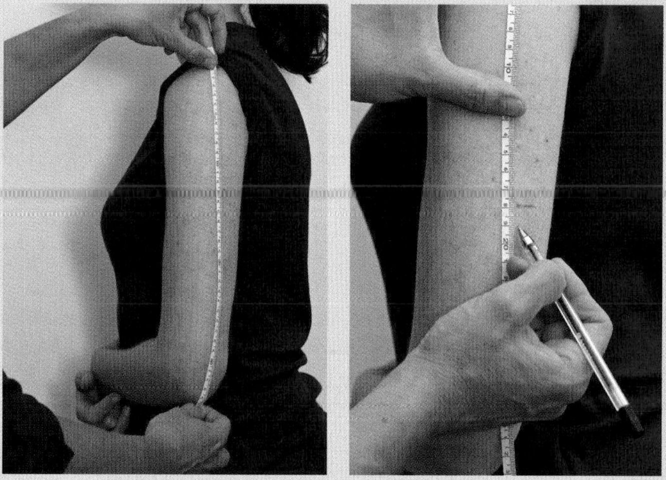

(a) (b)

Action Figure 13 Measure the mid-upper arm circumference (MUAC). (a) Identify the midpoint between the two points. (b) Mark the arm.

(continued)

Procedure guideline 8.8 Measuring the weight and height of a patient *(continued)*

Action	Rationale
Measuring waist circumference	
17 To measure waist circumference, ensure that a tape of adequate length is available. The correct position for measuring waist circumference is midway between the uppermost border of the iliac crest and the lower border of the costal margin (rib cage). The tape should be placed around the abdomen at the level of this midway point and a reading taken when the tape is snug but does not compress the skin (**Action figure 17**).	To obtain an accurate measurement of the waist circumference. Can be used to assess risk of heart disease, diabetes and some cancers (National Obesity Forum 2016, **C**).
Post-procedure	
18 Document height and weight, or estimated BMI, in the patient's notes.	To record the accurate measurement of the patient's height and weight (NMC 2018, **C**).

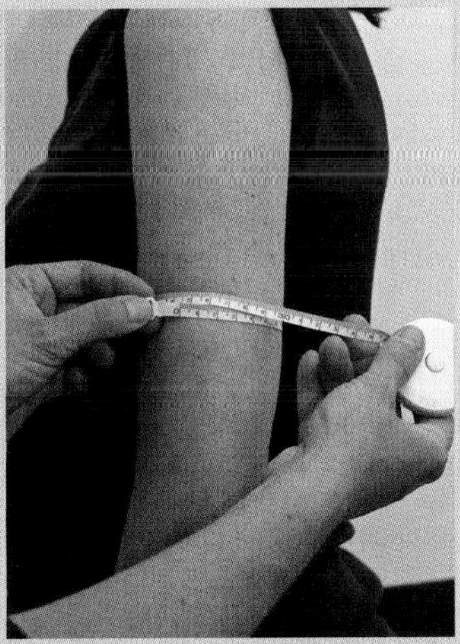

Action Figure 14 Measure the circumference of the arm.

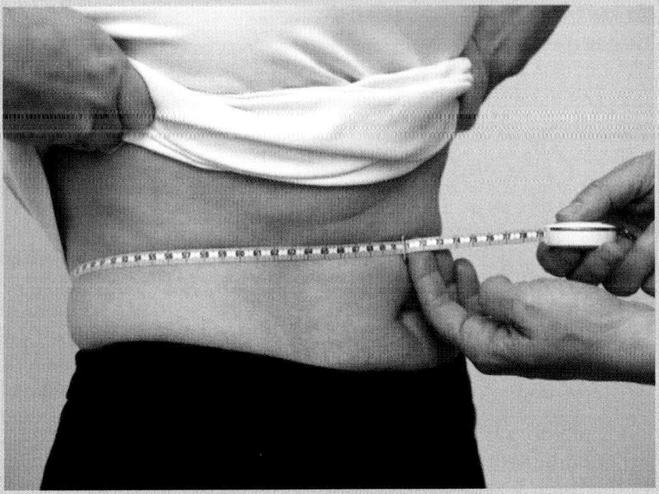

Action Figure 17 Measure the waist circumference.

Problem-solving table 8.2 Prevention and resolution (Procedure guideline 8.8)

Problem	Cause	Prevention	Action
Patient unable to stand on scale	Poorly positioned scales. Patient balance not sufficient.	Prior to asking the patient to stand on the scales, check with them whether they are able to do so. Offer sitting scales if necessary.	Ensure both sitting and standing scales are available in the hospital.
Weight obtained appears too low	Patient may have put pressure on the scales prior to them reaching zero.	Ensure zero is visible before patient touches scales.	Check weight with patient once obtained. Reweigh patient to check correct weight.
Weight obtained appears too high	Patient may be wearing outdoor clothes or shoes or be carrying a bag, drainage bag and so on. Patient may have fluid retention, for example oedema or ascites.	Ensure that the patient is wearing only light indoor clothes before standing on the scales. Check whether patient has fluid retention. Ask patient to empty any drainage bags.	Check weight with patient once obtained. Reweigh patient to check correct weight.
Patient is unable to stand for height measurement	Patient is unwell or has a physical disability.	Discuss the procedure with patient before undertaking height measurement.	Consider estimating height from ulna measurement.
Difficulty obtaining waist circumference in obese patients	Tape measure may not be long enough. Difficulty identifying the correct position to measure waist circumference.	Calculate BMI and if it exceeds 35 kg/m^2 then do not measure waist circumference.	Use BMI alone.

BMI, body mass index.

Post-procedural considerations

Consideration must be given to the patient's weight and whether this reflects a change in their clinical condition. The weight may be being used as part of a nutritional screening or for the planning of treatment, for example medication dosage. Any significant changes should be interpreted in light of potential changes in body composition and incorporated into the patient's care plan. For example, a loss of weight may require further questioning about dietary intake and the commencement of a nutritional care plan.

After taking a measurement of height, it is useful to check with the patient that the figure obtained is approximately the height expected. However, it is important to consider that patients may report a loss in height with increasing years. Cumulative height loss from ages 30 to 70 years may be about 3 cm for men and 5 cm for women, and by age 80 years it can increase to 5 cm for men and 8 cm for women (Sorkin et al. 1999).

Provision of nutritional support: Oral

Evidence-based approaches

Rationale

An essential part of providing diet for a patient is to ensure that they are able to consume the food and fluid in a safe and pleasant environment. Some patients may require assistance with feeding or drinking and a system should be in place to ensure that these patients receive the required attention at each mealtime and beverage service, as well as adapted cutlery or crockery if appropriate. Clear guidance on menu design and content is available via *The Nutrition and Hydration Digest* (BDA 2019). Menus are the ideal way to ensure a patient has choice. Either a cyclical or an à la carte menu can be used. It is important to remember when planning the menu that patients who have long stays may develop menu fatigue, so variety is key. In the UK, *The Eatwell Guide* (PHE 2016) is used to design menus. The standard menu should meet the needs of everybody, from those who are nutritionally well to those who are vulnerable. Coding should be used to assist patients to select suitable options; in the UK this should follow the following format:

- Healthier Eating (H or heart symbol)
- High Energy (E)
- Softer or Easier to Chew (S)
- Vegetarian (V).

Meals should also be available for patients requiring diets based on religious, cultural and lifestyle considerations, those who have allergies; and those who for therapeutic reasons need a modified diet. The International Dysphagia Diet Standardisation Initiative (IDDSI 2018) (Figure 8.13) provides a standardized approach to the assessment and care of patients experiencing dysphagias. This initiative offers toolkits to enable the guidance to be implemented.

It is essential that meals are appetizing and strictly comply with any dietary restriction relevant to the patient. For example, those

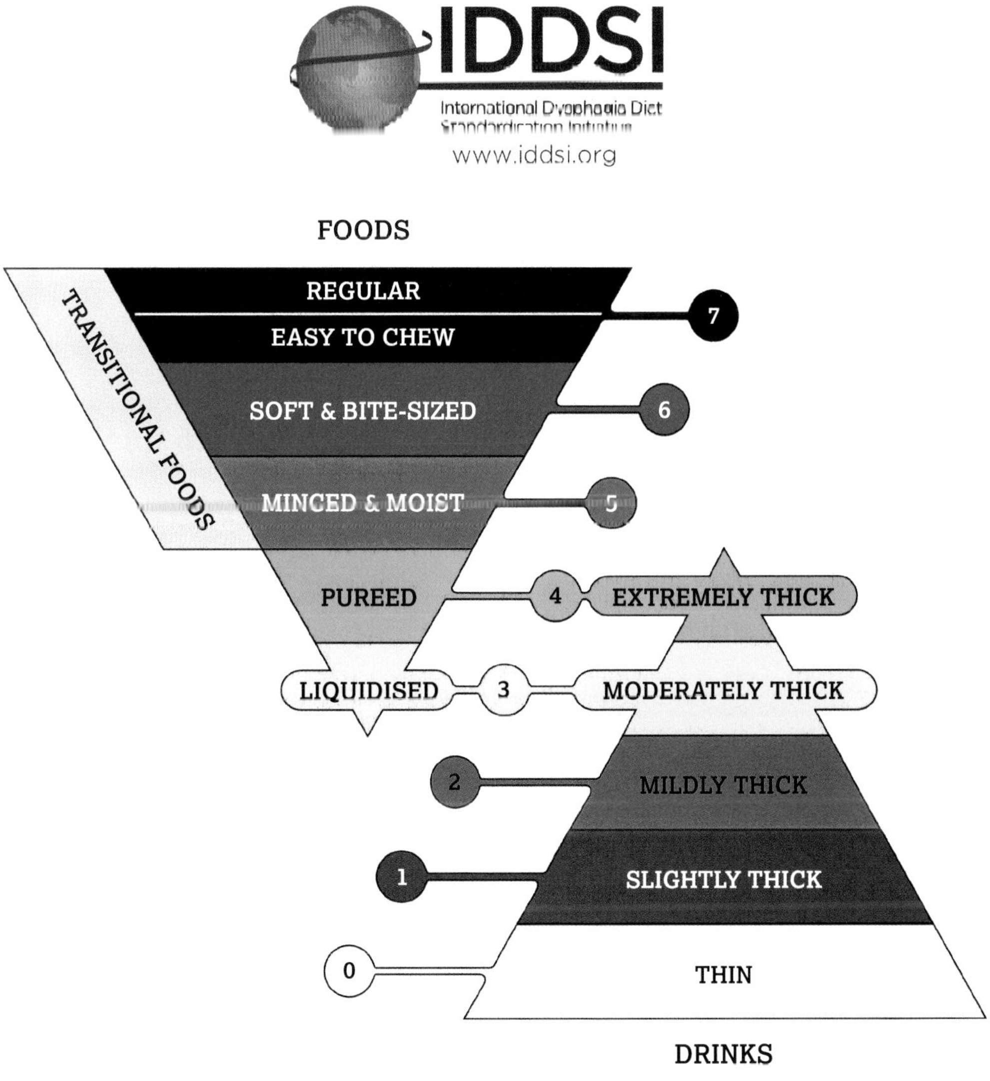

Figure 8.13 The IDDSI framework.

with food allergies, texture modifications, or religious or cultural dietary requirements need to be clearly identified with the senior ward nurse before assistance with feeding commences. Eating and drinking are pleasurable experiences and the psychosocial aspect of this cannot be overestimated. The inability to participate in mealtimes can be socially isolating (Nund et al. 2014a). Research has highlighted that dysphagia also affects carers due to its impact on eating and social activity, and it can lead to permanent changes in lifestyle for both patient and carer (Nund et al. 2014b).

Supporting the patient with feeding requires a patient-centred approach and involving the patient throughout the process (DH 2014).

Provision of food and nutrition in a hospital setting

Good nutritional care, adequate hydration and enjoyable mealtimes can dramatically improve the general health and wellbeing of patients who are unable to feed themselves, and can be particularly relevant to older people (Young et al. 2018). Unfortunately, it is evident that assistance with meals for those who require it does not always occur. In the summary of the results of the 2011 National Inpatients Survey, 15% described the hospital food as 'poor', an increase from 13% in 2010. Of those needing help to eat their meals, 14% did not receive this (NICE 2018).

There are many factors, including being in hospital, that need to be taken into consideration when planning nutritional support. For those in the UK, the Hospital Food Standards Panel published a report (DH 2014) that identified five food standards with which all hospitals should comply, in order to provide the highest quality and nutritional value of food for NHS patients, staff and visitors. The standards are:

- *10 Key Characteristics of 'Good Nutrition and Hydration Care'* (NHS England 2015a)
- *The Nutrition and Hydration Digest* (BDA 2019)
- *The MUST Toolkit* (or equivalent) (BAPEN 2018b)
- *Healthier and More Sustainable Catering: Nutrition Principles* (for staff and visitor catering) (PHE 2017)
- *Sustainable Procurement: The Government Buying Standards for Food and Catering Services* (DEFRA 2015).

Ten factors affecting intake and benchmarks of best practice have been identified to support optimal provision and monitoring of food and drink. These are shown in Box 8.3. The Department of Health and the Nutrition Summit Stakeholder Group have worked together to produce an action plan based on the 10 key characteristics of good nutritional care in hospitals. These are outlined in Box 8.4.

Box 8.3 Food and nutrition benchmark ('food' includes drinks)

Agreed patient-focused outcome

Patients are enabled to consume food (orally) that meets their individual needs.

Indicators/information that highlights concerns that may trigger the need for benchmarking activity

- Patient satisfaction surveys
- Complaints figures and analysis
- Audit results, including catering audit, nutritional risk assessments, documentation audit and environmental audit (including dining facilities)
- Contract monitoring, for example wastage of food, food handling and/or food hygiene training records
- Ordering of dietary supplements and special diets
- Audit of available equipment and utensils
- Educational audits and student placement feedback
- Litigation and the Clinical Negligence Scheme for Trusts
- Professional concern
- Media reports

Source: Adapted from Council of Europe Committee of Ministers (2003) with permission of the Council of Europe.

Box 8.4 10 key characteristics of 'good nutrition and hydration care'

1 All patients are screened on admission to identify the patients who are malnourished or at risk of becoming malnourished. All patients are re-screened weekly.
2 All patients have a care plan which identifies their nutritional care needs and how they are to be met.
3 The hospital includes specific guidance on food services and nutritional care in its clinical governance arrangements.
4 Patients are involved in the planning and monitoring for food service provision.
5 The ward implements protected mealtimes to provide an environment conducive to patients enjoying and being able to eat their food.
6 All staff have the appropriate skills and competencies needed to ensure that patients' nutritional needs are met. All staff receive regular training on nutritional care and management.
7 Hospital facilities are designed to be flexible and patient centred with the aim of providing and delivering an excellent experience of food service and nutritional care 24 hours a day, every day.
8 The hospital has a policy for food service and nutritional care which is patient centred and performance managed in line with governance frameworks.
9 Food service and nutritional care are delivered to the patient safely.
10 The hospital supports a multidisciplinary approach to nutritional care and values the contribution of all staff groups working in partnership with patients and users.

Source: Adapted from NHS England (2015a) with permission of the NHS.

Modification of diet

Various publications provide initial advice for people requiring modification of diet, such as *Have You Got a Small Appetite?* (NDRUK 2016). See also Table 8.8.

Dietary supplements

If patients are unable to meet their nutritional requirements with food alone then they may require dietary supplements. These may be used to improve an inadequate diet or as a sole source of nutrition if taken in sufficient quantity. Table 8.9 summarizes the key features of nutritional supplements currently available.

Specialist supplements

Supplements designed for specific patient groups are also available. For example, there are some aimed at patients with dementia, chronic obstructive pulmonary disease, renal problems or dysphagia.

Vitamin and mineral supplements

When dietary intake is poor, a vitamin and mineral supplement may be required. This can often be given as a one-a-day tablet supplement that provides 100% of the dietary reference values. Care should be taken to avoid unbalanced supplements and those containing amounts larger than the dietary reference value (FSA and Expert Group on Vitamins and Minerals 2003). Excessive doses of vitamins and minerals may be harmful, particularly as some vitamins and minerals are not excreted by the body when taken in amounts exceeding requirements. Additionally, vitamins and minerals may interact with medication to influence its efficacy; for example, vitamin K may influence anticoagulants such as warfarin (NICE 2018).

Patients being discharged from hospital on nutritional supplements

It is important to ensure that patients who require continued oral nutritional supplements in the community are discharged with a suitable supply. The decision on choice of supplement will usually be made by the prescriber and should be based on

Table 8.8 Suggestions for modification of diet

Eating difficulty	Dietary modification
Anorexia	• Serve small meals and snacks, for example twice-daily snack options • Make food look attractive with garnish • Fortify foods with butter, cream or cheese to increase the energy content of meals • Encourage food that patient prefers • Offer nourishing drinks between meals; in hospital, consider a 'cocktail' drinks round
Sore mouth	• Offer foods that are soft and easy to eat • Avoid dry foods that require chewing; choose moist, soft foods • Avoid citrus fruits and drinks • Avoid salty and spicy foods • Allow hot food to cool before the patient eats
Dysphagia	• Refer to or liaise with the speech and language therapy team regarding safe swallowing and modified diet/ fluid recommendations (IDDSI 2018)
Nausea and vomiting	• Offer cold foods in preference to hot as these emit less odour • Keep patient away from cooking smells • Encourage patient to sip fizzy, glucose-containing drinks • Offer small, frequent meals and snacks that are high in carbohydrate (e.g. biscuits and toast) • Offer ginger drinks and ginger biscuits or peppermint sweets or tea
Early satiety	• Offer small, frequent meals; in hospital, access an out-of-hours meal service • Avoid high-fat foods, which delay gastric emptying • Encourage the patient to avoid drinking large quantities when eating • Consider prokinetics, for example metoclopramide, to encourage gastric emptying

Table 8.9 Oral nutritional supplements

Type of supplement	Description	Indications for use*	Practical usage
Nutritionally complete/ supplementary	• Whole protein, milk-based supplements containing vitamins and minerals • Usually 1.5–2.4 kcal/mL and 6–10 g protein/100 mL • Some contain dietary fibre	Standard criteria: • Disease-related malnutrition • Intractable malabsorption • Pre-operative preparation for malnourished patients • Dysphagia • Proven inflammatory bowel disease • Following total gastrectomy • Short bowel syndrome • Bowel fistula	• Usually liquid and available in a bottle; milkshake or yoghurt style • Used to increase energy and protein intake • Used in addition to food or as main source of nutrition, e.g. in dysphagia
	• Fruit-juice-style supplements • Whole protein, generally low in fat • Not full complement of vitamins and minerals • Usually low in fat-soluble vitamins	Standard criteria (as above)	• Liquid available in a bottle • Used to increase protein and energy intake • Used in addition to food • Can be used in recipes, e.g. jelly, and can be blended with other drinks, e.g. lemonade, ginger ale, soda water or tonic water
High protein and energy	• Protein and carbohydrate supplement • Usually small volume, e.g. 30 mL	Biochemically proven hypoproteinaemia	• Liquid available in bottles or sachets • Can be drunk as a 'shot' or added to food and drinks
Protein and fat	• Protein and fat supplement • Usually taken as a small volume, e.g. 40 mL • Contains vitamins and minerals	• Disease-related malnutrition • Malabsorption states • Other conditions requiring fortification with a high-fat or high-carbohydrate (with protein) supplement	• Can be drunk as a 'shot' or added to food and drinks
Protein, fat and carbohydrate	• Protein (cows' milk) • Fat and carbohydrate supplement as a powder • Not full complement of vitamins and minerals	• Disease-related malnutrition • Malabsorption states • Other conditions requiring fortification with a high-fat or high-carbohydrate (with protein) supplement	• Usually presented as a powder that is reconstituted with whole milk and provides approximately 2 kcal/mL • Often has a sweet flavour and is made into a milkshake, but manufacturers' recipes include ice cream, and fortification of soup, desserts and cakes • Some savoury flavours available

* UK Advisory Committee on Borderline Substances (ACBS) criteria (BAPEN 2016a)

Source: Adapted from Shaw and Eldridge (2015).

clinical need and patient acceptability. Where more than one suitable option is available, the ease of use in a community setting, likely compliance and the impact on primary care budgets may be factors to be weighed up in the choice of supplement. Clear guidance should be given to the prescriber in the community, including on the anticipated outcome and duration of need. Monitoring should also be put in place to ensure that the use of oral nutritional supplements remains appropriate, that they are being tolerated and that the nutritional status of the patient is changing in accordance with the goals set by the patient and healthcare professional.

Anticipated patient outcomes

It is anticipated that feeding an adult will ensure safe delivery of the meal in a comfortable environment such that the patient has a pleasurable and positive experience, promoting adequate nutritional care.

Clinical governance

Protected mealtimes should be in place on wards, whereby all non-essential clinical activities are discontinued and a calm environment exists (Age UK 2016). The use of protected mealtimes within hospitals is strongly encouraged and trusts should have an appropriate policy in place to monitor and audit its implementation on wards. The Care Quality Commission carried out a dignity and nutrition inspection programme in 2012 and found that protected mealtimes was one of the contributing factors in encouraging support for patients to eat and drink sufficient amounts in hospitals, achieving the standard of 'meeting people's nutritional needs' (Care Quality Commission 2013). However, research suggests that the UK requirement for protected mealtimes may not have an impact on energy and protein intake as it was designed to do, and further reviews are required (Porter et al. 2017).

Pre-procedural considerations

Sufficient staff need to be available to support those who need help with eating and drinking. Patients who require assistance should be identified through screening and a discreet signal should be evident to identify that further assistance is required, for example a red tray, a coloured serviette or a red sticker (BDA 2016).

Specific patient preparation

Before commencing assistance, discuss this with the patient in order that they understand and consent to assistance being provided. When verbal communication is not possible, non-verbal agreement needs to be obtained wherever possible. Try to engage the patient in the feeding process and interpret and record any preferences or dislikes they may express regarding the meal process.

Prior to eating, make sure the patient has the opportunity to visit the bathroom, to wash or clean their hands with an antiseptic wipe, and to undertake any appropriate mouth care. Establish whether any medication is to be administered prior to or after feeding that will facilitate the feeding and digestive process.

Individual symptoms should be assessed; for example, if patients are nauseous they may benefit from the prescribing and administering of antiemetics or prokinetic agents. Patients who have pancreatic insufficiency may require pancreatic enzyme replacements. The timing in relation to feeding is important and antiemetics should be given approximately 30 minutes prior to meal service. Any special equipment, such as cutlery or non-slip mats, that is required to assist the patient with the meal should be provided. This may require referral to an occupational therapist for an assessment.

If the patient has dysphagia, ensure that the diet textures are as recommended for the patient by the speech and language therapy team as per the International Dysphagia Diet Standardisation Initiative (IDDSI 2018) (see Figure 8.13). This is in line with National Patient Safety Alert NHS/PSA/RE/2018/004 (NHSI 2018).

Procedure guideline 8.9 Feeding an adult patient

Essential equipment

- Personal protective equipment
- A clean table or tray
- Equipment required to assist the patient, such as adequate drinking water, adapted cups, cutlery and napkin
- A chair

Action	Rationale
Pre-procedure	
1 Ascertain whether the patient has dysphagia and is on a modified diet.	All foods and fluids given must comply with diet modification recommendations from the International Dysphagia Diet Standardisation Initiative (IDDSI 2018, **C**), which has developed a standard terminology with a colour and numerical index to describe texture modification for food and drink to reduce risk to patient safety (NHSI 2018, **C**).
2 Introduce yourself to the patient, explain and discuss the procedure with them, and gain their consent to proceed.	To ensure that the patient feels at ease, understands the procedure and gives their valid consent (NMC 2018, **C**).
3 Wash hands or clean them with an alcohol-based gel, and apply personal protective equipment.	To ensure that the procedure is as clean as possible and prevent cross-infection (NHS England and NHSI 2019, **C**).
4 Ensure that the patient is comfortable – that is, that they have an empty bladder, clean hands, a clean mouth and, if applicable, clean dentures. Ensure there are no unpleasant sights or smells that would put the patient off eating.	To make the mealtime a pleasant experience (Age UK 2016, **E**).
5 Position yourself in front of the patient or to their side and seated at the patient's level to assist with feeding.	To enable the patient and helper to see each other and to assist communication. **E**
6 Ensure that the patient is sitting upright in a supported midline position, preferably in a chair (if it is safe and appropriate) and at a table.	To facilitate swallowing and protect the airway. **E**
7 Protect the patient's clothing with a napkin.	To maintain dignity and cleanliness. **E**

Procedure		
8	Assist the patient to take appropriate portions of food at the correct temperature but encourage self-feeding. Tailor the size of each mouthful to the individual patient. If possible, each hot course of a meal should be served individually and items that may change in consistency, such as ice cream, served separately.	To make the mealtime a pleasant experience. To maintain textures of foods. To ensure that swallowing is not compromised if the patient feels that they must hurry with the meal (Young et al. 2018, **E**).
9	Allow the patient to chew and swallow foods before the next mouthful. Avoid hovering with the next spoonful.	To maintain the dignity of the patient and prevent them from rushing. **E**
10	Avoid asking questions when the patient is eating, but check between mouthfuls that the food is suitable and that the patient is able to continue with the meal.	To reduce the risk of the patient aspirating, which may be increased if they speak while eating. **E**
11	Use the napkin to remove particles of food or drink from the patient's face.	To maintain dignity and cleanliness. **E**
12	Ask the patient when they wish to have a drink. Assist the patient to take a sip. Support the glass or cup gently so that the flow of liquid is controlled or use a straw if this is helpful. Take care with hot drinks to avoid offering these when too hot to drink.	To give the opportunity for the patient to swallow. Hot liquids may scald the patient. **E**
13	If the food appears too dry, ask the patient whether they would like some additional gravy or sauce added to the dish (except when a modified diet is recommended and additional gravy or sauce is not permitted).	To facilitate chewing and swallowing (Wright et al. 2008, **E**). All foods and fluids given must comply with diet modification recommendations (IDDSI 2018, **C**).
14	Observe the patient for coughing, choking, wet or gurgly voice, nasal regurgitation or effortful swallow. See Table 8.10 for details of problems that may be experienced by patients.	May indicate aspiration, laryngeal penetration or weakness in the muscles required for swallowing (Langmore et al. 1998, **E**; Leslie et al. 2003, **E**).
15	Encourage the patient to take as much food as they feel able to eat, but do not press them if they indicate that they have eaten enough.	To improve nutritional intake but also maintain patient dignity and choice (Wright et al. 2008, **E**).
Post-procedure		
16	After the meal, assist the patient to meet their hygiene needs, for example wash hands and face and clean teeth.	To maintain cleanliness and dignity. **E**
17	If intake is being monitored then record what food was eaten on a food chart.	To provide essential monitoring of intake (BDA 2019, **C**).

Post-procedural considerations

Education of the patient and relevant others

It is important that volunteers, family members and visitors who wish to assist the patient with feeding are familiar with and trained in the processes listed in Procedure guideline 8.9: Feeding an adult patient. This is to ensure they are confident and can safely and effectively assist the patient.

Assessment, recording tools and plate wastage

Food waste must be monitored at all stages of production and service. Waste audits, both qualitative and quantitative, can be used to measure cost, food acceptability and nutritional intake. Standard audits can be devised and acceptable levels of waste set locally (BDA 2019). There should be regular patient satisfaction questionnaires on the quality of food as evidence for the Care Quality Commission (Care Quality Commission 2013).

Food and dietary intake record charts can be used to monitor a patient's intake. These will provide essential information that forms the basis of a nutritional assessment and will determine subsequent nutritional care. It is frequently not evident how much a patient is eating, particularly on busy wards with regular staff changes. Record charts are therefore a valuable resource for dietitians, nurses and ultimately the patient (BDA 2019). They can be used to assess whether the patient is eating and drinking enough, thereby enabling action to be taken to encourage intake in those who have a reduced dietary intake.

Intake changes as a result of disease, symptoms, medication, unfamiliar surroundings and food availability can be further compounded if there are difficulties observed with eating and drinking. Close monitoring of oral intake is essential, especially if weight loss is evident or concerns are expressed by the patient, staff and/or relatives regarding the patient's nutritional intake. An exception to this is when a patient is receiving end-of-life care and it has been clarified with the clinical team that active nutritional support is not appropriate.

The objective is to quantify the amount of food and drink (including oral nutritional supplements) consumed by a patient over an agreed time period.

Key points that should be considered include the following:

- All screening, including food charts, should be linked to a care plan and documented in the patient's notes (BDA 2019, DH 2014).
- Food charts should be available on all wards and should be simple to complete. Household measures (such as tablespoons, slices of bread or hospital portions) can assist with the speed of completion.
- Training should be given on how the chart should be completed; this training should preferably be provided by the dietitian or specialist nutrition nurse. This will facilitate understanding of the rationale and continuity of recording and improve accuracy.
- Institutions must decide whose responsibility it is to complete the charts (nurse, nursing associate, healthcare assistant or ward catering staff) to avoid confusion. Some patients may be able to complete the record themselves if given guidance on what is required.

Table 8.10 Difficulties that may be experienced by patients during eating and drinking and their potential implications

Difficulty experienced	Implications
Coughing and choking during and after eating and/or drinking	Indicates laryngeal penetration or aspiration (Langmore et al. 1998; Smith Hammond [illegible]).
Wet or gurgly voice quality	Indicates laryngeal penetration or aspiration (Langmore et al. 1998).
Drooling/excess oral secretions	Indicates less frequent swallowing and is associated with dysphagia (Langmore et al. 1998). May result from poor lip seal.
Nasal regurgitation	Indicates impaired velopalatal seal (Leslie et al. 2003).
Food/drink pooling in mouth	Indicates lack of oral sensation from intraoral flaps or may be a sign of cognitive impairment (Logemann 1998).
Swallow is effortful	May indicate weakness in muscles required for swallowing (Logemann et al. 1997).
Respiration rate on eating/drinking is increased	Increased respiration rate may be associated with risk of aspiration (Leslie et al. 2003).
Signs of recurrent chest infections and pyrexia	This may indicate aspiration pneumonia as a consequence of dysphagia (Leslie et al. 2003).
Patient reports swallowing problems	Patient-reported outcome (PRO) measures are commonly used to capture patient experience with dysphagia and to evaluate treatment effectiveness (Patel et al. 2017).
Patient reports food sticking	Patient-reported outcome (PRO) measures are commonly used to capture patient experience with dysphagia and to evaluate treatment effectiveness (Patel et al. 2017).
Additional time required to eat a meal	Taking a long time to eat may indicate dysphagia (Leslie et al. 2003).
Avoidance of certain foods	Patients will avoid food items that they find difficult to swallow (Leslie et al. 2003).
Weight loss	Patients may eat less due to difficulty swallowing (Leslie et al. 2003).
Poor oral hygiene	Aspiration of secretions in those with poor oral hygiene may result in aspiration pneumonia (Langmore 2001).

- Charts need to be carefully completed over a minimum of 2–3 consecutive days, or longer if requested by the dietitian.
- All food record charts that have been reviewed by a healthcare professional should be signed and dated on completion of review.
- If there is strong concern about the quantity of food that has been consumed by the patient, this must be verbally relayed to the nurse in charge, ward dietitian and managing team.
- Difficulties arise when food chart data are not accurately completed or reviewed, during which time malnutrition and its consequences continue, rather than being quickly identified and addressed.

Nutritional management of patients with dysphagia

Definition

Dysphagia is an impairment of swallowing that may involve any structure from the lips to the gastric cardia (Espitalier et al. 2018).

Evidence-based approaches

Rationale

Indications

Patients who are at high risk of dysphagia are summarized in Box 8.5.

Goals of clinical assessment

It is important to correctly ascertain the presence of dysphagia and the factors contributing to its possible aetiology. Such patients may be at risk of aspiration and subsequent chest infections and therefore require a referral to a speech and language therapist (SLT) for a full assessment ([illegible] 2018). These patients also require a nutritional assessment from a dietician to ascertain the need for enteral tube feeding if they are unable to maintain an adequate nutritional intake or are at risk of aspiration. A suitable swallowing rehabilitation programme should be developed.

Box 8.5 Patient groups at high risk of dysphagia

- Head and neck cancer patients undergoing surgery and/or radiotherapy/chemoradiotherapy. The risk of dysphagia is increased with multimodal therapy. Swallow function may be affected by side-effects of treatment, such as xerostomia (dry mouth), odynophagia (pain on swallowing), thick oral secretions, nausea, candidiasis, taste changes, mucositis, fatigue, fibrosis and trismus (reduced mouth opening). Nutritional support with enteral tube feeding may be required.
- Patients with neurological involvement including brain tumours or metastases, or other co-morbid neurological disorders, for example cerebrovascular accident, multiple sclerosis, motor neurone disease, Parkinson's disease or myasthenia gravis. Such patients may also have cognitive or behavioural issues that can affect their mood, motivation, feeding and appetite.
- Patients with lung cancer and vocal cord paralysis and respiratory disorders such as chronic obstructive pulmonary disease, including mechanically ventilated patients.
- Tracheostomy patients may present with swallowing problems, although frequently their medical diagnosis is the primary cause of dysphagia.
- Gastrointestinal patients may present with oropharyngeal or oesophageal dysphagia.
- Any other patient with significant generalized weakness or other co-morbidities, including critical care and palliative care patients.
- Patients with psychogenic dysphagia.
- Laryngectomy patients and particularly pharyngolaryngectomy and pharyngo-laryngo-oesophagectomy patients. Some patients may experience dysphagia due to altered anatomy after surgery.

Source: Adapted from Brady et al. (2015), Brodsky et al. (2014), Coffey and Tolley (2015), Groher and Crary ([illegible]), Patterson et al. ([illegible]).

Patients undergoing surgery or radiotherapy for head and neck cancer should have a baseline clinical swallowing evaluation before treatment (Jones et al. 2016).

Principles of care

Care will be influenced by the timing of the patient's referral, depending on their disease and treatment status. Management of dysphagic patients will be tailored to individual needs and they will require regular reviews to ensure that intervention and management decisions remain appropriate. The nature of the dysphagia may persist, recur or worsen depending on the patient's treatment or disease.

Treatment options may include normal diet with specifically targeted therapy techniques, modified diet, combination of alternative feeding and limited oral intake, or nil by mouth. For patients with oropharyngeal dysphagia, dysphagia food texture descriptors have been developed and updated to provide industry and in-house caterers with detailed guidance on categories of food texture, thereby enhancing patient safety (Cichero et al. 2017). For patients undergoing radiotherapy for head and neck cancer, it may be appropriate to implement a programme of prophylactic swallowing exercises (Cappell et al. 2009, Paleri et al. 2014).

Close liaison between the nursing staff, dieticians and members of the multidisciplinary team is essential. The SLT may recommend that the patient adopts certain compensatory swallow techniques to reduce the risk of aspiration or eliminate discomfort. Exercises or swallow techniques may be given to the patient to rehabilitate their swallow (Groher and Crary 2015). It is important for nurses to participate in educational programmes for patients and carers in order to improve awareness of the implications of dysphagia. Nurses may be required to supervise patients with oral intake and encourage their participation with regard to therapy exercises, and reduce other risk factors by encouraging good mouth care and independent feeding.

Methods of assessment

Clinical swallow assessment

In any patient presenting with a new onset of dysphagia, a medical review is necessary as this may be the first indicator of a change in disease or condition. A subsequent specialist SLT referral is then necessary. The SLT will take a comprehensive case history including subjective reports as well as medical, physical and mental status. Surgical and/or disease details will be determined, including where the patient is on the care pathway, for example pre-operative, post-operative, or receiving treatment, medication or palliative care. An examination of the oral cavity and cranial nerve assessment will be carried out to evaluate motor and sensory function associated with swallowing (Figure 8.14). Food and drink trials may be carried out by the SLT. The clinical swallowing evaluation may include tests such as the 100 mL Water Swallow Test (Patterson and Wilson 2011).

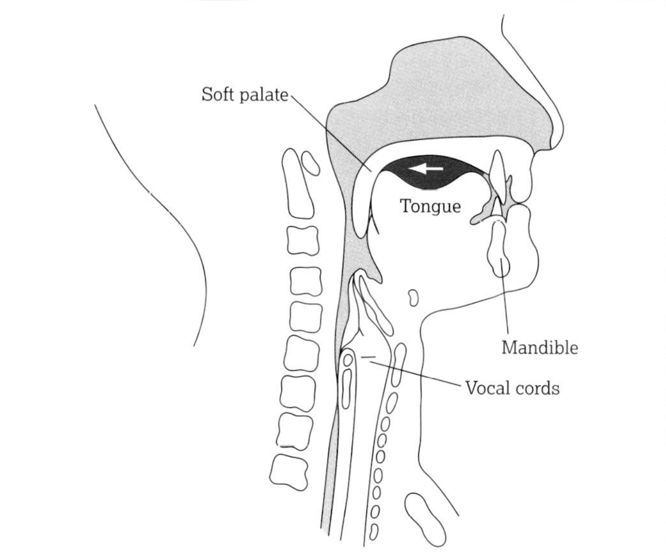

Figure 8.14 The oral stage of swallowing.

Instrumental swallowing evaluation

Following an initial assessment, the SLT may recommend instrumental assessments to evaluate in detail the nature and extent of any swallowing disorder. Silent aspiration is a particular issue and, in the absence of any overt clinical signs of aspiration or relevant medical history (such as frequent chest infections), instrumental evaluation will be the most appropriate way to identify the problem and its cause. The SLT can implement a range of compensatory strategies during these assessments to optimize swallowing function and minimize the risk of aspiration where possible. By observing swallowing biomechanics, SLTs will be able to define rehabilitation targets. A number of instrumental assessments of swallowing are available but videofluoroscopy (modified barium swallow) and fibreoptic endoscopic evaluation of swallowing (FEES) are the most commonly used (Roe 2012). Videofluoroscopy takes place in the X-ray department and involves the use of radio-opaque contrast mixed with food (Logemann 1998). FEES involves the use of an endoscope passed transnasally, allowing a view of the swallow process while a patient eats and drinks (Langmore 2001). These assessments should be selected on a patient-by-patient basis and in the knowledge that each method has its own particular advantages and limitations (Roe 2012).

Anticipated patient outcomes

Early identification of dysphagia and appropriate management are essential parts of patient care. Appropriate management aims to reduce the incidence of aspiration and the risk of aspiration pneumonia and to help maintain adequate nutrition. Potential complications of poorly managed dysphagia include malnutrition, weight loss and dehydration, aspiration and aspiration pneumonia, low mood, reduced quality of life and increased length of hospital stay (Groher and Crary 2015). Ensuring the patient has a clear understanding of their swallowing difficulty is essential and may help them to become a motivated rehabilitation partner (Roe and Ashforth 2011).

Enteral tube feeding

Definition

Enteral tube feeding refers to the delivery of a nutritionally complete feed (containing protein, fat, carbohydrate, vitamins, minerals, fluid and possibly dietary fibre) directly into the gastrointestinal tract via a tube. The tube is usually placed into the stomach, duodenum or jejunum via either the nose or a direct percutaneous route (NCCAC 2006).

Related theory

Enteral feeding tubes allow direct access to the gastrointestinal tract for the purposes of feeding. A nasogastric or nasojejunal tube is placed via the nose and passed down the oesophagus with the feeding tip ending in the stomach (gastric) or small intestine (jejunum) respectively. A gastrostomy tube is placed directly into the stomach, allowing infusion of nutrients into the stomach or, alternatively, such tubes may have a jejunal extension passing through the pylorus, allowing feeding into the jejunum (small intestine). A jejunostomy tube allows direct access to the jejunum for feeding.

The choice of tube should be based on the method of insertion and the associated risks, the length of time feeding is required, the function of the gastrointestinal tract, the physical condition of the patient and body image issues relating to the visibility of the feeding tube. The feeding regimen, care of the tube and stoma will depend on the enteral feeding tube inserted and should be undertaken within the care of a multiprofessional team (Majka et al. 2013, NCCAC 2006).

Evidence-based approaches

Rationale

While the majority of patients will be able to meet their nutritional requirements orally, there is a group of individuals who will require enteral tube feeding either in the short term or on a longer term basis (Hickson and Smith 2018, Weimann et al. 2017).

The primary aim of enteral tube feeding is to:

- meet nutritional requirements
- avoid further loss of bodyweight or improve nutritional status
- correct significant nutritional deficiencies
- maintain hydration
- stop the related deterioration of quality of life of the patient due to inadequate oral nutritional intake.

Indications

Indications for enteral tube feeding are as follows:

- patient is unable to meet nutritional needs through oral intake alone
- the gastrointestinal tract is accessible and functioning
- it is anticipated that intestinal absorptive function will meet all nutritional needs (NCCAC 2006).

Pre-procedural considerations

Equipment

Types of enteral feeding tube

Nasogastric/nasojejunal

Nasogastric feeding is the most commonly used type of enteral tube feeding and is suitable for short-term feeding – that is, 2–4 weeks (NCCAC 2006). Nasogastric and nasojejunal tubes (Figures 8.15 and 8.16) must be radio-opaque throughout their length and have externally visible length markings. Fine-bore feeding tubes should be used whenever possible as these are more comfortable for the patient than wide-bore tubes. They are also less likely to cause complications such as rhinitis, oesophageal irritation and gastritis. Polyurethane or silicone tubes are preferable to polyvinyl chloride (PVC) tubes as they withstand gastric acid and can stay in position longer than the 10 to 14 day lifespan of the PVC tube (Payne-James et al. 2001).

Gastrostomy

A gastrostomy may be more appropriate than a nasogastric tube when enteral tube feeding is anticipated to last longer than 4 weeks. It avoids delays in feeding and discomfort associated with tube displacement (NCCAC 2006).

A gastrostomy tube may be placed endoscopically (percutaneous endoscopically placed gastrostomy (PEG)) or radiologically (radiologically inserted gastrostomy (RIG)). PEG tubes may be placed while the patient is sedated, thereby avoiding the risks associated with general anaesthesia.

Certain groups of patients are not suitable for endoscopy; in these cases a RIG can be used. They are indicated for patients with oesophageal cancer with bulky tumours where it would be difficult to pass an endoscope and also for patients with a head and neck cancer whose airway would be obstructed by an endoscope. There is also a documented risk of the endoscope seeding the tumour to the gastrostomy site when it pulls the tube past a bulky tumour, although this is a rare complication (Cruz et al. 2005).

The tubes are made from polyurethane or silicone and are therefore suitable for short- and long-term feeding. A flange, flexible dome, bumper, inflated balloon or pigtail sits within the stomach and holds the tube in position (Figure 8.17). Post insertion, T-fasteners (Figure 8.18) are used to anchor the abdominal wall to the gastric wall until the gastrostomy tract is formed. For guidance on how to remove these, see Procedure guideline 8.14: Removal of T-fasteners.

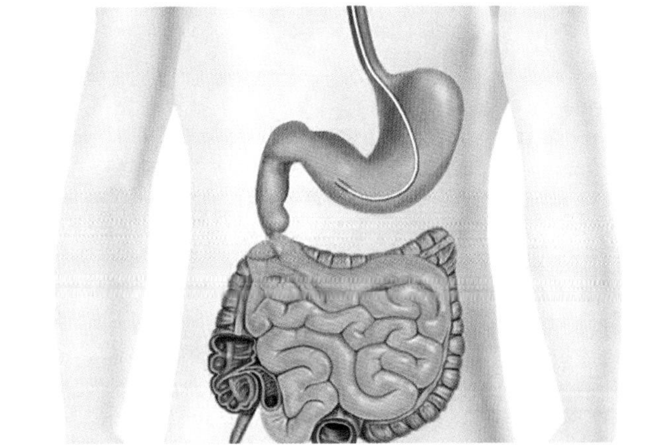

Figure 8.15 Nasogastric tube *in situ*. *Source*: Lord (2018).

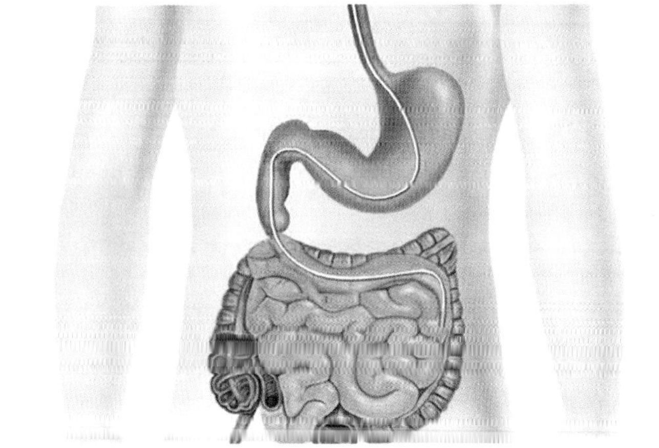

Figure 8.16 Nasojejunal tube *in situ*. *Source*: Lord (2018).

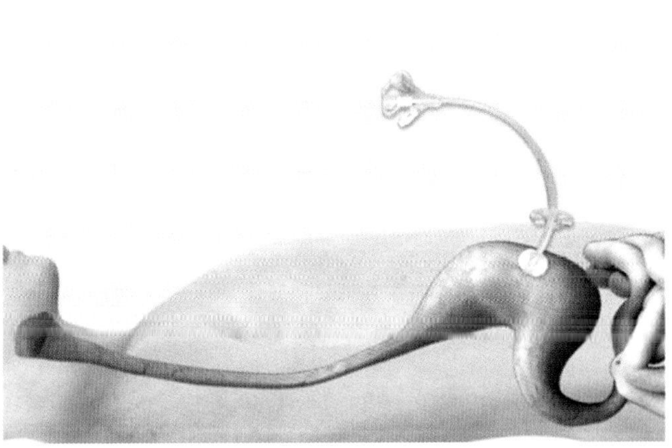

Figure 8.17 Gastrostomy tube *in situ*. *Source*: Lord (2018).

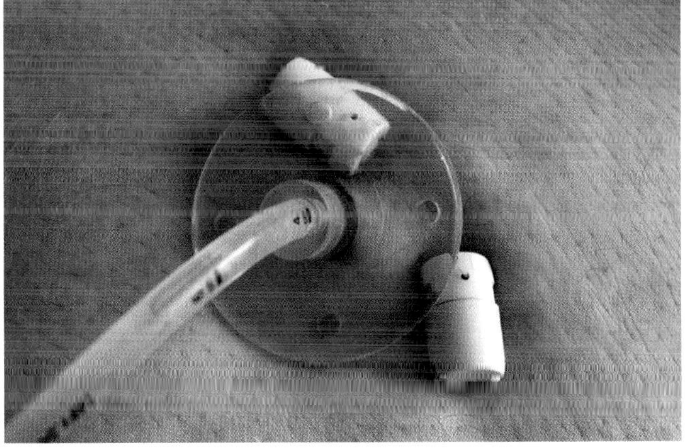

Figure 8.18 Radiologically inserted gastrostomy (RIG) with T-fasteners in place.

For longer-term feeding, a low-profile gastrostomy (Figure 8.19) or 'button' may be considered. This has the advantage of being less bulky and is therefore easier to conceal under clothing. A low-profile device contains a valve to prevent reflux of gastric contents through the device. Access through the device is obtained by an extension set that opens the valve, allowing administration of fluids or feed via a syringe or giving set. If the button has a balloon retention device then this must be checked regularly in line with the manufacturer's recommendations to ensure that any leaked fluid is replaced and that the balloon has maintained its integrity.

Jejunostomy

A jejunostomy is preferable to a gastrostomy if a patient has undergone upper gastrointestinal surgery or has severe delayed gastric emptying; in some cases it can be used to feed a patient with pyloric obstruction (Gandy 2014). Fine-bore feeding jejunostomy tubes may be inserted surgically or laparoscopically with the use of a jejunostomy kit, which consists of a needle-fine catheter. The use of needles and an introducer wire allows a fine-bore polyurethane catheter to be inserted into a loop of jejunum. Alternatively, some gastrostomy tubes allow the passage of a fine-bore tube through the pylorus and into the jejunum. A double-lumen tube allows aspiration of stomach contents while feed is administered into the small intestine. This is known as transgastric feeding (Toh Yoon et al. 2016).

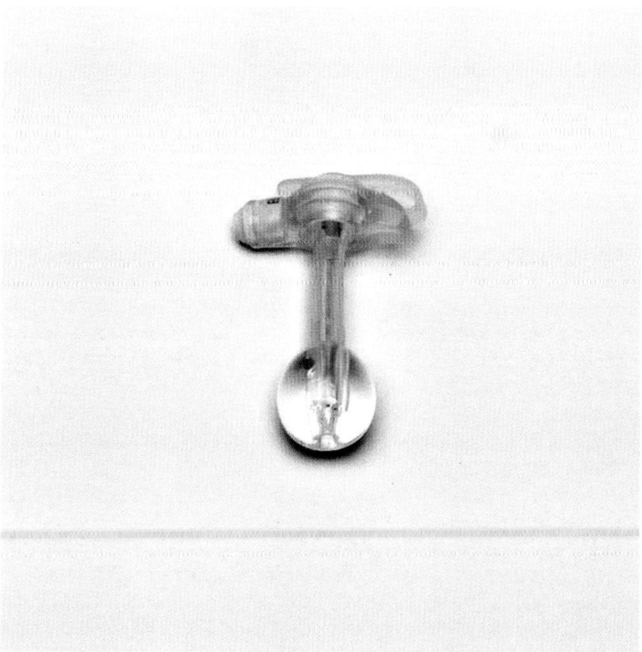

Figure 8.19 Low-profile gastrostomy. *Source*: Lord (2018).

Enteral feeding equipment

The administration of enteral feeds may be as a bolus, via intermittent or continuous infusion, via gravity drip or pump assisted (Table 8.11). There are many enteral feeding pumps available and they vary in their flow rates from 1 to 300 mL per hour. The following systems may be used for feeding via a pump or gravity drip:

- The 'ready-to-hang' system has a plastic bottle or pack attached directly to the administration set. The bottles and packs are available in different types of feeds and sizes for flexibility. This is a closed sterile system and it has been shown to be successful in preventing exogenous bacterial contamination (NICE 2012).
- For powdered feeds that require reconstitution with water, the feed is decanted into plastic bottles or PVC bags. The administration set may be an integral part of the bag or may be supplied separately. The feed is sterile until opened, and decanting feed into these bottles or PVC bags may increase the risk of contamination of the feed from handling (Payne-James et al. 2001). Malnourished and immunocompromised patients are particularly at risk from contamination and infection so this method of administration should be avoided in those patients where possible (NICE 2012).

ENFit

ENFit is an international safety initiative (ISO 80369-3) (Figure 8.20) applicable to all enteral feeding devices (e.g. feeding tubes, giving sets, enteral syringes and some Ryles tube drainage bags) that makes the connections of these devices incompatible with intravenous devices (EPSG 2016). A charitable organization (Global Enteral Device Supplier Association) has been set up to introduce the change and set international standards. This global change should reduce the risk of wrong route administration.

There is currently a period of transition where some patients who have long-term indwelling feeding tubes still have a non-ENFit connection. For these tubes an adapter is required to enable connection with feeding ancillaries such as giving sets and syringes. The adapters are a temporary step and will be withdrawn from the market at some stage. The dietitian responsible for the overall management of the patient must ensure that a suitable ENFit connection replaces any old connections still in use. This should be done before the manufacturers stop supplying adapters to the market.

Enteral feeds

Commercially prepared feeds should be used for nasogastric, gastrostomy and jejunostomy feeding. Available in liquid or powder form, they have the advantage of being of known composition and are sterile when packaged. Enteral feeds can be nutritionally complete when given in the advised quantity and can be used as a sole source of nutrition or to supplement the patient's oral intake.

Whole protein/polymeric feeds

These contain protein, lipids in the form of long-chain triglycerides (LCTs) and carbohydrate and so require digestion. As the energy density of the feed increases, so does the osmolarity. Hyperosmolar

Table 8.11 Methods of administering enteral feeds

Feeding regimen	Advantages	Disadvantages
Continuous feeding via a pump	• Easily controlled rate • Reduction of gastrointestinal (GI) complications	• Patient connected to the feed for majority of the day • May limit patient's mobility
Intermittent feeding via gravity or a pump	• Periods of time free of feeding • Flexible feeding routine • May be easier than managing a pump for some patients	• May have an increased risk of GI symptoms, for example early satiety • Difficult if outside carers are involved with the feed
Bolus feeding	• May reduce time connected to feed • Easy to administer via a syringe • Minimal equipment required	• May have an increased risk of GI symptoms • May be time consuming

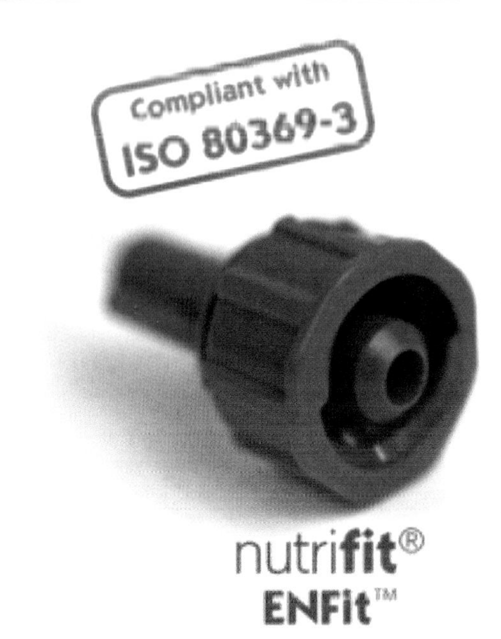

Figure 8.20 ENFit connector.

feeds tend to draw water into the lumen of the gut from the bloodstream and can contribute to diarrhoea if given too rapidly. Fibre may be beneficial for maintaining gut ecology and function, rather than promoting bowel transit time (Lever et al. 2019).

Feeds containing medium-chain triglycerides

In some whole-protein feeds, a proportion of the fat or LCTs may be replaced with medium-chain triglycerides (MCTs). These feeds often have a lower osmolarity and are therefore less likely to draw fluid from the plasma into the gut lumen. MCTs are transported via the portal vein rather than the lymphatic system. These feeds are suitable for patients with fat malabsorption and perhaps steatorrhoea (Hilal et al. 2013).

Elemental/peptide feeds

These contain free amino acids, short chain peptides or a combination of both as the nitrogen source. They are often low in fat or may contain some fat as MCTs. Glucose polymers provide the main energy source. These feeds require little or no digestion and are suitable for patients with impaired gastrointestinal function, maldigestion or malabsorption (Gandy 2014). They are hyperosmolar and low in residue.

Special application feeds

These feeds have altered nutrients for particular clinical conditions. Low-protein and low-mineral feeds may be used for patients with renal failure. High-fat, low-carbohydrate feeds may be used for ventilated patients because less carbon dioxide is produced per calorie of intake compared with a low-fat, high-carbohydrate feed. Very high-energy and high-protein feeds may be used where nutritional requirements are exceptionally high, for example in patients with burns or severe sepsis. These feeds contain approximately double the amount of energy and protein compared to standard whole-protein feeds.

Paediatric feeds

These are designed for children aged 1–12 years and/or 8–45 kg in weight. The protein, vitamin and mineral profile is suitable for children. Generally they are lower in osmolarity than adult feeds. The whole-protein/polymeric feeds are based on cows' milk but are lactose free. Some of these feeds contain dietary fibre. These feeds provide 1.0–1.5 kcal/mL for children who require additional energy and protein in a smaller volume. Hydrolysed protein feeds and elemental feeds are used in conditions such as food allergies and malabsorption. The osmolarity of these feeds is higher than whole protein feeds. They need to be introduced carefully (Gandy 2014).

Immune-modulating feeds

There is evidence to show that the addition of glutamine, arginine or omega-3 fatty acids, if given pre-operatively, may benefit post-surgical gastrointestinal patients by reducing the risk of post-operative infections (Arends et al. 2017). These specialized liquids may be given pre- or post-operatively. Up-to-date information on the exact composition of dietary supplements and enteral feeds can be obtained from the manufacturers.

Nasogastric tube insertion

Evidence-based approaches

Rationale

It is essential that the position of the nasogastric tube is confirmed prior to feeding to ensure that it has been placed safely in the gastrointestinal tract and has not been inadvertently placed in the lungs. Inadvertent placement of the tube would result in the risk of fluid or feed being administered to the lungs – a potentially life-threatening situation.

Indications

Nasogastric tube insertion is indicated for patients who require short-term enteral tube feeding (2–4 weeks) as a sole source of nutrition or for supplementary feeding.

Contraindications

Nasogastric tube insertion is contraindicated for:

- patients who require long-term enteral tube feeding, in whom it may be more appropriate to use a gastrostomy tube
- patients with an altered anatomy that would make it impossible to pass a nasogastric tube comfortably.

Careful consideration should also be given to patients with coagulation disorders, who should have their blood clotting checked by the medical team and appropriate blood products administered if required prior to insertion.

Anticipated patient outcomes

The patient has a nasogastric tube inserted comfortably and safely. The position is checked and it is confirmed that the tube is placed in the stomach.

Clinical governance

In law, enteral feeding is regarded as a medical treatment and should therefore not be started without considering all related ethical issues. Valid consent to treatment is essential in the placement of enteral feeding tubes.

In the management of those with an eating disorder, feeding against their will should be a last resort. It should be considered in the context of the Mental Health Act (1983), the Mental Capacity Act (2005) and the Children Act (1989) (and their respective Codes of Practice), as appropriate.

Where the Mental Capacity Act (2005) is used to authorize enteral feeding, the patient should be assessed to see whether additional authorization is required under the Deprivation of Liberty Safeguards. All mental capacity assessments must be Mental Capacity Act compliant.

Those passing a nasogastric tube should have achieved competencies set by the local trust (NHSI 2016, NNNG 2016a). Introduction of fluids or medication into the respiratory tract or pleura via a misplaced nasogastric or orogastric tube is a 'Never Event' (NHS England 2015b). Placement devices for nasogastric tube insertion do not replace initial position checks (NHS England 2013). All equipment used to support enteral feeding should be ENFit compliant (see the section above on ENFit) (NHSI 2016). Documentation of enteral tube placement should be rigorous and in line with local policy (e.g. care bundles or passport). Such documentation may include pre-insertion assessments, date and time of insertion, appropriate monitoring post-insertion and guidance for healthcare professionals on post-insertion care.

Pre-procedural considerations

Specific patient preparation

The planned procedure should be discussed with the patient so that they are aware of the rationale for the insertion of a nasogastric tube. The decision to insert a nasogastric tube must be made by at least two healthcare professionals, including the senior doctor responsible for the patient's care. Verbal consent for the procedure must be obtained from the patient if they are conscious and able to give it.

Prior to performing this procedure, the patient's medical and nursing notes should be consulted to check for potential complications. For example, anatomical alterations due to surgery, such as a flap repair, or the presence of a cancerous tumour or nasal polyps can prevent a clear passage for the nasogastric tube, resulting in pain and discomfort for the patient and further complications such as bleeding or tissue damage. Patients who have recurrent retching or vomiting, have swallowing dysfunction or are comatose have a high risk of placement error or migration of the tube so care must be taken when placing a nasogastric tube under these circumstances (NHSI 2016). It may be more appropriate for such patients to have a nasojejunal tube placed endoscopically to reduce the risks of vomiting, regurgitation and potential aspiration of feed, and tube misplacement. The assessment of the patient, the risks and the obtained patient consent should be clearly documented.

Social and psychological impact

For some patients a nasogastric tube can be distressing. This is not only due to physical discomfort but also perceptions of body image, particularly as this type of feeding tube is highly visible. Some people find that the tube limits their social activity due to embarrassment, which can lead to feelings of isolation. Others see it as a reminder of ill health, which can have an impact on mood. These issues should be discussed with the patient prior to tube insertion.

Procedure guideline 8.10 Nasogastric intubation with tubes using an internal guidewire or stylet

Essential equipment

- Personal protective equipment
- Clinically clean tray
- Hypoallergenic tape
- Adherent dressing tape
- Fine-bore ENFit-compliant nasogastric tube with internal guidewire or stylet that is radio-opaque through its entire length and has externally visible length markings (NHSI 2016)
- Adhesive patch if available (to secure device)
- Glass of water (if the patient can swallow and is not nil by mouth)
- Receiver
- Lubricating jelly (if required; some nasogastric tubes have a lubricated coating that is activated with water)
- Water
- CE-marked indicator strips with a pH range of 0–6 or 1–11 with gradations of 0.5
- 60 mL ENFit-compatible syringe
- Permanent marker pen or tape to mark tube

Action	Rationale
Pre-procedure	
1 Introduce yourself to the patient, explain and discuss the procedure with them, and gain their consent to proceed.	To ensure that the patient feels at ease, understands the procedure and gives their valid consent (NMC 2018, **C**).
2 Arrange a signal by which the patient can communicate if they want the nurse to stop, for example by raising their hand.	The patient is often less frightened if they feel that they have some control over the procedure. **E**
3 Assist the patient to sit in a semi-upright position in the bed or chair. Support the patient's head with pillows. *Note*: the head should not be tilted backwards or forwards (Rollins 1997).	To allow for easy passage of the tube. This position enables easy swallowing and ensures that the epiglottis is not obstructing the oesophagus (NCCAC 2006, **C**).
4 Decontaminate hands and apply personal protective equipment.	To reduce the risk of cross-contamination (NHS England and NHSI 2019, **C**).
5 Select the appropriate distance mark on the tube by measuring performing a NEX measurement: using the tube, measure the distance from the patient's nose to their earlobe plus the distance from the earlobe to the bottom of the xiphisternum (**Action figure 5**). Mark this position on the tube with a permanent pen or a piece of tape.	To ensure that the appropriate length of tube is passed into the stomach (NHSI 2016, **C**).
Procedure	
6 Wash hands with soap and water or an alcohol-based handrub, and assemble the equipment required.	Hands must be cleansed before and after patient contact to minimize cross-infection (NHS England and NHSI 2019, **C**).
7 Follow manufacturer's instructions to activate the lubricant on the tip of the tube, for example dip the end in tap water or lubricate the proximal end of the tube with lubricating jelly.	To lubricate the tube, assisting its passage through the nasopharynx. **E**

(continued)

Procedure guideline 8.10 Nasogastric intubation with tubes using an internal guidewire or stylet *(continued)*

Action	Rationale
8 Check that the nostrils are patent by asking the patient to sniff with one nostril closed. Repeat with the other nostril.	To identify any obstructions liable to prevent intubation. **E**
9 Insert the rounded end of the tube into the clearer nostril and slide it backwards and inwards along the floor of the nose to the nasopharynx. If any obstruction is felt, withdraw the tube and try again in a slightly different direction or use the other nostril.	To facilitate the passage of the tube by following the natural anatomy of the nose. **E**
10 As the tube passes down into the nasopharynx, unless swallowing is contraindicated, ask the patient to start swallowing and sipping water. If the patient is unable to drink safely but has capacity, ask them to perform a dry swallow.	To focus the patient's attention on something other than the tube. A swallowing action closes the glottis and the cricopharyngeal sphincter opens, enabling the tube to pass into the oesophagus (Lamont et al. 2011, **E**; NNNG 2016a, **C**).
11 Advance the tube through the pharynx as the patient swallows until the predetermined mark has been reached (NEX measurement). If the patient shows signs of distress, for example gasping or cyanosis, remove the tube immediately. *Do not* flush any fluid down the nasogastric tube until the position has been checked.	The tube may have accidentally been passed down the trachea instead of the pharynx. Distress may indicate that the tube is in the bronchus. However, absence of distress is not a reliable indicator of a correctly placed tube. (NHSI 2016, **C**). There is a risk of introducing fluid into the lungs if the tube is incorrectly positioned (NHSI 2016, **C**).
12 Secure the tube to the nose with either adherent dressing tape or an adhesive nasogastric stabilization/securing device. Alternatively, hypoallergenic tape can be applied to the cheek to secure the nasogastric tube. Ensure the nasogastric tube is not putting pressure on the nares.	To hold the tube in place. To ensure patient comfort. **E** Prolonged pressure from the tube to the nasal tissues could cause medical-device-related pressure damage. **E**
Post-procedure	
13 Measure the external (visible) part of the tube from the tip of the nose and record this and the NEX measurement in the care plan. Mark the tube at the exit site (nares) with a permanent marker pen or piece of tape.	To provide a record to assist in detecting movement of the tube (Metheny and Titler 2001, **E;** NHSI 2016, **C**). It is good practice to measure the external length in the case the markings become faded. **E**
14 Check the position of the tube to confirm that it is in the stomach by using the following methods. *Note*: placement devices (e.g. nasoendoscope or electromagnetic technology) do not replace the following checks (NHS England 2013).	No fluids must be given via the tube until the correct position of the tube has been confirmed (NHSI 2016, **C**). To confirm that the tube is in the correct position (NHS England 2013, **C**). *Note:* the following methods *must not* be used to test the position of a nasogastric feeding tube: auscultation (introducing air into the nasogastric tube and checking for a bubbling sound via a stethoscope, also known as the 'whoosh test'), use of litmus paper or absence of respiratory distress.

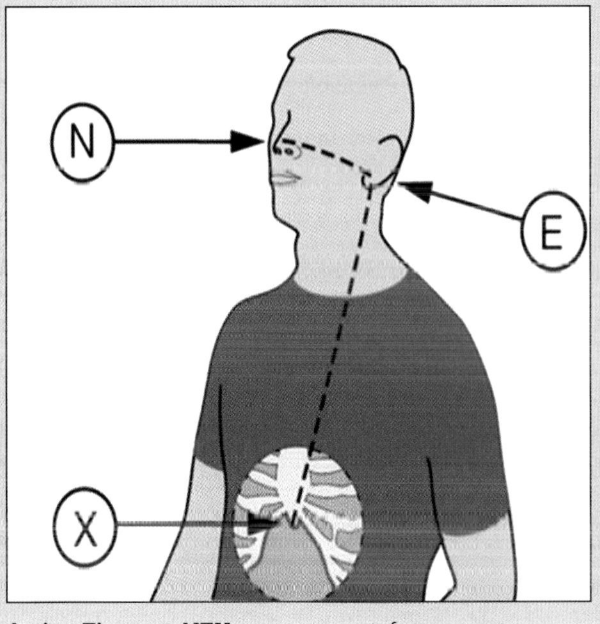

Action Figure 5 NEX measurement: from **n**ose to **e**ar lobe to the bottom of the **x**iphisternum.

First-line test method: pH paper. aspirate 0.5–1 mL of stomach contents and test its pH on indicator strips (NHSI 2016) (see Box 8.6 for methods of aspiration). When aspirating fluid for pH testing, wait at least 1 hour after a feed or medication has been administered (either orally or via the tube). Before aspirating, flush the tube with 20 mL of air to clear other substances. A pH level of between 1 and 5.5 is unlikely to be pulmonary aspirates and it is considered appropriate to proceed to feed through the tube (NHSI 2016). Regular proton pump inhibitors or altered anatomy (e.g. gastric sleeve) may affect readings of aspirates. Risk management should be taken in these cases to ensure safe feeding. See Problem-solving table 8.3.	pH indicator strips should have gradations of 0.5 or paper with a range of 0–6 or 1–11 to distinguish between gastric acid and bronchial secretions. They must be CE marked and intended to check gastric aspirate (NHSI 2016, **C**). To prove an accurate test result because the feed or medication may raise the pH of the stomach (NHSI 2016, **C**).
If a pH of 6 or above is obtained or there is doubt over a result in the range of pH 5–6 then feeding *must not* commence until a second competent person has checked the reading or retested the aspirate. The nasogastric tube may need to be repositioned or checked with an X-ray.	There is less certainty over the correct placement of the tube if the pH is above 6 (NHSI 2016, **C**).
Second-line test method: X-ray confirmation: take an X-ray of the chest and upper abdomen. The X-ray request form should clearly state that the purpose of the X-ray is to establish the position of the nasogastric tube for the purpose of feeding (NHSI 2016).	X-ray of radio-opaque tubes is the most accurate way of confirming position and is the second-line method of choice in patients for whom it is not possible to confirm correct placement with gastric aspirate and pH indicator strips (NHSI 2016, **C**). Clearly stating the purpose of the X-ray will ensure the correct image is obtained by the radiographer. **E**
15 X-rays must only be interpreted and the position confirmed by someone assessed as competent to do so. When the position is confirmed, the person interpreting the X-ray must document the tip's position in the patient's notes in an entry that is signed with the date and time.	To record the position and document that it is safe to feed through the nasogastric tube (NHSI 2016, **C**; NMC 2018, **C**).
16 Once placement of the nasogastric tube is confirmed, the guidewire/stylet can be removed following the manufacturer's guidelines; this can include the need to activate the internal lubricant of the tube immediately before removal.	To facilitate easy removal of the guidewire/stylet (NHS England 2013, **C**).
17 Remove and dispose of any equipment.	To reduce the risk of cross infection. **E**
18 Record the procedure in the patient's notes.	To maintain accurate records (NMC 2018, **C**).

Problem-solving table 8.3 Prevention and resolution (Procedure guideline 8.10)

Problem	Cause	Prevention	Action
Unable to place the nasogastric tube	The patient has altered anatomy.	Seek expert help for any altered anatomy	The nasogastric tube should be placed under X-ray guidance or via endoscopy.
	The patient is distressed or not compliant with the procedure.	Ensure the procedure is fully explained to the patient and try and reassure them as much as possible.	
Unable to obtain aspirate from the nasogastric tube	The tip of the tube is not sitting in gastric contents, is against the stomach wall or is not advanced sufficiently into the stomach.	Measure the tube correctly as shown in Procedure guideline 8.10 Action figure 5.	See Box 8.6.
A pH of greater than 5.5 is obtained	The nasogastric tube may be placed in the lungs. The patient may be on acid-inhibiting medication and this may contribute to a higher gastric pH.	Check the pH of the gastric aspirate just before the time of administration of acid-inhibiting medication, when gastric pH is likely to be at its lowest.	If initial confirmation cannot be obtained from pH aspirate then the tube may need to be X-rayed as it may be in the lungs.
Initial correct placement is confirmed but subsequently unable to obtain an aspirate	The nasogastric tube may not be positioned in gastric contents or may have become misplaced.	Check the length of tube against the NEX measurement; then, using the NEX measurement as a reference point, advance or withdraw the tube by 5–10 cm. Give mouth care to patients who are nil by mouth (this stimulates the secretion of gastric acid). Try and obtain an aspirate again (BAPEN 2012b).	Undertake risk assessment and document action. The nasogastric tube may need to be repositioned and rechecked with an X-ray.

Box 8.6 Methods to obtain an aspirate from a nasogastric tube

Try the following either one at a time or in combination:

- Turn patient onto their left side.
- Inject 10–20 mL of *air* (*do not use water to flush the tube until the position has been confirmed*) into the tube using a 60 mL ENFit syringe; wait 15–30 minutes.
- Advance or withdraw the tube by 10–20 cm.
- Check the NEX measurement and external length to assess whether the tube has moved (advance the tube 5–10 cm over NEX measurement if safe to do so).
- Provide mouth care (doing so may stimulate the secretion of gastic acid).
- Then try aspirating again.

Box 8.7 The clinical importance of the pH scale

The pH scale is a convenient way of recording large ranges of hydrogen ion concentrations without using the cumbersome numbers that are needed to describe the actual concentrations. That is why each step *down* the scale is a 10-fold *increase* in acidity (or a 10-fold *decrease* if going *up* the scale). This means that stomach contents of pH 5 have 10 times more acidity than lung fluid of pH 6. Not knowing this could place a patient in harm's way.

The midpoint of the scale is 7. This number is related directly to the actual concentration of hydrogen ions in water, which is one ten-millionth units per litre – an extremely small number. One ten-millionth is the same as 1 divided by 10^7. So a liquid of pH 6 has one-millionth units per litre – that is, 1 divided by 10^6 – and has 10 times the concentration of hydrogen ions as does pure water. This example shows why as the pH decreases, the hydrogen ion concentration, and thus the acidity, increases. For example, lemon juice and vinegar are acidic with pHs of 2.2 and 3 respectively, whereas bleach is alkaline with a low concentration of hydrogen ions and a pH of 11.

In the body, the pH of cells, body fluids and organs is usually tightly controlled in a process called 'acid-base homeostasis'. Without this careful regulation of pH or 'buffering', the normal body chemistry processes cannot take place successfully and illness, or in extreme cases death, can occur (Aoi and Marunaka 2014).

The pH of blood is slightly basic (slightly more alkalotic than acidic), with a value of 7.4, whereas gastric acid can range from 5.5 to the highly acidic 0.7 and pancreatic secretions are measured at 8.1. When the pH in the body decreases – that is, it becomes more acidic – 'acidosis' can occur, leading to symptoms such as shortness of breath, muscular seizure and coma.

pH also influences the structure and function of many enzymes in living systems. These enzymes usually only work satisfactorily within narrow pH ranges. Thus, pepsin, a stomach enzyme, works best at pH 2. In the duodenum, trypsin functions best at around pH 7.5–8.0. Generally, most human cell enzymes work best in a slightly alkaline medium of about 7.4.

Keeping the cellular pH at the correct level is very important. In the case of unregulated diabetes, high blood sugar levels occur, leading to acidic conditions that rapidly destroy enzymes and cells. Consequently, regular blood sugar monitoring is crucial for diabetics.

In living systems, pH is therefore more than just a measure of hydrogen ion concentration as it is critical to life and the many biochemical reactions that have to take place to maintain a person in optimum health.

Post-procedural considerations

Immediate care

The position of the nasogastric tube must be checked at initial placement and again prior to the administration of all medication and feeds. Failure to confirm the position of the tube in the stomach can lead to the administration of fluid, medication or feed directly into the lungs, resulting in aspiration pneumonia.

The position of the nasogastric tube can be checked using two methods:

- *First-line method: testing of gastric aspirate with pH indicator paper*: the use of pH to check the position of the tube is based on an understanding of the pH of body fluids, particularly gastric contents, and the pH scale (Box 8.7). This should have a pH less than 5.5 (NHSI 2016).
- *Second-line method: X-ray*: an X-ray must be used to confirm the position of the tube in patients for whom it has not been possible to confirm the position of the tip of the nasogastric tube by gastric aspirate and pH indicator strips. The X-ray must be read by medical staff with appropriate training and competence (NHSI 2016).

See Procedure guideline 8.10 for details on how to conduct these tests.

In accordance with NHS Improvement guidance, the following methods are outdated and unreliable, and should *not* be used to confirm the position of a feeding tube (NHSI 2016):

- auscultation of air insufflated through the feeding tube ('whoosh test')
- testing the pH of the aspirate using blue litmus paper
- interpreting the absence of respiratory distress as an indicator of the correct positioning
- monitoring bubbling at the end of the tube
- observing the appearance of feeding tube aspirate
- use of placement devices for nasogastric tube insertion.

In addition to the initial confirmation, the tube should be checked on a daily basis if not in use and/or prior to the administration of any medication or feed (see 'Ongoing care' below for further details).

When the nasogastric tube is confirmed to be in the stomach, a mark should be made on the tube at the exit site from the nostril with a permanent marker pen. The length of tube visible from the exit of the nostril to the end of the tube should be measured in centimetres and recorded along with the NEX measurement. This is to help detect whether the nasogastric tube has become displaced. See Figure 8.21 for an X-ray of a correctly inserted nasogastric tube, Figure 8.22 for information on test precision and test risk when checking the position of a nasogastric tube, and Figure 8.23 for checks to carry out when using pH indicator sticks.

Ongoing care

Once the nasogastric tube has been confirmed to be in the stomach and the guidewire or stylet removed, feeding may commence. The tube should be kept patent by regular flushing before and after administering feed and medication. Preferably only liquid medication should be used as tablets may block the lumen of the tube (BAPEN 2017). Tablets should only be used if no alternative liquid or soluble preparation is available, and they should be crushed before administration. Always check with a pharmacist as some medication should not be crushed. See also Procedure guideline 8.16: Jejunostomy feeding tube care including dressing change.

The position of the tube must be verified by checking the pH of aspirate from the tube and recorded on a chart kept at the patient's bedside (NHSI 2016):

- before administering each feed
- before giving medication
- following episodes of vomiting, retching or coughing as it is likely the tube will have become displaced
- following evidence of tube displacement (e.g. the measured length of the tube is longer).

If a pH of below 5.5 is not obtained then it is highly likely that the tube has become displaced. The medical team should be contacted as the tube may need to be replaced. For further details on checking nasogastric tubes, refer to the full NHS Improvement guidance or local policy (NHSI 2016).

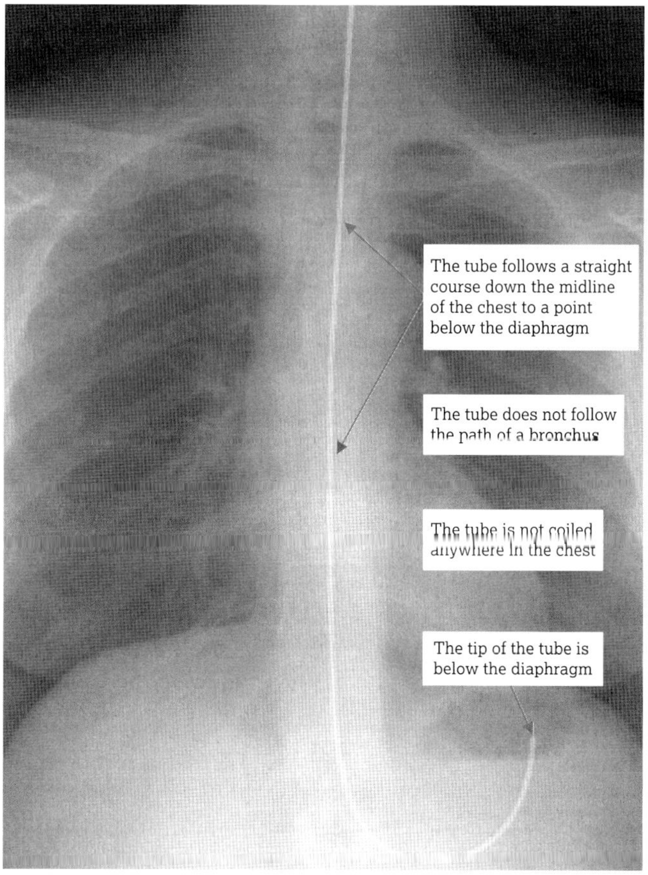

Figure 8.21 X-radiograph of a correctly inserted nasogastric tube. *Source*: Reproduced from PPSA (2006) with permission of the ECRI Institute (ecri.org.uk).

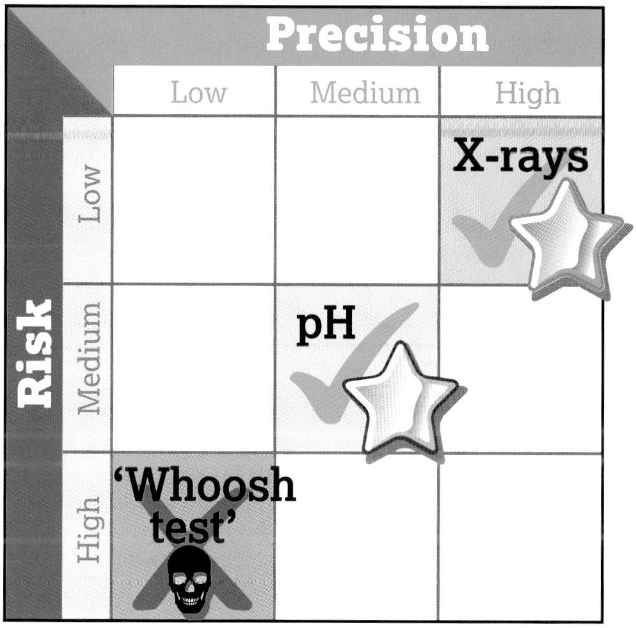

Figure 8.22 Test precision and test risk: the connection. *Source*: Reproduced from PPSA (2006) with permission of the ECRI Institute (ecri.org.uk).

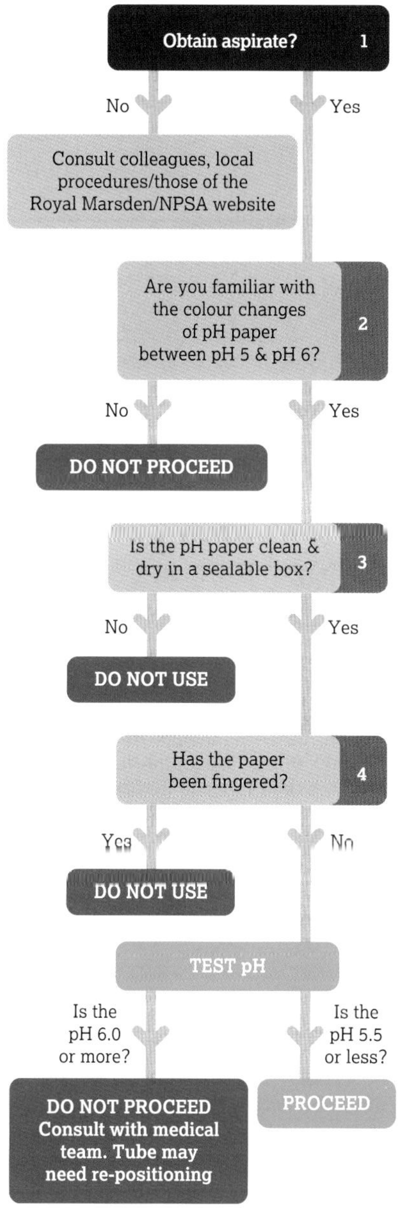

Figure 8.23 Four key checks to carry out when using the pH tests. *Source*: Reproduced with permission of the ECRI Institute (www.ecri.org.uk) and The Royal Marsden NHS Foundation Trust.

Education of the patient and relevant others

If appropriate, the patient may be taught how to check the position of the nasogastric tube. They should be made aware that if they feel the tube has moved, it must not be used for feeding or medication administration until its position has been confirmed by one of the methods described.

Complications

Nasal erosion

Prolonged nasogastric feeding or use of a wide-bore tube can lead to nasal erosion (NNNG 2016a). To reduce the risk of this occurring, it is important to use appropriate tape and assess the skin in this area on a regular basis. If erosion occurs, it is advised that the tube is removed and replaced in the other nostril. If feeding is to be long term then a gastrostomy or jejunostomy should be considered.

Displacement of tube

A tube can accidentally be pulled out or displaced, particularly if a patient is restless or distressed. It can also be coughed or vomited out of place. In this situation the position of the tube should be checked. If it is not possible to confirm that the tube remains within the stomach then it should be removed and a new tube placed (NHSI 2016).

Enteral tube removal

Pre-procedural considerations

A nasogastric tube may be removed because it has become dislodged or displaced or if it is no longer required for feeding. If it is being removed and not being replaced then it is essential that the multidisciplinary team is in agreement that the patient is able to meet their fluid and dietary requirements through the oral route and that they have the ability to swallow safely and without risk of aspiration.

Post-procedural considerations

Once the nasogastric tube has been removed then oral intake of food and fluids should be monitored on a fluid balance chart and a food record chart to ensure that the patient is meeting their daily requirements.

Enteral tube care

Evidence-based approaches

Percutaneous endoscopically placed gastrostomy (PEG) tube care

The first change of dressing should be performed 24 hours after PEG placement or earlier if indicated, for example if the site is bleeding (Loser et al. 2005, Soscia and Friedman 2011). Until granulation of the stoma canal has taken place, the dressing should be changed daily using aseptic technique. The wound should be inspected for bleeding, erythema, secretion, induration, allergic skin reaction and so on (Loser et al. 2005). This will help to maintain skin integrity and detect any problems early, for example infection or skin breakdown.

Radiologically inserted gastrostomy (RIG) tube care

After 24 hours and during the initial daily change of the dressing, the wound should be inspected and skin changes should be carefully noted. The site should be checked for bleeding, erythema, secretion or allergic skin reaction. For the first 10 days after the gastrostomy has been inserted, the site should be checked daily to ascertain skin integrity and detect any problems early, for example infection or skin breakdown. Most forms of local infection can be readily treated by cleaning the stoma site using aseptic technique and daily change of dressings (NNNG 2013). Antibiotics may be required in some instances. This procedure should be done by a nurse or nursing associate in hospital or by a suitably trained individual in the community (e.g. a community or practice nurse or a GP). For those patients who have a balloon gastrostomy inserted, the water content of the balloon should be topped up weekly to check the integrity of the balloon with the aim of preventing accidental dislodgement of the tube.

Jejunostomy feeding tube care

Care of the exit site should be performed daily to maintain skin integrity and detect any problems early, for example infection or skin breakdown. Most forms of local infection can be readily treated by cleaning the stoma site using aseptic technique and changing dressings daily (NNNG 2013). Antibiotics may be required in some instances.

Percutaneous endoscopically placed gastrostomy (PEG) placement and care

Pre-procedural considerations

Prior to performing PEG care the patient's medical and nursing notes should be consulted to identify the tube placement date and method, and any infection control issues. The endoscopist's instructions should be noted, including any specific detail with regard to post-placement care, for example suture removal, tube rotation, checking the volume of the balloon (if appropriate) and dressing changes.

The integrity of the water-filled balloon is important in ensuring that the balloon gastrostomy remains in place. This is usually done 1 week post-insertion and on a weekly basis while the balloon gastrostomy tube is *in situ*. The balloon is deflated and reinflated using an ENFit syringe via the balloon inflation valve.

Procedure guideline 8.11 Removal of a nasogastric tube

Essential equipment

- Personal protective equipment
- Dressing pack containing gauze and sterile gloves

Action	Rationale
Pre-procedure	
1 Introduce yourself to the patient, explain and discuss the procedure with them, and gain their consent to proceed.	To ensure that the patient feels at ease, understands the procedure and gives their valid consent (NMC 2018, **C**).
2 Assist the patient to sit in a semi-upright position in a bed or in a chair. Support the patient's head with pillows.	To allow for easy removal of the tube. **E**
3 Wash hands with soap and water or an alcohol-based handrub, and assemble the equipment required. Apply apron and clean gloves.	Hands must be cleansed before and after patient contact to minimize the risk of cross-infection (NHS England and NHSI 2019, **C**).
Procedure	
4 Remove any tape securing the nasogastric tube to the nose.	To assist in the removal of the nasogastric tube. **E**
5 Using a steady and constant motion, gently pull the tube until it has been completely removed.	To remove the nasogastric tube. **E**
Post-procedure	
6 Remove gloves and dispose of waste.	To reduce the chance of equipment being reused. **E**
7 Clean the nose and face to remove any traces of tape.	To maintain skin integrity and ensure patient comfort and dignity. **E**
8 Document the removal of the nasogastric tube in the care plan and the patient's notes.	To ensure adequate records and to enable continued care of the patient (NMC 2018, **C**).

Procedure guideline 8.12 Percutaneous endoscopically placed gastrostomy (PEG) tube care

Essential equipment

- Personal protective equipment
- Sterile procedure pack containing gallipot and low-linting gauze
- Dressing (absorbent, e.g. Lyofoam)
- 0.9% sodium chloride solution

Action	Rationale
Pre-procedure	
1 Introduce yourself to the patient, explain and discuss the procedure with them, and gain their consent to proceed.	To ensure that the patient feels at ease, understands the procedure and gives their valid consent (NMC 2018, **C**).
2 Wash hands with soap and water or an alcohol-based handrub, and assemble the equipment required. Apply apron and clean gloves.	Hands must be cleansed before and after patient contact to minimize cross-infections (NHS England and NHSI 2019, **C**).
Procedure	
3 Remove the existing dressing. Observe the peristomal skin and stoma site for signs of infection, erythema, irritation or excoriation. Observe the tube and consider how it is being kept in place, and note the presence of any sutures, external fixation plates, clamps or balloon ports.	To gain access to the stoma site. To detect complications early and instigate appropriate treatment (NNNG 2016b, **R**). To minimize the risk of accidental displacement of the tube. **E**
4 Note the number of the measuring guide on the tube closest to the end of the external fixation device. If the stoma tract has formed (14 days post-insertion), loosen the tube from the fixation device and ease the device away from the abdomen. The external fixation plate should be subjected to very low traction, without tension, to maintain contact of the stomach with the abdominal wall. If the tube is less than 14 days post-insertion then *do not* loosen the fixation device.	To ensure the gastrostomy tube is reattached to the fixation device in the correct position (Loser et al. 2005, **C**).
5 Clean the stoma site with a sterile solution, such as 0.9% sodium chloride, using a circular outward motion. Use low-linting gauze to dry the area thoroughly.	To minimize the risk of cross-infection and ensure the stoma site is thoroughly cleaned (Fraise and Bradley 2009, **E**; Lynch and Fang 2004, **R**).
6 If the stoma tract has formed (14 days post-insertion), rotate the gastrostomy tube 360°. If the tube is less than 14 days post-insertion then *do not* rotate the tube.	To prevent the tube adhering to the sides of the stoma tract (NNNG 2016b, **R**).
7 Gently push the external fixation device against the abdomen, checking the measurement guide.	To enable the gastrostomy tube to be reattached to the fixation device. **E**
8 Gently but firmly pull the gastrostomy tube and attach it to the fixation device. Consult the patient's medical and nursing notes for the correct numbered position mark at the gastrostomy exit site. The fixation device should remain at the same length, so that gentle traction on the tube allows 0.5 cm give but no more for the first 14 days.	To ensure that the tube is correctly secured. **E**
9 Ensure the correct point on the measuring guide on the tube is placed closest to the end of the fixation device.	To ensure that the tube is correctly secured. If the patient gains weight, the external fixation device should be released slightly to prevent pressure necrosis of the stoma site (Loser et al. 2005, **C**).
Post-procedure	
10 The dry dressing should be replaced daily using aseptic technique until the stoma site has no erythema or exudates or any other signs of infection. Most forms of infection can be readily treated by means of antiseptic measures and daily change of dressing using an aseptic technique (Loser et al. 2005). Do not replace the dressing with an occlusive type. *Do not* use bulky dressings, particularly under the external fixation device.	To encourage wound healing. **E** To prevent air getting to the stoma as this may cause infection (Lynch and Fang 2004, **R**) or abdominal discomfort. Using non-bulky dressings avoids increasing the pressure on the internal retention disc or retention balloon and increasing the risk of tissue necrosis and ulceration occurring in the stomach (Cappell et al. 2009, **E**).
11 Make the patient aware of and monitor them for red flag symptoms. In the immediate recovery period, ensure regular observations of temperature, blood pressure, pulse respirations and pain score. *Red flag* symptoms include pain on feeding, prolonged or severe pain, and external leakage of gastric contents. If the patient complains of pain or discomfort, administer analgesia. If this is persistent, liaise with the medical team and/or request a gastroenterology review (Healey et al. 2010).	To monitor for signs of peritonitis or potential complications following insertion of the gastrostomy tube (NNNG 2016b, **C**).
12 Remove and dispose of any equipment.	To reduce the risk of cross-infection. **E**
13 Record the procedure in the patient's notes.	To maintain accurate records (NMC 2018, **C**).

Problem-solving table 8.4 Prevention and resolution (Procedure guideline 8.12)

Problem	Cause	Prevention	Action
Displaced PEG tube	Excessive tension being applied to the tube, either when moving the external fixator or by over-tightening	Support the tube beneath the fixator when moving.	Liaise with medical team.
Tube cracked	Prolonged use of clamp without repositioning	Regular tube care and review. Change position of clamp regularly.	Liaise with medical team to arrange replacement.
Tube blockage	Inadequate tube flushing or overuse for administering medications	Regular tube flushing. Avoid/minimize use of tube for medications. Use appropriate medication formulation.	See Procedure guideline 8.20: Enteral feeding tubes: unblocking.

PEG, percutaneous endoscopically placed gastrostomy.

Procedure guideline 8.13 Radiologically inserted gastrostomy (RIG) tube care

Essential equipment

- Personal protective equipment
- Sterile procedure pack containing gallipot and low-linting gauze
- Dressing (absorbent, e.g. Lyofoam)
- 0.9% sodium chloride solution

Action	Rationale
Pre-procedure	
1 Explain and discuss the procedure with the patient.	To ensure that the patient understands the procedure and gives their valid consent (NMC 2018, **C**).
2 Wash hands with soap and water or an alcohol-based handrub, and assemble the equipment required. Apply apron and clean gloves.	Hands must be cleansed before and after patient contact to minimize the risk of cross-infection (NHS England and NHSI 2019, **C**).
Procedure	
3 Remove the post-procedural dressing if in place. Observe the peristomal skin and stoma site for signs of infection, erythema, irritation or excoriation.	To gain access to the stoma site. To detect complications early and instigate appropriate treatment (Healey et al. 2010, **R**).
4 Observe the tube and consider how it is being kept in place, and note the presence of any sutures, external fixation plates, clamps or balloon ports.	To minimize the risk of accidental displacement of the tube. **E**
5 Check that the T-fasteners are intact. These will stay in place for approximately 10–14 days after RIG insertion. The timing should be checked with the radiologist. For removal see Procedure guideline 8.14: Removal of T-fasteners.	To stabilize the stomach against the abdominal wall and allow the tract to form without complications (Lang et al. 2013, **E**).
6 Pull back the RIG flange and clean the stoma site with sterile solution, such as 0.9% sodium chloride, using a circular outward motion.	To minimize the risk of cross infection and ensure the stoma site is thoroughly cleaned (Loveday et al. 2014, **R**; NNNG 2013, **R**).
7 Use low-linting gauze to dry the area thoroughly.	To ensure the stoma site is thoroughly dried (NNNG 2013, **R**).
8 If it is 10–14 days after insertion, remove the T-fasteners and secure the fixation plate 1–2 cm away from the skin (if applicable). Refer to the manufacturer's guidelines as to whether the tube should be rotated.	To prevent the RIG tube moving into the stomach (Lang et al. 2013, **E**).
9 Secure the tube to the skin with hypoallergenic tape. Do not secure near the stoma site.	To prevent the weight of the tube pulling on the exit site. Tape near the stoma site will make it difficult to clean. **E**
10 Advise the patient not to use moisturizing creams or talcum powder around the stoma.	To prevent infection and/or irritation to the skin. **E**
11 If this is a balloon gastrostomy, change the water in the balloon on a weekly basis. See Procedure guideline 8.15: Changing the balloon water and checking the volume of a balloon gastrostomy.	To prevent tube displacement. **E**

Action	Rationale
Post-procedure	
12 After T-fasteners have been removed, do not cover the gastrostomy site with a new dressing unless there is a heavy discharge or leakage from the stoma site.	To encourage wound healing. **E**
13 Remove and dispose of any equipment.	To reduce the risk of cross-infection. **E**
14 Record the procedure in the patient's notes.	To maintain accurate records (NMC 2018, **C**).

Procedure guideline 8.14 Removal of T-fasteners

This usually takes place 10 days post-gastrostomy insertion unless dissolvable fasteners have been used, and it should be done after inspection of the gastrostomy site.

Essential equipment

- Personal protective equipment
- Sterile procedure pack containing gallipot, low-linting gauze, sterile gloves and sterile field
- 0.9% sodium chloride solution
- Sterile metal forceps
- Stitch cutter

Action	Rationale
Pre-procedure	
1 Introduce yourself to the patient, explain and discuss the procedure with them, and gain their consent to proceed.	To ensure that the patient feels at ease, understands the procedure and gives their valid consent (NMC 2018, **C**).
2 Wash hands with soap and water or alcohol-based handrub and apply personal protective equipment.	Hands should be cleaned before and after each patient contact (NHS England and NHSI 2019, **C**).
3 Assist the patient into a supine position if the patient is able.	To ensure patient comfort. **E**
4 Perform the procedure using aseptic technique.	To prevent infection (Loveday et al. 2014, **R**).
Procedure	
5 Prepare a tray or trolley and take it to the bedside. Clean hands as above. Open the sterile pack and prepare the equipment.	To reduce the risk of contamination of the contents (NICE 2012, **C**).
6 Decontaminate hands and apply sterile gloves.	To reduce the risk of cross-infection (NHS England and NHSI 2019, **C**).
7 Clean the surrounding skin with an appropriate sterile solution such as 0.9% sodium chloride.	To prevent infection and remove excess debris. **E**
8 Check the condition of the surrounding skin.	To assess for any excoriation of the skin. **E**
9 Lift the external knot of the T-fastener with metal forceps and cut the suture underneath the cuff, close to the skin. Remove the cuff and the metallic/plastic tag. Repeat on each T-fastener.	To remove the suture; plastic forceps tend to slip against nylon sutures. **E** To ensure removal of each fastener. **E**
10 Clean the skin with appropriate sterile solution such as 0.9% sodium chloride.	To prevent infection and remove excess debris. **E**
11 After T-fasteners have been removed, secure the fixation plate 1–2 cm away from the skin (if applicable). Do not cover the gastrostomy site with a new dressing unless there is a heavy discharge or leakage from the stoma site.	To encourage wound healing. **E**
Post-procedure	
12 Record the condition of the skin surrounding the gastrostomy site.	To document care and enable evaluation of the gastrostomy site (NMC 2018, **C**).
13 Remove and dispose of any equipment.	To reduce the risk of cross-infection. **E**
14 Record the procedure in the patient's notes.	To maintain accurate records (NMC 2018, **C**).

Procedure guideline 8.15 Changing the balloon water and checking the volume of a balloon gastrostomy

Essential equipment

- Personal protective equipment
- Sterile procedure pack containing gallipot, low-linting gauze, sterile gloves and sterile field
- Two 10 mL ENfit syringes (20 mL syringe required if balloon volume is greater than 10 mL)
- Sterile water

Action	Rationale
Pre-procedure	
1 Introduce yourself to the patient, explain and discuss the procedure with them, and gain their consent to proceed.	To ensure that the patient feels at ease, understands the procedure and gives their valid consent (NMC 2018, **C**).
2 Assist the patient to sit in a semi-upright position in the bed or in a chair. Support the patient's head with pillows.	To allow for easy access to the gastrostomy tube. **E**
3 Wash hands with soap and water or alcohol-based handrub, and assemble the equipment required. Apply personal protective equipment.	Hands must be cleansed before and after patient contact to minimize the risk of cross-infection (NHS England and NHSI 2019, **C**).
4 Discontinue the feed.	To ensure that the procedure can be undertaken without spillage of feed. **E**
5 Obtain an aspirate from the gastrostomy tube and test pH. If the result is below 5.5, proceed. If it is above 5.5, seek medical advice. For further information see Procedure guideline 8.10: Nasogastric intubation with tubes using an internal guidewire or stylet. If unable to obtain the correct pH then the gastrostomy tube change may need to be done under radiological guidance to ensure it remains in the stomach.	To ensure that the balloon is inflated in the stomach and not in the tract or another part of the stomach. **E**
6 Prepare a tray or trolley and take it to the bedside. Clean hands as above, open sterile pack and prepare equipment.	To reduce the risk of contamination of contents (NICE 2012, **C**).
7 Decontaminate hands and apply sterile gloves.	To reduce the risk of cross-infection (NHS England and NHSI 2019, **C**).
Procedure	
8 Providing the pH is under 5.5, proceed to slide the external retention flange up the tube, away from the abdomen, and push the tube 2–3 cm into the abdomen.	To ensure that the balloon is inflated in the stomach and not in the tract. **E**
9 Following the manufacturer's guidelines, attach an ENFit syringe to the inflation valve of the balloon gastrostomy. Withdraw all the water from the balloon. Discard the water and syringe.	To ensure that the balloon is completely deflated. **E**
10 Note the volume on the side of the inflation valve of the balloon gastrostomy. Draw up the required volume of sterile water in a new ENFit syringe.	To ensure that the correct volume of fluid is inserted into the balloon. **E**
11 Attach a syringe containing sterile water and reinflate the balloon with the appropriate volume (volume is indicated on the side of the inflation valve).	To ensure that the balloon is not over- or underfilled. **E**
12 Gently pull back the gastrostomy tube until the balloon can be felt against the stomach wall. Slide the external retention device along the tube until it sits comfortably against the abdomen.	To ensure that the balloon and the external retention device are returned to the correct position. **E**
Post-procedure	
13 Ensure that the skin surrounding the tube is clean and dry.	To promote patient comfort. **E**
14 Dispose of all equipment in accordance with local policy.	To reduce the chance of equipment being reused. **E**
15 Record the condition of the skin surrounding the gastrostomy site.	To document care and enable evaluation of the gastrostomy site (NMC 2018, **C**).
16 After refilling the balloon, check the pH by aspirating from the gastrostomy (pH should be below 5.5).	To confirm placement in the stomach (Fletcher 2011, **E**).

Procedure guideline 8.16 Jejunostomy feeding tube care including dressing change

Essential equipment

- Personal protective equipment
- Sterile procedure pack containing gallipot and low-linting gauze
- 0.9% sodium chloride solution

Action	Rationale
Pre-procedure	
1 Introduce yourself to the patient, explain and discuss the procedure with them, and gain their consent to proceed.	To ensure that the patient feels at ease, understands the procedure and gives their valid consent (NMC 2018, **C**).
2 Decontaminate hands and apply personal protective equipment.	To minimize the risk of cross-infection (NHS England and NHSI 2019, **C**).
Procedure	
3 Remove the existing dressing if in place. Observe the peristomal skin and stoma for signs of infection, erythema, irritation or excoriation. Observe the tube and consider how it is being kept in place, and note the presence of any sutures or external fixation plates. Refer to guidance from gastroenterologists for care of sutures.	To gain access to the stoma site. To detect complications early and instigate appropriate treatment (Lynch and Fang 2004, **R**). To minimize the risk of accidental displacement of the tube. **E**
4 Clean the stoma site with sterile solution, such as 0.9% sodium chloride, using a circular outward motion.	To minimize the risk of cross-infection and ensure the stoma site is thoroughly cleaned (Healey et al. 2010, **R**; Loveday et al. 2014, **R**).
5 Use low-linting gauze to dry the area thoroughly.	To ensure the stoma site is thoroughly dry (NNNG 2013, **R**).
6 Secure the jejunostomy tube to the skin with hypoallergenic tape. The site may be covered with a dry dressing or left uncovered.	To prevent the weight of the tube pulling on the exit site. **E**
Post-procedure	
7 Remove and dispose of any equipment.	To reduce the risk of cross infection. **E**
8 Record the procedure in the patient's notes.	To maintain accurate records (NMC 2018, **C**).

Local policy and guidelines (where available) should be identified and followed when managing the usage of these tubes.

Post-procedural considerations

Immediate care

Local protocols should specify the observations to be taken in the immediate post-operative recovery period. These should include observation of blood pressure, heart rate, respiration rate and pain score in addition to checks of the stoma site for bleeding, leakage of gastric contents or tube displacement (NHSI 2016). If the patient is complaining of pain or there are signs of peritonitis or tube displacement, contact the medical team immediately. Peritonitis manifests as abdominal pain, fever and a raised white cell count in the initial days after placement. Transient external leakage of the stomach contents from the puncture canal can also suggest that internal leakage is occurring (NHSI 2016).

If there is pain on feeding, prolonged or severe pain post-procedure or fresh bleeding, or external leakage of gastric contents then the feed should be stopped immediately. The patient should be reviewed by a senior clinician and the following considered: computed tomography (CT) scan, contrast study or surgical review (NHSI 2016).

Additional complications that may occur in the immediate period after gastrostomy insertion include aspiration pneumonia, haemorrhage and wound infection (Taheri et al. 2011). Colonic perforation is rare but may occur during the procedure and is likely to lead to peritonitis.

All assessments and care given should be clearly documented, including details of any observations noted and dressings used. The timing of future assessments should be planned to ensure that relevant aspects of care are followed up: for example, if a swab is taken to ascertain whether there is an infection, this needs to be followed up in order to act on the results of microbiology culture.

The patient should be advised not to use moisturizing creams or talcum powder around the stoma site. The grease in creams can cause the external retention device to slip, allowing movement of the tube and increasing the risk of hypergranulation, leakage and infection (Haywood 2012). Creams and talcs can affect the tube material, causing it to stretch or leak.

Once the stoma site has healed (approximately 10 days post-insertion), it is no longer necessary to perform an aseptic technique. Use soap and water to clean the stoma site and ensure the area around the stoma is dried thoroughly. The tube tip should be cleaned daily using water and a small brush (Loser et al. 2005).

Where the enteral feeding tube has been placed to allow nutritional support, the patient's feeding regimen should be checked. If there is no feeding regimen, liaise with dietetic staff as needed or contact the medical team.

Ongoing care

To reduce the risk of tube blockage, the patient's medication should be reviewed where the tube is required for drug administration. Liaise with both the medical team and the pharmacist to discuss the patient's prescription and alternative routes and medications (NICE and BNF 2019).

Education of the patient and relevant others

The need for patient and/or carer teaching should be considered in patients with newly inserted enteral feeding tubes, and discharge planning should be initiated. If a patient is discharged within 72 hours of gastrostomy insertion, the patient and their carers must be provided with appropriate local and out-of-hours contacts for urgent aftercare advice and warned of the danger signs that need urgent attention. These include pain on feeding, new bleeding and external leakage of gastric contents (NHSI 2016).

Complications

Infection

Infection can occur at the time of placement or be due to inappropriate site care, particularly prior to tract maturation. Patients who are immunocompromised may be at increased risk of infection. Initial care after insertion should be carried out using an aseptic technique until the tract is fully mature. If there are any signs of reddened skin or infection then a swab should be taken and sent off for microbiology culture and sensitivity. Appropriate antibiotic prescribing may be required depending on the condition of the stoma site and the microbiology results from the swab (Warriner and Spruce 2012).

Pressure necrosis

Excessive tightening of the external fixator device may cause pressure necrosis around the stoma site. The external fixator should be adjusted while the patient is sitting up, where possible. If the external fixator is adjusted while the patient is lying down then it is necessary to ensure that it is applied 1–2 cm from the skin surface.

The stoma site should be reviewed regularly and the patient and carer taught how to adjust and reposition the external fixator. This is particularly important if the patient has gained weight as this may cause pressure on the fixator.

Buried bumper

In enteral feeding tubes that have a bumper as the retention device, the retention bumper may become buried in the intestinal wall. The external fixator should be released and the tube pushed in approximately 5 cm and rotated fully both clockwise and anticlockwise. Ensure it is rotated regularly according to the manufacturer's instructions (NNNG 2013).

Peristomal leakage

It is important to examine the tube site for causes of peristomal leakage. Contributory factors include delayed gastric emptying, buried bumper and infection. Ensure correct management of the stoma area, including checking the internal balloon weekly if this is the method of tube retention. If there is delayed gastric emptying, investigate and treat the cause of this. Avoid use of bulky dressings under the external fixator. Consider skin care and use protective cream or spray if necessary. Liaise with medical colleagues and consider the need for antacid medication to reduce skin excoriation (Westaby et al. 2010).

Pneumoperitoneum

This is a known complication of the insertion procedure when air is present in the abdominal cavity. The patient's medical team must be contacted immediately if the patient is complaining of increased pain or pyrexia or has signs of an acute abdomen.

Unplanned removal of tube

A gastrostomy or jejunostomy that is accidentally removed within 14 days of insertion requires immediate attention (Westaby et al. 2010). It should be replaced endoscopically or radiologically as soon as possible as a mature tract will not have developed in this period (Lynch and Fang 2004).

The patient's medical team or nutrition nurse must be contacted immediately, as the stoma site can heal over within 2 hours. The leakage of gastric contents into an immature tract carries the risk of infection. See the section on enteral silicone plugs (below) for advice on how to minimize the risk of stoma occlusion.

Hypergranulation

There is a lack of high-quality evidence in the management of hypergranulation and so the treatment of this condition can be difficult. It is recognized as a common problem but classed as minor in the literature and so there is no standard practice of care (Warriner and Spruce 2012).

Excess movement of the enteral feeding tube within the tract may stimulate the growth of granulation tissue. Ensure that the fixation plate is firm but not too tight on the abdomen to minimize movement of the tube. If the tube does not have an external fixator plate then consider placing one to stop excessive movement of the tube (NNNG 2013). Other factors that may influence the formation of hypergranulation include excess moisture, critical colonization or true infection, and the presence of foreign material (NNNG 2013).

Local guidance on the management of hypergranulation should be agreed and be based on current evidence and the patient population.

Tube inspection

The tube should also be inspected for damage, such as splitting or cracking, during routine daily hygiene. Any damage to the tube could enable a leaking of gastric content onto the surrounding skin, resulting in skin breakdown or excoriation. Adherence to these principles is thought to contribute to the prevention or early detection of problems associated with enterostomal feeding.

Silicone gastrostomy stoma plugs

Definition

Silicone gastrostomy stoma plugs are designed for emergency use to keep stomas from closing when a gastrostomy device has fallen out. They are a temporary measure to minimize the risk of the stoma closing completely and come in several lengths and gauges to fit the need of the patient.

Procedure guideline 8.17 Insertion of a silicone gastrostomy stoma plug

Essential equipment

- Personal protective equipment
- Silicone gastrostomy stoma plug
- Tape

Action	Rationale
Pre-procedure	
1 Introduce yourself to the patient, explain and discuss the procedure with them, and gain their consent to proceed.	To ensure that the patient feels at ease, understands the procedure and gives their valid consent (NMC 2018, **C**).
2 Assist the patient to sit in a semi-upright position in the bed or chair. Support the patient's head with pillows.	To allow for access to the gastrostomy. **E**
3 Wash hands with soap and water or alcohol-based handrub, and assemble the equipment required. Apply apron and clean gloves.	Hands must be cleansed before and after patient contact to minimize the risk of cross-infection (NHS England and NHSI 2019, **C**).
Procedure	
4 Open the packet containing the different coloured silicone plugs. Select the plug that is the same size or closest in size to the current tube. Attempt to push it into the stoma.	To assist in keeping the stoma tract patent. **E**

If the first plug chosen goes in easily	
5 Leave the plug in place and secure with tape over the top.	To ensure the plug does not slip out. **E**
6 Contact the relevant health professional as soon as possible to have a new tube inserted.	A plug is a temporary measure to maintain the stoma tract. **E**
If you cannot insert the first plug chosen	
7 Try the next smallest size.	To ensure that the stoma is filled with the appropriate gauge of plug. **E**
Post-procedure	
8 Once the stoma has been successfully plugged, leave the plug in place and secure it with tape to cover the top.	To prevent movement or the plug falling out. **E**
9 Document which plug was inserted.	To ensure adequate records and to enable continued care of the patient (NMC 2018, **C**).

Administration of enteral tube feed

Pre-procedural considerations

Prior to using enteral feeding tubes for medication or feed administration, it is vital to know where in the gastrointestinal tract the tube tip lies. This may be difficult in patients who have tubes placed in other organs or where there is little visible difference externally between gastrostomy, transgastric or jejunostomy tubes. Where possible, the tube size, type, insertion date and method should be clearly documented. If this information is unavailable, the tube should be aspirated and the pH used to differentiate between gastric and small bowel placement. The pH in the jejunum is usually between 7 and 9 (neutral or slightly alkaline) whereas the pH of the stomach is below 5.5. If there are sutures securing the external fixator to the patient's abdomen, these should not be removed until it has been confirmed that they are not required to keep the tube in position.

Procedure guideline 8.18 Enteral feeding tubes: administration of feed using an enteral feeding pump

Essential equipment

- Personal protective equipment
- 60 mL ENFit-compatible syringe
- Enteral feeding pump
- ENfit-compliant giving set
- Commercial ready-to-hang feed

Optional equipment

- Freshly drawn tap water for patients who are not immunosuppressed, and either cooled freshly boiled water or sterile water from a freshly opened container for patients who are immunosuppressed (NICE 2012) (keep water covered)

Action	Rationale
Pre-procedure	
1 Introduce yourself to the patient, explain and discuss the procedure with them, and gain their consent to proceed.	To ensure that the patient feels at ease, understands the procedure and gives their valid consent (NMC 2018, **C**).
2 Decontaminate hands either by washing with soap and water or with an alcohol-based handrub. Apply personal protective equipment.	To minimize the risk of cross-contamination (NHS England and NHSI 2019, **C**).
Procedure	
3 Check the date on the feed container.	To ensure that the feed has not passed its expiry date. **E**
4 Shake the feed container gently.	To ensure the feed is evenly dispersed, thereby reducing the risk of blocking the giving set. **E**
5 Take a new giving set from a sealed package and ensure that the roller clamp/tap is closed.	To avoid accidental spillage of feed from the end of the administration set. **E**
6 Screw the giving set tightly onto the feed container.	To pierce the seal on the container and maintain a sealed system (Matlow et al. 2006, **C**).
7 Hang the container upside down from the hook on a drip stand.	To avoid backflow of intestinal contents into the feed container (Matlow et al. 2006, **E**).
8 Feed the giving set into the pump as directed by the manufacturer's instructions.	To connect the giving set to the pump device. **E**
9 Open the roller clamp/tap and prime the feed to the end of the giving set. (Follow instructions for individual pump.)	To ensure that air is not fed into the stomach when feeding commences. **E**
10 Set the rate of the feed as directed by the manufacturer's instructions and according to the patient's feeding regimen.	To ensure the correct rate of feed is administered. **E**

(continued)

Procedure guideline 8.18 Enteral feeding tubes: administration of feed using an enteral feeding pump (continued)

Action	Rationale
11 Set the dose of the feed as directed by the manufacturer's instructions and according to the patient's feeding regimen.	To ensure that the correct dose of feed is administered. E
12 Flush the feeding tube with a minimum of 30 mL of water or sterile water in an ENFit syringe by attaching the syringe to the end of the feeding tube. Depress the plunger on the syringe slowly.	To ensure the patency of the feeding tube (BAPEN 2017, **C**).
13 Remove the end cover from the giving set and connect it to the feeding tube.	To ensure that the feed is delivered via the enteral feeding tube. **E**
14 Commence administration of the feed.	To ensure that the feed is delivered via the enteral feeding tube. **E**
Post-procedure	
15 Dispose of any equipment that is no longer required.	To reduce the chance of equipment being reused and to reduce the risk of cross-contamination with new equipment. **E**
16 Document the time that the feed commenced and the rate of administration.	To ensure accurate documentation of nutritional and fluid intake (NMC 2018, **C**).

Problem-solving table 8.5 Prevention and resolution (Procedure guideline 8.18)

Problem	Cause	Prevention	Action
Pump alarm states 'occlusion' or 'empty'	The feed may have finished. There may be a blockage in the giving set or feeding tube.	Ensure the feed container was shaken well before feeding. Ensure the giving set was not kinked when feeding was commenced. Ensure that the roller clamp/tap is fully open. Flush the feeding tube as directed before commencing.	Straighten any kinks in the giving set. Ensure that the giving set is fixed correctly around the rotor. Open the roller clamp/tap fully. Check that the feeding tube is not blocked. Disconnect from the feeding tube and run the feed into a container; if feed runs and there is no alarm, this indicates that the pump is working properly and the feeding tube is probably blocked.
Pump alarm states 'low battery'	This indicates that the pump battery needs to be recharged.	Keep pump plugged in and charged.	Connect to the mains power and continue to feed.
Unable to prime giving set	The roller clamp/tap may not be fully open. There may be a fault with the giving set. If a drip chamber is present then feed may not have run into this. Also check the pump is functioning correctly to initiate the prime.	Ensure that the roller clamp/tap is fully open when beginning to prime the giving set.	Open the roller clamp/tap fully. Squeeze some feed into the drip chamber if applicable. Try with a new giving set.

Post-procedural considerations

Immediate care

As soon as the feed commences, check that it appears to be running without problems and at the correct rate. Monitor this regularly throughout the feed administration.

Monitor the patient for signs of nausea or abdominal discomfort within the first hour and every 2–4 hours during feed administration. This may not be possible if the feed is given overnight and the patient is asleep.

Ongoing care

In order to avoid complications and ensure optimal nutritional status, it is important to monitor the following in patients requiring enteral tube feeding.

- oral intake
- bodyweight
- urea and electrolytes
- blood glucose
- full blood count
- fluid balance
- tolerance to feed, for example nausea, fullness and bowel activity
- quantity of feed taken
- care of tube
- care of stoma site (where appropriate).

If appropriate, the patient should be taught how to follow the procedure of setting up the enteral feeding equipment. They should be confident with the maintenance of the equipment and be aware of how to troubleshoot.

Complications

Aspiration

This may occur due to regurgitation of feed, poor gastric emptying or incorrect placement of a nasogastric tube. The risk of this can be reduced by:

- the use of prokinetics (e.g. metoclopramide), which encourage gastric emptying
- checking the position of the tube before feeding
- ensuring the patient has their head at a 45° angle during feeding; if the patient is in bed then this can be achieved through raising the head of the bed and ensuring the patient has sufficient pillows for support (Gandy 2014).

Nausea and vomiting

This can be caused by a number of factors. It can be related to disease, a side-effect of treatment or a medication such as antibiotics or analgesia. A combination of poor gastric emptying and rapid infusion rates can also stimulate nausea and vomiting. Nausea and vomiting can best be controlled through the use of antiemetics, a reduction in the infusion rate or a change from bolus to intermittent feeding.

Diarrhoea

This could be a result of:

- medications such as antibiotics, chemotherapy or laxatives
- disease or treatment, for example pancreatic insufficiency or bile acid malabsorption
- gut infection, for example *Clostridioides difficile*
- poor tolerance to the feed.

Antidiarrhoeal agents can be used if a person is experiencing diarrhoea as a side effect of medication. If possible, an alternative medication should be found that does not cause diarrhoea. When the diarrhoea is disease related, the underlying problem should be treated; that is, if a person has pancreatic insufficiency, they should be provided with a pancreatic enzyme supplement and/or peptide-based feed.

Avoiding microbiological contamination of the feed and equipment will help to reduce the risk of diarrhoea. This will involve keeping the equipment clean and, when feeding, maintaining a sealed system.

A stool sample should be sent to microbiology to test for cultures and sensitivities to check for any gut infection. If the sample is found to be positive then the infection should be treated appropriately. Refer to Chapter 6: Elimination for further information on the diagnosis and treatment of diarrhoea.

If all of the above have been ruled out, the dietitian can review the osmolarity, fibre content and infusion rate (Todorovic and Mafrici 2019).

Constipation

Constipation can be caused by inadequate fluid intake, immobility, bowel obstruction, or the use of opiates or other medications causing gut stasis. Methods to improve symptoms of constipation include:

- checking fluid balance and increasing fluid intake if necessary
- providing laxatives or bulking agents
- if possible, encouraging mobility
- if there is a bowel obstruction, discontinuing enteral feeding (Todorovic and Mafrici 2019).

Abdominal distension

This can be caused by poor gastric emptying, rapid infusion of feed, constipation or diarrhoea. Possible ways to improve distension include:

- gastric motility agents
- reducing the rate of infusion
- encouraging mobility if possible
- treating constipation or diarrhoea.

Blocked tube

Blockage can be a result of inadequate flushing, failure to flush the feeding tube or administration of inappropriate medications via the tube. For ways to unblock a feeding tube refer to Procedure guideline 8.20: Enteral feeding tubes: unblocking.

Enteral feeding tubes: administration of medication

Evidence-based approaches

Rationale

Indications

Use of an enteral feeding tube for the administration of medication is indicated for patients requiring medications who are not able to take oral preparations due to dysphagia. Where possible, medications should be administered in liquid or soluble form. Alternatively, some preparations can be given in sublingual form.

Contraindications

There are no absolute contraindications to the use of enteral feeding tubes. However:

- Do not instil any medication that poses a risk of blocking the feeding tube.
- Enteric coated or slow-release medications should not be crushed and are therefore not suitable for administration down an enteral tube.

Other considerations when deciding whether to use the tube for medication administration are as follows:

- If the preparation would be harmful to the administrator, seek advice from a pharmacist.
- It is not advisable to mix different medications prior to administration unless advised to do so by a pharmacist.
- 60 mL ENFit syringes must *not* be used to measure drugs where the required drug volume is below 10 mL as they are not sufficiently accurate at such volumes. A 10 mL oral syringe must be used to measure drug volumes and the dose then transferred to an appropriate ENFit syringe for administration. Drug volumes of 10 mL and above can be measured using the ENFit syringe that is going to be used to administer the drug.

Post-procedural considerations

Immediate care

The tube's patency should be checked to ensure that the medication has not caused a blockage. This can be done by flushing the tube. The patient should be monitored to ensure that there are no unanticipated side-effects of the medication administered.

Education of the patient and relevant others

If the patient is going home with the enteral tube in place, it should be ensured that the patient is educated and confident with administering their feed and medication. If this is not possible then the patient should be referred to a healthcare professional, such as a community nurse, who can undertake this aspect of care.

Home enteral feeding

Some patients who are established on tube feeding in hospital also require enteral tube feeding at home. A multidisciplinary approach is needed for a successful discharge, usually involving a dietician, doctor, ward nurse, community nurse and GP. The patient's circumstances and the ability of the patient or carers to manage the feed must be considered when discharge is being planned. Adequate time should be allowed in the hospital setting for patients to become fully accustomed to the techniques of feed administration and care of the feeding tube, prior to discharge home. Patients should also be given written information to reinforce the education they receive prior to discharge (BAPEN 2016a).

Support in the form of the GP, community nurse and community dietetic services should be established before discharge. A multidisciplinary discharge meeting may be of benefit to both the patient and the professionals involved. Many of the commercial feed companies can organize for a patient's feed and equipment to be delivered to their home, after consultation with the local community services (BAPEN 2016a). The hospital or community dietician can arrange this. Early notification of discharge is essential to facilitate this transition of care.

Procedure guideline 8.10 Enteral feeding tubes: administration of medication

Essential equipment

- Personal protective equipment
- 60 mL ENfit enteral syringe
- 5 mL, 10 mL and 20 mL ENfit syringes (if required)
- 10 mL oral syringe (if required)
- Mortar and pestle or tablet crusher if tablets are being administered (BAPEN 2017)

Optional equipment

- Freshly drawn tap water for patients who are not immunosuppressed, and either cooled freshly boiled water or sterile water from a freshly opened container for patients who are immunosuppressed (NICE 2012) (keep water covered)

Action	Rationale
Pre-procedure	
1 Check whether the patient can take medication orally, whether medication is necessary or whether it can be temporarily suspended.	If the patient can take medication orally this reduces the risk of tube blockage (BAPEN 2017, **C**).
2 Consider whether an alternative route can be used, for example buccal, transdermal, topical, rectal or subcutaneous.	If the patient can take medication via an alternative route this reduces the risk of tube blockage (BAPEN 2017, **C**).
3 Check the drug is absorbed from the site of delivery.	Some drugs may not be absorbed directly from the jejunum (BAPEN 2017, **C**).
4 Introduce yourself to the patient, explain and discuss the procedure with them, and gain their consent to proceed.	To ensure that the patient feels at ease, understands the procedure and gives their valid consent (NMC 2018, **C**).
5 Clean hands with soap and water or alcohol-based handrub and apply personal protective equipment.	To minimize the risk of cross-infection and protect the practitioner from gastric/intestinal contents (NHS England and NHSI 2019, **C**).
Procedure	
6 Stop the enteral feed and flush the tube with at least 30 mL of water (sterile water for jejunostomy administration), using an enteral syringe. *Next, where there is an absolute contraindication for medicine to be taken with feed, follow steps 7 and 8. If not, skip to step 9.*	To clear the tube of enteral feed as this may cause a blockage or interact with medications. Sterile water should be used for jejunostomy tubes as the water is bypassing the protective acidic environment of the stomach. **E**
7 Stop the feed 1–2 hours before and leave the feed off for up to 2 hours after administration (this will depend on the drug); for example, for phenytoin administration, stop feed 2 hours before and for 2 hours after.	To avoid interaction with enteral feed. **E**
8 Consult with the dietitian to prescribe a suitable feeding regimen.	To ensure that the patient's nutritional requirements are met in the time available around medicine administration (BAPEN 2017, **C**).
9 Prior to preparation, check with the pharmacist which medicines should never be crushed.	Some medications are not designed to be crushed. These include: • *modified-release tablets*: absorption will be altered by crushing, possibly causing toxic side-effects • *enteric-coated tablets*: the coating is designed to protect the drug against gastric acid • *cytotoxic medicines*: crushing will risk exposing the practitioner to the drug (BNF 2019, **C**).
10 Prepare each medication to be given separately. Volumes greater than 2.5 mL may be drawn up in a 5 mL, 10 mL, 20 mL or 60 mL ENFit syringe according to the volume required and administered via the tube. Always choose the smallest syringe that will accommodate the volume of drug. For smaller volumes (less than 2.5 mL) follow step 13. *Either:* • *Soluble tablets*: dissolve in 10–15 mL water. *Or:* • *Liquids*: shake well. For thick liquids mix with an equal volume of water. *Or:* • *Tablets*: crush using a mortar and pestle or tablet crusher and mix with 10–15 mL water.	To avoid interaction between different medications and to ensure solubility (BAPEN 2017, **C**). To improve accuracy of measurement of the drug. **E**
11 Never add medication directly to the enteral feed.	To avoid interaction between medicines and feed (BAPEN 2017, **C**).
12 Administer the medication through the tube via a 60 mL ENFit enteral syringe.	To ensure the whole dose is administered (BAPEN 2017, **C**). To ensure that intravenous syringes are not connected to an enteral feeding system (NHSI 2017, **C**).

13 Rinse the tablet crusher or mortar with 10 mL water, draw the water up in a 60 mL ENFit syringe, and flush this through the tube.	To ensure the whole dose is administered (BAPEN 2017, **C**).
14 If volumes of less than 2.5 mL are required, the dose should be measured in a 10 mL oral syringe – *not* an ENFit syringe. The plunger of a 60 mL ENfit syringe should be removed and the 60 mL ENfit syringe connected with the enteral tube. The dose should then be administered into the barrel of the 60 mL ENFit syringe and the 10 mL syringe rinsed with water, and this water should also be administered via the barrel of the 60 mL ENFit syringe.	To avoid interactions between medicines (BAPEN 2017, **C**). To ensure that the whole dose is administered. **E**
15 Flush the tube with at least 30 mL of water between administrations of different drugs and following the administration of the last drug.	To avoid medicines blocking the enteral tube (BAPEN 2017, **C**).
16 If the patient is on fluid restriction or for a paediatric patient, consult the dietician and pharmacist about the quantity of water to be given before and after medication.	To ensure that the patient does not exceed their fluid restriction or requirements (BAPEN 2017, **C**).
Post-procedure	
17 Remove and dispose of any equipment.	To reduce the risk of cross-infection. **E**
18 Record the administration on the prescription chart. Record fluid intake on the fluid chart if applicable.	To maintain accurate records (NMC 2018, **C**). To ensure accuracy of fluid balance monitoring. **E**

Problem-solving table 8.6 Prevention and resolution (Procedure guideline 8.19)

Problem	Cause	Prevention	Action
Tube blocked with medication	Medication was not administered in the correct composition and/or the tube was not flushed adequately	Ensure that the guidance from the pharmacist is followed correctly. Ensure that the tube is flushed before and after administration.	See Procedure guideline 8.20: Enteral feeding tubes: unblocking.
Unable to administer required medication	Medication is in a form that cannot be crushed or dissolved	Ensure that the pharmacist and medical team are aware that all medications need to be administered via an enteral tube.	Contact the medical team or pharmacist to seek advice on an alternative medication.

Termination of enteral tube feeding

It is important to ensure that an individual is able to meet their nutritional requirements orally prior to termination of the feed. Enteral tube feeding may be discontinued when oral intake is established (NCCAC 2006). It may be useful to maintain an overnight feed while the patient is establishing oral intake (Pearce and Duncan 2002).

Parenteral nutrition

Definition

Parenteral nutrition is the direct infusion into a vein of solutions containing essential nutrients in quantities to meet the nutritional needs of a person who has an inaccessible or non-functioning gastrointestinal tract (intestinal failure) (Klek et al. 2016, NCEPOD 2010).

Related theory

The basic components of a parenteral nutrition regimen are provided by solutions including the following:

- *Amino acids (nitrogen source)*: commercially available solutions provide both essential amino acids, usually in proportions to meet requirements, and non-essential amino acids, such as alanine and glycine.
- *Glucose (carbohydrate energy source)*. Glucose is the carbohydrate source of choice. It provides 3.75 kcal/g (15.5 kJ/g) and usually provides 50% of non-nitrogen energy.
- *Fat emulsion (fat energy source)*: fat generates 9 kcal/g (37 kJ/g) and its inclusion in parenteral nutrition is necessary to provide essential fatty acids. Fat usually provides 50% of non-nitrogen energy.
- *Nitrogen*: non-nitrogen energy is usually provided in the ratio of 1:150–200. An insufficient energy supply from carbohydrate and fat will encourage the use of nitrogen for energy.
- *Electrolytes*: for example sodium, potassium, calcium, magnesium and phosphate.
- *Vitamins and minerals*: both water-soluble and fat-soluble vitamins are required as part of a standard bag.
- *Trace elements*: for example zinc, copper, chromium and selenium (Singer et al. 2018).

Evidence-based approaches

Rationale

Parenteral nutrition should only be used when it is not possible to meet nutritional requirements via the gastrointestinal tract. Parenteral

Procedure guideline 8.20 Enteral feeding tubes: unblocking

Essential equipment

- Personal protective equipment
- 60 mL ENFit enteral syringe
- Freshly drawn tap water for patients who are not immunosuppressed, and either cooled freshly boiled water or sterile water from a freshly opened container for patients who are immunosuppressed (NICE 2012) (keep water covered)
- To obtain lukewarm water (40–45°C), put approximately 120 mL of cold drinking tap water (sterile water for jejunostomy and for immunosuppressed patients) into a plastic cup and add about 40 mL of boiling water

Optional equipment

- Sterile water (for jejunostomy tubes)

Action	Rationale
Pre-procedure	
1 Introduce yourself to the patient, explain and discuss the procedure with them, and gain their consent to proceed.	To ensure that the patient feels at ease, understands the procedure and gives their valid consent (NMC 2018, **C**).
2 Always flush the enteral tube before and after administration of feed and medication with at least 30 mL of water (sterile water for jejunostomy and for immunosuppressed patients).	To avoid the tube blocking. Sterile water should be used for jejunostomy tubes as the water is bypassing the protective acidic environment of the stomach. **E**
3 Examine the tube for kinks.	To ensure that this is not the cause of the blockage (BAPEN 2016a, **E**).
Procedure	
4 Draw up 30 mL of water (lukewarm) in a 60 mL ENFit enteral syringe and attempt to flush/withdraw fluid from the tube. Boiling or hot water must *not* be used to flush an enteral feeding tube.	To dissolve any medication or soften any feed plugs in the tube. To prevent hot water being administered via the feeding tube (BAPEN 2016a, **C**). To remove blockage and acidic fluids such as carbonated drinks that may cause feed to clot (BAPEN 2016a, **C**).
5 If the tube is still blocked, consider use of a proprietary product designed to unblock tubes. Follow the manufacturer's instructions.	To break down the plug. Such products contain digestive enzymes, which may break down a protein plug, but they may not unblock a tube blocked with medication (manufacturer's recommendation, **C**).
6 If all of the above are unsuccessful then the enteral tube will need to be replaced.	To ensure continued enteral access for the administration of feed, fluids and medication. **E**
Post-procedure	
7 Document the procedure in the patient's notes.	To record actions and outcome (NMC 2018, **C**).

Problem-solving table 8.7 Prevention and resolution (Procedure guideline 8.20)

Problem	Cause	Prevention	Action
Cracked/split tube	Too much pressure applied while flushing tube	Avoid applying too much pressure while flushing the tube and take care with a syringe smaller than 50 mL.	If the tube cracks or splits then it must be replaced.

nutrition is an invasive and relatively expensive form of nutrition support and, in inexperienced hands, can be associated with risks from catheter placement, catheter infections, thrombosis and metabolic disturbance. Careful consideration is therefore needed when deciding to whom, when and how this form of nutrition support should be given (Klek et al. 2016, NCCAC 2006). It should be planned and managed by healthcare professionals with the relevant expertise (NCEPOD 2010). Whenever possible, patients should be made aware of why this form of nutrition support is needed and its potential risks and benefits.

Parenteral nutrition may be used in combination with enteral nutrition where some gut function is present but this is insufficient to meet nutritional requirements, for example in intestinal failure, where the patient can eat but absorptive capacity may be insufficient to maintain nutritional status.

Intestinal failure (IF) can be categorized as follows.

- *Type 1*: this type of IF is short term, self-limiting and often perioperative in nature. Type 1 IF is common and these patients are managed successfully in a multitude of healthcare settings, especially surgical wards, including all units that perform major (particularly abdominal) surgery. Some patients on high-dependency units and intensive care units will also fall into this category.
- *Type 2*: this occurs in metabolically unstable patients in hospital and requires prolonged parenteral nutrition over periods of weeks or months. It is often associated with sepsis and may be associated with renal impairment. These patients often need the facilities of an intensive care or high-dependency unit for some or

much of their stay in hospital. This type of IF is rarer and needs to be managed by a multiprofessional specialist IF team. Poor management of type 2 IF increases mortality and is expected to increase the likelihood of later development of type 3 IF.

- *Type 3*: this is a chronic condition requiring long-term parenteral feeding. The patient is characteristically metabolically stable but cannot maintain their nutrition adequately by absorbing food or nutrients via the intestinal tract. These are, in the main, the group of patients for which home parenteral nutrition or electrolytes are indicated.

Indications

The indications for parenteral nutrition are:

- failure of gut function (e.g. with obstruction, ileus, dysmotility, fistulae, surgical resection or severe malabsorption) to a degree that definitely prevents adequate gastrointestinal absorption of nutrients
- inaccessible gastrointestinal tract (e.g. unable to insert enteral feeding tube)
- the consequent intestinal failure has either persisted for several days (e.g. > 5 days) or is likely to persist for many days (e.g. 5 days or longer) before significant improvement (NICE 2017c).

Examples of the use of parenteral nutrition include for patients with prolonged gastrointestinal ileus, intractable vomiting or high-output gastrointestinal fistula where requirements cannot be met by the enteral route.

Contraindications

If the gut can be used or an attempt to use it has not yet been considered, then parenteral nutrition should be withheld pending the outcome of using the enteral system. Parenteral nutrition should also not be used if the perceived risk to the patient outweighs the benefits anticipated (NCCAC 2006).

Contents of parenteral nutrition

Parenteral nutrition provides nutrients in a form that can be used directly by the body when they are infused intravenously. Nitrogen (protein) is provided as free amino acids in a ratio designed to meet the requirements for essential amino acids. Specific amino acid profiles may be used for some disease states. Energy is usually provided from carbohydrate and fat. Carbohydrate is present as glucose and fat is provided as a lipid emulsion of essential fatty acids. The lipid source may be provided by long-chain, medium-chain triglycerides or fish oil containing omega-3 fatty acids, with different manufacturers using different lipid blends. Fluid, electrolytes, vitamins, minerals and trace elements are also provided by parenteral nutrition (Singer et al. 2018).

Choice of a parenteral nutrition regimen

Parenteral nutrition is usually administered from a single infusion container in which all the requirements for a 24-hour feed are premixed. Such infusions are available as standard ready-prepared bags that require mixing, and vitamins, minerals, and trace elements or individual bags may be added to a particular prescription and purchased from a compounding unit.

The regimen for a particular patient should be formulated according to their needs for energy, nitrogen, electrolytes and fluid. The majority of commercial vitamin and mineral preparations aim to meet both short- and long-term requirements although appropriate monitoring is required to ensure that nutritional requirements are met in the longer term as clinically indicated by the monitoring guidelines. Standard parenteral nutrition regimens may be suitable for some patients who require short-term nutritional support or do not appear to have excessively altered nutritional requirements.

The choice of such regimens depends on the patient's bodyweight and nutritional requirements. To allow for the possible need to vary the constituents of the infusion in response to changes in the patient's electrolyte or nutritional requirements, parenteral nutrition solutions should be ordered daily. Once compounded, parenteral nutrition has a limited lifespan determined by the manufacturers. Bags of parenteral nutrition that have been compounded with vitamins and minerals need to be stored in a refrigerator. However, some triple-chamber parenteral nutrition bags can be stored at ambient temperatures and require mixing prior to administration. These bags generally require the addition of vitamins, minerals and trace elements under aseptic conditions.

Parenteral nutrition should be introduced slowly in the seriously ill or injured, with no more than 50% of requirements given in the first 24–48 hours due to the risk of refeeding syndrome (NCCAC 2006).

Methods of administration

The traditional method of access is via a central venous catheter. Central venous access is required because parenteral nutrition solutions are hyperosmolar and there is a risk of thrombophlebitis associated with feeding into peripheral veins. However, it has been shown that, with care and attention, peripheral veins can be used to provide short-term parenteral nutrition (NCCAC 2006). This would be via a midline or peripheral cannula. For the administration of parenteral nutrition, the device should be placed in the largest vein possible, usually in the forearm away from a joint, with rotation of the site every 48–72 hours (Shaw 2008).

A skin-tunnelled catheter is the first choice for long-term nutrition but peripherally inserted central cannulas (PICCs), non-tunnelled central venous catheters or venous access ports can also be used in the short term. The number of lumens will depend on the patient's peripheral venous access and the number of additional therapies required. It is recommended that the minimum number of lumens is used but if additional intravenous access is required then a double- or triple-lumen catheter should be inserted and then one lumen should be dedicated for use with parenteral nutrition. If using a single-lumen device, routine blood sampling and additional infusions should be carried out independently, using a separate cannula if necessary (Das and Bowling 2018).

For setting up an infusion, see Procedure guideline 15.23: Medication: continuous infusion of intravenous drugs.

Post-procedural considerations

Ongoing care

Administration sets should always be changed every 24 hours (Loveday et al. 2014, NICE 2012, O'Grady et al. 2011). Existing injection sites on the administration set should never be used to give additional medications as parenteral nutrition is incompatible with numerous medications. Drugs may bind to the nutrients or the parenteral nutrition bag, reducing their availability. If any additional medications, blood products or central venous pressure (CVP) readings are required then they should be given or taken via a separate lumen or via an alternative device (NCEPOD 2010).

A volumetric infusion pump must be used to ensure accurate delivery of parenteral nutrition. No bag should be used for longer than 24 hours (BNF 2019).

If the infusion must be discontinued, the catheter should be flushed to maintain patency. The risk of infection increases if the infusion is disconnected from the central venous device; therefore, it is not advisable to disconnect parenteral nutrition until the whole daily requirement has been administered (NCEPOD 2010).

During intravenous feeding, monitoring is necessary to detect and minimize complications. Once feeding is established and the patient is biochemically stable then the frequency of monitoring may be reduced if the clinical condition of the patient permits (Table 8.12).

Home parenteral nutrition

There are a few indications for home parenteral nutrition. It may be necessary in patients who have complete intestinal failure or insufficient bowel function to maintain an adequate nutritional status via the enteral route, for example short bowel syndrome due to Crohn's disease or a high-output fistula. It may also be required if it is not possible to access the gastrointestinal tract, although all possible enteral routes should be explored.

Table 8.12 Monitoring in nutrition support

Parameter	Frequency of monitoring	Rationale	Interpretation
Catheter entry site	Daily	Signs of infection or inflammation	Interpret with knowledge of infection control
Skin over insertion site and tip of cannula or midline catheter	Daily	Signs of thrombophlebitis	
General condition	Daily	To check tolerance of feed and that feed and route continue to be appropriate	
Temperature/blood pressure	Daily, then as needed	Sign of infection, fluid balance	
Sodium, potassium, urea, creatinine	Baseline, then daily until stable, then one or two times a week	Assessment of renal function, fluid status	Interpret with knowledge of fluid balance and medication; urinary sodium may be helpful in complex cases with gastrointestinal fluid loss
Glucose	Baseline, then one or two times daily until stable (more if needed), then weekly	Glucose intolerance is common	Good glycaemic control is necessary
Magnesium, phosphate	Baseline, then daily if risk of refeeding syndrome, then three times a week until stable, then weekly	Depletion is common and under-recognized	Low concentrations indicate poor status
Liver function tests	Baseline, then twice weekly until stable, then weekly	Abnormalities common during PN	Complex; may be due to sepsis, other disease or nutritional intake
Calcium, albumin	Baseline, then weekly	Low or high levels may occur	Correct measured serum calcium concentration for albumin; hypocalcaemia may be secondary to magnesium deficiency; low albumin reflects disease, not protein status
C-reactive protein	Baseline, then two or three times a week until stable	Assists interpretation of protein, trace element and vitamin results	To assess the presence of an acute-phase reaction; the trend of results is important
Zinc, copper	Baseline, then every 2–4 weeks depending on results	Deficiency is common, especially with increased losses	Patients are most at risk when anabolic zinc decreases and copper increases in acute-phase reaction
Selenium	Baseline if risk of depletion, further testing depending on this	Deficiency is likely in severe illness and sepsis, and in long-term nutrition support	Decreases in acute-phase reaction; long-term status better assessed by glutathione peroxidase
Full blood count	Baseline, then one or two times a week until stable, then weekly	Anaemia due to iron or folate deficiency is common	Effects of sepsis may be important
Iron, ferritin	Baseline, then every 3–6 months	Iron deficiency is common in long-term PN	Iron status is difficult to assess in acute-phase reaction; iron decreases while ferritin increases
Folate, vitamin B_{12}	Baseline then every 2–4 weeks	Iron deficiency is common	Serum folate/B_{12} sufficient with full blood count
Manganese	Every 3–6 months if on home PN	Excess provision to be avoided, more likely in liver disease	Red blood cell or whole blood better measure of excess than plasma
Vitamin D	Six-monthly if on long-term PN	Low levels if housebound	Requires normal kidney function for effect
Bone densitometry	On starting home PN, then every 2 years	Diagnosis of metabolic bone disease	Together with lab tests for metabolic bone disease

PN, parenteral nutrition.

Source: Adapted from NCCAC (2006) with permission of NICE.

This is a complicated and specialist treatment, requiring 24-hour access to advice and support, and should be co-ordinated through a specialist intestinal failure centre.

No patient should be considered for home parenteral nutrition without a multidisciplinary discussion with the patient and the formulation of a clear management plan. If continuation of hospital-initiated parenteral nutrition is considered essential, the implications must be discussed with the multiprofessional team, including the medical consultant, dietetics, pharmacy, intravenous therapy team, complex discharge co-ordinator and patient (BAPEN 2016b).

Patients require an extensive period of specialized training to manage parenteral nutrition in the home environment. This should only be undertaken by specialist intestinal failure units or home parenteral nutrition (HPN) designated units with a multidisciplinary nutrition support team with the appropriate expertise (BAPEN 2016b).

It is important that all members of the multidisciplinary team, including the dietician, nurse, doctor, pharmacist and community services, are involved in the patient's nutritional care to ensure a thorough and co-ordinated approach to nutritional management.

Termination of parenteral nutrition

Parenteral nutrition should not be terminated until oral or enteral tube feeding is well established (NICE 2017c). Parenteral nutrition may require weaning at a reduced rate if there is concern about rebound hypoglycaemia or management of concurrent insulin, as well as to ensure adequate nutritional intake via an alternative route. It is important that all members of the multidisciplinary team are involved in the decision to terminate parenteral nutrition and that enteral intake is monitored sufficiently.

Complications

Metabolic complications should be detected by appropriate monitoring. Some of the more common complications are as follows.

Fluid overload

This may occur when other blood products and fluids are given concurrently. It may be possible to reduce the volume of a bag of parenteral nutrition while maintaining the nutritional content. A pharmacist and dietician can advise on the feasibility of creating such regimens.

Impaired liver function

Long-term parenteral nutrition and the lack of enteral nutrition may contribute to altered liver function and cholestasis. Liver function may be influenced by the total amount of glucose that is administered, the quantity and composition of lipid in parenteral nutrition, the type of administration (e.g. over 24 hours), and any underlying hepatic pathology (Das and Bowling 2018).

Hyperglycaemia

This may occur due to stress-induced insulin resistance or carbohydrate overload. A simultaneous sliding scale insulin infusion may be required. Failure to recognize hyperglycaemia may result in osmotic diuresis.

Hypoglycaemia

Abrupt cessation of parenteral nutrition may result in rebound hypoglycaemia. A reduction in infusion to half the rate prior to stopping the infusion may help to prevent this occurring.

Websites

Age Concern
www.ageuk.org.uk

Age UK, *Healthy Eating*
https://www.ageuk.org.uk/information-advice/health-wellbeing/healthy-eating

Age UK, *Still Hungry to Be Heard*
https://www.ageuk.org.uk/bp-assets/globalassets/london/documents/campaigns/still-hungry-to-be-heard.pdf

BAPEN
https://www.bapen.org.uk

BAPEN, *Hospital Services*
https://www.bapen.org.uk/nutrition-support/good-practice-in-nutritional-care/examples-of-good-practice-in-nutritional-care/hospital-services

British Dietetic Association, *Policy Statement: The Management of Malnourished Adults in All Community and All Health and Care Settings*
https://www.bda.uk.com/improvinghealth/healthprofessionals/policy_statements/policy_statement_-_management_malnourished_adults

ESPEN, *Guidelines and Consensus Papers*
https://www.espen.org/guidelines-home/espen-guidelines

NHS England, Commissioning Excellent Nutrition and Hydration 2015–2018
https://www.england.nhs.uk/wp-content/uploads/2015/10/nut-hyd-guid.pdf

Patients on Intravenous and Nasogastric Nutrition Therapy (PINNT)
https://pinnt.com

References

Adam, S., Osborne, S. & Welch, J. (2017) *Critical Care Nursing*, 3rd edn. Oxford: Oxford University Press.

Age UK (2016) *Policy Position Paper: Nutrition and Hydration (England)*. Available at: https://www.ageuk.org.uk/globalassets/age-uk/documents/policy-positions/health-and-wellbeing/ppp_nutrition_and_hydration england.pdf

Alexander, L. & Allen, D. (2011) Establishing an evidence-based inpatient medical oncology fluid balance measurement policy. *Clinical Journal of Oncology Nursing*, 15(1), 23–25.

Aoi, W. & Marunaka, Y. (2014) Importance of pH homeostasis in metabolic health and diseases: Crucial role of membrane proton transport. *BioMed Research International*, 2014, 1–8.

Arends, J., Bachmann, P., Baracos, V., et al. (2017) ESPEN guidelines on nutrition in cancer patients. *Clinical Nutrition*, 36(1), 11–48.

Atkinson, M. & McHanwell, S. (2002) *Basic Medical Science for Speech and Language Therapy Students*. London: Whurr.

Aya, H.D., Ster, I.C., Fletcher, N., et al. (2016) Pharmacodynamic analysis of a fluid challenge. *Critical Care Medicine*, 44(5), 880–891.

Bak, A. & Tsiami, A. (2016) Review on mechanisms, importance of homeostasis and fluid imbalances in the elderly. *Current Research in Nutrition and Food Science*, 4. DOI: 10.12944/CRNFSJ.4.Special-Issue-Elderly-November.01.

BAPEN (British Association for Parenteral and Enteral Nutrition) (2012a) *Nutrition Screening Survey in the UK and Republic of Ireland in 2011: Hospitals, Care Homes and Mental Health Units – A Report by BAPEN*. Available at: www.bapen.org.uk/pdfs/nsw/nsw-2011-report.pdf

BAPEN (2012b) *Decision Tree on Insertion of Nasogastric Tube*. Available at: https://www.bapen.org.uk/pdfs/decision-trees/naso-gastric-tube-insertion.pdf

BAPEN (2016a) *Oral Nutritional Supplements (ONS)*. Available at: www.bapen.org.uk/nutrition-support/nutrition-by-mouth/oral-nutritional-supplements

BAPEN (2016b). *British Intestinal Failure Alliance (BIFA) Position Statement 2016: Home Parenteral Nutrition (HPN)*. Available at: www.bapen.org.uk/images/pdfs/position-statements/position-statement-on-hpn.pdf

BAPEN (2017) *Medications: Administering Medicines via Enteral Feeding Tubes*. Available at: https://www.bapen.org.uk/nutrition-support/enteral-nutrition/medications

BAPEN (2018a) *The MUST Report: Nutritional Screening of Adults: A Multidisciplinary Responsibility*. Available at: https://www.bapen.org.uk/screening-and-must/must/must-report

BAPEN (2018b) *The MUST Toolkit*. Available at: https://www.bapen.org.uk/screening-and-must/must/must-toolkit

Baraz, S., Parvardeh, S., Mohammadi, E. & Broumand, B. (2009) Dietary and fluid compliance: An educational intervention for patients having haemodialysis. *Journal of Advanced Nursing*, 66(1), 60–68.

Barrett, K.E. (2014) *Gastrointestinal Physiology*, 2nd edn. New York: Lange Medical Books / McGraw Hill.

Bass, N.H. (1997) *The Neurology of Swallowing*, 3rd edn. Boston, MA: Butterworth-Heinemann.

Bauer, J., Capra, S. & Ferguson, M. (2002) Use of scored patient-generated subjective global assessment (PG-SGA) as a nutritional assessment tool in patients with cancer. *European Journal of Clinical Nutrition*, 56(8), 779–785.

Baumberger-Henry, M. (2008) *Quick Look Nursing: Fluids and Electrolytes*, 2nd edn. Sudbury, MA: Jones & Bartlett.

BDA (British Dietetic Association) (2019) *The Nutrition and Hydration Digest*, 2nd edn. Available at: https://www.bda.uk.com/publications/professional/NutritionHydrationDigest.pdf

Benítez Brito, N., Suárez Llanos, J.P., Fuentes Ferrer, M., et al. (2016) Relationship between mid-upper arm circumference and body mass index in inpatients. *PLOS ONE*, 11(8), e0160480.

BNF (British National Formulary) (2019) *British National Formulary*. National Institute for Health and Care Excellence. Available at: https://bnf.nice.org.uk

Brady, G.C., Carding, P.N., Bhosle, J. & Roe, J.W. (2015) Contemporary management of voice and swallowing disorders in patients with advanced lung cancer. *Current Opinion in Otolaryngology & Head and Neck Surgery*, 23(3), 191–196.

Brodsky, M.B., Gellar, J.E., Dinglas, V.D., et al. (2014) Duration of oral endotracheal intubation is associated with dysphagia symptoms in acute lung injury patients. *Journal of Critical Care*, 29(4), 574–579.

Bryant, H. (2007) Dehydration in older people: Assessment and management. *Emergency Nurse*, 15(4), 22–26.

Butler, C. & Leslie, P. (2012) *Anatomy and Physiology of Swallowing*. San Diego: Plural.

Cappell, M.S., Inglis, B. & Levy, A. (2009) Two case reports of gastric ulcer from pressure necrosis related to a rigid and taut percutaneous endoscopic gastrostomy bumper. *Gastroenterology Nursing*, 32(4), 259–263.

Care Quality Commission (2013) *Time to Listen in NHS Hospitals: Dignity and Nutrition Inspection Programme 2012 – National Overview*. Available at: https://www.cqc.org.uk/sites/default/files/documents/time_to_listen_-_nhs_hospitals_main_report_tag.pdf

Carlsson, M., Haglin, L., Rosendahl, E. & Gustafson, Y. (2013) Poor nutritional status is associated with urinary tract infection among older people living in residential care facilities. *Journal of Nutrition, Health & Aging*, 17(2), 186–191.

Cecconi, M., De Backer, D., Antonelli, M., et al. (2014) Consensus on circulatory shock and hemodynamic monitoring: Task force of the European Society of Intensive Care Medicine. *Intensive Care Medicine*, 40(12), 1795–1815.

Cederholm, T., Barazzoni, R., Austin, P., et al. (2017) ESPEN guidelines on definitions and terminology of clinical nutrition. *Clinical Nutrition*, 36(1), 49–64.

Chan, H.Y.L., Cheng, A., Cheung, S.S., et al. (2018) Association between dehydration on admission and postoperative complications in older persons undergoing orthopaedic surgery. *Journal of Clinical Nursing*, 27, 679–686.

Children Act (1989) Available at: https://www.legislation.gov.uk/ukpga/1989/41/contents

Chioncel, O., Collins, S.P., Ambrosy, A.P., et al. (2015) Pulmonary oedema: Therapeutic targets. *Cardiac Failure Review*, 1(1), 38–45.

Cichero, J.A., Lam, P., Steele, C.M., et al. (2017) Development of international terminology and definitions for texture modified foods and thickened fluids used in dysphagia management: The IDDSI framework. *Dysphagia*, 32(2), 293–314.

Clarkson, D.M. (2012) Patient weighing: Standardisation and treatment. *Nursing Standard*, 26(29), 33–37.

Coffey, M. & Tolley, N. (2015) Swallowing after laryngectomy. *Current Opinion in Otolaryngology & Head and Neck Surgery*, [illegible].

COMA (Committee on Medical Aspects of Food Policy) & DH (Department of Health) (1991) *Dietary Reference Values for Food Energy and Nutrients for the United Kingdom: Report of the Panel on Dietary Reference Values of the Committee on Medical Aspects of Food Policy*. London: HM Stationery Office.

Cooke, K., Sharvill, R., Sondergaard, S. & Aneman, A. (2018) Volume responsiveness assessed by passive leg raising and a fluid challenge: A critical review focused on mean systemic filling pressure. *Anaesthesia*, [illegible].

Council of Europe Committee of Ministers (2003) *Resolution ResAP(2003)3 on Food and Nutritional Care in Hospitals*. Available at: https://search.coe.int/cm/Pages/result_details.aspx?ObjectID=09000016805de855

Cruz, I., Mamel, J.J., Brady, P.G. & Cass-Garcia, M. (2005) Incidence of abdominal wall metastasis complicating PEG tube placement in untreated head and neck cancer. *Gastrointestinal Endoscopy*, 62(5), 708–711.

Das, R. & Bowling, T. (2018) Parenteral nutrition to prevent and treat undernutrition. In: Hickson, M. & Smith, S. (eds) *Advanced Nutrition and Dietetics in Nutrition Support*. Oxford: Wiley Blackwell, pp.207–216.

Davies, H., Leslie, G. & Morgan, D. (2015) Effectiveness of daily fluid balance charting in comparison to the measurement of body weight when used in guiding fluid therapy for critically ill adult patients: A systematic review protocol. *JBI Database of Systematic Reviews and Implementation Reports*, 13(3), 111–123.

DEFRA (Department for Environment, Food and Rural Affairs) (2015) *Sustainable Procurement: The GBS for Food and Catering Services*. Available at: https://www.gov.uk/government/publications/sustainable-procurement-the-gbs-for-food-and-catering-services

DH (Department of Health) (2014) *The Hospital Food Standards Panel's Report on Standards for Food and Drink in NHS Hospitals*. Available at: https://assets.publishing.service.gov.uk/government/uploads/system/uploads/attachment_data/file/523049/Hospital_Food_Panel_May_2016.pdf

Durnin, J.V. & Womersley, J. (1974) Body fat assessed from total body density and its estimation from skinfold thickness: Measurements on 481 men and women aged from 16 to 72 years. *British Journal of Nutrition*, 32(1), 77–97.

ECOG-ACRIN Cancer Research Group (2019) *ECOG Performance Status*. Available at: https://ecog-acrin.org/resources/ecog-performance-status

EPSG (Enteral Plastic Safety Group) (2016) *ISO 80369-3: ENFit Implementation*. Available at: https://www.bapen.org.uk/nutrition-support/enteral-nutrition/enfit

Espitalier, F., Fanous, A., Aviv, J., et al. (2018) International consensus (ICON) on assessment of oropharyngeal dysphagia. *European Annals of Otorhinolaryngology, Head and Neck Diseases*, 135(1), S17–S21.

European Medicines Agency (2013) Hydroxyethyl-starch solutions (HES) should no longer be used in patients with sepsis or burn injuries or in critically ill patients: CMDh endorses PRAC recommendations [Press Release EMA/640658/2013]. Available at: https://www.ema.europa.eu/en/news/hydroxyethyl-starch-solutions-hes-should-no-longer-be-used-patients-sepsis-burn-injuries-critically

Finfer, S., Liu, B., Taylor, C., et al. (2010) Resuscitation fluid use in critically ill adults: An international cross-sectional study in 391 intensive care units. *Critical Care*, 14(5), R185.

Fletcher, J. (2011) Nutrition: Safe practice in adult enteral tube feeding. *British Journal of Nursing*, 20(19), 1234–1239.

Fraise, A.P. & Bradley, T. (2009) *Aycliffe's Control of Healthcare-Associated Infections: A Practical Handbook*, 5th edn. London: Hodder Arnold.

Frost, J. (2015) Intravenous fluid therapy in adult inpatients. *BMJ*, 350, g7620.

FSA (Food Standards Authority) & Expert Group on Vitamins and Minerals (2003) *Safe Upper Levels for Vitamins and Minerals*. Available at: https://cot.food.gov.uk/sites/default/files/vitmin2003.pdf

Fuller, S., Beck, E., Salman, H. & Tapsell, L. (2016) New horizons for the study of dietary fiber and health: A review. *Plant Foods for Human Nutrition*, 71(1), 1–12.

Gandy, J. (2014) *Manual of Dietetic Practice*. Chichester: Wiley Blackwell.

Georgiades, D. (2016) A balancing act: Maintaining accurate fluid balance charting. *Australian Nursing & Midwifery Journal*, 24(6), 28–31.

Goldstein, S.L. (2014) Fluid management in acute kidney injury. *Journal of Intensive Care Medicine*, 29(4), 183–189.

Gonzalez, M.C. & Heymsfield, S.B. (2017) Bioelectrical impedance analysis for diagnosing sarcopenia and cachexia: What are we really estimating? *Journal of Cachexia, Sarcopenia and Muscle*, 8(2), 187–189.

Groher, M.E. & Crary, M.A. (2015) *Dysphagia: Clinical Management in Adults and Children*, 2nd edn. St Louis, MO: Elsevier Health Sciences.

Gross, W., Samarin, M. & Kimmons, L.A. (2017) Choice of fluids for resuscitation of the critically ill: What nurses need to know. *Critical Care Nursing*, 40(4), 309–322.

Guidelines and Protocols Advisory Committee (2017) *PRISMA-7 Questionnaire*. Available at: https://www2.gov.bc.ca/assets/gov/health/practitioner-pro/bc-guidelines/frailty-prisma7.pdf

Haywood, S. (2012) PEG feeding tube placement and aftercare. *Nursing Times*, 108(42), 20–22.

Healey, F., Sanders, D., Lamont, T., et al. (2010) Early detection of complications after gastrostomy: Summary of a safety report from the National Patient Safety Agency. *BMJ*, 340, c2160.

Hickson, M. & Smith, S. (2018) *Advanced Nutrition and Dietetics in Nutrition Support*. Oxford: Wiley Blackwell.

Hilal, M.A., Layfield, D.M., Di Fabio, F., et al. (2013) Postoperative chyle leak after major pancreatic resections in patients who receive enteral feed: Risk factors and management options. *World Journal of Surgery*, 37, 2918–2926.

IDDSI (International Dysphagia Diet Standardisation Initiative) (2018) *The IDDSI Framework*. Available at: https://iddsi.org

Jaffee, W., Hodgins, S. & McGee, W.T. (2018) Tissue edema, fluid balance, and patient outcomes in severe sepsis: An organ systems review. *Journal of Intensive Care Medicine*, 33(9), 502–509.

Jensen, G.L., Hsiao, P.Y. & Wheeler, D. (2012) Adult nutrition assessment tutorial. *Journal of Parenteral and Enteral Nutrition*, 36(3), 267–274.

Jevon, P. (2010) How to ensure patient observations lead to effective management of oliguria. *Nursing Times*, 106(7), 18–19.

Jevon, P. & Ewens, B. (2012) *Monitoring the Critically Ill Patient*, 2nd edn. Oxford: Wiley Blackwell.

Jones, T.M., De, M., Foran, B., et al. (2016) Laryngeal cancer: United Kingdom national multidisciplinary guidelines. *Journal of Laryngology and Otology*, 130(Suppl. 2), S75–S82.

KDIGO (Kidney Disease: Improving Global Outcomes) (2012) KDIGO clinical practice guideline for acute kidney injury. *Kidney International Supplements*, 2(1), 124–183.

Klek, S., Forbes, A., Gabe, S., et al. (2016) Management of acute intestinal failure: A position paper from the European Society for Clinical Nutrition and Metabolism (ESPEN) Special Interest Group. *Clinical Nutrition*, 35(6), 1209–1218.

Kondrup, J., Allison, S.P., Elia, M., et al. (2003) ESPEN guidelines for nutrition screening 2002. *Clinical Nutrition*, 22(4), 415–421.

Lamont, T., Beaumont, C., Fayaz, A., et al. (2011) Checking placement of nasogastric feeding tubes in adults (interpretation of X-ray images): Summary of a safety report from the National Patient Safety Agency. *BMJ*, 342, d2586.

Lang, E.K., Allaei, A., Abbey-Mensah, G., et al. (2013) Percutaneous radiologic gastrostomy: Results and analysis of factors contributing to complications. *Journal of the Louisiana State Medical Society*, 165, 254–259.

Langmore, S.E. (2001) *Endoscopic Evaluation and Treatment of Swallowing Disorders*. New York: Thieme.

Langmore, S.E., Terpenning, M.S., Schork, A., et al. (1998) Predictors of aspiration pneumonia: How important is dysphagia? *Dysphagia*, 13(2), 69–81.

Leahy, S., O'Neill, C., Sohun, R. & Jakeman, P. (2012) A comparison of dual energy X-ray absorptiometry and bioelectrical impedance analysis to measure total and segmental body composition in healthy young adults. *European Journal of Applied Physiology*, 112(2), 589–595.

Leslie, P., Carding, P.N. & Wilson, J.A. (2003) Investigation and management of chronic dysphagia. *BMJ*, 326(7386), 433–436.

Lever, E., Scott, S.M., Louis, P., et al. (2019) The effect of prunes on stool output, gut transit time and gastrointestinal microbiota: A randomised controlled trial. *Clinical Nutrition*, 38(1), 165–173.

Levi, R. (2005) Nursing care to prevent dehydration in older adults. *Australian Nursing Journal*, 13(3), 21–23.

Liaw, Y.Q. & Goh, M.L. (2018) Improving the accuracy of fluid intake charting through patient involvement in an adult surgical ward: A best practice implementation project. *JBI Database of Systematic Reviews and Implementation Reports*, 16(8), 1709–1719.

Logemann, J.A. (1998) *Evaluation and Treatment of Swallowing Disorders*, 2nd edn. Austin, TX: PRO-ED.

Logemann, J.A., Pauloski, B.R., Rademaker, A.W. & Colangelo, L.A. (1997) Super-supraglottic swallow in irradiated head and neck cancer patients. *Head & Neck*, 19(6), 535–540.

Lord, L.M. (2018) Enteral access devices: Types, function, care, and challenges. *Nutrition in Clinical Practice*, 33(1), 16–38.

Loser, C., Aschl, G., Hebuterne, X., et al. (2005) ESPEN guidelines on artificial enteral nutrition: Percutaneous endoscopic gastrostomy (PEG). *Clinical Nutrition*, 24(5), 848–861.

Loveday, H.P., Wilson, J.A., Pratt, R.J., et al. (2014) Epic3: National evidence-based guidelines for preventing healthcare-associated infections in NHS hospitals in England. *Journal of Hospital Infection*, 86(Suppl. 1), S1–S70.

Lynch, C.R. & Fang, J.C. (2004) Prevention and management of complications of percutaneous endoscopic gastrostomy (PEG) tubes. *Practical Gastroenterology*, 28(11), 66–76.

Madden, A.M., Tsikoura, T. & Stott, D.J. (2008) The estimation of body height from ulnar length in adults from different ethnic groups. *Journal of Human Nutrition and Dietetics*, 21(4), 394.

Majka, A.J., Wang, Z., Schmitz, K.R., et al. (2013) Care co-ordination to enhance management of long-term enteral tube feeding: A systematic review and meta-analysis. *Journal of Parenteral and Enteral Nutrition*, 38(1), 40–52.

Makizako, H., Shimada, H., Doi, T., et al. (2017) Predictive cutoff values of the Five-Times Sit-to-Stand Test and the Timed 'Up & Go' Test for disability incidence in older people dwelling in the community. *Physical Therapy*, 97(4), 417–424.

Marieb, E.N. & Hoehn, K. (2018) *Human Anatomy and Physiology*, 11th edn. San Francisco: Pearson.

Matlow, A., Jacobson, M., Wray, R., et al. (2006) Enteral tube hub as a reservoir for transmissible enteric bacteria. *American Journal of Infection Control*, 34(3), 131–133.

McGloin, S. (2015) The ins and outs of fluid balance in the acutely ill patient. *British Journal of Nursing*, 24(1), 14–18.

Mental Capacity Act (2005) Available at: https://www.legislation.gov.uk/ukpga/2005/9/contents

Mental Health Act (1983) Available at: https://www.legislation.gov.uk/ukpga/1983/20/contents

Mentes, J.C. & Kang, S. (2013). Evidence-based practice guideline: Hydration management. *Journal of Gerontological Nursing*, 39(2), 11–19.

Metheny, N.A. & Titler, M.G. (2001) Assessing placement of feeding tubes. *American Journal of Nursing*, 101(5), 36–45, quiz 45–46.

Michard, F. (2016) Hemodynamic monitoring in the era of digital health. *Annals of Intensive Care*, 6(1), 15.

Monnet, X., Marik, P. & Teboul, J.L. (2016) Passive leg raising for predicting fluid responsiveness: A systematic review and meta-analysis. *Intensive Care Medicine*, 42(12), 1935–1947.

Mor, V., Laliberte, L., Morris, J.N. & Wiemann, M. (1984) The Karnofsky performance status scale: An examination of its reliability and validity in a research setting. *Cancer*, 53(9), 2002–2007.

National Obesity Forum (2016) *Waist circumference*. Available at: www.nationalobesityforum.org.uk/index.php/healthcare-professionals/assessment-mainmenu-168/171-waist-circumference.html

Nazli, A., Brigham-Chan, F., Fernandes, M. & Anjum, A. (2016) Adequacy of fluid balance chart documentation on wards. *Clinical Medicine*, 16(Suppl. 3), S21.

NCCAC (National Collaborating Centre for Acute Care) (2006) *Nutrition Support in Adults: Oral Nutrition Support, Enteral Tube Feeding and Parenteral Nutrition* [CG32]. Available at: www.nice.org.uk/guidance/cg032

NCEPOD (National Confidential Enquiry into Patient Outcome and Death) (2009) *Adding Insult to Injury*. Available at: www.ncepod.org.uk/2009report1/Downloads/AKI_report.pdf

NCEPOD (2010) *A Mixed Bag: An Enquiry into the Care of Hospital Patients Receiving Parenteral Nutrition*. Available at: https://www.ncepod.org.uk/2010pn.html

NDRUK (Nutrition and Diet Resources United Kingdom) (2016) *Do You Have a Small Appetite? Your Guide to Eating Well*. Available at: https://www.ndr-uk.org/item/39/FoodFortification/Do-You-Have-a-Small-Appetite.html

NHS England (2013) *Patient Safety Alert: Placement Devices for Nasogastric Tube Insertion DO NOT Replace Initial Insertion Checks* [NHS/PSA/W/2013/001]. Available at: https://www.england.nhs.uk/wp-content/uploads/2013/12/psa-ng-tube.pdf

NHS England (2015a) *10 Key Characteristics of 'Good Nutrition and Hydration Care'*. Available at: https://www.england.nhs.uk/commissioning/nut-hyd/10-key-characteristics

NHS England (2015b) *Never Events List 2015/16*. Available at: https://www.england.nhs.uk/wp-content/uploads/2015/03/never-evnts-list-15-16.pdf

NHS England and NHSI (NHS Improvement) (2019) *Standard Infection Control Precautions: National Hand Hygiene and Personal Protective Equipment Policy*. Available at: https://improvement.nhs.uk/documents/1957/National_policy_on_hand_hygiene_and_PPE_2.pdf

NHSI (NHS Improvement) (2016) *Resource Set Initial Placement Checks for Nasogastric and Orogastric Tubes*. Available at: https://improvement.nhs.uk/resources/resource-set-initial-placement-checks-nasogastric-and-orogastric-tubes

NHSI (2017) *Small Bore Connectors: An Introduction to Safe Use*. Available at: https://improvement.nhs.uk/resources/small-bore-connectors-safety-introduction

NHSI (2018) *Patient Safety Alert: Resources to Support Safer Modification of Food and Drink* [NHS/PSA/RE/2018/004]. Available at: https://improvement.nhs.uk/documents/2955/Patient_Safety_Alert_-_Resources_to_support_safer_modification_of_food_and_drink_v2.pdf

NICE (National Institute for Health and Care Excellence) (2012) *Nutrition Support in Adults*. Available at: https://www.nice.org.uk/guidance/qs24

NICE (2013) *Acute Kidney Injury: Prevention, Detection and Management of Acute Kidney Injury up to the Point of Renal Replacement Therapy* [CG169]. Available at: www.nice.org.uk/guidance/cg169

NICE (2017a) *Healthcare-Associated Infections: Prevention and Control in Primary and Community Care*. Available at: https://www.nice.org.uk/guidance/cg139/chapter/1-Guidance

NICE (2017b) *Intravenous Fluid Therapy in Adults in Hospital* [CG174]. Available at: www.nice.org.uk/guidance/cg174

NICE (2017c) *Nutrition Support for Adults: Oral Nutrition Support, Enteral Tube Feeding and Parenteral Nutrition Clinical Guideline* [CG32]. Available at: https://www.nice.org.uk/guidance/cg32

NICE (2018) *Patient Experience in Adult NHS Services: Improving Experience of Care for People Using Adult NHS Services* [CG138]. Available at: https://www.nice.org.uk/guidance/cg138/uptake

NICE & BNF (British National Formulary) (2019) *Interactions*. Available at: https://bnf.nice.org.uk/interaction

NMC (Nursing and Midwifery Council) (2018) *The Code: Professional Standards of Practice and Behaviour for Nurses, Midwives and Nursing Associates*. Available at: https://www.nmc.org.uk/standards/code

NNNG (National Nurses Nutrition Group) (2013) *Good Practice Consensus Guideline: Exit Site Management for Gastrostomy Tubes in Adults and Children*. Available at: www.nnng.org.uk/wp-content/uploads/2013/10/Gastrostomy-Exit-site-guidelines-Final.pdf

NNNG (2016a) *Safe Insertion and Ongoing Care of Nasogastric (NG) Feeding Tubes in Adults*. Available at: www.nnng.org.uk/wp-content/uploads/2016/06/NNNG-Nasogastric-tube-Insertion-and-Ongoing-Care-Practice-Final-Aprill-2016.pdf

NNNG (2016b) *Changing of a Balloon Gastrostomy Tube (BGT) into the Stomach for Adults and Children*. Available at: www.nnng.org.uk/wp-content/uploads/2016/06/Good-practice-changing-a-gastrostomy-tube-Final-June-20161.pdf

Nund, R.L., Ward, E.C., Scarinci, N.A., et al. (2014a) Carers' experiences of dysphagia in people treated for head and neck cancer: A qualitative study. *Dysphagia*, 29(4), 450–458.

Nund, R.L., Ward, E.C., Scarinci, N.A., et al. (2014b) The lived experience of dysphagia following non-surgical treatment for head and neck cancer. *International Journal of Speech-Language Pathology*, 16(3), 282–289.

O'Grady, N.P., Alexander, M., Burns, L.A., et al. (2011) Guidelines for the prevention of intravascular catheter-related infections. *Clinical Infectious Diseases*, 52(9), e162–e193.

Paleri, V., Roe, J.W., Strojan, P., et al. (2014) Strategies to reduce long-term postchemoradiation dysphagia in patients with head and neck cancer: An evidence-based review. *Head & Neck*, 36(3), 431–443.

Patel, D.A., Sharda, R., Hovis, K.L., et al. (2017) Patient-reported outcome measures in dysphagia: A systematic review of instrument development and validation. *Diseases of the Esophagus*, 30(5), 1–23.

Patterson, J. & Wilson, J.A. (2011) The clinical value of dysphagia preassessment in the management of head and neck cancer patients. *Current Opinion in Otolaryngology & Head and Neck Surgery*, 19, 177–181.

Patterson, J.M., Brady, G.C. & Roe, J.W. (2016) Research into the prevention and rehabilitation of dysphagia in head and neck cancer: A UK [illegible] 24(3), 208–214.

Payne-James, J., Grimble, G. & Silk, D. (2001) Enteral nutrition: Tubes and techniques of delivery. In: Payne-James, J., Grimble, G. & Silk, D. (eds) *Artificial Nutrition Support in Clinical Practice*, 2nd edn. London: Greenwich Medical Media, pp.301–303.

Pearce, C.B. & Duncan, H.D. (2002) Enteral feeding: Nasogastric, nasojejunal, percutaneous endoscopic gastrostomy, or jejunostomy – its indications and limitations. *Postgraduate Medical Journal*, 78, 198–204.

Perner, A., Prowle, J., Joannidis, M., et al. (2017) Fluid management in acute kidney injury. *Intensive Care Medicine*, 43(6), 807–815.

PHE (Public Health England) (2016) *The Eatwell Guide*. Available at: https://www.gov.uk/government/publications/the-eatwell-guide

PHE (2017) *Healthier and More Sustainable Catering: Nutrition Principles*. Available at: https://www.gov.uk/government/publications/healthier-and-more-sustainable-catering-a-toolkit-for-serving-food-to-adults

Pickett, J.D., Bridges, E., Kritek, P.A. & Whitney, J.D. (2017) Passive leg-raising and prediction of fluid responsiveness: Systematic review. *Critical Care Nurse*, 37(2), 32–47.

Pinnington, S., Ingleby, S., Hanumapura, P. & Waring, D. (2016) Assessing and documenting fluid balance. *Nursing Standard*, 31(15), 46–54.

Polderman, K.H. & Varon, J. (2015) Do not drown the patient: Appropriate fluid management in critical illness. *American Journal of Emergency Medicine*, 33(3), 448–450.

Porter, J., Ottrey, E. & Huggins, C.E. (2017) Protected mealtimes in hospitals and nutritional intake: Systematic review and meta-analyses. *International Journal of Nursing Studies*, 65, 62–69.

Powell-Tuck, J., Gosling, P., Lobo, D.N., et al. (2011) *British Consensus Guidelines on Intravenous Fluid Therapy for Adult Surgical Patients*. Available at: https://www.bapen.org.uk/pdfs/bapen_pubs/giftasup.pdf

PPSA (Pennsylvania Patient Safety Authority) (2006) *Confirming Feeding Tube Placement: Old Habits Die Hard*. Harrisburg, PA: Pennsylvania Patient Safety Authority.

Raeder, H., Kværner, A.S., Henriksen, C., et al. (2018) Validity of bioelectrical impedance analysis in estimation of fat-free mass in colorectal cancer patients. *Clinical Nutrition*, 37(1), 292–300.

Reid, J., Robb, E., Stone, D., et al. (2004) Improving the monitoring and assessment of fluid balance. *Nursing Times*, 100(20), 36–39.

Resuscitation Council (2015) *Advanced Life Support*, 7th edn. London: Resuscitation Council.

Rhoda, K.M., Porter, M.J. & Quintini, C. (2011) Fluid and electrolyte management: Putting a plan in motion. *Journal of Parenteral and Enteral Nutrition*, 35(6), 676–685.

Rhodes, A., Evans, L.E., Alhazzani, W., et al. (2017) Surviving Sepsis Campaign: International guidelines for management of sepsis and septic shock – 2016. *Intensive Care Medicine*, 43(3), 304–377.

Robertson, C.E. (2018) Dietary assessment in undernutrition. In: Hickson, M. & Smith, S. (eds) *Advanced Nutrition and Dietetics in Nutrition Support*. Oxford: Wiley Blackwell, pp.82–90.

Roe, J.W. (2012) *Alternative Investigations*. San Diego: Plural.

Roe, J.W. & Ashforth, K.M. (2011) Prophylactic swallowing exercises for patients receiving radiotherapy for head and neck cancer. *Current Opinion in Otolaryngology & Head and Neck Surgery*, 19(3), 144–149.

Rollins, H. (1997) A nose for trouble. *Nursing Times*, 93(49), 66–67.

Santanasto, A.J., Goodpaster, B.H., Kritchevsky, S.B., et al. (2017) Body composition remodeling and mortality: The health aging and body composition study. *Journals of Gerontology Series A: Biological Sciences and Medical Sciences*, 72(4), 513–519.

Scales, K. & Pilsworth, J. (2008) The importance of fluid balance in clinical practice. *Nursing Standard*, 22(47), 50–57, quiz 58, 60.

Schol, P.B., Terink, I.M., Lance, M.D. & Scheepers, H.C. (2016) Liberal or restrictive fluid management during elective surgery: A systematic review and meta-analysis. *Journal of Clinical Anesthesia*, 35, 26–39.

Self, W., Semler, M., Wanderer, J., et al. (2018) Balanced crystalloids versus saline in non-critically ill adults. *New England Journal of Medicine*, 378, 819–828.

Semler, M.W., Self, W.H., Wanderer, J.P., et al. (2018) Balanced crystalloids versus saline in critically ill adults. *New England Journal of Medicine*, 378, 829–839.

Shachar, S.S., Williams, G.R., Muss, H.B. & Nishijima, T.F. (2016) Prognostic value of sarcopenia in adults with solid tumours: A [illegible] 57, 58–67.

Shaw, C. (2008) Parenteral nutrition. In: Dougherty, L. & Lamb, J. (eds) *Intravenous Therapy in Nursing Practice*, 2nd edn. Oxford: Blackwell, pp.395–407.

Shaw, C. (2011) *Nutrition and Palliative Care*. Chichester: John Wiley & Sons.

Shaw, C. & Eldridge, L. (2015) Nutritional considerations for the palliative care patient. *International Journal of Palliative Nursing*, 21(1), 7–8, 10, 12–15.

Shaw, C., Fleuret, C., Pickard, J.M., et al. (2015) Comparison of a novel, simple nutrition screening tool for adult oncology inpatients and the Malnutrition Screening Tool (MST) against the Patient-Generated Subjective Global Assessment (PG-SGA). *Supportive Care in Cancer*, 23(1), 47–54.

Shaw, V. & McCarthy, H. (2014) Nutritional assessment, dietary requirements and feed supplementation. In: Shaw, V. (ed) *Clinical Paediatric Dietetics*, 4th edn. Chichester: Wiley Blackwell, pp.3–23.

Shepherd, A. (2011) Measuring and managing fluid balance. *Nursing Times*, 107(28), 12–16.

Sheppard, M. & Wright, M.M. (2006) *Principles and Practice of High Dependency Nursing*, 2nd edn. Edinburgh: Baillière Tindall.

Silva, F.M. & Figueira, L. (2017) Estimated height from knee height or ulna length and self-reported height are no substitute for actual height in inpatients. *Nutrition*, 33, 52–56.

Singer, P., Blaser, A.R., Berger, M.M., et al. (2018) ESPEN guideline on clinical nutrition in the intensive care unit. *Clinical Nutrition*, 38, 48–79.

Smith, J. & Roberts, R. (2011) *Vital Signs for Nurses*. Oxford: Blackwell.

Smith Hammond, C. (2008) Cough and aspiration of food and liquids due to oral pharyngeal dysphagia. *Lung*, 186(Suppl. 1), S35–S40.

Sorkin, J.D., Muller, D.C. & Andres, R. (1999) Longitudinal change in height of men and women: Implications for interpretation of the body mass index – The Baltimore Longitudinal Study of Aging. *American Journal of Epidemiology*, 150(9), 969–977.

Soscia, J. & Friedman, J.N. (2011) A guide to the management of common gastrostomy and gastrojejunostomy tube problems. *Paediatrics & Child Health*, 16(5), 281–287.

Sumnall, R. (2007) Fluid management and diuretic therapy in acute renal failure. *Nursing in Critical Care*, 12(1), 27–33.

Taheri, M., Singh, H., & Duerksen, D. (2011) Peritonitis after gastrostomy tube replacement: Case series and review of literature. *Journal of Parenteral and Enteral Nutrition*, 35, 56–60.

Thibault, R., Genton, L. & Pichard, C. (2012) Body composition: Why, when and for who? *Clinical Nutrition*, 31(4), 435–447.

Thomsen, G., Bezdjian, L., Rodriguez, L. & Hopkins, R.O. (2012) Clinical outcomes of a furosemide infusion protocol in edematous patients in the intensive care unit. *Critical Care Nurse*, 32(6), 25–34.

Tidy, C. (2018) *Acute pulmonary oedema. Patient*. Available at: https://patient.info/doctor/acute-pulmonary-oedema

Todorovic, V.E. & Mafrici, B. (2019) *A Pocket Guide to Clinical Nutrition*, 5th edn. London: Parenteral and Enteral Nutrition Group of the British Dietetic Association.

Toh Yoon, E.W., Yoneda, K., Nakamura, S., et al. (2016) Percutaneous endoscopic transgastric jejunostomy (PEG J): A retrospective analysis on its utility in maintaining enteral nutrition after unsuccessful gastric feeding. *BMJ Open Gastroenterology*, 3, e000098corr1.

Tortora, G.J. & Derrickson, B.H. (2017) *Principles of Anatomy & Physiology*, 15th edn. Hoboken, NJ: John Wiley & Sons.

van den Berg, M.M.G.A, Kok, D.E., Posthuma, L., et al. (2019) Body composition is associated with risk of toxicity-induced modifications of treatment in women with stage I–IIIB breast cancer receiving chemotherapy. *Breast Cancer Research and Treatment*, 173(2), 475–481.

Warriner, L. & Spruce, P. (2012) Managing overgranulation around gastrostomy sites. *British Journal of Nursing*, 21(5 Suppl.), S14–S16.

Weimann, A., Braga, M., Carli, F., et al. (2017) ESPEN guideline: Clinical nutrition in surgery. *Clinical Nutrition*, 36, 623–650.

Welch, K. (2010) Fluid balance. *Learning Disability Practice*, 13(6), 33–38.

Westaby, D., Young, A., O'Toole, P., et al. (2010) The provision of a percutaneously placed enteral tube feeding service. *Gut*, 59(12), 1592–1605.

Wright, L., Cotter, D. & Hickson, M. (2008) The effectiveness of targeted feeding assistance to improve the nutritional intake of elderly dysphagic patients in hospital. *Journal of Human Nutrition and Dietetics*, 21(6), 555–562.

Young, A.M., Banks, M.D. & Mudge, A.M. (2018) Improving nutrition care and intake for older hospital patients through system-level dietary and mealtime interventions. *Clinical Nutrition ESPEN*, 24, 140–147.

Chapter 9

Patient comfort and supporting personal hygiene

Suzanna Argenio-Haines with Helena Aparecida de Rezende and Rhiannon Llewelyn

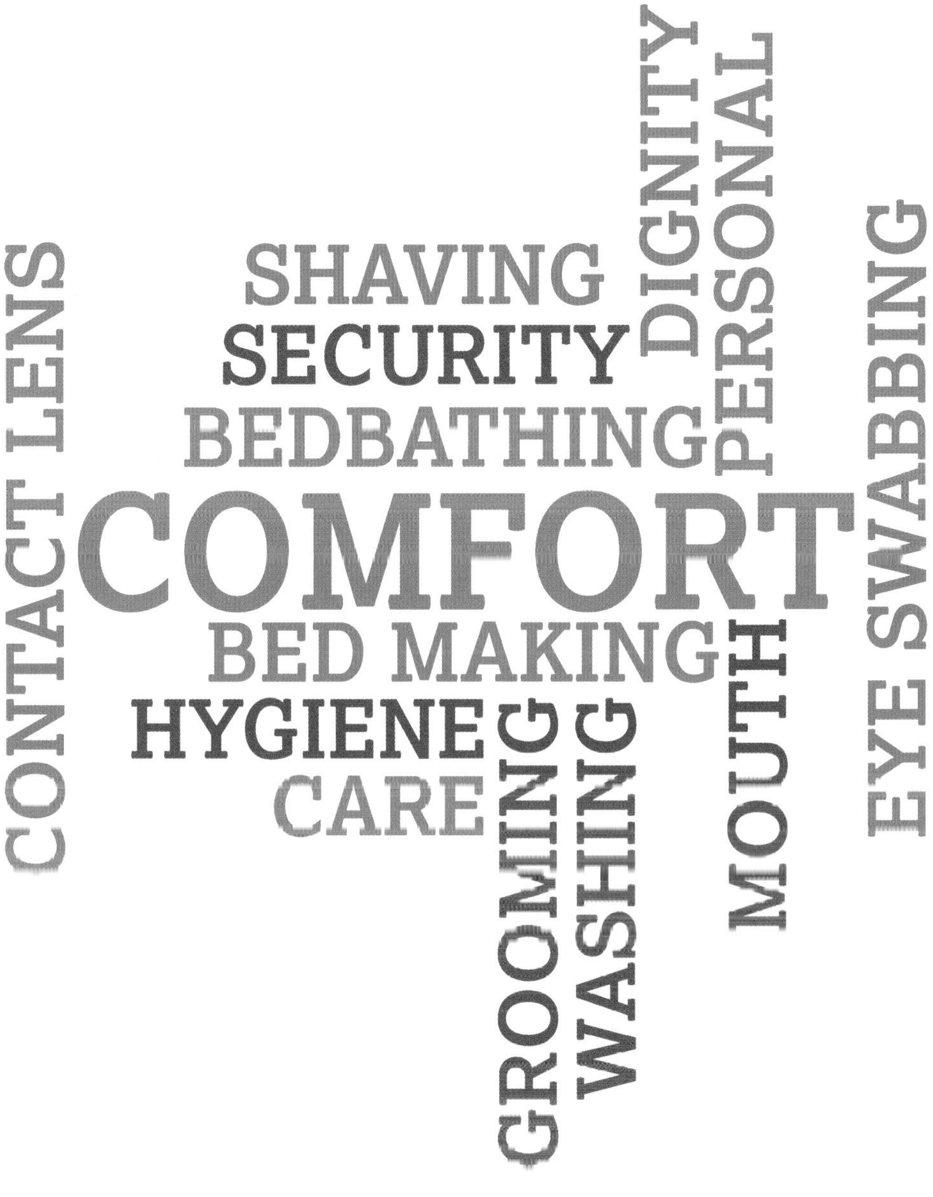

The Royal Marsden Manual of Clinical Nursing Procedures: Professional Edition, Tenth Edition. Edited by Sara Lister, Justine Hofland and Hayley Grafton.

Procedure guidelines

Being an accountable professional

At the point of registration, the nurse will:

3. Use evidence based, best practice approaches for meeting needs for care and support with rest, sleep, comfort and the maintenance of dignity, accurately assessing the person's capacity for independence and self-care and initiating appropriate interventions

4. Use evidence based, best practice approaches for meeting the needs for care and support with hygiene and the maintenance of skin integrity, accurately assessing the person's capacity for independence and self-care and initiating appropriate interventions

Future Nurse: Standards of Proficiency for Registered Nurses (NMC 2018)

Overview

The aim of this chapter is to present the many and varied procedures that contribute towards the comfort of patients at all times. This includes the many specific procedures that promote comfort and hygiene, such as bathing, hair care and shaving, as well as procedures that enhance care of the eye, ear and mouth.

Comfort will mean different things to different patients. It may relate to a state of wellbeing, security or contentment. It may involve being in a relaxed state, having tolerable pain, or perhaps having feelings of satisfaction or physical wellbeing due to the care provided. For the nurse or allied health professional delivering personal care to the patient, the goal should be to contribute to and enhance the patient's state of comfort.

Personal hygiene

Definition

Hygiene is defined as the practices involved in maintaining health and preventing disease (O'Connor 2016b). Personal hygiene is the self-care by which people attend to functions such as bathing, toileting, general body hygiene and grooming. Hygiene is a highly personal matter determined by individual values and practices. It involves care of the skin, hair, nails, teeth, oral and nasal cavities, eyes, ears, and perianal and perineal–genital areas (Berman et al. 2015). Maintaining a good level of personal hygiene is essential for all patients during their stay in hospital (O'Connor 2016b).

Anatomy and physiology

Skin

Skin is the largest organ of the body and maintaining its integrity is essential to the prevention of infection and the promotion of both physical and psychological health. The skin has several functions:

- regulation of temperature
- physical and immunological protection
- excretion and preservation of water balance
- sensory perception
- communication of feelings
- synthesis: vitamin D and melanin production (Hussain et al. 2013).

The skin is made up of three layers: epidermis, dermis and deep subcutaneous layer (Figure 9.1).

Epidermis

The epidermis is the outer layer of the skin and contains no blood vessels or nerve endings. The cells on the surface are gradually shed and replaced by new cells that have developed from the deeper layers; this process takes approximately 28 days. The epidermis has hairs, sweat glands and the ducts of sebaceous glands passing through it. It provides a protective barrier for the internal organs (Farage et al. 2013) and an efficient natural barrier against the potential threats posed by the external environment, such as pathogens and physical trauma (Jones 2014, Marks and Miller 2013, Maurer et al. 2016).

Dermis

The dermis is the thickest layer of skin and contains blood and lymph vessels, nerve fibres, sweat and sebaceous glands. It is made up of white fibrous tissue and yellow elastic fibres, which give the skin its toughness and elasticity. It provides the epidermis with structural and nutritional support (Jones 2014).

Subcutaneous layer

The subcutaneous layer contains the deep fat cells (areolar and adipose tissue) and provides heat regulation for the body. It is also the support structure for the outer layers of the skin. Maintaining skin integrity, through good personal hygiene, will

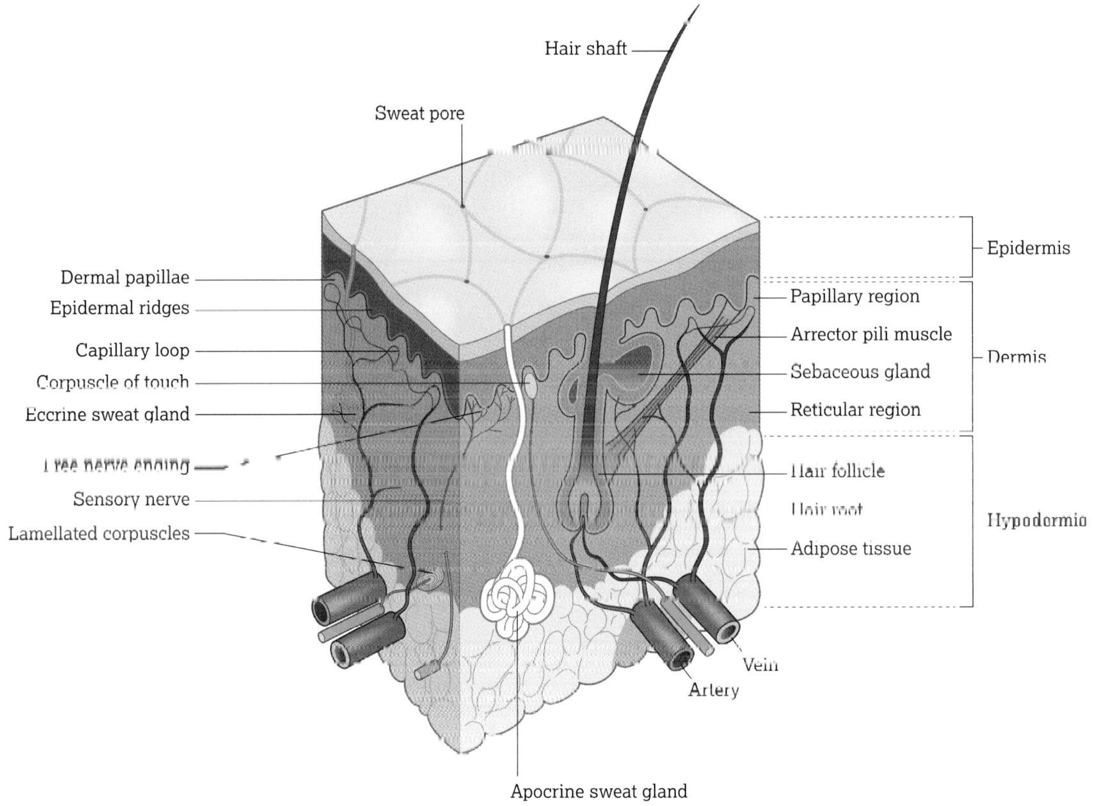

Figure 9.1 Skin and subcutaneous layer. *Source:* Reproduced from Peate et al. (2014) with permission of John Wiley & Sons, Ltd.

allow this complex system to provide an efficient natural barrier against the external environment.

Skin health

It is important to remember that the skin is an adaptive organ, affected by internal and external factors such as temperature, air humidity and age (Slominski et al. 2012). It has great ability to adapt to changes in the environment and stimuli but is affected by ill health, immobility and malnutrition (Dunk 2015, Leaker 2013). Its integrity, continuity and cleanliness are essential to maintaining its physiological functions.

The ageing process can adversely affect the skin's structure (Farage et al. 2013). Skin tissue becomes thinner, less elastic and less resistant to trauma and shearing forces. The blood supply is reduced as cells are replaced more slowly, which can adversely affect healing. Transmission of stimuli from sensory receptors slows, so reaction to warning stimuli produced by the sensory receptors can be delayed and result in damage. The production of natural oils declines and can lead to dry skin, which increases the risk of infection and tissue breakdown (Kottner et al. 2013). Nursing interventions for skin care can protect, maintain and promote skin integrity (Cowdell and Steventon 2015, Farage et al. 2013).

Evidence-based approaches

Personal cleanliness is a fundamental value in society. Often, when an individual becomes unwell, they depend on others to assist them with meeting their personal hygiene needs. Within the healthcare setting, they will depend upon nursing and support staff. Although the provision of personal hygiene is a fundamental aspect of nursing care, the nursing workforce is changing and quite often the delivery of personal hygiene care is delegated to support staff team members. Personal hygiene is considered part of the essence of care and should never be treated as ritualistic. It is recommended that all professionals involved – nurses, student nurses, nursing associates, assistant practitioners and healthcare support workers – should be appropriately trained, so that they can question and evaluate care (HEE 2015). It is recommended that the personal hygiene care of patients be performed under the supervision of a qualified nurse to protect the best interests of the patient and maintain patient safety (NMC 2018b, RCN 2017).

Hygiene is a personal issue and everyone will have their own individual requirements and standards of cleanliness (Spencer 2016). It is important that the nurse or other professional delivering care observes and assesses the patient's needs on an individual basis. The nurse should not impose their own standards of cleanliness on the patient or even assume that theirs will match those of the patient.

Some patients may have a long-term need for personal care support, such as those with dementia or a severe physical or learning disability. If a patient is unable to communicate their needs and preferences, then their family and carers may be able to advise on how best to provide such personal care.

When the patient has any degree of cognitive impairment, the approach taken to provide any personal care must consider how the patient is likely to experience that care. For example, a patient who has dementia may not retain the knowledge of who is delivering the care or what the person is doing, so they may need to be repeatedly orientated and talked through the process to prevent them from becoming distressed.

Within the patient assessment, religious and cultural beliefs that relate to and have an impact on personal care practices and the maintenance of personal hygiene should be taken into account and incorporated into care. For some religions such as Hinduism, Islam and Judaism, modesty is important (Fowler 2017a, 2017b, 2017c) and can be challenging to manage in the hospital setting (Mujallad and Taylor 2016). In Western culture, privacy is of the utmost importance and considered to be a basic human right (Human Rights Act 1998). There are patients who may feel a great deal of embarrassment having to depend on another person to help them with an extremely private act. It is therefore surprising that so little reference is made to this in the literature. However, in the clinical situation, it is best to discuss this directly with the patient if possible, exploring with them how they want their hygiene needs to be met and identifying any specific requests they may have relating to their culture or religion (Mendes 2018).

Florence Nightingale (1860) was the first to note the importance of good personal hygiene and the essential role nurses have in maintaining this in order to prevent infection and increase wellbeing (Boge et al. 2013). During the delivery of personal hygiene care, the nurse is able to demonstrate a wide range of skills such as assessment, communication and observation. Within the activity, opportunities may arise for the patient to discuss issues, concerns or fears regarding admission, treatment, discharge planning or prognosis (El-Soussi and Asfour 2017). This can be the most significant social interaction of the day for the patient, as the nurse develops a deeper understanding of the patient's personality and needs, which serves to build a personal bond between the nurse and patient (Morrison and Korol 2014). This relationship offers the nurse opportunities to encourage the patient to reclaim autonomy and independence within the care need through participation, which can increase patients' feelings of self worth and dignity.

Principles of care

Skin care is particularly important to prevent the colonization of gram-positive and gram-negative micro-organisms on the skin, which lead to healthcare-associated infections (Septimus and Schweizer 2016). By implementing simple personal hygiene measures such as regular bathing and changing of clothing and bed linen, the risk of infection can be reduced.

An initial assessment of the skin using observational skills is essential to ascertain the skin's general condition, colour, texture, smell and temperature (Voegeli 2012b). Factors that may influence the appearance of the skin are outlined in Box 9.1 and specific considerations for the care of the skin are outlined in Table 9.1.

Methods of care

Perineal and perianal care

Meticulous care of the perineal and perianal areas is vital, especially for people who are prone to infection. Problems can also arise from treatment modalities that can cause fistulas, diarrhoea, constipation and urinary tract infections. Whenever possible, and if able, patients should be encouraged and assisted to perform this care themselves (Butcher et al. 2018). If a nurse is performing the care of this area, it is important that informed consent is sought, where possible, and privacy is maintained throughout. Nurse and patient should discuss this procedure together, ensuring that the patient agrees to care (NMC 2018a).

Ideally, perineal and perianal hygiene should be attended to at the end of the general bath or wash. If using a bowl of water and wipes, these should be changed after attending to this area due to the large colonies of bacteria that tend to live in and around it (Nicol et al. 2012, Peate and Lane 2015). It is generally acknowledged that soap and lotions administered incorrectly to the perineum or perianal area can cause irritation and infection (Swamiappan 2016). Female patients should be washed from the front to the back (towards the anus), thus reducing the translocation of bacteria. Male uncircumcised patients should have the foreskin of the penis drawn back during washing and then returned to cover the glans of the penis (Lloyd Jones 2014, Peate and Lane 2015).

Hair care

The way a person feels is often related to their appearance; hair condition and style are usually pertinent to this. Hair care can be complex and so it should be planned and carried out according to the patient's personal preferences (Peate 2015). Washing the hair of a bed-bound patient can be challenging, but there are several ways to manage this, as follows:

- using a special bed tray water aid
- using an inflatable shampoo basin
- using a dry or no-rinse shampoo
- using a no-rinse shampoo cap (Peate 2015, Travis 2014).

Box 9.1 Factors that influence the appearance of the skin

Nutritional and hydration status

Imbalances will cause loss of elasticity and drying of the skin. Oedema will cause stretching and thinning of the skin (Everett and Sommers 2013).

Incontinence

The presence of urine and/or faeces on the skin increases the normal pH of 4.0–5.5 and makes the skin wet, which increases the risk of tissue breakdown and infection (Woo et al. 2017).

Age, health and mobility status

Reduced mobility in age, in ill health or with mobility problems can lead to the development of pressure ulcers (NICE 2015a).

Treatment therapies

Many medications can adversely affect the skin. For example:
- Steroids may cause the skin to become papery and fragile.
- Treatments such as radiotherapy may cause the skin to become moist and cracked.
- Systemic anti-cancer therapies can cause side-effects relating to the hair and nails (e.g. alopecia or paronychia), on the skin barrier (e.g. skin rash or skin dryness) and on the mucosa. They can also cause a condition known as palmar-plantar erythrodysaesthesia syndrome, which presents with cracking and epidermal sloughing of the palms and soles (Chirdharla and Kasi 2017).

Treatments that result in a low platelet count can lead to an increased risk of bruising, and a decrease in white blood cells can influence the rate of healing.

Any concurrent conditions

Eczema, psoriasis, diabetes and stress (for example) can affect the ability of the skin to maintain its integrity (Okonkwo and DiPietro 2017).

Source: Adapted from Attum and Shamoon (2018), Fosarelli (2014), Fowler (2017a).

Table 9.1 Considerations for the care of the skin

Skin condition	Special considerations
Frail and papery skin	Take extra gentle care in the bathing process, using soft cloths to wash the skin. Ensure that correct and/or preferred products and methods are used to cleanse and moisturize, thus not disrupting or impairing the skin barrier (Voegeli 2012b). This will maintain the integrity of the skin surface and prevent the skin integrity from being compromised.
Areas of red skin	If erythema or redness is noted, wound prevention measures need to be implemented to prevent sores and ulcers from developing. These include good pressure-relieving positioning and repositioning and the use of barrier products in the form of creams, ointments and films (NICE 2014, 2015a).
Open wounds	When open wounds are present, such as pressure ulcers, abrasions or cuts, preventive measures such as pressure relieving mattresses and seat cushions should be used to prevent further breakdown (NICE 2014, 2015a). Appropriate cleaning solutions should be used to clear the area; soaps and perfumed creams should be avoided. Dressings should be used where appropriate to promote wound healing (NICE 2014, 2015a).
Medical devices and drains	Frequently, patients have medical devices and wound drains inserted as part of their therapy and these should be handled with care to prevent the introduction of infection or the pulling of the tubes and devices (Young 2018).

The patient's condition must always be assessed before performing this task as it would not be appropriate for patients with head, neck or spinal injuries. Shampooing frequency depends on the patient's wellbeing and their hair condition. Referral to a hairdresser may be appropriate.

Grooming the hair provides an ideal opportunity to observe for dandruff, psoriasis, flaky skin and head lice. Head lice are extremely infectious so if they are present it is imperative to treat the hair with a medicated shampoo as soon as possible. Hospital policy should be followed regarding the disposal of infected linen. Towel drying of hair should occur and hairdryers can be used with the consent of the patient (Peate 2015). However, use of a hairdryer may not be appropriate if the patient has had recent alopecia (loss of hair). Hairdryers should be checked for safety in accordance with local policy.

Care of the beard and moustache is also important. Excess food can often become lodged here so regular grooming is essential for hygiene and comfort purposes. Shaving or beard trimmers can be used as appropriate.

Care of the nails and feet

The feet and nails require special care in order to avoid pain and infection. Poor toenail condition can affect mobility, compromise independence and increase the risk of localized infection (King and Callaghan 2011, Stockert 2017). Fingernails and toenails should be kept short and neat; nail clippers are recommended for the trimming of nails and emery boards for filing to prevent jagged edges (Soliman and Brogan 2016). Patients with visual impairment or dexterity problems and those with learning disabilities may require assistance with the trimming and filing of nails.

Some conditions (such as peripheral vascular disease, toe infections and diabetes) carry an increased risk of peripheral complications (such as neuropathy, ischaemia and foot ulcers). Such patients must therefore be assessed by a chiropodist and/or podiatrist (Soliman and Brogan 2016).

Special attention should be paid to cleaning the feet and in between the toes to avoid any fungal infection (Forbes and Watt 2015). Fungal infections of the skin can be subdivided into two distinct categories: dermatophytes (moulds) and *Candida* (yeasts). A fungal infection occurs where moulds or yeasts begin to live on the keratin of the host individual. This can include the keratin of the nail plate, leading to onychomycosis (fungal nail infection). The term 'athlete's foot' – which describes a condition caused by poor foot hygiene and is associated with excess sweating, infrequent changes of shoes and ineffective washing – is a common misnomer for a fungal foot infection. However, it is a precursor to infection as it provides the ideal environment for dermatophytes and yeasts. In general, fungal infections present as red, itchy, dry and flaky areas of skin and, depending on location, there may also be associated maceration and fissuring. Onychomycosis presents as thickened, discoloured nails that are also crumbly, elevated from the nailbed and malodorous (NICE 2018a, Watkins 2015). Topical drugs are available for the treatment of infections and odour management (Ameen et al. 2014, Watkins 2015).

Diabetic footcare

Chronic diseases such as diabetes and the long-term use of steroids can result in problems such as pressure ulcers, breakdown of skin integrity and delays in healing. A patient's whole body is affected by diabetes but, in particular, this chronic disease can cause foot complications. Damage to the nerves and blood supply to the feet causes lack of sensation and ischaemia. These problems can lead to diabetic foot ulceration, which, if left untreated, can result in amputation or even death (Bowling et al. 2015).

The Diabetes UK (2013) campaign 'Putting Feet First' highlighted the increasing number of amputations caused by diabetes and called for better awareness and improved standards of care for people with the disease. The organization suggests that all healthcare professionals should know how to carry out foot checks, make people aware of the risks and know how to refer patients to specialist advice appropriately. The importance of nurses recognizing and acting on a diabetic foot ulcer cannot be overestimated (Corl et al. 2014, Powers et al. 2017).

Guidelines published by the National Institute for Health and Care Excellence (NICE 2015b) recommend that all people with diabetes have an annual foot examination. It is important to remove patients' shoes, socks, bandages and dressings so as to be able to examine both feet for evidence of risk factors (outlined in Table 9.2). Based on the findings of the foot examination, the person can then be classified as low risk, increased risk or high risk of developing a foot ulcer (Table 9.2). By having this information, patients can be given the appropriate education, care and screening to avoid any acute diabetic foot episodes (Bus et al. 2016).

When a patient with diabetes has a foot with complications, such as sensory neuropathy or poor blood supply, it can be damaged easily. It would be prudent for them not to walk barefooted, and use open sandals or shoes with caution, as even a small graze or bruise can lead to the development of a foot ulcer. Some potential causes of foot ulceration are:

- animal hair and scratches
- corn/verruca treatment containing salicylic acid
- footwear – friction caused by creases, seams and stitching in or on the shoe
- foreign body in shoe
- hot water bottle used in bed
- ill-fitting hosiery, for example due to pressure from sock seams
- elastic on stockings
- resting feet on or near a heater or radiator
- scald from bath water (Moakes 2012).

The formation of a foot ulcer is multifactorial. The underlying features of diabetes predispose the person to ulceration. Any altered sensation in the foot may impair recognition of injury to the skin, particularly in individuals who are unable to cut their toenails adequately. A mycotic nail may damage the nailbed or the skin of an adjacent toe, leading to subungual ulceration. Older people with diabetes may suffer from age-related changes to vision, which makes nail care more difficult; bending down to carry out self-checks of the foot may be hampered by reduced mobility, being overweight and/or loss of dexterity (Crews at al. 2013, Turns 2015).

Daily foot care checks should be undertaken either by the person or by a relative or carer, reviewing the whole of the foot and footwear. If the person with diabetes requires help reviewing the underside of the foot independently, then a mirror can be placed either on the floor or propped in a position to assist with viewing the sole of the foot. Daily checks should include the following:

- Check top of foot, bottom of foot, tips of toes, in between toes and back of heels. Feel the foot to assess its temperature and assess sensation, ideally using a 10 g monofilament.
- Be aware of fragile skin, especially in those who are very old, and of pressure areas if the person is spending a lot of time in one position, for example in bed or seated.
- Check for pain, but remember that absence of pain in those with neuropathy does not mean that all is well.
- Check for changes in the skin's colour and look for ulcers, sores and areas of hard skin and any signs of inflammation or infection.
- Check footwear for any foreign bodies and evidence of any blood, which could indicate injury to the foot.
- Apply emollient all over the feet but not in between the toes because this may predispose the person to fungal infection as this is already a moist and warm area.
- Refer for specialist help if needed (Moakes 2012, NICE 2015b).

When the person is in a healthcare setting, these checks can be undertaken by a competent healthcare professional. By performing these checks and by touching the feet when applying emollient, problems are likely to be detected and treated promptly.

Table 9.2 Risk factors and the level of risk for developing foot ulcers (NICE 2015b)

Risk factors	Risk level
No risk factors present except callus alone	Low risk
Deformity Neuropathy Non-critical limb ischaemia	Moderate risk
Previous ulceration, previous amputation, on renal replacement therapy, neuropathy and non-critical limb ischaemia together, neuropathy in combination with callus and/or deformity, non-critical limb ischaemia in combination with callus and/or deformity	High risk
Ulceration, spreading infection, critical limb ischaemia, gangrene, suspicion of an acute Charcot arthropathy, or an unexplained hot, red, swollen foot with or without pain	Active diabetic foot problem

Source: Adapted from NICE (2015b), Turns (2015).

Methods of care of the ears and nose

Lack of attention to cleaning the ears and nose can lead to impairment of the senses of smell and hearing. Usually these small organs require minimal care, but observation for a build-up of wax in the ears and deposits in the nose is essential to ensure patency. The outer ear can be cleaned with cotton wool or gauze and warm water. Cotton buds must be avoided; they can damage the ear canal and eardrum, and push the wax further down into the ear (NICE 2018b, Poulton et al. 2015).

Patients with a nasogastric tube *in situ* and/or oxygen therapy should have regular nasal care to avoid excessive drying, excoriation of the delicate air passages, pressure damage and skin breakdown (Asti et al. 2017, Young 2018). Gentle cleaning of the nasal mucosa with cotton wool or gauze and water is recommended.

Coating the area with a thin water-based lubricant to prevent discomfort can be beneficial, but petroleum jelly is not recommended when oxygen therapy is in progress, as it is highly flammable. These interventions will remove debris and maintain a moist environment (Bauters et al. 2016).

Patients who have piercings to the ears or nose will require cleaning of the holes to avoid the risk of infection. Gently cleaning around the pierced area with cotton wool or gauze and warm water and then towel drying is recommended. Observe for inflammation or oozing; if this occurs, inform the patient and doctor and seek permission from the patient to remove the device (Smith 2016).

Pre-procedural considerations

Prior to undertaking the procedures that contribute to the maintenance of personal care and comfort, preparations should include attention to the patient's immediate environment to promote the safety of the patient and the healthcare professional, and a holistic assessment of the patient to gain an insight into their personal preferences and specific needs. Discussing the procedure with the patient, offering explanations and allowing questions will assist in gaining the patient's informed consent. This is imperative to ensuring the maintenance of the patient's autonomy.

Maintaining the privacy and dignity of the patient throughout the procedure should be a principal consideration. Ensuring the patient's comfort and instigating appropriate pain control measures, as required, are necessary in ensuring the patient can tolerate the procedure. For some patients with additional needs – for instance, those with dementia or learning disabilities – ensuring patient comfort may rely on additional skills such as observation, non-verbal communication, or working closely with family and carers to help identify and meet the patient's needs.

Non-pharmacological support

Soap

Persistent use of some soaps can alter the pH of the skin and remove the natural oils, leading to drying and cracking of the skin; this compromise of the skin barrier can create an ideal environment for bacteria to multiply (Lichterfeld et al. 2015). Patients with dry skin have a greater likelihood of skin breakdown (Andriessen 2013). Care should be taken with skinfolds and crevices, paying particular attention to thorough drying of the areas and observing for any breaks in the skin. It is recommended that the skin is patted and not rubbed, to reduce damage caused by friction (Guenther et al. 2012).

Emollient therapy

Current evidence recommends a move away from traditional washing using soap and water, and recent research demonstrates that the surfactants found in soap are irritants to the skin (Andriessen 2013, Moncrieff et al. 2013). The use of emollient therapy for washing and moisturizing to seal the skin has therefore been recommended. In a literature review of hygiene practices, the use of soap and water remained common practice but several studies suggest that emollient creams, followed by moisturizing, are less likely to disrupt the skin barrier and have a therapeutic benefit (Moncrieff et al. 2013).

Washbowls

Conventional plastic washbowls can harbour bacteria and fungi if they are not cleaned and dried effectively. Research indicates that reusable washbowls, washcloths and water can all pose serious risks of cross-infection (Danielson et al. 2013, Martin et al. 2017, McGoldrick 2016). Inadequate storage of reusable washbowls can contribute to the presence of microbial biofilms and place patients at risk of cross infection (Phua et al. 2016). Many organizations now utilize single-use maceratable pulp washbowls.

Pre-packaged cloths

Bacteria exist in hospital water supplies and hospital staff can transmit bacteria both into and via water. In addition, reusable washcloths can spread harmful bacteria when they are transferred to the basin and returned to the patient. Due to the risk of transmission of meticillin-resistant *Staphylococcus aureus* and deterioration of the skin, Martin et al. (2017) suggest that organizations should consider utilizing single-use wipes.

Pre-packaged cloths impregnated with cleanser and moisturizers are an alternative to soap and water and may offer advantages (Craven et al. 2017). Pre packaged cloths are soft and soap free with impregnated emollients, so the likelihood of causing skin irritation and dryness during cleaning is reduced (Martin et al. 2017). These wipes are designed for single use straight from the packet and the cleansers and emollients delivered via the wipe are formulated to nourish and hydrate the skin without the need for rinsing and drying after use. To enhance patient comfort, the wipes can be warmed before use.

Chlorhexidine-impregnated washcloths are available and some are designed specifically for the bedbath. There is limited evidence to support or dispute their use within the general patient population; however, they have been advocated for use with high-risk patients such as those in intensive care (Frost et al. 2016) and those about to undergo surgery.

Cultural and religious factors

The nurse must respect and consider the patient's cultural and religious values and beliefs, while maintaining privacy and dignity at all times; for example, some people prefer to wash under running water rather than sitting in a bath (Fowler 2017a, Pols 2013). Some religions do not allow hair washing or brushing, while others may require the hair to be covered (Peate 2015). Similarly, in some cultures facial hair is significant and should never be removed without the patient's or their relatives' consent. Always establish any preferences before beginning care (Mujallad and Taylor 2016; Padela et al. 2012) (Box 9.2).

Clothing

Effort should be made to encourage and empower patients to dress in their own clothing during the day, where possible, and in their own nightwear to sleep. This increases independence and wellbeing, encourages normality and promotes dignity. This approach was championed by NHS England with the #EndPJparalysis campaign (NHS England 2018), which aimed to get patients up, dressed and moving, citing the many benefits relating to reduced immobility and expedited recovery (Oliver

Box 9.2 Religion-specific considerations relating to personal hygiene

Hinduism

Hindus place importance on washing using running water before prayer; they believe the left hand should dominate in this process and therefore do not eat with the left hand as it is deemed unclean (Fowler 2017a).

Islam

Those following Islam must perform ablution (*wudhu*, to use the Islamic term) before the daily prayer, which is the formal washing of the face, hands and forearms. One of the criteria for cleanliness is washing after using the lavatory. Any traces of urine or faeces must be eliminated by washing with running water (at a minimum), and additional products can be used according to the patient's personal preference. If a bedpan or commode is used, fresh water must be provided for cleaning. The use of toilet tissues for cleaning is not sufficient (Attum and Shamoon 2018).

Sikhism

Sikhs place great importance on not shaving or cutting hair, choosing to comb their hair twice a day and washing it regularly. Male Sikhs wear their hair underneath a turban as a sign of respect for God (Fosarelli 2014).

2017, Peate 2018). If the patient is too unwell or does not have their own clothing, hospital provision should be made available to protect their modesty (Fitzgerald 2017).

Bedbathing

A bedbath is not the most effective way of washing patients, and wherever possible patients should be encouraged and supported to shower or bathe. However, a bedbath can be performed if it is the only way to meet a patient's hygiene needs (Lopes et al. 2013).

Before commencing this procedure, read the patient's care plan and manual handling risk assessment to gain knowledge of safe practice. Prior to each part of the procedure, explain and obtain verbal consent from the patient where possible (NMC 2018a). It is important that the nurse engages in appropriate conversation with the patient. If two nurses are present during bedbathing, the patient should not be excluded from any conversation. Where necessary, complex language and terminology should be adapted to meet the needs of the patient and ensure that they understand the procedure (O'Hagan et al. 2014).

Planned care should be negotiated with the patient and based on assessment of their individual needs; this should be documented and changed according to the patient's needs. Prior to commencing each step, the patient should be offered the opportunity to participate if able, to encourage dignity, independence and autonomy. Privacy and dignity must be maintained throughout; doors and curtains should be kept closed and only opened when absolutely necessary, with the patient's permission.

Procedure guideline 9.1 Bedbathing a patient

Essential equipment

- Personal protective equipment
- Clean bed linen
- Bath towels
- Laundry skip, applying local guidelines for soiled and/or infected linen
- Flannels, preferably disposable wipes
- Toiletries, as preferred by patient
- Comb and/or brush
- Equipment for oral hygiene
- Clean clothes
- Washbowl

Optional equipment

- Antiembolic stockings
- Razor (see Procedure guideline 9.3: Shaving the face: wet shave and Procedure guideline 9.4: Shaving the face: dry electric shaver)
- Scissors and/or nail clippers
- Emery boards
- Manual handling equipment
- Urinal, bedpan or commode

Action	Rationale
Pre-procedure	
1 Introduce yourself to the patient, explain and discuss the procedure with them, and gain their consent to proceed. Assess and plan care with the patient. Note personal preferences, addressing religious and cultural beliefs.	To ensure that the patient feels at ease, understands the procedure and gives their valid consent, and to plan care and encourage participation and independence (Alpers and Hanssen 2014, **R**; NMC 2018a, **C**; Tobiano et al. 2015, **R**).
2 Offer the patient analgesia as appropriate. During the procedure, observe for any non-verbal cues, such as grimacing or frowning, that may suggest that the patient is experiencing pain or discomfort.	To maintain patient comfort throughout the procedure (O'Hagan et al. 2014, **R**).
3 Clear the area of any obstacles, ensuring that the environment is warm. Draw the curtains around the bed or close the doors to ensure privacy and dignity. Use available signage as appropriate.	To maintain comfort and a safe environment and promote privacy and dignity (NMC 2018a, **C**).
4 Offer the patient the opportunity to use a urinal, bedpan or commode.	To reduce any disruption to the procedure and prevent any discomfort (NMC 2018a, **C**).
5 Collect all the equipment listed and place it by the bedside.	To minimize time away from the patient during the procedure. **E**
6 Clean the washbowl with hot soapy water before use if a non-disposable bowl is being used. Fill the bowl with warm water as close to the patient's bedside as possible. Check the temperature of the water with the patient and adjust it as necessary.	To minimize cross-infection (Rebeiro et al. 2013, **E**). To promote patient comfort. **E**
7 Check that the bed brakes are on and adjust the bed to an appropriate height for you to carry out care comfortably.	To prevent the bed moving unexpectedly and to avoid back strain or injury (Davis and Kotowski 2015, **R**).
8 Wash your hands and put on disposable gloves and apron in accordance with local guidelines.	To minimize the risk of cross-infection (NHS England and NHSI 2019, **C**).

(continued)

Procedure guideline 9.1 Bedbathing a patient (continued)

Action	Rationale
Throughout the procedure	
9 The linen skip should be positioned and kept near to the bed throughout the procedure.	To reduce the potential dispersal of micro-organisms, dust and skin cells from the linen into the environment (DH 2016, **C**).
10 The water used to wash the patient may be changed at any stage during the procedure – for example, if the patient feels the temperature is too hot or too cold. Very soapy or dirty water must be changed before proceeding with the wash, and the water should be changed after washing the genitalia and surrounding area. Ideally utilize single-use wipes for this area.	To promote patient comfort. **E** To minimize the risk of cross-infection or translocation of micro-organisms (Peate and Lane 2015, **E**; Rebeiro et al. 2013, **E**). Disposable flannels or wipes are preferable as this reduces the risk of infection (Martin et al. 2017, **C**).
11 Avoid wetting drains, dressings and intravenous devices.	To reduce the risk of infection and prevent any drains or intravenous catheters from becoming dislodged (Peate and Lane 2015, **E**).
12 Check skin and pressure areas throughout the procedure for evidence of damage.	To ensure any potential or actual damage is identified and treated early. **E**
Procedure	
13 Check for hearing aids, spectacles and wrist watches and (with permission) remove these from the patient, putting them in a safe place.	To ensure that the patient's face is washed thoroughly and to avoid damage to such devices. **E**
14 Place a towel across the patient's chest.	To protect the patient from splashes and to prepare for drying. **E**
15 Ask the patient whether they use soap on their face. The face, neck and ears should be washed, rinsed and dried.	To promote cleanliness and to ensure that the patient's preferences are acknowledged. **E**
16 Hearing aids and spectacles should be cleaned and returned to the patient.	To ensure that the prostheses are in good working order and free from debris and contaminants (Peate and Lane 2015, **E**).
17 Assist the patient with the removal of their upper clothing. The patient should be covered with a bath towel or sheet before folding back the bedclothes. Areas of the body that are not being washed should remain covered.	To maintain the patient's modesty and sustain body temperature (Rebeiro et al. 2013, **E**).
18 Wash, rinse and pat dry the top half of the patient's body, starting with the side furthest away from you.	To avoid any spills on parts of the body that have already been washed and dried (Rebeiro et al. 2013, **E**).
19 If pyjama trousers are worn, these should be removed while keeping the patient covered. If worn, antiembolic stockings should also be carefully removed.	To allow access to the lower half of the body and to assess the skin beneath stockings. **E**
20 Wash the patient's legs, rinse and pat them dry, starting with the leg furthest away from you.	To avoid any spills on parts of the body that have already been washed and dried (Rebeiro et al. 2013, **E**).
21 Tell the patient that the next step is to wash around the genitalia. Ask the patient whether they wish to wash this area themselves or gain verbal consent from the patient to do it for them.	To reduce the risk of infection and to maintain a safe environment (NMC 2018a, **C**; Rebeiro et al. 2013, **E**).
22 Using a new disposable wipe, wash around the area and then dry it. • *Female patients*: wash from the front to the back. • *Male patients*: the foreskin needs to be drawn back gently when washing the penis of uncircumcised male patients.	To ensure the area is cleaned and dried. **E** To prevent the translocation of bacteria (Lloyd Jones 2014, **E**; Peate and Lane 2015, **E**).
23 *If the patient has an indwelling catheter*: put on clean gloves and wash the tubing, moving the disposable cloth down the tube away from the genital area, then dry the tubing. Remove your gloves and dispose of them as per hospital policy.	To reduce the risk of catheter-associated urinary tract infection (RCN 2019, **C**).
24 Ensure the patient is covered and has a call bell within easy reach. Change the water and put on clean gloves.	To maintain cleanliness and to preserve dignity and privacy (NMC 2018a, **C**).
25 Request assistance as necessary to roll the patient onto their side. Cover the areas of the patient that are not being washed. Wash their back, assessing the skin and pressure areas accordingly.	To prevent and treat pressure ulcers. **E** Disposable flannels or wipes are preferable as this reduces the risk of infection (Martin et al. 2017, **C**).
26 Using a disposable flannel or wipe, wash the sacral area, then rinse and dry the area. Gloves should be removed and hands decontaminated.	To minimize the risk of cross-infection (NHS England and NHSI 2019, **C**).

27 Keep the patient on their side while changing the bottom bed sheet. Return the patient onto their back, ensuring that they remain covered. Roll the patient onto the other side as required (to change the bottom sheet). Apply toiletries as required.	To enable the sheets to be changed with minimal disruption to the patient. **E**
28 Allow the patient to choose what clothing they would like to wear.	To enhance patient comfort, to promote positive body image and to promote the #EndPJparalysis campaign (NHS England 2018, **C**).
29 Encourage the patient to do as much for themselves as they are able. For patients who require help in dressing, it is advised to put clothing on the weak or paralysed side first.	To encourage self-care, independence and rehabilitation. **E**
30 Inspect the patient's fingernails. If necessary, clean under the nails. Cut or clip fingernails to the top level of the finger, shaping the edges with an emery board if necessary.	To enhance positive body image and patient comfort and reduce the risk of infection (NMC 2018a, **C**).
31 Check the feet for any areas of skin dryness, inflammation or calluses. The need for podiatry referral should be assessed. Refit antiembolic stockings as necessary, measuring according to local policy (see Procedure guideline 16.1: Measuring and applying antiembolic stockings).	To ensure adequate foot care. **E** To maintain venous thromboembolism (VTE) prophylaxis (as determined by a VTE risk assessment) (Roberts and Lawrence 2017, **E**).
32 Provide appropriate equipment and assist the patient to brush their teeth and/or rinse their mouth (see Procedure guideline 9.14: Mouth care).	To maintain good oral hygiene and prevent infection (Rebeiro et al. 2013, **E**).
33 Style the patient's hair as desired.	To enhance patient comfort and to promote a positive body image (NMC 2018a, **C**).
34 Assist male patients with facial shaving if required, using either a disposable razor (see Procedure guideline 9.3: Shaving the face: wet shave) or an electric shaver (see Procedure guideline 9.4: Shaving the face: dry electric shaver).	To enhance patient comfort and to promote a positive body image (NMC 2018a, **C**).
35 Remake the top bedclothes.	To ensure the patient is adequately covered, maintaining comfort and dignity (NMC 2018a, **C**).
36 Help the patient to sit or lie in their desired position, considering the previous position.	To enhance patient comfort and reduce the risk of pressure area breakdown (NMC 2018a, **C**).
Post-procedure	
37 Remove your apron and gloves, disposing of them according to local regulations.	To prevent cross-infection (NHS England and NHSI 2019, **C**).
38 Remove the equipment from the patient's bedside and replace the patient's possessions. Place the locker, bedside table and call bell within the reach of the patient.	To maintain a safe environment and promote patient independence (NMC 2018a, **C**).
39 Document any changes in planned care.	To provide recorded documentation of care and aid communication to the multiprofessional team (NMC 2018a, **C**).

Procedure guideline 9.2 Washing a patient's hair in bed

Essential equipment

- Personal protective equipment
- Comb and brush
- Plastic sheet or pad
- Two large towels
- Shampoo tray
- Receptacle for the shampoo water, e.g. bucket
- Basin and jug
- Shampoo and conditioner
- Hairdryer if required
- Washcloth or pad

(continued)

Procedure guideline 9.2 Washing a patient's hair in bed (continued)

Action	Rationale
Pre-procedure	
1 Introduce yourself to the patient, explain and discuss the procedure with them, and gain their consent to proceed. Assess and plan care with the patient. Note personal preferences, addressing religious and cultural beliefs.	To ensure that the patient feels at ease, understands the procedure and gives their valid consent, and to plan care and encourage participation and independence (NMC 2018a, **C**; Tobiano et al. 2015, **R**).
2 Determine the type of shampoo to be used. Arrange for any prescribed care, e.g. medicated shampoo, to be administered.	To ensure the necessary products are utilized. **E**
3 Assess the patient's ability to lie flat throughout the procedure.	To ensure patient stability, comfort and safety. **E**
4 Collect all the equipment listed and place it by the bedside.	To minimize time away from the patient during the procedure. **E**
5 Clear the area of any obstacles, ensuring that the environment is warm. Draw the curtains around the bed or close the doors to ensure privacy and dignity. Use available signage as appropriate.	To maintain comfort and a safe environment and promote privacy and dignity (NMC 2018a, **C**).
6 Wash your hands and put on disposable gloves and apron in accordance with local guidelines.	To minimize the risk of cross-infection (NHS England and NHSI 2019, **C**).
Procedure	
7 Remove the pillows from under the patient's head, and lower or remove the bed head.	To gain access to the patient and give the nurse more control during the procedure, thus reducing the risk of water entering the patient's eyes and ears (Seray-Wurie 2017, **E**).
8 Place the plastic sheet under the patient's head and tuck a bath towel around their shoulders, bringing it towards their chest.	To keep the bed and patient dry. To prevent unnecessary disruption to the patient by having to change bed linen and clothes. **E**
9 Gently lift the patient's head and slide in the shampoo tray with the U opening under the neck. Place a towel underneath the patient's neck for support.	The shampoo tray allows water drainage into a receptacle and prevents spills onto the floor. Padding supports the muscles of the neck and prevents undue strain and discomfort (Seray-Wurie 2017, **E**; Windle 2014, **E**).
10 Fold the top bedding down to the waist and cover the upper part of the patient with a towel.	To maintain patient dignity and prevent them from becoming cold (Seray-Wurie 2017, **E**; Windle 2014, **E**).
11 Place the receptacle for the shampoo water on the floor with an absorbent sheet underneath. Put the spout of the shampoo basin over the receptacle.	The receptacle must be lower than the bed to collect used water. Not using an absorbent sheet increases the risk of spills and slips (Peate 2015, **R**).
12 Protect the patient's eyes and ears. Place a washcloth over the patient's eyes. Place cotton balls in the patient's ears if indicated.	The washcloth protects the eyes from soapy water (Spencer 2016, **E**). The cotton balls keep water from collecting in the ear canals (Peate 2015, **E**; Seray-Wurie 2017, **E**).
13 Ensure the patient is covered and has a call bell within easy reach. Fill the basin with warm water. Check the temperature of the water with the patient and adjust it as necessary.	To preserve dignity, privacy and patient safety, and to promote patient comfort (NMC 2018a, **C**).
14 Fill a jug with water from the basin, carefully wet the patient's hair and make sure the water drains into the receptacle.	To ensure there is minimal spillage of water. **E**
15 Apply a small amount of shampoo to the hair and scalp, and gently massage with your fingertips.	Massaging stimulates the blood circulation in the scalp. The pads of the fingers are used so that fingernails cannot scratch the scalp (Windle 2014, **E**).
16 Using fresh water from the basin, rinse the hair thoroughly. Start at the top of the head and let the water work its way down to the bottom of the head.	To ensure all the shampoo is removed (Windle 2014, **E**).
17 Apply conditioner if desired and rinse using warm water until the water runs clear.	Soapy residue causes the appearance of soap scum in the hair and the scalp will become irritated and dry. **E**
18 Squeeze excess water from the hair into the shampoo tray before removal. Gently rub the hair dry with a towel. Dry the patient's face.	To facilitate optimal drying of the hair. **E** To ensure patient comfort. **E**
19 Remove any equipment and return the patient back to a comfortable position.	To ensure patient comfort (Seray-Wurie 2017, **E**; Spencer 2016, **E**).
20 Replace any wet linen and ensure that the patient is appropriately clothed.	To ensure patient comfort and warmth. **E**

21 Style the patient's hair. Use a hairdryer on a cool or warm setting if the patient wishes and if it has had all appropriate safety checks.	To prevent drying of the scalp. To prevent the discomfort of prolonged heat on the scalp (Seray-Wurie 2017, **E**; Windle 2014, **E**).
Post-procedure	
22 Clear away the equipment from the patient's bedside. Place the call bell within the reach of the patient.	To maintain a safe environment and promote patient independence (NMC 2018a, **C**).
23 Remove your apron and gloves, disposing of them according to local regulations.	To prevent cross-infection (NHS England and NHSI 2019, **C**).
24 Document any changes in planned care.	To provide recorded documentation of care and aid communication to the multiprofessional team (NMC 2018a, **C**).

Also available are commercial dry shampoos and disposable shampoo caps. They can make shampooing easier to accomplish and less of a physical stress for the patient (Spencer 2016). Be sure to follow the manufacturer's instructions and local policies (Peate 2015, Treas and Wilkinson 2014).

Shaving

Shaving to remove hair is a common cosmetic practice for men to maintain a well-groomed appearance (Maurer et al. 2016). The process of shaving to remove facial hair is one more commonly associated with men; however, it should be remembered that there may be some instances when female patients wish to remove unwanted facial hair (Bloomfield et al. 2017), although in females the hair of the axilla and legs is more frequently shaved (Burton and Ludwig 2014).

If a patient requires help to shave, then the nurse should make themselves aware of personal preferences with regard to shaving as well as any religious and/or cultural considerations. Some religions (e.g. Sikhism) do not permit the removal of any body or facial hair and so for male Sikh patients, beards will require rolling and netting (Peate 2015).

An assessment of the patient's history and blood results should be carried out prior to shaving to ascertain the risk of bleeding. Patients at risk of bleeding should use an electric razor to shave (Spencer 2016). The skin functions as an important barrier to external pathogens (Jones 2014, Marks and Miller 2013, Maurer et al. 2016). Compromising this barrier by cutting the skin while shaving, coupled with the fact that male skin displays slower wound-healing rates than female skin (Maurer et al. 2016), could lead to an infection. The patient's immunity and infection status should also be reviewed prior to shaving with a razor; it may be advisable to use an electric razor to minimize the risk of cutting the skin. Only the patient's own razor or a new disposable razor should be used to shave the patient; this is to prevent the risk of cross-infection (Bloomfield et al. 2017).

Procedure guideline 9.3 Shaving the face: wet shave

Essential equipment

- Personal protective equipment
- Towels
- Bowl or basin
- Mirror
- Razor – patient's own or disposable razor
- Shaving product – foam, soap or gel
- Shaving brush (if appropriate)
- Washcloth or pad

Action	Rationale
Pre-procedure	
1 Prior to shaving the patient with a razor, it is essential that the patient is assessed for their risk of bleeding. Clinical history and laboratory blood tests (including full blood count, clotting times and platelet count) should be reviewed. It would also be prudent to check the patient's immunity status as any breach in the skin integrity could lead to an infection. If there is a risk of bleeding or infection, an electric razor should be used to shave the patient.	To ensure that the patient is safe to have a wet shave and that the possible risks associated with cutting the patient are mitigated (Bloomfield et al. 2017, **E**; Moore and Cunningham 2017, **E**).
2 Introduce yourself to the patient, explain and discuss the procedure with them, and gain their consent to proceed. Determine their preferences with regard to shaving and the type of shaving products to be used (e.g. gel or foam).	To ensure that the patient feels at ease, understands the procedure and gives their valid consent (NMC 2018a, **C**). Shaving is individual to the patient (Maurer et al. 2016, **E**). To arrange for any prescribed care (e.g. medicated product) to be administered. **E**

(continued)

Procedure guideline 9.3 Shaving the face: wet shave *(continued)*

Action	Rationale
3 Assess the patient's ability to be in a comfortable position throughout the procedure: either sitting or lying (if confined to bed) or sitting in a chair.	To ensure patient stability, comfort and safety. **E**
4 Collect all the equipment listed and place it by the bedside. Only use the patient's own razor or a disposable razor. If using the patient's razor, check the condition of the blades to ensure they are not blocked or corroded.	To minimize time away from the patient during the procedure. **E** To prevent cross-infection (Bloomfield et al. 2017, **E**; Moore and Cunningham 2017, **E**). To ensure that the razor can cut the beard hair, which reduces the risk of skin irritation from repeated strokes. **E**
5 Clear the area of any obstacles, ensuring that the environment is warm. Draw the curtains around the bed or close the doors to ensure privacy and dignity. Use available signage as appropriate.	To maintain comfort and a safe environment and promote privacy and dignity (NMC 2018a, **C**).
6 Wash your hands and put on disposable gloves and apron in accordance with local guidelines.	To minimize the risk of cross-infection (NHS England and NHSI 2019, **C**).
Procedure	
7 Drape a towel over the patient's chest, around the neck.	To allow the patient to be kept clean and dry during the procedure. **E**
8 Wet the patient's face and beard by applying a warm, moist cloth.	This will soften the beard hair, which may result in less force being required during shaving (Maurer et al. 2016, **E**).
9 Apply shaving cream or gel to the patient's face as per the patient's preference, using hands or the patient's shaving brush, if available.	To soften the patient's beard hair and skin (Draelos 2018, **E**). To provide lubrication for the razor, causing less friction. **E**
10 With the non-dominant hand, hold the skin of the face taut.	To remove skin creases, providing a smoother surface and pathway for the razor, thus maintaining patient comfort (Moore and Cunningham 2017, **E**; Spencer 2016, **E**).
11 Holding the razor at a 45° angle to the skin, shave the hair in short, firm strokes in the direction of the hair growth. Rinse the razor in the water regularly to remove accumulated shaving foam on the blade.	To remove the hair effectively and promote comfort, avoiding the risk of skin irritation and ingrowing hairs (Bloomfield et al. 2017, **E**; Burton and Ludwig 2014, **E**; Spencer 2016, **E**).
12 After shaving the whole of the beard and moustache area, wipe the patient's face using moist wipes.	To remove any remaining shaving cream and hair. **E**
13 Dry the face using the towel and apply any aftershave products the patient desires. Lotions should be patted onto the skin.	To avoid excess rubbing, which can cause skin irritation (Kozier et al. 2008, **E**).
14 Remove the equipment and return the patient to a comfortable position.	To ensure patient comfort (Delay-Wurie 2017, **E**; Windle 2014, **E**).
15 Remove any wet linen and ensure that the patient is appropriately clothed.	To ensure patient comfort and warmth. **E**
Post-procedure	
16 Clear away the equipment from the patient's bedside. Place the call bell within the reach of the patient.	To maintain a safe environment and promote patient independence (NMC 2018a, **C**).
17 Dispose of the disposable razor in the sharps bin. Remove apron and gloves, disposing of them according to local regulations. Undertake hand hygiene.	For the safe disposal of sharps. To prevent injury and cross-infection (Moore and Cunningham 2017, **C**; NHS England and NHSI 2019, **C**).
18 Document any changes in planned care.	To provide recorded documentation of care and aid communication to the multiprofessional team (NMC 2018a, **C**).

Procedure guideline 9.4 Shaving the face: dry electric shaver

Essential equipment

- Personal protective equipment
- Mirror
- Towel
- Razor – patient's own electric razor
- Shaving product – pre-shave lotion and aftershave if desired

Action	Rationale
Pre-procedure	
1 Introduce yourself to the patient, explain and discuss the procedure with them, and gain their consent to proceed. Determine their preferences with regard to electric shaving. Only use the patient's own razor. Examine the electric razor to ensure that it is clean and in optimal condition, ready for use. If it is battery operated, check the batteries are working; if it is mains operated, check that any electrical cables are safe and intact before plugging the razor into the mains.	To ensure that the patient feels at ease, understands the procedure and gives their valid consent (NMC 2018a, **C**). To ensure the preferences of the patient are adhered to and that the equipment is safe and ready for purpose. **E** To prevent cross-infection (Bloomfield et al. 2017, **E**; Moore and Cunningham 2017, **E**). To ensure that the razor can cut the beard hair, so as to reduce the risk of skin irritation from repeated strokes. **E**
2 Determine whether the patient would like full removal or a trim.	To ensure the patient's preferences are considered and individuality maintained. **E**
3 Determine the type of shaving products to be used (e.g. pre-shave lotion, aftershave lotion).	To arrange for any prescribed care (e.g. medicated products) to be administered and/or apply any products as per the patient's preference. **E**
4 Assess the patient's ability to be in a comfortable position throughout the procedure: either sitting or lying (if confined to bed) or sitting in a chair.	To ensure patient stability, comfort and safety. **E**
5 Collect all the equipment listed and place it by the bedside.	To minimize time away from the patient during the procedure. **E**
6 Clear the area of any obstacles, ensuring that the environment is warm. Draw the curtains around the bed or close the doors to ensure privacy and dignity. Use available signage as appropriate.	To maintain comfort and a safe environment and promote privacy and dignity (NMC 2018a, **C**).
7 Wash hands and put on disposable gloves and apron in accordance with local guidelines.	To minimize the risk of cross-infection (NHS England and NHSI 2019, **C**).
Procedure	
8 Drape a towel over the patient's chest, around the neck	To allow the patient to be kept clean during the procedure. **E**
9 Apply any desired pre-shaving products to the face, massage them into the beard hair.	To soften the beard hair (Burton and Ludwig 2014, **E**, Maurer et al. 2016, **E**).
10 After turning the electric razor on, shave the cheeks in a circular motion, going over the same area a few times to cut the hair adequately. Shave the upper lip area in a downward direction following the direction of the hair growth and shave the neck area in an upward direction.	To remove the hair effectively and promote comfort, avoiding the risk of skin irritation and ingrowing hairs (Bloomfield et al. 2017, **E**; Burton and Ludwig 2014, **E**; Spencer 2016, **E**).
11 Apply any aftershave products as per the patient's preference. Lotions should be patted onto the skin.	To avoid excess rubbing, which can cause skin irritation (Kozier et al. 2008, **E**).
12 Return the patient to a comfortable position.	To ensure patient comfort (Seray-Wurie 2017, **E**; Windle 2014, **E**).
13 Remove and dispose of any used towels according to local policy and ensure that the patient is appropriately clothed.	To ensure patient comfort and warmth. **E**
Post-procedure	
14 Clear away the equipment from the patient's bedside. Brush the razor to clean it, and store it in an appropriate safe place. Place the call bell within the reach of the patient.	To maintain a safe environment and promote patient independence (NMC 2018a, **C**).
15 Remove apron and gloves, disposing of them according to local regulations. Undertake hand hygiene.	To prevent cross-infection (Moore and Cunningham 2017, **C**; NHS England and NHSI 2019, **C**).
16 Document and report any changes in planned care.	To provide recorded documentation of care and aid communication to the multiprofessional team (NMC 2018a, **C**).

Sleep promotion in a hospitalized patient

Definition

Sleep is a recurring restorative process characterized by altered consciousness, inhibited sensory activity, inhibition of voluntary muscles and reduced interactions with external stimuli (National Institute of Neurological Disorders and Stroke 2017).

Anatomy and physiology

Sleep has an underlying structure composed of an alternating cycle of rapid eye movement (REM) and non-REM (NREM) sleep (Assefa et al. 2015) and is actively regulated by two separate biological mechanisms: sleep–wake homeostasis and the circadian rhythm, which is entrained to the 24 hour clock (Carley and Farabi 2016). The recommended sleep time for adults aged 18–64 is

7–9 hours, and the recommended time is 7–8 hours in adults over 64 (Hirshkowitz et al. 2015).

Related theory

Sleep is a fundamental component in maintaining good health (Pilkington 2013). Sleep deprivation can have a number of detrimental physiological effects, including fatigue, irritability, confusion, decreased pain tolerance, delayed wound healing (Radtke et al. 2014), and declines in immune function, memory and strength (Tamarat et al. 2014).

Inadequate sleep, either in length or quality, can therefore contribute to poor health, further complicate existing illnesses, prolong recovery and therefore increase length of hospital stay. Sleep promotion should be a nursing priority (Clark and Mills 2017).

The hospital environment is often poorly conducive to sleep (Auckely et al. 2018). Factors contributing to this can be external or internal (Honkavuo 2018). External factors include noise caused by alarms, equipment, or movements or conversations; care interventions by healthcare staff, such as nocturnal vital sign monitoring or pressure relief; temperature and comfort issues; and light exposure (Dobing et al. 2016, Fillary et al. 2015, Honkavuo 2018). Internal factors can be physical, such as pain, hunger, thirst and toilet needs (Honkavuo 2018), or psychological, such as anxiety, restlessness, poor communication and being in a new environment (Salzmann-Erikson et al. 2016). As the primary caregivers, nurses are strategically placed to minimize these factors and support patients to achieve and sustain sleep (Hoey et al. 2014).

Evidence-based practice

Promoting sleep

Noise and light

Given that noise and light are stimuli that can disrupt sleep, nurses should make efforts to reduce these as much as possible and as appropriate. Straightforward measures include:

- reducing volumes on pumps, monitors and alarms
- talking in hushed voices when necessary
- maintaining a dark environment via the use of torches overnight instead of turning on overhead lights for patient care
- positioning equipment with bright screens or flashing lights to face away from the patient.

Measures to block external stimuli, such as providing earplugs and eye-masks, can provide a simple and inexpensive way of promoting sleep (Dubose and Hadi 2016). In particular, these are useful when efforts to reduce light or noise are not successful, or when it is impractical to reduce noise levels caused by equipment (Darbyshire and Young 2013) – for example, in the intensive care unit (ICU). The use of earplugs in patients admitted to the ICU has been associated with a significant reduction in the risk of delirium (Litton et al. 2016).

Daytime bright-light therapy has been shown to aid sleep at night, the rationale being that it helps to regulate the patient's circadian rhythms by maintaining a dark–light cycle (Tamarat et al. 2014). In hospitals, a similar effect can be achieved by opening blinds or curtains during the day in order to facilitate sleepiness at night. In addition, this can be complemented by encouraging daytime physical activity, for example a walk outside, serving food in a separate room or even bed exercises. Avoiding daytime napping can promote sleep at night; however, a short nap in the daytime may compensate for less sleep at night (Tan et al. 2018) and so should be considered in context.

Communication

Clear and effective communication is integral to the quality of patients' experience in hospital (Barber 2016) and should not be overlooked in aiding sleep promotion. Conversations and planning regarding overnight interventions can aid sleep promotion. By preparing the patient about what to expect, feelings of safe care can be established – for example, warning the patient that they have antibiotics due at midnight, or that the nurse will be entering the room to record vital signs (Salzmann-Erikson et al. 2016). Involving patients in this way allows them to have more control in their care and is therefore more likely to achieve a 'home like' experience in line with their normal routine that is conducive to sleep (Gellerstedt et al. 2014). The way that information is communicated is also relevant; Gellerstedt et al. (2014) reported that open body language, kind facial expressions and gentle tone of voice evoked feelings of security, made patients feel relaxed and therefore facilitated better sleep. On the other hand, a lack of bedside manner awakened feelings of abandonment and insecurity, creating a disturbing factor for sleep.

Cluster care

The idea of 'cluster care' involves clustering several routine or nursing care events together rather than spacing them out over time, the main goal being that the patient has fewer disruptions and longer periods of rest (Valizadeh et al. 2014). For example, continence care can be combined with recording vital signs. Patient interactions should be limited during typical sleep hours to those that are truly necessary for patient care (Auckely et al. 2018). Reviewing timing of medications, taking samples at appropriate times and avoiding routine checks can all be considered to avoid unnecessary interruptions during the night.

Sleep rounds

Sleep-promoting interventions can be formalized into a 'sleep checklist' based on the concept of 'intentional rounding', which is carried out in the majority of hospitals and is a formal means of carrying out and documenting regular checks of patients' fundamental care needs. Box 9.3 provides an example checklist.

Carrying out a sleep assessment aims to address the patient's normal sleep routine and identify any reasonable adjustments that can be made to improve their experience of sleep while in hospital. Questions can include (Gilsenan 2017):

- How many hours of sleep do you usually get?
- Where do you usually sleep (e.g. bed or chair)?
- Do you have any bedtime routines (e.g. warm drink, book)?
- Do you usually take any medications to aid sleep?

It is important that care is planned with the multidisciplinary team so that interventions can be clustered to minimize the number of times the patient is disturbed, allowing longer periods of rest. The results of the sleep assessment, any techniques used to promote sleep and the effectiveness of these should be documented within the patient's notes, together with the amount and quality of sleep experienced. This will assist in the continuity of this aspect of patient care and comply with the Nursing and Midwifery Council's documentation standards (NMC 2018a).

Box 9.3 Summary of interventions to promote sleep in a hospitalized patient

- Undertake a 'sleep assessment' with the patient or the next of kin.
- Communicate with the patient (if able) and explain the plan for the night, including anticipated interruptions. Give them the opportunity to negotiate the timings of interventions.
- Encourage bright light exposure and physical activity during daytime hours and avoid prolonged daytime napping.
- Perform sleep round, ensuring the following:
  - encourage patient to use the bathroom
  - patient comfort (positioning, pillows, nightwear, bedclothes)
  - consider analgesia and/or medications to aid sleep
  - administer any due medications and review the timing of others due throughout the night
  - adjust lights and noise accordingly
  - offer ear plugs and eye mask
  - ensure table, drinks and call bell are near by
  - discuss care needs overnight and prepare the patient for potential disruptions.

Patient environment

Providing a safe, clean, comfortable area where patients can rest and recuperate can add to the patient's sense of wellbeing and is vital for maintaining health and promoting healing (Dubose and Hadi 2016). The area should be free from clutter, so that it can be properly maintained, cleaned and decontaminated, thus reducing the risk of hospital-acquired infection (Cullen and Thomas 2018).

Related theory

The bed is an important piece of hospital equipment used by patients to rest, although there is currently a drive to reduce the amount of time patients unnecessarily stay in bed (Oliver 2017).

Hospital beds are generally composed of a metal frame (some are divided into three sections to assist with positioning) and set on castors or wheels to aid mobility. Hospital beds have become more sophisticated. Many have electrical or battery-powered motors that are operated via a control panel attached to the bed; these can help to alter the patient's position or alter the height of the bed. This assists nurses by reducing the strain of altering a patient's position, and it assists patients by giving them some autonomy in altering their own position independently (Ghersi et al. 2016). Common bed positions are highlighted in Table 9.3 and shown in Figure 9.2.

Standard healthcare mattresses are usually constructed of supportive foam with a waterproof lining to aid with cleaning (Spencer 2016). There are a number of more sophisticated mattresses available that use variable air pressures; these can offer pressure relief to patients who are at risk of developing pressure damage while in bed for extended periods.

Pre-procedural considerations

Equipment

Linen

Bed linen will require changing frequently as it is in regular contact with the patient. Humans produce and shed fungi and bacteria from skin cells, sputum and sweat as well as vaginal and anal excretions while they are in bed (Tierno 2017). Bed linen needs to be regarded as a potential vehicle for pathogen transfer. Skin flora and pathogens such as *Escherichia coli* (*E. coli*), *Clostridioides difficile* (*C. diff*), *Staphylococcus aureus* and meticillin-resistant *Staphylococcus aureus* (MRSA) have been isolated from linen (Bloomfield et al. 2015). Regular changing and laundering of linen is important in preventing the spread of these pathogens (Bloomfield et al. 2015). Soiled linen should never be shaken in the air because shaking can disseminate secretions, excretions and micro-organisms into the atmosphere to contaminate the surrounding environment (Tierno 2017). For this reason, many healthcare settings change bed linen daily. Linen will always require prompt changing when the patient is incontinent (Spencer 2016).

Making a bed

Making a hospital bed is considered an essential technical and practical nursing skill requiring considerations of safety, moving and handling, and infection prevention and control (Bloomfield et al. 2015). As the hospital bed is the piece of equipment most frequently used by patients, making up a hospital bed is fundamental to promoting an environment that is comfortable for the patient (Spencer 2016). There are a number of ways that a bed can be prepared, depending on its specific purpose: surgical, post-operative or inpatient. Beds are frequently made while unoccupied, but there are also circumstances when the bed will be made while it is occupied by the patient.

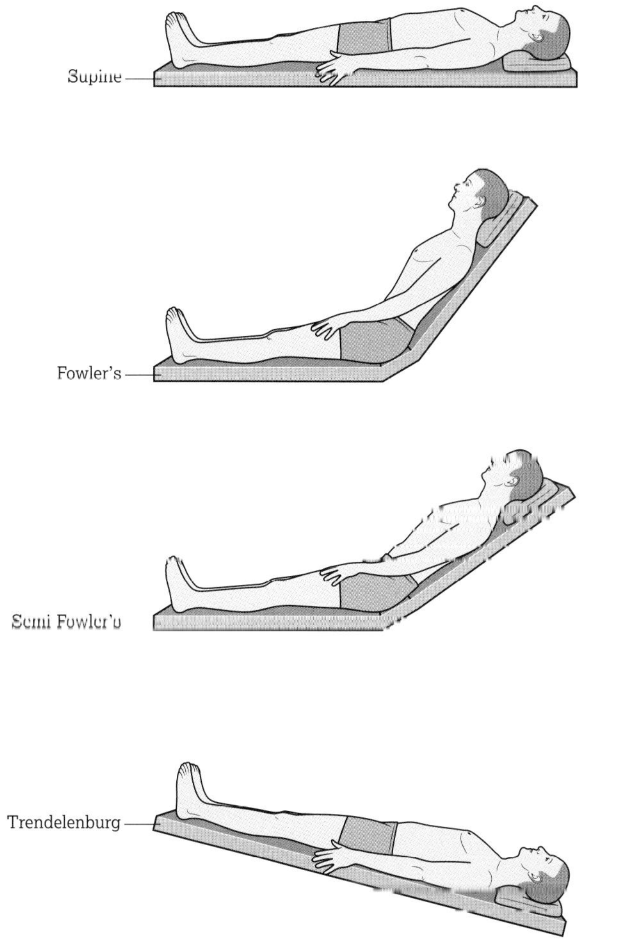

Figure 9.2 Bed positions.

Table 9.3 Common bed positions

Supine/flat	Mattress flat and parallel to the floor	• Generally adopted position for sleeping patients • For patients who are hypotensive • For patients in cervical traction due to vertebral injuries
Fowler's position	Head of the bed raised to 45° or more; the end of the bed may be raised at the knee to stop the patient sliding down the bed	• Positioning for procedures such as nasogastric tube insertion and nasotracheal suctioning • Position to assist with eating
Semi-Fowler's position	Head of bed raised, but to a lesser degree than the Fowler's position	• Reduces risk of aspiration and regurgitation • Promotes lung expansion
Trendelenburg	Mattress in the level position, entire bed tilted with the head of the bed down and feet elevated	• Positioning for procedures such as central venous catheter removal to assist in increase of intra-abdominal pressure • Improves venous return • For postural draining

Source: Spencer (2016).

Procedure guideline 9.5 Making an unoccupied bed

Essential equipment

- Personal protective equipment
- Clean bed linen: sheets (bottom and top), pillowcases, blankets
- Laundry skip (apply local guidelines for segregation and disposal of soiled and/or infected linen)

Action	Rationale
Pre-procedure	
1 Collect all of the equipment listed and place it by the bedside. If available, use the linen tray at the end of the bed, or a clean chair beside the bed within comfortable reach. If the patient is in the bed, offer assistance to them to transfer to a chair	To ensure efficient time use and reduce the need to leave the bedside. **E**
2 Carry out hand hygiene and apply personal protective equipment (apron and gloves).	To protect against the transfer of contaminants on the hands of the healthcare worker causing cross-contamination. Linen could be contaminated with body fluids (Bloomfield et al. 2015, **E**; NHS England and NHSI 2019, **C**).
3 Clear the area of any obstacles; be aware of any items of clinical equipment – e.g. call bell cords, drip stand, electrical cords. If necessary, move the bed to gain adequate space to move freely to carry out the procedure.	To maintain a safe environment (NMC 2018a, **C**).
4 Reposition the bed as required and then check that the bed brakes are on. Adjust the bed to an appropriate height to maintain a comfortable posture during the procedure.	To prevent the bed moving unexpectedly and to avoid back injury (Davis and Kotowski 2015, **R**).
5 The linen skip should be positioned and kept near to the bed throughout the procedure.	To reduce the potential dispersal of micro-organisms, dust and skin cells from the linen into the environment (Bloomfield et al. 2015, **E**; DH 2016, **C**).
Procedure	
6 Check the bed linen for the presence of any personal articles belonging to the patient. Remove any call bells attached to the linen.	To ensure that personal belongings are not lost when the soiled linen is disposed. To promote patient comfort. **E**
7 Remove and fold unsoiled, reusable linen. Place on the pull-out tray at the foot end of the bed (if available).	To ensure reusable linen is stored for reuse. **E**
8 Loosen the linen, moving methodically from the head of the bed to the foot end of the bed. Remove pillowcases and place them with the soiled sheets. Place pillows on the pull-out tray at the foot end. Avoid shaking the soiled linen.	To avoid stretching across the bed, causing back injury (Davis and Kotowski 2015, **R**). To minimize the risk of cross-infection (Peate and Lane 2015, **E**; Roboiro et al. 2013, **E**).
9 Fold the soiled linen into the centre of the bed and secure it into a roll. Avoid putting any soiled linen on the floor or holding it against your uniform. Gather it together and place it directly in a linen skip.	To prevent the spread of micro-organisms to the environment via airborne or contact means (Bloomfield et al. 2015, **E**; DH 2016, **C**; Lynn 2018, **E**; Potter et al. 2016, **E**).
10 If soiled, clean the mattress as per local policy. Check the mattress to ensure integrity of the covering.	To maintain a clean environment and prevent the spread of micro-organisms (Fraise and Bradley 2009, **C**; Spencer 2016, **E**).
11 Remove gloves and dispose of them in an appropriate receptacle. Carry out hand hygiene. Replace gloves if the patient's infection status necessitates.	To avoid cross-contamination of clean bed linen from soiled gloves (NHS England and NHSI 2019, **C**).
12 *Make a mitred 'hospital corner'*: stand at the head of the bed. Tuck the top of the sheet under the top (short) end of the mattress. Then move to stand alongside the long side of the mattress. At the head end of the mattress, pick up the edge of the sheet approximately 50 cm from the head of the bed. Lift the sheet to make a triangle-shaped fold in the sheet. Lay the formed triangle of sheet on the bed, Lift the corner of the mattress and tuck the hanging straight edge of the sheet under the mattress. Lift the triangle fold down over the tucked-in sheet and tuck it under the mattress. This should form a triangle at the corner of the bed (**Action figure 12**). *Note*: it is advised that pressure-relieving mattresses should have their sheets left untucked. *If working in pairs*: work from the head of the bed to the foot end. *If working alone*: make up the linen on one side of the bed before moving to the other side and completing the bed.	To secure the position of the sheet so that it does not move when the bed is occupied by the patient. **E** To work in the most time-efficient way. **E**

13 Ensure the sheet is pulled tight to ensure a smooth surface under the patient.	To reduce the discomfort caused by wrinkles in the sheet. To ensure a smooth, comfortable surface for the patient. **E**
14 Place the top sheet on the bed and open it out so that the centre crease is running down the middle of the mattress and the top hem is approximately 20–30 cm from the top of the mattress. The foot end of the top sheet can either be folded over to form a horizontal cuff or tucked under with a mitred corner. Leave the sides of the sheet hanging freely.	Follow local guidance or patient preference. A cuffed top sheet can provide more room for the patient's feet. **E**
15 Place the blanket on the bed. Open it out so that the centre seam is in the centre of the mattress and the top seam is approximately 20–30 cm from the top of the mattress.	To ensure the blanket is placed in the middle of the bed. **E**
16 At the head end of the bed, fold the blanket and sheet down together to form a cuff.	To ensure that the sheet rather than the blanket is in contact with the patient's skin, as the blanket could cause irritation. **E**
17 Tuck the blanket under the foot end of the mattress, mitring the corners as before but leaving the sides of the blanket to hang free.	To enable the patient to fold back the sheet and blanket with ease. **E**
18 Lay pillows on the bed and replace all pillowcases.	Applying pillowcases while the pillows are on the bed reduces the chance of neck, arm and back strain for the nurse (Lynn 2018, **E**)
19 Place the pillows at the head end of the bed.	For patient comfort. **E**
20 Return the bed to its original position and height.	To maintain a safe environment and promote safety (NMC 2018a, **C**).

Post-procedure

21 Dispose of soiled linen as per local policy.	To prevent cross-infection (Bloomfield et al. 2015, **E**; Loveday et al. 2014, **R**; Moore and Cunningham 2017, **E**).
22 Dispose of apron and gloves and perform hand hygiene.	To prevent cross-infection (Bloomfield et al. 2015, **E**; Moore and Cunningham 2017, **E**; NHS England and NHSI 2019, **C**).

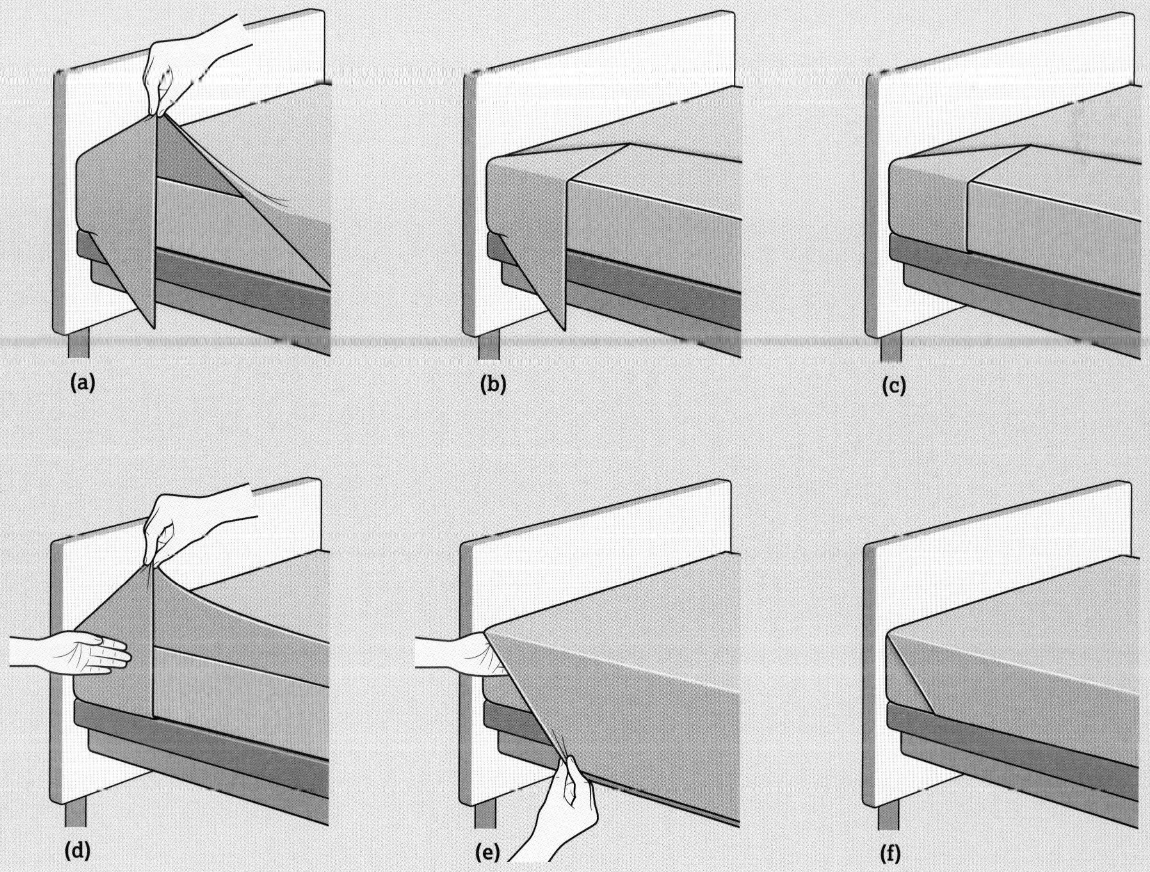

Action Figure 12 Bed making: mitring corners.

Procedure guideline 9.6 Making an occupied bed

This procedure assumes that two nurses are delivering care to the bed-bound patient.

Essential equipment

- Personal protective equipment
- Clean bed linen: sheets (bottom and top), pillowcases, blankets
- Laundry skip (apply local guidelines for segregation and disposal of soiled and/or infected linen)

Action	Rationale
Pre-procedure	
1 Collect all the equipment listed and place it by the bedside. If available, use the linen tray at the end of the bed to store the clean linen, or a clean chair beside the bed within comfortable reach. Introduce yourself to the patient, explain and discuss the procedure with them, and gain their consent to proceed.	To ensure efficient time use, reducing the need to leave the bedside (Bloomfield et al. 2015, **E**). To ensure that the patient feels at ease, understands the procedure and gives their valid consent (NMC 2018a, **C**).
2 Assess the patient for any mobility restrictions and pain to be sure that the patient is able to tolerate movement. Analgesia may be required.	To promote patient comfort (Spencer 2016, **E**).
3 Carry out hand hygiene and apply personal protective equipment (apron and gloves).	To protect against the transfer of contaminants on the hands of the healthcare worker causing cross-contamination. Linen could be contaminated with body fluids (NHS England and NHSI 2019, **C**; Pegram and Bloomfield 2015, **E**).
4 Clear the area of any obstacles; be aware of any items of clinical equipment – e.g. call bell cords, drip stand, electrical cords. If necessary, move the bed to gain adequate space to move freely to carry out the procedure.	To maintain a safe environment (NMC 2018a, **C**).
5 Reposition the bed as required and then check that the bed brakes are on. Adjust the bed to an appropriate height to maintain a comfortable posture during the procedure.	To prevent the bed moving unexpectedly and to avoid back injury (Davis and Kotowski 2015, **R**).
6 The linen skip should be positioned and kept near to the bed throughout the procedure.	To reduce the potential dispersal of micro-organisms, dust and skin cells from the linen into the environment (Bloomfield et al. 2015, **E**; DH 2016, **C**).
Procedure	
7 Check the bed linen for the presence of any personal articles belonging to the patient. Remove any call bells attached to the linen.	To ensure that personal belongings are not lost when the soiled linen is disposed. To promote patient comfort. **E**
8 Remove unsoiled, reusable linen (blankets etc.) and fold them over a chair or place them on the tray at the end of the bed. Ensure that the patient remains covered with a top sheet. Apply a clean top sheet if required.	To keep these items near to hand so they can easily be used later in the bed-making process. **E** To preserve dignity and privacy (NMC 2018a, **C**).
9 If it is raised, lower the bed side nearest you. Loosen the bottom sheet by moving methodically around the bed from the head to the foot. Ask the patient to roll on to their side (side rails can be used if available). Ensure that the second nurse is on that side to offer assistance if the patient is unable to roll independently. Adjust the pillow and ensure that any tubing attached to the patient is not being pulled or stretched.	To avoid the nurse stretching across the bed, potentially causing back injury (Davis and Kotowski 2015, **R**).
10 Roll the soiled sheet into the centre of the bed towards the patient and tuck it under the patient's shoulder and buttocks as much as possible. Avoid shaking the soiled linen.	To prevent the spread of micro-organisms to the environment via airborne or contact means (DH 2016, **C**; Lynn 2018, **E**; Pegram and Bloomfield 2015, **E**; Potter et al. 2016, **E**).
11 If soiled, clean the mattress as per local policy. Check the mattress to ensure integrity of the covering.	To ensure the mattress is in good condition and avoid cross-contamination of the clean linen (NHS England and NHSI 2019, **C**; Windle 2014, **E**).
12 Place the bottom sheet on the mattress and open it out so that the centre crease is running down the middle of the mattress. Cover half of the mattress and ensure that the sheet is smooth. Tuck in the sheet to the mattress, mitring the corners (see Procedure guideline 9.5: Making an unoccupied bed for how to do this). Fan-fold the remainder of the sheet vertically and place it alongside the patient, keeping the clean and soiled sheets apart.	To avoid cross-contamination of clean bed linen from the soiled sheet (NHS England and NHSI 2019, **C**; Pegram and Bloomfield 2015, **E**; Wolfensberger et al. 2018, **E**).

13 Keeping the patient covered, ask the patient to roll back and onto their other side. Advise that they will feel that they will be a rolling over a roll of linen when they do so.	To preserve dignity and privacy (NMC 2018a, **C**).
14 Remove the soiled bottom sheet. Gather it into a ball, rolling the soiled area into the centre of the ball. Clean and dry the mattress if soiled as per local policy. Dispose of soiled linen in the linen skip, holding it away from your uniform. Change gloves if soiled.	To prevent the spread of micro-organisms to the environment via airborne or contact means (Bloomfield et al. 2015, **E**; DH 2016, **C**; Lynn 2018, **E**; NHS England and NHSI 2019, **C**; Potter et al. 2016, **E**).
15 Pull the fan-folded clean linen from beneath the patient towards you and spread it out to provide a smooth surface across the mattress.	To provide a smooth surface for the patient to sleep on, avoiding discomfort for the patient and the potential formation of pressure damage (Bloomfield et al. 2015, **E**; Lynn 2018, **E**).
16 Mitre the top and bottom corners of the sheet and tuck the remaining sheet under the mattress.	To secure the position of the sheet so that it does not move. **E**
17 Place a clean top sheet lengthwise over the patient with the centre fold vertically down the centre of the bed. Open the sheet from the patient's head to their feet.	To maintain patient dignity. **E**
18 Ask the patient for their preference: the foot end of the top sheet can either be folded over to form a horizontal cuff or tucked under with a mitred corner. Leave the sides of the sheet hanging freely.	Follow local guidance or patient preference. A cuffed top sheet can provide more room for the patient's feet. **E**
19 If required, place the blanket on the bed. Open it out so that the centre seam is in the centre of the mattress and the top seam is placed as per the patient's preference.	To promote patient comfort. **E**
20 Fold the blanket and sheet down over together to form a cuff.	To ensure that the sheet rather than the blanket is in contact with the patient's skin, as the blanket could cause irritation. **E**
21 Change the pillowcases. Ask the patient to raise their head; supporting the patient's head with your hand, remove the pillow. Lower the patient's head to the mattress. Remove the soiled pillowcase and dispose of it directly into the linen bag. Clean and dry the pillow if soiled, and replace the pillowcase. Ask the patient to raise their head, support their head with your hand and replace the pillow.	To promote patient comfort. **E**
22 Adjust the position of the bed to suit the patient's preference and/or any clinical requirements.	To promote patient comfort. **E**
23 Return the bed to its original location (if moved) and height. Ensure that the call bell cord is available to the patient and position the bedside table to be accessible to the patient.	To ensure a safe environment for the patient (Bloomfield et al. 2015, **E**).
Post-procedure	
24 Dispose of soiled linen as per local policy.	To prevent cross-infection (Bloomfield et al. 2015, **E**; Loveday et al. 2014, **R**; Moore and Cunningham 2017, **E**).
25 Dispose of apron and gloves and perform hand hygiene.	To prevent cross-infection (Bloomfield et al. 2015, **E**; Moore and Cunningham 2017, **E**; NHS England and NHSI 2019, **C**).

Eye care

Definition

Eye care is the process of assessing, cleaning and/or irrigating the eye, including the instillation of prescribed ocular preparations where applicable. Eye care also includes patient education (Ehrlich 2018; Shaw and Lee 2016a).

Anatomy and physiology

The eye consists of three main parts: the orbit, the globe (eyeball) and the extrinsic structures.

The orbit

The orbit, or socket, is formed by seven bones of the skull and is lined with fat; it supports and protects the globe and its accessory structures (blood vessels and nerves) and provides attachments for the ocular muscles (Shaw and Lee 2016b).

The globe

The globe is approximately 2.5 cm in diameter and can be divided into three layers (Figure 9.3).

- The *outer layer or fibrous tunic* is composed of the transparent cornea and the white sclera. The primary function of the outer layer, in particular the sclera, is protective and it gives shape to the eyeball. The cornea is a transparent tissue that forms a window at the front of the eye and its main function is to protect the eye by providing a physical barrier against pathogens. It is also responsible for refracting or bending light rays, focusing them as they pass through on their route to the retina (Eghrari et al. 2015, Marsden 2017).

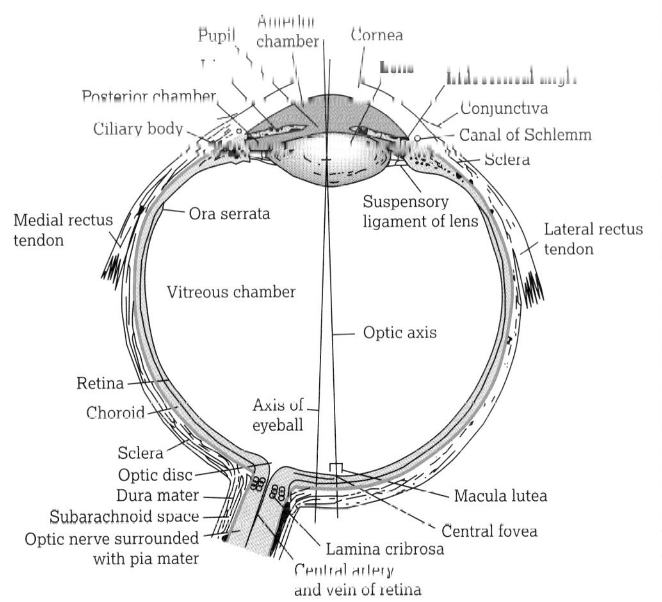

Figure 9.3 Horizontal cross-section through the eyeball at the level of the optic nerve. The optic axis and axis of the eyeball are included.

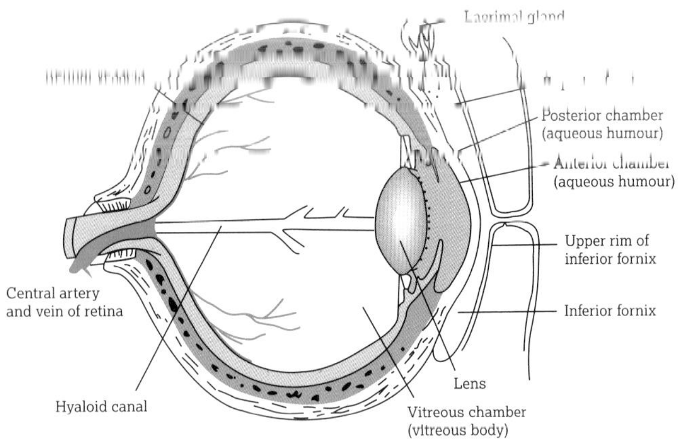

Figure 9.4 The anterior cavity in front of the lens is incompletely divided into the anterior chamber (anterior to the iris) and the posterior chamber (behind the iris), which are continuous through the pupil. Aqueous humour, which fills the cavity, is formed by ciliary processes and reabsorbed into the venous blood via the canal of Schlemm.

- The *middle layer or vascular tunic* is composed of the choroid, ciliary body and iris; the globe's vascular supply is provided by the choroid.
- The *inner layer or nervous tunic* is composed of the retina, which contains light-sensitive cells called rods and cones. It is responsible for converting light rays into electrical signals, which are transmitted to the brain via the optic nerve. This area contains the macula lutea, also known as the yellow spot. The central fovea, the area of highest visual acuity, is also located here, as is the blind spot, the area of no visual field (Overby-Canon 2014).

The internal part of the globe

The globe is divided into two chambers by the lens (Figure 9.4): the anterior cavity (in front of the lens) and the vitreous chamber (behind the lens). The anterior cavity is divided into the anterior chamber and the posterior chamber by the iris. It contains a clear, watery fluid called the aqueous humour. The vitreous chamber is filled with a clear, jelly-like substance called the vitreous body or vitreous humour. The vitreous humour fills the vitreous chamber, which, unlike the aqueous humour, is produced during foetal development and is never replaced (Tortora and Derrickson 2017). Together, these two fluid-filled cavities help to maintain the shape of the eyeball and the intraocular pressure (Tortora and Derrickson 2017).

The aqueous humour is continuously secreted by the ciliary process (a part of the ciliary body), which is located behind the iris. This fluid then permeates the posterior chamber, passing between the lens and the iris, and flows through the pupil into the anterior chamber. From the anterior chamber, the aqueous humour drains into the scleral venous sinus (canal of Schlemm) and is absorbed back into the bloodstream (Figure 9.4).

The aqueous humour is the principal source of nutrients and waste removal for the lens and cornea, as these structures have no direct blood supply. If the outflow of aqueous humour is blocked, excessive intraocular pressure may develop, leading to the disease process known as glaucoma. This excessive pressure can cause degeneration of the retina, which may result in blindness (Lee 2015).

Extrinsic structures

The extrinsic structures of the eye protect the globe from external injury (Shaw and Lee 2016b):

- *Eyelashes*: protect the eye from debris.
- *Eyebrows*: prevent moisture, in particular sweat, from flowing into the eye.
- *Eyelids*: the eyelid is made up of complex muscles for eye movement, glands for the production of tears and oil (which serve as a cleansing mechanism against dirt and foreign objects), and sensitive nerves for defence. The eyelids also protect the eyes from excess light (Rehman et al. 2018).
- *Lacrimal (tear) apparatus*: tears are produced in the lacrimal glands, located at the upper, outer edges of the eyes. They are excreted onto the upper surface of the globe and wash over the ocular surface by the action of blinking. The function of tears is to clean, moisten and lubricate the ocular surface and eyelids. Tears also provide antisepsis as they contain an enzyme called lysozyme, which is able to rupture the cell membranes of some bacteria, leading to their lysis and death (Forrester et al. 2016). The tears collect in the nasal canthus (inner, medial aspect of the eye), from which they drain into the upper and lower lacrimal puncta, which drain into the lacrimal sac. From here, the tears pass into the nasolacrimal duct and empty into the nasal cavity (Figure 9.5) (Tortora and Derrickson 2017).

Optic nerve

The optic nerve, which is responsible for vision (cranial nerve II), exits the eye to the side of the macula lutea at an area called the optic disc. This area is sometimes referred to as the anatomical blind spot. The optic nerve passes from the orbit through the optic foramen and into the brain. The two separate optic nerves meet at the optic chiasma and some optic nerve fibres cross over here to the opposite side of the brain. The nerves then continue along the optic tracts and terminate in the thalamus. From there, projections extend to the visual areas in the occipital lobe of the cerebral cortex (Tortora and Derrickson 2017) (Figure 9.6).

An additional blind spot or area of depressed vision, called a scotoma, may be indicative of a brain tumour. In pituitary gland tumours, for example, it is common for patients to develop bilateral defects in the field of vision due to invasion of the optic chiasm (O'Leary and Birkbimer 2016).

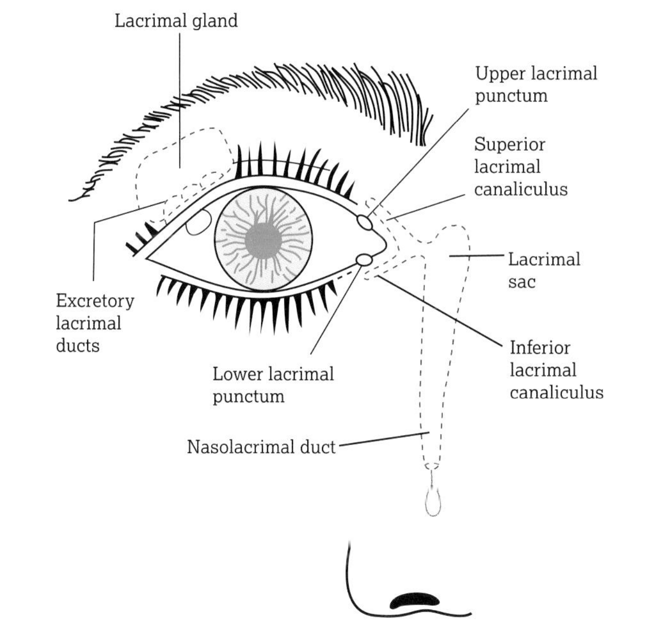

Figure 9.5 Lacrimal apparatus.

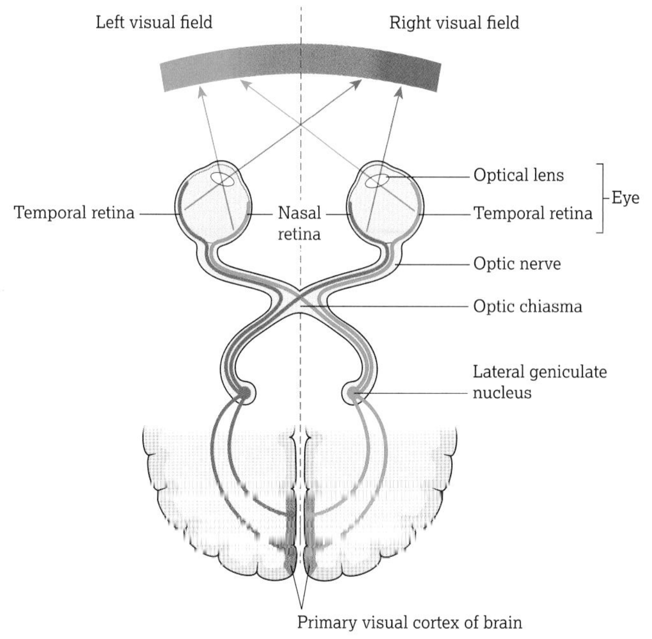

Figure 9.6 Visual pathways and visual fields. *Source*: Reproduced from MRI Questions (2019) with permission of Elster LLC.

Table 9.4 Effects of ageing on the eye

Anatomical changes	Physiological changes	Eye conditions common in the older population
• The retro-orbital fat atrophies. • The eyelid tissues become weak. • The levator muscle weakens, causing the eyelid to droop, which can occlude the upper visual field.	• *Presbyopia*: the distance from which print can be read increases. • Reduced flexibility of the lens means it can no longer change shape to focus on close objects quickly. • *Cataracts*: the lens becomes dense and yellow, affecting colour perceptions; it can become so dense that the lens proteins precipitate, creating a halo effect around bright lights. • Night vision reduces. • Cells within the retina die, causing diminished central vision. • Reduced tear production leads to dry eyes.	• *Glaucoma*: the optic nerve is damaged by increased pressure in the eye, resulting in a reduced visual field and pain • *Cataract:* see physiological changes. • *Diabetic retinopathy*: blood vessels connected to the retina are damaged by the disease and sight becomes blurred and patchy, and can be totally lost. • *Age-related macular degeneration*: this is a chronic disorder of the macula cells in the centre of the retina, a highly sensitive area responsible for detailed central vision. As this degenerates, central vision declines, which can lead to blindness.

Source: Adapted from Aldwin et al. (2017), Lin et al. (2016).

The ageing process

The eye changes with age. This process can start in the third decade of life, with most anatomical and physiological changes becoming more prevalent the older a person gets (Aldwin et al. 2017) (Table 9.4).

Related theory

Sight provides us with important sensory input to enable self-care and pleasurable activities such as reading. Early diagnosis and treatment of eye diseases and conditions can improve the course of vision impairment by either slowing the progression of the disease or conditions, or correcting the vision impairment itself (National Academies of Sciences, Engineering, and Medicine et al. 2016).

Evidence-based approaches

Rationale

Indications

Eye care may be necessary under the following circumstances:

- after eye surgery to prevent post-operative complications
- in the care of unconscious patients to maintain eye integrity
- to relieve pain and discomfort
- to prevent or treat infection
- to prevent or treat injury to the eye, for example to remove sharp objects
- for eye tests such as refraction

- for screening to detect disease such as glaucoma
- to treat existing problems such as conjunctivitis
- to detect drug-induced toxicity at an early stage
- to maintain contact lenses and care for false eye prostheses
- to optimize the eyes' visual function, especially with age-related degeneration (Astbury 2016, Gelston 2013, Raizman et al. 2017, Shaw and Lee 2016a, Stevens 2013).

These indications may present singularly or in combination.

Eye care includes patient education about the eye and surrounding structures as well as health promotion and safety advice to promote quality of life (Shaw and Lee 2016a).

Principles of care

Eye care is performed to maintain healthy eyes that are moist and infection free. The eye is an important organ, and inadequate care techniques can lead to the transmission of infection from one eye to the other or the development of irreversible damage to the eye, which can lead to loss of sight (Marsden 2015). If an infection is present in one eye, this should be cleaned and/or treated last to prevent transmission of infection to the uninfected eye (Tollefson and Hillman 2016).

A clean technique should be used for eye care procedures and an aseptic technique, if deemed necessary, should be used for vulnerable exposed eyes or to reduce the risk of infection (Pickering and Marsden 2015). The eye area must be treated gently and unnecessary pressure avoided, especially to the globe (Pickering and Marsden 2015). Low-linting swabs are generally used as lint from other types of swab can become detached and scratch the cornea (Marsden 2016). The fluids most commonly used for eye care procedures are sterile 0.9% sodium chloride and sterile water for irrigation; however, sterile 0.9% sodium chloride can irritate and sting the sensitive eye area so where possible it is recommended that sterile water is used (Marsden 2016).

If they are able, and after appropriate instruction, patients should be encouraged to carry out eye care procedures themselves. However, in the case of post-operative patients, physically limited or unconscious patients, it is often the nurse who is responsible for eye care.

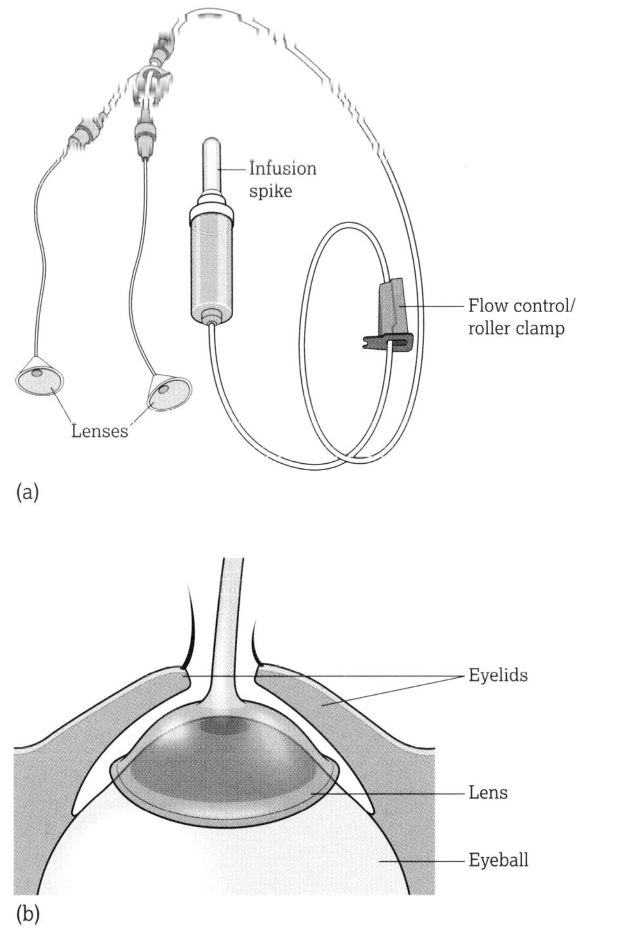

Figure 9.7 (a) The Morgan irrigation lens. (b) The Morgan lens *in situ*.

Methods of care

Eye assessment

Examine and assess the eye and surrounding structures prior to and then again after any intervention. Begin by examining the eye closed, looking carefully at the eyelids and noting asymmetry as well as any bruising, spasms, inflammation, discharge or crusting (Marsden 2015). Look for signs that the eyelids are closed properly, as an inability to close completely could indicate (for instance) the presence of a cyst or lump that would require further investigation (Marsden 2015).

Ask the patient to open their eyes and, using a pen torch, look for abnormalities in the conjunctiva, such as inflammation, a foreign body, redness or the presence of a discharge; the eye should be clear of clouding and redness (Marsden 2015). Ask the patient whether they are experiencing any pain or photophobia. Any abnormalities need to be reported to the patient's doctor immediately, as eye complications can develop quickly. Any changes should also be documented (Marsden 2015, NMC 2018a).

Eye swabbing

Eye swabbing is performed to clear the outer eye structures of foreign bodies, which could be infected matter, as well as discharges. The swab should be moistened with sterile water for irrigation and lightly wiped over the eyelid from the nose outward. This process should be repeated with clean gauze until the area is clean of discharge and encrustation (Stevens 2010).

Eye irrigation

Eye irrigation is usually performed to remove foreign bodies or caustic substances from the eye, for example domestic cleaning agents or medications, particularly cytotoxic material; it should be performed as soon as possible to minimize damage (Marsden 2016). The procedure is also used for pre-operative preparation and to remove infected material.

The volume required will vary depending on the degree of contamination; copious amounts (at least 1 L) are needed for corrosive chemicals. Irrigation should be carried out for 15–30 minutes until a pH of between 7–8 is obtained (College of Optometrists 2018).

Smaller volumes of irrigation fluid will be required for removal of eye secretions. The solution may be directed to the affected area by using an intravenous fluid-giving set to ensure a controllable, direct flow of fluid (Marsden 2016). To avoid physical damage, the tubing should be held approximately 2.5 cm from the eye (Shaw and Lee 2016c) and directed to the inner canthus. The Morgan lens (Figure 9.7) is an irrigating contact lens that is attached to a giving set to enable hands-free irrigation.

Care of contact lenses

Contact lenses are thin, curved discs made of hard or soft plastic or a combination of both. Hard contact lenses are made of a rigid plastic that does not absorb water or saline solutions and can be worn for a maximum of 12–14 hours continuously. Gas-permeable lenses are a combination of both hard and soft plastic; these permit oxygen to reach the cornea, providing greater comfort (Olver et al. 2014). Soft contact lenses are more pliable as they retain more water. Soft lenses can be used daily and be disposed of after use; alternatively, some are reusable and can worn for up to 30 days but will require regular removal for cleaning and disinfecting. Ill-fitting lenses may reduce the tear film between lens and cornea, which may result in oxygen deprivation of the cornea, leading to corneal oedema and blurred vision. Further damage to the corneal epithelial cells may lead to corneal abrasion and pain. Poor hygiene practices with either the contact lens or the contact lens case can lead to the build-up of biofilms containing bacteria, such as *Pseudomonades* and *Staphylococci*, causing eye infections such as microbial keratitis, which can lead to corneal ulceration and can threaten vision (Tzu-Ying et al. 2015).

Most people look after their own contact lenses. Cleaning and storage solutions depend on the type of lens used; manufacturers provide specific instructions for the care of their products. The lenses should be stored in an appropriate contact lens storage container with slots for the right (R) and left (L) eyes, so they can be worn in the correct eyes. Seriously ill patients should have their lenses removed and stored correctly until they can reinsert them. Contact lenses are stored in a sterile solution when they are not in the eye; this helps to lubricate the lens and enable it to glide over the cornea, reducing the risk of injury.

Care and attention should also be given to the cleanliness of the lens storage case, as this can harbour microbial sources of infection, such as *Staphylococci*, if not cleaned regularly (Tzu-Ying et al. 2015). Lens storage solution should be emptied from the case daily, once lenses have been removed for use. The case should be rinsed with saline and left to air dry daily (Lakhani 2018a, 2018b, Tzu-Ying et al. 2015). Contact lens cases and lenses should never be rinsed with tap water, as contaminants and micro-organisms, such as *Acanthamoeba*, can reside in them (Carnt et al. 2018). Contamination of the lens or case by these micro-organisms can lead to serious eye infections and potentially a degree of permanent vision loss (Moorfields Eye Hospital 2019). For this reason, contact lenses should not be worn while showering or bathing (Carnt et al. 2018, Lakhani 2018a, 2018b).

Artificial eyes

Artificial eyes are made of glass or plastic; some are permanently implanted. Most people who have artificial eyes care for them themselves. If the patient is unable to do this, it is recommended that the eye is removed once daily for cleaning; the patient will be able to advise how they would like this done (Stevens 2013). However, if they are unable to do so, advice should be sought from the local ophthalmology service or the nursing team in the ophthalmology unit.

Pre-procedural considerations

Equipment

A good light source (such as a minor procedure light, a bright pen torch or lamp, or a bright ophthalmoscope) is necessary to enable careful assessment of the eyes and to avoid damage to the delicate structures (Marsden 2015). The light source should be positioned above and behind the nurse. It is important to inform the patient that a bright light will be shone in their eyes and that this may be painful. Topical anaesthetic drops can be used to alleviate pain before examination, eye irrigation and other procedures (Marsden 2015, Stevens 2016).

Position of the patient

The patient should be sitting or lying with their head tilted backwards and chin pointing upwards. This allows for easy access to the eyes and is usually a good position for patient comfort and compliance (Shaw and Lee 2016c).

Procedure guideline 9.7 Eye swabbing

Essential equipment

- Personal protective equipment
- Sterile low-linting or lint-free swabs
- Sterile water
- Light source

Optional equipment

- Sterile or non-sterile powder-free gloves

Action	Rationale
Pre-procedure	
1 Introduce yourself to the patient, explain and discuss the procedure with them, and gain their consent to proceed. Ask the patient to explain how their eyes feel, if they are able to do so.	To ensure that the patient feels at ease, understands the procedure and gives their valid consent (NMC 2018a, **C**). To obtain a baseline prior to the procedure. **E**
2 Assist the patient into the correct position: • head well supported and tilted back • preferably the patient should be in bed or lying on a couch.	The patient needs to be discouraged from flinching or making unexpected movements and so should be in the most comfortable, pain-free position possible at the start of the procedure (Shaw 2017, **E**). To enable access to and assessment of the eyes. **E** To enable patient comfort. **E**
3 Ensure an adequate light source, taking care not to dazzle the patient.	To enable maximum observation of the eyes without causing the patient harm or discomfort (Shaw 2017, **E**).
4 Wash hands or use an alcohol-based handrub and put on personal protective equipment.	To reduce the risk of cross-infection (NHS England and NHSI 2019, **C**).
Procedure	
5 Always treat the uninfected or uninflamed eye first.	To reduce the risk of cross-infection (Tollefson and Hillman 2016, **C**).
6 Always bathe the lids with the eyes closed first.	To reduce the risk of damaging the cornea and to remove any crusted discharge. **E**
7 Ask the patient to look up. Using a slightly moistened swab, gently swab the lower lid from the inner canthus outwards. Use an aseptic technique for the damaged or post-operative eye.	If the swab is too wet, the solution will run down the patient's cheek. This increases the risk of cross-infection and causes the patient discomfort. Swabbing from the nasal corner outwards avoids the risk of swabbing discharge into the lacrimal punctum or even across the bridge of the nose into the other eye. Aseptic technique reduces the risk of cross-infection (Loveday et al. 2014, **R**).

(continued)

Procedure guideline 9.7 Eye swabbing (continued)

Action	Rationale
8 Ensure that the edge of the swab is not above the lid margin.	To avoid touching the sensitive cornea. E
9 Using a new swab each time, repeat the procedure until all the discharge has been removed.	To reduce the risk of cross-infection (Shaw 2016, E).
10 Gently swab the upper lid by slightly everting the lid margin and asking the patient to look down. Swab from the nasal corner outwards and use a new swab each time until all discharge has been removed.	To effectively remove any foreign material from the eye. **E** To reduce the risk of cross-infection (Stevens 2016, **R**).
11 Once both eyelids have been cleaned and dried, make the patient comfortable.	To ensure patient comfort. **E**
12 Remove and dispose of equipment, and decontaminate hands.	To keep the environment clean and reduce the risk of cross-infection (NHS England and NHSI 2019, **C**).
Post-procedure	
13 Discuss with the patient any changes post-procedure; report any adverse effects to the patient's doctor. Record the procedure in the appropriate documents.	To monitor the effectiveness of the procedure as well as any trends and fluctuations (NMC 2018a, **C**).

Procedure guideline 9.8 Eye irrigation

Essential equipment

- Personal protective equipment
- Sterile water for irrigation (in an emergency, tap water may be used)
- Receiver (kidney dish or plastic receptacle)
- Towel
- Plastic cape
- Intravenous fluid-giving set and drip stand
- Warm water in a bowl to warm irrigating fluid to tepid temperature
- Low-linting or lint-free swabs
- Light source

Optional equipment

- Anaesthetic drops
- Sterile or non-sterile powder-free gloves

Action	Rationale
Pre-procedure	
1 Introduce yourself to the patient, explain and discuss the procedure with them, and gain their consent to proceed. Ask the patient to explain how their eyes feel, if they are able to do so.	To ensure that the patient feels at ease, understands the procedure and gives their valid consent (NMC 2018a, **C**). To have a baseline understanding of current problems or changes the patient is experiencing (Marsden 2016, **E**).
2 Wash hands and put on personal protective equipment.	To reduce the risk of cross-infection (NHS England and NHSI 2019, **C**).
3 If possible, remove any contact lenses (see Procedure guideline 9.11: Contact lens removal: hard lenses and Procedure guideline 9.12: Contact lens removal: soft lenses)	To ensure no reservoir of chemicals remains in the eye (Marsden 2016, **E**).
4 Instil anaesthetic drops if required.	To relieve pain and aid irrigation (Marsden 2015, **E**).
5 The patient should sit upright with their head supported and tilted to the affected side.	To avoid the solution running either over the nose into the other eye or down the side of the cheek (Marsden 2016, **E**).
6 Drape the patient's shoulders with a towel or, if available, a waterproof cape. Ask the patient to hold the receiver (kidney dish or plastic receptacle) against the cheek below the eye being irrigated.	To protect the patient from getting wet and to collect irrigation fluid as it runs away from the eye (Marsden 2016, **E**).

7 Prepare the irrigation fluid to the appropriate temperature by placing it in a bowl of water until warmed. Hang the irrigation fluid on the drip stand, connect the fluid to the intravenous fluid-giving set and prime the line. Pour the solution across the inner aspect of your wrist to test the temperature.	Tepid fluid will be more comfortable for the patient (Stevens 2016, **E**). To ensure that the irrigation fluid is ready for the procedure (Marsden 2016, **E**).
Procedure	
8 If there is any discharge from the eye, proceed as for eye swabbing (see Procedure guideline 9.7: Eye swabbing).	To remove any infected material. **E**
9 Hold the patient's eyelids apart, using your first and second fingers, against the orbital ridge. Do not press on the eyeball.	The patient will be unable to hold the eye open once irrigation commences (Marsden 2016, **E**). To avoid causing the patient discomfort or pain (Stevens 2016, **E**).
10 Warn the patient that the flow of solution is going to start and pour a little onto the cheek first.	To allow time to adjust to the feeling of water flowing (Marsden 2016, **E**).
11 Direct the flow of the fluid from the nasal corner outwards (**Action figure 11**). Keep the fluid flow constant by adjusting the giving set roller clamp.	To wash away from the lacrimal punctum and prevent contaminating the other eye. **E** To ensure a constant flow (Stevens 2016, **E**).
12 Ask the patient to look up, down and to either side while irrigating.	To ensure that the whole area, including the fornices, is irrigated (Stevens 2016, **E**).
13 Evert the upper and lower lids while irrigating.	To ensure complete removal of any foreign body (Stevens 2016, **E**).
14 When the eye has been thoroughly irrigated, ask the patient to close their eyes and use a new swab to dry the lids.	For patient comfort (Marsden 2016, **E**).
15 Take the receiver from the patient and dry the cheek.	To prevent spillage of receiver contents and promote patient comfort (Marsden 2016, **E**).
16 Make the patient comfortable.	To promote comfort and dignity (NMC 2018a, **C**).
Post-procedure	
17 Remove and dispose of equipment as per local policy, and decontaminate hands.	To keep the environment clean and reduce the risk of cross-infection (NHS England and NHSI 2019, **C**).
18 Document the intervention in the patient's notes.	To maintain accurate records. To provide a point of reference in the event of any queries. To prevent any duplication of treatment (NMC 2018a, **C**).
19 Discuss with the patient any changes post-procedure; report any adverse effects to the patient's doctor.	To monitor the effectiveness of procedure as well as any trends and fluctuations (NMC 2018a, **C**; RCN 2016, **C**).

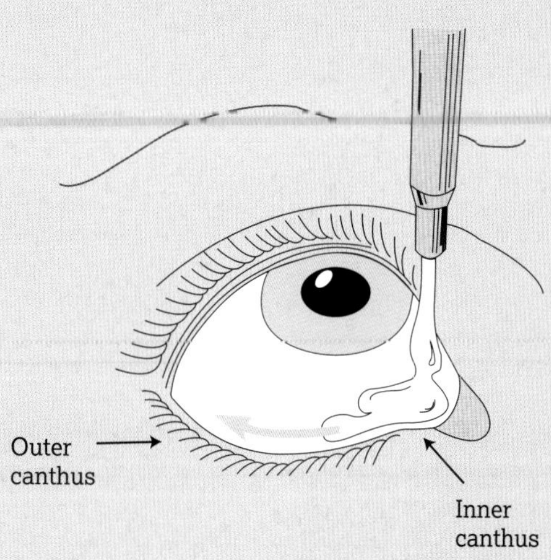

Action Figure 11 Irrigation of the eye from inner to outer canthus.

Procedure guideline 9.9 Artificial eye care: insertion

Essential equipment
- Personal protective equipment
- Sterile water for irrigation
- Low linting or lint-free swabs
- Non-sterile powder-free gloves

Action	Rationale
Pre-procedure	
1 Introduce yourself to the patient, explain and discuss the procedure with them, and gain their consent to proceed.	To ensure that the patient feels at ease, understands the procedure and gives their valid consent (NMC 2018a, **C**).
2 Wash hands or use an alcohol-based handrub and put on personal protective equipment.	To reduce the risk of cross-infection (NHS England and NHSI 2019, **C**).
Procedure	
3 Wearing non-sterile gloves and with the dominant hand, gently lift up the upper eyelid and pull down the lower eyelid. With the other hand, hold the prosthesis between the thumb and index finger and gently insert it.	To minimize patient discomfort and ensure correct insertion. **E**
Post-procedure	
4 Remove gloves, dispose of equipment and decontaminate hands.	To keep the environment clean and reduce the risk of cross-infection (NHS England and NHSI 2019, **C**).
5 Document the intervention in the patient's notes.	To maintain accurate records. To provide a point of reference in the event of any queries. To prevent any duplication of treatment (NMC 2018a, **C**).

Procedure guideline 9.10 Artificial eye care: removal

Essential equipment
- Personal protective equipment
- Sterile water for irrigation
- Low-linting or lint-free swabs
- Non-sterile powder-free gloves

Optional equipment
- Extractor

Action	Rationale
Pre-procedure	
1 Introduce yourself to the patient, explain and discuss the procedure with them, and gain their consent to proceed.	To ensure that the patient feels at ease, understands the procedure and gives their valid consent (NMC 2018a, **C**).
2 Wash hands or use an alcohol-based handrub and put on personal protective equipment.	To reduce the risk of cross-infection (NHS England and NHSI 2019, **C**).
Procedure	
3 Wearing non-sterile gloves and with the dominant hand, gently pull the bottom eyelid downwards and exert slight pressure below the eyelid to overcome the suction, enabling the prosthesis to be removed. An extractor may be necessary to gently lever the eye out.	To minimize patient discomfort and trauma to the area (Stevens 2013, **E**)
4 Rinse and drain the eye socket with sterile water for irrigation.	To remove any loose debris and to minimize damage caused by touch. **E**
5 Clean the eye with sterile water for irrigation.	To prevent the build-up of debris and to reduce the risk of infection (Stevens 2013, **E**).
Post-procedure	
6 Remove gloves, dispose of equipment and decontaminate hands.	To keep the environment clean and reduce the risk of cross-infection (NHS England and NHSI 2019, **C**).
7 Document the intervention in the patient's notes.	To maintain accurate records. To provide a point of reference in the event of any queries. To prevent any duplication of treatment (NMC 2018a, **C**).

Procedure guideline 9.11 Contact lens removal: hard lenses

Essential equipment

- Personal protective equipment
- Non-sterile powder-free gloves
- Contact lens cleaning solution
- 0.9% saline solution
- Contact lens case
- Low-linting or lint-free swabs

Action	Rationale
Pre-procedure	
1 Introduce yourself to the patient, explain and discuss the procedure with them, and gain their consent to proceed.	To ensure that the patient feels at ease, understands the procedure and gives their valid consent (NMC 2018a, **C**).
2 Wash hands or use an alcohol-based handrub and put on apron.	To reduce the risk of cross-infection (NHS England and NHSI 2019, **C**).
Procedure	
3 Wearing non-sterile gloves and using thumb and forefinger, separate the eyelids. *Method 1*: keeping the eyelid stationary, place an index finger on the lower eyelid. Press the edge of the lower eyelid against the eyeball beneath the bottom of the contact lens. Lift the upper lid above the top of the lens and then push the lid down over the eyeball until the eyelid is shut – the lens should come out (**Action figure 3**). *Method 2*: placing the index finger at the outer corner of the eye, pull the eyelids tight by pulling out towards the ear. Get the patient to blink – the lens should come out. If neither method is successful, a suction device may be required to remove the lens.	To remove the lens with minimal pain and trauma to the cornea (Lakhani 2018a, **C**; Shaw and Lee 2016c, **E**).
4 Place the lens in the palm of the hand, apply some drops of cleaning solution to the lens and gently rub the lens with the little finger.	To clean the lens of debris and contaminants (Lakhani 2018a, **C**).
5 Apply 0.9% saline solution to the lens and rinse the lens by rubbing the lens gently between the index finger and thumb.	To remove residues of cleaning solution and debris loosened during cleaning (Lakhani 2018a, **C**).
6 Fill the clean storage case with new lens storage solution. Store the lenses in the contact lens storage case, in appropriate solution as recommended by the manufacturer, and ensure the lenses are placed in the correct storage pots (left and right).	To prevent deterioration and contamination (Lakhani 2018a, **C**).
7 Refer to the manufacturer's instructions for further storage information, particularly if the patient will not be using the lenses for a lengthy period of time.	To prevent deterioration of the lenses and growth of organisms. **E**
Post-procedure	
8 Remove and dispose of personal protective equipment, and decontaminate hands.	To keep the environment clean and reduce the risk of cross-infection (NHS England and NHSI 2019, **C**).
9 Document the intervention in the patient's notes.	To maintain accurate records. To provide a point of reference in the event of any queries. To prevent any duplication of treatment (NMC 2018a, **C**; RCN 2016, **C**).

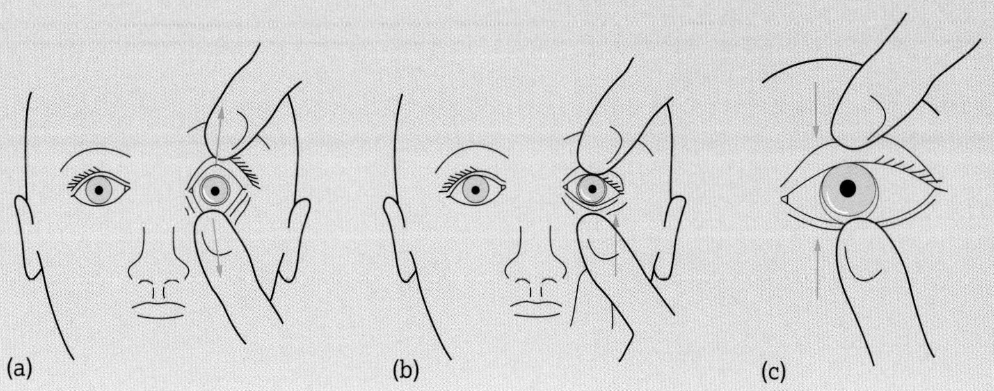

Action Figure 3 Removing hard contact lenses.

Procedure guideline 9.12 Contact lens removal: soft lenses

Essential equipment

- Personal protective equipment
- Contact lens cleaning solution
- 0.9% saline solution
- Low-linting or lint-free swabs
- Non-sterile powder-free gloves

Action	Rationale
Pre-procedure	
1 Introduce yourself to the patient, explain and discuss the procedure with them, and gain their consent to proceed.	To ensure that the patient feels at ease, understands the procedure and gives their valid consent (NMC 2018a, **C**).
2 Wash hands or use an alcohol-based handrub and put on personal protective equipment.	To reduce the risk of cross-infection (NHS England and NHSI 2019, **C**).
Procedure	
3 Wearing non-sterile gloves and using thumb and forefinger, separate the eyelids. Slide the contact lens onto the conjunctiva (white) of the eye. Gently pinch the lens between the thumb and index finger and lift away from the eye (**Action figure 3**).	To encourage the lens to fold together, allowing air to enter underneath the lens for easy removal. (Lakhani 2018b, **C**).
4 If the lens is a daily disposable, dispose of it immediately in appropriate waste.	Disposable lenses should not be reused. For the appropriate disposal of waste. To reduce the risk of cross-infection (Loveday et al 2014, **R**).
5 If the lens is reusable, place the lens in the palm of the hand, apply some drops of cleaning solution to the lens and gently rub the lens with the little finger.	To clean the lens of debris and contaminants (Lakhani 2018a, **C**).
6 Apply 0.9% saline solution to the lens and rinse the lens by rubbing the lens gently between the index finger and thumb.	To remove residues of cleaning solution and debris loosened during cleaning (Lakhani 2018a, **C**).
7 Fill the clean storage case with new lens storage solution. Store the lenses in the contact lens storage case, in appropriate solution as recommended by the manufacturer, and ensure the lenses are placed in the correct storage pots (left and right).	To prevent deterioration and contamination (Lakhani 2018a, **C**).
8 Refer to the manufacturer's instructions for further storage information, particularly if the patient will not be using the lenses for a lengthy period of time.	To prevent deterioration and growth of organisms. **E**
Post-procedure	
9 Remove and dispose of personal protective equipment, and decontaminate hands.	To keep the environment clean and reduce the risk of cross-infection (NHS England and NHSI 2019, **C**).
10 Document the intervention in the patient's notes.	To maintain accurate records. To provide a point of reference in the event of any queries. To prevent any duplication of treatment (NMC 2018a, **C**; RCN 2016, **C**).

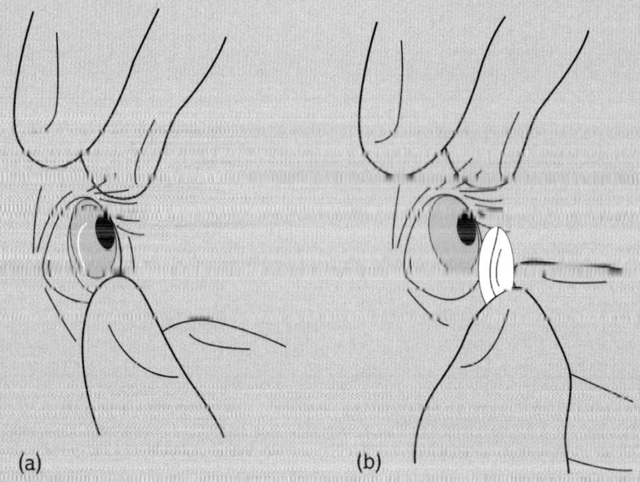

Action Figure 3 (a) Moving a soft lens down the inferior part of the sclera. (b) Removing a soft lens by pinching it between the pads of the thumb and index finger.

Ear care

Definition

Ear care encompasses the assessment and cleaning of the ears, including the instillation of prescribed ear drops. The monitoring and maintenance of hearing are also included.

Anatomy and physiology

The ears capture sounds for hearing and maintain balance for equilibrium (Knight et al. 2017, Millward 2017a). The ear has three parts: external, middle and inner (Figure 9.8).

External ear

The external ear is a protective funnel made up of the cartilaginous pinna, the external acoustic canal and the eardrum (Figure 9.8). The external acoustic canal is lined with small hairs and next to it lie the ceruminous glands, which produce cerumen, or ear wax. The amalgamation of cerumen and hairs help to prevent foreign objects from entering the ear.

The pinna collects sound waves and delivers them via the external acoustic canal to the tympanic membrane or eardrum, which vibrates in harmony (Millward 2017a). The eardrum separates the external and middle ear; it has a slightly conical shape and the pointed end sits within the inner ear to assist the funnelling of sounds.

Middle ear

The middle ear is an air-filled chamber. It contains the three smallest bones in the body: the malleus, incus and stapes, collectively known as the auditory ossicles. To one side, it has a thin bony partition that holds two small membrane-covered apertures which are the oval and round windows (Tortora and Derrickson 2017). The auditory ossicles receive vibrations from the tympanic membrane. Vibrations are passed on to the oval window and through to the cochlea in the inner ear; within this process the sound waves are magnified (Balkany and Brown 2017).

At the bottom of the chamber lies the eustachian tube, which connects to the nasopharynx and regulates the pressure in the ear. It is usually closed but yawning or swallowing briefly opens it, allowing air to enter or leave until the pressure in the middle ear equalizes with the external air pressure (Balkany and Brown 2017). When the pressures are equalized, the tympanic membrane vibrates freely as the sound waves hit it. However, if the pressures are not balanced, the individual may experience pain, hearing impairment, tinnitus and/or vertigo (Tortora and Derrickson 2017).

Inner ear

The inner ear is very small and includes the organ of Corti (which is situated inside the snail-shaped cochlea), the three semi-circular canals and the vestibular apparatus (Figure 9.8) and is the organ for hearing. It is filled with fluid and has a membranous layer that connects to the end of the auditory nerve; the membrane is covered in tiny cells with hair like projections (Eggermont 2014). Sound waves travel through the fluid and are distributed to the hair cells. At this point, the sound waves change to impulses, which pass along the auditory nerve to the brainstem and cortex, where they are interpreted as sound.

The semi-circular canals and vestibular apparatus maintain balance. These canals are highly sensitive; they contain fluid and hair cells that recognize when the head moves and send signals to the brain to maintain equilibrium. The brain interprets these messages along with visual input from the eyes (Balkany and Brown 2017). Adjustments to the muscles and joints are made in response to the information received (Balkany and Brown 2017, Tortora and Derrickson 2017).

Disorders of the inner ear structures can lead to the patient developing symptoms of vertigo or hearing loss (Balkany and

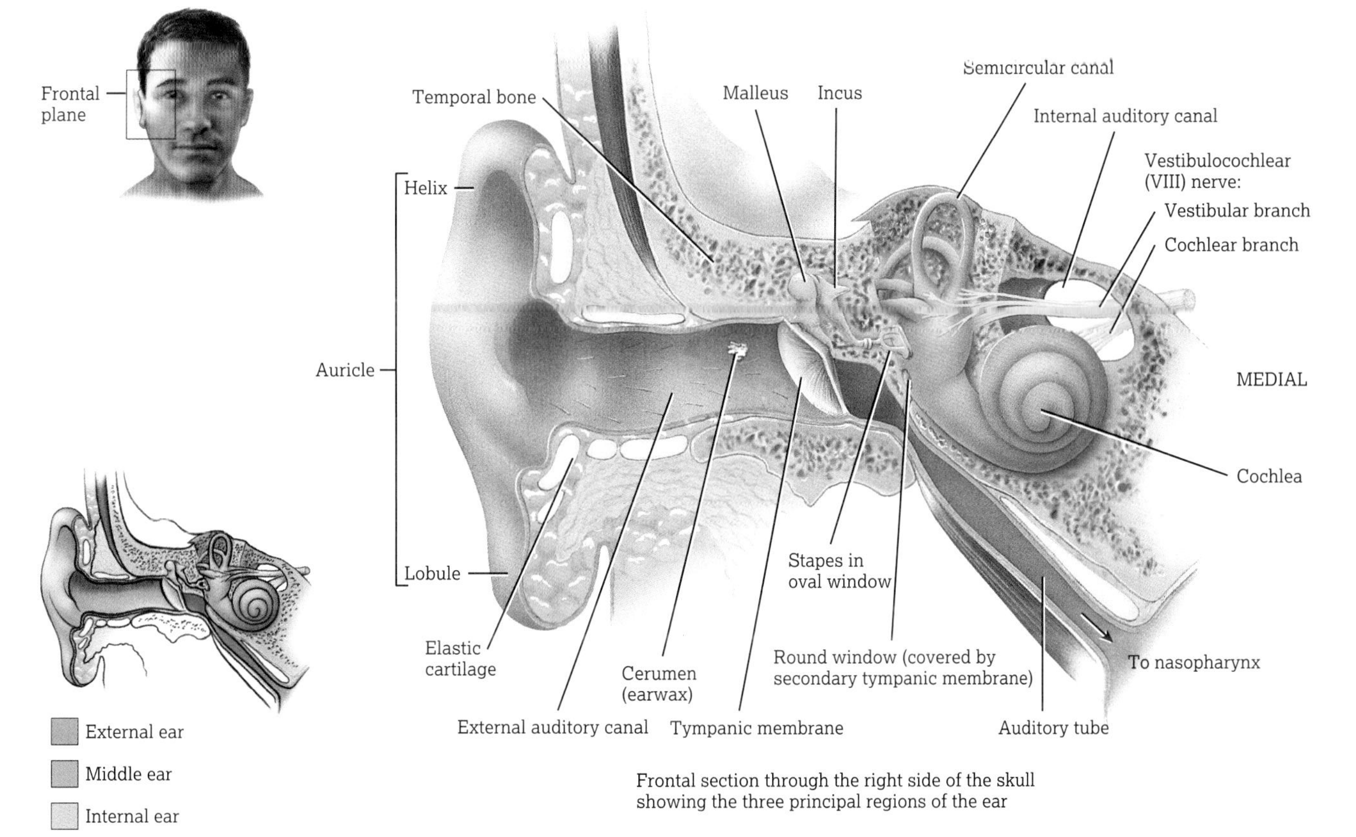

Figure 9.8 Internal structure of the ear. *Source*: Reproduced from Tortora and Derrickson (2017) with permission of John Wiley & Sons, Ltd.

Brown 2017). Vertigo is a sensation of the environment around the patient moving or spinning; other potential symptoms include loss of balance, feeling sick or being sick, and dizziness (NHS Inform Scotland 2019).

Ear wax impaction

Ear wax (cerumen) is a waxy secretion from glands within the auditory canal, combined with skin scales and hair. As the cerumen dries, it usually falls out of the ear canal but in some circumstances the wax can become impacted (Schwartz et al. 2017). A build-up of wax is more likely to occur in older adults and patients who use hearing aids, people with learning difficulties, people who have a narrow exterior auditory meatus and people who insert implements into the ear (RPECCAS 2016) (Box 9.4). Communication and balance can be affected by poor ear hygiene; for example, using cotton buds to clean the ears can result in ear wax impaction, which can dull hearing.

Cerumen impaction occurs in up to 6% of the general population, affecting 10% of children and over 30% of the elderly and cognitively impaired populations (Sevy and Singh 2017). Excessive wax should be removed before it becomes impacted, to avoid symptoms of ear wax impaction. The symptoms of ear wax impaction are:

- hearing loss
- blocked ears
- ears discomfort
- feeling of fullness in the ear
- tinnitus
- earache
- itchiness in the ear
- reflex cough
- vertigo or disturbed balance (NICE 2016a).

Box 9.4 Individuals prone to ear wax impaction

- Older adults
- Men
- People with learning disabilities
- People with narrow ear canals
- Hearing aid users
- People who frequently use ear plugs
- People who frequently use in-ear headphones
- People who use cotton buds to clean the ear as this causes the wax to be pushed further down the canal and can cause injury to the surface of the canal

Source: Adapted from Aaron et al. (2018), Wright (2015).

Related theory

Hearing loss can develop over time and become less noticeable to the individual and those close to them, as they find alternative ways to cope. Hearing impairment can cause frustration, stress, social isolation, paranoia and depression (NHS England 2017b).

There is a high overall incidence of hearing difficulties in people with learning disabilities (McClimens et al. 2014). These difficulties can be due to a variety of factors including genetic tendencies to deafness, fragile X syndrome, structural abnormalities within the organ and neural complications; this can further complicate communication difficulties for this population (McClimens et al. 2014).

Nurses should be aware of how ear problems occur so they are able to explore these with patients to identify problems early and provide appropriate patient education. All findings should be documented and handed over to the patient's doctor for further investigation, such as a hearing assessment (Box 9.5).

Evidence-based approaches

The ear canal is self-cleaning through jaw movement and epithelial migration action, which moves wax and debris up to the outer ear. Therefore, it should not be necessary to remove the wax manually (Mills 2017).

Box 9.5 Hearing tests for adults

Pure tone audiometry

Pure tone audiometry (PTA) tests the hearing of both ears. During PTA, a machine called an audiometer is used to produce sounds at various volumes and frequencies (pitches).

Speech perception

The speech perception test, sometimes known as a speech discrimination test or speech audiometry, involves testing the ability to hear words without using any visual information. The words may be played through headphones or a speaker, or spoken by the tester.

Tympanometry

The eardrum should allow as much sound as possible to pass into the middle ear. If sound is reflected back from the eardrum, hearing will be impaired. During tympanometry, a small tube is placed at the entrance of the ear and air is gently blown down it into the ear. The test can be used to confirm whether the ear is blocked, most commonly by fluid.

Whispered voice test

The whispered voice test is a very simple hearing test. It involves the tester blocking one of the patient's ears and testing their hearing by whispering words at varying volumes.

Tuning fork test

A tuning fork produces sound waves at a fixed pitch when it is gently tapped. It can be used to test various aspects of hearing. The tester will tap the tuning fork on their elbow or knee to make it vibrate, before holding it at different places around the patient's head.

Bone conduction test

A bone conduction test is often carried out as part of a routine PTA test in adults. A bone conduction test involves placing a vibrating probe against the mastoid bone behind the ear. It tests how well sounds transmitted through the bone are heard. Bone conduction is a more sophisticated version of the tuning fork test. When used together with PTA, it can help to determine whether hearing loss comes from the outer and middle ear, the inner ear, or both (NHS Direct Wales 2015).

Principles of care

Ear hygiene should be carried out carefully to avoid causing damage to the ear. Public awareness of this is low and leads to attempts to remove wax with instruments such as cotton swabs and hairpins (NICE 2016a). As well as traumatizing the skin, these actions often contribute to increased wax production and impaction (see Box 9.4) and can also impair the self-cleansing mechanism of the organ. Fundamentals of ear hygiene include the following:

- To dry or clean the outside of the ear, use a dry tissue or alcohol-free baby wipe around and behind the ear after the patient has showered or bathed.
- Use a soft disposable damp cloth to gently wipe around the cartilaginous area of the ear.
- *Never insert any implements, such as cotton buds, into the ear.*

If there are any signs of inflammation or the patient is complaining of any discomfort:

- keep the ears dry, avoiding any entry of water; shampoo and soaps may be irritating to the skin
- when washing hair, use cotton wool coated in petroleum jelly or ear plugs placed at the entrance to both ear canals.

Assessment

A good light source and an operating lamp positioned above and behind the nurse are necessary prior to commencing ear care procedures to enable careful assessment of the ears (RPECCAS 2016). The patient and nurse should be sitting at the same height to examine the outer ear and pinna (NICE 2016a). Any alteration to the appearance of the ear must be reported to the doctor.

Before proceeding with any form of invasive ear care, it is important to undertake careful examination of the ear, taking note of any discharge, redness or swelling, and the amount and texture of any ear wax present, as this will give an indication of the general health of the ear. A small amount of wax should be expected in the ear canal. Its absence may be a sign of a dry skin condition, infection or excessive cleaning that has interfered with the normal wax production (Millward 2017b).

The nurse should discuss with the patient their current level of hearing and after the procedure they should ask the patient whether there are any changes, so as to monitor the effectiveness of the intervention. Consideration should always be given to a patient's hearing aids and assistance should be given, as required, to clean these. Advice regarding the most appropriate method should be sought, preferably from the patient. Irrigation of the inner ear is sometimes necessary to remove foreign bodies or to clear excessive build-up of ear wax (cerumen) (Millward 2017a).

Poor ear care can cause:

- otitis media (middle ear infection)
- trauma to the external meatus
- tinnitus
- deafness
- perforation of the tympanic membrane.

Special care should be taken to avoid damage to the aural cavity and eardrum.

Methods of ear wax softener use

Due to the invasive nature of ear irrigation, it is advised that the patient first tries using wax softeners such as olive oil, which may avoid the need for irrigation (BSA 2017, Millward 2017a). It is advised that this should be administered two to four times daily for a minimum of three to five days, following the manufacturer's guidance. The British Society of Audiology advocates that if the ear wax remains very firm, the softening oil or spray can continue to be applied for up to a maximum of 10 days (BSA 2017).

Ear irrigation

Ear irrigation should only be carried out by healthcare professionals who have had specialist training and have demonstrated theoretical and practical competence to carry out the procedure. Physical fitness to practise should also be considered, as this procedure requires manual dexterity and good vision (BSA 2017). The BSA (2017) recommends that the audiology, nursing or medical professional usually undertaking this procedure should be registered with the Health and Care Professions Council (HCPC) or the Registration Council for Clinical Physiologists (RCCP). It goes on to recommend that non-registered professionals, such as assistant audiologists, hearing care assistants and healthcare assistants who are trained in the removal of ear wax, should ensure that their employers make their procedural and professional scope clear, and they must demonstrate theoretical and practical competence (BSA 2017).

Ear irrigation should not be carried out using a syringe. The traditional method of irrigation using a metal water-filled, hand-held syringe is no longer recommended practice due to the high risk of infection and the potential to cause trauma to the ear and the delicate structures within the ear; these syringes are also difficult to decontaminate after use (Millward 2017b, NICE 2016a, NICE 2018b). There are a number of electronic ear irrigators available. NICE (2016a) recommends that an approved electronic irrigator fitted with an ear probe is used for ear irrigation. It should have a variable pressure control to enable the water pressure to be controlled more precisely so that the ear irrigation can commence at the minimum pressure and so that the direction of the water can be better controlled (Millward 2017a). The water temperature should be 37°; if too hot or cold, it can cause dizziness or vertigo (RPECCAS 2016).

Procedure guideline 9.13 Irrigation of the external auditory canal using an electronic irrigator

Essential equipment

- Personal protective equipment
- Otoscope/auriscope
- Headlight or direct light source
- Electronic ear irrigator and new irrigation tips
- Receiver or Noots tank
- Water heated to approximately 37°C
- Receiver for soiled instruments
- Waste bag for disposal of soiled swabs
- Disposable waterproof cape
- Tissues
- Cotton wool carrier (Jobson Horne Probe or ProScoop)
- Low-linting, high-quality cotton wool

(continued)

Procedure guideline 9.13 Irrigation of the external auditory canal using an electronic irrigator *(continued)*

Action	Rationale
Pre-procedure	
1 Collect the equipment listed. Introduce yourself to the patient, explain and discuss the procedure with them, and explain all the potential risks, ensuring their comprehension and gaining their consent to proceed. Check whether irrigation has been previously performed and assess the patient to determine whether this procedure is appropriate and whether there are any contraindications to performing irrigation (see Box 9.6).	To ensure efficient time use, reducing the need to leave the bedside. To ensure patient safety. **E** To ensure that the patient feels at ease, understands the procedure and gives their valid consent, and to ensure the appropriateness of the procedure (BSA 2017, **C**; Millward 2017a, **E**; NMC 2018a, **C**).
2 Prepare the irrigator as per the manufacturer's instructions, ensuring that it is in good working order and that a new irrigation tip is attached for the procedure.	To ensure the equipment is used according to the manufacturer's guidance. **E**
3 Carry out hand hygiene and apply personal protective equipment (apron and gloves).	To prevent the spread of micro-organisms and infection (Millward 2017a, **E**; NHS England and NHSI 2019, **C**).
4 Both the healthcare professional and the patient should be sitting in upright positions in chairs. Ensure that the patient is in a comfortable position that can be sustained throughout the procedure.	To ensure patient stability, comfort and safety during the procedure (BSA 2017, **C**; RPECCAS 2016, **C**).
5 Positioning the light source as necessary, examine both of the patient's ears. Commence with examining the pinna and adjacent scalp, then inside the auditory canal. Check for any evidence of skin defects or scarring that could indicate previous surgery.	To ensure a thorough assessment of the ear prior to commencing irrigation (RPECCAS 2016, **C**).
6 Place the disposable waterproof cape around the shoulders of the patient, taking particular care to ensure it covers the area under the ear to be irrigated.	To protect the patient's clothing from irrigation fluid and debris (BSA 2017, **C**).
7 If they are able, ask the patient to hold the receiver or Noots tank under the ear to be irrigated close to their head; if they are unable, a colleague or relative can assist.	To collect the irrigation fluid and debris (BSA 2017, **C**).
8 Heat the irrigation fluid to 40°C and fill the irrigator reservoir to 500 mL. Check the temperature of the fluid: the temperature of the fluid irrigated into the ear should be approximately 37°C.	Irrigation fluid should be at body temperature to avoid triggering the vestibular reflex – i.e. symptoms of nausea, vomiting and vertigo (BSA 2017, **C**; NICE 2016a **C**).
9 Securely attach the new applicator irrigation tubing and probe, and set the irrigator machine pressure to minimum.	To ensure that the probe will not dislodge from the irrigator under pressure from the water, potentially causing damage to the auditory canal. To ensure the pressure used is the minimum necessary, reducing the potential for damage (RPECCAS 2016, **C**).
10 Direct the irrigator into the receiver and switch on the machine. Let it run for 15–20 seconds. Discard any water in the receiver.	To check the functioning of the machine and the water temperature. To eliminate any trapped air or cold water in the irrigator. To allow the patient to become accustomed to the noise of the irrigator (RPECCAS 2016, **C**).
Procedure	
11 Inform the patient that you are about to start the procedure. Advise them to inform you of any pain or dizziness immediately. Gently pull the pinna upwards and outwards.	To stretch and straighten the external auditory canal and hold the ear steady (BSA 2017, **C**; NICE 2016a, **C**).
12 Place the tip of the probe at the exterior auditory canal entrance at the posterior wall of the exterior auditory membrane. Direct the irrigator probe to the posterior wall.	Aiming the stream of water incorrectly at the anterior wall risks stimulating the vagus nerve (Millward 2017a, **E**; RPECCAS 2016, **C**).
13 *If the patient experiences any symptoms of nausea, dizziness or pain, stop the procedure immediately.* It is recommended to seek immediate advice from ENT (ear, nose and throat) specialists if severe pain, deafness or vertigo occur during or after the irrigation procedure or if perforation is seen.	To prevent further triggering of the vestibular reflex and prevent further damage to the tympanic membrane (NICE 2016a, **C**; RPECCAS 2016, **C**).
14 Direct a steady stream of water along the top of the external auditory canal, aiming towards to the posterior wall. The perimeter of the exterior auditory canal can be compared to a clock face: • For the left ear: aim the jet of fluid towards the 1 o'clock position. • For the right ear: aim the jet of fluid towards the 11 o'clock position.	Fluid should not be directed at the tympanic membrane as this can cause perforation, nor should it be aimed directly at the wax plug as this can cause further impaction. It should flow behind the plug of wax and along the canal to wash out the wax plug (Millward 2017a, **E**).

15 Inspect and monitor the ear canal (with the otoscope/auriscope) and the fluid draining into the receiver or Noots tank for traces of wax.	To evaluate the effect of the irrigation and to determine whether the wax has been removed (RPECCAS 2016, **C**).
16 Further irrigation may be necessary. If the patient is comfortable, the pressure of the irrigator may, with caution, be gradually increased if there is difficulty in removing the wax plug. No more than 500 mL of water per ear should be used for irrigation (NICE 2016a).	To remove remaining ear wax while irrigating the ear on the lowest pressure setting to reduce the risk of complications (BSA 2017, **C**; RPECCAS 2016, **C**).
17 Examine the ear with the otoscope/auriscope to check that all of the wax plug has been removed and that the tympanic membrane is intact.	To monitor the condition of the ear and the success of the irrigation (NICE 2016a, **C**).
18 If wax remains, seek further advice from ENT specialists.	Medical advice should be sought if further treatment is required to remove impacted wax (NICE 2016a, **C**).
19 *Aural toilet*: under direct vision using the otoscope/auriscope and the light source, dry the external auditory canal using the cotton wool carrier (Jobson Horne Probe or ProScoop tip wrapped in cotton wool) in a gentle rotation action. Change the cotton wool frequently and immediately if it is soiled. Avoid touching the tympanic membrane.	Removal of stagnated water reduces the risk of maceration of the skin and infection. Abrasion increases the risk of perforation of the tympanic membrane (BSA 2017, **C**; RPECCAS 2016, **C**).
Post-procedure	
20 Remove the waterproof (potentially contaminated) covering from the patient and dispose of it as per local policy. Dispose of single-use used consumable equipment in the appropriate waste bag following local policy.	To ensure correct disposal of contaminated material (Loveday et al. 2014, **R**).
21 Remove personal protective equipment and decontaminate hands.	To reduce the risk of cross-infection (NHS England and NHSI 2019, **C**).
22 Advise the patient to return promptly if they develop symptoms of earache, itching, ear discharge, odour, swelling or disruption of hearing. Provide verbal and written advice on complications and details of how to contact medical advice (if they occur).	These symptoms may be signs of infection and further treatment may be required. So that inspection and appropriate referral and treatment can be instigated (BSA 2017, **C**; NICE 2016a, **C**).
23 Document the procedure and its outcome.	To provide recorded documentation of care and aid communication to the multiprofessional team (NMC 2018a, **C**).
24 Clean, disinfect and calibrate the irrigator according to the manufacturer's guidelines and local policy. Perform hand hygiene.	To reduce the risk of cross infection (NHS England and NHSI 2019, **C**; RPECCAS 2016, **C**).

Following irrigation, the patient's symptoms should resolve. If the symptoms continue, further treatment may be required and in some cases referral to ENT (ear, nose and throat) specialists may be appropriate. Irrigation is not the only method of removing excess earwax. Those patients who have contraindications to ear irrigation (Box 9.6) still require wax removal, and this can be done via instrumentation or microsuction. This must only be carried out by a nurse trained in the procedure. This procedure is not readily accessible in primary care so patients are usually referred to local ENT clinics.

Mouth care

Definition

Mouth care is the care given to the oral mucosa, lips, teeth and gums in order to promote health and prevent or treat disease. It involves assessment, care and patient education to promote independence (Croyère et al. 2012).

Anatomy and physiology

Structure of the oral cavity

The mouth consists of the vestibule and the oral cavity (Figure 9.9). The vestibule is the space between the lips and cheeks on the outside and the teeth and gingivae (gums) on the inside. The palate forms the roof of the oral cavity with the base of the tongue forming the floor of the mouth. It is bordered by the alveolar arches, teeth and gums at either side (Long et al. 2016). The lips and cheeks are formed of skeletal muscle; the inner part of the cheeks is known as the buccal mucosa and consists of columnar epithelium. The lips are involved in speech and facial expression and keep food within the oral cavity. The cheeks control the location of food as the teeth break it down.

Teeth

Teeth are formed of the crown (the visible part) and the root. The crown is covered in enamel – a hard, dense material that cannot repair itself once damaged. Below the enamel cap, the tooth is formed of a bone-like material called dentine. This extends into the

Box 9.6 Contraindications and cautions regarding ear irrigation

Contraindications

- Perforated eardrums or recently healed perforation
- Previous complications from ear irrigation (e.g. vertigo, pain, tinnitus)
- Middle ear infection in the previous 6 weeks
- Perforation
- Mucus discharge
- Acute otitis externa with pain and tenderness to the pinna
- History of ear surgery
- Presence of a foreign body, including vegetable matter in the ear (hygroscopic matter, such as lentils and peas, can swell in the presence of water)

Cautions

- Tinnitus
- Gromets *in situ*
- Healed perforation
- Dermatological conditions (e.g. seborrheic dermatitis, eczema)
- Dizziness or vertigo
- Patient taking anticoagulants
- Cleft palate (repaired or not)
- Previous head or neck radiotherapy
- Immunocompromise
- Diabetes
- Permanent hearing loss in the non-affected ear

Source: Adapted from BAS (2017), Millward (2017a), NICE (2016a), RPECCAS (2016), Schwartz et al. (2017).

root and surrounds the pulp cavity, which contains nerve fibres, blood vessels and connective tissue. Where the pulp cavity extends into the root, it is known as the root canal. Teeth are embedded in alveoli (sockets) in the maxilla and mandible and are held in place by periodontal ligaments and a substance known as cementum. Teeth are important in breaking down and grinding food and are also involved in producing sounds in speech (Marieb and Keller 2017).

Tongue

The tongue is a muscular structure that extends from its tip (apex) to the posterior attachment in the oropharynx. It houses taste buds and is involved in taste, forming food into a bolus and pushing it to the back of the mouth for swallowing. It is also involved in the articulation of sounds in speech.

Palate

The palate consists of the hard palate anteriorly and the soft palate, which is a muscular structure leading to the palatoglossal arches and the uvula. The hard and soft palates are involved in mastication, swallowing and production of speech (Hand and Frank 2014).

Saliva

Saliva is produced by the parotid glands (in front of the ears), which are rich in amylase; the submandibular glands (in the lower part of the floor of the mouth), which produce mucinous saliva; and the sublingual glands (in the floor of the mouth between the sides of the tongue and the teeth), which produce viscous saliva. There are also minor salivary glands in the buccal mucosa (Hand and Frank 2014). On average, 1000–1500 mL can be produced daily, consisting mainly of water with electrolytes, amylase, proteins (such as mucin, lysozyme and immunoglobulin A), and metabolic wastes (Tortora and Derrickson 2017). It is important for mastication, taste and speech. Saliva is also slightly acidic and can act as a buffer; it acts as a defence against infection by physically washing debris off teeth, and saliva proteins have an antibacterial action (Hand and Frank 2014).

Related theory

The World Health Organization defines oral health as consisting of an oral cavity that is free from tooth decay; tooth loss; disease and disorders, such as birth defects (cleft lip and palate); chronic mouth and facial pain; oral and throat cancer; and oral sores (WHO 2018). Mouth care is an integral and essential part of personal care (NHS HEE 2016). Good oral hygiene is essential, as

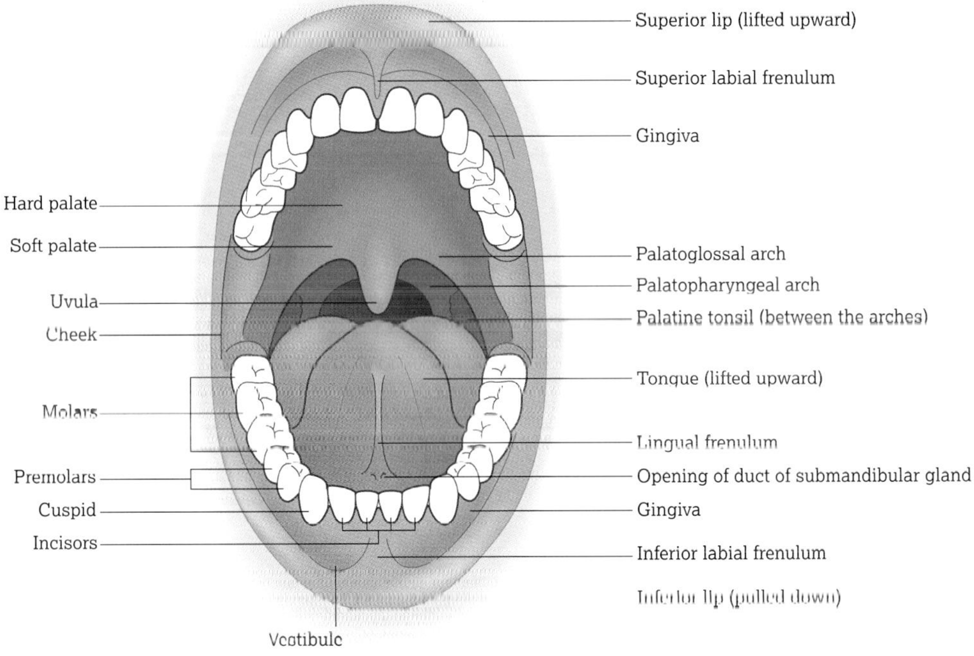

Figure 9.9 Structures of the mouth (the oral cavity). *Source*: Reproduced from Peate et al. (2014) with permission of John Wiley & Sons, Ltd.

poor oral health can have a profound impact on the individual, affecting their ability to eat or taste food and to communicate; it can also lead to pain and/or infection, and in some cases life-threatening illness (Jablonski 2012). Knowledge and attitudes of caregivers are integral to the delivery of effective oral care. Oral health is often seen as a low priority, and issues relating to the intimacy of having another person working inside one's mouth can compound ineffective mouth care (Croyère et al. 2012).

Dental decay

Dental decay begins with the formation of a biofilm known as plaque, which is made up of sugar, bacteria and other debris on the teeth. Tooth enamel can be damaged due to bacterial action, resulting in a drop in pH around the tooth. Once there is damage to the enamel, the inner dentine can also decay (Ozdemir 2013). Areas of decay in teeth are known as caries. Plaque can be physically removed by brushing and flossing teeth. If it is not regularly removed, it can harden to form calculus (tartar), which requires dental treatment for removal. Calculus can also disrupt the seal between the gingiva and the tooth, resulting in red, swollen and bleeding gums (gingivitis). This inflammation can progress to the formation of deep pockets of infection, damaging the teeth and underlying bone (periodontitis) (Marieb and Keller 2017). Smoking is known to be a risk factor for periodontitis; other factors include xerostomia.

Xerostomia

Xerostomia is the subjective sensation of a dry mouth; it is not always correlated with a reduction in saliva production (Anil et al. 2014). It can be associated with thickened saliva or discomfort, which may be burning in nature, leading to difficulty eating or speaking. The prevalence of xerostomia increases with age, and it can be caused by dehydration, systemic health conditions, certain medications and treatments (Anil et al. 2014, NHS HEE 2016).

Where possible, the cause should be treated; sips of water normally only relieve the problem briefly. Viscous solutions and gels such as Caphosol or Xerotin should be considered to moisten and protect the mucosa (UKOMiC 2019) (see also the section below on artificial saliva). Production of saliva may be stimulated by the use of sugar free chewing gum but acidic sweets should be avoided as they increase the risk of dental caries (NICE 2018c). Salivary stimulants such as pilocarpine can be useful (NICE 2018c). Studies have also demonstrated that acupuncture may be helpful (Homb et al. 2014, RD-UK 2016).

Patients with xerostomia must pay careful attention to oral hygiene regimes and require good education about mouth care and the associated risks of xerostomia. Xerostomia can cause difficulty in chewing and swallowing food, putting the patient at increased risk of choking as well as oral complications such as caries and periodontitis due to loss of the protective effect of saliva (Plemons et al. 2014).

Evidence-based approaches

Principles of care

The aims of oral care are to:

- keep the oral mucosa and lips clean, soft, moist and intact
- keep natural teeth free from plaque and debris
- maintain denture hygiene and prevent disease related to dentures
- prevent oral infection
- prevent oral discomfort
- maintain the mouth in a state of normal function (Coker et al. 2013, Peate and Gault 2013).

Box 9.7 lists the recommendations for maintaining oral health.

Within a variety of care settings, patients can find themselves at risk of poor oral health. Patients who may need extra care with their oral health include:

- patients who are nil by mouth (including unconscious and ventilated patients)
- patients who mouth breathe (including those on oxygen therapy or with a nasogastric tube)
- cancer patients receiving radiotherapy to the head and neck
- patients receiving systemic anti-cancer therapy, which can result in reduced immunity to infection
- patients receiving targeted therapy or immunotherapy, which can directly affect the oral cavity
- patients having oral surgery or who have traumatic injury to the head and/or neck
- older patients
- patients with diabetes
- patients unable to maintain their own oral hygiene due to physical disability or psychological disorders that could affect motivation
- patients with clotting disorders
- patients who have dry mouth or gum overgrowth as side-effects of medication (Binks et al. 2017, Carpenito 2017, WHO 2018).

Box 9.7 Oral health advice

- Brush teeth at least twice daily with fluoridated toothpaste; spit out toothpaste but do not rinse
- Ideally brush teeth before bed and at least on one other occasion with a manual or powered toothbrush
- Clean between teeth using appropriate appliance or tool daily
- Reduce risk factors by:
  - eating a healthy diet, and limiting sugary foods and drinks (including sugar-containing medicines)
  - stopping smoking (to reduce the risk of gum disease and oral cancer)
  - limiting alcohol consumption (to reduce the risk of oral cancer)
- Have regular dental check-ups
- Change toothbrush regularly

Source: Adapted from PHE (2017).

Every patient should have a thorough assessment of their oral cavity. This should begin with a detailed nursing history of the patient's usual oral hygiene practices. This will help the nurse or allied healthcare professional to determine the patient's needs and preferences when planning oral care, and will also establish the level of nursing care required. Examples of those who may need assistance include:

- patients with dexterity problems (where hand co-ordination may be impaired)
- patients with cognitive impairment
- patients whose illness may cause them to feel fatigued
- patients whose illness imposes restrictions on activities (O'Connor 2016a, PHE 2017).

Good assessment is vital before a care plan can be formulated. Assessment of the oral cavity should always include a thorough visual inspection. Many factors should be considered when carrying out a full oral assessment (Box 9.8).

Assessment should include lips, tongue, gums, saliva, natural teeth or dentures, oral cleanliness, and the presence of any dental pain (O'Connor 2016a). This is especially important if the patient has cognitive impairment or a learning disability that may prevent them from self-reporting any oral or dental symptoms.

Inspection should be undertaken in good light, gloves should be worn, a pen torch must be used, and any dentures or plates should be removed and gums inspected. It is helpful to have a set order in which areas are examined so nothing is missed (PHE 2017):

1. *The lips*: are they dry, cracked or bleeding?
2. *The upper and lower labial sulci* (inner part of the lip towards the vestibule): the lip should be retracted with a gloved finger or tongue depressor; is it intact, soft, moist, coated, ulcerated or inflamed?

3 *The buccal mucosa on the right and left sides*: is it intact, soft, moist, coated, ulcerated or inflamed?
4 *The dorsal surface of the tongue (ask the patient to stick out the tongue)*: is it dry, fissured, coated or ulcerated?
5 *The ventral surface of the tongue (ask the patient to lift the tongue up and move it from side to side)*: can the patient move it normally?
6 *The floor of the mouth*: is the normal saliva pool present? Is the saliva watery?
7 *The hard and soft palates*: are they intact, ulcerated or red?
8 *The gums*: are they inflamed or bleeding?
9 *The teeth*: are they present, cared for, loose or stained? Is debris present?

Patients with dentures

Patients with dentures should be encouraged or assisted to remove and clean the dentures daily (Bartlett et al. 2018). The dentures should be cleaned over a towel or a water-filled sink to reduce the risk of damage if they are dropped. They should be brushed with a toothbrush and a specialized non-abrasive denture paste or cleaner. Toothpaste should never be used as it is too abrasive for dentures (HEE 2016). The dentures should be rinsed with water before being replaced in the mouth.

Denture wearers should be advised not to keep their dentures in the mouth overnight, unless there are specific reasons for keeping them in. This is particularly important for people at a higher risk of developing stomatitis. Denture wearers are at risk of fungal infections developing under the denture and spreading to the hard palate. Soaking the dentures in a denture cleanser solution after mechanical cleaning is beneficial in assisting the breakdown of plaque, preventing denture stomatitis and reducing the risk of pneumonia (Bartlett et al. 2018).

If it is suspected that a denture-wearing patient has an oral infection, the dentures should be soaked in 0.2% chlorhexidine for 15 minutes and rinsed thoroughly (HEE 2016, Voegeli 2012a). Denture wearers should also clean any remaining teeth and their gums and tongue with a soft toothbrush and fluoride toothpaste. Finally, they should have regular dental check-ups as ill-fitting dentures can cause ulcers and irritation (Bartlett et al. 2018, Burns 2012).

Losing dentures while in hospital can be very distressing to the individual and can have serious effects on their nutrition, ability to communicate, self-image and overall wellbeing. Furthermore, the financial implications for reimbursement for denture loss are relatively significant for the NHS (Mann and Doshi 2017). Any denture storage container should be clearly marked with the wearer's personal identification details (HEE 2016). An incident report form must be completed by the clinical unit for every lost denture (HEE 2016).

Box 9.8 Factors to consider when carrying out an oral assessment

- Usual oral hygiene practice and frequency
- Regularity of dental visits
- Oral discomfort or pain
- Dry mouth
- Difficulty chewing
- Difficulty swallowing
- Difficulty speaking
- Halitosis (malodorous breath)
- Drooling
- Presence of dentures and normal care routine
- Current and past dental problems
- Other risk factors, for example diabetes, steroid treatment, oral fluid intake, altered nutritional status, smoking, alcohol consumption, mental health diseases, learning difficulties and palliative care

Source: Adapted from Burns (2012), HEE (2016).

Assessment and recording tools

The mouth should be examined as part of the initial nursing assessment and should be reassessed regularly thereafter (Brooker et al. 2013, HEE 2016, Steel 2017). Every adult hospitalized for more than 24 hours should have a mouth care risk assessment completed to identify high risk patients. High risk patients should have a mouth care assessment daily and low-risk patients should have their mouth reassessed every 7 days (HEE 2016). The use of an oral assessment tool (Figure 9.10) is recommended to ensure consistency between assessors and to monitor changes.

There is a variety of other guidance that can be used to assist with mouth care assessments:

- In 2016, Health Education England published a guide for hospital healthcare professionals: *Mouth Care Matters*. An assessment tool has been developed in line with this guidance. The Mouth Care Pack is a comprehensive assessment tool and includes a mouth care screening tool, mouth care assessment tool and daily recording sheet (Figure 9.11).
- For adults in care homes, the National Institute for Health and Care Excellence's *Oral Health for Adults in Care Homes* (Guideline 48) is a useful resource and covers oral health, including dental health and daily mouth care (NICE 2016b).
- The UK Oral Management in Cancer Care Group has developed mouth care guidance and support for cancer and palliative care (UKOMiC 2019). This is expert guidance for oral care for all health professionals involved in care of patients with cancer, and it can be adapted to other clinical settings, including elderly care and care of patients with dementia.

Patients needing assistance

A variety of patient groups may need assistance with mouth care. Patients with mental health issues or learning disabilities may need encouragement or assistance to maintain their oral hygiene (HEE 2016, Leroy and Declerck 2013, Petrovic et al. 2016). Patients with conditions affecting mobility, sight or dexterity may find it difficult to carry out oral hygiene without assistance. Practical aids (such as a mirror) and sitting down rather than standing can aid independence. Patients can also find it easier to use a foam handle aid (to make the toothbrush easier to hold) (Figure 9.12) or a pump-action toothpaste (HEE 2016). Critically ill, unconscious and disabled patients may be completely dependent on healthcare professionals or carers to deliver effective oral care regularly.

Older patients may be at risk of oral problems due to a natural decline in salivary gland function, wear and tear of teeth, and taking medication with side-effects that can cause oral problems, such as increased risk of infection, dry mouth and taste changes (Anil et al. 2014, Burns 2012, Hewson and Lee 2017). Regular assessment and assistance with maintaining oral hygiene is recommended (Royal College of Surgeons 2017). For those patients who require assistance, it is recommended that the nurse or carer stands behind or to the side of them and supports the lower jaw (Brocklehurst et al. 2016).

Unconscious patients

Unconscious patients require particular interventions to maintain oral hygiene and comfort. For patients who are at the end of life, there is a lack of evidence relating to oral care and the focus should be on patient comfort. Any interventions that cause distress should be reviewed, and the frequency with which mouth care is offered should be dependent on the needs of the individual (AACCN 2017, Brooker et al. 2013, Riley 2018). Gentle cleaning with a soft toothbrush is recommended and a lubricant should be applied to the lips (Brooker et al. 2013).

In critically ill patients who are unconscious and require mechanical ventilation, oral care management is different (Box 9.9). It is well documented that aspiration of oropharyngeal flora can cause bacterial pneumonia (Brooker et al. 2013). Ventilator-associated pneumonia (VAP) is a serious complication that can

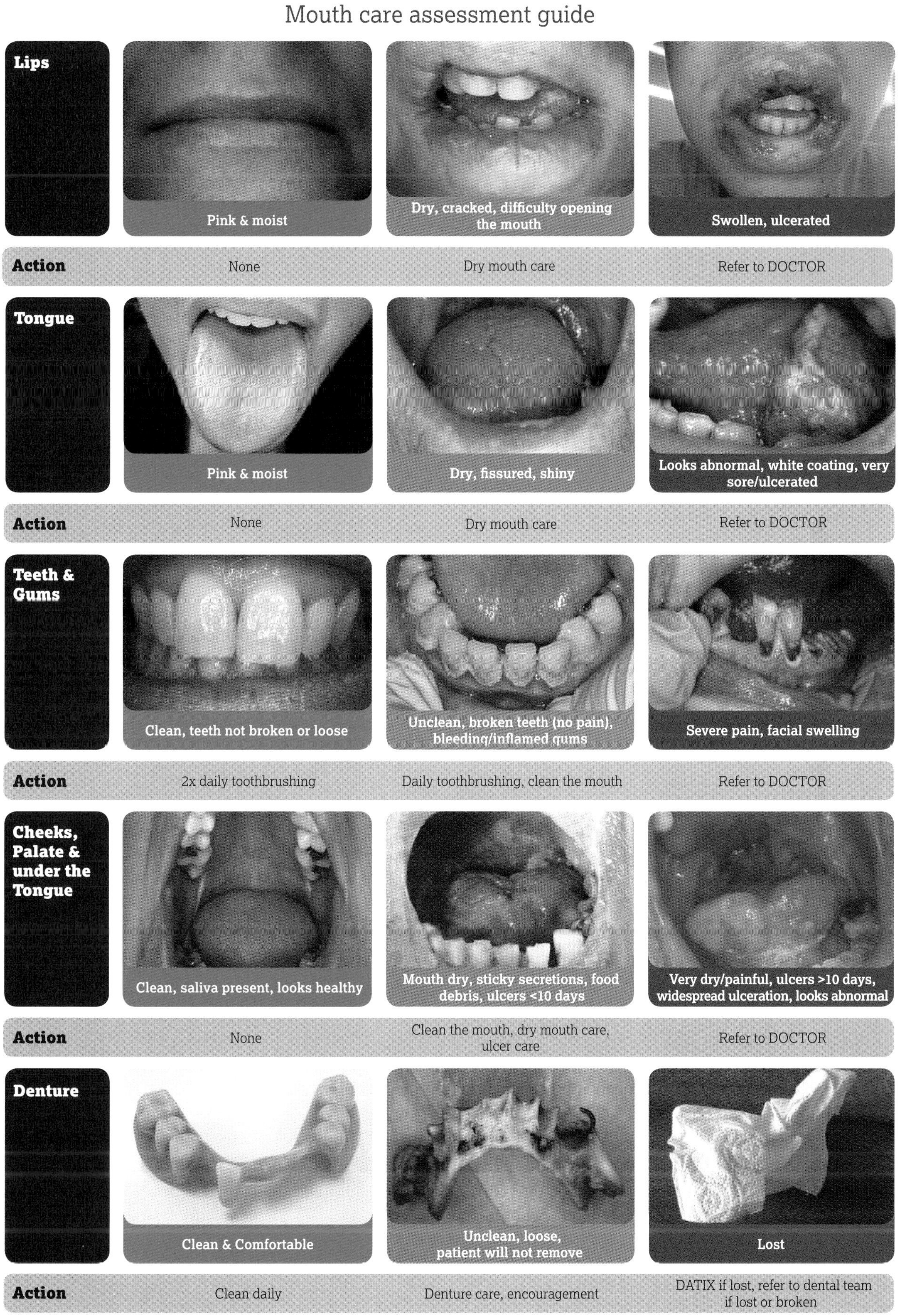

Figure 9.10 Mouth Care Assessment Guide. *Source*: Reproduced from HEE (2016) with permission of the NHS. Image created and owned by Public Health England (www.mouthcarematters.hee.nhs.uk).

Mouth Care Matters

NHS Health Education England

Mouth Care Pack

To be completed for every patient 24 hours after admission

Mouth care screening sheet

Patient name	
DOB	
MRN Number	
NHS Number	

Any tick in a red highlighted box indicates a **MOUTH CARE ASSESSMENT** is required

1. Patient has:

Toothbrush	Y ☐	N ☐	Provided ☐
Toothpaste	Y ☐	N ☐	Provided ☐
Upper denture	Y ☐	N ☐	At home ☐
Lower denture	Y ☐	N ☐	At home ☐
Denture pot	Y ☐	N ☐	Provided ☐
No teeth	Y ☐	(Patient will still require mouth care)	

If 'Y' to dentures, place the sunflower sign at the bedside

2. Does the patient have any pain or discomfort in the mouth?

Severe dry mouth	Y ☐	N ☐
Ulcers	Y ☐	N ☐
Painful mouth	Y ☐	N ☐
Painful teeth	Y ☐	N ☐
Sore tongue	Y ☐	N ☐
Other ☐ (please specify):		

3. Patients with any of the following will require a mouth care assessment:

☐ Chemotherapy	☐ Learning difficulties
☐ Delirium	☐ Nil by mouth
☐ Dementia	☐ Palliative care
☐ Dependent on oxygen use	☐ Refusing food or drink
☐ Dysphagia	☐ Severe mental health
☐ Frail	☐ Stroke
☐ Head & neck radiation	☐ Unable to communicate
☐ ICU / HDU	☐ Uncontrolled diabetes

4. Level of support: ☐ Requires risk assessment ☐ Unable to get to a sink/needs assistance

Patient is fully dependent on others for mouth care ☐
Mouth care assessment required. Record all mouth care on the daily recording sheet

Patient requires some assistance ☐
Unable to get to a sink or needs help with mouth care. Record all mouth care on the daily recording sheet
Please state the assistance patient requires: (i.e: bowl, encouragement, reminder, remove dentures etc)

Patient is independent ☐
Able to walk to a sink and needs **NO** assistance with mouth care

Signed:	Name:	Date:	Job title:

Figure 9.11 Mouth Care Pack. *Source:* Reproduced from HEE (n.d.) with permission of the NHS.

{Mouth Care Matters

NHS Health Education England

Mouth care assessment

Complete **WEEKLY** if the patient has a red box ticked on the mouth care screening sheet or if their condition deteriorates during their stay.

Patient name	
D.O.B	
MRN Number	
NHS Number	

Look in the patients mouth using a light source and carry out a weekly mouth care assessment. Mark as L, M or H in the white box.

	Low risk (L)	Medium risk (M)	High risk (H)*	Date	Date	Date	Date	Date
Lips	• Pink & moist	• Dry/cracked • Difficulty opening the mouth	• Swollen • Ulcerated					
Action	None	Dry mouth care	Refer to DOCTOR					
Tongue	• Pink & moist • Clean	• Dry • Fissured/shiny	• Looks abnormal • White coating • Very sore • Ulcerated					
Action	None	Dry mouth care	Refer to DOCTOR					
Teeth & gums	• Clean • Teeth not broken • Teeth not loose • Gums not bleeding • Gums not inflamed	• Unclean • Broken teeth (no pain) • Bleeding gums • Inflamed gums	• Severe pain • Facial swelling					
Action	2 x daily tooth brushing	2x daily toothbrushing & clean the mouth	Refer to DOCTOR or DENTAL TEAM	Advise the patient to visit their dentist on discharge if there are any problems with their teeth that do not require urgent treatment in hospital				
Cheeks, Palate & under the tongue	• Clean • Saliva present • Looks healthy	• Mouth dry • Sticky secretions • Food debris • Ulcer < 10 days	• Very dry/painful • Ulcer > 10 days • Widespread ulceration • Looks abnormal					
Action	None	• Clean the mouth • Dry mouth care • Ulcer care	Refer to DOCTOR	An ulcer present for more than **2 weeks** must be referred to the doctor				
Dentures	• Clean • Comfortable	• Unclean • Loose • Patient will not remove	• Lost • Broken and unable to wear					
Action	Clean daily	• Denture care • Denture fixative • Encourage removal	DATIX if lost or refer to the DENTAL TEAM if broken	Remember to place the denture sunflower at the patients bedside. Advise the patient to visit their dentist if the denture is loose				
			Signed:					

*For patients who are unable to communicate or cooperate with a mouth care assessment, some signs of a mouth related problem may include; not eating/drinking, facial swelling & behavioural changes

Dry mouth care

Frequent sips of water unless nil by mouth

Moisturise dry mouth gel onto the tongue, cheeks and palate

Hydrate with a moist toothbrush

Apply lip balm to dry lips

Keep mouth clean

Ulcer care

Rinse mouth with saline

Anti-inflammatory mouth spray – discuss with doctor

ULCER PRESENT FOR MORE THAN **2 WEEKS**; REFER TO DOCTOR

Denture care

Advise the patient to leave denture out at night in a named denture pot with a lid

If the patient has oral thrush, soak in chlorhexidine (0.2%) mouthwash for 15 minutes twice a day, rinse thoroughly and encourage the patient to leave the denture out whilst the mouth heals

Figure 9.11 *Continued*

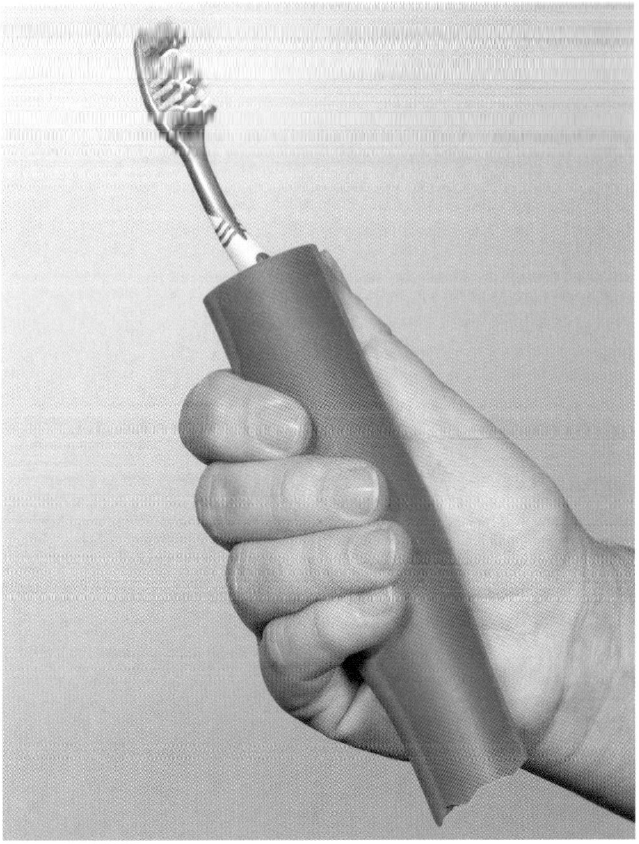

Figure 9.12 Foam handle to assist with holding a toothbrush.

Box 9.9 Recommendations for oral care in critically ill patients

- Reassess the patient at least every 8 hours.
- Brush teeth, gums and tongue at least twice a day using a soft, compacted-head (paediatric or adult) toothbrush or a suction toothbrush and an antiseptic mouthwash, such as chlorhexidine, diluted as appropriate.
- Using an oral chlorhexidine mouthwash, rinse the mouth twice a day in intubated patients to reduce the risk of ventilator-associated pneumonia.
- Apply oral moisturizer to the oral mucosa and lip balm to the lips every 2 to 4 hours.
- Minimize traumatic ulceration caused by endotracheal tubes using specifically designed fasteners and bite block, and alternating tubing from side to side.
- Use suction to prevent aspiration as required.

Source: Adapted from AACCN (2017), Brooker et al. (2013), HEE (2016).

occur in up to a quarter of ventilated patients and has an overall mortality of 13% (Melsen et al. 2013). In critically ill patients, the mouth can become colonized within 48 hours of admission to hospital with bacteria that tend to be more virulent than those normally found in the mouth (Hua et al. 2016). The oropharynx can become colonized, as can an artificial airway, allowing pathogens to travel to the respiratory tract, resulting in pneumonia (Brooker et al. 2013). Good oral care is essential in critically ill patients to reduce the incidence of VAP (Hua et al. 2016).

Dry mouth related to mouth breathing, the patient being nil by mouth and the use of oxygen can make oral care challenging. The presence of tubes and/or securing tapes can make it difficult to view and clean the oral cavity.

Clinical governance

Nurses should provide a high standard of care to patients, based on the best evidence available, ensuring they have the necessary skills (NMC 2018a). A number of documented studies have found that nurses feel they lack knowledge and training about providing oral care (Croyere et al. 2012, Gibney et al. 2015, Steel 2017). Although a number of training tools are available, the provision of adequate training before and after registration requires further attention (HEE 2016).

As is the case for all procedures, a full explanation must be given to the patient and verbal consent obtained (NMC 2018a). If patients refuse oral care, nurses should try to explore their reasons for refusal. If a nurse suspects that a patient lacks the capacity to understand the outcome of refusing oral care, they should follow the guidance in the most current version of the Mental Capacity Act (2005).

Pre-procedural considerations

Equipment

Toothbrush

The toothbrush is recognized as the most effective means of removing plaque and debris from the teeth and gums. A small-headed, medium-textured brush is most effective at reaching all areas of the mouth. Aids such as foam handles (available from occupational therapists) can make a manual toothbrush easier to hold (see Figure 9.12), and powered toothbrushes may be easier for patients with limited dexterity to use and have been shown to be as effective as manual toothbrushes (HEE 2016). For patients with a sore mouth, a soft or baby toothbrush can be used. The toothbrush should be allowed to air dry to reduce bacterial contamination, and in hospitals the toothbrush should be covered, ideally with a container for air circulation, rather than a plastic bag (HEE 2016).

Moistened mouth care sticks and foam sticks

Pre-moistened mouth care sticks are impregnated with moisturizers and can be effective in aiding mouth comfort. The dry foam stick is one of the most common pieces of equipment used in hospital to moisten the mouth or soak up saliva secretions, although it is not effective to remove dental plaque (Binks et al. 2017), so they should not be used as an alternative to tooth brushing (Steel 2017). A national alert on their use was issued following a choking incident: it stated that prior to using them, care should be taken to ensure that the foam head is securely attached, to avoid risk of accidental detachment and aspiration (MHRA 2012). If used, sticks should not be left to soak in liquid but moistened immediately prior to being used and immediately discarded after use. Soaking sticks in liquid may detrimentally affect the strength of the foam head attachment. Patients and relatives using foam swabs should be made aware of their proper use (MHRA 2012).

Interdental cleaning

The use of dental floss or other equipment is recommended to clean areas between the teeth that may be difficult to reach with a toothbrush (Birchenall and Streight 2013). Correct dental flossing or use of interdental cleaners once a day may help with plaque reduction, although these should be used with caution for patients with thrombocytopaenia or clotting disorders (UKOMiC 2019). A variety of equipment is available, such as dental floss, dental tape, wooden sticks and interdental brushes (Figure 9.13). For patients who have limited dexterity, this kind of cleaning may be difficult or impossible to carry out. Similarly, in patients with painful mouths or bleeding gums, this type of equipment can cause further discomfort, trauma and bleeding, and should be avoided. Oral irrigation devices such as the Waterpik® can be used for interdental cleaning. Oral irrigation uses a jet of water to remove debris and plaque and can be useful for people who find it difficult to use dental floss or tape, such as those with braces. Daily use of oral irrigation is safe and effective in addition to tooth brushing to remove biofilm from tooth surfaces and bacteria from periodontal pockets (Johnson et al. 2015, Jolkovsky and Lyle 2015).

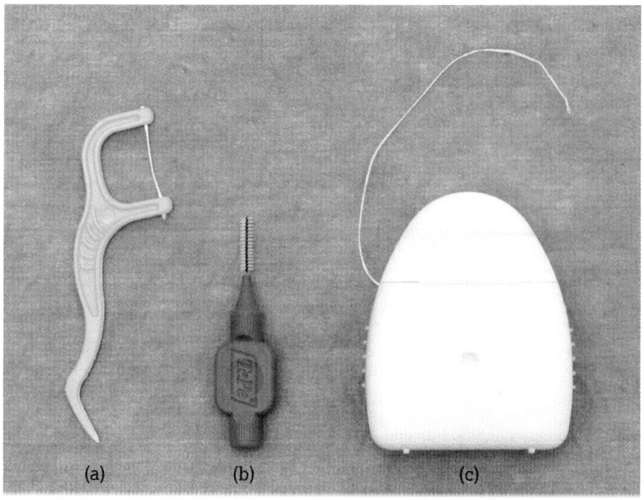

Figure 9.13 Examples of interdental cleaning products. (a) Disposable flosser. (b) Interdental brush. (c) Dental floss.

Pharmacological support

The choice of an oral care agent depends on the aim of care. The agent may be used to remove debris and plaque, prevent superimposed infection, alleviate pain, provide comfort, stop bleeding, provide lubrication or treat specific problems (HEE 2016, UKOMiC 2019). A wide variety of agents are available and the choice of which to use should be determined by the individual needs of the patient, the clinical situation and a detailed nursing assessment.

Toothpaste

Toothpaste is a paste or gel used with a toothbrush (mechanical or powered) to clean and maintain the health of teeth and gums. It is an abrasive substance that aids in the removal of food from the teeth and dental plaque. Most of the cleaning is achieved by the mechanical action of the toothbrush and not by the toothpaste. Most toothpastes have active ingredients to help prevent tooth and gum disease. Toothpastes are composed of 20–42% water with abrasive components (to remove plaque and stains from the tooth surface), fluoride (to prevent cavities) and detergents (surfactants used mainly as foaming agents). Different types are listed in the *Dental Practitioners' Formulary* (NICE 2019).

A pea-sized amount of fluoride toothpaste should be used, and patients should be advised to 'spit not rinse' (spit out excess toothpaste but do not rinse out the mouth with water) to ensure that a film of toothpaste is left in contact with the teeth, allowing it to be absorbed. After tooth brushing, it is recommended that patients wait at least 30 minutes before eating or drinking (HEE 2016).

Commercial mouthwash

Mouthwashes are an adjunct to brushing and not a replacement. For those with active caries (decaying or crumbling teeth), dry mouth, orthodontic appliances or other risk factors, 0.05% (225 ppm) fluoride mouthwash is recommended (PHE 2017).

Bland rinses

Several agents can be used to rinse the mouth, moisten the mucosa, and loosen and remove debris. Normal saline mouthwashes and saline sprays may provide some relief for dry mouth (UKOMiC 2019). Additional studies have shown some benefit in the use of saline for mouth care in cancer and elderly patients (Kim and Kim 2014, McGuire et al. 2013). For patients with severe dry mouth, water-based mouth-moisturizing gels or sprays can be applied before mouth cleaning and eating so that these activities are less painful (HEE 2016); these gels and sprays are also helpful for tenacious secretions. Sodium bicarbonate has been used in some centres and oral hygiene regimes and can provide a good effect in dental decay prevention and have significant bactericidal activity (Giancio 2017). However, it can affect the mucosa, so its use should be reviewed after 48 hours.

Chlorhexidine gluconate

Chlorhexidine gluconate is an effective antibacterial and anti-plaque agent. For patients who are unable to use a toothbrush, it can provide a chemical method of stopping plaque build-up. Chlorhexidine gluconate mouthwash used as an adjunct to mechanical oral hygiene can reduce dental plaque (HEE 2016, James et al. 2017). Chlorhexidine mouthwash or gel reduces the risk of critically ill patients developing VAP from 25% to about 19% (Hua et al. 2016, Veitz-Keenan and Ferraiolo 2017). Longer-term use is associated with altered taste, reversible staining of the teeth and parotid gland enlargement (Steel 2017). It should be avoided in patients receiving radiotherapy to the head and neck regions or patients who have mucositis; in these cases, preparations such as Caphosol®, Difflam®, Gelclair® and MuGard® are advocated (RD-UK 2016, UKOMiC 2019).

Contraindicated agents

A number of agents widely used in the past for mouth care have been found to have detrimental effects and are no longer recommended. Glycerine and lemon swabs dehydrate the mucosa and exhaust salivary secretion, which acts to dry the mouth (NICE 2016c). Hydrogen peroxide is also not recommended as it can cause mucosal abnormalities and pain (Consolaro 2013).

Specific patient pharmacological preparations

Fluoride

Fluoride helps to prevent and arrest tooth decay (HEE 2016), especially radiation caries, demineralization and decalcification. High dose fluoride toothpaste may be recommended for patients with current active caries, dry mouth or other predisposing factors, such as during and after receipt of radiotherapy treatment (PHE 2017, RD-UK 2016, UKOMiC 2019).

Artificial saliva

For patients with salivary dysfunctions and dry mouth, saliva substitutes may help to alleviate these symptoms (Jawad et al. 2015). There are a variety of products available, such as artificial saliva replacements and salivary stimulants (Jawad et al. 2015, NHS HEE 2016). Current recommendations suggest avoiding artificial saliva products with an acidic pH due to the increased risk of dental decay, and instead choosing preparations with fluoride (RD-UK 2016, UK Medicines Information 2015, UKOMiC 2019).

Coating agents

A coating agent can be used to coat the surface of the mouth, forming a thin protective film over painful oral lesions or for patients with mucositis. Oral lesions and mucositis can be caused by medication, disease, oral surgery, stress, traumatic ulcers caused by dental braces and dentures, radiotherapy and chemotherapy. Examples of coating agents include Caphosol®, Difflam®, Episil®, GelClair® and MuGard® (RD-UK 2016, UKOMiC 2019). These products should be rinsed around the mouth to form a protective layer over the sore areas, and generally applied 1 hour before eating. Several agents can be used to coat the oral mucosa and they are thought to have a protective effect although there is limited evidence to support their use (Saunders et al. 2013). Sucralfate has not been shown to be effective in preventing or treating chemotherapy- or radiotherapy-associated oral mucositis (Saunders et al. 2013).

Antifungal agents

Colonization of the mouth with yeast occurs in one-third of the population. In patients receiving steroids or antibiotics, the balance of the oral flora can be altered and oral candidiasis (oral thrush) can occur. Predisposing factors also include xerostomia, poor oral health and the presence of dentures. These infections can be treated with either topical or systemic antifungal medications. In debilitated or immunocompromised patients, candidiasis can become a systemic infection.

Antifungal agents are a group of drugs specifically used for the treatment of fungal infections. A number of preparations are available. Selection should be based on location and severity of infection (HEE 2016). Oropharyngeal candidiasis can be treated with either topical antifungal agents (e.g. nystatin, clotrimazole or amphotericin B oral suspension) or systemic oral azoles (fluconazole, itraconazole or posaconazole). Length of treatment depends on the pharmacological agent chosen and recommendations regarding their relevant pharmacology. Local prescribing guidelines should be followed.

Procedure guideline 9.14 Mouth care

Essential equipment

- Personal protective equipment
- Small torch
- Clean receiver or bowl
- Gauze
- Wooden spatula
- Small-headed, medium-texture toothbrush
- Toothpaste
- Dental floss

Action	Rationale
Pre-procedure	
1 Introduce yourself to the patient, explain and discuss the procedure with them, and gain their consent to proceed. Where possible, encourage patients to carry out their own oral care.	To ensure that the patient feels at ease, understands the procedure and gives their valid consent (NMC 2018a, **C**). To enable patients to gain confidence in managing their own symptoms (NHS England 2017a, **C**).
2 Wash hands with soap and water and dry with a paper towel, or use alcohol-based handrub. Put on disposable gloves.	To reduce the risk of cross-infection (NHS England and NHSI 2019, **C**).
Procedure	
3 Carry out an oral assessment using an approved oral assessment tool. See Figure 9.11.	To provide a baseline to enable monitoring of mucosal changes and evaluate the patient's response to treatment and care (HEE 2016, **C**).
4 a Inspect the patient's mouth, including the teeth, with the aid of a torch, spatula and gauze, paying special attention to the lips, buccal mucosa, lateral and ventral surfaces of the tongue, floor of the mouth and soft palate (**Action figure 4**).	The mouth is examined for changes in condition with respect to moisture, cleanliness, infected or bleeding areas, ulcers and so on. These areas are known to be particularly susceptible to cytotoxic damage (HEE 2016, **C**).
b Ask the patient whether they have any of the following: taste changes, change in saliva production or composition, oral discomfort or difficulty swallowing.	To assess nutritional deficits, salivary changes and pain secondary to oral changes (HEE 2016, **C**).
5 Using a small-headed, medium-texture toothbrush and toothpaste, begin to brush the patient's natural teeth, gums and tongue. Small circular brushing movements are recommended.	To control gum disease. The physical removal of plaque is the important element of tooth brushing as it reduces the inflammatory response of the gingivae and its sequelae (HEE 2016, **C**; PHE 2017, **C**). Small circular brushing movements enhance plaque removal (Peterson et al. 2015, **C**; PHE 2017, **C**).
6 Hold the brush against the teeth with the bristles at a 45° angle. The tips of the outer bristles should rest against and penetrate under the gingival sulcus. Using the tips of the bristles, vibrate back and forth with short, light strokes for a count of 10, allowing the tips of the bristles to enter the sulcus and cover the gingival margin. Lift the brush and continue on to the next area or group of teeth until all areas have been cleaned. After the vibratory motion has been completed in each area, sweep the bristles over the crowns of the teeth, towards the biting surface. The toe bristles of the brush can be used to clean the lingual (tongue) anterior area in the arch.	Brushing loosens and removes debris trapped on and between the teeth and gums (HEE 2016, **C**). This reduces the growth medium for pathogenic organisms and minimizes the risk of plaque formation and dental caries (PHE 2017, **C**).
7 Ask the patient to spit out excess toothpaste into the receiver or bowl but do not allow them to rinse the mouth out with water.	To ensure that a film of toothpaste is left in contact with the teeth, allowing it to be absorbed (HEE 2016, **C**).
8 Floss teeth (unless contraindicated due to conditions such as clotting abnormality or thrombocytopenia) once every 24 hours using lightly waxed floss.	Flossing helps to remove debris between teeth (UKOMiC 2019, **C**).
a To floss the upper teeth, use your thumb and index finger to stretch the floss and wrap one end of the floss around the third finger of each hand. Move the floss up and down between the teeth from the tops of the crowns to the gum and along the gum lines wherever possible (**Action figure 8**).	Flossing when a patient has abnormal clotting or low platelets may lead to bleeding and predispose the oral mucosa to infection (American Cancer Society 2017, **C**; Elad et al. 2015, **C**).
b To floss the lower teeth, use the index fingers to stretch the floss.	

Post-procedure

9 Discard remaining mouthwash solutions.	To prevent infection (Bullock and Manias 2014, **E**).
10 Clean the toothbrush and allow it to air dry.	To reduce the risk of contamination (HEE 2016, **C**).
11 Remove gloves. Decontaminate hands.	To reduce the risk of cross-infection (NHS England and NHSI 2019, **C**).
12 Ensure the patient is comfortable.	To maintain patient comfort and dignity (NMC 2018a, **C**).
13 Advise the patient not to eat or drink within 30 minutes of brushing (HEE 2016).	To ensure that a film of toothpaste is left in contact with the teeth, allowing it to be absorbed (HEE 2016, **C**).

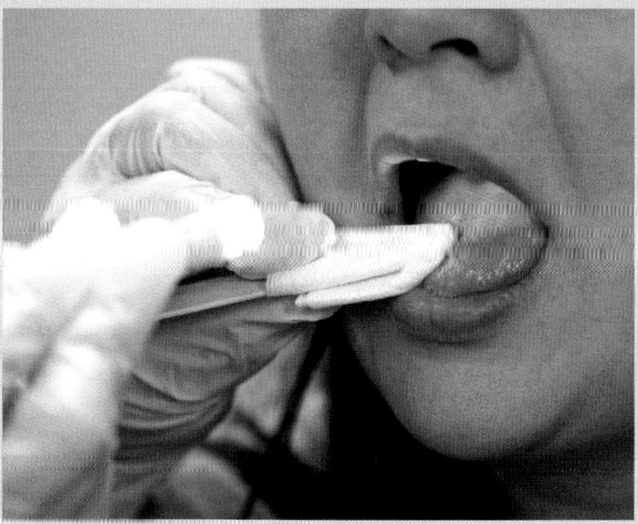

Action Figure 4 Oral assessment using a torch, spatula and gauze.

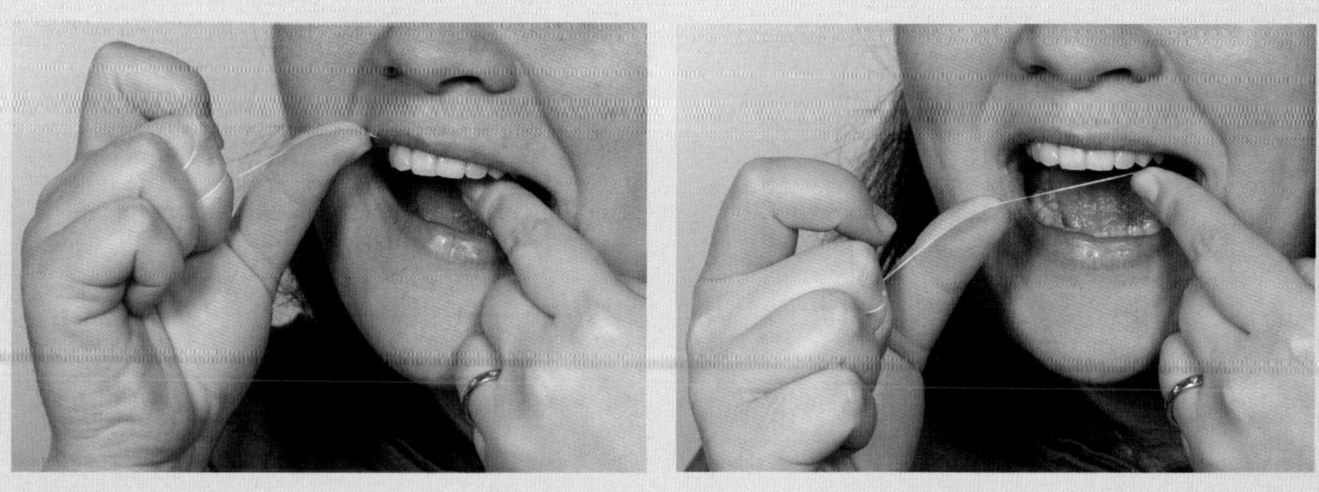

Action Figure 8 Interdental cleaning using dental floss.

Procedure guideline 9.15 Mouth care for a patient with dentures

Essential equipment

- Personal protective equipment
- Small torch
- Plastic cups
- Gauze
- Wooden spatula
- Cleaning solutions
- Clean receiver or bowl
- Tissues
- Small-headed, soft toothbrush or a denture brush
- Denture pot

(continued)

Procedure guideline 9.15 Mouth care for a patient with dentures *(continued)*

Action	Rationale
Pre-procedure	
1 Introduce yourself to the patient, explain and discuss the procedure with them, and gain their consent to proceed. Where possible, encourage patients to carry out their own oral care.	To ensure that the patient feels at ease, understands the procedure and gives their valid consent (NMC 2018a, **C**). To enable patients to gain confidence in managing their own symptoms (NHS England 2017a, **C**).
2 Wash hands with soap and water and dry with a paper towel, or use alcohol-based handrub. Put on disposable gloves.	To reduce the risk of cross-infection (NHS England and NHSI 2019, **C**).
Procedure	
3 Prepare solutions required.	Solutions must always be prepared immediately before use to maximize their efficacy and minimize the risk of microbial contamination (Bullock and Manias 2014, **E**).
4 If the patient cannot remove their own dentures, remove the lower denture first. a *Lower denture*: grasp it in the middle and lift it, rotating it gently to remove it from the mouth. Place it in the denture pot. b *Upper denture*: remove the upper denture by grasping it firmly in the middle and tilting the denture forward while putting pressure on the front teeth to break the seal with the palate. Rotate the denture from side to side to remove it from the mouth and place it in the denture pot.	Removal of dentures is necessary for cleaning of underlying tissues and all surfaces of the dentures themselves (Birchenall and Streight 2013, **E**).
5 Carry out an oral assessment using an approved oral assessment tool. See Figure 9.11.	To provide a baseline to enable monitoring of mucosal changes and evaluate the patient's response to treatment and care (HEE 2016, **C**).
6 a Inspect the patient's mouth with the aid of a torch, spatula and gauze, paying special attention to the lips, buccal mucosa, lateral and ventral surfaces of the tongue, floor of the mouth and soft palate (see Action figure 4 in Procedure guideline 9.14: Mouth care). b Ask the patient whether they have any of the following: taste changes, change in saliva production or composition, oral discomfort or difficulty swallowing.	The mouth is examined for changes in condition with respect to moisture, cleanliness, infected or bleeding areas, ulcers and so on. These areas are known to be particularly susceptible to cytotoxic damage (HEE 2016, **C**). To assess nutritional deficits, salivary changes and pain secondary to oral changes (HEE 2016, **C**).
7 Give a cup of water to the patient. Encourage the patient to rinse their mouth vigorously then spit the contents into a receiver. Paper tissues should be on hand to dry any spillage of water or dribbling.	Rinsing removes loosened debris and makes the mouth taste fresher (Birchenall and Streight 2013, **E**).
8 Clean the patient's dentures on all surfaces with a toothbrush and soap and water or a denture cleaner. Check the dentures for cracks, sharp edges and missing teeth. Dentures should be removed for at least 1 hour but ideally overnight and placed in a suitable cleaning solution. Rinse them well and return them to the patient.	Cleaning dentures removes accumulated food debris, which could be broken down by salivary enzymes to products that irritate and cause inflammation of the adjacent mucosal tissue (HEE 2016, **C**). Dentures can easily become colonized by bacteria. Soaking can disinfect the dentures, discouraging bacterial growth (HEE 2016, **C**).
Post-procedure	
9 Discard remaining mouthwash solutions.	To prevent infection (Bullock and Manias 2014, **E**).
10 Clean the toothbrush or denture brush and allow it to air dry.	To prevent contamination (HEE 2016, **C**).
11 Remove gloves. Wash hands with soap and water and dry with a paper towel, or use alcohol-based handrub.	To reduce the risk of cross-infection (NHS England and NHSI 2019, **C**)
12 Ensure the patient is comfortable.	To maintain patient comfort and dignity (NMC 2018a, **C**).
13 Ensure the dentures and container are clearly labelled.	To ensure the dentures are kept safe. **E**

Problem-solving table 9.1 Prevention and resolution (Procedure guidelines 9.14 and 9.15)

Problem	Cause	Prevention	Action
Dry mouth (xerostomia)	Oxygen therapy, mouth breathing, nil by mouth	Humidified oxygen	Swab the mouth with a moistened foam stick or encourage the patient to rinse the mouth with water and spit it out.
	Salivary gland hypofunction due to disease, drugs or side-effects of radiotherapy or chemotherapy	Not always possible to prevent; if due to a side-effect of medication, then medical advice should be sought to swap the patient to a different drug that may not have that side-effect.	Try one or more of the following: • Encourage the patient to sip water or suck on ice chips. • Conduct a daily review of the oral cavity to identify signs of infection. • Encourage good oral hygiene to prevent complications. • Use salivary stimulants, e.g. sugar-free chewing gum, pilocarpine or saliva substitutes/replacements. • Use steam inhalation and saline nebulizers to manage thickened secretions.
Patient unable to tolerate toothbrush	Pain (e.g. post-surgery), mucositis.	Consider using anaesthetic mouth spray or mouthwash before mouth care. Give analgesia regularly or as needed.	0.9% sodium chloride rinse can be used if the patient cannot tolerate any form of oral care.
Toothbrush inappropriate or ineffective	Infectious stomatitis; accumulation of dried mucus, new lesions, blood or debris	See 'Patient unable to tolerate toothbrush'.	See 'Patient unable to tolerate toothbrush'. Also take a swab of any infected areas for culture before giving mouth care.

Post-procedural considerations

Comfort and personal hygiene preferences are individual to each patient; each procedure should be carried out with consideration of these preferences. Furthermore, the preferences, along with assessments and outcomes of procedures, should be documented and communicated to other health professionals involved in the patient's care to ensure continuity and effective evaluation of the care provided.

Websites

British Tinnitus Association
www.tinnitus.org.uk

College of Optometrists
www.college-optometrists.org

Diabetes UK
www.diabetes.org.uk/professionals

Health Education England
www.hee.nhs.uk

Moorfields Eye Hospital
www.moorfields.nhs.uk

Mouth Care Matters
www.mouthcarematters.hee.nhs.uk

National Institute of Health and Care Excellence
www.nice.org.uk

National Institute of Neurological Disorders and Stroke
www.ninds.nih.gov

Rotherham Primary Ear Care Centre and Audiology Services
www.earcarecentre.com

World Health Organization: Oral Health
www.who.int/oral_health/en

References

AACCN (American Association of Critical-Care Nurses) (2017) Oral care for acutely and critically ill patients. *Critical Care Nurse*, 37(3), e19–e21.

Aaron, K., Cooper, T.E., Warner, L. & Burton, M.J. (2018) Ear drops for the removal of ear wax. *Cochrane Database of Systematic Reviews*, 7, CD012171.

Aldwin, C.M., Igarashi, H., Gilmer, D.F. & Levenson, M.R. (2017) Aging of the sensory and nervous systems. In: *Health, Illness, and Optimal Aging: Biological and Psychosocial Perspectives*, 3rd edn. New York, NY: Springer, pp.163–188.

Alpers, L.M. & Hanssen, I. (2014) Caring for ethnic minority patients: A mixed method study of nurses' self-assessment of cultural competency. *Nurse Education Today*, 34(6), 999–1004.

Ameen, M., Lear, J.T., Madan, V., et al. (2014) British Association of Dermatologists' guidelines for the management of onychomycosis 2014. *British Journal of Dermatology*, 171(5), 937–958.

American Cancer Society (2017) *Bleeding or Low Platelet Count*. Available at: https://www.cancer.org/treatment/treatments-and-side-effects/physical-side-effects/low-blood-counts/bleeding.html

Andriessen, A. (2013) Prevention, recognition and treatment of dry skin conditions. *British Journal of Nursing*, 22(1), 26–30.

Anil, S., Vellappally, S., Hashem, M., et al. (2014) Xerostomia in geriatric patients: A burgeoning global concern. *Journal of Investigative and Clinical Dentistry*, 5, 1–8.

Assefa, S., Diaz-Abad, M., Wickwire, E. & Scharf, S. (2015) The functions of sleep. *AIMS Neuroscience*, 2(3), 155–171.

Astbury, N. (2016) Improving cataract outcomes though good postoperative care. *Community Eye Health*, 29(94), 21–22.

Asti, E., Sironi, A., Milito, P., et al. (2017) Prevalence and risk factors of nasal pressure ulcers related to nasogastric intubation: An observational study. *European Surgery*, 49(4), 171–174.

Attum, B. & Shamoon, Z. (2018) Cultural competence in the care of Muslim patients and their families. *StatPearls*. Available at: https://www.ncbi.nlm.nih.gov/books/NBK499933

Auckley, D., Benca, R. & Eichler, A. (2010) Poor sleep in the hospital: Contributing factors and interventions. *UpToDate*. Available at: https://www.uptodate.com/contents/poor-sleep-in-the-hospital-contributing-factors-and-interventions

Balkany, T.J. & Brown, K.D. (2017) Understanding your ears. In: *The Ear Book: A Complete Guide to Ear Disorders and Health*. Baltimore: Johns Hopkins University Press, pp.3–20.

Barber, C. (2016) Communication and the 6Cs: Patient experience. *Nursing Times*, 112(online issue 1), 4–5.

Bartlett, D., Carter, N., de Baat, C., et al. (2018) *White Paper on Optimal Care and Maintenance of Full Dentures for Oral and General Health*. Global Task Force for Care of Full Dentures. Available at: https://www.dentalhealth.org/Handlers/Download.ashx?IDMF=81d96249-f307-4e21-aaea-1c861730710e

Bauters, T., Schandevyl, G.V. & Laureys, G. (2016) Safety in the use of Vaseline during oxygen therapy: The pharmacist's perspective. *International Journal of Clinical Pharmacy*, 38, 1032–1034.

Berman A., Snyder, J. & Frandsen, G. (2015) *Kozier & Erb's Fundamentals of Nursing: Concepts, Process and Practice*, 10th edn. Harlow: Pearson, pp.695–743.

Binks, C., Doshi, M. & Mann, J. (2017) Standardising the delivery of oral health care practice in hospitals. *Nursing Times*, 113(11), 18–21.

Birchenall, J.M. & Streight, E. (2013) Personal care. In: *Mosby's Textbook for the Home Care Aide*, 3rd edn. St Louis, MO: Elsevier Mosby, pp.232–263.

Bloomfield, J., Pegram, A., Wilson, R., et al. (2017) Facial shaving. In: *Clinical Nursing Skills: An Australian Perspective*. Cambridge: Cambridge University Press, pp.168–169.

Bloomfield, S., Exner, M., Flemming, H.C., et al. (2015) Lesser-known or hidden reservoirs of infection and implications for adequate prevention strategies: Where to look and what to look for. *GMS Hygiene and Infection Control*, 10, 4.

Boge, J., Kristoffersen, K. & Martisen, K. (2013) Body cleanliness in modern nursing. *Nursing Philosophy*, 14, 78–85.

Bowling, F.L., Rashid, S.T. & Boulton, A.J.M. (2015) Preventing and treating foot complications associated with diabetes mellitus. *Nature Reviews Endocrinology*, 11, 606–616.

Brocklehurst, P., Williams, L., Hoare, Z., et al. (2016) Strategies to prevent oral disease in dependent older people (protocol). *Cochrane Database of Systematic Reviews*, 10, CD012402.

Brooker, S., Murff, S., Kitko, L. & Jablonski, R. (2013) Mouth care to reduce ventilator associated pneumonia. *AJN*, 113(10), 24–30.

BSA (British Society of Audiology) (2017) *Practice Guidance: Aural Care (Ear Wax Removal)*. Seafield: British Society of Audiology.

Bullock, S. & Manias, E. (2014) Antiseptics and disinfectants. In: *Fundamentals of Pharmacology*, 7th edn. Frenchs Forrest, Australia: Pearson, pp.960–968.

Burns, B. (2012) Oral care for older people in residential care. *Nursing & Residential Care*, 14(1), 26–31.

Burton, M.A. & Ludwig, L.J.M. (2014) Shaving: Personal care. In: *Fundamentals of Nursing Care: Concepts, Connections and Skills*, 2nd edn. Philadelphia: F.A. Davis, pp.277–308.

Bus, S.A., Netten, J.J., Lavery, L.A., et al. (2016) IWGDF guidance on the prevention of foot ulcers in at-risk patients with diabetes. *Diabetes/Metabolism Research and Reviews*, 32(1), 16–24.

Butcher, H.K., Bulecheck, G.M., McCloskey Dochterman, J.M. & Wagner, C. (2018) *Nursing Interventions Classification*, 7th edn. St Louis, MO: Mosby Elsevier.

Carley, D. & Farabi, S. (2016) Physiology of sleep. *Diabetes Spectrum*, 29(1), 5–9.

Carnt, N., Hoffman, J., Verma, S., et al. (2018) Acanthamoeba keratitis: Confirmation of the UK outbreak and a prospective case-control study identifying contributing risk factors. *British Journal of Ophthalmology*, 102(12), 1621–1628.

Carpenito, L.J. (2017) Oral mucous membrane. In: *Nursing Diagnosis: Application to Clinical Practice*, 15th edn. Philadelphia: Wolters Kluwer, pp.624–629.

Chidharla, A. & Kasi, A. (2019) Cancer, chemotherapy acral erythema (palmar-plantar erythrodysesthesia, palmoplantar erythrodysesthesia, hand-foot syndrome). *StatPearls*. Available at: https://www.ncbi.nlm.nih.gov/books/NBK459375

Clark, A. & Mills, M. (2017) Can a sleep menu enhance the quality of sleep for the hospitalised patient? *MEDSURG Nursing*, 26(4), 253–258.

Coker, E., Ploeg, J., Kaasalainen, S. & Fisher, A. (2013) A concept analysis of oral hygiene care in dependent older adults. *Journal of Advanced Nursing*, 69(10), 2360–2371.

College of Optometrists (20[illegible]) *Chemical Trauma Guidelines*. Available at: www.college-optometrists.org/guidance/clinical-management-guidelines/trauma-chemical-.html

Consolaro, A. (2013) Mouthwashes with hydrogen peroxide are carcinogenic, but are freely indicated on the internet: Warn your patients! *Dental Press Journal of Orthodontics*, 18(6), 5–12.

Corl, D.E., McCliment, C.D.E., Sean, M.H.A., et al. (2014) Efficacy of diabetes nurse expert team program to improve nursing confidence and expertise in caring for hospitalized patients with diabetes. *Journal for Nurses in Professional Development*, 30(3), 134–142.

Cowdell, F. & Steventon, K. (2015) Skin cleansing practices for older people: A systematic review. *International Journal of Older People Nursing*, 10(1), 3–13.

Crews, R.T., Yalla, S.V., Fleischer, A.E. & Wu, S.C. (2013) A growing troubling triad: Diabetes, aging, and falls. *Journal of Aging Research*, 2013, 1–6.

Croyère, N., Belloir, M.N., Chantler, L. & McEwan, L. (2012) Oral care in nursing practice: A pragmatic representation. *International Journal of Palliative Care*, 18(9), 435–440.

Cullen, D. & Thomas, Y. (2018) The impact of clutter on healthcare acquired infections in a long-term acute care hospital. *American Journal of Infection Control*, 46(6), S71.

Danielson, B., Willanson, S., Johnson, N. & Danielson, B. (2013) Patient's bath basin: Friend or foe. *American Journal of Infection Control*, 41(6), S93.

Darbyshire, J. & Young, D. (2013) An investigation of sound levels on intensive care units with reference to the WHO guidelines. *Critical Care*, 17(5), R187.

Davis, K.G. & Kotowski, S.E. (2015) Role of bed design and head-of-bed articulation on patient migration. *Journal of Nursing Care Quality*, 30(3), E1–E9.

DH (Department of Health) (2016) *Health Technical Memorandum 01-04: Decontamination of Linen for Health and Social Care – Management and Provision*. Available at: https://assets.publishing.service.gov.uk/government/uploads/system/uploads/attachment_data/file/527542/Mgmt_and_provision.pdf

Diabetes UK (2013) *Putting Feet First: Diabetes UK Position on Preventing Amputations and Improving Foot Care for People with Diabetes*. Available at: https://www.diabetes.org.uk/professionals/position-statements-reports/specialist-care-for-children-and-adults-and-complications/putting-feet-first-diabetes-foot-care

Dobing, S., Frolova, N., McAlister, F. & Ringrose, J. (2016) Sleep quality and factors influencing self-reported sleep duration and quality in the general internal medicine inpatient population. *PLOS ONE*, 11(6), e0156735.

Draelos, Z. (2018) Cosmeceuticals for male skin. *Dermatologic Clinics*, 36(1), 17–20.

Dubose, J. & Hadi, K. (2016) Improving inpatient environments to support patient sleep. *International Journal for Quality in Health Care*, 28(5), 540–553.

Dunk, A.M. (2015) Importance of the microclimate in maintaining skin integrity. *Australian Nursing & Midwifery Journal*, 23(3), 43.

Eggermont, J. (2014) Introduction. In: *Noise and the Brain*. London: Academic Press, pp.1–21.

Eghrari, A.O., Riazuddin, S.A. & Gottsch, J.D. (2015) Overview of the cornea: Structure, function and development. *Progress in Molecular Biology and Translational Science*, 134, 7–23.

Ehrlich, J.R. (2018) What is the value of preference values for patient-centered eye care? *JAMA Ophthalmology*, 136(6), 664–665.

Elad, S., Raber-Durlacher, J.E., Brennan, M.T. & Saunders, D.P. (2015) Basic oral care for hematology–oncology patients and hematopoietic stem cell transplantation recipients: A position paper from the joint task force of the Multinational Association of Supportive Care in Cancer/International Society of Oral Oncology (MASCC/ISOO) and the European Society for Blood and Marrow Transplantation (EBMT). *Journal of Supportive Care in Cancer*, 23(1), 223–236.

El-Soussi, A.H. & Asfour, H.I. (2017) A return to the basics: Nurses' practices and knowledge about interventional patient hygiene in critical care units. *Intensive Care Nurse*, 40, 11–17.

Everett, J.S. & Sommers, M.S. (2013) Skin viscoelasticity: Physiologic mechanisms, measurement issues, and application to nursing science. *Biological Research for Nursing*, 15(3), 338–346.

Farage, M.A., Miller, K.W., Elsner, P. & Maibach, H.I. (2013) Characteristics of the aging skin. *Advances in Wound Care*, 2(1), 5–10.

Fillary, J., Chaplin, H., Jones, G., et al. (2015) Noise at night in hospital general wards: A mapping of the literature. *British Journal of Nursing*, 24(10), 536–540.

Fitzgerald, C. (2017) Modernising patient clothing: A Florence Nightingale Foundation project. *British Journal of Nursing*, 26(8), 472–473.

Forbes, H. & Watt, E. (2015) Peripheral vascular assessment. In: Jarvis, C. (ed) *Jarvis's Physical Examination & Health Assessment*. Sydney: Elsevier, pp.312–335.

Forrester, J.V., Dick, A.W., McMenamin, P.G., et al. (2016) Physiology of vision and the visual system. In: *The Eye: Basic Sciences in Practice*, 4th edn. Edinburgh: Saunders, pp.269–337.

Fosarelli, P.M. (2014) Professionalism, medicine and religion. In: De Angelis, C.D. (ed) *Patient Care and Professionalism*. New York: Oxford University Press, pp.148–162.

Fowler, J. (2017a) From staff nurse to nurse consultant: Spiritual care part 6 – Hinduism. *British Journal of Nursing*, 26(17), 998.

Fowler, J. (2017b) From staff nurse to nurse consultant: Spiritual care part 7 – Islam. *British Journal of Nursing*, 26(19), 1082.

Fowler, J. (2017c) From staff nurse to nurse consultant: Spiritual care part 9 – Judaism. *British Journal of Nursing*, 26(22), 1262.

Fraise, A.P. & Bradley, C. (2009) *Ayliffe's Control of Healthcare-Associated Infection: A Practical Handbook*, 5th edn. London: Hodder Arnold.

Frost, S.A., Alogso, M.-C., Metcalfe, L., et al. (2016) Chlorhexidine bathing and health care-associated infections among adult intensive care patients: A systematic review and meta-analysis. *Critical Care*, 20(1), 379.

Gellerstedt, L., Medin, J. & Karlsonn, M. (2014) Patients' experiences of sleep in hospital: A qualitative interview study. *Journal of Research in Nursing*, 19(3), 176–188.

Gelston, C.D. (2013) Common eye emergencies. *American Family Physician*, 88(8), 515–519.

Ghersi, I., Mariño, M. & Miralles, T. (2016) From modern push-button hospital-beds to 20th century mechatronic beds: A review. *Journal of Physics (Conference Series)*, 705.

Giancio, S.G. (2017) Baking soda dentifrices and oral health. *JADA*, 148(11), 1S–3S.

Gibney, J., Wright, C., Sharma, A. & Naganathan, V. (2015) Nurses' knowledge, attitudes, and current practice of daily oral hygiene care to patients on acute aged care wards in two Australian hospitals. *Special Care in Dentistry*, 35(6), 285–293.

Gilsenan, I. (2017) How to promote patients' sleep in hospital. *Nursing Standard*, 31(28), 42–44.

Groven, F.M.V., Zwakhalen, S.M.G., Oderkerken-Schröder, G., et al. (2017) How does washing without water perform compared to the traditional bed bath: A systematic review. *BMC Geriatrics*, 17(31), 1–16.

Guenther, L., Lynde, C.W., Andriessen, A., et al. (2012) Pathway to dry skin prevention and treatment. *Journal of Cutaneous Medicine and Surgery*, 16(1), 23–31.

Hand, A.R. & Frank, M.E. (2014) Oral structures and tissues. In: *Fundamentals of Oral Histology and Physiology*. Oxford: Wiley Blackwell, pp.1–12.

HEE (Health Education England) (2015) *Shape of Caring: A Review of the Future Education and Training of Registered Nurses and Care Assistants*. Available at: https://www.hee.nhs.uk/sites/default/files/documents/2348-Shape-of-caring-review-FINAL.pdf

HEE (2016) *Mouth Care Matters: A Guide for Hospital Healthcare Professionals*. Available at: www.mouthcarematters.hee.nhs.uk/wp-content/uploads/2019/04/MCM-GUIDE-2016_100pp_OCT-16_v121.pdf (Figure 9.10 is created and owned by Public Health England: www.mouthcarematters.hee.nhs.uk)

HEE (n.d.) *Mouth Care Pack*. Available at: www.mouthcarematters.hee.nhs.uk/wp-content/uploads/2016/10/MCM_PACK_KB_V4_sp.pdf

Hewson, V. & Lee, A. (2017) Addressing the oral health needs of older people in care. *Nursing & Residential Care*, 19(1), 23–28.

Hirshkowitz, M., Whiton, K., Albert, S.M., et al. (2015) National Sleep Foundation's sleep time duration recommendations: Methodology and results summary. *Sleep Health*, 1(1), 40–43.

Hoey, L.M., Fulbrook, P. & Douglas, J.A. (2014) Sleep assessment of hospitalised patients: A literature review. *International Journal of Nursing Studies*, 51, 1281–1288.

Homb, K.A., Wu, H., Tarima, S. & Wang, D. (2014) Improvement of radiation-induced xerostomia with acupuncture: A retrospective analysis. *Acupuncture & Related Therapies*, 2(2), 34–38.

Honkavuo, L. (2018) Nurses' experiences of supporting sleep in hospitals: A hermeneutical study. *International Journal of Caring Studies*, 11(1), 4–10.

Hua, F., Xie, H., Worthington, H.V., et al. (2016) Oral hygiene care for critically ill patients to prevent ventilator-associated pneumonia. *Cochrane Database of Systematic Reviews*, 10, CD008367.

Human Rights Act (1998) Available at: https://www.legislation.gov.uk/ukpga/1998/42/contents

Hussain, S.H.H., Limthongkul, B., & Humphreys, T. (2013) The biomechanical properties of the skin. *Dermatologic Surgery*, 39, 193–213.

Jablonski, R.A. (2012) Oral health and hygiene content in nursing fundamentals textbooks. *Nursing Research and Practice*, 2012, 1–7.

James, P., Worthington, H., Parnell, C., et al. (2017) Chlorhexidine mouthrinse as an adjunctive treatment for gingival health. *Cochrane Database of Systematic Reviews*, 3(3), CD008676.

Jawad, H., Hodson, N.A. & Nixon, P.J. (2015) A review of dental treatment of head and neck cancer patients, before, during and after radiotherapy: Part 2. *British Dental Journal*, 218(2), 69–74.

Johnson, T.M., Worthington, H.V., Clarkson, J.E., et al. (2015) Mechanical interdental cleaning for preventing and controlling periodontal diseases and dental caries (protocol). *Cochrane Database of Systematic Reviews*, 12, CD012018.

Jolkovsky, D. & Lyle, D.M. (2015) Safety of a water flosser: A literature review. *Compendium of Continuing Education in Dentistry*, 36(2), 146–149.

Jones, M.L. (2014) Personal hygiene 3.2: Anatomy and physiology (A&P) of the skin. *British Journal of Healthcare Assistants*, 8(8), 374–376.

Kim, J.O. & Kim, N.C. (2014) Effects of 4% hypertonic saline solution mouthwash on oral health of elders in long term facilities. *Journal of Korean Academy of Nursing*, 44(1), 13–20.

King, T. & Callaghan, T. (2011) Basic nail care: To cut or not to cut. *British Journal of Health Care Assistants*, 5(2), 86–88.

Knight, J., Wigham, C. & Nigam, Y. (2017) Anatomy and physiology of ageing 6: The eyes and ears. *Nursing Times*, 113(7), 39–42.

Kottner, J., Lichterfeld, A. & Blume-Peytavi, U. (2013) Maintaining skin integrity in the aged: A systematic review. *British Journal of Dermatology*, 169, 528–542.

Kozier, B., Erb, G., Berman, A., et al. (2008) Beard and moustache care. In: *Fundamentals of Nursing: Concepts, Process and Practice*. London: Pearson Educational, pp.285–290.

Lakhani, S. (2018a) *Patient Information Leaflet: Care of Your Rigid Gas Permeable Contact Lenses*. Moorfields Eye Hospital NHS Foundation Trust. Available at: https://www.moorfields.nhs.uk/sites/default/files/Care%20of%20your%20rigid%20gas%20permeable%20%28RGP%29%20contact%20lenses.pdf

Lakhani, S. (2018b) *Patient Information Leaflet: Care of Your Soft Contact Lenses*. Moorfields Eye Hospital NHS Foundation Trust. Available at: www.moorfields.nhs.uk/sites/default/files/Care%20of%20your%20soft%20contact%20lenses.pdf

Leaker, S.H. (2013) The role of nutrition in preventing pressure ulcers. *Nursing Standard*, 28(7), 66–70.

Lee, A. (2015) The angle and aqueous. In: Marsden, J. (ed) *Ophthalmic Care*. Hoboken, NJ: John Wiley & Sons, pp.443–440.

Leroy, R. & Declerck, D. (2013) Objective and subjective oral health care needs among adults with various disabilities. *Clinical Oral Investigations*, 17, 1869–1878.

Lichterfeld, A., Hauss, A., Surber, C., et al. (2015) Evidence-based skin care: A systematic literature review and the development of a basic skin care algorithm. *Journal of Wound, Ostomy and Continence Nursing*, 42(5), 501–524.

Lin, J.B., Tsubota, K. & Apte, R.S. (2016) A glimpse at the aging eye. *NPJ Aging and Mechanisms of Disease*, 2(16003), 1–7.

Litton, E., Carnagie, V., Elliot, R. & Webb, S. (2016) The efficacy of earplugs as a sleep hygiene strategy for reducing delirium in the ICU: A systematic review and meta-analysis. *Critical Care Medicine*, 44(5), 992–999.

Lloyd Jones, M. (2014) Bed bathing [illegible]. *British Journal of Healthcare Assistants*, 8(10), 476–478.

Long, B.W., Rollins, J.H. & Smith, B.J. (2016) [illegible]. In: *Merrill's Atlas of Radiographic Positioning and Procedures*. St Louis, MO: Elsevier Mosby, pp.57–68.

Lopes, J.L., Nogueira, L.A. & Barros, A.L.B.L. (2013) Bed and shower baths: Comparing the perceptions of patients with acute myocardial infarction. *Journal of Clinical Nursing*, 22(5/6), 733–740.

Loveday, H.P., Wilson, J.A., Pratt, R.J., et al. (2014) Epic3: National evidence-based guidelines for preventing healthcare-associated infections in NHS hospitals in England. *Journal of Hospital Infection*, 8651, S1–S70.

Lynn, P. (ed) (2018) *Clinical Nursing Skills. A Nursing Process Approach*, 5th edn. Philadelphia: Lippincott Williams & Wilkins / Wolters Kluwer.

Mann, J. & Doshi, M. (2017) An investigation into denture loss in hospitals in Kent and Sussex. *British Dental Journal*, 223, 435–438.

Marieb, E.W. & Keller, S.M. (2017) *Essentials of Human Anatomy & Physiology*, 12th edn. Harlow: Pearson Education.

Marks, J.G. Jr. & Miller, J.J. (2013) Structure and function of the skin. In: *Lookingbill & Marks' Principles of Dermatology*, 5th edn. Philadelphia: Saunders, pp.2–10.

Marsden, J. (2015) How to examine an eye. *Nursing Standard*, 30(13), 34–37.

Marsden, J. (2016) How to perform irrigation of the eye. *Nursing Standard*, 30(23), 36–39.

Marsden, J. (2017) Preserving vision and promoting visual health in older people. *Nursing Older People*, 29(6), 22–26.

Martin, E.T., Haider, S., Palleschi, M., et al. (2017) Bathing hospitalized dependent patients with prepackaged disposable washcloths instead of traditional bath basins: A case-crossover study. *American Journal of Infection Control*, 45(9), 990–994.

Maurer, M., Rietzler, M., Burghardt, R. & Siebenhaar, F. (2016) The male beard and facial skin: Challenges of shaving. *International Journal of Cosmetic Surgery*, 38(Suppl. 1), 3–9.

McClimens, A., Brennan, S. & Hargreaves, P. (2014) Hearing problems in the learning disability population: Is anybody listening? *British Journal of Learning Disabilities*, 43(3), 153–160.

McGoldrick, M. (2016) Reducing the risk of infection when using a bath basin. *Home Healthcare Now*, 34(6), 339.

McGuire, D.B., Fulton, J.S., Park, J., et al. (2013) Systematic review of basic oral care for the management of oral mucositis in cancer patients. *Supportive Care in Cancer*, 21(11), 3165–3177.

Melsen, W.G., Rovers, M.M., Groenwold, R.H.H., et al. (2013) Attributable mortality of ventilator-associated pneumonia: A meta-analysis of individual patient data from randomised prevention studies. *Lancet Infectious Diseases*, 13(8), 665–671.

Mendes, A. (2010) Personal beliefs, culture and religion in community nursing care. *British Journal of Community Nursing*, 23(1), 46–47.

Mental Capacity Act (2005) Available at: https://www.legislation.gov.uk/ukpga/2005/9/contents

MHRA (Medicines and Healthcare products Regulatory Agency) (2012) *Medical Device Alert: Oral Swabs with a Foam Head*. Available at: https://www.gov.uk/drug-device-alerts/medical-device-alert-oral-swabs-with-a-foam-head-heads-may-detach-during-use

Mills, L. (2017) *Ear Wax Removal & Tinnitus*. British Tinnitus Association. Available at: https://www.tinnitus.org.uk/ear-wax

Millward, K. (2017a) Ear care: An update for nurses (part 1). *Practice Nursing*, 28(4), 154–160.

Millward, K. (2017b) Ear care: An update for nurses (part 2). *Practice Nursing*, 28(8), 332–337.

Moakes, H. (2012) An overview of foot ulceration in older people with diabetes. *Nursing Older People*, 24(7), 14–19.

Moncrieff, G., Cork, M., Lawton, S., et al. (2013) Use of emollients in dry-skin conditions: Consensus statement. *Clinical and Experimental Dermatology*, 38, 231–238.

Moore, T. & Cunningham, S. (eds) (2017) *Clinical Skills for Nursing Practice*. Oxford: Routledge.

Moorfields Eye Hospital (2019) *Acanthamoeba Keratitis*. Available at: https://www.moorfields.nhs.uk/condition/acanthamoeba-keratitis

Morrison, K.B. & Korol, A. (2014) Nurses' perceived and actual caregiving roles: Identifying factors that can contribute to job satisfaction. *Journal of Clinical Nursing*, 23, 3468–3477.

MRI Questions (2018) [illegible]. Available at: http://mriquestions.com/ocular.html

[illegible] & Taylor, E.J. (2016) [illegible] Muslim women: Implications for nursing care. *MEDSURG Nursing*, 25(3), 169–172.

National Academies of Sciences, Engineering, and Medicine; Health and Medicine Division; Board on Population Health and Public Health Practice; Committee on Public Health Approaches to Reduce Vision Impairment and Promote Eye Health; Welp, A., Woodbury, R.B., McCoy, M.A., et al. (eds) (2016) *Making Eye Health a Population Health Imperative: Vision for Tomorrow*. National Academies Press. Available at: https://www.ncbi.nlm.nih.gov/books/NBK385157

National Institute of Neurological Disorders and Stroke (2017) *Brain Basics: Understanding Sleep*. Available at: https://www.ninds.nih.gov/Disorders/Patient-Caregiver-Education/Understanding-Sleep

NHS Direct Wales (2015) *Hearing Tests*. Available at: www.nhsdirect.wales.nhs.uk/encyclopaedia/h/article/hearingtests

NHS England (2017a) *Involving People in Their Own Health and Care: Statutory Guidance for Clinical Commissioning Groups and NHS England*. Available at: https://www.england.nhs.uk/publication/involving-people-in-their-own-health-and-care-statutory-guidance-for-clinical-commissioning-groups-and-nhs-england

NHS England (2017b) *What Works: Hearing Loss and Health Ageing*. Available at: https://www.england.nhs.uk/wp-content/uploads/2017/09/hearing-loss-what-works-guide-healthy-ageing.pdf

NHS England (2018) *70 Days to End Pyjama Paralysis*. Available at: https://www.england.nhs.uk/2018/03/70-days-to-end-pyjama-paralysis

NHS HEE (Health Education England) (2016) *Mouth Care Matters: A Guide for Hospital Healthcare Professionals*. London: Health Education England.

NHS Inform Scotland (2019) *Vertigo*. Available at: https://www.nhsinform.scot/illnesses-and-conditions/ears-nose-and-throat/vertigo

NHS England and NHSI (NHS Improvement) (2019) *Standard Infection Control Precautions: National Hand Hygiene and Personal Protective Equipment Policy*. Available at: https://improvement.nhs.uk/documents/4957/National_policy_on_hand_hygiene_and_PPE_2.pdf

NICE (National Institute for Health and Care Excellence) (2014) *Pressure Ulcers: Prevention and Management: Clinical Guideline* [CG179]. Available at: nice.org.uk/guidance/cg179

NICE (2015a) *Pressure Ulcers: Quality Standard* [QS89]. Available at: nice.org.uk/guidance/qs89

NICE (2015b) *Diabetic Foot Problems: Prevention and Management* [NG19]. Available at: https://www.nice.org.uk/guidance/ng19

NICE (2016a) *Bunions*. London: National Institute for Health and Care Excellence.

NICE (2016b) *Oral Health for Adults in Care Homes* [NG 48]. London: National Institute for Health and Care Excellence.

NICE (2016c) *Palliative Care: Oral*. London: National Institute for Health and Care Excellence.

NICE (2018a) *Clinical Knowledge Summaries: Fungal Nail Infections*. Available at: http://cks.nice.org.uk/fungal-nail-infection

NICE (2018b) *Hearing Loss in Adults: Assessment and Management* [NG98]. Available at: https://www.nice.org.uk/guidance/ng98/chapter/Recommendations#removing-earwax

NICE (2018c) *Treatment of Dry Mouth*. Available at: https://bnf.nice.org.uk/treatment-summary/treatment-of-dry-mouth.html

NICE (2019) *Dental Practitioners' Formulary*. Available at: https://bnf.nice.org.uk/dental-practitioners-formulary

Nicol, M., Bavin, C., Cronin, P., et al. (2012) Patient hygiene. In: *Essential Nursing Skills*, 4th edn. London: Mosby Elsevier, pp.313–337.

Nightingale, F. (1860) *Notes on Nursing: What It Is and What It Is Not*. London: Harrison.

NMC (Nursing and Midwifery Council) (2018a) *The Code: Professional Standards of Practice and Behaviour for Nurses, Midwives and Nursing Associates*. Available at: https://www.nmc.org.uk/standards/code

NMC (2018b) *Delegation and Accountability: Supplementary Information to the NMC Code*. Available at: https://www.nmc.org.uk/globalassets/sitedocuments/nmc-publications/delegation-and-accountability-supplementary-information-to-the-nmc-code.pdf

O'Connor, L.J. (2016a) Oral health care. In: Boltz, M., Capezuti, E., Fulmer, T. & Zwicker, D. (eds) *Evidence-Based Geriatric Nursing: Protocols for Best Practice*, 5th edn. New York: Springer, pp.103–110.

O'Connor, O.P. (2016b) Hygiene. In: Potter, P.A., Perry, A.G. & Stockert, P. (eds) *Fundamentals of Nursing*, 9th edn. St Louis, MO: Elsevier, pp.821–870.

O'Hagan, S., Manias, E., Elder, C., et al. (2014) What counts as effective communication in nursing? Evidence from nurse educators' and clinicians' feedback on nurse interactions with simulated patients. *Journal of Advanced Nursing*, 70(6), 1344–1355.

Okonkwo, U.A. & DiPietro, L.A. (2017) Diabetes and wound angiogenesis. *International Journal of Molecular Sciences* 18(7), 1419.

O'Leary, C. & Birkbimer, D. (2016) Endocrine malignancies. In: Yarbro, C.H., Wujcik, D. & Gobel, B.H. (eds) *Cancer Nursing: Principles and Practice*, 8th edn. Burlington, MA: Jones & Bartlett, pp.1487–1514.

Oliver, D. (2017) Fighting pyjama paralysis in hospital wards. *BMJ*, 357, j2096.

Olver, J., Cassidy, L., Jutley, G. & Crawley, L. (2014) Correction of refractive errors. In: *Ophthalmology at a Glance*. Oxford: Wiley Blackwell, pp.28–31.

Overby-Canon, J. (2014) Care of a patient with a sensory disorder. In: Cooper, K. & Gosnell, K. (eds) *Foundations and Adult Health Nursing*, 7th edn. St Louis, MO: Elsevier, pp.1847–1894.

Ozdemir, D. (2013) Dental caries: The most common disease worldwide and preventive strategies. *International Journal of Biology*, 5(4), 55–61.

Padela, A.I., Gunter, K., Killawi, A. & Heisler, M. (2012) Religious values and healthcare accommodations: Voices from the American Muslim community. *Journal of General Internal Medicine*, 27(6), 708–715.

Peate, I. (2015) Washing a patient's hair in bed: A care fundamental. *British Journal of Health Care Assistants*, 9(3), 114–118.

Peate, I. (2018) Putting an end to pyjama paralysis: The benefits. *British Journal of Nursing*, 27(9), 471.

Peate, I. & Gault, C. (2013) Clinical skills series/6: Oral hygiene. *British Journal of Healthcare Assistants*, 7(7), 330–335.

Peate, I. & Lane, L. (2015) Bed bathing: How good cleaning turns into great care. *British Journal of Healthcare Assistants*, 9(4), [illegible].

Peate, I., Nair, M. & Wild, K. (2014) *Nursing Practice: Knowledge and Care*. Chichester: Wiley Blackwell.

Pegram, A. & Bloomfield, J. (2015) Infection prevention and control. *Nursing Standard*, 29(29), 37–42.

Peterson, D.E., Boers-Doets, C.B., Bensadoun, R.J. & Herrstedt, J. (2015) Management of oral and gastrointestinal mucosal injury: ESMO clinical practice guidelines for diagnosis, treatment and follow-up. *Annals of Oncology*, 26(Suppl. 5), v139–v151.

Petrovic, B.B., Peric, T.O., Markovic, D.L., et al. (2016) Unmet oral health needs among persons with intellectual disability. *Research in Developmental Disabilities*, 59, 370–377.

PHE (Public Health England) (2017) *Delivering Better Oral Health: An Evidence-Based Toolkit for Prevention*, 3rd edn. Available at: https://assets.publishing.service.gov.uk/government/uploads/system/uploads/attachment_data/file/605266/Delivering_better_oral_health.pdf

Phua, M.Y., Salmon, S., Straughan, P. & Fisher, D. (2016) Disposable single-use receptacles in a tertiary hospital: A large survey of staff after a hospital-wide implementation. *American Journal of Infection Control*, 44(9), 1041–1043.

Pickering, D. & Marsden, J. (2015) Techniques for aseptic dressing and procedures. *Community Eye Health*, 28(89), 17.

Pilkington, S. (2013) Causes and consequences of sleep deprivation in hospitalised patients. *Nursing Standard*, 27(49), 35–42.

Plemons, J.M., Al-Hashimi, I. & Marek, C.L. (2014) Managing xerostomia and salivary gland hypofunction: Executive summary of a report from the American Dental Association Council on Scientific Affairs. *American Dental Association Council on Scientific Affairs*, 145(8), 867–873.

Pols, J. (2013) Washing the patient: Dignity and aesthetic values in nursing care. *Nursing Philosophy*, 14(3), 186–200.

Potter, P.A., Perry, A.G., Stockert, P. & Hall, A.M. (eds) (2016) *Fundamentals of Nursing*, 9th edn. St Louis, MO: Elsevier.

Poulton, S., Yau, S., Anderson, D. & Bennett, D. (2015) Ear wax management. *Australian Family Physician*, 44(10), 731–734.

Powers, M.A., Bardsley, J.B., Cypress, M., et al. (2017) Diabetes self-management education and support in type 2 diabetes: A joint position statement of the American Diabetes Association, the American Association of Diabetes Educators, and the Academy of Nutrition and Dietetics. *Diabetes Educator*, 43(1), 40–53.

Radtke, K., Obermann, K. & Teymer, L. (2014) Nursing knowledge of physiological and psychological outcomes related to patient sleep deprivation in the acute care setting. *MEDSURG Nursing*, 23(3), 178–184.

Raizman, M.B., Hamrah, P., Holland, E.J., et al. (2017) Drug-induced corneal epithelial changes. *Survey of Ophthalmology*, 62(3), 286–301.

RCN (Royal College of Nursing) (2016) *The Nature, Scope and Value of Ophthalmic Nursing*. London: Royal College of Nursing.

RCN (2017) *Accountability and Delegation: A Guide for the Nursing Team*. Available at: https://www.rcn.org.uk/-/media/royal-college-of-nursing/documents/publications/2017/september/pub-006465.pdf

RCN (2019) *Catheter Care*. London: Royal College of Nursing.

RD-UK (2016) *Predicting and Managing Oral and Dental Complications of Surgical and Non-surgical Treatment for Head and Neck Cancer: A Clinical Guideline*. Available at: www.restdent.org.uk/uploads/RD-UK%20H%20and%20N%20guideline.pdf

Rebeiro, G., Jack, L., Scully, N. & Wilson, D. (2013) Skill 34–1: Bathing a patient. In: *Fundamentals of Nursing: Clinical Skills Workbook*, 2nd edn. Sydney: Elsevier, pp.164–169.

Rehman, U., Mahabadi, N. & Patel, B.C. (2018) Anatomy, head, eye. In: *StatPearls*. Available at: https://www.ncbi.nlm.nih.gov/books/NBK482428

Riley, E. (2018) The importance of oral health in palliative care patients. *Journal of Community Nursing*, 32(3), 57–61.

Roberts, H.S. & Lawrence S.M. (2017) CE: Venous thromboembolism. *American Journal of Nursing*, 117(5), 38–47.

Royal College of Surgeons (2017) *Improving Older People's Oral Health*. Available at: https://www.rcseng.ac.uk/-/media/files/rcs/fds/media-gov/fds-improving-older-peoples-oral-health-2017.pdf

RPECCAS (Rotherham Primary Ear Care Centre and Audiology Services) (2016) *Ear Irrigation Guideline*. Available at: www.earcarecentre.com/uploadedFiles/Pages/Health_Professionals/Protocols/Ear%20irrigation%20Guideline.pdf

Salzmann-Erikson, M., [illegible] (2016) Keep calm and have a good night: Nurses' strategies to improve inpatients' sleep in the hospital environment. *Scandinavian Journal of Caring Sciences*, 30(2), 356–364.

Saunders, D.P., Epstein, J.P., Elad, S., et al. (2013) Systematic review of antimicrobials, mucosal coating agents, anesthetics, and analgesics for the management of oral mucositis in cancer patients. *Supportive Care in Cancer*, 21(11), 3191–3207.

Schwartz, S.R., Magit, A.E., Rosenfeld, R.M., et al. (2017) Clinical practice guideline (update): Earwax (cerumen impaction). *Otolaryngology: Head and Neck Surgery*, 156(1), S1–S29.

Septimus, M.L. & Schweizer, M.L. (2016) Decolonization in prevention of health care-associated infections. *Clinical Microbiology Reviews*, 29(2), 201–222.

Seray-Wurie, M. (2017) Personal care. In: Moore, T. & Cunningham, S. (eds) *Clinical Skills for Nursing Practice*. Oxford: Routledge, pp.47–72.

Sevy, J.O. & Singh, A. (2017) Cerumen impaction. In: *StatPearls*. Available at: https://www.ncbi.nlm.nih.gov/books/NBK448155

Shaw, M. (2016) How to administer eye drops and eye ointment. *Nursing Standard*, 30(39), 34–36.

Shaw, M.E. (2017) Examination of the eye. In: Marsden, J. (ed) *Ophthalmic Care*. Cumbria: M&K Publishing, pp.71–92.

Shaw, M.E. & Lee, A. (2016a) The ophthalmic nurse. In: Shaw, M.E. & Lee, A. (eds) *Ophthalmic Nursing*, 5th edn. Boca Raton, FL: CRC Press, pp.5–18.

Shaw, M.E. & Lee, A. (2016b) The globe: A brief overview. In: Shaw, M.E. & Lee, A. (eds) *Ophthalmic Nursing*, 5th edn. Boca Raton, FL: CRC Press, pp.89–92.

Shaw, M.E. & Lee, A. (2016c) The protective structures, including removal of an eye. In: Shaw, M.E. & Lee, A. (eds) *Ophthalmic Nursing*, 5th edn. Boca Raton, FL: CRC Press, pp. 93–114.

Slominski, A.T., Zmijewski, M.A., Skobowiat, C., et al. (2012) Introduction. In: *Sensing the Environment: Regulation of Local and Global Homeostasis by the Skin's Neuroendocrine System*. Berlin: Springer, pp.1–6.

Smith, F.D. (2016) Caring for surgical patients with piercings 2.2. *AORN Journal*, 103(6), 583–596.

Soliman, A. & Brogan, M. (2016) Foot assessment and care for older people. *Nursing Times*, 110(50), 12–15.

Spencer, A. (2016) Bathing and personal hygiene. In: Perry, A.G., Potter, P. & Ostendorf, W.R. (eds) *Nursing Interventions & Clinical Skills*, 6th edn. St Louis, MO: Elsevier, pp.243–269.

Steel, B.J. (2017) Oral hygiene and mouth care for older people in acute hospitals: Part 2. *Nursing Older People*, 29(10), 20–25.

Stevens, S. (2013) Management of an eye prosthesis or conformer. *Community Eye Health*, 26(81), 16.

Stevens, S. (2016) Cleaning and dressing the eye after surgery. *Community Eye Health*, 29(94), 36.

Stockert, P. (2017) Health assessment and physical examination. In: Potter, P.A., Stockert, P.A., Perry, A.G. & Hall, A.M. (eds) *Fundamentals of Nursing*. St Louis, MO: Elsevier, pp.533–608.

Swamiappan, M. (2016) Anogenital pruritus: An overview. *Journal of Clinical and Diagnostic Research*, 10(4), WE01–WE03.

Tamarat, R., Huynh-Le, M. & Goyal, M. (2014) Non-pharmacologic interventions to improve the sleep of hospitalized patients: A systematic review. *Journal of General Internal Medicine*, 29(5), 788–795.

Tan, X., Egmond, L., Partinen, M., et al. (2018) A narrative review of interventions for improving sleep and reducing circadian disruption in medical inpatients. *Sleep Medicine*, 59, 42–50.

Tierno, P. (2017) *Changing the Bed Linens in Sickness and in Health*. Available at: https://cdifffoundation.org/2017/07/18/changing-the-bed-linens-in-sickness-and-in-health

Tobiano, G., Bucknall, T., Marshall, A., et al. (2015) Nurses' views of patient participation in nursing care. *Journal of Advanced Nursing*, 71(12), 2741–2752.

Tollefson, J. & Hillman, E. (2016) Medication administration: Eye drops or ointment. In: *Clinical Psychomotor Skills: Assessment Tools for Nurses*, 6th edn. Melbourne: Cengage Learning, pp.156–160.

Tortora, G.J. & Derrickson, B.H. (2017) *Principles of Anatomy & Physiology*, 15th edn. Hoboken, NJ: John Wiley & Sons.

Travis, L. (2014) Hygiene and care of the patient's environment. In: Cooper, K. & Gosnell, K. (eds) *Foundations and Adult Health Nursing*, 7th edn. St Louis, MO: Elsevier, pp.185–227.

Treas, L.S. & Wilkinson, J.M. (2014) Hygiene. In: *Basic Nursing: Concepts, Skills & Reasoning*. Philadelphia: F.A. Davis, pp.683–743.

Turns, M. (2015) Prevention and management of diabetic foot ulcers. *British Journal of Community Wound Care*, 20(Suppl. 3), S30, S32, S34–S37.

Tzu-Ying, Y.W., Willcox, M., Zhu, H. & Stapleton, F. (2015) Contact lens hygiene compliance and lens case contamination: A review. *Contact Lens & Anterior Eye*, 38(5), 307–316.

UK Medicines Information (2015) *Saliva Substitutes: Choosing and Prescribing the Right Product*. Available at: https://www.sps.nhs.uk/wp-content/uploads/2015/07/NW-QA190.8-Saliva-substitutes-.pdf

UKOMiC (UK Oral Management in Cancer Care Group) (2019) *Oral Care Guidance and Support in Cancer and Palliative Care*, 3rd edn. Available at: http://www.ukomic.co.uk/guidelines.html

Valizadeh, L., Avazeh, M., Hosseini, M. & Jafarabad, M. (2014) Comparison of clustered care with three and four procedures on physiological responses of preterm infants: Randomized crossover clinical trial. *Journal of Caring Sciences*, 3(1), 1–10.

Veitz-Keenan, A. & Ferraiolo, D.M. (2017) Oral care with chlorhexidine seems effective for reducing the incidence of ventilator-associated pneumonia. *Evidence-Based Dentistry*, 18(4), 113–114.

Voegeli, D. (2012a) Managing hygiene. In: Bullock, I. & Rycroft-Malone, J. (eds) *Adult Nursing Practice: Use Evidence in Care*. Oxford: Oxford University Press, pp.343–357.

Voegeli, D. (2012b) Understanding the main principles of skin care in older adults. *Nursing Standard*, 27(11), 59–68.

Watkins, J. (2015) Understanding and diagnosing nail infections. *Practice Nursing*, 26(3), 134–139.

WHO (World Health Organization) (2018) *Oral Health Information Sheet*. Available at: https://www.who.int/news-room/fact-sheets/detail/oral-health

Windle, P.E. (2014) Personal hygiene and bed making. In Perry, A.G., Potter, P.A. & Ostendorf, W.R. (eds) *Clinical Nursing Skills and Techniques*, 8th edn. St Louis, MO: Elsevier Mosby, pp.391–432.

Wolfensberger, A., Clack, L., Kuster, S.P., et al. (2018) Transfer of pathogens to and from patients, healthcare providers, and medical devices during care activity: A systematic review and meta-analysis. *Infection Control & Hospital Epidemiology*, 39(9), 1093–1107.

Woo, K.Y., Beeckman, D. & Chakravarthy, D. (2017) Management of moisture-associated skin damage: A scoping review. *Advances in Skin & Wound Care*, 30(11), 494–501.

Wright, T. (2015) Ear wax. *BMJ Clinical Evidence*, 351, h3601.

Young, M. (2018) Medical device-related pressure ulcers: A clear case of iatrogenic harm. *British Journal of Nursing*, 27(15 Suppl.), S6–S12.

Chapter 10

Pain assessment and management

Suzanne Chapman with Farzana Carvalho and Caroline Dinen

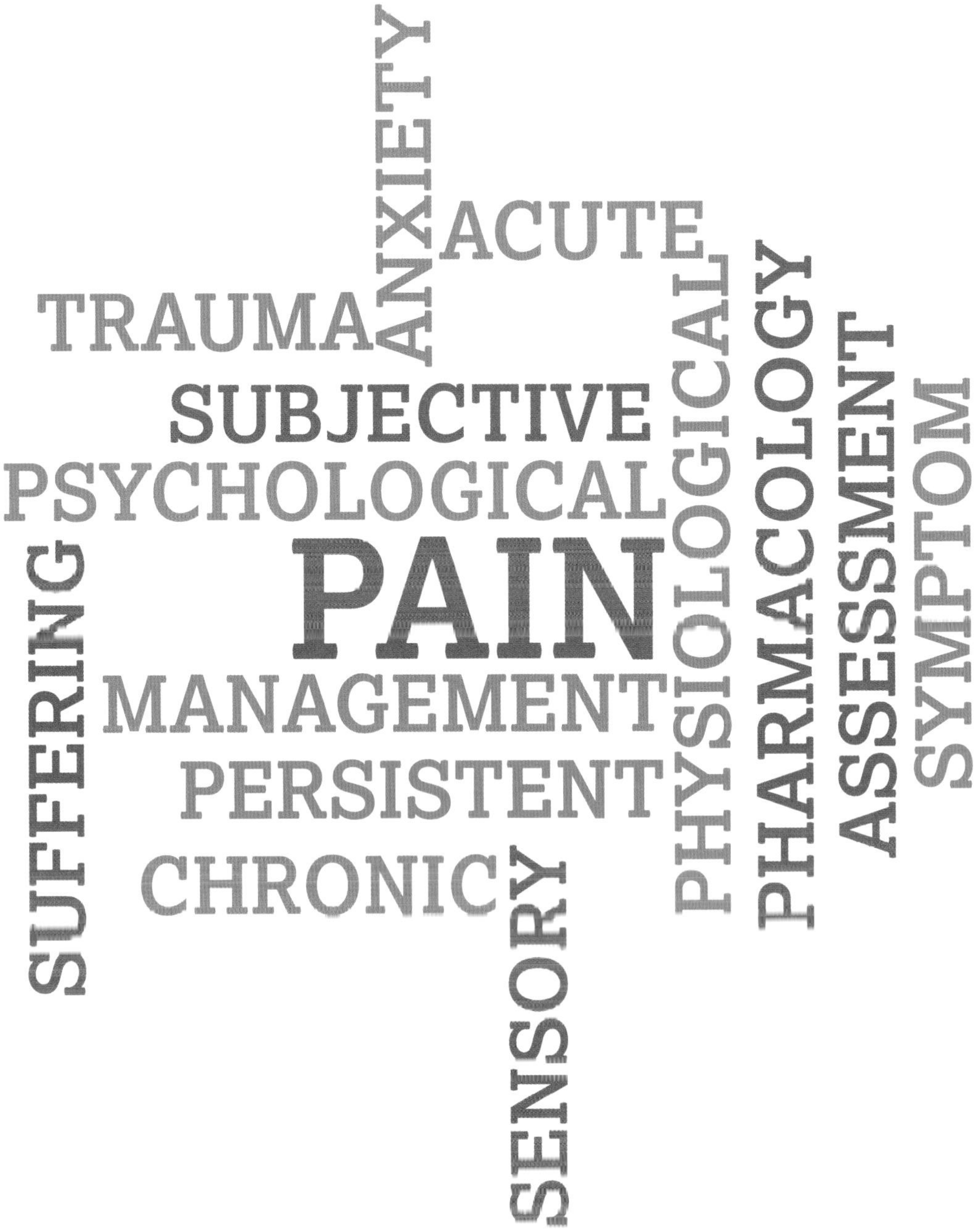

The Royal Marsden Manual of Clinical Nursing Procedures: Professional Edition, Tenth Edition. Edited by Sara Lister, Justine Hofland and Hayley Gratton.

Procedure guidelines

Overview

Pain is a symptom that is often experienced by patients seeking healthcare. It can be the presenting symptom that prompts patients to seek medical attention, initiating the first contact with healthcare professionals.

Pain can be experienced suddenly and unexpectedly as a result of acute conditions such as trauma, acute illness or surgery. This is referred to as acute pain.

Pain can also be experienced as a result of longer-term conditions such as osteoarthritis, rheumatoid arthritis, low back pain and sciatica, headaches or migraines, endometriosis, or irritable bowel syndrome. Pain may also be present in the absence of a diagnosis or identifiable cause. In these conditions, pain is often referred to as chronic, persistent or long term.

Pain is a complex subjective multidimensional experience. Effective assessment and management of pain can relieve suffering and can help to reduce patient anxiety associated with pain. While technological advances in other areas of nursing continue to refine the assessment and management of patients, to assess and manage pain effectively nurses will be required to utilize knowledge, interviewing skills and physical assessment skills due to the subjective nature of pain and pain assessment.

This chapter focuses on definitions of pain, anatomy and physiology related to pain, pain assessment, and pharmacological and non-pharmacological approaches to pain management. It focuses primarily on acute and chronic pain. For the comprehensive management of cancer pain, see the chapter on pain assessment and management in *The Royal Marsden Manual of Cancer Nursing Procedures* (Lister et al. 2019).

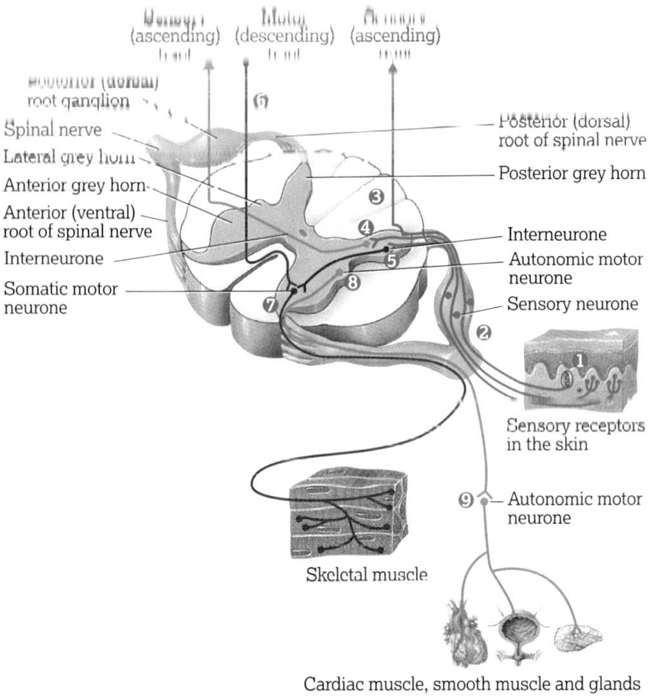

Figure 10.1 Processing of sensory input and motor output by the spinal cord. *Source*: Reproduced from Tortora and Derrickson (2017) with permission of John Wiley & Sons.

Pain

Definition

Pain is a complex phenomenon that has physiological (biological), psychological and social factors that influence the individual patient's experience. It is subjective, so it is important to understand the patient's perspective. It has both physical and affective (emotional) components. Pain is an emotion experienced in the brain; it is not like touch, taste, sight, smell or hearing. It is categorized into acute pain (less than 12 weeks' duration) and chronic pain (more than 12 weeks' duration). Pain can be perceived as a warning of potential damage, but it can also be present when no actual harm is being done to the body (British Pain Society 2014).

To reflect this, the International Association for the Study of Pain (IASP 1994) published the following definition of pain: 'an unpleasant sensory and emotional experience associated with actual or potential tissue damage, or described in terms of such damage'. As pain is subjective, another favoured definition for use in clinical practice, proposed originally by McCaffery (1968, p.95), is: 'Pain is whatever the experiencing person says it is, existing whenever the experiencing person says it does.'

In each individual, the 'pain experience' will be a result of the interaction of biological, psychological, environmental and social factors. Nurses are therefore encouraged to adopt an integrated, multidisciplinary approach to management that also considers patients' preferences and prior experience (Schug et al. 2015).

Anatomy and physiology

Pain mechanisms (anatomy and physiology) are usually described in terms of nociceptive pain or neuropathic pain. As with acute and chronic pain, it may be common for pain to be both nociceptive and neuropathic in origin rather than purely one or the other.

Nociceptive pain

Nociceptive pain is the 'normal' pain pathway that occurs in response to tissue injury or damage. Figure 10.1 demonstrates the normal pathway for sensory input and motor output through the spinal cord. As an example, if a person touches a hot plate, this causes pain and this sensory input travels through the spinal cord to the brain and the motor output. In response, the person withdraws their hand from the painful heat source.

The pain pathway consists of four components: transduction, transmission, perception and modulation. Nociceptors are free nerve endings found at the end of pain neurones. Nociceptive primary afferents are widely distributed throughout the body (skin, muscle, joints, viscera and meninges) and comprise both medium-diameter lightly myelinated A delta fibres and small-diameter, slow-conducting unmyelinated C fibres (Schug et al. 2015). Nociceptors respond to noxious thermal stimuli (heat and cold) and mechanical stimuli (stretching, compression and infiltration) and to the chemical mediators released as part of the inflammatory response to tissue injury (Steeds 2016). These chemical mediators include prostaglandins, bradykinin, histamine, hydrogen ions (protons), 5-hydroxytryptamine (5-HT), cytokines and leukotrienes (Steeds 2016). As a result of this stimulation process, an action potential is generated in the nerve (*transduction*).

The pain signal is then transmitted along the peripheral nervous system (A delta and C fibres) to the central nervous system, arriving at the dorsal horn of the spinal cord. Neurotransmitters are released to allow the pain signal to be transmitted from the endings of the peripheral nerves to the receptors in the dorsal horn and onwards through the central nervous system. These include substance P, galanin, glutamate, GABA (γ-aminobutyric acid), cholecystokinin and others (Steeds 2016). The message is then transmitted to the brain, where perception of the pain occurs (*transmission*). *Perception* is the end result of the neuronal activity of pain transmission. The perception of pain includes behavioural, psychological and emotional components as well as physiological processes.

Modulation occurs when the transmission of pain impulses in the spinal cord is changed or inhibited. Modulatory influences on pain perception are complex, involving a gating system that is linked to a descending modulatory pathway. Modulation can occur as a result of a natural release of inhibitory neurotransmitter chemicals (noradrenaline and 5-HT) that inhibit transmission of pain impulses and therefore produce analgesia. Other interventions, including distraction, relaxation, sense of wellbeing, heat and cold

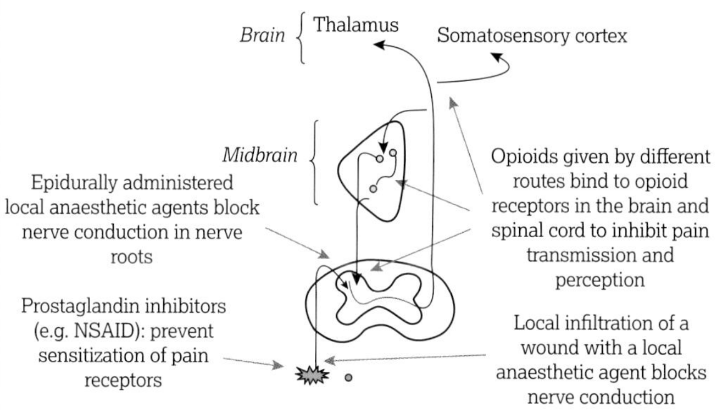

Figure 10.2 The pain pathway, showing key sites for particular analgesic interventions.

therapy, massage and TENS, can also help to modulate pain perception. Analgesic medications work by inhibiting some of the chemicals involved in pain transduction and transmission and thus modulating pain perception (Figure 10.2). Pain signals can also be increased by certain factors such as anxiety, fear, and low mood or depression.

Neuropathic pain

Neuropathic pain is not pain that originates as part of 'normal' pain pathways. It has been described as pain related to abnormal processing within the nervous system. Although distinct definitions of neuropathic pain have been used over the years, its most recent and widely accepted definition is pain or abnormal sensation caused by a primary lesion or disease of the nervous system (Colloca et al. 2017). This can consist of motor, sensory or autonomic dysfunction (Steeds 2016).

The somatosensory system allows for the perception of touch, pressure, pain, temperature, position, movement and vibration. The somatosensory nerves arise in the skin, muscles, joints and fascia and include thermoreceptors, mechanoreceptors, chemoreceptors, pruriceptors and nociceptors, which send signals to the spinal cord and eventually to the brain for further processing. Lesions or diseases of the somatosensory nervous system can lead to altered and disordered transmission of sensory signals into the spinal cord and the brain (Colloca et al. 2017).

Common conditions associated with neuropathic pain include postherpetic neuralgia, trigeminal neuralgia, painful radiculopathy, diabetic neuropathy, HIV infection, leprosy, amputation, peripheral nerve injury pain, stroke (in the form of central post-stroke pain), trauma (such as surgery or acute injury), and nerve compression or infiltration (such as degenerative joint and spinal disease or tumours) (Colloca et al. 2017, Mann 2009).

The following theories are currently thought to explain the mechanisms by which neuropathic pain is generated and maintained (Baron et al. 2010, Nickel et al. 2012):

- Damage or abnormalities in the nerves change the way that nerves communicate with each other.
- Pain receptors require less stimulation to initiate pain signals both in the peripheral nerves and in the central nervous system; this is often referred to as 'central sensitization'.
- Pain transmission is altered from its normal sequence.
- There may be an increase in the release of chemical neurotransmitters.
- There can be increased and chaotic firing of nerves.
- Damaged nerves spontaneously generate impulses in the absence of any stimulation.
- The descending inhibitory systems may be reduced or lost.

The nervous system changes its structure and function in response to the input it receives – in other words, it is plastic. Plasticity is evident at all levels from the nociceptors to the brain (cortex). These mechanisms result in increased activity or transmission of pain signals despite less input from the peripheral nervous system. Pain may be spontaneous, may be triggered by non-painful stimuli such as touch (allodynia) or may consist of an exaggerated pain response (hyperalgesia). Patients may also experience non-painful sensations such as pins and needles and tingling (paraesthesia).

Related theory

Many factors influence the expression of pain; these may be associated with the patient, the nurse or the clinical environment. Pain can have many dimensions, including physical/biological, psychological, spiritual and sociocultural.

Pain can be described in the following ways:

- acute pain
- chronic (or persistent) pain
- referred pain
- cancer pain.

There are several ways to categorize the types of pain that occur – for example, nociceptive (somatic or visceral) or neuropathic. It is increasingly recognized that acute and chronic pain may represent a continuum rather than being distinct, separate entities (Macintyre and Schug 2015) and may combine different pain mechanisms and vary in duration.

There may be wide variation in the way that individuals experience pain and the meanings they attribute to it. The perception of pain can be influenced by many things, including (Mann 2009):

- the *meaning* of the pain (does the patient know the cause or are they still waiting for it to be explained?)
- the *significance* of the pain (does it represent a significant, life-changing or life-threatening event for the patient?)
- whether the pain was *expected* (did the patient have time to prepare themselves for it?)
- whether the patient can *distract* themselves and what else is going on around them (e.g. pain is often reported as worse at night due to the lack of distracting stimulation)
- the patient's *cultural or family background* (do they openly express and discuss their pain, or do they maintain control with minimal expression of pain?)
- the patient's *spiritual faith* (a strong belief system may enable some people to endure pain and discomfort with calm and serenity).

Acute pain

Acute pain is short-term pain of less than 12 weeks' duration (British Pain Society 2014). Acute pain serves a purpose by alerting the individual to a problem and acting as a warning of tissue damage or potential tissue damage. If left untreated, it may result in severe consequences; for example, not seeking help for acute abdominal pain may result in an emergency, such as appendicitis progressing to peritonitis. Acute pain occurs in response to any type of injury to the body and resolves when the injury heals.

Common causes of acute pain include:

- surgery (e.g. upper or lower abdominal surgery, colorectal surgery, gynaecological surgery, appendicectomy or orthopaedic surgery)
- acute trauma (e.g. work-related injuries, road traffic accidents, sports injuries, head injury, spinal and neck injuries, and burns or scalds)
- acute musculoskeletal pain (e.g. acute low back pain or acute joint pain)
- procedural pain or incident pain (e.g. related to a painful procedure such as venepuncture or insertion of a catheter or drain, or pain as a consequence of a movement or an event, e.g. defaecation after anal surgery or ischaemic leg pain associated with intermittent claudication on walking)
- acute visceral pain (e.g. ischaemic heart disease, pancreatitis, cholecystitis, ulcerative colitis, Crohn's disease or cystitis).

Chronic pain

Chronic pain is defined as persistent or recurrent pain lasting longer than 12 weeks (Treede et al. 2019). It is often associated with major changes in personality, lifestyle and functional ability (Orenius et al. 2013).

Chronic pain disorders can be categorized into the following seven groups (Treede et al. 2019):

- chronic primary pain
- chronic cancer pain
- chronic post-traumatic and post-surgical pain
- chronic neuropathic pain
- chronic headache and orofacial pain
- chronic visceral pain
- chronic musculoskeletal pain.

Chronic pain is often associated with significant emotional distress and functional disability. It can be associated with many different types of disease processes and tissue injuries. Pain has a significant impact on individuals and their family, affecting mood, sleep, mobility, role within the family, ability to work and other aspects of life (NICE 2018).

Referred pain

In many instances of visceral pain, the pain is either perceived deep within the skin that overlies the affected organ or experienced at a location distant from the site of the painful stimulus or organ; the latter is known as referred pain (Tortora and Derrickson 2017). One explanation for the phenomenon of referred pain is that the visceral organ involved and the area to which the pain is referred are served by the same segment of the spinal cord, and the sensory fibres enter the spinal cord at the same level. Referred pain is presumed to occur because the information from multiple nociceptor afferents converges onto individual spinothalamic tract neurons, and the brain therefore interprets the information coming from visceral receptors as having arisen from receptors on the body surface, since this is where nociceptive stimuli originate most frequently. Examples of referred pain include pain in the left arm during a myocardial infarction, pain from pancreatic pathology experienced as pain in the back, and pain from irritation of the diaphragm experienced as shoulder tip pain (see Figure 10.3).

Cancer pain management

Pain is a common symptom in patients with cancer (Chapman 2012). Causes of cancer pain can be multifactorial and often are related to the effects of cancer treatments such as surgery, radiotherapy, chemotherapy, hormone therapy or immunotherapy. In some instances, pain can be caused by the cancer itself, such as in patients with bone metastases or where the cancer has caused injury to nerves. Cancer pain has been reported as being present in a third of patients undergoing active anticancer treatment with a curative intent. It has also been suggested that patients who have treatment with curative intent or for palliation report pain prevalence rates of 39.3% after curative treatment, 55.0% during anti-cancer treatment, and 66.4% in advanced, metastatic or terminal disease (van den Beuken-van Everdingen et al. 2016). Cancer pain can be both acute and chronic and requires careful assessment and attention to detail, including a detailed history of previously tried medications and responses to these pharmacological interventions. Assessment, the treatment plan and reviews are key in the management of cancer pain, particularly as the nature and severity of pain can change rapidly in response to treatment or progression of the cancer itself. For the comprehensive management of cancer pain, see the chapter on pain assessment and management in *The Royal Marsden Manual of Cancer Nursing Procedures* (Lister et al. 2019).

Evidence-based approaches

The emphasis of this section will be based on acute and chronic pain management.

Rationale for effective acute pain control

The relief of acute pain is primarily a humanitarian matter, but effective pain management may also result in improved clinical outcomes and reduced complication rates (RCA 2017).

There are many short-term and long-term consequences of inadequately treated acute pain. These include hyperglycaemia, insulin resistance, increased risk of infection, decreased patient comfort

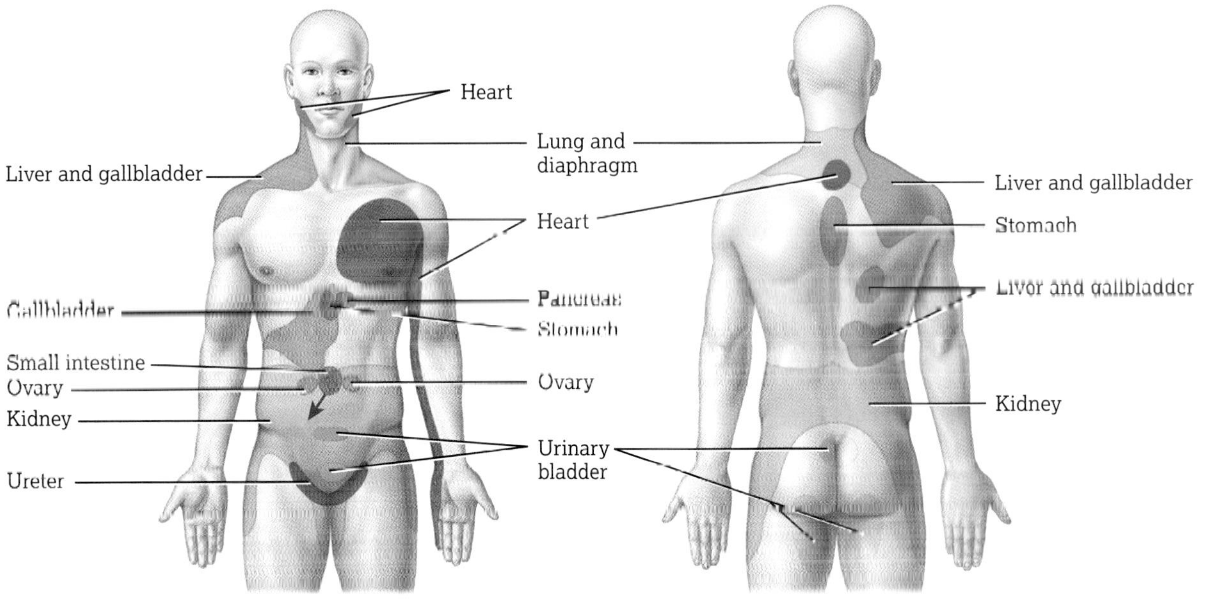

Figure 10.3 Distribution of referred pain. *Source*: Reproduced from Tortora and Derrickson (2017) with permission of John Wiley & Sons.

and satisfaction, and the development of chronic pain (Reardon et al. 2015). The transition of acute post-operative or post-traumatic pain to pathological chronic pain is a complex and poorly understood process (Shipton 2014). Uncontrolled pain can lead to increased anxiety, fear, sleeplessness and muscle tension, which further exacerbate pain. It can delay the recovery process by hindering mobilization and deep breathing, which increases the risk of a patient developing a deep vein thrombosis, chest infection or pressure damage. The accumulating evidence that a range of psychological factors (anxiety, depression and catastrophizing) can contribute to the experience and impact of acute pain, as well as the development and impact of persisting or chronic pain, has potentially important implications for pain management in the acute pain setting (Schug et al. 2015). There is huge variability between individuals concerning the contribution these psychological factors make to pain intensity and interference with function. It is important that these factors are assessed. There is evidence to suggest that, in the long term, poorly controlled acute pain may lead to the development of chronic pain (Shipton 2014).

Assessment of pain

Pain assessment is a key step in the process of managing pain, and pain should be assessed before any intervention takes place. The aim of assessment is to identify all of the factors, physical and non-physical, that affect the patient's perception of pain. Pain should be assessed within a biopsychosocial model that recognizes that physiological, psychological and environmental factors influence the overall pain experience. A comprehensive clinical assessment is essential to gain a thorough understanding of the patient's pain. This then assists in eliciting the likely cause of the pain. A thorough clinical assessment will also assist in selecting the appropriate analgesic therapy and non-pharmacological approaches; evaluating the effectiveness of interventions, and modifying therapy according to the patient's response, recent therapy, and potential risks and side-effects. Additionally, any management plan should consider the patient's preferences (Schug et al. 2015). Box 10.1 lists criteria for an effective pain assessment tool.

Assessment of acute pain

The key components of acute pain assessment are the pain history, the measurement of the pain and the response to any intervention (Macintyre and Schug 2015). A pain history, in addition to a physical examination, can provide important information that will help in understanding the cause of the pain and should be repeated when there is any sign of an alteration in the nature and intensity of the pain. In acute pain management, the assessment should be repeated at frequent intervals, as evidence demonstrates that regular assessment of pain leads to improved acute pain management (Schug et al. 2015). As pain is by definition a subjective experience, self-reporting of pain utilizing appropriate assessment and screening tools should be used whenever appropriate (Schug et al. 2015). A comprehensive pain assessment includes pain location and quality, aggravating and alleviating factors, timing, duration and intensity of the pain, pain relief, and functional goals (Pasero and McCaffery 2011). The effectiveness of any previous pain treatment, as well as the effects of pain on quality of life, should also be assessed (Wuhrman and Cooney 2011).

Box 10.1 Criteria for an effective pain assessment tool

The most commonly used pain assessment tools meet the following criteria:

- *Simplicity*: all patient groups can easily understand the tool.
- *Reliability*: the tool is reliable when used in similar patient groups; the results are reproducible and consistent.
- *Valid*: the tool measures the patient's perception of pain.
- *Sensitivity*: the tool is sensitive enough to detect changes in the patient's pain.
- *Accuracy*: the tool allows for the accurate and precise recording of data.
- *Interpretable*: meaningful pain scores or data are produced.
- *Feasibility/practicality*: the degree of effort involved in using the tool is acceptable; a practical tool is more likely to be used by patients.

Assessment of location of pain

Assessing the location of the pain and whether it radiates to any other areas of the body is one key part of the initial pain assessment and measurement. It is fundamental to the process of diagnosing the cause of the pain and developing a pain management plan (Schug et al. 2015). Patients can describe the location of the pain verbally or they can use a body map diagram (Figure 10.4) to indicate the areas where they are experiencing pain.

Many patients presenting with acute pain will have more than one site of pain; for example, complex surgical procedures may involve more than one incision site and/or multiple drain sites, and the nature and extent of pain at each site may vary. A careful assessment of the location and type of pain is required, because each pain problem may respond to different pain management techniques.

Assessment of intensity of pain

As part of the assessment process, it is important to assess the intensity of pain. Only then can the effects of any intervention be evaluated and care modified as appropriate. The simplest and most commonly used techniques for pain intensity measurement involve the use of unidimensional assessment tools such as verbal descriptor scales, numerical rating scales, faces scales or visual analogue scales. Patients are asked to match their pain intensity to the scale:

- *Verbal descriptor scales (VDSs)* are based on numerically ranked words such as 'none', 'mild', 'moderate', 'severe' and 'very severe' for assessing both pain intensity and response to analgesia.
- *Numerical rating scales (NRSs)* have both written and verbal forms. The written forms consist of either a vertical or a horizontal line with '0' (indicating no pain) located at one end of the line and '10' (indicating severe pain) located at the other end. This type of scale is easily used as a verbal scale of 0–10 if patients are unable to see or focus on a written scale. Although originally published as a line with a scale of 0–10, there are many versions of this type of scale.

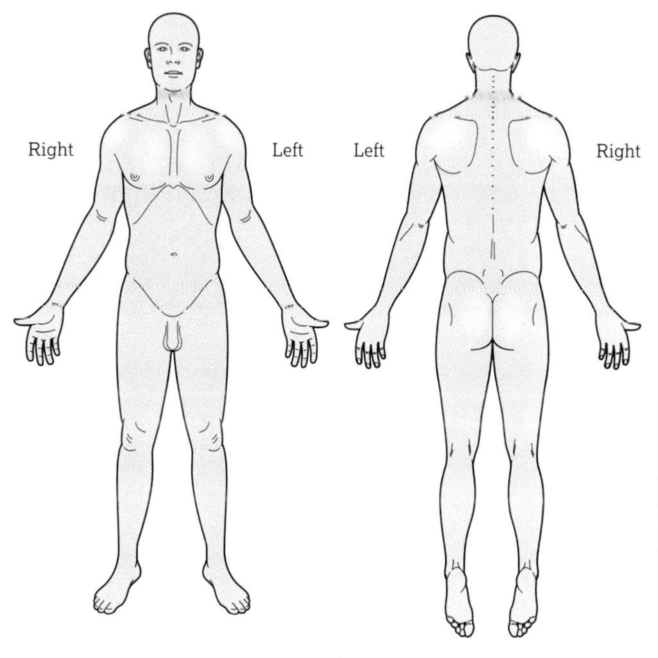

Figure 10.4 Body diagram used for pain assessment.

- *Faces scales*: one example is the Wong-Baker FACES Pain Rating Scale, which was originally developed for children. It is useful for children because they may not understand the idea of rating their pain on a scale of 0–10. However, they are likely to be able to understand the cartoon faces and the emotions they represent, and be able to point to the one that 'best matches their level of pain'. This type of pain scale is also appropriate for adult patients who do not know how to count, and those who have known or suspected mild to moderate impaired cognitive or brain function.
- *Visual analogue scales (VASs)* consist of a 100 mm horizontal line with verbal anchors at both ends (such as 'no pain' on the left and 'worst pain imaginable' on the right) and no tick marks along the line. The patient is asked to mark the line, and the 'score' is the distance in millimetres from the left-hand side of the scale to the mark. These are most commonly used to rate pain intensity for research. They can also be used to measure other aspects of the pain experience (e.g. patient satisfaction, affective components or adverse effects).

See Figure 10.5 for examples of unidimensional assessment tools.

Since many of these scales focus on assessing the intensity of pain, it is important that nurses remember to combine their use of these tools with an assessment of the patient's psychosocial needs. Regardless of which tool is used, the intensity of pain should be assessed both at rest (important for comfort) and during movement (important for function) (Gordon 2015). Most pain intensity measurement scales and tools follow these principles:

- The patient must be involved in scoring their own pain intensity. This provides the patient with an opportunity to express their pain intensity and also what it means to them and the effect it has on their life. This is important because healthcare professionals frequently underestimate the intensity of a patient's pain and overestimate the effectiveness of pain relief (Gordon 2015, Wuhrman and Cooney 2011).
- Pain intensity assessment should incorporate various components of pain. It should include assessment of static pain (at rest) and dynamic pain (on sitting, coughing or moving the affected part). For example, in a post-operative patient, this is important to prevent complications relating to delayed recovery such as chest infections and emboli (deep vein thrombosis or pulmonary embolism) and to determine whether the current level of analgesia is adequate for the return of normal function (Macintyre and Schug 2015).
- It is important to remember that a complete picture of a patient's pain cannot be derived solely from the use of a pain scale. Ongoing communication with the patient is required to uncover and manage any psychosocial factors that may be affecting the patient's pain experience. It is likely that multiple tools and outcome measures will be required to fully appreciate the complexity of the pain experience and how it can be modified by pain management (Schug et al. 2015).

Descriptors

Noting the words that patients use to describe their pain is a key part of the assessment process. This may help to distinguish the underlying type of pain, such as nociceptive pain (visceral or somatic) or neuropathic pain.

Somatic pain may be described as sharp, hot or stinging; is generally well localized; and is associated with local and surrounding tenderness. By contrast, visceral pain may be described as dull, cramping or colicky; is often poorly localized; and may be associated with tenderness locally or in the area of referred pain, or with symptoms such as nausea, sweating and cardiovascular changes (Schug et al. 2015).

Features that may suggest a diagnosis of neuropathic pain include (Schug et al. 2015):

- pain descriptors such as 'burning', 'shooting' and 'stabbing'
- spontaneous nature of the pain, which may have no clear precipitating factors

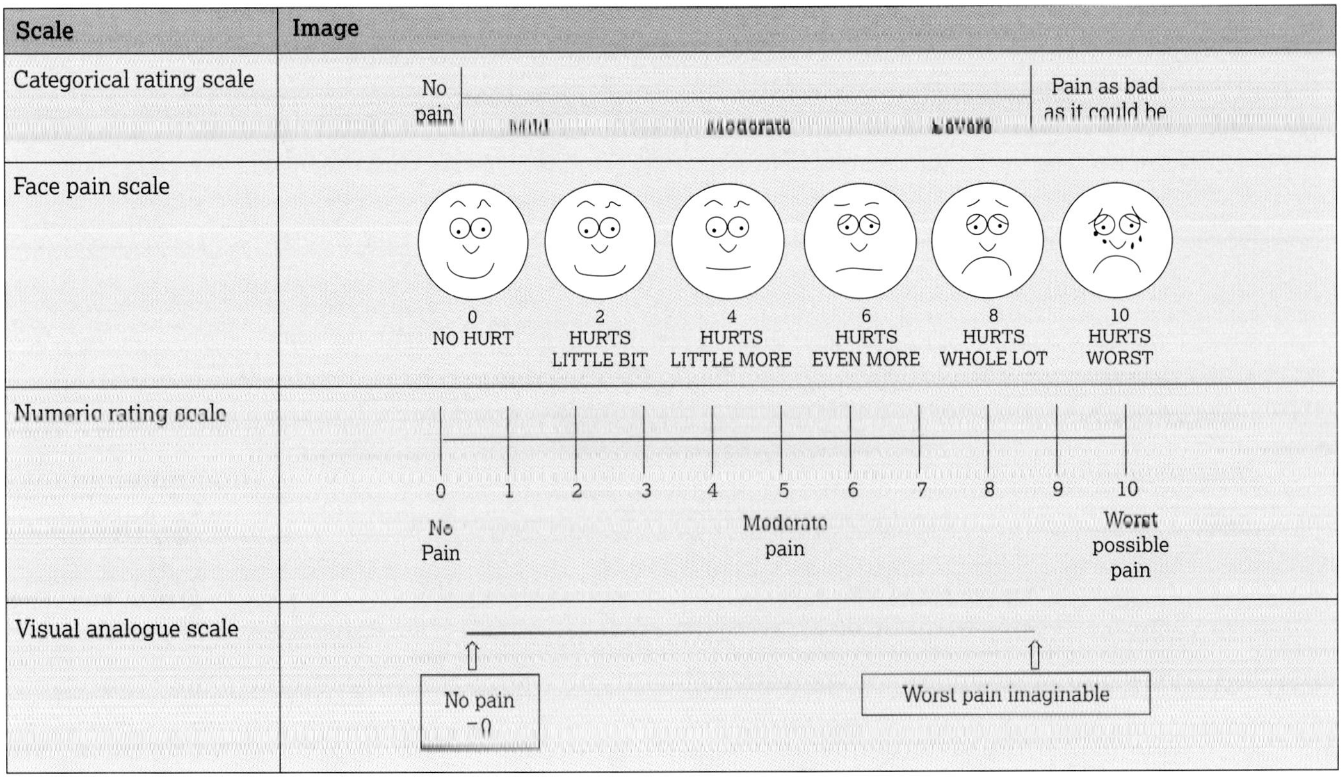

Figure 10.5 Examples of universal pain assessment tools. *Source*: Reproduced from Rhodes and Branham (2016) with permission of *Pharmacy Times*.

- the presence of dysaesthesias (spontaneous or evoked unpleasant abnormal sensations), hyperalgesia (increased response to a normally painful stimulus), allodynia (pain due to a stimulus that does not normally evoke pain, such as light touch) or areas of hypoaesthesia (reduced sense of touch or sensation, numbness)
- procedures associated with a high risk of nerve injury (e.g. thoracic or chest wall procedures, amputations or hernia repairs).

Neuropathic pain may require a specific assessment tool. Patients may describe spontaneous pain (arising without detectable stimulation) and evoked pain (abnormal responses to stimuli) (Bennett 2001). The Leeds Assessment of Neuropathic Symptoms and Signs (LANSS) pain scale (Bennett 2001) was developed to more accurately assess this type of pain.

The SOCRATES and PQRST frameworks are pain assessment mnemonic tools commonly used by healthcare professionals to guide pain assessment. The SOCRATES framework has the following components:

S – *severity*: none, mild, moderate, severe
O – *onset*: when and how did it start?
C – *characteristic*: is it shooting, burning, aching – ask the patient to describe it
R – *radiation*: does it radiate anywhere else?
A – *additional factors*: what makes it better?
T – *time*: is it there all the time, is there a time of day when it is worse?
E – *exacerbating factors*: what makes it worse?
S – *site*: where is the pain?

The components of the PQRST framework are as follows:

P – provoking or precipitating factor
Q – quality of pain
R – region (location) and radiation
S – severity or associated symptoms
T – temporal factors and timing

Assessment of pre-existing opioid use

Patients who have been taking regular opioid analgesics for a pre-existing chronic pain problem or those who take recreational opioid drugs may require higher doses of analgesia to manage an acute pain episode. This is due to opioid tolerance, which is a physiological decrease in the effect of a drug over time so that a progressive increase in the amount of the drug is required to achieve the same effect (Schug et al. 2015). Additionally, patients already taking opioids are physically dependent, whereby the abrupt discontinuation or a sudden reduction in its dose leads to a withdrawal (abstinence) syndrome (Schug et al. 2015). It is therefore important to take a history of pre-existing pain and analgesic use or recreational drug use so that appropriate analgesic measures can be planned in advance of surgery. In cases of acute trauma, undertaking a pain and/or drug history as soon as possible will help to plan appropriate analgesia. This is important for opioid-tolerant patients irrespective of whether opioid tolerance is due to analgesic therapy or recreational opioid drug use as the pain management intervention needs to both manage pain and prevent a withdrawal syndrome. Such patients are complex and early referral to a specialist pain management service is recommended.

The key components of a pain assessment are displayed in Box 10.2.

Box 10.2 Key components of a pain assessment

1 Site of pain
  - primary location: description with or without body map diagram
  - radiation
2 Circumstances associated with pain onset
  - including details of trauma or surgical procedures
3 Character of pain
  - sensory descriptors, e.g. sharp, throbbing, aching
  - consider using pain assessment tool, e.g.:
    - McGill Pain Questionnaire (MPQ): includes sensory and affective descriptors*
    - Neuropathic Pain Questionnaire (NPQ), Douleur Neuropathique (DN4), Leeds Assessment of Neuropathic Symptoms and Signs (LANSS), PainDETECT or ID Pain: these assess neuropathic pain characteristics**
4 Intensity of pain
  - at rest
  - on movement
  - temporal factors
    - duration
    - current pain, highest level of pain and lowest level of pain
    - continuous or intermittent
  - exacerbating or relieving factors
5 Associated symptoms (e.g. nausea)
6 Effect of pain on activities and sleep
7 Treatment
  - current and previous medications: dose, frequency of use, efficacy and adverse effects
  - other treatments currently using or tried in the past, e.g. transcutaneous electrical nerve stimulation (TENS) or acupuncture
  - other health professionals consulted
8 Relevant medical or surgical history
  - prior and co-existing pain conditions and treatment outcomes
  - prior and co-existing medical conditions
9 Factors influencing the patient's symptomatic treatment
  - beliefs concerning the causes of pain
  - knowledge, expectations and preferences for pain management
  - expectations of outcome of pain treatment
  - reduction in pain required for patient satisfaction or to resume 'reasonable activities'
  - typical coping response for stress or pain, including presence of anxiety or psychiatric disorders (e.g. depression or psychosis)
  - family expectations and beliefs about pain, stress and post-operative course

*MPQ: Melzack (1975).
**NPQ: Krause (2003); DN4: Bouhassira et al. (2005); LANSS: Bennett (2001), PainDETECT: Freynhagen et al. (2006); ID Pain: Portenoy (2006)
Source: Adapted from Schug et al. (2015) with permission of the Australian and New Zealand College of Anaesthetists.

Assessment of chronic pain

There are many pain assessment tools that have been developed specifically for patients with chronic pain (Dansie and Turk 2013). Pain assessment tools should be used to support diagnosis and to determine the effectiveness of any treatment for the pain. Assessment tools should be easy to use and understand by patients and healthcare professionals (Cox 2010). Assessment tools for chronic pain need to be able to define the pain as well as assess the impact the pain is having on the patient's wellbeing and lifestyle. One-dimensional tools can be suitable for the assessment of acute pain; however, in chronic pain, more holistic tools are required to facilitate a better understanding of the nature of the pain. Assessment of chronic pain needs to take these limitations into account and particular attention must be paid to factors that will modulate pain sensitivity (Table 10.1).

Other pain assessment tools have been developed to capture the multidimensional nature of pain. These specifically measure several features of the pain experience, including the location and intensity of pain, the pattern of pain over time, the effect of pain on the patient's daily function and activities, and the effect of pain on the patient's mood and ability to interact and socialize with others. Examples of these tools include the McGill Pain Questionnaire (MPQ) (Melzack 1975) and the Brief Pain Inventory, which has been validated for use in chronic non-cancer pain (Tan et al. 2004). These are most commonly used in chronic pain assessment. Accurate pain assessment and reassessment are crucial in developing an understanding and baseline measurement of the pain, and the key is to ask appropriate questions. Particularly, questions relating to the following psychosocial elements should be addressed:

- the effect of the pain on the patient's mood
- whether the patient's relationships are affected by the pain
- whether the patient has any physical limitations caused by the pain
- whether the pain has resulted in a loss of work or loss of role (social effects)
- whether the patient is affected by any other types of pain
- whether the patient has previously had any treatments for the pain, and what their effects were
- whether the patient has any co-morbidities
- whether the patient has any allergies.

Assessment in vulnerable and older adults

Pain assessment in vulnerable adults, for example those with cognitive impairment or dementia, and older adults may require careful consideration. There will be an increase in the older population in the UK over the next 30 years. This is anticipated to bring an increase in the prevalence of chronic pain, and with this will come the challenge of assessment of pain in many and varied settings (Schofield 2018). Older people form the population most likely to have their pain inadequately assessed, and this is especially so for patients who are elderly and have dementia (Ni Thuathail and Welford 2011). Barriers to effective pain relief for this group of patients include issues such as lack of recognition by the staff that the patient is in pain, insufficient education about pain in this group, misdiagnosis of pain and the lack of use of appropriate assessment tools (McAuliffe et al. 2009). A multidisciplinary approach to the assessment and treatment of pain is essential, but assessment in this group is a complex process that is hampered by many communication issues, including cognitive ability and sociocultural factors (Schofield 2018). A number of valid and reliable self-report measures are available and can be used even when moderate dementia exists. The Numeric Pain Rating Scale or verbal descriptors can be used with people who have mild to moderate cognitive impairment. For people with severe cognitive impairment, the Pain in Advanced Dementia (PAINAD) (Warden et al. 2003) and Doloplus-2 (Lefebvre-Chapiro 2001) scales are recommended (Schofield 2018). These two scales show positive results in terms of reliability and validity. Another scale that is widely used throughout the UK is the Abbey Pain Scale, but it has not been evaluated recently (Schofield 2018).

Table 10.1 Factors affecting pain sensitivity

Sensitivity increased	Sensitivity lowered
Discomfort	Relief of symptoms
Insomnia	Sleep
Fatigue	Rest
Anxiety	Sympathy
Fear	Understanding
Anger	Companionship
Sadness	Diversional therapy and/or activities
Depression	Reduction in anxiety
Boredom	Elevation of mood

Assessment in adults with learning or intellectual disabilities

People with learning or intellectual disabilities experience the same acute and chronic conditions as the general population, and chronic pain is often highly prevalent in this group due to associated physical disabilities and/or co-morbidities (McGuire et al. 2010). It is not uncommon for assumptions to be made that people with learning disabilities do not experience pain and for their pain to go unassessed (Beacroft and Dodd 2010, Doody and Bailey 2017), and for pain relief to be inadequate (McKenzie et al. 2012). Self-report tools (such as describing the location and intensity of pain with numeric rating scales, verbal descriptor scales or visual analogue scales) may or may not be difficult for people with a learning or intellectual disability to use. It is important to understand that many people with mild learning or intellectual disability will be able to use these self-report measures. However, some will lack the ability to communicate their pain in this way or lack the cognitive ability to convert their pain experience into expressive language (Doody and Bailey 2017). Assessing pain in people with more severe learning or intellectual disabilities may require the use of non-verbal pain assessment tools and working closely with family and carers, who may recognize indicators that the person with a learning disability is in pain. Specialist pain assessment tools may need to be used, such as the Disability Distress Assessment Tool (DisDAT) (Regnard et al. 2007) or the Pain and Discomfort Scale (PADS) (Bodfish et al. 2001), which are intended to help identify distress cues in people who have severely limited communication because of cognitive impairment or physical illness.

Assessment in unconscious patients

Tools also exist for the assessment of pain in unconscious patients. Examples include the Critical-Care Pain Observational Tool (CPOT) (Gélinas et al. 2011) and the Behavioural Pain Scale (BPS) (Ahlers et al. 2010), which provide a score based on observations such as facial expressions, muscle tension and compliance with mechanical ventilation.

Culture and effects on pain assessment

Individuals are greatly influenced by each other and by the cultural groups to which they belong. Ethnic, religious and socio-economic factors all affect the way we live in society. Pain is greatly influenced by cultural factors. Some groups are stoical regarding expressions of pain while others are more expressive, and these are behaviours that may have been learned in childhood. Disparities in assessment, analgesic requirements and effective treatment of pain exist across ethnic groups (Schug et al. 2015). The key in nursing is to ensure patients are cared for in a way that they feel comfortable with according to their cultural background. The principles that can be applied in this situation include the following (Schug et al. 2015):

- Pain assessment and management should be done on an individual patient basis. Differences between ethnic and cultural groups should not be used to stereotype patients, but rather used to inform the nurse of possible cultural preferences.

- Health outcomes for culturally and linguistically diverse patients are improved when healthcare professionals are supported by cultural competency training.
- An accredited medical interpreter should be involved when language proficiency poses a barrier to conducting a pain assessment; this will facilitate a positive outcome for the patient.
- The ethnic and cultural backgrounds of both the healthcare professional and the patient can affect the outcome of the assessment and the treatment of pain.
- Multilingual printed information and pain measurement scales are useful in managing patients from different cultural backgrounds.

Pre-procedural considerations

Assessment and recording tools

Accurate pain assessment is a prerequisite of effective control and is an essential component of nursing care. In the assessment process, the nurse gathers information from the patient that allows an understanding of their experience and its effect on their life. The information obtained guides the nurse in planning and evaluating strategies for care. Pain is rarely static; therefore, its assessment is not a one-time process but is ongoing.

The sections above outline several tools that can be effective with different patient groups. However, some degree of caution must be exercised with the use of pain assessment tools. The nurse must be careful to select the tool that is most appropriate for a particular type of pain experience; for example, it would not be appropriate to use a pain assessment tool designed for use with patients with chronic pain to assess acute trauma or post-operative pain.

In Procedure guideline 10.1: Pain assessment, fixed times for reviewing the pain have intentionally been omitted to allow for flexibility. It is suggested that, initially, the patient's pain is reviewed by the patient and nurse every 4 hours. However, this may need to be done more frequently if acute pain persists or if the nurse is evaluating the effects of an intervention. When a patient's level of pain has stabilized, recordings may be made less frequently, for example 12-hourly or daily. The chart should be discontinued if the patient's pain becomes totally controlled.

Procedure guideline 10.1 Pain assessment

Essential equipment

An appropriate assessment tool – e.g.:

- in acute pain, consider the use of a verbal or numerical rating
- in chronic pain, consider the use of the Brief Pain Inventory (BPI)
- in adults with severe cognitive impairment, consider the use of the Abbey Pain Scale (see the section above on assessment in vulnerable and older adults)
- in unconscious patients, consider the use of the Critical-Care Pain Observational Tool (CPOT) (see the section above on assessment in unconscious patients)

Action	Rationale
Pre-procedure	
1 Introduce yourself to the patient, explain and discuss the procedure with them, and gain their consent to proceed.	To ensure that the patient feels at ease, understands the procedure and gives their valid consent (NMC 2018, **C**).
Procedure	
2 Encourage the patient, where appropriate, to identify the pain themselves and to describe the character of the pain, if possible.	The body outline (see Figure 10.4) is a tool that a patient can use to describe their own pain experience (Macintyre and Schug 2015, **E**).
3 Ensure that the patient's own description of their pain is recorded.	To reduce the risk of misinterpretation (Schug et al. 2015, **R**).
4 a Record any factors that influence the intensity of the pain, for example activities or interventions that reduce or increase the pain, such as distractions or a heat pad. b Record whether or not the patient is pain free at night, at rest or on movement. c Record the frequency of the pain, what helps to relieve the pain, what makes the pain worse and how the patient feels when they are in pain. d Determine whether there are any associated symptoms when the pain is present (e.g. nausea and vomiting).	Ascertaining how and when the patient experiences pain enables the nurse to plan realistic goals. For example, relieving the patient's pain during the night and while they are at rest is usually easier to achieve than relief from pain on movement. **E** To gain an understanding of the experience of pain for the patient (Schug et al. 2015, **R**). To ensure all elements of a pain assessment are explored (Macintyre and Schug 2015, **E**).
5 Index each site (see Figure 10.4) in whatever way seems most appropriate, for example shading or colouring areas, or using arrows to indicate shooting pains.	To enable individual pain sites to be located (Dansie and Turk 2013, **E**).
6 Give each pain site a value according to the pain intensity or the pain scale and note the time recorded where possible. If cognitive impairment is present, complete an appropriate tool so that the patient does not need to verbalize a pain score.	To indicate the intensity of the pain at each site (Gordon 2015, **E**). To ensure that the patient's pain is assessed as well as possible (Doody and Bailey 2017, **E**; Schofield 2018, **E**).
7 Record any analgesia given and note the route, dose and response.	To monitor the efficacy of prescribed analgesia. **E**

(continued)

Procedure guideline 10.1 Pain assessment *(continued)*

Action	Rationale
Post-procedure	
8 Record any significant activities that are likely to influence the patient's pain.	Because extra pharmacological or non-pharmacological interventions might be indicated (Gordon 2015, **E**).
9 Discuss with the patient an ongoing reassessment plan for their pain.	To ensure that the patient is informed regarding ongoing pain assessment and understands when to alert the nurse if they need additional help (e.g. when there is a change in the nature of the pain, when the pain is not responding to the planned treatment or when activities of daily living are being inhibited that previously could be maintained) (Macintyre and Schug 2015, **E**).

Pain management

Evidence-based approaches

Pain management uses a multidisciplinary approach that matches therapy to the individual patient. In some instances, simple analgesia can be sufficient to control pain. Simple or non-opioid analgesics include paracetamol and non-steroidal anti-inflammatory drugs (NSAIDs), used either individually or in combination. Other incidences may require a multimodal approach.

Multimodal analgesia

Multimodal analgesia is the administration of two or more drugs that act by different mechanisms (via the same or different routes) to provide analgesia. This allows for lower doses of individual drugs. It combines different analgesics that act by different mechanisms and at different sites in the nervous system. The aim is to achieve greater analgesia than each of the individual drugs could provide alone and to reduce the patient's opioid requirements and any related side effects (Polomano et al. 2017, Rosero and Goshi 2014).

Opioids, non-opioids (such as paracetamol, NSAIDs, and cyclo-oxygenase-2-selective inhibitors (COX-2)), local anaesthetics and anticonvulsants are all examples of drugs that may be used as part of a multimodal analgesic approach. An example of multimodal analgesia to manage acute post-operative pain would be a continuous epidural infusion of a combined opioid and local anaesthetic solution along with paracetamol and an NSAID (if not contraindicated). Another example would be a continuous peripheral nerve block with paracetamol and a NSAID. Both of these approaches combine different analgesic compounds and analgesic approaches (oral route, epidural route and peripheral nerve block).

A multimodal approach may also include non-pharmacological approaches, such as relaxation therapy, guided imagery, transcutaneous electrical nerve stimulation (TENS) and heat therapy. During the process of devising a multimodal analgesic plan, it is good practice for the prescriber to be aware of any Medicines and Healthcare products Regulatory Agency alerts that may influence their prescribing and management strategy (see https://www.gov.uk/government/organisations/medicines-and-healthcare-products-regulatory-agency).

Management of persistent chronic and cancer pain

It has been suggested that despite progress in pain management, chronic non-cancer pain still represents a clinical challenge, with data demonstrating that chronic pain affects between one-third and one-half of the population of the UK – a figure that is likely to increase further, with time, in line with the ageing of the population (Fayaz et al. 2015). Chronic pain has negative impacts on quality of life, interferes with work and causes increased mortality (Moore et al. 2013).

The management of pain is directed by the 'analgesic ladder' (also known as the 'pain ladder'), which was published by the World Health Organization (WHO) in 1986 as a guide to the management of persistent cancer pain (Figure 10.6). Although the analgesic ladder was originally published for the management of cancer pain, it is now widely used by medical professionals for the management of all types of pain, including chronic persistent non-cancer pain (Balding 2013). It involves a stepwise approach to the use of analgesics, including non opioids (step 1), opioids for mild to moderate pain (step 2) and opioids for moderate to severe pain (step 3). Adjuvant drugs are those that contribute to pain relief but are not primarily indicated for pain management. They can be used at all steps of the ladder. Examples include antidepressant and anticonvulsant drugs, corticosteroids, benzodiazepines, antispasmodics and bisphosphonates.

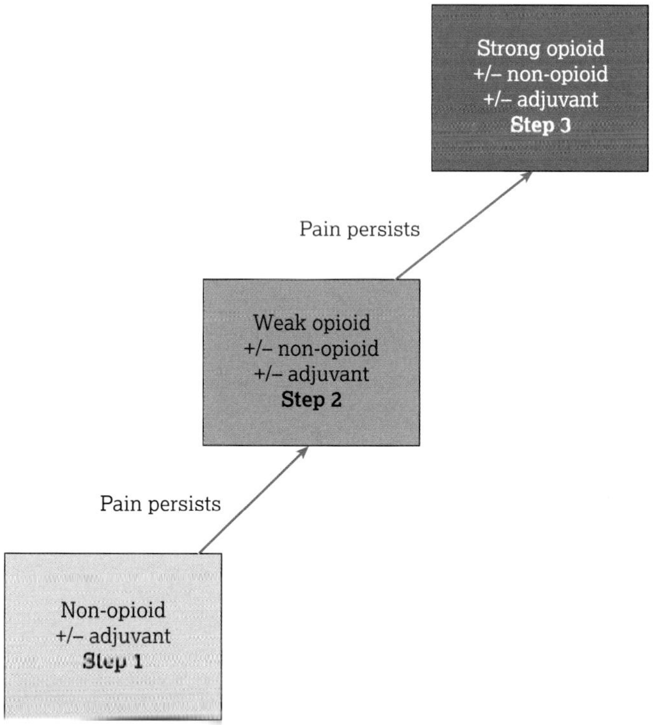

Figure 10.6 The WHO analgesic ladder.

The WHO treatment guide recommends the following five points for the correct use of analgesics (WHO 1986):

- They should be administered orally if appropriate.
- They should be given at regular intervals.
- They should be prescribed according to an assessment of pain intensity evaluated using a pain intensity scale.
- The dose of the analgesic should be adapted to the individual. There is no standard dose to treat certain types of pain.
- Analgesia should be prescribed with ongoing review, monitoring for effectiveness and side-effects.

Some patients who present with severe pain will need to start on step 3 of the ladder; it is frequently not appropriate for patients to progress through each step in these circumstance. Raffa and Pergolizzi (2014) discuss how adaptations could potentially be made to the WHO analgesia ladder due to advancements that have been made in the basic science around pain anatomy and physiology, advancements in the breadth of therapeutic treatments available, and a societal shift that has occurred in attitudes toward pain management. They note, however, that it is still a useful construct in devising a pain management strategy, as it provides a series of review points in a clinician's ongoing assessment, although they caution that it should not act as a substitute for evidence-based guidelines. Carlson (2016) supported the use of the WHO analgesics ladder, indicating that at least 20% and potentially 100% of patients with cancer pain can be provided with adequate pain relief across the span of their illness, via the application of the WHO's guidelines.

It is important to remember that each patient will experience different types of pain, and individual patients may experience various types of pain, due to aetiological and physiological differences. Each pain needs to be assessed separately, since an individual's pain may need to be managed in various ways and one analgesic intervention or route will rarely be sufficient. Often the best practice is to combine different types of analgesia in order to achieve maximum pain control (Table 10.2). It is also important to use non-pharmacological interventions at all stages of the treatment plan. And, finally, accurate ongoing assessment is imperative for efficient and effective pain control.

Using the WHO analgesic ladder

The analgesic ladder (see Figure 10.6) was designed as a framework for the pharmacological management of cancer pain and is also often used to manage chronic pain. There are several pharmacological agents available to manage pain and the analgesic ladder allows the flexibility to choose from this range according to the patient's requirements and tolerance. In 2010, new guidance on the analgesic ladder promoted its bidirectional use with a 'step up, step down' approach, proposing an upward pathway for the treatment of cancer pain and a downward pathway for the treatment of intense acute pain, uncontrolled chronic pain and breakthrough pain (Vargas-Schaffer 2010).

For acute pain management, the WHO ladder can be used as a guide in reverse, starting at step 3 for immediate post-operative pain and moving down through step 2 and then step 1 as post-operative pain improves.

The principles of the WHO analgesic ladder are to provide a therapeutic effect alongside all other interventions (both pharmacological and non-pharmacological), to guide the patient's treatment and help in managing their underlying condition, to prevent avoidable complications, and to maintain or improve quality of life (Vargas-Schaffer and Cogan 2014).

Step 1: non-opioid drugs

Examples of non-opioid drugs include paracetamol, aspirin and NSAIDs. NSAIDs are especially effective for pain from inflammation. All of the examples of non-opioid drugs given in Table 10.2 are used to manage mild to moderate pain and can also be used as adjuncts to opioid analgesia to manage moderate to severe pain (Polomano et al. 2017).

Step 2: opioids for mild to moderate pain

Examples of opioids for mild to moderate pain include codeine, dihydrocodeine, tramadol and low dose oxycodone (steps 2 and 3). These drugs are used when non-opioids are unable to achieve adequate pain control and are usually used in combination formulations. It is not recommended to administer another step 2 analgesic if pain remains uncontrolled. Uncontrolled pain needs to be assessed and managed with the titration of an opioid by moving up the ladder. The exception to this would be if the patient was experiencing intolerable side-effects on the weak opioid and an alternative drug might be beneficial.

Step 3: opioids for moderate to severe pain

Examples of opioids for moderate to severe pain include morphine, oxycodone, fentanyl, diamorphine, methadone, buprenorphine, hydromorphone and alfentanil.

Methods of drug delivery

Oral analgesia

Oral opioids are used less frequently in the immediate post-operative period because many patients are nil by mouth or on restricted oral

Table 10.2 The use of adjuvant drugs (co-analgesics)

Type	Use	Examples
Non-steroidal anti-inflammatory drugs (NSAIDs)	Bone pain Muscular pain Inflammation Visceral pain	Diclofenac Naproxen Ibuprofen
Steroids	Pressure Bone pain Inflammation Raised intracranial pressure	Dexamethasone Prednisolone
Tricyclic antidepressants	Neuropathic pain	Amitriptyline
Anticonvulsants	Neuropathic pain	Sodium valproate Carbamazepine Gabapentin Pregabalin
Antibiotics	Infection	Flucloxacillin Trimethoprim
Benzodiazepines	Anxiety	Diazepam Clonazepam
Antispasmodics	Spasms	Baclofen
Bisphosphonates	Bone pain	Sodium clodronate Disodium pamidronate Zoledronic acid

intake for a period of time. Often this route is used if patients require strong analgesics following discontinuation of epidural or intravenous analgesia. Morphine is an ideal oral preparation because it is available as a tablet (Sevredol) or an elixir (Oramorph). Oxycodone can be given as a second-line opioid treatment if patients are allergic or sensitive to morphine, or fail to respond to it.

Intravenous analgesia

Continuous intravenous infusions of opioids such as morphine, diamorphine and fentanyl are effective for controlling pain in the immediate post-operative period. Their use is often restricted to critical care units, where patients can be closely monitored, because of the potential risk of respiratory depression (Macintyre and Schug 2015). The need for this restriction is reinforced by Lee et al. (2015), who found that 88% of respiratory depression events occurred within 24 hours of a surgical procedure. A meta-analysis found that compared with patient-controlled analgesia (PCA) using bolus only, the addition of a continuous or background infusion was associated with an increased risk of respiratory depression (George et al. 2010).

Patients may control post-operative pain via self-administration of intravenous opioids using devices designed for this purpose (i.e. PCA). In a Cochrane review, McNicol et al. (2015) found evidence that PCA is an efficacious alternative to non-patient-controlled systemic analgesia for post-operative pain control, with patients demonstrating lower visual analogue scale pain intensity scores versus patients not using PCA over most time intervals. When in pain, the patient presses a button connected to the pump and a set dose of opioid is delivered (usually intravenously but it may also be given subcutaneously or via epidural) (Macintyre and Schug 2015).

There are a number of advantages to using PCA:

- PCA is more likely than non-patient-controlled systemic analgesia to maintain reasonably constant blood concentrations of the drug within the analgesic corridor (the blood level where analgesia is achieved without significant side-effects). The flexibility of PCA helps to overcome the wide inter-patient variation in opioid requirements (Macintyre and Schug 2015).
- PCA allows for intra-patient variability in analgesic needs, allowing patients to titrate analgesia according to daily variations in their pain stimulus (Hurley et al. 2010). By using a PCA pump, patients can administer analgesia as soon as pain occurs and titrate the dose according to increases and decreases in the pain stimulus. This is particularly helpful for controlling more intense pain during movement or other activities that can trigger pain.
- PCA gives patients better autonomy and control over the amount of medication used (Garimella and Cellini 2013).

While PCA may be very effective for controlling pain for a number of patients, particularly those who have undergone surgery (Macintyre and Schug 2015), it is not suitable for the groups listed in Box 10.3.

Epidural analgesia

Epidural analgesia refers to the provision of pain relief by continuous administration of analgesic pharmacological agents (usually low concentrations of local anaesthetics and opioids) into the epidural space via an indwelling catheter (Schug et al. 2015). Giving analgesia epidurally is a particularly valuable technique for the prevention of post-operative pain in patients undergoing major thoracic, abdominal or lower limb surgery, and can sometimes be used to manage the pain associated with trauma. Commonly used opioids for epidural analgesia include fentanyl and morphine (Mariano 2010). Combinations of low concentrations of local anaesthetic agents and opioids have been shown to provide consistently superior pain relief compared with either drug alone (Macintyre and Schug 2015).

Box 10.3 Patients unsuitable for PCA

- Those with poor manual dexterity or severe visual impairment, who may be physically incapable of activating the demand button
- Those with cognitive impairment (such as confusion) or learning difficulties who are unable to understand the concept of PCA and how to use the device

Source: Adapted from Elliott (2016), Stewart (2017).

Subcutaneous analgesia

Opioids are often given subcutaneously to manage chronic cancer pain. More recently, there has been an increase in the use of subcutaneous opioids for post-operative pain control. Both PCA and nurse-administered opioid injections of morphine, diamorphine or oxycodone via an indwelling subcutaneous cannula have been used successfully to manage post-operative pain (Macintyre and Schug 2015). An advantage of giving analgesia subcutaneously is that it avoids the problems associated with maintaining intravenous access.

Intramuscular analgesia

Until the early 1990s, regular (every 3–4 hours) intramuscular injections of opioids, such as pethidine and morphine, were routinely used for the management of post-operative pain. Because alternative techniques, such as PCA and epidural analgesia, are now available, intramuscular analgesia is used less frequently. Some useful algorithms have been developed to give guidance on titrating intramuscular analgesia (Harmer and Davies 1998, Macintyre and Schug 2015). Absorption via this route may be impaired in conditions of poor perfusion (e.g. in hypovolaemia, shock, hypothermia or immobility). This may lead to inadequate early analgesia (where the drug cannot be absorbed properly and reach the systemic circulation and so forms a drug depot) and late absorption of the drug depot (where the drug has remained in the muscular tissue and is absorbed only once perfusion is restored) (Schug et al. 2015).

Transdermal analgesia

Transdermal analgesia is a simple method of giving analgesia. It is convenient and often very acceptable to patients, particularly those who dislike tablets or have many to take. A number of patch formulations have been developed to allow the delivery of drugs across the skin (such as fentanyl, buprenorphine or local anaesthetics). Disadvantages of giving strong opioids such as fentanyl by this route include inflexibility (the patient usually has to be on a stable dose of an opioid and it takes a long time for a dose increase to take effect), and breakthrough doses must be given by another route (oral, buccal or sublingual). Transdermal fentanyl (except for iontophoretic patient-controlled transdermal devices) should not be used in the management of acute pain because of safety concerns and difficulties in the short-term dose adjustments needed for titration (Schug et al. 2015).

Buccal and sublingual analgesia

Buccal means the analgesia is placed between the upper lip and the lining of the upper gum. A sublingual drug is placed under the tongue. Drugs given by this route pass directly into the systemic circulation and bypass first pass hepatic metabolism. Their speed of onset is often rapid as this method avoids the harsh acidic environment of the stomach and the enzymatic milieu of the small intestine (Sattar et al. 2014).

Pre-procedural considerations

Pharmacological support

Non-opioid analgesics

Paracetamol and paracetamol combinations

The use of non-opioid analgesics, such as paracetamol or paracetamol combined with a weak opioid such as codeine, has been shown to decrease acute pain after various surgical procedures

(Mahajan et al. 2017). Paracetamol can be given rectally if the oral route is contraindicated. An intravenous preparation of paracetamol offers the ability to achieve therapeutic blood concentrations more readily and more reliably (Chiam et al. 2015). It is more effective and has a faster onset than the same dose given enterally. The use of the intravenous form should be limited to patients in whom the enteral route cannot be used. With regard to dosing schedules for parenteral administration of paracetamol, the dose should be reduced for those who weigh 50 kg or under. For example, patients who weigh between 33 and 50 kg should not exceed a maximum daily dose of 60 mg/kg (up to a limit of 3 g). For patients over 50 kg with an additional risk factor for hepatotoxicity, the maximum daily dose should be 3 g in 24 hours, and for patients over 50 kg with no risk factor then the maximum daily dose can be up to 4 g (Bristol-Myers Squibb 2012).

Paracetamol taken in the correct dose of not more than 4 g per day is relatively free of side-effects. When used in combination with codeine preparations, the most frequent side-effect is constipation.

Non-steroidal anti-inflammatory drugs

Non-steroidal anti-inflammatory drugs (NSAIDs) have been shown to provide superior pain relief over paracetamol alone (Moore et al. 2015). These drugs can be used alone or in combination with both opioid and non-opioid analgesics as part of a multimodal approach. Two commonly used NSAIDs are diclofenac, which can be administered by the oral, parenteral, enteral or rectal routes, and ibuprofen, which is available only as an oral or enteral preparation.

Although aspirin confers cardioprotective effects, most other NSAIDs are associated with an increased risk of adverse cardiovascular events, including hypertension, myocardial infarction, cerebrovascular accident (CVA) and heart failure (Brune and Patrignani 2015). A meta-analysis has suggested that there is little evidence to suggest that any of these drugs are safe in cardiovascular terms (Trelle et al. 2011). Compared with placebo, rofecoxib was associated with the highest risk of myocardial infarction and ibuprofen with the highest risk of CVA followed by diclofenac. Diclofenac and lumiracoxib were associated with the highest risk of cardiovascular death. Naproxen is viewed as the least harmful for cardiovascular safety but this advantage should be weighed against gastrointestinal toxicity (Trelle et al. 2011). Newer COX-2-specific NSAIDs such as parecoxib, celecoxib and etorocoxib (BNF 2019) have the advantage that they have similar analgesic and anti-inflammatory effects but also provide a potential reduction in gastrointestinal toxicity. Results of a 2012 meta-analysis of 28 observational studies by Castellsague et al. (2012) showed a low risk (relative risk (RR) <2) of upper gastrointestinal complications for aceclofenac, celecoxib and ibuprofen; an intermediate risk (RR 2–4) for diclofenac, meloxicam and ketoprofen, among others; a high risk (RR 4–5) for tenoxicam, naproxen, indomethacin and diflunisal; and the highest risk (RR >5) for piroxicam, ketorolac and azapropazone.

Each patient's clinical background, including gastrointestinal and cardiovascular risk factors, should be taken into account when selecting appropriate NSAIDs (Brune and Patrignani 2015).

Opioid analgesics

Opioids remain the mainstay of acute pain related to trauma and post-operative pain management (Rawal 2016) and can also be prescribed for cancer- and non-cancer-related chronic pain. Opioid doses need to be titrated carefully to achieve a level of pain relief that suits each individual patient while minimizing any unwanted side-effects (Vargas-Schaffer and Cogan 2014).

A number of opioids are used for controlling pain following surgery. These include morphine, diamorphine, fentanyl and oxycodone. The most common routes of opioid administration are intravenous, epidural, subcutaneous, intramuscular and oral.

Rotating several different WHO level III opioid drugs is a therapeutic option for patients with chronic cancer-related pain who suffer from inadequate analgesia and/or intolerable side-effects (Schuster et al. 2018). This may also be a useful strategy to consider in the management of acute pain.

Opioids for the management of mild to moderate pain

Tramadol

Tramadol is a centrally acting opioid analgesic (Wolkerstorfer et al. 2016). The main advantages of tramadol over other conventional opioids are less sedation, less opioid-induced respiratory impairment and potentially less constipation (Macintyre and Schug 2015).

Tramadol acts at mu opioid receptors but also inhibits the reuptake of norepinephrine and serotonin at the nerve terminals, and this latter effect may explain its efficacy in neuropathic pain (Gupta 2014). It is metabolized in the liver and excreted by the kidneys. There is a potential risk that tramadol can lower seizure threshold, and therefore care needs to be taken in patients who have a history of epilepsy and in patients who are taking any other medications that may contribute to the lowering of the seizure threshold, for example tricyclic antidepressants and selective serotonin reuptake inhibitors (SSRIs) (Mu et al. 2017). Tramadol can also cause serotonin syndrome (due to drug-induced inhibition of serotonin reuptake, which may induce excess serotonin release), a life-threatening complication that can have a good prognosis if managed early (Beakley et al. 2015). Symptoms include changes in mental status (agitation, anxiety, disorientation, restlessness and excitement), autonomic hyperactivity function (hypertension, tachycardia, tachpnoea, hyperthermia, vomiting, diarrhoea, arrhythmias and shivering) and neuromuscular activity (tremor, clonus, hyperreflexia and muscle rigidity) and can range in severity from mild to life threatening (Beakley et al. 2015).

Few patients with severe pain will achieve a satisfactory level of pain control with tramadol. It can be administered by the oral, rectal, intravenous and intramuscular routes. It is available in immediate and modified-release preparations.

Codeine phosphate

Codeine is metabolized by the hepatic cytochrome CYP2D6 to morphine. Approximately 7% of Caucasians and 1–3% of the Asian population are poor CYP2D6 metabolizers and therefore do not experience effective analgesia with codeine.

Codeine is available in tablet and syrup formulations. Doses of 30–60 mg via the oral route, four times daily, are generally prescribed to a maximum of 240 mg in 24 hours. Codeine is also available in combination preparations with a non-opioid. The combination preparations are available in varying strengths of codeine and paracetamol, including co-codamol 8 mg/500 mg, 15 mg/500 mg and 30 mg/500 mg. One of the most common side-effects is constipation (BNF 2019).

Opioids for the management of chronic non-cancer pain

Opioids are increasingly being used to treat persistent pain. They have a well-established role in the management of acute pain and for those with cancer and palliative care needs. There is also evidence from research that opioids can be helpful in the short and medium term in providing symptomatic pain relief from other non-cancer pain conditions (FPM 2019). Opioids are prescribed to reduce pain intensity. Rarely is pain completely relieved by opioids alone (FPM 2019). In approximately 80% of cases, patients will experience at least one adverse side-effect from opioids. Opioids should be given careful consideration before they are commenced and patients should be informed that the effects of long-term use of opioids are unknown in terms of endocrine and immune function (FPM 2019). When opioid therapy is commenced, a plan to review the patient in terms of opioid effects must be in place. From a palliative care perspective, there is guidance available from the National Institute for Health and Care Excellence (NICE) to support safe prescribing of opioids (NICE 2016). There are various opioid analgesics available and they can be given by a variety of routes. Selection is based on a thorough clinical assessment.

Morphine

A large amount of information and research is available concerning morphine and therefore it tends to be the first-line opioid. It is available in oral, rectal, parenteral and intra-spinal preparations.

All strong opioids require careful titration by an expert practitioner. When possible, modified-release preparations should be [illegible] in the management of [illegible] (FPM 2019). Oral morphine should be the drug of choice according to the Faculty of Pain Medicine (2019). Patients should be informed of potential side-effects, such as constipation, nausea and increased sleepiness, in order to allay any fears. Patients should also be told that nausea and drowsiness are transitory and normally improve within 48 hours but that constipation can be an ongoing problem; it is recommended that a laxative is prescribed when the opioid is started. The most effective laxative for this group of patients is a combination of both a softening and a stimulating laxative (Boland and Boland 2017).

Patients often have many concerns about commencing strong drugs such as morphine. Fears frequently centre around addiction and abuse. Time should be taken to reassure patients and their families and provide verbal and written information (NICE 2016).

Fentanyl transdermal patches

Fentanyl is a strong opioid, available in a patch, which is recommended in patients who have stable pain requirements. Transdermal patches are available in doses of 12, 25, 50, 75 or 100 μg per hour. It is reported to have an improved side-effect profile in comparison to morphine in relation to constipation, nausea, vomiting and dizziness (Dima et al. 2017, Reddy et al. 2016). Use of the patch has increased because it frees patients from taking tablets.

A transdermal fentanyl patch produces 72 hours of systemic drug delivery through the skin, so the patch is changed every 3 days. Occasionally the duration of analgesia does not last more than 48 hours (Vellucci et al. 2014), and patients may need to change the patch every 2 days. The patch should be applied to skin that is free from excess hair and any form of irritation, and it should not be applied to irradiated areas. It is advisable to change the location on the body when a new patch is applied to avoid an adverse skin reaction. Occasionally, difficulties arise relating to the titration of the patch as each patch is equivalent to a range of morphine (Table 10.3). This may require the use of additional breakthrough analgesia until an appropriate dose and pain efficacy have been established.

Methadone

Methadone is used for the treatment of opioid addiction and for the treatment of chronic pain. Methadone is a synthetic opioid that was introduced as an analgesic in the mid-1940s but soon lost favour because of its side-effect profile. A better understanding of pharmacokinetics and dynamics resulted in the re-emergence of methadone in the 1980s. Oral methadone as an analgesic was included in the 21st edition of the WHO model list of essential medicines in 2019 (WHO 2019; see also Palat and Charyy 2018). It is available in oral, rectal and parenteral preparations. There has been some reluctance among professionals to use methadone arising from the difficulties experienced in titrating the drug due to its long half-life. The half-life of methadone is usually assumed to be approximately 1 day, and is rarely outside a range of 15 to 60 hours (Chou et al. 2014).

When methadone is used to treat chronic pain and when a patient is switched to methadone from higher doses of another [illegible] therapy at a dose of 75–90% less than the calculated equianalgesic dose and no higher than 30 to 40 mg per day, with initial dose increases of no more than 10 mg per day every 5 to 7 days. Methadone should be withheld if there is evidence of sedation.

Titration is recommended in a hospital setting to ensure accurate administration. This can be difficult for patients because they have to experience pain before they are administered a dose of methadone in the titration period.

Mercadante and Bruera (2018) highlight the enormous advantage of methadone in developing countries due to its limited cost. It is particularly useful in patients with renal failure. Morphine is excreted via the kidneys, and, if renal failure occurs, this may lead to the patient experiencing severe drowsiness as a result of the accumulation of morphine metabolites. Methadone is lipid soluble and is metabolized mainly in the liver. About half of the drug and its metabolites are excreted by the intestines and half by the kidneys. Methadone should be used with the advice of a pain specialist.

Oxycodone

Oxycodone is available as an immediate or modified release preparation and titration should occur in the same way as for morphine. It has similar properties to morphine and can be administered orally, rectally or parenterally. Oxycodone is usually given 4–6 hourly. It has an analgesic potency 1.5–2.0 times higher than morphine. It has similar side-effects to morphine, most commonly constipation, dizziness, drowsiness, dry mouth, euphoric mood, flushing, hallucination, headache, hyperhidrosis, hypotension (with high doses), miosis and nausea (more common on initiation) (BNF and NICE 2019). A study by Riley et al. (2012) identified that on a population level there is no difference between morphine and oxycodone in terms of analgesia efficacy and tolerability.

Targinact is a combination of modified-release oxycodone and naloxone. The aim of this combination is to prevent the potential negative effects of opioid-induced constipation. It has been suggested that approximately 97% of the naloxone is eliminated by first pass metabolism in a healthy liver, preventing it from significantly affecting analgesic effects (Vellucci et al. 2014).

Tapentadol

Tapentadol is a centrally acting opioid analgesic supported by evidence for the management of acute and severe chronic pain (Schwartz et al. 2011, Wild et al. 2010). It has been shown to provide potent and efficacious analgesia in various rodent models of nociceptive and neuropathic pain (Wolkerstorfer et al. 2016). It is available in oral preparations in immediate- and modified-release forms. The conversion factor for tapentadol from oral morphine is 2.5:1. Therefore, 10 mg oral morphine is equivalent to 25 mg of tapentadol. The side-effects associated with tapentadol are similar to those associated with other opioids, including dizziness, headaches, somnolence, nausea and constipation.

Diamorphine

Diamorphine is used parenterally in a syringe pump or PCA pump for the control of moderate to severe pain when patients are unable to take the oral form of morphine. The dose is calculated by dividing the total daily dose of oral morphine by three. Breakthrough doses are calculated by dividing the 24-hour dose of diamorphine by six and administering on an as-required basis (Fallon et al. 2010).

Buprenorphine

Buprenorphine is an alternative strong opioid available in patch form. The patch has similar advantages to fentanyl but does not contain a reservoir of the drug. Instead, it is contained in a matrix form with effective levels of the drug being reached within 24 hours. Titration is recommended with an alternative opioid initially, and then the patient should be transferred to the patch when

Table 10.3 Recommended conversion rate guide from oral morphine to 72-hour fentanyl patch

Morphine dose in 24 hours (mg)	Fentanyl TTS (μg per hour)
30	12
60	25
120	50
180	75
240	100

TTS, transdermal therapeutic system.
Source: Reproduced from BNF (2019) with permission of Pharmaceutical Press.

stable requirements have been reached. A lower dose patch (BuTrans) is available in strengths of 5, 10 and 20 µg/h and should be worn continuously by the patient for 7 days. A higher dose patch (Transtec) of 35, 52.5 and 70 µg/h is now licensed to be used for up to 96 hours or twice weekly for patient convenience. Conversion is based on the chart supplied by the pharmaceutical company, which demonstrates equivalent doses. Buprenorphine is also available as a sublingual tablet, which is titrated from 200 to 800 µg every 6 hours. Conversion is based on multiplying the total daily dose of buprenorphine by 100 to give the total daily dose of morphine (i.e. 200 µg buprenorphine every 8 hours = 600 µg buprenorphine every 24 hours = 60 mg morphine every 24 hours). Transdermal buprenorphine patches are commonly used in the management of cancer and chronic pain. Due to their slow onset and offset they are considered unsuitable for the management of acute pain (Macintyre and Schug 2015).

Oral transmucosal fentanyl citrate (Actiq)

Transmucosal opioids, such as fentanyl citrate (Actiq), Abstral, Effentora and intranasal preparations such as PecFent, are licensed to be used for the treatment of cancer breakthrough pain. There are some circumstances when these agents are used off licence but they should always be used under the guidance of a specialist.

Licensed for the management of breakthrough pain in patients who are already on an established maintenance dose of opioid for cancer pain, oral transmucosal fentanyl citrate (OTFC) is a lozenge that is rubbed against the oral mucosa on the side of the cheek, which leads to the lozenge being dissolved by the saliva. The advantages of OTFC are its fast onset via the buccal mucosa (5–15 minutes) and its short duration (up to 2 hours). It is available in a range of doses (200–1600 µg) but there is no direct relationship between the baseline analgesia and the breakthrough dose. Titration can be difficult and lengthy as the recommended starting dose is 200 µg with titration upwards (Portenoy et al. 1999). It is recommended that the lozenge be removed from the mouth if the pain subsides before it has completely dissolved. The lozenge should not be reused but should be dissolved under running hot water.

Fentanyl buccal or sublingual tablet (Effentora or Abstral)

Effentora is a licensed medication for breakthrough pain in adults with cancer who are already receiving a maintenance opioid for chronic cancer pain. Patients receiving maintenance opioid therapy are those who are taking at least 60 mg of oral morphine daily, at least 25 µg of transdermal fentanyl per hour, at least 30 mg of oxycodone daily, at least 8 mg of oral hydromorphone daily, or an equianalgesic dose of another opioid for a week or longer. This buccal tablet is available in five dosing strengths: 100, 200, 400, 600 and 800 µg. It is placed on the oral mucosa above the third upper molar, which leads to the tablet being dissolved by the saliva. It usually takes 15–25 minutes for the tablet to dissolve. It is recommended that if the tablet has not completely dissolved within 30 minutes then the remainder of the tablet should be swallowed with water as it is thought that the tablet will then only be likely to consist of inactive substances rather than active fentanyl (Darwish et al. 2007).

Abstral is an oral transmucosal delivery formulation of fentanyl citrate indicated for the management of breakthrough pain in patients using opioid therapy for chronic cancer pain (Rauch et al. 2009). The tablet is administered sublingually and it rapidly disintegrates, ensuring the fentanyl dissolves quickly. Abstral is available in six dosing strengths: 100, 200, 300, 400, 600 and 800 µg fentanyl citrate. Zeppetella et al. (2014) found in their evidence review of all breakthrough cancer pain analgesia that transmucosal fentanyl medications achieve a greater level of pain relief in a shorter time frame than placebo or oral morphine.

Adjuvant drugs (co-analgesics)

Most chronic pain has elements of neuropathic pain. Patients with nociceptive pain are likely to gain some benefit from conventional medications such as NSAIDs but these drugs come with a strong side-effect profile. Individuals with neuropathic pain are likely to gain some relief from co-analgesics such as tricyclic antidepressants (e.g. amitriptyline and nortriptyline) and anticonvulsant drugs (e.g. gabapentin and pregabalin). Pregabalin has been shown to have beneficial effects on symptoms of neuropathic pain, but it increases the risk of a number of adverse effects (weight gain, dizziness, somnolence, peripheral oedema, vertigo and euphoria) as well as the risk of subsequent discontinuation due to these adverse effects (Onakpoya et al. 2019).

The WHO analgesic ladder recommends the use of these drugs in combination with non-opioids for mild to moderate pain and with opioids for moderate to severe pain (see Figure 10.6).

Nitrous oxide (Entonox)

Inhaled nitrous oxide provides analgesia that is short acting and works quickly. It has a special role in managing pain associated with procedures such as wound dressings and drain removal, and in acute trauma (see the section on Entonox administration later in this chapter for further details).

Local anaesthetics

In addition to epidural analgesia, local anaesthetics may be used to block individual or groups of peripheral nerves during surgical procedures and to infiltrate surgical wounds at the end of an operation. Wound catheter local anaesthetic injections have been shown to provide minor analgesic benefits for up to 48 hours and reduced length of hospital stay only in patients undergoing obstetric and gynaecological surgery (Schug et al. 2015). Occasionally, these techniques may be used to extend the duration of post-operative analgesia beyond the finite period that a single injection technique provides (Schug et al. 2015). Techniques include regular intermittent bolus doses or continuous infusions of local anaesthetic.

A topical preparation (lidocaine patch 5%) containing local anaesthetic is also available to manage acute or chronic neuropathic pain in areas of intact skin with hypersensitivity. There are also multiple topical creams available that can provide benefit – for example, Topical EMLA cream (eutectic mixture of local anaesthetics: lignocaine and prilocaine) has been shown to be effective in reducing the pain associated with venous ulcer debridement (Schug et al. 2015).

Cannabis

The UK government announced on 1 November 2018 that 'cannabis-derived medicinal products of appropriate standard' will be moved from Schedule 1 into Schedule 2 of the Misuse of Drugs Act (1971) and the Misuse of Drugs Regulations (2001) after a commissioned two-part review.

Separately, NICE has been commissioned to produce a clinical guideline on the prescribing of cannabis-based products for medicinal use in humans. The draft scope of NICE guidance includes use in people with chronic pain, people with intractable nausea and vomiting, people with spasticity and people with severe treatment-resistant epilepsy.

The British Paediatric Neurology Association (2018) has developed clinical advice on the use of cannabis-based medicinal products in paediatric patients with certain forms of severe epilepsy. This guidance covers use in rare epilepsies and multiple-sclerosis-related spasticity. The recommendations were jointly produced with the Royal College of Physicians and the Royal College of Radiologists, and in liaison with the Faculty of Pain Medicine of the Royal College of Anaesthetists. The guidance covers cannabis-based products for medicinal use for chemotherapy-induced nausea and vomiting and chronic pain (cancer pain and chronic neuropathic pain). It recommends that for chemotherapy-induced nausea and vomiting, cannabis-based products for medicinal use should remain an option for patients for whom standard therapies have not been successful. They should not be used as a first-line treatment. The guidance does not recommend the use of cannabis-based medicinal products for chronic pain as there is no robust evidence supporting this at present.

Hill et al. (2017) acknowledge that with the increased use of medical cannabis as pharmacotherapy for pain, there is a need for comprehensive risk–benefit discussions that take into account cannabis' significant possible side-effects. As cannabis use increases in the context of medical and recreational cannabis policies, additional research is essential to support or refute the current evidence base. See DH and NHS England (2018) for further information on using cannabis-products for medicinal purposes.

Anaesthetic interventions for managing complex pain

Sometimes it is difficult to attain and maintain adequate pain control without significant side-effects. In such situations, anaesthetic interventions may be of benefit.

Effective control can be achieved by epidural or intrathecal (spinal) infusions as single injections for simple nerve blocks or as regional nerve blocks that target individual nerves, plexi or ganglia (Hicks and Simpson 2004). An example is the use of a lumbar sympathetic block in the management of inoperable peripheral vascular disease, herpes zoster or diabetic neuropathy (Cherny et al. 2015).

These interventions can be useful but careful consideration and assessment must take place to ensure that any potential side-effects are discussed with the patient (anaesthetic interventions may severely limit the patient's activities). Additionally, future planning must be addressed with the patient and their family as an epidural or intrathecal infusion may limit discharge options for a patient who is dying.

Post-procedural considerations

Education of the patient and relevant others

Opioids and driving

In the UK, patients who are prescribed opioids are permitted to drive. However, the Faculty of Pain Medicine (2018) has suggested that, under certain circumstances, patients who are taking opioids should not drive. These circumstances include:

- the condition for which they are being treated has physical consequences that might impair their driving ability
- they feel unfit to drive
- they have just started opioid treatment
- the dose of opioid has recently been adjusted upwards or downwards (withdrawal from opioids can also have an impact on driving)
- they have consumed alcohol or drugs, which can produce an additive effect.

The Driving and Vehicle Licensing Agency (DVLA) is the only body that can legally advise a patient about their right to hold a driving licence. Patients starting opioids should be advised to inform the DVLA that they are now taking opioids and prescribers should document that this advice has been given. In March 2015 (section 5A of the Road Traffic Act 1988 as amended in 2013) the law on drugs and driving changed; if a person's driving is impaired for any reason, including taking medicines, it is illegal to drive (Gov.uk 2015).

Complications

The use of opioids in renal failure

Renal failure can cause significant and dangerous side-effects due to the accumulation of opioids. A systematic review in patients with cancer pain concluded that fentanyl, alfentanil and methadone, with caveats, are the medications likely to cause least harm in patients with renal impairment when used appropriately (King et al. 2011). Basic guidelines for pain management in renal failure include the following:

- reduce analgesia dose and/or dose frequency (8-hourly instead of 4-hourly)
- select a more appropriate drug (not renally excreted)
- avoid modified release preparations
- seek advice from a specialist pain or palliative care team and/or pharmacist (Farrell and Rich 2000).

Endocrine system

Long-term administration of opioids is associated with endocrine abnormalities (FPM 2018):

- Influences on both the hypothalamic–pituitary–adrenal axis and the hypothalamic–pituitary–gonadal axis have been demonstrated in patients taking oral opioids, with consequent hypogonadism and adrenal insufficiency in both sexes.
- Hypogonadism and decreased levels of dehydroepiandrosterone sulphate have been reported in men and women.

Immune system

Opioids have also been shown to affect the immune system (FPM 2018):

- Both animal and human studies have demonstrated that opioids have an immunomodulating effect. These effects are mediated via opioid receptors both on immune effector cells and in the central nervous system.
- In animals, opioids have been demonstrated to have effects on antimicrobial response and anti-tumour surveillance. Opioids may differ in their propensity to cause immunosuppression.
- In animal studies, buprenorphine has been demonstrated to have no impact on immune function. The relevance of these findings to the clinical use of opioids is not known.

Fractures and falls

Opioids have a number of implications for the risk of fractures and falls (FPM 2018):

- Opioids increase the risk and incidence of falls. This is of particular importance in elderly patients.
- In a systematic review of observational studies, the relative risk of any fracture in patients on opioids compared to non-using patients was 1.38.
- The relative risk of falls associated with opioids was similar to the risks associated with benzodiazepines (1.34 compared to non-using patients) and antidepressants (1.60 compared to non-using patients).

Opioid-induced hyperalgesia

Finally, opioids can have implications for pain sensitivity (FPM 2018):

- Both animal and human studies have demonstrated that prolonged use of opioids can lead to a state of abnormal pain sensitivity sometimes called opioid-induced hyperalgesia (OIH).
- The prevalence of OIH in clinical practice is unknown.

Regional analgesia: local anaesthetic nerve blocks and infusions

Definition

The term 'regional analgesia' includes peripheral nerve blocks (arm, leg or head) and spinal blocks. The term 'spinal analgesia' refers to both the epidural and intrathecal routes (discussed in the next section).

Regional analgesia can be used for acute post-operative pain, trauma pain and chronic pain. It can take the form of either a single injection ('single shot') or a continuous infusion such as a continuous peripheral nerve block (CPNB). A CPNB can also be delivered as an ambulatory service where patients are discharged home with the infusion.

Anatomy, physiology and related theory

Regional analgesia blocks transmission of pain impulses through a nerve by depositing an analgesic drug (usually local anaesthetic with or without an opioid) close to the nerve, cutting off sensory innervation to the region it supplies. This can target either peripheral or central (spinal) nerves. Pain impulses are inhibited but some sensations of touch and muscle functions are intact. Regional analgesia gives relief of pain on movement. This facilitates early post-operative mobilization of patients, even after major surgery in frail patients. Infiltration of the wound with local anaesthetics followed by optimally dosed non-opioid and opioid analgesics is a good alternative for some types of surgery.

Specific regional analgesia nerve blocks

Specific types of regional analgesia nerve blocks can be used for different types of acute or chronic pain. Table 10.4 lists examples of different regional nerve blocks and the procedures they can be used for.

Evidence-based approaches

Rationale

Regional analgesia approaches can be used for several reasons. The ability to provide selective analgesia with minimal adverse effects can be beneficial, particularly in older patients, who may have co-existing conditions (Macintyre and Schug 2015, Parizkova and George 2009a, 2009b). A nerve block or a continuous infusion of local anaesthetic can provide pain relief that is superior to the use of opioids alone, and the use of opioids can be minimized in the post-operative setting, resulting in fewer adverse effects, such as nausea, vomiting, sedation and pruritus (D'Arcy 2011). Pain relief and functionality may also be improved. Ilfeld (2011) found that, in comparison with systemic opioid analgesia (including PCA), CPNB leads to better pain relief and fewer opioid-related side-effects. Humble et al. (2015) found during their systematic review of perioperative interventions that regional analgesia was beneficial for reducing perioperative pain and subsequent chronic symptoms.

Contraindications

Contraindications for regional analgesia nerve blocks and infusions include the following:

- *Bleeding*: the risk of bleeding may be increased due to patient age, routine thromboprophylaxis and frequent use of anti-haemostatic drugs, including platelet inhibitors. Caution should be exercised in all patients with impaired coagulation, particularly around the timing of catheter removal.
- *Discharge planning*: if a patient is unable to physically or cognitively care for the continuous infusion at home when used in the ambulatory care setting, then it is contraindicated.

Methods of administration

Regional analgesia can be administered as a single-shot injection where the effects last for several hours after the procedure or as a continuous infusion (CPNB). CPNB can be used in both the inpatient and ambulatory care settings. CPNB analgesia infusion pumps can also be programmed to allow patients the option of bolus dosing in addition to the baseline continuous infusion rate.

Classes of drugs used in regional analgesia and mechanism of action

In peripheral nerve blocks, the most frequently used drug is a local anaesthetic. Commonly used local anaesthetic agents include bupivacaine, levobupivacaine and ropivacaine. Local anaesthetics bind directly within the intracellular portion of voltage-gated

Table 10.4 Examples of regional analgesia blocks

Type of block	Remarks
Brachial plexus block	The brachial plexus is the major nerve bundle going to the shoulder and arm. This block can be used to manage pre-operative pain in shoulder injuries and intractable cancer pain from tumours invading the brachial plexus, such as those involving the breast and chest wall. Depending on the level of surgery, the anaesthetist will decide at what level to block the brachial plexus – e.g. for surgery at the shoulder, an interscalene or cervical paravertebral block performed at a location above the clavicle may be used. For surgeries below the shoulder joint or clavicle, an intraclavicular or axillary block may be used.
Paravertebral block	Paravertebral blocks can be used to numb a specific area in one part of the body, depending on where the block is performed. For example, paravertebral blocks at the level of the neck can be used for thyroid gland or carotid artery surgery; blocks at the level of the chest and abdomen can be used for many types of breast, thoracic and abdominal surgery; and blocks at the level of the hip can be used for surgeries involving the hip, the knee and the front of the thigh.
Femoral nerve block	The femoral nerve provides sensation and motor function to the front of the thigh and knee. This block is commonly used for procedures that cover this area (such as surgery of the knee). It can also be used to provide analgesia for patients with hip fractures pre-operatively while they are waiting to go to theatre.
Sciatic and popliteal nerve block	The sciatic nerve provides sensation and motor function to the back of the thigh and most of the leg below the knee. This block is commonly used for surgery on the knee, calf, Achilles tendon, ankle or foot.
Lumbar plexus block	The lumbar nerves join to form the lumbar plexus. An anterior or posterior approach can be used. This block is commonly used for lower limb surgery such as hip and knee surgery, and for femoral shaft and neck fractures.
Spinal (intrathecal) central nerve blocks	Spinal blocks are forms of anaesthesia that temporarily interrupt sensation from the chest, abdomen and legs by injection of local anaesthetic medication in the vertebral canal, which contains the spinal cord, spinal nerves and cerebrospinal fluid. They can be used as a form of anaesthesia and are typically given as a single injection that will last for 2–6 hours, depending on the type and volume of local anaesthetic given. If an opioid is given, such as morphine, this can produce analgesia lasting 12 hours (Schug et al. 2015).
Intercostal and interpleural block	This block is used to provide somatosensory and motor blockade to the chest and abdominal wall. It is often used in thoracotomy, mastectomy and rib fractures. Continuous local anaesthetic infusion analgesia can be achieved using a subpleural catheter placed in the space posterior to the parietal pleura alongside the paravertebral area, or more laterally in the intercostal region (Schug et al. 2015).

Source: Adapted from Schug et al. 2015.

sodium channels. The degree of block produced by local anaesthetics is dependent on how the nerve has been stimulated and on its resting membrane potential. Local anaesthetics are only able to bind to sodium channels in their charged form and when the sodium channels are open. They cause numbness and loss of sensation and there may also be some loss of muscle function depending on the purpose of the block.

The dose of a local anaesthetic agent will also determine which nerves are blocked. Low concentrations of bupivacaine (e.g. 0.100–0.125%) preferentially block nerve impulses in the smallest-diameter nerve fibres, which include the pain and temperature sensory fibres. As the larger-diameter motor fibres are less likely to be blocked with concentrations of 0.100–0.125% bupivacaine, the incidence of motor weakness is reduced and patients are able to mobilize.

Clinical governance

There should be formal induction courses and regular updates for doctors, nurses, theatre staff and recovery staff who will be responsible for supervising patients receiving CPNBs. The acute pain service or a clearly designated consultant anaesthetist from the anaesthesia department will be responsible for the immediate supervision of patients receiving local anaesthetic infusions. The National Patient Safety Agency (NPSA) (2007) recommends that in addition to routine training and regular updates, additional training should occur when changes are made to protocols, medicinal products or medical devices.

Competencies

Nurses who monitor patients with a CPNB should have knowledge of:

- the anatomy and physiology of the spinal cord and column and the neurological system
- the purpose of the peripheral nerve catheter for pain management
- the CPNB process and signs and symptoms of peripheral nerve catheter misplacement
- the effects of medication administered for a CPNB
- untoward reactions to medication and management of complications.

Nursing care responsibilities include:

- observation [illegible] dressings or catheter removal)
- an understanding of the infusion pump in use
- documentation of care
- removal of the catheter once treatment has been discontinued.

Pre-procedural considerations

Equipment

CPNB catheters are inserted using a hollow Tuohy-type needle connected to a nerve stimulator or an ultrasound that identifies the nerve and allows the correct placement of the catheter (D'Arcy 2011, Parizkova and George 2009a, 2009b). Once correct placement has been confirmed, the catheter is threaded down the hollow centre of the needle to the area that needs analgesia. All products should now be NRFit compatible, following a nationwide conversion from the Luer connector to NRFit for intrathecal procedures, epidural procedures and delivery of regional blocks in accordance with NPSA (2017). For more information, see the section on clinical governance within the section below on epidural analgesia.

Dressings

The dressing over the CPNB catheter exit site needs to fulfil the following three functions:

- help to secure the CPNB catheter
- minimize the risk of infection
- allow observation of the site without disturbing the dressing.

A transparent moisture-responsive occlusive dressing (e.g. Tegaderm, OPSITE or IV3000) fulfils these functions. The CPNB catheter site should be inspected daily.

Pharmacological support

In CPNBs, local anaesthetic infusions are used. Rarely are other drugs combined with this approach.

Procedure guideline 10.2 Peripheral nerve catheter removal

Essential equipment

- Personal protective equipment
- Sterile dressing pack including gloves
- Sodium chloride 0.9% ampule
- Transparent occlusive dressing

Action	Rationale
Pre-procedure	
1 Introduce yourself to the patient, explain and discuss the procedure with them, and gain their consent to proceed.	To ensure that the patient feels at ease, understands the procedure and gives their valid consent (NMC 2018, **C**).
2 Wash hands with soap and water or use an alcohol-based handrub and apply personal protective equipment.	To reduce the risk of cross-infection (NHS England and NHSI 2019, **C**).
3 Clean the trolley or plastic tray following local guidelines for an aseptic procedure.	To reduce the risk of cross-infection (Loveday et al. 2014, **R**).
4 Open dressing pack using an aseptic technique.	To reduce the risk of cross-infection (Loveday et al. 2014, **R**).
5 Ensure the patient is in a comfortable position whereby the catheter is accessible.	To maintain dignity and comfort (RCN 2016, **E**).
Procedure	
6 Remove the tape and dressing from the catheter insertion site.	To gain access to the catheter for removal. **E**
7 Observe the site for any evidence of infection, such as redness, swelling or purulent discharge.	If infection is suspected, the tip of the catheter should be sent to microbiology for culture and sensitivity analysis, as per local policy. **E**

8 If the exit site appears clean and dry, it is not necessary to clean the skin prior to removal. If the site does require cleaning (e.g. due to exudate or dried blood), use an aseptic non-touch technique with sodium chloride 0.9% solution and sterile gauze.	To assess the site and ensure it is clean of any exudate or residue prior to catheter removal. **E**
9 Decontaminate hands and apply clean gloves.	To reduce the risk of cross-infection (NHS England and NHSI 2019, **C**).
10 Grasp the catheter as close as you can to where it enters the skin and gently, in one swift movement, remove the catheter. There should be little discomfort or resistance to the removal. A small amount of blood or fluid drainage is normal.	To ensure the catheter is removed intact with minimum discomfort to the patient. **E**
11 Inspect the catheter, ensuring it is intact by observing the markings at the tip (usually blue or black) and checking that the 1 cm markings along the catheter are all intact.	To ensure the catheter has been removed whole and intact and that part of the catheter has not been left in the patient. **E**
12 If required (if an infection is suspected) and as per local policy, send the tip to microbiology for further investigation.	To assess the catheter as a potential source of infection. **E**
13 Apply a transparent occlusive dressing (unless there is exudate, in which case use an occlusive dressing with absorbent pad) and leave it *in situ* for 24 hours.	To ensure all bleeding has stopped. To prevent inadvertent access of micro-organisms along the tract. **E**
14 Remove gloves and apron and dispose of all materials as per local policy. Decontaminate hands.	To prevent cross-infection (NHS England and NHSI 2019, **C**).
Post-procedure	
15 Observe the site for signs of infection, such as redness, tenderness, swelling or pus-like drainage at the insertion site. Also observe for any signs of bleeding at the site.	To ensure any adverse signs of infection or bleeding are identified and treated early to prevent any further complications. **E**

Post-procedural considerations

Immediate and ongoing care

When caring for a patient receiving regional analgesia, it is important to monitor them for the following at regular intervals (Macintyre and Schug 2015):

- pain score, functional activity score, sedation score and respiratory rate
- blood pressure and heart rate
- motor block: motor function should be assessed and any decreasing motor function should also be noted
- sensory block: any increasing sensory deficit should be noted as it may reflect the development of complications; however, routine monitoring of sensory block is not required and may not be helpful with a CPNB.

Education of the patient and relevant others

Patients in the ambulatory setting with a CPNB must accept a degree of responsibility for self-management of the catheter and infusion pump at home as they will not have clinician support 24 hours a day. Patient education needs to start in the pre-operative setting and extend to and be reinforced in the post-operative setting.

Instructions must be both verbal and written, and they should include key contact numbers of healthcare professionals who are available around the clock in case problems occur. Patient and family general education should include information on:

- medical equipment, i.e. patient guidelines on how to manage the infusion system at home
- observing for drug-related side-effects
- observing for procedure-related side-effects
- what to do if they have pain
- whom to contact if they have any problems, including details of the pain service and out-of-hours contact details
- when to call for further advice and help and how to clamp the tubing
- how to use supplemental oral analgesics if they have pain
- whether the catheter will be removed at home by the patient, at home by the nurse or on return to the hospital.

Additionally, all patients discharged with a CPNB should receive the following general instructions:

- Do not drive or operate machinery, equipment (including for sports or hunting) or tools for the duration of the block.
- Protect the operative limb (due to motor loss and loss of feeling) for the duration of the block.
- Keep the catheter site clean and dry.
- Observe for warning signs such as infection, haematoma, compartment syndrome and local anaesthetic toxicity.

Table 10.5 outlines the principles of care for a patient receiving a CPNB infusion.

Complications

Complications can:

- be drug related
- arise from the insertion of the needle or the presence of the indwelling catheter.

Drug related: local anaesthetic systemic toxicity

Systemic toxicity results from the effects of local anaesthetic drugs on the central nervous system and the cardiovascular system. This may occur if excessive doses are given or if the CPNB catheter has migrated into a blood vessel and the dose of local anaesthetic reaches the systemic circulation, which can cause very serious effects on the neurological, respiratory and cardiovascular systems. Management of severe toxicity is outlined in Figure 10.7.

Table 10.5 Care of a patient receiving a continuous peripheral nerve block infusion (CPNB)

Observations and care	Comments
Observe for the warning signs of: • infection • haematoma (nerve compression) • nerve trauma • compartment syndrome	These include: • increase in pain or continuous pain • fever, chills or sweats • bowel or bladder changes • difficulty breathing • redness, warmth, discharge or excessive bleeding from the catheter site • pain, swelling or a large bruise around the catheter site
Observe for signs and symptoms of local anaesthetic systemic toxicity	These include: • dizziness or light-headedness • blurred vision • ringing or buzzing in the ears • metallic taste in the mouth • numbness and/or tingling of the fingers or toes, or around the mouth • drowsiness • confusion
Dressing maintenance	Do not remove the dressing as this may move or remove the catheter. The catheter dressing may be reinforced with a clear occlusive dressing as needed, taking care not to move or remove the catheter.
Monitoring and care of the infusion pump system	This includes: • The infusion pump should be labelled as per the prescription. • The infusion pump should be running at the prescribed rate. • Check for kinks in the tubing. If the tubing is kinked, massage that area of the tubing to facilitate flow. • Troubleshoot any pump alarms.
Other monitoring and care	This includes: • assessment of the catheter site • assessment of the integrity of the dressing • assessment of the sensory, motor and vascular condition of the limb (capillary refill, colour and motor function of the affected extremity will help to differentiate intended block from potential nerve compromise or ischaemic pain) • limb positioning (maintain a neutral position) • assessment of the skin with attention to the 'hot spots': the heel should be free from continuous contact with the pillow or bed • patients may have difficulty with weight bearing if the lower limb has been blocked; care should be taken to prevent falls and provide assistance when mobilizing
Patient/family education	This includes: • Ensure the patient or their carer is competent to continue care of the CPNB at home. • Provide both written and verbal information; check the patient's understanding of the information provided. • Document the information provided.
Peripheral nerve catheter removal (see Procedure guideline 10.2: Peripheral nerve catheter removal and follow local guidelines)	Indications for catheter removal: • end of infusion • infection • failure to control pain • catheter leaking

Source: Adapted from Schug et al. 2015

The signs and symptoms of systemic local anaesthetic toxicity are:

- light-headedness
- circumoral numbness or numbness of the tongue
- tinnitus or visual disturbances
- muscular twitching
- drowsiness
- unconsciousness
- convulsions
- coma
- respiratory depression
- cardiovascular depression.

Insertion of the needle or catheter

Other complications can be related to the insertion of the needle or catheter (Box 10.4).

There are currently no national guidelines on the care and monitoring of patients who have received a single-injection regional analgesia block rather than a continuous infusion. Nurses are advised to follow local guidelines on monitoring these patients post procedure. Considerations should include the following.

- Has the patient received an opioid? If so, what is the drug, what is the dose and what is the expected duration of effect?

AAGBI Safety Guideline

Management of Severe Local Anaesthetic Toxicity

1 Recognition

Signs of severe toxicity:

- Sudden alteration in mental status, severe agitation or loss of consciousness, with or without tonic-clonic convulsions
- Cardiovascular collapse: sinus bradycardia, conduction blocks, asystole and ventricular tachyarrhythmias may all occur
- Local anaesthetic (LA) toxicity may occur some time after an initial injection

2 Immediate management

- Stop injecting the LA
- Call for help
- Maintain the airway and, if necessary, secure it with a tracheal tube
- Give 100% oxygen and ensure adequate lung ventilation (hyperventilation may help by increasing plasma pH in the presence of metabolic acidosis)
- Confirm or establish intravenous access
- Control seizures: give a benzodiazepine, thiopental or propofol in small incremental doses
- Assess cardiovascular status throughout
- Consider drawing blood for analysis, but do not delay definitive treatment to do this

3 Treatment

IN CIRCULATORY ARREST

- Start cardiopulmonary resuscitation (CPR) using standard protocols
- Manage arrhythmias using the same protocols, recognising that arrhythmias may be very refractory to treatment
- Consider the use of cardiopulmonary bypass if available

GIVE INTRAVENOUS LIPID EMULSION

(following the regimen overleaf)

- Continue CPR throughout treatment with lipid emulsion
- Recovery from LA-induced cardiac arrest may take >1 h
- Propofol is not a suitable substitute for lipid emulsion
- Lidocaine should not be used as an anti-arrhythmic therapy

WITHOUT CIRCULATORY ARREST

Use conventional therapies to treat:

- hypotension,
- bradycardia,
- tachyarrhythmia

CONSIDER INTRAVENOUS LIPID EMULSION

(following the regimen overleaf)

- Propofol is not a suitable substitute for lipid emulsion
- Lidocaine should not be used as an anti-arrhythmic therapy

4 Follow-up

- Arrange safe transfer to a clinical area with appropriate equipment and suitable staff until sustained recovery is achieved
- Exclude pancreatitis by regular clinical review, including daily amylase or lipase assays for two days
- Report cases as follows:

  in the United Kingdom to the National Patient Safety Agency (via **www.npsa.nhs.uk**)

  in the Republic of Ireland to the Irish Medicines Board (via **www.imb.ie**)

If Lipid has been given, please also report its use to the international registry at **www.lipidregistry.org**. Details may also be posted at **www.lipidrescue.org**

Your nearest bag of Lipid Emulsion is kept ....

This guideline is not a standard of medical care. The ultimate judgement with regard to a particular clinical procedure or treatment plan must be made by the clinician in the light of the clinical data presented and the diagnostic and treatment options available.

Figure 10.7 Safety guideline: management of severe local anaesthetic toxicity. *Source*: Reproduced from AAGBI (2010) with permission of the Association of Anaesthetists of Great Britain and Ireland.

IMMEDIATELY

Give an initial intravenous bolus injection of 20% lipid emulsion **1.5 ml.kg^{-1}** over 1 min

AND

Start an intravenous infusion of 20% lipid emulsion at **15 ml.kg^{-1}.h^{-1}**

AFTER 5 MIN

Give **a maximum of two** repeat boluses (same dose) if:

- cardiovascular stability has not been restored **or**
- an adequate circulation deteriorates

Leave **5 min** between boluses

A maximum of **three** boluses can be given (including the initial bolus)

AND

Continue infusion at same rate, but:

Double the rate to **30 ml.kg^{-1}.h^{-1}** at any time after 5 min, if:

- cardiovascular stability has not been restored or
- an adequate circulation deteriorates

Continue infusion until stable and adequate circulation restored or maximum dose of lipid emulsion given

Do not exceed a maximum cumulative dose of 12 ml.kg^{-1}

An approximate dose regimen for a 70 kg patient would be as follows:

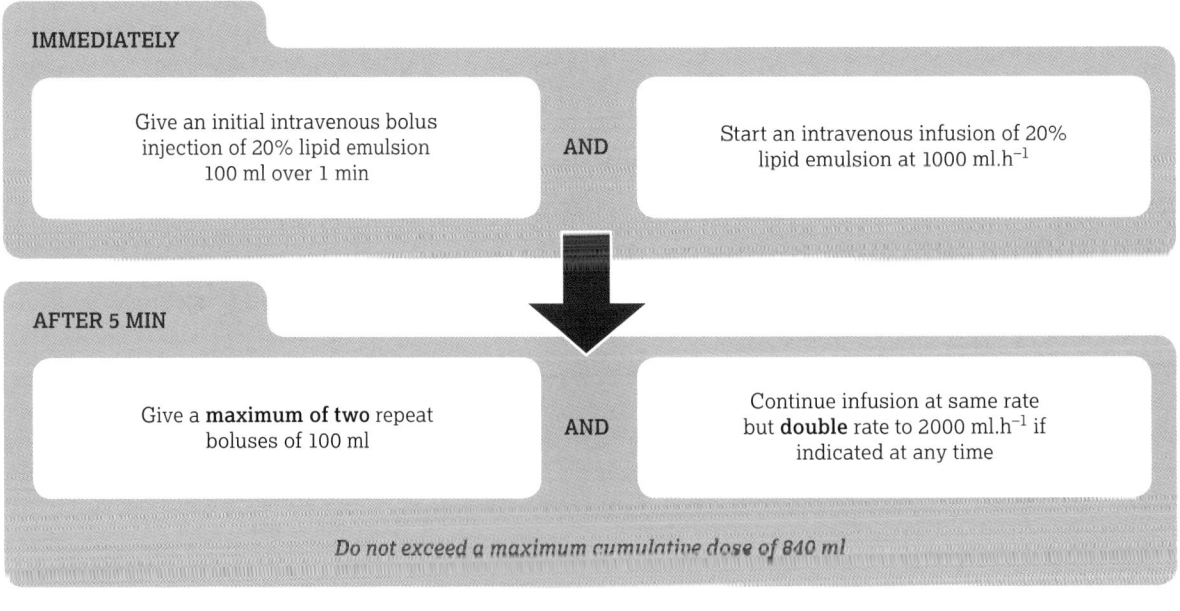

IMMEDIATELY

Give an initial intravenous bolus injection of 20% lipid emulsion 100 ml over 1 min

AND

Start an intravenous infusion of 20% lipid emulsion at 1000 ml.h^{-1}

AFTER 5 MIN

Give a **maximum of two** repeat boluses of 100 ml

AND

Continue infusion at same rate but **double** rate to 2000 ml.h^{-1} if indicated at any time

Do not exceed a maximum cumulative dose of 840 ml

This AAGBI Safety Guideline was produced by a Working Party that comprised:

Grant Cave, Will Harrop Griffiths (Chair), Martyn Harvey, Tim Meek, John Picard, Tim Short and Guy Weinberg.

This Safety Guideline is endorsed by the Australian and New Zealand College of Anaesthetists (ANZCA).

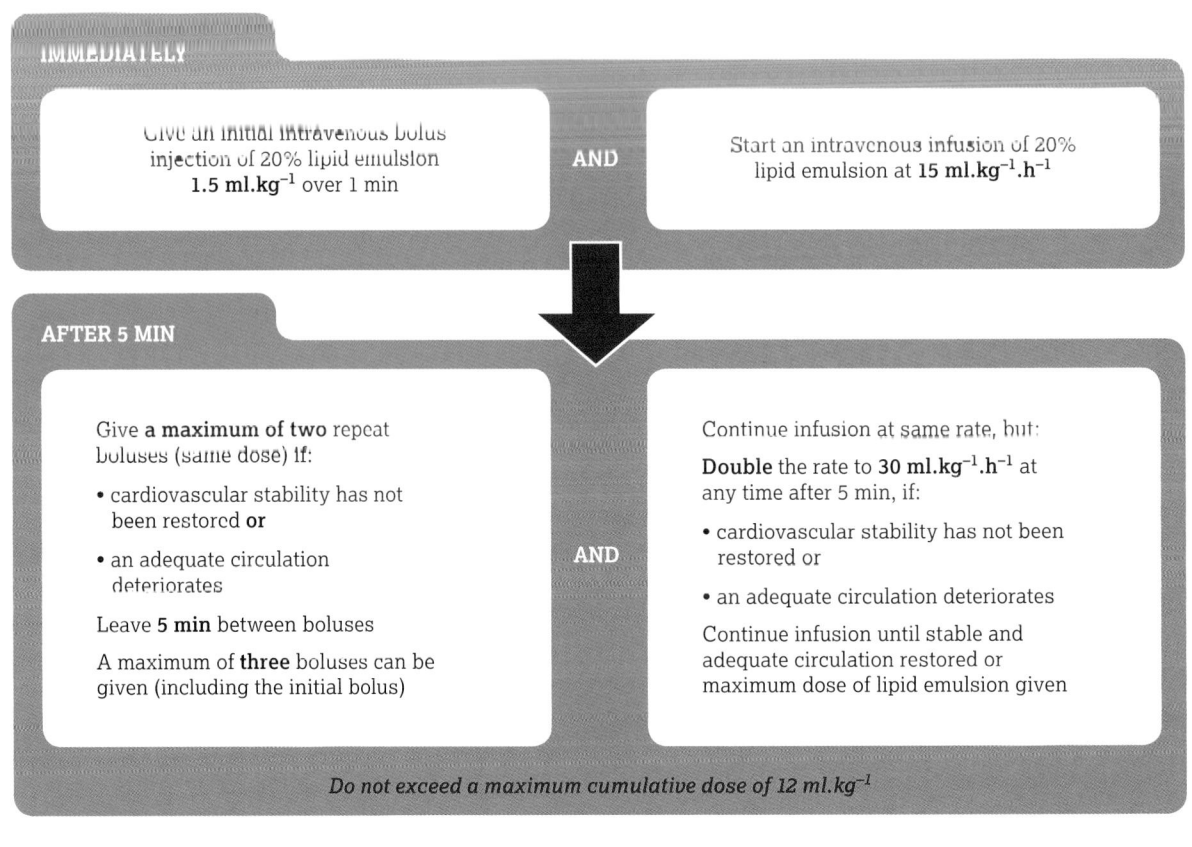

Figure 10.7 *Continued*

Box 10.4 Complications relating to continuous peripheral nerve blocks (CPNB)

Bleeding

The risk of bleeding increases with the age of the patient, routine thromboprophylaxis and frequent use of antihaemostatic drugs, including platelet inhibitors. Caution should be exercised in all patients with impaired coagulation, particularly around the timing of catheter removal.

Nerve injury

This may occur as a result of insertion of the needle or catheter during the CPNB. Most nerve injury results in residual paraesthesia only, and most of these resolve over time. However, there can be a more significant and often permanent injury. Examples include:

- spinal cord damage following injection of local anaesthetic into the cord during interscalene blocks under general anaesthesia
- pneumothorax following brachial plexus blockade

Infection

CPNB indwelling catheters carry a risk of infection. The risk increases with duration of use.

Catheter or pump related

Problems with equipment may occur at any time. Simple problems include a kinked catheter or tubing. More complex problems may also occur, such as pump errors, or the catheter breaking and leaving a residual portion in the patient.

- Assessment of the injection site for evidence of bleeding or haematoma.
- Assessment of the limb or affected area for sensory function and, if appropriate, motor function, and evidence of return to normal baseline function.

Epidural analgesia

This section focuses on epidurals used for acute pain.

Definition

Epidural analgesia

Epidural analgesia is the administration of medication via a catheter inserted into the epidural space at the thoracic or lumbar level (Macintyre and Schug 2015). Epidural analgesia is an effective method of providing sustained and effective pain relief following surgery, such as thoracic or orthopaedic surgeries, or major abdominal procedures (Argoff 2014, Pöpping et al. 2014).

Intrathecal analgesia

Intrathecal (spinal) analgesia is the administration of analgesic drugs via a catheter inserted into the intrathecal space and cerebrospinal fluid (CSF) (Vayne-Bossert et al. 2016). This method is most commonly used for cancer pain; see the chapter on pain assessment and management in *The Royal Marsden Manual of Cancer Nursing Procedures* (Lister et al. 2019) for further information.

Anatomy and physiology

The spinal cord (Figures 10.8 and 10.9) is covered by the meninges; the pia mater is closely applied to the cord and the arachnoid mater lies closely with the outer, tough covering called the dura mater (Tortora and Derrickson 2017). The epidural space lies outside all three membranes, encasing the spinal cord between the spinal dura and ligamentum flavum. The contents of the epidural space include a rich venous plexus, spinal arterioles, lymphatics and extradural fat.

The intrathecal space (also termed the subarachnoid space) lies between the arachnoid mater and pia mater and contains the CSF (Tortora and Derrickson 2017). There are 31 pairs of spinal nerves of varying size that pass out through the intervertebral foramina between each vertebra (Tortora and Derrickson 2017). There are two main groups of nerve fibres:

- *Myelinated*: myelin is a thin, fatty sheath that protects and insulates the nerve fibres and prevents impulses from being transmitted to adjacent fibres.
- *Unmyelinated*: these are delicate fibres that are more susceptible to hypoxia and toxins than myelinated fibres.

The spinal nerves are each composed of a posterior and an anterior root, which join to form the nerve:

- *Posterior root*: this transmits ascending sensory impulses from the periphery to the spinal cord.
- *Anterior root*: this transmits descending motor impulses from the spinal cord to the periphery by means of its corresponding spinal nerve (Gélinas and Arbour 2014).

Specific skin surface areas are supplied or innervated by each of the spinal nerves. These skin areas are known as 'dermatomes' (Figure 10.10).

Evidence-based approaches

Epidural analgesia is the administration of analgesics (local anaesthetics and opioids with or without adjuvants such as corticosteroids and clonidine) into the epidural space via an indwelling catheter (Macintyre and Schug 2015). This technique enables analgesics to be injected close to the spinal cord and spinal nerves, where they exert a powerful analgesic effect. Epidural analgesia can provide longer-lasting pain relief with less dosing of opioids (Chou et al. 2016). It is one of the most effective techniques available for the management of acute pain (Chou et al. 2016) and is deemed the gold standard technique for managing pain after surgery (Bashandy and Elkholy 2014).

Intrathecal (spinal) analgesia is the administration of analgesic drugs directly into the CSF in the intrathecal space (Gélinas and Arbour 2014). Analgesic drugs given via this route are 10 times as potent as those given into the epidural space so the doses given are much smaller.

Spinal blocks are forms of anaesthesia that temporarily interrupt sensation from the chest, abdomen and legs by injection of local anaesthetic medication into the vertebral canal, which contains the spinal cord, spinal nerves and CSF. They are typically given as a single injection, which will last for 2–6 hours depending on the type and volume of local anaesthetic given. If an opioid is given, such as morphine, this can produce analgesia lasting 12 hours (Macintyre and Schug 2015). See the previous section for more information on spinal blocks.

In chronic cancer pain, intrathecal drug delivery (ITDD) can be used for the delivery of continuous infusions of analgesia in patients with spasticity and in patients with cancer pain that is uncontrolled with appropriate systemic opioids or when analgesia leads to intolerable side-effects (British Pain Society 2015, NHS England 2015).

In 2015, NHS England stopped commissioning ITDD fully implantable systems for patients with non-cancer pain. Healthcare professionals should note that patients with chronic non-cancer pain may have had an ITDD inserted prior to 2015 and they may continue to be managed by their specialist chronic pain service today (NHS England 2015). See the chapter on pain assessment and management in *The Royal Marsden Manual of Cancer Nursing Procedures* (Lister et al. 2019) for further information about using this device for cancer pain.

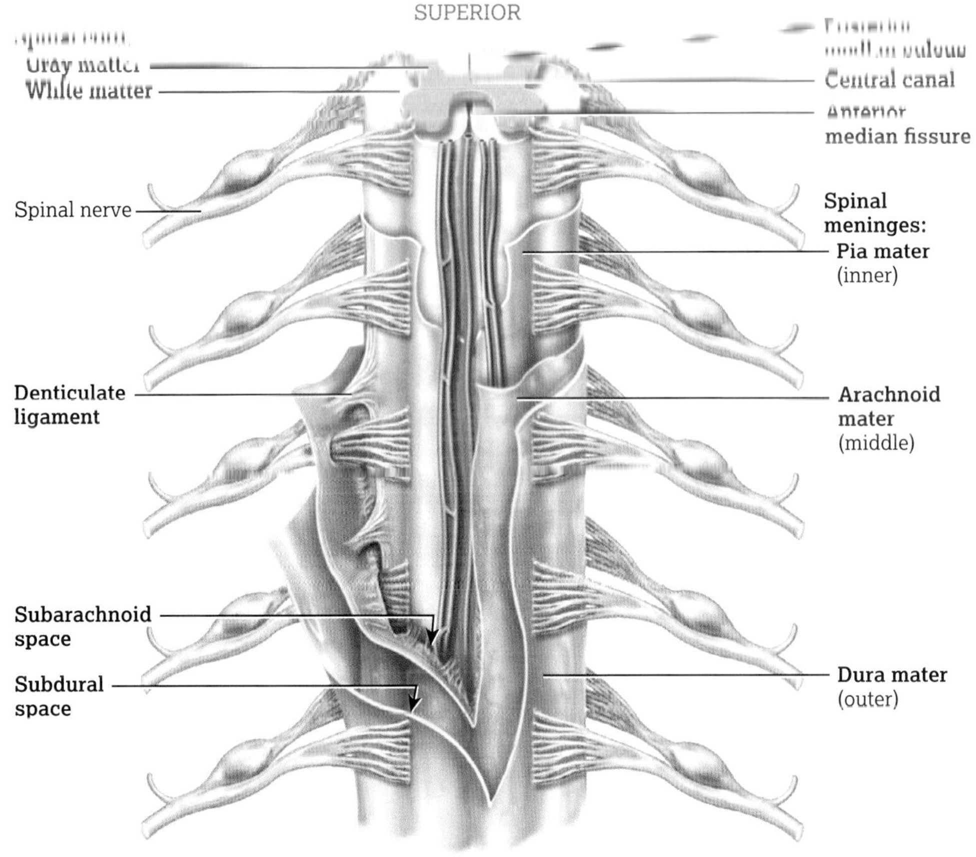

(a) Anterior view and transverse section through spinal cord

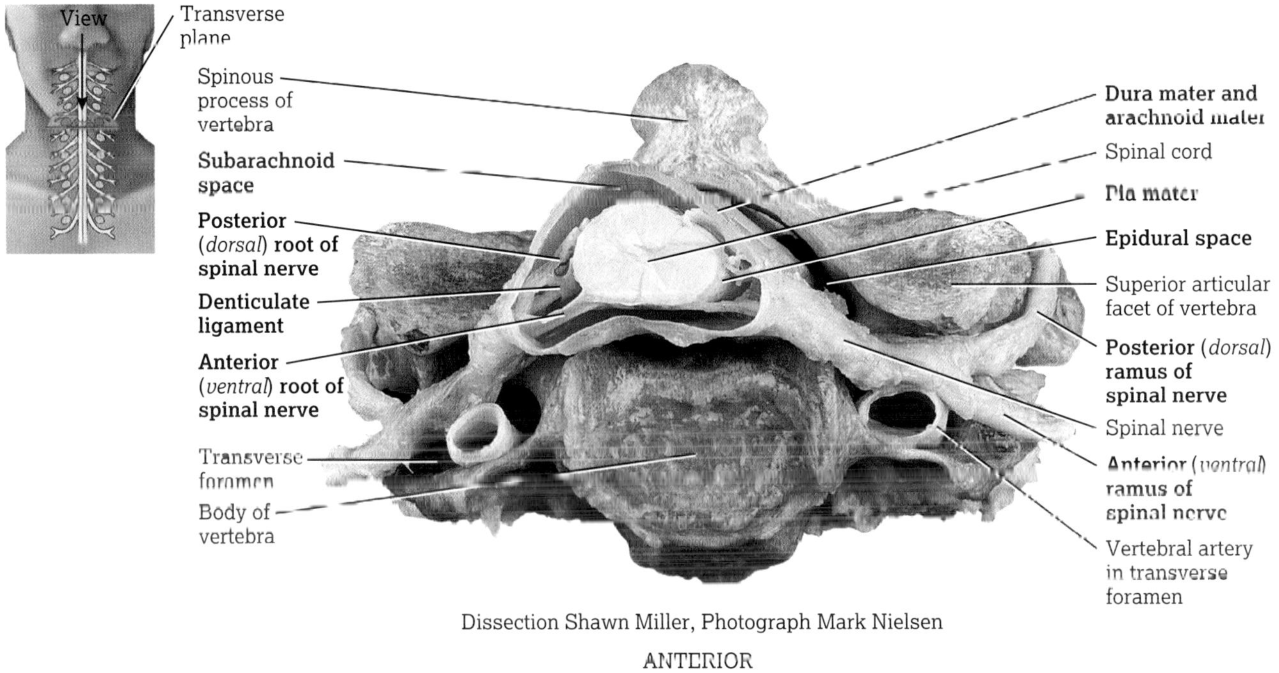

(b) Transverse section of the spinal cord within a cervical vertebra

Figure 10.8 Gross anatomy of the spinal cord. (a) Anterior view and transverse section through the spinal cord. (b) Transverse section of the spinal cord within a cervical vertebra. *Source:* Reproduced from Tortora and Derrickson (2017) with permission of John Wiley & Sons.

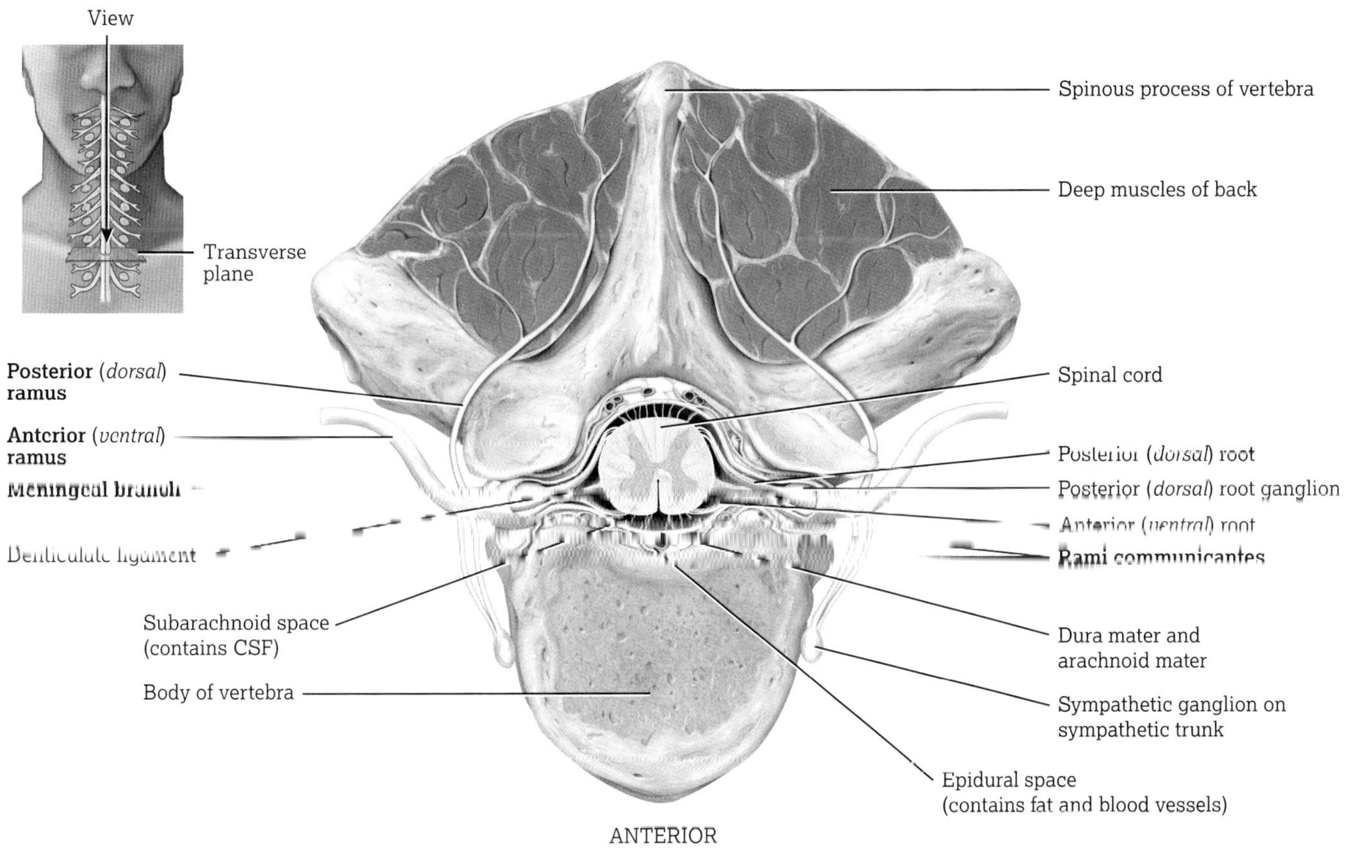

Figure 10.9 Branches of a typical spinal nerve, shown in cross-section through the thoracic portion of the spinal cord: transverse section. *Source*: Reproduced from Tortora and Derrickson (2017) with permission of John Wiley & Sons.

Rationale

There are three main advantages to using epidural analgesia:

- It has the potential to provide effective dynamic pain relief for many patients (Rosero et al. 2014).
- The combination of local anaesthetic agents with opioids has a synergistic action that allows the concentration of each drug to be reduced. This limits the unwanted side-effects of each drug (McClymont and Celnick 2018).
- There is evidence that the use of epidural analgesia may reduce the stress response (McClymont and Celnick 2018) to surgery or trauma, thereby reducing morbidity, recovery time and duration of hospital stay (Rosero et al. 2014).

Indications

Indications for epidural analgesia include the following:

- provision of analgesia during labour
- as an alternative to general anaesthesia, for example in severe respiratory disease or for patients with malignant hyperthermia
- provision of post-operative analgesia: epidural analgesia has been used since the late 1940s as a method of controlling post-operative pain (Toledano and Tsen 2014)
- provision of analgesia for pain resulting from trauma, for example fractured ribs, which may result in respiratory impairment due to pain on breathing
- management of chronic intractable pain in patients with chronic or cancer-related pain who experience the following:
  - unacceptable side-effects with systemic opioids
  - unsuccessful treatment with opioids via other routes despite escalating doses
  - severe neuropathic pain due to tumour invasion or compression of nerves (McSwain et al. 2014)
- to relieve muscle spasm and pain resulting from lumbar cord pressure due to disc protrusion or local oedema and inflammation.

Contraindications

These may be absolute or relative.

Absolute

Absolute contraindications for epidural analgesia include the following:

- patients with coagulation defects, which may result in haematoma formation and spinal cord compression, for example iatrogenic (anticoagulated patient) or congenital (haemophiliacs), or thrombocytopenia due to disease (Harrop-Griffiths et al. 2013, Schug et al. 2015)
- local sepsis at the site of proposed epidural; the result might be meningitis or epidural abscess formation (Vayne-Bossert et al. 2016)
- proven allergy to the intended drug
- unstable spinal fracture
- patient refusal to consent to the procedure.

Relative

Relative contraindications for epidural analgesia include the following:

- unstable cardiovascular system
- spinal deformity
- raised intracranial pressure (a risk of herniation if a dural tap occurs)
- certain neurological conditions, for example multiple sclerosis, where an epidural may result in an exacerbation of the disease (McSwain et al. 2014)

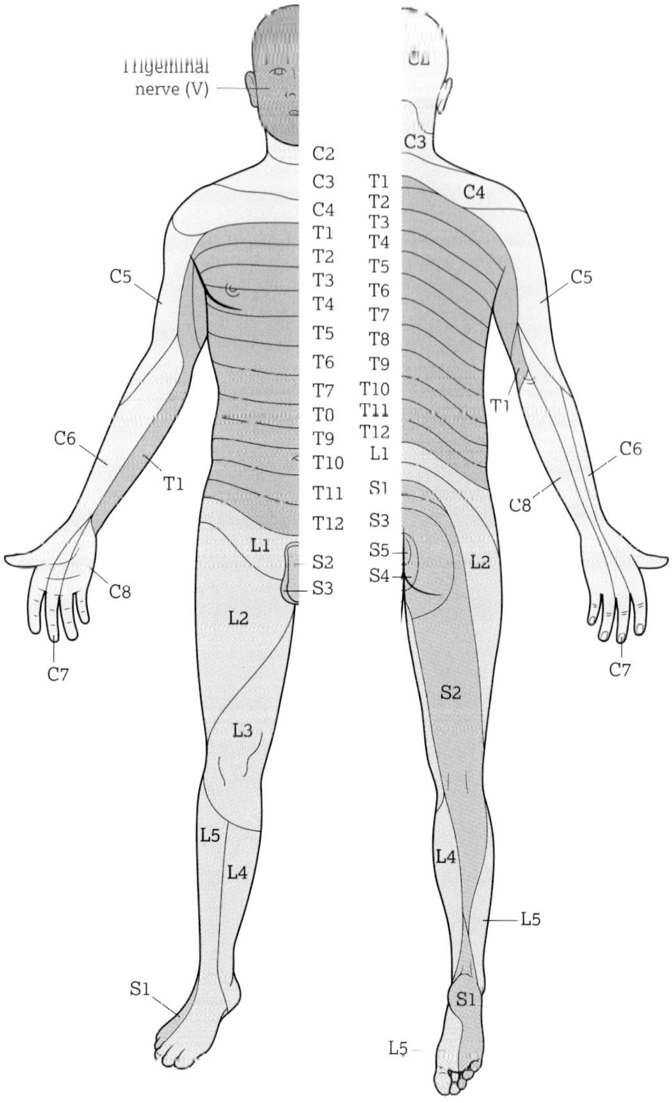

Levels of principal dermatomes

C5	Clavicles
C5, 6, 7	Lateral parts of upper limbs
C8; T1	Medial sides of upper limbs
C6	Thumb
C6, 7, 8	Hand
C8	Ring and little fingers
T4	Level of nipples
T10	Level of umbilicus
T12	Inguinal or groin regions
L1, 2, 3, 4	Anterior and inner surfaces of lower limbs
L4, 5; S1	Foot
L4	Medial side of great toe
L5; S1, 2	Outer and posterior sides of lower limbs
S1	Lateral margin of foot and little toe
S2, 3, 4	Perineum

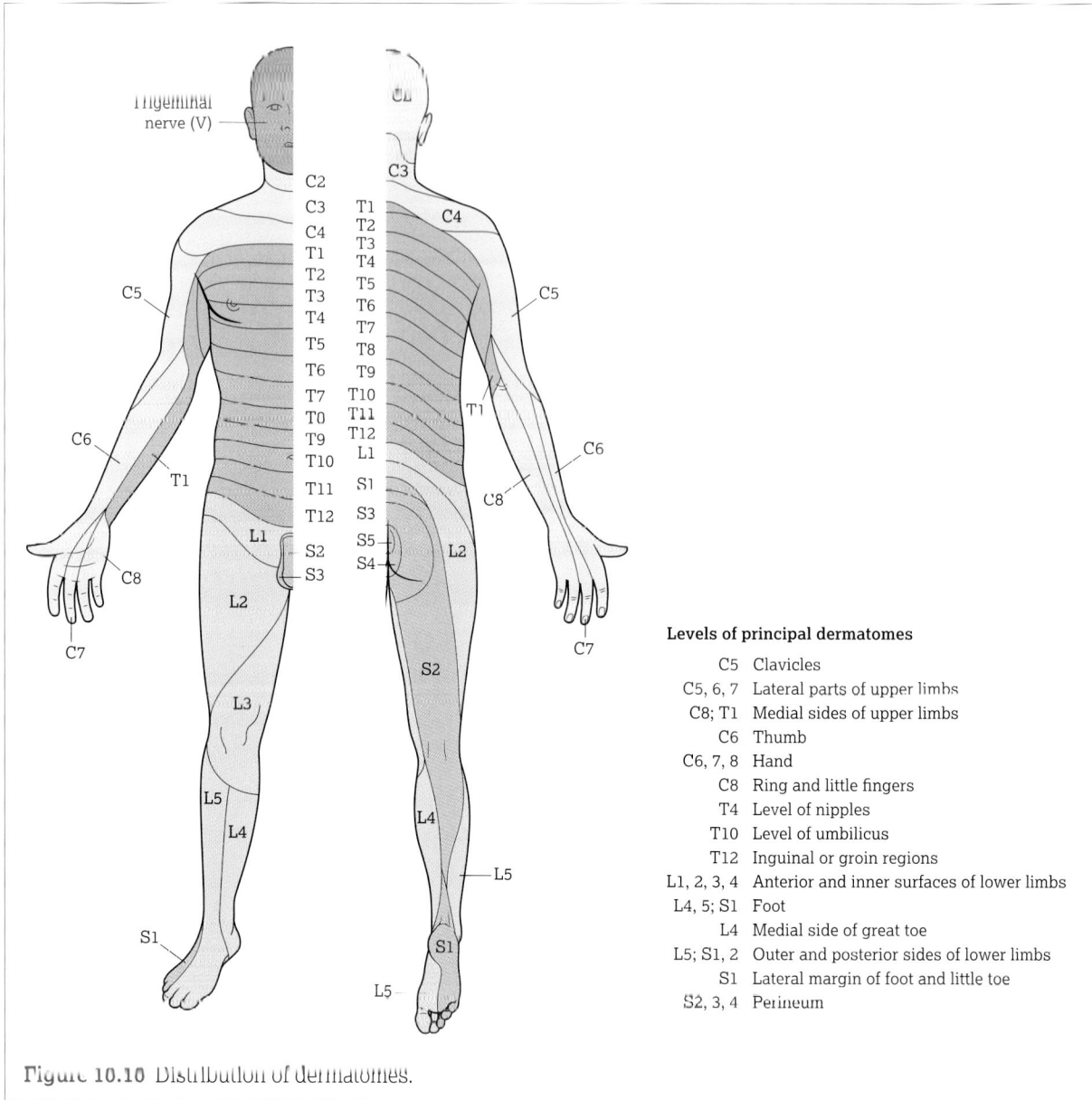

Figure 10.10 Distribution of dermatomes.

- unavailability of staff trained in the management of epidural analgesia (Macintyre and Schug 2015): it is identified that epidural analgesia carries specific risks and it is recommended that staff undertake a period of formal training in this area to enable them to care for patients safely and competently (Schug et al. 2015).

Methods of administration

Continuous infusion

Continuous infusions of epidural drugs are the most effective way of providing dynamic pain relief after major surgical procedures (Argoff 2014). The epidural is placed near to the site of the surgery to achieve the optimum analgesic effect (RCA 2015).

Continuous infusions can be given via either a syringe pump or a dedicated infusion pump system. The effectiveness of this method of administering drugs is dependent on a number of factors, including the combination of drugs used, whether the catheter is positioned at a level appropriate to the site of the surgery or pain (Kooij et al. 2014, RCA 2015) and the volume of the local anaesthetic agent infused (Chou et al. 2016).

Patient-controlled epidural analgesia

The use of patient-controlled epidural analgesia (PCEA) enables patients to control their analgesia (Schug et al. 2015, Tiippana et al. 2014). For post-operative patients, PCEA can provide greater analgesia efficacy in combination with a low-dose background infusion (Jules-Elysee et al. 2015, Tiippana et al. 2014). This ensures a baseline level of analgesia, which can then be supplemented by the patient when required (Jules-Elysee et al. 2015).

Bolus injections

Bolus injections of local anaesthetic agents and/or opioids are used infrequently to manage post-operative pain but are more commonly used for managing labour pain (Bujedo 2014). This procedure is usually performed by a doctor. However, bolus doses of low-dose concentrations may be given by nursing or midwifery staff as part of an advanced practice role, according to local policy. This should follow an agreed period of education and supervised practice, which must be documented.

This is a clean, aseptic procedure. Most epidural infusion pumps allow a bolus dose to be programmed and delivered from the pump. This prevents the administration line and bacterial filter being accessed and thus minimizes the risk of introducing infection.

Classes of epidural and intrathecal drugs and mechanism of action

Three classes of drugs are commonly used to provide epidural analgesia: opioids, local anaesthetic agents, and adjuvant drugs such as corticosteroids and clonidine.

Opioids

The two opioids most commonly used for epidurals are diamorphine and fentanyl (Gorlin et al. 2016). When either of these opioids is injected into the *epidural* space, part of the opioid dose:

- crosses the dura and arachnoid membrane and enters the CSF; from the CSF, a proportion of the drug is taken up into the spinal cord and reaches the opioid receptors in the spinal cord; once bound to the opioid receptors, pain impulses are blocked
- enters the systemic circulation and contributes to analgesia
- binds to the epidural fat and does not contribute to analgesia.

In contrast, when opioids are placed directly into the CSF in the *intrathecal* space, they attach directly to the opioid spinal cord receptor sites ([illegible] 2010). In acute pain, spinal intrathecal analgesia is usually given in a monitored environment (e.g. critical care or a high-dependency unit).

Fentanyl differs from diamorphine in that it is more lipid soluble (Gorlin et al. 2016). This means that it passes more easily into the CSF, and so gains faster access to the opioid receptors and has a more rapid onset of action. Fentanyl also has a shorter duration of action (1–4 hours) compared to diamorphine (6–12 hours) (Macintyre and Schug 2015).

Local anaesthetic drugs

As for regional blocks, commonly used local anaesthetic agents for epidural analgesia include bupivacaine, levobupivacaine and ropivacaine. They inhibit pain transmission by blocking sodium ion channels, which are involved in the propagation of electrical impulses along the spinal nerves. In epidural analgesia, these drugs gain access to the nerve roots and the spinal cord by crossing the dura and subarachnoid membrane (O'Neill and Arbour 2014).

The dose of a local anaesthetic agent will also determine which nerves are blocked. Low concentrations of bupivacaine (e.g. 0.100–0.125%) preferentially block nerve impulses in the smallest-diameter nerve fibres, which include the pain and temperature sensory fibres. As the larger-diameter motor fibres are less likely to be blocked with concentrations of 0.100–0.125% bupivacaine, the incidence of leg weakness is reduced and patients are able to mobilize.

Adjuvant drugs

Clonidine is an example of an adjuvant drug that can be used to provide epidural analgesia. It is a mixed alpha-adrenergic agonist. Alpha-2 adrenoceptor agonists act as analgesics at the level of the dorsal horn of the spinal cord, although there may be peripheral effects as well (Nguyen et al. 2017). Clonidine is believed to enhance analgesia provided by spinal opioids and local anaesthetic drugs, and additionally may reduce post-operative systemic opioid requirements (Gallagher and Grant 2018, Schug et al. 2015). Systemic adverse effects predominantly consist of centrally mediated sedation and hypotension.

Clinical governance

There should be formal induction courses and regular updates for doctors, nurses, theatre staff and recovery staff who will be responsible for supervising patients receiving continuous epidural analgesia (RCA 2019). The acute pain service or a clearly designated consultant anaesthetist from the anaesthesia department will be responsible for the immediate supervision of patients receiving local anaesthetic infusions. The NPSA (2007) recommends that in addition to routine training and regular updates, additional training should occur when changes are made to protocols, medicinal products or medical devices. Routine training should include a programme to help healthcare staff gain competence and confidence in using infusion devices employed to deliver epidural or intrathecal analgesia, a theoretical understanding of how the drugs work, and the monitoring required to detect both drug- and procedure-related side-effects and complications. Table 10.6 contains an example of learning outcomes and essential skills that could be included in a work-based competency outline for all healthcare professionals caring for patients with epidural analgesia.

There have been reports of fatal cases when epidural medicines were administered by the intravenous route and intravenous medicines were administered by the spinal route. In response, the NPSA (2009) issued a Patient Safety Alert recommending that all epidural, spinal (intrathecal) and regional anaesthesia infusions and bolus doses should be given with devices with connectors that will not connect with intravenous equipment – so-called 'safer connectors'. As a consequence, in 2017, international connectors known as NRFit, which include a dedicated connector for neuraxial devices, were released (NHS Improvement 2017). Therefore, all NHS organizations have had to review their transition plans and start using this new, safer device.

Pre-procedural considerations

Equipment

Epidural catheters are inserted using:

- a spinal (Tuohy) needle (a bevelled, curved-tip needle to reduce the risk of accidental dural puncture, with 1 cm length markings), either 16 or 18 G
- an epidural or intrathecal catheter (a relatively stiff catheter made of polyamide, length 1000 mm with clear blue markings completely embedded in the catheter material)
- a bacterial filter (filters provide an additional degree of safety and control to prevent bacterial infections; minimal dead space enables accurate dosing; a high-pressure resistance up to 7 bar enhances safety during manual injection)
- a connector (to ensure safe catheter fixation)
- a loss-of-resistance device (to aid clear identification of the epidural space).

This equipment often comes in prepared sterile disposable epidural trays or packs (McClymont and Celnick 2018) (Figure 10.11).

Dressings

The dressing over the epidural exit site needs to fulfil the following three functions:

- help secure the epidural catheter
- minimize the risk of infection
- allow observation of the site without disturbing the dressing.

A transparent moisture-responsive occlusive dressing (e.g. Tegaderm, OPSITE or IV3000) fulfils these functions. The epidural site should be inspected daily and the dressing changed at least once per week or more frequently if there is any serous discharge from the site (see Procedure guideline 10.4: Epidural exit site dressing change).

Pharmacological support

Combination of drugs used

Epidural infusions of local anaesthetic and opioid combinations are commonly used (McClymont and Celnick 2018, Tosounidis et al. 2015). The rationale behind their combined use is based on the observation that better analgesia is achieved with lower doses of each drug, as this minimizes the drug-related side-effects produced by higher concentrations (Duncan et al. 2014). Although the solutions used will vary with the clinical situation, combinations of fentanyl and a local anaesthetic (such as levobupivacaine) are often used. The use of premixed bags is recommended to

Table 10.6 An example of a competency role development profile for epidural analgesia for acute pain: intended learning outcomes and elements of practitioner competency

Knowledge and understanding	Skills
You are expected to possess knowledge and understanding of the following: • The normal anatomy of the spinal cord • The physiology of pain and measures of pain management • Education and information needs of the patient/family/carer with regard to the implications of having an epidural, to ensure valid consent is given • Contraindications for epidural analgesia • Infection control considerations before, during and after insertion of an epidural • Principles of epidural care and management including side-effects and complications of epidural insertion and epidural analgesia • Observations required during the administration of epidural analgesia and the rationale for the frequency of: – respiratory rate/sedation levels – cardiovascular status – temperature – epidural site – dermatomal blockade – pain assessment • The standard prescription for epidural analgesia for acute pain management • Deviations from the standard prescription available and situations in which they may be used • Pharmacology of epidurally administered local anaesthetics and opioids and their side-effects • The optimum infusion rate • When to stop and remove an epidural catheter • Implications of anticoagulant therapy prior to removing the epidural catheter • Considerations for analgesia once epidural analgesia is stopped	You are expected to possess the following skills: • Ability to care for the patient before, during and immediately after epidural insertion • Ability to check the epidural site, along with knowledge of appropriate frequency of checks and what problems to look for • Ability to re-dress the epidural site, along with knowledge of appropriate frequency of epidural site dressing changes • Ability to assess pain, along with knowledge of appropriate frequency of assessment • Ability to carry out a dermatomal blockade assessment, along with knowledge of where to document it • Ability to change the epidural infusion rate • Ability to change an epidural infusion bag and awareness of the frequency of infusion bag changes • Ability to change and prime the infusion administration set and awareness of the frequency of change • Ability to deal with equipment problems: – proximal occlusion alarm – distal occlusion alarm – cassette not fitted – low battery • Ability to deal with administration problems: – catheter disconnection from bacterial filter – catheter occlusion – catheter leakage – the patient still has pain – side-effects of analgesia – complications of epidural catheter insertion • Procedure for removing an epidural catheter • Safe disposal of unused epidural infusion bags after discontinuing therapy

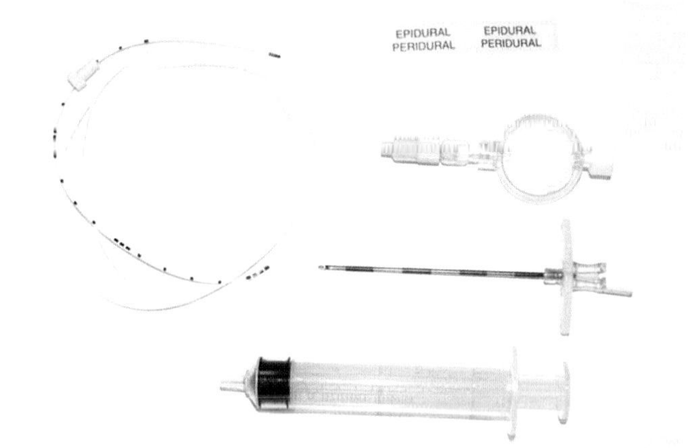

Figure 10.11 Epidural insertion kit. *Source*: Reproduced with permission of Vygon.

minimize medication errors involving the epidural and intrathecal routes (Grissinger 2012, NPSA 2007).

Specific patient preparation

Patients undergoing an epidural should always have a venous access device *in situ* before the procedure. This is because, although rare, a reaction to the opioid or local anaesthetic solution (e.g. respiratory depression or sympathetic blockade) may require immediate access to the venous system. The procedure should be performed in a clinical area with access to a full set of resuscitation equipment.

Position of the epidural catheter

Local anaesthetic drugs block nerve fibres at spinal segments adjacent to their site of administration. To ensure the local anaesthetic agent spreads to the dermatomes or nerves supplying the area of pain (i.e. the surgical site), the tip of the spinal catheter should be placed within the mid-dermatomal distribution of the pain site (Table 10.7). This achieves optimal analgesia using the smallest possible amount of drugs (FPM 2015). If the catheter is placed below the dermatomes supplying the pain site, then analgesia is likely to be inadequate (Macintyre and Schug 2015).

Effectiveness of the blockade

The spinal nerves supply specific areas of skin known as dermatomes (see Figure 10.10). Sensitivity to changes in temperature (ethyl chloride spray) along the sensory dermatome can be used to assess the level of epidural block (see Procedure guideline 10.3: Epidural sensory blockade: assessment). This level should be checked to ensure that the epidural is providing pain relief by covering the area of the site of pain, but it is also necessary to maintain safety during the administration of epidural infusions.

Table 10.7 Optimal catheter locations for different surgical sites

Surgical site	Catheter location
Thoracic	T6–T9
Upper abdominal	T7–T10
Lower abdominal	T9–L1
Hip or knee	L1–L4

Procedure guideline 10.3 Epidural sensory blockade: assessment

Essential equipment

- Personal protective equipment
- Ethyl chloride spray (check local policy for alternative options)
- Copy of a dermatome distribution figure or chart (see Figure 10.10)

Action	Rationale
Pre-procedure	
1 Introduce yourself to the patient, explain and discuss the procedure with them, and gain their consent to proceed.	To ensure that the patient feels at ease, understands the procedure and gives their valid consent (NMC 2018, **C**).
2 Decontaminate hands and apply personal protective equipment	To reduce the risk of cross-infection (NHS England and NHSI 2019, **C**).
Procedure	
3 Explain to the patient that they need to report: • if the temperature of the spray changes or becomes warmer • if they cannot feel the cold sensation at all.	This will indicate the dermatome level at which the epidural analgesia is working. **E**
4 Remove any clothing that may restrict the assessment.	The spray needs to be applied directly to the skin to undertake the assessment. **E**
5 Test the spray on an area of the body that should not be affected by the epidural infusion (the face or the back of the hand).	To ensure the patient can feel the cold sensation and to provide a point of comparison. **P**
6 Starting at the top of the chest on one side of the torso (start at T1; see Figure 10.10), spray the ethyl chloride and ask the patient whether this feels as cold as when it was sprayed on the test area. Continue this procedure down one side of the torso and the leg (if appropriate for the level of epidural analgesia). Repeat on the opposite side of the body. Take note of the point at which the patient feels the stimulus become warmer or is unable to feel it at all.	To ensure the highest and lowest points of the epidural block are assessed. **E**
Post-procedure	
7 Document at what level the patient can detect a change as per the dermatome chart (see Figure 10.10).	Good record keeping will reveal a trend or pattern of the block that will help with the pain assessment of the patient. **E**

Procedure guideline 10.4 Epidural exit site dressing change

Essential equipment

- Personal protective equipment
- Sterile dressing pack including gloves
- Skin-cleaning agent, for example normal saline 0.9%.
- Transparent occlusive dressing

Action	Rationale
Pre-procedure	
1 Introduce yourself to the patient, explain and discuss the procedure with them, and gain their consent to proceed.	To ensure that the patient feels at ease, understands the procedure and gives their valid consent (NMC 2018, **C**).
2 Wash hands with soap and water. Clean trolley or plastic tray following local guidelines for aseptic procedure.	To minimize cross-infection (NHS England and NHSI 2019, **C**).
3 Position the patient comfortably on their side or sitting forward so that the site is easily accessible without undue exposure of the patient.	To maintain the patient's dignity and comfort (RCN 2016, **E**).
4 Prepare the trolley or tray with a sterile field and cleaning solution.	To minimize the risk of infection and ensure the equipment is available (Preston 2005, **C**).
Procedure	
5 Remove the old dressing and place it in a disposable bag.	To prevent cross-infection (Fraise and Bradley 2009, **E**).
6 Decontaminate hands with soap and water or with an alcohol-based handrub. Put on gloves and apron.	To minimize the risk of microbial contamination (NHS England and NHSI 2019, **C**).

(continued)

Procedure guideline 10.4 Epidural exit site dressing change *(continued)*

Action	Rationale
7 Observe the site for any signs of infection, such as redness, swelling or purulent discharge.	To ensure careful monitoring of the site to minimize the chance of infection (FPM 2010, **C**).
8 Clean the site with a skin-cleaning agent (e.g. aseptic non-touch technique with normal saline 0.9%).	To minimize the risk of infection (Hebl 2006, **R**).
9 Apply transparent occlusive dressing over the whole area.	To anchor the epidural or intrathecal catheter, minimize the risk of infection, and allow observation of the epidural or intrathecal site (FPM 2010, **E**).
10 Ensure that the patient is comfortable.	To maintain patient comfort and dignity on completion of the procedure. **P**
Post-procedure	
11 Remove gloves and apron and dispose of all material in the clinical waste bag. Decontaminate hands.	To prevent environmental contamination (NHS England and NHSI 2019, **C**).

Post-procedural considerations

Immediate care

Volume of infusion

The medication 'spread' within the epidural space is determined by the site of the epidural catheter, the patient's age and the volume of the drug being infused (Macintyre and Schug 2015). It is therefore important to maintain the hourly infusion rate at a volume that keeps the appropriate nerves blocked.

If the sensory block is too low, it may not provide sufficient pain relief or blockade of the intended site (e.g. surgical site). If the sensory block is too high (above T4) then there is an increased risk of respiratory and cardiac symptoms as a result of the local anaesthetic effects on nerves at this level, and if it is too dense it will cause unnecessary motor blockade.

Ongoing care

When caring for a patient receiving epidural analgesia, it is important to monitor the patient for the following:

- drug-related side-effects
- pain intensity
- signs of complications caused by the procedure (see Problem-solving table 10.1)
- equipment-related problems, such as with the catheter or infusion pump (see Problem-solving table 10.1).

Drug-related side-effects

There are a number of drug-related side-effects associated with epidural opioids and local anaesthetic agents.

Opioids

For opioids, the side-effects include the following:

- *Respiratory depression*: this is due to the action of opioids on the respiratory centre. Respiratory depression may occur at two different time intervals:
  - *Early*: usually within 2 hours of the opioid injection. This may occur if high blood levels of the opioid follow absorption from the epidural space into the systemic circulation (Macintyre and Schug 2015).
  - *Late*: this may not be seen for 6–12 hours after an opioid is given. It results from rostral migration of the drug in the CSF to the brainstem and respiratory centre (Macintyre and Schug 2015). This is less likely to occur with lipid-soluble opioids such as fentanyl.
- *Sedation*: although there may be many different causes of sedation, epidural opioids can cause sedation owing to their effect on the central nervous system. Opioid-induced sedation is often an early warning sign of respiratory depression.
- *Nausea and vomiting*: nausea and vomiting are caused by the action of opioids on the vomiting centre in the brainstem and stimulation of the chemoreceptor trigger zone in the fourth ventricle of the brain.
- *Pruritus*: although the exact mechanism is unknown, pruritus is presumed to be centrally mediated and a consequence of activation of opioid receptors in the spinal cord (Schug et al. 2015).
- *Urinary retention*: this is due to opioid inhibition of the micturition reflex, which is evoked by increases in bladder volume (Schug et al. 2015).

Local anaesthetic agents

For local anaesthetic agents, the side-effects include the following:

- *Hypotension*: this can be caused by two mechanisms. Firstly, local anaesthetic agents can spread outside the epidural space, blocking the sympathetic nerves. This results in peripheral vasodilation and hypotension. It is most likely to occur if a bolus dose of local anaesthetic agent (e.g. 10 mL of 0.25% bupivacaine) is given to improve pain control (Macintyre and Schug 2015). Secondly, if the local anaesthetic agent spreads above the T4 dermatome (nipple line), the cardio-accelerator nerves may become blocked, leading to bradycardia and hypotension (Macintyre and Schug 2015).
- *Motor blockade*: this will depend on the concentration and total dose of local anaesthetic agent used and the position of the epidural or intrathecal catheter (Schug et al. 2015). Motor blockade occurs when the local anaesthetic agent blocks the larger-diameter motor nerves. Leg weakness will occur if the motor nerves supplying the legs are blocked.
- *Urinary retention*: as with epidural opioids, blockade of the nerves supplying the bladder sphincter can cause urinary retention.

Patient monitoring

Routine monitoring of patients for these side-effects must be carried out to facilitate early management. The patient's blood pressure, respiratory rate and peripheral tissue oxygenation should be monitored continuously initially and then according to local policy and as the patient's condition dictates.

For guidance on managing the side-effects associated with epidural opioids and local anaesthetic agents, see Table 10.8.

Table 10.8 Epidural infusions of local anaesthetic agents and opioids: management of side-effects

Problem	Cause	Suggested action
Respiratory depression	Increasing age: elderly patients are more susceptible to the side-effects of opioids due to age-related alterations in the distribution, metabolism and excretion of drugs.	If respiratory rate falls to eight breaths a minute or below: 1 Stop the epidural infusion. 2 Summon emergency assistance. 3 Commence oxygen via face-mask and encourage the patient to take deep breaths. 4 Review current analgesic prescription and consider reducing opioid and local anaesthetic doses before resuming the infusion (Macintyre and Schug 2015).
	Concurrent use of systemic opioids or sedatives: patients receiving opioids by epidural infusion should not be given opioids by any other route unless given in the palliative care setting for breakthrough pain	Take the following steps: 1 Stop the epidural infusion. 2 Stay with the patient and monitor their respiratory rate, sedation score and peripheral tissue oxygenation (using a pulse oximeter) continuously. 3 Commence oxygen therapy. 4 Consider giving naloxone if prescribed and if the patient is unrousable. 5 Review analgesia: stop any other opioids prescribed and consider changing the parameters of the epidural infusion (Schug et al. 2015).
Sedation: • *Mild*: patient drowsy but easy to rouse • *Severe*: patient difficult to rouse	See 'Respiratory depression' above.	Take the following steps according to the patient's level of sedation: • If the patient has mild sedation, consider reducing the rate of the infusion or the dose of opioid or taking the opioid out of the infusion. • If the patient is difficult to rouse and opioid toxicity/overdose is suspected, follow the management steps for respiratory depression (above).
Hypotension	Patients with hypovolaemia. Patients with a high thoracic epidural in whom the concentration of local anaesthetic agent and volume of infusion causes blockade of the cardio-accelerator nerves.	If blood pressure falls suddenly: 1 Stop the epidural infusion. 2 Summon emergency assistance. 3 Administer oxygen via face-mask or nasal cannula. 4 Stay with the patient and monitor their blood pressure at 5-minute intervals. 5 Administer intravenous fluids with or without vasopressors as appropriate (Macintyre and Schug 2015).
Motor blockade	This is more likely to occur when higher concentrations of local anaesthetic agents are given by continuous infusion. If a high concentration of a local anaesthetic agent is administered via a low lumbar epidural catheter then the lumbar motor nerves are likely to be blocked, causing leg weakness.	Do not attempt to mobilize the patient if leg weakness is evident. Contact the pain or anaesthetic team for advice: reducing the concentration of the local anaesthetic agent or the rate of the epidural infusion may help to resolve this problem (Schug et al. 2015).
Nausea and vomiting	Previous episodes of nausea and vomiting with opioids. Exacerbated by low blood pressure.	Consider the following: • Regular administration of antiemetics (Schug et al. 2015). • Treat other causes, for example low blood pressure. • Consider use of non-pharmacological methods (e.g. stimulation of the PC6 acupressure point) (White et al. 2018).
Pruritus (usually more marked over the face, chest and abdomen)	Previous pruritus with opioids.	Administer an antihistamine such as chlorphenamine (may be contraindicated in patients who are becoming increasingly sedated) or a small dose of naloxone (administer with caution as this can easily reverse analgesia). If pruritus does not resolve, consider switching to another opioid or removing the opioid from the infusion (Schug et al. 2015).
Urinary retention	More likely to occur if opioids and local anaesthetic agents are infused in combination.	If the patient is in retention, they may require an indwelling urinary catheter. Patients should return to normal bladder function once the epidural has been discontinued (Macintyre and Schug 2015).

Table 10.9 Epidural safety checklist

Check	Rationale
Check the prescription and rate of the epidural infusion	To ensure epidural drugs are being administered correctly
Check the epidural extension set is connected to the NRFit epidural catheter and not to any other access device	To ensure drugs are administered via the correct route
Check the bacterial filter is securely attached to the epidural catheter	To prevent accidental disconnection of the catheter from the filter
Check that the dressing over the epidural catheter exit site is secure	To prevent catheter dislodgement and minimize the risk of contamination of the catheter site

Assessment of pain for patients with epidural analgesia

Pain should be assessed (at rest and on movement) at the same time that the patient's routine observations are carried out. Refer to Procedure guideline 10.1: Pain assessment.

Equipment and prescription safety checks

When a patient is receiving a continuous infusion of epidural analgesia, it is advisable to carry out the safety checks listed in Table 10.9 at least once per shift.

Discharge planning

In rare circumstances, patients with intractable cancer pain can be considered to go home with a continuous epidural infusion. See *The Royal Marsden Manual of Cancer Nursing Procedures* (Lister et al. 2019) for further detail about discharge planning with an epidural.

Complications

If pain is not controlled and the infusion has already been titrated according to hospital guidelines, the pain or anaesthetic team should be contacted for advice after checking the following:

- the catheter is still *in situ*
- the catheter is still connected to the bacterial filter
- there are no leaks within the system
- the height of the epidural block is appropriate: this will indicate whether the block has fallen below the upper limit of the incision or pain site (to check the height of the block, see Procedure guideline 10.3: Epidural sensory blockade: assessment).

If the height of the block has fallen below the upper limit of the incision or pain site, the pain or anaesthetic team may give the patient a bolus dose of local anaesthetic agent to re-establish the block or they may reposition the epidural catheter. If either of these measures fails, other methods of analgesia need to be considered.

Haematoma

An epidural haematoma can arise from trauma to an epidural blood vessel during catheter insertion or removal. Although the incidence of a haematoma occurring is extremely rare, particular care must be taken in patients receiving thromboprophylaxis. Initial symptoms include back pain and tenderness. As the haematoma expands to compress the nerve roots or the spinal cord, symptoms proceed to sensorimotor weakness (Lagerkranser and Lindquist 2017).

Dural puncture

This usually occurs when the dura mater is inadvertently punctured during the placement of the epidural catheter. The main symptom is a headache, which arises from leakage of CSF through the dura (Schug et al. 2015).

Catheter migration

In extremely rare cases, the catheter may migrate into either a blood vessel or the CSF. If it migrates into a blood vessel, opioid or local anaesthetic toxicity will occur. Opioid toxicity results in sedation and respiratory depression. Local anaesthetic toxicity results in circumoral tingling, numbness, twitching, convulsions and apnoea (Macintyre and Schug 2015). If the catheter migrates into the CSF, the epidural opioids and local anaesthetic agents may reach as high as the cranial intrathecal space. If this occurs, the respiratory muscles are paralysed together with the cranial nerves, resulting in apnoea, profound hypotension and unconsciousness (Macintyre and Schug 2015).

Meningitis

Meningitis is a rare complication of epidural analgesia (Macintyre and Schug 2015). The epidural route is often considered safer than the intrathecal route as the intact dura serves as an effective barrier to the spread of infection to the intrathecal space. The incidence of infection is in the range of 1–5 in 10,000 (Macintyre and Schug 2015). If the patient presents with headaches, fever, neck stiffness or photophobia, they must be reviewed as a matter of urgency by the medical or anaesthetic team; if meningitis is suspected, CSF samples can be obtained and sent to microbiology for analysis, and antibiotic therapy initiated promptly (Schug et al. 2015).

Abscess formation

Bos et al. (2017) note that infection can be introduced into the epidural space from an exogenous source via contaminated equipment or drugs or from an endogenous source, leading to bacteraemia that seeds to the insertion site or catheter tip. Alternatively, the catheter can act as a wick through which the infection tracks down from the entry site on the skin to the epidural or intrathecal space. Symptoms include back pain and tenderness accompanied by redness with a purulent discharge from the catheter exit site (Schug et al. 2015). Effective site care is therefore essential; see Procedure guideline 10.4: Epidural exit site dressing change.

Removal of an epidural catheter

Pre-procedural considerations

Before an epidural or intrathecal catheter is removed, it is essential to consider the clotting status of the patient's blood. If the patient is fully anticoagulated, a clotting profile must be performed and advice sought from the medical staff as to when the catheter can be removed. If the patient is receiving a prophylactic anticoagulant, the following guidelines are recommended (Harrop-Griffiths et al. 2013).

Low-dose, low-molecular-weight heparin

If this is given once daily, the epidural catheter should be removed at least 12 hours after the last injection and several hours prior to the next dose. The timing will depend on the manufacturer's recommended guidelines; for example, for tinzaparin (Leo Laboratories Ltd), it is recommended that epidural or spinal catheters are removed a minimum of 4 hours before the next dose.

Unfractionated heparin

The epidural catheter should be removed following local guidelines and the advice of the anaesthetic or pain management team.

Procedure guideline 10.5 Epidural catheter removal

Essential equipment

- Personal protective equipment
- Sterile dressing pack including gloves
- Skin-cleaning agent, for example normal saline 0.9%
- Specimen container (if epidural catheter needs to be sent for bacterial culture)
- Occlusive dressing

Action	Rationale
Pre-procedure	
1 Check the patient's anticoagulation status and time of last administered dose of anticoagulant. For patients receiving prophylactic anticoagulant (e.g. low-molecular-weight heparin), wait at least 12 hours post-dose but commence the procedure at least 4 hours prior to the next dose. Seek medical advice if the clotting profile is deranged.	To ensure the patients coagulation is not deranged and it is safe to remove the catheter (Harrop-Griffiths et al. 2013, **C**).
2 Introduce yourself to the patient, explain and discuss the procedure with them, and gain their consent to proceed.	To ensure that the patient feels at ease, understands the procedure and gives their valid consent (NMC 2018, **C**).
3 Wash hands with bactericidal soap and water or an alcohol-based handrub, apply personal protective equipment, and clean the trolley or plastic tray following local guidelines for aseptic procedure. Open the dressing pack.	To minimize the risk of cross infection (NHS England and NHSI 2019, **C**).
Procedure	
4 Remove the tape and dressing from the catheter insertion site; dispose of them as per local policy.	To minimize the risk of cross-infection (Loveday et al. 2014, **R**).
5 Decontaminate hands and apply fresh gloves.	To minimise the risk of cross-infection. **C**
6 Gently, in one swift movement, remove the catheter. Check that the catheter is intact. This can be done by observing that the tip of the catheter is marked blue and that the 1 cm marks along the length of the catheter are all intact.	To ensure the catheter is removed intact with the minimum of discomfort to the patient. **E**
7 Clean around the catheter exit site using a skin-cleaning agent (e.g. aseptic non-touch technique with normal saline 0.9%).	To minimize contamination of the site by micro-organisms. **E**
8 Apply an occlusive dressing and leave it *in situ* for 24 hours.	To prevent inadvertent access of micro-organisms along the tract. **E**
Post-procedure	
9 The epidural catheter tip may be sent for culture and sensitivity if infection is suspected, or according to local policy.	To assess the catheter as a potential source of infection. **E**
10 Remove gloves and apron and dispose of all material in the clinical waste bag. Decontaminate hands.	To minimize the risk of cross-infection (NHS England and NHSI 2019, **C**).
11 Document that the catheter was removed successfully and intact in the nursing notes.	To ensure accurate documentation of care (NMC 2018, **C**).
12 Conduct post-removal observations for 48 hours.	Epidural observations of motor and sensory function must continue for 48 hours after removal of the epidural catheter to detect any signs of developing epidural haematoma (Macintyre and Schug 2015, **E**).

Post-procedural considerations

Catheter-associated spinal epidural haematomas can occur during catheter placement or removal. Their incidence has been reported to range from 2 to 20 cases per 100,000 epidural procedures (Li et al. 2010; Rosero and Joshi 2016). The development and progression of haematomas associated with epidural anaesthesia are relatively slow and are generally characterized by symptoms such as impaired motor function (paraplegia) and sensory abnormalities, and moderate to severe back pain also occurs in many cases (Umegaki et al. 2016). The time course of spinal epidural haematoma development after catheter removal is variable, and it is reported that paraplegia can occur as early as 1 hour after catheter removal, with some patients developing symptoms after more than 24 hours (Ladha et al. 2013, Mahapatra et al. 2016). The consequences of an epidural haematoma may be permanent paralysis below the level of the haematoma.

For this reason, it is recommended that patients continue to be vigilantly monitored after the epidural catheter has been removed so that prompt action can be taken if there is any evidence of haematoma development (see step 12 in Procedure guideline 10.5: Epidural catheter removal).

Problem-solving table 10.1 Prevention and resolution (Procedure guidelines 10.2, 10.3 and 10.6)

Problem	Cause	Prevention	Action
Headache	Dural puncture caused during the insertion procedure	Expertise of practitioner inserting the epidural	Bedrest: headache will be less severe if patient lies flat. Provide replacement fluids either intravenously or orally to encourage formation of CSF. Administer analgesics for headache. If headache does not settle, contact the anaesthetic team, who may consider an epidural blood patch to seal the puncture (Sachs and Smiley 2014).
Sedation and respiratory depression (opioid toxicity) Circumoral tingling and numbness, twitching, convulsions and apnoea (local anaesthetic toxicity)	If the catheter migrates into a blood vessel, signs of opioid or local anaesthetic toxicity can occur.	Expertise of practitioner inserting the epidural. Careful monitoring of the patient to detect early symptoms.	Stop epidural infusion. Contact pain or anaesthetic team, or summon emergency assistance. Treat the patient for complications of opioid or local anaesthetic overdose. If necessary, give oxygen.
Apnoea, profound hypotension and unconsciousness	If an epidural catheter migrates from the epidural space into the intrathecal space to the CSF, the analgesic solution may reach as high as the cranial intrathecal space. If this occurs, the respiratory muscles are paralysed together with the cranial nerves, resulting in apnoea, profound hypotension and unconsciousness. This is because intrathecal doses are calculated as one-tenth of the epidural dose and migration from the epidural space to the intrathecal space leads to a drug overdose.	Expertise of practitioner inserting the epidural. Careful monitoring of the patient to detect early symptoms.	Stop the epidural infusion. Summon emergency assistance. Prepare emergency equipment to support respiration and ventilate lungs. Prepare emergency drugs and intravenous fluids and administer as directed. Prepare equipment for intubation.
Back pain and tenderness and nerve root pain with sensory and motor weakness	Epidural haematoma.	Assessment of coagulation status before insertion and removal of the epidural/intrathecal catheter.	Urgent neurological assessment. Carry out an MRI or CT scan to accurately diagnose whether there is nerve or spinal cord compression. If a haematoma is diagnosed, urgent surgery may be required to relieve the pressure (Hewson et al. 2018). To avoid haematoma on removal of epidural in patients treated with prophylactic anticoagulants, see local guidelines for timing of removal.
Back pain and tenderness May have redness and purulent discharge from catheter exit site May also develop nerve root signs with neuropathic pain and sensory/motor weakness	Epidural abscess.	Maintain aseptic technique when accessing the epidural/intrathecal analgesic system. Monitor temperature regularly and check insertion site for evidence of infection.	If the epidural catheter is still *in situ*, remove the tip and send it for culture and sensitivity. Treat the patient with antibiotics. Carry out an MRI or CT scan and refer the patient for urgent neurosurgery to prevent paraplegia (Hewson et al. 2018).
Headaches, fever, neck stiffness and/or photophobia	Meningitis.	Maintain aseptic technique when accessing the epidural analgesic system. Monitor temperature regularly.	Assist the anaesthetist or doctor to obtain a CSF sample for microbiology analysis. Initiate antibiotic therapy as per hospital policy. Consider non-pharmacological measures for symptom management, for example dim lights (Macintyre and Schug 2015)
Low block	Catheter potentially dislodged. The height of the block has fallen below the upper limit of the surgical incision or pain site.	Regular assessment of sensory block.	Increase the rate if prescribed. Contact the anaesthetic team or acute pain team for review and consideration of a bolus to re-establish the block or to reposition the epidural catheter.

Problem	Cause	Prevention	Action
High block (i.e. T4 or above)	The rate may be too high. The position of the catheter may have moved.	Regular assessment of sensory block.	Stop the epidural. Contact the anaesthetic team, acute pain team or emergency team if the patient is unable to breathe. Sit the patient upright. Administer oxygen if needed. The pain or anaesthetic team will provide advice on when to restart the epidural infusion.
Unilateral block	The position of the catheter may have moved.	Regular assessment of sensory block.	Roll the patient onto their side with no block (the analgesia may move with gravity). Contact the pain or anaesthetic team to review the epidural for consideration of adjusting the epidural catheter or giving a bolus dose.
No block	The catheter may have been dislodged	Regular assessment of sensory block	Contact the pain or anaesthetic team to review the epidural. They can consider adjusting the epidural catheter or giving a bolus dose. The patient may need to have an alternative method of analgesia if a block cannot be established and/or pain becomes an issue (note that patients may have no pain if they have an opioid running alongside a local anaesthetic; therefore, it can be possible for the patient to have no block and have minimal pain).

CSF, cerebrospinal fluid; CT, computed tomography; MRI, magnetic resonance imaging.

Entonox administration

Definition

Entonox (BOC Healthcare 2019), a gaseous mixture of 50% nitrous oxide (N_2O) and 50% oxygen (O_2), is a patient-controlled, inhaled analgesic that is used for the short-term relief of acute pain (Young et al. 2012). Nitrous oxide is a colourless, sweet-smelling gas with powerful analgesic properties and is supplied in premixed cylinders (Brown and Sneyd 2015). The gas is inhaled and self-administered by the patient using a demand valve system attached to a face mask or mouthpiece (Collins 2018). The nitrous oxide component of the gas acts as a powerful analgesic, producing similar physiological effects to opioids, while the oxygen component has an anti-hypoxic effect (Bonafé-Monzó et al. 2015).

Related theory

Although the exact mechanism of action of nitrous oxide is unknown, its effects take place within the pain centres of the brain and spinal cord and are related to the release of endogenous neurotransmitters such as opioid peptides and serotonin and the activation of certain opioid receptors (Huang and Johnson 2016). N-methyl-D-aspartate (NMDA) receptor currents are inhibited by nitrous oxide and it is known that these receptors are involved with many central nervous system pathways (Huang and Johnson 2016). The release of these neurotransmitters is thought to activate descending pain pathways that modulate pain transmission in the spinal cord (Huang and Johnson 2016). Pulmonary transfer of nitrous oxide is rapid, with onset of effect in seconds and full analgesic effect within 2–3 minutes (BOC Healthcare 2015). It is also rapidly eliminated from the blood, via the lungs, when inhalation ceases (Collins 2018).

Special precautions for storage

To ensure that Entonox is suitable for immediate use, cylinders of it should be maintained at a temperature above 10°C for at least 24 hours before use. If Entonox cylinders are allowed to get too cold (below 6°C) the nitrous oxide component of the gas will start to separate out of the gas mixture, changing the concentration of the gas delivered to the patient (BOC Healthcare 2013) – that is, the cylinders will initially deliver a high concentration of oxygen but then will deliver nearly pure nitrous oxide.

Evidence-based approaches

Rationale

There are several advantages to using Entonox:

- As the gas is inhaled, it is painless, in contrast to systemic methods of administering analgesia (such as injections).
- It has a rapid onset of effect.
- The side-effects are few and are self-limiting as the gas is self-administered.
- It does not depress respiratory or cardiovascular function when used as directed.
- Effects wear off rapidly, usually within 5 minutes.
- The patient is in full control, which provides reassurance that they have instant, self-regulated access to analgesia. This also provides a focus or distraction from the procedure taking place. These factors can both help to reduce anxiety. Entonox also has sedative properties, which means it can act as an anxiolytic (BOC Healthcare 2011).

Because of these properties, Entonox is an ideal agent for short-term pain relief following injury or trauma and during therapeutic and investigative procedures. It is used in a variety of settings, including accident and emergency (Huang and Johnson 2016), obstetrics (Collins 2018), paediatrics (BOC Healthcare 2015) and endoscopy, and for biopsy procedures (Wang et al. 2016) and dental procedures (Bonafé-Monzó et al. 2015).

Indications

Entonox is indicated for the following:

- [illegible]
- normal labour
- changing or removing of packs and drains
- removal of sutures from sensitive areas, for example the vulva
- invasive procedures such as catheterization and sigmoidoscopy
- removal of radioactive intracavity gynaecological applicators
- altering the position of a patient who experiences incident pain
- manual evacuation of the bowel in severe constipation
- acute trauma, for example applying orthopaedic traction following pathological fracture or in reduction of joint dislocation
- physiotherapy procedures, particularly post-operatively.

Contraindications

Entonox should not be used in any of the following conditions:

- maxillofacial injuries (BOC Healthcare 2019), as the patient may not be able to hold the mask tightly to the face or use the mouthpiece adequately, there is a risk of causing further damage to facial wounds, and there may also be a significant risk of blood inhalation
- head injuries with impairment of consciousness
- heavily sedated patients, as they would be unable to breathe in the Entonox on demand, and to potentiate sedation further may be hazardous
- intoxicated patients, as drowsiness and aspiration would be a hazard in the event of vomiting
- laryngectomy patients, as they would be unable to use the apparatus.

Additionally, Entonox should not be used in any condition in which gas is entrapped within the body and where its expansion may be dangerous. This is because the nitrous oxide constituent of Entonox passes into any air-filled cavity within the body faster than nitrogen passes out. As the gas expands, this is likely to result in a build-up of tension, which will increase the patient's symptoms. These conditions include:

- pneumothorax (artificial, traumatic or spontaneous)
- air embolism
- severe bullous emphysema
- abdominal distension or bowel obstruction
- decompression sickness
- following a recent dive
- following air encephalography
- during myringoplasty
- bowel obstruction
- in patients who have received recent intraocular injection of gas (BOC Healthcare 2015).

Use during pregnancy and lactation

Entonox is not absolutely contraindicated for use during pregnancy and lactation. However, it has been suggested that prolonged exposure to high levels of nitrous oxide may affect a woman's ability to become pregnant (Boiano et al. 2017). Mild skeletal teratogenic changes have been observed in pregnant rat embryos when the dam (pregnant mother) is exposed to high levels of nitrous oxide during the period of organogenesis. However, no increased incidence of foetal malformation has been discovered in eight epidemiological studies and case reports in humans (BOC Healthcare 2011). No published material shows that nitrous oxide is toxic to the human foetus. Therefore, there is no absolute contraindication to its use in the first 16 weeks of pregnancy. There are no known adverse effects to using Entonox during the breast-feeding period (BOC Healthcare 2016).

Principles of care

Cautions

[illegible]

- The high level of oxygen (50%) in Entonox may depress respiration in patients who have chronic obstructive pulmonary disease and are carbon dioxide (CO_2) retainers.
- Entonox should not be used as a replacement for intravenous analgesia or general anaesthesia in procedures requiring increased levels of medical intervention.
- Concomitant administration of Entonox in patients who are already on opioids and/or benzodiazepines may result in increased sedation and affect respiration; in this situation, the use of Entonox should take place under close supervision (BOC Healthcare 2015).
- BOC Healthcare (2016) states that when Entonox is used as a sole analgesic or sedative agent, driving or operating complex machinery is not recommended until all of the following are true:
  - the healthcare professional has judged that the patient has returned to normal mental status (Entonox can cause psychotropic effects)
  - the patient feels they are competent to drive or operate the machinery after the relevant procedure is completed
  - at least 30 minutes have elapsed after the administration of Entonox has ceased.

Clinical governance

Healthcare professionals involved in the assessment, administration and continuing care of patients receiving Entonox should have undergone training to do so. To maintain patient safety, healthcare professionals need to understand the properties, applications and prescribing practices for any medicinal product, which includes all medical gases (BOC Healthcare 2015). They should be able to demonstrate knowledge of the properties of the gas, precautions to be taken, actions in the event of an emergency and the correct operating procedures for the equipment. Training should cover:

- physical properties of the medical gas Entonox
- indications for its use
- protocols and policies for safe administration
- known side-effects and contraindications
- any other safety precautions
- methods of safe operation of the gas.

Training can be supplied by BOC Healthcare or a designated trainer and certificated.

Prescribing of Entonox

In a number of healthcare settings, nurses, midwives and physiotherapists may be able to administer Entonox without a written prescription from a doctor providing there is a local Patient Group Direction to allow this. Where this is the case, Entonox can be used more readily and time is not wasted waiting for a medical prescription. Non-medical prescribers who have completed the relevant training as independent prescribers may also prescribe Entonox if this is within their area of competence.

Pre-procedural considerations

Equipment

Cylinders

Entonox cylinders are available from BOC Healthcare in a variety of sizes. All cylinders have blue and white markings on their

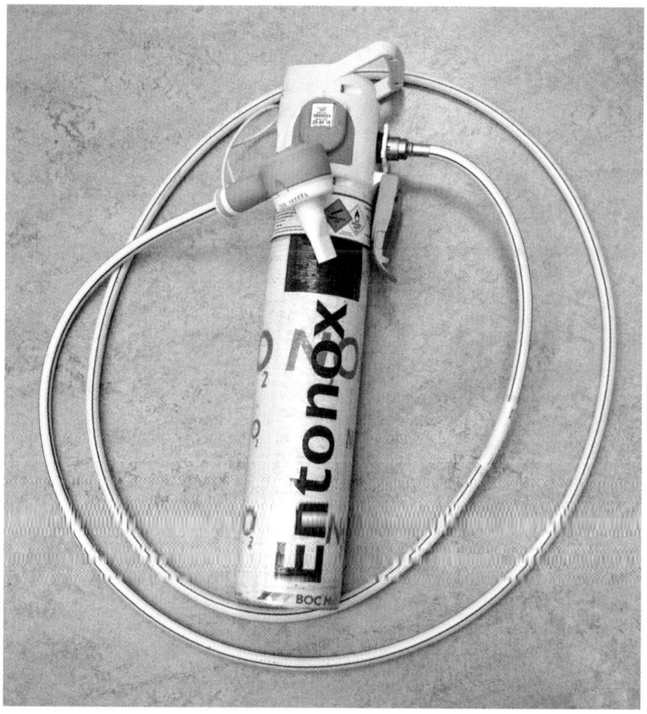

Figure 10.12 Entonox cylinder and hose.

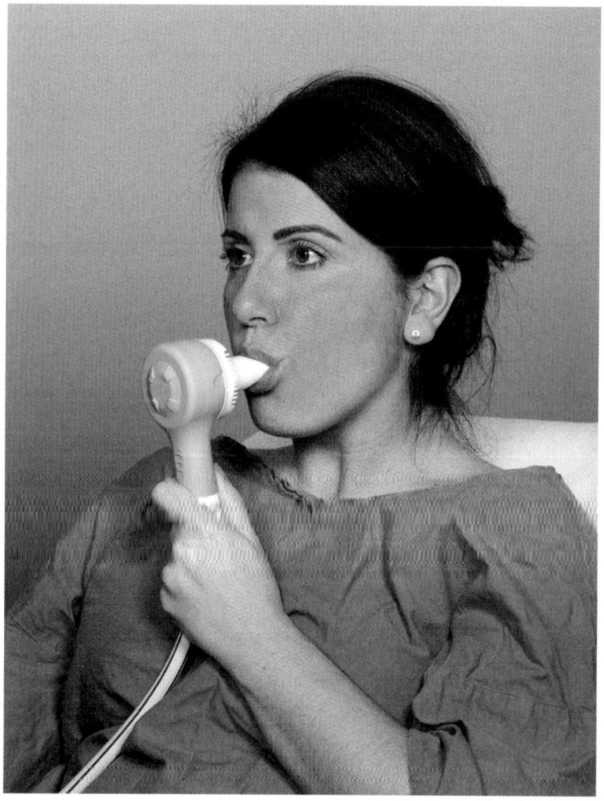

Figure 10.13 Patient using an Entonox demand valve.

shoulder (Figure 10.12). The lightweight, smaller cylinders have the following advantages:

- They are easier to carry.
- They have a live contents gauge.
- Changing an empty cylinder is simple because it is not necessary to fit a regulator or use a cylinder key.

The smaller cylinders tend to be used in ambulances and by midwives due to their portability in home births. Some clinical areas may have piped Entonox, such as accident and emergency departments, high-dependency units and critical care units. The larger cylinders, which require a trolley to move them around, are more suitable for ward areas.

Demand apparatus

There are a number of different companies that supply the demand apparatus for self-administered Entonox use. The face mask or mouthpiece is connected to an Entonox supply through a demand valve system. The demand valve allows the Entonox gas to flow when the patient inhales, and then the valve closes when the patient stops inhaling the gas (BOC Healthcare 2015) (Figure 10.13). This method of administration makes use of a demand unit, which safeguards the patient from excessive inhalation of Entonox. Thus, patients are able to self-regulate the dose of Entonox (a method of patient-controlled analgesia). The patient must hold the mask firmly over the face or hold the mouthpiece to the lips to produce an airtight fit and breathe in before the gas will flow. Expired gases escape via the expiratory valve on the hand piece (BOC Healthcare 2016). It is essential to adhere to this method of self-administration as it is then impossible for patients to overdose themselves because, if they become drowsy, they will relax their grip on the handset and the gas flow will cease when no negative pressure is applied. However, should inhalation continue, light anaesthesia supervenes and the mask drops away as the patient relaxes.

Entonox has an oxygen content 2.5 times that of air and is therefore a good way of giving extra oxygen as well as providing analgesia.

Bacterial filters and mouthpieces or face-masks

Because Entonox equipment is a potential source of cross-infection, bacterial filters (single use only) should be fitted between the face-mask or mouthpiece and the demand valve if the demand valve is not for single use (BOC Healthcare 2016). Face-masks and mouthpieces must also be single use only and disposed of once therapy ceases. Local policies must be followed for the cleaning and sterilization of non-disposable equipment between patient use.

Assessment

The patient's ability to administer Entonox safely and effectively (particularly in the very young or very old) must be assessed prior to use. Patients should be able to:

- understand the instructions for Entonox use
- hold the demand valve to self-administer the gas
- inhale the gas through the mask or mouthpiece while breathing normally (patients who have impaired lung function may not be able to inhale the gas sufficiently to provide adequate analgesia).

Duration and frequency of administration

The duration and frequency of Entonox administration should always be tailored to individual patient needs. Because prolonged exposure to Entonox causes inactivation of vitamin B_{12}, impaired folate metabolism and pernicious anaemia (BOC Healthcare 2015), it is recommended that:

- Entonox is used on a short-term rather than a long-term basis.
- When Entonox is used for more than a total of 24 hours, or more frequently than every 4 days, it must be used with close clinical supervision and haematological monitoring for vitamin B_{12} deficiency (BOC Healthcare 2015).
- If daily use is required for more than 4 days, this should be accompanied by close supervision and haematological monitoring (blood tests) (BOC Healthcare 2015). Consideration should also be given to the administration of B_{12} and folate supplements.

Procedure guideline 10.6 Entonox administration

Essential equipment

- Personal protective equipment
- Entonox cylinder and head
- Sterile bacterial filter
- Face-mask and/or mouthpiece
- Method of documentation

Action	Rationale
Pre-procedure	
1 Introduce yourself to the patient, explain and discuss the procedure with them, and gain their consent to proceed. Obtain a medical history.	To ensure that the patient feels at ease, understands the procedure and gives their valid consent (NMC 2018, **C**). To reduce patient anxiety (RCA 2006, **C**). To ensure the patient has no underlying medical problems that contraindicate the use of Entonox (BOC Healthcare 2015, **C**).
2 Turn on the Entonox supply from the cylinder.	To ascertain whether there is any Entonox in the cylinder. **E**
3 Examine the gauge to determine how much gas is in the cylinder.	To ensure an adequate supply of gas throughout the procedure (BOC Healthcare 2013, **C**).
4 Ensure that the patient is in as comfortable a position as possible.	To promote patient comfort. **P**
5 Demonstrate how to use the apparatus by holding the mask or mouthpiece to your own face or mouth (replace the mask or mouth piece before handing the equipment to the patient). Explain to the patient that they should breathe in and out regularly and deeply. Advise them that a hissing sound will be heard, indicating that the gas is being inhaled.	To ensure that the patient understands what to do and what to expect. **E**
6 Allow the patient to practise using the apparatus (with the gas turned on).	To enable the patient to adopt the correct technique (BOC Healthcare 2013, **C**).
Procedure	
7 Encourage the patient to breathe gas in and out for at least 2–3 minutes, as this is the time it takes for the analgesic effect to take place (BOC Healthcare 2013). If the gas is being used before a painful procedure, allow the patient to breathe the gas in for about 2 minutes before starting (BOC Healthcare 2013).	To allow sufficient time for an adequate circulatory level of nitrous oxide to provide analgesia. When the patient inhales, gas first enters the lungs and then the pulmonary and systemic circulations. It takes 2–3 minutes to build up reasonable concentrations of nitrous oxide in the brain (BOC Healthcare 2015, **C**).
8 While they are using Entonox, encourage the patient to breathe in and out regularly and deeply.	To maintain adequate circulatory levels, thus providing adequate analgesia (BOC Healthcare 2015, **C**).
9 Evaluate the effectiveness of the Entonox by verbally questioning the patient and/or conducting a pain assessment, and encouraging the patient to self-assess the analgesic effect. This should then be documented.	To establish whether the Entonox has been a useful analgesic. **E**
Post-procedure	
10 Turn off the Entonox supply from the cylinder.	To avoid potential seepage of gas from the apparatus (BOC Healthcare 2016, **C**).
11 Depress the diaphragm under the demand valve.	To remove residual gas from the tubing (BOC Healthcare 2013, **C**).
12 Follow local policies and guidelines for the cleaning and sterilization of expiratory valves and tubing, and face-masks (or dispose of the equipment if it is single use). Filters and mouthpieces should be discarded after use.	To reduce the risk of cross-infection (BOC Healthcare 2011, **C**)
13 At the end of the procedure, observe the patient for up to 30 minutes until the gases have worn off.	Some patients may feel transient drowsiness or giddiness and should be discouraged from getting out of bed until these effects have worn off (BOC Healthcare 2016, **C**). Adverse psychometric effects will normally cease shortly after the administration of Entonox has stopped due to the rapid elimination of the nitrous oxide component of the medical gas mixture from the body (BOC Healthcare 2011, **C**).
14 Record the administration on the appropriate documentation.	To promote continuity of care, maintain accurate records and provide a point of reference in the event of any queries (NMC 2018, **C**).

Problem-solving table 10.2 Prevention and resolution (Procedure guideline 10.6)

Problem	Cause	Prevention	Action
Patient not experiencing adequate analgesic effect	Entonox cylinder empty. Apparatus not properly connected.	Check equipment before use.	Change to a full cylinder.
	Patient not inhaling deeply enough (BOC Healthcare 2016).	Educate patient prior to use.	Encourage the patient to breathe in until a hissing noise can be heard from the cylinder. Reassess the suitability of the patient for Entonox use. The patient may not be strong enough to inhale deeply or may have reduced lung capacity.
	Patient inhaling pure oxygen – that is, cylinder has been stored below −6°C and nitrous oxide has liquified and settled at the bottom of the cylinder.	To ensure that the gas is suitable for immediate use, all cylinders should be stored horizontally at a temperature of 10°C or above for 24 hours before use (BOC Healthcare 2016).	Initially this is safe, but later the patient may inhale pure nitrous oxide and be asphyxiated. Discontinue the procedure. Ensure adequate warming and inversion of the cylinder to remix the gases adequately.
	Not enough time has been allowed for nitrous oxide to exert its analgesic effect.	Allow at least 2 minutes of Entonox use before evaluating any analgesic effect or before commencing the procedure.	Stop the procedure. Allow 2 minutes of Entonox use. Restart the procedure.
Patient experiencing generalized muscle rigidity	Hyperventilation during inhalation (BOC Healthcare 2011).	Educate patient prior to starting procedure.	Discontinue Entonox and allow the patient to recover. Explain the procedure again, stressing deep and regular inspiration. Use a mouthpiece in place of a mask.
Patient unable to tolerate a mask	Smell of rubber. Feeling of claustrophobia.	Assess patient preference to use either mask or mouthpiece before Entonox use.	Use a mouthpiece in place of a mask.
Patient feels nauseated, drowsy or dizzy	Effect of nitrous oxide accumulation (BOC Healthcare 2015).		Discontinue Entonox administration; the effect will rapidly subside after removal of the gas. Restart Entonox use; if the same effect occurs, stop using Entonox and use an alternative form of analgesia.
Patient afraid to use Entonox	Patient associates gases with previous hospital procedures, for example anaesthesia before surgery (BOC Healthcare 2011).	Assess suitability of patient for Entonox use. Address fear and anxiety issues before starting Entonox use.	Reassure the patient and reiterate instructions for use and short-term effects.

Complications

Effects such as euphoria, disorientation, sedation, nausea, vomiting, dizziness and generalized tingling are commonly described. These are generally minor and rapidly reversible (BOC Healthcare 2016). If the patient experiences any of these complications, ask them to stop inhaling the gas (BOC Healthcare 2016).

Inappropriate inhalation (if patient already has an altered state of consciousness) of Entonox will ultimately result in unconsciousness, with the patient passing through stages of increasing light-headedness and intoxication. The treatment is moving to fresh air or using bag valve mask resuscitation (BOC Healthcare 2016). Inappropriate inhalation can be avoided by conducting a thorough assessment of the patient prior to Entonox administration.

Safety in the environment

Inhalation of a gas has the potential to contaminate the working environment (BOC Healthcare 2016). The manufacturer (BOC Healthcare) and the UK Health and Safety Executive recommend that Entonox should only be administered in a well-ventilated area to limit the average occupational exposure level of the healthcare professional to less than 100 ppm (over an 8-hour period) (BOC Healthcare 2015, Health and Safety Executive 2002).

Non-pharmacological methods of managing pain

Optimal pain control is more likely to be achieved by combining non-pharmacological with pharmacological techniques. Despite the lack of robust research evidence to support the effectiveness of many non-pharmacological techniques, their benefits to patients and families should not be underestimated.

Non-pharmacological approaches can help to reduce pain by (El Geziry et al. 2018):

- increasing the patient's ability to control their feelings
- reducing the feeling of weakness
- enhancing function and activity levels

- reducing anxiety and stress
- decreasing pain behaviour (e.g. guarding, bracing, rubbing, grimacing and sighing) and focused pain level.

Non-pharmacological interventions can be categorized into the following:

- psychological interventions
- physical interventions.

Psychological interventions

A number of simple psychological interventions can contribute to improving a patient's pain management. These include:

- *Providing information*: this includes procedural information summarizing what will happen during the treatment, and sensory information describing the sensory experiences that the patient can expect during treatment. This demonstrates the most benefit when both types of information are combined (Schug et al. 2015).
- *Stress or tension reduction*: relaxation, guided imagery and hypnosis strategies have been shown to reduce pain intensity in a number of chronic pain studies, but the evidence is less robust for acute pain (El Geziry et al. 2018, Schug et al. 2015).
- *Attentional strategies*: these involve strategies that provide distraction from the pain, and those that divert the attention to an imagined scene (e.g. mindfulness meditation or virtual reality) or to external stimuli (e.g. music or smells) (El Geziry et al. 2018, Schug et al. 2015).
- *Cognitive–behavioural therapy (CBT) and acceptance and commitment therapy (ACT)*: these interventions involve the application of a range of behaviour-change principles to target cognitive responses to pain. They may involve identification and modification of unhelpful thoughts, changing responses to negative thoughts to improve outcomes, positive reinforcement of desired behaviours, and goal setting in order to achieve a change in targeted behaviours (El Geziry et al. 2018, Schug et al. 2015).

Some of these interventions need to be delivered by healthcare professionals trained in the specific techniques (e.g. psychological therapists, counsellors or specialist nurses). However, some can be delivered easily to improve patients' sense of wellbeing and reduce pain by nurses working in clinical environments. Some simple interventions include the following.

Creating trusting therapeutic relationships

By creating trusting relationships with patients, nurses are instrumental in reducing anxiety and helping patients to cope with pain. Establishing rapport with patients and helping them to find a degree of acceptance of pain is often the first step (Schug et al. 2015). Nurses may underestimate the benefits and comfort they bring by staying with a patient who is experiencing pain. Nurses can help to create a trusting relationship by:

- listening to the patient
- believing the patient's pain experience
- acting as a patient advocate
- providing patients with appropriate physical and emotional support.

The use of gentle humour

Several mechanisms have been postulated to explain the association between humour and mental and physical health. Evidence supports numerous positive physiological effects of humour on several bodily systems, including the musculoskeletal, respiratory, cardiovascular, endocrine, immune and nervous systems. Positive humour has been shown to decrease negative and increase positive emotions and coping (DeKeyser Ganz and Jacobs 2014). Humour has also been found to be significantly associated with social support and self-efficacy (DeKeyser Ganz and Jacobs 2014). Tse et al. (2010) report that many older patients find gentle humour to be an effective way of reducing pain; they also found that it reduced patients' perception of loneliness and that patients reported significant increases in happiness and life satisfaction. DeKeyser Ganz and Jacobs (2014) found that attendance at a humour therapy workshop was associated with positive effects upon subsequent depression, anxiety and general wellbeing. Humour may be particularly helpful prior to a painful procedure as it can have a lasting effect. In the clinical setting, humorous recordings and books can be made available for patient use.

Information and education

Patient information and education can make all the difference between effective and ineffective pain relief. Information and education help to reduce anxiety (Macintyre and Schug 2015, Schug et al. 2015) and enable patients to make informed decisions about their care. Patients should be given specific information about why pain control is important, what to expect in terms of pain relief, how they can participate in their management and what to do if pain is not controlled. Some caution is required, however, because not all patients respond positively to the same level of information. Patients with high levels of anxiety may find that detailed information can increase their anxiety and negatively influence their pain control.

Relaxation

While scientific evidence for the effectiveness of relaxation techniques is limited for acute pain management, a number of studies have shown benefits for patients experiencing chronic pain (El Geziry et al. 2018). Techniques can range from simple breathing techniques to progressive muscle relaxation (PMR) and more complex techniques. PMR is a technique where the patient tightens and relaxes different muscle groups throughout the body in a progressive manner, provoking a sense of relaxation and comfort (El Geziry et al. 2018).

Music

Music therapy employs specific musical elements to encourage or facilitate movement, positive interactions, and/or improved emotional or cognitive states (Bernatzky et al. 2011). The use of music in the healthcare setting can provide relaxation and distraction from pain. Theories suggest that music works by influencing the physical and psychological factors of pain. Cognitive activities such as listening to music affect the perceived intensity and unpleasantness of pain, enabling the sensation of pain to be reduced. Another mechanism by which music therapy is advantageous is reducing autonomic nervous system activity, such as reducing heart and respiratory rates and decreasing blood pressure (Hole et al. 2015). Setting up a library of music (e.g. easy listening, classical) and having personal listening devices available for patient use is a simple way to provide patients with relaxing music. Vaajoki et al. (2012) reported significantly lower pain intensity and pain distress on the second post-operative day in a music-listening group compared with a control group after elective abdominal surgery. Hole et al. (2015) suggest that music played in the peri-operative period can reduce post-operative pain, anxiety and analgesia needs, and improve patient satisfaction.

Art

Art therapy is a form of psychotherapy that combines visual art-making and psychotherapy to promote self-exploration and understanding (Angheluta and Lee 2011). It can be used in chronic pain management, where a biopsychosocial approach is needed to address the impact of living with chronic pain. Art therapies can assist patients in moving the focus of their attention away from the physical sensation of pain, it can also resolve conflicts and problems, develop interpersonal skills, manage behaviour, reduce stress, increase self-esteem and self-awareness, and achieve insight (American Art Therapy Association 2017). The skills of an art therapist are required to ensure the successful use of this intervention through active art-making, creative process, applied psychological theory, and human experience within a psychotherapeutic relationship. A key component of this form of psychotherapy is the development of a strong working relationship between client and therapist (Angheluta and Lee 2011).

Physical interventions

In addition to psychological interventions, a number of physical interventions can be helpful in reducing pain.

Positioning and comfort measures

Positioning as an intervention involves the maintenance of proper body alignment to reduce stress and anxiety. Simple comfort measures such as positioning pillows and bed linen appropriately and positioning the patient correctly (such as supporting a painful limb) can help to reduce pain (El Geziry et al. 2018). Patients can feel more relaxed and these measures can improve patient comfort by reducing muscle tension and discomfort. Other comfort measures include ensuring that interruptions and noise are minimized to promote rest and ensuring the ambient temperature is comfortable.

Exercise

Joint stiffness and muscle wasting may further compound pain problems, and preventing or minimizing this is a key approach in pain management. The aim of physical exercise is to improve function and prevent any current disability from getting worse (Shipton 2018). This can apply to both acute and chronic pain. Exercise should always be tailored to the patient's tolerance and stamina. A simple exercise regimen that is practised regularly and supervised by a therapist can help patients to feel better and more in control, and it can also have benefits in terms of pain relief. In patients with chronic pain, it can increase mobility and flexibility while restoring confidence and challenging fear-avoidance behaviour (Shipton 2018).

Transcutaneous electrical nerve stimulation

Transcutaneous electrical nerve stimulation (TENS) is a non-pharmacological intervention that makes use of a complex neuronal network to reduce pain by activating descending inhibitory systems in the central nervous system. It uses an electrical device (Figure 10.14) to deliver an electrical current through the intact surface of the skin to stimulate the sensory nerve endings. It is thought to work by activating the large myelinated fibres, which in turn block small pain-transmitting nerve fibres (El Geziry et al. 2018). It is also thought to work by stimulating the release of natural pain-relieving chemicals (endogenous opioids) in the brain and spinal cord (Johnson 2014). TENS is recognized as a treatment modality with minimal contraindications.

Evidence for the use of TENS is variable. In a summary of systematic reviews by Vance et al. (2014), it was suggested that TENS, when applied at adequate intensities, is effective for post-operative pain, osteoarthritis, painful diabetic neuropathy and some acute pain conditions. When compared to sham TENS (where a medical device with the only purpose of acting as a placebo is used in controlled clinical trials), TENS has been shown to reduce acute pain (procedural and non-procedural), including pain after thoracic surgery, and it is also effective in primary dysmenorrhoea (Schug et al. 2015).

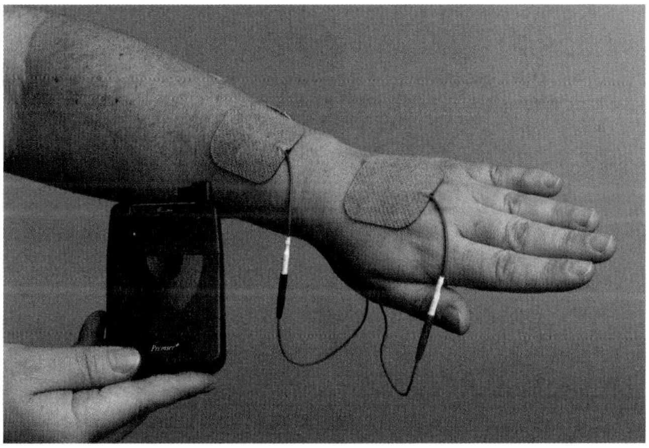

Figure 10.14 TENS machine.

Thermotherapy

Thermotherapy has for many years been advocated as a useful adjunct to pharmacological therapies. Ice is used for acute injuries and warmth is used for sprains and strains.

Heat therapies

For decades, superficial heat therapy has been used to relieve a variety of muscular and joint pains, including arthritis, back pain and period pain. There is much anecdotal and some scientific evidence to support the usefulness of heat as an adjunct to other pain treatments. The physiological effects of heat therapy include pain relief and increases in blood flow, metabolism and elasticity of connective tissues (Malanga et al. 2015). Heat therapy works by:

- stimulating thermoreceptors in the skin and deeper tissues, thereby reducing sensitivity to pain by closing the gating system in the spinal cord
- reducing muscle spasm
- reducing the viscosity of synovial fluid, which alleviates painful stiffness during movement and increases joint range (El Geziry et al. 2018).

In the home environment, people use a variety of different methods for applying heat therapies, such as warm baths, hot water bottles, wheat-based heat packs and electrical heating pads. In the hospital setting, caution is required with equipment as many devices do not reach health and safety standards (e.g. they may have uneven and irregular temperature distribution) and there have been incidences of burns (El Geziry et al. 2018). Heat therapy should not be used immediately following tissue damage as it will increase swelling. All devices used in the hospital should include instructions on their safe use in order to prevent harm to patients.

Cold therapies

Cold therapies can also be used to stimulate nerves and modulate pain. The physiological effects of cold therapy include reductions in pain, blood flow, oedema, inflammation, muscle spasm and metabolic demand (Malanga et al. 2015). Cold may be particularly valuable following an acute bruising injury, where it can help to reduce inflammation and limit further damage. Cold can be applied in the form of crushed ice or gel-filled cold packs, which should be wrapped in a towel to protect the skin from an ice burn.

NICE recommendation on thermotherapy

NICE (2014) concluded that the evidence base on thermotherapy is limited. All the thermotherapy studies in osteoarthritis have explored the application of cold rather than heat and there was no significant difference in pain between cold thermotherapy and the control groups. The results of randomized controlled trials (RCTs) assessing physical function are mixed when compared with controls. There is no economic evidence available on the subject. Malanga et al. (2015) also concluded that there remains an ongoing need for more high-quality RCTs on the effects of cold and heat therapy on recovery from acute musculoskeletal injury.

Despite the scarcity of evidence, local heat and cold are widely used as part of self-management. They may not always take the form of packs or patches, with some patients simply using hot baths to the same effect. As an intervention, this has a very low cost and is extremely safe as long as all safety instructions for the bathing equipment are followed. NICE (2014) therefore concluded that a positive recommendation was justified and the use of local heat or cold should be considered as an adjunct to core treatments.

Acupuncture

Definition

Acupuncture is a therapeutic technique that involves the insertion of fine needles into the skin and underlying tissues at specific points for therapeutic or preventative purposes (White et al. 2018). In the UK, there are two main types of approach to acupuncture: Chinese medical acupuncture and conventional (sometimes termed Western) medical acupuncture. In the NHS, conventional medical acupuncture is most commonly used for the treatment of chronic pain. The selection of acupuncture points is based on the region affected and there is minimal needle manipulation (as is the practice in Chinese acupuncture) except for in the use of electro-acupuncture. This section focuses on conventional (Western) medical acupuncture.

Anatomy and physiology

Acupuncture has been used in China for over 2000 years. The history of Western medical acupuncture started in the 1970s when a medically qualified doctor took a rational, scientific approach to exploring acupuncture and its benefits (White et al. 2018).

There is evidence to show that acupuncture works on the nervous system and the muscles. Electro-acupuncture activates the endogenous opioid system, causing analgesia and mediating anti-hyperalgesia effects (Yap 2016). Acupuncture also affects the endocrine system, leading to an increased release of adrenocorticotropic hormone (ACTH), producing an anti-inflammatory effect (Yap 2016). However, how and why insertion of needles can cause such physiological responses is still largely unknown (Yap 2016), and the variability in individual responses is also not well understood.

Five mechanisms have been identified, although these can overlap: local effects, segmental effects, extra-segmental effects, central effects and myofascial trigger point effects (White et al. 2018).

Local effects

Action potentials in nerve fibres in the skin and muscle are activated by the acupuncture needles. Various substances are released as a result and this causes an increase in local blood flow. This can often be seen as a red mark around the acupuncture needle during treatment. The local effect can also cause an increase in the blood supply in the deeper tissue, which can aid wound healing.

Segmental effects

The action potentials activated by the local effects continue to travel up the nerve to the spinal cord and reduce the painful stimuli by reducing activity at the dorsal horn. This is the main mechanism by which acupuncture relieves pain.

Extra-segmental effects

This is a response in which the effect of acupuncture is not restricted to a single area. This is due to the action potentials continuing to the brainstem, with the result that every segment of the spinal cord is affected (White et al. 2018).

Central effects

Acupuncture affects other structures in the brain, such as the hypothalamus and the limbic system. In these areas, acupuncture can have a regulatory effect; this can be used to treat nausea, hormone imbalances and drug addiction. These effects have been shown on MRI scans.

Myofascial trigger point effects

People can experience pain due to 'tight bands' or 'pressure or trigger points' in their muscles. Acupuncture is effective in treating this pain; the needles are inserted directly into the painful area and often the patient experiences instant pain relief. It is thought that acupuncture was originally developed for this type of pain (White et al. 2012).

Evidence-based approaches

Rationale

Acupuncture is used for a number of different conditions; both acute and chronic pain, nausea (post operative and chemotherapy induced), fatigue, addiction and infertility. There are a number of Cochrane reports (e.g. Lee and Ernst 2011) indicating the effectiveness of the use of acupuncture in various conditions. They concluded that acupuncture is effective for migraines, neck disorders, tension-type headaches and peripheral joint osteoarthritis. There have also been numerous RCTs showing the effectiveness of acupuncture (White et al. 2012).

Indications

Acupuncture is indicated for:

- pain – both acute and chronic
- xerostomia
- nausea and vomiting (post-operative, secondary to chemotherapy and in pregnancy)
- intractable fatigue
- breathlessness
- anxiety
- vasomotor symptoms (e.g. hot flushes)
- encouragement of wound healing
- addiction (e.g. to help patients stop smoking and to aid treatment of alcohol dependence)
- infertility and dysmenorrhoea
- asthma
- urological conditions (e.g. irritable bladder).

Clear evidence for the effectiveness of acupuncture in treating pain conditions has been obtained through high-quality sources such as RCTs (Molsberger et al. 2010, Shin et al. 2013) and through other sources such as individual patient data meta-analysis (Vickers et al. 2012). Figures 10.15, 10.16 and 10.17 show some common acupuncture points used in practice.

Contraindications

Acupuncture is contraindicated in patients who:

- refuse (e.g. in cases of extreme needle phobia)
- have pain originating from an unknown cause
- are unable to give informed consent or co-operate with treatment
- have severe clotting dysfunction or bruise spontaneously.

Needling should be avoided:

- directly onto a tumour nodule or into an area of ulceration
- in lymphoedematous limbs or limbs prone to lymphoedema
- in the ipsilateral arm in patients who have undergone axillary dissection (because there is a risk of the development of swelling and lymphoedema after insertion of any needle)
- in areas of spinal instability because of the risk of cord compression (due to acupuncture's muscle-relaxing properties)
- into a prosthesis (could cause leakage of saline or silicone)
- over intracranial deficits following neurosurgery.

Caution should be taken with:

- patients who are underweight (so as not to needle too deeply over the chest wall)
- patients who are confused
- patients who are agitated
- patients with a metal allergy
- patients receiving anticoagulation therapy
- patients who are immunocompromised
- patients with peripheral vascular disease

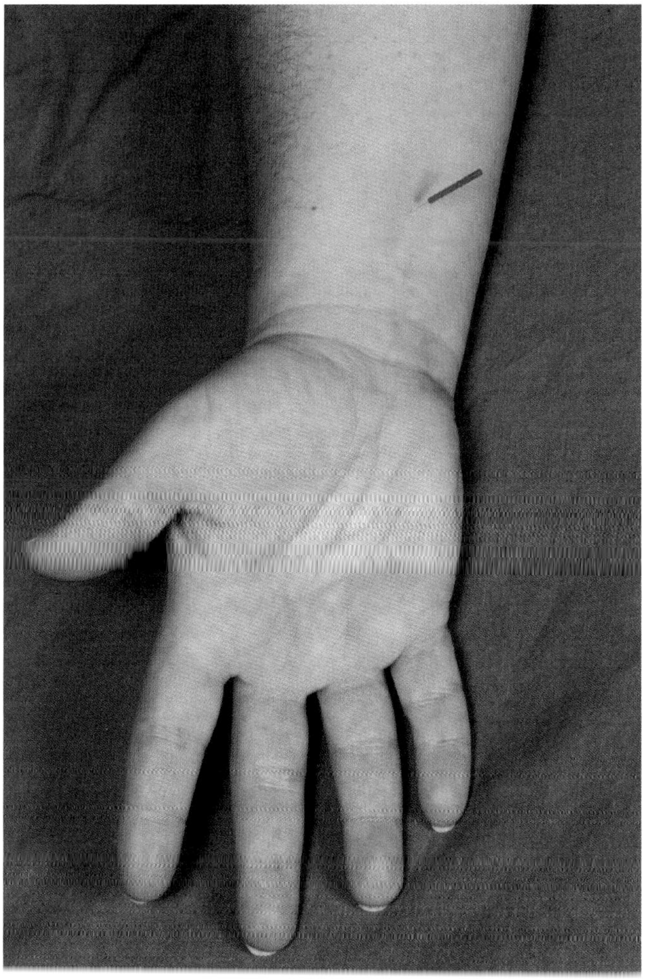

Figure 10.15 A generic acupuncture point (PC6) often used for nausea and pain.

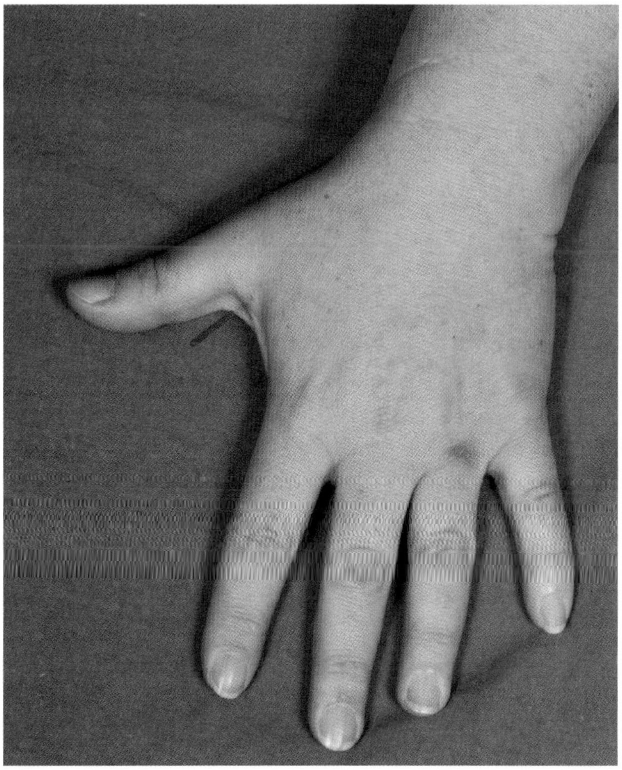

Figure 10.16 A point (LI4) used for relief of pain such as headaches and toothache, for relief of sinus infections, or as a generic point in conjunction with other points specific to the painful area.

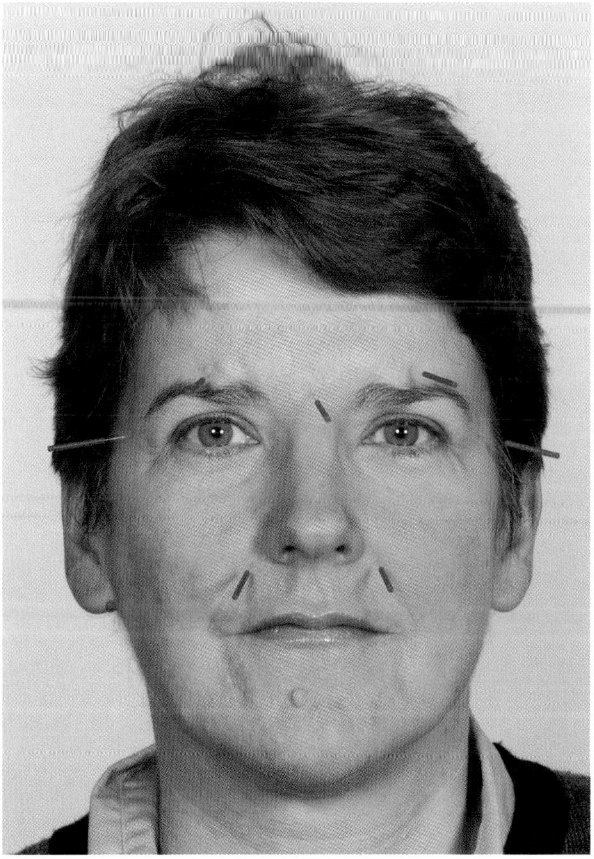

Figure 10.17 Points used to treat migraines and headaches.

- patients with blood-borne infections (e.g. HIV)
- patients who are pregnant
- patients who are prone to keloid scar formation
- all cancer patients as they may be very sensitive to acupuncture, so close supervision is advised, especially during the first treatment.

Various authors have reviewed the safety aspects of acupuncture for palliation of symptoms. Reported adverse effects of acupuncture have been categorized as follows:

- delayed or missed diagnosis (i.e. orthodox diagnostic categories)
- deterioration of disorder under treatment
- vegetative reactions (e.g. syncope, vertigo or sweating)
- bacterial and viral infections (e.g. hepatitis B and C, and HIV infection)
- trauma of tissues and organs.

Clinical governance

All acupuncture practitioners must have completed a recognized, validated, formal training course within their scope of professional practice (e.g. the Foundation Course in acupuncture provided by the British Medical Acupuncture Society (BMAS)). Any nurses who practise acupuncture should check with their union to ensure they have appropriate indemnity cover.

Date of first presentation	Ref.	Age	Sex	Diagnosis or presenting complaint (PC)	Duration of PC (months)	No. of Rx	Response

Figure 10.18 A sample acupuncture treatment record chart. Rx, prescription. *Source*: Adapted from BMAS (2013).

Pre-procedural considerations

Equipment

Acupuncture needles consist of a shaft and a handle. The handle is made of either plastic or metal. The needles are single use and disposable and are covered by a safety guide tube.

There are various dimensions of needles available. However:

- 0.25 or 0.30 mm diameter needles are standard.
- 25 or 40 mm length needles are standard.

Assessment and recording tools

Record the patient's treatment in the hospital notes or hospital computer system. Documentation should include the patient's condition, the acupuncture points used and the outcome (Figure 10.18).

Specific patient preparation

Patients should be treated in a comfortable, well-supported position on a couch, either lying down or sitting with the facility to lie down quickly in case they feel faint during or after the procedure. A healthcare professional should remain with the patient throughout their first treatment as their reaction to acupuncture will be unknown.

Consent

All patients must sign a consent form to agree to treatment, as per local policy. An example of a consent form to use can be found on the BMAS website (BMAS 2013).

Procedure guideline 10.7 Preparation for acupuncture and actions post-treatment

Essential equipment

- Personal protective equipment
- Hand-washing facilities
- Couch and pillows to support the patient
- Cotton wool swabs
- Sharps bin
- Tray to hold needles
- Needles
- Facilities for record keeping

Action	Rationale
Pre-procedure	
1 Take a full medical history from the patient.	To ensure acupuncture is not contraindicated and to ascertain which treatment points need to be used. **E**
2 Introduce yourself to the patient, explain and discuss the procedure with them, and gain their consent to proceed.	To ensure that the patient feels at ease, understands the procedure and gives their valid consent (NMC 2018, **C**).
Procedure	
3 Ask the patient to lie down.	To reduce the risk of the patient fainting (White et al. 2018, **E**).
4 Decontaminate hands and apply personal protective equipment.	To minimize the risk of infection (NHS England and NHSI 2019, **C**).
5 Give treatment.	
6 Count the needles used (use the empty introducers on the tray as a reminder).	To ensure no needles are lost or miscounted (White et al. 2018, **E**).
7 Leave the needles *in situ* for 20 minutes; remove them if the patient cannot tolerate them. Stay with the patient throughout.	To ensure safe treatment. **E**
8 Remove the needles and count them as they are removed.	To ensure no needles are lost or miscounted (White et al. 2018, **E**).
9 Ensure the patient feels okay; let the patient rest on the couch if they feel dizzy or otherwise affected.	To reduce the risk of the patient fainting (White et al. 2018, **E**).
Post-procedure	
10 Document the needling points used on the patient's record.	To ensure that the treatment can be replicated or adjusted at the next appointment according to the patient's response (White et al. 2018, **E**).

Post-procedural considerations

If the patient is having treatment in an outpatient setting, they can travel home immediately after treatment. If the patient feels dizzy or faint, they should rest and drink fluids until the feeling passes.

Complications

Although rare, there can be some complications when practising acupuncture:

- Fainting can occur in some patients who are tired, nervous or stressed. This occurs in 5–10% of patients. To avoid this, all patients should be treated while lying down.
- Pain can be felt during insertion of the needles, but this is due to clumsy technique. It can also occur if a patient moves during treatment, and therefore patients should be treated on a stable bed.
- Pneumothorax: this is very rare in practice and is caused by practitioners having poor anatomical knowledge (Park et al. 2010).

References

AAGBI (Association of Anaesthetists of Great Britain and Ireland) (2010) *AAGBI Safety Guideline: Management of Severe Local Anaesthetic Toxicity.* Available at: https://www.aagbi.org/sites/default/files/la_toxicity_2010_0.pdf

Ahlers, S.J.G.M., van der Veen, A.M., van Dijk, M., et al. (2010) The use of the Behavioral Pain Scale to assess pain in conscious sedated patients. *Anesthesia & Analgesia*, 110(1), 127–133.

American Art Therapy Association (2017) *About Art Therapy.* Available at: https://arttherapy.org/about-art-therapy

Angheluta, A.M. & Lee, B.K. (2011) Art therapy for chronic pain: Applications and future directions. *Canadian Journal of Counselling and Psychotherapy*, 45(2), 112–131.

Argoff, C.E. (2014) Recent management advances in acute postoperative pain. *Pain Practice*, 14(5), 477–487.

Balding, L. (2013) The World Health Organisation analgesic ladder: Its place in modern Irish medical practice. *Irish Medical Journal*, 106(4), 122–124.

Baron, R., Binder, A. & Wasner, G. (2010) Neuropathic pain: Diagnosis, pathophysiological mechanisms, and treatment. *Lancet Neurology*, 9(8), 807–819.

Bashandy, G.M.N. & Elkholy, A.H.H. (2014) Reducing postoperative opioid consumption by adding an ultrasound-guided rectus sheath block to multimodal analgesia for abdominal cancer surgery with midline incision. *Anesthesiology and Pain Medicine*, 4(3), 1–6.

Beacroft, M. & Dodd, K. (2010) Pain in people with learning disabilities in residential settings: The need for change. *British Journal of Learning Disabilities*, 38(3), 201–209.

Beakley, B.D., Kaye, A.M. & Kaye, A.D. (2015) Tramadol, pharmacology, side effects, and serotonin syndrome: A review. *Pain Physician*, 18, 395–400.

Bennett, M. (2001) The LANSS pain scale: The Leeds Assessment of Neuropathic Symptoms and Signs. *Pain*, 92(1–2), 147–157.

Bernatzky, G., Presch, M., Anderson, M. & Panksepp, J. (2011) Emotional foundations of music as a non-pharmacological pain management tool in modern medicine. *Neuroscience & Biobehavioral Reviews*, 35(9), 1989–1999.

BMAS (British Medical Acupuncture Society) (2013) *Treatment Record Chart.* Available at: www.medical-acupuncture.co.uk/Default.aspx?tabid=64

BNF (British National Formulary) (2019) *British National Formulary.* National Institute for Health and Care Excellence. Available at: https://bnf.nice.org.uk

BNF & NICE (National Institute for Health and Care Excellence) (2019) *Oxycodone Hydrochloride.* Available at: https://bnf.nice.org.uk/drug/oxycodone-hydrochloride.html

BOC Healthcare (2011) *Summary of Product Characteristics: Entonox.* Guildford: BOC Healthcare.

BOC Healthcare (2013) *ENTONOX® (50% Nitrous Oxide/50% Oxygen): Integral Valve Cylinders (ED, EX).* Manchester: BOC Healthcare.

BOC Healthcare (2015) *Entonox®: The Essential Guide.* Available at: www.bochealthcare.co.uk/en/images/entonox_essential_guide_hlc401955_Sep10_tcm409-64836.pdf

BOC Healthcare (2016) *ENTONOX®: Essential Safety Information.* Guildford: BOC Healthcare.

BOC Healthcare (2019) *ENTONOX® (Medical Nitrous Oxide and Oxygen Mixture).* Available at: www.bochealthcare.co.uk/en/products-and-services/products-and-services-by-category/medical-gases/entonox/entonox.html

Bodfish, J., Harper, V., Deacon, J.M. & Symonds, F. (2001) *Identifying and Measuring Pain in Persons with Developmental Disabilities: A Manual for the Pain and Discomfort Scale (PADS).* Morganton, NC: Western Carolina Center.

Boiano, J.M., Steege, A.L. & Sweeney, M.H. (2017) Exposure control practices for administering nitrous oxide: A survey of dentists, dental hygienists, and dental assistants. *Journal of Occupational and Environmental Hygiene*, 14(6), 409–416.

Boland, J.W. & Boland, E. (2017) Pharmacological therapies for opioid induced constipation in adults with cancer. *BMJ*, 358, j3313.

Bonafé-Monzó, N., Rojo-Moreno, J. & Catalá-Pizarro, M. (2015) Analgesic and physiological effects in conscious sedation with different nitrous oxide concentrations. *Journal of Clinical and Experimental Dentistry*, 7(1), 63–68.

Bos, E., Hollmann, M., Markus, W. & Philipp, L. (2017) Safety and efficacy of epidural analgesia. *Current Opinion in Anesthesiology*, 30(6), 736–742.

Bouhassira, D., Attal, N., Alchaar, H., et al. (2005) Comparison of pain syndromes associated with nervous or somatic lesions and development of a new neuropathic pain diagnostic questionnaire (DN4). *Pain*, 114, 29–36.

Bristol-Myers Squibb (2012) *Perfalgan: Dosing Tool.* Uxbridge: Bristol-Myers Squibb.

British Paediatric Neurology Association (2018) *Guidance on the Use of Cannabis-Based Products for Medicinal Use in Children and Young People with Epilepsy.* Available at: https://bpna.org.uk/userfiles/BPNA_CBPM_Guidance_Oct2018.pdf

British Pain Society (2014) *Useful Definitions and Glossary: Pain.* Available at: https://www.britishpainsociety.org/people-with-pain/useful-definitions-and-glossary/#pain

British Pain Society (2015) *Intrathecal Drug Delivery for the Management of Pain and Spasticity in Adults: Recommendations for Best Clinical Practice.* London: British Pain Society.

Brown, S.M. & Sneyd, J.R. (2015) Nitrous oxide in modern anaesthetic practice. *BJA Education*, 16(1), 87–91.

Brune, K. & Patrignani, P. (2015) New insights into the use of currently available non-steroidal anti-inflammatory drugs. *Journal of Pain Research*, 8, 105–118.

Bujedo, B.M. (2014) Current evidence for spinal opioid selection in post-operative pain. *Korean Journal of Pain*, 27(3), 200–209.

Carlson, C.L. (2016) Effectiveness of the World Health Organization cancer pain relief guidelines: An integrative review. *Journal of Pain Research*, 9, 515–534.

Castellsague, J., Riera-Guardia, N., Calingaert, B., et al. (2012) Individual NSAIDs and upper gastrointestinal complications: A systematic review and meta-analysis of observational studies (the SOS project). *Drug Safety*, 35(12), 1127–1146.

Chapman, S. (2012) Cancer pain part 2: Assessment and management. *Nursing Standard*, 26(48), 44–49.

Cherny, N., Fallon, M., Kaasa, S., et al. (2015) *Oxford Textbook of Palliative Medicine*, 5th edn. Oxford: Oxford University Press.

Chiam, E., Weinberg, L. & Bellomo, R. (2015) Paracetamol: A review with specific focus on the haemodynamic effects of intravenous administration. *Heart Lung Vessel*, 7(2), 121–132.

Chou, R., Cruciani, R.A., Fiellin, D., et al. (2014) Methadone safety: A clinical practice guideline from the American Pain Society and College on Problems of Drug Dependence, in collaboration with the Heart Rhythm Society. *Journal of Pain*, 15(4), 321–337.

Chou, R., Gordon, D.B., de Leon-Cassasola, O.A., et al. (2016) Management of postoperative pain: A clinical practice guideline from the American Pain Society, the American Society of Regional Anesthesia and Pain Medicine, and the American Society of Anesthesiologists' Committee on Regional Anesthesia, Executive Committee, and Administrative Council. *Journal of Pain*, 17(2), 131–157.

Collins, M. (2018) Use of nitrous oxide in maternity care: AWHONN practice brief number 6. *Nursing for Women's Health*, 22(2), 195–198.

Colloca, L., Ludman, T., Bouhassira, D., et al. (2017) Neuropathic pain. *Nature Reviews: Disease Primers*, 3, 17002.

Cox, F. (2010) Basic principles of pain management: Assessment and intervention. *Nursing Standard*, 25(1), 36–39.

[illegible] & Turk, D.C. (2013) Assessment of patients with chronic pain. *British Journal of Anaesthesia*, [illegible]

[illegible] (2011) *Compact Clinical Guide to Acute Pain Management: An Evidence-Based Approach*. New York: Springer.

Darwish, M., Kirby, M. & Giang, J.D. (2007) Effect of buccal dwell time on the pharmacokinetic profile of fentanyl buccal tablet. *Expert Opinion in Pharmacotherapy*, 8, 2011–2016.

DeKeyser Ganz, F. & Jacobs, J.M. (2014) The effect of humor on elder mental and physical health. *Geriatric Nursing*, 35(3), 205–211.

DH (Department of Health) & NHS England (2018) *Supplementary Information on Cannabis-Based Products for Medicinal Use*. Available at: https://www.england.nhs.uk/wp-content/uploads/2018/11/letter-additional-guidance-on-cannabis-based-products-for-medicinal-use.pdf

Dima, D., Tomuleasa, C., Frinc, I., et al. (2017) The use of rotation to fentanyl in cancer-related pain. *Journal of Pain Research*, 10, 341–348.

Doody, O. & Bailey, M.E. (2017) Pain and pain assessment in people with intellectual disability: Issues and challenges in practice. *British Journal of Learning Disability*, 45, 157–195.

Duncan, F., Day, R., Haigh, C., et al. (2014) First steps toward understanding the variability in acute pain service provision and the quality of pain relief in everyday practice across the United Kingdom. *Pain Medicine*, 15(1), 142–153.

El Geziry, A., Toble, Y., Al Kadhi, F., et al. (2018) Non-pharmacological pain management. In: Shallik, N. (ed) *Pain Management in Special Circumstances*. Available at: https://www.intechopen.com/books/pain-management-in-special-circumstances/non-pharmacological-pain-management

Elliott, J.A. (2016) Patient controlled analgesia in the management of acute pain. In: Elliott, J.A. & Smith, H.S. (eds) *Handbook of Acute Pain Management*. n.p.: CRC Press, pp.110–127.

Fallon, M., Cherny, N.I. & Hanks, G. (2010) Opioid analgesia therapy. In: Doyle, D., Cherny, N.I., Christakis, N.A., et al. (eds) *Oxford Textbook of Palliative Medicine*, 4th edn. Oxford: Oxford University Press, pp.599–625.

Farrell, A. & Rich, A. (2000) Analgesic use in patients with renal failure. *European Journal of Palliative Care*, 7(6), 201–205.

Fayaz, A., Croft, P., Langford, R.M., et al. (2015) Prevalence of chronic pain in the UK: A systematic review and meta-analysis of population studies. *BMJ Open*, 6(6), e010364.

FPM (Faculty of Pain Medicine) (2010) *Best Practice in the Management of Epidural Analgesia in the Hospital Setting*. Royal College of Anaesthetists. Available at: https://www.rcoa.ac.uk/system/files/FPM-EpAnalg2010_1.pdf

FPM (2015) *Core Standards for Pain Management Services in the UK*. Royal College of Anaesthetists. Available at: https://www.rcoa.ac.uk/system/files/CSPMS-UK-2016-v2-white.pdf

FPM (2018) *Opioids Aware: A Resource for Patients and Healthcare Professionals to Support Prescribing of Opioid Medicines for Pain*. Royal College of Anaesthetists. Available at: www.rcoa.ac.uk/faculty-of-pain-medicine/opioids-aware

FPM (2019) *The Effectiveness of Opioids for Long Term Pain*. Available at: https://www.rcoa.ac.uk/faculty-of-pain-medicine/opioids-aware/clinical-use-of-opioids/effectiveness-for-long-term-pain

Fraise, A.P. & Bradley, T. (eds) (2009) *Ayliffe's Control of Healthcare-Associated Infection: A Practical Handbook*, 5th edn. London: Hodder Arnold.

Freynhagen, R., Baron, R., Gockel, U., & Tölle, T.R. (2006) painDETECT: A new screening questionnaire to identify neuropathic components in patients with back pain. *Current Medical Research and Opinion*, 22(10), 1911–1920.

Gallagher, M. & Grant, C.R. (2018) Adjuvant agents in regional anaesthesia. *Anaesthesia & Intensive Care Medicine*, 9(11), 615–618.

Garimella, V. & Cellini, C. (2013) Postoperative pain control. *Clinical Colon Rectal Surgery*, 26(3), 191–196.

Gélinas, C. & Arbour, C. (2014) Pain and pain management. In: Urden, L.D., Stacy, K.M. & Lough, M.E. (eds) *Critical Care Nursing: Diagnosis and Management*, 7th edn. St Louis, MO: Mosby Elsevier, pp.143–169.

Gélinas, C., Tousignant-Laflamme, Y., Tanguay, A. & Bourgault, P. (2011) Exploring the validity of the bispectral index, the Critical-Care Pain Observation Tool and vital signs for the detection of pain in sedated and mechanically ventilated critically ill adults: A pilot study. *Intensive and Critical Care Nursing*, 27(1), 46–52.

George, J.A., Lin, E.E., Hanna, M.N., et al. (2010) The effect of intravenous opioid patient controlled analgesia with and without background infusion on respiratory depression: A meta-analysis. *Journal of Opioid Management*, 6(1), [illegible]

[illegible] (2015) Acute pain assessment tools: Let us move beyond simple pain ratings. *Current Opinion in Anesthesiology*, [illegible]

Gorlin, A.W., Rosenfeld, D., Maloney, J., et al. (2016) Survey of pain specialists regarding conversion of high-dose intravenous to neuraxial opioids. *Journal of Pain Research*, 9, 693–700.

Gov.uk (2015) *Drugs and Driving: The Law*. Available at: https://www.gov.uk/drug-driving-law

Grissinger, M. (2012) Reducing the risk of deadly mixups with epidural and intravenous drugs. *Pharmacy & Therapeutics*, 37(8), 432–434.

Gupta, R. (2014) Opioids: Clinical use. In: *Pain Management: Essential Topics for Examination*. Berlin: Springer, pp.41–43.

Harmer, M. & Davies, K.A. (1998) The effect of education, assessment and a standardised prescription on postoperative pain management: The value of clinical audit in the establishment of acute pain services. *Anaesthesia*, 53(5), 424–430.

Harrop-Griffiths, W., Cook, T., Gill, H., et al. (2013) *Regional Anaesthesia and Patients with Abnormalities of Coagulation*. London: Association of Anaesthetists of Great Britain and Ireland.

Health and Safety Executive (2002) *Control of Substances Hazardous to Health (COSHH)*. Available at: www.hse.gov.uk/coshh

Hebl, J.R. (2006) The importance and implications of aseptic techniques during regional anesthesia. *Regional Anesthesia & Pain Medicine*, 31(4), 311–323.

Hewson, D.W., Bedforth, N.M. & Hardman, J.G. (2018) Spinal cord injury arising in anaesthesia practice. *Anaesthesia*, 73(1), 43–50.

Hicks, F. & Simpson, K.H. (2004) Regional nerve blocks. In Hicks, F. & Simpson, K.H. (eds) *Nerve Blocks in Palliative Care*. Oxford: Oxford University Press, pp.53–55.

Hill, K.P., Palastro, M.D., Johnson, B. & Ditre, J.W. (2017) Cannabis and pain: A clinical review. *Cannabis and Cannabinoid Research*, 2(1), 96–104.

Hole, J., Hirsch, M., Ball, E. & Meads, C. (2015) Music as an aid for postoperative recovery in adults: A systematic review and meta-analysis. *Lancet*, 386, 1659–1671.

Huang, C. & Johnson, N. (2016) Nitrous oxide, from the operating room to the emergency department. *Current Emergency and Hospital Medicine Reports*, 4(1), 11–18.

Humble, S.R., Dalton, A.J., & Li, L. (2015) A systematic review of therapeutic interventions to reduce acute and chronic post surgical pain after amputation, thoracotomy or mastectomy. *European Journal of Pain*, 19, 451–465.

Hurley, R.W., Cohen, S.P. & Wu, C.L. (2010) Acute pain in adults. In: Fishman, S., Ballantyne, J. & Rathmell, J.P. (eds) *Bonica's Management of Pain*, 4th edn. Philadelphia: Lipincott Williams & Wilkins, pp.699–723.

IASP (International Association for the Study of Pain) (1994) *IASP Terminology*. Available at: https://www.iasp-pain.org/Education/Content.aspx?ItemNumber=1698

Ilfeld, B.M. (2011) Continuous peripheral nerve blocks: A review of the published evidence. *Anesthesia & Analgesia*, 113(4), 904–925.

Johnson, M.I. (2014) Mechanism of action of TENS. In: *Transcutaneous Electrical Nerve Stimulation (TENS): Research to Support Clinical Practice*. Oxford: Oxford University Press, pp.712–103.

Jules-Elysee, K.M., Goon, A.K., Westrich, G.H., et al. (2015) Patient-controlled epidural analgesia or multimodal pain regimen with periarticular injection after total hip arthroplasty: A randomized, double-blind, placebo-controlled study. *Journal of Bone and Joint Surgery*, 97(10), 789–798.

King, S., Forbes, K., Hanks, G.W., et al. (2011) A systematic review of the use of opioid medication for those with moderate to severe cancer pain and renal impairment: A European Palliative Care Research Collaborative opioid guidelines project. *Palliative Medicine*, 25(5), 525–552.

Kooij, F.O., Schlack, W.S., Preckel, B. & Hollmann, M.W. (2014) Does regional analgesia for major surgery improve outcome? Focus on epidural analgesia. *Anesthesia & Analgesia*, 119(3), 740–744.

Krause, S. (2003) Development of a neuropathic pain questionnaire. *Clinical Journal of Pain*, 19(5), 306–314.

Ladha, A., Alam, A., Idestrup, C., et al. (2013) Spinal haematoma after removal of a thoracic epidural catheter in a patient with coagulopathy resulting from unexpected vitamin K deficiency. *Anaesthesia*, 68, 856–860.

Lagerkranser, M. & Lindquist, C. (2017) Neuraxial blocks and spinal haematoma: Review of 166 cases published 1994–2015. Part 2: Diagnosis, treatment, and outcome. *Scandinavian Journal of Pain*, 15, 130–136.

Lee, L., Caplan, R., Stephens, L., et al. (2015) Postoperative opioid-induced respiratory depression: A closed claims analysis. *Anesthesiology*, 122, 659–665.

Lee, M.S. & Ernst, E. (2011) Acupuncture for pain: An overview of Cochrane reviews. *Chinese Journal of Integrated Medicine*, 17, 187–189.

Lefebvre-Chapiro, S. (2001) The DOLOPLUS 2 scale: Evaluating pain in the elderly. *European Journal of Palliative Care*, 8, 191–194.

Li, S.L., Wang, D.X. & Ma, D. (2010) Epidural hematoma after neuraxial blockade: A retrospective report from China. *Anesthesia & Analgesia*, 111, 1322–1324.

Lister, S., Dougherty, L. & McNamara, L. (eds) (2019) *The Royal Marsden Manual of Cancer Nursing Procedures*. Oxford: Wiley-Blackwell.

Loveday, H.P., Wilson, J.A., Pratt, R.J., et al. (2014) epic3: National evidence-based guidelines for preventing healthcare-associated infections in NHS hospitals in England. *Journal of Hospital Infection*, 86(Suppl. 1), S1–S70.

Macintyre, P.E. & Schug, S.A. (2015) *Acute Pain Management: A Practical Guide*. 4th edn. Boca Raton, FL: CRC Press.

Mahajan, L., Mittal, V., Gupta, R., et al. (2017) Study to compare the effect of oral, rectal, and intravenous infusion of paracetamol for postoperative analgesia in women undergoing cesarean section under spinal anesthesia. *Anesthesia Essays and Researches*, 11(3), 594–598.

Mahapatra, S., Chandrasekhara, N.S. & Upadhyay, S.P. (2016) Spinal epidural haematoma following removal of epidural catheter after an elective intra-abdominal surgery. *Indian Journal of Anaesthesia*, 60, 355–357.

Malanga, G.A., Yan, N. & Stark, J. (2015) Mechanisms and efficacy of heat and cold therapies for musculoskeletal injury. *Postgraduate Medicine*, 127(1), 57–65.

Mann, E. (2009) Pain management. In: Glasper, A., McEwing, G. & Richardson, J. (eds) *Foundation Studies for Caring: Using Student Centred Learning*. Basingstoke: Palgrave Macmillan, pp.259–284.

Mariano, E.R. (2018) Management of acute perioperative pain. *UpToDate*. Available at: https://www.uptodate.com/contents/management-of-acute-perioperative-pain

McAuliffe, L., Nay, R., O'Donnell, M. & Fetherstonhaugh, D. (2008) Pain assessment in older people with dementia: Literature review. *Journal of Advanced Nursing*, 65(1), 2–10.

McCaffery, M. (1968) *Nursing Practice Theories Related to Cognition, Bodily Pain and Man-Environment Interactions*. Los Angeles: University of California, Los Angeles.

McClymont, W. & Celnick, D. (2018) Techniques of epidural block. *Anaesthesia & Intensive Care Medicine*, 19(11), 600–606.

McGuire, B.E., Daly, P. & Smythe, F. (2010) Chronic pain in people with an intellectual disability: Under-recognised and under-treated. *Journal of Learning Disability Research*, 54, 240–245.

McKenzie, K., Smith, M. & Purcell, A. (2012) The reported expression of pain and distress by people with intellectual disability. *Journal of Clinical Nursing*, 22, 1833–1842.

McNicol, E.D., Ferguson, M.C., & Hudcova, J. (2015) Patient controlled opioid analgesia versus non-patient controlled opioid analgesia for postoperative pain. *Cochrane Database of Systematic Reviews*, 6, CD003348.

McSwain, J.R., Doty, J.W. & Wilson, S.H. (2014) Regional anesthesia in patients with pre-existing neurologic disease. *Current Opinion in Anesthesiology*, 27(5), 538–543.

Melzack, R. (1975) The McGill Pain Questionnaire: Major properties and scoring methods. *Pain*, 1(3), 277–299.

Mercadante, S. & Bruera, E. (2018) Methadone as a first-line opioid in cancer pain management: A systematic review. *Journal of Pain and Symptom Management*, 55(3), 998–1003.

Misuse of Drugs Act (1971) Available at: https://www.legislation.gov.uk/ukpga/1971/38/contents

Misuse of Drugs Regulations (2001) Available at: www.legislation.gov.uk/uksi/2001/3998/pdfs/uksi_20013998_en.pdf

Molsberger, A.F., Schneider, T., Gotthardt, H. & Drabik, A. (2010) German randomized acupuncture trial for chronic shoulder pain (GRASP): A pragmatic, controlled, patient-blinded, multi-center trial in an outpatient care environment. *Pain*, 151(1), 146–154.

Moore, R.A., Derry, S., Taylor, R.S., et al. (2013) Review article: The costs and consequences of adequately managed chronic non-cancer pain and chronic neuropathic pain. *Pain Practice*, 14(1), 79–94.

Moore, R.A., Derry, S., Wiffen, P.J., et al. (2015) Overview review: Comparative efficacy of oral ibuprofen and paracetamol (acetaminophen) across acute and chronic pain conditions. *European Journal of Pain*, 19, 1213–1223.

Mu, A., Weinberg, E., Moulin, D.E. & Clarke, H. (2017) Clinical review: Pharmacologic management of chronic neuropathic pain – Review of the Canadian Pain Society consensus statement. *Canadian Family Physician*, 63, 844–852.

Nguyen, V., Tiemann, D., Park, E. & Salehi, A. (2017) Alpha-2 agonists. *Anesthesiology Clinics*, 35(2), 233–245.

NHS England (2015) *Clinical Commissioning Policy: Intrathecal Pumps for Treatment of Severe Chronic Pain*. Available at: https://www.england.nhs.uk/commissioning/wp-content/uploads/sites/12/2015/10/d08pa-intrathecal-pumps-oct15.pdf

NHS England and NHSI (NHS Improvement) (2019) *Standard Infection Control Precautions: National Hand Hygiene and Personal Protective Equipment Policy*. Available at: https://improvement.nhs.uk/documents/4957/National_policy_on_hand_hygiene_and_PPE_2.pdf

NHS Improvement (2017) *Patient Safety Alert: Resources to Support Safe Transition from the Luer Connector to NRFit™ for Intrathecal and Epidural Procedures, and the Delivery of Regional Blocks*. Available at: https://improvement.nhs.uk/documents/1550/Patient_Safety_Alert_-_resources_to_support_transition_to_NRFit_Aug_2017v2.pdf

Ni Thuathail, A. & Welford, C. (2011) Pain assessment tools for older people with cognitive impairment. *Nursing Standard*, 26(6), 39–46.

NICE (National Institute for Health and Care Excellence) (2014) *Osteoarthritis Care and Management* [Clinical Guideline CG177]. Available at: www.nice.org.uk/guidance/CG177

NICE (2016) *Controlled Drugs: Safe Use and Management* [NICE Guideline NG46]. Available at: www.nice.org.uk/guidance/NG46

NICE (2018) *NICE Guideline Final Scope: Chronic Pain – Assessment and Management*. Available at: https://www.nice.org.uk/guidance/gid-ng10069/documents/final-scope

Nickel, F.T., Seifert, F., Lanz, S. & Maihöfner, C. (2012) Mechanisms of neuropathic pain. *European Neuropsychopharmacology*, 22, 81–91.

NMC (Nursing and Midwifery Council) (2018) *The Code: Professional Standards of Practice and Behaviour for Nurses, Midwives and Nursing Associates*. Available at: https://www.nmc.org.uk/standards/code

Nolan, J.P. (2018) Anaesthesia and neuromuscular block. In: Brown, M., Sharma, P., Mir, F. & Bennett, P. (eds.) *Clinical Pharmacology*, 12th edn. Edinburgh: Elsevier, pp.308–323.

NPSA (National Patient Safety Agency) (2007) *Recognising and Responding Appropriately to Early Signs of Deterioration in Hospitalised Patients*. Available at: https://www.patientsafetyoxford.org/wp-content/uploads/2018/03/NPSA-DeteriorPatients.pdf

NPSA (2009) *Safer Spinal (Intrathecal), Epidural and Regional Devices – Part B*. Available at: https://www.sps.nhs.uk/wp-content/uploads/2018/02/2011-NRLS-0972B-Safer-spinal-dpart-B-2009.11.24-v1.pdf

NPSA (2017) *Resources to Support Safe Transition from the Luer Connector to NRFit for Intrathecal and Epidural Procedure and Delivery of Regional Blocks*. Available at: https://improvement.nhs.uk/documents/1550/Patient_Safety_Alert_-_resources_to_support_transition_to_NRFit_Aug_2017v2.pdf

Onakpoya, I.J., Thomas, E.T., Lee, J.J., et al. (2019) Benefits and harms of pregabalin in the management of neuropathic pain: A rapid review and meta-analysis of randomized clinical trials. *BMJ Open*, 9(1), e023600.

Orenius, T., Koskela, T., Koho, P., et al. (2013) Anxiety and depression are independent predictors of quality of life of patients with chronic musculoskeletal pain. *Journal of Health Psychology*, 18(2) 167–175.

Palat, G. & Charyy, S. (2018) Practical guide for using methadone in pain and palliative care practice. *Indian Journal of Palliative Care*, 24(1), 21–29.

Parizkova, B. & George, S. (2009a) Regional anaesthesia and analgesia, Part 1: Peripheral nerve blockade. In: Cox, F. (ed) *Perioperative Pain Management*. Oxford: John Wiley & Sons, pp.127–143.

Parizkova, B. & George, S. (2009b) Regional anaesthesia and analgesia, Part 2: Central neural blockade. In: Cox, F. (ed) *Perioperative Pain Management*. Oxford: John Wiley & Sons, pp.144–160.

Park, J.E., Lee, M.S., Choi, J.Y., et al. (2010) Adverse events associated with acupuncture: A prospective survey. *Journal of Alternative and Complementary Medicine*, 16(9), 959–963.

Pasero, C. & McCaffery, M. (2011) Misconceptions that impede assessment and treatment of patients who report pain. In: Pasero, C. & McCaffery, M. (eds) Pain Assessment and Pharmacologic Management. St Louis, MO: Mosby Elsevier, pp.20–48.

Polomano, R.C., Fillman, M., Giordano, N.A., et al. (2017) Multimodal analgesia for acute postoperative and trauma-related pain. *American Journal of Nursing*, 117(3), S12–S26.

Pöpping, D.M., Elia, N., Van Aken, H.K., et al. (2014) Impact of epidural analgesia on mortality and morbidity after surgery: Systematic review and meta-analysis of randomized controlled trials. *Annals of Surgery*, 259(6), 1056–1067.

Portenoy, R. (2006) Development and testing of a neuropathic pain screening questionnaire: ID Pain. *Current Medical Research and Opinion*, 22(8), 1555–1565.

Portenoy, R.K., Payne, R., Coluzzi, P., et al. (1999) Oral transmucosal fentanyl citrate (OTFC) for the treatment of breakthrough pain in cancer patients: A controlled dose titration study. *Pain*, 79(2–3), 303–312.

Preston, R.M. (2005) Aseptic technique: Evidence-based approach for patient safety. *British Journal of Nursing*, 14(10), 540–542, 544–546.

Raffa, R.B. & Pergolizzi, J.V. (2014) A modern analgesics pain 'pyramid'. *Journal of Clinical Pharmacy and Therapeutics*, 39, 4–6.

Rauch, R.L., Tark, M., Reyes, E., et al. (2009) Efficacy and long term tolerability of sublingual fentanyl oral disintegrating tablet in the treatment of breakthrough cancer pain. *Current Medical Research and Opinion*, 25(12), 2877–2885.

Rawal, N. (2016) Current issues in postoperative pain management. *European Journal of Anaesthesiology*, 33(3), 160–171.

RCA (Royal College of Anaesthetists) (2006) Section 1: Key issues in developing new materials. In: Lack, J.A., Rollin, A.M., Thoms, G., et al. (eds) *Raising the Standard: Information for Patients*, 2nd edn. London: Royal College of Anaesthetists, pp.14–29.

RCA (2015) *Core Standards for Pain Management in the UK*. Available at: www.rcoa.ac.uk/system/files/CSPMS-UK-2015-v2-white.pdf

RCA (2017) *Section 12: Nerve Damage Associated with a Spinal or Epidural Injection*. Available at: https://www.rcoa.ac.uk/system/files/12-NerveDamageSpinalEpidural2017.pdf

RCA (2019) *Guidelines for the Provision of Anaesthesia Services for Inpatient Pain Management 2019*. Available at: https://www.rcoa.ac.uk/system/files/GPAS-2019-11-PAIN.pdf

RCN (Royal College of Nursing) (2016) *Preserving People's Dignity*. Available at: https://rcni.com/hosted-content/rcn/first-steps/preserving-peoples-dignity

Reardon, D.P., Anger, K.E. & Szumita, P.M. (2015) Pathophysiology, assessment, and management of pain in critically ill adults. *American Journal of Health System Pharmacy*, 72(18), 1531–1543.

Reddy, A., Tayjasanant, S., Haider, A., et al. (2016) The opioid rotation ratio of strong opioids to transdermal fentanyl in cancer patients. *Cancer*, 122(1), 149–156.

Regnard, C., Reynolds, J., Watson, B., et al. (2007) Understanding distress in people with severe communication difficulties: Developing and assessing the Disability Distress Assessment Tool (DisDAT). *Journal Intellectual Disability Research*, 51(Pt. 4), 277–292.

Rhodes, L. & Branham, A. (2016) Acute pain: Considerations in geriatric patients. *Pharmacy Times*. Available at: https://www.pharmacytimes.com/publications/health-system-edition/2016/july2016/acute-pain-considerations-in-geriatric-patients

Riley, J., Branford, R., Droney, J., et al. (2015) Morphine or oxycodone for cancer pain? A randomized, open-label, controlled trial. *Journal of Pain and Symptom Management*, 49(2), 161–172.

Road Traffic Act (1988) Available at: www.legislation.gov.uk/ukpga/1988/52/contents

Rosero, E.B., Cheng, G.S., Khatri, K.P. & Joshi, G.P. (2014) Evaluation of epidural analgesia for open major liver resection surgery from a US inpatient sample. *Proceedings (Baylor University Medical Center)*, 27(4), 305–312.

Rosero, E.B. & Joshi, G.P. (2014) Preemptive, preventive, multimodal analgesia: What do they really mean? *Plastic and Reconstructive Surgery*, 134(4), 85–93.

Rosero, E.B. & Joshi, G.P. (2016) Nationwide incidence of serious complications of epidural analgesia in the United States. *Acta Anaesthesiologica Scandinavica*, 60, 810–820.

Sachs, A. & Smiley, R. (2014) Post-dural puncture headache: The worst common complication in obstetric anesthesia. *Seminars in Perinatology*, 38(6), 386–394.

Sattar, M., Sayed, O.M. & Lane, M.E. (2014) Oral transmucosal drug delivery – Current status and future prospects. *International Journal of Pharmaceutics*, 471, 498–506.

Schofield, P. (2018) The assessment of pain in older people: UK national guidelines. *Age and Ageing*, 47(Suppl. 1), i1–i22.

Schug, S.A., Palmer, G.M., Scott, D.A., et al. (2015) *Acute Pain Management: Scientific Evidence*, 4th edn. Melbourne: Australian and New Zealand College of Anaesthetists and Faculty of Pain Medicine.

Schuster, M., Bayer, O., Heid, F. & Laufenberg-Feldmann, R. (2018) Opioid rotation in cancer pain treatment. *Deutsches Ärzteblatt International*, 115(9), 135–142.

Schwartz, S., Etropolski, M., Shapiro, D.Y., et al. (2011) Safety and efficacy of tapentadol ER in patients with painful diabetic peripheral neuropathy: Results of a randomized-withdrawal, placebo-controlled trial. *Current Medical Research Opinion*, 27(91), 151–162.

Shin, J.S., Ha, I.H., Lee, J., et al. (2013) Effects of motion style acupuncture treatment in acute low back pain patients with severe disability: A multicenter, randomized, controlled, comparative effectiveness trial. *Pain*, 154(7), 1030–1037.

Shipton, E.A. (2014) The transition of acute postoperative pain to chronic pain: Part 1 – Risk factors for the development of postoperative acute persistent pain. *Trends in Anaesthesia and Critical Care*, 4, 67–70.

Shipton, E.A. (2018) Physical therapy approaches in the treatment of low back pain. *Pain Therapy*, 7(2) 127–137.

Steeds, C.E. (2016) The anatomy and physiology of pain. *Surgery*, 34(2), 55–59.

Stewart, D. (2017) Pearls and pitfalls of patient controlled analgesia. *US Pharmacist*, 42(3), HS24–HS27.

Tan, G., Jensen, M.P., Thornby, J.I. & Shanti, B.F. (2004) Validation of the Brief Pain Inventory for chronic nonmalignant pain. *Journal of Pain*, 5(2), 1331–1337.

Tiippana, E., Nelskylä, K., Nilsson, E., et al. (2014) Managing post-thoracotomy pain: Epidural or systemic analgesia and extended care – A randomized study with an "as usual" control group. *Scandinavian Journal of Pain*, 5(4), 240–247.

Toledano, R.D. & Tsen, L.C. (2014) Epidural catheter design history, innovations, and clinical implications. *Anesthesiology*, 121(1), 9–17.

Tortora, J. & Derrickson, B. (2017) *Principles of Anatomy & Physiology*, 15th edn. Hoboken, NJ: John Wiley & Sons.

Tosounidis, T.H., Sheikh, H., Stone, M.H. & Giannoudis, P.V. (2015) Pain relief management following proximal femoral fractures: Options, issues and controversies. *Injury*, 46, 52–58.

Treede, R.-D., Rief, W., Barke, A., et al. (2019) Chronic pain as a symptom or a disease: The IASP classification of chronic pain for the *International Classification of Diseases* (ICD-11). *Pain*, 160(1), 19–27.

Trelle, S., Reichenbach S., Wandel S., et al. (2011) Cardiovascular safety of non-steroidal anti-inflammatory drugs: Network meta-analysis. *BMJ*, 342, c7086.

Tse, M.M.Y., Lo, A.P.K., Cheng, T.L.Y., et al. (2010) Humor therapy: Relieving chronic pain and enhancing happiness for older adults. *Journal of Aging Research*, 2010, 1–9.

Umegaki, T., Hirota, K., Ohira, S., et al. (2016) Rapid development of a spinal epidural hematoma following thoracic epidural catheter removal in an esophageal carcinoma surgical patient: A case report. *JA Clinical Reports*, 2(1), 37.

Vaajoki, A., Pietilä, A.M., Kankkunen, P. & Vehviläinen-Julkunen, K. (2012) Effects of listening to music on pain intensity and pain distress after surgery: An intervention. *Journal of Clinical Nursing*, 21(5–6), 708–717.

van den Beuken-van Everdingen, M.H.J., Hochstenbach, L.M.J., Joosten, E.A.J., et al. (2016) Update on prevalence of pain in patients with cancer: Systematic review and meta-analysis. *Journal of Pain and Symptom Management*, 51(6), 1070–1090.

Vance, C.G., Dailey, D.L., Rakel, B.A. & Sluka, K.A. (2014) Using TENS for pain control: The state of the evidence. *Pain Management*, 4(3), 197–209.

Vargas-Schaffer, G. (2010) Is the WHO analgesic ladder still valid? Twenty-four years of experience. *Canadian Family Physician*, 56, 514–517.

Vargas-Schaffer, G. & Cogan, J. (2014) Patient therapeutic education. Placing the patient at the centre of the WHO analgesic ladder. *Canadian Family Physician*, 59, 235–241.

Vayne-Bossert, P., Afsharimani, B., Good, P., et al. (2016) Interventional options for the management of refractory cancer pain: What is the evidence? *Supportive Care in Cancer*, 24(3), 1429–1438.

Vellucci, R., Mediati, R.D. & Ballerini, G. (2014) Use of opioids for treatment of osteoporotic pain. *Clinical Cases in Mineral Bone Metabolism*, 11(3), 173–176.

Vickers, A.J., Cronin, A.M., Maschino, A.C., et al. (2012). Acupuncture for chronic pain: Individual patient data metaanalysis. *Archives of Internal Medicine*, 172(19), 1444–1453.

Wang, C.X., Wang, J., Chen, Y.Y., et al. (2016) Randomized controlled study of the safety and efficacy of nitrous oxide-sedated endoscopic ultrasound-guided fine needle aspiration for digestive tract diseases. *World Journal of Gastroenterology*, 22(46), 10242–10248.

Warden, V., Hurley, A.C., & Volicer, V. (2003) Development and psychometric evaluation of the Pain Assessment in Advanced Dementia (PAINAD) scale. *Journal of the American Medical Directors Association*, 4, 9–15.

White, A., Hinton, S., Kwee, S.H., et al. (2012) Acupuncture research update: Summaries of recent papers. *Acupuncture in Medicine*, 30, 354–361.

White, A., Cummings, M. & Filshie, J. (2018) *An Introduction to Western Medical Acupuncture*, 2nd edn. London: Elsevier.

WHO (World Health Organization) (1986) *Cancer Pain Relief.* Geneva: World Health Organization.

WHO (2019) *World Health Organization Model List of Essential Medicines: 21st List.* Available at: https://apps.who.int/iris/bitstream/handle/10665/325771/WHO-MVP-EMP-IAU-2019.06-eng.pdf?ua=1

Wild, J.E., Grond, S., Kuperwasser, B., et al. (2010) Long-term safety and tolerability of tapentadol extended release for the management of chronic low back pain or osteoarthritis pain. *Pain Practice*, 10(5), 416–427.

Wolkerstorfer, A., Handler, N. & Buschmann, H. (2016) New approaches to treating pain. *Bioorganic & Medicinal Chemistry Letters*, 26, 1103–1119.

Wuhrman, E. & Cooney, M.F. (2011) Acute pain: Assessment and treatment. *Medscape*, 3 January. Available at: www.medscape.com/viewarticle/735034

Yap, S.H. (2016) Acupuncture in pain management. *Anaesthesia & Intensive Care Medicine*, 17(9), 448–450.

Young, A., Ismail, M., Papatsoris, A.G., et al. (2012) Entonox® inhalation to reduce pain in common diagnostic and therapeutic outpatient urological procedures: A review of the evidence. *Annals of The Royal College of Surgeons of England*, 94(1), 8–11.

Zeppetella, G., Davies, A., Eijgelshoven, I. & Jansen, J.P. (2014) A network meta-analysis of the efficacy of opioid analgesics for the management of breakthrough cancer pain episodes. *Journal of Pain and Symptom Management*, 47(4), 772–785.

Chapter 11

Symptom control and care towards the end of life

Anna-Marie Stevens with Anne Doerr, Alistair McCulloch, Pedro Mendes, Jodie Rawlings and Laura Theodossy

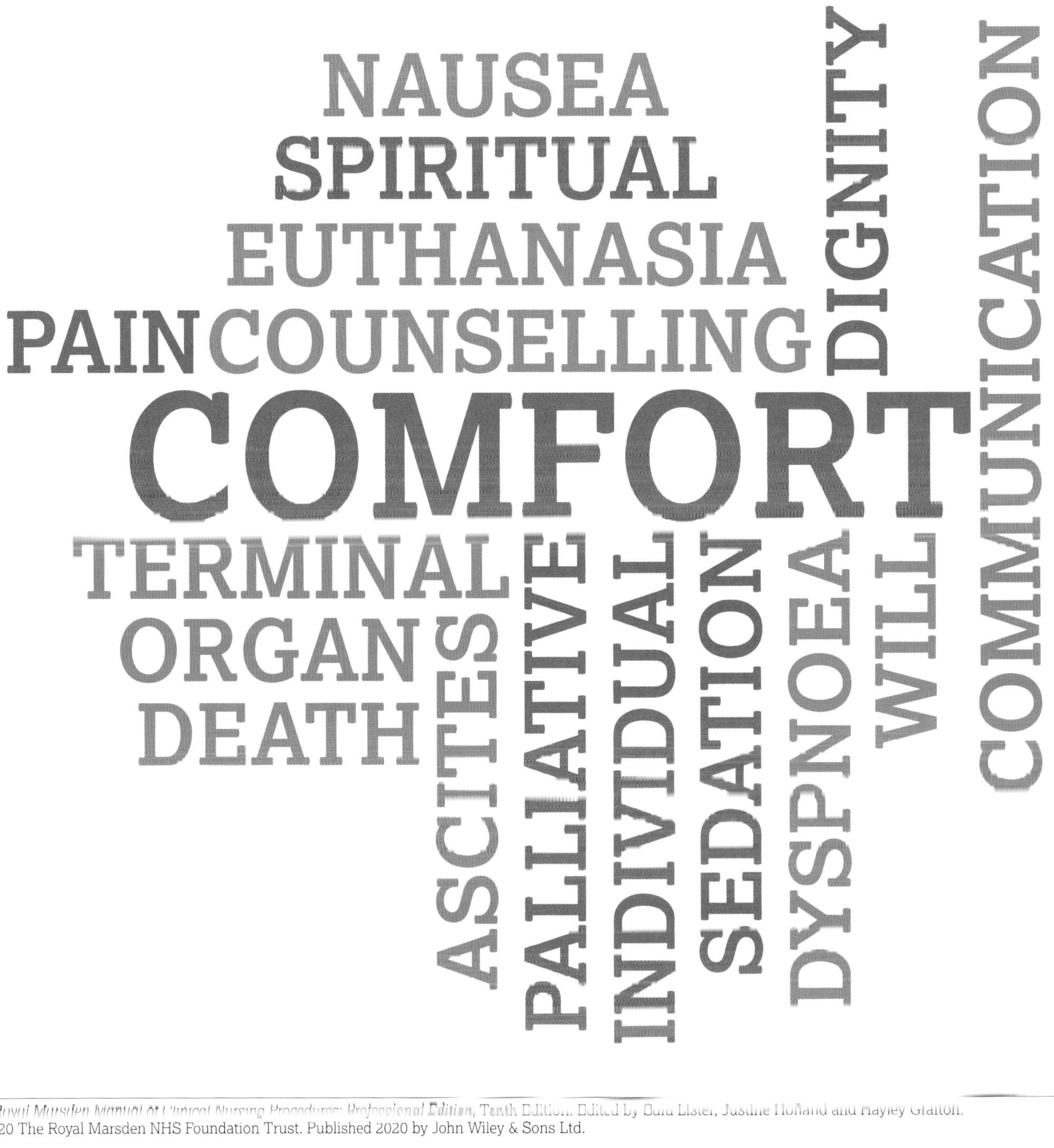

The Royal Marsden Manual of Clinical Nursing Procedures: Professional Edition, Tenth Edition. Edited by Sara Lister, Justine Hofland and Hayley Grafton.

Procedure guidelines

Being an accountable professional

At the point of registration, the nurse will:

10. Use evidence-based, best practice approaches for meeting needs for care and support at the end of life, accurately assessing the person's capacity for independence and self-care and initiating appropriate interventions

Future Nurse: Standards of Proficiency for Registered Nurses (NMC 2018)

Overview

This chapter presents procedures that contribute towards the comfort of patients approaching the end of life and those required following death. It covers considerations relating to symptom control at the end of life, including the management of ascites and procedures that contribute to the delivery of compassionate end-of-life care. The focus of this chapter is on patients who are primarily being cared for in the hospital setting. It also sets out the procedures to be followed once death has occurred.

Caring for patients who are reaching the end of their life can present both challenges and rewards. In addition to physical symptoms such as pain, breathlessness, nausea and increasing fatigue, people who are approaching the end of life may experience anxiety, depression, and social and spiritual difficulties. Individualized management of these issues requires collaborative, multidisciplinary working and effective channels of communication.

End-of-life care

Definition

There is considerable ambiguity surrounding the terms 'palliative care', 'terminal care' and 'end-of-life care'. They are often used interchangeably but are not synonymous.

Palliative care

Palliative care is the active, total care of a patient whose disease is not responsive to curative treatment. Control of pain, other symptoms, and social, psychological and spiritual problems is paramount. Palliative care affirms life and regards dying as a normal process: it neither hastens nor postpones death (WHO 2002). Recent advances in healthcare mean that many people now live with advanced, incurable illness for many years. This has been acknowledged by the World Health Organization (WHO), which in 2002 reviewed its definition of palliative care to advise that this type of care may be applicable earlier in the disease trajectory:

> Palliative care:
> - provides relief from pain and other distressing symptoms;
> - affirms life and regards dying as a normal process;
> - intends neither to hasten or postpone death;
> - integrates the psychological and spiritual aspects of patient care;
> - offers a support system to help patients live as actively as possible until death;
> - offers a support system to help the family cope during the patient's illness and in their own bereavement;
> - uses a team approach to address the needs of patients and their families, including bereavement counselling, if indicated;
> - will enhance quality of life, and may also positively influence the course of illness;
> - is applicable early in the course of illness, in conjunction with other therapies that are intended to prolong life, such as chemotherapy or radiation therapy, and includes those investigations needed to better understand and manage distressing clinical complications. (WHO 2002, p.1)

Palliative care, with its gradual shift in transition from curative and life-prolonging treatment towards managing quality of life, can relieve significant medical burdens such as unwanted interventions that may have no ongoing benefit to the patient. It can also maintain a patient's dignity and comfort.

End-of-life care

End-of-life care is defined as care of patients who are likely to die within 12 months. It refers to patients who have advanced, progressive, incurable conditions and patients with life-threatening acute conditions. It also ensures support for their families and carers (NICE 2017b).

The term 'families and carers' is used throughout this chapter, although it is acknowledged that not all family are carers and not all carers are family. The term 'family' or 'families' is also used to describe anyone close to the patient, who may or may not be related.

Terminal care

The 'terminal phase' is defined as a period of irreversible decline in functional status prior to death. It can last from hours to days and on some occasions weeks.

Anatomy and physiology

In the days and hours leading up to an expected death, many physiological changes occur that signify the closing down of the body before death (Box 11.1). It is important for healthcare professionals to have an understanding of this process so that they can provide information and reassurance for patients and families. Cheyne–Stokes breathing and cardiovascular changes (e.g. peripheral vasoconstriction) are common. For the patient and their family to have sufficient time to express their preferences for end-of-life care, recognition of dying must occur as early as possible.

The last weeks of life for most people are characterized by a progressive physical decline, frailty, lethargy, worsening mobility, reduced oral intake, and little or no response to medical interventions. These changes can be subtle and can first be identified by nursing staff, allied health professionals or family members. In cancer, which characteristically has a smooth downward trajectory in the last few weeks, death can be easier to predict than in non-cancer diseases such as chronic obstructive pulmonary disease and heart failure, which are characterized by relapses and remissions. Similarly, death from frailty or dementia can be difficult to predict because patients can live for a long time with a very poor level of function, making the dying phase difficult to distinguish (Sleeman 2013).

Related theory

Enabling people to die in comfort and with dignity is hugely important for the patient and their family and is a core function of the NHS (DH 2008, NEoLCP 2015, NICE 2017a). End-of-life care has come to the forefront of international government health policies. The Care Quality Commission has included end-of-life care as one of its key areas of assessment (CQC 2015).

The *End of Life Care Strategy* (DH 2008) set out guidance aimed at improving care and choices for all people regardless of their diagnosis and place of care. The principal aims are to improve the quality of care for those approaching the end of their life and to enable greater choices and control about their place of care and

Box 11.1 Physiological changes at the end of life

- Decreased blood perfusion that may result in discolouration of skin and pressure points
- Weight loss
- Profound weakness
- Social withdrawal
- Disinterest in food and drink
- Dysphagia (difficulty swallowing)
- Refractory delirium, confusion and/or agitation
- Depression and/or anxiety
- Extended periods of drowsiness
- Reduced urine output
- Changes in skin temperature
- Dyspnoea (shortness of breath)
- Retained chest secretions
- A waxy look to the skin
- Incontinence

Source: Adapted from Hui et al. (2014), Lacey (2015).

death. The strategy, which focuses on the role of health and social care, states that high-quality end-of-life care should be available wherever the person may be: at home, in a care home, in hospital, in a hospice or elsewhere (DH 2008). In 2015, the document *Ambitions for Palliative and End of Life Care* set out six ambitions (Figure 11.1) that offer further guidance on caring for this group of patients and their families (NEoLCP 2015). Each of the six ambitions includes a statement to describe the ambition in practice, primarily from the point of view of a person nearing the end of life. Although the focus of this document is related to the experience of the dying person, its reach is much broader. The document suggests that each statement should be read as an ambition for carers, families, those important to the dying person, and (where appropriate) people who have been bereaved.

Evidence-based approaches

Palliative care is a relatively new speciality in nursing and medicine; its services operate in various ways and vary in funding (voluntary or NHS), team composition, staff-to-patient ratio, out-of-hours care and treatment regimens used. Palliative care's evidence base is comparatively small and, consequently, applying an evidence-based approach is not always easy. Higginson (1999) points out that an absence of evidence does not necessarily mean that a service or treatment is not effective, just that its efficacy has not been validated. More recently, there has been a focus of interest in the development of research in palliative and end-of-life care, including promoting earlier referrals and access to palliative care services based on the needs of patients (Hui et al. 2014).

Outcomes such as quality-of-life measures are extremely hard to determine, especially when patients are frail and ill. Thus, many studies exclude quality of life as an outcome variable or include only patients who can complete questionnaires. However, in order to promote greater use of clinical protocols, of best-practice guidelines within services and of guidance on the most effective models of care, more research evidence is undoubtedly needed.

Evidence suggests that patients and carers who have had an opportunity to discuss end-of-life care about 3 months before the patient's death:

- are significantly less likely to receive inappropriate aggressive medical treatment
- have significantly reduced levels of depression
- have significantly better adjustment after bereavement (Temel et al. 2010).

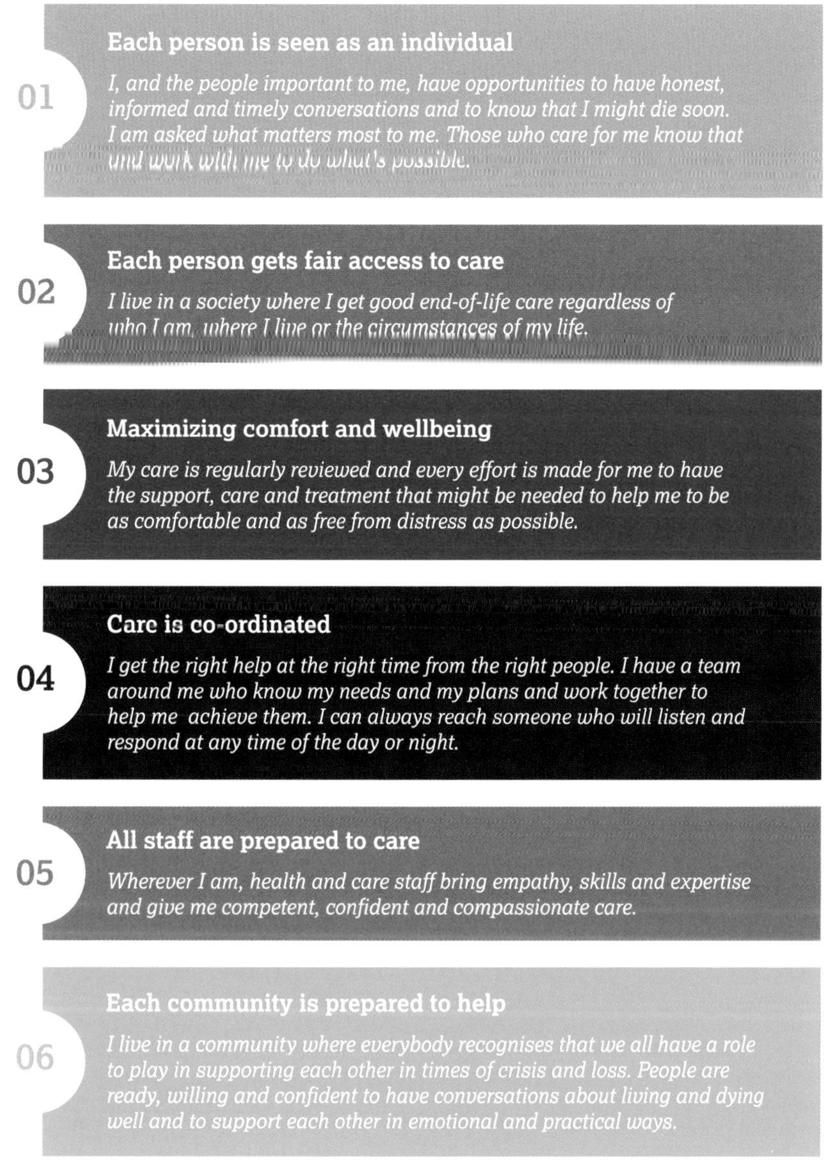
01
Each person is seen as an individual
I, and the people important to me, have opportunities to have honest, informed and timely conversations and to know that I might die soon. I am asked what matters most to me. Those who care for me know that and work with me to do what's possible.
02
Each person gets fair access to care
I live in a society where I get good end-of-life care regardless of who I am, where I live or the circumstances of my life.
03
Maximizing comfort and wellbeing
My care is regularly reviewed and every effort is made for me to have the support, care and treatment that might be needed to help me to be as comfortable and as free from distress as possible.
04
Care is co-ordinated
I get the right help at the right time from the right people. I have a team around me who know my needs and my plans and work together to help me achieve them. I can always reach someone who will listen and respond at any time of the day or night.
05
All staff are prepared to care
Wherever I am, health and care staff bring empathy, skills and expertise and give me competent, confident and compassionate care.
06
Each community is prepared to help
I live in a community where everybody recognises that we all have a role to play in supporting each other in times of crisis and loss. People are ready, willing and confident to have conversations about living and dying well and to support each other in emotional and practical ways.

Figure 11.1 Six ambitions of palliative and end-of-life care. *Source:* NEoLCP (2015).

Recognition of the dying phase

Care of a dying patient starts with the multiprofessional team recognizing and accepting that the terminal phase has begun. This has been cited as perhaps the single most important factor in enabling the achievement of all the elements associated with a 'good death' (Lacey 2015).

Early identification that a patient is dying is a key element in quality end-of-life care. A major challenge for all staff is knowing how and when to open up a discussion with individuals and their families about what they wish for as the patient nears the end of life. Nurses are ideally placed to identify the various clinical triggers. One tool that supports professionals in recognizing those patients who need supportive and palliative care is the Supportive and Palliative Care Indicators Tool (SPICT) (see www.spict.org.uk/the-spict). The SPICT™ is a guide to identifying people with one or more advanced illnesses, deteriorating health and a risk of dying (Highet et al. 2013).

It is important that healthcare professionals recognize that sometimes the individual and their family and carers may struggle to consider the future. Therefore, conversations and care should be guided and planned sensitively (NEoLCP 2015). This planned approach can lead to improved outcomes in terms of both patient care and best use of NHS resources. Early discussion enables the patient to have more control over their care and should result in the more frequent use of advance care planning (discussed further below) (NEoLCP 2015).

The National Palliative and End of Life Care Partnership (2015) has clarified the most important issues in facilitating and optimizing end-of-life care. These are:

- honest conversations
- clear expectations
- skilled assessment and symptom control
- shared records
- support for staff.

Recognizing dying can be challenging for health and social care professionals. There is often uncertainty about how long a person has left to live, and the signs that suggest that someone is dying are complex and often subtle (NICE 2015). Nursing care during this period does not simply represent a continuation of previously given care, or, necessarily, the complete cessation of all 'active treatment' measures. Assessment of the individual patient and their family will help to determine the appropriate next steps, which can vary greatly from person to person. It is important that family members and carers of people approaching the end of life are involved in the provision of care and decision making, and it is vital to recognize that they have their own needs (DH 2008, NEoLCP 2015).

Individualized preferences and wishes of patients

Treating patients as individuals with differing needs is pivotal to the delivery of optimum palliative and end of life care. Included in this is enabling patients to be cared for and to die in a place of their choice, which is a central tenet of the delivery of good-quality end-of-life care (DH 2008, NEoLCP 2015). Nurses play a key role in assessing the patient's complex needs relating to preferred place of care and death. Discussions must be sensitive and taken at the patient's pace. Ahearn et al. (2013) performed a retrospective study which revealed that the preferred place of death was not discussed with 92% of patients. It also revealed that if advance care planning had taken place, a number of the patients included in the study could have avoided a hospital admission and died in their normal place of residence. A number of barriers to achieving patients' individualized preferences and wishes have been recognized, such as lack of recognition of patients entering the last year of life and therefore limited advance care planning as well as issues surrounding communication (DH 2013, NHS England 2013).

National documentation, including the *End of Life Care Strategy* (DH 2008) and *Ambitions for Palliative and End of Life Care* (NEoLCP 2015), identified the need to improve co-ordination of care, recognizing that people at the end of life frequently receive care from many different organizations. The subsequent national development of locality registers (now known as 'electronic palliative care co-ordination systems') came about as a mechanism for enabling coordination between health and social care professionals involved in a patient's care. One such system, Co-ordinate My Care, has shown that in areas where these records are used, the successful achievement of preferred place of death has increased for those patients who have expressed a preference (Petrova et al. 2016). Consent to use these systems should be sought from patients who are being discharged for end-of-life care at home, in order to ensure that their wishes are effectively communicated and adhered to.

For individuals who wish to be discharged to their home or a care home, access to specialist palliative care and 24/7 advice and support is vital (NEoLCP 2015). Proactive working and a combination of services across many different settings and providers are crucial; prior to discharge, nurses should ensure that appropriate referrals are made to specialists within the team who will work in partnership with primary and community care services to facilitate the patient's safe discharge. The community nurses and/or hospice teams must be provided with all the necessary documentation and information relating to the patient's condition and discharge form or checklist (an example discharge checklist is shown in Figure 11.2). Anticipatory medications for pain, agitation, nausea and additional chest secretions should be planned, with the medications prescribed in advance.

> To ensure people receive the care they need, end of life care has to be considered as everybody's business and all paid carers and clinicians at every level of expertise need to be trained, supported and encouraged to bring a professional ethos to that care. They should know how to listen to people and to help them make decisions. (NEoLCP 2015, p.30)

For care home and home settings, it is essential that the GP is notified immediately of any patient who is being discharged for end-of-life care. This will enable them to make arrangements to review the patient as soon as possible; it is crucial that the GP reviews the person regularly and at least every 14 days, as this ensures that, when the patient dies, a Medical Certificate of Cause of Death (MCCD) can be appropriately issued without involving the coroner.

Advance care planning

Advance care planning is 'the process by which patients, together with their families and healthcare practitioners, consider their values and goals and articulate their preferences for future care' (Tulsky 2005, p.360). This planning allow adults (over the age of 18) to make a legal decision to refuse, in advance, a proposed treatment (or the continuation of a treatment) if at the relevant time the person lacks the capacity to consent to it. Comprehensive advance care planning can help to avoid inappropriate interventions and/or readmission to hospital. Guidance on decision making and mental capacity (NICE 2018) clearly highlights the importance of advance care planning at the beginning of a long-term or life-limiting condition to better support patients and co-ordinate their care.

An Advance Decision to Refuse Treatment (ADRT) can only be made by those who are deemed to have the mental capacity to do so, and it allows only for the refusal of treatments – it cannot enforce the provision of specified treatments (DH 2012). The Mental Capacity Act (2005) contains statutory guidance about ADRTs. If an ADRT complies with all the tests set out in the Mental Capacity Act, it is legally binding, so it must be respected as if the person who made the ADRT had capacity and refused the treatment at the time the treatment was required.

ADRTs must be made in writing, must be signed and witnessed, and must expressly state that the decision stands even if the person's life is at risk (DH 2012). They can be withdrawn verbally or in writing and are not considered valid if the person has conferred

The ROYAL MARSDEN
NHS Foundation Trust

Name: **Hospital No:**

**Patients Being Discharged Home for Complex/Urgent Palliative Care:
Checklist for Discharge**

This form should be used to assist with planning an urgent/complex discharge home for a patient with terminal care needs. It should be used in conjunction with the Discharge Policy.
Sign and date to confirm when arranged and equipment given. Document relevant information in the discharge planning section of the nursing documentation. Document if item or care is not applicable. Appoint a designated discharge lead:

Name: .... Designation: .... Contact No: ....

	Date and time	Signature and print name
Patient/Family Issues		
Meeting with patient/family to discuss plans for discharge.		
Continuing Healthcare funding discussed and information leaflet given.		
Level of care required has been discussed and agreed.		
Role of community services (district nurses and community palliative care team) has been discussed and consent obtained for referral if needed.		
Consent obtained if in area and Coordinate My Care record created or updated. Upload DNACPR form onto CMC record if this has been discussed with patient and there is a DNACPR form on EPR.		
Continuing Healthcare application/Fast Track form commenced by Discharge Team and completed by MDT. Fast Track form can be found on the intranet under Discharge support/NHS continuing healthcare and can be accessed on T-drive under each ward/Dept. Contact Discharge team when complete for form to be sent to relevant CCG.		
Communication with District Nurse		
Referral made to District Nurses using the Community Services Referral Form		
Equipment has been requested (delete as appropriate): - Electric, profiling hospital bed - Pressure relieving mattress - Pressure relieving seat cushion - Commode/urinal/bed pan - Hoist/sling/sliding sheets - Other		
Communication with Community Palliative Care Team		
Referral made to Community Palliative Care Team		
Communication with GP and Community Palliative Care Medical Team: Medical Responsibilities (hospital medical team to organise; the nurse to confirm when arranged)		
Registrar to discuss patient's condition with GP and request home visit for as soon as possible after discharge.		
Oxygen: HOOF and IHORM (Consent) forms to be completed by the medical team and faxed to relevant company. Please access website below for a list of the oxygen companies and their geographical area. https://www.pcc-cic.org.uk/article/home-oxygen-order-form.		
Registrar or Specialist Nurse to discuss with the Community Palliative Care team the patient's needs and proposed plan of care.		

Figure 11.2 Palliative care discharge checklist. *Source:* Reproduced with permission of The Royal Marsden NHS Foundation Trust.

The ROYAL MARSDEN
NHS Foundation Trust

	Date and time	Signature and print name
Adequate supply of drugs prescribed for discharge (TTOs) including crisis drugs e.g. s/c morphine, midazolam.		
Authorisation for drugs to be administered by community nurses. Please refer to Subcutaneous Drugs policy and complete the discharge checklist for the McKinley T34 syringe pump.		
'Ambulance transfer of palliative care patients' document completed for Ambulance Crew.		

Equipment		
Has confirmation been received from a family member or the community equipment service provider that the equipment has been delivered to the discharge address?		
Provide an adequate supply of:		
- dressings		
- water/sodium chloride for injection (if going home with end-of-life care medications for subcutaneous use)		
- sharps bin		
- continence aids		
- supply of needles and syringes		
Transport (confirm by ticking appropriate boxes)	**CHECK OTHER DISCHARGE DOCUMENTATION**	
Escort (family/nurse).		
Discussed with family that if the patient dies during the journey, the ambulance crew will not attempt resuscitation. Discharge destination in this event has been agreed.		
Written Information and Documentation		
A discharge summary will need to be completed prior to discharge. The discharge letter must be printed and given to a pharmacist to check the medication list is complete and accurate. Medical summary given to patient or relative.		
Medical discharge summary sent to GP, Community Palliative Care Team and District Nursing Team.		
Prescription sheet of authorisation for drugs to be administered by community nurses. Faxed to District Nurse, GP and Community Palliative Care Team.		
Copies of HOOF and IHORM faxed to GP for information only.		
Patient/carer given list of contact numbers of community services **(including night service): Discharge information sheet.**		
Medication list, stating reasons for drugs, given and explained to patient/relative.		
All documentation sent to community services is scanned onto EPR and filed in patient's medical records.		

Signature/print name of designated ward-based discharge lead: ....
Date/time ....

File this form in the patient's records on discharge.

Figure 11.2 *Continued*

lasting power of attorney on another person. Equally, they can be invalidated if the person has done anything that is clearly inconsistent with the original ADRT, for example if there has been any change in their religious faith.

Organ donation

Organ donation is an important consideration at the end of life. From spring 2020, the law changed from an 'opt-in' system (where individuals are required to register as potential donors) to an 'opt-out' system. This means that everybody can be considered a potential donor unless they have added their details to the NHS Organ Donor Register to say that they do not wish to donate their organs, or unless they are in one of the excluded groups (NHS Blood and Transplant 2019). However, this new law recognizes that the dying person's wishes regarding organ, tissue and body donation should be taken into consideration, and consultation with the patient and/or their family should be sought. There are some restrictions on the organs that some people can donate, such as patients with cancer; however, this does not mean that they cannot donate anything. Some might be able to donate parts of the eyes (the cornea), and other tissue can be considered; this should be discussed with local transplant services.

Patients who wish to donate and are able to do so may require specific preparation before and after death. Specialist advice and guidance should be sought from the local organ transplant specialist nurses or service by contacting NHS Blood and Transplant directly (www.organdonation.nhs.uk).

Needs of carers

It is possible for carers to become tired or ill, and informal carers may need particular support to understand the complexity of looking after dying patients (NEoLCP 2015). Often, discussions relating to the patient's preferences and wishes are extremely sensitive and need to be facilitated by an objective outsider who is able to voice the fears and concerns of all those involved. Identifying the needs of carers is an important aspect of nursing care, and one tool that can be helpful is the Carer Support Needs Assessment Tool (CSNAT) (Ewing et al. [illegible]). The CSNAT is an evidence-based tool that facilitates tailored support for family members and friends (carers) of adults with life-limiting condition. It comprises 14 domains (broad topic areas) in which carers commonly say they require support. Carers may use this tool to indicate further support they need in relation to enabling them to care for someone at home, as well as support for their own health and wellbeing within their caregiving role. The use of the CSNAT requires training and a licence.

Clinical governance

Marriages at the end of life

Patients whose illnesses are terminal often reflect on the meaning of their lives (Stanley and Hurst 2011). This can often involve deepening connections with loved ones, planning financially and completing personal goals (Arthur et al. 2012, Seaman et al. 2014). On occasion, critically or terminally ill patients may request support in arranging a marriage or civil partnership. For those patients who are deemed too ill to move to a venue licensed for marriage (such as a registry office), the ceremony can take place at the bedside in an establishment where they are being cared for, such as a hospital or hospice.

Where people wish to marry in hospital, a Registrar General's Licence must be obtained in order for the marriage to be performed. The intended spouse or partner of the patient must give notice of the marriage or civil partnership personally to the superintendent registrar at the local Registry Office. In all circumstances, the registrar will require a letter signed by the registered medical practitioner stating that the patient is too ill to be moved and is not expected to recover. The letter should also confirm that the patient has capacity and understands the nature and purpose of the marriage or civil partnership ceremony. The registrar will also need a letter giving permission for the marriage or civil partnership to take place on hospital grounds. Most hospitals will have existing templates that they use for such occasions. There is no fixed waiting period for a Registrar General's Licence. Once the licence has been granted, the ceremony may take place at any hour of the day or night, within a month of the notice being taken (Marriage (Registrar General's Licence) Act 1970).

From a legal perspective, the following are necessary for a marriage or civil partnership to go ahead:

- proof of name (e.g. valid passport)
- proof of age (e.g. birth certificate)
- proof of nationality (e.g. valid passport or national identity card)
- proof of address (e.g. valid driving licence or recent utility bill)
- decree absolute or final order (if applicable)
- death certificate of the former partner (if applicable)
- entry visa (if applicable)
- details of where and when the individuals intend to get married.

Last will and testament

A patient may wish to make a will in hospital, and some patients will not be able to complete this process independently. Healthcare staff must ensure that a doctor has reviewed the patient to assess that they have capacity to make decisions (Mental Capacity Act 2005) and ensure this is recorded in the patient's medical notes.

Where possible, wills should be drawn up professionally and patients should be encouraged to seek the assistance of a solicitor, particularly if there are complex property or financial matters. Nurses may be approached to witness a will; the Royal College of Nursing (2019a) states that although there is nothing in law preventing a nurse from witnessing a will, it is not advisable for nurses to sign legal documents as this could lead to involvement in legal cases should there be a later dispute. This advice is endorsed by the Nursing and Midwifery Council, which reminds nurses of the importance of maintaining clear professional boundaries and being impartial at all times (NMC 2018). All healthcare professionals should consult their hospital's local policy relating to the signing of last wills or any other legal documents.

Euthanasia and assisted suicide

Euthanasia is the act of deliberately, by act or omission, ending a person's life to relieve suffering. Assisted suicide is the act of deliberately assisting or encouraging another person to die by suicide (or attempt to do so). If the relative of a person with a terminal illness were to obtain powerful sedatives knowing that the person intended to take an overdose of sedatives to kill themselves, the relative would be assisting suicide (DH 2013).

Both euthanasia and assisted suicide are illegal in the UK (Suicide Act 1961), and euthanasia carries a maximum penalty of life imprisonment. There are campaigns ongoing to change the law, and since 2003 there have been over 10 attempts to legalize assisted suicide (Care n.d.). Nurses must not participate in either process. However, they should be aware that those patients who approach healthcare professionals with a request for assisted suicide or euthanasia will be doing so from a position of significant vulnerability and must be treated with respect, care and compassion. Commonly, these requests stem from a fear of pain, indignity and dependence, and it is imperative to ensure that patients are offered adequate opportunities to express these fears (Dowler 2011) and that they are reassured as much as possible. Nurses have a duty of care to ensure that patients' concerns are communicated to the multidisciplinary team in order that the appropriate specialist physical, psychosocial and spiritual support is offered to minimize their distress.

Artificial hydration

In the last few days to weeks of life, anorexia, weight loss and swallowing difficulties are common (Lacey 2015). Reduced oral intake can be hard for the family to accept and it is not uncommon for them to request artificial hydration and/or feeding via enteral or parenteral routes. It is always important to discuss the risks versus benefits of these measures with the patient and their family (Lacey 2015). Signs of dehydration should be assessed regularly (at least 12-hourly) and regular mouth care should be offered to keep the patient's mouth and lips moist. People who do want to drink should be given help to carry on drinking if they can still swallow safely; assessment of their ability to swallow should be performed regularly as difficulties in swallowing and dysphasia can occur towards the end of life (Lacey 2015).

For some patients it may be necessary to consider artificial hydration. The decision around hydration needs to be in line with discussions regarding ceilings of care and potential benefits and risks addressed with the patient and family (Lanz et al. 2019). There is some evidence to suggest that dehydration can cause patients to experience increased symptoms, such as confusion and restlessness in patients who are not in the final stages of life; however, these are issues that can also be experienced by patients who are dying (Fritzson et al. 2013). Providing artificial hydration at the end of life may have no benefit for symptoms; one study recognized that there was no difference in hydration after 7 days between patients with advanced cancer who were given 1 L per day versus 100 mL per day (Bruera et al. 2013). Risks of overhydration include increasing shortness of breath and fluid retention. This study also suggests that patients who receive more than 1 L of fluid in 24 hours may have increased bronchial secretions in the last 48 hours of life compared to patients who receive less artificial hydration. It is important to view the evidence on this subject with a critical eye, being careful to interpret any findings. Currently, there is insufficient high-quality evidence to say categorically that in the palliative care setting fluids improve symptomatology (Lanz et al. 2019); however, it is of paramount importance to ensure individualized care of the patient and support for their family, and to engage in conversations regarding the use of fluids.

The preferred route for the administration of fluids in patients at the end of life is often subcutaneously; in this way, 1.0–1.5 L of normal saline can be delivered over 24 hours (Dalal et al. 2009). The use of permanent access devices that are already in place may be suitable for the delivery of fluid intravenously. Absorption has been found to be as effective when fluid is delivered subcutaneously as when it is delivered intravenously (Vidal et al. 2016).

Pre-procedural considerations

Communication

Excellent communication is vital in all areas of nursing practice but arguably more so when dealing with dying patients and their relatives. If patients and their family and carers are to make educated end-of-life decisions, they need to have nurses who can engage with them and have open, honest and unambiguous dialogue (Wilson 2015). Nurses must have the confidence to raise the issue of planning for future care and death, and they must also be able to respond to issues and concerns raised by the patient and/or their family and carers (Henry and Wilson 2012).

Do Not Attempt Cardiopulmonary Resuscitation

Do Not Attempt Cardiopulmonary Resuscitation (DNaCPR) discussions with patients and their families have been subjected to intense ethical and legal debate in recent years (Hall et al. 2018). In October 2014, the Resuscitation Council, the British Medical Association and the Royal College of Nursing reviewed their guidance for doctors making decisions about DNaCPR orders (BMA, RC & RCN 2016, Etheridge and Gatland 2015). This revised guidance followed the Court of Appeal decision in 2014 in the case of *Traccy v Cambridge University Hospitals* – a case that resulted in two important amendments to resuscitation guidelines. The first change relates to the fact that patient distress is no longer a good enough reason not to discuss DNaCPR with patients unless it is deemed likely to cause the patient physical or psychological harm. The second change is that even if doctors feel resuscitation would be futile, a discussion should still occur; futility is not seen as an argument for not discussing DNaCPR (Etheridge and Gatland 2015).

Timing of discussions should be individualized, although discussions earlier in the illness are often preferable, in line with other discussions relating to advance care planning. Discussions held in the acute setting are suboptimal. DNaCPR decisions should be part of a wider discussion about future care and adequate communication skills training is important (Mockford et al. 2015).

The Resuscitation Council endorses the ReSPECT document (https://www.respectprocess.org.uk) (Figure 11.3). ReSPECT is a process that creates personalized recommendations for clinical care in a future emergency in which individuals are unable to make or express choices. It provides health and social care professionals responding to that emergency with a summary of recommendations to help them make immediate decisions about the person's care and treatment. ReSPECT can be complementary to a wider process of advance care planning. The plan is created through conversations between a person and their health professionals. The plan is recorded on a form and includes the person's own priorities for care and agreed clinical recommendations about care and treatment that could help to:

- achieve the outcome that they would want
- avoid outcomes that would not help them
- avoid outcomes that they would not want.

ReSPECT can be used for anyone, but it has particular relevance for people who have complex health needs, people who are likely to be nearing the end of their lives, and people who are at risk of sudden deterioration or cardiac arrest.

Prognosis

There are tools available to guide clinicians in making prognoses in palliative care. Prognostat is one such tool and is available online (Glare et al. 2015). The clinical act of prognostication in advanced cancer is often based on two approaches. The first involves clinical prediction of survival by an appropriate clinician. The second approach, referred to as 'actuarial prognostication' relies on statistical data such as median survival rates (Glare et al. 2015). Clinicians must be able to communicate the prognosis to the patient in a meaningful way and at the pace of the patient.

The principles of breaking potentially bad news should be adhered to in undertaking discussions about prognosis.

Breaking potentially bad news

Bad news may be defined as 'any information which adversely and seriously affects an individual's view of his or her future' (Buckman 1992, p.15). Bad news is always, however, in the eye of the beholder, because the impact of the news cannot be estimated until the recipient's expectations or understanding have been determined. There is some evidence to suggest that inappropriate delivery of potentially bad news can heighten a patient's anxiety and distress. It has also been found to impact their perception of their condition and adversely affect their relationship with the healthcare team (Baile and Parker 2017). Additionally, when professionals are uncomfortable about these difficult conversations, they may avoid discussing distressing information, such as a poor prognosis, or convey unwarranted optimism to the patient (Maguire 1985).

There are some key points in a patient's disease trajectory when breaking potentially bad news may be necessary. Baile and Parker (2017) give the following examples:

- confirming the diagnosis of a disease
- giving a prognosis for an illness
- prescribing treatments
- confirming disease recurrence or relapse
- communicating unexpected side-effects
- letting the patient know they are not responding to treatment
- discussing end of possible treatment/DNaCPR

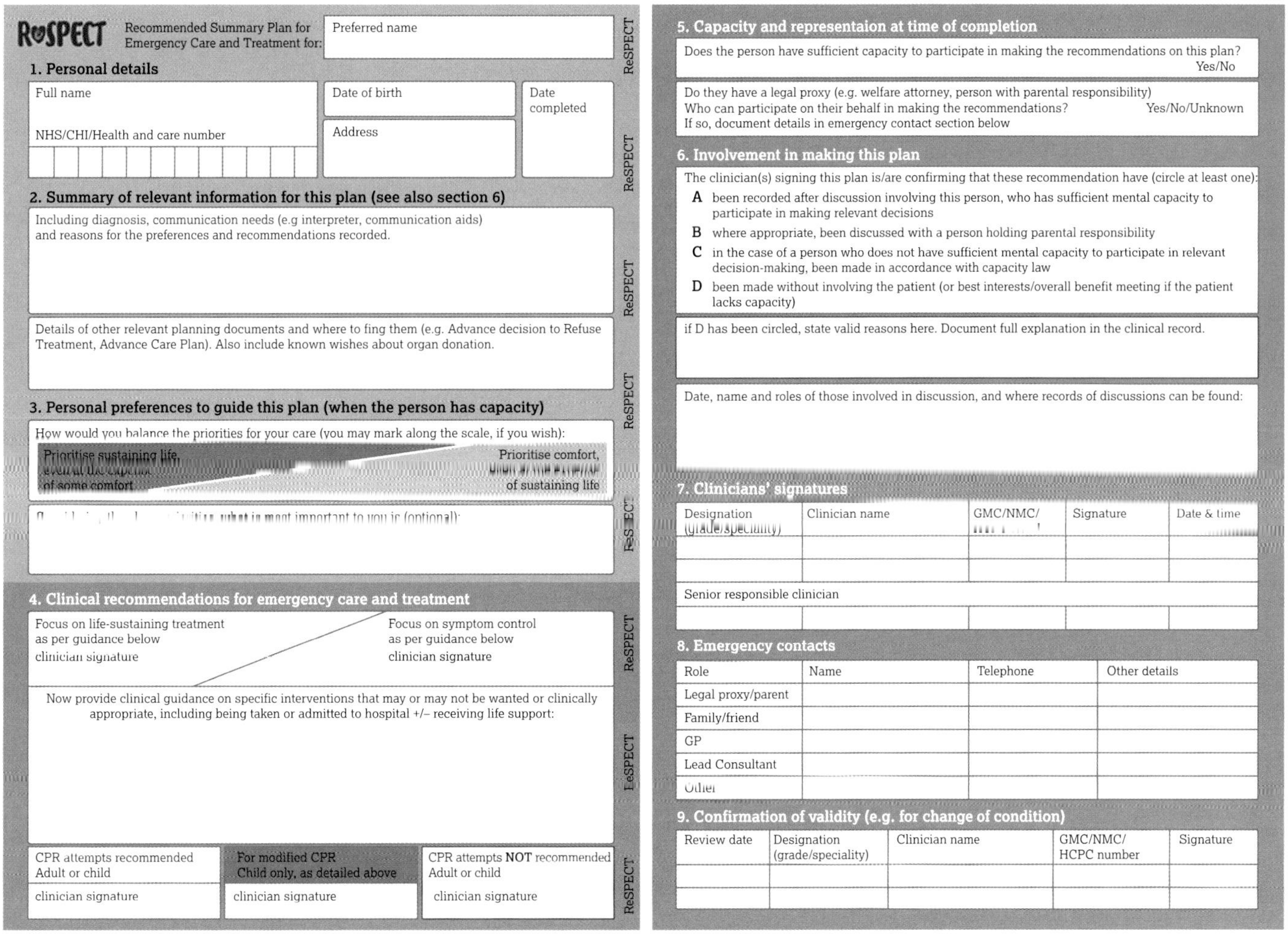
ReSPECT Recommended Summary Plan for Emergency Care and Treatment for: Preferred name

1. Personal details

Full name | Date of birth | Date completed

NHS/CHI/Health and care number | Address

2. Summary of relevant information for this plan (see also section 6)

Including diagnosis, communication needs (e.g interpreter, communication aids) and reasons for the preferences and recommendations recorded.

Details of other relevant planning documents and where to fing them (e.g. Advance decision to Refuse Treatment, Advance Care Plan). Also include known wishes about organ donation.

3. Personal preferences to guide this plan (when the person has capacity)

How would you balance the priorities for your care (you may mark along the scale, if you wish):

Prioritise sustaining life, even at the expense of some comfort | Prioritise comfort, even at the expense of sustaining life

Considering the above priorities, what is most important to you is (optional):

4. Clinical recommendations for emergency care and treatment

Focus on life-sustaining treatment as per guidance below clinician signature | Focus on symptom control as per guidance below clinician signature

Now provide clinical guidance on specific interventions that may or may not be wanted or clinically appropriate, including being taken or admitted to hospital +/– receiving life support:

CPR attempts recommended Adult or child	For modified CPR Child only, as detailed above	CPR attempts NOT recommended Adult or child
clinician signature	clinician signature	clinician signature

5. Capacity and representaion at time of completion

Does the person have sufficient capacity to participate in making the recommendations on this plan? Yes/No

Do they have a legal proxy (e.g. welfare attorney, person with parental responsibility) Who can participate on their behalf in making the recommendations? Yes/No/Unknown
If so, document details in emergency contact section below

6. Involvement in making this plan

The clinician(s) signing this plan is/are confirming that these recommendation have (circle at least one):

A been recorded after discussion involving this person, who has sufficient mental capacity to participate in making relevant decisions
B where appropriate, been discussed with a person holding parental responsibility
C in the case of a person who does not have sufficient mental capacity to participate in relevant decision-making, been made in accordance with capacity law
D been made without involving the patient (or best interests/overall benefit meeting if the patient lacks capacity)

if D has been circled, state valid reasons here. Document full explanation in the clinical record.

Date, name and roles of those involved in discussion, and where records of discussions can be found:

7. Clinicians' signatures

Designation (grade/speciality)	Clinician name	GMC/NMC/HCPC no.	Signature	Date & time
Senior responsible clinician				

8. Emergency contacts

Role	Name	Telephone	Other details
Legal proxy/parent			
Family/friend			
GP			
Lead Consultant			
Other			

9. Confirmation of validity (e.g. for change of condition)

Review date	Designation (grade/speciality)	Clinician name	GMC/NMC/ HCPC number	Signature

Figure 11.3 Recommended summary plan for emergency care and treatment. Source: Reproduced from Resuscitation Council (2015) with permission of ReSPECT.

- discussing ceilings of care and/or discontinuation of treatments/ support
- sudden or unexpected death
- genetic test results.

A strategy listed as a mnemonic (SPIKES) has been developed (Baile et al. 2000) to help support clinicians with breaking bad news. The idea is to split the conversation up into sections. The principles are shown in Box 11.2. Communication at the end of life needs to be honest, direct and delivered in a compassionate way. The concerns of the family also need to be heard and acknowledged, and the likely course of the patient's illness should be explained (Lacey 2015).

Principles of care

The importance of individually tailored care for those in the terminal phase of their lives, and their relatives, cannot be overemphasized. No framework, pathway or care plan is a substitute for careful assessment, information giving, listening, referral and skilled intervention. Each person will require slightly different care in one way or another, and assumptions should never be made solely on the basis of previous preferences, or sociocultural or religious stereotypes.

However, some principles and interventions are important and should be routinely considered. These are outlined in Figure 11.4, which provides an algorithm for the principles of care for dying patients. These principles should reflect the ethos of palliative care and integrate the physical, psychological, social and spiritual aspects of care (Watts 2013). In addition, Figure 11.5 provides a sample care plan that can act as a supportive document or framework. Both examples were developed by the London Cancer Alliance (2013) and can be customized and used in the hospital setting or modified for other areas. Both prompt clinical teams to remember to address the personalized needs of the patient and their family.

Symptoms at the end of life

In the final stages of life, the focus is on optimizing symptom control and relieving distress. Common symptoms experienced at the end of life include pain, dyspnoea, nausea and vomiting, and sometimes an increase in respiratory secretions (leading to the 'death rattle'). Bowel obstruction and ascites are also distressing symptoms that may need management. Delirium may be apparent with some patients and can be distressing for both the patient and their family. Appropriate treatment regimens should be in place to manage these symptoms. Some of these are discussed below.

It is important to remember that as a patient begins to die, swallowing may become increasingly difficult. Therefore, the route of medication administration may need to be altered (Lacey 2015).

Pharmacological support

Pharmacological support can be used in various ways to improve the quality of life of patients with severe, life-limiting illness. Depending on a person's position on the disease trajectory and their goals of care, drugs, including chemotherapy, may be prescribed to actively treat the disease; prevent, reduce or eliminate symptoms; or slow the disease process. Antibiotics may also still have a place in the terminal phase – for example, a patient may choose to have antibiotics to

Box 11.2 The SPIKES strategy for breaking significant news

S	**Setting up**	• Arrange for privacy. • Involve significant others, sit down, make connection and establish rapport with the patient. • Manage time constraints and interruptions.	What time would suit you and your family members for a chat about your diagnosis?
P	**Perception of condition/ seriousness**	• Determine what the patient knows about the medical condition. • Listen to the patient's level of comprehension; accept any denial but do not confront it at this stage.	Explain to me what you understand of your recent diagnosis.
I	**Invitation from the patient to give information**	• Ask the patient if they wish to know the details of the medical condition. Accept the patient's right not to know. • Offer to answer questions later if the patient wishes.	Would you like me to explain exactly what your diagnosis means?
K	**Knowledge: giving medical facts**	• Use language intelligible to the patient (consider educational level, socioeconomic background and current emotional state). • Give information in small chunks. • Check whether the patient understands what you have said. Respond to the patient's reactions as they occur.	When we examined your chest X-ray, we saw a small visible mass. This is usually an indication of cancer. Is this all making sense to you?
E	**Explore emotions and sympathize**	• Prepare to give an empathetic response. • Identify emotion expressed by the patient. • Identify the cause or source of the emotion, and give the patient time to express their feelings.	Has your diagnosis come as a shock to you? Explain to me how you are feeling.
S	**Strategy and summary**	• Close the interview. • Ask whether the patient wants to clarify anything else. • Offer an agenda for the next meeting.	Has this all made sense to you? Have you got any more questions? When do you wish to arrange our next meeting?

Source: Adapted from Baile et al. (2000).

treat a symptomatic urinary tract infection but may decline to have antibiotics to treat a recurring episode of severe pneumonia.

Various medications and combinations of medications are used for the control of symptoms during end-of-life care. These are discussed in more detail in each individual section below and a summary of recommended medications is outlined in Table 11.1.

Choice of medication for pain should be guided by current and previously tried analgesics, adjuncts and techniques. Further information is detailed in Chapter 10: Pain assessment and management.

Currow et al. (2013) report that 20% of people take at least eight medications at the time of referral to a specialist palliative service, adding that many people admitted to palliative care services have an increase in prescribed medications as death approaches. They point out that frail and vulnerable patients have diminished capacity for withstanding adverse drug reactions, which increases the risk of iatrogenic harm. There is, therefore, a greater responsibility on those prescribing medication to palliative patients to optimize all medications, balancing benefit and risk, monitoring and adjusting for each individual in the context of a changing clinical picture (Currow et al. 2013). Cessation of long-term medications often occurs as a result of suspected adverse drug reaction or loss of the oral route of administration. However, cessation of long-term medications without careful discussion with patients or their families carries the potential for both physiological and psychological harm (Lacey 2015). It can be extremely difficult for patients or families who for a lifetime have monitored blood glucose levels to suddenly let go of this practice.

However, in the terminal phase of the patient's life, all medications will be reviewed. At this time only essential medications should be administered, and this should be done through the least invasive route possible (Lacey 2015). As a person enters the terminal phase, there may also be changes to their renal function. Careful monitoring and adjustment of medications is required – for example, there may be signs of opioid toxicity and an alternative renal-sparing opioid may be considered.

Continuous syringe pump

Continuous (24-hour) subcutaneous infusions include a portable battery-operated syringe pump to administer medications to the patient (Figure 11.6). While this chapter refers to end-of-life care, it is important to note that starting a subcutaneous syringe pump is not a sign of impending death. There are other occasions when the oral route for a patient may be impaired, and the continuous subcutaneous route of drug administration can offer temporary relief to patients; these are outlined in Box 11.3. The subcutaneous route is advantageous over the intravenous route in this setting as it negates the need for a painful cannula and the risks associated with this, or the need for an IV-competent nurse.

Advantages of a 24-hour subcutaneous infusion include the following:

- acceptability and reliability
- reduced need for injections
- maintenance of a person's mobility
- constant therapeutic drug levels over a 24-hour period
- only needs to be refilled every 24 hours.

Disadvantages include the following:

- potential source of infection
- skin site reactions
- in emaciated people or those on long-term infusions, skin site availability may become an issue
- need for daily visit in the community.

It is essential to regularly check the 24-hour pump and assess the effectiveness of the drugs being administered to ensure adequate function and symptom control. Figure 11.7 gives an example of an assessment chart.

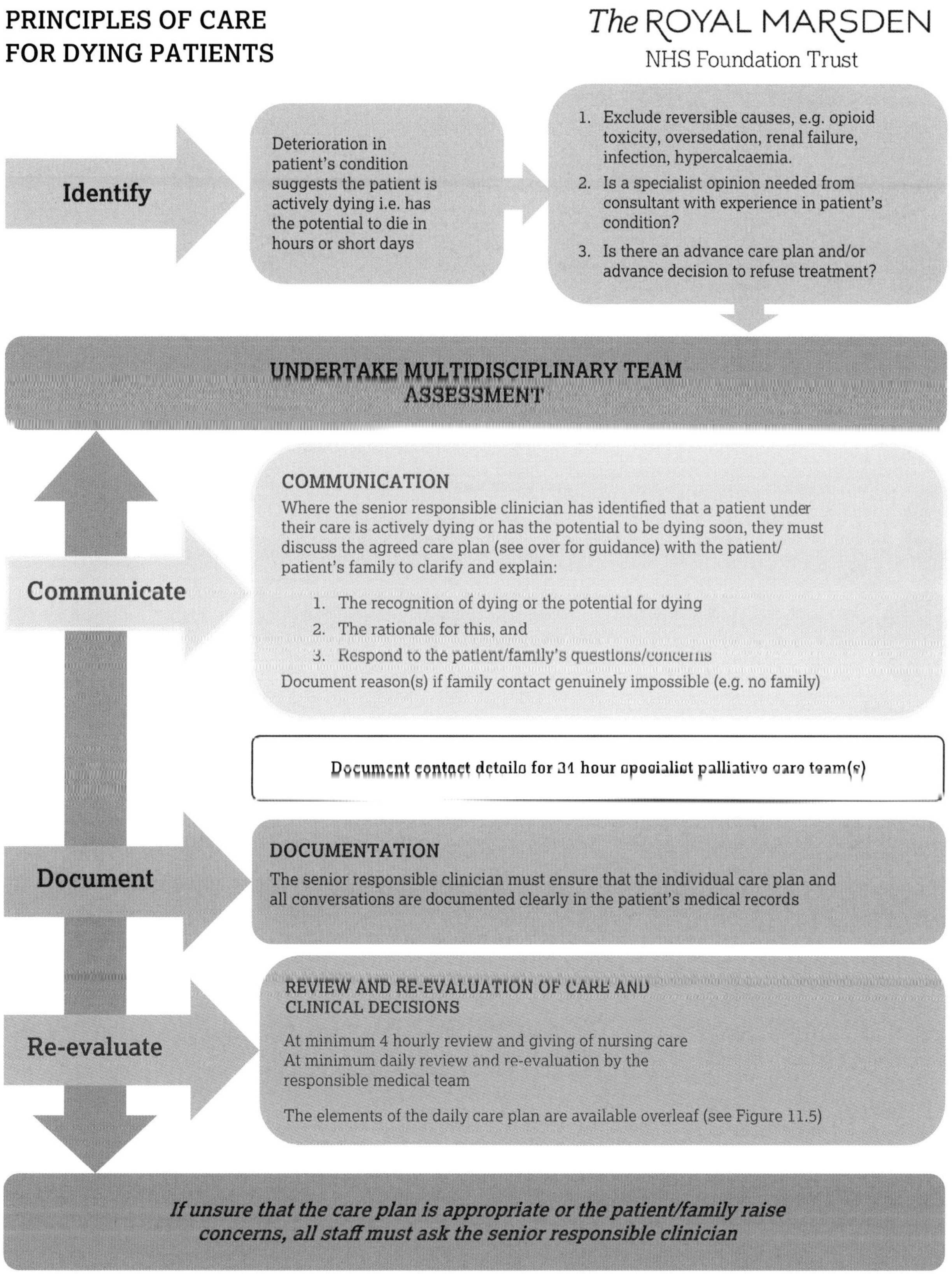
PRINCIPLES OF CARE
FOR DYING PATIENTS
The ROYAL MARSDEN
NHS Foundation Trust
Identify
Deterioration in patient's condition suggests the patient is actively dying i.e. has the potential to die in hours or short days
1. Exclude reversible causes, e.g. opioid toxicity, oversedation, renal failure, infection, hypercalcaemia.
2. Is a specialist opinion needed from consultant with experience in patient's condition?
3. Is there an advance care plan and/or advance decision to refuse treatment?
UNDERTAKE MULTIDISCIPLINARY TEAM ASSESSMENT
Communicate
COMMUNICATION
Where the senior responsible clinician has identified that a patient under their care is actively dying or has the potential to be dying soon, they must discuss the agreed care plan (see over for guidance) with the patient/ patient's family to clarify and explain:
1. The recognition of dying or the potential for dying
2. The rationale for this, and
3. Respond to the patient/family's questions/concerns
Document reason(s) if family contact genuinely impossible (e.g. no family)
Document contact details for 24 hour specialist palliative care team(s)
Document
DOCUMENTATION
The senior responsible clinician must ensure that the individual care plan and all conversations are documented clearly in the patient's medical records
Re-evaluate
REVIEW AND RE-EVALUATION OF CARE AND CLINICAL DECISIONS
At minimum 4 hourly review and giving of nursing care
At minimum daily review and re-evaluation by the responsible medical team
The elements of the daily care plan are available overleaf (see Figure 11.5)
If unsure that the care plan is appropriate or the patient/family raise concerns, all staff must ask the senior responsible clinician

Figure 11.4 Royal Marsden NHS Foundation Trust principles of care for dying patients. *Source*: Adapted from LCA (2013).

Symptoms most commonly controlled with a syringe pump include:

- pain
- agitation
- respiratory secretions
- nausea and vomiting
- convulsions.

A variety of medications can be administered via a syringe pump, but the exact medications to use should be checked with local

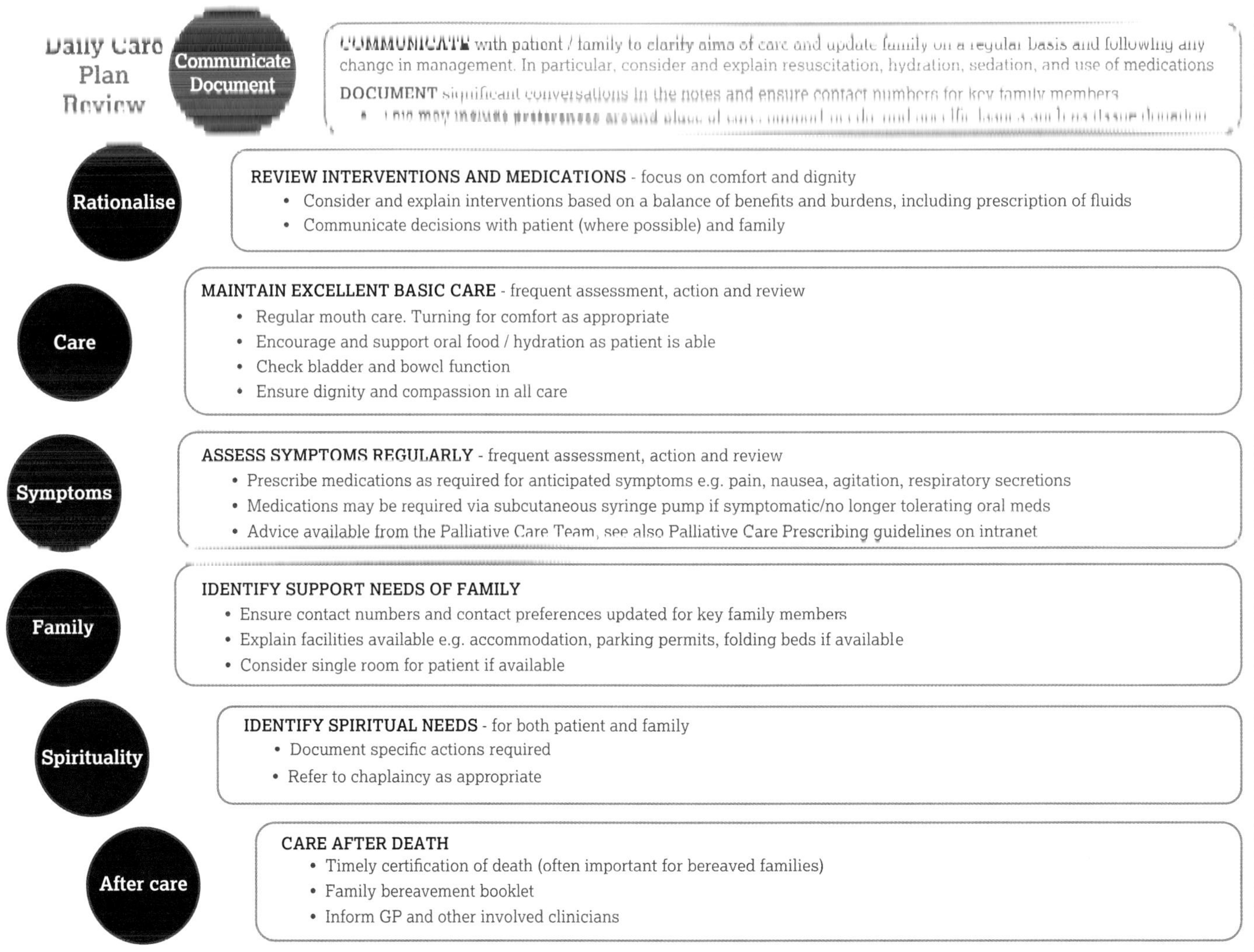

Daily Care Plan Review
Communicate Document
COMMUNICATE with patient / family to clarify aims of care and update family on a regular basis and following any change in management. In particular, consider and explain resuscitation, hydration, sedation, and use of medications
DOCUMENT significant conversations in the notes and ensure contact numbers for key family members
Rationalise
REVIEW INTERVENTIONS AND MEDICATIONS - focus on comfort and dignity
• Consider and explain interventions based on a balance of benefits and burdens, including prescription of fluids
• Communicate decisions with patient (where possible) and family
Care
MAINTAIN EXCELLENT BASIC CARE - frequent assessment, action and review
• Regular mouth care. Turning for comfort as appropriate
• Encourage and support oral food / hydration as patient is able
• Check bladder and bowel function
• Ensure dignity and compassion in all care
Symptoms
ASSESS SYMPTOMS REGULARLY - frequent assessment, action and review
• Prescribe medications as required for anticipated symptoms e.g. pain, nausea, agitation, respiratory secretions
• Medications may be required via subcutaneous syringe pump if symptomatic/no longer tolerating oral meds
• Advice available from the Palliative Care Team, see also Palliative Care Prescribing guidelines on intranet
Family
IDENTIFY SUPPORT NEEDS OF FAMILY
• Ensure contact numbers and contact preferences updated for key family members
• Explain facilities available e.g. accommodation, parking permits, folding beds if available
• Consider single room for patient if available
Spirituality
IDENTIFY SPIRITUAL NEEDS - for both patient and family
• Document specific actions required
• Refer to chaplaincy as appropriate
After care
CARE AFTER DEATH
• Timely certification of death (often important for bereaved families)
• Family bereavement booklet
• Inform GP and other involved clinicians

Figure 11.5 Daily care plan review for patients at the end of life. *Source:* Adapted from LCA (2013).

Table 11.1 Recommendations for the pharmacological management of patients who are actively dying

Symptom	Medication
Pain	Morphine or other opioid
Breathlessness	Morphine or other opioid
Breathlessness with anxiety	Lorazepam
Refractory breathlessness	Midazolam
Nausea	Haloperidol (centrally acting) Levomepromazine Cyclizine
	Prokinetics can be used in the short term if required; however, they should be avoided if the patient has a bowel obstruction with associated cramps (EMA 2013)
Gastrointestinal obstruction	Hyoscine butylbromide Octreotide
Terminal restlessness	See Procedure guideline 11.4 Terminal sedation
Audible respiratory secretions	Glycopyrronium

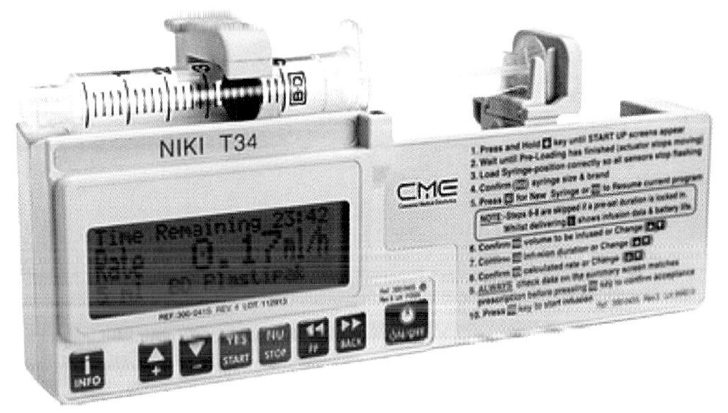

Figure 11.6 Example of a continuous syringe pump: the McKinley T34 Syringe Pump. *Source:* Reproduced with permission of BDB.

Box 11.3 Rationales for changing the administration route of medications from oral to subcutaneous

- Patient no longer able to swallow
- Poor absorption (e.g. bowel obstruction)
- Nausea and vomiting
- Tablet burden for the patient
- Uncontrolled symptoms via the oral route

The ROYAL MARSDEN
NHS Foundation Trust

SUBCUTANEOUS SYRINGE PUMP CHART FOR USE IN THE HOSPITAL

SURNAME:	HOSPITAL NO: NHS NO:
FORENAMES:	D.O.B:
WARD:	CONSULTANT:

THIS IS NOT A PRESCRIPTION – refer to the patient's prescription chart.

For advice regarding combinations of dilution of drugs see the last page of this chart, *The Syringe Driver* (3rd Edn) (2011) by Andrew Dickman and Jennifer Schneider or www.pallcare.info

If a patient has TWO syringe pumps, use a separate box/page for each syringe pump.

REFER TO RM POLICY: Subcutaneous Drugs: The Safe Administration for Adults and Children and the Use of the McKinley T34 and Alaris GH Plus Syringe Pumps

IMPORTANT: *Please make sure you know which* ***pump*** *is being used*

McKinley T34 Syringe Pump

Infuses drugs at a rate of mL/hr.
Syringe pump set and locked to infuse over 24 hours ONLY.
Use with 20, 30 or 50 ml **BD Plastipak Luer Lock syringes ONLY.**
When load/reload syringe do not use previous settings – **set NEW PROGRAMME for each syringe**
i.e. Press YES to resume **Press NO for new programme.**
The syringe pump registers the syringe size and the content and works out the appropriate rate.
Draw volume according to the syringe size:

20 mL syringe **must** be drawn up to **17 mL** – approximate rate would be 0.71 mL per 24 hours
30 mL syringe **must** be drawn up to **22 mL** – approximate rate would be 0.92 mL per 24 hours
50 mL syringe **must** be drawn up to **32 mL** – approximate rate would be 1.33 mL per 24 hours

Alaris GH plus Syringe Pump

Infuses drugs at a rate of **mL/hr.**
Draw volume up to **48 mL** and **set rate to 2 mL/hour** to infuse over 24 hours.
Use 50 mL **Luer Lock** syringes ONLY.

PROBLEMS	ACTIONS
1. Won't start: pump alarming	See alarm message to identify specific problem. For McKinley T34 pump – 'pump unattended' – left in STOP programme mode for 2 minutes without a key press – check programme settings and press start.
2. Light stops flashing	See alarm message to identify specific problem.
3. Infusion too fast	Check rate setting and calculation.
4. Infusion too slow or stopped	Check tube for kinking/blockage/trapped. Check syringe/tubing is still connected. Check that syringe plunger clamp is correctly positioned. Check clamp released.
5. Some medications occasionally crystallize, e.g. cyclizine	Change syringe and extension set and re-site. Consider diluting in a large volume of diluent. Consider change of drug.
6. Inflammation of needle site	Irritation or infection – re-site. Treat local infection. Inappropriate drugs given – review drugs/dilution.

Figure 11.7 Example of a subcutaneous infusion chart. *Source:* The Royal Marsden.

NAME:

HOSPITAL NO:
NHS NO:

BOX A Cannula for syringe pump sited in ....

Medication in Syringe	**Dose**	**Duration**	McKinley T34 Pump **mL/hr**	AlarisGH plus Pump mL/hr Volume in **48 mL** **Rate: 2 mL/hour**
		24 hours	**Record Serial Number**	

REVIEW patient's symptoms before refilling the pump – have any breakthrough doses been required?

Check infusion site, rate and volume remaining and the battery/pump working: please write time, volume remaining and initial

The label on the syringe and the information above should always be checked against the original prescription on the Inpatient Medication Prescription and Administration Chart

	Infusion Checks	Start	15 min	1 hrs	02 14 06 18 10 22 am pm	02 14 06 18 10 22 am pm	02 14 06 18 10 22 am pm	02 14 06 18 10 22 am pm	02 14 06 18 10 22 am pm	02 14 06 18 10 22 am pm
Date:	Site									
Commenced by (Signature):	Rate									
	Vol. remaining									
	Battery status %									
....	Initials									

	Infusion Checks	Start	15 min	1 hrs	02 14 06 18 10 22 am pm	02 14 06 18 10 22 am pm	02 14 06 18 10 22 am pm	02 14 06 18 10 22 am pm	02 14 06 18 10 22 am pm	02 14 06 18 10 22 am pm
Date:	Site									
Commenced by (Signature):	Rate									
	Vol. remaining									
	Battery status %									
....	Initials									

	Infusion Checks	Start	15 min	1 hrs	02 14 06 18 10 22 am pm	02 14 06 18 10 22 am pm	02 14 06 18 10 22 am pm	02 14 06 18 10 22 am pm	02 14 06 18 10 22 am pm	02 14 06 18 10 22 am pm
Date:	Site									
Commenced by (Signature):	Rate									
	Vol. remaining									
	Battery status %									
....	Initials									

Move to a new page each time a change is made (see below)

Circle reason for change of page and cross through old box with black ink for clarity.

Reason for change: (Please circle)	Change/ Addition of Drug	Change of Dose	Change of Rate/Pump	Site

Figure 11.7 *Continued*

guidelines, specialist palliative care teams, GPs or local medical information departments, as appropriate. *The Syringe Driver* (Dickman and Schneider 2016) contains information on all aspects of the use of the pump. Local units may well have guidelines to support starting doses or conversions of oral medications to subcutaneous medications.

Non-pharmacological support

Non-pharmacological approaches to physical and psychological symptoms may be of benefit to patients receiving end of life care (Booth et al. 2011). Non-pharmacological measures can help to empower patients at a time when the majority of their symptom management is prescriptive. As an example, there is a body of literature concerning the non-pharmacological management of breathlessness (Booth et al. 2011, Chin and Booth 2016, Corner et al. 1996). This literature advocates the involvement of the multidisciplinary team to draw on all resources available – for example, using the physiotherapist to give advice on breathing exercises and the occupational therapist to teach relaxation techniques; this is discussed further later.

Florence Nightingale (1859) wrote of the effect that the environment had on health, highlighting the negative effects of factors such as noise as well as lack of air, light and sleep. Booth et al. (2011) also advocate assessment of the environment, acknowledging the benefits of a bright, well-ventilated room.

The essence of non-pharmacological interventions is both holistic and heuristic (Taylor 2007). Nurses, who often spend more time than other healthcare professionals with patients during end-of-life care, are often best placed to assist patients with non-pharmacological interventions. The element of reassurance or 'presence' is very important – for example, knowing when to touch or not to touch a patient or relative, when to simply sit quietly with the patient or when draw up a chair for a deeply anxious relative. Nursing routines, performed in a calm and reassuring manner, bring normality to interactions, providing a sense of safety and security. These fundamental aspects of care are often extremely simple but are not always evident to those who do not have experience or specialist skills in relation to caring for patients receiving end-of-life care. Other examples of non-pharmacological interventions and support at the end of life are relaxation techniques, counselling, music therapy, art and pet therapy (Clements-Cortés 2016, Engelman 2013, Safari 2013).

Physical care

Physical discomfort can be one of the greatest concerns as patients with a terminal illness anticipate dying (NICE 2015). National guidance advises that patients expect to be offered optimal symptom management at the end of life and recommends that this should be achieved in all healthcare settings (NEoLCP 2015).

There should be a holistic assessment of the patient's needs followed by comprehensive care planning and regular reviews of symptoms (NEoLCP 2015). Nurses should be competent to build on this assessment in a dynamic, sensitive, consistent manner and to observe and record subtle changes (NEoLCP 2015). Some of the physiological changes that occur at the end of life are outlined in Box 11.1.

Changes in blood perfusion, increased weakness and reduced mobility increase the risk of pressure area injury. Consider a pressure-relieving mattress and cushion (if appropriate) (Langemo et al. 2015).

Decreased urinary output may occur in relation to the reduced oral intake (if artificial hydration is not being administered) as well as reduced perfusion to the kidneys. Incontinence may also ensue; planning for this with the use of pads or catheterization may need to be considered. Inability of the patient to urinate can often contribute to agitation at the end of life, so there is a need to assess for possible urinary retention.

A reduced interest in food and fluid coupled with profound weakness is not uncommon at the end of life; however, this can be distressing for families and loved ones. As a patient's level of consciousness reduces, the risk of dysphasia and possible aspiration is higher (Lacey 2015). The use of artificial fluids is addressed above. At this point, discontinuing non-essential medications should be considered, as should an alternative route for medications (e.g. converting from oral to subcutaneous).

Retained chest secretions may become evident in the last hours to days of life (Hui et al. 2014). This symptom has been found to occur in approximately 50% of patients at the end of life (Hui et al. 2014). Medications can be considered with the aim of reducing secretions in the upper airway that can occur as a result of pooling of saliva, with reduced swallowing reflexes and an inability to expectorate (Lacey 2015).

Delirium (presenting as confusion and agitation) should initially be managed by excluding any causative factors, such as urinary retention, faecal impaction, medications, electrolyte disturbances, organ failure or sepsis (Lacey 2015); treat these as appropriate. Once these have been excluded or if their treatment would be inappropriate, manage the delirium by optimizing the patient's environment and reorientating them to time and place regularly. Consider haloperidol for any patient who displays distress. Midazolam or lorazepam may be required if haloperidol is ineffective (Hosker and Bennett 2016).

Meeting the physical needs of patients at the end of life is aimed at providing as much comfort as possible. The change from acute active management to end-of-life care often requires a larger focus towards providing comfort with the least invasive procedures, and maintaining privacy and dignity becomes paramount.

Addressing psychosocial and existential concerns at the end of life

Psychosocial issues can greatly impact those who are dying. Establishing how to best support a patient and their family through this time requires an understanding of these issues (Detering et al. 2010, Lacey 2015, Steinhausser et al. 2000).

Provision of psychosocial care and support may need to be adjusted according to the changing needs of the patient – many will experience increasing anxiety and distress, increased feelings of social isolation and, alongside this, a decrease in physical energy available to them for dealing with these concerns (Hudson et al. 2012). Relatives will naturally be distressed by the deterioration of the patient and may exhibit signs of grief even before death occurs. Nurses should ensure that, wherever possible, the physical environment is conducive to patients and relatives being able to express their thoughts and emotions, and that appropriately trained staff are available to listen and support them (Hudson et al. 2012, NEoLCP 2015).

Alleviating distress when patients no longer feel connected with the world and are angry that their body has failed them can be challenging for healthcare professionals. Patients may find it difficult to discuss threats to their personhood and it is only through effective communication and interpersonal skills that nurses can address these issues (Lacey 2015).

The importance of psychosocial care should never be underestimated, and psychological management should be considered just as important as physical management across primary, acute and tertiary care (Lacey 2015). All healthcare professionals need to understand and recognize patients with complex psychosocial needs and be able to make comprehensive assessments of the distressing issues that patients may face. Nurses should be aware of their own limitations in this area and seek the support of specialists when needed.

Psychological, social and spiritual factors may exacerbate physical suffering. For instance, depression amplifies pain and other somatic symptoms (Goesling et al. 2013). When physical, psychological and spiritual sources of distress are inseparably intermixed, causing 'total pain' (Saunders 1976), a fully integrated clinical approach that addresses the multiple dimensions of suffering is required, looking at the individual needs of the patient from all perspectives.

Spiritual and religious care

Considerable energy and debate continue to be devoted to defining and exploring the concept of spirituality and its relationship to religion (NEoLCP 2015). Spiritual care has risen in visibility in health services over the past three decades, from a position where it was equated with religious care and regarded as the sole province of chaplains to one where a broad concept of spirituality is employed and spiritual care is recognized as having relevance for all sectors. However, this perceptual shift has not necessarily occurred at the level of practice and there is evidence of continuing uncertainty and ambiguity over how, when and where spiritual need should be addressed (Phelps et al. 2012).

In the UK, the *Guidelines for Hospice and Palliative Care Chaplaincy* affirm that assessment of spiritual and religious need should be available to all patients and carers, including those of no

Table 11.2 Cultural and religious considerations in the care of dying patients and their care after death

	Beliefs about death	Cultural and religious routines	Preparing the body	Post-mortem and transplantation	Specific burial requirements	Contact for further information
Baha'i	Baha'is have great respect for life and a belief in the afterlife. During life, the spiritual attributes are acquired for the next stage of existence that follows death.	The body is to be treated with great respect as it is considered to be the vehicle of the soul. Friends and relatives may say prayers for the dead.	The body is to be washed and wrapped in plain cotton or silk, by the family or observed by the family. A special ring is placed on one of the patient's fingers and is not to be removed.	There is no objection to necessary post-mortems. Organ donation is considered praiseworthy.	Embalming and cremation are forbidden. The burial should take place no more than an hour's journey from the place of death.	UK Baha'i: www.bahai.org.uk
Buddhism	Death is viewed as very important as it is a time of transition before rebirth as the person moves towards Nirvana, a state of enlightenment.	There is no one specific ritual, as different traditions have developed over time, but death should ideally take place in an atmosphere of peace, calm and sensitivity. In some traditions, a monk may be called to recite prayers or lead meditation. The family may want the body to remain in one place for up to 7 days for the rebirth to take place, but it is recognized that this is not possible in a healthcare setting.	At all times the body should be treated with the greatest care and respect. When washing has taken place, the body should be wrapped in a plain white sheet.	Approaches may vary.	Cremation is preferred as it is a symbol of the impermanence of the body.	The Buddhist Centre: https://thebuddhistcentre.com/tags/buddhist-healthcare-chaplaincy-group
Christians (including Church of England, Roman Catholic, Free Churches, non-denominational churches and Orthodox Churches)	There are different Christian churches with differing structures, beliefs and rituals but the concept of one God who reveals Himself as a Father, a Son and a Holy Spirit (the Trinity) is central to almost all Christian teaching. Christians believe in eternal life.	Christians have a range of pastoral needs. A priest, minister or chaplain may attend to say prayers with the patient and to pray with and support their relatives and friends. Roman Catholic patients should be offered the ministry of a Catholic priest. The sacrament of the sick with anointing is of particular importance, as are last rites when a patient is dying.	No specific customs.	No religious objection to post-mortems or organ donation.	No preference.	Refer to chaplain or patient's church for additional advice.
Christian Scientist	Christian Science teaches a reliance on God for healing, and patients will often seek care at home or in a Christian Science nursing home.	There are no specific rituals associated with death.	Only females can touch a female body.	Post-mortems are only permitted if required by law. Organ donation is an individual decision.	Cremation is preferred.	For details of local Christian Science Churches and Reading Rooms www.christianscience.org.uk

Church of Jesus Christ of Latter-Day Saints (LDS) (Mormon Church)	Earthly life is viewed as a test to see if individuals are fit to return to God on death. Death is viewed as a temporary separation from loved ones and is a purposeful part of eternal existence.	At the patient's request, two members of the LDS priesthood may be asked to visit.	The body should be washed and dressed in a shroud. Some patients may wear a religious undergarment, which must remain in place after the patient has died.	No religious objection to post-mortems or organ donation.	Burial is preferred.	Church of Jesus Christ of Latter-Day Saints: www.lds.org
Hinduism	Hindus believe that all human beings have a soul that passes through successive cycles of birth, death and rebirth governed by karma (a complex belief relating to cause and effect). Hinduism allows a great deal of freedom in matters of faith and worship.	Relatives may wish to perform last rites and keep vigil by the bedside.	Always consult the family, asking them if they wish to be involved in preparing the body, as distress could be caused if the body is touched by non-Hindus. A female must only be touched by a female and a male by a male. The body should be covered by a plain white sheet. All religious objects should remain in place.	Post-mortems are only permitted if required by law. Organ donation is an individual decision.	Hindus are always cremated.	National Council of Hindu Temples: www.nchtuk.org
Islam	Death is a mark of transition from one state of being to another. Muslims are encouraged to accept death as part of the will of Allah.	The time before death is important for extending forgiveness to family and friends, and so large numbers of visitors may arrive. Familiar people can give comfort by reading from the Qur'an until the point of death.	The body should be turned to the right to face Mecca if this has not happened before the patient dies. If relatives are available, the body should be prepared according to the wishes of the family. If not, a female must be handled by female nursing staff and a male by male staff. The whole body must be covered in a sheet and handled as little as possible. Maintaining modesty and dignity is essential.	Post-mortems are only permitted if required by law. Organ donation may be refused.	Burial will take place as quickly as possible. Cremation is forbidden.	Muslim Council of Great Britain: https://mcb.org.uk
Jehovah's Witness	Jehovah's Witnesses believe that when a person dies, their existence completely stops. However, death is not the end of everything: each person can be remembered by God and eventually be resurrected.	There are no special rituals or practices to perform.	No special requirements are to be observed.	There are no religious objections to either post-mortems or transplants, but advice should be sought.	No preference.	The Jehovah's Witnesses have established a countrywide network of Hospital Liaison Committees: www.jw.org

(continued)

Table 11.3 Cultural and religious considerations in the care of dying patients and their care after death *(continued)*

	Beliefs about death	Cultural and religious routines	Preparing the body	Post-mortem and transplantation	Specific burial requirements	Contact for further information
Judaism	There is a wide spectrum of observance among Jews: Orthodox, Liberal and Reform Communities.	It is important to consult the family and /or a rabbi acceptable to the family for advice, as there are specific Jewish laws and customs that need to be observed according to the beliefs of the patient. After death, someone from the Jewish community may sit with the body and psalms may be recited.	The body will be ritually washed by either trained members of the synagogue or the Jewish Burial Society. If the rabbi cannot be contacted, essential procedures can be performed by healthcare staff, but the body should not be washed. Traditionally, the body is covered by a plain white sheet with the feet facing the door.	Post-mortems should only be carried out if required by law. Organ donation is a complex issue in Jewish law but is usually permitted However, it is advisable to consult with a rabbi before making a decision.	Orthodox Jews are buried, and the burial usually takes place within 24 hours. Cremation may be permitted for non-Orthodox Jews.	Burial Society of the United Synagogue (Orthodox): www.theus.org.uk Liberal Judaism https://www.liberaljudaism.org Reform Judaism https://www.reformjudaism.org.uk
Sikhism	Life and death are a continuous cycle of rebirth: the person's soul is their essence.	The family will normally be present and say prayers for the dying patient. They may read from the holy book (the Guru Granth Sahib). The body should be released as soon as possible to enable the funeral to take place.	Relatives should be asked whether they wish to prepare the body. The five Ks should be left on the body: • Kesh – uncut hair, symbolic of sanctity and a love of nature • Kangha – a wooden comb symbolizing cleanliness • Kara – a steel band worn on the right wrist, symbolic of strength and restraint • Kirpan – a sword or dagger symbolizing the readiness to fight against injustice • Kacha – unisex under-shorts symbolizing morality The body must be touched only by staff of the same sex as the patient. The eyes and mouth must be closed, the face straight and clean.	There is no objection on religious grounds to organ donation or post-mortems.	Sikhs are always cremated.	Sikh Chaplaincy http://www.sikhchaplaincy.org.uk/~sikhchap/images/publications/a_guide_to_sikhism_key_issues_in_healthcare_practices.pdf

This list is not exhaustive. The Inter Faith Network for the UK works to promote understanding, cooperation and good relations between organizations and persons of different faiths in the UK, and is a helpful resource for the above and other faith communities (https://www.interfaith.org.uk/members/list).
Source: Adapted from information about dying and death on the faith-group websites listed within the table.

faith (AHPCC 2013). Exploring spiritual needs is defined as exploring the individual's sense of meaning and purpose in life. This involves attitudes, beliefs, ideas, values and concerns around life and death issues; affirming life and worth by encouraging reminiscence about the past; and exploring the individual's hopes and fears regarding the present and future. Each patient and their relatives should have the opportunity to express, in advance, any religious, cultural or practical needs they have for the time of death or afterwards, particularly regarding urgent release for burial or cremation. This can be done as part of the advance care planning process or it can be completed nearer the point of death (Wilson 2015). It is important to try to discuss these issues with the patient, as even where relatives share a common faith, as there may be differences in the way each person practises. It is vital that assumptions are not made on the basis of a previously disclosed religious preference. Further information about religious and cultural perspectives and practices is given in Table 11.2. A person's religion and culture is central to their well-being and patients will receive great comfort from practising their faith and from having their religious and cultural needs recognized and respected.

Symptom control

Dyspnoea (shortness of breath)

Definition

Breathlessness, or dyspnoea, is an unpleasant sensation defined as 'a subjective experience of breathing discomfort that consists of qualitatively distinct sensations that vary in intensity' (Parshall et al. 2012, p.435). Some of the causes of breathlessness are listed in Box 11.4.

Approximately 70% of patients experience dyspnoea in the last 6 weeks of life and the distress associated with this symptom increases as death approaches (Ben-Aharon et al. 2008, Kamal et al. 2012). The causes of dyspnoea are often multifactorial (Ekstrom et al. 2015). In a prospective study, 50.65% of almost 600 patients attending a specialized palliative care unit had more frequent incidence of dyspnoea during the last 3 months of life (Ekstrom et al. 2015). Both patients and their families and carers report breathlessness to be a distressing symptom that can result in reduced quality of life, largely due to measures taken to manage this symptom (such as undertaking less physical activity), increased anxiety and depression, and the increased likelihood of hospital admissions (Simon et al. 2010). As death approaches, it still may be appropriate to try to manage reversible causes of breathlessness to manage the distress of this symptom, but dyspnoea can become refractory to intervention (Lacey 2015).

Pharmacological management with oral or parenteral opioids has been shown to help with the sensation of dyspnoea (Ben-Aharon et al. 2008, Chin and Booth 2016, Dudgeon 2018, Ekstrom et al. 2015, Jennings et al. 2002). Benzodiazepines may be useful for reducing panic and anxiety but have not been evidenced to show an improvement in breathing (Simon et al. 2010). Oxygen therapy has been found to improve dyspnoea in patients who have been found to be hypoxic. In one study, approximately 10% of patients used oxygen therapy to help them with the distress of dyspnoea (Campbell et al. 2013).

Box 11.4 Causes of dyspnoea

- Obstructing lung tumour
- Weakness and frailty
- Chest wall disease
- Lymphangitis carcinomatosis
- Diffuse lung pathology
- Infection
- Anaemia
- Heart failure

Table 11.3 Common medications used in the management of dyspnoea

Drug	Use
Oxygen	Reduce risk of hypoxia
Salbutamol or terbutaline	Short-acting bronchodilators
Furosemide	Bronchodilator and diuretic
Tiotropium or ipratropium bromide	Long-acting bronchodilators
Carbocisteine	Mucolytic – loosens secretions
Theophylline	Bronchodilator – added if not getting benefit from optimum doses of inhaled bronchodilators
Salmeterol	Long-acting bronchodilator – may be used in combination with inhaled steroids
Opioids	Reduce sensation of breathlessness
Steroids	Reduce inflammation
Lorazepam	Relaxant
Nebulized saline	Loosen secretions

Any reversible causes should be treated initially; however, if symptomatic relief is the aim of treatment, combining both pharmacological (Table 11.3) and non-pharmacological interventions will improve symptom burden and quality of life (Currow et al. 2013). In patients who have low haemoglobin, a blood transfusion can help with the symptom of breathlessness. However, in some instances receiving a blood transfusion does not make the patient feel any better. Any ongoing interventions (such as blood transfusions) should only be considered if they are providing symptom relief and/or improving quality of life.

Evidence-based approaches

Anticipated patient outcomes

The patient will be free of symptoms that are distressing and/or having an impact on their quality of life.

Non-pharmacological interventions

Non-pharmacological interventions can give patients control and independence. Fan therapy creates air flow across the face, stimulating the skin and mucosa and causing activation of the second and third branches of the trigeminal nerve, resulting in relief of the sensation of breathlessness (Booth et al. 2016). Breathing retraining, different positioning, and cognitive–behavioural and self-management techniques can all also help with breathlessness (Chin and Booth 2016).

Systematic reviews show limited evidence that acupuncture or acupressure are beneficial in dyspnoea (Towler et al. 2013). One study demonstrated that the use of acupuncture alone or in combination with morphine could offer some benefit to patients (Minchom et al. 2016). The Cambridge-based Breathlessness Intervention Service recognizes key issues in the non-pharmacological management of breathlessness including breathing techniques, mindfulness and relaxation (Booth et al. 2011, Dudgeon 2018). While these techniques may be helpful, it may be difficult for patients to engage with them at the end of life. However, playing music is becoming increasingly common within holistic care delivered to those at the end of life (Clements-Cortés 2016).

Non-invasive ventilation (NIV) delivers respiratory support without the need for intubation. NIV usually provides positive pressure via a tight-fitting mask, nasal mask or helmet, to aid inspiration, help lung expansion and improve gaseous exchange. Modes and methods are discussed in detail in Chapter 12: Respiratory care, CPR and blood transfusion. NIV can be useful to support the patient's respiratory function during recovery from exacerbations of chronic conditions, during infective processes or in progressive respiratory disease. The aim would be to avoid intubation and invasive mechanical ventilation, which would be inappropriate for most patients at the end of life; therefore, NIV is often the 'ceiling' of treatment for advanced respiratory disease (Stevens and Laverty 2018).

Pre-procedural considerations

It is useful to explore the extent of their breathlessness with the patient; how this is impacting them physically and psychologically; and how this is affecting their quality of life. Assessing previous effective methods used to control dyspnoea is useful as these can be implemented.

Procedure guideline 11.1 Management of dyspnoea (breathlessness)

Essential equipment

- Personal protective equipment
- Fan
- Oxygen and a variety of administration interfaces (e.g. mask, nasal cannula)
- Pillows
- Mouth care equipment

Action	Rationale
Pre-procedure	
1 Introduce yourself to the patient, explain and discuss the procedure with them, and gain their consent to proceed.	To ensure that the patient feels at ease, understands the procedure and gives their valid consent (NMC 2018, **C**).
2 Explore the meaning of breathlessness to the patient, their family and carers.	To ascertain fears and anxieties (Chin and Booth 2016, **E**).
3 Involve the multidisciplinary team.	To ensure clinicians, the physiotherapist and the occupational therapist help to optimize symptom control (Chan et al. 2015, **E**).
4 Help the patient into a high side-lying position (using pillows or the electric bed head) and forward lean onto pillows.	To support the patient's position in bed, optimizing air entry (Booth et al. 2011, **R**).
5 Offer a lubricant (such as lip balm) for lips if they become dry due to mouth breathing. If the patient is having oxygen therapy, avoid products containing petroleum jelly or oil-based emollients. Use water-based products (such as vitamin E or Surgilube) instead.	To prevent dry, cracked lips (Cancer Research UK 2018, **C**). Petroleum jelly and oil-based products are fire hazards. **E**
Procedure	
6 Reassure the patient and try to ensure someone stays with them during the dyspnoea episode, especially if this is a new or acute episode.	To help with fear and anxiety (Lacey 2015, **C**).
7 Ensue the call bell is within reach.	To ensure the patient can call for help if their symptoms worsen or if they feel particularly anxious. **P**
8 Offer a fan (if appropriate to the clinical area).	To reduce subjective sensation of dyspnoea (Chin and Booth 2016, **E**; Dudgeon 2018, **E**; Ekstrom et al. 2015, **E**)
9 Optimize positioning: help the patient to sit upright, well supported with pillows.	Specific positions can help with breathing exercises to optimize air entry and are often taken up instinctively by patients (Booth et al. 2011, **E**).
10 Offer guidance on breathing techniques, such as breathing through pursed lips, diaphragmatic breathing and pacing techniques. *Note:* some of these techniques may not be appropriate as the patient approaches the last days to hours of life.	Specific breathing techniques (including the recovery breathing method, breathing control and pacing techniques) can help patients to regain (and maintain) some control over their breathing (Booth et al. 2016, **R**; Chan et al. 2015, **R**).
11 Encourage relaxation, using techniques suitable to the individual patient (such as breathing techniques, music or mindfulness).	Relaxation can help the patient to feel less anxious and more in control of their breathing. They can also apply these techniques when needed to reduce anxiety (Booth et al. 2016, **R**).
12 Consider acupuncture (delivered by an appropriately trained practitioner).	To help with the sensation of breathlessness (Minchom et al. 2016, **R**).
13 Consider and implement required pharmacological interventions, such as: • antibiotics • inhaled or nebulized bronchodilators • steroids • cough suppressants	To help optimize symptom control (Chan et al. 2015, **R**; Ekstrom et al. 2015, **E**; Jennings et al. 2002, **R**): • Use antibiotics if dyspnoea is caused by infection. • Use bronchodilators to reduce any bronchoconstriction or wheeze. • Use steroids to reduce any inflammation.

• systemic opioids • oxygen therapy (if patient is hypoxic) • heliox • benzodiazepines.	• Use cough suppressants to ease a persistent cough. • Use opioids to relieve the sensation of dyspnoea (Barnes et al. 2016, **R**; Jennings et al. 2002, **R**). • Use oxygen to treat hypoxia. • Use heliox because helium has a low density and the potential to reduce the work of breathing. • Use benzodiazepines to relax the patient and help address issues of panic and anxiety (Chan et al. 2015, **R**).
14 Assess and intervene if chest secretions are audible. Suctioning may be appropriate in some patients; however, this is an invasive procedure that causes discomfort and sometimes distress, and therefore it requires careful consideration as to its suitability in this setting. Consider an anticholinergic medication.	Suctioning should only be used where clinically appropriate to enhance patient comfort (Lacey 2015, **C**). Anticholinergic medication helps to dry out secretions (Twycross et al. 2017, **C**).
15 Review current artificial hydration; assess the need for it and ascertain whether it could be contributing to chest secretions and therefore increasing dyspnoea.	To ensure additional fluid is not adding to additional chest secretions (Lanz et al. 2019, **C**).
16 Consider diuretic medications to offload some fluid from the chest and lungs.	To optimize symptoms and reduce breathlessness (Dudgeon 2018, **E**).
17 Request the input of physiotherapy.	To help the patient get into a supportive position that is comfortable and optimized for breathing, and to request advice on chest physiotherapy if suitable (Chan et al. 2015, **R**).
Post-procedure	
18 Evaluate the effectiveness or ineffectiveness of any interventions and document them accordingly.	To ensure the interventions are reviewed and communicated to the multidisciplinary team. This will also help to avoid the repeated implementation of any interventions that were ineffective. **E**

For patients with refractory dyspnoea and severe distress in the terminal phase, sedation may need to be considered as an option to adequately control the symptom and to relieve suffering (Lacey 2015). Terminal sedition is explored further below.

Nausea and vomiting

Definition

Nausea

Sanger and Andrews (2018) describe nausea as a 'warning' to inhibit any further ingestion of potentially harmful substances. Nausea (and vomiting) is primarily a defence mechanism; however, it also occurs as a side-effect of both disease and treatment.

Vomiting

Vomiting (or emesis) is an objective experience that involves the forceful movement and elimination of the contents of the stomach by the constant action of the abdominal muscles with the opening of the gastric cardia (Sanger and Andrews 2018). Vomiting and the associated sensation of nausea are significant and distressing symptoms that patients may experience as a result of either disease or treatment (Bennett 2009). Vomiting can also be a warning sign of deterioration (Frese et al. 2011), a defence mechanism against ingested toxins or poisons, or a symptom of bowel obstruction. The most common causes are outlined in Table 11.4.

Anatomy and physiology

The pathophysiology of nausea and vomiting is complex (Figure 11.8); two main centres within the brainstem are involved: the chemoreceptor trigger zone (CTZ) and the vomiting centre (Kelly and Ward 2013). Vomiting is ultimately controlled by the vomiting centre, which receives input from a wide range of sources. Some of these inputs are directly connected to the vomiting centre but most are directed through the CTZ (Kelly and Ward 2013). The CTZ is an area of the brain that is not fully separated from the blood by the blood–brain barrier, allowing it to detect chemicals in the blood and cerebrospinal fluid and initiate vomiting where necessary. It is also stimulated by the vagus and vestibular nerves, which receive signals from the gut and inner ear respectively (Bennett 2009, Kelly and Ward 2013).

Table 11.4 Common causes of nausea and vomiting in palliative care

Cause	Examples
Toxins	• Medications/drugs (e.g. cytotoxics, opioids, NSAIDs, antibiotics, anticonvulsants, iron and many others) • Poisoning • Substance abuse
Metabolic conditions	• Hypercalcaemia • Hyponatremia • Ketoacidosis
Organ failure/ disorders of viscera	• Liver • Renal • Obstruction (e.g. gastric outlet, bowel, biliary, pancreatic) • Severe constipation • Gastroparesis • Inflammation or irritation (e.g. gastroenteritis, hepatitis, cholecystitis, NSAID, chemotherapy, radiation) • Malignancy • Ascites
Neurological conditions	• Increased intracranial pressure (e.g. malignancy, haemorrhage, cranial irradiation or abscess) • Meningeal infiltration • Vestibular (e.g. labyrinthitis or effects of medications or drugs) • Anxiety • Pain

NSAIDs, non-steroidal anti-inflammatory drugs.

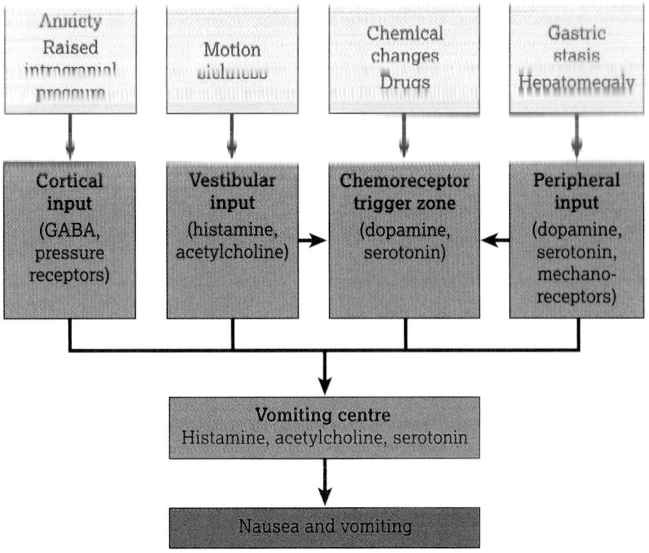

Figure 11.8 The emetic pathway. *Source*: Reproduced from Kelly and Ward (2013) with permission of EMAP Publishing Ltd.

The causes of vomiting are often multifactorial and therefore thorough assessment of the risk factors, precipitating factors and alleviating factors is key to identifying effective strategies for managing this symptom.

Related theory

Post-operative nausea and vomiting affect up to 30% of surgical patients (Gan et al. 2014) (this is further described in Chapter 16: Perioperative care). Around 40–80% of cancer patients receiving chemotherapy experience nausea and vomiting (dependent on the regime and agents used) (Del Fabbro et al. 2019). Nausea and vomiting are unpleasant symptoms and a systematic review demonstrated that in patients with advanced disease the prevalence of this symptom is between 6% and 68%. Less is known about the prevalence of vomiting; however, while these symptoms are separate, they often occur together (Hardy et al. 2015, Solano et al. 2006). Twycross et al. (2009) report that nausea and vomiting are experienced by up to 70% of patients in their last week of life.

Evidence-based approaches

Anticipated patient outcomes

The patient will be free of symptoms that are distressing and/or having an impact on their quality of life.

Assessment

Assessment may either focus on risk factors (in the case of post-operative nausea and vomiting, in order to prevent or minimize the symptom occurring) or focus on identifying causative factors. Risk assessment tools for post-operative nausea and vomiting consider a range of factors relating to the patient themselves (e.g. gender, age, history of motion sickness, smoker status), the surgical procedure (e.g. duration, open versus laparoscopic, type of surgery) and the anaesthetic (e.g. type of agent, duration, premedication, use of opioids) (Hambridge 2013). In those patients who are experiencing nausea and vomiting associated with other causes, a consistent and systematic approach should be used to assess symptoms and determine the cause (Kelly and Ward 2013). It is helpful to consider reversible causes alongside goals of care to determine the right treatment actions (Walsh et al. 2017). Anticipatory, acute or delayed chemotherapy-induced nausea and vomiting can be reported using self-assessment tools (Molassiotis et al. 2016), although strict adherence to pharmacological guidelines is paramount for optimal management irrespective of the phase (Molassiotis et al. 2016).

Assessment of nausea and vomiting at the end of life primarily requires detailed history taking and physical assessment. The most common causes of nausea and vomiting at the end of life are outlined in Table 11.4. Further diagnostic tests may be required to confirm the cause; however, the risks and benefits of carrying out such tests should be considered, especially at the end of life. Del Fabbro et al. (2019) suggest that, when the cause of nausea and vomiting cannot be confirmed, an empirical approach (treatment initiated based on a 'best guess' of the cause) may be more suitable.

Vomiting is a significant yet complex symptom that requires a multifactorial approach to assess, prevent and manage it effectively.

Non-pharmacological approaches

There are a range of non-pharmacological strategies available to manage nausea and vomiting. First, consideration needs to be given to any precipitating factors that can be controlled or removed, such as exposure to food smells or malodour, or large meals. Complementary therapies, such as acupressure and acupuncture (Abraham 2008, Lee et al. 2015) and aromatherapy (Hines et al. 2018), may be used but the evidence base for their effectiveness is relatively weak. Interventions including progressive muscle relaxation techniques (Charalambous et al. 2016) and hypnosis (Richardson et al. 2007) have been found to be effective in reducing nausea and vomiting associated with chemotherapy, but more research is required to establish the wider effectiveness of these approaches.

Pharmacological approaches

There is a wide variety of antiemetic drugs available, all of which act on one or more type of neuroreceptor, resulting in a central and/or peripheral effect. Antiemetics and their receptor affinity sites can be found in Table 11.5. A Cochrane review in 2015 looked into the use of cannabinoids for chemotherapy-induced nausea and vomiting, and it confirmed that the use of cannabinoids may be helpful in the management of this refractory symptom (Smith et al. 2015). Bennett (2009) identifies nine categories of antiemetics, a summary of which can be found in Box 11.5.

Table 11.5 Receptor affinity sites of selected anti-emetics

Drug	D2	H1	Muscarinic	5HT2	5HT3	NK1	5HT4	CB1	GABAmimetic
Aprepitant and fosaprepitant	–	–	–	–	–	+++	–	–	–
Chlorpromazine	+++	+++	++	++	–	–	–	–	–
Cyclizine	–	++	++	–	–	–	–	–	–
Domperidone (does not normally cross the blood–brain barrier)	++	–			–	–	–	–	–
Haloperidol	+++	–	–	–	+/–		–	–	–
Hyoscine hydrobromide	–	–	+++	–	–	–	–	–	–
Levomepromazine	++	+++	++	+++	–	–	–	–	–
Lorazepam	–	–	–	–	–	–	–	–	+++

Drug	D2	H1	Muscarinic	5HT2	5HT3	NK1	5HT4	CB1	GABAmimetic
Metoclopramide	++	–	–	–	+	–	++	–	–
Nabilone	–	–	–	–	–	–	–	+++	–
Ondansetron and granisetron	–	–	–	–	+++	–	–	–	–
Olanzapine	++	+	++	++	+	–	–	–	–
Prochlorperazine	+++	++	+	+/++	–	–	–	–	–
Promethazine	+/++	++	++	–	–	–	–	–	–

+++, marked pharmacological activity; ++, moderate; +, slight; –, no or insignificant activity.
Source: Adapted from Twycross et al. (2017).

Box 11.5 Classes of antiemetics

Antihistamines

Antihistamines block the histamine H1 receptor and are widely used. The main side-effects are the sedative potential and anticholinergic effects (e.g. dry mouth, constipation). Cyclizine tends to be less sedating than other antihistamines and is commonly used as a first line treatment for post-operative nausea and vomiting or motion sickness.

Dopamine antagonists

These act by blocking the dopamine D2 receptors in the chemoreceptor trigger zone (CTZ). Some antipsychotic drugs, such as the phenothiazines, have a strong affinity for these receptors but also block D2 receptors elsewhere, leading to side-effects such as restlessness and tremors, which may limit their use as antiemetics, particularly in very young or older patients (Bennett 2009). Metoclopramide and domperidone act on D2 receptors in the CTZ but also on receptors in the gastrointestinal tract, which can reduce abdominal bloating. There is a particular risk of neurological side-effects with longer-term use and higher doses (BNF 2019). Levomepromazine is a broad-spectrum antiemetic, which means it acts on a range of receptors; it also has sedating and analgesic effects and so is often used in the palliative care setting.

5-HT3 antagonists

These are regarded as highly effective antiemetics that block 5-HT3 receptors in the CTZ and the gastrointestinal tract. They are commonly used to prevent chemotherapy-induced nausea and vomiting.

Steroids

Dexamethasone, a corticosteroid, is recognized for its antiemetic effect (Warren and King 2008), and is often used in conjunction with other antiemetics, although its mechanism of action is not clear.

Other antiemetics

Other categories of antiemetic include:

- benzodiazepines, which work in the central nervous system to inhibit the GABA (gamma-aminobutyric acid) neurotransmitter
- anticholinergics, such as hyoscine hydrobromide, which acts directly on the vomiting centre
- cannabinoids, which inhibit nausea and vomiting caused by substances that irritate the CTZ, although the precise mechanism of action is not clearly understood.

Neurokinin-1 antagonists are a relatively new category of antiemetic that act on NK1 receptors in the CTZ. They have been found to be most effective in the treatment of chemotherapy-induced nausea and vomiting when used in conjunction with an HT3 antagonist and dexamethasone (BNF 2019, Dikken and Wildman 2013).

Source: Adapted from Bennett (2009), BNF (2019).

Procedure guideline 11.2 Care of a patient who is vomiting

Essential equipment

- Personal protective equipment
- 2 vomit bowls
- Tissues/wipes
- Bowl of warm water
- Wipes
- Towel

Action	Rationale
Pre-procedure	
1 Introduce yourself to the patient, explain and discuss the procedure with them, and gain their consent to proceed.	To ensure that the patient feels at ease, understands the procedure and gives their valid consent (NMC 2018, **C**).
2 Ensure the patient is in a safe place and position to avoid an unnecessary injury or fall.	To maintain patient safety (NMC 2018, **C**).

(continued)

Procedure guideline [illegible] Care of a patient who is vomiting (continued)

Action	Rationale
3 Decontaminate hands and apply personal protective equipment.	To ensure the procedure is as clean as possible (NHS Improvement 2019, **C**)
Procedure	
4 Close the door or draw the curtains around the patient's bed area.	To maintain privacy and dignity and avoid any unnecessary embarrassment for the patient (NMC 2018, **C**).
5 Provide the patient with a vomit bowl and tissues.	To reduce the risk of spillage and cross-infection (NHS Improvement 2019, **C**).
6 Remain with the patient.	To provide reassurance and maintain safety (Kelly and Ward 2013, **E**).
7 Once the patient has stopped vomiting, remove the used vomit bowl and offer warm water and towels for them to wash their face and hands.	For infection prevention and control and for patient comfort (Kelly and Ward 2013, **E**).
8 Assist the patient to find a comfortable position and leave the second, clean vomit bowl with them.	To ensure comfort following the procedure (Kelly and Ward 2013, **E**).
9 Take the first vomit bowl to the dirty utility (sluice) room and, where necessary, measure the volume and note the characteristics (colour, consistency and smell) of the vomit.	The characteristics of the vomit may help to determine the cause (Kelly and Ward 2013, **E**).
Post-procedure	
10 Dispose of the contents safely and place the vomit bowl in the washer or disposal unit.	For infection prevention and control (Fraise and Bradley 2009, **E**).
11 Remove personal protective equipment. Wash hands using soap and water or use an alcohol based handrub.	For infection prevention and control (NHS Improvement 2019, **C**).
12 Record the volume and any notable characteristics of the vomit in the patient's notes.	To maintain accurate documentation (NMC 2018, **C**).
13 Administer any prescribed antiemetics.	To prevent any further episodes of nausea or vomiting and to help control symptoms (Bennett 2009, **E**).
14 Return to the patient and assess them at regular intervals, evaluating the effectiveness of any interventions.	To monitor the patient and maintain their safety and comfort. **E**

Insertion of a nasogastric drainage tube

For some patients it may be appropriate to insert a nasogastric drainage tube in order to decompress the stomach (following surgery or to conservatively treat a bowel obstruction and associated nausea and vomiting). This avoids any unnecessary trauma from the retching associated with vomiting and allows more effective monitoring of fluid output.

Due to the invasive nature of this procedure, it is not often advocated for patients at the end of life. However, it remains a treatment option for those experiencing vomiting due to a bowel obstruction for which antiemetics are unsuccessful (NHS Scotland 2019, Walsh et al. 2017). Details of how to insert a drainage nasogastric tube can be found in Chapter 6: Elimination.

Ascites

Definition

Ascites is an accumulation of fluid (above 25 mL) in the peritoneal cavity (Pedersen et al. 2015). Abdominal paracentesis is a simple bedside or clinic procedure in which a needle is inserted into the peritoneal cavity and ascitic fluid is removed. Diagnostic paracentesis refers to the removal of a small quantity of fluid for testing. Therapeutic paracentesis refers to the removal of 5 L or more of fluid to reduce intra-abdominal pressure and relieve the associated dyspnoea, abdominal pain and early satiety (Runyon 2018).

Anatomy and physiology

The peritoneum is a semi-permeable serous membrane consisting of two separate layers: the parietal layer and the visceral layer. The parietal layer covers the abdominal and pelvic walls and the undersurface of the diaphragm. The visceral layer lines and supports the abdominal organs and the parietal peritoneum (Figure 11.9). The space between the parietal and visceral layers is known as the peritoneal cavity (Marieb and Hoehn 2018). The normal peritoneal cavity has a small amount of free fluid of approximately 50 mL (Zhou et al. 2015).

In a healthy individual, fluid is produced from the capillaries lining the peritoneal cavity and is drained by lymphatic vessels under the diaphragm. The fluid is collected by the right lymphatic duct, which drains into the vena cava. The peritoneum forms the largest serous membrane in the body (Tortora and Derrickson 2017) (Box 11.6). However, in patients with malignant ascites, this balance of production and drainage is disrupted and ascitic fluid collects in the peritoneal cavity.

Related theory

Ascites can be caused by non-malignant conditions such as cirrhosis of the liver, advanced congestive heart failure, chronic pericarditis and nephrotic syndrome. Cirrhosis of the liver is the most common cause of ascites in the Western world and in this clinical condition the development of ascites indicates a poor prognosis (Tasneem et al. 2015).

Malignant conditions such as metastatic cancer of the ovary, stomach, colon or breast can also cause ascites. If a definitive diagnosis is needed to establish cause, to aid staging and possible surgical intervention, then a peritoneal tap and analysis of fluid will be useful (Runyon 2019). It is not possible to distinguish between malignant and benign ascites by physical examination or radiographic techniques so invasive testing is necessary to differentiate the two types (Sangisetty and Miner 2012).

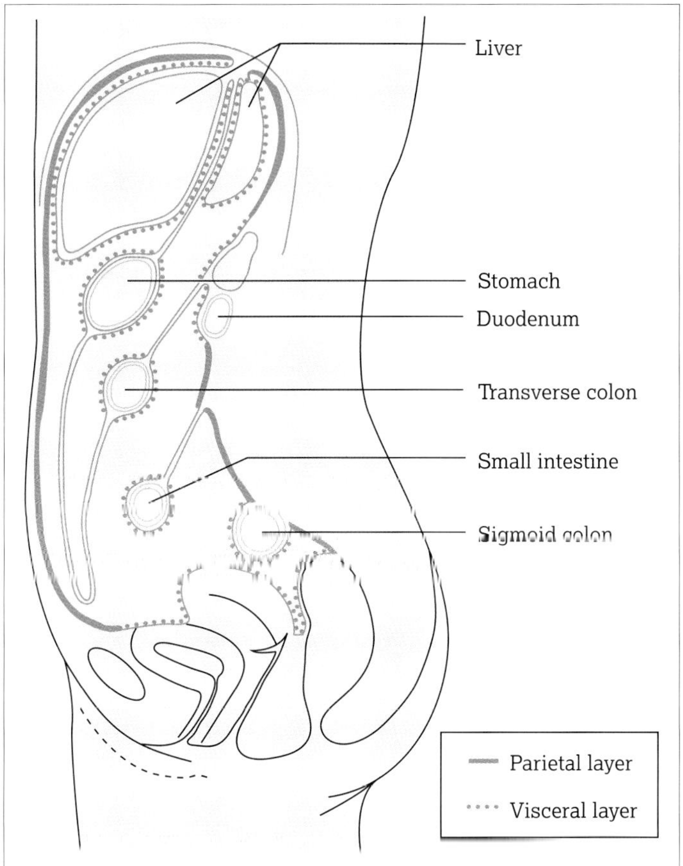

Figure 11.9 Peritoneum of female in lateral view.

Box 11.6 Functions of the peritoneum

- The peritoneum is a serous membrane that enables the abdominal contents to glide over each other without friction.
- It forms a partial or complete cover for the abdominal organs.
- It forms ligaments and mesenteries, which help to keep the organs in position.
- The mesenteries contain fat and act as a store for the body.
- The mesenteries can move to engulf areas of inflammation and this prevents the spread of infection.
- The peritoneum has the power to absorb fluids and exchange electrolytes.

Source: Adapted from Marieb and Hoehn (2016), Thibodeau and Patton (2010).

The pathogenesis of ascites differs depending on its primary related factors:

- Cirrhotic ascites is believed to be directly related to portal hypertension (Pedersen et al. 2015).
- The increased pressure caused by fibrosis and lesions of the liver from chronic liver disease causes obstruction to venous flow.
- Heart failure and constrictive pericarditis can cause an increase in pressure on the portal venous system, leading to portal hypertension and ascites (Tasneem et al. 2015).

The pathogenesis of malignant ascites is more complex than that of non-cancer-related ascites. Cytokines, mechanical obstruction and hormonal influence are thought to be related. Cytokines, such as vascular endothelial growth factor (VEGF) and vascular permeability factor (VPF), regulate vascular permeability. The obstruction of lymphatic drainage by the disseminating malignant cells in the peritoneal cavity reduces absorption of peritoneal exudates (Chopra et al. 2017). This reduction activates the renin–angiotensin–aldosterone system and leads to sodium retention, which then further exacerbates the ascites.

Ascites is often accompanied by debilitating symptoms as large amounts of fluid collect in the peritoneal cavity, causing an increase in intra-abdominal pressure and resulting in pressure on internal structures (Kipps et al. 2013). The fluid accumulation may occur over several weeks or rapidly over a few days (Lee and Grap 2008). Symptoms initially include vague abdominal discomfort, which can go on to affect the respiratory and gastrointestinal systems, depending on the amount of fluid present. Pressure on the diaphragm decreases the intrathoracic space and causes shortness of breath. Gastric pressure may cause anorexia, indigestion or hiatus hernia. Intestinal pressure may result in constipation, bowel obstruction or decreased bladder capacity. Patients also become increasingly fatigued, finding simple daily tasks difficult (Slusser 2014). Additionally, body image can be affected even when minimal distension is present.

Cytological confirmation of malignant cells is the gold standard although its sensitivity is only around 60% (Jung et al. 2016).

Evidence-based approaches

Rationale

There is much debate about whether it is safe to drain large volumes of fluid rapidly from the abdomen. One concern is that profound hypotension may follow because of the sudden release of intra-abdominal pressure and consequent possible vasodilation (Lindsay et al. 2014). However, some studies suggest that total paracentesis – that is, removal of all ascites (even more than 20 L) – can usually be performed safely (Pericleous et al. 2016). In cases of cirrhosis, however, Moore (2015) suggests that when a large volume paracentesis is performed, it should be completed as rapidly as possible once started but at least within 6 hours, with the use of albumin to prevent hemodynamic consequences.

Martin et al. (2018) have shown that continuous paracentesis with an indwelling peritoneal catheter can be a safe and effective means to manage patients in the hospital with large-volume, tense ascites. This can be used for up to 72 hours and it is suggested that an intravenous albumin infusion is used to maintain optimal perfusion and renal function.

To avoid exposing patients to blood products, the use of terlipressin rather than albumin has been proposed for the prevention of paracentesis-induced circulatory dysfunction (PICD) after large-volume paracentesis (Annamalai et al. 2016). Initial studies suggest that terlipressin is as effective as albumin for this purpose (Shah 2017).

The literature suggests the use of ultrasound-guided paracentesis to confirm the presence of ascites and to identify the best site to perform the procedure, particularly when a small amount of fluid is present (Montgomery and Leitman 2014).

Indications

Paracentesis may be performed:

- to obtain a specimen of fluid for analysis for diagnostic purposes (diagnostic paracentesis)
- to relieve the symptoms associated with ascites, both physical and psychological (therapeutic paracentesis)
- to administer substances such as cytotoxic drugs (e.g. bleomycin, cisplatin) or other agents into the peritoneal cavity, to achieve regression of malignant deposits (Chmielowski 2017).

Contraindications

There are a number of relative contraindications for paracentesis (Runyon 2018):

- clinically apparent disseminated intravascular coagulation
- primary fibrinolysis
- massive ileus with bowel distension
- surgical scars at the proposed paracentesis site
- symptomatic disseminated intravascular coagulation
- symptomatic hyperfibrinolysis.

An elevated international normalised ratio (INR) or thrombocytopenia is not a contraindication to paracentesis, and there is no published data supporting blood product administration prior to the procedure (Runyon 2016).

Preparatory investigations

The patient's clinical condition and the purpose of the procedure must be taken into account when deciding which investigations are necessary, but most pre-procedural investigations include a blood screen (full blood count, coagulation screen, urea and electrolytes, liver function tests and plasma proteins) and an ultrasound examination (Runyon 2012). To keep intrusion to a minimum for palliative patients, fewer investigations may be performed. In the case of a diagnostic paracentesis or a large-volume therapeutic paracentesis (>5 L), the ascitic fluid should be analysed for cell count, bacterial culture, total protein and albumin (Pedersen et al. 2015).

Methods of managing ascites

The development of ascites is secondary to many different conditions, and the prognosis and outlook for patients will depend on the underlying cause. Ascites can be managed, but sometimes the underlying problem cannot be resolved. For patients and families, ascites is associated with poorer quality of life and increased risk of infection (Mortimore 2018). Treatment for ascites may include use of diuretics, paracentesis, diet low in sodium, instillation of peritoneal agents or the insertion of long-term catheters. However, the literature available is mostly generated from studies with patients suffering from acute or chronic liver failure; this should be taken into account when managing patients with non-malignant ascites.

Paracentesis

Paracentesis is the most common way of managing ascites in a fast and effective way, as long as the loss of ascitic fluid is compensated with a low-sodium diet, diuretic therapy and/or plasma expanders (Annamalai et al. 2016).

Sodium-restricted diet

The amount of fluid retained in the body depends on the balance between sodium ingested in the diet and sodium excreted in the urine. The ideal sodium restriction is between 20 and 30 mEq per day or 460 and 690 mg of sodium per day (Shah 2017), or between 1.2 and 1.7 grams per day of common salt or sodium chloride.

Diuretics

Diuretics are useful mainly in cirrhotic-type ascites. These may be used for malignant ascites together with a restriction of salt and fluid intake, and have been found to be effective in about 43% of patients (Sangisetty and Miner 2012). Additionally, they appear to be more effective for management of patients with small-volume ascites (only diagnosed by ultrasound). Spironolactone is the diuretic of choice (Pedersen et al. 2015). The most effective way of monitoring the fluid loss is by weighing the patient daily (Evans and Best 2014).

Chemotherapy

Instillation of heated intraperitoneal chemotherapy has successfully been used in reducing and eventually eliminating malignant ascites (Sangisetty and Miner 2012).

Long-term catheters

There are three types of catheter that can be used for long-term management of ascites:

- *Peritoneovenous shunt*: these are generally used in patients with a long-term prognosis. These shunts drain ascitic fluid into the superior vena cava and require general anaesthesia for insertion (Christensen et al. 2016).
- *PleurX drain*: this is a tunnelled catheter placed under ultrasound and fluoroscopic guidance. This device is associated with low rates of serious adverse clinical events, catheter failure, discomfort and electrolyte imbalance (Narayanan et al. 2014). Additionally, it may allow patients to avoid spending added time in hospital for repeated paracentesis.
- *Peritoneal port-catheter*: this is similar to but larger than a central venous catheter. It allows long-term drainage with reduced infection risk (Ghattar et al. 2014). A limited number of studies support its use.

Anticipated patient outcomes

Patients' comfort and quality of life will be improved by relieving the symptoms caused by ascites (Slusser 2014). Thoughtful and sympathetic support should be offered (Mortimore 2018).

Clinical governance

Competencies

The procedure is performed by a doctor or a practitioner trained in paracentesis, assisted by a nurse throughout. There is no accredited pathway or course for learning this clinical skill and specific training has to be negotiated and developed locally (Vaughan 2013).

Pre-procedural considerations

Equipment

The equipment should be prepared by the health professional performing the paracentesis or by a colleague familiar with the technique. Nurses should describe the equipment to be used during paracentesis to the patient. This may be more relevant when looking after a patient undergoing the procedure for the first time, to whom the size of the catheter used may be concerning.

Assessment and recording tools

A detailed nursing assessment is important when caring for patients requiring paracentesis. Nurses should pay particular attention to the cause of the ascites and the frequency with which the procedure is occurring. The involvement of the palliative care team can at this stage be indicated. As well as assessing the patient's psychological wellbeing, nurses must pay attention to the skin condition and pain levels.

In preparation for the paracentesis, nurses should measure the patient's girth around the umbilicus and check the patient's weight before the procedure. The same chart should be used to record all subsequent measurements so a comparison can be made.

Pharmacological support

The health professional performing the paracentesis must use a local anaesthetic, and lidocaine at the concentration of 1% is often the drug of choice. The lidocaine is injected subcutaneously initially with a 25 G needle and subsequently with a 23 G needle until optimal pain control is achieved, not to exceed the maximum dose of 4.5 mg/kg (or 200 mg). Optimal pain control can take between 2 and 5 minutes after the drug is injected and it is important for the practitioner to assess the effectiveness of the local anaesthetic before starting the procedure. Lorazepam at a dose of 1 mg can be of benefit prior to the procedure for patients who are anxious, due to its muscle relaxant and anxiolytic effects.

Non-pharmacological support

Nurses should enquire about the patient's fears and concerns regarding paracentesis. For some patients, music, relaxation and visualization techniques are of great benefit so the use of these approaches should be considered, if available.

Specific patient preparation

Education

Nursing interventions for patients undergoing abdominal paracentesis include education about the nature of the procedure, what results can realistically be expected, and the risks and benefits. Information should also be given about post-procedure care of the puncture site and about the importance of diet and fluid intake to replace proteins and fluid lost in the ascitic fluid. It is essential that the patient, their family and their carers are involved in the discussion so that an informed and joint decision may be made in order to achieve the best possible outcome.

Procedure guideline 11.3 Abdominal paracentesis

Essential equipment

- Personal protective equipment (including sterile gloves, sterile drapes and sterile gown)
- Sterile abdominal paracentesis set (Figure 11.10) containing forceps, scalpel blade and blade holder, swabs, towels, suturing equipment, trocar access needle and cannula (or other approved catheter and introducer), connector to attach to the cannula to direct the fluid into the container (Figure 11.10)
- Sterile dressing pack
- Sterile receiver
- Sterile specimen pots
- Local anaesthetic
- Needles and syringes
- Chlorhexidine 0.5% in 70% alcohol
- Adhesive dressing
- Large sterile drainage bag or container (with connector if appropriate to attach to cannula)
- Gate clamps
- Sharps bin
- Weighing scales
- Tape measure

Action	Rationale
Pre-procedure	
1 Introduce yourself to the patient, explain and discuss the procedure with them, and gain their consent to proceed.	To ensure that the patient feels at ease, understands the procedure and gives their valid consent (NMC 2018, **C**).
2 Ask the patient to empty their bladder.	If the bladder is full there is a chance of it being punctured when the trocar access needle is introduced (McGibbon et al. 2007, **E**).
3 Weigh the patient before the procedure and record their weight.	To assess weight changes and fluid loss. **E**
4 Ensure privacy.	To maintain dignity (NMC 2018, **C**).
5 Measure the patient's girth around the umbilicus before the procedure and record it. Mark the position on the abdomen where the drain will be inserted using a skin marker.	To provide an indication of fluid shift and how much fluid has reaccumulated. **E**
6 Help the patient to lie supine in bed with their head raised 45–50 cm with a backrest.	Normally the pressure in the peritoneal cavity is no greater than atmospheric pressure; however, when fluid is present, pressure becomes greater than atmospheric pressure. This position will aid gravity in the removal of fluid and the fluid will drain of its own accord until the pressure is equalized. **E**

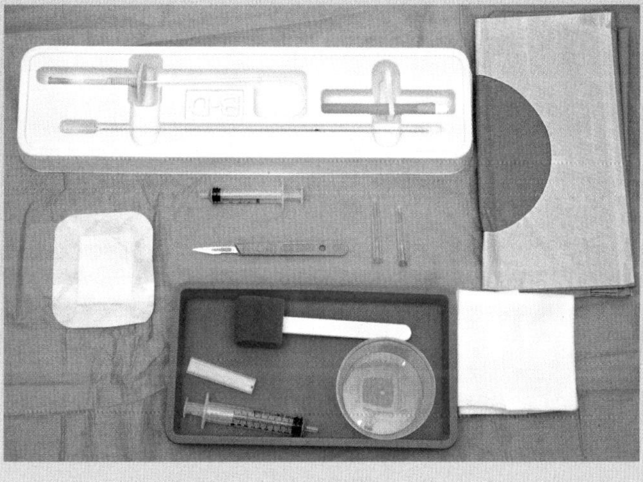

Figure 11.10 Example of sterile equipment tray for abdominal paracentesis.

(continued)

Procedure guideline 11.3 Abdominal paracentesis (continued)

Action	Rationale
Procedure	
7 Decontaminate hands.	To minimize the risk of contamination (NHS Improvement 2019, **C**).
8 Perform the procedure using an aseptic technique. Always perform the procedure in hospital with a second, appropriately trained person.	To minimize the risk of contamination. **E** To ensure patient safety at all times. **E**
9 Bring the equipment to the bedside on a clean trolley. Remove the sterile abdominal paracentesis pack from its outer wrapping and open it on the trolley.	To minimize the risk of infection. **E**
10 Lay out the remaining equipment except the personal protective equipment.	To facilitate access to the equipment. **E** To create a clean working area. **E**
11 Put on sterile personal protective equipment.	To protect the professional and patient from the risks of cross-infection (NHS Improvement 2019, **C**).
12 Clean hands with an alcohol-based handrub.	To minimize the risk of infection. (NHS Improvement 2019, **C**).
13 Clean the skin thoroughly at the marked site for the paracentesis with an antiseptic or alcohol solution, and allow it to dry. Drape the area with sterile towels.	To reduce the risk of local and/or systemic infection. The peritoneal cavity is normally sterile. **E**
14 Administer a local anaesthetic.	To minimize pain during the procedure. **E**
15 Once the anaesthetic has taken effect, the practitioner performing the procedure should make an incision into the skin of the abdomen where previously marked.	To minimize pain during the procedure and thus maximize patient comfort and facilitate co-operation. **E**
16 The trocar and cannula are inserted via the incision.	To ensure correct insertion of the trocar and cannula. **E**
17 The trocar is removed and disposed of in a sharps container.	To reduce the risk of accidental needle stick injury (NHS Employers 2015, **C**).
18 Attach the closed drainage system to the cannula using a connector if appropriate. Apply a dry dressing to ensure the drain exit site is protected and the drain is taped firmly in position.	A sterile container with a non-return valve is necessary to maintain sterility. **E**
19 Collect ascitic fluid from the cannula with a syringe (20–100 mL as instructed by the practitioner) and send it for cytology.	If necessary, in order to diagnose the cause of ascites (Huang et al. 2014, **E**).
20 If the cannula is to remain in position, sutures may be inserted, by the practitioner, adjacent to the cannula and looped around it to prevent it becoming dislodged and to prevent local trauma to the patient.	To ensure the cannula remains *in situ*. To reduce the risk of trauma to the patient. **E**
Post-procedure	
21 Dispose of equipment as per local policy.	To reduce the risk of environmental contamination (Loveday et al. 2014, **R**).
22 Monitor the patient's blood pressure, pulse and respirations hourly.	To observe for signs of shock and/or infection. **E**
23 Weigh the patient after the procedure and record their weight.	To assess weight changes and fluid loss. **E**
24 Measure the patient's girth around the umbilicus after the procedure and record it.	This provides an indication of fluid shift and how much fluid has reaccumulated. **E**
25 Observe the rate and nature of the drainage. Reduce the flow of fluid by clamping the drain if the patient complains of abdominal pain.	To ensure safe and unobstructed drainage. **E**
26 Monitor the patient's fluid balance daily, reviewing the intake and output. Review biochemistry results daily.	After removal of large amounts of peritoneal fluid, fluid moves from the vascular space and reaccumulates in the peritoneal cavity. Ascitic fluid contains protein in addition to sodium and potassium. Problems relating to dehydration and electrolyte imbalance may be present. **E**

Problem-solving table 11.1 Prevention and resolution (Procedure guideline 11.3)

Problem	Cause	Prevention	Suggested action
Patient exhibits shock	Major circulatory shift of fluid or sudden release of intra-abdominal pressure, vasodilation and subsequent lowering of blood pressure	Monitor blood pressure and consider administration of intravenous fluid if volumes larger than 5 L are expected to drain.	Clamp the drainage tube with a gate clamp to prevent further fluid loss. Record the patient's vital signs. Refer to the medical staff for immediate intervention.
Cessation of drainage of ascitic fluid	Abdomen is empty of ascitic fluid		Check the total output of ascitic fluid given on the patient's fluid balance chart. Measure the patient's girth; compare this measurement with the pre-abdominal paracentesis measurement. Suggest to the medical staff that the cannula should be removed. Discontinue the drainage system.
	Patient's position is inhibiting drainage	Teach the patient to avoid exerting pressure on the drainage tubing.	Assist the patient to change position – ideally to sit upright or to lie on their side to encourage flow by gravity. Encourage the patient to mobilize.
	The ascitic fluid has clotted in the drainage system	Keep the drainage bag on a stand and lower than the puncture site to facilitate drainage by gravity.	'Milk' the tubing. If this is unsuccessful, change the drainage system aseptically. Refer to the medical staff.
Cannula becomes dislodged	Ineffective sutures or trauma at the puncture site	Collaborate with medical staff when applying the suture or alternatively apply a secure dressing. The tube can be taped to the skin further down to prevent pulling with movement at the puncture site.	Apply a secure, dry dressing. Reassure the patient. Inform the medical staff.
Pain	Pressure of ascites or position of drain	Offer analgesia 30 minutes prior to the procedure. Apply the dressing in such a way as to allow enough padding around the puncture site but avoid drain movement within the abdomen.	Identify the cause. Anchor the drain securely to avoid pulling at the insertion site or movement within the abdomen. Assist the patient with repositioning. Administer an appropriate prescribed analgesic; monitor the patient's response and inform medical staff.

Post-procedural considerations

Immediate care

Observations must be carried out every 30 minutes for 2 hours and hourly for 4 hours to detect early signs of shock, cardiovascular compromise and infection so that medical staff can be informed and action can be taken promptly. Drainage of the fluid must be monitored regularly, volumes recorded on a fluid balance chart and blockages detected and managed. Patients may require assistance to move and position themselves, and they may experience pain, requiring careful repositioning or appropriate analgesia.

All paracentesis should be completed as rapidly as possible and all ascetic drains should be removed within 4 to 6 hours of commencing the paracentesis to prevent infection (Moore 2015). The patient's renal function should be checked following this procedure to ensure that any signs of dehydration or pre-renal failure are treated as early as possible.

Patients should be informed that leakage following removal of the drain may happen and should be reported promptly.

Complications

Bleeding

Haemorrhagic complications of paracentesis are generally divided into three groups: abdominal wall hematoma, pseudoaneurysm and haemoperitoneum. The likelihood of requiring a transfusion following paracentesis is about 0.3% (Sharzehi et al. 2014).

Abdominal wall hematoma is the most frequently occurring haemorrhagic complication. Pseudoaneurysms of the inferior epigastric artery represent two-thirds of all of these haemorrhagic complications. Haemoperitoneum, which is usually the result of injury to a mesenteric varix, is responsible for close to one-third of these complications (Sharzehi et al. 2014).

Paracentesis-induced circulatory dysfunction

The removal of large fluid volumes may result in impaired circulatory function for up to 6 days after paracentesis. Paracentesis-induced circulatory dysfunction (PICD) is clinically silent and not spontaneously reversible. The occurrence of PICD is associated with rapid recurrence of ascites, renal failure and a significant decrease in the probability of survival (Annamalai et al. 2016).

Local infection or peritonitis

There is the risk of introducing infection into the ascitic fluid, which can be minimized by the use of sterile technique. A swab from the site of the cannula should be obtained for culture review and a dry dressing applied.

Bowel or bladder perforation

This risk is decreased by ensuring the patient has an empty bladder and avoiding sites of scarring on the abdomen when inserting the cannula, as these may indicate internal adhesions between the bowel and peritoneum.

Terminal sedation

Definition

Palliative sedation can be defined as a controlled induction of sedation, sometimes to the point of unconsciousness, to relieve the severe, refractory suffering of a terminally ill patient (Krakauer 2015, Twycross 2019). It is important to distinguish between normal palliative sedation and deep sedation. Normal sedation occurs commonly at the end of life for a variety of reasons. Deep sedation is for severe suffering that is refractory to all reasonable and aggressive treatment including normal sedation (Prado et al. 2018, Twycross 2019).

Evidence-based approaches

The most fundamental task of palliative medicine is to relieve suffering (Cassel 1982). For some patients, suffering continues to be uncontrolled despite specialist measures employed to relieve it. Controlled sedation can on rare occasions be the only effective way to relieve the patient's anguish (Krakauer 2015).

Pre-procedural considerations

Recognition that the patient is dying and is in the final hours or days of life is paramount to providing effective terminal sedation. For a patient to be considered for sedation, they must be deemed to be suffering from one or more severe physical or neuropsychiatric symptoms, including but not limited to pain, dyspnoea, vomiting, seizures, agitated delirium, anxiety or depression. The symptoms must be refractory to standard palliative interventions such as medications, nerve blocks, palliative radiotherapy or other treatments offered by specialists in pain and psychiatry. Comfort must be the most important goal of the patient's care (Krakauer 2015). A DNaCPR order should be in place and the decision to sedate should be discussed with the patient where possible, as well as the family. It is also imperative to consult the wider multidisciplinary team in order to ensure any concerns are discussed. This procedure involves the support of a specialist palliative care team. Where deep sedation is considered, the expertise of an anaesthetist may be necessary.

Procedure guideline 11.4 Terminal sedation

Essential equipment

- Personal protective equipment
- Sedatives
- Necessary administration equipment (e.g. needles, syringes, appropriate flushing agents, subcutaneous cannula)
- Syringe pump (if applicable)

Action	Rationale
Pre-procedure	
1 Consider and exclude any physiological issues that may be causing agitation (such as urinary retention, constipation or pain). Treat any issues identified; if agitation continues, consider this to be terminal agitation and continue to step 2.	To ensure distress cannot be attributed to any other cause and to confirm it is terminal restlessness (Krakauer 2015, **C**).
2 Consider a single room if the patient is in hospital depending on the previous wishes of the patient.	To ensure privacy and dignity is maintained and the ambience in the room remains peaceful (NICE 2017a, **C**). A single room may allow a family member to stay, and it may be reassuring for the patient to hear a familiar voice (Krakauer 2015, **C**; Williams and Gardiner 2015, **P**).
3 Perform a mental capacity assessment and (if appropriate) make a best interest decision (see Chapter 5: Communication, psychological wellbeing and safeguarding).	To ensure that the patient's capacity is assessed and documented and that any best interest decisions are clearly documented (NICE 2018a, **C**).
4 If appropriate, introduce yourself to the patient (if not then to their family). Explain and discuss the procedure and the need for terminal sedation with the patient and/or their family, and gain their consent to proceed. Discussions with the wider multidisciplinary team caring for the patient may also be necessary.	To ensure the patient's wishes are met and to involve them in decision making and giving consent where possible (NMC 2018, **C**). Clear communication with the family will also aid their understanding and acceptance (Krakauer 2015, **C**).
Procedure	
5 Administer sedative medications as prescribed. Common medications include benzodiazepines (e.g. lorazepam, midazolam, clonazepam) and/or antipsychotics (e.g. levomepromazine, haloperidol, olanzapine). In deep sedation, medications such as phenobarbital and propofol may be considered by a specialist palliative care team.	To ensure agitation is controlled as quickly as possible (Krakauer 2015, **C**; Lacey 2015, **C**).
Post-procedure	
6 Evaluate the effectiveness of the medications and review the dose regularly.	To implement adequate dosing to ensure patient comfort (Krakauer 2015; **C**, Lacey 2015, **C**).

Verification and certification of death

Definition

Verification of death involves determining whether a person is deceased (RCN 2019b), formally documenting this, and notifying the necessary parties of any infectious illnesses and/or implantable devices. The time the death is verified is recognized as the official time of death (Wilson 2015).

Certification of death is the legal recording of a death and is achieved by the completion of the Medical Certificate of Cause of Death (MCCD). This is done by a medical practitioner in accordance with the Births and Deaths Registration Act (1953). The medical practitioner completing the certificate must have seen the patient in the 14 days preceding the death or seen the body after death (Wilson 2015).

Clinical governance

Only medical practitioners can certify a death; however, specifically trained nursing staff can confirm or verify an expected death. National guidance and competencies are available. Once they have been deemed competent, a nurse is able to undertake this procedure independently (Hospice UK 2019, Laverty et al. 2018). It is hoped that this guidance will prevent untimely delays in the verification process and thus help to support the family and loved ones at a difficult time.

Pre-procedural considerations

Verification of expected death will require the nurse to assess the patient for a minimum of 5 minutes to establish that irreversible cardiorespiratory arrest has occurred. Any spontaneous return of cardiac or respiratory activity during this period of observation should prompt a further 5 minutes of observation (Hospice UK 2019).

Procedure guideline 11.5 Verification of death

Essential equipment

- Personal protective equipment
- Magnet (if required; to deactivate an implanted cardiac defibrillator)
- Stethoscope
- Pen torch

Action	Rationale
Pre-procedure	
1 Check for completed DNaCPR documentation.	To ensure cardiopulmonary resuscitation should not be commenced (Hospice UK 2019, **C**).
2 Correctly identify the patient by cross-referencing the details on the patient's wristband with clinical records.	To correctly identify the deceased (Hospice UK 2019, **C**).
3 Identify from the clinical notes any infectious diseases, radioactive implants or implantable medical devices.	To ensure the safety of any staff involved in care after death (Hospice UK 2019, **C**).
4 Instigate the process for deactivation of any implanted cardiac defibrillator (ICD) if not already deactivated.	To ensure the timely deactivation of the ICD and to avoid it delivering defibrillation to the deceased patient (Beattie 2013, **C**).
5 Apply personal protective equipment.	To ensure the protection of the caregiver and to comply with infection control procedures (NHS Improvement 2019, **C**).
Procedure	
6 Lie the patient flat. Leave all tubes, lines, drains, medication patches and infusions *in situ*. Switch off pumps.	To ensure the patient is flat ahead of rigor mortis and that all treatments are *in situ* ahead of verifying death (Hospice UK 2019, **C**).
7 Assess for cessation of the circulatory system; feel for a carotid (or central) pulse for at least 1 full minute.	To ensure there are no signs of cardiac output (Hospice UK 2019, **C**; WHO 2017, **C**).
8 Listen to heart sounds with a stethoscope for at least 1 full minute.	To ensure there are no signs of cardiac output (Hospice UK 2019, **C**; WHO 2017, **C**).
9 Assess for cessation of the respiratory system; auscultate the lungs with a stethoscope for at least 1 full minute to verify there are no breath sounds or respiratory effort.	To ensure there are no visible respirations (Hospice UK 2019, **C**; WHO 2017, **C**).
10 Assess for cessation of cerebral function; using a pen torch, assess the pupils for reactivity to light. Both pupils should be fixed (not reacting to light or to any other stimulus) and dilated.	To ensure there is no cerebral activity (Hospice UK 2019, **C**; WHO 2017, **C**).
11 Apply painful stimuli by performing a trapezius squeeze; there should be no response to this.	To ensure no cerebral activity (Hospice UK 2019, **C**; WHO 2017, **C**).
12 Wait with the patient for at least 5 minutes.	To ensure no spontaneous return of cardiac or respiratory function (WHO 2017, **C**).
13 If the patient has an unexpected response to the tests above or there are any signs of life, repeat the procedure and assess the patient for a further 5 minutes.	To ensure or confirm that death has occurred (WHO 2017, **C**).
Post-procedure	
14 Once verification has been made, this should be documented according to local trust guidance. Time of death is recorded when verification of death is completed (i.e. not when the death is first reported).	To ensure legible documentation and legal requirements are met (Hospice UK 2019, **C**; NMC 2018, **C**).
15 Follow trust guidance on who to inform of the death (this will usually include the patient's family or next of kin, the consultant, the GP, the community nursing teams and patient liaison).	To ensure consistent communication. **E**

Source: Reproduced with permission of the authors: Jo Wilson, Dr Di Laverty and Marie Cooper.

Post-procedural considerations

Unexpected deaths must be confirmed by a medical doctor (and usually a senior medical doctor). Confirmation of death must be recorded in the clinical notes. If the death is suspicious or unexplained, a special forensic post-mortem may be required, in which case the family and carers will only be able to view the body with the agreement of the police and coroner. In many instances the restrictions will be minimal; however, if the death is thought to be suspicious, it is important that forensic evidence is not contaminated; there should therefore be no removal of indwelling devices or other such equipment from the patient (Wilson 2015).

Infectious patients

The practitioner who verified the death is responsible for ascertaining whether the person had a known or suspected infection and whether this is notifiable. Guidance is available from the Health and Safety Executive (HSE 2018).

Care after death (last offices)

Definition

'Care after death' has historically been referred to as 'last offices', a term related to the Latin *officium*, meaning 'service' or 'duty', which was associated with the military. This term also has religious connotations from its association with 'last rites', a Christian sacrament and prayer administered to the dying (Quested and Rudge 2003). It is used to refer to the final act performed on a person's body.

Related theory

Care after death is the final act a nurse will carry out for a patient and remains associated with ritual (Wilson 2015). Nursing care for a patient who has died has historical roots dating back to the 19th century (Wolf 1988). However, contemporary nursing practice has moved away from the ritualistic practices of cleansing, plugging, packing and tying the patient's orifices (to prevent the leakage of body fluids) to encompass much more than simply dealing with a dead body (Wilson 2015).

Consideration must be given to legal issues surrounding death, the removal (or non-removal) of equipment, washing and grooming, and ensuring correct identification of the patient (Wilson 2015). National guidance emphasizes the importance of care after a patient has died, and in particular highlights the value of managing the necessary paperwork and procedure following the patient's death as well as psychosocial care (NEoLCP 2015). Being treated with dignity is an underlying premise of achieving a 'good death', and a 'good death' encompasses all stages of dying and death (Wilson 2015); this principle, therefore, continues after death.

Carrying out such an intimate act, which in many cultures would be carried out only by certain family or community members, requires careful consideration by nurses and adequate preparation. This can include family members, religious leaders and/or others, depending on patient and family wishes and religion. Every effort should be made to accommodate the wishes of the patient's relatives (Wilson 2015).

For nurses, care after death is a continuation of the care delivered in life (Martin and Bristowe 2015); it should be seen as a privilege and treated with the utmost sensitivity. There is only one chance to get it right so it is imperative that nurses ensure the wishes of the family and carers are, where possible, adhered to. Guidance is available to assist nurses with this complex aspect of care (Wilson 2015). This guidance encourages nurses to honour the integrity of the person who has died and places the deceased and their carers central to the care being delivered while taking into consideration any legal aspects at this time (Wilson 2015). Personal care after death should be carried out within 2–4 hours of the person dying to preserve their appearance, condition and dignity (unless the death has been referred to the coroner or for religious reasons this should not occur).

Care after death can have symbolic meaning for nurses, often providing a sense of closure. It can be a fulfilling experience as it is the final demonstration of respectful, sensitive care given to a patient (Olausson and Ferrell 2013).

Many parts of the nursing procedures relating to care after death are based on principles of infection prevention and control. Care of the patient who has died must therefore take into account health and safety guidelines to ensure families, healthcare workers, mortuary staff and undertakers are not put at risk. Local guidelines should be adhered to with respect to ensuring safety for staff involved in care after death.

Evidence-based approaches

Rationale

Indications

Care after death is indicated:

- when a patient's death has been verified and documented
- for adult patients who have died in hospital or in a hospice.

Contraindications

There are no absolute contraindications. However, in the following circumstances, seek further guidance before undertaking care after death:

- if the patient who has died is referred to the coroner and/or for post-mortem (Box 11.7)
- if the patient who has died is a candidate for organ donation.

Clinical governance

Nurses should be aware of the legal requirements for care of patients after death as it is essential that correct procedures are followed (Wilson 2015). It is particularly important that nurses are aware of deaths that require referral to the coroner (Box 11.7) as this will facilitate the correct personal care and enable nurses to prepare the family for both a potential delay in the processing of the Medical Certificate of Cause of Death (MCCD) and the possibility of a post-mortem examination (Wilson 2015). If the death is going to be referred to the coroner, the patient's body should remain untouched. This includes leaving invasive lines and devices in situ. The patient must not be washed in case evidence is destroyed (Wilson 2015).

If the death was expected and there is no need for a referral to the coroner, local guidance should be sought as to the most appropriate person to proceed to remove lines and tubes from the patient. In some areas this will be the healthcare staff at the bedside during care after death; however, in some areas this is the responsibility of the mortician.

Guidance relating to vulnerable adults is available (Mental Capacity Act 2005). If after death safeguarding issues are raised, it is important to follow local policy and ensure that concerns are communicated with relevant agencies, such as Social Services, the police and the coroner.

Box 11.7 Reasons for referral to a coroner

A post-mortem examination, also known as an autopsy, is the examination of a body after death. The aim of a post-mortem is to determine the cause of death. In most cases, a doctor or the police refer a death to the coroner if:

- the death was unexpected, such as the sudden death of a baby (cot death)
- the cause appears violent, unnatural or suspicious, such as a suicide or drug overdose
- the death is the result of an accident or injury
- the death occurred during or soon after a hospital procedure, such as surgery, and the cause of death is unknown.

Out-of-hours death

Where a death is expected to occur out of hours and for religious reasons the funeral will need to take place immediately after death, it is the responsibility of the medical team to ensure that the on-call doctor is notified so that they can review the dying patient at the start of their shift and be able to complete the Medical Certificate of Confirmation of Death when death occurs. It is hoped that any cultural and religious guidance needed will have been ascertained with the patient and family through advance care planning in the event of an expected death (Wilson 2015).

In some exceptional cases, a family member or next of kin may be unable to wait over a weekend to meet with regular staff who would support the administrative process and guide the family. In these circumstances, the family or next of kin should be offered the following:

- Medical Certificate of Cause of Death (MCCD)
- any information the organization or trust has on what to do in the event of someone dying
- directions to the Register Office
- information on how to register a death
- hospital documentation to give to the undertakers formalizing release of the patient's body from the hospital
- information regarding bereavement support.

Infectious diseases

The Health and Safety Executive has issued guidelines on the handling of the deceased with infections; nurses, doctors and other healthcare professionals should be aware of related local infection-control policies and reporting responsibilities (HSE 2018). It is vital that processes are in place to protect confidentiality, which continues after death, but this does not prevent the use of sensible rules to safeguard the health and safety of all those who care for the deceased.

Families and carers should also be supported in adhering to infection prevention and control procedures if they wish to assist in personal care after the death of an infectious patient. There are a few, very rare, exceptions when it is not possible for families to participate.

Porters, mortuary staff, undertakers and those involved with the care of patients who have died must also be informed if there is a possibility of infection. In all cases, local policies and guidelines should be followed.

Pre-procedural considerations

Family involvement

Some families and carers may wish to assist with personal care after death, and within certain cultures it may be unacceptable for anyone other than a family member or religious leader to wash the patient (Wilson 2015). It may also be necessary for somebody of the same sex as the patient to undertake personal care after death (Henry and Wilson 2012, Martin and Bristowe 2015, Rodgers et al. 2016). Families and carers should be supported and encouraged to participate if possible as this may help to facilitate the grieving process. If children are involved, nurses should be mindful of their needs and should consider the physical environment.

Families may request specific items to accompany the patient who has died to the mortuary and funeral home. These might be items of sentimental value or items of jewellery. This should be discussed with the family and next of kin, documented and witnessed in accordance with local policy.

Additional considerations

It is important to inform other patients of the death, particularly if the person has died in an area where other people are present (such as a bay or open ward) and might know the patient. Residents in communal settings, such as care homes and prisons, have often built significant relationships with other residents (Wilson 2015). It is important to consider how to address their needs within the boundaries of patient confidentiality, being careful not to provide information about the cause and reason for death (Wilson 2015).

Finally, carry out all personal care after death in accordance with safe manual handling guidance and where possible within 4 hours of death. This is because rigor mortis can occur relatively soon after death, and this time is shortened in warmer environments (Wilson 2015). It is best practice to do this with two people, to ensure privacy and dignity are maintained and manual handling guidance is followed.

Procedure guideline 11.6 Care after death

Essential equipment

- Personal protective equipment
- Bowl of warm water, soap, patient's own toiletries, disposable washcloths and two towels
- Comb and equipment for nail care
- Equipment for mouth care including equipment for cleaning dentures
- Two identification labels
- Documents required by law and by organization/institution policy, for example Notification of Death cards
- Shroud or patient's personal clothing, such as night-dress, pyjamas, clothes previously requested by patient or clothes that comply with the deceased patient's wishes, the wishes of their family and any cultural wishes
- Body bag if required (if there is actual or potential leakage of body fluids and/or if there is infectious disease)
- Gauze, tape, dressings and bandages if there are wounds, puncture sites or intravenous or arterial devices
- Valuables/property book
- Plastic bags for clinical and domestic (household) waste
- Laundry skip and appropriate bags for soiled linen
- Clean bed linen
- Documentation for personal belongings
- Bags for the patient's personal possessions
- Disposable receptacle for collecting urine, if appropriate
- Sharps bin, if appropriate

Optional equipment

- Caps/spigots for urinary catheters (if catheters are to be left *in situ*)
- Additional equipment as needed for infectious diseases (per organizational policy)
- Suction equipment and absorbent pads (where there is the potential for leakage)

(continued)

Procedure guideline 11.6 Care after death (continued)

Action	Rationale
Pre-procedure	
1 Apply personal protective equipment. If the patient has an infectious disease, additional equipment such as gowns, masks or goggles may be required.	To ensure staff are protected from soiled sheets and body fluids (NHS Improvement 2019, **C**).
2 If the patient is on a pressure-relieving mattress or device, consult the manufacturer's instructions before switching it off.	If the mattress deflates too quickly, it may cause a manual handling challenge to the nurses carrying out care after death. **E**
Procedure	
3 Lay the patient on their back with their arms lying by their side. Straighten any limbs as far as possible (adhering to local manual handling policy and procedure). This should ideally be undertaken by two nurses.	To maintain the patient's privacy and dignity (NMC 2018, **C**). Stiff, flexed limbs can be difficult to fit into a mortuary trolley, mortuary fridge or coffin and can cause additional distress to any family or carers who wish to view the body. If there is a problem with straightening the limbs then the mortuary staff should be notified (Wilson 2015, **C**).
4 Remove all but one pillow. Close the mouth and support the jaw by placing a pillow or rolled-up towel on the chest or underneath the jaw. Do not bind the patient's jaw with bandages.	To avoid leaving pressure marks on the face, which can be difficult to remove (Wilson 2015, **C**).
5 When the death is *not* being referred to the coroner as per local policy *Either*: Remove mechanical aids such as syringe pumps, tubes, drains and venous access devices; dress any oozing sites; and document disposal of medication *Or*: Leave devices *in situ* (if this is the role of the mortician locally).	To minimize the number of healthcare-related devices with the aim of restoring the patient's usual appearance (as far as possible). **E**
6 Spigot any urinary catheters (if not removed already). Do not tie the penis. Use pads and pants to absorb any leakage from the urethra, vagina or rectum.	To prevent or manage any leakage (Wilson 2015, **C**).
7 Close the patient's eyes by applying light pressure to the eyelids for 30 seconds.	To maintain the patient's dignity (NMC 2018, **C**) and for aesthetic reasons. Closure of the eyelids will also provide tissue protection in case of corneal donation (Wilson 2015, **C**).
8 a Remove, prepare and/or bung lines and tubes (in some clinical areas this will be completed by the mortician) b Contain leakages from the oral cavity or tracheostomy sites by suctioning and positioning. c Suction and spigot nasogastric tubes (if not already removed). Cover exuding wounds or unhealed surgical incisions with a clean absorbent dressing and secure with an occlusive dressing. d Leave stitches and clips intact. e Cover stomas with a clean bag. Clamp drains (remove the bottles), pad around wounds and seal with an occlusive dressing. f Avoid waterproof, strongly adhesive tape as this can be difficult to remove at the funeral home and can leave a permanent mark.	Leaking orifices pose a health hazard to staff coming into contact with the patient's body (HSE 2018, **C**). Ensuring that the patient's body is clean will demonstrate continued respect for the patient's dignity. **E** It is the role of the mortuary staff to pack orifices, not the nurse. If the body continues to leak, place it on absorbent pads in a body bag and advise the mortuary or funeral director.
9 Exuding wounds and unhealed surgical scars should be covered with a clean, absorbent occlusive dressing. Stitches and clips should be left intact. Consider leaving intact recent surgical dressings for wounds that could potentially leak, for example large amputation wounds. Reinforcement of the dressing should be sufficient.	To aid the absorption of any leakage. **E**
10 Consider whether the family may wish to be involved in personal care of the deceased.	It can be an expression of respect and affection, and part of the process of adjusting to loss and expressing grief (Wilson 2015, **C**).
11 Wash the patient, unless requested not to do so for religious or cultural reasons; because the patient is being referred to the coroner; or because of the preferences of the patient, their family or carer. The deceased should not be shaved when still warm; this can be undertaken by the funeral director and it may be necessary to discuss this sensitively with the family.	To ensure dignity and respect for the deceased (NICE 2017b, **C**). Shaving when the deceased is still warm can cause bruising to the skin (Wilson 2015, **C**).

12 Clean the mouth to remove debris and secretions. Clean and replace dentures as soon as possible after death. If they cannot be replaced, send them with the body in a clearly identified receptacle.	To ensure the patient's dignity and to show respect. **E**
13 Tidy the hair as soon as possible after death and arrange it in the preferred style (if known).	This will guide the funeral director for final presentation (Wilson 2015, **C**).
14 Remove jewellery (in the presence of another member of staff) unless specifically requested by the family to do otherwise, and document this according to local policy. Secure any jewellery left on the patient with tape, documenting this according to local policy.	To ensure the patient's culture and wishes are respected (NICE 2017b, **C**).
15 Consider any religious ornaments that need to remain with the deceased (see Table 11.2).	To ensure the patient's culture and wishes are respected (NICE 2017b, **C**).
16 Dress the deceased appropriately, whether in pyjamas, hospital gowns or something they have chosen themselves. Be aware that soiling can occur.	For aesthetic reasons and to maintain dignity (NICE 2017b, **C**).
17 Clearly identify the deceased person with a name band on their wrist and/or ankle (avoid toe tags). As a minimum this needs to identify their name, date of birth, address, ward (if a hospital inpatient) and ideally their NHS number. The person responsible for identification is the person who verifies the death. Nurses should refer to local policies for the identification of deceased patients within their organization.	To ensure correct and easy identification of the patient's body in the mortuary (Wilson 2015, **C**).
18 Provided no leakage is expected and there is no notifiable disease present, the body can be wrapped in a sheet and taped lightly to ensure it can be moved safely. Do not bind the sheet or tape too tightly as this can cause disfigurement.	To maintain dignity without causing damage or disfigurement. **E**
19 Place the patient's body in a body bag if leakage of body fluids may be anticipated or if the patient has a known infectious disease.	To ensure the safe transfer of the patient to the mortuary, protecting any handlers (HSE 2018, **C**).
Post-procedure	
20 Request the portering staff to remove the patient's body from the hospital ward and transport it to the mortuary within 4 hours of death.	To allow refrigeration to take place (Henry and Wilson 2012, **C**).
21 Screen off the beds and area that will be passed as the patient's body is removed.	To ensure the privacy and dignity of the deceased on transfer from the place of death and to avoid causing unnecessary distress to other patients, relatives and staff (King's Fund 2008, **E**).
22 Remove personal protective equipment. Dispose of equipment according to local policy and wash hands.	To minimize the risk of cross-infection and contamination (NHS Improvement 2019, **C**).
23 Record all aspects of care after death in the nursing and medical documentation and identify the professionals involved. Update and organize the medical and nursing records as quickly as possible so they are available to the bereavement team and other relevant professionals, such as pathologists.	To record the time of death, the names of those present and the names of those informed (NMC 2018, **C**).
24 Transfer property and patient records to the appropriate administrative department.	To enable the administration process of giving the medical death certificate and to enable the patient's property to be returned to their family or friends. **E**

Problem-solving table 11.2 Prevention and resolution (Procedure guideline 11.6)

Problem	Cause	Prevention	Action
The family are not prepared for how the body will look and feel	Possible changes in how the patient may look following death	Prepare the family for how the person may look and feel. If the patient has died some time before the family views the body, advising them regarding how the skin may feel (cold) before they touch the patient will prepare them for this.	Meet with the family prior to reviewing the patient. Ensure the deceased has been checked before the family enter the room.

(continued)

Problem-solving table 11.2 Prevention and resolution (Procedure guideline 11.6) *(continued)*

Problem	Cause	Prevention	Action
Relatives or next of kin not contactable by telephone or by the GP	Out-of-date or missing contact information	Ensure next of kin contact information is documented and up to date.	Within the UK, local police will go to the next of kin's house. Abroad, the relevant British embassy will assist.
Death occurs within 24 hours of an operation		Ensure the patient is cared for and monitoring in the most appropriate setting following their surgery. If death occurs, ensure information around the circumstances of the death is documented and handed over to relevant healthcare staff (to prevent miscommunication).	All tubes and/or drains must be left in position. Spigot or cap off any cannulas or catheters. Treat stomas as open wounds. Leave any endotracheal or tracheostomy tubes in place. Machinery can be disconnected (discuss with coroner) but settings must be left untouched. Post-mortem examination will be required to establish the cause of death. Any tubes, drains and so on may have been a major contributing factor to the death.
Unexpected death		As above.	As above. Post-mortem examination of the patient's body will be required to establish the cause of death.
Unknown cause of death		As above.	As above.
Patient brought into hospital who is already deceased		Not preventable but where possible ensure patients' families are prepared for all eventualities, particularly for palliative care patients whose death is expected, and that family know who to call and what to do in the event of death.	As above, unless the patient has been seen by a medical practitioner within 14 days before their death. In this instance, the attending medical officer may complete the death certificate if they are clear as to the cause of death.
Patient dies after receiving systemic radioactive iodine	There is a potential risk of exposure to radiation (IPEM 2002)	Radiation protection should be undertaken.	Ensure those in contact with the patient's body are aware. Pregnant nurses should not carry out care after death for these patients.
Patient dies after insertion of gold grains, colloidal radioactive solution, caesium needles, caesium applicators, iridium wires or iridium hair pins	There is a potential risk of exposure to radiation (IPEM 2002)	Radiation protection should be undertaken when removing wires. The physicist may remove radioactive wires/needles and so on themselves, depending on source.	Inform the physics department as well as the appropriate medical staff. Once a doctor has verified death, the sources should be removed and placed in a lead container. A Geiger counter should be used to check that all sources have been removed. This reduces the radiation risk when completing care after death. Record the time and date of removal of the sources. Ensure those in contact with the patient's body are aware. Pregnant nurses should not carry out care after death for these patients.
Patient and/or relative wishes to donate organs or tissues for transplantation		Discussion around transplantation should occur with families or next of kin wherever appropriate (as deemed by clinical team). Exceptions apply.	Contact the local transplant co-ordinator as soon as the decision is made to donate organs or tissue and before care after death is attempted. Obtain verbal and written consent from the next of kin, as per local policy. Prepare the patient who has died as per the transplant co-ordinator's instructions. For further guidance see www.organdonation.nhs.uk.
Patient to be moved straight from ward to undertakers			Contact senior nurse for hospital. Contact local Register Office as a certificate for burial or cremation (often called the 'green document') needs to be obtained. Liaise with chosen funeral directors and the deceased's family. Perform care after death as per religious, cultural and family wishes. Obtain written authority from the next of kin for removal of the person by the funeral directors. Document all actions and proceedings (Travis 2002).

Problem	Cause	Prevention	Action
Relatives want to see the person who has died after removal from the ward			Inform the mortuary staff in order to allow time for them to prepare the body. Occasionally nurses might be required to undertake this preparation in institutions where there are no mortuary staff. The patient's body will normally be placed in the hospital viewing room. A nurse should accompany the family and stay in the area to support the family.
The patient has an implantable cardiac device (deactivation of implantable cardiac defibrillators needs to be considered when the patient is recognized as entering the end-of-life phase)		Knowledge of device being *in situ* prior to death.	Nurses must inform funeral directors and mortuary staff about patients with an implantable cardiac device and ensure it is clearly documented (Wilson 2015, **C**).

Post-procedural considerations

Ensure that all the information outlined in Box 11.8 is available for the mortuary staff and funeral directors.

Immediate care

Since there is a time limit on how long a patient should remain in the heat of a ward (there could potentially be early onset of rigor mortis), nurses will have to exercise discretion over when to organize the transfer of the patient to the mortuary. This will vary according to family circumstances (there could be a delay in a relative travelling to the ward or area) and the ward situation (e.g. the availability of beds). As a general rule, 4 hours would be considered the upper limit for a patient to remain in the ward area once care after death has been completed (Wilson 2015).

Viewing the patient

Families may wish to view the patient in a viewing room. It is important to ensure that the patient is in a presentable state before taking the family to see them.

Bereavement support

The bereaved family may find it difficult to comprehend the death of their family member and it can take great sensitivity and skill to support them at this time. Explaining all procedures as fully as possible can help families to understand the practices that happen at the end of life. Offering bereavement care services may be useful to families for that difficult period immediately after death and in the future. National services such as Cruse Bereavement Care (www.cruse.org.uk) can be useful if local services are not known. There may be extreme distress; this is a difficult situation to handle and other family members are likely to be of most comfort and support at this point. Distressed family members may wish for their GP to be contacted.

Box 11.8 Information required by mortuary staff and funeral directors

- Identifying information, including the patient's name, date of birth, address and NHS number
- Date and time of death
- Any implantable devices that are present
- Any current radioactive treatments
- Any notifiable infections
- Any jewellery or religious mementoes left on the deceased
- Name and signature of registered nurse responsible for the care after death
- Name and signature of any second healthcare professional who assisted with the care

Source: Adapted from Wilson (2015).

Education of the patient and relevant others

Helping the family to understand procedures after death in the role of many people in hospital but primarily this will fall upon those who first meet with the family after their relative has died. Most hospitals and other healthcare settings will have developed local guidance around informing families and friends regarding the process that is followed after death. If the family suggest that they feel the death was unnatural or even that it was interfered with, professionals have a responsibility to explore these feelings and even outline the family's legal entitlement to request a post-mortem.

Before taking the family and friends to see the patient, prepare them for what they might see. Then, proceed to:

- Invite the family into the bed space or room.
- Accompany the family but respect their need for privacy should they require it.
- Anticipate questions.
- Offer the family the opportunity to discuss care (at that time or in the future).
- Offer to contact relatives on behalf of the family.
- Advise the family about the bereavement support services that can be accessed.
- Arrange an appointment with facilities or the patient liaison service.
- Provide the family with a point of contact with the hospital.

Some families may wish for a memento of the patient, such as a lock of hair. Try to anticipate and accommodate these wishes as much as possible.

Nominated next of kin requirements post-death

Local administrative processes following the death of a patient will vary and local policy and procedures should be followed. For patients who die in hospital, the next of kin to whom the medical certification of death has been given should then proceed to register the death. Once this is completed, they can proceed to make contact with an undertaker depending on the wishes of the patient in terms of burial or cremation. In some circumstances a family may wish for the body to be repatriated home. Most hospital trusts will offer written guidance on this with additional support services that may be available for bereavement support.

In the event of no next of kin being identified by the patient, healthcare staff should notify those identified in their local policy who will be responsible for registering the death at the Registry Office and liaising with the appropriate funeral directors to organize a contract funeral, if necessary. Contract funerals are organized by the local authority. Under Section 46 of the Public Health (Control of Disease) Act (1984), the council has a statutory obligation to carry out the funeral arrangements of a person who dies within the local area where there is no one else willing or able to deal with the funeral arrangements, for whatever reason.

Support of nursing staff and others

End-of-life care has been described as challenging, complex and emotionally demanding but, if staff have the necessary knowledge, skills and attitudes, it can be one of the most important and rewarding areas of care (Lacey 2015). Providing end-of-life care can expose staff to risks of emotional burnout and psychological stress (Lacey 2015). To prevent this, a supportive and nurturing environment for all those who provide end-of-life care is necessary. Pattison (2011) agrees, stating that the practical and emotional support needed by staff cannot be overestimated. She advises that this can be provided by mentorship and clinical supervision as well as staff counselling but warns that consideration needs to be given to workload and skill mix to enable this to take place. This support should extend to doctors and all members of the multidisciplinary team because the emotional implications of dealing with end-of-life care affect all (Lacey 2015).

The palliative care team can be a useful resource in providing informal teaching and educational support for staff relating to end-of-life care issues. This is often achieved via joint patient care or meetings with family members. This experiential learning can be valuable, especially for junior team members, who may have more confidence to ask questions on a one-to-one basis.

Websites

Citizens Advice Bureau
www.citizensadvice.org.uk

Coordinate My Care
https://www.coordinatemycare.co.uk

Cruse Bereavement Care
www.cruse.org.uk

NHS Organ Donation
www.organdonation.nhs.uk

References

Abraham, J. (2008) Acupressure and acupuncture in preventing and managing postoperative nausea and vomiting in adults. *Journal of Perioperative Practice*, 18(12), 543–551.

Ahearn, D.J., Nidh, N., Kallat, A., et al. (2013) Offering older hospitalised patients the choice to die in their preferred place. *Postgraduate Medical Journal*, 89, 30–34.

AHPCC (Association of Hospice and Palliative Care Chaplains) (2013) *Guidelines for Hospice and Palliative Care Chaplaincy*. Available at: www.ahpcc.org.uk/wp-content/uploads/2013/03/guidelines2012.pdf

Annamalai, A., Wisdom, L., Herada, M., et al. (2016) Management of refractory ascites in cirrhosis: Are we out of date? *World Journal of Hepatology*, 8(8), 1182–1193.

Arthur, J., Hui, D., Reddy, S. & Bruera, E. (2012) Till death do us part: Getting married at the end of life. *Journal of Pain and Symptom Management*, 44(3), 466–470.

Baile, W., Buckman, R., Lenzi, R., et al. (2000) SPIKES: A six-step protocol for delivering bad news – Application to the patient with cancer. *Oncologist*, 5(4), 302–311.

Baile, W. & Parker, P.A. (2017) Breaking bad news. In: Kissane, D., Bultz, B., Butow, C., et al. (eds) *Oxford Textbook of Communication in Oncology and Palliative Care*, 2nd edn. Oxford: Oxford University Press, pp.71–76.

Barnes, H., McDonald, J., Smallwood, N. & Manser, R. (2016) Opioids for the palliation of refractory breathlessness in adults with advanced disease and terminal illness. *Cochrane Database of Systematic Reviews*, 31(3), CD011008.

Beattie, J. (2013) *ICD Deactivation at the End of Life: Principles and Practice.* British Heart Foundation. Available at: https://www.bhf.org.uk/-/media/files/publications/hcps/icd-deactivation.pdf

Ben Aharon, I., Paul, M., Leibovici, L. & Stemmer, S.M. (2008) Interventions for alleviating cancer-related dyspnea: A systematic review. *Journal of Clinical Oncology*, 26(14), 2396–2404.

Bennett, S. (2009) Antiemetics: Uses, mode of action and prescribing rationale. *Nurse Prescribing*, 7(2), 63–70.

Births and Deaths Registration Act (1953) Available at: www.legislation.gov.uk/ukpga/Eli2/1-2/20

BMA (British Medical Association), RC (Resuscitation Council) & RCN (Royal College of Nursing) (2016) *Decisions Relating to Cardiopulmonary Resuscitation*, 3rd edn, rev. Available at: https://www.resus.org.uk/dnacpr/decisions-relating-to-cpr

BNF (British National Formulary) (2019) *British National Formulary.* National Institute for Health and Care Excellence. Available at: https://bnf.nice.org.uk

Booth, S., Galbraith, S., Ryan, R., et al. (2016) The importance of the feasibility study: Lessons from a study of the hand-held fan used to relieve dyspnoea in people who are breathless at rest. *Palliative Medicine*, 30(5), 504–509.

Booth, S., Moffat, C., Burkin, J., et al. (2011) Non-pharmacological interventions for breathlessness. *Current Opinion in Supportive and Palliative Care*, 5(2), 77–86.

Bruera, E., Hui D., Dalal, S., et al. (2013) Parenteral hydration in patients with advanced cancer: A multicentre double blind placebo controlled randomised trial. *Journal of Clinical Oncology*, 31(1), 111–118.

Buckman, R. (1992) *How to Break Bad News: A Guide for Health Care Professionals.* Baltimore: Johns Hopkins University Press.

Campbell, M.L., Yarandi, H. & Dove-Medows, E. (2013) Oxygen is nonbeneficial for most patients who are near death. *Journal of Pain and Symptom Management*, 45, 517–523.

Cancer Research UK (2018) *Oxygen at Home.* Available at: https://www.cancerresearchuk.org/about-cancer/coping/physically/breathing-problems/treatment/oxygen-at-home

Care (Christian Action Research and Education) (n.d.) *Euthanasia: The History & the Law.* Available at: https://www.care.org.uk/our-causes/sanctity-life/euthanasia-history

Cassel, E.J. (1982) The nature of suffering and the goals of medicine. *New England Journal of Medicine*, 306(11), 693–645.

Chan, W.L., Ng, C.W., Lee, C., et al. (2015) Effective management of breathlessness in advanced cancer patients with a program-based, multidisciplinary approach: The 'SOB Program' in Hong Kong. *Journal of Pain and Symptom Management*, 51, 623–627.

Charalambous, A., Giannakopoulou, M., Bozas, E., et al. (2016) Guided imagery and progressive muscle relaxation as a cluster of symptoms management intervention in patients receiving chemotherapy: A randomized control trial. *PLOS ONE*, 11(6), e0156911.

Chin, C. & Booth, S. (2016) Managing breathlessness: A palliative care approach. *Postgraduate Medical Journal*, 92, 393–400.

Chmielowski, B. (2017) *Manual of Clinical Oncology*, 8th edn. Philadelphia: Lippincott Williams & Wilkins.

Chopra, N., Kumar, S. & Chandra, A. (2017) Malignant ascites: A review of pathogenesis and management. *Nature Reviews Cancer*, 13(4), 273–282.

Christensen, L., Wildgaard, L. & Wildgaard, K. (2016) Permanent catheters for recurrent ascites: A critical and systematic review of study methodology. *Supportive Care in Cancer*, 24(6), 2767–2779.

Clements-Cortés, A. (2016) Development and efficacy of music therapy techniques within palliative care. *Complementary Therapies in Clinical Practice*, 23, 125–129.

Corner, J., Plant, H., A'Hern, R. & Bailey, C. (1996) Non-pharmacological intervention for breathlessness in lung cancer. *Palliative Medicine*, 10(4), 299–305.

CQC (Care Quality Commission) (2015) *Core Service: End of Life Care, NHS Acute Hospitals.* Available at: https://www.cqc.org.uk/sites/default/files/20160120_End_of_life_care_core_service_framework_Latest_net_version.pdf

Currow, D.C., Agar, M. & Abernethy, A.P. (2013) Hospital can be the actively chosen place for death. *Journal of Clinical Oncology*, 31, 651–652.

Dalal, S., Del Fabbro, E. & Bruera, E. (2009) Is there a role for hydration at the end of life? *Current Opinion in Supportive and Palliative Care*, 3(1), 72–78.

Del Fabbro, E., Bruera, E., Givens, J., et al. (2019) Palliative care: Assessment and management of nausea and vomiting. *UpToDate.* Available at: https://www.uptodate.com/contents/palliative-care-assessment-and-management-of-nausea-and-vomiting

Detering, K.M., Hancock, A.D., Reade, M.C., et al. (2010) The impact of advance care planning on end of life care in elderly patients: Randomised controlled trial. *BMJ*, 340, c1345.

DH (Department of Health) (2008) *End of Life Care Strategy: Promoting High Quality Care for All Adults at the End of Life*. London: Department of Health.

DH (2012) *End of Life Care Strategy: Fourth Annual Report*. Available at: www.gov.uk/government/uploads/system/uploads/attachment_data/file/136486/End-of-Life-Care-Strategy-Fourth-Annual-report-web-version-v2.pdf

DH (2013) *More Care, Less Pathway: A Review of the Liverpool Care Pathway*. Available at: www.gov.uk/government/uploads/system/uploads/attachment_data/file/212450/Liverpool_Care_Pathway.pdf

Dickman, A. & Schneider, J. (2016) *The Syringe Driver*, 4th edn. Oxford: Oxford University Press.

Dikken, C. & Wildman, K. (2013) Control of nausea and vomiting caused by chemotherapy. *Cancer Nursing Practice*, 12(8), 24–29.

Dowler, C. (2011) Nurses must not 'ignore' patients' requests for assisted suicide, RCN advises. *Nursing Times*, 20 October. Available at: www.nursingtimes.net/nursing-practice/clinical-zones/end-of-life-andpalliative-care/nurses-must-not-ignore-patients-requests-for-assistedsuicide-rcn-advises/5036758.article#

Dudgeon, D. (2018) Assessment and management of dyspnea in palliative care. *UpToDate*. Available at: https://www.uptodate.com/contents/assessment-and-management-of-dyspnea-in-palliative-care

Ekstrom, M., Abernethy, A. & Currow, D. (2015) The management of chronic breathlessness in patients with advanced cancer and terminal illness. *BMJ*, 349, 1–7.

EMA (European Medicines Agency) (2013) *European Medicines Agency Recommends Changes to the Use of Metoclopramide*. London: European Medicines Agency.

Engelman, S. (2013) Palliative care and the use of animal assisted therapy. *Omega*, 67(1/2), 63–67.

Etheridge, Z. & Gatland, E. (2015) When and how to discuss 'do not resuscitate' decisions with patients. *BMJ*, 350, H2640.

Dunn, L. & Beal, C. (2011) Accurate assessment of patient weight. *Nursing Times*, 14 March. Available at: https://www.nursingtimes.net/clinical-archive/assessment-skills/accurate-assessment-of-patient-weight/5068941.article

Ewing, G., Brundle, C., Payne, S. & Grande, G. (2013) The Carer Support Needs Assessment Tool (CSNAT) for use in palliative and end of life care at home: A validation study. *Journal of Pain and Symptom Management*, 46(3), 395–405.

Fraise, A.P. & Bradley, T. (eds) (2009) *Ayliffe's Control of Healthcare-Associated Infection: A Practical Handbook*, 5th edn. London: Hodder Arnold.

Frese, T., Klauss, S., Hermann, K. & Sandholzer, H. (2011) Nausea and vomiting as the reasons for encounter in general practice. *Journal of Clinical Medicine Research*, 3(1), 23–29.

Fritzson, A., Tavelin, B. & Axelsson, B. (2013) Association between parenteral fluids and symptoms in hospital end-of-life care: An observational study of 280 patients. *BMJ Supportive & Palliative Care*, 5(2), 160–168.

Gan, T.J., Diemunsch, P., Habib, A.S., et al. (2014) Consensus guidelines for the management of postoperative nausea and vomiting. *Anesthesia & Analgesia*, 118(1), 85–113.

Ghaffar, M.K.A., Hassan, M.S. & Mostafa, M.Y. (2014) Value of implantable peritoneal ports in managing recurrent malignant ascites. *Egyptian Journal of Radiology and Nuclear Medicine*, 45(2), 417–422.

Glare, P., Sinclair, C., Stone, P. & Clayton, J. (2015) Predicting survival in patients with advanced disease. In: Cherny, N., Fallon, M., Kaasa, S., et al. (eds) *Oxford Textbook of Palliative Medicine*, 5th edn. Oxford: Oxford University Press, pp.65–76.

Goesling, J., Clauw, D.J. & Hassett, A.L. (2013) Pain and depression: An integrative review of neurobiological and psychological factors. *Current Psychiatry Reports*, 15(12), 421.

Hall, C.C., Lugton, J., Spiller, J.A. & Carduff, E. (2018) CPR decision-making conversations in the UK: An integrative review. *BMJ Supportive & Palliative Care*, 9(1), 1–11.

Hambridge, K. (2013) Assessing the risk of post-operative nausea and vomiting. *Nursing Standard*, 27(18), 35–43.

Hardy, J., Glare, P., Yates, P. & Mannix, K.A. (2015) Palliation of nausea and vomiting. In: Cherny, N., Fallon, M., Kaasa, S., et al. (eds) *Oxford Textbook of Palliative Medicine*, 5th edn. Oxford: Oxford University Press, pp.661–674.

Henry, C. & Wilson, J. (2012) Personal care at the end of life and after death. *Nursing Times*, 108. Available at: https://www.nursingtimes.net/Journals/2012/05/08/h/i/z/120805-Innov-endoflife.pdf

Higginson, I.J. (1999) Evidence based palliative care. *BMJ*, 319, 462–463.

Highet, G., Crawford, D., Murray, S.A. & Boyd, K. (2013) Development and evaluation of the Supportive and Palliative Care Indicators Tool (SPICT): A mixed-methods study. *BMJ Supportive & Palliative Care*, 4(3), 285–290.

Hines, S., Steels, E., Chang, A. & Gibbons, K. (2018) Aromatherapy for treatment of postoperative nausea and vomiting. *Cochrane Database of Systematic Reviews*, 18(4), CD007598.

Hosker, M.G. & Bennett, M.I. (2016) Delirium and agitation at the end of life. *BMJ*, 353, i3085.

Hospice UK (2019) *Care after Death: Registered Nurse Verification of Expected Adult Death (RNVoEAD) Guidance*, 2nd edn. London: Hospice UK.

HSE (Health and Safety Executive) (2018) *Managing Infection Risks when Handling the Deceased*. Available at: www.hse.gov.uk/pUbns/priced/hsg283.pdf

Huang, L.L., Xia, H.H. & Zhu, S.L. (2014) Ascitic fluid analysis in the differential diagnosis of ascites: Focus on cirrhotic ascites. *Journal of Clinical and Translational Hepatology*, 2(1), 58–64.

Hudson, P.L., Lobb, E.A., Thomas, K., et al. (2012) Psycho-educational group intervention for family caregivers of hospitalized palliative care patients: Pilot study. *Journal of Palliative Medicine*, 15, 277–281.

Hui, D., Kim, S.H., Roquemore, J., et al. (2014) Impact of timing and setting of palliative care referral on quality of end-of-life care in cancer patients. *Cancer*, 120(11), 1743–1749.

IPEM (Institute of Physics and Engineering in Medicine) (2002) *Medical and Dental Guidance Notes: A Good Practice Guide on All Aspects of Ionising Radiation Protection in the Clinical Environment*. York: Institute of Physics and Engineering in Medicine.

Jennings, A.L., Davies, A.N., Higgins, J.P., et al. (2002) A systematic review of the use of opioids in the management of dyspnoea. *Thorax*, 57(11), 939–944.

Jung, M., Pützer, S., Gevensleben, H., et al. (2016) Diagnostic and prognostic value of *SHOX2* and *SEPT9* DNA methylation and cytology in benign, paramalignant, and malignant ascites. *Clinical Epigenetics*, 8, 24.

Kamal, A.H., Maguire, J.M., Wheeler, J.L., et al. (2012) Dyspnoea review for the palliative care professional: Treatment goals and therapeutic options. *Journal of Palliative Medicine*, 15, 106–114.

Kelly, B. & Ward, K. (2013) Nausea and vomiting in palliative care. *Nursing Times*, 109(39), 16–19.

King's Fund (2008) *Improving Environments for Care at End of Life*. London: King's Fund.

Kipps, E., Tan, D.S.P. & Kaye, S.B. (2013) Meeting the challenge of ascites in ovarian cancer: New avenues for therapy and research. *Nature Reviews Cancer*, 13(4), 273–282.

Krakauer, E. (2015) Sedation at the end of life. In: Cherny, N., Fallon, M., Kaasa, S., et al. (eds) *Oxford Textbook of Palliative Medicine*, 5th edn. Oxford: Oxford University Press, pp.1134–1141.

Lacey, J. (2015) Management of the actively dying patient. In: Cherny, N., Fallon, M., Kaasa, S., et al. (eds) *Oxford Textbook of Palliative Medicine*, 5th edn. Oxford: Oxford University Press, pp.1125–1133.

Langemo, D., Haesler, E., Naylor, W., et al. (2015) Evidence-based guidelines for pressure ulcer management at the end of life. *International Journal of Palliative Nursing*, 21(5), 225–232.

Lanz, K.M., Gabriel, M.S. & Tschanz, J.A. (2019) Medically administered nutrition and hydration. In: Rolling Ferrell, B. & Paice, J.A. (eds) *Oxford Textbook of Palliative Nursing*, 5th edn. Oxford: Oxford University Press, pp.206–216.

Laverty, D., Wilson, J. & Cooper, M. (2018) Registered nurse verification of expected adult death: New guidance provides direction. *International Journal of Palliative Nursing*, 24(4), 178–183.

LCA (London Cancer Alliance) (2013) *Principles of Care for Dying Patients*. Available at: www.londoncanceralliance.nhs.uk/news,-events-publications/news/2013/10/lca-develops-principles-for-care-of-the-dying

Lee, A., Chan, S.K. & Fan, L.T. (2015) Stimulation of the wrist acupuncture point PC6 for preventing postoperative nausea and vomiting. *Cochrane Database of Systematic Reviews*, 11, CD003281.

Lee, L. & Grap, M.J. (2008) Care and management of the patient with ascites. *MEDSURG Nursing*, 17(6), 376–381.

Lindsay, A.J., Burton, J. & Ray, C.E. Jr. (2014) Paracentesis-induced circulatory dysfunction: A primer for the interventional radiologist. *Seminars in Interventional Radiology*, 31(3), 276–278.
Loveday, H.P., Wilson, J.A., Pratt, R.J., et al. (2014) epic3: National evidence-based guidelines for preventing healthcare-associated infections in NHS hospitals in England. *Journal of Hospital Infection*, 86(1), S1–S70.
Maguire, P. (1985) Barriers to psychological care of the dying. *BMJ*, 291(6510), 1711–1713.
Marieb, E.N. & Hoehn, K. (2016) *Human Anatomy & Physiology*, 10th edn. Harlow: Pearson.
Marieb, E.N. & Hoehn, K. (2018) *Human Anatomy & Physiology*, 11th edn. Harlow: Pearson.
Marriage (Registrar General's Licence) Act 1970. Available at: https://www.legislation.gov.uk/ukpga/1970/34/section/8
Martin, D.K., Walayat, S., Jinma, R., et al. (2016) Large-volume paracentesis with indwelling peritoneal catheter and albumin infusion: A community hospital study. *Journal of Community Hospital Internal Medicine Perspectives*, 6(5), 32421.
Martin, S. & Bristowe, K. (2015) Last offices: Nurses' experiences of the process and their views about involving significant others. *International Journal of Palliative Nursing*, 21(4), 173–178.
McGibbon, A., Chen, G.I., Peltekian, K.M. & van Zanten, S.V. (2007) An evidence-based manual for abdominal paracentesis. *Digestive Diseases & Sciences*, 52(12), 3307–3315.
Mental Capacity Act (2005) Available at: https://www.legislation.gov.uk/ukpga/2005/9
Minchom, A., Punwani, R., Filshie, J., et al. (2016) What is the evidence for the use of acupuncture as an intervention for symptom management in cancer supportive and palliative care: An integrative overview of reviews. *Supportive Care in Cancer*, 21, 102–110.
Mockford, C., Fritz, Z., George R., et al. (2015) Do not attempt cardiopulmonary resuscitation (DNaCPR) orders: A systematic review of the barriers and facilitators of decision making and implementation. *Resuscitation*, 88, 99–113.
Molassiotis, A., Lee, P.H., Burke, T.A., et al. (2016) Anticipatory nausea, risk factors, and its impact on chemotherapy-induced nausea and vomiting: Results from the Pan European Emesis Registry Study. *Journal of Pain and Symptom Management*, 6, 987–993.
Montgomery, M.M. & Leitman, I.M. (2014) Endoscopic ultrasound and paracentesis in the evaluation of small volume ascites in patients with intra-abdominal malignancies. *World Journal of Gastroenterology*, 20(30), 10219–10222.
Moore, K. (2015) Managing ascites: Hazards of fluid removal. *PSNet*. Available at: https://psnet.ahrq.gov/webmm/case/363/managing-ascites-hazards-of-fluid-removal
Mortimore, G. (2018) Management of ascites in patients with liver disease. *Nursing Times*, 114, 10, 36–40.
Narayanan, G., Pezeshkmehr, A., Venkat, S., et al. (2014) Safety and efficacy of the PleurX catheter for the treatment of malignant ascites. *Journal of Palliative Medicine*, 17(8), 906–912.
NEoLCP (National Palliative and End of Life Care Partnership) (2015) *Ambitions for Palliative and End of Life Care: A National Framework for Local Action 2015–2020*. Available at: http://endoflifecareambitions.org.uk/wp-content/uploads/2015/09/Ambitions-for-Palliative-and-End-of-Life-Care.pdf
NHS Blood and Transplant (2019) *Organ Donation Laws*. Available at: https://www.organdonation.nhs.uk/uk-laws
NHS Employers (2015) *Managing the Risks of Sharps Injuries*. Available at: https://www.nhsemployers.org/-/media/Employers/Documents/Retain-and-improve/Health-and-wellbeing/Managing-the-risks-of-sharps-injuries-v7.pdf
NHS England (2013) *Leadership Alliance for the Care of Dying People*. Available at: https://www.engage.england.nhs.uk/consultation/care-dying-ppl-engage/supporting_documents/lacdpengage.pdf
NHS Improvement (2019) *Standard Infection Control Precautions: National Hand Hygiene and Personal Protective Equipment Policy*. Available at: https://improvement.nhs.uk/resources/national-hand-hygiene-and-personal-protective-equipment-policy
NHS Scotland (2019) *Bowel Obstruction: Scottish Palliative Care Guidelines*. Available at: https://www.palliativecareguidelines.scot.nhs.uk/guidelines/symptom-control/bowel-obstruction.aspx
NICE (National Institute for Health and Care Excellence) (2015) *Care of Dying Adults in the Last Days of Life* [NICE Guideline 31]. Available at: https://www.nice.org.uk/guidance/ng31
NICE (2017a) *Care of Dying Adults in the Last Days of Life* [Quality Standard 144]. Available at: https://www.nice.org.uk/guidance/QS144
NICE (2017b) *End of Life Care for Adults* [Quality Standard 13]. Available at: https://www.nice.org.uk/guidance/qs13
NICE (2018) *Decision Making and Mental Capacity* [NICE Guideline 108]. Available at: https://www.nice.org.uk/guidance/ng108
Nightingale, F. (1859) *Notes on Nursing: What It Is and What It Is Not*. London: Churchill Livingstone.
NMC (Nursing and Midwifery Council) (2018) *The Code: Professional Standards of Practice and Behaviour for Nurses, Midwives and Nursing Associates*. Available at: https://www.nmc.org.uk/standards/code
Olausson, J. & Ferrell, B.R. (2013) Care of the body after death. *Clinical Journal of Oncology Nursing*, 17(6), 647–651.
Parshall, M.B., Schwartzstein, R.M., Adams, L., et al. (2012) An official American Thoracic Society statement: Update on the mechanisms, assessment and management of dyspnea. *American Journal of Respiratory and Critical Care Medicine*, 185(4), 435–452.
Pattison, N. (2011) End of life in critical care: An emphasis on care. *Nursing in Critical Care*, 16(3), 113–115.
Pedersen, J.S., Bendtsen, F. & Møller, S. (2015) Management of cirrhotic ascites. *Therapeutic Advances in Chronic Disease*, 6(3), 124–137.
Pericleous, M., Sarnowski, A., Moore, A., et al. (2016) The clinical management of abdominal ascites, spontaneous bacterial peritonitis and hepatorenal syndrome: A review of current guidelines and recommendations. *European Journal of Gastroenterology & Hepatology*, 28(3), e10–e18.
Petrova, M., Riley, J., Abel, J. & Barclay, S. (2016) Crash course in EPaCCS (Electronic Palliative Care Coordination Systems): 8 years of successes and failures in patient data sharing to learn from. *BMJ Supportive & Palliative Care*, 8(4), 447–455.
Phelps, A.C., Laudersale, K.E., Alcorn, S., et al. (2012) Addressing spirituality within the care of patients at the end of life: Perspectives of patients with advanced cancer, oncologists, and oncology nurses. *Journal of Clinical Oncology*, 30(20), 2538–2544.
Prado, B.B., Gomes, D., Serrano, P., et al. (2018) Continuous palliative sedation for patients with advanced cancer at a tertiary care cancer center. *BMC Palliative Care*, 17(1), 1.
Public Health (Control of Disease) Act (1984) Available at: https://www.legislation.gov.uk/ukpga/1984/22
Quested, B. & Rudge, T. (2003) Nursing care of dead bodies: A discursive analysis of last offices. *Journal of Advanced Nursing*, 41(6), 553–560.
RCN (Royal College of Nursing) (2019a) *Gifts and Wills*. Available at: https://www.rcn.org.uk/get-help/rcn-advice/gifts-and-wills
RCN (2019b) *Confirmation or Verification of Death by Registered Nurses*. Available at: https://www.rcn.org.uk/get-help/rcn-advice/confirmation-of-death
Resuscitation Council (2015) *ReSPECT: Recommended Summary Plan for Emergency Care and Treatment*. Available at: https://www.respectprocess.org.uk
Richardson, J., Smith, J.E., McCall, G., et al. (2007) Hypnosis for nausea and vomiting in cancer chemotherapy: A systematic review of the research evidence. *European Journal of Cancer Care*, 16(5), 402–412.
Rodgers, D., Calmes, B. & Grotts, J. (2016) Nursing care at the time of death: A bathing and honouring practice. *Oncology Nursing Forum*, 43(3), 363–371.
Runyon, B.A. (2012) *Management of Adult Patients with Ascites Due to Cirrhosis: Update 2012*. American Association for the Study of Liver Diseases. Available at: http://unmhospitalist.pbworks.com/w/file/fetch/115070379/AASLD%20ascites%20guidelines.pdf
Runyon, B.A. (2018) *Diagnostic and Therapeutic Abdominal Paracentesis*. Available at: https://www.uptodate.com/contents/diagnostic-and-therapeutic-abdominal-paracentesis
Runyon, B.A. (2019) *Evaluation of Adults with Ascites*. Available at: https://www.uptodate.com/contents/evaluation-of-adults-with-ascites
Safari, M.B. (2013) Art therapy in hospice: A catalyst for insight and healing. *Journal of the American Art Therapy Association*, 30(3), 122–129.
Sanger, G.J. & Andrews, P.L.R. (2018) A history of drug discovery for treatment of nausea and vomiting and the implications for future research. *Frontiers in Pharmacology*, 9, 913.

Sangisetty, S.L., & Miner T. J. (2012) Malignant ascites: A review of prognostic factors, pathophysiology and therapeutic measures. *World Journal of Gastrointestinal Surgery*, 4(4), 87–95.

Saunders, C. (1976) Care of the dying – 4: Control of pain in terminal cancer. *Nursing Times*, 72, 1133–1135.

Seaman S., Pengelly, M. & Noble, S. (2014) Tying the knot: Helping patients who want to get married in hospital. *British Journal of Hospital Medicine*, 75(1), 35–38.

Shah, R. (2017) Ascites treatment & management. *Medscape*. Available at: https://emedicine.medscape.com/article/170907-treatment#d6

Sharzehi, K., Jain, V., Naveed, A. & Schreibman, I. (2014) Hemorrhagic complications of paracentesis: A systematic review of the literature. *Gastroenterology Research and Practice*, 2014, 1–6.

Simon, S.T., Higginson, I.J., Booth, S., et al. (2010) Benzodiazepines for the relief of breathlessness in advanced malignant and non-malignant disease in adults. *Cochrane Database of Systematic Reviews*, 1, CD007354.

Sleeman, K. (2013) Caring for a dying patient in hospital. *BMJ*, 346, f2174.

Slusser, K. (2014) Malignant ascites. In: Yarbro, C., Wujcik, D. & Gobel, B.H. (eds) *Cancer Symptom Management*, 3rd edn. Sudbury, MA: Jones & Bartlett, pp.241–262.

Smith, L., Azariah, F., Lavender, V., et al. (2015) Cannabinoids for nausea and vomiting in adults with cancer receiving chemotherapy. *Cochrane Database of Systematic Reviews*. DOI: 10.1002/14651858.CD009464.pub2.

Solano, J.P., Gomes, B. & Higginson, I.J. (2006) A comparison of symptom prevalence in far advanced cancer, AIDS, heart failure, chronic obstructive airway disease and renal disease. *Journal of Pain and Symptom Management*, 31, 58–69.

Stanley, P. & Hurst, M. (2011) Narrative palliative care: A method for building empathy. *Journal of Social Work in End-of-Life Palliative Care*, 7(1), 39–55.

Steinhausser, K.E., Christakis, N.A., Clipp, E.X., et al. (2000) Factors considered important at the end of life by patients, family, physicians and other care providers. *JAMA*, 284(19), 2476–2482.

Stevens, A. & Laverty, D. (2018) Physical symptom management, with a focus on nursing interventions for complex symptoms. In: Walshe, C., Preston, N. & Johnston, B. (eds) *Palliative Care Nursing: Principles and Evidence for Practice*, 3rd edn. London: Open University Press, pp.134–157.

Suicide Act (1961) Available at: www.legislation.gov.uk/ukpga/Eliz2/9-10/60

Tasneem, H., Shahbaz, H. & Ali Sherazi, B. (2015) Causes, management and complications of ascites: A review. *International Current Pharmaceutical Journal*, 4(3), 370–377.

Taylor, J. (2007) The non-pharmacological management of breathlessness. *End of Life Care*, 1, 20–27.

Temel, J.S., Greer, J.A., Muzikansky, A., et al. (2010) Early palliative care for patients with metastatic non-small-cell lung cancer. *New England Journal of Medicine*, 363, 733–742.

Thibodeau, G. & Patton, K. (2010) Anatomy of the digestive system. In: Thibodeau, G. & Patton, K. (eds) *Anatomy and Physiology*, 7th edn. St Louis, MO: Mosby, pp.837–876.

Tortora, G.J. & Derrickson, B.H. (2017) *Principles of Anatomy & Physiology*, 15th edn. Hoboken, NJ: John Wiley & Sons.

Towler, P., Molassiotis, A. & Brearley, S.G. (2013) What is the evidence for the use of acupuncture as an intervention for symptom management in cancer supportive and palliative care: An integrative overview of reviews. *Supportive Care Cancer*, 21, 2913–2923.

Travis, S. (2002) *Procedure for the Care of Patients Who Die in Hospital.* London: Royal Marsden NHS Foundation Trust.

Tulsky, J.A. (2005) Beyond advance directives: Importance of communication skills at the end of life. *JAMA*, 294(3), 359–365.

Twycross, R. (2019) Reflections on palliative sedation. *Palliative Care: Research and Treatment*, 12, 1178224218823511.

Twycross, R., Wilcock, A. & Howard, P. (2017) *Palliative Care Formulary*, 6th edn. London: Pharmaceutical Press.

Twycross, R.G., Wilcock, A. & Stark Toller, C. (2009) *Symptom Management in Advanced Cancer*, 4th Revised edn. Nottingham: Palliativedrugs.com Ltd.

Vaughan. J. (2013) Developing a nurse-led paracentesis service in an ambulatory care unit. *Nursing Standard*, 28(4), 44–50.

Vidal, M., Hui, D., Williams, J. & Bruera, E. (2016) Prospective study of hypodermoclysis performed by caregivers in the home setting. *Journal of Pain and Symptom Management*, 52, 570–574.e9.

Walsh, D., Davis, M., Ripamonti, C., et al. (2017) 2016 Updated MASCC/ESMO consensus recommendations: Management of nausea and vomiting in advanced cancer. *Supportive Care in Cancer*, 25(1), 333–340.

Warren, A. & King, L. (2008) A review of the efficacy of dexamethasone in the prevention of postoperative nausea and vomiting *Journal of Clinical Nursing*, 17(1), 58–68.

Watts, T. (2013) End-of-life care pathways and nursing: A literature review. *Journal of Nursing Management*, 21, 47–57.

WHO (World Health Organization) (2002) *WHO Definition of Palliative Care*. Available at: https://www.who.int/cancer/palliative/definition

WHO (2017) *Clinical Criteria for the Determination of Death*. Geneva: World Health Organization.

Williams, C. & Gardiner, C. (2015) Preference for a single or shared room in a UK inpatient hospice: Patient, family and staff perspectives. *BMJ Supportive & Palliative Care*, 5(2), 169–174.

Wilson, J. on behalf of Hospice UK and the National Nurse Consultant Group (Palliative Care) (2015) *Care after Death: Guidance for Staff Responsible for Care after Death*, 2nd edn. Available at: https://www.hospiceuk.org/what-we-offer/publications?cat=72e54312-4ccd-608d-ad24-ff0000fd3330

Wolf, Z. (1988) *Nurses' Work: The Sacred and the Profane.* Philadelphia: University of Pennsylvania Press.

Zhou, J., Pi, H. & Zheng, Y. (2015) Characteristics of abdominal cavity drainage fluid in Chinese patients without postoperative complications after surgery for gastrointestinal or retroperitoneal tumours. *Clinical Interventions in Aging*, 10, 367–370.

Chapter 12

Respiratory care, CPR and blood transfusion

Louise Davison and Wendy McSporran with Grainne Brady, Catherine Forsythe and Olivia Ratcliffe

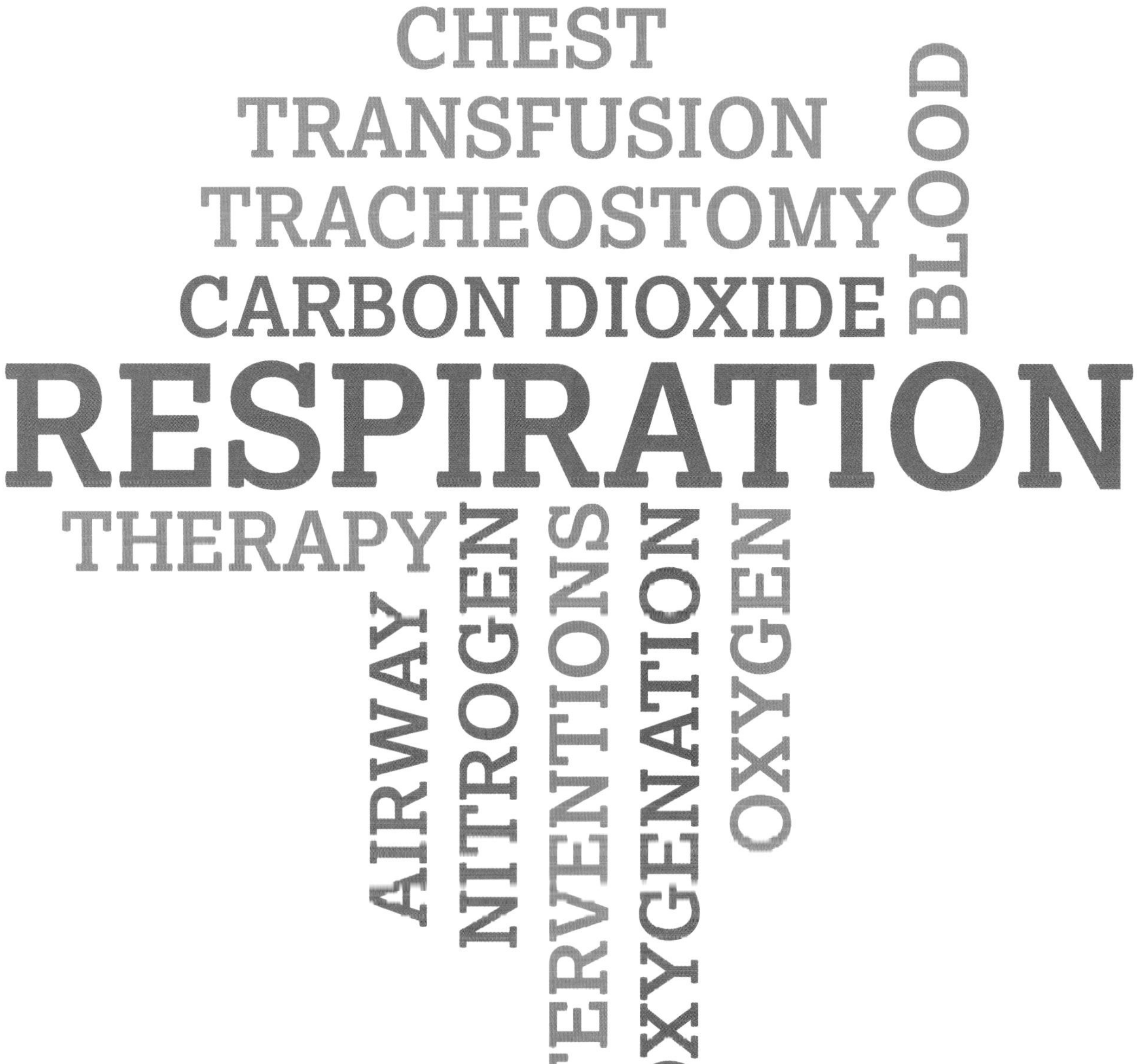
CHEST
TRANSFUSION
TRACHEOSTOMY
CARBON DIOXIDE
BLOOD
RESPIRATION
THERAPY
AIRWAY
NITROGEN
INTERVENTIONS
OXYGENATION
OXYGEN

The Royal Marsden Manual of Clinical Nursing Procedures: Professional Edition, Tenth Edition. Edited by Sara Lister, Justine Hofland and Hayley Grafton

Procedure guidelines

Being an accountable professional

At the point of registration, the nurse will:

2. Use evidence-based, best practice approaches to undertake the following procedures:
- **2.2** undertake venepuncture and cannulation and blood sampling, interpreting normal and common abnormal blood profiles and venous blood gases
- **2.4** manage and monitor blood component transfusions
- **2.7** undertake a whole body systems assessment including respiratory, circulatory, neurological, musculoskeletal, cardiovascular and skin status
- **2.15** administer basic physical first aid
- **2.16** recognise and manage seizures, choking and anaphylaxis, providing appropriate basic life support

8. Use evidence-based, best practice approaches for meeting needs for respiratory care and support, accurately assessing the person's capacity for independence and self care and initiating appropriate interventions

Future Nurse: Standards of Proficiency for Registered Nurses (NMC 2018)

Overview

This chapter explains the assessment and nursing management of patients with respiration problems. This includes the administration of different types of oxygen therapy and respiratory support, and the management of patients with chest drains and altered airways, in particular tracheostomies. Basic life support is explored and guidance is offered on how best to deliver it.

Blood transfusion can also be life saving and is certainly life supporting in some conditions. This chapter discusses blood component transfusion, and the relevant procedures offer guidance on how to deliver a blood transfusion safely.

Respiratory therapy

Definition

The principle of respiratory therapy is the application of pharmacological and non-pharmacological means to improve breathing and therefore gaseous exchange. This requires a thorough assessment of the patient prior to the implementation of interventions in an attempt to identify and treat the underlying cause, or optimize and support respiratory function (Brady 2018).

Anatomy and physiology

The respiratory system is a complex system that is responsible for the efficient delivery and exchange of respiratory gases, primarily oxygen (O_2) and carbon dioxide (CO_2). The respiratory system is composed of the following structures, some of which are illustrated in Figure 12.1:

- the respiratory centres in the medulla oblongata and pons of the brain
- the nose, mouth and connecting airways
- the trachea, main bronchus, bronchioles and alveoli
- the respiratory muscles (diaphragm and intercostal muscles)
- the respiratory nerves (subphrenic and intercostal nerves)
- the bone structures of the thorax (ribs, vertebrae and sternum)
- the lung parenchyma
- the pleura and pleural fluid (Tortora and Derrickson 2017).

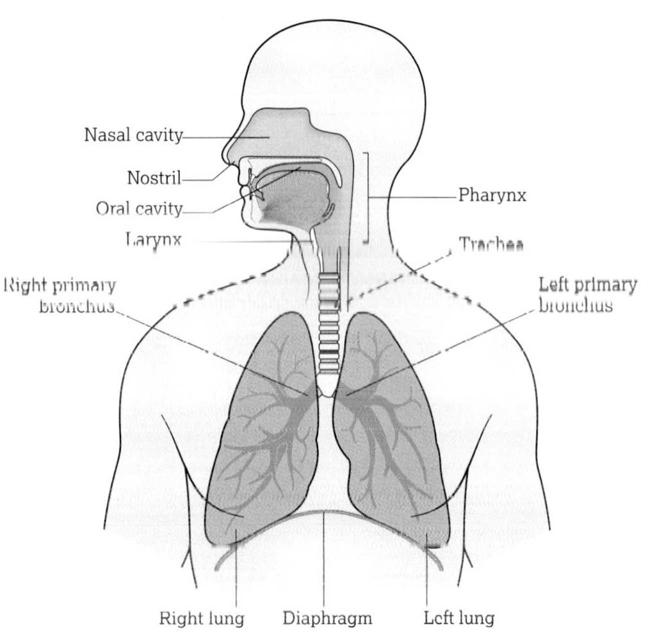

Figure 12.1 The major respiratory organs in relation to surrounding structures. *Source:* Marieb and Hoehn (2016).

Alteration, damage or blockage to any of the structures listed above may result in respiratory impairment or failure. It is essential when considering respiratory function to remember the close association between the cardiovascular, neurological, musculoskeletal and respiratory systems (Marieb and Hoehn 2018).

Tissue oxygenation

Every cell of the body requires a continuous supply of oxygen for the growth and repair of tissues, and to ensure optimum metabolism. Oxygen is drawn into the body through the nose and mouth; it then travels down the trachea and into the smaller airways and alveoli of the lungs. Once it has reached the alveoli, oxygen is able to diffuse into the network of capillaries that surround the lung. The oxygenated blood travels via the pulmonary vein from the lungs to the heart, where it is then pumped to all cells of the body via the arterial system (Tortora and Derrickson 2017). 'Hypoxia' is the term used to describe a lack of tissue oxygenation.

Within the cell mitochondria, oxygen and glucose are used to produce energy in the form of adenosine triphosphate (ATP), and carbon dioxide is produced as a waste product. This is known as aerobic 'cellular respiration'. In low-oxygen conditions, cellular respiration becomes anaerobic, generating less ATP and producing the by-product lactic acid. If the low-oxygen state is allowed to continue, lactic acid will accumulate, leading to metabolic acidosis and cell death (Lenihan and Cormac 2013).

There are three components of cellular oxygenation: oxygen uptake, oxygen transportation and oxygen utilization. *Oxygen uptake* is the process of extracting oxygen from the environment. *Oxygen transportation* is the mechanism by which the uptake of oxygen results in the delivery of oxygen to the cells. *Oxygen utilization* is the metabolic need for molecular oxygen by the cells of the body (Tortora and Derrickson 2017).

Oxygen uptake

The air that we breathe in from the atmosphere is composed of the following gases:

- oxygen: 21%
- carbon dioxide: 0.03%
- nitrogen: 78%
- argon: >0.9%
- other gases: 0.07%.

Inspired air at sea level has a total atmospheric pressure of 101.3 kPa (760 mmHg). According to Dalton's law, where there is a mixture of gases, each gas exerts its own pressure as if there were no other gases present (Jones and Berry 2015). The pressure of an individual gas in a mixture is called the 'partial pressure' and is denoted as Pa. This is followed by the symbol of the gas. For example, the partial pressure of oxygen is written as PaO_2 (Tortora and Derrickson 2017). The partial pressures of the three main gases in the air are as follows:

- oxygen: 0.21 × 101.3 = 21.3 kPa (159.8 mmHg)
- carbon dioxide: 0.03 × 101.3 = 3.0 kPa (22.8 mmHg)
- nitrogen: 0.78 × 101.3 = 79.0 kPa (592.6 mmHg)

The partial pressure controls the movement of oxygen and carbon dioxide between the atmosphere and the lungs, the lungs and the blood, and finally the blood and the cells.

Gaseous exchange

Gases move by diffusion. Diffusion is the movement of gas molecules from an area of relatively high partial pressure to an area of low partial pressure (Tortora and Derrickson 2017). Oxygen diffuses from the alveoli, where the partial pressure is highest, into the pulmonary capillaries, where it is lower. From here it continues to travel, and as the partial pressure changes it diffuses into the tissues and finally the mitochondria of the cells. The waste product carbon dioxide diffuses in the same way back from the cells to

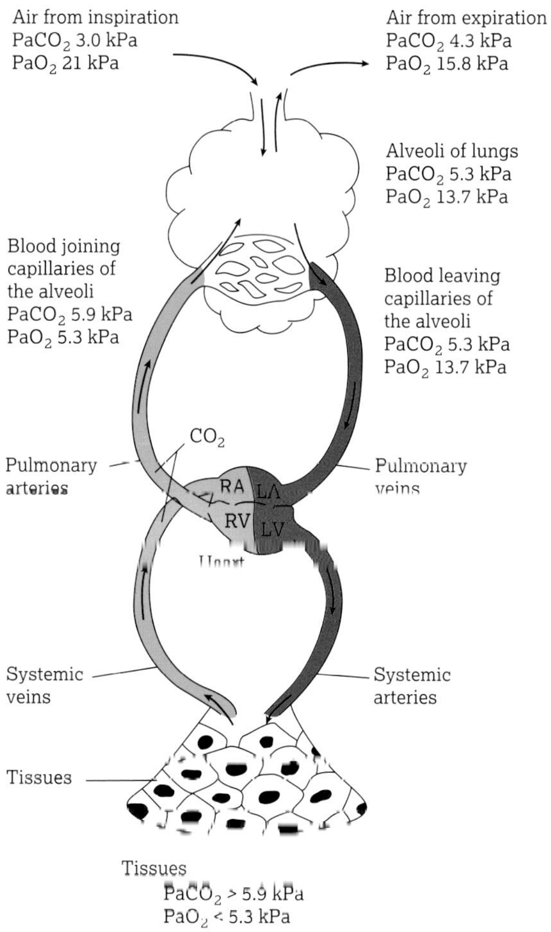

Figure 12.2 Gas movement in the body is facilitated by partial pressure differences. Top of figure illustrates pressure gradients that facilitate oxygen (O_2) and carbon dioxide (CO_2) exchange in the lungs. Bottom of figure shows pressure gradients that facilitate gas movements from systemic capillaries to tissues. LA, left atrium; LV, left atrium; RA, right atrium; RV, right ventricle.

Oxygen transportation

Oxygen is carried in the blood in two ways:

- *Dissolved in the plasma (serum)*: only 2–3% (0.03 mL O_2 per 100 mL of plasma) is carried in this way as oxygen is not very soluble (Marieb and Hoehn 2018). It is expressed as the PaO_2.
- *Bound to the haemoglobin of the red blood cells*: 95–98% of oxygen is carried in this way; it is measured as the percentage of haemoglobin saturated with oxygen. Each gram of haemoglobin can carry 1.34 mL of oxygen per 100 mL blood (Thomas and Lumb 2012). It is expressed as the SaO_2 when measured from arterial blood gas. When pulse oximetry is used, it is expressed as SpO_2.

Haemoglobin is composed of haem (iron) and globulin (protein). Each haemoglobin molecule has four binding sites, each able to carry one molecule of oxygen. A haemoglobin molecule is said to be fully saturated when oxygen is bound to all four molecules. When fewer than four are attached, the haemoglobin is said to be partially saturated (Jones and Berry 2015). The bond between haemoglobin and oxygen is represented by the oxygen disassociation curve and is affected by various physiological factors that shift the curve to the right or left (Figure 12.3).

Oxyhaemoglobin curve shift to the right

When a shift occurs to the right, there is reduced binding of oxygen to haemoglobin and oxygen is given up more easily to the tissues. Oxygen saturation of the haemoglobin molecule will be lower (Collins et al. 2015, Kaufman and Dhamoon 2018). Increases in the following cause the curve to shift to the right:

- body temperature (due to infection or sepsis)
- hydrogen ion content (acidaemia), known as the Bohr effect (due to sepsis or other shock conditions)
- carbon dioxide (due to sepsis or pulmonary disease)
- 2,3-diphosphoglycerate (2,3-DPG) (an enzyme found in the red bloods cells that affects haemoglobin and oxygen binding).

Oxyhaemoglobin curve shift to the left

When a shift occurs to the left, there is an increase in the binding of oxygen to the haemoglobin, oxygen is given up less easily to the tissues and cellular hypoxia can occur (Jones and Berry 2015,

the alveoli, where the partial pressure of carbon dioxide is lowest (Figure 12.2)

Inspired air encounters water vapour as it is warmed and humidified in the upper airways of the respiratory tract. Water vapour exerts its own partial pressure of 6.3 kPa (47 mmHg), which must be subtracted from the total atmospheric pressure to give the corrected total atmospheric pressure (Brady 2018):

- corrected total atmospheric pressure: 101.3 − 6.3 = 95 kPa (713 mmHg)

This figure of 95 kPa is then used to find the partial pressures of each gas:

- oxygen: 0.21 × 95 = 20.0 kPa (150.0 mmHg)
- carbon dioxide: 0.03 × 95 = 2.9 kPa (21.8 mmHg)

As oxygen continues to pass down the respiratory tract to the alveoli, it encounters carbon dioxide leaving the respiratory tract. This exerts a partial pressure of approximately 5.3 kPa (40.0 mmHg). This in turn must be subtracted to determine the correct value for oxygen (Jones and Berry 2015, O'Driscoll et al. 2017). For example:

- corrected partial pressure of oxygen: 20.0 kPa (150.0 mmHg) − 5.3 kPa (40.0 mmHg) = 14.7 kPa (110 mmHg)

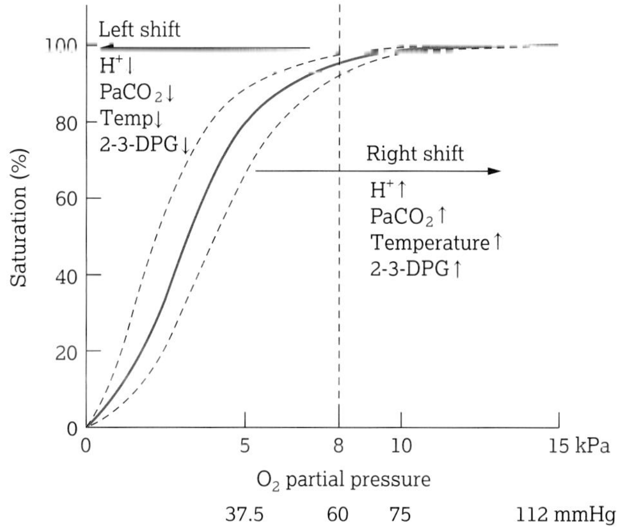

Figure 12.3 Oxyhaemoglobin dissociation curve. With a PaO_2 of 8 kPa and more, saturations will remain high (flat portion of curve). The middle red line is the normal position of the curve. 2,3-DPG, 2,3-diphosphoglycerate.

Kaufman and Dhamoon 2018). Decreases in the following cause the curve to shift to the left:

- body temperature (due to exposure to cold, near drowning or immersion)
- hydrogen ion content (due to alkalaemia)
- carbon dioxide (due to hyperventilation)
- 2,3-DPG.

Oxygen utilization

Oxygen uptake in the lungs is shown by the upper flat part of the curve. When the PaO_2 is between 8.0 and 13.3 kPa (60–100 mmHg), the haemoglobin molecule is saturated with more than 90% oxygen. At this point of the curve, large changes in the PaO_2 lead to small changes in the SaO_2 because the haemoglobin is almost completely saturated. The lower part of the curve shows the release of oxygen from the haemoglobin molecule to the tissues. Oxygen is given up very easily to the tissues and small changes in the PaO_2 cause major changes to the SaO_2 (Marieb and Hoehn 2018). A patient's PaO_2 must therefore be kept above 8 kPa (60 mmHg) to prevent hypoxia and cell death (Jones and Berry 2015). 'Hypoxaemia' is the term used to describe a low partial pressure of oxygen within the blood.

In addition to measuring the partial pressure of oxygen within the arterial blood, the fraction of inspired oxygen is also considered (FiO_2). This represents the percentage of oxygen participating in gas exchange. Room air has a FiO_2 of 0.21 (21%); therefore, any additional oxygen inhaled will increase the FiO_2. If a patient is receiving large concentrations of oxygen therapy and is hypoxaemic, this may indicate a problem within the lungs caused by a ventilation/perfusion mismatch, a shunt, alveolar hypoventilation, decreased partial pressure of oxygen or decreased diffusion (Sarkar et al. 2017).

Oxygen consumption

At rest, the normal oxygen consumption rate is approximately 200–250 mL per minute. As the available oxygen per minute in an average-sized man is about 700 mL, this means there is an oxygen reserve of 450–500 mL per minute (MacIntyre 2014). Factors that increase the consumption of oxygen include fever, sepsis, shivering, restlessness and increased metabolism (Semenza 2012). It is difficult to say at which absolute level oxygen therapy is necessary, as each situation should be judged by the clinical condition of the patient and their oxygen requirements. Generally speaking, additional oxygen will be required when the PaO_2 has fallen to 8 kPa (60 mmHg) or less (O'Driscoll et al. 2017), as measured on an arterial blood gas sample.

Carbon dioxide excretion

The second function of the respiratory system is to excrete carbon dioxide from the lungs during expiration in order to maintain a normal level of carbon dioxide in the blood (4.5–6.0 kPa or 34–45 mmHg). Carbon dioxide has a direct effect on the respiratory centre in the brain (Marhong and Fan 2014). As the carbon dioxide level rises and diffuses from the blood into the cerebrospinal fluid (CSF), it is hydrated and carbonic acid is formed. The acid then dissociates and hydrogen ions are liberated. Because there is no bicarbonate in the CSF to buffer the hydrogen ions, the pH of the CSF falls, which excites the central chemoreceptors, resulting in an increased respiratory rate (Cheng and Jusof 2018, Marieb and Hoehn 2018).

Evidence-based approaches

Respiratory assessment

During normal respiration, eating, drinking and speaking in full sentences are effortless. The first stage of a respiratory assessment is to observe the patient for the following:

- general colour and appearance (ashen, cyanosis, pallor or sweating)
- position adopted by the patient to assist breathing
- use of accessory muscles
- work of breathing at rest and on movement
- respiratory rate
- respiratory pattern
- ability to speak in full sentences
- additional audible breath sounds (Wild and Poole 2013).

A thorough patient history and physical assessment will help to determine what the underlying cause of the respiratory concern may be. Additional investigations such as a chest X-ray, arterial blood gas analysis, and a computed tomography (CT) scan or ventilation/perfusion (V/Q) scan may also be necessary to aid diagnosis.

Having made a comprehensive assessment, the immediate cause of respiratory insufficiency should be corrected where possible. The cause may be directly related to respiratory function or a secondary effect of another process. For example, the patient may be in severe pain and good pain management may allow them to breathe deeply and cough more effectively, improving respiratory function. Conversely, an opioid overdose may result in decreased or absent respiration, and treatment will include supporting respiration and administering the antidote to the opioid. Regardless of the cause, respiratory function needs to be supported while the underlying condition is being treated (O'Driscoll et al. 2017).

Respiratory therapy therefore includes a variety of interventions, such as:

- pharmacological management, including oxygen therapy
- bronchodilators
- analgesia
- antidotes to drug toxicity
- antimicrobials for infections of the respiratory tract
- support and guidance on smoking cessation.

Surgery may be indicated to repair a ruptured diaphragm or to manage trauma of the thoracic cavity. Some patients may require insertion of a tracheostomy tube or chest drain, or a stent or shunt for superior vena cava obstruction (for example). Finally, positioning (see Chapter 7: Moving and positioning) and physiotherapy play a major role in improving respiratory function (English 2015). Any person who is unable to maintain tissue oxygenation requires supplemental oxygen until they are able to manage again on room air.

Oxygen therapy

Definition

Oxygen therapy is the administration of oxygen at concentrations greater than that in ambient air (21%), with the intention of treating or preventing the symptoms and manifestations of hypoxia (McCoy 2013).

Evidence-based approaches

Rationale

Indications

Oxygen is indicated for any condition that causes hypoxaemia. For example:

- during cardiac or respiratory arrest
- for initial treatment during critical illness (anaphylaxis, shock, sepsis, carbon monoxide poisoning, major head injury, status epilepticus, major pulmonary haemorrhage, near drowning etc.)
- during serious illness when hypoxaemia is suspected or has been confirmed (e.g. acute asthma, pneumonia, pulmonary embolism, pulmonary oedema, pleural effusion lung cancer or worsening lung fibrosis)

Table 12.1 Common causes of respiratory failure

Type 1 respiratory failure (hypoxaemic)	Type 2 respiratory failure (hypercapnic)
• COPD • Pneumonia • Pulmonary oedema • Pulmonary fibrosis • Asthma • Pneumothorax • Pulmonary embolism • Pulmonary arterial hypertension • Pneumoconiosis • Granulomatous lung diseases • Cyanotic congenital heart disease • Atelectasis • ARDS • Fat embolism syndrome • Kyphoscoliosis • Obesity	• COPD • Severe asthma • Drug overdose or sedative drugs • Poisoning • Myasthenia gravis • Polyneuropathy • Poliomyelitis • Primary muscle disorders • Porphyria • Cervical cordotomy • Head and cervical cord injury • Primary alveolar hypoventilation • Obesity hypoventilation syndrome • Pulmonary oedema • ARDS • Myxoedema • Tetanus

ARDS, acute respiratory distress syndrome; COPD, chronic obstructive pulmonary disease.
Source: Adapted from Feller-Kopman and Schwartzstein (2017), Kayner (2012).

- during and after conscious sedation or anaesthesia if the patient is unable to maintain their own airway or maintain oxygen saturations between 94% and 98% (or 88–92% if at risk of hypercapnic respiratory failure) (O'Driscoll et al. 2017).

Any of the above conditions can lead to respiratory failure, of which there are two types (Brady 2018):

- *Type 1* is referred to as 'hypoxaemic respiratory failure' (failure to oxygenate the tissues), where the PaO_2 is less than 8 kPa (60 mmHg) while the carbon dioxide ($PaCO_2$) is normal or low.
- *Type 2* is referred to as 'hypercapnic respiratory failure' (raised carbon dioxide) or 'respiratory pump failure', where the $PaCO_2$ is greater than 6 kPa (45 mmHg). Alveolar ventilation is insufficient to excrete carbon dioxide and this is accompanied by hypoxaemia.

Table 12.1 outlines some of the common causes of the different types of respiratory failure.

Contraindications

No specific contraindications to oxygen therapy exist (Bein et al. 2016), but the following precautions need to be considered (GOLD 2017, Moore 2016, NICE 2018a, O'Driscoll et al. 2017):

- Patients at risk of hypercapnic respiratory failure (e.g. those with chronic obstructive pulmonary disease) should receive prescribed titrated oxygen to maintain oxygen saturations of 88–92%.
- The administration of high concentrations of fractional inspired oxygen (FiO_2) for prolonged periods of time can cause absorption atelectasis (incomplete lung inflation) and oxygen toxicity.
- Supplemental oxygen should be administered with caution to patients with paraquat poisoning and those who have previously received bleomycin chemotherapy due to the risk of pulmonary toxicity and bleomycin-induced pneumonitis.
- Bacterial contamination associated with certain nebulization and humidification systems is a possible hazard.
- Fire hazard is increased in the presence of increased oxygen concentrations.

Anticipated patient outcomes

The patient will achieve the desired oxygen saturations with the least amount of supplementary oxygen necessary.

Clinical governance

Competencies

NHS Improvement (2018a) highlights the concerns surrounding delivery of oxygen therapy via cylinders. The valve mechanism in place to address fire prevention has led to an unintended consequence in that staff may believe oxygen is flowing when it is not. It has also been reported that staff have been unable to turn the oxygen flow on in an emergency. In a recent 3-year period, over 400 incidents involving incorrect operation of oxygen cylinder controls were reported to the National Reporting and Learning System (NHS Improvement 2018a).

It follows that nursing staff must be adequately trained to administer oxygen therapy and their competency should be assessed. They should check and document that a device is being used appropriately and that the flow and/or concentration of oxygen is as prescribed and appropriate to the patient's need (O'Driscoll et al. 2017).

Nursing and physiotherapy staff may assess patients and may initiate and monitor oxygen therapy within the prescribed parameters; an exeception to this would be in an emergency, when oxygen should be given first and prescribed later (Dhruve et al. 2015).

Governance

Clinical governance leads should audit current practice and develop local policies and evidence-based guidelines (Dixon and Jones 2017) to ensure that:

- oxygen is administered and prescribed according to national guidance from the British Thoracic Society (O'Driscoll et al. 2017)
- all equipment is regularly checked for safety
- staff are adequately trained to use equipment and troubleshoot it when problems occur.

Risk management

The use of medical equipment relating to oxygen therapy should be monitored as identified within local medical equipment policies. All incident reports relating to oxygen therapy and equipment should be reviewed by local risk management committees to identify themes and trends, and propose appropriate risk reduction measures to prevent reoccurrence and improve patient safety (MHRA 2013).

Pre-procedural considerations

Ensure a prescription is in place before administering any oxygen (unless in an emergency situation). Pulse oximetry monitoring equipment must be readily available in all clinical areas where oxygen may be administered (O'Driscoll et al. 2017).

Equipment

Oxygen is an odourless, tasteless, colourless and transparent gas that is slightly heavier than air. Oxygen supports combustion so there is always a danger of fire in the presence of a spark or naked flame when oxygen is being used. The following safety measures should be remembered (Dhruve et al. 2015):

- Oil or grease around oxygen connections should be avoided.
- Alcohol, ether and other inflammable liquids should be used with caution near oxygen.
- No electrical device should be used in or near an oxygen tent.
- Oxygen cylinders should be kept secure, in an upright position and away from heat.
- There must be no smoking in the vicinity of oxygen.
- A fire extinguisher should be readily available.

- Care should be taken with high concentrations of oxygen when using a defibrillator in a cardiorespiratory arrest or during elective cardioversion.
- All oxygen delivery systems should be checked at least once per day.

Oxygen delivery

Any oxygen delivery system will include these basic components:

- *oxygen supply*: from either a piped supply or a portable cylinder (portable cylinders range from size C to size J and contain compressed gas held at high pressure; size C is for ambulatory use whereas size J is for use at the bedside when a piped supply is not available)
- *reduction gauge*: to reduce the pressure to atmospheric pressure
- *flowmeter*: a device that controls the flow of oxygen in litres per minute (L/min)
- *tubing*: disposable tubing of varying diameters and lengths
- *mechanism for delivery*: a mask or nasal cannula
- *humidifier* (optional): to warm and moisten the oxygen before administration.

Nasal cannula

A nasal cannula (Figure 12.4) consists of two plastic prongs that are inserted inside the anterior nares and supported on a light frame. A nasal cannula can be used when the patient requires a low concentration of oxygen (between 24% and 35%) with flow rates of 1–4 L/min. While Table 12.2 shows oxygen concentrations in relation to flow when oxygen is delivered via a nasal cannula, the actual uptake of oxygen and its subsequent effect on blood oxygen and carbon dioxide levels cannot be accurately predicted due to the variation in a patient's rate and pattern of breathing (O'Driscoll et al. 2017). Medium concentrations of oxygen up to 44% (6 L/min) can be used but are often not well tolerated due to nasal irritation of the mucous membranes.

As an alternative to a mask, the nasal cannula may seem less claustrophobic; is generally more comfortable; and does not interfere with eating, drinking or communication. There is also no risk of rebreathing carbon dioxide (Brill and Wedzicha 2014).

Simple face-mask

Simple face-masks (Figure 12.5) are medium-concentration masks that entrain the air from the atmosphere, delivering a variable oxygen concentration (anything from 40% to 60%; Table 12.3). These masks are useful for patients with type 1 respiratory failure who need a higher percentage of oxygen temporarily while the cause of their hypoxia is treated.

As with the nasal cannula, the actual oxygen concentration delivered is not accurate as it differs depending on the set flow rate and the patient's rate and depth of breathing (O'Driscoll et al. 2017). Using less than 5 L/min is not recommenced due to the possible build-up and rebreathing of carbon dioxide, caused by the low flow and resistance to breathing against the mask (Brill and Wedzicha 2014, Herren et al. 2017). If the patient requires more than 60% oxygen (10 L/min), expert help should be sought as the patient may require more invasive respiratory support.

Reservoir mask (non-rebreathing mask)

Reservoir masks (Figure 12.6) are similar to simple face-masks with the addition of a reservoir bag. They allow oxygen to be delivered at concentrations between 60% and 90% when used at a flow rate of 10–15 L/min. Oxygen flows into the bag (the bag should be inflated with oxygen prior to use) and mask during inhalation while, on exhalation, air is diverted out of the mask's side valves. A separate one-way valve prevents expired air from flowing back into the reservoir bag and the rebreathing of carbon dioxide.

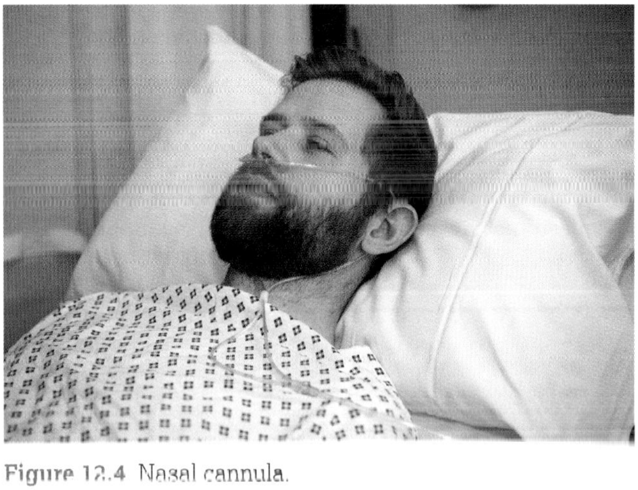

Figure 12.4 Nasal cannula.

Table 12.2 Approximate oxygen concentrations related to flow rates of nasal cannulas

Oxygen flow rate (L/min)	Oxygen concentration delivered (%)
1	24
2	28
3	32
4	36
5	40
6	44

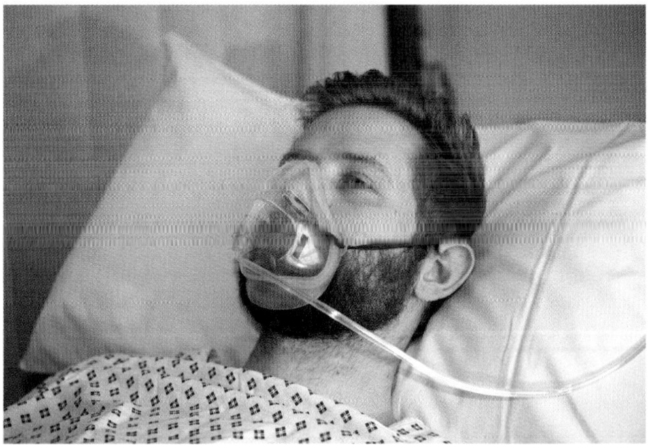

Figure 12.5 Simple face-mask.

Table 12.3 Approximate oxygen concentrations related to flow rates of simple face-masks

Oxygen flow rate (L/min)	Oxygen concentration delivered (%)
2	24
4	35
6	50
8	55
10	60
12	65
15	70

As with the nasal cannula and simple face-mask, the actual concentration of oxygen delivered varies depending on the patient's breathing rate and pattern, as well as the mask fit (O'Driscoll et al. 2017).

Note that if the oxygen flow is less than 10 L/min, carbon dioxide can accumulate in the reservoir bag, resulting in an increase in carbon dioxide inhalation (Herren et al. 2017) and a failure to meet the patient's oxygen requirements. This device is usually used during an emergency situation and in the presence of expert nursing and medical support. It may also be used as a short-term measure before more invasive respiratory support is instituted.

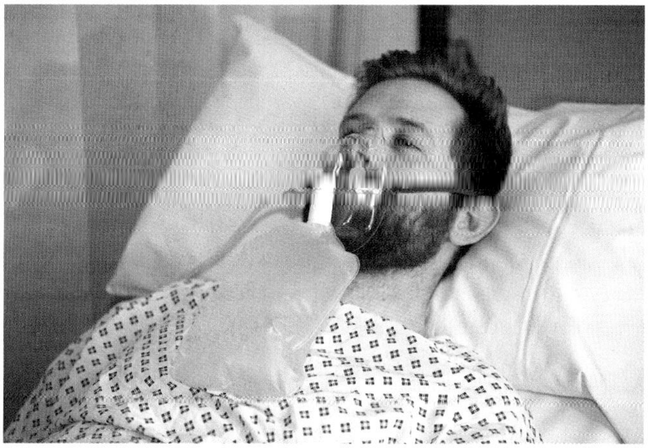

Figure 12.6 Reservoir mask (non-rebreathe mask)

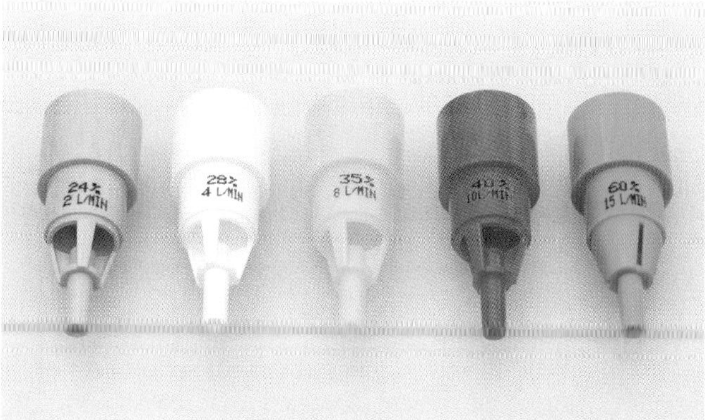

Figure 12.7 Venturi attachments.

Venturi mask (fixed performance mask or high-flow mask)

The Venturi mask (composed of a simple face-mask and a Venturi adaptor) delivers high-flow oxygen when the oxygen flow rate is set above the minimum rate printed on the side of the attachment (Figure 12.7). The adaptors are colour coded according to the percentage of oxygen they deliver and are available in the following concentrations: 24%, 28%, 35%, 40% and 60%. The Venturi effect ensures an accurate concentration of oxygen is delivered regardless of the proportion of air drawn into the attachment and the flow of oxygen delivered (providing it is above the minimum stated). Unlike in the devices mentioned previously, the oxygen concentration delivered is not affected by the patient's rate and depth of breathing. Because of the accuracy in oxygen delivery offered by these masks, the 24% and 28% Venturi masks are suited to patients at risk of hypercapnic respiratory failure (Brill and Wedzicha 2014, O'Driscoll et al. 2017).

Venturi masks are also suitable for patients with an increased respiratory rate (more than 30 breaths per minute) who require an increased inspiratory flow. It is suggested that for such patients the flow rate is increased by 50% from the minimum printed on the side of the attachment to help overcome this demand (O'Driscoll et al. 2017). For example, increasing the oxygen flow from 2 to 4 L/min on a 24% Venturi mask doubles the total inspiratory flow from 51 L/min to 102 L/min. As shown in Table 12.4, when a high oxygen flow is used with a higher oxygen concentration adaptor, the total flow decreases dramatically, which may not be suitable for a patient in extremis. In this scenario, a different type of oxygen delivery (such as high-flow oxygen via a nasal cannula, non-invasive ventilation, or use of continuous positive airway pressure) may be preferred.

Tracheostomy mask

Tracheostomy masks (Figure 12.8) perform in a similar way to the simple face-mask. The mask is placed over the tracheostomy tube or laryngectomy stoma. Oxygen needs to be humidified to prevent drying of airways and secretions since the patient's natural mechanisms of humidification have been bypassed (NTSP 2013). For more information, see the section below on humidification.

A summary of the oxygen devices discussed and their advantages and disadvantages can be found in Table 12.5.

Pharmacological and non-pharmacological support

The following measures should be prescribed or offered to help improve a patient's respiratory status (GOLD 2017, NICE 2018b, O'Driscoll et al. 2017), where relevant:

- antimicrobials if pneumonia is suspected or during exacerbations of chronic obstructive pulmonary disease (COPD) associated with purulent sputum
- oral or inhaled therapy (such as bronchodilators, steroids and mucolytics) for patients with asthma and COPD
- opioid analgesia for patients with intractable breathlessness caused by their underlying disease
- pharmacological products and nicotine replacement therapies to aid smoking cessation

Table 12.4 Total gas flow from Venturi masks at different oxygen flow rates

Set oxygen flow (L/min)	24% Venturi (L/min)	28% Venturi (L/min)	35% Venturi (L/min)	40% Venturi (L/min)	60% Venturi (L/min)
15			84	82	30
12			67	50	24
10			56	41	
8		89	46		
6		67			
4	102	44			
2	51				

Source: Adapted from O'Driscoll et al. (2017) with permission of BMJ Publishing Group, Ltd.

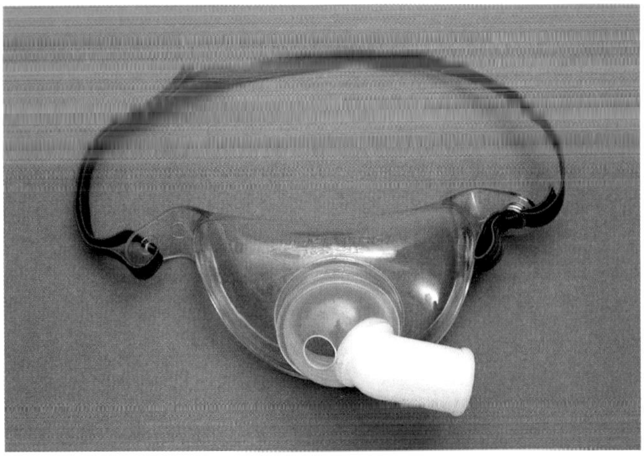

Figure 12.8 Tracheostomy mask.

- pneumococcal vaccination and annual influenza vaccination for susceptible and immunocompromised patients
- physiotherapy and pulmonary rehabilitation for patients with COPD to aid physical mobility, clearance of secretions and deep breathing exercises

Specific patient preparation

The patient should be provided with an explanation as to why oxygen therapy is indicated, what device is to be used (such as a mask or nasal cannula) and the importance of keeping the device in place. If the patient is mobile, portable cylinders should be readily available to allow oxygen therapy to continue while the patient attends to toileting and personal care away from their bed space. The patient should be educated about the hazards of oxygen and the dangers of smoking, naked flames, aerosol sprays and petroleum-based products used within their immediate vicinity. The nurse should instruct the patient to report symptoms such as increasing shortness of breath, difficulty breathing, anxiety, distress, nausea, or a dry mouth, nose or throat.

Table 12.5 Summary of oxygen devices

	Oxygen concentration				
Device	Low	Medium	High	Advantages	Disadvantages
Nasal cannula	✓	×	×	Comfortable and well tolerated. Patient can eat, drink and communicate easily. No risk of rebreathing carbon dioxide.	Can cause drying and irritation of airways when higher flow rates are used.
Simple face-mask	×	✓	×	Generally well tolerated when used for a short period of time (hours rather than days).	Can cause build-up of carbon dioxide when used at a flow rate of <5 L/min. Inaccurate oxygen concentration delivery. Patients may find the mask claustrophobic.
Reservoir mask	×	×	✓	Provides a high concentration of oxygen to critically unwell patients in an emergency situation.	Not suitable for weaning oxygen flow or concentration.
Venturi mask	✓	✓	×	Safe to use for patients at risk of hypercapnic respiratory failure. Accurate delivery of prescribed/desired oxygen concentration. Suitable for patients with a respiratory rate above 30 breaths per minute who have an increased inspiratory flow requirement.	Patients may find the mask claustrophobic.
Tracheostomy mask	×	✓	×	Provides oxygen at varying concentrations (best used for medium concentrations). Placed directly over the tracheostomy tube.	Oxygen concentration delivery can vary (depending on the patient's rate and depth of breathing). If required for prolonged periods, the oxygen should be humidified and ideally warmed, as upper airways are bypassed.

Procedure guideline 12.1 Oxygen therapy

Essential equipment

- Personal protective equipment
- Piped or wall oxygen
- Oxygen flow meter or regulator
- Portable oxygen cylinders (for use during ambulation or when transporting the patient)
- Selection of oxygen masks, nasal cannulas and Venturi attachments
- Oxygen tubing of varying lengths
- Emergency equipment, including reservoir mask and bag valve mask (used during resuscitation)

Action	Rationale
Pre-procedure	
1 Introduce yourself to the patient, explain and discuss the procedure with them, and gain their consent to proceed.	To ensure that the patient feels at ease, understands the procedure and gives their valid consent (NMC 2018, **C**).
2 Decontaminate hands with an alcohol-based handrub. Hands should be cleansed before and after each patient contact.	To minimize the risk of healthcare-associated infection (NHS England and NHSI 2019, **C**).
3 Monitor the patient's oxygen saturations and respiratory rate to determine whether a low-, medium- or high-flow device is required. Take into consideration the advantages and disadvantages (as described in Table 12.5) to help guide the choice of device. Seek expert help if required.	To ensure that the most appropriate device for oxygen delivery is chosen to suit the patient's condition and requirements (O'Driscoll et al. 2017, **C**).
4 Except in emergency situations, ensure an oxygen prescription is in place with clear target oxygen saturations.	Medical oxygen is a drug and so requires a prescription (Brill and Wedzicha 2014, **C**). Patients at risk of hypercapnic respiratory failure should have target saturations of 88–92% (GOLD 2017, **C**). Those not at risk should have target saturations of 94–98% (O'Driscoll et al. 2017, **C**). Oxygen can be administered in an emergency without a prescription; however, it should be prescribed at the earliest opportunity (Dhruve et al. 2015, **C**).
Procedure	
5 Attach oxygen tubing to the port on the wall or cylinder (and not to the medical air port).	To ensure oxygen will be delivered. **E** The administration of air rather than oxygen will cause hypoxia (NHS Improvement 2016, **C**).
6 If a cylinder is used, remove the plastic side cap and turn the valve before adjusting the flow to the desired setting. If wall oxygen is used, set the flow meter to the desired setting. Check oxygen is flowing through the system by using fingertips.	To ensure the system is turned on and oxygen is being delivered (NHS Improvement 2018a, **C**).
7 *Either:*	
Apply a *nasal cannula* by gently placing the nasal prongs of the cannula into the patient's nostrils. Drape the tubing over the patient's ears and slide the fit connector up under the chin to hold the tubing securely in place.	To ensure the cannula is correctly applied and to ensure maximum oxygen delivery. **E**
Or:	
Apply an *oxygen mask* by placing the mask over the patient's mouth and nose, then pull the elastic strap over the head and adjust the strap on both sides to secure the mask in a position that seals it against the face.	To ensure the mask is correctly fitted and is comfortable for the patient. **E**
Or:	
On a *reservoir mask*, first cover the one-way valve with fingers until the reservoir bag is fully inflated. Then apply the mask as described above.	To ensure the reservoir is fully inflated before applying the reservoir mask onto the patient. **E**
Post-procedure	
8 Record what device has been used, as well as the flow rate and concentration (if applicable). Record what time the therapy was commenced.	To maintain accurate records (NMC 2018, **C**). To help guide treatment. **E**
9 Check patient observations and National Early Warning Score (NEWS) 5 minutes and again 1 hour after starting oxygen therapy as a minimum.	To observe for any deterioration in the patient's condition, to assess the effectiveness of the intervention and to help guide treatment (O'Driscoll et al. 2017, **C**).
10 Increase or reduce oxygen flow and/or concentration to achieve the target oxygen saturations.	Oxygen should be titrated up to overcome hypoxia but avoid hyperoxia, especially in patients with known chronic obstructive pulmonary disease (Brill and Wedzicha 2014, **C**).
11 Provide continued reassurance to the patient and allow them the opportunity to ask questions.	To minimize apprehension and anxiety and to improve concordance with treatment. **E**
12 Inspect the patient's skin regularly around the face, ears and back of head.	To ensure pressure sores are not developing where the oxygen device comes into contact with the patient's skin. **E**

Problem-solving table 12.1 Prevention and resolution (Procedure guideline 12.1)

Problem	Cause	Prevention	Action
Inability to maintain an airway	Position of patient	Place the patient in the Fowler position (Figure 12.9) by elevating the head of the bed and using pillows to support the patient.	Reposition the patient sitting up at an angle of greater than 45°.
	Reduced consciousness level	Assess the patient's consciousness level routinely (see Chapter 14: Observations).	Call for expert help immediately. If worried, call for the cardiac arrest or medical emergency team. Perform the head tilt, chin lift manoeuvre to open up the patient's airway.
	Airway secretions	Humidify the oxygen. Consider regular saline nebulizers if prescribed to help loosen secretions. Refer to physiotherapy for assistance with breathing techniques, to aid deep breathing and expectoration of secretions. Ensure the patient is well hydrated. Encourage mobility. Provide tissues and a sputum pot.	Add humidification to the oxygen therapy if able. Give saline nebulizers. Encourage the patient to cough and expectorate secretions. If the patient is unable to clear their own secretions, consider suctioning. Hydrate by the most suitable route (oral, enteral or intravenous).
Inability to maintain target saturations	Oxygen not turned on or delivery system not patent	Ensure the oxygen is turned on at the wall or portable cylinder. Ensure the oxygen delivery system is properly set up with no breaks or leaks.	Turn on oxygen. Inspect the oxygen delivery system to determine where the break or leak is. Connect the system or replace parts as required.
	Inadequate oxygen flow/concentration being delivered	Ensure the most appropriate oxygen device is selected depending on the patient's condition and oxygen requirement.	Titrate up the oxygen flow/concentration until the target oxygen saturations have been met.
	Patient's condition deteriorating	Monitor observations/NEWS frequently and escalate urgently if total NEWS is ≥5 or 3 in one parameter.	Call immediately for expert help (as per local policy). If worried, call cardiac arrest or medical emergency team. Commence 15 L/min reservoir mask until expert help arrives. Attach pulse oximetry and monitor observations continuously. Titrate oxygen flow/concentration down to meet the saturation target, or in response to the patient's clinical condition.
Nasal irritation or dry mucous membranes	Oxygen therapy can lead to irritated and dry nasal passages and mucous membranes	Provide regular mouth care or artificial saliva if prescribed. Give as low a flow rate as possible to prevent drying of airways (while still meeting the saturation target).	Add humidification to the system if able. Give regular mouth/nasal care.
	Patient dehydrated	Ensure the patient is well hydrated.	Hydrate the patient by the most suitable route (oral, enteral or intravenous).
Nasal cannula or mask discomfort	Position or prolonged use of nasal cannula or oxygen mask	Ensure correct size and placement of mask used. Alternate the devices used.	Ensure correct placement of the device used. Use pressure-relieving foam, tape or dressings to minimize discomfort on the face and around the ears and head. Alternate the devices used if able.
Intolerance of oxygen therapy	Fear and anxiety	Explain the need/benefit of oxygen therapy. Allow the patient to express their fears/concerns. Offer reassurance and support.	Reassure the patient and offer support. Try an alternative oxygen delivery device.
	Confusion and/or hypoxia	Treat the underlying cause of confusion or hypoxia. Give oxygen as soon as hypoxia is detected. Frequently reorientate the patient to the environment and oxygen device.	If the patient is hypoxic, oxygen may need to be increased, or the device changed. Seek expert help immediately to determine and treat the underlying cause of confusion and/or hypoxia.

Problem	Cause	Prevention	Action
Inability of patient to communicate	Mask can make communication difficult	Provide the patient with non-verbal means of communication (e.g. mobile phone to text, pen and paper, or symbol board). Ensure the patient's call bell is to hand.	Encourage the patient to keep the mask on and use alternative means of communication. Consider changing the device to a nasal cannula or high-flow oxygen therapy if a higher oxygen flow/concentration is required.
Inability of patient to maintain personal hygiene and elimination independently	Oxygen therapy restricting patient's mobility and preventing them from being able to carry out usual daily activities independently	Give the patient a nurse call bell and encourage them to ask for help with daily activities. Promote patient independence where able.	Enable the patient to mobilize to the toilet using a portable oxygen cylinder. If the patient's condition is too unstable for them to mobilize, consider using urinals, bedpans a or commode by the bedside, or transfer the patient to the toilet or washroom in a wheelchair. Assist the patient to carry out personal care at the bedside if required.
Inability to maintain safe environment	Patient confused, hypoxic or acutely unwell	Check on the patient at regular intervals. Monitor observations and NEWS frequently. Check the patency of the oxygen delivery system and set flow rate with each set of patient observations. Ensure the oxygen device is not removed by the patient. Ensure the patient has a nurse call bell to hand and encourage them to call if they have any concerns or a change in breathing pattern.	Seek expert help immediately if the patient's condition worsens. Ensure the oxygen delivery system is properly set up and the correct flow/concentration is being delivered. Reapply the oxygen device if removed. Attend to the patient promptly if the nurse call bell is activated. Consider one-to-one nursing if the patient requires constant supervision or nursing care.

NEWS, National Early Warning Score.

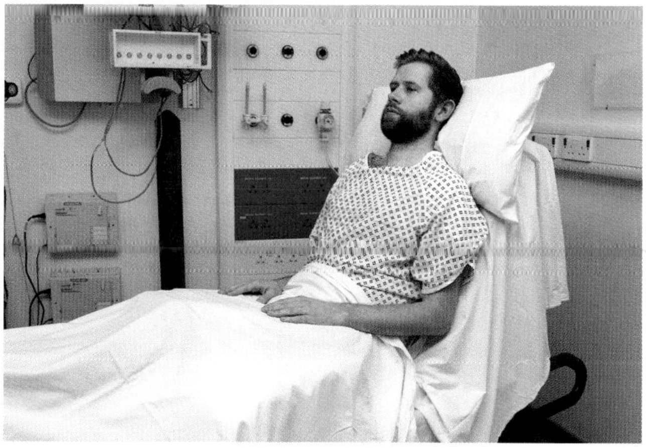

Figure 12.9 Fowler position.

Post-procedural considerations

Immediate care

The patient should be educated regarding the necessity of keeping the oxygen cannula or mask on to prevent periods of hypoxaemia. This includes during periods of mobilization. Reassurance should be given and the patient should be allowed opportunities to ask questions and express any concerns or discomfort.

Document the device, flow rate and concentration of oxygen administered, in addition to the patient's observations, within 5 minutes of commencing oxygen therapy (O'Driscoll et al. 2017). Monitor for changes in consciousness level, especially if the patient is at risk of hypercapnic respiratory failure, and escalate any concerns immediately.

All patients should be assessed and monitored using the National Early Warning Score (NEWS) (RCP 2017). The device, flow and/or concentration delivered should also be documented on the patient's observation chart (see Table 12.6 for the approved abbreviations for recording oxygen delivery on the observation chart).

Patients who are hypoxaemic must be assessed by an experienced clinician to determine the cause of their hypoxaemia so the underlying cause can be treated (O'Driscoll et al. 2017). The clinician should also determine what the target saturations for the patient are and document this on the observation chart, on the drug chart, and in the nursing and medical records (Brill and Wedzicha 2014, O'Driscoll et al. 2017).

Arterial blood gas (ABG) analysis should be undertaken as soon as possible in all critically ill patients and situations involving hypoxaemic patients. It also forms part of the essential assessment in patients who are at risk of hypercapnic respiratory failure (GOLD 2017). Interpretation of the results must take into account the amount of supplementary oxygen being administered at the time of ABG sampling. ABG sampling should be repeated after 30 minutes in accordance with the patient's clinical response to treatment, and in all cases where the patient is found to be both hypercapnic and acidotic (GOLD 2017, O'Driscoll et al. 2017).

Ongoing care

Recheck the patient's condition, observations and NEWS 1 hour after starting oxygen therapy and then a minimum of every 4 hours thereafter (O'Driscoll et al. 2017). Patients with a NEWS of 5 or more will require more frequent observations (RCP 2017). This will

Table 12.6 Abbreviations for recording oxygen delivery on an observation chart

Abbreviation	Meaning
A	Air (not requiring oxygen)
CP	CPAP system
H28	Humidified oxygen 28% (also H35, H40 and H60 for humidified oxygen at 35%, 40% and 60% respectively)
HFN	High-flow oxygen via nasal cannula
N	Nasal cannula
NIV	Non-invasive ventilation system
RM	Reservoir mask/non-rebreathing mask
SM	Simple mask
TM	Tracheostomy mask
V24	Venturi 24%
V28	Venturi 28%
V35	Venturi 35%
V40	Venturi 40%
V60	Venturi 60%

Source: Adapted from O'Driscoll et al. (2017) with permission of BMJ Publishing Group, Ltd.

allow for early identification and escalation of patients at risk of clinical deterioration.

For patients requiring high-flow oxygen therapy for more than 24 hours, or when a patient reports discomfort due to dryness, humidification should be commenced to protect airway defences and optimize patient comfort.

Encouraging patients to sit out in a chair and mobilize frequently will help to prevent atelectasis (incomplete lung inflation) and aid removal of secretions. Ensuring that post-operative patients have effective pain relief will allow them to carry out deep breathing exercises and aid early ambulation, reducing the risk of post-operative atelectasis.

Weaning and discontinuing oxygen therapy

Reduce oxygen flow/concentration or stop oxygen therapy if the patient is clinically stable and their peripheral oxygen saturations have been within the target range for two consecutive observations (O'Driscoll et al. 2017). Observe the patient 5 minutes after stopping or lowering the dose of oxygen therapy and document the observations. Repeat observations again after 1 hour; if saturations remain within the desired target range, oxygen therapy has been successfully weaned or stopped (O'Driscoll et al. 2017).

Patients should be observed for signs and symptoms of hypercapnia. These include anxiety, mild dyspnoea, headache, hypersomnolence, delirium, confusion, facial flushing, bounding pulse, tachycardia, warm peripheries, drowsiness and flapping tremor (Feller-Kopman and Schwartzstein 2017, Patel and Majmundar 2018). If hypercapnia is suspected, reduce the oxygen concentration down slowly. Do not stop oxygen completely as this may cause rebound hypoxia (Feller-Kopman and Schwartzstein 2017).

Documentation

Accurate documentation of patient observations and the oxygen device, flow and concentration administered will assist healthcare professionals in determining whether a patient is clinically improving or deteriorating, and help to guide future treatments. Clear documentation of the events that led up to a patient requiring oxygen therapy, in addition to any other relevant information, must be available for all healthcare professionals to review if required, as this will improve communication and reduce patient risk (NMC 2010).

Domiciliary oxygen and patient education

Long-term oxygen therapy at home may be required if the patient is chronically hypoxaemic and requires oxygen for more than 15 hours per day (Hardinge et al. 2015). Relevant conditions include COPD, cystic fibrosis, interstitial lung disease, neuromuscular and skeletal disorders, pulmonary hypertension, obstructive sleep apnoea and heart failure. Palliative oxygen therapy may also be required for patients with intractable breathlessness caused by their underlying lung disease (O'Driscoll et al. 2017). A full clinical assessment should be performed before a referral is made to the home oxygen assessment team.

The patient and their family should be formally educated and provided with written information on the hazards of oxygen use at home. Healthcare providers must be sure that the patient and their family members understand the dangers of smoking (including e-cigarettes) in an oxygen-enriched environment. An increased amount of oxygen in the environment increases the speed at which things burn once a fire starts. Oxygen can saturate clothing, fabric, hair and beards. Even flame-retardant clothing can burn when oxygen content increases. It is important to keep all naked flames and heat sources away from oxygen systems. Patients should be advised never to smoke or light a match while using oxygen, or allow others in the same room to do so. The local fire brigade should be informed of any home with an oxygen system (Hardinge et al. 2015) and every home should have at least one working smoke detector on every level and near all bedrooms. When transported in a car, oxygen cylinders should be adequately secured, a warning triangle should be displayed and the car insurance company should be informed.

The oxygen supplier in the community has a responsibility to carry out a detailed risk assessment of the patient's home and ensure the environment is safe, as well as educate the patient and provide written information on the use of oxygen equipment. The patient should also be followed up by a specialist home oxygen assessment team at least 4 weeks after hospital discharge to ensure safe use and compliance with oxygen therapy (Hardinge et al. 2015). Oxygen may be supplied in cylinders or in an oxygen concentrator, which is more economical for patients requiring long-term oxygen therapy. For more guidance see the British Thoracic Society's guidelines for home oxygen use in adults (Hardinge et al. 2015).

Complications

Carbon dioxide narcosis

Carbon dioxide is the chemical that most directly influences respiration via its effect on the efficiency of alveolar ventilation. The normal partial pressure of carbon dioxide in the blood is 4.0–6.0 kPa (30–45 mmHg). When this level rises, the pH of the CSF drops, which in turn causes excitation of the central chemoreceptors, and hyperventilation occurs (Patel and Majmundar 2018, Tortora and Derrickson 2017).

Patients with COPD often retain carbon dioxide due to a change in the normal ventilation/perfusion ratio of the lungs and reduced alveolar ventilation. Chemoreceptors are no longer sensitive to a raised carbon dioxide level, so the falling PaO_2 becomes the principal respiratory stimulus. Giving high levels of supplementary oxygen can reduce the patient's stimulus to breathe, resulting in a fall in minute ventilation, which leads to respiratory depression, coma and death (Feller-Kopman and Schwartzstein 2017). The link between giving high concentrations of oxygen and hypercapnia is complex and related to several processes in addition to reducing the patient's hypoxic drive.

Patients with known COPD should aim for target saturations of 88–92% and acute exacerbations treated with a 24–28% Venturi mask (GOLD 2017).

Absorption atelectasis

Nitrogen within the alveoli help to splint the air sacs open and prevent them from collapsing. Hyperoxia should therefore be avoided as high concentrations of oxygen wash out alveolar nitrogen, causing atelectasis (Hafner et al. 2015).

Oxygen toxicity

Prolonged hyperoxygenation and hyperoxia can result in pulmonary toxicity and lung injury. Hyperoxia increases the level of reactive oxygen-derived free radicals, which causes an imbalance between oxidants and antioxidants, disrupting homeostasis at the cellular level (Hafner et al. 2015). A complex process ultimately results in lung fibrosis, which is permanent and irreversible (Mach et al. 2011). However, the degree of injury is related to the length of time and concentration of oxygen to which the individual is exposed. Where possible, long periods (i.e. 24 hours or more) of oxygen therapy above 50% FiO_2 should be avoided. However, treating hypoxia is the priority; use as little oxygen as possible to achieve the target oxygen saturations.

Oxygen is hazardous to patients with paraquat poisoning as it worsens pneumonitis and lung fibrosis. It should also be avoided in patients who have received bleomycin chemotherapy due to the risk of pulmonary toxicity; oxygen should only be given if the patient's saturations fall below 85% (O'Driscoll et al. 2017).

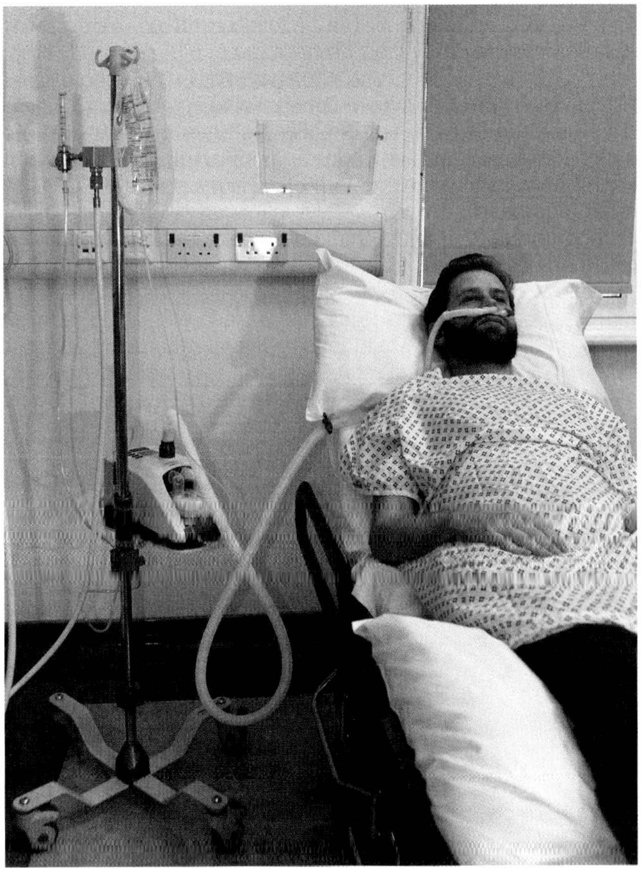

Figure 12.10 High-flow oxygen via a nasal cannula.

High-flow oxygen via a nasal cannula

Definition

High-flow oxygen via a nasal cannula (Figure 12.10) is the provision of high flow, warmed and humidified oxygen to the patient via nasal prongs.

Evidence-based approaches

High-flow nasal (HFN) oxygen allows delivery of an oxygen concentration of up to 100% at a flow rate of 60 L/min (system dependent). It is an alternative to giving high-flow oxygen via a reservoir mask in patients with respiratory failure who are not at risk of hypercapnic respiratory failure (O'Driscoll et al. 2017). Because patients with hypoxaemic respiratory failure have greater inspiratory flow requirements, HFN oxygen can meet or exceed the patient's demand while minimizing the risks of air dilution and the inaccurate delivery of oxygen (Nishimura 2015, Papazian et al. 2016). Invariably, oxygenation and the work of breathing improve.

Although research on the effects and outcomes of HFN oxygen is limited, several studies have shown that high-flow oxygen helps to increase alveolar ventilation by flushing out the anatomical dead space of CO_2 (Dysart et al. 2009, Nishimura 2015). It also provides low levels of positive end-expiratory airway pressure (PEEP), which aids alveolar recruitment and reduces atelectasis (Möller et al. 2015, Nishimura 2015).

HFN oxygen emulates the temperature and humidity of a healthy adult lung (37°C and 44 mg/L H_2O), providing the physiological benefits of humidification (see the section on humidification below). In addition to increased patient comfort, the nasal cannula allows the patient to eat, drink and communicate freely, increasing compliance (Cuquemelle et al. 2012).

HFN oxygen can be used as a step between conventional oxygen therapy and mechanical ventilation, or as an alternative to non-invasive ventilation (NIV) (Frat et al. 2015, Sztrymf et al. 2011). This may allow the patient to receive care on the ward setting and possibly prevent admission to a high-dependency or intensive therapy unit. It may also help to wean patients off NIV or mechanical ventilation, and reduce the need for reintubation (Frat et al. 2015, Hernández et al. 2016).

High-flow oxygen can also be delivered via a tracheostomy with an attachment, to give warmed and humidified high-flow oxygen. However, the other benefits listed above may not apply as no studies have looked at the outcome of using high-flow oxygen therapy with this patient group.

Rationale

Indications

HFN oxygen is indicated in the following circumstances:

- mild to moderate hypoxaemic respiratory failure
- difficulty clearing secretions
- respiratory wean
- cardiogenic pulmonary oedema
- symptomatic breathlessness.

Contraindications

There are no documented absolute contraindications to HFN oxygen but relative contraindications may include:

- upper gastrointestinal or head and neck surgery and cancers
- obstructed nasopharynx
- haemoptysis or uncontrolled oral or nasal bleeding
- deranged clotting.

Procedure guideline 12.2 High-flow oxygen therapy

Essential equipment

- Personal protective equipment
- Oxygen supply
- Drip stand
- High-flow oxygen delivery system
- High-flow breathing circuit and water humidification chamber
- High-flow oxygen nasal cannula or tracheostomy attachment
- Bag of sterile water

Action	Rationale
Pre-procedure	
1 Introduce yourself to the patient, explain and discuss the procedure with them, and gain their consent to proceed.	To ensure that the patient feels at ease, understands the procedure and gives their valid consent (NMC 2018, **C**).
2 Decontaminate hands with an alcohol-based handrub.	To minimize the risk of healthcare-associated infection (NHS England and NHSI 2019, **C**).
3 Assess patient observations and/or National Early Warning Score (NEWS). Perform physical assessment and arterial blood gas (ABG) measurement.	To determine whether the patient is hypoxaemic (O'Driscoll et al. 2017, **C**) and whether high-flow oxygen via a nasal cannula (HFN oxygen) is indicated.
4 Document patient observations/NEWS prior to commencing HFN oxygen.	To provide baseline observations/NEWS. **E**
5 Ensure the patient is sitting upright and in a comfortable position, e.g. the Fowler position (Figure 12.9).	To promote comfort and aid lung expansion. **E**
Procedure	
6 Set up HFN oxygen as per the manufacturer's instructions, and attach a sterile water bag to water the humidification chamber.	Adhering to the manufacturer's guidelines ensures the safe and correct use of equipment. **E**
7 Turn the system on and allow it to reach the optimum temperature (37°C).	To warm the water in the chamber. **E**
8 Correctly place the nasal cannula onto the patient and tighten the straps around the patient's head.	To ensure the fit is snug and comfortable. An ill-fitting cannula may result in poor oxygenation. **E**
9 Monitor the patient's condition and observations/NEWS for the first 5 minutes after HFN oxygen is commenced.	To detect any deterioration in the patient's condition (O'Driscoll et al. 2017, **C**).
10 Titrate up the oxygen concentration.	To achieve target saturations of 94–98% (or 88–92% if the patient is at risk of hypercapnic respiratory failure) (O'Driscoll et al. 2017, **C**).
11 Titrate up the flow rate (L/min).	Until a reduction in respiratory rate and target saturations is achieved. **E**
12 Document the indication for HFN oxygen, the patient's observations/NEWS, the target oxygen saturations, and the set oxygen concentration and flow rate.	To maintain accurate records (NMC 2018, **C**) and ensure continuity of care.
Post-procedure	
13 Monitor and document the patient's observations/NEWS 1 hour after commencing HFN oxygen, and a minimum of 4-hourly thereafter.	To monitor for signs of clinical deterioration (O'Driscoll et al. 2017, **C**).
14 Escalate any concerns to an appropriate member of staff (e.g. senior nursing staff, critical care outreach team, medical staff or physiotherapist).	To prevent patient deterioration (NICE 2007, **C**).
15 Monitor the patient's response to HFN oxygen and titrate the flow or oxygen concentration to meet the target saturations, or as per senior nursing/medical staff advice.	To ensure the patient is not being over- or under-oxygenated. **E**
16 Check the equipment regularly (e.g. 4-hourly) to ensure the correct flow and oxygen concentration are being administered.	To ensure the equipment is working properly and the patient is not being over- or under-oxygenated. **E**
17 Check the tubing regularly to ensure it is free from trapped water. If trapped water is found, lift the tubing and drain the water back into the water humidification chamber.	Trapped water will result in the inaccurate delivery of oxygen. **E**
18 Replace the bag of sterile water approximately every 12 hours or as required so that the water humidification chamber does not dry out.	The delivery of un-humidified high-flow oxygen may dry out or damage the patient's airway. **E** Drying out of the water chamber may damage the equipment. **E**
19 Replace the HFN oxygen breathing circuit and water humidification system as instructed by the manufacturer (usually once to twice weekly). All parts should be changed more frequently if they are damaged or discoloured.	To maintain good infection control practice (Fisher & Paykel Healthcare 2013, **C**).

Problem-solving table 12.2 Prevention and resolution (Procedure guideline 12.2)

Problem	Cause	Prevention	Action
The display shows fluctuating oxygen concentrations	The tubing is water-logged	Check the tubing at least 4-hourly.	Hold tubing upright to allow any logged water to flow back into the water chamber.
The patient is unable to tolerate the high flow	High flow of oxygen/air	Explain the rationale for the high flow to the patient as this may aid compliance.	Reduce the flow by 5–10 L/min. Continue to monitor patient's observations, in particular SpO_2, respiratory rate and work of breathing. Escalate any concerns to a senior member of nursing/medical staff.
The patient cannot tolerate the warm oxygen	Warming of gases by the device	Explain to the patient the benefits of warmed oxygen as this may aid compliance.	Consider reducing the temperature if patient is not able to tolerate the oxygen when set at 37°C.
The humidifier/ high-flow system alarms sounds	The nasal cannula has been removed and the HFN oxygen system has been left on	Switch the system off if no longer required.	Replace the nasal cannula on the patient and tighten the straps to ensure a snug fit. Switch the system off if no longer required.
	Part of the system has become disconnected	Check the system set-up at least 4-hourly.	Correct any accidental disconnections.
	The bag of sterile water is empty	Replace the bag of sterile water when near empty.	Replace the bag of sterile water.

Humidification

Definition

Humidity is the amount of water vapour present in a gas. The terms used to define humidity are 'absolute humidity', 'maximum capacity' and 'relative humidity'. *Absolute humidity* is the mass of water vapour that a given volume of gas can carry at a set temperature. When a gas is at its *maximum capacity*, it is said to be fully saturated. *Relative humidity* is the ratio of the absolute humidity to the maximum capacity. The warmer the gas, the more water vapour it can hold. Therefore, if the temperature of the gas falls, water will condense out of the gas into the surrounding atmosphere (Al Ashry and Modrykamien 2014).

Anatomy and physiology

The mucosa of the respiratory tract is lined with pseudostratified columnar epithelial cells, which are covered in hair-like structures known as cilia. Mucous secreted by goblet cells in the mucosa traps inhaled particles and pathogens, and the mucous is swept by the cilia from the distal to the proximal airways to be either swallowed or coughed up. Airway mucous therefore defends the airways and forms part of our innate immune system (Tortora and Derrickson 2017).

Normal room air has an approximate temperature of 22°C with a relative humidity of 50% and a water content of 10 mgH_2O per litre. For effective gas exchange to occur in the lungs, the air needs to be at a temperature of 37°C with 100% humidity and a water content of 44 mgH_2O per litre by the time it reaches the bifurcation in the trachea (McNulty and Eyre 2015). This is referred to as the 'isothermic point'. In normal circumstances, inspired air is mainly conditioned (optimally heated and humidified) in the nose and oropharynx (Doctor et al. 2017).

Related theory

Less-than-optimal heat and humidification cause several changes within the airways: mucous begins to thicken and the mobility of the cilia is affected, reducing mucociliary clearance (Doctor et al. 2017). If there is a continuing lack of humidity, the mucosal lining of the respiratory tract is damaged and cilia can break off. The isothermic point of saturation moves from the bifurcation of the trachea to a lower point in the lungs, causing collapse of the alveoli (atelectasis), decreased lung function and hypoxaemia (McNulty and Eyre 2015).

Evidence-based approaches

Many devices can be used to supply humidification. The best of these will fulfil the following requirements (Al Ashry and Modrykamien 2014, McNulty and Eyre 2015):

- The inspired gas must be delivered to the trachea at a temperature of 32–37°C with 100% humidity and should have a water content of 33–44 g/m^3.
- The appliance should not increase resistance or affect the compliance of respiration.
- Electrical humidifiers should have a safety alarm system to guard against overheating and overhydration. The set temperature should also remain constant; temperature and humidification should not be affected by large ranges in flow.

Rationale

The provision of humidification and heat in high-flow oxygen therapy (>5 L/min) can minimize symptoms of dryness and improve patient tolerance. Although there is no evidence to support the use of humidification in patients receiving low-flow oxygen therapy or those receiving it in the short term, it should always be considered for patients where the natural pathway of humidification is bypassed (those with an altered airway such as a tracheostomy, laryngectomy or endotracheal tube) (McNulty and Eyre 2015). Adequately heated and humidified oxygen therapy reduces the tenacity of secretions, improves the clearance of secretions, and reduces atelectasis, thus improving lung ventilation and gas exchange (McNulty and Eyre 2015, Nishimura 2015).

Indications

Humidification is indicated for:

- patients who are intubated and mechanically ventilated
- patients who have an altered airway
- patients with COPD to aid expectoration of viscous secretions
- patients who report upper airway discomfort due to dryness.

Contraindications

Humidification should not be used for patients requiring open system (mask) ventilation when their infective status determines that 'droplet contact' isolation precautions are required.

Anticipated patient outcomes

Secretions will be cleared and the patient's lung function and gas exchange will be improved through the provision of humidified gases.

Pre-procedural considerations

Equipment

Heat and moisture exchanger (HME)

A heat and moisture exchanger (HME) performs the function of the upper airways in conditioning the inspired air and filtering out dust and large airborne particles. It works passively by retaining heat and moisture from the expired air and returns it to the patient in the next inspired breath (Doctor et al. 2017, Wong et al. 2016). HMEs may contain a bacterial filter and consist of spun, pleated, highly thermal conductive material. There are several types of HMEs; they can be attached directly onto a tracheostomy tube (Figure 12.11) or within a laryngectomy stoma (Figure 12.12), or used in a ventilator breathing circuit (Figure 12.13) for patients who are intubated and mechanically ventilated. HMEs are portable, simple to use and a cost effective means of providing humidification (Ari et al. 2016, McNulty and Eyre 2015, NTSP 2013).

Cold water bubble humidifier

A cold water bubble humidifier delivers gas, which is bubbled through water at room temperature and delivers partially humidified oxygen at about 50% relative humidity. They are no longer advised as there is no evidence to suggest they are of clinical benefit to patients, and they may be an infection risk (O'Driscoll et al. 2017).

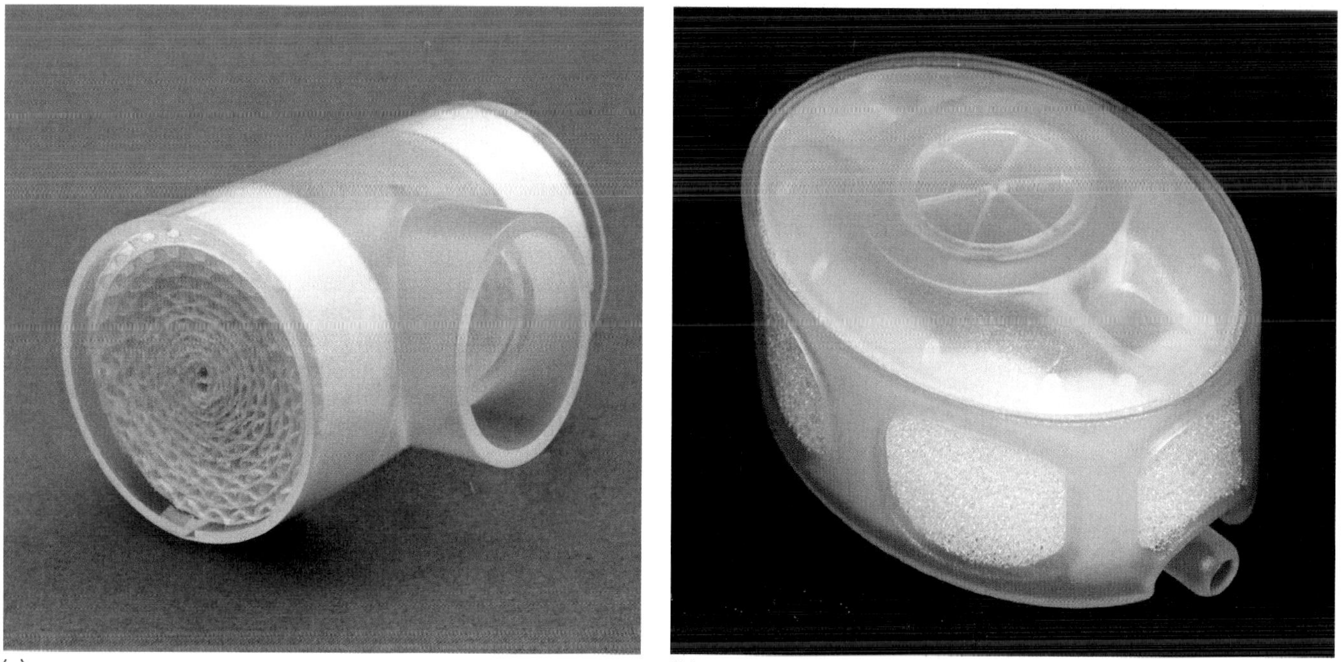

(a) (b)

Figure 12.11 Heat and moisture exchanger for a tracheostomy tube. (a) Swedish nose. (b) Trachphone.

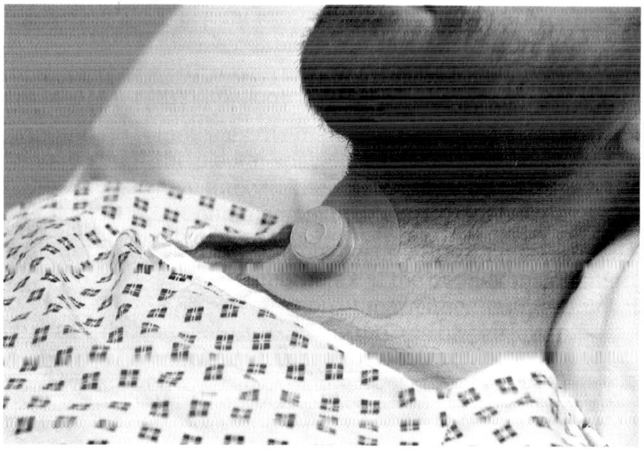

Figure 12.12 Heat and moisture exchanger for a laryngectomy.

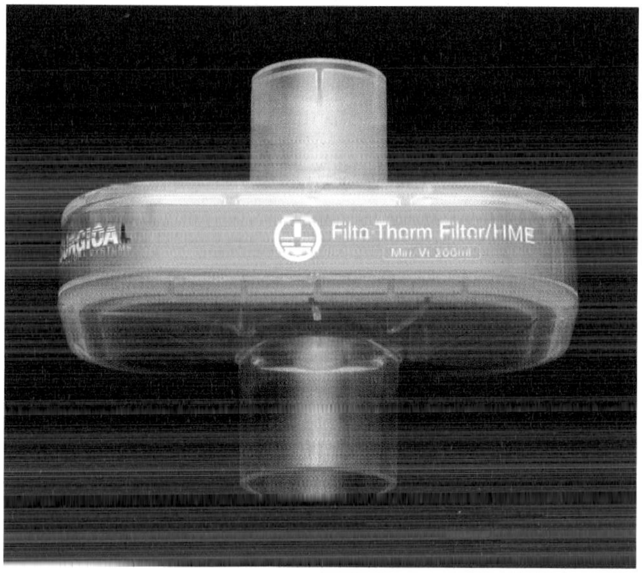

Figure 12.13 Heat and moisture exchanger for a ventilation circuit.

Water humidification chamber

In a water humidification chamber, inspired gas is forced over a heated reservoir of water, actively humidifying the oxygen or air. Hot water bath humidifiers are more efficient for providing humidification in patients who are mechanically ventilated or who are on high-flow oxygen therapy (McNulty and Eyre 2015, NTSP 2013). However, they are associated with higher costs and potential hazards (Gaffney and Dalton 2018).

Aerosol generators

While they are not true humidification devices, aerosol generators create highly saturated micro-droplets of water, which are suspended in the gas to be delivered, through an aerosol device (McNulty and Eyre 2015). These devices are particularly useful for spontaneously breathing patients with COPD to aid expectoration of viscous secretions or to deliver bronchodilatory drugs. If an electrical compressor or ultrasonic nebulizer is not available, a jet nebulizer can be given via compressed air. Care must be taken to ensure the nebulizer is not delivered using oxygen in patients who are at risk of hypercapnic respiratory failure.

Non-invasive ventilation

Definition

Non-invasive ventilation (NIV) is the application of positive airway pressure using a mechanical device via an external (i.e. non-invasive) interface such as a face-mask, nasal mask or helmet. It has become a standard of care in many forms of acute respiratory failure and can provide more immediate relief of respiratory symptoms when compared to standard therapy (Brill 2014, Davison et al. 2016). Maintenance of positive pressure throughout the respiratory cycle can have numerous benefits, such as relieving dyspnoea, improving oxygenation, optimizing gas exchange and reducing the work of breathing (Ireland et al. 2014).

The term NIV is often used interchangeably to refer to both a method of respiratory support and a mode of ventilation. For the purpose of this section, NIV is used in the context of a method of respiratory support unless otherwise specified.

Related theory

NIV has been established as a useful and safe method of respiratory support in individuals with a variety of aetiologies of respiratory compromise, such as acute respiratory failure, exacerbations of COPD and acute cardiogenic pulmonary oedema (Corrêa et al. 2015). If initiated in a timely manner and competently managed, NIV may be used as a strategy to prevent tracheal intubation and mechanical ventilation in appropriately selected patients and may thus reduce mortality and morbidity (NCEPOD 2017).

NIV may be indicated for patients with respiratory compromise if they are conscious, co-operative and able to tolerate the interface used to deliver this type of ventilation (i.e. face-mask, nasal mask or helmet). Patients who present with acute respiratory failure, especially in the presence of hypercapnia, may have symptoms of drowsiness; however, providing they have the ability to protect their airway, NIV can be a useful and effective management strategy (Vadde and Pastores 2016).

Evidence-based approaches

NIV as a method of respiratory support is the maintenance of positive pressure throughout the respiratory cycle when the patient is breathing spontaneously. It provides an additional option of therapy between conventional oxygen therapy and controlled, invasive ventilation. Advances in NIV devices, the development of more comfortable interfaces, and improvements in patient monitoring and care during NIV delivery have contributed to the increased use of NIV within a variety of clinical settings (Corrêa et al. 2015).

The aims of NIV therapy are to improve gas exchange, reduce the work of breathing, relieve dyspnoea and prevent atelectasis (incomplete lung inflation). These outcomes are achieved by:

- *Increasing functional residual capacity (FRC)*, which is the amount of gas left in the lungs at the end of normal expiration available for pulmonary gas exchange. In acute lung injury where gaseous exchange is severely inhibited, NIV increases the FRC by reopening collapsed alveoli and improving ventilation and oxygenation (Chowdhury et al. 2012).
- *Improving the ventilation/perfusion ratio*: under-ventilation of the lungs can lead to intrapulmonary shunting (blood passing through the lungs without being oxygenated). NIV helps to decrease this by improving the ventilation/perfusion mismatch (Davison et al. 2016).
- *Improved lung compliance (elasticity) of the lungs*: in respiratory failure, the lungs become much stiffer and less compliant and breathing can become more difficult. Reduction in lung volume below a certain level results in airway collapse, hypoventilation and reduced gaseous exchange. The increase in transpulmonary pressure required to overcome this can be achieved by NIV (Demoule et al. 2016).
- *Increasing lung volume (alveolar volume)*: NIV maximizes alveolar recruitment, leading to an increase in the surface area of the alveoli available for gaseous exchange (Demoule et al. 2016). Therefore, oxygen requirements can be reduced and the work of breathing relieved.

Other benefits include the preservation of the ability to speak, cough, clear secretions and swallow while warming and humidifying inspired air via natural upper airway mechanics (Davison et al. 2016).

Rationale

Indications

NIV methods are usually commenced to improve lung expansion and are indicated in the presence of clinically significant pulmonary atelectasis when other forms of therapy, such as high-flow oxygen therapy, incentive spirometry, chest physiotherapy and deep breathing exercises, have been unsuccessful. Success of NIV will be influenced by patient selection, underlying pathology, severity of respiratory compromise, interface tolerance and presence of other organ dysfunction (Brill 2014).

The clinical presentations that may benefit from NIV therapy are outlined in Box 12.1.

Box 12.1 Clinical presentations that may require non-invasive ventilation (NIV)

- Acute respiratory failure (Beitler et al. 2016, Ozsancak Ugurlu et al. 2016, Vadde and Pastores 2016)
- Acute exacerbation of COPD (Schnell et al. 2014)
- Post-surgical respiratory failure (Cammarota et al. 2011, Ferrer and Torres 2015), except in cases of laryngeal trauma or recent tracheal anastomosis
- Immunocompromised patients (Cortegiani et al. 2017, Ferreira et al. 2015, Huang et al. 2017, Schnell et al. 2014)
- Obstructive sleep apnoea (Gulati et al. 2015)
- Obesity hypoventilation syndrome (Bry et al. 2018)
- Acute cardiogenic oedema (Masa et al. 2016)
- Neuromuscular disease (NICE 2016)
- Cystic fibrosis (Rodriguez-Hortal et al. 2017)
- Chest wall deformities (Davies et al. 2018)
- Post-extubation difficulties (Lin et al. 2014)
- Weaning difficulties (Yeung et al. 2018)
- Patients 'not for intubation' but who still have a need for aggressive or supportive interventions for reversible respiratory clinical presentations (Vadde and Pastores 2016)

Contraindications

Contraindications to the use or application of NIV include:

- recurrent pneumothoraces or untreated pneumothorax
- inability to maintain own airway (Corrêa et al. 2015)
- upper airway obstruction secondary to tumour involvement (Vadde and Pastores 2016)
- recent facial or head and neck surgery (not necessarily a contraindication if using helmet NIV or CPAP)
- facial burns
- epitaxis
- excessive secretions or ineffective cough (Olivieri et al. 2015)
- vomiting or high risk of aspiration (Vadde and Pastores 2016)
- haemodynamic instability or shock
- cardiac arrhythmias
- any condition where an elevated intracranial pressure is undesirable or where reduction in cerebral blood flow is inappropriate (Backhaus et al. 2017).

Assessment

Patient assessment and early escalation to NIV are paramount in ensuring the success of the therapy and avoiding further deterioration in respiratory function (which may result in the patient requiring intubation). A trial period of NIV is often useful to predict its effectiveness (Demoule et al. 2016).

Patients who meet the criteria for NIV should have therapy initiated within 60–120 minutes of an acute presentation or deterioration (Davison et al. 2016). A comprehensive initial assessment and timely review following NIV initiation can help to identify predictors for patients who may fail a NIV trial and allow for prompt intubation. NIV failure can be identified by (Corrêa et al. 2015):

- lack of improvement in gas exchange within 2 hours (Olivieri et al. 2015)
- inability to correct dyspnoea
- increased fatigue
- incapacity to manage copious secretions
- interface discomfort and/or intolerance
- agitation
- anxiety
- haemodynamic instability
- progression of respiratory failure.

Anticipated patient outcomes

The anticipated patient outcomes of NIV include:

- increased capillary oxygen saturations (SpO_2): oxygen should be prescribed to achieve a target saturation of 94–98% for most acutely ill patients or 88–92% for those at risk of hypercapnic respiratory failure (e.g. patients with COPD) (Davison et al. 2016)
- decreased administration of supplementary oxygen to achieve targeted oxygen saturation range (Davison et al. 2016)
- reduced dyspnea, aiming for a respiratory rate of under 30 breaths per minute (Brill and Wedzicha 2014)
- achievement of exhaled tidal volumes (Vt) of 6 mL/kg of ideal bodyweight (Corrêa et al. 2015)
- effective secretion clearance as a consequence of humidification, deep breathing and coughing
- improvement of breath sounds on auscultation
- increased peak flow
- improvement in chest radiography
- ability to wean the patient off the NIV mask or helmet and maintain an improvement of respiratory status with lower oxygen requirements.

Clinical governance

Competencies

NIV respiratory support is being delivered in an increasingly wide variety of hospital settings, such as (Masa et al. 2016):

- critical care units
- high-dependency units
- step-down units
- intermediate-care units
- recovery departments
- emergency departments
- respiratory wards

Close and thorough clinical assessment is of paramount importance when caring for a patient receiving NIV. It is recommended that staff caring for these patients have formal education and training, with a competency-based assessment to ensure safe standards of care (NCEPOD 2017). Physiological monitoring is not a substitute for clinical assessment, and patients should be observed regularly.

Pre-procedural considerations

Equipment

Non-invasive ventilation devices

Non-invasive devices provide a specific level of positive pressure during the respiratory cycle to prevent alveolar collapse and increase lung volume (Vargas et al. 2018). Devices that generate NIV support can broadly be divided into two categories:

- continuous flow with a continuous level of pressure (e.g. CPAP)
- variable flow with two levels of pressure (e.g. BiPAP).

It is recommended that settings are started at low pressures and titrated to physiological parameters, patient comfort and device synchronicity (Vadde and Pastores 2016).

Continuous positive airway pressure (CPAP)

In this mode, pressure is delivered at a constant level throughout the respiratory cycle through the use of a fixed or adjustable exhalation valve (known as a 'PEEP valve') (Figure 12.14). PEEP (positive end-expiratory pressure) prevents alveoli from collapsing and thus increases lung diffusion area and gas exchange, and reduces the work of breathing (Roth et al. 2018).

Bilevel positive airway pressure (BiPAP)

BiPAP devices provide two levels of support during the respiratory cycle. An inspiratory pressure (higher pressure) is delivered on inhalation (IPAP), while an expiratory pressure (lower pressure) is provided on exhalation (EPAP).

This mode of ventilation is a common choice for patients with hypercapnic respiratory failure, patients with COPD and patients with sleep disorders such as obstructive sleep apnoea (OSA). The upper airways are splinted and the respiratory muscles are assisted during inspiration, thereby reducing the work of breathing and dyspnoea (Demoule et al. 2016, Stickle 2018).

Patients who use NIV in the long term for chronic conditions such as COPD and OSA will often have their own devices at home, which they can bring in with them if a stay in the acute setting is necessitated, for example in the presence of acute exacerbations of COPD (Davies et al. 2018). When NIV is used in conjunction with usual care, such as bronchodilators, there is an overall reduction in the likelihood of these patients requiring intubation by up to 50% (Stickle 2018).

Within the hospital setting, in the presence of an acute clinical presentation of respiratory compromise, BiPAP modes of ventilation are often delivered using mechanical ventilator devices that have the option of supporting invasive and non-invasive modes, often within a critical care unit or high-dependency unit.

NIV interface options

There are a variety of interfaces available for delivering NIV therapy, including nasal masks, face-masks, full face-masks (Figure 12.15) and helmets (Figure 12.16). The ideal interface should ensure a good seal to optimize effectiveness while maintaining patient comfort and compliance.

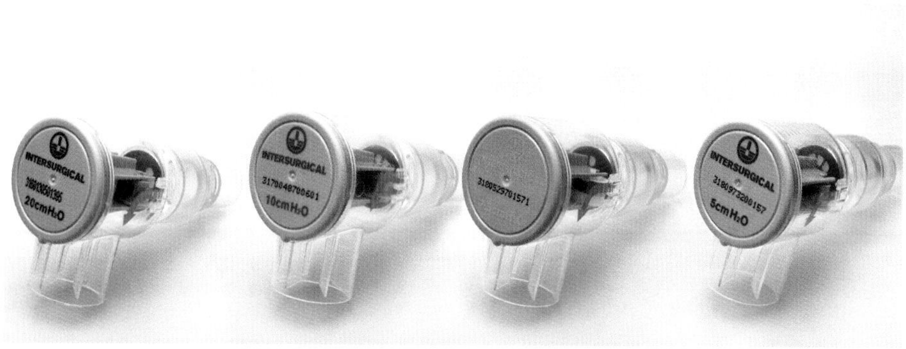

Figure 12.14 Positive end-expiratory pressure (PEEP) valves.

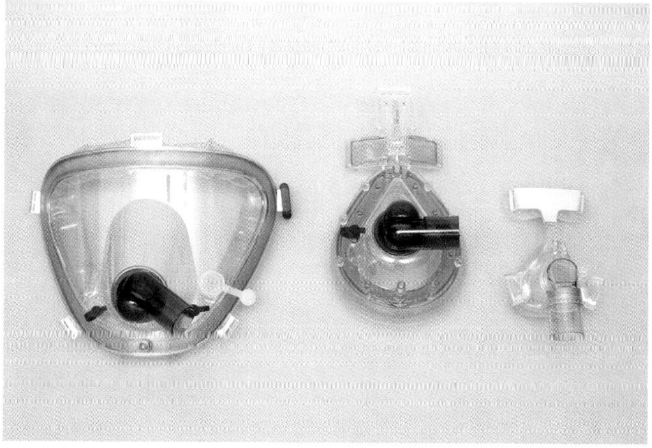

Figure 12.15 Non-invasive ventilation (NIV) patient interfaces.

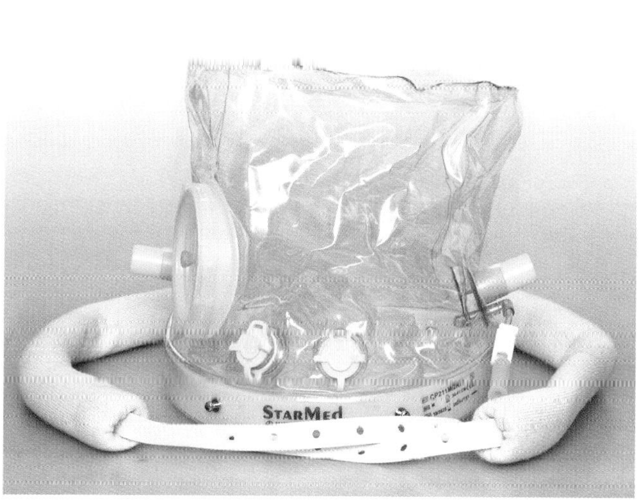

Figure 12.16 Non-invasive ventilation (NIV) helmet.

The first few hours of NIV are extremely important and continuous application is crucial in increasing the likelihood of success of NIV. Some of the issues that patients may experience include (Patel et al. 2016):

- discomfort
- pressure intolerance with difficulty exhaling
- air leaks
- claustrophobia
- skin breakdown (particularly over the bridge of the nose when using masks)
- upper airway dryness
- eye irritation.

Interface-related problems are common reasons for poor adaptation and NIV intolerance. This can cause an increase in respiratory rate and minute volume, which can lead to poor synchronicity with the device (Spoletini and Hill 2016). Good nursing and multidisciplinary care are essential to improving interface tolerance.

Non-invasive masks

Non-invasive masks are made from a combination of a soft material (polyvinyl chloride, polypropylene, silicone, silicone elastomer or hydrogel) that forms the seal against the patient's face and a transparent mask made of polyvinyl chloride, polycarbonate or thermoplastic.

Unintentional leaks around the interface can interfere with the effectiveness of the therapy and cause irritation to the eyes. Most interfaces come with a fitting gauge to ensure correct sizing and minimize this issue. Other strategies include tightening the straps, adjusting the position of the mask, adjusting the volume of air in the mask and optimizing the patient's head position.

A certain amount of pressure is required when fitting the mask to keep it in place and form a seal (Brill 2014). Too much pressure can lead to discomfort, intolerance and skin integrity issues, particularly on the nasal bridge and ears. This can be minimized by ensuring the patient's skin is clean and dry, applying pressure-relieving dressings and relieving the pressure of the mask, where possible.

Non-invasive helmets

Non-invasive helmets or hoods are transparent devices made from latex-free polyvinyl chloride with a soft collar neck seal; they do not come in contact with the patient's face (Figure 12.16). Helmets have the advantage of avoiding skin integrity issues and improving patient comfort independent of face morphology (Liu et al. 2016). Patients are also able to drink freely, communicate and expectorate.

CPAP

The set-up and use of CPAP is described in Procedure guideline 12.3: Continuous positive airway pressure (CPAP). Its use should be considered only with a co-operative patient who can maintain their airway and control secretions with an adequate cough reflex. The patient should be able to co-ordinate their breathing with the ventilator and breathe unaided for several minutes if CPAP is delivered via a ventilator (Stickle 2018).

CPAP requires the following equipment:

- A *ventilation device* that can generate a flow of pressurized breathable gas and oxygen at variable rates – for example, Dräger's CPAP bellows (Figure 12.17), Breas Medical Ltd's NIPPY or Philips' Respironics.

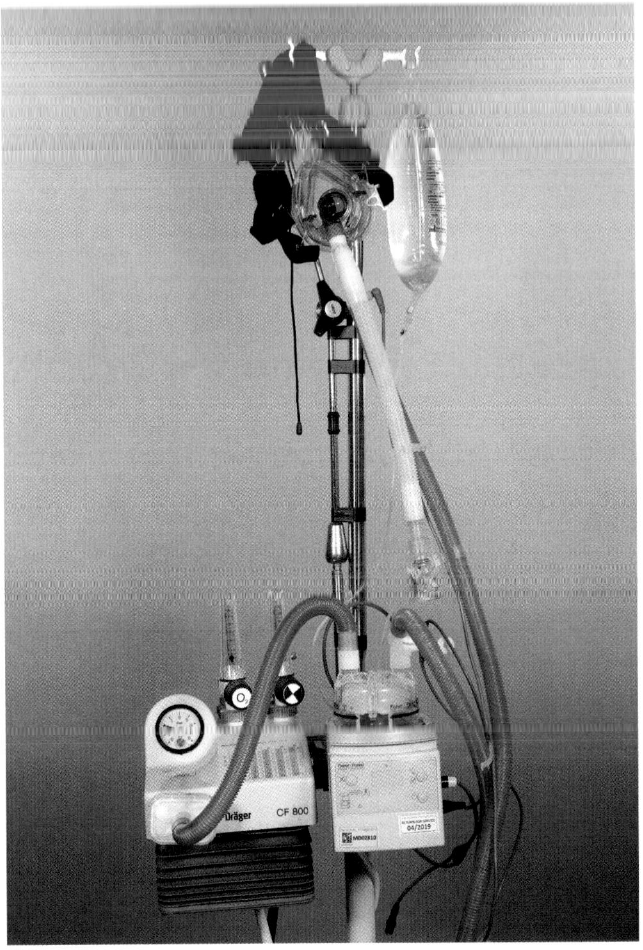

Figure 12.17 Continuous positive airway pressure (CPAP) bellows.

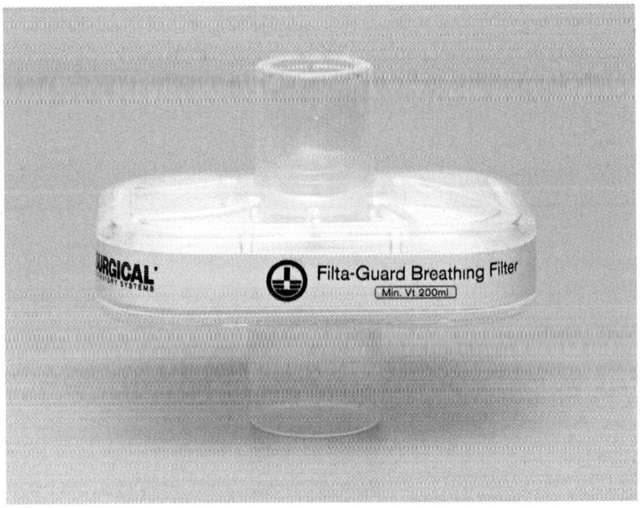

Figure 12.18 Bacterial–viral filter.

- A *bacterial–viral filter* (not a heat and moisture exchanger) (Figure 12.18). This filter provides protection against various particles including bacteria, viruses and water droplets. It also helps to protect the patient, the equipment and the breathing circuit from contamination.
- *Ventilation device tubing.* Consider active humidification if delivering NIV or CPAP through a face mask or nasal mask, to optimize mucocillary clearance.
- A *CPAP mask (face mask or nasal mask)* or *CPAP helmet* with securing straps (see Figures 12.15 and 12.16).
- A *positive end-expiratory pressure (PEEP) valve* of the prescribed level. Available fixed PEEP valves range from 5 cmH$_2$O to 20 cmH$_2$O (see Figure 12.14).

Assessment and recording tools

While a patient is on CPAP, it is essential to monitor their respiratory rate, cardiovascular status (blood pressure and heart rate), pulse oximetry (SpO$_2$) and fluid balance at least hourly. It is also vital to carry out regular arterial blood gas (ABG) sampling.

Clinical features that should be assessed are:

- chest wall movement
- co-ordination of respiratory effort with the ventilator
- accessory muscle recruitment
- general assessment – whether the patient is sweating, clammy or dyspnoeic
- auscultation of the chest for air entry and additional breath sounds
- patient comfort
- neurological status – signs of confusion or tiredness.

Although patients may need a few hours of therapy to achieve the full benefit, there should be a noticeable improvement in the above physiological parameters within 2 hours if the NIV (in this case CPAP) is likely to be effective (Cortegiani et al. 2017, Davison et al. 2016). If there is no improvement within 2–4 hours, NIV should be discontinued and invasive ventilation considered.

Pharmacological support

Depending on the clinical presentation necessitating the use of NIV or CPAP, and also the patient's ability to tolerate the chosen interface, pharmacological support may increase the success rate of NIV management:

- *Diuretics* may be given if pulmonary oedema is present (Schnell et al. 2014).
- *Bronchodialators* may be given in patients with COPD or asthma, or in the presence of acute respiratory distress (Masa et al. 2016).
- *Antimicrobials* may be given if patients have suspected or confirmed clinical indicators of a respiratory infection (Masa et al. 2016).
- *Steroids* may be given in patients with acute or chronic exacerbations of COPD (Olivieri et al. 2015).
- In some cases, *small* doses of *sedatives* or *anxiolytics* may be a valuable option if patients are overly distressed, tachypnoeic, uncomfortable or experiencing claustrophobia that may lead them to refuse ongoing NIV or CPAP despite adequate explanation and reassurance (Hilbert et al. 2015). *This must be done with caution as it may lead to loss of airway protection and/or depression of respiratory drive.* Therefore, this will require increased levels of monitoring to ensure patient safety and may warrant transferring the patient to a critical care or high-dependency area (Liu et al. 2016).

Non-pharmacological support

There are a number of measures that can be initiated to help support patients during the use of NIV, such as:

- For some patients, the presence of a relative, a nurse or another healthcare professional may help to relieve the distress caused by NIV or CPAP.
- Optimizing patient positioning in bed by sitting the patient upright or in a semi-recumbent position to at least 30° can relieve the symptoms of breathlessness (Corrêa et al. 2015).
- It is important to ensure the most favourable type, size and fit of the chosen interface (Hilbert et al. 2015).
- If appropriate and clinically feasible, patients can be offered a break from the chosen interface by switching them to an alternative level of respiratory support, such as high-flow oxygen therapy (Brill 2014).

- Ensuring the trigger sensitivity, pressurization level and compatibility of the device tubing are appropriate will optimize synchronicity (Brill 2014).

Specific patient preparation

Education

CPAP can cause distress to patients, especially due to the tight-fitting mask, while the hood can seem claustrophobic. If possible, a clear and concise description of how the therapy works should be provided either verbally or via an information leaflet. Time spent fitting the interface and building the patient's confidence is well invested (Brill 2014). As with any procedure, consent needs to be gained before treatment can commence. Allow time for the patient to express any concerns or fears they have regarding treatment. Acutely hypoxic patients may not comprehend the relevance of the therapy and so it should be explained to their relatives or carers so they can reassure the patient.

Procedure guideline 12.3 Continuous positive airway pressure (CPAP)

Essential equipment

- Personal protective equipment
- Dräger bellows or similar device (see Figure 12.17)
- Compressed medical gas supply (air with or without oxygen, depending on the particular device)
- CPAP helmet or mask
- CPAP circuit and/or tubing
- Humidification system (mask only) with temperature control
- Pulse oximeter

Action	Rationale
Pre-procedure	
1 Introduce yourself to the patient, explain and discuss the procedure with them, and gain their consent to proceed.	To ensure that the patient feels at ease, understands the procedure and gives their valid consent (NMC 2018, **C**).
2 Assess the patient's consciousness level.	To obtain a baseline and be able to assess the patient for changes in condition (see Chapter 14: Observations). **E** A reduction in level of consciousness or altered mental status may indicate hypoxaemia. **E**
3 Observe and record the following: a respiratory function b respiratory rate c work of breathing d colour, skin and mental status e oxygen saturation (SpO_2).	To obtain a baseline of respiratory function. **E** To observe for any change in respiratory function. **E**
4 Explain the principles of CPAP to the patient and their family and demonstrate the system to them.	To minimize anxiety, increase knowledge and aid in patient compliance. **E**
5 Decide whether it is appropriate to insert an arterial cannula for ongoing assessment of arterial blood gases (ABGs).	In order to monitor the partial pressures of serum oxygen and carbon dioxide and the acid/base balance, to evaluate the effectiveness of the intervention. **E**
6 Observe and record the patient's cardiovascular function, including: a heart rate b blood pressure c temperature d central venous pressure (if patient has a central venous access device).	To obtain a baseline in order to assess any change in conditions (see Chapter 14: Observations). **E**
7 Assess and record the patient's fluid balance: a input b output c accumulative balance d overall fluid balance e daily weight.	To obtain a baseline of fluid balance (see Chapter 8: Nutrition and fluid balance). **E** To enable an assessment of dehydration, fluid overload and renal function (Beitler et al. 2016, **E**).
8 Assess the patient's level of anxiety and compliance with treatment (the patient's ability to cope with the treatment).	To enable an assessment to be made and an evaluation of the suitability of CPAP therapy (Dres and Demoule 2016, **E**).
Procedure	
9 Set up the CPAP circuit as per the manufacturer's instructions.	To prepare the equipment for use. **E**
10 Ensure the patient is comfortable, sitting in a semi-recumbent position, ideally with their head elevated to a 30–45° angle (or sitting in a supportive chair).	To promote comfort and aid lung expansion and breathing (Brill 2014, **E**).

(continued)

Procedure guideline 12.3 Continuous positive airway pressure (CPAP) (continued)

Action	Rationale
11 Explain to the patient how the mask or helmet is to be applied.	To relieve anxiety and to reassure the patient. **E** To aid the patient's compliance with CPAP. **E**
If using a mask	
12 Ensure the correct size is selected for the patient by using the manufacturer's guide or measurement device.	To relieve anxiety and to reassure the patient. **E** To aid the patient's compliance with CPAP. **E**
13 Connect the mask to the circuit and ensure the settings are correct. Commence the flow of gases.	To ensure the correct set-up of the circuit and to check gases are flowing through the circuit prior to initiation of treatment. **E**
14 Place the mask over the patient's nose and mouth; applying a little pressure, hold the mask in place, ensuring there are no leaks. Allow the patient a short time to get used to the pressure and mask.	To allow the patient time to adapt to the change in pressure and the feeling of the tight-fitting mask. **E**
15 Once the patient is comfortable and settled, apply the straps.	To retain the mask in place and aid patient comfort (Vargas et al. 2018, **E**).
16 Apply tissue protective dressings around vulnerable pressure points as required, e.g. nose, ears, back of head and neck.	To alleviate pressure and prevent tissue breakdown (Scott 2017, **E**).
If using a helmet	
17 Using a two-person technique, stretch the seal around the bottom of the helmet and lower the helmet over the patient's head.	Two people are usually required to stretch the seal enough to lower the helmet over the patient's head comfortably. **E**
18 Attach the straps, ensuring patient comfort.	The helmet will begin to lift once pressure is applied. **E**
19 Close the safety valve or outlet and allow the pressure to build up within the helmet until the valve remains closed.	The helmet requires time to fill and expand. Once the helmet is full, the pressure within it will keep the valve closed. **E**
20 Ensure a good seal and that no leaks are present. Inflate the inner neck cuff if applicable.	To ensure a tight seal in order for the system to function optimally (Vargas et al. 2018, **E**).
Post-procedure	
21 Give further explanation to the family or next of kin of how CPAP works and the importance of their presence and participation in communication.	To relieve anxiety and support and reassure the family and patient. **E**
22 Reassure the patient constantly.	To relieve patient anxiety and promote co-operation. **E**
23 Discuss with the medical team the use of medication that might aid patient compliance with CPAP therapy and administer it as necessary.	Prophylactic administration of small doses of anxiolytic can aid compliance with CPAP therapy (Hilbert et al. 2015, **E**).
24 Continue observation of vital signs and work of breathing. If patient is tiring, notify the doctor.	To prevent acute respiratory deterioration and to inform the doctor in a timely manner in order to intubate the patient to avoid a respiratory arrest (Davison et al. 2016, **C**).

Problem-solving table 12.3 Prevention and resolution (Procedure guideline 12.3)

Problem	Cause	Prevention	Action
Airway is not maintained	Deteriorating respiratory or neurological function and/or the patient is tiring	Use NEWS scoring to identify deterioration early. Insert a nasopharyngeal airway (Figure 12.19).	Regular monitoring of respiratory function including skin colour, breathing pattern, respiratory rate, oxygen saturation and blood gases. Discuss changes with medical or anaesthetic staff.
Aspiration	Inability to maintain own airway	Request speech and language therapy (SLT) assessment.	Observe and assess the patient closely. After discussion with medical staff, a nasogastric tube may be inserted to reduce gastric distension.

Problem	Cause	Prevention	Action
	Continuous pressure from the CPAP system can lead to insufflation of air into the stomach, causing aspiration	Keep the patient nil by mouth and insert a nasogastric tube.	As above.
Mask or helmet incorrectly sealed	Incorrect size of mask or helmet	Use appropriate size of mask or helmet.	Alter mask or helmet position to correct the issue and ensure comfort. Ensure the mask or helmet is the correct size. Alter the position to ensure a correct seal.
Helmet not inflating or patient finding it difficult to breathe with mask	Disconnection of tubing Not connected to piped oxygen	Switch on all audible alarms on equipment. Clarify alarm parameters with medical or senior nursing staff. Keep bed space tidy and free from clutter. If possible, ensure bed space is close to or visible from the nurse station.	Ensure a nurse is present with the patient at all times. Observe the patient and CPAP system closely to ensure the equipment is working optimally and that there is no failure of the system.
Eyes are dry or sore, or patient develops conjunctival oedema (all three issues only apply to face-mask CPAP)	Air leak from mask High-flow oxygen causing the eyes to dry out Facial pressure from mask causing oedema	Protect eyes from drying out. Use correct size of mask or helmet for patient.	Ensure the mask or helmet is well sealed with no leaks. Apply pressure-relieving padding around the mask. Carry out regular eye care (see Chapter 9: Patient comfort and supporting personal hygiene). Adjust the mask to the patient's facial contours. Alter and position the mask as comfortably as possible. Position padding around the head strap to relieve pressure.
Dry mouth	CPAP system uses a very high oxygen flow, which has a drying effect	Provide adequate oral hydration	Carry out regular mouth care. Give the patient regular sips of water, ice to suck or drinks (as much as the patient is able to take). Humidify the oxygen if using a face-mask.
Non-compliance with CPAP equipment	Anxiety	Calm, informative communication.	Inform the patient of any changes taking place. Communicate with the patient's family, keep them informed and involve them in care and communication with the patient. Inform the doctor of the patient's anxiety level. Administer prescribed anxiolytic agent if required.
Inability to eat	Gastric distension due to CPAP Loss of appetite Distress caused by respiratory status and CPAP Nausea and vomiting	Provide small but regular easily managed (soft) oral diet or supplement drinks.	Encourage dietary intake and oral supplementary fluids. If patient is unable to take these orally, refer to dietician as an alternative method of feeding may be considered, for example enteral feeding via nasogastric or jejunal tube or intravenous feeding (parenteral nutrition). Administer an antiemetic. Encourage and reassure the patient.
Inability to communicate effectively	Mask or helmet restriction.	Provide means of non-verbal communication.	Reassure the patient and ensure they are comfortable.
Feelings of isolation		Ask a relative, carer or healthcare assistant to stay with the patient.	Encourage the patient to communicate, and explain how they can use non-verbal means of communicating (e.g. letter board, tablets). Reassure the patient.

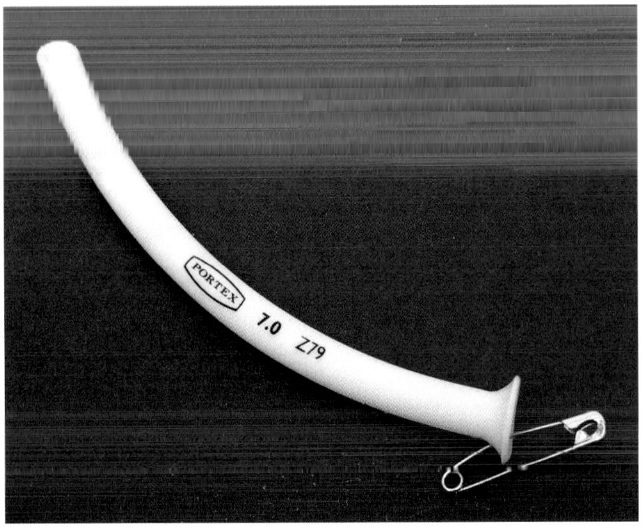

Figure 12.19 Nasopharyngeal airway and safety pin.

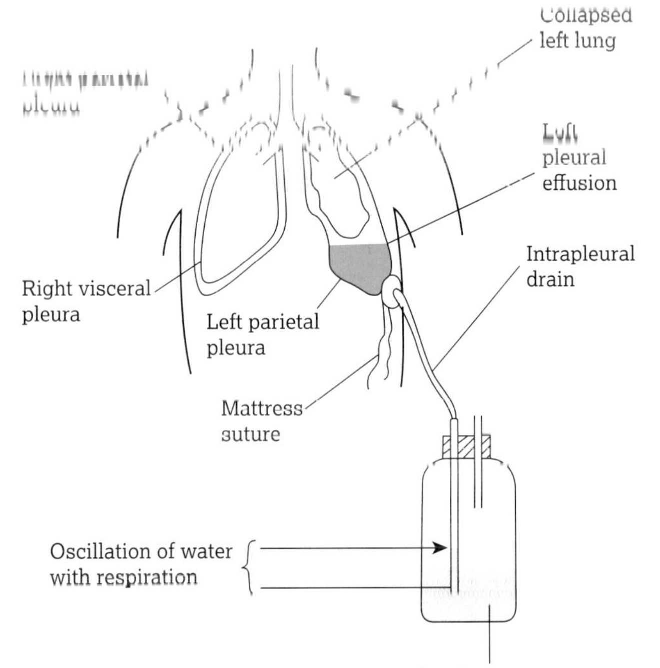

Figure 12.20 A chest drain and underwater seal bottle are used to drain a left pleural effusion.

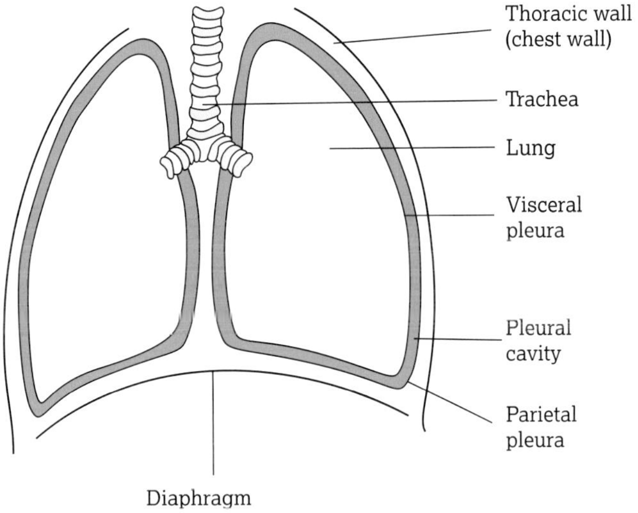

Figure 12.21 The relationship between the pleural membranes, chest wall and lungs.

Post-procedural considerations

Immediate care

It is important to maintain a high level of monitoring while encouraging the patient to maintain good lung expansion by sitting upright and expectorating as required. CPAP can cause the oral mucosa to dry out with prolonged use, leading to an increased risk of infection, so it is essential that regular mouth care is provided. Regular ABG sampling can be used to assess the effectiveness of the treatment as well as to guide any changes required to either oxygen concentration or PEEP. As with all patients requiring an increased level of support, an accurate fluid balance chart should be maintained to ensure that fluid overload does not occur (Beitler et al. 2016).

Documentation

Document all the vital signs and monitoring as well as the patient's response to CPAP or NIV treatment.

Education of the patient and relevant others

It is worth discussing with the patient and their family or carer that intermittent use of CPAP is sometimes beneficial and that if it is required again, this does not necessarily indicate deterioration.

Complications

With any circuit that includes the use of PEEP, there is the possibility of reduction in cardiac output due to an increase in intrathoracic pressure. However, spontaneous ventilation decreases both the incidence and the severity of this complication if patients have had their fluid balance optimized (Cortegiani et al. 2017).

There is also a risk of gastric insufflation (blowing of air causing gastric distension), which can lead to vomiting and aspiration, although the risk is minimized when PEEP is used in awake patients or by the insertion of an orogastric or nasogastric tube (Vadde and Pastores 2016).

Preventative pressure dressings should be considered in underweight patients or those with bony facial prominences. There should also be regular skin checks to ensure that the tight-fitting face-mask required for CPAP is not compromising the skin integrity of vulnerable areas on the bridge of the nose and over the ears (Scott 2017).

Chest drain management

Definition

A chest drain is a length of flexible tubing commonly made from PVC or silicone. Chest drains come in a variety of sizes ranging from 6 to 40 French (Fr) and often incorporate a radio-opaque strip that enables X-ray detection. The proximal end is inserted into the pleura and has a number of holes, which facilitate drainage. The distal end is connected to the drainage system (Figure 12.20).

Anatomy and physiology

Each lung is surrounded by a double membrane called a pleura. The outer membrane is the parietal pleura, which is attached to the thoracic (chest) wall and contains nerve receptors that detect pain. The inner membrane is the visceral pleura, which adheres to the lung and covers the lung fissures, hilar bronchi and blood vessels (Figure 12.21) (Tortora and Derrickson 2017).

The pleurae help to maintain the negative pressure required to prevent the lung from collapsing. Before inspiration, the pressure within the pleural space is equal to −5 cmH_2O. During inspiration, there is a decrease in intrapleural pressure due to the diaphragm being drawn down and the outward expansion of the chest. The pressure falls to −7.5 cmH_2O, which causes air to be drawn in for gaseous exchange. During expiration, the lung returns to its pre-inspiratory state by elastic recoil, with collapse of the chest wall and diaphragm and the exhalation of gas. The intrapleural pressure subsequently rises to −4 cmH_2O (Noorani and Abu-Omar 2018). If either of the pleura is damaged, partial or total lung collapse will occur due to loss of the normally negative pressure (Woodrow 2013).

The space that exists between the parietal and visceral pleurae is commonly known as the pleural space, pleural cavity or potential space. While approximately 1 to 2 L of serous fluid moves across the thin and porous pleural membranes each day, only 3–5 mL of fluid actually fills the space. The serous fluid allows the pleurae to move in unison with the chest wall on inspiration and enables the membranes to be held closely together by surface tension forces (George and Papagiannopoulos 2016). The amount of fluid present in the pleural space is maintained by the oncotic and hydrostatic pressures across the pleurae and lymphatic drainage network (Chadwick et al. 2015). Disruption in this balance results in an accumulation of fluid within the pleural space.

Related theory

Drainage is required for patients who are symptomatic of excess air (pneumothorax) or fluid (pleural effusion) within the pleural space. Chest drains may also be inserted to drain blood (haemothorax), lymph (chylothorax) or pus (empyema), or a combination of air and fluid (Mao et al. 2015).

Pleural effusion

The mechanisms by which pleural effusions develop are complex, but they generally occur when the rate of filtration overwhelms the rate of lymphatic clearance resulting in an excessive amount of fluid in the pleural space (Chadwick et al. 2015).

Pleural effusions are classified as either transudative or exudative. A *transudative pleural effusion* occurs when the balance of hydrostatic forces influencing the formation and absorption of pleural fluid is altered to favour pleural fluid accumulation. The permeability of the capillaries to proteins is normal. In contrast, an *exudative pleural effusion* develops when the pleural surface and/or the local capillary permeability are altered. There are many causes of transudative and exudative effusions, as outlined in Box 12.2.

Pleural effusion develops in nearly half of all patients with metastatic disease. The most common cancers that cause malignant pleural effusions are adenocarcinomas; other carcinomas of the lung, breast and ovaries; and lymphoma (Egan et al. 2014).

Patients with pleural effusion usually present with a number of symptoms and signs (Na 2014, Saguil et al. 2014). Symptoms include the following:

- dyspnoea
- chest pain (may be mild or severe and is often worse on deep inspiration; it is typically described as a sharp or stabbing pain)
- cough (usually dry and unproductive).

Signs include the following:

- unequal chest expansion
- tracheal deviation may be seen with a very large pleural effusion
- decreased tactile and vocal fremitus
- dull to percussion
- diminished air entry on auscultation.

Pneumothorax

Pneumothorax can be defined as air in the pleural cavity that causes the lung to collapse due to a loss in negative pressure (Tschopp et al. 2015). A pneumothorax occurs as the result of the processes described in Table 12.7. Pneumothoraces can therefore be classified as iatrogenic, traumatic, primary spontaneous and secondary spontaneous (Tschopp et al. 2015).

The symptoms of a pneumothorax are proportional to its size and depend on the degree of pulmonary reserve. Common signs and symptoms are listed in Box 12.3.

Box 12.2 Causes of transudative and exudative pleural effusions

Transudative pleural effusion

- Left ventricular failure
- Liver cirrhosis
- Nephrotic syndrome
- Peritoneal dialysis or continuous ambulatory peritoneal dialysis
- Hypoproteinaemia (e.g. severe starvation)
- Hypothyroidism
- Mitral stenosis

Causes of exudative pleural effusion

- Malignant disease
- Infectious diseases, including tuberculosis
- Parapneumonic effusions
- Pulmonary embolism
- Pancreatitis
- Collagen vascular diseases: rheumatoid arthritis, systemic lupus erythematosus, benign asbestos effusion
- Drug-induced primary pleural disease: nitrofurantoin, amiodarone, procarbazine, methotrexate, bleomycin, metronidazole, phenytoin or beta blockers
- Injury after cardiac surgery, pacemaker implantation, myocardial infarction, blunt chest trauma or angioplasty

Source: Adapted from Na (2014), Saguil et al. (2014).

Table 12.7 Causes of pneumothorax

Cause	Notes
Breach of the integrity of either pleural layer, causing direct or indirect communication between the atmosphere and the pleural space	Many procedures performed in an intensive care or emergency setting can result in an iatrogenic pneumothorax. Examples of these procedures include incorrect chest tube insertion, mechanical ventilation therapy, central venous catheterization, cardiopulmonary resuscitation, lung or liver biopsy, or surgery. A blunt or penetrating trauma to the chest wall, diaphragm or bowel may cause a traumatic pneumothorax.
Communication between the alveolar spaces and the pleura	This can occur spontaneously and is most common in tall, thin males (primary spontaneous pneumothorax). It can also occur secondarily to underlying lung conditions such as asthma, chronic bronchitis, tuberculosis, pneumonia, cystic fibrosis or carcinoma of the lung (secondary spontaneous pneumothorax).
Gas-producing organisms in the pleural space	Micro-organisms that produce gas will cause an increase in the amount of air within the pleura and subsequent pneumothorax.

Source: Adapted from Cardillo et al. (2016), Hassan and Shaarawy (2018).

Box 13.3 Signs and symptoms of pneumothorax and tension pneumothorax

Symptoms of a pneumothorax	Signs of a pneumothorax
• Dyspnoea • Acute pleuritic chest pain • Shoulder tip pain • Restlessness, anxiety	• Tachypnoea • Tachycardia • Subcutaneous emphysema • Decreased tactile and vocal fremitus • Hyper-resonance on percussion • Absent or diminished breath sounds

Signs and symptoms of a tension pneumothorax (in addition to those listed above)

- Acute respiratory distress
- Hypoxia
- Hypotension
- Tracheal deviation away from the affected side
- Asymmetrical chest expansion
- Engorged neck veins
- Reduced breath sounds

Source: Adapted from Cardillo et al. (2016), Tschopp et al. (2015).

Tension pneumothorax

A tension pneumothorax is the complete collapse of a lung as the intrapleural pressure becomes greater than the atmospheric pressure during both inspiration and expiration (Tschopp et al. 2015). A breach in the pleura creates a one-way valve, which allows air to progressively accumulate within the pleural space with each inspiration (Woodrow 2013). As the amount of air in the pleural space increases, the lung becomes compressed, the mediastinum shifts and venous return to the heart decreases, causing cardiac arrest (Woodrow 2013). A tension pneumothorax is therefore a life-threatening emergency that requires immediate treatment (RCUK 2015).

Diagnosis of a simple pneumothorax can be confirmed on a chest X-ray, which should be taken during inspiration (MacDuff et al. 2010). However, diagnosis of a tension pneumothorax is based on clinical history and examination alone. It is a medical emergency and should be treated urgently without the need for diagnostic imaging. Ultrasound can be performed at the bedside so long as it does not delay treatment (MacDuff et al. 2010, RCUK 2015). Supportive therapy should be given until needle decompression or chest drain insertion is performed. This may include sitting the patient upright and giving oxygen therapy to maintain saturations between 94% and 98% (O'Driscoll et al. 2017, Woodrow 2013).

Haemothorax

Haemothorax is a collection of blood within the pleural space, usually as a result of injury to the heart, lungs or major vessels within the thoracic cavity, or in a patient who has bled on anticoagulation therapy (Patrini et al. 2015).

Haemopneumothorax

Haemothorax may also be associated with pneumothorax, in which case it is called 'haemopneumothorax'. Depending on the amount of blood or air in the pleural cavity, a collapsed lung can lead to respiratory and haemodynamic compromise (Patrini et al. 2015).

Empyema

Empyema is defined as pus in the pleural space. It may occur following rupture of an abscess within the lung, pneumonia, pulmonary tuberculosis or an infection following thoracic surgery (McCauley and Dean 2015).

Chylothorax

Chylothorax is a collection of lymphatic fluid within the pleural space, usually resulting from disruption of the thoracic duct or its tributaries (Alamdari et al. 2018). The fluid is usually milky and contains a high level of triglycerides (>110 mg/dL), an essential feature for its diagnosis (Bender et al. 2016). Chylothorax can be split into traumatic (thoracic surgery or penetrating trauma) and non-traumatic/spontaneous (congenital, neoplastic, infectious or obstructive) classifications (Bender et al. 2016).

Chest drain: insertion

Evidence-based approaches

Management of excess fluid or air within the pleural space is dependent on the size and complexity of the effusion or pneumothorax, the patient's symptoms and the presence of any underlying disease (Tschopp et al. 2015). Fine needle aspiration using a needle and syringe is recommended by the British Thoracic Society for primary spontaneous pneumothoraces or small free-flowing effusions (Davies et al. 2010, Hassan and Shaarawy 2018, MacDuff et al. 2010) and this would be carried out by an appropriately trained clinician. Chest drain insertion is recommended for patients with secondary spontaneous pneumothoraces, failed fine needle aspiration for primary spontaneous pneumothoraces, malignant effusions, or complicated accumulations of fluid that are causing the patient to be symptomatic (Davies et al. 2010, MacDuff et al. 2010, Mahmood and Wahidi 2013); this would again be carried out by an appropriately trained clinician with the assistance of a nurse. While both are common procedures, they are not without risk. Chest drain insertion should be carried out in a clean area using a strict aseptic technique and with adequate monitoring available (Adlakha et al. 2016, Havelock et al. 2010). The sections below relate to chest drain insertion; needle aspiration would only be carried out by a doctor or highly trained nurse and is beyond the scope of this manual.

Rationale

Ventilation and the normal mechanics of breathing become compromised as the abnormal collection of fluid or air compresses the lung, or as the negative pressure within the chest cavity is altered, causing partial or complete collapse of the affected lung (Tschopp et al. 2015). Needle aspiration and chest drain insertion are methods used to remove the collection of air, serous fluid, pus, lymph or blood from the pleural space, restoring the negative pressure within the chest cavity and allowing the lung to re-expand (Noorani and Abu-Omar 2018).

Indications

Chest drain insertion is indicated in the following circumstances (Noorani and Abu-Omar 2018, Porcel 2018a, Yousuf and Rahman 2018):

- pneumothorax
- pleural effusion
- empyema
- traumatic haemopneumothorax
- chylothorax
- post-operatively following thoracotomy, oesophagectomy or cardiac surgery
- bronchopleural fistula.

Contraindications

No contraindications exist for a patient with a tension pneumothorax (MacDuff et al. 2010). The risks and benefits should be weighed up for all other patients, and expert advice and guidance sought if required. The procedure should be carried out by a healthcare professional with extensive and relevant ultrasound skills (Havelock et al. 2010). Depending on the nature of the problem (e.g. a loculated pleural effusion), it may be preferential for the procedure to be carried out by an experienced radiologist.

Absolute contraindications

Chest drain insertion is absolutely contraindicated if the patient does not consent to the procedure and they are not at risk of imminent cardiac arrest.

Relative contraindications

Chest drain insertion has the following relative contraindications (Havelock et al. 2010, Porcel 2018b, Ravi and McKnight 2018):

- abnormal blood clotting screen or low platelet count; it is good practice to correct any coagulopathy or thrombocytopenia prior to chest drain insertion; ideally, international normalized ratio (INR) should be less than or equal to 1.5 and platelets above 50×10^9/L
- differential diagnosis between pneumothorax and bullous lung disease needs to be investigated
- any previous surgery involving the thoracic cavity on the side of the proposed intervention
- diaphragmatic hernia
- localized skin infection, or cutaneous metastatic cancerous deposits at the site of the drain insertion.

Principles of care

The following principles should be adhered to (Havelock et al. 2010, Porcel 2018b, Woodrow 2013):

- Maintain sterility of the chest drainage system and avoid introduction of bacteria into the pleural space.
- Maintain a negative intrapleural pressure by keeping the system patent and airtight.
- Keep the system upright and below chest level, and prevent water and/or pleural fluid re-entering the pleural space.
- Drain the fluid slowly and prevent pain and/or re-expansion pulmonary oedema.
- Monitor the patient's observations/NEWS and pain score, and escalate any change or concerns regarding the patient's condition.
- Monitor the drain for swinging, bubbling, and the amount and type of fluid drained.
- Remove the drain as soon as it has reached the predefined therapeutic goal, or when it has become non-functioning.

Clinical governance

Pleural aspiration and chest drain insertion should only be inserted by healthcare professionals who have had relevant training and are deemed competent, or who have adequate supervision by an experienced clinician (Havelock et al. 2010). The use of ultrasound guidance is advocated when performing pleural aspiration or inserting a chest drain to prevent injury to adjacent organs. Practitioners must be competent in the use of the ultrasound equipment (Adlakha et al. 2016, Havelock et al. 2010). It is also advisable that there should be a clinical lead identified for the training of all staff involved in chest drain insertion.

Clinical policies regarding chest drain insertion and management should be implemented and followed by both medical and nursing staff. Incidents regarding chest drain insertion and management should be reported to risk management teams, and processes should be reviewed regularly.

Consent

Prior to commencing chest tube insertion, the procedure should be explained fully to the patient and written consent gained and recorded in accordance with national guidelines (Havelock et al. 2010). The General Medical Council guidelines for consent state that it is the responsibility of the doctor carrying out a procedure, or an appropriately trained individual with sufficient knowledge of the procedure, to explain its nature and the risks associated with it. The exception to this is during an emergency when chest drain insertion is indicated to prevent further clinical deterioration and cardiac arrest. In this scenario, verbal consent should be gained if possible and documented (GMC 2008). Associated risks include visceral injury, pneumothorax, pain, haemorrhage, infection, drain blockage, drain dislodgment and procedure failure (Havelock et al. 2010, Yousuf and Rahman 2018).

Competencies

All staff caring for patients undergoing chest drain insertion and those managing a patient with an exisiting chest drain should have undertaken the relevant local training and be deemed competent. The basis of these competencies should include the following (Mallet et al. 2013):

- knowledge of the indications for chest drain insertion
- knowledge of the potential complications regarding insertion and having a chest drain *in situ*
- knowledge of how to manage any potential complications
- familiarity with the equipment and the ability to set it up for insertion, change the chest drain bottle while *in situ*, and remove the drain effectively and safely.

Pre-procedural considerations

Equipment

Drain size

In the past, the use of a large-bore chest drain (>14 Fr) (Figure 12.22) was recommended to prevent blockage of the drain by viscous malignant or infected fluid. Although there is currently no consensus on the optimal chest drain size, the British Thoracic Society advocates the use of small, flexible catheters (10–14 Fr) for the drainage of most simple effusions and pneumothoraces, and recommends that they are inserted using the Seldinger technique (Mahmood and Wahidi 2013, Porcel 2018b). Small-bore drains may be straight, angled or coiled at the end (pigtail; Figure 12.23). Pigtail drains have the advantage of a thread that, when pulled, creates the pigtail effect to hold the drain firmly in place. Small-bore drains can easily be flushed to prevent blockage, have fewer complication rates, and are generally more comfortable and tolerable for patients (Mahmood and Wahidi 2013).

Large-bore chest drains (>20 Fr) may be inserted for ongoing air leaks, pneumothoraces caused by mechanical ventilation, haemothoraces and post-operative drainage of the chest cavity (Porcel 2018a). Drains larger than 24 Fr should be inserted using a blunt dissection technique. Trocars should no longer be used as they are associated with high complication rates and leave patients with an unsightly scar (Havelock et al. 2010).

Drainage systems

There is a wide variety of drainage systems available to drain effusions or pneumothoraces; however, the single-bottle, underwater-seal drainage system can be used for the majority of situations

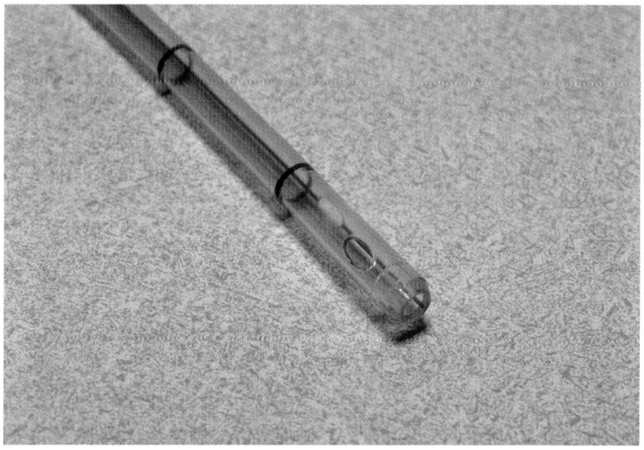

Figure 12.22 Large-bore chest drain.

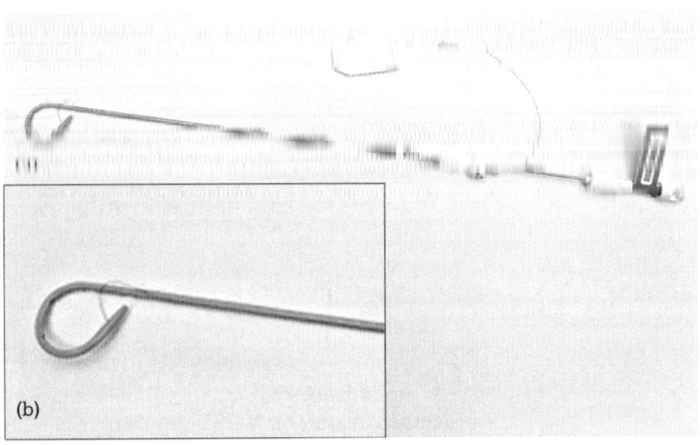

Figure 12.23 (a) Pigtail drain with (b) magnification of the end.

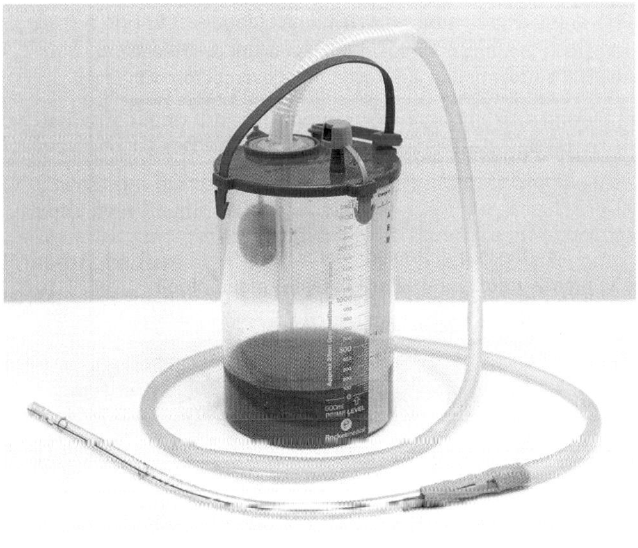

Figure 12.24 Underwater chest drainage system.

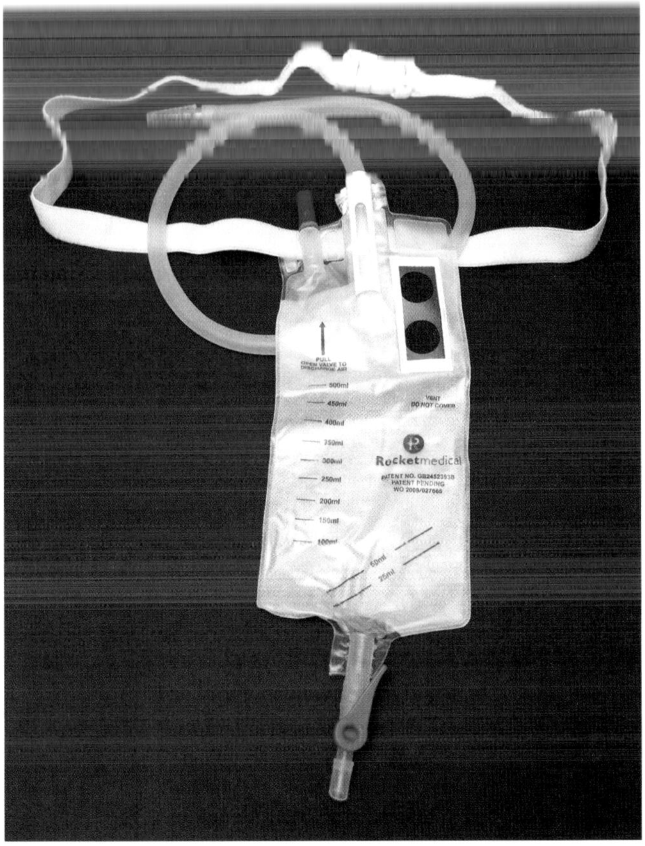

Figure 12.25 Ambulatory chest drain bag with Heimlich valve.

(Figure 12.24). The underwater seal occurs when the screw-top lid is removed and sterile water is poured into the chest drain bottle up to the fluid line. The long length of tubing supplied in the pack is attached to the distal end of the chest drain, and the other end is inserted into the screw-top port and immersed 2–3 cm below the level of the water (Havelock et al. 2010).

There is a second port, which acts as a venting aid and is either exposed to air or attached to a suction unit. Venting prevents the build-up of pressure in the chest drainage system and aids evacuation of air or fluid from the lungs. The underwater seal maintains the negative intrapleural pressure and acts as a one-way valve, preventing the backflow of air into the pleural space (George and Papagiannopoulos 2016).

Other multi-chamber or digital drainage systems may also be used. The three-chamber system consists of a collection chamber, a water-seal chamber and a suction chamber, all of which are interconnected. Suction can be applied to assist in the management of an ongoing air leak. Digital systems are able to monitor for air leaks and can maintain and adjust the negative pressure accordingly without the use of external suction (Porcel 2018a). Manufacturers' instructions should be followed to guide set up and aid maintenance of the system.

A dry drainage system that incorporates a one-way Heimlich valve can also be used to facilitate early discharge home in ambulatory patients (Woodrow 2013). The ambulatory bag (Figure 12.25) must be primed prior to use to ensure that the Heimlich valve is working. This can be done by flushing air through the valve using a 50 mL syringe and inspecting for slight bag inflation.

Pharmacological support

Surrounding tissue and nerve fibres are damaged during chest drain insertion, which may cause the patient significant pain throughout and after the procedure. Supportive treatment in the form of oxygen and analgesia should therefore be given before and after drain insertion, and prior to drain removal. Unless contraindicated, opioid analgesia should be prescribed and administered to ensure the patient is able to tolerate the drain and subsequent drainage of fluid, and also to allow them to breathe deeply and cough effectively ([illegible] and Abu-Omar 2010, Woodrow 2013).

Specific patient preparation

The patient's baseline observations and NEWS must be recorded prior to the procedure. A chest X-ray should be performed and reviewed by the practitioner to confirm the site of the pneumothorax or effusion to be drained. CT (computed tomography) imaging may also be required for uncertain or complex cases (Davies et al. 2010, Hooper et al. 2010). The exception to this is for patients who have signs and symptoms of a tension pneumothorax when immediate needle decompression or chest drain insertion is required (MacDuff et al. 2010). The British Thoracic Society strongly advocates the use of ultrasound guidance during chest drain placement (Havelock et al. 2010).

To minimise the risk of bleeding, patients should temporarily stop their usual anticoagulation therapy, and drain insertion

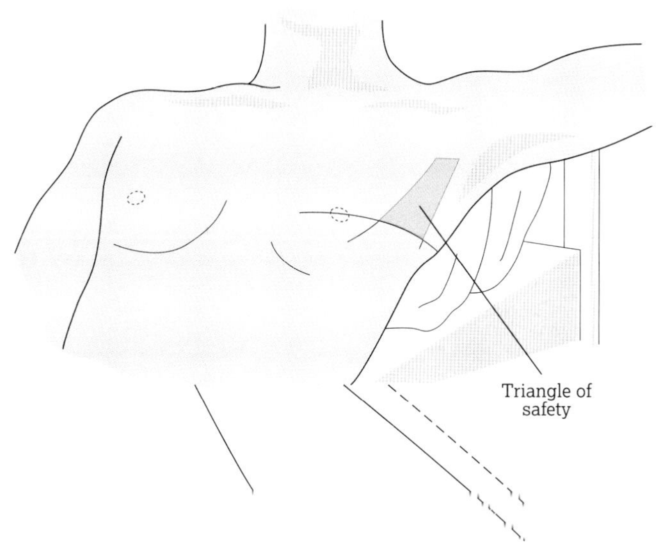

Figure 12.26 Triangle of safety. *Source*: Laws et al. (2003). Reproduced with permission of BMJ Publishing Group, Ltd.

should be delayed until their INR is below 1.5 (Havelock et al. 2010, Porcel 2018b). Platelet and coagulation abnormalities should be corrected as per local policy or as advised by a haematologist.

Chest drains are usually inserted in an area known as the 'triangle of safety' (Figure 12.26). This is the triangle outlined by the anterior border of the latissimus dorsi, the lateral border of the pectoralis major, a line superior to the horizontal level of the nipple, and an apex below the axilla. Drains may be placed outside this area under ultrasound or radiology guidance (Mahmood and Wahidi 2013). Depending on the area for insertion, patients may be placed in a supine, 45° position with the arm on the affected side abducted, externally rotated and placed behind their head (Figure 12.27a). Alternatively, patients may sit upright on the side of the bed leaning over an adjacent table, with arms resting on a pillow in front of them (Figure 12.27b), or lie on their side (Figure 12.27c) (Adlakha et al. 2016).

Education

Nurses caring for patients with chest drains must be familiar with their management and keep up to date with current guidelines, local policies and protocols (Havelock et al. 2010, Noorani and Abu-Omar 2018).

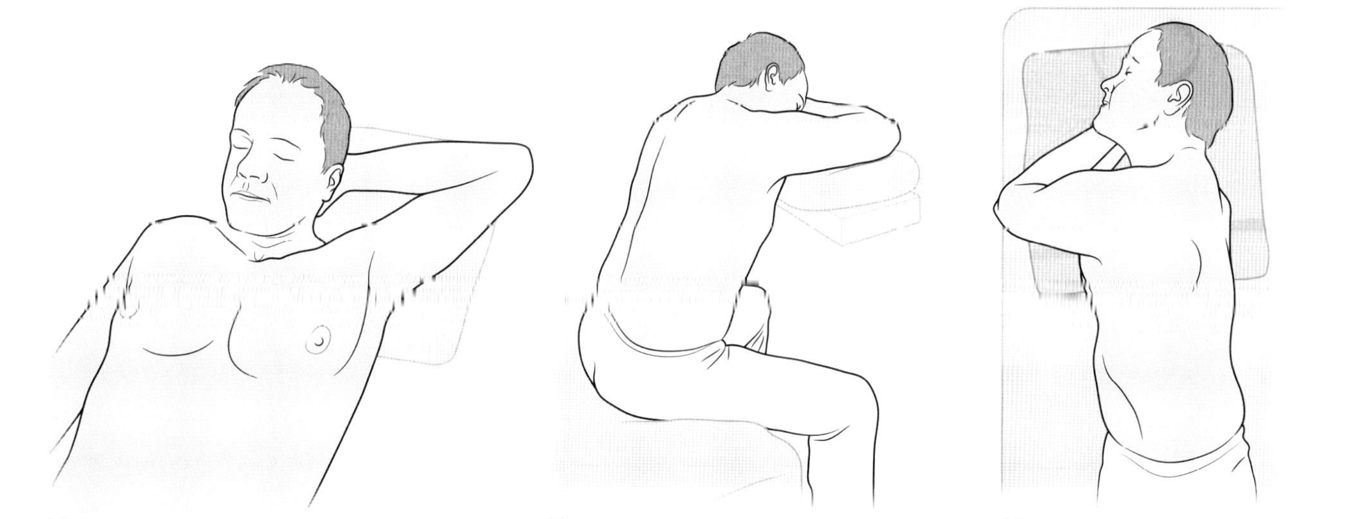

Figure 12.27 Alternative positions for chest drain insertion. (a) Supine on the bed with the arm on the affected side placed behind the head away from the chest wall or abducted to 90°. (b) Resting over an adjacent table supported by a pillow in front. (c) On the side with the lung to be drained uppermost.

Procedure guideline 12.4 Chest drain: assisting insertion

For the purpose of this chapter, only the procedure for inserting small-bore chest drains using the Seldinger technique shall be discussed. Only trained and competent personnel should carry out the procedure; however, nurses should be familiar with the process as they are often required to assist.

Essential equipment

Some of the equipment below may be available in kit form.

- Personal protective equipment, including sterile gloves, gown, mask and hat
- Portable ultrasound machine, sterile ultrasound jelly and sterile ultrasound probe cover
- Sterile chest drain pack containing gallipot, disposable towel and forceps
- Skin antiseptic solution, for example 2% alcoholic chlorhexidine
- Ideally a split fenestrated sterile drape design with a large clear plastic window surrounding the aseptic field to allow optimal views of the hemithorax
- Sterile gauze swabs

(continued)

Procedure guideline 12.4 Chest drain: assisting insertion *(continued)*

- A selection of syringes (5, 10 and 20 mL) and safety needles (21–25 G)
- Local anaesthetic
- Scalpel and blade
- Suture (e.g. Mersilk 2.0 or 3.0)
- Instrument for blunt dissection (e.g. curved clamp)
- Guidewire with dilators (in most Seldinger drain packs)
- Chest drain
- Connecting tubing
- Closed drainage system (including 500 mL sterile water if underwater seal bottle is being used)
- Occlusive dressing
- Chest drain clamps × 2

Medicinal products

- Local anaesthetic, such as lidocaine 1% (up to 3 mg/kg), is usually infiltrated. In addition, epinephrine may be used to aid homeostasis and allow larger doses of lidocaine to be administered. Levobupivacaine 0.25% may also be used to prolong post-procedure anaesthesia.
- Conscious sedation may be considered for certain patients if it is unlikely that they will be able to tolerate the procedure with oral analgesia and local anaesthetic alone. Titrated doses of intravenous midazolam and opioid analgesia may be given by practitioners experienced in conscious sedation to achieve the desired effect. The aim is for the patient to be able to tolerate the procedure but remain conscious throughout. Practitioners should be trained in immediate life support and ideally have airway skills. Patients must be appropriately monitored throughout the procedure and drug reversal agents (flumazenil and naloxone) should be readily available in case required (Academy of Medical Royal Colleges 2013, American Society of Anesthesiologists 2018, Havelock et al. 2010).

Action	Rationale
Pre-procedure	
1 Introduce yourself to the patient, explain and discuss the procedure with them, and ensure the operator has gained their consent to proceed (if the patient is conscious and able to consent).	To ensure that the patient feels at ease, understands the procedure and gives their valid consent (NMC 2018, **C**).
2 Decontaminate hands.	To minimize the risk of healthcare-associated infection (NHS England and NHSI 2019, **C**).
3 Ensure the patient has intravenous access that is patent.	For patient safety in the event of an acute deterioration (Yousuf and Rahman 2018, **C**).
4 Administer analgesia at least half an hour before the procedure.	To minimize pain during the procedure and to ensure the patient is able to co-operate (Noorani and Abu-Omar 2018, **C**).
5 Clean and prepare a trolley, placing the equipment on the bottom shelf.	To ensure the trolley is clean and all equipment required is available. **E**
6 Prime the underwater seal drainage bottle with sterile water and fill to the fluid line.	To create negative pressure and prevent the backflow of fluid or air into the pleural space (Woodrow 2013, **C**).
7 Decontaminate hands with an alcohol-based handrub again.	To minimize the risk of infection (NHS England and NHSI 2019, **C**).
8 Assist the operator by opening up packs/equipment as instructed, maintaining a sterile environment throughout.	To minimize the risk of infection. **E**
9 Assist the operator to scan the chest using real-time ultrasound.	To confirm the side of the effusion or pneumothorax (Yousuf and Rahman 2018, **C**).
10 Position the patient in preparation for the procedure. The patient may be positioned supine on the bed with the arm on the affected side placed behind their head away from the chest wall, or abducted to 90° (see Figures 12.26 and 12.27a). Alternatively, position the patient on their side with the lung to be drained uppermost (see Figure 12.27c). If the patient is able to sit upright, they can be positioned resting over an adjacent table supported by a pillow in front (see Figure 12.27b).	To facilitate insertion of the chest drain and prevent injury to adjacent organs (Adlakha et al. 2016, **C**). To ensure optimal patient comfort. **E**
Procedure	
11 Assist the practitioner as requested.	To ensure the procedure is carried out as smoothly and quickly as possible. **E**
12 Observe the patient throughout the procedure, paying attention to their respiratory and cardiovascular status. Monitor the patient's respiratory rate and pattern, movement of the chest wall, oxygen saturations, colour, blood pressure and heart rate. Inform the practitioner inserting the drain of any concerns or change in the patient's condition.	To monitor for signs of acute deterioration and complications associated with the procedure (Woodrow 2013, **C**).

13 Communicate with the patient during the procedure and explain what is happening at each stage.	To minimize anxiety (Woodrow 2013, **C**).

During the procedure

Using a sterile procedure throughout, the practitioner prepares the skin using a cleansing solution before infiltrating the surrounding area with local anaesthetic. Using ultrasound guidance, the drain is inserted into the pleural space using a Seldinger technique. Prior to unclamping the drain, the distal end is attached to the drainage system (tubing, bottle and sterile water) and the proximal end is secured to the skin and subcutaneous tissue using an anchor suture. For large-bore drains, a mattress suture may also be required (see Figure 12.28). The drain site should be cleaned and dressed using a specifically designed adhesive-dressing-based fixation system, or covered with gauze and an occlusive dressing. The drain can then be unclamped (Havelock et al. 2010, Woodrow 2013).

Post-procedure

14 Check the drain is well secured at the exit site using an anchor suture and occlusive dry dressing.	To prevent accidental disconnection or removal of the drain (Havelock et al. 2010, **C**; Jeffries 2017, **C**).
15 Check the whole drainage system and ensure all connections are secure. Tape the connection between the chest drain and tubing with an H-shaped dressing (see Figure 12.30).	To secure the connection and prevent accidental disconnection. **E** To ensure there are no leaks that will prevent re-expansion of the lung, or accidental introduction of a pneumothorax (Woodrow 2013, **C**).
16 Assist the patient into a comfortable position in bed, ensuring the drain and tubing are not occluded or kinked.	To optimize patient comfort and ensure the system is not occluded or limited, which would prevent drainage (Woodrow 2013, **C**).
17 Check the patient's observations/NEWS and document.	To observe for any change or deterioration in the patient's condition (RCP 2017, **C**).
18 Give further analgesia if required.	To ensure patient comfort (Woodrow 2013, **C**).
19 Monitor for bubbling in the chest drain bottle. Report any unexpected bubbling immediately to the practitioner who inserted the drain, or a senior member of staff.	Bubbling is to be expected with a pneumothorax but should not be present with a pleural effusion (Woodrow 2013, **C**). Bubbling may indicate an air leak or introduction of a pneumothorax and should be urgently investigated (Woodrow 2013, **C**).
20 Record either the presence or absence of bubbling on the chest drain observation chart. Inform medical or surgical staff when the bubbling ceases.	To keep an accurate record of the status of the chest drain (Woodrow 2013, **C**). A chest drain inserted for drainage of a pneumothorax will stop bubbling once all the excess air has been dispensed and the lung has reinflated (Porcel 2018b, **C**).
21 Do not clamp a bubbling chest drain.	Clamping a bubbling chest drain could cause a life-threatening tension pneumothorax (Porcel 2018b, **C**).
22 Monitor for swinging of fluid in the tubing and record its presence or absence on the chest drain observation chart.	To keep an accurate record of the status of the chest drain (Woodrow 2013, **C**). The absence of fluid swinging within the tube may indicate a blocked drain (Chadwick et al. 2015, **C**).
23 Monitor the amount and appearance of any fluid drained and record this on the chest drain observation chart.	To keep an accurate record of the status of the chest drain, and the amount and type of fluid drained (Woodrow 2013, **C**).
24 If the drain has been inserted to drain fluid, allow a maximum of 1.5 L of fluid to be drained in the first hour then clamp. It may be advisable to drain smaller volumes, especially if the patient is petite or frail. Stop draining if the patient begins to cough, complains of chest pain or has vasovagal symptoms.	To prevent re-expansion pulmonary oedema (Havelock et al. 2010, **C**).
25 Dispose of waste appropriately.	To reduce the risk of sharps injury and cross-infection (NICE 2017, **C**).
26 Educate the patient on the need to keep the drainage bottle upright and below chest level, and to avoid any pulling of the drain.	To prevent drained fluid re-entering the pleural space, or any accidental disconnection or removal of the chest drain (Woodrow 2013, **C**).
27 Advise the patient to report any concerns or change in breathing.	To detect any change or deterioration in the patient's condition early. **E**
28 Record chest drain status and patient observations/NEWS 5 minutes and 1 hour after drain insertion, then to a minimum of 4-hourly thereafter. Repeat observations before and after drainage.	To detect any change or deterioration in the patient's condition and ensure timely escalation to senior staff if required (RCP 2017, **C**).
29 Escort the patient to radiology for a post-drain insertion chest X-ray.	To rule out any post-procedural complications and observe the position of the drain (Porcel 2018b, **C**).
30 Cleanse hands with an alcohol-based handrub.	To minimize the risk of cross-infection (NHS England and NHSI 2019, **C**).

Post-procedural considerations

Immediate care

The nurse should monitor the patient's observations and NEWS immediately after insertion to check for any signs of respiratory or cardiovascular compromise. The patient should also be observed for changes in their breathing pattern or increasing shortness of breath (Woodrow 2013). Any change in condition or deterioration in the patient's observations or NEWS warrants immediate escalation and review by a senior member of staff (RCP 2017). This may include the practitioner who inserted the chest drain or members of the clinical team. Radiological imaging (chest X-ray) should be performed to determine where the drain is placed and the status of the pneumothorax or effusion (Porcel 2018b). The drain should be monitored for the features outlined in Table 12.8, and the monitoring should be documented on the relevant chart.

As described in Table 12.8, ongoing bubbling indicates the presence of an air leak, which should be investigated immediately (Woodrow 2013). The drain and tube should be inspected thoroughly down to the level of the underwater seal to eliminate any external problems such as loose tubing connections, poor seal around the drain insertion site or tube migration outside the chest wall. If no loose connections are found, a chest X-ray or CT scan will be required to determine the position of the chest drain and rule out a pleural tear (Havelock et al. 2010, Porcel 2018b). Depending on the cause of the leak, the chest drain may need to be removed and another reinserted. An ongoing air leak may also warrant low-pressure thoracic suction (see Procedure guideline 12.5: Chest drainage: suction). See Problem-solving table 12.4 for further guidance on the prevention and recommended actions for problems associated with a chest drain.

Table 12.8 Chest drain observations

Observation	Detail
Bubbling	Indicates air is still present in the pleural space. Bubbling should decrease and eventually stop as the pneumothorax resolves and the lung reinflates. If bubbling continues, an air leak may be present. Causes of air leaks include: • un-resolving pneumothorax • an eyelet on the drain may be outside the chest wall, allowing air to be drawn into the system on inspiration • inadequate drain size inserted • disconnection at the connection site between the drain and tubing • poor seal around the entry site to the lung • pleural tear. *Note*: a bubbling chest drain should never be clamped (even during intra-hospital transfer to the radiology department, for example).
Swinging	Indicates the drain is patent and sitting within the pleural space. If swinging is absent, this may indicate that the drain is blocked, kinked or sitting up against the pleural wall.
Draining	Drainage will not occur if the drain is inserted for a pneumothorax. If the drain stops draining a pleural effusion, it may either require removal or indicate that the drain is blocked and requires flushing.

Source: Adapted from Chadwick et al. (2015), Havelock et al. (2010), Mohammed (2015), Porcel (2018b), Woodrow (2013).

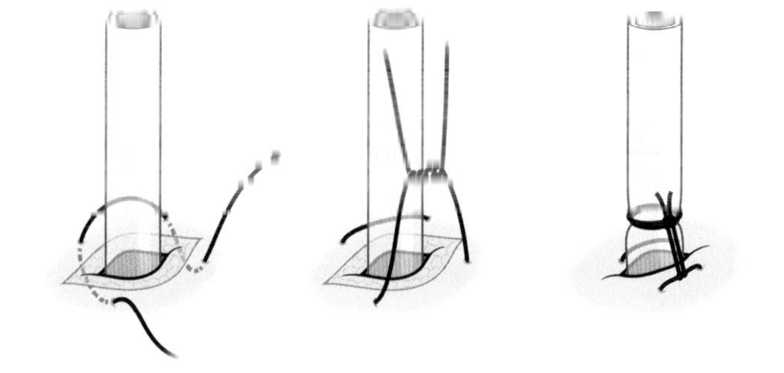

Figure 12.28 Mattress suture.

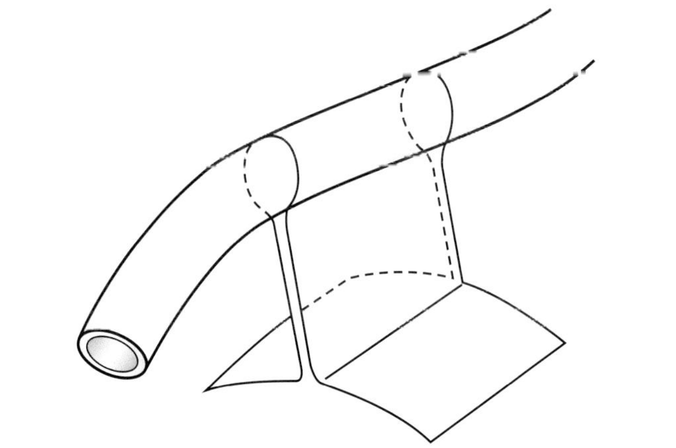

Figure 12.29 Omental tag.

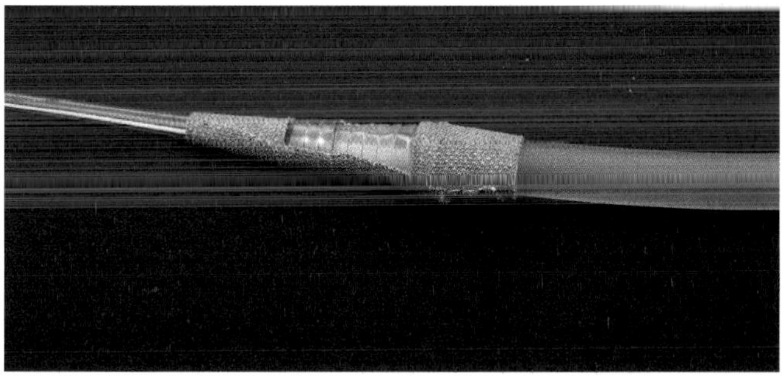

Figure 12.30 H-shaped securing tape.

Securing the drain

Purse string sutures are no longer advised due to the skin trauma and unsightly scar that they cause. A mattress suture (Figure 12.28) is preferred as it offers a more natural closure once the drain is removed and ultimately less scarring. It is recommended that all drains, regardless of size, should have an anchor suture inserted to prevent them pulling and falling out (Havelock et al. 2010, Porcel 2018b). The drain may also be secured to the surrounding skin with a specifically designed adhesive fixation dressing or an omental tag (Figure 12.29) (Havelock et al. 2010).

The drains and connections should be checked to ensure that they are secure and the drain tubing is not kinked or looped. An 'H' dressing (Figure 12.30) should be applied to reinforce the connection between the drain and the tubing while allowing the connection to be visualized at regular intervals.

Dressing the insertion site

If a specifically designed adhesive fixation dressing is not available, a simple dry dressing (low-linting gauze) may be applied around the drain and secured with adhesive tape or an occlusive dressing. Strapping should be avoided as it can restrict chest movement. The dressing should be kept dry and clean, and changed daily or as required. The skin around the drain site should be inspected daily to ensure it is clean, dry, and free from maceration and infection (Havelock et al. 2010, Jeffries 2017).

Ongoing care

Clamping of chest drains

Pneumothorax

A bubbling chest drain should never be clamped, as clamping will prevent air leaving the pleural space, which has the potential to cause a tension pneumothorax (Woodrow 2013). The drain should remain unclamped even when patients are mobilizing or being transported to other departments within the hospital. The only time a bubbling chest drain should be momentarily clamped is in the event of accidental disconnection, if there is damage to the drainage bottle or to locate a leak in the drainage system (Mohammed 2015, Woodrow 2013).

Pleural effusion

Drainage of a pleural effusion should be controlled by clamping the chest drain intermittently. Davies et al. (2010) recommend draining off a maximum of 1500 mL in the first hour after insertion, then 1500 mL every 2 hours thereafter. Draining large volumes may cause re-expansion pulmonary oedema as the lung rapidly re-expands. It may therefore be advisable to drain off smaller volumes (500 to 1000 mL), especially if the patient is petite or frail. Drainage can either be slowed down or clamped temporarily if the patient experiences pain, starts coughing, experiences vasovagal symptoms or has a drop in blood pressure. Coughing usually subsides within 15 minutes, analgesia can be administered to help with pain, and an IV fluid bolus can be given if the patient becomes haemodynamically unstable. The chest drain should be unclamped in the event of an acute clinical deterioration (Havelock et al. 2010) and expert help sought immediately.

Stripping and milking of chest drains

Stripping and milking of chest tubes to keep tubing patent increases the negative pressure in the intrathoracic cavity to −100 to −400 cmH_2O. Such an increase in negative pressure may harm lung tissue; therefore, milking or stripping of chest tubes on a

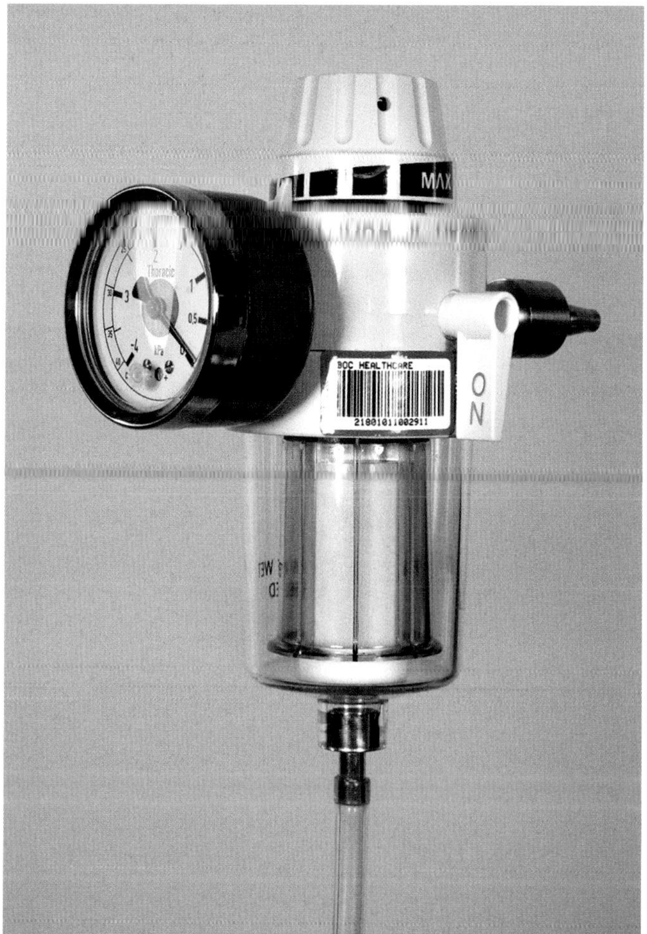

Figure 12.31 High-volume, low-pressure suction unit (thoracic suction adaptor).

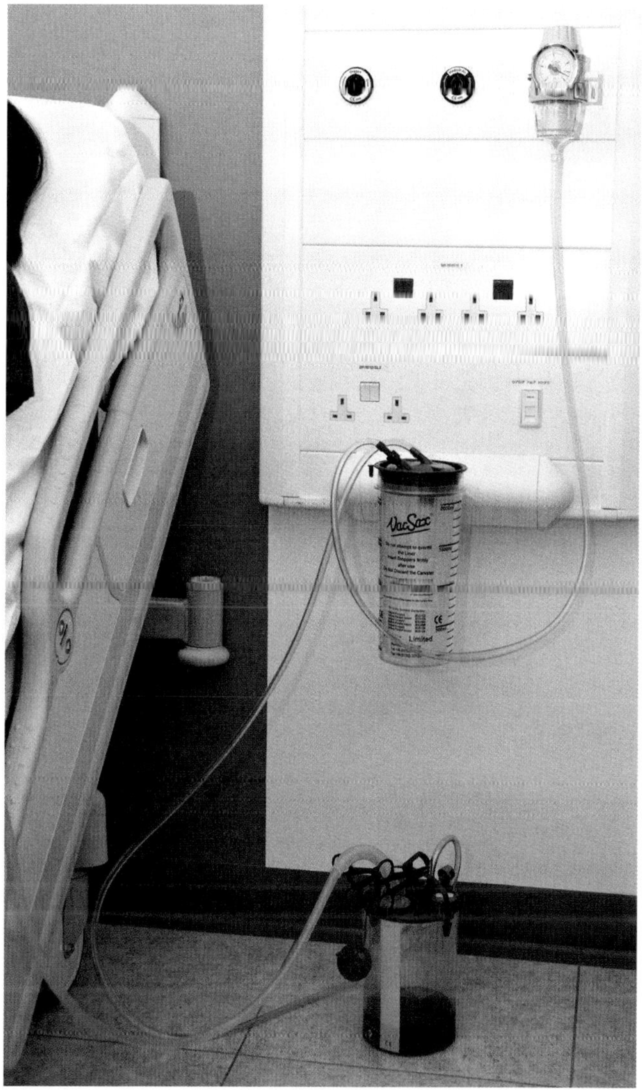

Figure 12.32 Chest drain on suction.

routine basis should be avoided (Mohammed 2015). If a chest drain becomes blocked, the tubing should be flushed or replaced.

Chest drain: suction

Evidence-based approaches

The evidence for connecting low pressure thoracic suction to an underwater-seal chest-drain bottle to assist in the management of a pneumothorax is controversial, despite the widespread use of this technique in clinical practice (Havelock et al. 2010). While 70% of pneumothoraces resolve within 3 days after chest drain insertion, up to 30% continue to have an ongoing air leak. Thoracic suction may be indicated for this group of patients (Tschopp et al. 2015).

If indicated, appropriately trained staff should set up the system and advice should be sought from a specialist if required. The addition of suction to the drainage system increases the negative pressure, enhancing lung re-expansion. A high-volume, low-pressure thoracic suction unit (Figure 12.31) should be applied to a single-chamber chest-drain bottle, using pressure in the range of 10–20 cmH_2O (1–2 kPa) (Havelock et al. 2010, Zisis et al. 2015). Suction should be applied and the pressure increased gradually to prevent lung tear (George and Papagiannopoulos 2016).

When the tubing is attached to the suction port of the chest drain bottle, the suction must remain on at all times. However, the suction tubing can be disconnected from the port to allow the patient to mobilize away from the bed space. Once suction has been discontinued, the tubing must be disconnected from the port before the suction is turned off. Turning off the suction and leaving the tubing attached to the port of the underwater-seal chest-drain bottle could potentially cause a tension pneumothorax (Havelock et al. 2010).

Most suction units are fitted with a disposable air filter capsule between the vacuum connector and the filter capsule mount. The filter prevents cross-infection and should be changed after use in each patient. Direct connection between the chest drain bottle and the high-flow, low-pressure suction unit without an intermediate suction jar or canister can lead to patient injury, loss of effective suction, and contamination of the hospital vacuum system, posing an infection control risk. An intermediate suction canister must therefore be attached between the thoracic suction unit and the underwater-seal chest-drain bottle to prevent contamination of the thoracic suction unit filter (MHRA 2010) (Figure 12.32).

While ambulatory chest drainage bags with a built-in Heimlich valve cannot be attached to suction, ambulatory digital chest drainage systems monitor the negative pressure within the thoracic space and adjust the suction pressure accordingly. Multi-chamber chest drain bottles have a built-in suction control compartment that is controlled by either an underwater seal or external suction. The manufacturer's instructions must be followed.

Procedure guideline 12.5 Chest drainage: suction

Essential equipment

- Personal protective equipment
- Thoracic high-volume, low-pressure suction unit (see Figure 12.31)
- Two lengths of suction tubing measuring 1–2 metres each
- Suction canister
- Portable suction unit to be kept at the patient's bedside in the event of clinical deterioration and need for emergency/resuscitation equipment (if only one suction port available)

Action	Rationale
Pre-procedure	
1 Introduce yourself to the patient, explain and discuss the procedure with them, and gain their consent to proceed.	To ensure that the patient feels at ease, understands the procedure and gives their valid consent (NMC 2018, **C**).
2 Cleanse hands with an alcohol-based handrub.	To minimize the risk of infection (NHS England and NHSI 2019, **C**).
Procedure	
3 Remove the usual high-pressure suction unit from the wall suction outlet. Insert the specifically designed high-volume, low-pressure thoracic suction unit into the wall suction outlet instead.	To ensure the correct unit is used. Using the wrong suction unit at high pressures will cause trauma to the lung tissues (Woodrow 2013, **C**).
4 Attach one end of a length of suction tubing to the high-volume, low pressure thoracic suction unit and attach the other end to the suction canister.	To prevent contamination of the thoracic suction unit filter with pleural fluid. **E** A wet filter could block the system, which has the potential to cause a tension pneumothorax (MHRA 2010, **C**).
5 Attach a length of suction tubing from the suction canister and turn the suction on. Occlude the end of the tubing and check for the presence of low-pressure suction.	To check the suction unit is working properly. **E**
6 Connect the suction tubing (leave one end attached to the suction canister) to the suction port of the chest drain bottle. Adjust the suction pressure to 10 cmH_2O.	To allow the lung to slowly re-expand without damaging the lung tissues or causing the patient pain or distress (George and Papagiannopoulos 2016, **C**).
7 Monitor for bubbling, swinging and draining of fluid (see Table 12.8), and document.	To monitor and record the chest drain status (Woodrow 2013, **C**).
8 Check the patient's observations/NEWS and document.	To detect any change or deterioration in the patient's condition and ensure timely escalation to senior staff if required (RCP 2017, **C**).

9 Slowly titrate the suction up to the pressure prescribed, or to a pressure that the patient can tolerate (maximum of 20 cmH_2O)	To allow the lung to slowly re-expand without damaging the lung tissues or causing the patient pain or distress (George and Papagiannopoulos 2016, **C**).
Post-procedure	
10 If the patient needs to leave their bed space, disconnect the suction tubing from the chest drain suction port. Reconnect it when the patient is back at their bed space. Ensure the tubing is properly reconnected and the suction unit is on at the prescribed pressure.	To ensure a patent and safe system. If the tubing is reattached but suction is not turned on, air is unable to escape from the bottle, which could result in a tension pneumothorax. **E**
11 Record the addition of suction and the set pressure on the chest drain observation chart and in the nursing documentation.	To keep an accurate record of the amount of pressure applied. **E**
12 Observe for any change in the patient's respiratory status and recheck the patient's observations/NEWS. Escalate any concerns or deterioration immediately.	To identify any concerns or clinical deterioration early and ensure timely escalation to senior staff if required (RCP 2017, **C**; Woodrow 2013, **C**).

Chest drain: changing the bottle

Evidence-based approaches

The drainage bottle should be changed when it is three-quarters full, if there is any damage to the container, or if the tubing has been accidentally disconnected from the chest drain (Woodrow 2013). If there are any concerns about atmospheric air entering the system during the bottle or tubing change, ask the patient to gently cough to get rid of any air within the pleural space. The drainage bottle and hazardous waste contents should be disposed of as per local infection control policy (Woodrow 2013).

Procedure guideline 12.6 Chest drain: changing the bottle

Essential equipment

- Personal protective equipment
- Cleaning solution (e.g. chlorhexidine in 70% alcohol)
- Tape
- Sterile chest drain bottle
- Sterile water
- Chest drain non-toothed clamps x 2
- Procedure pack

Action	Rationale
Pre-procedure	
1 Introduce yourself to the patient, explain and discuss the procedure with them, and gain their consent to proceed.	To ensure that the patient feels at ease, understands the procedure and gives their valid consent (NMC 2018, **C**).
2 Cleanse hands with soap and water or an alcohol-based handrub.	To minimize the risk of cross-infection (NHS England and NHSI 2019, **C**).
Procedure	
3 Follow the manufacturer's instructions for opening and filling the bottle with sterile water up to the fluid line.	To ensure the drainage system is properly set up with enough water to fully immerse the drainage tube and create an underwater seal (Woodrow 2013, **C**).
4 Undo the taping that secures the chest drain to the chest drain tubing. Do not disconnect at this stage.	To allow disconnection of the tubing from the chest drain. **E**
5 Clamp the chest drain close to the chest wall with two clamps. Clamp the drain for the shortest possible period of time needed to change the tubing and bottle.	To prevent air entering the chest cavity (Woodrow 2013, **C**). Clamping the drain for long periods of time may increase the risk of pneumothorax (Woodrow 2013, **C**).
6 Remove the old tubing and bottle and clean the chest drain connection. Attach the new tubing to the chest drain.	To prevent bacterial contamination of the new tubing. **E**
7 Immerse the distal end of the tubing into the new chest drain bottle and ensure it is 2–3 cm below the level of the water.	To create an underwater seal (Havelock et al. 2010, **C**).
8 Ensure all connections are secure before removing the clamps.	To prevent accidental disconnection. **E**
9 Tape the connection between the chest drain and tubing with an H-shaped dressing (see Figure 12.30).	To secure the connection and prevent accidental disconnection. **E**
10 Cleanse hands with soap and water or an alcohol-based handrub.	To minimize the risk of cross-infection (NICE 2017, **C**).

(continued)

Procedure guideline 12.6 Chest drain: changing the bottle (continued)

Action	Rationale
Post-procedure	
11 Record the addition of the new bottle on the chest drain observation chart and in the nursing documentation.	To keep an accurate record of the amount of fluid drained since insertion (Woodrow 2013, **C**).
12 Observe for any change in the patient's respiratory status and recheck the patient's observations/NEWS. Escalate any concerns or deterioration immediately.	To identify any concerns or clinical deterioration early and ensure timely escalation to senior staff if required (RCP 2017, **C**; Woodrow 2013, **C**).

Problem-solving table 12.4 Prevention and resolution (Procedure guidelines 12.4, 12.5 and 12.6)

Problem	Cause	Prevention	Action
Lack of drainage	Kinking, looping or pressure on the tubing may block and impede drainage	Educate the patient on care of the drain and how to position themselves to prevent occlusion or kinking of the drain tubing. Secure the tubing to the patient to prevent kinking or looping using an omental tag.	Check the tubing and unkink or unloop as required. Reposition the patient.
	Excess fluid in the pleural space may have fully drained	None necessary.	Perform a chest X-ray to check if excess fluid has been adequately drained. Remove drain if required.
Drain is not swinging	Drain or tubing blocked by viscous fluid or tissue	Flush drain on a regular basis if fluid is viscous and likely to block the drain or tubing.	Gently flush the chest drain with sterile normal saline 0.9% to unblock.
Underwater seal drain not bubbling as expected	Drain occluded	Monitor for bubbling post-insertion. Ensure the tubing is not kinked or looped, and that the system is patent. Ensure the drain is open and not clamped.	Check the tubing and unkink or unloop it as required. Flush the drain to ensure it is patent and not blocked. Unclamp the drain if it is found to be clamped.
	Drain not correctly placed	The practitioner inserting the drain should ensure correct landmarking and effective drain insertion.	Perform a chest X-ray to check the position of drain. Discuss with radiology if the drain requires repositioning, or if removal and reinsertion of the drain is required.
Continuous bubbling in chest drain bottle	Air leak in system	Check the bottle for bubbling and swinging, and check integrity of the chest drain system regularly. Ensure all connections are secure.	Check for any loose connections throughout the chest drain system. Check the drain insertion site to determine whether the drain has moved. The eyelets of the drain may be exposed to the atmosphere, allowing air to enter. Perform a chest X-ray to check the position of the drain and status of the effusion or pneumothorax. Prepare for drain removal and reinsertion if required.
Ooze from drain site	Bleeding or infection	Remove the dressing at least once daily, clean and re-dress, and document any concerns. Review the need for the drain daily with senior staff, and remove it as soon as possible.	Remove the dressing, observe the site and take a wound swab. Clean and re-dress the site. Discuss with medical/surgical team whether antimicrobial therapy is indicated. Remove the drain as soon as it is no longer required (if the lung has reinflated or the effusion has been adequately drained).

Problem	Cause	Prevention	Action
Fluid leaking from around the drain site	Bypassing of fluid from around the drain site due to blockage of the drain	Flush the chest drain regularly if the fluid is viscous and likely to block the drain.	Gently flush the chest drain using sterile normal saline 0.9% to unblock it. If unable to unblock, removal and reinsertion of a new drain may be required.
Accidental disconnection of the drainage tubing from the chest drain	Connections not secure	Secure the connection using an H-shaped dressing (see Figure 12.30).	Immediately apply a clamp to the drain above the site of disconnection. Re-establish the connection as soon as possible. The tubing may need to be changed if it was contaminated during disconnection. As soon as the drain and tubing are connected, remove the clamp and ask the patient to cough gently to aid removal of air. If a pneumothorax is present and the bottle was bubbling prior to disconnection, the drain can be unclamped and temporarily submerged in a sterile bottle of water until a new system is set up. Reassure the patient. Report the incident to the clinical team and ask them to review the patient. Consider performing a chest X-ray to assess whether a pneumothorax is present. Record the incident in the relevant records and nursing documentation.
Chest drain falls out	Drain not secure	Check the drain insertion site regularly. Ensure the anchoring stitch is still intact. Apply a clear dressing over the chest drain site and consider the use of an omental tag to secure the tubing onto the patient's surrounding skin	Immediately pull the mattress suture closed (if present) and cover it with an occlusive sterile dressing. Check the patient's observations/NEWS and escalate immediately if the patient is clinically deteriorating or there are any concerns. Inform the clinical team and ask for an immediate review. If the patient is stable, perform a chest X-ray to determine whether a pneumothorax has been caused. If the patient is clinically deteriorating and has signs and symptoms of a pneumothorax or tension pneumothorax, call the medical emergency team and prepare for urgent drain reinsertion or needle decompression. Reassure the patient.
Patient complains of pain	Drain pulling at site	Secure the drain to the patient's skin using an omental tag to prevent pulling. Administer appropriate analgesia on a regular basis.	Reposition the tube and secure it using an omental tag to prevent the drain pulling. Administer analgesia as prescribed. Escalate to the clinical team if prescribed analgesia is not sufficient.

Post-procedural considerations

Documentation

Clearly document in the patient's nursing notes the date, type and size of drain inserted, and for what indication. The status of the drain should be documented at least 4-hourly to determine whether there is evidence of bubbling, swinging or draining of fluid. The type and volume of fluid should also be recorded on a specific chest drain observation chart (Havelock et al. 2010). If low-pressure thoracic suction is used, regularly check and document the suction pressure used (Woodrow 2013). Bottle changes and drain removals should also be recorded in both the nursing notes and the chest drain observation chart.

Monitor patient observations/NEWS regularly to ensure the patient is stable and there are no signs of clinical deterioration. Observations should be recorded every 5 minutes for the first 15 minutes following drain insertion and then reduced slowly over the next few hours to a minimum frequency of 4-hourly (Woodrow 2013). The patient's pain score should also be recorded and analgesia given as required (Woodrow 2013).

Education of the patient and relevant others

Educate the patient as to why the chest drain is required and, if possible, teach the patient how to look after the drain. They should be taught to keep the drain below chest level at all times and ensure the bottle is kept upright and does not fall over (Havelock et al. 2010, Woodrow 2013). If suction is indicated, the patient can be taught how to disconnect the suction tubing from the suction port on the underwater-seal chest-drain bottle, to allow them to mobilize away from the bed space. They should be instructed to reconnect it or call the nurse to assist with reconnection on their return. When resting in bed, the patient should be encouraged to lie in a position that prevents the tubing being occluded or kinked. The patient should also be encouraged to report any change in their breathing while the chest drain is in place.

Complications

Complications of chest drains include (Mao et al. 2015, Ravi and McKnight 2018):

- incorrect placement (extrapleural, intrapulmonary or sub-diaphragmatic)
- drain dislodgement
- puncturing of adjacent organs: lung, stomach, spleen, liver, heart or great vessels
- pulmonary laceration (haemorrhage or fistula)
- pneumothorax
- haemorrhage
- infection
- mechanical obstruction
- surgical emphysema
- re-expansion pulmonary oedema.

Chest drain removal

Evidence-based approaches

The decision to remove a drain is usually made by a clinician based on the following criteria:

- There is an absence of air bubbling in the underwater seal chest drain bottle, usually noted when the patient exhales forcibly or coughs. This will coincide with expiration in a patient who is being mechanically ventilated with positive pressure.
- The volume of fluid draining into the chest-drain bottle is minimal, usually between 100 and 300 mL per day (Chadwick et al. 2015).
- There is no evidence of respiratory compromise or failure.
- There is no coagulation deficit or increased risk of bleeding (check the latest coagulation results prior to removal).
- In many cases, radiological evidence of the absence of air or fluid within the pleural space will be required before removal.

The patient should be offered analgesia at least 30 minutes prior to chest drain removal (Woodrow 2013) before being placed in a comfortable position in bed that allows the nurse to gain access to the drain insertion site. The Valsalva manoeuvre (asking the patient to hold their breath, bear down and breathe against a closed glottis) should be taught and practised before the drain is removed (Mohammed 2015).

Small-bore pigtail drains should have the holding thread cut or released (depending on the make and manufacturer) so as to uncoil the drain within the pleural space and allow removal. Both large-bore and small-bore drains will have an anchor suture, which should be cut prior to removal. Large-bore chest drains may also have an additional mattress suture to help seal the incision site immediately after the drain is removed.

After removing the anchor suture, the chest drain should be removed with a brisk, firm movement while the patient performs the Valsalva manoeuver on the third expiratory breathe. If a mattress suture is present, a second nurse should tie this closed at the same time as the drain is removed (Havelock et al. 2010). Chest drains inserted for pneumothorax do not need to be clamped during the removal process.

A follow-up post-removal chest X-ray is required to ensure no air has been allowed to enter during the removal process with formation of a subsequent pneumothorax (Woodrow 2013).

Procedure guideline 12.7 Chest drain: removal

The removal technique is dependent on the type of chest drain used. While only one nurse is required to remove a small-bore chest drain, two nurses are required to facilitate safe removal of a large-bore chest drain. One is required to remove the drain while the other ties the mattress suture to close and seal the site.

Essential equipment

- Personal protective equipment
- Sterile dressing pack containing gallipot, gauze and a sterile towel
- Cleaning solution, for example 0.9% sodium chloride
- Stitch cutter
- Sterile occlusive dressing

Action	Rationale
Pre-procedure	
1 Introduce yourself to the patient, explain and discuss the procedure with them, and gain their consent to proceed.	To ensure that the patient feels at ease, understands the procedure and gives their valid consent (NMC 2018, **C**).
2 Cleanse hands with soap and water or an alcohol-based handrub.	To minimize the risk of infection (NHS England and NHSI 2019, **C**).
3 Encourage the patient to practice the Valsalva manoeuvre before the chest drain is removed. The Valsalva manoeuvre requires the patient to hold their breath, bear down and breathe against a closed glottis at the end of expiration.	To ensure the patient understands and is able to perform the Valsalva manoeuvre prior to drain removal. **E** To increase the intrathoracic pressure, reducing the possibility of air re-entering the pleural space during drain removal (Cerfolio et al. 2013, **C**).
4 Administer analgesia at least half an hour before the procedure.	To minimize any pain during the procedure (Woodrow 2013, **C**).
5 Discontinue suction if in use and disconnect the suction tubing from the suction port.	To reduce the number of tubes and amount of equipment in the surrounding area. **E**

6 Cleanse hands with soap and water or an alcohol-based handrub.	Hands need to be cleansed before and after each patient contact to minimize the risk of infection (NHS England and NHSI 2019, **C**).
7 Prepare a trolley for the procedure. Open the sterile procedure pack onto the top of a clean trolley using aseptic technique, then open the stitch cutter, gallipot and occlusive dressing onto the sterile field. Pour the cleaning solution into the gallipot.	To ensure all equipment required is prepared prior to starting the procedure. **E**
8 Assist the patient into a position that facilitates drain removal while ensuring patient comfort.	To aid patient comfort and ensure easy removal of the chest drain (Woodrow 2013, **C**).
9 Place a protective pad underneath the patient.	To absorb any leakage from the drain during removal. **E**
Procedure	
10 Cleanse hands with an alcohol-based handrub and apply apron and gloves.	Hands need to be cleansed before and after each patient contact to minimize the risk of infection (NHS England and NHSI 2019, **C**).
11 Remove the dressing from around the drain site. Examine what size of drain has been used and which sutures are present: either a large bore drain with a mattress suture and anchor suture (requires two nurses) or a fine-bore drain with only an anchor suture (requires one nurse).	To prepare for drain removal and determine how many nurses are required to perform the procedure. **E**
Large-bore drain	
12 To remove a large-bore drain, two nurses are required: one to remove the drain and the other to seal the site. The first nurse loosens the mattress suture, exposing the ends to be tied on removal of the drain.	To prepare the drain and ensure it is ready for removal. **E**
13 The second nurse cuts the anchor suture and ensures the drain is mobile and ready to be removed.	To prepare the drain and ensure it is ready for removal. **E**
14 The second nurse asks the patient to take two deep breaths and then perform the Valsalva manoeuvre at the end of expiration on the third breath. While the patient performs the Valsalva manoeuvre, the second nurse pulls out the drain steadily and smoothly.	Performing the Valsalva manoeuvre at the end of expiration increases intrathoracic pressure, preventing air flowing into the intrathoracic cavity and the formation of a new pneumothorax (Cerfolio et al. 2013, **C**).
15 The first nurse pulls and ties the mattress suture while the drain is simultaneously removed.	To close and seal the drain site, preventing the entry of air and formation of a pneumothorax (Havelock et al. 2010, **C**).
16 Ask the patient to breathe normally after the drain is removed.	To assess if there is any air escaping from suture/drain site. **E**
Fine-bore drain	
17 One nurse is required to remove a fine-bore drain. The anchor suture should be cut and the drain prepared ready for removal. If a pigtail drain is in place, the nurse will need to follow the manufacturer's instructions to unlock the device, usually by either cutting or unlocking the thread.	Following the manufacturer's instructions ensures correct removal and reduces the risk of pain, trauma and the formation of a pneumothorax secondary to incorrect removal technique. **E**
18 The nurse should remove the drain in a smooth but brisk fashion while the patient performs the Valsalva manoeuvre (see above) on the third expiratory breath.	Performing the Valsalva manoeuvre at the end of expiration increases intrathoracic pressure and prevents air flowing into the intrathoracic cavity and the formation of a new pneumothorax (Cerfolio et al. 2013, **C**).
19 The drain site should immediately be covered with sterile gauze until an occlusive dressing can be applied.	To close and seal the drain site, preventing the entry of air and formation of a pneumothorax (Havelock et al. 2010, **C**).
20 Ask the patient to breathe normally after the drain is removed.	To assess if there is any air escaping from suture/drain site. **E**
Post-procedure	
21 Clean around the site with 0.9% sodium chloride and apply an occlusive dressing.	To clean the site and prevent air entry by forming an airtight seal. **E**
22 Dispose of waste appropriately, remove gloves and clean hands.	To ensure safety and reduce the risk of infection (NICE 2017, **C**).
23 Assist the patient into a comfortable position.	To ensure patient comfort and aid respiration. **E**
24 Monitor the patient's respiratory status and observations/NEWS. Escalate any concerns or deterioration immediately.	To identify any concerns or clinical deterioration early, and ensure timely escalation to senior staff if required (RCP 2017, **C**; Woodrow 2013, **E**).
25 Document removal of the drain on the chest drain chart and in the nursing documentation.	To maintain accurate patient records (NMC 2018, **C**).
26 Escort the patient for a chest X-ray following drain removal.	To check that a pneumothorax has not reformed or been introduced during removal (Porcel 2018a, **C**).
27 Monitor the wound site and change the dressing as required.	To monitor for signs of infection (Havelock et al. 2010, **C**).

Tracheostomy and laryngectomy care

Definition

A tracheostomy is the creation of a permanent or temporary opening (stoma) in the anterior wall of the trachea to facilitate ventilation (Figure 12.33). The opening is commonly made at the level of the second or third cartilaginous rings and is usually maintained by the use of a tracheostomy tube (Adam et al. 2017). A tracheostomy may be created surgically or percutaneously, and as either an elective (planned) or non-elective (unplanned/emergency) procedure.

A total laryngectomy is the surgical removal of the larynx (Figure 12.33). The end of the trachea is stitched to the skin of the anterior neck and forms a permanent and irreversible stoma. The upper airway is no longer connected to the trachea and lungs, and all ventilation takes place via the laryngectomy stoma (Bonvento et al. 2017). Because the larynx has been removed, the patient is unable to phonate using their vocal cords so alternative methods of communication and voice facilitation must be used instead (Ward and Van As-Brooks 2014).

Regardless of whether the newly created stoma is permanent or temporary, a patient with a tracheostomy or laryngectomy may be referred to as a 'neck breather' or as having an 'altered airway'.

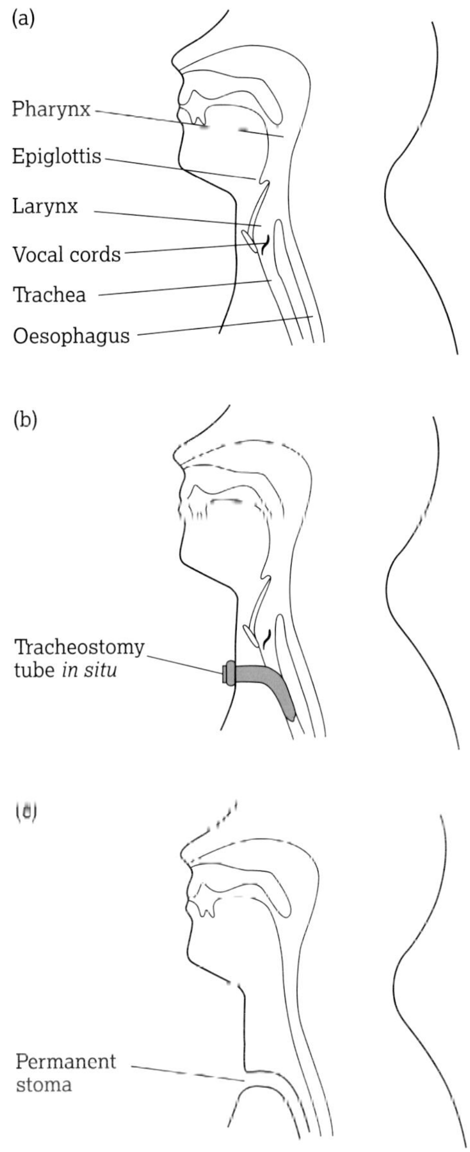

Figure 12.33 (a) Anatomy of the head and neck. (b) Tracheostomy. (c) Laryngectomy.

Anatomy and physiology

Figure 12.33a shows the anatomy of the neck. The larynx, situated at the top of the trachea, houses the vocal cords and is the point of transition between the upper (mouth, nose and pharynx) and lower airways. It is made up of nine cartilage segments, the largest of which is called the thyroid cartilage. Attached to the entrance of the larynx is the epiglottis, a large elastic cartilage that closes over the glottis during swallowing, protecting the lower airway from aspiration. At the inferior end is the cricoid cartilage, which attaches to the trachea, a large cylindrical structure approximately 11 cm long. The trachea is made up of C-shaped hyaline cartilage anteriorly and a membranous portion posteriorly; this composition provides reinforcement and protection while allowing the trachea to collapse slightly as food passes down the oesophagus. The trachea then divides at the carina to form the right and left main stem bronchi of the lungs (Tortora and Derrickson 2017).

Related theory

Approximately 5000 surgical tracheostomies and 15,000 percutaneous tracheostomies are performed each year in England (Wilkinson et al. 2014). Despite the increasing numbers of altered airways being performed, several reports recognize key themes of poor tracheostomy care and a lack of care pathways, resulting in harm to patients, prolonged hospital stay and poor survival to hospital discharge (Bonvento et al. 2017, Mortimer and Kubba 2017, Wilkinson et al. 2014). While nurses carry out a significant amount of care for patients with an altered airway, a multidisciplinary team approach is essential to co-ordinate and plan safe and effective care before and after stoma formation (Bonvento et al. 2017, Wilkinson et al. 2014).

Speech and language therapists (SLTs) play a pivotal role in the assessment and management of patients' impaired swallowing and speech, especially in patients who have undergone a total laryngectomy (Bonvento et al. 2017). Specialized physiotherapists are skilled in mobilization, rehabilitation, humidification techniques and the general care of tracheostomies. Patients may have difficulty with an altered body image and need psychological support, not only from the professionals closely involved in their care but also potentially from a formal psychological support team. Other key support teams include ENT (ear, nose and throat) and head and neck clinical nurse specialists, rehabilitation teams, dieticians, critical care outreach teams, anaesthetists (in the event of an airway emergency), and discharge co-ordinators and community teams (for patients with altered airways who are going home).

Evidence-based approaches

Types of tracheostomy

A *temporary tracheostomy* may be performed surgically in theatre or percutaneously in a critical care environment. The tracheostomy may be formed because the patient is unable to maintain their own airway and/or clear their own secretions, because they are expected to require ventilator support for longer than 7–10 days, or because they are expected to be a slow respiratory wean from the mechanical ventilator (Cosgrove and Carrie 2015). It may also be formed during certain head and neck surgeries to allow access to the upper airways. The tracheostomy tube will be removed as soon as the patient has recovered and can safely maintain their own airway again.

A *permanent tracheostomy* is required when it is unlikely that the patient will be able to maintain their own airway or manage their own secretions because of an underlying disease or condition that is likely to be progressive or irreversible. Examples of such conditions include certain cancers of the head and neck, a neuromuscular disorder, a cerebral vascular accident or following a traumatic head injury (Cheung and Napolitano 2014). In these examples, other than the creation of the tracheostomy stoma, the patient's anatomy is not surgically altered and the upper airway remains connected to the trachea.

Following complete surgical removal of the larynx (total laryngectomy), the trachea is sutured in position to form a permanent stoma, known as a laryngectomy stoma. Because the patient's anatomy has been permanently altered, there is no longer any connection between the upper airways and the trachea, and the patient will breathe through the laryngectomy stoma for the remainder of their life (Ceachir et al. 2014).

Percutaneous tracheostomy

The percutaneous method most commonly used is known as percutaneous dilatational tracheostomy (PDT). It enables the pretracheal tissues to be incised under local anaesthesia. A sheath is inserted into the trachea between the cricoid and the first tracheal ring, or between the first and second rings. A series of conical dilators are slipped over a guidewire, progressively dilating the trachea until the stoma is dilated enough to allow insertion of a tracheostomy tube (Cheung and Napolitano 2014).

Percutaneous tracheostomies are more cost-effective and are associated with fewer complications than surgical tracheostomies and so are becoming increasingly popular (Cheung and Napolitano 2014). They also have the additional benefits of rapid stoma closure and healing following decannulation (tracheostomy tube removal), with patients being left with a smaller and less visible scar (Batuwitage et al. 2014). They are frequently performed in the critical care setting as an early intervention after initiation of mechanical ventilation (Cosgrove and Carrie 2015).

Surgical tracheostomy

Surgical tracheostomy is ideally performed in the operating theatre under a general anaesthetic. The procedure is usually elective (planned) and performed during head and neck surgery, or during surgery for other conditions where the patient is expected to have a prolonged period of mechanical ventilation post-operatively (e.g. gastro-oesophagectomy). A surgical tracheostomy can also be performed in a critical care environment under local anaesthetic during a life-threatening airway emergency as a non-elective procedure (unplanned).

The tracheostomy is usually sited over the second and third, or third and fourth tracheal cartilages. Depending on the type of incision made, temporary stay sutures may be placed to ensure the trachea can easily be recannulated if the tracheostomy tube is accidentally dislodged before an adequate tract has formed. Traction of the sutures helps to keep the trachea open and prevents soft tissues from obscuring the stoma, facilitating recannulation (Lee et al. 2015).

Rationale

Indications

Tracheostomies and laryngectomies are carried out to maintain a patent airway and facilitate effective ventilation. Indications for both are listed in Tables 12.9 and 12.10 respectively.

Table 12.9 Indications for a tracheostomy

Indication	Detail
Airway maintenance or protection	Acute upper airway obstruction (e.g. by a foreign object or oedema of the soft tissues) may make emergency short-term tracheostomy essential. More lasting damage to the upper airway (e.g. from chemical or inhalation burns) may require long-term tracheostomy.
Laryngeal pathology or prolonged upper airway obstruction (e.g. head and neck surgery)	Some maxillofacial and head and neck procedures make it necessary to secure the patient's airway without obstructing the mouth and pharynx.
Tracheal toilet	A patient who has a poor cough and cannot clear their secretions may require a tracheostomy.
Prolonged intubation (>7–10 days)	Prolonged endotracheal intubation carries a high risk of damage to the soft tissues of the mouth, pharynx and trachea. It reduces the patient's ability to communicate and increases the work of breathing by extending the dead space. Tracheostomy reduces or removes the risk of tissue damage, facilitates lip reading and reduces the work of breathing by shortening the dead space, so promoting the process of weaning from mechanical ventilation.
Delayed return of glottic reflexes	Patients with reduced function in cranial nerves V, VII, IX, X or XII, with damage to the brain stem or a reduced consciousness level, may be unable to maintain a patent airway or protect their airway from aspiration of food, drink and saliva. Short- or long-term tracheostomy may be indicated.

Source: Adapted from Bonvento et al. (2017), Cheung and Napolitano (2014), Hyzy and McSparron (2018), NTSP (2013).

Table 12.10 Indications for a laryngectomy

Indication	Detail
Malignancy	Laryngectomy can be a curative treatment for laryngeal cancer or malignancy of adjacent structures.
Non-functioning larynx	A functional laryngectomy may be performed if the larynx is no longer functioning and where aspiration is severe and life threatening. This may occur following previous treatments for head and neck cancers.
Post-trauma laryngeal stenosis	Laryngectomy may be performed for severe laryngeal trauma or stenosis when other surgical techniques have not been effective.

Source: Adapted from Ceachir et al. (2014).

Contraindications

Relative contraindications for tracheostomy include:

- severe localized skin infection
- uncorrected coagulopathies
- tracheomalacia
- an inability to extend the neck due to an underlying condition (e.g. cervical fusion or cervical spine instability).

They may also include conditions that obscure or distort the neck anatomy, such as a short and/or obese neck, previous neck surgery, tumour, haematoma or thyromegaly (Hyzy and McSparron 2018, ICS 2014).

Clinical governance

Competencies

NCEPOD recommends that all nurses involved in the care of patients with an altered airway should be competent in the management of the tracheostomy or laryngectomy, including the actions to take in an emergency (Wilkinson et al. 2014). All procedures should be undertaken in accordance with local policies and protocols, and only after approved training, supervised practice and competency assessment. The core skills related to caring for a patient with an artificial airway are detailed in Box 12.4.

In addition, NCEPOD recommends that nurses are trained in the recognition and management of common airway complications

Box 12.4 Core skills required to care for a patient with an artificial airway

Tracheostomy	Laryngectomy
• Maintaining airway (monitoring tube placement and patency) • Humidification • Tube tie (tube holder) change • Suctioning • Inner cannula change • Cuff pressure measurement • Psychological support and education • Discharge planning	• Maintaining airway (monitoring stoma patency) • Humidification • Care of the stoma • Changing baseplate, laryngectomy tube or heat moisture exchanger cassette • Caring for the voice prosthesis (cleaning and testing for leakage) • Caring for the tracheo-oesophageal puncture (emergency dislodgement of the voice prosthesis or stoma gastric tube) • Psychological support and education • Discharge planning

Source: Adapted from NTSP (2013), Wilkinson et al. (2014).

including tracheostomy tube dislodgement, and airway obstruction in tracheostomy and laryngectomy. Written algorithms to support the emergency management of a laryngectomy airway and a blocked or dislodged tracheostomy tube (Figure 12.34) should be available at the patient's bedside, along with signage detailing the patient's current airway status (Figure 12.35). Emergency equipment should also be readily available at the bedside (NTSP 2013); this is discussed further below. The algorithms should not only include the practical steps required to manage the airway emergency but also details of who to call to assist. This may include teams or individuals specialized in anaesthetics and airway management; critical care and resuscitation; and ENT or head and neck surgery.

Risk management

Tracheostomy tube information should be readily available detailing the type, size and date of tube insertion, in addition to any other information that may be required in an emergency (Wilkinson et al. 2014). This is often referred to as either the 'tracheostomy passport' or 'altered airway passport'. Similar information should be available regarding laryngectomy stoma patency and method of communication. Signage for the bedside is useful to provide instant recognition of the presence of an altered airway and its type and duration (Figure 12.35).

Each altered airway or head and neck ward should have at least one altered airway trained nurse (band 5+) on duty who has passed a trust-approved altered airway competency standard. At the beginning of each shift, each patient with an altered airway should be assessed to determine:

- why the patient has an altered airway
- whether the patient's anatomy has been surgically altered so that ventilation via the upper airways is no longer possible (i.e. laryngectomy)
- in the case of tracheostomy, when it was performed and whether the stoma was performed surgically or percutaneously
- the type and size of the tracheostomy tube or laryngectomy stoma (the latter of which may or may not have a tube)
- the appearance of the stoma site
- the amount and consistency of secretions
- the patient's swallowing and cough reflexes
- the patient's weaning plan
- the patient's method of communication

Pre-procedural considerations

Equipment

Caring for a patient with a tracheostomy requires the availability of a number of pieces of equipment, outlined in Box 12.5. These should be readily available at the patient's beside. Additional equipment required for patients with a laryngectomy is listed in Box 12.6.

Tracheostomy tubes

Tracheostomy tubes are made of silicone, plastic or metal, and therefore differ considerably in rigidity, durability and kink resistance. However, the majority of tracheostomy tubes are manufactured from plastics of varying types, some of which become softer at body temperature (e.g. polyvinyl chloride construction). Most tracheostomy tubes come in a sterile pack with an obturator to assist with insertion. The obturator should be removed as quickly as possible after insertion as it completely occludes the tracheostomy tube when in place (NTSP 2013).

The main components of a tracheostomy tube are predominantly universal. Most are dual lumen incorporating an outer tube and inner cannula, with a universal diameter of 15 mm at the upper aspect to allow connection to other equipment. Most tubes also have a neck flange to which tube ties or tapes can be attached; the ties or tapes are then fitted around the patient's neck to secure the tracheostomy.

The outer tube of a dual-lumen tracheostomy maintains the patency of the airway, while the inner tube (which fits snugly inside the outer tube) can be removed for cleaning or changing without disturbing the stoma site. Removal of the inner cannula allows immediate relief of life-threatening airway obstruction in the event of a blocked tracheostomy tube due to tenacious secretions. For this reason, dual-lumen tubes are recommended as they are inherently safer (Wilkinson et al. 2014). Disposable single-use inner tubes are available from certain manufacturers; these minimize the risk of cross-infection as no cleaning is required.

Tubes vary in their length and shape, and are sized according to their internal diameter in millimetres. The type of tube chosen will depend on the size of the trachea and the needs of the individual patient. A selection of commonly used tube types are described below and grouped in the following categories:

- the presence or absence of a cuff
- the presence or absence of a hole or 'fenestration'
- specialist-function tubes.

Cuffed tracheostomy tubes

Cuffed tracheostomy tubes (Figures 12.38 and 12.39) are single-use tracheostomy tubes that when inflated provide an airtight seal, facilitating effective ventilation and protecting the lower respiratory tract against aspiration. Some are of a 'high-volume, low-pressure' design, which distributes the pressure evenly on the tracheal wall and aims to minimize the risks of tracheal ulceration, necrosis and stenosis at the cuff site (Cipriano et al. 2015). To further reduce these risks, the cuff pressure should not exceed 25 cmH_2O (NTSP 2013). The pressure should be checked at least once per shift or more regularly if there is any change in the patient's clinical condition or if there are concerns regarding the patient's airway (Wilkinson et al. 2014). The cuff is kept inflated in the immediate post-operative phase, during mechanical ventilation, if the patient has a reduced consciousness level or if there are concerns regarding aspiration (NTSP 2013). Once the patient is awake and able to follow commands, the cuff can be deflated as part of the weaning plan. The cuff should always be deflated when a speaking valve or decannulation plug is in place (Mitchell et al. 2013).

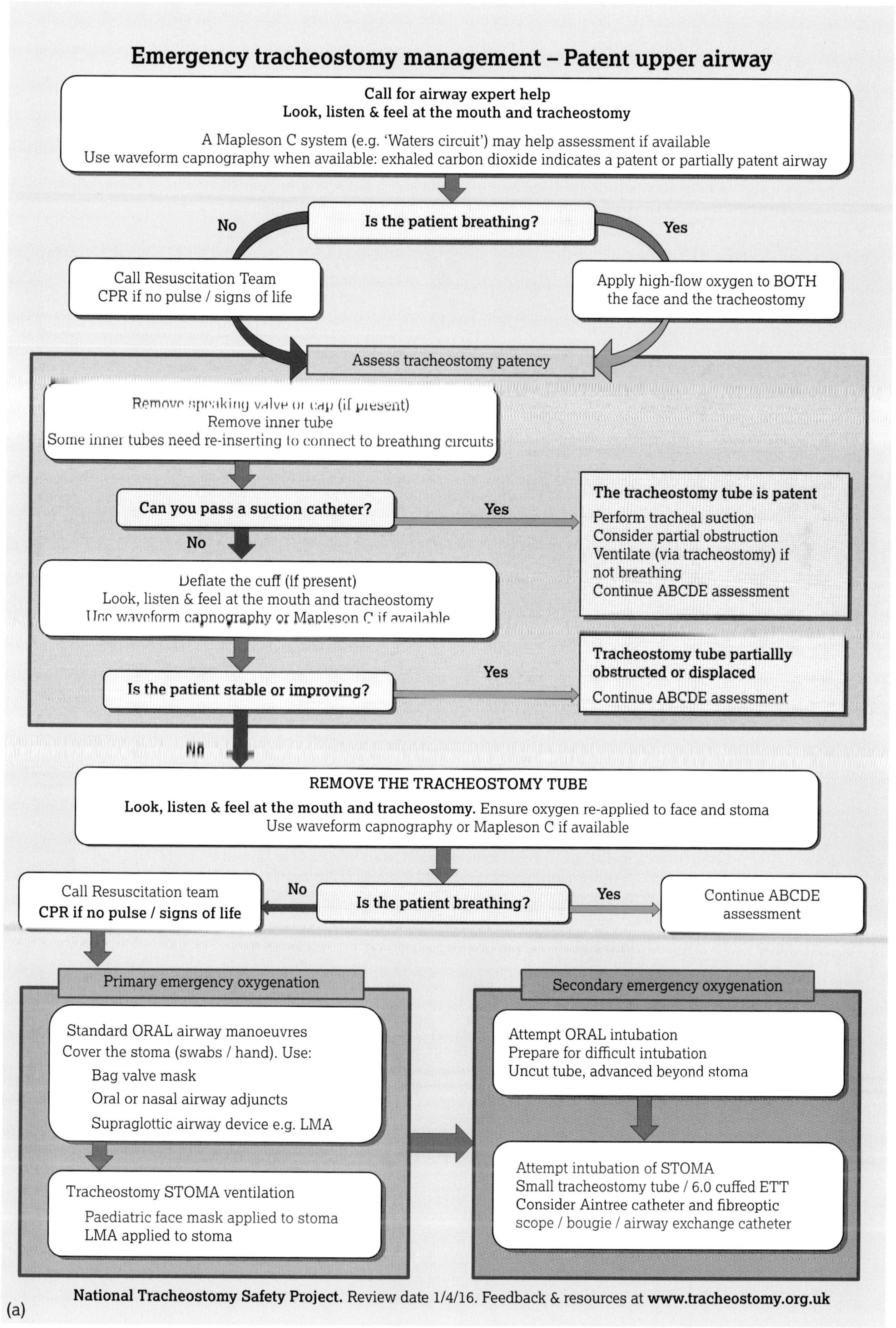
Emergency tracheostomy management – Patent upper airway
Call for airway expert help
Look, listen & feel at the mouth and tracheostomy
A Mapleson C system (e.g. 'Waters circuit') may help assessment if available
Use waveform capnography when available: exhaled carbon dioxide indicates a patent or partially patent airway
Is the patient breathing?
No
Yes
Call Resuscitation Team
CPR if no pulse / signs of life
Apply high-flow oxygen to BOTH the face and the tracheostomy
Assess tracheostomy patency
Remove speaking valve or cap (if present)
Remove inner tube
Some inner tubes need re-inserting to connect to breathing circuits
Can you pass a suction catheter?
Yes
No
The tracheostomy tube is patent
Perform tracheal suction
Consider partial obstruction
Ventilate (via tracheostomy) if not breathing
Continue ABCDE assessment
Deflate the cuff (if present)
Look, listen & feel at the mouth and tracheostomy
Use waveform capnography or Mapleson C if available
Is the patient stable or improving?
Yes
Tracheostomy tube partiallly obstructed or displaced
Continue ABCDE assessment
No
REMOVE THE TRACHEOSTOMY TUBE
Look, listen & feel at the mouth and tracheostomy. Ensure oxygen re-applied to face and stoma
Use waveform capnography or Mapleson C if available
Call Resuscitation team
CPR if no pulse / signs of life
No
Is the patient breathing?
Yes
Continue ABCDE assessment
Primary emergency oxygenation
Standard ORAL airway manoeuvres
Cover the stoma (swabs / hand). Use:
Bag valve mask
Oral or nasal airway adjuncts
Supraglottic airway device e.g. LMA
Tracheostomy STOMA ventilation
Paediatric face mask applied to stoma
LMA applied to stoma
Secondary emergency oxygenation
Attempt ORAL intubation
Prepare for difficult intubation
Uncut tube, advanced beyond stoma
Attempt intubation of STOMA
Small tracheostomy tube / 6.0 cuffed ETT
Consider Aintree catheter and fibreoptic scope / bougie / airway exchange catheter
National Tracheostomy Safety Project. Review date 1/4/16. Feedback & resources at www.tracheostomy.org.uk
(a)

Figure 12.34 (a) Emergency tracheostomy management algorithm. (b) Emergency laryngectomy management algorithm. *Source*: Reproduced with permission from the National Tracheostomy Safety Project (www.tracheostomy.org.uk).

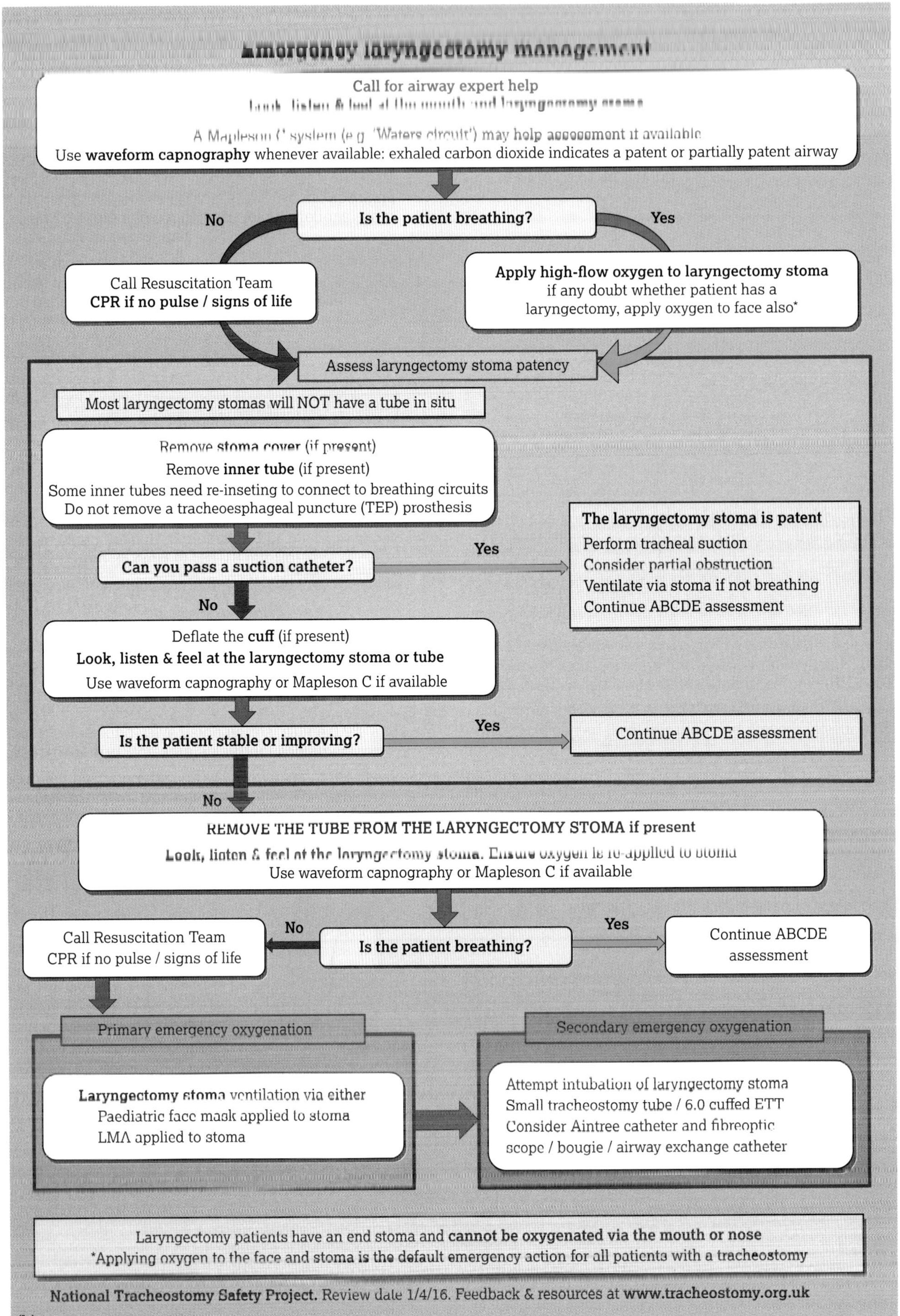
Emergency laryngectomy management
Call for airway expert help
Look, listen & feel at the mouth and laryngectomy stoma
A Mapleson C system (e.g. 'Waters circuit') may help assessment if available
Use waveform capnography whenever available: exhaled carbon dioxide indicates a patent or partially patent airway
Is the patient breathing?
No
Yes
Call Resuscitation Team
CPR if no pulse / signs of life
Apply high-flow oxygen to laryngectomy stoma
if any doubt whether patient has a laryngectomy, apply oxygen to face also*
Assess laryngectomy stoma patency
Most laryngectomy stomas will NOT have a tube in situ
Remove stoma cover (if present)
Remove inner tube (if present)
Some inner tubes need re-inseting to connect to breathing circuits
Do not remove a tracheoesphageal puncture (TEP) prosthesis
Can you pass a suction catheter?
Yes
No
The laryngectomy stoma is patent
Perform tracheal suction
Consider partial obstruction
Ventilate via stoma if not breathing
Continue ABCDE assessment
Deflate the cuff (if present)
Look, listen & feel at the laryngectomy stoma or tube
Use waveform capnography or Mapleson C if available
Is the patient stable or improving?
Yes
Continue ABCDE assessment
No
REMOVE THE TUBE FROM THE LARYNGECTOMY STOMA if present
Look, listen & feel at the laryngectomy stoma. Ensure oxygen is re-applied to stoma
Use waveform capnography or Mapleson C if available
Call Resuscitation Team
CPR if no pulse / signs of life
No
Is the patient breathing?
Yes
Continue ABCDE assessment
Primary emergency oxygenation
Laryngectomy stoma ventilation via either
Paediatric face mask applied to stoma
LMA applied to stoma
Secondary emergency oxygenation
Attempt intubation of laryngectomy stoma
Small tracheostomy tube / 6.0 cuffed ETT
Consider Aintree catheter and fibreoptic scope / bougie / airway exchange catheter
Laryngectomy patients have an end stoma and cannot be oxygenated via the mouth or nose
*Applying oxygen to the face and stoma is the default emergency action for all patients with a tracheostomy
National Tracheostomy Safety Project. Review date 1/4/16. Feedback & resources at www.tracheostomy.org.uk

(b)

Figure 12.34 *Continued*

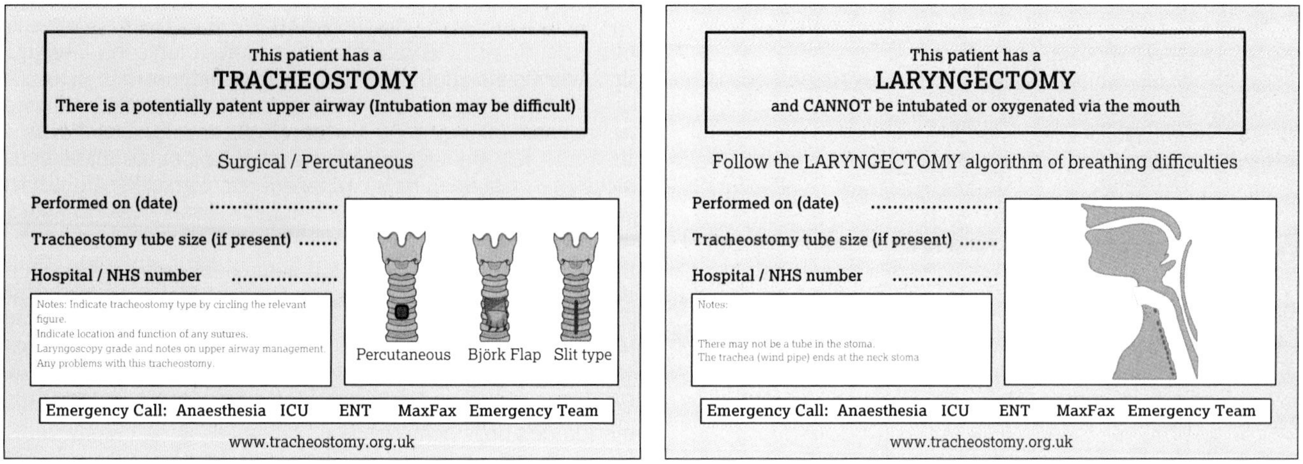

(a) (b)

Figure 12.35 Bed signage. (a) Tracheostomy. (b) Laryngectomy. *Source:* Reproduced with permission from the National Tracheostomy Safety Project (www.tracheostomy.org.uk).

Box 12.5 Essential equipment required for tracheostomy care

In an emergency

- Personal protective equipment: gloves, aprons and eye protection
- Resuscitation equipment/trolley: bag valve mask, endotracheal tubes, laryngeal mask airway (LMA), laryngoscope and blade, bougie and Cook exchange catheter
- Advanced airway equipment/trolley
- Fibreoptic scope
- Waveform capnography

At the patient's bedside

- Oxygen supply and equipment: tracheostomy mask, reservoir mask and tubing
- Suction device with a selection of fine-bore suction catheters and Yankauer suction tips
- Bottle of sterile water

In a 'tracheostomy box' at the patient's bedside (and to accompany the patient on any transfers)

- Cuffed tracheostomy tube of the same size as the patient's current tube
- Cuffed tracheostomy tube at least half a size smaller
- 10 mL syringe
- Tracheal dilator (Figure 12.36)
- Suture cutter
- Scissors
- Water-soluble lubricating gel
- Spare tracheostomy tapes
- Cuff pressure manometer (Figure 12.37)
- Catheter mount
- Inner cannula(s)

Source: Adapted from McGrath et al. (2012), NTSP (2013).

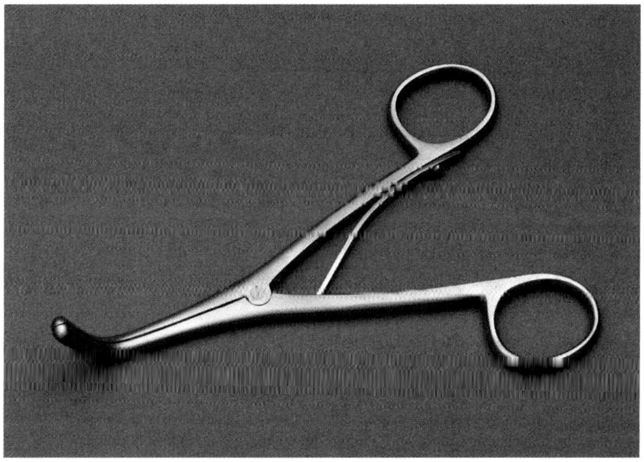

Figure 12.36 Tracheal dilator.

Cuffed tubes with subglottic port

These are single-use tracheostomy tubes that have an additional port for aspiration of subglottic secretions (above the cuff) (Figure 12.40). They are often used for the prevention of ventilator-associated pneumonia in critically ill patients but are also indicated for some patients to enable effective clearance of secretions accumulating above the tracheostomy tube (Hess and Altobelli 2014).

Uncuffed tracheostomy tubes

Uncuffed tubes (Figure 12.41) are predominantly used for long-term patients who are able to protect their own airway due to having an adequate cough and gag reflex (Hess and Altobelli 2014). An uncuffed tube removes the risk of tracheal damage and can be used in the weaning and decannulation process and to aid swallowing and communication with the concomitant use of a speaking valve.

Fenestrated tracheostomy tubes

Tubes may also be fenestrated or non-fenestrated. A fenestrated uncuffed tube (Figure 12.42) is a double-lumen tracheostomy tube with holes or fenestrations midway down the outer tube. If a fenestrated inner tube (often a different colour to highlight the fenestration) is used, air can move through the fenestrations and past the vocal cords within the larynx (Figure 12.43), facilitating voice production (Hess and Altobelli 2014).

Fenestrated cuffed tubes

A fentestrated tube that incorporates a cuff is particularly useful for weaning as it provides the benefits of both the cuffed tube and the fenestrated uncuffed tube. These are most suited to patients who require periods of both cuff inflation (to protect the airway) and cuff deflation (to enable a speaking valve to be used).

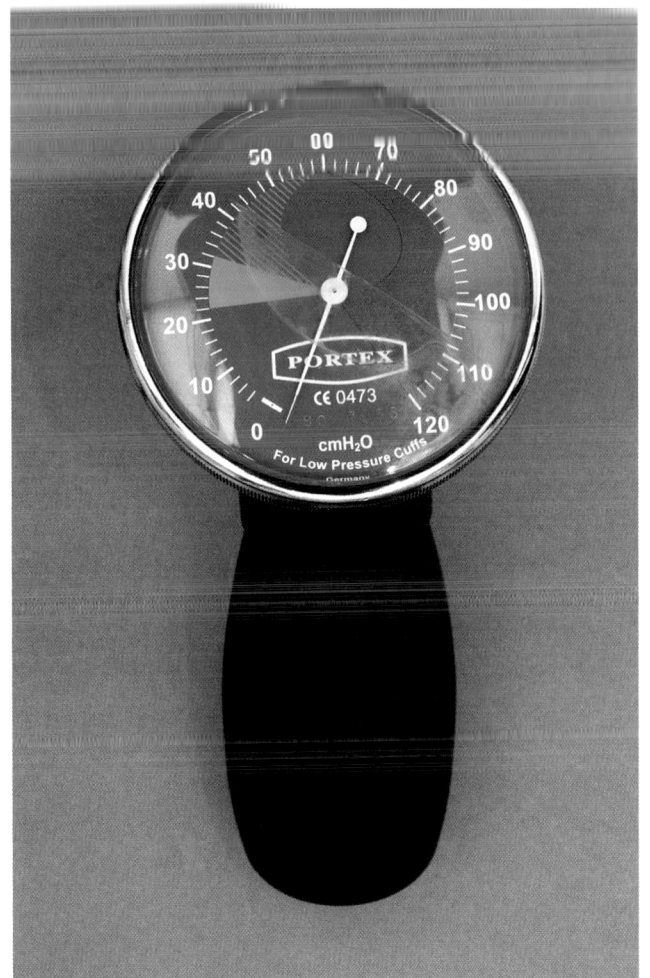

Figure 12.37 Cuff pressure manometer.

Box 12.6 Additional equipment required for laryngectomy

In a 'laryngectomy box' at the patient's bedside

- The contents kept in a 'tracheostomy box' (see Box 12.5)
- Spare laryngectomy tube
- Tilley's forceps (angled forceps used to remove crusts or plugs of mucus from in and around the stoma)
- Pen torch (or access to a light source)
- Micropore or Elastoplast tape for patients with a tracheo-oesophageal puncture, to secure the catheter keeping the puncture patent
- 14 Fr red rubber catheter to be used in the event of accidental voice prosthesis dislodgement

Source: Adapted from NTSP (2013)

Specialist-function tracheostomy tubes

Longer length tracheostomy tubes

The standard design of tracheostomy tube may be unsuitable for some patients because of the short length and angulation of the tube. Extra proximal length is needed for patients with a deep-set trachea (i.e. large neck due to obesity, goitre or neck mass). Extra distal length may be needed for patients with tracheal problems but who have normal neck anatomy (i.e. tracheomalacia or tracheal stenosis). For these types of patient, a flexible (reinforced) tracheostomy tube with an adjustable flange (Figure 12.41) can be used (Hess and Altobelli 2014). It is important that the length of

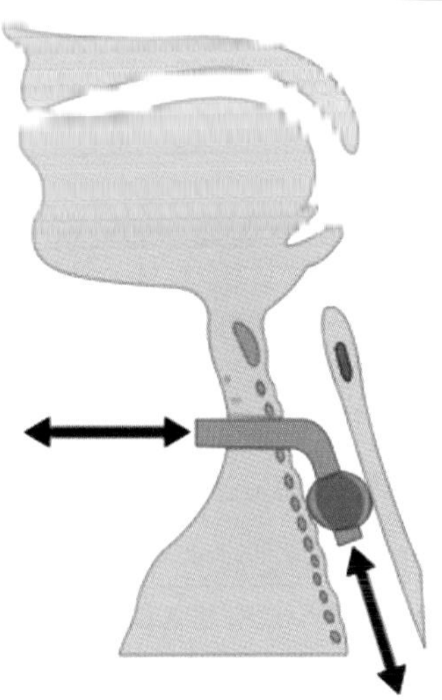

Figure 12.38 Cuffed tracheostomy tube *in situ*. *Source*: Reproduced with permission from the National Tracheostomy Safety Project (www.tracheostomy.org.uk).

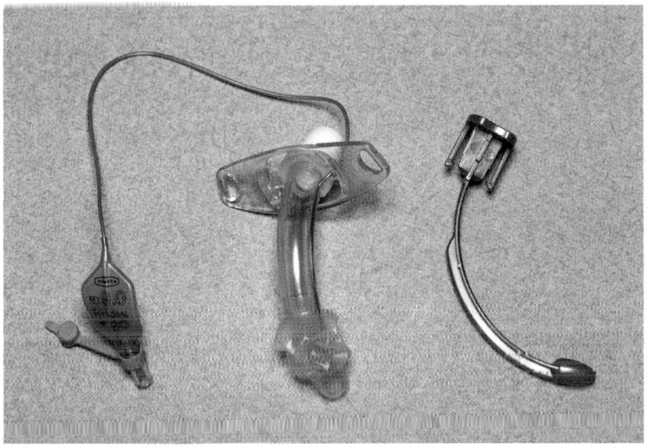

Figure 12.39 Portex® Blue Line Ultra® tracheostomy tube shown with introducer.

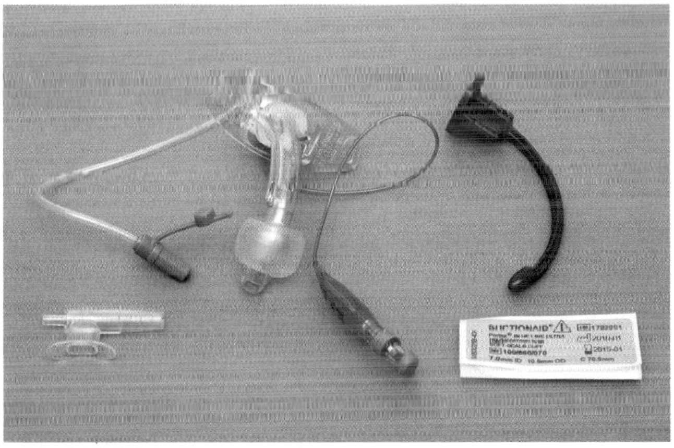

Figure 12.40 Portex® Blue Line Ultra® Suctionaid tracheostomy tube.

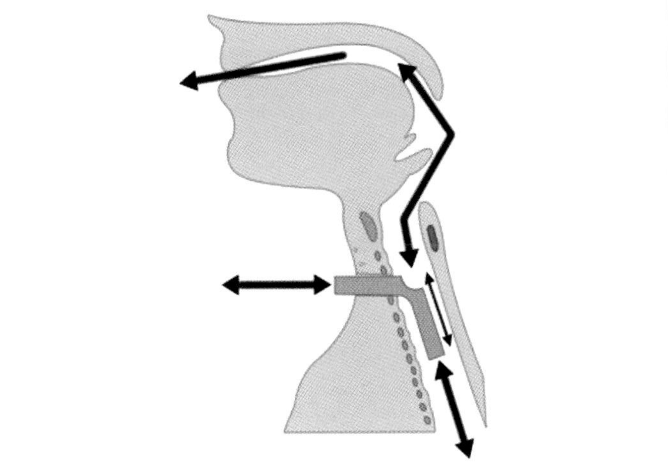

Figure 12.41 Uncuffed tracheostomy tube *in situ*. *Source*: Reproduced with permission from the National Tracheostomy Safety Project (www.tracheostomy.org.uk).

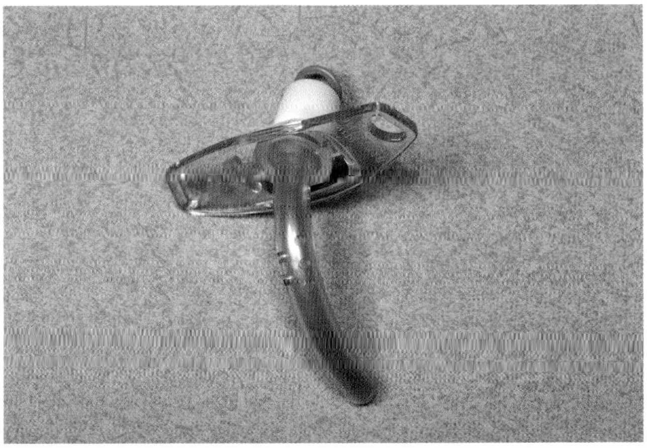

Figure 12.42 Portex® uncuffed fenestrated tracheostomy tubes with red inner tube to highlight that the inner tube is also fenestrated.

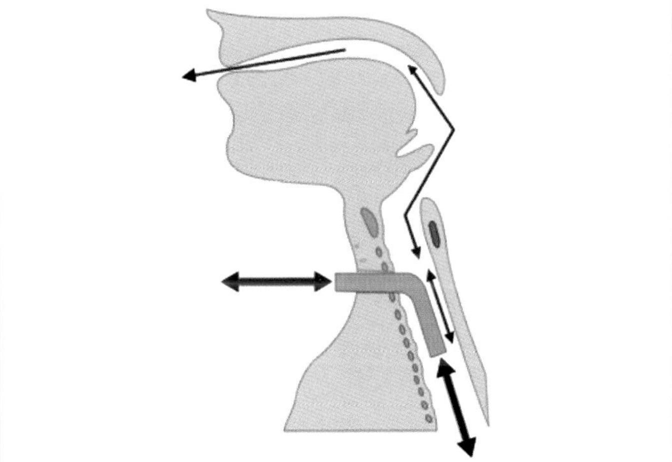

Figure 12.43 Fenestrated uncuffed tube *in situ*. *Source*: Reproduced with permission from the National Tracheostomy Safety Project (www.tracheostomy.org.uk).

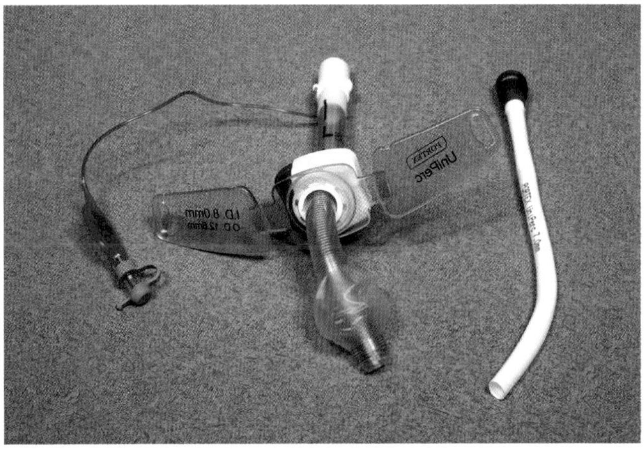

Figure 12.44 Portex® Uniperc® adjustable flange tracheostomy tube with Soft Seal® cuff and inner cannula.

the adjustable flange is documented in the patient's tracheostomy passport on insertion and after any adjustments are made. Additionally, the position of the flange should be checked and documented daily (NTSP 2013).

Metal tubes

Metal tubes are not commonly used but may still be seen in older patients who have had a permanent tracheostomy (Figure 12.45).

Tracheostomy sutures

Sutures are usually applied to either side of the tracheostomy tube flange and attached to the patient's skin for at least 7 days after tracheostomy insertion (7–10 days if percutaneous) (Hess and Altobelli 2014). The sutures help to secure the tube until the stoma has formed around the tracheostomy, increasing safety and preventing accidental decannulation. As described earlier, a stay suture may also be placed when a surgical tracheostomy is formed to increase safety and allow rapid reintubation in the event of an accidental decannulation. The ends of the stay sutures are normally taped onto the patient's chest and labelled 'DO NOT REMOVE'. The stay sutures can be removed by a suitably trained professional either after decannulation or during the first tube change (Mitchell et al. 2013).

Tracheostomy humidification

Humidification of an altered airway is essential since the natural mechanisms of humidification, warming and filtration normally provided by the upper airways are bypassed. A lack of humidification will cause drying of the airway, depressed mucociliary function and increased viscosity of mucous secretions (Tortora and Derrickson 2017). As well as being uncomfortable for the patient, it can impair secretion removal and cause infection, micro-atelectasis (collapse of the alveoli) or tracheostomy tube occlusion (NTSP 2013). Providing adequate humidification to patients with a tracheostomy tube is therefore imperative in maintaining a safe airway and preventing acute deterioration (Wilkinson et al. 2014).

Humidification can be provided to patients using a disposable nebulizer set with sterile 0.9% sodium chloride (approximately 5 mL). It can be delivered using an aerosol-driven nebulizer, or it can be attached to the oxygen or air supply with a flow rate high enough for the liquid to form humidification droplets. The nebulizer is administered using a specific tracheostomy mask every 2–4 hours, or more frequently in patients with more tenacious secretions (NTSP 2013). Where possible, a heated circuit should be used to provide humidification to patients who require continual oxygen therapy.

A heat and moisture exchanger (HME) such as a 'Swedish nose' (see Figure 12.11a) can be connected directly onto the tracheostomy tube to provide humidification. A humidification bib can also

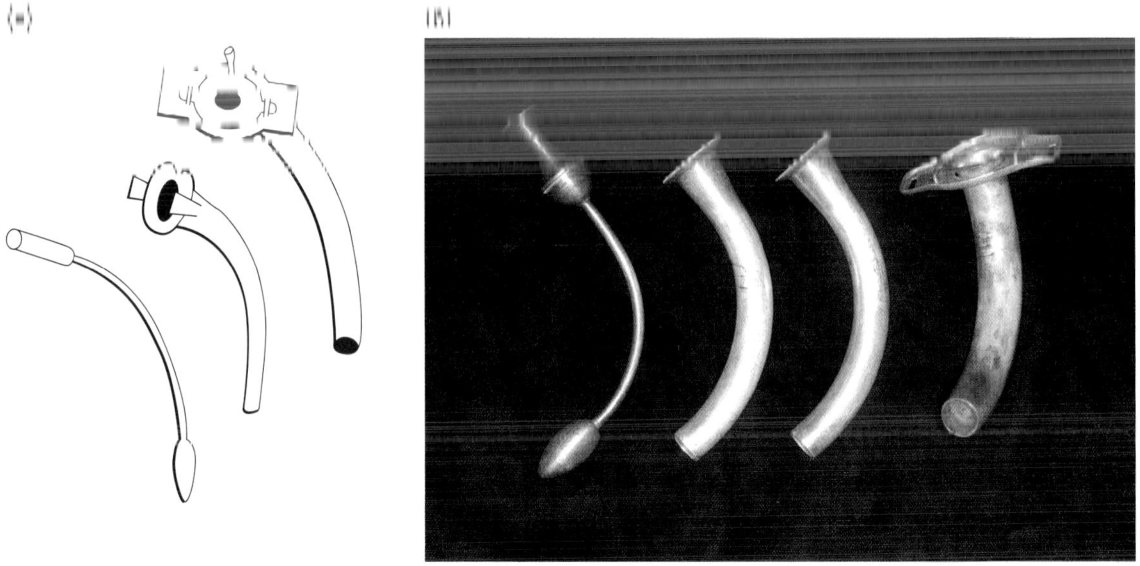

Figure 12.45 (a) Jackson silver tube. (b) Negus silver tube.

be worn by a patient with a well-established tracheostomy. Both of these devices mimic the function of the upper airways by helping to filter and warm inspired air (Wong et al. 2016). Some devices, such as the TrachPhone and ProTrach DualCare valve, assist with both communication and humidification. The cuff should be disposed of every 24 hours, or sooner if saturated with secretions (NTSP 2013).

Tracheostomy adaptations for communication

Since the larynx is bypassed in patients with a tracheostomy, phonation is not typically possible unless some adaptations are made to the tube. This can often be one of the most difficult aspects for a patient with an altered airway, causing significant angst and frustration. Alternative methods of communication should be facilitated as soon as possible; one or more of the methods listed in Box 12.7 can be used (Bonvento et al. 2017, Tang and Sinclair 2015).

Tracheostomy speaking valves

There are a range of speaking valves (Figures 12.46 and 12.47) available that, when placed on the end of the tracheostomy tube, will redirect air on expiration from the lungs through the larynx, facilitating voice production. If a cuffed tracheostomy is in place, the cuff must be fully deflated before a speaking valve is placed, otherwise there will no longer be a patent airway and the patient will not be able to breathe (Hess and Altobelli 2014).

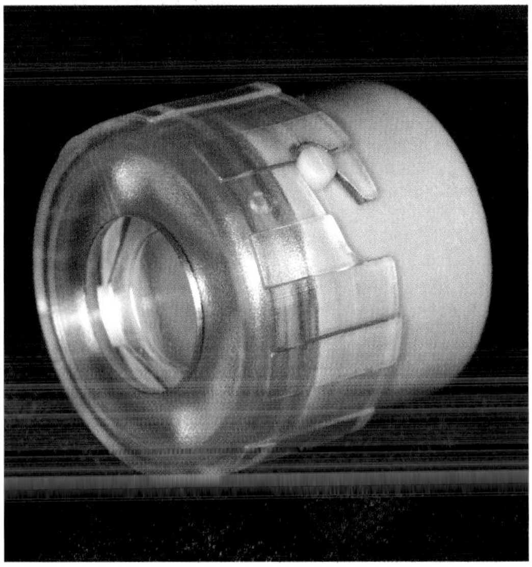

Figure 12.46 Rusch speaking valve.

Box 12.7 Methods of communication for patients with a tracheostomy

Non-verbal methods of communication

- Lip reading
- Facial expression and gestures
- Coded eye blink or hand gestures
- Alphabet board, picture board or phrase book
- Notepad or wipeable board and pen
- Tablet or smartphone

Verbal methods of communication for patients with a tracheostomy tube

- Cuff deflation with speaking valve, with or without the insertion of a fenestrated tube

Source: Adapted from NTSP (2013), Tang and Sinclair (2015).

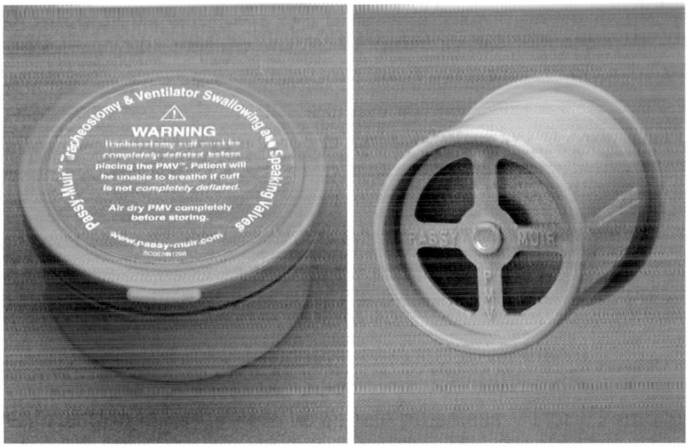

Figure 12.47 Passy Muir valve.

Specific patient preparation

Education

Patient education is paramount to providing quality care. In the initial post-operative or post-procedure phase, this may be purely to aid comfort and relaxation, explaining and stressing the rationale and importance of suctioning, positioning and strengthening the patient's cough.

For patients with long-term tracheostomy needs, early education is vital. Supporting an individual with a tracheostomy of any type requires an understanding of the impact the tracheostomy tube has on the patient's airway, communication and swallowing, and knowing how to manage potential complications. Education will be both practical (i.e. through demonstration with the patient's own tracheostomy, possibly using mirrors) and provided through the use of leaflets, posters and pictures. Practical tracheal suctioning on a specialized mannequin and examining tracheostomy tubes can also be beneficial. As with all elements of tracheostomy care, a multidisciplinary approach is advocated (Wilkinson et al. 2014). Patient education will come from various sources, including clinical nurse specialists, nursing, medical and surgical staff, SLTs, physiotherapists and community teams.

Tracheostomy: dressing and tube tape or tie change

Evidence-based approaches

Rationale

Tracheostomy dressing and tube tie or tape change is carried out to keep the surrounding skin clean and dry and free from infection and pressure damage. It also helps to keeps the tracheostomy tube secure, preventing accidental decannulation.

Indications

The tracheostomy stoma directly exposes the trachea to the environment and so is a potential route for infection. Secretions can cause irritation and maceration of the surrounding skin, and the tracheostomy tube itself may cause pressure damage to the patient's neck area. To prevent tissue damage and wound breakdown, the site should be inspected regularly and cleaned and dried as required (Everitt 2016a). A specific foam tracheostomy dressing may be used to help absorb secretions, prevent pressure sores and increase patient comfort. The dressing should be changed at least every 24 hours or more frequently if required (Dawson 2014).

All tracheostomy tubes must be secured with the use of tube tapes or ties (ICS 2014, Mitchell et al. 2013). These are attached to either side of the flange and connected at the side or back of the patient's neck. They should be changed if they become soiled or wet.

Contraindications

Occasionally the ENT surgical team may request that the original dressing be left and not changed for a specific period of time. This is usually due to the increased risk of bleeding associated with new stoma formation.

They may also request that tube tapes or dressings are not used if a surgical flap has been made and there is concern that any pressure from the dressing or tapes may restrict blood flow and cause the flap to fail (Mitchell et al. 2013). In this scenario, the tube must be sutured in place and great care taken that the tube is not accidentally dislodged.

Principles of care

Changing a tracheostomy dressing requires two people: one to hold and secure the tracheostomy tube while the other removes, cleans and then reapplies the tube tapes and new dressing (Dawson 2014). The stoma site should be cleaned thoroughly with 0.9% sodium chloride and allowed to air dry before an appropriate tracheostomy dressing is applied. This should be a foam dressing with a cross-shaped incision to fit around the tracheostomy tube (ICS 2014). For patients with secretions that tend to accumulate around the stoma, a specialized barrier product can be used to protect the skin and prevent tissue breakdown (Dawson 2014). Once the dressing is in place, the tube tapes should be reapplied (or renewed if soiled or wet). The tapes should be tight enough that they keep the tube secure, but not so tight that they are uncomfortable for the patient. As a guide, two fingers should fit comfortably between the patient's neck and the tapes (Dawson 2014, NTSP 2013).

Anticipated patient outcomes

The skin around the stoma and neck area will remain clean and dry, and free from infection and tissue damage. Additionally, the tube will remain firmly in place, reducing the risk of accidental decannulation.

Procedure guideline 12.8 Tracheostomy: dressing and tube tape/tie change

Essential equipment

- Personal protective equipment
- Dressing tray or trolley
- Sterile procedure pack
- Cleaning solution, such as 0.9% sodium chloride
- Tracheostomy dressing
- Tracheostomy tube tapes or ties
- Gauze

Medicinal products

- Analgesia (if the patient finds the procedure painful)
- Barrier cream

Action	Rationale
Pre-procedure	
1 Introduce yourself to the patient, explain and discuss the procedure with them, and gain their consent to proceed.	To ensure that the patient feels at ease, understands the procedure and gives their valid consent (NMC 2018, **C**).
2 Ensure enough nurses are present. This is a clean procedure and requires two nurses.	To ensure patient safety and reduce the risk of accidental decannulation or loss of the patient's airway (Dawson 2014, **C**).
3 Cleanse hands with soap and water or an alcohol-based handrub.	To minimize risk of infection (NHS England and NHSI 2019, **C**).

(continued)

Procedure guideline 12.8 Tracheostomy: dressing and tube tape/tie change *(continued)*

Action	Rationale
4 Help the patient to sit in a semi-recumbent position with the neck slightly extended.	To ensure patient comfort and allow easy access to the neck area (NTSP 2013, C).
5 Prepare the dressing tray or trolley for the procedure. Open the sterile procedure pack and open the tracheostomy dressing and tapes/ties onto the sterile sheet. Pour the cleaning solution over the gauze.	To ensure all equipment required is available and prepared prior to starting the procedure. **E**
Procedure	
6 Cleanse hands with an alcohol-based handrub and put on disposable plastic apron, gloves and eye protection.	To minimize the risk of cross-infection (NHS England and NHSI 2019, **C**). Manipulation of the patient's airway may cause the patient to cough. Eye protection should therefore be worn (NICE 2017, **C**).
7 The first nurse holds onto the tracheostomy tube while the second nurse removes the tracheostomy tube tapes/ties.	To ensure the tracheostomy tube is not accidentally dislodged during the procedure (Dawson 2014, **C**).
8 The first nurse continues to hold onto the tracheostomy tube (until the end of step 12) while the second nurse removes the soiled dressing from around the tube and disposes of it directly into the clinical waste bag.	To minimize the risk of cross-infection (NICE 2017, **C**).
9 The second nurse cleans around the stoma with 0.9% sodium chloride using gauze, and allows it to air dry.	To remove wet or dried secretions from the stoma site (ICS 2014, **C**).
10 The second nurse applies barrier cream if required.	To protect the skin (Dawson 2014, **C**).
11 The second nurse replaces the tracheostomy dressing.	To increase patient comfort and protect the skin (Everitt 2016a, **C**).
12 The second nurse reapplies or replaces the tracheostomy tapes/ties, checking that one or two fingers can be placed between the tapes/ties and the neck once the tapes/ties are secure.	To secure the tracheostomy tube, ensuring it is not too loose or too tight (Dawson 2014, **C**).
13 Ask the patient whether the tracheostomy dressing and tapes/ties are comfortable.	To ensure patient comfort. **E**
14 Remove apron, gloves and eye protection and dispose of them in a clinical waste bag. Cleanse hands with soap and water or an alcohol-based handrub.	To minimize the risk of infection (NHS England and NHSI 2019, **C**).
Post-procedure	
15 Monitor the patient's respiratory status and observations/NEWS. Escalate any concerns or deterioration in condition or NEWS immediately.	To identify any concerns or clinical deterioration early, and ensure timely escalation to senior staff if required (RCP 2017, **C**).

Tracheostomy: suctioning

Evidence-based approaches

Rationale

An effective cough requires closure then reopening of the glottis once an adequate intrathoracic pressure has been achieved. The mechanism of closing the glottis is compromised in patients with a tracheostomy tube, and so these patients are unable to generate the high flows required for coughing (Barnett 2012). In addition, the lack of natural warmth and humidification usually provided by the upper airways can increase sputum load or make secretions tenacious and difficult to expectorate (McNulty and Eyre 2015). Thick and dry secretions can block the tracheostomy tube and cause airway obstruction. Tracheal suction is therefore a critical part of tracheostomy care and all professionals caring for patients with altered airways should be competent in the procedure (Wilkinson et al. 2014).

Indications

Suctioning can cause significant patient distress and is associated with airway changes and cardiovascular instability. It should therefore only be performed when indicated and not at fixed intervals (Barnett 2012). Frequency should be determined on an individual patient basis with the aim of clearing airway secretions when the patient is not able to do so themselves, ensuring airway patency. A careful assessment of the patient should be carried out to determine the following:

- whether the patient is able to clear their own secretions through the use of a good, strong cough
- the location of any secretions
- whether these secretions could be reached by the suction catheter
- how detrimental these secretions might be for the patient.

Suctioning may be indicated if the following are present (Everitt 2016a, NTSP 2013):

- prominent audible or visible secretions
- reduced oxygen saturations
- increased respiratory rate or effort
- increased or ineffective cough
- use of accessory muscles for breathing
- restlessness
- patient request

Contraindications

While there are no absolute contraindications, suctioning may be painful and distressing for the patient and can be complicated by (Bonvento et al. 2017, ICS 2014, Pathmanathan et al. 2014):

- hypoxaemia
- bradycardia and cardiovascular compromise
- alveolar collapse and atelectasis (incomplete lung inflation)
- tracheal mucosal damage
- bleeding
- possible introduction of infection.

Infection risk

Standard precautions must be used at all times when suctioning; this includes wearing an apron, gloves and eye protection (NICE 2017). As with all procedures, hands should be decontaminated with soap and water or an alcohol-based handrub before and after contact with the patient, and all equipment disposed of in the clinical waste. All disposable equipment used for suctioning (e.g. suction tubing and canister) presents an infection control risk due to the presence of bacteria. Equipment should therefore be dated and changed regularly, as per the manufacturer's recommendations or local policy (Wilkinson et al. 2014).

Method of suctioning

Suctioning should be performed with an inner tube (non fenestrated) in place (Morris et al. 2015) using a fine bore suction catheter of the appropriate size (Figure 12.48). Instillation of 0.9% sodium chloride to 'aid' suctioning is not recommended (Pathmanathan et al. 2014). The routine use of 'deep suctioning' is also discouraged due to the risk of hypoxia, mucosal damage, inflammation, bleeding and airway occlusion (Barnett 2012, Greenwood and Winters 2014, NTSP 2013). If deep suctioning is required, the patient should be pre-oxygenated (see the section on specific patient preparation below) and the whole procedure should take no longer than 10 seconds to prevent hypoxia and patient distress (NTSP 2013).

Shallow suctioning, where the catheter is inserted no further than the distal end of the tracheostomy tube, is preferred (Dawson 2014). Patients should be encouraged to cough secretions up to the tracheostomy tube if they are able, and these are then cleared through the use of shallow suctioning (ICS 2014). Any difficulty in passing the suction catheter should prompt further investigation as it may be that the tube is blocked or misplaced and requires immediate attention (Cosgrove and Carrie 2015, ICS 2014, NTSP 2013). Oral suctioning may also be required; this can be achieved by using a rigid Yankauer suction catheter tip (Figure 12.49).

Anticipated patient outcomes

The patient's airway will remain patent through the use of suction to help clear excess secretions that the patient is not able to expectorate. Suctioning should be performed in a manner that causes the least possible amount of distress for the patient.

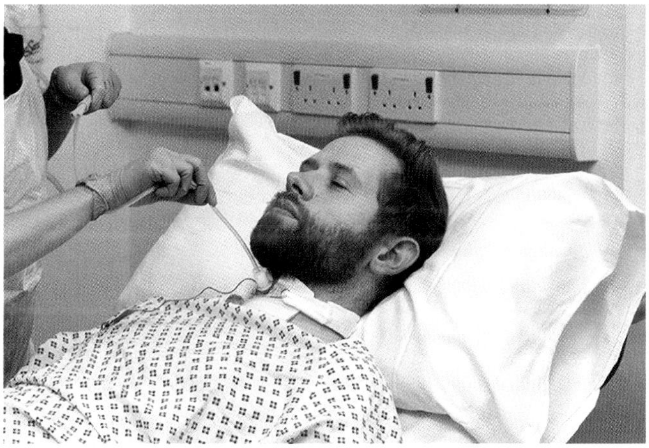

Figure 12.48 Tracheal suction using a fine-bore suction catheter.

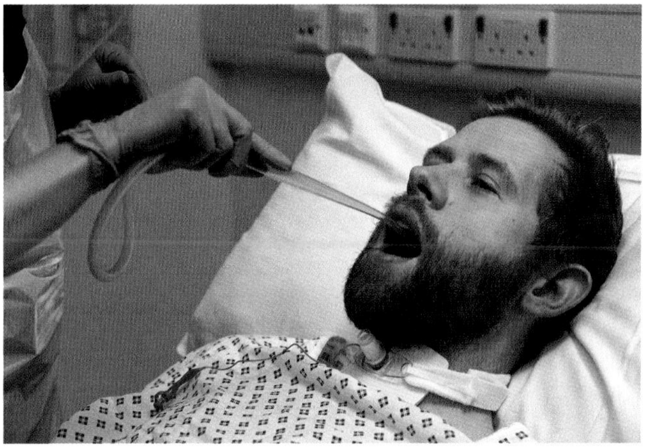

Figure 12.49 Oral suction using a Yankauer suction tip.

Clinical governance

Competencies

All staff caring for patients with an altered airway should be aware of the indications and risks of suctioning. They should be trained and assessed as competent in doing so safely before performing the procedure unsupervised (Wilkinson et al. 2014). They should also be aware of the different types of suction device available, and be able to assemble, maintain and use them safely.

Pre-procedural considerations

Equipment

Suction unit

A low-volume, high-pressure suction unit should be used for tracheal suctioning, with the pressure set between 13 and 20 kPa (100–150 mmHg) (NTSP 2013). The lowest possible suction pressure should be used to prevent hypoxia, mucosal trauma and atelectasis. Prior to the procedure being performed, the suction unit should be turned on at the correct suction pressure and the system checked to ensure the suction is working prior to use.

A suction canister should be placed in between the suction unit and the suction tubing to collect the fluid and secretions suctioned. After the procedure, a small amount of sterile water should be suctioned to clear the tubing of secretions. The canister, tubing and bottle of sterile water should be changed every 24 hours to prevent bacterial growth and contamination, and all equipment should be dated and checked daily, even when not in regular use.

Suction catheters

Choosing the correct suction catheter size depends on the size of the tracheostomy tube. As a guide, the diameter of the suction catheter should not exceed half of the internal diameter of the tracheostomy tube. The formula in Box 12.8 can be used to determine the correct size catheter.

Most suction catheters are single use and should be disposed of immediately after each use in the clinical waste. However, within a critical care setting, a closed-circuit suction system may be used for patients being mechanically ventilated. In a closed-circuit system, the catheter is sealed in a protective plastic sleeve (Figure 12.50) and is connected to the ventilator circuit, and can remain within the circuit unit until it requires changing. A closed-circuit system helps to reduce the risk of infection caused by bacterial contamination of the catheter (Pathmanathan et al. 2014). In addition, it reduces the risk of hypoxia and the loss of positive end-expiratory pressure (PEEP) by removing the need to break or disconnect the ventilator circuit. These circuits are usually changed every 72 hours or as per the manufacturer's recommendation (NTSP 2013).

Box 12.8 Formula used to determine the correct suction catheter size

In the following, Fr (French) refers to the size of the catheter.

$2 \times$ (*size of tracheostomy tube in mm − 2*) = *suction catheter size in Fr*

For example:

$2 \times (8-2) = 12$ Fr suction catheter

Source: Adapted from Greenwood and Winters (2014), NTSP (2013), Pathmanathan et al. (2014).

Specific patient preparation

Patients who are mechanically ventilated and are receiving high concentrations of oxygen may benefit from being pre-oxygenated prior to the procedure (Greenwood and Winters 2014, NTSP 2013). This involves the delivery of 100% FiO_2 to the patient for 1 minute prior to passing the suction catheter.

The procedure should always be explained to the patient and verbal consent gained (if the patient is conscious). If required, the patient should be repositioned to ensure their comfort and allow easy access to the tracheostomy tube.

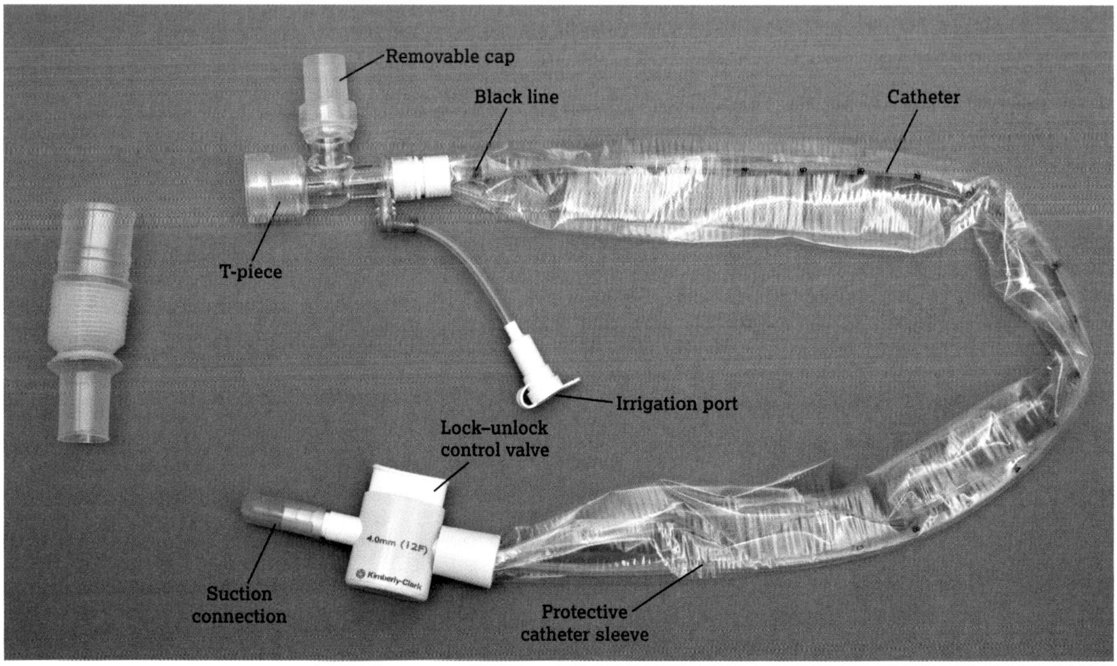

Figure 12.50 Components of a closed-circuit catheter. The control valve locks the vacuum on or off. The catheter is protected inside an airtight sleeve. A T-piece connects the device to the tracheal tube.

Procedure guideline 12.9 Tracheostomy: suctioning a patient (single-use suction catheter)

Essential equipment

- Personal protective equipment
- Suction unit (wall or portable)
- Suction canister and tubing
- Sterile suction catheters of assorted sizes
- Sterile bottled water (labelled 'suction' with opening date)

Action	Rationale
Pre-procedure	
1 Introduce yourself to the patient, explain and discuss the procedure with them, and gain their consent to proceed.	To ensure that the patient feels at ease, understands the procedure and gives their valid consent (NMC 2018, **C**).
2 This is a clean procedure.	To ensure patient safety (NTSP 2013, **C**).
3 Cleanse hands with soap and water or an alcohol-based handrub.	To minimize the risk of infection (NHS England and NHSI 2019, **C**).
4 Help the patient to sit in a semi-recumbent position with the neck slightly extended.	To ensure patient comfort and allow easy access to the neck area (NTSP 2013, **C**).
5 Ensure the following are readily available in case required: • oxygen supply and masks/tubing • resuscitation trolley • emergency airway trolley • bedside tracheostomy box • additional staff.	To ensure patient safety in the event of an airway emergency (NTSP 2013, **C**).

6 If the secretions are tenacious, consider nebulizing 0.9% sterile sodium chloride or other prescribed mucolytic agents.	To loosen dry and thick secretions (Bonvento et al. 2017, **C**).
7 If the patient is oxygen dependent, pre-oxygenate them for a period of 1 minute.	To minimize the risk of hypoxia (Greenwood and Winters 2014, **C**).
8 If the patient has a fenestrated outer tube, ensure that a plain (non-fenestrated) inner tube is inserted prior to suctioning.	Suctioning via a fenestrated inner and outer tube may cause trauma to the tracheal wall (Morris et al. 2015, **C**).
Procedure	
9 Cleanse hands with an alcohol-based handrub and put on disposable plastic apron, gloves and eye protection.	To minimize the risk of cross-infection (NHS England and NHSI 2019, **C**). Manipulation of the patient's airway may cause the patient to cough. Eye protection should therefore be worn (NICE 2017, **C**).
10 a Turn the suction on and ensure that the pressure is set to an appropriate level. It should not exceed 20 kPa (150 mmHg).	To minimize the risk of atelectasis and mucosal trauma (ICS 2014, **C**; NTSP 2013, **C**).
b Select the correct size of catheter (see Box 12.8).	A catheter that is too small a diameter may not be effective in removing thick secretions. A catheter that is too big will occlude the tube, cause hypoxia and distress the patient (NTSP 2013, **C**).
11 Keeping the suction catheter in the sterile pack, open the end and attach it onto the suction tubing. The suction catheter should not be removed from the sterile pack until ready.	To keep the catheter as sterile as possible, minimizing the risk of cross-infection. **E**
12 Apply an additional clean disposable glove onto the dominant hand.	To facilitate easy disposal of the suction catheter after use and minimize the risk of cross-infection. **E**
13 Remove oxygen therapy (if applicable).	To allow access to the tracheostomy tube. **E**
14 *If performing a shallow suction*: remove the catheter from the sterile pack and introduce it into the tracheostomy tube. Ask the patient to cough, then apply suction as secretions meet the catheter. Suction is created by placing a thumb over the suction port. *If performing a deep suction*: introduce the catheter to about one-third of its length (approximately 10–15 cm) or until the patient coughs. If resistance is felt, withdraw the catheter 1–2 cm before applying suction then slowly withdraw the catheter out.	Suction is only applied on withdrawal and never on insertion to reduce the risk of mucosal trauma (NTSP 2013, **C**). The catheter should go no further than the carina and should be withdrawn slightly before suction is applied to prevent trauma (Greenwood and Winters 2014, **C**).
15 Suction the patient for no more than 10 seconds.	Prolonged suctioning may result in acute hypoxia, cardiac arrhythmias, mucosal trauma and significant distress for the patient (NTSP 2013, **C**).
16 Wrap the catheter around the dominant hand and then pull the glove back over the soiled catheter. Discard immediately into the clinical waste.	Wrapping the soiled catheter up in the glove minimizes the risk of cross-infection. **E** Catheters are single use and should be disposed of as per infection control guidelines. **E**
17 Repeat the procedure until the airway is clear. No more than three suction passes should be made during any one suction episode (unless in an emergency, such as tube occlusion). A new suction catheter should be used each time, and the patient should be allowed sufficient time to recover in between each suction.	To minimize the risk of hypoxia, minimize the risk of infection, and cause minimal distress for the patient (NTSP 2013, **C**).
Post-procedure	
18 Reapply oxygen therapy (if applicable).	To prevent hypoxia. **E**
19 Clear the suction tubing of secretions by dipping it into the sterile water bottle and applying suction until the solution has rinsed the tubing through.	To loosen and flush secretions that have adhered to the inside of the suction tubing (NTSP 2013, **C**).
20 Remove apron, gloves and eye protection and dispose of them in the clinical waste. Cleanse hands with soap and water or an alcohol-based handrub.	To minimize the risk of infection (NHS England and NHSI 2019, **C**).
21 Monitor the patient's respiratory status and observations/ NEWS. Escalate any concerns or deterioration in condition/ NEWS immediately.	To identify any concerns or clinical deterioration early, and ensure timely escalation to senior staff if required (RCP 2017, **C**).

Complications

Hypoxia

The act of suctioning reduces vital volume from the lungs and upper airways. Each suctioning procedure should last no longer than 10 seconds to decrease the risk of tracheal damage and hypoxia (NTSP 2013). Ventilator disconnection or removal of the oxygen supply will also add to the risk of hypoxia prior to suctioning. This risk can be reduced by pre-oxygenating the lungs with 100% oxygen, either manually or via a ventilator (Greenwood and Winters 2014).

Cardiac arrhythmias

Arrhythmias may be brought about by the onset of hypoxaemia, or a vagal reflex due to tracheal stimulation by the suction catheter (Bonvento et al. 2017).

Raised intracranial pressure

This may occur if the suction catheter causes excessive tracheal stimulation and results in coughing and an increase in the patient's intrathoracic pressure, both of which can compromise cerebral venous drainage (Greenwood and Winters 2014).

Tracheal mucosal damage

Damage may be caused by using a catheter that is too big, using too high a suction pressure or passing a suction catheter down through a fenestrated inner tube (NTSP 2013). Unnecessary 'deep' suctioning may also contribute to mucosal damage.

Tracheostomy: changing an inner cannula

Evidence-based approaches

Rationale

Tracheostomy tubes with an inner cannula are inherently safer than ones without an inner cannula and are therefore advocated (NTSP 2013). Regular checking and changing of the inner cannula allows for visual inspection of secretions and assists in assessment regarding humidification, reducing the risk of airway obstruction.

Indications

The inner cannula should be removed regularly and inspected for patency (Cosgrove and Carrie 2015). Indications for inspection include:

- signs of respiratory distress
- increased work of breathing

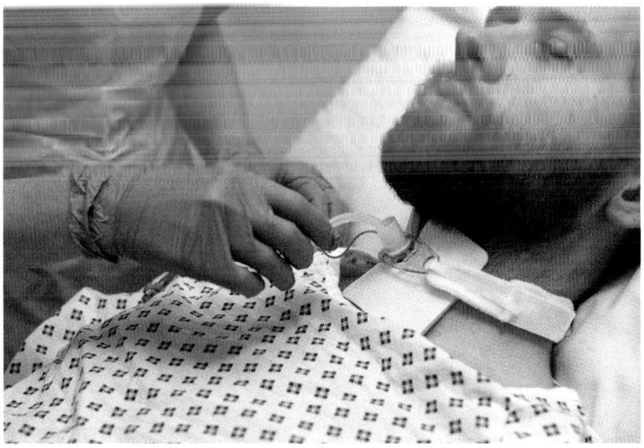

Figure 12.51 Tracheostomy inner tube change.

- a drop in oxygen saturations
- any other sign of clinical deterioration (NTSP 2013).

Contraindications

There are no contraindications for inspecting or changing an inner tube. However, inner cannulas should only be used with the tracheostomy they are designed for.

Principles of care

The inner cannula should be removed (Figure 12.51), inspected and changed if required. Although this should be done at regular intervals, the frequency of inspection will depend on the volume and tenacity of the patient's secretions. Patients with copious secretions may require 2-hourly inner tube changes, while a patient with a good cough and minimal secretions will require much less frequent checks. The timing should be determined following assessment of the patient and their secretions, and documented in the tracheostomy passport. Inner cannulas should either be cleaned or disposed of after each use according to the manufacturer's recommendations.

Anticipated patient outcomes

The altered airway will remain patent and free from secretions, which have the potential to obstruct the tracheostomy tube. The inner cannula change will be done confidently and efficiently, causing the patient minimal distress and anxiety.

Procedure guideline 12.10 Tracheostomy: changing an inner cannula

Essential equipment

- Personal protective equipment
- Sterile dressing pack
- Cleaning solution, such as 0.9% sodium chloride
- Inner cannula of the same size as the tracheostomy tube
- Tracheostomy tube brush cleaner (if the patient has a reusable inner tube)
- Gallipot

Action	Rationale
Pre-procedure	
1 Introduce yourself to the patient, explain and discuss the procedure with them, and gain their consent to proceed.	To ensure that the patient feels at ease, understands the procedure and gives their valid consent (NMC 2018, **C**).
2 This is a clean procedure.	To ensure patient safety (NTSP 2013, **C**).
3 Cleanse hands with soap and water or an alcohol-based handrub.	To minimize the risk of infection (NHS England and NHSI 2019, **C**).

4 Ensure the following are readily available in case required: • emergency oxygen and equipment (masks, tubing) • suction and equipment (suction catheters and Yankauer suction tips) • resuscitation trolley • emergency airway trolley • bedside tracheostomy box • additional staff.	To ensure patient safety if unable to secure the airway with the new tube (NTSP 2013, **C**).
5 Help the patient to sit in a semi-recumbent position with the neck slightly extended.	To ensure patient comfort and allow easy access to the neck area (Dawson 2014, **C**).
6 Pre-oxygenate the patient if they are known to desaturate off oxygen.	To minimize the risk of hypoxia (Greenwood and Winters 2014, **C**).
7 Prepare a dressing tray or trolley for the procedure. Open the sterile procedure pack and empty the tracheostomy inner tube onto the sterile sheet. If a reusable inner tube is being used, pour normal saline 0.9% into a gallipot and open a tracheostomy tube brush cleaner.	To ensure all equipment required is prepared prior to starting the procedure. **E**
Procedure	
8 Cleanse hands with an alcohol-based handrub and put on disposable plastic apron, gloves and eye protection.	To minimize the risk of cross-infection (NICE 2017, **C**).
9 Remove the inner cannula and dispose of it in the clinical waste. If non-disposable inner tube is used, remove it and place it on the sterile sheet.	To minimize the risk of cross-infection (NICE 2017, **C**).
10 Immediately place the new inner tube in position and ensure it is secured in the 'locked' position.	To re-establish the airway and ensure the inner cannula is secure. **E**
11 Check that the patient is comfortable and they are at ease with their breathing.	To ensure patient comfort. **E**
12 If a reusable inner tube is used, clean the old tube with normal saline 0.9% and the brush cleaner. Do not leave the inner tube to soak. The tube should be dried thoroughly then placed in a clean container for future use.	Soaking tubes in stagnant cleaning solutions may cause bacterial colonization and subsequent cross infection (Cosgrove and Carrie 2015, **C**).
13 Remove apron, gloves and eye protection and dispose of them in the clinical waste, along with the old procedure pack. Cleanse hands with an alcohol-based handrub.	To minimize the risk of infection (NICE 2017, **C**).
Post-procedure	
14 Monitor the patient's respiratory status and observations/ NEWS. Escalate any concerns or deterioration in condition/ NEWS immediately.	To identify any concerns or clinical deterioration early, and ensure timely escalation to senior staff if required (RCP 2017, **C**). Changing an inner tube is potentially hazardous and may cause respiratory problems. **E**
15 Document the inner cannula change time, in addition to the tenacity and volume of the secretions.	To ensure all staff are aware of the tracheostomy care that has been performed and how often the inner tube requires checking or changing. **E**

Complications

If the patient has any difficulty breathing or shows any signs of clinical deterioration during or after the procedure, expert help should be called immediately and the emergency algorithm for an altered airway followed (see Figure 12.34). The same applies if the inner cannula cannot be advanced.

Tracheostomy: changing a tube

Evidence-based approaches

Rationale

Changing a tracheostomy tube involves the removal of the old tracheostomy tube and its replacement with a new device.

Indications

Changing a tracheostomy tube is indicated as follows (Greenwood and Winters 2014, Hess and Altobelli 2014, NTSP 2013):

- when the tracheostomy tube has been in place for 30 days, or as per the manufacturer's recommendations (Hess and Altobelli 2014)
- changing from a non-fenestrated to a fenestrated tracheostomy tube to facilitate weaning and improve communication
- downsizing the tracheostomy tube if the patient is clinically improving
- changing from an uncuffed tube to a cuffed tube if the patient requires mechanical ventilation
- to replace a faulty, ill-fitting or displaced tube.

Contraindications

The decision to change a tracheostomy tube will be made after weighing up the risks and benefits and after discussion and agreement with the multidisciplinary team. Contraindications may include (NTSP 2013):

- time since formation: changing a tracheostomy tube too soon after formation is contraindicated as the tract may not have healed adequately and can create a false passage

- poor visualization of the tracheostomy tract and inadequate lighting or exposure
- lack of emergency equipment
- practitioner inexperience or lack of availability of staff competent in airway management
- patient is on high ventilator settings or has high oxygen requirements
- patient is receiving radiotherapy to the neck or has done in the past 2 weeks
- patient is nearing the end of their life
- patient refuses or is not co-operative.

Principles of care

The first tracheostomy tube change must be performed by a practitioner who is not only competent in tracheostomy tube placement but also has advanced airway management and intubation skills (ICS 2014). Except in emergencies, the first change should not be performed for 72 hours following a surgical tracheostomy or for 7–10 days following a percutaneous tracheostomy (Mitchell et al. 2013). This is to allow the tract between the skin and the trachea to develop. Removal of the tracheostomy tube before this time may result in complete loss of the patient's airway if there is difficulty recannulating the tracheostomy. This procedure requires the presence of a second practitioner who is trained in tracheostomy care and who is able to summon more expert help if required. Subsequent changes should be performed by practitioners trained in tube changes, and always with a second practitioner present who is competent in tracheostomy care (ICS 2014).

Unless it is an emergency situation, the procedure should be well planned in advance. All equipment, including emergency equipment and intubation drugs, should be immediately accessible. Appropriate medical support should also be readily available if the tube change does not go to plan.

The tube change may be performed using a 'blind insertion' technique for well-established stomas, or it may be guided using a bougie, an exchange catheter or a guidewire. A guided technique allows the tube to be exchanged over the guide, reducing the risk of creating a false passage (ICS 2014). It is particularly useful for newly created stomas and for patients with a large neck (NTSP 2013). A fibreoptic scope may also be used to assist with the insertion and confirm the correct placement of the new tube (NTSP 2013). The tube change should be documented in the patient's records along with any adverse events and when the next tube change is due.

Anticipated patient outcomes

The procedure will be well planned with all the necessary equipment immediately available and suitably trained personnel present to ensure patient safety. The tracheostomy tube will be changed confidently and efficiently, causing the patient minimal distress and anxiety.

Pre-procedural considerations

Prior to tube change, the following questions should be asked:

- Is this the best time to be doing this procedure?
- Am I the best person to do it?
- Have I got all the essential equipment required?
- Is there appropriate support available if required?

If the answer to all of the questions above is 'yes', then it is safe to proceed with the procedure. The practitioner should talk through the details of the procedure with all staff involved and ensure all members are familiar with what to do if the exchange does not go to plan. The procedure should always be explained to the patient and verbal consent gained (if the patient is conscious). The patient should be repositioned to allow easy access to the tracheostomy stoma. This can be achieved by lying the patient supine or at 45°, with a towel or pillow under their shoulders and the neck extended (NTSP 2013).

Procedure guideline 12.11 Tracheostomy: changing a tube

Essential equipment

- Personal protective equipment
- Sterile dressing pack
- New tracheostomy tube for insertion
- Lubricating gel
- Stitch cutter (if flange sutures are still present)
- 10 mL syringe
- Bougie, exchange catheter or guidewire (if a guided technique is to be used)
- Cleaning solution, such as 0.9% sodium chloride
- Tracheostomy foam-based dressing
- Tracheostomy tapes/ties
- Cuff manometer
- Gauze

Emergency equipment

- Oxygen and masks/tubing
- Suction, suction catheters and Yankauer suction tips
- Resuscitation trolley
- Emergency airway trolley
- Fibreoptic scope
- Bedside tracheostomy box
- Intubation drugs
- Additional staff

Action	Rationale
Pre-procedure	
1 The first tracheostomy change should be carried out by a practitioner trained in advanced airway and intubation skills. Subsequent changes should be carried out by practitioners competent in tube change. In both cases, a second appropriately trained person should assist.	To ensure that the most appropriately trained member of staff performs the procedure, ensuring patient safety (ICS 2014, **C**).

2 The patient should be nil by mouth for 6 hours (solids) and for 2 hours (fluids) prior to the tube change. If the patient has a nasogastric tube, this should be aspirated prior to the procedure.	Any manipulation of the airway may cause the patient to vomit, increasing the risk of aspiration. Keeping the patient nil by mouth will reduce this risk (NTSP 2013, **C**).
3 Introduce yourself to the patient, explain and discuss the procedure with them, and gain their consent to proceed.	To ensure that the patient feels at ease, understands the procedure and gives their valid consent (NMC 2018, **C**).
4 Cleanse hands with an alcohol-based handrub.	To minimize the risk of infection (NHS England and NHSI 2019, **C**).
5 Ensure all emergency equipment is immediately available.	In case it is not possible to secure the airway with the new tube (ICS 2014, **C**).
6 Help the patient to sit in a semi-recumbent position with the neck extended. It may be necessary to place a rolled towel under the patient's shoulders to further extend the neck.	To allow easy access to the neck area. **E** To bring the trachea closer to the skin and stretch the stoma opening to aid tube reinsertion (NTSP 2013, **C**).
7 Pre-oxygenate the patient if they are known to desaturate off oxygen.	To reduce the risk of hypoxia (NTSP 2013, **C**).
8 Prepare a dressing tray or trolley for the procedure. Open the sterile procedure pack and open the new tracheostomy tube and its contents onto the sterile sheet.	To ensure all equipment required is prepared prior to starting the procedure. **E**
9 If the new tracheostomy is cuffed, fully inflate the cuff using a 10 mL syringe. Once satisfied the cuff is functioning correctly, deflate the cuff prior to insertion.	To ensure there is no air leak and the cuff does not spontaneously deflate. **E**
10 Insert the obturator into the new tube, checking that it can be easily removed.	To become familiar with removing the obturator prior to insertion. **E**
11 Lubricate the new tube sparingly with a lubricating jelly and place it onto the sterile sheet.	To facilitate insertion and maintain sterility (Hess and Altobelli 2014, **C**).

Procedure

12 Cleanse hands using an alcohol-based handrub and apply disposable plastic apron, gloves and eye protection.	To minimize the risk of infection (NHS England and NHSI 2019, **C**).
13 Encourage the patient to cough and suction any secretions as required from the oral cavity (see Figure 12.49). Aspirate the subglottic port if present.	To reduce the risk of pooled secretions sitting above the cuff entering the lungs when the cuff is deflated (NTSP 2013, **C**).
14 Remove the inner cannula.	To assist with the outer tube removal. **E**
15 While one practitioner holds the tube, the other practitioner should unfasten the tube tapes and remove the sutures (if applicable).	To secure the tube and ensure it is not accidentally removed before the right time (NTSP 2013, **C**).
16 If the tracheostomy tube is cuffed, gently deflate the cuff, providing additional suctioning if required.	To prevent secretions from entering the lungs when the cuff is deflated (NTSP 2013, **C**).
17 Check both practitioners and the patient are happy to proceed prior to removing the tube. Provide reassurance to the patient as required.	To ensure patient safety at all times. **E** To reassure the patient and ease any anxiety. **E**
18 Administer conscious sedation as required and as prescribed.	Conscious sedation relaxes the patient and reduces the risk of coughing (NTSP 2013, **C**). Coughing can result in unwanted closure of the tracheostomy stoma. **E**
19 If a guided technique is being used, insert the guide into the tracheostomy tube.	To maintain the patency of the stoma (NTSP 2013, **C**).
20 Gently remove the old tube from the patient's neck while asking the patient to exhale. Remove it using a brisk, 'out and downwards' movement. Place it directly into the clinical waste bag.	To reduce the risk of cross-infection (NICE 2017, **C**).
21 Put traction on the stay sutures if present, or use tracheal dilators if required.	To maintain the patency of the trachea and prevent soft tissues from obstructing the stoma (Lee et al. 2015, **C**).
22 Quickly clean around the stoma with 0.9% sodium chloride and dry it gently with gauze. Apply barrier cream if required.	To clean the skin, reducing the risk of infection and tissue damage (ICS 2014, **C**).
23 *If using a blind technique*: insert the clean tube with the obturator in place using an 'up and over' action. Remove the obturator immediately.	Introduction of the tube is less traumatic if directed along the contour of the trachea (Greenwood and Winters 2014, **C**). The patient cannot breathe while the obturator is in place as it completely occludes the tracheostomy tube (NTSP 2013, **C**).

(continued)

Procedure guideline 12.11 Tracheostomy: changing a tube (continued)

Action	Rationale
24 *If using a guided technique*: **railroad** (thread) the new tracheostomy tube over the guide and into the stoma. Once satisfied, remove the guide as quickly as possible.	To guide insertion of the new tube into the stoma and prevent the creation of a false passage (NTSP 2013, **C**). The patient cannot breathe properly while the guide is in place. **E**
25 *Whether using a blind technique or a guided technique*: insert the inner tube and ensure it is in a 'locked' position.	The presence of an inner tube increases safety as it can be quickly removed and replaced if it becomes obstructed with tenacious secretions or a sputum plug (NTSP 2013, **C**).
26 If the tube is cuffed, gently inflate the cuff and check the pressure using a cuff manometer. The cuff pressure should be 15–25 cmH_2O (10–18 mmHg).	Too low a pressure will cause a cuff leak, resulting in ineffective ventilation and protection from aspiration. Too high a pressure may cause tracheal stenosis, tracheomalacia, tracheo-oesophageal fistula or an arterial fistula (ICS 2014, **C**; NTSP 2013, **C**).
27 Insert the tracheostomy dressing around the tube if required.	A foam dressing will protect the skin and prevent tissue damage (Everitt 2016a, **C**).
28 Secure the tracheostomy tube with the tapes/ties. Ensure one or two fingers can be comfortably inserted between the tapes and the patient's skin.	To secure the tube without causing the patient discomfort (Dawson 2014, **C**).
29 Check that the patient is comfortable and they are at ease with their breathing.	To ensure patient comfort and to assess for any signs of incorrect tube placement. **E**
30 Remove apron, gloves and eye protection and dispose of them in the clinical waste bag, along with the procedure pack and all other disposable equipment used. Cleanse hands with an alcohol-based handrub.	To minimize the risk of infection (NHS England and NHSI 2019, **C**).
Post-procedure	
31 Assess the airway by checking the following: • no evidence of breathing problems • bilateral chest movement • exhaled air felt through the end of the tracheostomy • air entry heard on auscultation • suction catheter able to pass though tube • for difficult procedures, capnography or a fibreoptic scope can be used to confirm placement.	To ensure the new tracheostomy is sitting in the trachea and the patient is being ventilated or oxygenated (NTSP 2013, **C**).
32 Monitor the patient's respiratory status and observations/NEWS. Escalate any concerns or deterioration in condition/NEWS immediately.	To identify any concerns or clinical deterioration early, and ensure timely escalation to senior staff if required (RCP 2017, **C**).
33 Document the tracheostomy tube change, including the new tube make and size. Document any problems observed during the procedure.	To ensure all staff are aware of the new tube size and type (NMC 2018, **C**).

Complications

Changing a tracheostomy tube is a high-risk procedure and may result in the loss of an airway. All staff involved should stay calm and reassure the patient as necessary. There should be no delay in seeking expert or additional help if required, or in following the emergency algorithm for an altered airway if necessary (see Figure 12.34) (ICS 2014, NTSP 2013). The patient should be oxygenated in between attempts and the stoma kept open using dilators or by putting traction on the stay sutures (Lee et al. 2015). If there is difficulty recannulating the stoma then insertion of a tube half a size smaller should be attempted (Mitchell et al. 2013). The tube should never be forced, and blind insertion of a guide into the stoma after the tube has been removed should only be considered in an emergency. The NTSP (2013) recommends the use of a fibreoptic scope and airway exchange catheter as a second line if recannulation using a tube one size smaller is unsuccessful.

Tracheostomy: applying a speaking valve

Evidence-based approaches

Rationale

The inability to communicate verbally can be extremely frustrating and upsetting a patient. Following initial formation of the tracheostomy, the patient may have a period of being nursed with the cuff up if they require mechanical ventilation. As the patient weans from the ventilator and the stoma becomes established, the cuff can be intermittently deflated and a speaking valve attached. In addition to restoring the patient's voice, the presence of a speaking valve helps to restore a more normalized physiology for respiration, can enhance swallowing, promotes the clearance of secretions through the mouth, and facilitates weaning and decannulation (Sutt et al. 2015). The speaking valve trial should be discussed and agreed by the multidisciplinary team, with a clear plan regarding how long and how often the speaking valve should be in place in a 24-hour period.

Indications

Inserting a speaking valve is indicated where (Morris et al. 2015):

- the patient's secretion load is minimal and they have an effective cough
- the patient does not require positive pressure mechanical ventilation.

Contraindications

Inserting a speaking valve may be contraindicated in patients who (Hess and Altobelli 2014, Morris et al. 2015):

- are at high risk of aspiration
- have a high secretion load
- have severe upper airway obstruction
- have a decreased consciousness level
- cannot tolerate having their cuff down.

Principles of care

Depending on why the tracheostomy has been formed and the status of the patient, they may cope with having the cuff down and a speaking valve may be attached fairly quickly and for long periods of time. Some may actually feel their breathing is easier and prefer this set-up. It can, however, cause a significant increase in a patient's work of breathing, and some patients with a large tube or narrow trachea may find it difficult to cope with the speaking valve due to reduced airflow around the tube (Bonvento et al. 2017). In this situation, consider downsizing the tracheostomy tube or changing it to an appropriate tube with a fenestrated inner cannula (Morris et al. 2015).

Anticipated patient outcomes

The patient will be able to tolerate having the cuff down and the speaking valve on for the prescribed length of time. The presence of the speaking valve will aid communication and facilitate weaning.

Pre-procedural considerations

Specific patient preparation

The procedure should always be explained to the patient and verbal consent gained. The patient should be counselled prior to the procedure and warned that their breathing may feel very different and that they may cough considerably when the cuff is deflated initially.

If required, the patient should be repositioned to ensure their comfort and allow easy access to the tracheostomy tube. Prior to the cuff being deflated, the patient should be encouraged to cough and clear secretions. Suction may also be required. If a patient has a subglottic port, secretions should be aspirated using a 10 mL syringe prior to the cuff being deflated (Morris et al. 2015).

Procedure guideline 12.12 Tracheostomy: insertion and removal of a speaking valve

Essential equipment

- Personal protective equipment
- Sterile dressing pack
- Speaking valve
- 10 mL syringe
- Cuff manometer
- Suction, suction catheters and Yankauer suction tips
- normal saline 0.9%

Action	Rationale
Pre-procedure	
1 Discuss the possibility of a speaking valve trial with the multidisciplinary team.	To ensure the multidisciplinary team agree to the speaking valve trial. **E**
2 This is a clean procedure and requires the presence of two nurses.	To ensure patient safety (NTSP 2013, **C**).
3 Introduce yourself to the patient, explain and discuss the procedure with them, and gain their consent to proceed.	To ensure that the patient feels at ease, understands the procedure and gives their valid consent (NMC 2018, **C**).
4 Cleanse hands with soap and water or an alcohol-based handrub.	To minimize the risk of infection (NHS England and NHSI 2019, **C**).
5 Help the patient to sit in a semi-recumbent position with neck slightly extended.	To ensure patient comfort and allow easy access to the neck area (NTSP 2013, **C**).
Procedure	
6 Cleanse hands using an alcohol-based handrub and apply disposable plastic apron, gloves and eye protection.	To minimize the risk of infection (NHS England and NHSI 2019, **C**).
7 Prepare a dressing tray or trolley for the procedure. Place the speaking valve and a 10 mL syringe onto the sterile sheet.	To ensure all equipment required is prepared prior to starting the procedure. **E**
8 Encourage the patient to cough and suction secretions in the mouth or from above the cuff if necessary. If the tube has a subglottic port, aspirate gently using a 10 mL syringe.	To prevent pooled secretions entering the lungs when the cuff is deflated (NTSP 2013, **C**).
9 If the tracheostomy tube is cuffed, gently deflate the cuff using a clean 10 mL syringe on expiration while simultaneously providing suction.	Providing suction while the cuff is deflated helps to clear any secretions that remain, reducing the risk of aspiration (Morris et al. 2015, **C**; NTSP 2013, **C**).
10 Reassure the patient as required.	The patient may cough for a period of time after cuff deflation, which may cause them to panic and worsen their breathing. **E**

(continued)

Procedure guideline 12.12 Tracheostomy: insertion and removal of a speaking valve *(continued)*

Action	Rationale
11 Apply the speaking valve directly onto the tracheostomy tube. Ask the patient to inhale through the tracheostomy tube and exhale through their mouth.	To encourage air to flow past the vocal cords and aid phonation. **E**
12 Ask the patient to say 'ah' or count from one to five. If the patient's voice sounds wet, ask them to cough and clear secretions. If the problem persists, remove the speaking valve and ask them to cough and clear secretions again. Provide suction as required.	Deflating the cuff can move secretions into the upper airways; these need to be cleared (Morris et al. 2015, **C**).
13 Monitor the patient closely during the speaking valve trial. Remove the speaking valve if: • the patient shows signs of respiratory distress • the patient's oxygen saturations fall • there is an evident wheeze or stridor • the patient is unable to vocalize • the patient looks fatigued • the patient requests it.	A change in breathing or evidence of clinical deterioration requires immediate removal of the speaking valve and reinflation of the cuff (Morris et al. 2015, **C**).
14 Depending on how the patient copes with the speaking valve, make a weaning plan with the multidisciplinary team.	To ensure a collaborative approach to weaning. **E**
15 At the end of the speaking valve trial, re-perform steps 2–6, then remove the speaking valve.	As above. To end the speaking valve trial. **E**
16 Use the 10 mL syringe to reinflate the cuff and check the pressure using the cuff manometer. The pressure should be between 15 and 25 cmH_2O (10–18 mmHg).	To ensure the cuff is sufficiently inflated to prevent aspiration, but not overinflated so as to cause damage to the trachea (NTSP 2013, **C**).
17 Check that the patient is comfortable and they are at ease with their breathing.	To ensure patient comfort. **E**
Post-procedure	
18 Monitor the patient's respiratory status and observations/NEWS. Escalate any concerns or deterioration in condition/NEWS immediately.	To identify any concerns or clinical deterioration early, and ensure timely escalation to senior staff if required (RCP 2017, **C**).
19 Clean the speaking valve using normal saline 0.9% and leave it to air dry. Store it in an airtight container.	To minimize bacterial colonization and prevent infection (Everitt 2016a, **C**).
20 Document how long the cuff was down and if the speaking valve was tolerated. Document any other concerns or details that may assist the multidisciplinary team.	To communicate to the multidisciplinary team the details of the cuff-down speaking valve trial. **E**

Complications

Deflating the cuff and inserting a speaking valve may cause respiratory distress. If at any time the patient experiences difficulty in breathing, is unable to vocalize, or begins to sound wheezy or stridulous, the speaking valve should be removed immediately and the patient reassessed (Hess and Altobelli 2014, Morris et al. 2015). The speaking valve should also be removed if there is any evidence of aspiration or if the patient cannot cope with their secretions.

Tracheostomy: decannulation

Evidence-based approaches

Rationale

Prior to decannulation, the patient should have been appropriately weaned and be able to tolerate having the cuff down with either a speaking valve or a heat and moisture exchanger on permanently. It may also be appropriate to trial an occlusion or decannulation plug for 12–24 hours (NTSP 2013). This is a small plastic plug or cap that fits onto the outer tube of either a fenestrated or a non-fenestrated tracheostomy tube (Figure 12.52). It completely blocks off the tracheostomy tube and diverts air around the tube and into the patient's nose and mouth instead. Patients may find this stage difficult as airway resistance is high, and so it may not be well tolerated. As with all care pathways related to tracheostomies, a multidisciplinary approach is required and all members should be involved in the decision to decannulate (Bonvento et al. 2017).

Indications

Decannulation can be considered if there are no concerns regarding the patient's ability to maintain their own airway once the tracheostomy tube is removed and if the patient meets the following criteria (Cheung and Napolitano 2014, Global Tracheostomy Collaborative 2013, NTSP 2013, Singh et al. 2017):

- the airway is patent above the level of the stoma
- the pathological process necessitating the insertion of the tracheostomy tube has been resolved
- the patient is conscious and able to follow commands

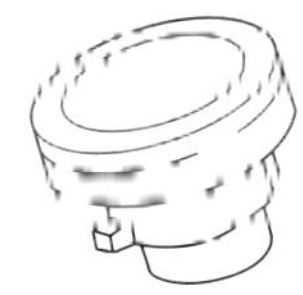

Figure 12.52 Decannulation plug.

- the patient is able to tolerate having the cuff down for long periods of time
- the patient does not have copious secretions
- the patient can cough and clear their secretions effectively
- the patient has an effective swallow
- the patient is cardiovascularly stable
- no new lung infiltrates appear on chest X-ray
- the multidisciplinary team agrees to decannulation.

Contraindications

Decannulation is contraindicated if any of the above criteria have not been met.

Principles of care

The process should be undertaken or supervised by a practitioner who is competent in recannulation and airway management. The procedure should be well planned and performed at an appropriate time of the day when experienced staff are present (Dawson 2014, ICS 2014).

Undiagnosed damage to the trachea – including stenosis, tracheomalacia and granuloma – may result in a failed decannulation (Cipriano et al. 2015, ICS 2014). It is important, therefore, that the patient is closely monitored for a period of time after decannulation, to ensure they remain stable and are able to maintain their own airway.

Anticipated patient outcomes

The patient will be able to maintain their own airway once the tracheostomy tube has been removed and will show no signs of clinical deterioration, in particular respiratory distress or tiring.

Pre-procedural considerations

Equipment

A tracheostomy box, with a new tracheostomy tube and all emergency equipment (oxygen, suction and a fibreoptic scope), should be available at the bedside and in working order. A resuscitation and advanced airway trolley should be easily accessible if required.

Specific patient preparation

The procedure should always be explained to the patient and verbal consent gained. If required, the patient should be repositioned to ensure their comfort and allow easy access to the tracheostomy tube.

The patient should be nil by mouth for at least 6 hours after eating solids and 2 hours after consuming fluids (NTSP 2013). This is to minimize the risk of vomiting and aspiration.

Procedure guideline 12.13 Tracheostomy: decannulation

Essential equipment

- Personal protective equipment
- Sterile dressing pack
- 10 mL syringe
- Stitch cutter (if sutures are present)
- Occlusive dressing
- Tracheostomy box
- Oxygen, mask and tubing
- Suction, suction catheters and Yankauer suction tips
- Stethoscope
- Resuscitation trolley
- Advanced airway trolley
- Fibreoptic scope
- Normal saline 0.9% solution
- Gallipot
- Gauze

Action	Rationale
Pre-procedure	
1 Discuss decannulation with the multidisciplinary team.	To ensure the multidisciplinary team agree to the patient being decannulated and are readily available if required. **E**
2 This procedure requires the presence of two nurses.	To ensure patient safety (NTSP 2013, **C**).
3 Introduce yourself to the patient, explain and discuss the procedure with them, and gain their consent to proceed.	To ensure that the patient feels at ease, understands the procedure and gives their valid consent (NMC 2018, **C**).
4 Cleanse hands with soap and water or an alcohol-based handrub.	To minimize the risk of infection (NHS England and NHSI 2019, **C**).
5 Help the patient to sit in a semi-recumbent position with the neck slightly extended.	To ensure patient comfort. **E** Extending the neck will make removal of the tube easier (NTSP 2013, **C**).
6 Apply oxygen therapy via either a nasal cannula or a face-mask (if required).	To reduce the risk of hypoxia (O'Driscoll et al. 2017, **C**).
7 Prepare a dressing tray or trolley for the procedure. Open the procedure pack and pour normal saline 0.9% solution into a gallipot. Prepare the dressing to be applied over the tracheostomy stoma.	To ensure all equipment required is prepared prior to starting the procedure. **E**
Procedure	
8 Cleanse hands using an alcohol-based handrub and apply disposable plastic apron, gloves and eye protection.	To minimize the risk of infection (NHS England and NHSI 2019, **C**).

(continued)

Procedure guideline 12.13 Tracheostomy: decannulation (continued)

Action	Rationale
9 Encourage the patient to cough and suction any secretions as required.	To minimize the risk of aspiration (Morris et al. 2015, **C**).
10 While one nurse holds onto the tracheostomy tube, the second nurse removes the tapes and any sutures present at the flange, and deflate the cuff (if still inflated).	To ensure the tube is not accidentally dislodged before the right time. **E** To prepare the tube for decannulation. **E**
11 Check both practitioners and the patient are happy to proceed prior to removing the tube. Provide reassurance to the patient as required.	Good communication increases patient safety. **E** To minimize patient anxiety. **E**
12 Remove the tube on maximal inspiration.	To reduce the risk of alveolar collapse (Global Tracheostomy Collaborative 2013, **C**).
13 Clean the stoma site using normal saline 0.9% soaked gauze then allow it to air dry.	To clean the skin and minimize the risk of infection (Global Tracheostomy Collaborative 2013, **C**).
14 Bring together the top and bottom of the stoma to ensure an optimal seal is achieved. Secure with gauze and an occlusive dressing.	To encourage the stoma to close and ensure all ventilation takes place via the upper airways. **E** Covering the stoma also reduces the risk of infection by ensuring dust and particles are not inhaled directly into the respiratory tract. **E**
15 Check that the patient is comfortable and is at ease with their breathing.	To ensure patient comfort. **E**
Post-procedure	
16 Monitor the patient's respiratory status and observations/ NEWS. Escalate any concerns or deterioration in condition/ NEWS immediately.	Removal of a tracheostomy tube is a high-risk procedure. The patient may not be able to maintain their own airway and may require emergency recannulation or intubation. Patients should be monitored closely and the situation escalated immediately if there are any concerns (NTSP 2013, **C**).
17 Encourage the patient to hold their hand over the stoma dressing when they speak or cough.	To prevent the occlusive dressing being dislodged and to divert air through the vocal cords, aiding phonation and communication (NTSP 2013, **C**).
18 Inform the patient that the stoma may take 7–14 days to heal over and close.	To increase patient understanding and appreciation of how long the stoma will take to heal. **E**
19 Document what date and time the patient was decannulated, and any issues or concerns arising during or after the procedure.	To ensure all members of the multidisciplinary team are aware of when the patient was decannulated and to help plan future care. **E**
20 Renew the dressing every 24 hours or more frequently if required. Monitor the size of the stoma daily.	To minimize infection, promote wound healing and monitor stoma closure (Global Tracheostomy Collaborative 2013, **C**).
21 Keep the tracheostomy box at the patient's bedside for a further 48 hours post-decannulation.	To allow easy access to the emergency equipment if the patient deteriorates and requires emergency recannulation (Global Tracheostomy Collaborative 2013, **C**).

Complications

The main complication that can arise post-decannulation is the patient's inability to maintain their own airway, which may not become evident until a few hours after decannulation. For this reason, the tracheostomy box and emergency equipment should be kept by the patient's bedside for at least 24 hours (Global Tracheostomy Collaborative 2013). If there are any concerns, the patient should be escalated immediately and preparations made for recannulation.

Tracheostomy: emergency care and recannulation

Evidence-based approaches

Rationale

Patients with an altered airway (or who have recently been decannulated) who present with signs of airway, breathing or circulatory problems should be escalated immediately and assessed by an experienced and appropriate practitioner.

Indications

The following indications would give cause for concern and necessitate immediate management (ICS 2014, NTSP 2013):

- a dislodged tracheostomy
- overt signs of respiratory distress (pale, sweaty, clammy, cyanosed, increased work of breathing, tachypnoea, using accessory muscles)
- silent breathing, or grunting, snoring or stridor
- reduced or falling oxygen saturations
- restlessness, agitation or confusion
- tachycardia or hypotension
- blood stained secretions (haemoptysis).

Contraindications

There are no contraindications to managing a patient who has airway compromise and subsequent breathing problems.

Principles of care

A patient's airway may become compromised for a variety of reasons. The compromise may be secondary to an underlying condition or disease, such as cancer of the head and neck. It may be that the patient already has an altered airway that has occluded due to tenacious secretions, and requires suctioning or change of the inner cannula. It may be that the tracheostomy tube has become partially or completely dislodged, or the patient may have failed decannulation due to an underlying problem such as tracheomalacia and require recannulation. All of the above require immediate management and escalation to an expert practitioner versed in airway management. Algorithms produced by the NTSP (2013) can be used to guide practitioners in the emergency management of altered airways (see Figure 12.34).

Anticipated patient outcomes

The patient will have a patent airway and be able to ventilate and oxygenate, preventing further deterioration or cardiopulmonary arrest.

Pre-procedural considerations

All staff should remain calm and reassure the patient as required. Staff should work together but with clear leadership, communicating what actions need to be taken and when. There should be no delay in escalating the situation to the relevant teams, and staff should be encouraged to call the resuscitation team if the patient is deteriorating or expert help is delayed. The resuscitation and advanced airway trolley should be brought to the patient's bedside along with a fibreoptic scope in order to deal with the emergency (NTSP 2013).

Procedure guideline 12.14 Tracheostomy: emergency management

Essential equipment

- Personal protective equipment
- Oxygen supply plus bag valve mask and a selection of oxygen masks and tubing
- Suction, suction catheters and Yankauer suction tips
- Resuscitation trolley
- Advanced airway trolley
- Tracheostomy box
- Fibreoptic scope

Action	Rationale
Pre-procedure	
1 Introduce yourself to the patient, explain the situation and reassure them as much as possible.	To ensure the patient is kept informed and reassured. **E**
2 Cleanse hands using an alcohol-based handrub and apply personal protective equipment.	To minimize the risk of infection (NHS England and NHSI 2019, **C**).
Procedure	
3 Assess whether the patient is breathing. If not, call the resuscitation team and commence cardiopulmonary resuscitation (CPR).	A patient who is not breathing requires immediate CPR (RCUK 2015, **C**).
4 If the patient is breathing, apply high-flow oxygen therapy (reservoir mask at 15 L/min to both the face and the stoma or tube).	To reduce the risk of hypoxia (O'Driscoll et al. 2017, **C**).
5 Call for expert help.	To get additional and expert help early (NTSP 2013, **C**).
6 Assess the patency of the tracheostomy tube, if present. If there is not a tracheostomy tube in place, proceed to step 8.	To determine whether there is any air flow in or out of the tracheostomy tube (NTSP 2013, **C**).
7 Remove the decannulation cap, speaking valve, or heat and moisture exchanger (if present).	To remove any potential source of obstruction (Morris et al. 2015, **C**).
8 Remove the inner tube (if present).	To determine whether an occluded inner tube is the source of the obstruction (Cosgrove and Carrie 2015, **C**).
9 Pass a suction catheter down the tracheostomy tube or stoma and apply suction.	To determine the patency of the tube and remove a sputum plug if present (NTSP 2013, **C**).
10 If the suction catheter can be passed, the tube is patent. Repeat suction if a sputum plug is the likely cause.	To remove any secretions that may be obstructing the airway (NTSP 2013, **C**).
11 If the suction catheter cannot be passed, deflate the cuff (if present) and reassess the patient.	Deflating the cuff will allow air to flow past the cuff in the event of a completely obstructed tracheostomy tube (NTSP 2013, **C**). This will also help to assess whether it is the tube that is causing the problem. **E**
12 Ventilate the patient using either a bag valve mask or a Mapleson C system (water circuit). These can either be applied directly onto the patient's face using an anaesthetic mask or attached directly onto the tracheostomy tube.	To ventilate the patient while the cause is being investigated or treated. By attempting to 'bag' or ventilate via the tracheostomy tube, its patency can simultaneously be assessed (ICS 2014, **C**; NTSP 2013, **C**).
13 If the patient stabilizes or improves, continue to ventilate and oxygenate until expert help arrives and the tracheostomy tube can be assessed.	To prevent hypoxia (NTSP 2013, **C**; O'Driscoll et al. 2017, **C**).
14 If the patient continues to deteriorate, the tracheostomy tube needs to be removed.	It is safer to remove the tracheostomy tube and ventilate the patient by other means if there is no ventilation via the altered airway (NTSP 2013, **C**).

(continued)

Procedure guideline 12.14 Tracheostomy: emergency management *(continued)*

Action	Rationale
15 Prepare to remove the tracheostomy tube by removing any external sutures and tube tapes.	To allow removal of the tube (NTSP 2013, **C**).
16 Quickly remove the tube and cover the stoma with gauze and an occlusive dressing, or with a gloved hand.	To allow effective ventilation of the upper airway. **E**
17 Continue to ventilate using any of the methods described in step 12.	To prevent hypoxia (ICS 2014, **C**; NTSP 2013, **C**).
18 Prepare to either intubate the patient orally or recannulate the stoma using an endotracheal tube or a size smaller tracheostomy tube.	To secure an appropriate airway in the patient (Mitchell et al. 2013, **C**).
19 Use a fibreoptic scope and perform a guided insertion if able.	To minimize the risk of causing a false passage, especially if the patient's airway is known to be difficult (NTSP 2013, **C**).
20 Once the airway has been inserted, inflate the cuff and secure the endotracheal tube or tracheostomy tube in place with tapes or ties.	To secure the airway. **E**
21 Continue to ventilate using a bag valve mask or water circuit until the patient is able to ventilate spontaneously and stabilizes. Administer supplemental oxygen as required.	To ensure the patient is being ventilated and oxygenated (NTSP 2013, **C**).
22 Check the patient's observations/NEWS and document. Aim for oxygen saturations of 94–98% (or 88–92% if the patient is at risk of hypercapnic respiratory failure).	To ensure the patient is not being over- or under-oxygenated (O'Driscoll et al. 2017, **C**).
23 Consider performing an arterial blood gas and chest X-ray.	To ensure the post-event patient assessment is thorough. **E**
24 Assess how the patient is ventilating and oxygenating and determine whether they require further respiratory support in a high-dependency or intensive care unit.	To ensure the patient is being cared for in the most appropriate clinical area. **E**
Post-procedure	
25 Monitor the patient's respiratory status and observations/NEWS frequently until they are stable. Escalate any concerns or deterioration in condition/NEWS immediately.	To identify any concerns or clinical deterioration early, and ensure timely escalation to senior staff if required (RCP 2017, **C**).

Problem-solving table 12.5 Prevention and resolution (Procedure guideline 12.14)

Problem	Cause	Prevention	Action
Profuse tracheal secretions	Local reaction to tracheostomy tube or infection (as below)	Ensure vigilant care of the tracheostomy or stoma. Keep the patient well hydrated. Ensure good infection control practice and take standard precautions at all times when carrying out any aspect of care for a patient with an altered airway.	Suction frequently and ensure secretions are kept thin and loose. Check inner tube frequently and change if required. Consider use of saline or mucolytic nebulizers if secretions are tenacious. Ensure vigilant care of the surrounding skin to keep it as clean and dry as possible. Use a foam dressing and change it frequently. Send a sputum sample to microbiology to ensure it is not infected. Give antimicrobials if indicated and prescribed.
Lumen of tracheostomy tube occluded	Tenacious or dried sputum or blood occluding tube	Provide humidification via an HME or warmed and humidified oxygen therapy. Check and change inner tubes frequently. Suction the patient as required. Encourage the patient to report if they notice any change or difficulty with their breathing.	Call for help from the resuscitation team. Apply high-flow oxygen over the nose and mouth and over the tracheostomy tube. Remove the speaking valve or HME immediately. Remove the inner tube. Suction the patient. Deflate the cuff (if applicable). Remove the tracheostomy if the above interventions have failed and the patient is deteriorating. Ventilate and oxygenate the patient using a bag valve mask or water circuit until a new altered airway has been inserted.

Problem	Cause	Prevention	Action
Tracheostomy tube accidentally dislodged	Tracheostomy tapes not adequately secured Tracheostomy tube not secured by staff during procedures or moving and handling of the patient	Ensure the tracheostomy tapes are secure at all times with a maximum of one or two finger spaces between the skin and tapes. Always hold the tracheostomy tube while turning, moving or mobilizing the patient. Educate the patient and staff about safe mobilization and manual handling of patients with an altered airway. The person who holds and secures the tube should lead the manoeuvre and give clear commands regarding when it is safe to move.	Call for expert help or the resuscitation team, depending on how newly formed the tracheostomy tube is and the condition of the patient. Oxygenate the patient via the nose and mouth and via the stoma. Prepare a new tracheostomy tube and promptly insert it. If there are any concerns regarding the risk of forming a false passage, the tube should be checked by an appropriate clinician using a fibreoptic scope.
Unable to insert a clean tracheostomy tube during tube change or after accidental dislodgment	Unpredicted shape or angle of stoma	Emergency equipment with spare tubes, lubricant, tracheostomy dilators etc. should always be readily available at the patient's bedside, in the tracheostomy box. Ensure the resuscitation trolley, the advanced airway trolley and the fibreoptic scope are readily available. Ensure an appropriately trained practitioner changes the tube and a second competent practitioner assists. Discuss the plan of action for the team to take if recannulation is not possible. Ensure all members are aware of their role and actions to be taken	Remain calm and summon expert help or call the resuscitation team. Apply high-flow oxygen over the patient's stoma site and the nose and mouth. Lubricate the tube well and attempt to reinsert it at various angles. If unsuccessful, attempt to insert a smaller-size tracheostomy tube. If this is impossible, keep the tracheostomy tract open using tracheal dilators or put traction on the stay sutures if present. Do so until expert help arrives. Monitor the patient and observations continuously. If the patient's condition deteriorates, begin ventilation using a bag valve mask over the patient's nose and mouth while occluding the stoma with a dressing or gloved hand. Once the tube has been successfully inserted, it may be necessary for an expert to look via a fibreoptic scope and check no false passage was created during the procedure and the tube is cannulating the trachea.
Tracheal bleeding	Trauma to the trachea during tube change or from suctioning, bleeding from a tumour, erosion into a blood vessel, or uncorrected coagulopathies	Ensure vigilant care of the tracheostomy or stoma. Avoid frequent and multiple suctions if not indicated. Correct any coagulopathies.	Minimal bleeding should be monitored and reported to the multidisciplinary team. The tracheostomy cuff should be inflated to protect the airway if there is perfuse bleeding, and the patient escalated immediately. Perform suction as required.
Infection	Upper airway defences are bypassed in patients with a tracheostomy, predisposing patients to a higher risk of lower respiratory tract infection	Ensure good infection control practice and take standard precautions at all times when carrying out any aspect of care for patients with an altered airway.	Obtain a sputum sample or swab the stoma site and send the sample to microbiology. Give empirical antibiotics as per local microbiology guidelines.

HME, heat and moisture exchanger.

Laryngectomy

Related theory

Patients who have undergone a total laryngectomy may require a cuffed tracheostomy tube for the first 24 hours following their operation or until they have been weaned off ventilation. Once the tracheostomy tube has been removed, the ear, nose and throat (ENT) surgeon will decide whether a laryngectomy tube is required for stoma patency. For patients with no laryngectomy tube in place, the nurse must be extremely vigilant, assessing the bare stoma frequently to ensure that it is not at risk of stenosis. A stenosed stoma will restrict the patient's breathing and hinder the removal of secretions (Sharma et al. 2016). The stoma should be sufficiently large, ideally 15 × 15 mm in diameter. Less than 10 mm is deemed critical (Sharma et al. 2016). There are various stoma patency devices available, including laryngectomy tubes, stoma studs and stoma buttons (Figure 12.53). The ENT surgical team, clinical nurse specialist and speech and language therapist (SLT) can help to guide which device should be used.

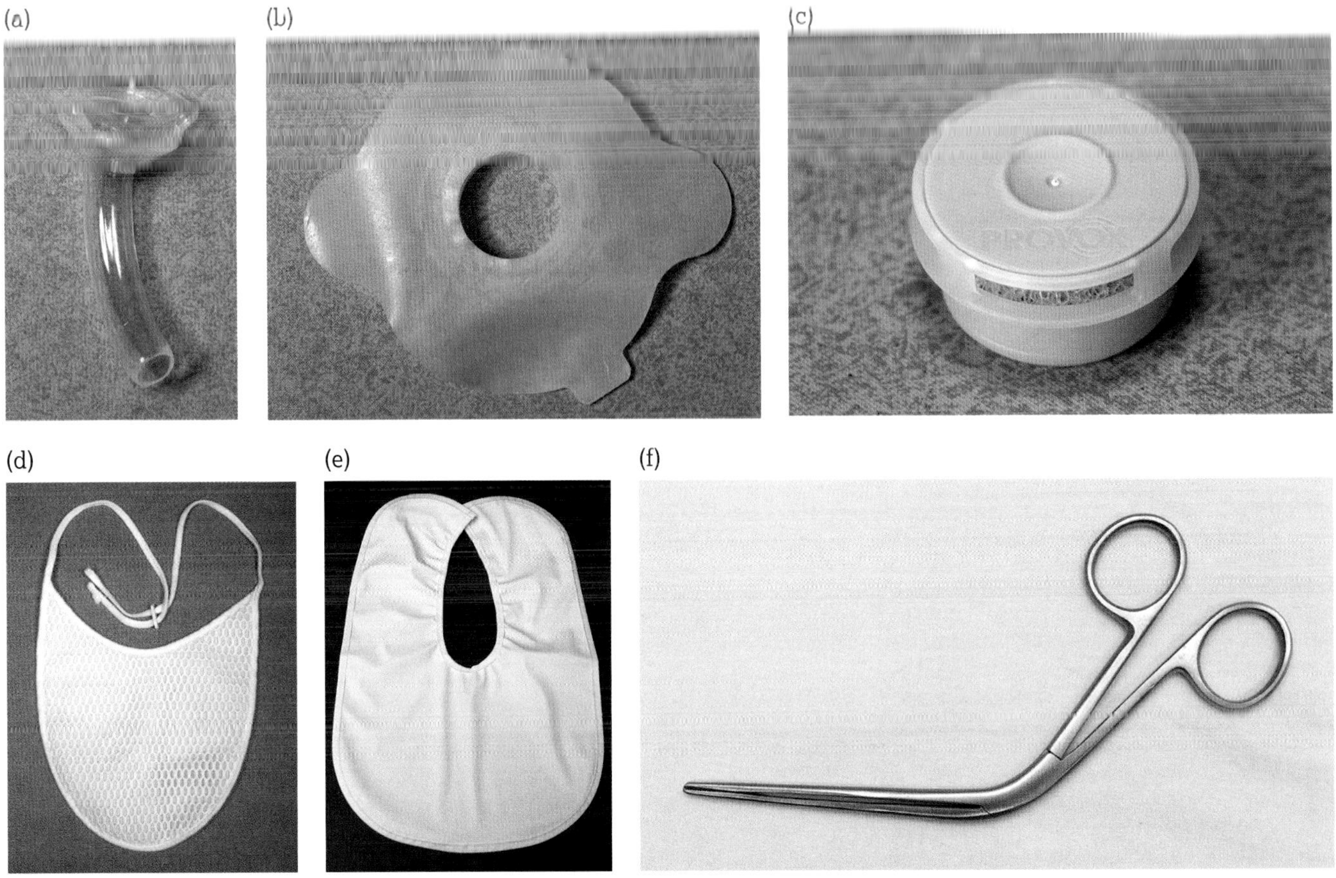

Figure 12.53 Larnyngectomy devices. (a) Laryngecomy tube. (b) Baseplate. (c) Filter cassette. (d) Stoma covers. (e) Shower aid. (f) Tilley's forceps.

Laryngectomy: humidification

Evidence-based approaches

As with patients who have a tracheostomy, humidification for laryngectomy patients is essential since the natural mechanisms of humidification, warming and filtration of inspired air normally provided by the upper airways are permanently bypassed (Clarke et al. 2016).

The following choices are available:

- *Humidification systems*: a heat and moisture exchanger (HME) consists of a laryngectomy tube or baseplate/housing that attaches to the neck and contains a filter cassette (Figure 12.53b and c). This system is highly recommended as it provides maximum protection and humidification of the airway. There are a range of types of filter and baseplate.
- *Stoma covers*: these filter and humidify inhaled air and are available in a variety of sizes and attachments (Figure 12.53d).

Laryngectomy: communication

Evidence-based approaches

The following options are available (Everitt 2016c, NTSP 2013, Zenga et al. 2018):

- *Surgical voice restoration* (SVR) allows communication to be restored via the use of a voice prosthesis, which may also be referred to as a valve. See below for further information.
- *Oesophageal voice* involves moving air into the oesophagus either by inhaling or injecting air into the back of the mouth. Instead of the vocal cords vibrating, the walls of the pharynx vibrate. Sound then moves into the mouth, where recognizable speech is produced by the articulators (i.e. the tongue, lips and palate). Patients are asked to imagine gulping air into their mouth, beginning to swallow but returning the air to their mouth in a controlled manner. Oesophageal voice has previously been described as 'burped speech' and usually the patient can achieve a small number of words in one breath.
- An *artificial larynx* involves using a battery-powered device that is placed against the neck or cheek, or intraorally. When a button is pushed, a vibration occurs in the head of the device and it is this vibration through the tissues that creates sound as the patient mouths words.

SVR has become the most popular means of restoring communication, with success rates of up to 90% reported (Zenga et al. 2018). SVR entails creating a puncture between the posterior wall of the trachea and the anterior wall of the oesophagus, into which a one-way voice prosthesis is placed. By occluding the stoma, pulmonary air is diverted through the prosthesis into the oesophagus, where the walls vibrate to make sound (Ward and Van As-Brooks 2014).

The prosthesis is a silicone device that fits into the tracheo-oesophageal puncture (TEP) and acts as a one-way valve, preventing food and drink from entering the trachea from the oesophagus (Zenga et al. 2018). Patients can have the puncture created during their laryngectomy operation, in which case it is called a 'primary puncture'. Post-operatively, patients with a primary puncture may have a catheter or a stoma gastric tube in place in the TEP, which enables the puncture to remain patent. Once healing has occurred, the stoma gastric tube is removed and the prosthesis can be placed into the TEP (secondary voice prosthesis placement). Alternatively, a voice prosthesis may be placed at the time of TEP creation: however, it will not be used for a period of time, until adequate healing has occurred (primary voice prosthesis placement).

If patients are required to wait for their puncture following the laryngectomy surgery – for example, due to an extended laryngectomy – they are likely to have a 'secondary puncture'. A secondary puncture may involve primary or secondary placement and can be done in the operating theatre under general anaesthetic or in the outpatient setting under local anaesthetic (Noel et al. 2016).

Laryngectomy: care and emergency management

Evidence-based approaches

Rationale

The aim of routine and emergency laryngectomy care is to (Everitt 2016b, NTSP 2013):

- maintain the patency of the laryngectomy stoma
- provide humidification
- keep the stoma clean and free from infection
- aid voice restoration.

Indications

The patient's laryngectomy stoma should be cleaned regularly and any crusts removed to ensure they are not aspirated and to ensure that the stoma remains unobstructed and patent. An HME or humidification bib should be used to heat and humidify inspired air.

Contraindications

There are no contraindications to providing laryngectomy care, especially in the initial post-operative phase, when the patient may not yet be able to care for their stoma independently.

Procedure guideline 12.15 Laryngectomy care

Essential equipment

- Personal protective equipment
- Sterile dressing pack
- Tilley's forceps (see Figure 12.53)
- Ruler
- Laryngectomy tube (see Figure 12.53)
- Heat and moisture exchanger (HME) or humidification bib
- Suction, suction catheters and Yankauer suction tips
- 0.9% sodium chloride
- Low-linting gauze

Optional equipment

- Baseplate

Action	Rationale
Pre-procedure	
1 This is a clean procedure.	To ensure patient safety (NTSP 2013, **C**).
2 Introduce yourself to the patient, explain and discuss the procedure with them, and gain their consent to proceed.	To ensure that the patient feels at ease, understands the procedure and gives their valid consent (NMC 2018, **C**).
3 Cleanse hands with soap and water or an alcohol-based handrub.	To minimize the risk of infection (NHS England and NHSI 2019, **C**).
4 Help the patient to sit in a semi-recumbent position with the neck slightly extended.	To ensure patient comfort. Extending the neck will allow easy access to the laryngectomy stoma (NTSP 2013, **C**).
5 Prepare a dressing tray or trolley for the procedure. Open the sterile procedure pack and any additional equipment required (tube, baseplate etc.). Pour the cleaning solution over the low-linting gauze.	To ensure all equipment required is prepared prior to starting the procedure. **E**
Procedure	
6 Cleanse hands using an alcohol-based handrub and apply disposable plastic apron, gloves and eye protection.	To minimize the risk of infection (NHS England and NHSI 2019, **C**).
7 Clean around the stoma with 0.9% sodium chloride using low-linting gauze. If required, use Tilley's forceps to remove any dried secretions or crusts from around the stoma. Allow the stoma to air dry.	To remove wet or dried secretions from the stoma site. **E**
8 Measure the laryngectomy stoma and document the size in the patient's laryngectomy passport.	To check for tracheal stenosis (Sharma et al. 2016, **C**).
9 If required, insert a laryngectomy tube. (The speech and language therapist will determine what size to use and document this in the patient's laryngectomy passport.)	To maintain patency or to help shape the laryngeal stoma (Everitt 2016b, **E**).
10 A baseplate may also be considered. This can be inserted around the stoma to house a HME cassette. A humidification bib or scarf is another alternative.	To facilitate phonation and/or humidification (Everitt 2016b, **E**; NTSP 2013, **C**).
11 Remove apron, gloves and eye protection and dispose of them in the clinical waste. Cleanse hands with soap and water or an alcohol-based handrub.	To minimize the risk of infection (NHS England and NHSI 2019, **C**).

(continued)

Action	Rationale
Post-procedure	
12 Monitor the patient's respiratory status and observations/NEWS. Escalate any concerns or deterioration in condition/NEWS2 immediately.	To identify any concerns or clinical deterioration early, and ensure timely escalation to senior staff if required (RCP 2017, **C**).
13 Discuss any concerns with the multidisciplinary team.	To ensure the multidisciplinary team is involved in all aspects of the care of patients with a laryngectomy (NTSP 2013, **C**).

Problem-solving table 12.6 Prevention and resolution (Procedure guideline 12.15)

Problem	Cause	Prevention	Action
Breathing difficulties	Mucus plug or reduced airflow due to secretions Reduction in stoma size	Regularly check and clean the stoma. Ensure adequate humidification over the stoma. Regularly administer nebulizers. Encourage the patient to carry out steam inhalation if the secretions are tenacious. Encourage regular mobilization to assist in the clearing of secretions. Regularly measure the stoma's size.	Check the stoma and clean it if mucus plugs or crusts have formed. If a laryngectomy tube is in place, remove it and clean the tube. Administer normal saline 0.9% nebulizer. Measure the stoma and consider insertion of a stoma button or laryngectomy tube (refer to SLT if required). Seek expert help if the patient is deteriorating and the above interventions have not helped with their breathing difficulties.
Bleeding from stoma	Bleeding may be caused by trauma to the trachea from cleaning or suctioning, or a lack of humidification	Check and clean the stoma as required. Suction the patient only when absolutely necessary. Encourage the patient to cough and wipe away secretions. Ensure humidification of the laryngectomy stoma. Regularly administer nebulizers.	If the bleeding is profuse and there is a risk of aspiration of blood into the lungs, a small tracheostomy tube should be inserted and the cuff inflated to protect the airway. Seek expert help and ask for an urgent review.
Chest infection	Possible aspiration if the patient has a transoesophageal puncture	Monitor for signs and symptoms of chest infection. Monitor the speaking valve for patency and size. Clean the speaking valve to reduce the risk of secretions accumulating.	Check for leakage from the voice prosthesis (see 'Voice prosthesis falls out accidentally' below). Contact the team or SLT for an urgent assessment if leakage is suspected. Keep the patient nil by mouth until reviewed.
Stoma shrinkage	Laryngectomy stoma reduced in size	Regularly measure the stoma's size.	Insert a laryngectomy tube or stoma button. Escalate to the team and SLT and ask for a patient review.
Voice prosthesis falls out accidentally	Voice prosthesis not adequately secured or accidentally removed	Ensure that care is taken when cleaning the stoma and valve to reduce the risk of it falling out.	Insert a red rubber tube (Figure 12.54) (14 Fr catheter) or dilator. If using a red rubber tube, tie a knot in the end of the tube and secure the end onto the neck or chest wall using tape. Check for leakage around the tube or dilator (encourage several sips of coloured liquid or milk and watch for leakage; use a good torch or light to see clearly). If leakage is noted, commence thickened drinks to reduce the risk of a chest infection. Contact the SLT for an urgent review. If unable to insert the red rubber tube or dilator, contact ENT team immediately. Check the patient has removed the voice prosthesis from the airway; if not, the patient should be seen by the ENT team to check the prosthesis is not still in the airway.
Voice difficulties	Voice prosthesis blocked or not working	Clean the voice prosthesis regularly	Clean the voice prosthesis with a brush. If this does not help, contact the SLT.

ENT, ear, nose and throat; SLT, speech and language therapist.

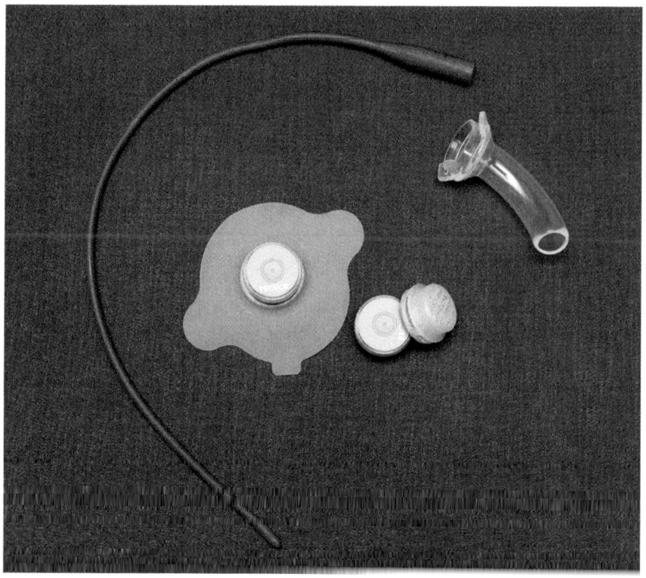

Figure 12.54 Red rubber tube, base plate with a heat and moisture exchanger, and a laryngectomy tube.

Basic life support

Definition

Cardiopulmonary resuscitation (CPR) is an emergency procedure involving cardiac compressions and manual ventilation. The aim of CPR is to preserve cardiac output and maintain oxygenation of the brain in a person in cardiac arrest until further measures can be taken to restore spontaneous breathing and blood circulation (RCUK 2015). Resuscitation is the emergency treatment of any condition in which the brain fails to receive enough oxygen.

CPR guidelines in the UK are produced and implemented by the Resuscitation Council UK (RCUK 2015). These are based on the European Resuscitation Council's guidelines, which were last updated and republished in 2015 (ERC 2015).

Anatomy and physiology

The heart

The heart is made up of four chambers: two upper atria and two lower ventricles. The right atrium receives deoxygenated blood from the systemic venous circulation. From the right atrium, blood flows into the right ventricle, which pumps it back to the lungs via the pulmonary artery. Carbon dioxide is released and oxygen is absorbed within the lungs. This blood, which is now oxygenated, returns to the heart via the pulmonary vein and empties into the left atrium. The blood then passes into the left ventricle, which pumps it into the aorta and the arterial systemic circulation (Waugh and Grant 2014).

The atrioventricular septum completely separates the right and left sides of the heart. From shortly after birth, the two sides of the heart never directly communicate, with blood flowing from the right side to the left side via the lungs only. However, the right and left atria and the right and left ventricles work together, contracting simultaneously (Marieb and Hoehn 2018). To prevent the backflow of blood, the heart has four valves. The valves open and close in response to pressure changes as the heart contracts and relaxes (Tortora and Derrickson 2017). The valve between the right atrium and ventricle is known as the tricuspid valve, while the valve between the left atrium and ventricle is called the mitral valve. The pulmonary valve prevents backflow of blood from the pulmonary artery into the right ventricle. Likewise, the aortic valve sits within the aorta and prevents regurgitation into the left ventricle.

The cardiac conduction system

The sinoatrial (SA) node is the natural pacemaker of the heart. It releases an electrical stimulus at a regular rate that will vary depending on whether the body is at rest or in action. As each stimulus passes through the myocardial cells, it creates a wave of contraction, which spreads rapidly through both atria and is known as 'atrial depolarization' (Tortora and Derrickson 2017).

The rapidity of atrial contraction is such that around 100 million myocardial cells contract in less than one-third of a second. When the electrical stimulus from the SA node reaches the atrioventricular (AV) node, within the septum, it is delayed briefly so that the contracting atria have enough time to pump the blood into the ventricles. Once the atria are empty of blood, the valves between the atria and ventricles close. At this point, the atria begin to refill and the electrical stimulus passes through the AV node and the bundle of His, along the left and right bundle branches, and finally terminates in the Purkinje fibres within the ventricles. In this way, all the myocardial cells (around 400 million) in the ventricles receive an electrical stimulus, which causes them to contract (Marieb and Hoehn 2018). This process is known as 'ventricular depolarization' and also happens in less than one-third of a second. As the ventricles contract, the right ventricle pumps blood to the lungs, where carbon dioxide is released and oxygen is absorbed, while the left ventricle pumps blood into the coronary and arterial circulation via the aorta. At this point the ventricles are empty, the atria are full and the valves between them are closed.

Prior to the process starting again, the SA and AV nodes must recharge. This process is known as 'atrial and ventricular repolarization'. The SA and AV nodes recharge while the atria and ventricles are refilling with blood (Herring and Paterson 2018). This process takes less than one-third of a second, resulting in a minimal pause in heart function. The times given for the three different stages are based on a heart rate of 60 beats per minute, or 1 beat per second.

The three stages of a single heart beat are therefore:

- atrial depolarization
- ventricular depolarization
- atrial and ventricular repolarization (Tortora and Derrickson 2017).

Pathophysiology of cardiopulmonary arrest

Cardiac arrest occurs when the cardiac output of the heart stops due to cessation of its mechanical activity. This is usually as a result of heart disease, such as coronary heart disease, cardiomyopathy, aortic valve stenosis, cardiac arrhythmias or congenital heart abnormalities.

Related theory

Cardiac arrest implies a sudden interruption of cardiac output. It may be reversible with appropriate treatment (RCUK 2015). The four arrhythmias that are found in cardiac arrest are:

- asystole (Figure 12.55a)
- pulseless electrical activity (PEA) (Figure 12.55b, although PEA can look like any rhythm that would normally be compatible with life)
- pulseless ventricular tachycardia (VT) (Figure 12.55c)
- ventricular fibrillation (VF) (Figure 12.55d).

For the purposes of resuscitation guidelines, these rhythms are divided into two groups:

- VF and pulseless VT require defibrillation (shockable rhythms).
- Asystole and PEA do not require defibrillation (non-shockable rhythms).

Potentially reversible causes of a cardiopulmonary arrest

During cardiac arrest, potential causes or aggravating factors for which specific treatment exists should be considered. There are

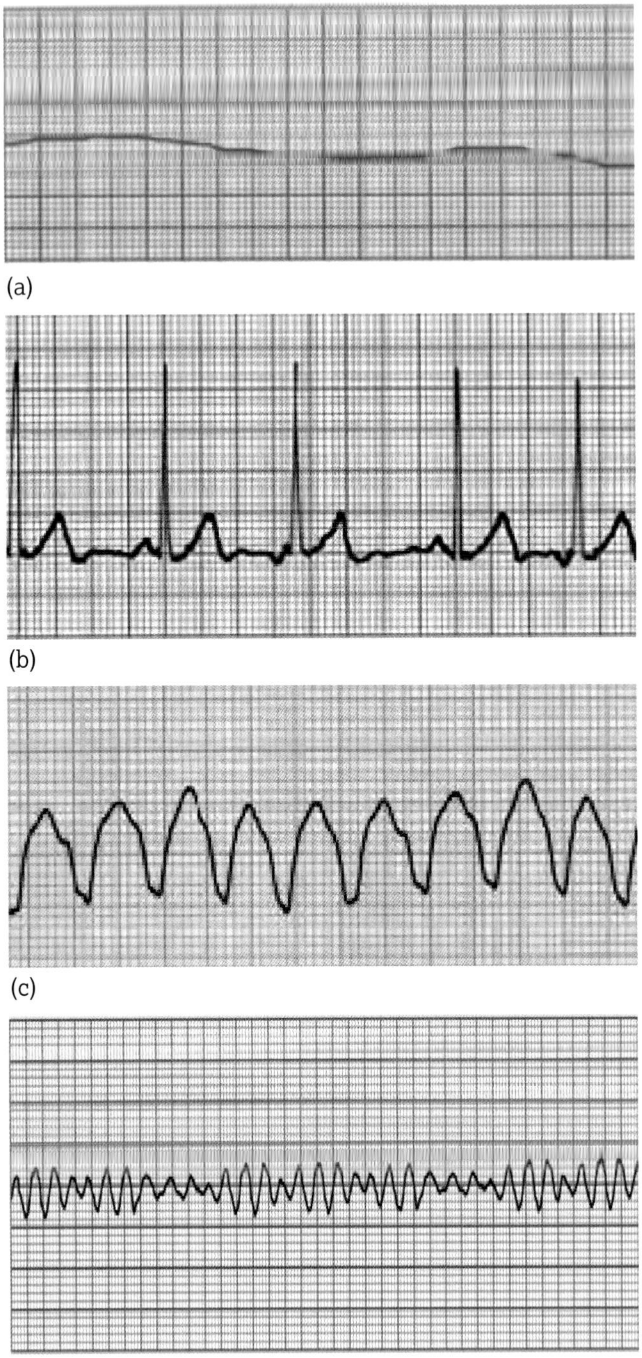

(a)

(b)

(c)

(d)

Figure 12.55 Cardiac arrest rhythms. (a) Asystole: non-shockable. (b) Pulseless electrical activity (PEA): non-shockable. (c) Pulseless ventricular tachycardia (VT): shockable. (d) Ventricular fibrillation (VF): shockable. *Source*: Reproduced from RCUK (2015).

eight reversible causes of arrest, four of which begin with the letter H and four of which begin with the letter T; this can be useful in aiding memory (Table 12.11).

Hypoxia

For normal cell respiration, the body requires a constant supply of oxygen. When this is interrupted for more than 3 minutes (except when there is severe hypothermia), lactic acidosis and cell death occur. This can rapidly lead to cardiorespiratory arrest if left untreated. Patients may become severely hypoxic due to acute respiratory failure, airway obstruction or acute lung injury.

Table 12.11 Reversible causes of cardiac arrest

Hs	Ts
• Hypoxia • Hypovolaemia • Hypokalaemia, hyperkalaemia and other metabolic disorders • Hypothermia	• Thrombosis: coronary or pulmonary • Tamponade • Toxicity: poisining and drug intoxication • Tension pneumothorax

Hypoxia in cardiac arrest is treated by ensuring that the patient's lungs are adequately ventilated with as near to 100% oxygen as possible. The patient also receives good-quality chest compressions, which deliver oxygenated blood to the major organs (RCUK 2015).

Hypovolaemia

Hypovolaemia in adults results in PEA and is usually caused by severe blood loss. The most common causes of severe blood loss are:

- trauma
- surgical procedure
- gastrointestinal mucosa erosion
- oesophageal varices
- clotting abnormality
- peripheral vessel erosion (e.g. by tumour).

Although blood loss may be overt, it may not become apparent until the patient collapses. The treatment for hypovolaemia is identifying and stopping the source of fluid or blood loss, and replacing the circulating volume with the appropriate fluid.

A large-scale Cochrane review found no evidence that the use of colloids improves a patient's survival compared to the use of crystalloids (Lewis et al. 2018). Both colloids and crystalloids are solutions used to restore circulating volume. Colloids have larger molecules than crystalloids and can be synthetic (e.g. starches, dextrans or gelatins) or naturally occurring (e.g. albumin or fresh frozen plasma). Crystalloids are salt based (e.g. saline or Hartmann's solution) and contain smaller molecules than colloids. Furthermore, due to the considerable expense of colloids, fluid resuscitation is normally started with a crystalloid (e.g. 0.9% sodium chloride or compound sodium lactate solution). An acute loss of 30–40% of total blood volume (1500–2000 mL) will require blood product replacement. This will become a life-saving therapy if more than 40% (>2000 mL) of the total blood volume is lost (Shander et al. 2013).

Hypokalaemia, hyperkalaemia and other metabolic disorders

An imbalance of potassium affects both the nerve conduction and the muscular function of the heart. A severe rise or fall in potassium can cause arrhythmias, which will cause cardiac arrest. Hypokalaemia is defined as plasma potassium below 3.5 mmol/L. It may be classified as (RCUK 2015):

- mild: <3.5 mmol/L
- severe: <2.5 mmol/L.

The causes of hypokalaemia are:

- gastrointestinal fluid losses
- polyuria
- fluid shifts between intra- and extracellular spaces
- drugs that affect cellular potassium, for example antifungal agents such as amphotericin.

The immediate treatment for hypokalaemia that has resulted in cardiac arrest is to give concentrated infusions of potassium while carefully monitoring serial potassium measurements. During cardiac arrest or in an emergency, potassium levels can be checked promptly via a venous or arterial blood gas. Prolonged CPR attempts may be required in order to allow for potassium replacement.

Hyperkalaemia is defined as plasma potassium in excess of 5.5 mmol/L. It may be classified as (Wilkinson et al. 2017):

- mild: 5.5–5.9 mmol/L
- moderate: 6.0–6.4 mmol/L
- severe: 6.5 mmol/L and above.

Patients who are most at risk of hyperkalaemia are those with renal failure, heart failure and/or diabetes (Adamson 2015). The immediate treatment for severe hyperkalaemia is to give intravenous calcium gluconate, which protects the myocardium (Wilkinson et al. 2017). Efforts should then move to the 'shifting' or removal of excess potassium. Methods for achieving this include administering a combination of insulin and glucose via rapid infusion in an attempt to move the potassium into the cells. Alternatively, removal via dialysis can be considered in specialist centres with the ability to do so.

Hypothermia

Hypothermia is defined as a core temperature below 35°C and is classified as (Malhotra et al. 2013):

- mild: 32–35°C
- moderate: 30–32°C
- severe: below 30°C.

Temperature is normally tightly regulated but is less well controlled in the very young, the elderly, and those with chronic disease, injury or intoxication. As the body cools, the metabolic rate falls and neural transmission is inhibited. Multiple derangements occur, which ultimately lead to reduced tissue oxygenation, including (Malhotra et al. 2013):

- depressed myocardial contractility
- leftward shift of the oxygen dissociation curve
- vasoconstriction
- ventilation/perfusion mismatch
- increased blood viscosity.

Initially, in an attempt to retain heat and body temperature, the sympathetic drive increases the heart rate and respiratory rate, and heat is produced via shivering. At around 30°C, this process ceases and ventilation, heart rate, blood pressure and cardiac output fall. Intravascular volume falls due to a cold diuresis and fluid shifts into the extravascular space. Sinus bradycardia develops followed by atrial fibrillation. Below 28°C, ventricular arrhythmias (including VF) may occur before the patient finally goes into asystole (Schober et al. 2014).

Hypothermia should be suspected in any submersion or immersion injury. Resuscitation in the presence of hypothermia should continue until the patient is warmed to normothermia or as near to it as possible. Resuscitation attempts in a patient who is hypothermic may therefore be prolonged. Conversely, it is important to be mindful that a prolonged resuscitation attempt may lead to a patient who was normothermic at the onset of cardiac arrest becoming hypothermic (RCUK 2015).

Thrombosis: coronary or pulmonary

The most common cause of thromboembolic or mechanical circulatory obstruction is a massive pulmonary embolus (Konstantinides et al. 2014). Options for definitive treatment include thrombolysis, cardiopulmonary bypass and operative removal of the clot (RCUK 2015).

Acute coronary syndromes (ACS) are a group of clinical conditions, all of which usually present with chest pain or discomfort resulting in myocardial ischaemia:

- ST segment elevation myocardial infarction (STEMI)
- non ST elevation myocardial infarction (NSTEMI)
- unstable angina.

Commonly, an ACS is initiated by the rupture or erosion of an atherosclerotic plaque within a coronary artery. This causes:

- acute thrombosis within the vessel lumen, often with haemorrhagic extension into the atherosclerotic plaque
- contraction of the smooth muscle cells within the artery wall, resulting in vasoconstriction and reducing the lumen of the artery
- associated partial or complete obstruction of the lumen, often with an embolism or thrombus in the distal part of the vessel.

The above process causes a rapid and critical reduction in blood flow to the myocardium. The degree and extent of this reduction in blood flow are largely determined by the clinical presentation and type of ACS (RCUK 2015).

Tamponade

Tamponade is where there is an acute effusion of fluid in the pericardial space, which is usually blood but can be malignant or infected fluid ([illegible] 2015). As the collection of fluid increases, the heart is splinted until it can no longer beat (tamponade).

The most common cause of a sudden tamponade is penetrating chest trauma, in which case resuscitative thoracotomy may be indicated. Otherwise, pericardiocentesis should be performed (Fitch et al. 2012). If resuscitation is successful, follow-up surgery may also be required (Harper 2010).

Toxicity: poisoning and drug intoxication

Poisoning rarely leads to cardiac arrest but it is a leading cause of death in patients less than 40 years old; self-poisoning with therapeutic or recreational drugs is the main reason for hospital admission in this group of patients (Truhlar et al. 2015). There are few specific therapeutic measures for poisons that are useful in the immediate situation. The emphasis must be on intensive supportive therapy, with correction of hypoxia, acid/base balance and electrolyte disorders. Specialist information and guidance can be obtained from pharmacists and the TOXBASE website (https://www.toxbase.org).

Tension pneumothorax

A tension pneumothorax can develop from either a spontaneous pneumothorax or a traumatic pneumothorax (RCUK 2015). The most common causes are:

- trauma
- acute lung injury
- mechanical ventilation with excessive positive pressure and/or volume.

A breach in the pleura allows air to flow into the pleural space during inhalation but it is retained in the pleural cavity during exhalation. Thus, the air cannot exit, and this leads to a gradual increase in the intrapleural cavity pressure, inducing an interthoracic shift. During tension pneumothorax, the affected lung completely collapses and the contralateral lung and heart are pressurized (Choi 2014). The result is severe dyspnoea and cyanosis due to hypoxia, in addition to hypotension caused by restriction of the venous return to the heart (Roberts et al. 2015). Ultimately, a tension pneumothorax is an acute emergency and can lead to death if it is not imminently treated. During cardiac arrest, a tension pneumothorax should be treated with immediate needle decompression (Choi 2014). The procedure involves insertion of a large-bore cannula into the second intercostal space at the mid-clavicular line on the affected side (RCUK 2015). The aim is to expel the pressure and create an outlet for trapped air. This should be followed up with the insertion of a chest drain.

Evidence-based approaches

Sudden death as a result of cardiac arrest is responsible for 60% of ischaemic heart disease deaths across Europe (RCUK 2015). The

British Heart Foundation (2018) also reports that of the 545 people who attend hospital within the UK each day with heart-attack-like symptoms, 180 people die.

Changes to adult basic life support (BLS) guidelines have been made to reflect the importance of performing high-quality chest compressions. The rescuer should minimise the number and duration of pauses during chest compressions (RCUK 2015). The duration of collapse is frequently difficult to estimate accurately, so CPR should be given before attempting defibrillation outside hospital, unless the arrest is witnessed by a healthcare professional or an automated external defibrillator is being used (RCUK 2015). Audit and reports of cardiac arrest demonstrate that 70% of in-hospital cardiac arrests are found to be in asystole and PEA; however, only 8–10% of those cardiac arrests are followed by survival to hospital discharge (Nolan et al. 2014).

Rationale

Changes to Resuscitation Council UK guidelines suggest that the BLS rescuer should make a rapid, simple assessment of the patient to determine they are in cardiorespiratory arrest and commence BLS immediately. The rescuer should not stop to check the patient or discontinue CPR unless the person starts to show signs of life, such as regaining consciousness, coughing, opening eyes, speaking or moving purposefully, and starts to breathe normally (RCUK 2015).

Indications

BLS is indicated if the patient is unconscious, has absent or agonal (gasping) respirations, and has no pulse.

Contraindications

BLS is contraindicated:

- if a valid Do Not Attempt Cardiopulmonary Resuscitation (DNaCPR) order is in place
- if the environment would place the rescuer at risk (in which case, do not attempt resuscitation until the environment is made safe).

Clinical governance

Do Not Attempt Cardiopulmonary Resuscitation

The rate of survival after an in-hospital cardiac arrest is still only in the region of 10%, depending on numerous factors, such as initial cardiac ECG (electrocardiogram) rhythm, co-morbidities, age, performance status (a measure of the patient's activity level and performance), reason for hospital admission and cause of cardiac arrest (Findlay et al. 2012, Meaney et al. 2010, Nolan et al. 2014). To reduce the number of futile resuscitation attempts, many hospitals and organizations have introduced formal DNaCPR policies, which can be applied to individual patients in specific circumstances. Healthcare professionals must be able to show that their decisions relating to CPR are compatible with the Human Rights Act (1998) as every person has the right to life, the right to be free from inhumane or degrading treatment, and freedom of expression (BMA et al. 2016). Where no such decision has been made and the wishes of the patient are unknown, CPR should be performed without delay (RCUK 2015).

The following guidelines are based on those provided in a joint statement by the British Medical Association, the Royal College of Nursing and the RCUK (BMA et al. 2016):

- An advance DNaCPR order should only be made after consideration of the likely clinical outcome, the patient's wishes and their human rights. Each individual case should take into consideration whether:
  - attempting CPR would restart the patient's heart and breathing
  - there would be no benefit to restarting the patient's heart and breathing
  - the expected benefit is outweighed by the burdens (RCUK 2015).
- The clinician has a duty to discuss the decision with the patient, even if the discussion is likely to upset and distress the patient. The exception to this is if such a discussion is thought likely to cause the patient significant physical or psychological harm, in which case it may not be appropriate (BMA et al. 2016). Neither patients nor those close to them can demand treatment that is clinically inappropriate. If the healthcare team believes that CPR will not be successful, this should be explained to the patient in a sensitive way. Written information explaining CPR should be available for patients and those close to them to read. The aforementioned joint statement may help patients and their families to discuss DNaCPR with medical and nursing staff (BMA et al. 2016).
- Patients who are deemed to have metal capacity are entitled to refuse CPR even when there is a reasonable chance of success (Mental Capacity (Amended) Act 2019).
- The overall responsibility for decisions about CPR and DNaCPR orders rests with the consultant in charge of the patient's care. Issues should, however, be discussed with other members of the healthcare team, the patient and people close to the patient where appropriate.
- The most senior members of the medical and nursing team available should clearly document any decisions made about CPR in the patient's medical and nursing notes. The decision should be dated and the reasons for it given. This information must be communicated to all other relevant healthcare professionals (BMA et al. 2016). Unless it is against the wishes of the patient, their family should also be informed.
- The DNaCPR order should be reviewed on each admission and reconsidered if the patient's condition changes (BMA et al. 2016).
- Finally, it should be noted that a DNaCPR order applies only to CPR and should not reduce the standard of medical or nursing care (Moffat et al. 2016). Any reversible conditions identified should be treated as deemed appropriate.

Each hospital should audit all CPR attempts and assess what proportion of patients should have had a DNaCPR decision in place prior to the cardiac arrest and should not have undergone CPR, rather than have the decision made after the patient has arrested. This will improve future patient care by avoiding undignified and potentially harmful CPR attempts during the dying process (Findlay et al. 2012).

Pre-procedural considerations

Assessment

There are two stages of assessment:

1 An immediate assessment is made by the rescuer to ensure that CPR may safely proceed (i.e. checking there is no immediate danger to the rescuer from any hazard, for example an electrical power supply).
2 The rescuer assesses the likelihood of injury being sustained by the patient as a result of CPR, particularly injury to the cervical spine. Although there may be no external evidence of injury, the immediate situation may provide the necessary evidence. For example, trauma to the cervical spine should be suspected in an accelerating or decelerating injury, such as a fall or road traffic accident.

Once these two aspects have been assessed, the patient's level of consciousness should be checked by shaking their shoulders and loudly asking whether they are alright (Figure 12.56). If there is no response, the rescuer should commence a rapid 'look, listen and feel' assessment.

Airway

The most likely obstruction in an unconscious person is the tongue. The head tilt, chin lift manoeuvre (Figure 12.57), which prevents the tongue from occluding the oropharynx, is an

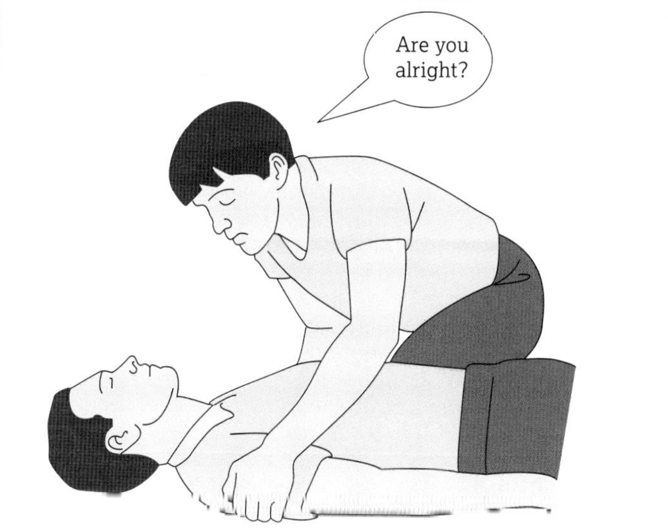

Figure 12.56 Assessing for signs of life.

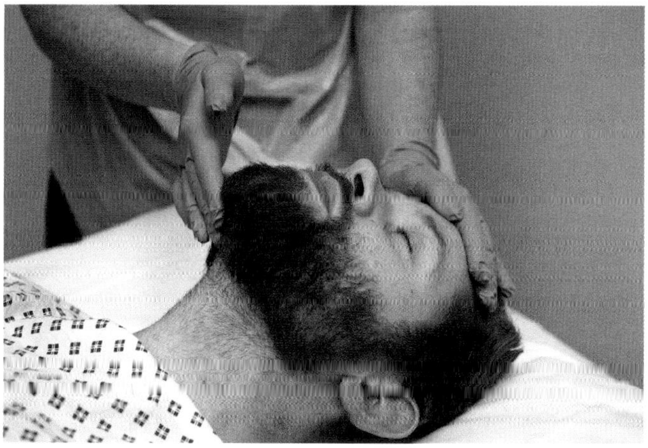

Figure 12.57 Head tilt, chin lift.

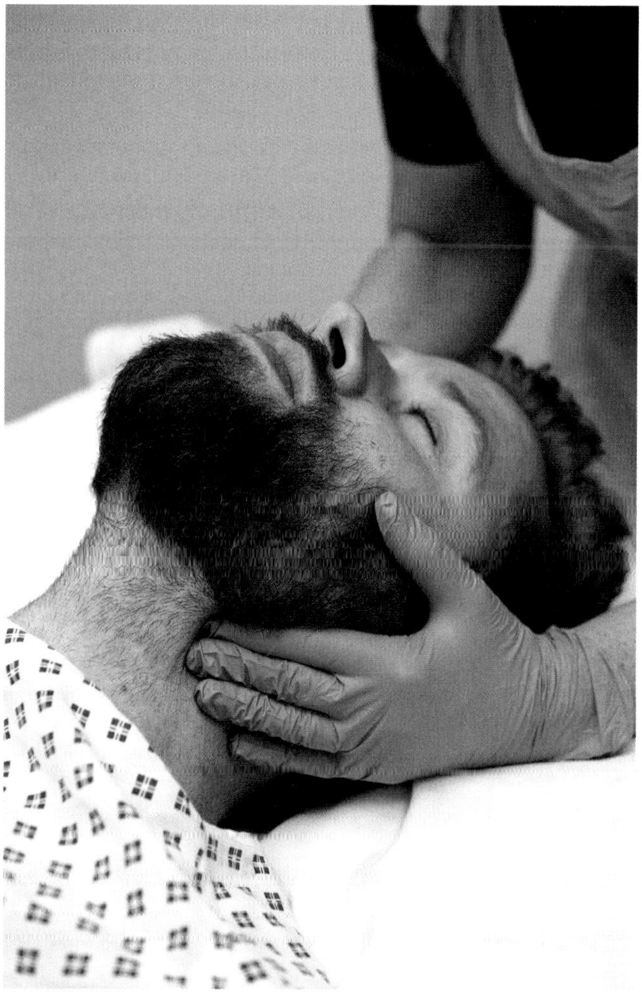

Figure 12.58 Jaw thrust.

effective method of opening an airway and relieving obstruction (Wittels 2018). If there is any suspicion of cervical spine injury, establish a clear upper airway by performing a jaw thrust (Figure 12.58) or chin lift with manual in-line stabilization (Prasarn et al. 2014).

The rescuer should look in the mouth and remove any visible obstruction (leave well-fitting dentures in place). A wide-bore suction catheter, such as a Yankauer, should be used to remove blood, saliva or gastric contents from the upper airway. This is best done under direct vision during intubation but should not result in any delay in achieving a definitive airway (RCUK 2015). If tracheal suction is necessary, it should be as brief as possible, preceded and followed by ventilation with 100% oxygen.

Breathing

Keeping the airway open, the rescuer should look, listen and feel for breathing (more than an occasional gasp or weak attempts at breathing) for up to 10 seconds. If the patient is breathing normally, they should be moved into the recovery position (Figure 12.59). If the patient is not breathing, an immediate call for the cardiac arrest team should be made. Normal breathing should not be confused with agonal respirations, which are infrequent, slow and noisy gaps, often seen within the first few minutes after cardiac arrest (RCUK 2015, Riou et al. 2018). If there is any doubt as to whether breathing is normal, prepare to start CPR.

Circulation

Circulation is assessed simultaneously with assessment of breathing. The rescuer should look for any signs of life, including movement, swallowing or breathing. If the rescuer is trained to do so, a pulse check should also be made by feeling the carotid pulse (Figure 12.60).

Conclusion of the assessment

The above assessment should take less than 10 seconds to complete. The rapid assessment will indicate whether the patient is critically unwell and in need of immediate help. In the event of poor respiratory effort where no circulation is detected, cardiac compressions are used to maintain blood flow and ultimately oxygen delivery.

Chest compressions

The action of chest compressions squeezes the blood from the heart into the circulation. The downward pressure on the heart closes the mitral and tricuspid valves, preventing the backflow of blood between the ventricles and the atria. The aortic and pulmonary valves open in response to forward blood flow from the ventricles into the systemic and pulmonary circulation. The rescuer should position themselves vertically above the patient with arms straight and elbows locked. The heel of one hand is placed in the centre of the lower half of the sternum. The opposite hand is then placed directly on top and fingers interlocked (Figure 12.61).

Compressions should be given at a rate of 100–120 per minute and to a depth of 5–6 cm. The chest should be allowed to completely recoil between compressions to enable the heart to refill

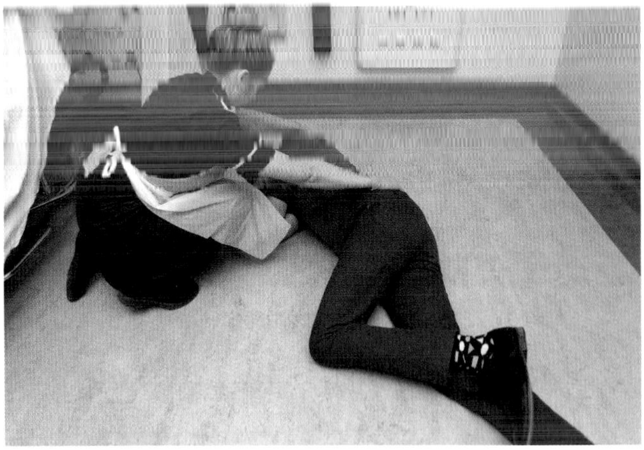

(a)

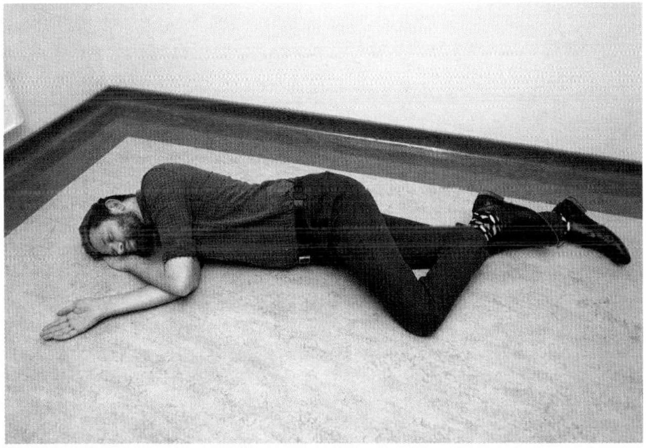

(b)

Figure 12.59 (a) Assisting the patient into the recovery position. (b) The patient in the recovery position.

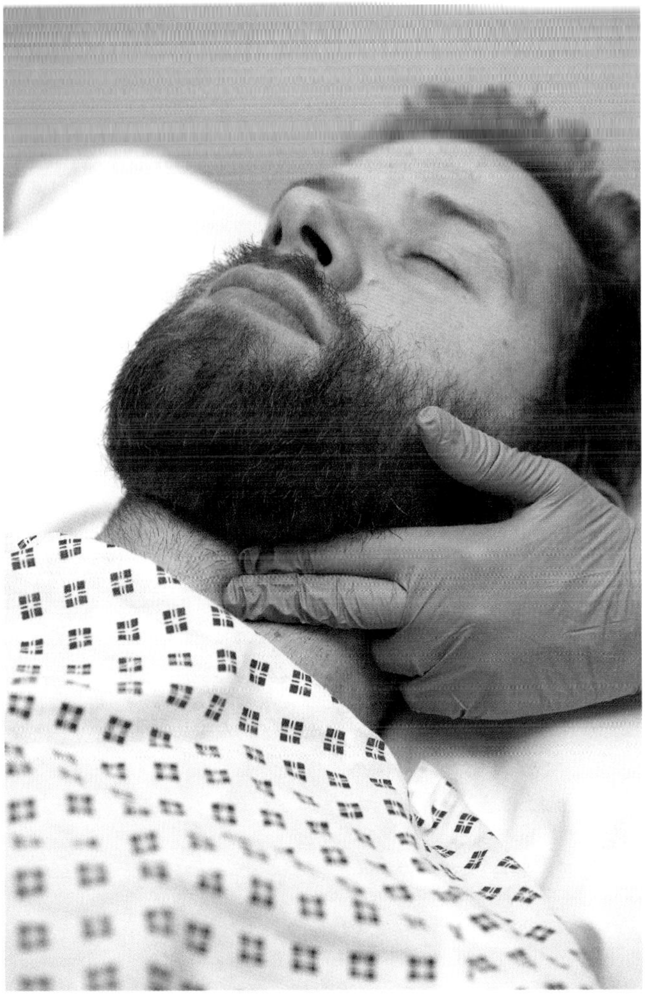

Figure 12.60 Feeling the carotid pulse.

with blood. The rescuer should give 30 compressions followed by two rescue breaths. The sequence of chest compressions to rescue breaths should then continue at a ratio of 30:2 (RCUK 2015). There is evidence recognizing that interruptions to the delivery of chest compressions are associated with a reduction in the chance of survival. Therefore, if chest compressions need to be interrupted, the pause should be pre-planned and last a few seconds only (RCUK 2015).

Rescue breaths

Mouth-to-mouth ventilation

Mouth-to-mouth ventilation should be considered only if there are no immediate aids available. There have been isolated reports of infections such as tuberculosis and severe acute respiratory syndrome following mouth-to-mouth ventilation but none resulting in the transmission of HIV (RCUK 2015). There is no evidence to quantify the degree of risk to the rescuer that arises from performing mouth-to-mouth ventilation, but it is widely acknowledged that many people may be reluctant, especially if the victim is not known to the rescuer. If mouth-to-mouth ventilation is given, the recommended length of each breath is 1 second.

Pocket mask or mouth-to-face-mask ventilation

Pocket mask or mouth-to-face-mask ventilation (Figure 12.62) can be used to avoid direct person to person contact. Some devices contain a filter that reduces the risk of cross-infection between patient and rescuer (RCUK 2015). The patient should be in the supine position with the head in the 'sniffing position' (head tilt, chin lift). Apply the mask to the patient's face using the thumbs of both hands. Lift the jaw into the mask with the remaining fingers by exerting pressure behind the angles of the jaw (jaw thrust) (Figure 12.63). Blow through the inspiratory valve and watch the chest rise. Stop inflation and allow the chest to fall before blowing in the second breath. The mask directs the patient's exhaled air and any fluid away from the rescuer, and the oxygen port allows attachment of oxygen with enrichment of up to 45%.

Oropharyngeal airway

An oropharyngeal airway is the recommended airway adjunct to be used in the event of a cardiac arrest (RCUK 2015). It is a curved plastic tube that is flanged and reinforced at the oral end, with a flattened shape to ensure that it fits neatly between the tongue and the hard palate. It is used to overcome backward tongue displacement in an unconscious patient (Wittels 2018). Oropharyngeal airways come in sizes 2, 3 and 4, for small, medium and large adults respectively. The right size is chosen by measuring the oropharyngeal airway against the patient's incisors to the angle of the jaw or mandible (see Procedure guideline 12.16: Insertion of an oropharyngeal airway, Action figure 4). The technique for inserting an oropharyngeal airway is outlined in Procedure guideline 12.16.

Bag valve mask

A bag valve mask (such as the Ambu bag) is the preferred means of delivering rescue breaths. When the device is attached to an oxygen supply, it can provide a patient with up to 85% oxygen. However, it should be emphasized that effective use of a bag valve mask requires two rescuers: one to hold the mask in place while

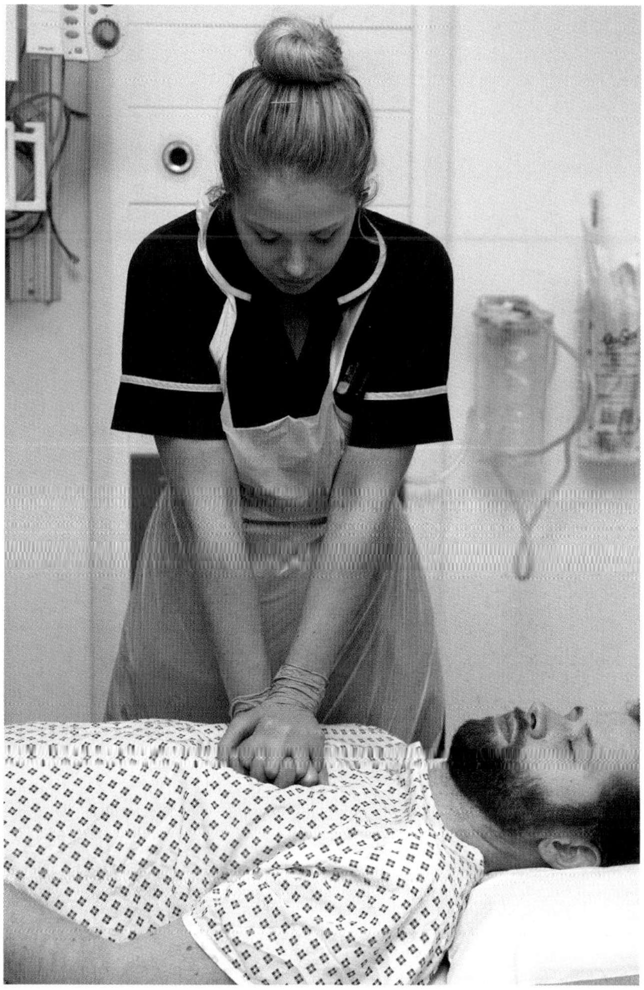

Figure 12.61 Correct hand and arm position for chest compressions.

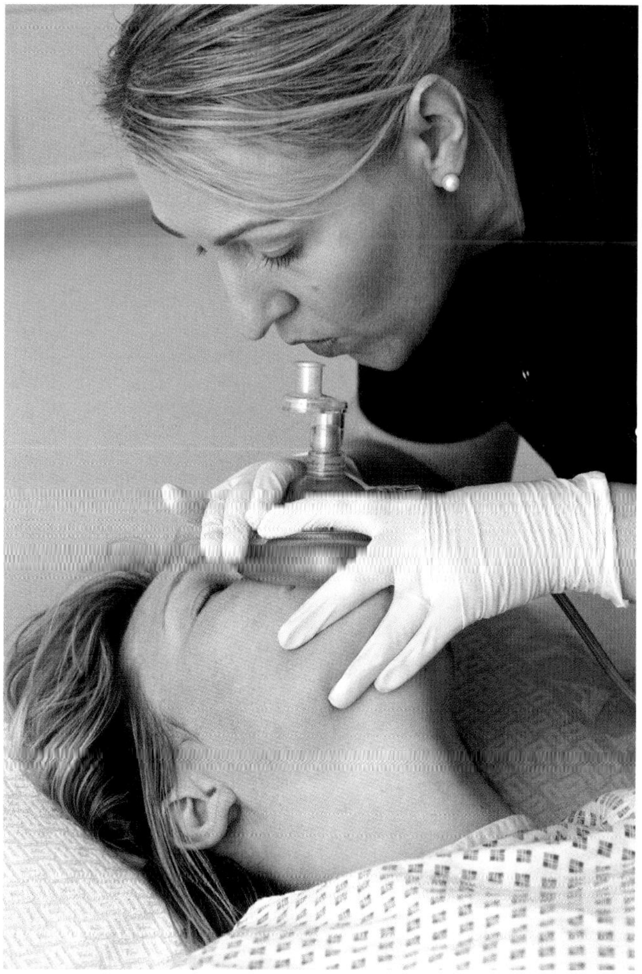

Figure 12.63 Mask with one way valve over patient's nose and mouth and rescuer giving breath.

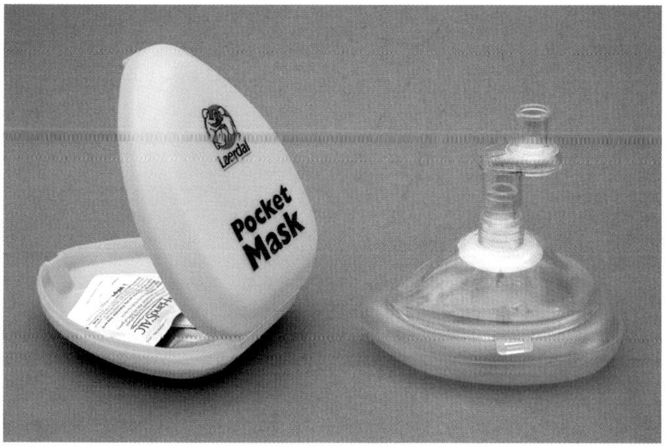

Figure 12.62 Pocket mask with oxygen port.

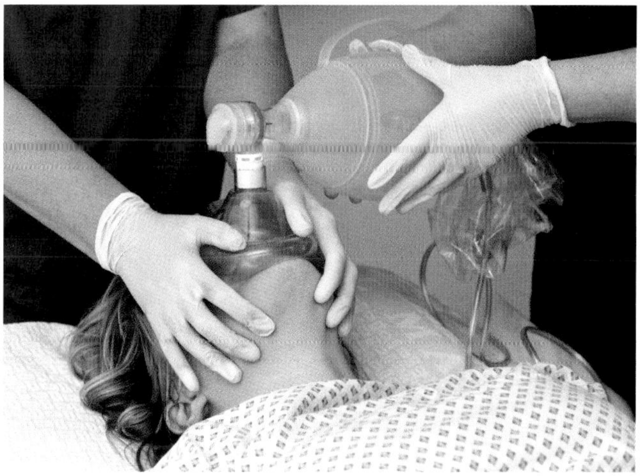

Figure 12.64 Two people ventilating a patient with a bag valve mask.

maintaining an open airway, while the second rescuer gently squeezes the bag (RCUK 2015) (Figure 12.64; see also Figure 12.65).

Defibrillation

Evidence-based approaches

Defibrillation causes a simultaneous depolarization of the myocardium and aims to restore a normal rhythm to the heart. This is the definitive treatment for VF and pulseless VT. It has been shown that 16% of adults who have a cardiac arrest in hospital are found to be in shockable VF or pulseless VT when first attached to a monitor or defibrillator (Nolan et al. 2014). Defibrillation can be delivered using either a manual defibrillator or an automated external defibrillator (AED).

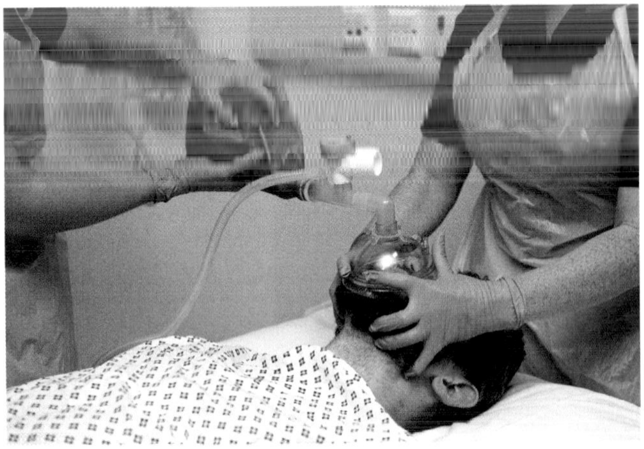

Figure 12.65 Two people ventilating a patient using a Mapleson C system.

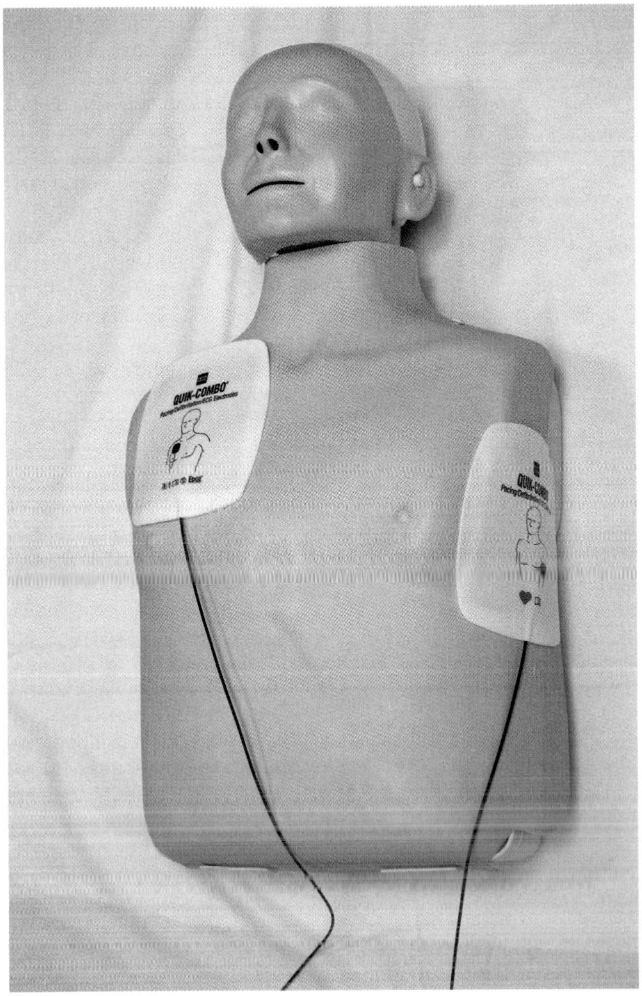

Figure 12.66 Standard position of self-adhesive electrodes.

The aim of an effective defibrillation strategy is to reduce the pre-shock pause to chest compressions to less than 5 seconds by planning ahead and continuing compressions while the defibrillator charges and a brief safety check is performed (RCUK 2015). Early defibrillation is a vital link in the chain of survival, hence the increase in public access to AEDs and first responder defibrillation by the public.

If an arrest is witnessed and monitored but a defibrillator is not immediately to hand, a single precordial thump (i.e. a sharp blow with a closed fist on the patient's sternum) should be administered. If this is delivered within 10 seconds of cardiac arrest, it may convert VF back to a perfusing rhythm (RCUK 2015).

Placement of self-adhesive electrodes (defibrillation pads)

The *standard positions* for electrode placement are the right (sternal) electrode to the right of the upper sternum below the clavicle, and the left (apical) electrode in the midaxillary line (Figure 12.66). The electrodes should be placed clear of any breast tissue.

Other acceptable electrode positions are:

- In *anteroposterior* placement, one electrode is placed anteriorly over the left precordium (Figure 12.67) and the other electrode is placed on the back, posterior to the heart. The posterior electrode should be placed inferior to the left scapula.
- In *biaxillary* placement, the electrodes are placed on the lateral chest walls, one on the right side and the other on the left (Figure 12.68).

Ensure good contact between the self-adhesive electrodes and the patient's skin. Ensure the skin is dry and consider shaving a very hairy chest; however, it should not delay placement of the electrodes and defibrillation. This also applies to the removal of jewellery and transdermal medication patches.

Safe defibrillation practice

High-flow oxygen in the presence of a spark or naked flame could present a danger to the patient and rescuers. It is therefore essential to ensure that oxygen tubing and equipment are moved away from the chest when defibrillation is performed. Using adhesive electrodes as opposed to defibrillation paddles may also minimize the danger (RCUK 2015).

A *metallic, wet or other conductive surface* does not usually compromise patient safety when defibrillation is performed. However, the nurse must ensure the self-adhesive electrodes are applied correctly and are in direct contact with the patient's skin. If the patient is wet, the chest should be dried so that the self-adhesive electrodes will stick securely (RCUK 2015).

Direct contact with the patient or bed must be avoided when a shock is delivered. This guarantees there is no direct pathway for electricity to take and so prevents the user and other rescuers from experiencing a shock (RCUK 2015). The person in charge of the defibrillator during cardiac arrest must order everyone to 'stand clear' while the shock is delivered.

Clinical governance

The use of an AED or shock advisory defibrillator (Perkins et al. 2015) is recommended to reduce mortality from cardiac arrests relating to ischaemic heart disease (Soar et al. 2015). While not all healthcare professionals are trained in manual defibrillation, the RCUK resuscitation guidelines suggest using an AED if one is available, as it can be used safely and effectively without previous training (RCUK 2015).

The administration of a defibrillator shock should not be delayed by waiting for more highly trained personnel to arrive. The same principle should apply to individuals whose period of qualification has expired (RCUK 2015).

To ensure best practice, make sure that practitioners' training in BLS – and, if appropriate, intermediate life support or advanced life support – is regularly updated (RCUK 2015).

Competencies

Cardiopulmonary resuscitation standards and training

The RCUK (2015) recommends the provision of an in-hospital resuscitation team and training for all staff, as outlined in Table 12.12.

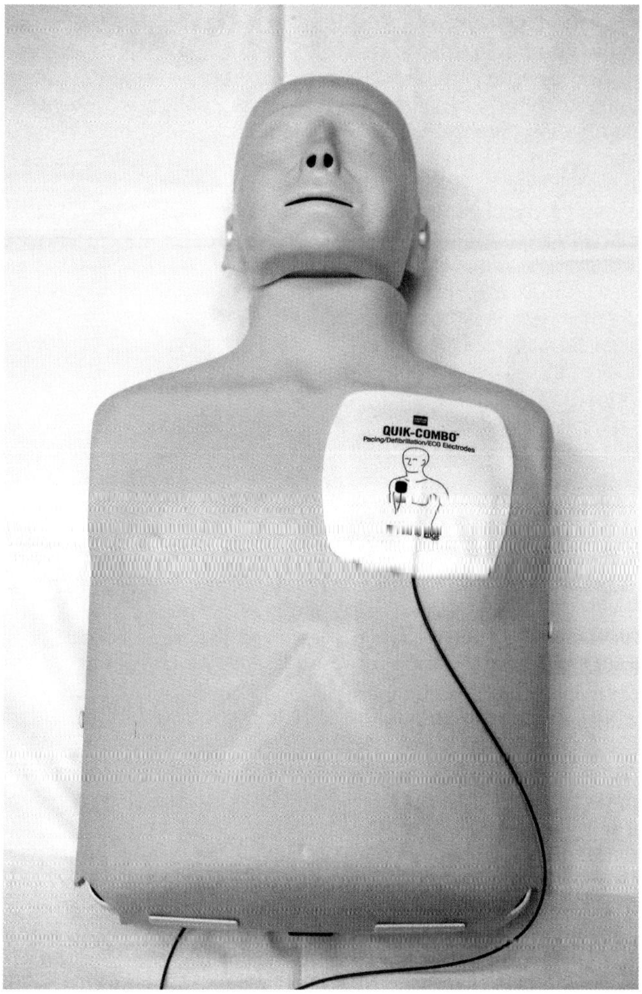

Figure 12.67 Anteroposterior position of self-adhesive electrodes.

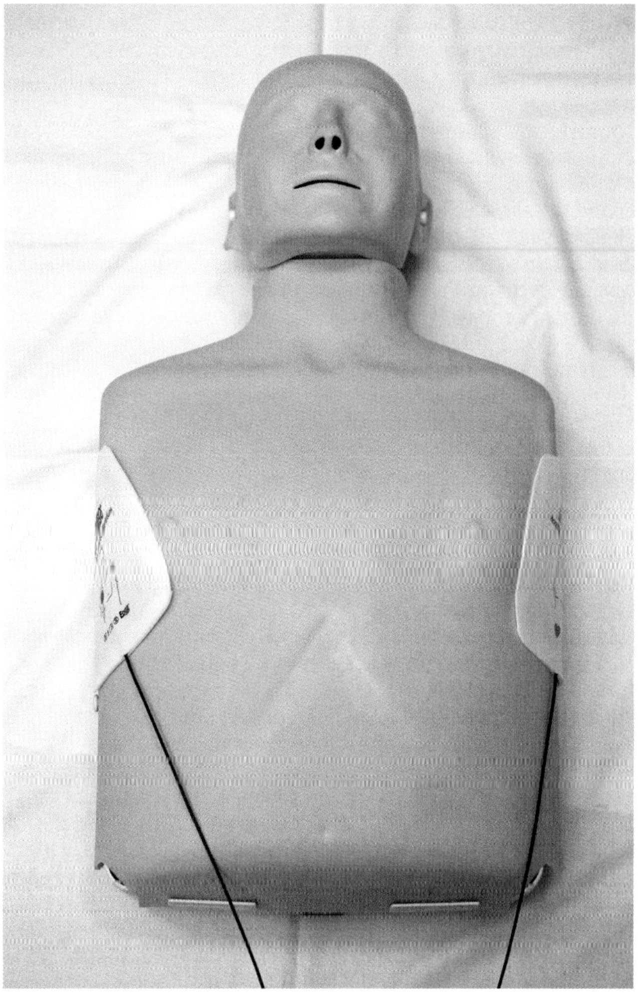

Figure 12.68 Biaxillary position of self-adhesive electrodes.

Table 12.12 Essential elements of an in-hospital resuscitation team

Element	Description
Resuscitation committee	The committee should consist of medical and nursing staff who advise on the role and composition of the cardiac arrest team, resuscitation equipment and resuscitation training equipment.
Resuscitation training officer (RTO)	The RTO should be responsible for all training in resuscitation, equipment maintenance, and the auditing of resuscitation and clinical trials.
Resuscitation training	Hospital staff should receive at least annual resuscitation training appropriate to their level and role. Medical and nursing staff should receive basic resuscitation training and should be encouraged to recognize patients who are at risk of having a cardiac arrest and to call for help early. This is the most effective method of improving outcomes (Harrison et al. 2014). All medical staff should have advanced resuscitation training, and senior nurses and doctors working in acute specialities (critical care units, intensive care units and A&E departments) should hold a valid RCUK intermediate life support (ILS) or advanced life support (ALS) certificate.
Cardiac arrest team	Each hospital should have a cardiac arrest team of approximately five people, including a minimum of two doctors (physician and anaesthetist), an ALS-trained nurse, the RTO and a porter when possible. Clear procedures should be available for calling the cardiac arrest team.
Medical emergency team	It is recommended that each hospital should have its own medical emergency or critical care outreach team to treat acutely deteriorating patients and avert cardiac arrest. Early warning scores and track-and-trigger systems such as NEWS (RCP 2017) have been established to assist nursing staff in the recognition of acutely deteriorating patients and provide guidelines regarding when to escalate and to whom (Tirkkonen et al. 2018).

Pre-procedural considerations

Equipment

All hospital wards and departments should have a standardized cardiac arrest trolley. Resuscitation equipment, including the AED or defibrillator, should be checked on a daily basis (RCUK 2015). A record of this check should be maintained.

Assessment and recording tools

Decisions relating to CPR ideally should have been documented prior to a cardiac arrest. Every hospital should have a DNaCPR policy based on national guidelines (RCUK 2015).

Procedure guideline 12.16 Insertion of an oropharyngeal airway

Equipment

- Personal protective equipment
- A range of oropharyngeal airways in a variety of sizes

Action	Rationale
Pre-procedure	
1 Assess the patient's consciousness level.	Only attempt the insertion of an oropharyngeal airway (OPA) in an unconscious patient, as vomiting and laryngospasm may otherwise occur (RCUK 2015, **C**).
2 Open patient's mouth and assess for loose dental fixtures. Remove any ill-fitting dentures. If foreign bodies are visible, remove with suction.	To minimize airway obstruction while avoiding injury to the soft palate (Soar et al. 2015, **C**).
3 Perform the head tilt, chin lift manoeuvre: place one hand on the patient's forehead and tilt the head back gently, then place the fingertips of the other hand under the point of the patient's chin and gently lift upwards to stretch the anterior neck structures. Alternatively, if there is a suspected injury to the cervical spine, use a jaw thrust. Approach the patient superior from their head. Identify the angle of the mandible, and provide upward and forward pressure with fingers to lift the mandible. Using thumbs, slightly open the mouth by downward displacement of the chin.	The position of the head and neck must be maintained to keep the airway patent and aligned (RCUK 2015, **C**). To protect the integrity of the cervical spine while ensuring a patent airway (RCUK 2015, **C**).
4 Select an OPA with a length that corresponds to the vertical distance between the patient's incisors and the angle of the jaw/mandible (**Action figure 4**).	An OPA that is too small will not maintain an open airway. An OPA that is too big may cause trauma, laryngospasm or worsening of the airway obstruction (Wittels 2018, **C**).
Procedure	
5 Insert the OPA into the oral cavity in the 'upside down' position. Advance to the junction of the hard and soft palates, then rotate the OPA through 180 degrees. Once it has been rotated, advance the OPA into the oropharynx (**Action figures 5a and 5b**).	The insertion technique avoids pushing the tongue back and downwards, potentially obstructing the airway (ERC 2015, **C**).
6 Ensure the flattened, reinforced section of the OPA is between the patient's teeth/gums and the flange is at the lips (**Action figure 6**).	This indicates correct positioning and improves airway patency (RCUK 2015, **C**).
Post-procedure	
7 Remove the OPA if the patient gags or strains.	This indicates that the patient is conscious and therefore unable to tolerate an airway adjunct. **E**

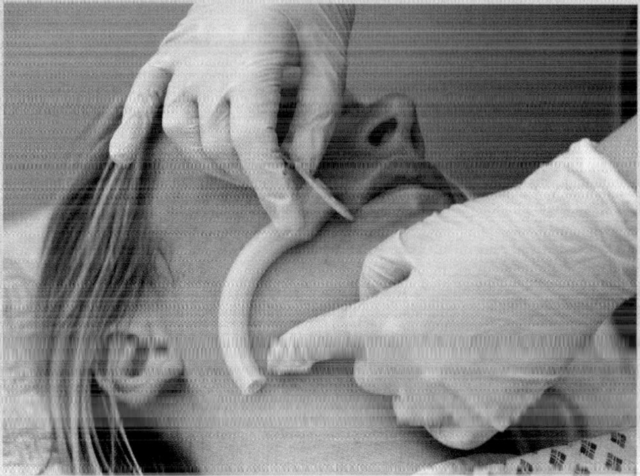

Action Figure 4 Sizing an oropharyngeal airway.

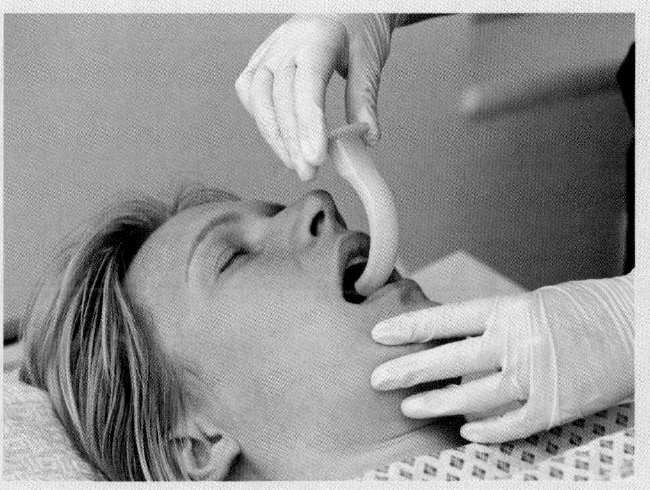
(a)

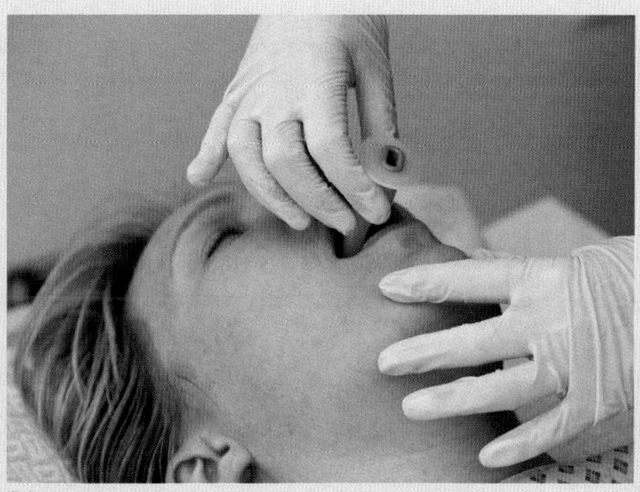
(b)

Action Figure 5 Insertion of an oropharyngeal airway.

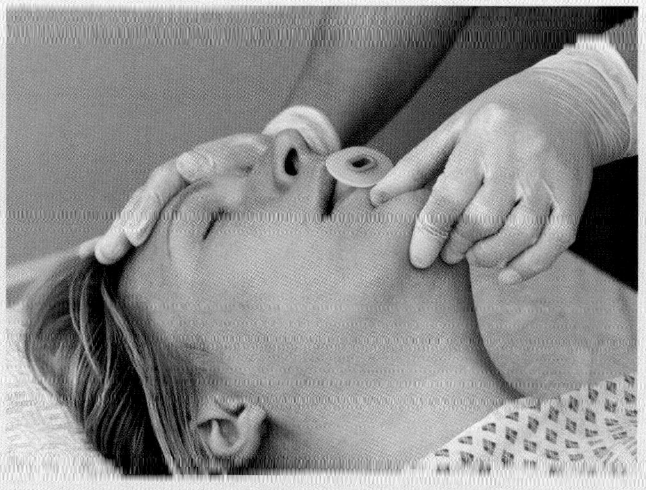

Action Figure 6 Correct placement of an oropharyngeal airway.

Procedure guideline 12.17 Basic life support

Essential equipment: airway and breathing management

- Oropharyngeal airways in sizes 2, 3 and 4
- Yankauer suckers × 2
- Suction (wall or portable)
- Oxygen supply or portable cylinders × 2 (if no wall oxygen)
- Reservoir mask
- Pocket masks with oxygen port
- Bag valve mask (BVM) with oxygen tubing
- Clear face-masks in sizes 4, 5 and 6

Essential equipment: circulation management

- Self-adhesive electrodes (defibrillator pads)
- ECG electrodes
- Intravenous cannulas: 18 G × 3, 14 G × 3
- Hypodermic needles: 21 G × 10
- Syringes: 2 mL × 6, 5 mL × 6, 10 mL × 6, 20 mL × 6
- Cannula securement dressings and tapes × 4
- Intravenous administration sets × 3
- 0.9% sodium chloride: 1000 mL bags × 2

Additional equipment

- Personal protective equipment
- Clock
- A sliding sheet or similar device (for safe handling)
- Cardiac arrest audit form

(continued)

Procedure guideline 12.17 Basic life support *(continued)*

Action	Rationale
Pre-procedure	
1 Shake the patient's shoulders and loudly ask whether they are okay.	To rouse the patient (if possible) and determine the need for emergency support (RCUK 2015, **C**).
2 If the above does not illicit a response, shout for help or press the emergency alarm bell.	The patient is acutely unwell and so requires immediate medical attention. **E**
Procedure	
3 Look, listen and feel for breathing. If trained to do so, palpate the carotid pulse.	To check that there are no signs of life to confirm cardiac arrest (RCUK 2015, **C**).
4 If no help is available, leave the patient and call/fast-bleep the cardiac arrest team before commencing CPR. If help is available, ask a member of staff to call/fast-bleep the cardiac arrest team. Another member of staff should bring the cardiac arrest trolley and screen off the area.	To ensure expert help is called prior to commencing CPR. **E** To ensure CPR starts as soon as possible after cardiac arrest is confirmed. **E**
5 Position the patient flat on a firm surface or bed. If the patient is in a chair, lower the patient to the floor while supporting their head. If the patient is nursed on a pressure-relieving mattress, pull the CPR cord to deflate the mattress.	Effective external cardiac massage can only be performed on a hard surface (RCUK 2015, **C**).
6 Note the time of cardiac arrest (if witnessed) or the time CPR is commenced.	Lack of cerebral perfusion for approximately 3–4 minutes can lead to irreversible brain damage; therefore, it is important to know the patient's 'down time' (RCUK 2015, **C**).
7 Stand directly over the patient's chest. Place the heel of one hand on the lower half of the sternum. Place the heel of the other hand on top and interlock the fingers. Keep arms straight and lock the elbows out (see Figure 12.61). If necessary, stand on a stool or kneel on the side of the patient's bed.	Performing direct chest compressions with a downward force improves patient outcome (ERC 2015, **C**). Positioning oneself at a height where effective chest compressions can be delivered improves patient outcome (RCUK 2015, **C**).
8 The sternum should be depressed sharply by 5–6 cm, with the chest allowed to fully recoil between each compression. Chest compressions should be sustained at a rate of 100–120 per minute.	Giving chest compressions at a depth of 5–6 cm and a rate of 100–120 per minute delivers an adequate cardiac output to the brain and other vital organs (RCUK 2015, **C**).
9 Do not remove well-fitted dentures.	Dentures help to create a mouth-to-mask seal during ventilation. **E**
10 The BVM should be attached to an oxygen source as soon as possible. The flow should be set at 15 L/min. If oxygen is not immediately available, the BVM can deliver ambient air.	An oxygen flow of 15 L/min and the use of a BVM (which incorporates a reservoir) delivers 85% oxygen to the patient during resuscitation (RCUK 2015, **C**).
11 Apply the face-mask with the BVM over the patient's nose and mouth and create a seal using the thumbs and forefingers to push the mask down onto the patient's face. The remaining fingers should pull the jaw up and into the mask.	A good seal around the mouth and nose ensures optimal ventilation of the lungs. **E**
12 Maintain cardiac compressions and ventilation at a ratio of 30:2. Allow a slight pause after each ventilator breath is delivered. Count aloud the number of chest compressions and BVM breaths delivered.	The delivery of chest compressions and ventilation at a ratio of 30:2 maintains circulation and oxygenation of the brain and other vital organs during cardiac arrest (RCUK 2015, **C**). A slight pause after each delivered breath allows the rescuer to observe whether the patient's chest rises. **E** Counting aloud will ensure co-ordination of compression and ventilation ratio, and minimize any delay in the delivery of effective CPR. **E**
Defibrillation	
13 As soon as an AED arrives, apply the electrodes/pads onto the patient's chest without disrupting CPR. It may be necessary to shave the chest if very hairy and adhesion of the electrode to the patient's skin is unlikely.	Timely defibrillation improves patient outcomes in patients who are in a shockable rhythm. To ensure the electrodes/pads are applied correctly and are in direct contact with the patient's skin, optimizing electrical conduction (RCUK 2015, **C**).
14 The person leading the cardiac arrest should advise the other practitioners to stop CPR to allow the AED to analyse the rhythm and determine whether the patient is in a shockable or non-shockable rhythm.	Any movement will interfere with the AED's ability to interpret the rhythm. **E**
15 The AED will advise whether a shock is appropriate. In the event of a shockable rhythm, the AED will advise that the shock button be pressed. A countdown will follow before a single shock is delivered to the patient.	Defibrillation is required to terminate pulseless VT or VF and restart the heart by depolarizing the electrical conduction system (ERC 2015, **C**).

16 While the AED analyses the rhythm, charges and delivers the shock, the team and any relatives/visitors must stand clear of the patient and bed. The person delivering the shock must ensure everyone is standing clear before pressing the shock button.	To ensure that no one is in contact with the patient or the bed, minimizing the risk of injury. **E**
17 Oxygen should be moved at least 1 metre away from the patient unless they are intubated.	To reduce the risk of sparks igniting the oxygen source (Sjoberg and Singer 2013, **C**).
18 If a shock is not advised by the AED, CPR should recommence for a further 2 minutes.	A patient who is in a non-shockable rhythm does not require defibrillation. CPR should recommence (RCUK 2015, **C**).
Intravenous access	
19 Venous access must be established through a large vein as soon as possible.	To allow the administration of emergency drugs and fluid replacement. **E**
20 The administration of drugs and solutions infused must be accurately recorded.	To maintain accurate records, provide a point of reference in the event of queries and prevent any duplication of treatment (NMC 2018, **C**).
Post procedure	
21 On the arrival of the cardiac arrest team, deliver a succinct and detailed handover and ensure roles are re-established.	To allow open communication of roles and responsibilities (RCUK 2015, **C**).
22 If the patient is in bed, remove the bed head and ensure adequate space between the back of the bed and the wall.	To allow easy access for the anaesthetist to facilitate intubation. **E**
23 Once the anaesthetist has established a definitive airway, the team must conduct cardiac compressions and ventilator breaths continually. Ventilations should continue at approximately 10–12 breaths per minute. CPR should be stopped every 2 minutes to re-analyse the rhythm using the AED.	To minimize interruptions and maximize the circulation of oxygenated blood (RCUK 2015, **C**).
24 Complete the cardiac arrest audit form.	To ensure all trust cardiac arrests are audited so services can be evaluated (RCUK 2015, **C**).

Problem-solving table 12.7 Prevention and resolution (Procedure guideline 12.17)

Problem	Cause	Prevention	Action
Inadequate chest compressions	Rescuer performing chest compressions tiring	Enable the rescuers performing chest compressions to change over every other cycle of CPR, or sooner if tiring.	The person leading the cardiac arrest should ensure the rescuer performing the chest compressions changes over every other cycle. This should be done with minimal interruption to CPR.
Chest not rising after attempted delivery of ventilation breath	Inadequate seal between the mask and the patient's face	Ensure two rescuers use the BVM to optimize the chance of delivering effective ventilation breaths.	Continue the next cycle of CPR if two ventilation breaths have already been attempted. Do not attempt to give a third ventilation breath.
Electrodes/pads not sticking	Excess hair Excess sweat Patient wet	Before attempting to stick the electrodes on, quickly remove excess hair with razor and towel dry the patient's chest to remove excess sweat or water.	Quickly shave the chest using a razor, or use spare adhesive electrodes/pads to swiftly rip out hair. Towel dry water or excess sweat.
Portable suction not working	Battery pack not charged	Ensure that the suction unit is plugged in so the battery can charge when not in use.	Ask another member of the team to locate an alternative portable suction unit.
	Tubing not connected correctly	Ensure the suction unit is properly set up and in working order.	Reconnect the tubing.
Equipment missing from resuscitation trolley	Removal of equipment without replacing or returning it	Maintain a checklist of all the equipment needed on the resuscitation trolley. Restock and recheck the trolley after each use. Perform regular checks of the trolley as per local policy. Seal or lock the trolley after use or the weekly check. Record the trolley checks.	Ask a member of the team to bring an alternative trolley or bag from another ward or department.

BVM, bag valve mask; CPR, cardiopulmonary resuscitation.

Post-procedural considerations

Immediate care

The patient should be handed over to the cardiac arrest team to provide ongoing advanced life support. If the patient has a return of spontaneous circulation, the cardiac arrest team will consider moving them to an appropriate intensive care or high dependency environment once they have been stabilized. The person leading the cardiac arrest should continue to do so after the return of spontaneous circulation, or if resuscitation has been unsuccessful. They should determine who is best to facilitate the transfer, who should update the patient's next of kin, and any other issues that need to be addressed. The pastoral needs of all those professionals involved in the arrest should not be forgotten (RCUK 2015) and a debrief session is advised, regardless of whether the resuscitation was successful or not.

Informing next of kin, families and carers

The Nursing and Midwifery Council (2018) is clear that nurses should only share information with the next of kin (NOK) when consent has been given to do so. Nurses must also uphold the Mental Capacity (Amended) Act (2019) and make sure that the rights and best interests of those who lack capacity are at the centre of the decision-making process (NMC 2018). In the event of a cardiac arrest, when the patient will lack capacity, nurses must immediately notify the NOK. If the NOK is not present, a phone call can be made. Best practice dictates to always try to speak to the NOK directly, without releasing information to whoever answers the phone if at all possible (DH 2003). High-quality communication is one of the most important aspects for families (Lautrette et al. 2007); therefore, while informing the patient's NOK of a cardiac arrest is a difficult task, it must be handled sensitively and with empathy. Information given should be relevant and communicated in a way that can be understood (NMC 2018).

In recent years, many hospital trusts have adopted policies that allow for family or the NOK to be present during resuscitation. The psychological benefits for the family or the NOK include enhancing acceptance and closure, and a reduction in the incidence of post-traumatic distress syndrome (Goldberger et al. 2015). Importantly, the above benefits stand even if the patient outcome is death (Jabre et al. 2013). However, despite the well-documented evidence and an increase in trust policies, barriers still exist. Reasons include healthcare professionals' perception that families might interrupt care, a lack of space to accommodate family members in the room and a perceived increased risk of litigation (Fernandez et al. 2009).

Documentation

Good record keeping is an integral part of nursing practice and is essential in the provision of safe and effective care (Griffith 2016, NMC 2018). Both nursing and medical staff should document the events leading up to the incident, details of the cardiac arrest, any decisions made and the patient outcome.

Hospitals should collect data regarding cardiac arrest for the National Cardiac Arrest Audit (NCAA), ideally using a nationally recognized template such as the Utstein template (RCUK 2015). Accurate recording of the time BLS commenced and the timings of each intervention, including any drugs (and dose) administered during cardiac arrest, is essential. The appointment of a scribe during the cardiac arrest is therefore recommended (RCUK 2015).

Education of the patient and relevant others

Education of patients and relevant others should be geared towards the promotion of healthy living and the prevention of cardiac disease. This includes eating a healthy, balanced diet low in sugar and saturated fat, as well as exercise, smoking cessation, and regular checkups to treat or control any underlying conditions such as hypertension and diabetes.

Complications

Table 12.13 lists some of the most prevalent complications that may arise from CPR.

Table 12.13 Complications of cardiac arrest

Complication	Description
Fractures of the ribs and/or sternum leading to punctured lungs	Fractures can occur as a result of chest compressions. The correct placement of hands during chest compression is vital in helping to prevent fracturing of the ribs and sternum. However, fractured rib(s) and/or sternum are often inevitable during cardiac arrest.
Gastric distension	Manual ventilation (via bag valve mask) during resuscitation causes air to enter the stomach. Excess air may cause the patient to vomit and aspirate gastric contents into their lungs (Afacan et al. 2014). It is therefore good practice to insert a nasogastric tube once the airway has been secured.
Brain injury	Brain injury is a leading cause of mortality and long-term neurological disability in survivors of cardiac arrest. Primary brain injury is related to hypoxia due to cessation of cerebral blood flow. Secondary brain injury is most commonly related to oedema, which causes an increase in intracranial pressure and a corresponding decrease in cerebral perfusion (O'Connor 2017). Other causes of secondary brain injury include reperfusion injury, microcirculatory dysfunction, impaired cerebral autoregulation, hypoxaemia, hyperoxia, hyperthermia, fluctuations in arterial carbon dioxide, and concomitant anaemia (Sekhon et al. 2017).

Transfusion of blood and blood components

Definition

'Blood transfusion' refers to the act of transferring blood or blood components from one person (the donor) into the blood stream of another person (the recipient). 'Transfusion' refers to the act of transferring donated blood, blood products, or other fluid into the circulatory system of a person or animal. Whole blood is rarely transfused; instead, blood is prepared into its constituent parts and the patient is given the specific component required (Norfolk 2013). The Blood Safety and Quality Regulations (2005) define blood components (red cells, white cells, platelets and plasma) as therapeutic constituents of human blood that can be prepared for transfusion by various methods.

Anatomy and physiology

ABO and Rh D blood groups

In 1901, Karl Landsteiner discovered that human blood groups existed and identified the ABO system; this marked the start of safe blood transfusion (Bishop 2008). There are four principal blood groups: A, B, AB and O. Each group relates to the presence or absence of surface antigens on the red blood cells and antibodies in the serum, and these antigens and antibodies dictate ABO compatibility (Table 12.14). A key recommendation of the 2017 Serious Hazards of Transfusion (SHOT) report was that all staff involved in the transfusion process, both laboratory and clinical, must have an understanding of the A, B, O and Rh D blood groups so that incompatibility will be recognized (Bolton-Maggs 2018). However, there are many more blood groups than the ones mentioned in this chapter.

Table 12.14 Red cell compatibility

Group	Antigens	Immunoglobulin M antibodies	Compatible donor for	Compatible recipient of
A	A	Anti-B	A and AB	A and O
B	B	Anti-A	B and AB	B and O
AB	A and B	None	AB	A, B, AB and O
O	No A or B	Anti-A and Anti-B	A, B, AB and O	O

People with the blood group AB have red cells with A and B surface antigens, but they do not have any anti-A or anti-B immunoglobulin M (IgM) antibodies in their serum. Therefore, they are able to receive blood from any group but can only donate to other people from group AB.

People with group O red cells do not have either A or B surface antigens but they do have anti-A and anti-B IgM antibodies in their serum. They are only able to receive blood from group O but can donate to people in the A, B, AB and O groups.

People with group A red cells have type A surface antigens and they have anti-B IgM antibodies in their serum. They are only able to receive blood from groups A or O and can only donate blood to people from the A and AB groups.

People with group B red cells have type B surface antigens and they have anti-A IgM antibodies in their serum. They are therefore only able to receive blood from groups B or O and can only donate blood to people from the B and AB groups.

In addition to the ABO system, the Rh blood group was discovered in 1940; again, Rh blood group antigens are surface antigens and they are another essential system used in transfusion therapy and safety (Klein and Anstee 2014). The Rh D antigen is the most immunogenic of the Rh antigens (Porth 2005). Approximately 85% of Caucasians have the D antigen and are therefore Rh positive, whereas approximately 15% lack the D antigen and are Rh negative (Daniels 2013). Several hundred red cell transfusion-related antigens have now been identified. Antibody production can happen after contact with 'non-self' blood antigens, usually due to transfusion or pregnancy (Zwaginga and van Ham 2013).

Related theory

Blood group incompatibility

The transfusion of ABO-incompatible red cells can lead to intravascular haemolysis, where the recipient's anti-A and/or anti-B IgM antibodies bind to the corresponding surface antigens of the transfused cells (Norfolk 2013). Complement activation results in lysis of the transfused cells and the haemoglobin that is released precipitates renal failure, with the fragments of the lysed cells activating the clotting pathways, which in turn leads to the development of disseminated intravascular coagulation (Klein and Anstee 2014).

Transfusion of Rh D-positive cells to a Rh D-negative individual will result in immunization and the appearance of anti-D antibodies in at least 30% of recipients (Daniels 2013). If the person is immunized and undergoes any subsequent exposure to D-positive red cells, extravascular haemolysis occurs as Rh antibody-coated red cells are destroyed by macrophages in the liver and spleen (McClelland 2007). This can present as a severe immediate or delayed haemolytic transfusion reaction (Daniels 2013).

A patient's Rh status is of particular importance if they are female and of child-bearing age or require a transfusion during pregnancy. Immunization can happen by two processes: transfusion of D-positive cells into someone who is D negative, or in pregnancy when transplacental passage of foetal red cells exposes the mother to D-positive cells. When the mother is Rh D negative and the developing foetus is Rh D positive, the exposure to foetal blood can stimulate anti-D activation in the mother. Anti-D is one of the red cell antibodies that can cross the placenta and cause haemolysis of the foetal blood, which results in what is known as 'haemolytic disease of the foetus and newborn' (HDFN) (Norfolk 2013).

Blood groups in haemopoietic stem cell transplantation

The human leucocyte antigen (HLA) is used to determine compatibility for organ transplantation, including bone marrow and peripheral blood stem cells. However, because the ABO blood groups and HLA tissue types are determined genetically, it is common to find a suitable HLA donor who is ABO and/or Rh incompatible with the recipient. Approximately 20–40% of allogeneic haemopoietic stem cell transplantation (HSCT) recipients receive grafts from ABO-mismatched donors (Tekgündüz and Özbek 2010). In such circumstances, major transfusion reactions can be avoided by red cell and/or plasma depletion of the donor cells in the laboratory before reinfusion (Mollison et al. 1997). However, collection of peripheral stem cells by apheresis usually results in a product that has a low red cell haematocrit and therefore further removal of mature red cells is not necessary before the product is cryopreserved (Mian et al. 2017).

Evidence-based approaches

The transfusion of blood components is a complex multistep process involving personnel from various professional backgrounds with differing levels of knowledge and understanding. Errors made in the process of transfusion present a significant risk to patients, and SHOT highlights that a team approach with good communication is essential (Narayan 2019). Every step should have the necessary checks carried out in full to ensure any errors in the steps prior are identified.

The evidence to support the efficacy of set procedures to manage this risk has been evaluated and provided in recommendations by the British Society for Haematology (BSH) and the SHOT reports (Bolton-Maggs 2018, Robinson et al. 2017). As a result of this guidance, every hospital should have a policy for the provision and administration of blood components that includes all steps of the process outlined in Figure 12.69. Furthermore, hospitals are required to manage and report any adverse events or near misses, and there is a statutory requirement to hold a record of every step of the transfusion process, including the final fate of each blood product, for 30 years (BSQR 2005, JPAC 2013). Only authorized staff should be involved at any stage in the transfusion process.

In the UK, nurses are usually the healthcare professionals ultimately responsible for the bedside check that is carried out before administering the blood component. The bedside check is the final opportunity to prevent patients from receiving the incorrect component, including recognizing any missing specific requirements (Bolton-Maggs 2018). Errors in the requesting, collection and administration of blood components have led to significant harm and sometimes fatal consequences. Since its launch in 1996, the SHOT scheme has continually shown that 'wrong blood into patient' episodes are a frequently reported transfusion hazard. These 'wrong blood' incidents are mainly caused by human error arising from misidentification of the patient during blood sampling, errors in blood component collection and delivery, and errors in administration; these can lead to life-threatening haemolytic transfusion reactions and other significant morbidity (Bolton-Maggs 2018). In the 2017 SHOT report, the cumulative data submitted since 1996 was analysed to assess the likelihood of preventability (Bolton-Maggs 2018). It was found that half of all reported incidents had been preventable, adverse events caused

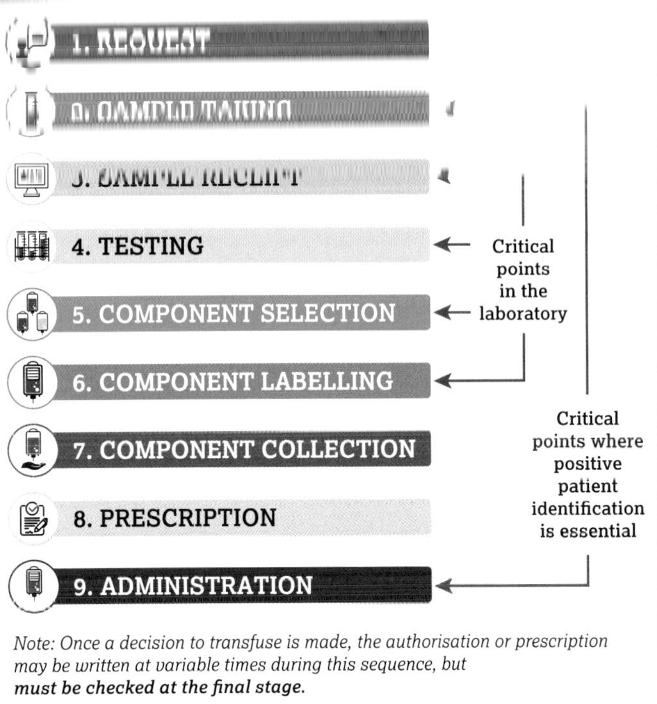

Figure 12.69 Vital steps involved in the transfusion of blood components. *Source*: Reproduced from Bolton-Maggs (2018) with permission of Serious Hazards of Transfusion.

by mistakes, such as assuming patient identity or not following the correct checking processes (Figure 12.70). Furthermore, the National Comparative Audit [illegible] shows that patients are placed at risk of avoidable complications of transfusion through misidentification and inadequate monitoring (NHSBT 2003, 2009, 2011a).

Due to the continuing risk of 'wrong blood' incidents, despite interventions such as competency assessments for transfusion, a Central Alerting System (DH 2017) has been issued mandating the use of a bedside checklist for transfusion administration (Figure 12.71).

Rationale

Blood transfusion is an essential part of modern medicine and potentially a life-saving intervention. However, the use of blood components should be appropriate and limited when possible, and alternative treatments – such as pharmacological interventions, and good surgical and anaesthetic techniques – should be considered (AAGBI 2016, NBTC 2014, NICE 2015, WHO 2011). The National Blood Transfusion Committee for England describes patient blood management as evidence based and multidisciplinary, encompassing measures to reduce the need for transfusion (NBTC 2014). These recommendations were further echoed by NICE (2015), which advocates measures to decrease the need for transfusion during surgery and to restrict the use of transfusion in all patients. Only when options to minimize the need for a transfusion have been implemented should a transfusion be considered. The pillars of patient blood management can be seen in Figure 12.72.

Recent publications and recommendations (Narayan 2019, NBTC 2014, NICE 2015) have created greater awareness of the need to continue to improve transfusion practice in many ways.

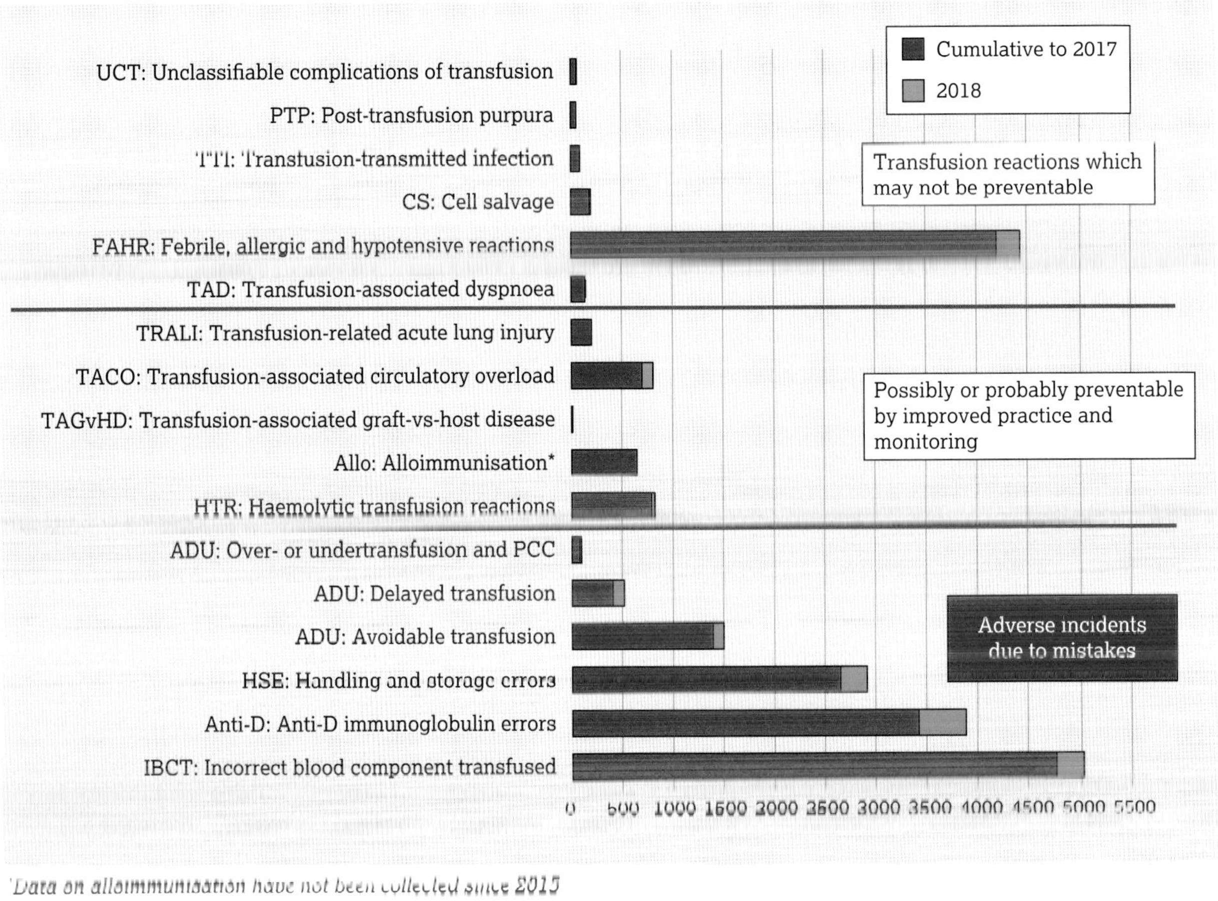

Figure 12.70 Cumulative data for SHOT categories 1996 to 2017, $n = 19{,}815$. *Source*: Adapted from Bolton-Maggs (2018) with permission of Serious Hazards of Transfusion.

Be safe! Use the bedside checklist

Check positive patient identification

- ask the patient to state first name, last name and date of birth
- must match exactly those on patient identification band

Check patient identification details on component pack

- against patient identification band and prescription

Check the prescription

- has this component been prescribed?

Check the component

- is this the correct component?
- is this component ABO-compatible with the recipient?
- expiry date
- donation number and blood group must match attached laboratory produced label
- for any signs of leakage or damage to packaging and inspect for any [illegible]

Check for specific requirements

- does the patient need irradiated components or specially selected units?

Signature:

Figure 12.71 Bedside checklist. *Source*: Reproduced from Bolton-Maggs (2018) with permission of Serious Hazards of Transfusion.

Blood components are no longer regarded as safe, unlimited resources. There are risks inherent in transfusion practice and therefore unnecessary exposure to blood components should be avoided. This is of particular importance for patients who may only have one transfusion in their lifetime, such as surgical patients. However, all patients should only receive a transfusion when it is absolutely necessary. Furthermore, the appropriate use of blood and its components is essential for the conservation of blood supplies. Regularly updated guidance on the safe and appropriate use of blood and blood components is available online at www.transfusionguidelines.org.uk and this should be consulted in collaboration with local hospital and national blood transfusion guidelines.

Red cells: indications

The WHO defines anaemia and its severity by the haemoglobin concentration in blood (Pasricha et al. 2018). A person is considered anaemic when their haemoglobin level is below the expected value, taking into consideration age, biological sex and pregnancy. In general, anaemia is a consequence of one or more of the following generic causes:

- increased loss of red blood cells
- decreased production of red blood cells
- increased destruction of red blood cells
- increased demand for red blood cells
- increased production of abnormal red blood cells.

The cause of anaemia should be ascertained and possible effective treatment options explored, such as treatment of iron deficiency before the patient is transfused with red cells (NBTC 2014).

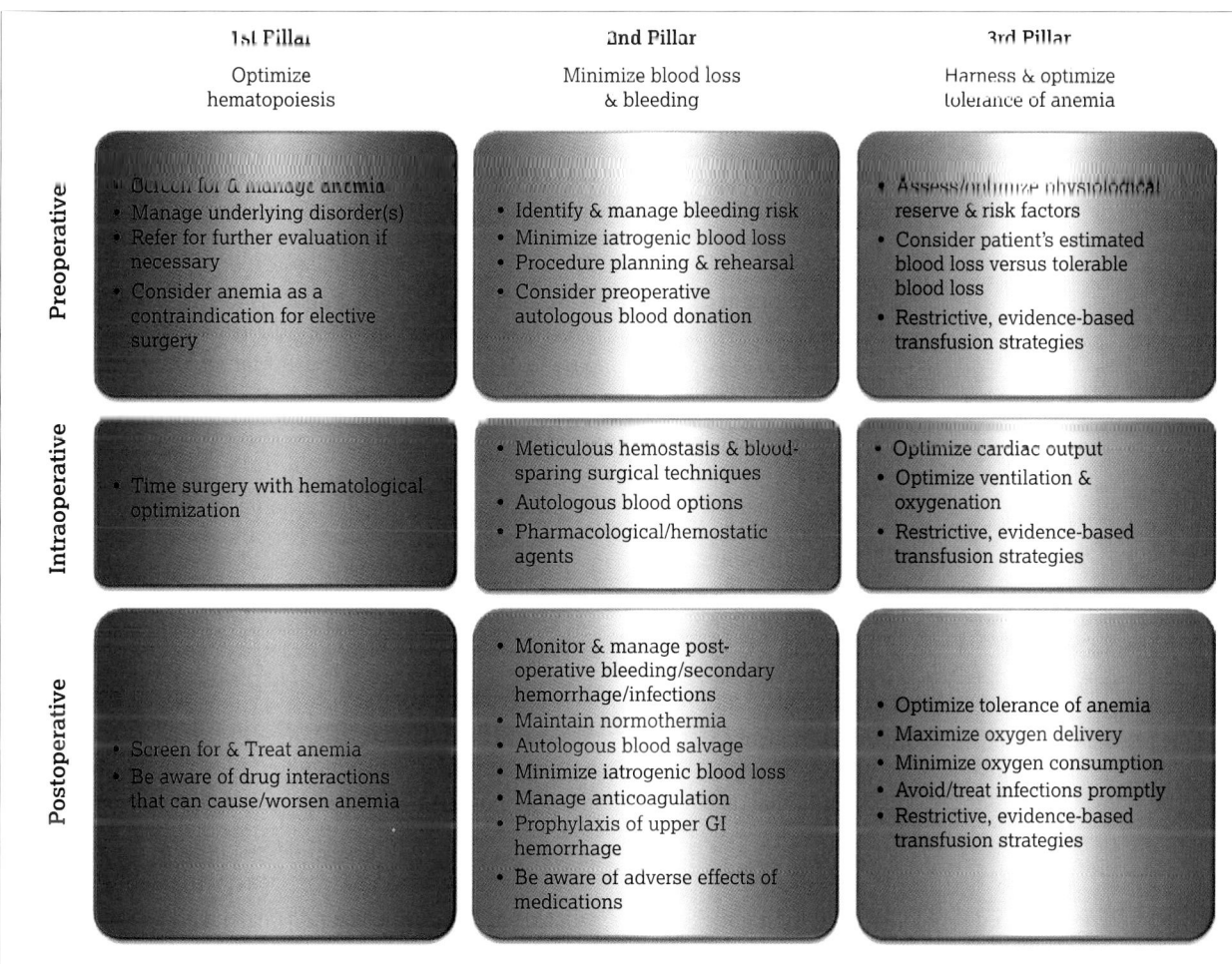

	1st Pillar Optimize hematopoiesis	2nd Pillar Minimize blood loss & bleeding	3rd Pillar Harness & optimize tolerance of anemia
Preoperative	• Screen for & manage anemia • Manage underlying disorder(s) • Refer for further evaluation if necessary • Consider anemia as a contraindication for elective surgery	• Identify & manage bleeding risk • Minimize iatrogenic blood loss • Procedure planning & rehearsal • Consider preoperative autologous blood donation	• Assess/optimize physiological reserve & risk factors • Consider patient's estimated blood loss versus tolerable blood loss • Restrictive, evidence-based transfusion strategies
Intraoperative	• Time surgery with hematological optimization	• Meticulous hemostasis & blood-sparing surgical techniques • Autologous blood options • Pharmacological/hemostatic agents	• Optimize cardiac output • Optimize ventilation & oxygenation • Restrictive, evidence-based transfusion strategies
Postoperative	• Screen for & Treat anemia • Be aware of drug interactions that can cause/worsen anemia	• Monitor & manage post-operative bleeding/secondary hemorrhage/infections • Maintain normothermia • Autologous blood salvage • Minimize iatrogenic blood loss • Manage anticoagulation • Prophylaxis of upper GI hemorrhage • Be aware of adverse effects of medications	• Optimize tolerance of anemia • Maximize oxygen delivery • Minimize oxygen consumption • Avoid/treat infections promptly • Restrictive, evidence-based transfusion strategies

Figure 12.72 The pillars of patient blood management. *Source*: Reproduced from Shander et al. (2012) with permission of John Wiley & Sons.

Pasricha et al. (2018) highlight that when choosing a treatment for anaemia it is important to take into consideration the severity of the patient's symptoms and the clinical effects of the anaemia as well as its chronicity.

Due to the variability of patient co-morbidities and anaemia tolerance, there is little evidence to support a generic 'transfusion trigger' (a haemoglobin level that requires subsequent blood transfusion). Evidence suggests that most patients can safely tolerate anaemia of 70 g/L of haemoglobin in the absence of active bleeding (NICE 2015). A systematic review exploring the evidence on haemoglobin thresholds for blood transfusion concluded that restrictive transfusion triggers were favourable in the majority of patients and that a haemoglobin threshold of 70 or 80 g/L lowers the number of red cell units transfused (Carson et al. 2012). The review also concluded that restrictive transfusion triggers had no adverse effects on cardiac morbidity, mortality or length of hospital stay (Carson et al. 2012).

Red cells: contraindications

NICE (2015) recommends that patients without acute coronary syndrome should have a restrictive transfusion approach and a post-transfusion target threshold of 70–90 g/L, and that those with acute coronary syndrome should have a post-transfusion threshold of 80–100 g/L. Patients who have cardiovascular disease, renal disease, low albumin concentration or are of low bodyweight (in particular, the elderly and children) may also be more susceptible to volume overload leading to congestive cardiac failure when blood and other fluids are infused (McClelland 2007, Norfolk 2013). SHOT (Bolton-Maggs 2018, Narayan 2019) has developed a checklist for risk factors for transfusion-associated circulatory overload (TACO) (Figure 12.73). In 2017, there were seven patient deaths reported to SHOT that were attributed to over-transfusion and TACO. The 2017 SHOT report (Bolton-Maggs 2018) and the BSH (Robinson et al. 2017) recommend a formal risk assessment for TACO prior to each transfusion. NICE (2015) and the BSH (Robinson et al. 2017) recommend that, to help mitigate the risk of TACO, single-unit transfusions should be given in stable, non-bleeding patients and then further assessment of the patient should be made prior to administering further units.

Red cell transfusions are contraindicated when the underlying cause of the anaemia has a non-transfusion treatment available. For example, iron deficiency anaemia should be treated with oral or intravenous iron infusion (NICE 2018c), or B_{12} treatment in the case of pernicious anaemia. Red cell transfusions are also limited in patients who are potential renal transplant recipients (Norfolk 2013) to limit the risk of alloimmunization and subsequent transplant rejection.

Platelets: indications

Platelet transfusions are indicated in the prevention and treatment of haemorrhage in patients with thrombocytopenia or platelet function defects (Estcourt et al. 2017). Thrombocytopenia can be defined as a platelet count below the normal range for the population, which is usually considered to be between 150 and 450 × 10^9/L (Weil et al. 2019). Thrombocytopenia is usually caused by either decreased platelet production or increased destruction. Not all thrombocytopenic patients require a platelet transfusion and in some cases it may be contraindicated. Patients who have chronic stable thrombocytopenia due to such conditions as myelodysplasia and aplastic anaemia often do not require a transfusion and do not experience haemorrhage even with platelet counts below 10 × 10^9/L (Estcourt et al. 2017). In prophylactic situations there are various thresholds, depending on the reason for the transfusion and the presence of risk factors for bleeding; see Table 12.15 for adult thresholds for transfusion.

In all cases of prophylactic platelet transfusions, the patient should receive one adult therapeutic dose (one pool or pack) and then be reassessed. Giving double-dose platelet transfusions does not decrease the risk of the patient bleeding (Slichter et al. 2010). There should be careful assessment of the need for a platelet transfusion

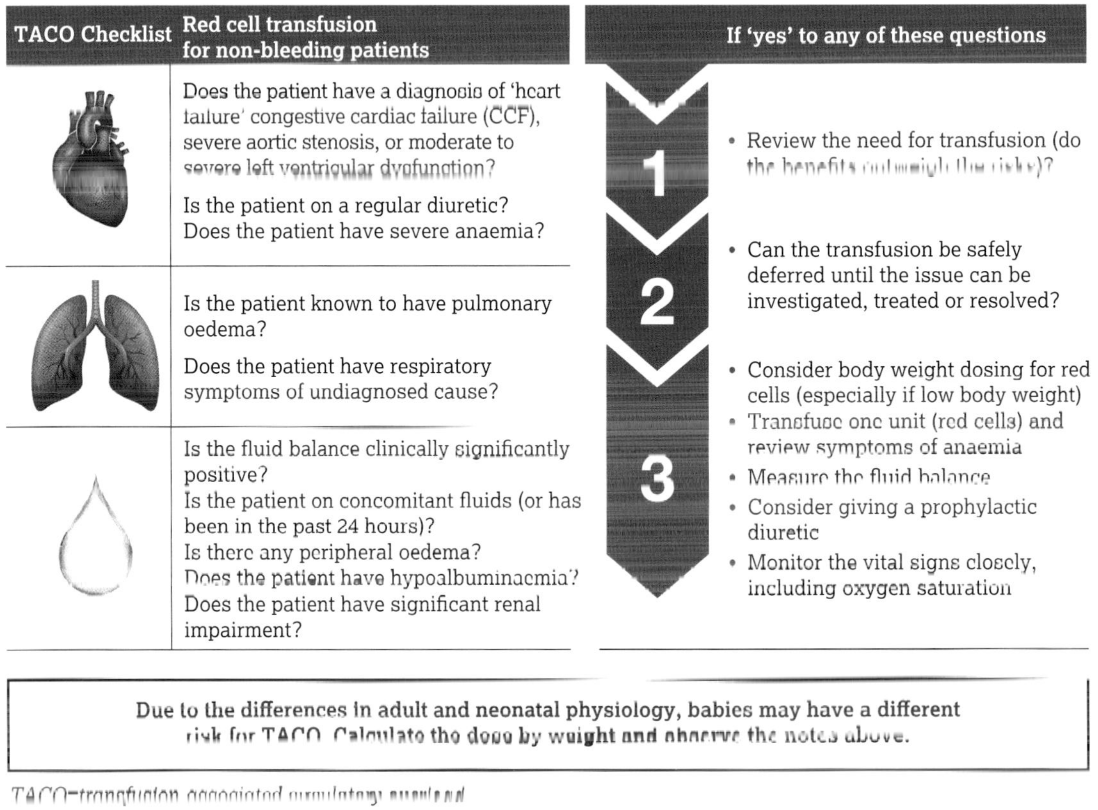
TACO Checklist
Red cell transfusion for non-bleeding patients
If 'yes' to any of these questions
Does the patient have a diagnosis of 'heart failure' congestive cardiac failure (CCF), severe aortic stenosis, or moderate to severe left ventricular dysfunction?
Is the patient on a regular diuretic?
Does the patient have severe anaemia?
Is the patient known to have pulmonary oedema?
Does the patient have respiratory symptoms of undiagnosed cause?
Is the fluid balance clinically significantly positive?
Is the patient on concomitant fluids (or has been in the past 24 hours)?
Is there any peripheral oedema?
Does the patient have hypoalbuminaemia?
Does the patient have significant renal impairment?
1
• Review the need for transfusion (do the benefits outweigh the risks)?
2
• Can the transfusion be safely deferred until the issue can be investigated, treated or resolved?
3
• Consider body weight dosing for red cells (especially if low body weight)
• Transfuse one unit (red cells) and review symptoms of anaemia
• Measure the fluid balance
• Consider giving a prophylactic diuretic
• Monitor the vital signs closely, including oxygen saturation
Due to the differences in adult and neonatal physiology, babies may have a different risk for TACO. Calculate the dose by weight and observe the notes above.
TACO=transfusion associated circulatory overload

Figure 12.73 Transfusion-associated circulatory overload (TACO) safety checklist. *Source*: Reproduced from Bolton-Maggs (2018) with permission of Serious Hazards of Transfusion.

Table 12.15 Indications for the use of platelet transfusions in adults

Indication	Transfusion indicated (threshold)/not indicated
Prophylactic use (no bleeding or WHO grade 1)	
One adult dose required	
Reversible BMF including allogeneic stem cell transplantation	10×10^9/L
Reversible BMF with autologous stem cell transplantation (consider no prophylaxis)	10×10^9/L
Critical illness	10×10^9/L
Chronic BMF receiving intensive therapy	10×10^9/L
Chronic BMF to prevent persistent bleeding of grade ≥2	Count variable
Chronic stable BMF, abnormal platelet function, platelet consumption/destruction (e.g. DIC, TTP) or immune thrombocytopenia (HIT, ITP, PTP)	Not indicated
Prophylactic use in the presence of risk factors for bleeding (e.g. sepsis, antibiotic treatment, abnormalities of haemostasis)	
Reversible/chronic bone marrow failure/critical care	$10–20 \times 10^9$/L
Abnormal platelet function, platelet consumption/destruction, immune thrombocytopenia	Not indicated
Platelet transfusion pre-procedure	
CVC excluding PICC line	20×10^9/L
Lumbar puncture	40×10^9/L
Percutaneous liver biopsy	50×10^9/L
Major surgery	50×10^9/L
Epidural anaesthesia, insertion and removal	80×10^9/L
Neurosurgery or ophthalmic surgery involving the posterior segment of the eye	100×10^9/L
Bone marrow aspirate or trephine biopsies, PICC line insertion, traction removal of CVCs, cataract surgery	Not indicated
Therapeutic use (bleeding WHO grade 2 or above)	
Severe bleeding	50×10^9/L
Multiple trauma, brain or eye injury, spontaneous intracerebral haemorrhage	100×10^9/L
Bleeding (WHO grade ≥2) but not severe	30×10^9/L
Bleeding in specific clinical conditions – see below for indications	
Specific clinical conditions	
Platelet function defect	Count variable
Congenital: pre-procedure or therapeutic use; when alternative therapy contraindicated or ineffective; directed by specialist in haemostasis	
Acquired (anti-platelet agents, uraemia): only indicated for severe bleeding	
Disseminated intravascular bleeding: pre-procedure or therapeutic use; consider threshold counts above but may not be achievable and individual case review required	Use pre-procedure/ therapeutic threshold as guide
Thrombotic thrombocytopenic purpura: platelet transfusion contraindicated unless life-threatening bleeding	Count variable
Immune thrombocytopenia (ITP, HIT, PTP): pre-procedure when other therapy ineffective or procedure urgent, or to treat severe bleeding; consider threshold counts above but may be unachievable or unnecessary and individual case review required	Use pre-procedure/ therapeutic threshold as guide

BMF, bone marrow failure; CVC, central venous catheter; DIC, disseminated intravascular coagulation; HIT, heparin-induced thrombocytopenia; ITP, primary immune thrombocytopenia; PICC, peripherally inserted central catheter; PTP, post-transfusion purpura; TTP, thrombotic thrombocytopenic purpura; WHO, World Health Organization. See Estcourt et al. (2017) for an explanation of the World Health Organization's bleeding scale.
Source: Adapted from Estcourt et al. (2017) with permission of John Wiley & Sons.

as the effectiveness and the platelet rise following the transfusion will start to reduce as the number of platelet transfusions increases (Slichter et al. 2010). Following the transfusion, the platelets' effectiveness should be evaluated by checking the increment; a sample should be taken 10 minutes after completion of the transfusion. One adult dose of platelets in a 70 kg adult typically gives a rise of $20–40 \times 10^9$/L (NHSBT 2011b, O'Connell et al. 1988).

Platelets: contraindications

Platelets are contraindicated in patients with microangiopathies such as thrombotic thrombocytopenic purpura and should only be used to treat life-threatening bleeding, as recommended in the BSH's 2017 guidelines (Estcourt et al. 2017). Prophylactic platelets are also not advised for patients with immune thrombocytopenia (Estcourt et al. 2017). Platelet transfusions should only be used in severe bleeding for patients with post-transfusion purpura (Eldin and Teruya 2012).

Fresh frozen plasma (FFP) and pathogen-inactivated FFP: indications

Plasma is mainly used for patients who are bleeding due to multiple clotting factor deficiencies such as disseminated intravascular coagulation or to replace clotting factors following massive haemorrhage (Hunt et al. 2015, Norfolk 2013). The BSH guidelines report that the evidence base to support the use of plasma to correct clotting in non-bleeding patients is lacking (Green et al. 2018); however, plasma is often given prior to invasive procedures to prevent bleeding, and abnormal clotting results do not predict bleeding risk (Green et al. 2018). In major haemorrhage episodes, FFP is recommended by the BSH to be given at a minimum ratio of 1 FFP to 2 red cells until coagulation results are available (Hunt et al. 2015).

Patients born after 1 January 1996 require imported and pathogen-inactivated plasma; this is to reduce the risk of infectious agents. The date is significant in that acquisition of vCJD (variant Creutzfeldt–Jakob disease) via diet is 'assumed to have ceased' by this time (Norfolk 2013, p.59). The component is imported from countries at low risk for vCJD.

Fresh frozen plasma (FFP) and pathogen inactivated FFP: contraindications

FFP is not indicated for warfarin reversal (Norfolk 2013). It is also not indicated in cases of hypervolaemia to support circulating volume (Green et al. 2018).

Further guidance on the use (in various patient groups) and handling of FFP and cryoprecipitate products can be found in the BSH guidelines (Green et al. 2018).

Cryoprecipitate and pathogen-inactivated cryoprecipitate: indications

The main constituents of cryoprecipitate are fibrinogen, factor VIII and von Willebrand factor (Norfolk 2013). It is clinically indicated in major haemorrhage when fibrinogen supplementation is required (Hunt et al. 2015). The BSH guidelines highlight that there is limited evidence for a threshold or level when cryoprecipitate would be beneficial, but a fibrinogen level of below 1.5 g/L in a bleeding patient is given to guide clinical practice (Hunt et al. 2015). In non-bleeding situations, such as an invasive procedure, there again is a lack of evidence to support recommendations. The recommendation is to assess patients' risk of bleeding by undertaking an assessment of previous bleeding episodes or any familial history of bleeding and, when a significant risk is identified, to consider transfusion when the fibrinogen level is below 1.0 g/L (Green et al. 2018).

Patients born after 1 January 1996 require imported and pathogen-inactivated cryoprecipitate for the same reason as they require imported and pathogen-inactivated plasma (see above).

Cryoprecipitate and pathogen inactivated cryoprecipitate: contraindications

Cryoprecipitate should not be used to treat clotting factor deficiencies when a clotting factor concentrate or pharmaceutical agent is available. For example, it should not be used to treat factor VIII deficiency in haemophilia, to treat von Willebrand factor deficiency, or for warfarin reversal (Eldin and Teruya 2012).

Methods

Blood donation and testing

All blood donated in the UK is given voluntarily and without remuneration. The successful selection of a donor involves protecting them from any harm that could be caused by the donation process and also protecting the possible recipient of components derived from the donor's blood. Donors of blood for therapeutic use should be in good health; if there is any doubt about their suitability, the donation should be deferred and they should be fully assessed by a designated medical officer. All donors of blood or its components (via apheresis) should be assessed in accordance with the Joint UK Blood Transfusion Services and National Institute for Biological Standards and Control Professional Advisory Committee (JPAC) donor selection guidelines (JPAC 2013). The assessment of fitness to donate includes a questionnaire relating to general health, lifestyle, past medical history and medication. Donation may be temporarily or permanently deferred for a variety of reasons, including cardiovascular disease, central nervous system diseases, malignancy and some infectious diseases, all of which are detailed in the JPAC (2013) guidelines. Donors are also screened for risk of exposure to transmissible infectious diseases, and specific guidance is provided for donors receiving therapeutic drugs.

Prevention of the transmission of infection is determined by donor selection criteria and laboratory testing. In the UK, all blood donations are tested for infections that could be passed on to the recipient. Transfusion-related vCJD transmission has been reported in four cases (Seed et al. 2018). Although in 2011 a prototype blood test for diagnosis of vCJD in symptomatic individuals was developed by the Medical Research Council's Prion Unit, there is still no available high-throughput and specific screening test (Seed et al. 2018). At present, donor exclusion criteria and leucodepletion remain as precautionary measures for all infection including vCJD (Seed et al. 2018). Since April 2004, all individuals who have received a blood component since January 1980 have been excluded from donating blood due to the risk of transmitting vCJD (DH 2013). When a donor has been successfully screened, they must validate the information they have provided and record that they have given consent to proceed.

Cell salvage and autologous transfusion

Since the 1980s, there has been interest in autologous transfusion (blood collected from an individual and intended solely for subsequent autologous transfusion to that same individual) (BSQR 2005). The objective of autologous transfusion is to decrease the need for allogeneic blood transfusion and the associated risks and costs (Sikorski et al. 2017). Autologous transfusion is used primarily for surgical patients, as explained below. It is not risk free, and SHOT reports the adverse reactions and events for the UK. In 2017, 17 cases were reported in relation to cell salvage; however, there was no major morbidity (Bolton-Maggs 2018). Autologous transfusion is contraindicated in certain circumstances; however, in cases of surgery with large anticipated blood loss, patients can benefit from the use of cell salvage (Sikorski et al. 2017). There have been concerns over using cell salvage in cancer surgery in case it leads to circulating tumour cells and causes tumour dissemination (Sikorski et al. 2017, Zaw et al. 2017). However, it is now known that this does not cause metastases (NICE 2008, Zaw et al. 2017). A Cochrane review of pre-autologous donation in 2002 concluded that it was difficult to say whether the benefit outweighs the harm (Henry et al. 2002) and it is now rarely undertaken by hospitals. Three principal methods of autologous transfusion exist: pre-operative autologous donation (PAD), acute normovolaemic haemodilution (ANH), and either intraoperative cell salvage (ICS) or post-operative cell salvage.

Pre-operative autologous donation

PAD is rarely undertaken and not currently recommended unless the clinical circumstances are exceptional – for example, if the patient has a rare blood group and allogeneic blood would be difficult to obtain (BCSH et al. 2007). It requires the patient to donate up to four units of blood while simultaneously taking iron supplements in the month preceding surgery. This technique can only be carried out in organisations licensed as blood establishments by the Medicines and Healthcare products Regulatory Agency (MHRA) under the Blood Safety and Quality Regulations (2005).

Acute normovolaemic haemodilution

ANH is not currently encouraged and the effectiveness of the procedure is unproven (Norfolk 2013). It involves the donation of up to three units of blood immediately prior to surgery. The patient is then given crystalloids to dilute the circulating volume. This method is only indicated for surgery where considerable blood loss is expected on the principle that the number of red cells lost will be reduced and the patient's autologous whole blood can be returned after surgery.

Intraoperative cell salvage

In ICS, blood loss during surgery is collected, anticoagulated, filtered and held in a sterile reservoir. The collected blood is then processed, washed and suspended in 0.9% sodium chloride for return. NICE (2015) recommends the use of cell salvage in conjuction with tranexamic acid for patients who are having surgery likely to result in high blood loss. Cell salvage has been shown to be effective in reducing the requirement for perioperative allogeneic blood transfusion in orthopaedic, cardiac and vascular surgery (Carless et al. 2010). The effectiveness of ICS to minimize a patient's exposure to allogeneic blood is dependent on the amount of blood lost during surgery, and better surgical techniques have resulted in less blood loss during surgery (NICE 2015).

Post-operative cell salvage

In post-operative cell salvage, where there is predictable blood loss following elective surgery, the blood is collected in the wound drain and then reinfused to the patient through special equipment. The blood can be passed through a filter incorporated into the cell salvage post-operative equipment or washed before being returned to the patient. This has become almost routine for some orthopaedic procedures, mainly hip and knee surgery (Norfolk 2013).

Several cases have been reported to SHOT (Bolton-Maggs 2012) where the autologous blood had not been labelled with the correct patient identification and in some cases this had not been noted by staff in the clinical area prior to reinfusion (Bolton-Maggs 2012). SHOT highlighted that it is still critical to maintain correct patient identification in autologous transfusion.

In 2006 a UK cell salvage group was founded to support the implementation of cell salvage; more information and advice can be found at JPAC (2019). The group produces a wide range of materials including training and competency documents, patient leaflets and guidance on the provision of cell salvage.

Blood component donation

Donors of blood components via automated apheresis are subject to the same selection criteria used for donating whole blood and any exception to this must be decided by a designated medical officer. Apheresis can be used to collect plasma, red cells and platelets. Leukapheresis procedures are used for the collection of granulocytes, lymphocytes and peripheral blood progenitor cells (JPAC 2013).

Appropriate use of donated blood components

Donated blood components are not a limitless resource and must be used appropriately. The BSH has guidelines in place for the use of red cell, platelet, FFP, cryoprecipitate and cryosupernatant transfusions (Estcourt et al. 2017, Green et al. 2018, Hunt et al. 2015, Retter et al. 2013). The decision to transfuse must be based on a thorough clinical assessment of the patient and their individual needs. Each blood component should only be given after careful consideration, when there is a valid clinical indication or when there are no alternative treatment options available (NICE 2015).

Blood and blood components have varying shelf lives and storage requirements. The range of components currently available, indications for their use and recommendations for their administration are listed in Table 12.16. Clinical indications for use are also provided by the BSH (Estcourt et al. 2017, Green et al. 2018, Hunt et al. 2015, Retter et al. 2013).

Anticipated patient outcomes

Blood component transfusion can be life saving; however, the focus is now on optimizing patients' own blood and trying to limit the need for transfusion (NBTC 2014). Liberal transfusion strategies (i.e. transfusing patients above the current recommended thresholds) have not been shown to add any benefit to patient outcomes (Holst et al. 2015)

If absolutely required, the patient will safely receive a blood product transfusion without adverse effect or incident.

Clinical governance

Blood safety and quality in the UK

Approximately 2.4 million blood components were administered in the UK in 2017 (Bolton-Maggs 2018). The transfusion of blood and its components is usually safe and uneventful; however, there are associated risks and there have been significant developments over recent years to improve the quality and safety of transfusion practice in the UK. The Blood Safety and Quality Regulations came into effect in 2005 and cover the collecting, testing, processing, storing and distributing of blood and blood components (BSQR 2005). The official government agency with jurisdiction for these regulations is the MHRA.

The principal requirements of the regulations in relation to transfusion practice are as follows.

- *Traceability*: there must be a full audit trail from the donor to the recipient, so hospitals must have a system to record and retain information on the fate of each unit of blood or blood component. These records must be kept for a period of 30 years.
- *Haemovigilance*: this is an organized surveillance procedure relating to serious adverse or unexpected events or reactions. The reporting of such events can be done via the online Serious Adverse Blood Reactions and Events (SABRE) system, which is maintained by the MHRA. This will usually be done by a designated member of laboratory staff or transfusion practitioner and therefore clinical staff must ensure that all incident reporting is conducted in line with hospital policy.

The Blood Safety and Quality Regulations (2005) define serious adverse or unexpected events or reactions as follows:

- A *serious adverse event* is defined as an unintended occurrence associated with the collection, testing, processing, storage and/or distribution of blood or blood components that might lead to death or life-threatening, disabling or incapacitating conditions for patients or that results in, or prolongs, hospitalization or morbidity.
- A *serious adverse reaction* is defined as an unintended response in a donor or a patient associated with the collection or transfusion of blood components that is fatal, life-threatening, disabling or incapacitating, or that results in or prolongs hospitalization or morbidity.

Prior to these regulations, 'Better Blood Transfusion' initiatives (still relevant today) aimed to ensure that such guidance became an integral part of NHS care, making blood transfusion safer, ensuring that all blood used in clinical practice is necessary, and improving the information both patients and the public receive about blood transfusion (DH 2007). Therefore, it is a key requirement that all staff involved in the process of transfusion maintain their awareness of all appropriate guidance.

Competencies

The transfusion of any blood component is not without risk and carries with it the potential for reaction (Bolton-Maggs 2018). All staff involved in the transfusion of blood and/or blood components must have the knowledge and skills to ensure the process is completed safely. Therefore, nurses caring for patients receiving transfusion therapy must do so within their sphere of competence, always acting to minimize risk to patients (NMC 2018).

Practitioners must understand the theory and reasoning behind transfusion procedures and practices (Pirie and Gray 2007). In November 2006, the National Patient Safety Agency (NPSA), the Chief Medical Officer's National Blood Transfusion Committee

Table 12.16 Blood, blood components and blood products used for transfusion

Type	Description	Indications	Cross-matching	Shelf life	Average infusion time	Technique	Special considerations
Red cells in optimal additive solutions (SAGM)*	Red cells with plasma removed: 100 mL additive fluid used as replacement to give optimal red cell preservation; haematocrit 60–65% leuco-depleted	Correction of anaemia	ABO and Rh compatible (not necessarily identical)	35 days at 2–6°C	1.5–2 hours/unit Transfusion to be completed within 4 hours of component's removal from storage Those patients at risk of TACO should have careful monitoring	Give via a blood administration set	If more than half blood volume is replaced with red cells in SAGM, use of FFP should be considered to replace clotting factors
Washed red blood cells	Red cells centrifuged and resuspended twice in 0.9% sodium chloride Leuco-depleted	Correction of anaemia where patient may react to plasma components, for example in IgA deficiency when the patient has formed an anti-IgA	As above	Prepared by non-sterile process, used within 24 hours Closed system preparation, used within 14 days	As above	As above	–
Frozen red blood cells	Red cells of very rare phenotype Leuco-depleted	To treat patients with very rare antibodies	As above	Stored frozen cells: up to 10 years Use within 24 to 72 hours depending on preparation	2–3 hours/unit	As above	–
White blood cells: granulocytes	Pooled granulocytes obtained by pooling the white cells from whole blood donations	To treat patients with life-threatening granulocytopenia	As above	Until midnight 1 day after donation	60–90 minutes/unit	Administer via a blood administration set	White blood cell infusion induces fever and may cause hypotension, rigors and confusion Treat symptoms and reassure patient White cell component is always irradiated to prevent initiation of TA-GVHD *Do not* give to patients receiving amphotericin B For the clinical indications and contraindications for granulocyte transfusions refer to the NHS Blood and Transplant guidelines ([illegible], 2016)

Platelets*	Platelets in 30–35% plasma and 65–70% platelet additive solution May be pooled from four whole blood donations or apheresed from a single donor Leuco-depleted	To treat thrombocytopenia either for prophylaxis to prevent bleeding or therapeutically to treat bleeding	No cross-matching necessary	Up to 7 days after collection Storage is at 22°C with continuous gentle agitation	30–60 minutes/unit	Administer using a platelet or blood component administration set Use a new set for each transfusion Do not use micro-aggregate filters	General guide to use: use in chronic bone marrow failure for routine prophylaxis is not indicated Platelets are not clinically indicated for a bone marrow aspirate and trephine regardless of the cause of thrombocytopenia See also Table 12.15
Fresh frozen plasma	Citrated plasma separated from whole blood	To treat multifactor deficiencies associated with severe bleeding and/or DIC FFP is not indicated in DIC without bleeding or for the immediate reversal of warfarin	No cross-matching necessary	3 years at <−25°C Once thawed, kept at 4°C and used as soon as possible but within 24 hours	10–20 mg/kg (approx. 250 mL); more rapid infusion may be indicated in major haemorrhage	Administer rapidly via a blood administration set	FFP should be considered if the patient has received more than half their blood volume in red cells, to prevent dilutional hypocoagulability The dose given is based on the patient's weight
Albumin 4.5% (HAS)	Solution of albumin from pooled plasma in a buffered, stabilized 0.9% sodium chloride diluent Supplied in 250 mL or 500 mL bottle	To treat hypovolaemic shock or hypoproteinaemia due to burns, trauma, surgery or infection Sourced outside the UK to reduce the risk of transmission of vCJD	No cross-matching necessary	5 years at room temperature Kept in the dark	30–60 minutes/unit	Administer via a standard solution administration set	The solution should be crystal clear with no deposits
Albumin 20% (HAS)	Heat-treated, aqueous, chemically processed fraction of pooled plasma	To treat hypovolaemic shock or hypoproteinaemia due to burns, trauma, surgery or infection To maintain appropriate electrolyte balance	No cross-matching necessary	5 years at room temperature Kept in the dark	30–60 minutes/unit	Administer via a blood administration set undiluted or diluted with 0.9% sodium chloride or 5% glucose solution Slower administration is advised if a cardiac disorder is present to avoid gross fluid shift	The solution should be crystal clear with no deposits

(continued)

Table 12.5 Blood, blood components and blood products used for transfusion *(continued)*

Type	Description	Indications	Cross-matching	Shelf life	Average infusion time	Technique	Special considerations
Cryoprecipitate	Cold-insoluble portion of plasma recovered from FFP: rich in factor VIII, von Willebrand factor and fibrinogen	To treat hypofibrinogenaemia, in acute DIC with bleeding and surgery prophylaxis with fibrinogen < 1.5 g/L To treat severe liver disease with bleeding and in cases of massive transfusion	No cross-matching necessary	3 years at <−25°C Use immediately after thawing	Available as single donor units or as pooled units (five single-donor units); typical adult dose is two pooled packs, administered at 10–20 mL/kg/hr, 30–60 minutes as a pooled unit	Administer via a blood administration set	–
Solvent detergent treated FFP Licensed medicinal product Octaplas	FFP prepared from pools of donations; the solvent detergent process inactivates bacteria and most encapsulated viruses	Guidelines recommend use in treating thrombotic thrombocytopenic purpura: patients are plasma-exchanged daily to reduce circulating von Willebrand factor	No cross-matching necessary	4 years at <−18°C Use immediately after thawing	Time depends on machine; average approximately 2.5 hours	Via apheresis machine	–

DIC, disseminated intravascular coagulation; FFP, fresh frozen plasma; HAS, human albumin solution; IgA, immunoglobin A; SAGM, saline, adenine, glucose and mannitol; TACO, transfusion-associated circulatory overload; TA-GVHD, transfusion-associated graft-versus-host disease; vCJD, variant Creutzfeldt–Jakob disease.
* Most commonly used blood components.

(NBTC) and SHOT, working in collaboration, developed strategies aimed at ensuring that blood transfusions are carried out safely, and issued Safer Practice Notice No. 14: *Right Patient, Right Blood* (NPSA 2006). One of the key action points in this notice was for all NHS and independent sector organizations involved in administering blood transfusions to develop and implement an action plan for competency-based training and assessments for all staff involved in blood transfusions. In 2017, the BSH stated that the evidence for recommending a frequency for training is low (Robinson et al. 2017). Robinson et al. (2017) highlight that since the SHOT scheme was launched (in 1996), it has continued to report that despite individuals being competency assessed, transfusion errors still occur. Transfusion committees across the UK have reviewed their practices and made their own recommendations, and the BSH (Robinson et al. 2017) has published a summary of training and competency assessments requirements in the UK by country (Table 12.17).

There are three key principles that underpin every stage of the blood component transfusion process:

- patient identification
- documentation
- communication (Robinson et al. 2017).

Non-medical written instruction to transfuse

Section 130 of the Medicines Act (1968) was amended by Regulation 25 of the Blood Safety and Quality Regulations (2005) and this has resulted in blood components being excluded from the Act (Green and Pirie 2009). In this way, blood components were removed from the legal definition of medicinal products and they can no longer be legally prescribed by any practitioner. Blood components are therefore authorized by a competent practitioner and a written instruction is completed for transfusion. The amendment to the Medicines Act also removed the legal barrier to nurses expanding their role to authorize blood components. This does not mean, however, that all nurses can make the decision to transfuse blood components or authorize their use with a written instruction. Green and Pirie (2009) developed a document for nurses and midwives who wish to expand their role. This framework contains clear guidance for the implementation of non-medical authorization of blood components while ensuring patient safety. The guidance includes advice on selecting the patient group, selection criteria for nurses and midwives, education and training required to support role development, clinical governance procedures, safe and appropriate practice, and how to review and monitor improvements to local services (Green and Pirie 2009).

Consent

In 2010 the Advisory Committee on the Safety of Blood, Tissues and Organs (SaBTO) undertook a public consultation on consent for blood transfusion. A total of 14 recommendations were published following the consultation (SaBTO 2011). They recommended that valid consent for transfusion should be obtained and documented in the patient's record by the healthcare professional. SaBTO also recommends that patients who cannot give consent before a transfusion should receive information retrospectively. The *Good Practice Guidance* (SaBTO 2011) states that retrospective information can be given at any point during the hospital stay but recommends that it is incorporated in the discharge procedure. The retrospective information should include the risk of a transfusion-transmitted infection and inform the patient that, as they have received a blood component, they can no longer donate blood (SaBTO 2011).

Providing the patient with information before a procedure and ascertaining that the patient understands the procedure and has consented to it is the responsibility of the healthcare professional carrying out the procedure as well as those ordering it (NMC 2018). A blood component transfusion must be treated like any prescribed medicine: that is, patients (or their guardian) must be informed of the indication for the transfusion, advised of the risks and benefits, and told about alternatives to blood transfusion, including autologous transfusion (Robinson et al. 2017). They should also be given the opportunity to ask questions and have the right to refuse to receive the transfusion in accordance with local and national guidance (NMC 2018). One of the key objectives of the Better Blood Transfusion initiative (DH 2007) was to improve information provided to patients and to ensure that those who are likely to receive a blood transfusion will be well informed of their choices. There are a number of information leaflets issued by the NHS Blood and Transplant Service for both patients and healthcare professionals. Guidance is also available from SaBTO (2011) to ensure that patients receive standardized information prior to a transfusion; this guidance outlines all the key information that should be provided.

Patients with mental capacity have the legal and ethical right to refuse transfusion (RCS 2016), and information regarding alternative treatment must be given. Staff must respect the patient's decision and their autonomy in making the decision; this is a legal duty (RCN 2017).

Jehovah's Witnesses and other patients who may refuse a blood transfusion

Patients may choose to refuse a blood transfusion for a variety of reasons. Principles in caring for patients remain the same regardless of the reason for refusal and there should be a local policy in place to expedite non-blood management for these patients.

The role of blood in Jehovah's Witnesses' spiritual belief is based on scripture and followers are usually well informed on both their beliefs and their rights. The need to ensure informed consent is very important. Jehovah's Witnesses' religious position leads them to refuse red cells, white cells, plasma and platelets. Derivatives of these are seen as a matter of individual patient choice. Staff caring for patients must ensure that they have clearly documented what the patient will accept or refuse and that decisions to consent to or refuse treatment are respected and recorded appropriately (Norfolk 2013). Furthermore, in individual circumstances, practitioners should endeavour to consider non-blood or autologous methods, as described previously, where appropriate (Norfolk 2013). Jehovah's Witness patients usually carry an advance directive listing which blood products and autologous procedures are acceptable or not acceptable to them (Norfolk 2013). The Jehovah's Witness community has a network of support called Hospital Liaison Committees and they are available at any time, night and day, to assist with communication between hospital teams and patients.

Management of massive blood loss

Massive blood loss has several definitions, such as loss of one blood volume within 24 hours, loss of 50% blood volume within 3 hours, or a loss rate of 150 mL/min. However, the BSH Transfusion Task Force suggests that these definitions are not particularly helpful in acute situations due to their retrospective nature (Hunt et al. 2015). Good patient outcomes are dependent on clinical staff recognizing the blood loss early, taking effective action and ensuring efficient communication between the clinical area and the transfusion laboratory (NPSA 2010). To aid the provision of blood in an emergency situation, the majority of hospitals will have an agreed major haemorrhage protocol in which all processes required in the provision of emergency blood are clearly stated. This includes how to activate the protocol, what blood component availability will be and how the blood components will be transferred from the laboratory to the clinical area.

In emergency situations, where the need for blood is immediate and the patient's blood group is unknown, it may be necessary to transfuse group O un-cross-matched red cells (Hunt et al. 2015). In major haemorrhage situations, there is still a need to use group O Rh D-negative blood judiciously as it is a scarce resource. At the earliest opportunity, a sample should be taken from the patient so that blood group determination can take place. Once the laboratory has received the sample and determined the blood group, it can issue group-specific blood (Hunt et al. 2015).

Table 12.17 Summary of training and competency assessment requirements in the UK by country

England	Wales	Scotland	Northern Ireland
Theory, training and knowledge assessment			
All staff involved in the transfusion process should receive training no less frequently than 3-yearly (2-yearly for blood collection). Knowledge and understanding assessment should be performed at least every 3 years (2 years for blood collection).	There should be annual competence-based educational updates for staff involved in collection of blood from the issue fridge/local storage facility, with assessment of competence as agreed locally in compliance with the Blood Safety and Quality Regulations (2005). There should be biennial training for other staff involved in sampling and/or administration of blood. There should be continued monitoring of the competence of all relevant staff through the appraisal process.	The NHS Quality Improvement Scotland (NHS QIS)* *Clinical Standards: Blood Transfusion* (2006) required 2-yearly theoretical knowledge training for all staff involved in the transfusion process. In 2015, NHS Healthcare Improvement Scotland (NHS HIS)* reviewed these improvement standards against current practice/guidance and archived the standards. It has been recognized that the 2-yearly training/updating requirement for all staff involved in the transfusion process is embedded in NHS Scotland's health boards, supported and reported on by Better Blood Transfusion to the Scottish Transfusion Advisory Committee.	Minimum training requirements for clinical and support staff involved in transfusion practice should be 3-yearly knowledge updates (RCN 2016). There should be 3-yearly training in blood components and their indications for use for doctors who authorize (prescribe) blood components. Healthcare staff should update their knowledge of transfusion that is relevant to their clinical practice and be able to demonstrate evidence of this in their appraisal documentation.
Practical observed competency assessment			
Following an individual's initial training a one-off practical competency assessment must be undertaken. This practical assessment need not be repeated if there is ongoing satisfactory performance but it should be repeated if there is a period of greater than 1 year out of a workplace where transfusion routinely takes place.	There must be a competency assessment of relevant staff (e.g. newly qualified staff). Review evidence of competence for new employees assessed elsewhere.	Staff involved in the collection and delivery of blood components should undertake competency-based assessment for this role at least every 2 years, as agreed locally in compliance with the Blood Safety and Quality Regulations (2005).	Practical competency assessment in the transfusion roles practised by staff must be done at a minimum of 3-yearly intervals. Staff involved in the collection and delivery of blood components should undertake competency-based assessment for this role at least every 2 years.
Sources			
National Blood Transfusion Committee (2016a, 2016b)	Welsh Blood Service (Shreeve, 2014)	Scottish Clinical Transfusion Advisory Committee (personal communication, 2017)	Northern Ireland Transfusion Committee (personal communication, 2016)

* NHS Quality Improvement Scotland (NHS QIS) was replaced by NHS Healthcare Improvement Scotland (NHS HIS) in April 2011.
Source: Adapted from Robinson et al. (2017).

Pre-procedural considerations

Equipment

Intravenous access

Blood components may be administered through a peripheral cannula or via a central venous access device. Where possible, one lumen should be reserved for the taking of blood specimens and blood component administration for the duration of therapy.

Administration sets

All blood components must be transfused through a sterile blood component administration set with an integral mesh filter (170–200 μm) that is CE marked. Blood administration sets should be changed at least every 12 hours or after every second unit for a continuing transfusion (Loveday et al. 2014; see also local guidance). Administration sets used for blood components must be changed immediately upon suspected contamination or when the integrity of the product or system has been compromised. Platelets and plasma components may be administered through a normal blood administration set or through a platelet set. Platelets should never be administered through an administration set that has previously been used for transfusion of red cells or other blood component as this may cause aggregation of platelets in the administration set (Norfolk 2013). Administration sets used for blood components must be changed using aseptic technique, observing standard precautions and in line with the manufacturer's instructions (RCN 2010).

Infusion devices

Either gravity or electronic infusion devices may be used for the administration of blood components. There are a variety of electronic infusion devices available and it is therefore essential that healthcare professionals using any type of infusion device are competent in their use. Only blood component administration sets compatible with the infusion device should be used. Rapid infusion devices that are CE marked may be used when large volumes have to be infused rapidly. Typically, devices can infuse from 6 to 30 L an hour and usually incorporate a blood-warming device (Norfolk 2013).

Blood-warming devices

In cases where there will be rapid transfusion of red cells, warming is recommended. Red cells removed from cold storage and then transfused rapidly can cause hypothermia (Norfolk 2013). The rapid transfusion of cold blood components is cautioned against as it may cause impaired coagulation and cardiac arrhythmias (Norfolk 2013).

However, whichever device is chosen, the temperature should be maintained below 38°C. Warming in excess of this can cause haemolysis of red cells and can denature proteins and increase the risk of bacterial infection. Blood warmers must always be used and maintained according to the manufacturer's guidelines. Blood components must *never* be warmed by improvisation, such as putting the pack into hot water, in a microwave or on a radiator, as uncontrolled heating can damage the contents of the pack (McClelland 2007, Norfolk 2013). The use of water baths also increases the risk of bacterial contamination. Therefore, certain safety measures must be adhered to:

- Water baths must be drained after each use and stored dry and empty.
- Blood warmers must be drained after each use and stored dry and empty.
- When needed, water baths and blood warmers should be refilled with sterile water.
- A protective sterile over-bag to thaw blood and blood products reduces the entry of contaminants through microscopic punctures or breaks in the seal.
- The product should be used immediately after it has been thawed.

All devices should be serviced as per hospital health and safety policies, MHRA guidance and manufacturers' guidelines.

Blood component request

The details on the blood component request form and the sample tube are the only direct contact between the clinical area and the blood transfusion laboratory. The accuracy and completeness of this information are therefore of vital importance (Estcourt et al. 2017). Incorrect or inadequate patient identification has the potential to result in blood being issued to the wrong patient, possibly leading to ABO-incompatible transfusions. In the 2017 SHOT report, there were 789 instances of 'wrong blood in tube' (WBIT) and one case where WBIT led to an incorrect blood component being transfused (Bolton-Maggs 2018).

Inadequately or mislabelled samples are up to 40 times more likely to contain blood from the wrong patient (BCSH 2009). A WBIT is usually identified in the laboratory by comparing the current patient group to previous group results, so the patients most at risk from this error are those who only have one sample sent and where blood is issued based on that sample. The British Committee for Standards in Haematology has produced guidelines advocating that when a patient has not had their blood group tested by the current blood transfusion laboratory on a previous occasion, they should have a second separate sample sent before the blood is issued (BCSH et al. 2013). This guidance does not apply to the emergency provision of blood or when waiting for a second sample to be processed would cause patient harm. It is also not necessary to implement the recommendation if the hospital has a secure electronic patient identification system (discussed below) in place (BCSH et al. 2013). The collection of the blood sample from the patient and the subsequent labelling of the sample tube should be performed as a continuous, uninterrupted event at the patient's side, involving one patient and one member of staff only (Robinson et al. 2017).

The NBTC (2016) has produced standardized adult indication codes (Box 12.9) for transfusion; these codes can also be used as an audit tool that can be incorporated into the transfusion request (Robinson et al. 2017).

Specific patient preparation

Wristbands for patient identification and transfusion

In 2007, the NPSA issued Safer Practice Notice No. 24: *Standardising Wristbands Improves Patient Safety*. This notice stated that only the following core identifiers should be used on patients' identification bands:

- last name
- first name
- date of birth
- NHS number.

Patients should have their identification confirmed on admission to the unit and one wristband attached to their wrist. If a wristband is removed for any reason, for example to gain intravenous access via a cannula, it is the responsibility of the person removing it to ensure that a correctly completed wristband is then reapplied.

Electronic systems for patient identification and transfusion

Wristbands can now hold patient information in an electronic format, such as in a bar code or a radiofrequency identification (RFID) tag. Electronic systems offer improved security and patient safety (Kaufman et al. 2019, Robinson et al. 2017) by removing the element of human error from the process. At the point of taking a sample for pre-transfusion testing, the patient is identified through the usual process of stating their name and date of birth, but there is the added safety of scanning the bar code or RFID tag on the wristband.

Box 12.9 National Blood Transfusion Committee clinical indication codes for transfusion

Red cell concentrates

Dose: in the absence of active bleeding, use the minimum number of units required to achieve the target level of haemoglobin (Hb). Consider the size of the patient, assume an increment of 10 g/L per unit for an average 70 kg adult.

R1: acute bleeding

Acute blood loss with haemodynamic instability. After normovolaemia has been achieved or maintained, frequent measurement of Hb (including via near-patient testing) should be used to guide the use of red cell transfusion (see suggested thresholds below).

R2: Hb 70 g/L stable patient

Acute anaemia. Use an Hb threshold of 70 g/L and a target Hb of 70–90 g/L to guide red cell transfusion. Follow local/specific protocols for indications such as following cardiac surgery, in traumatic brain injury or in acute cerebral ischaemia.

R3: Hb 80 g/L if cardiovascular disease

Use an Hb threshold of 80 g/L and a target Hb of 80–100 g/L.

R4: chronic transfusion-dependent anaemia

Transfuse to maintain an Hb that prevents symptoms. Try an Hb threshold of 80 g/L initially and adjust as required. Haemoglobinopathy patients require individualized Hb thresholds depending on age and diagnosis.

R5: maintain Hb >110 g/L in radiotherapy

There is limited evidence for maintaining an Hb of 110 g/L in patients receiving radiotherapy for cervical and possibly other tumours.

Source: Adapted from NBTC (2016).

These electronic systems can be used during collection and administration. During administration, the blood component and the wristband are scanned to confirm that the right component is being given to the right patient. Safer Practice Notice No. 14: *Right Patient, Right Blood* (NPSA 2006) recommended that all NHS trusts and independent sector organizations responsible for administering blood should risk assess their transfusion procedures and look at the feasibility of using bar codes and other electronic identification and tracking systems for patients, samples and blood components. In a key recommendation, SHOT stated

Box 12.10 Essential information for a blood transfusion request

- Patient core identifiers (see Procedure guideline 12.18: Blood product request)
- Date (and time if appropriate) the blood component is required
- Type of blood component to be administered
- Any clinical special transfusion requirements, for example irradiation or administration via a blood warmer
- Volume or number of units to be transfused (for paediatric transfusions, exact number in mL)
- Time over which each unit is to be transfused (for paediatric transfusions, exact rate or length of time over which the specified volume is to be transfused)
- Any special instructions, for example concomitant drugs required, such as diuretics
- Signature of the authorizer ('prescriber') (Robinson et al. 2017)

that electronic blood systems should be the standard towards which all trusts aim (Bolton-Maggs 2018).

Informed consent

Nurses must ensure that patients have been informed of the proposed transfusion, have had an opportunity to raise any concerns, understand the risks and benefits of the transfusion, have agreed to the transfusion, and are available for the transfusion. Pre-transfusion/baseline observations (including blood pressure, temperature, pulse and respiratory rate) must be undertaken and documented, and it must be ensured that there is patent venous access prior to administering the transfusion (Robinson et al. 2017).

Pre-transfusion/bedside check

While professional accountability measures must be taken at every stage by the personnel involved, the final barrier to wrong blood administration is at the bedside. The final bedside check is the last chance to ensure the right patient receives the right blood and it is therefore essential that this check is performed thoroughly prior to the transfusion of each component (Norfolk 2013, Robinson et al. 2017).

To ensure that each blood component is used to its full advantage, local hospital policy should be followed with regard to correct handling, storage, transportation and administration of blood components. If unused, the component should be returned to the transfusion laboratory as quickly as possible to maximize the opportunity for it to be used for another patient.

The written order for the blood component must be checked to ensure that it is correctly completed and that it contains all the information outlined in Box 12.10.

Procedure guideline 12.18 Blood product request

Essential equipment

- Blood request form – electronic or paper format

Action	Rationale
Procedure	
1 The following information must be completed on the request: • first name • surname • date of birth • NHS • hospital identification number • ward or department	Full identifiers are required to minimize the risk of patients with the same or similar names being given the incorrect blood component (Norfolk 2013, **E**; Robinson et al. 2017, **C**). To enable the laboratory staff to cross-reference the details on the request form with the details on the enclosed blood sample. Discrepant samples should not be processed ([illegible] 2013, **C**).

2 Complete the following clinical information: • diagnosis • reason for request: depending on local policy, this may include the National Blood Transfusion Committee indication code (see Box 12.9) (NBTC 2016); if relevant, state the surgical procedure • number and type of components requested • any special requirements, such as irradiated or cytomegalovirus-negative blood • if group and screen only • date and time required.	To enable laboratory staff to assess need against the surgical blood ordering schedule. **E** Some patient groups may have a fatal reaction to wrongly specified components, so non-irradiated or washed components may be required (Norfolk 2013, **E**; Robinson et al. 2017, **E**). To allow laboratory staff to plan ahead for stock management and to ensure the required products are available at the correct time (SNBTS 2004, **C**).
3 Each request should also include: • the name of the competent healthcare professional requesting the component(s) • the name and signature of the person who has taken the blood sample.	Every step of the transfusion must be fully traceable and the record held for 30 years (BSQR 2005, **C**).
4 The following information can also be included if it is available from the patient or in the patient's clinical record • presence of known blood group antibodies • date of last transfusion • transfusions within the past 3 months • any previous reactions to transfusions • current or recent pregnancy (within preceding 3 months) • anti-D administered in the previous 12 weeks • details of any drug treatments that interfere with the cross-match (e.g. daratumumab).	To facilitate the timely provision of blood components and interpretation of laboratory testing (Robinson et al. 2017, **C**)

Procedure guideline 12.19 Blood sampling: pre-transfusion

Essential equipment

- Personal protective equipment
- Antimicrobial skin cleanser (the recommended solution is 0.5% chlorhexidine in 70% alcohol)
- Safety needle or winged infusion device
- Appropriate tubes for blood sample collection
- Gauze
- Hypoallergenic tape
- Sharps container

Action	Rationale
Pre-procedure	
1 Introduce yourself to the patient, explain and discuss the procedure with them, and gain their consent to proceed.	To ensure that the patient feels at ease, understands the procedure and gives their valid consent (NMC 2018, **C**).
2 Note that pre-transfusion blood should be taken from one patient at a time and the whole procedure, including labelling, should be completed in one continuous event.	To ensure that samples from different patients are not confused, which can have fatal consequences (Bolton-Maggs 2018, **C**; Robinson et al. 2017, **C**).
3 Check all packaging before opening and preparing the equipment.	To ensure there has been no contamination and all equipment is in date. **E**
Procedure	
4 Before taking the sample, ask the patient to state their first name, surname and date of birth. Cross-check these details against the blood request form. For patients unable to identify themselves, verification can be obtained from a carer or relative if present.	To ensure that the sample obtained corresponds with the request (Robinson et al. 2017, **C**).
5 Check these details against the patient's identity wristband.	To ensure that the patient is positively identified before obtaining a blood sample (Robinson et al. 2017, **C**).
6 Check the patient's hospital number on the wristband against that on the blood request form.	To ensure that the sample obtained corresponds with the request (Robinson et al. 2017, **C**).
7 Obtain the blood sample by direct venepuncture or via central venous access device, in the appropriate tube.	To ensure the correct procedure is followed and an adequate sample is obtained. **E**

(continued)

Procedure guideline 12.19 Blood sampling: pre-transfusion *(continued)*

Action	Rationale
Post-procedure	
8 Hand-write the required information on the sample tube clearly and accurately, ensuring all names are spelled correctly. Alternatively, print an on-demand patient identification label. This should only be done once the sample has been successfully obtained and should be done at the patient's bedside. Information to include: • first name • surname • date of birth • sex • hospital identification number • ward or department • date.	To ensure the sample is labelled with the correct patient details. Robinson et al. (2017, **C**) state that only labels printed on demand next to the patient and immediately attached to the sample bottle are acceptable for transfusion samples. Blood tubes should never be pre-labelled in advance either by hand or electronically as this has been identified as a major cause of patient identification errors (Bolton-Maggs 2018, **C**).

Procedure guideline 12.20 Blood components: collection and delivery to the clinical area

Errors in blood collection remain a root cause of patients ultimately receiving a wrong blood component (Norfolk 2013). Only those staff who are authorized, trained and competent may remove blood components from storage. A guide to the necessary elements of blood pack labelling is shown in Figure 12.74.

Essential equipment

- Documentation containing the patient's three core identifiers – full name, date of birth and hospital number/unique identifying number – must be held by the person removing the component from storage

Action	Rationale
Pre-procedure	
1 Check that the reason for the transfusion has been documented in the patient's notes.	To ensure the transfusion is appropriate and necessary (Robinson et al. 2017, **C**).
2 Check that there is a valid written order for the administration of the component, including any special requirements.	To ensure the selected component meets the patient's individual requirements (Robinson et al. 2017, **C**).
3 Introduce yourself to the patient, explain and discuss the procedure with them, and gain their consent to proceed.	To ensure that the patient feels at ease, understands the procedure and gives their valid consent (NMC 2018, **C**).
4 Check the patient is wearing an identification wristband.	To avoid delays in confirming the patient's identity (BCSH 2009, **C**).
5 Check the patient is available.	To avoid delays once the component has been removed from storage. **E**
6 Take baseline observations to include blood pressure, temperature, pulse and respiratory rate.	To ensure that any transfusion reaction can be immediately identified via changes from the baseline (Robinson et al. 2017, **C**) and managed appropriately (Tinegate et al. 2012, **C**).
7 Check the patient has patent venous access. If not, ensure the appropriate device is inserted.	To avoid any delay in commencement of the transfusion when it has been removed from storage and prevent possible wastage. **E**
Procedure	
8 The collector must bring locally agreed documentation to collect the blood component and it must contain the core identifiers for the patient being transfused.	To minimize the risk of the wrong blood component being given to a patient (Robinson et al. 2017, **C**).
9 Remove the component (using an electronic or manual method) from storage in accordance with trust policy and ensure that the date, time and collector are recorded.	To ensure that only authorized, trained and competent staff collect blood components and cold chain requirements are met (BSQR 2005 **C**; Robinson et al. 2017, **C**). *Note.* the blood cold chain is a system for ensuring the blood (or blood product) is kept at the correct temperature during storage and when being transported.
10 Remove one component at a time, unless rapid transportation of large quantities is needed or if blood is being transported to remote areas in specifically designed and validated blood transport containers. If large quantities are required, this must be discussed with the transfusion laboratory and local procedures followed.	To meet cold chain requirements and ensure the components are stored and transported in the appropriate conditions (BSQR 2005, **C**).

Compatibility label or tie-on tag

The compatibility label is generated in the hospital transfusion laboratory. It is attached to the blood bag and contains the following patient information: *Surname, First Name(s), Date of Birth, Gender, Hospital Number/Patient Identification Number, Hospital* and *Ward*.
The *blood group, component type* and *date requested* are also included on the label. The *unique donation number* is printed on the compatibility label; this number must match exactly with the number on the blood bag label.

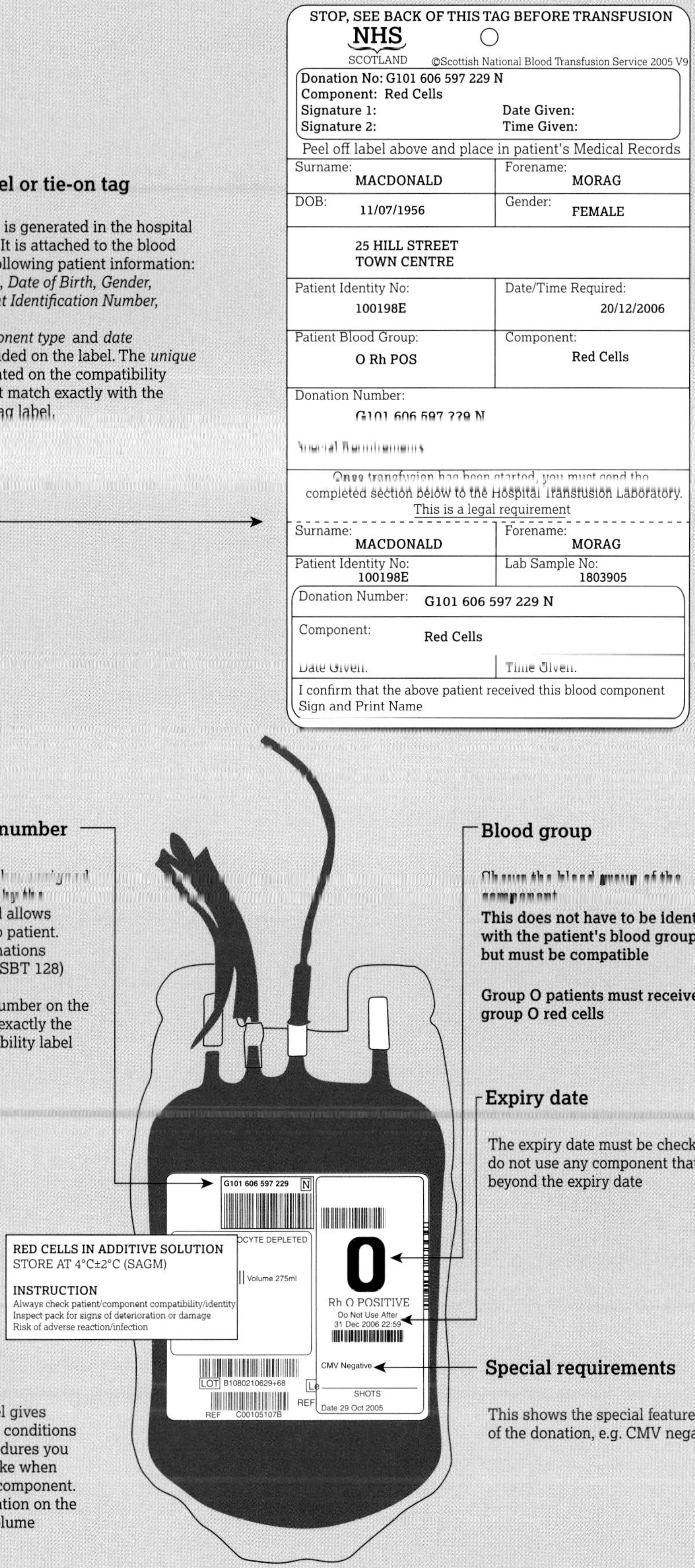

STOP, SEE BACK OF THIS TAG BEFORE TRANSFUSION
NHS
SCOTLAND
©Scottish National Blood Transfusion Service 2005 V9
Donation No: G101 606 597 229 N
Component: Red Cells
Signature 1:
Date Given:
Signature 2:
Time Given:
Peel off label above and place in patient's Medical Records
Surname: MACDONALD
Forename: MORAG
DOB: 11/07/1956
Gender: FEMALE
25 HILL STREET
TOWN CENTRE
Patient Identity No: 100198E
Date/Time Required: 20/12/2006
Patient Blood Group: O Rh POS
Component: Red Cells
Donation Number: G101 606 597 229 N
Once transfusion has been started, you must send the completed section below to the Hospital Transfusion Laboratory.
This is a legal requirement
Surname: MACDONALD
Forename: MORAG
Patient Identity No: 100198E
Lab Sample No: 1803905
Donation Number: G101 606 597 229 N
Component: Red Cells
Date Given:
Time Given:
I confirm that the above patient received this blood component
Sign and Print Name
G101 606 597 229 N
OCYTE DEPLETED
Volume 275ml
RED CELLS IN ADDITIVE SOLUTION
STORE AT 4°C±2°C (SAGM)
INSTRUCTION
Always check patient/component compatibility/identity
Inspect pack for signs of deterioration or damage
Risk of adverse reaction/infection
O
Rh O POSITIVE
Do Not Use After
31 Dec 2006 22:59
CMV Negative
LOT B1080210629+68
REF C00105107B
SHOTS
Date 29 Oct 2005

Unique donation number

This is the unique number assigned to each blood donation by the transfusion service and allows follow-up from donor to patient.
From April 2001 all donations bear the new 14 digit (ISBT 128) donation number
The unique donation number on the blood bag must match exactly the number on the compatibility label

Blood group

Shows the blood group of the component
This does not have to be identical with the patient's blood group but must be compatible

Group O patients must receive group O red cells

Expiry date

The expiry date must be checked – do not use any component that is beyond the expiry date

Cautionary notes

This section of the label gives instructions on storage conditions and the checking procedures you are required to undertake when administering a blood component. It also includes information on the component type and volume

Special requirements

This shows the special features of the donation, e.g. CMV negative

Figure 12.74 A guide to the necessary elements of blood pack labelling.

(continued)

Procedure guideline 12.20 Blood components: collection and delivery to the clinical area *(continued)*

Action	Rationale
11 Check the components at the point of removal for correct patient-identifying details. A visual inspection of the components should also be performed to check the expiry date and any signs of clumping, discolouration, damage or leaks. The laboratory compatibility label attached to the unit must also be checked with the NHS Blood and Transplant label for batch number.	In order to minimize the risk of administering the component to the wrong patient (Bolton-Maggs 2018, **C**; Robinson et al. 2017, **C**). Expired or damaged products must not be used. To ensure that the correct label has been attached to the blood component. **E**
Post-procedure	
12 Deliver the component to the clinical area.	To ensure the correct component has been received for the patient, to comply with traceability and cold chain requirements (Robinson et al. 2017, **C**).

Procedure guideline 12.21 Blood component administration

Essential equipment

- Personal protective equipment
- Written order for blood component transfusion
- Blood administration set with a 170–200 μm macroaggregate filter
- A bedside checklist (DH 2017)

Action	Rationale
Pre-procedure	
1 Introduce yourself to the patient, explain and discuss the procedure with them, and gain their consent to proceed.	To ensure that the patient feels at ease, understands the procedure and gives their valid consent (NMC 2018, **C**).
2 Check that the component has a correct written instruction, including any special requirements such as irradiated or cytomegalovirus (CMV)-negative blood, and if the patient requires any other medications, for example diuretic or premedication.	To prevent incorrect blood component transfused (IBCT) error and transfusion-associated circulatory overload (TACO): ABO incompatibility or non-irradiated CMV-positive products may cause a fatal reaction if transfused (Bolton-Maggs 2018, **C**; Robinson et al. 2017, **C**).
3 Check that the patient's baseline vital signs, temperature, pulse, blood pressure and respirations have been recorded within 60 minutes prior to the start of the transfusion.	To ensure that any transfusion reaction can be immediately identified due to changes from the baseline. **E** To ensure any such reaction can be managed appropriately (Robinson et al. 2017, **C**).
4 Conduct a visual inspection of the component to be used for signs of clumping, discolouration, damage or leaks.	Expired or damaged products can cause patient harm and must not be used (Robinson et al. 2017, **E**).
5 If there are any discrepancies at this point, do not proceed until they have been resolved.	To ensure an IBCT event does not occur (Bolton-Maggs 2018, **C**).
6 Positively identify the patient by asking them to state the following information: • first name • surname • date of birth. If the patient is unable to positively identify themselves, verification can be given by a carer or relative. This information must match the identity band exactly.	This is the final check of identity, which must be performed next to the patient prior to transfusion and is absolutely vital in minimizing the risk of IBCT errors (Robinson et al. 2017, **C**; SNBTS 2004, **C**).
7 Check the details given against the patient's identity band and the patient details on the blood component (see Figure 12.75).	To minimize the risk of giving the wrong blood to the patient (SNBTS 2004, **C**).
8 Check that the information on the compatibility label matches the details on the blood component, checking expiry date, unique component donation number and blood group on the component label against the laboratory-produced label. Check any special requirements have been met. If there are any interruptions during the checking procedure, the entire process should be restarted from the beginning.	To minimize the risk of error (Robinson et al. 2017, **C**).
9 If there are any discrepancies at any point during the bedside check, do not proceed until they have been resolved.	To ensure an IBCT event does not occur (Bolton-Maggs 2018, **C**).

Procedure	
10 Prime the set with the blood or blood components, unless there are concerns about the patency of the device, in which case prime with 0.9% sodium chloride.	Other agents may damage the product components and precipitate transfusion complications (SNBTS 2004, **C**). For example, dextrose should never be used to prime a set or flush the blood administration set following a transfusion as this can cause haemolysis (SNBTS 2004, **C**).
11 Set up the infusion either via gravity or via an infusion pump if appropriate. Check the infusion pump is appropriate for the administration of blood and blood components.	Some older infusion pumps can damage the red cells; check the manufacturer's instructions. Blood administration sets for specific infusion pumps must always be used. If none are available, the standard blood administration set should be used via gravity and the rate monitored as necessary. **E**
12 Set the desired infusion rate as indicated by the blood component being used and the patient's condition. Monitor to ensure the expected volume is given at the correct rate.	The rate of administration is indicated by the patient's clinical condition (Norfolk 2013, **E**; Robinson et al. 2017, **C**).
Either:	
Red cell administration can range from 5 to 10 minutes in acute blood loss and must be completed within a maximum of 4 hours of removal from storage. Typical transfusion time is 90–120 minutes in patients who are not at risk of TACO (Norfolk 2013, Robinson et al. 2017).	To minimize the risk of bacterial growth and transfusion-transmitted infection (Norfolk 2013, **E**; Robinson et al. 2017, **C**).
Or:	
Platelets, fresh frozen plasma and cryoprecipitate should be transfused over 30–60 minutes, with the process completed within 4 hours of removal from temperature-controlled storage.	To ensure the patient receives the optimum benefit from the component. **E**
13 Sign the written order ('prescription') as the person administering the component. The unique component donation number, date and start time should be recorded in the patient's clinical notes.	To ensure that documentation and traceability requirements are met (BSQR 2005, **C**; Norfolk 2013, **E**; Robinson et al. 2017, **C**).
14 Fifteen minutes after the commencement of each component, take and record patient observations – blood pressure, temperature, pulse and respiratory rate. Follow local hospital policy regarding how observations are documented, but they should be easily identifiable as being related to the transfusion.	Adverse reactions will often occur during the first 15 minutes of transfusion (Tinegate et al. 2012, **C**). Complaints of serious anxiety, transfusion site pain, loin pain, backache, fever, skin flushing or urticaria could be indicative of a serious transfusion reaction (NICE 2013, **C**; Norfolk 2013, **E**; Robinson et al. 2017, **C**; Tinegate et al. 2012, **C**).
15 Observe and monitor the patient throughout the transfusion episode. If there are any concerns, undertake additional observations as appropriate. If there are any signs or symptoms of a transfusion reaction, the transfusion should be stopped immediately and urgent medical advice sought (see Box 12.11).	To monitor for any adverse reactions (Norfolk 2013, **E**; Robinson et al. 2017, **C**; Tinegate et al. 2012, **E**).
16 Record the finish time of each unit. All units must be completed within 4 hours of removal from storage.	To minimize the risk of a bacterial transmission (Norfolk 2013, **E**).
17 Take and record the patient's observations on completion of each unit, ensuring that post-transfusion observations are performed within 60 minutes of completion of the unit.	To ensure the patient's progress is recorded, to detect delayed reactions and act as a baseline for subsequent units (Robinson et al. 2017, **C**).
Post-procedure	
18 Record the time the transfusion finished and the volume of the component transfused on the patient's fluid balance chart.	To ensure an accurate record of fluid is maintained as fluid balance monitoring can identify fluid overload in at-risk patients (Bolton-Maggs 2018, **E**).
19 Carefully file all transfusion documentation in the patient's clinical record. In line with local policy, return information on the final fate of each blood component to the hospital transfusion laboratory.	To ensure the transfusion episode has been recorded, maintaining the clinical record for patient safety. To comply with the Blood Safety and Quality Regulations (2005, **C**), which specify that the final fate of all blood components must be held for 30 years.
20 Return any unused blood components to the laboratory promptly, preferably within 30 minutes.	To allow unused components to be reallocated if returned in time. Refer to local guidelines. **E**
21 If there is any suspicion of a transfusion reaction, return the pack to the transfusion laboratory with full clinical details. If the transfusion is completed uneventfully, dispose of the empty pack and administration set according to local policy.	To ensure transfused bags are available for laboratory tests and investigation (Tinegate et al. 2012, **C**).
22 For patients receiving ongoing transfusion support, the blood administration set should be changed at least every 12 hours or in accordance with the manufacturer's instructions. Dispose of the used set in the clinical waste. refer to local guidelines and protocols.	To minimize the risk of bacterial contamination (Robinson et al. 2017, **C**).

Problem solving table 12.[illegible] Prevention and resolution (Procedure guidelines 12.18, 12.19, 12.20 and 12.21)

Problem	Cause	Prevention	Action
Unable to collect patient information	Unknown unconscious patient	Do not transfuse unless clinically essential. The patient must be allocated a unique patient identifier; NHS Improvement (2018b) mandates that trusts develop a system with an estimated date of birth and a 'name' based on a non-sequential phonetic alphabet. This information must be used in conjuction with the patient's sex for transfusion requests.	Assign the unique hospital identification number to all requests and samples (Robinson et al. 2017).
	Major incident	Do not transfuse unless clinically essential. As above if transfusion is essential.	Use unique major incident identification number for all requests and samples. The transfusion laboratory also needs patient sex, minimum identification ('unknown male/female') and patient incident or hospital number. Follow local policy for major incidents.
	Patient unable to communicate verbally	Follow hospital policy for identification of patients unable to confirm identity verbally. Consider the introduction of a photo identification card. Ensure interpreting services are available if appropriate.	Confirm identity with a relative or second member of staff (SNBTS 2004).
Patient does not have an identity band	Identity band has been removed or is no longer legible	Always follow local policy and *never* use secondary identifiers such as bed numbers, notes or request forms that the patient may be carrying (Murphy et al. 2009). If a member of staff removes a patient's identification band, they are responsible for ensuring that it is replaced.	All inpatients are required to wear an identity band; therefore, replace identity band and reconfirm identity (NPSA 2007).
	Patient is in an outpatient setting	Follow hospital policy for the identification of patients.	Ensure the patient has a correctly completed identification wristband prior to commencing a transfusion.
Unable to obtain verbal confirmation	Patient unconscious	Ensure hospital policy for the identification of unconscious patients is followed.	Confirm identity with a relative or second member of staff or use a unique patient identifier.
Patient unable to communicate verbally	Disease or language barrier	Follow hospital policy for the identification of patients unable to confirm their identity verbally. Consider the introduction of photo identification cards. Ensure interpreting services are available if appropriate.	Always follow local policy and *never* use secondary identifiers such as bed numbers, notes or request forms that the patient may be carrying (Murphy et al. 2009).
Infusion slows or stops	Venous spasm due to cold infusion	Apply a heat pad prior to the transfusion to reduce venous spasm.	Apply a warm compress to dilate the vein and increase blood flow.
	Occlusion	Check patency prior to administration. Always use a pulsatile flush ending with a positive pressure flush.	Flush gently with 0.9% sodium chloride and resume infusion. If occlusion persists, consider resiting cannula. For a central venous access device occlusion, see Chapter 17: Vascular access devices: insertion and management.
Elevation of the patient's temperature of less than 2°C after commencing a unit of blood with no other symptoms, and temperature falls if the blood is stopped	Febrile non-haemolytic transfusion reaction	Take a history to identify whether the patient has had a reaction previously.	Stop the transfusion and observe the patient's temperature, pulse and blood pressure. If the patient has no other signs or symptoms, give paracetamol and continue the transfusion at a slower rate and observe more frequently (Norfolk 2013).

Post-procedural considerations

Immediate care

Patients should be asked to inform a member of staff of any symptoms that may indicate a transfusion-related adverse event, such as feeling anxious, rigors (shivering), flushing, pain or shortness of breath. Patients should be cared for where they can be visually observed and should be shown how to use the nurse call system. Patients should have their vital signs monitored as indicated in Procedure guideline 12.21: Blood component administration. However, it may be necessary to take additional observations if clinically indicated, such as if the patient complains of feeling unwell or if they develop signs of a transfusion reaction (Tinegate et al. 2012). Guidance for the initial recognition of transfusion reactions is provided in Table 12.18.

Many drugs may cause a pyretic hypersensitivity reaction (BNF 2019). There is at present insufficient evidence to offer guidance on the co-administration of drugs with red blood cell transfusion. A lack of clinical reporting of reactions in patients cannot be taken to indicate safe practice; adverse reactions may be attributed to other causes; subclinical haemolysis or agglutination may occur undetected; and serious adverse effects may be masked by pre-existing illness in a patient (Murdock et al. 2009).

Ongoing care

On completion of a blood transfusion episode, observations (to include blood pressure, temperature, pulse and respiratory rate) should be taken and recorded. The patient's records should be updated to confirm that the transfusion has taken place, including the volume transfused, whether the transfusion achieved the desired effect (either post-transfusion increment rates or an improvement in the patient's symptoms) and the details of any reactions to the transfusion. If intravenous fluids are prescribed to follow the transfusion, these should be administered through a new administration set appropriate for the infusion. The traceability documentation confirming the fate of the component should be returned to the laboratory (BSQR 2005).

The 2017 SHOT annual report (Bolton-Maggs 2018) emphasizes that, on occasion, transfusion reactions can occur many hours and sometimes days after a transfusion is completed. Therefore, for patients receiving a transfusion as a day case, it is important to ensure that they are counselled on the possibility of later adverse reactions and that they have access to clinical advice at all times. SHOT and the BSH recommend that day case and short stay patients are issued with a contact card facilitating 24-hour access to appropriate clinical advice, similarly to patients receiving chemotherapy treatments on an outpatient basis (Bolton-Maggs 2014, Robinson et al. 2017).

Table 12.18 Recognition of transfusion reactions

Symptoms/signs	Mild	Moderate	Severe
Temperature	Temperature of ≥38°C *and* a rise of 1–2°C from baseline temperature	Temperature of ≥39°C *or* a rise of ≥2°C from baseline temperature	Sustained febrile symptoms or any new, unexplained pyrexia *in addition* to clinical signs
Rigors/shaking	None	Mild chills	Obvious shaking/rigors
Pulse	Minimal or no change from baseline	Rise in heart rate from baseline of 10 bpm or more not associated with bleeding	Rise in heart rate from baseline of 20 bpm or more not associated with bleeding
Respirations	Minimal or no change from baseline	Rise in respiratory rate from baseline of 10 or more	Rise in respiratory rate from baseline of 10 or more accompanied by dyspnoea/wheeze
Blood pressure (hypotension or hypertension)	Minor or no change to systolic or diastolic pressure	Change in systolic or diastolic pressure of ≤30 mmHg *not* associated with bleeding	Change in systolic or diastolic pressure of ≥30 mmHg *not* associated with bleeding
Skin	No change	Facial flushing, rash, urticaria, pruritus	Rash, urticaria *and* periorbital oedema; conjunctivitis
Pain	None	General discomfort or myalgia, pain at drip site	Acute pain in chest, abdomen or back
Urine	Clear normal output		Haematuria, haemoglobinuria, oliguria, anuria
Bleeding	No new bleeding		Uncontrolled oozing
Nausea	None		Nausea or vomiting
Actions			
All *mild* symptoms/signs present at the same time	*STOP the transfusion but leave connected.* Recheck the identity of the unit with the patient and inform doctor. If all well, continue at a reduced rate *for the next 30 minutes* and then resume at the rate of written instuction. Continue to monitor the patient carefully and be alert for other symptoms or signs of a transfusion reaction. Antipyretics may be required.		
One or more *moderate* symptom/sign	*STOP the transfusion but leave connected.* Request urgent clinical review, recheck identity of the unit with the patient, and give IV fluids. If symptoms stable or improving over the next 15 minutes, consider restarting the unit. Antihistamines and/or antipyretics may be required.		
One or more *severe* symptom/sign	*STOP the transfusion and disconnect.* Request immediate clinical review, recheck identity of the unit with the patient, give IV fluids, inform the transfusion laboratory, and contact the consultant haematologist.		

In all cases where a transfusion reaction is suspected and the transfusion is stopped and disconnected, the implicated unit, complete with giving set, must be returned to the laboratory for further investigation. Follow local transfusion policy and contact the transfusion laboratory for further instructions. bpm, beats per minute; IV, intraveous.
Source: Produced by Wales Transfusion Practitioner Group, V2: WBS BBT Team Oct 2012. Based on Tinegate et al. (2012), UK Blood Services (2007).

Complications: general

Reporting of adverse effects and reactions

In November 1996, the Serious Hazards of Transfusion (SHOT) scheme was launched. This voluntary and anonymised reporting [illegible] and Ireland. The purpose of SHOT is to collect data on serious morbidity related to the transfusion of blood and blood products. This data has since been used to inform education programmes, policy development and guideline development, ultimately improving hospital transfusion practice. SHOT also monitors the effect of its recommendations (Bolton-Maggs 2018).

Although the Blood Safety and Quality Regulations (2005) have now made the reporting of such events via SABRE mandatory, the SHOT scheme remains active and important and has presented yearly retrospective reports of data collected since its inception. These data demonstrate improved performance in recognizing reporting of transfusion-related incidents and continues to generate key recommendations to improve all transfusion practice. Despite significant improvement in the reduction of risk from transfusion-transmitted infection, human error that results in an incorrect blood component transfusion (IBCT) (i.e. the transfusion of a blood product that is not suitable for or not intended for the recipient) remains one of the greatest risks to patients. Figures from the 2017 SHOT report indicate that there were 307 cases in this category (Bolton-Maggs 2018). SHOT provided a risk assessment per 100,000 blood components issued: the risk of death was 1 in 114,000 and the risk of serious harm was 1 in 21,000 (Bolton-Maggs 2018).

The prompt management of any adverse transfusion reaction can reduce associated morbidity and can be life saving. Therefore, staff caring for patients receiving transfused products must be fully familiar with the immediate management of any suspected reaction (Box 12.11). However, specialist advice should always be sought regarding the diagnosis and ongoing management of transfusion reactions, such as haemolytic, anaphylactic and septic reactions (Robinson et al. 2017, Tinegate et al. 2012).

Transfusion-associated graft-versus-host disease

Although rare, transfusion-associated graft-versus-host disease (TA-GVHD) is a serious complication and is often fatal. TA-GVHD is usually caused by an IBCT incident where non-irradiated blood components containing immunocompetent T lymphocytes are given to severely immunocompromised recipients. The donor T lymphocytes engraft and multiply, reacting against the recipient's 'foreign' tissue, causing a graft-versus-host reaction (Norfolk 2013). Onset occurs 1–2 weeks after transfusion (maximum 30 days) and the condition is predominantly fatal (Norfolk 2013). Irradiation (25 gray) of blood and cellular blood components (not required for [illegible] cipitate), to inactivate T lymphocytes (Norfolk 2013), is essential in the prevention of TA-GVHD and is especially important in the following recipients:

- foetuses receiving intrauterine transfusions
- patients undergoing or having undergone blood or bone marrow progenitor cell transplantation
- immunocompromised recipients
- patients with Hodgkin's lymphoma
- patients who have received purine analogues, e.g. fludarabine.

At present, the guidelines are being reviewed for patients receiving T-cell-depleted agents such as alemtuzumab for non-haematological indications. However, while this review is underway, the British Committee for Standards in Haematology recommends that these patients receive irradiated blood components (Treleaven et al. 2011).

Box 12.11 Initial management of a suspected transfusion reaction

- Stop the transfusion and seek urgent medical help.
- Initiate appropriate emergency procedures, for example call the resuscitation team.
- Depending on venous access, withdraw the contents of the lumen being used and disconnect the blood product.
- Keep venous access patent.
- Confirm the patient's identity and recheck their details against the product compatibility label.
- Keep the patient and relatives informed of all progress and reassure them as indicated.
- Initiate close and frequent observations of temperature, pulse, blood pressure and fluid balance.
- Inform the transfusion laboratory and seek the urgent advice of the haematologist for further management.
- Return the transfused product to the laboratory with new blood samples (10 mL clotted and 5 mL ethylenediamine tetra-acetic acid from the patient's opposite arm) (Tinegate et al. 2012) with a completed transfusion reaction notification form (if available) or note the patient's details, the nature and timing of the reaction, and the details of the component transfused.

Bacterial infections

Contamination of blood and blood components can occur during donation, collection, processing, storage and administration. Despite strict guidelines and procedures, the risk of contamination remains. The most common contaminating organisms are skin contaminants such as staphylococci, diphtheroids and micrococci, which enter the blood at the time of venesection (Barbara and Contreras 2009, Provan et al. 2015). Bacterial contamination can lead to severe septic reaction. Two strategies have been implemented by NHS Blood and Transplant (NHSBT) to reduce bacterial infections: donor arm disinfection and the diversion of the first 30 mL of each donation to reduce contamination of the blood component by the skin plug from venepuncture. Since 1996, 44 confirmed bacterial infections have been reported to SHOT, 37 of these related to platelet transfusions (Narayan 2019). NHSBT implemented bacterial screening in January 2011, and aerobic and anaerobic cultures are performed on each platelet collection (NHSBT 2011b).

Viral infections

Many viral infections have been well controlled by combinations of screening the donor, improvements in testing and good manufacturing practice (Katz and Dodd 2019, Norfolk 2013). Despite a now low incidence, vigilance must remain for new viruses that may emerge and compromise transfusion safety (Katz and Dodd 2019, Norfolk 2013). Plasma-borne viruses include hepatitis A (rarely), hepatitis B, hepatitis C, hepatitis E, serum parvovirus B19, and human immunodeficiency viruses (HIV-1 and HIV-2). Cell-associated viruses include cytomegalovirus (CMV), Epstein–Barr virus, human T-cell leukaemia/lymphoma viruses (HTLV-1 and HTLV-2), and HIV-1 and HIV-2. Since 1996 there have been 34 viral transfusion-transmitted infections, involving 41 recipients, confirmed and reported to SHOT (Narayan 2019). In 2017, both the Scottish National Blood Transfusion Service and NHSBT implemented 100% screening of all blood donations for hepatitis E. SHOT reported one confirmed case of hepatitis E transmission from transfusion in 2018 (Narayan 2019).

Human T-cell leukaemia/lymphoma virus type 1 (HTLV-1)

HTLV-1 is an oncogenic retrovirus associated with the white cells that cause adult T-cell leukaemia and is connected with several degenerative neuromuscular syndromes. Screening using the enzyme-linked immunosorbent assay (ELISA) has been recommended because of concerns relating to the transmission of the virus via blood transfusion and the associated long incubation period of adult T-cell leukaemia. In 2017, NHSBT changed from universal HTLV screening to selective (for new donors and components that will not be leuco-depleted) (Bolton-Maggs 2018). Since the introduction of leucodepletion and screening, transmission of HTLV has been virtually eliminated (Norfolk 2013).

Cytomegalovirus (CMV)

CMV is classified as part of the herpes family and hence has the ability to remain latent within monocytes and dendritic cells and can then reactivate during periods of immunosuppression (Al-Omari et al. 2016). Approximately 50% of the UK population have antibodies to CMV. Therefore, it is recognized that the virus may be transmitted by transfusion. Although it poses little threat to immunologically competent recipients, in vulnerable patient groups CMV infection can cause significant morbidity and mortality. In March 2012, the Advisory Committee on the Safety of Blood, Tissues and Organs issued a position statement with guidance that the leucodepletion of blood components 'provides a significant degree of CMV risk reduction' (SaBTO 2012, p.11). This risk reduction is considered adequate protection against transmission of CMV to the majority of patients, including haemopoietic stem cell transplant patients. It is recommend that if an intrauterine, neonate and/or elective transfusion during pregnancy is required that these patients receive CMV-seronegative components (SaBTO 2012).

Hepatitis B virus (HBV)

Screening for hepatitis B (HBV) is conducted via nucleic acid testing (HBV NAT) (JPAC 2013). SHOT reported one probable and one indeterminate hepatitis B transfusion infection in 2018 (Narayan 2019).

Hepatitis C virus (HCV)

Screening for hepatitis C (HCV) is conducted via nucleic acid testing (HCV NAT) (JPAC 2013). HCV is transmitted primarily via contact with blood or blood products (Friedman 2001). The last reported HCV transfusion transmitted infection occurred in 1997 (Bolton-Maggs 2018).

Human immunodeficiency virus (HIV-1 and HIV-2)

HIV is a retrovirus that infects and kills helper T cells, also known as CD4 positive lymphocytes. The virus can be transmitted via most blood products, including red cells, platelets, FFP, and factor VIII and IX concentrates. These viruses are not known to be transmitted in albumin, immunoglobulins or antithrombin III products (Barbara and Contreras 2009). The retrovirus invades cells and slowly destroys the immune system, rendering the individual susceptible to opportunistic infections. Since 1983, when it was recognized that the virus could be transmitted via transfusion, actions have been developed to safeguard blood supplies from transmitting the virus that causes acquired immune deficiency syndrome (AIDS). These include the careful screening of donors and the testing of donated blood. The last transmission of HIV-1 or HIV-2 due to a blood transfusion occurred in 2002, before the introduction of NAT (nucleic acid testing) screening (Bolton-Maggs 2018).

Other infective agents

Parasites

Plasmodium falciparum is the most dangerous of the human malarial parasites (Barbara and Contreras 2009). Prevention is maintained by questioning donors about foreign travel, in particular travel to areas where the disease is prevalent (Bishop 2008). The last parasite transfusion-transmitted infection to be reported to SHOT occurred in 2003 (Bolton-Maggs 2018).

Prion diseases

Known as transmissible spongiform encephalopathies (TSEs), these are a rare group of conditions that cause progressive neurodegeneration in humans and some animal species (Box 12.12). Prion diseases are caused by the presence of an abnormal misfolded aggregated cellular protein (Sigurdson et al. 2019). Key characteristics of vCJD include an accumulation of protease-resisitant prion protein in lymphoid tissue and the presence of 'florid' plaques on neuropathology (Centers for Disease Control and Prevention 2019).

Box 12.12 Prion diseases

Prion diseases in animal species

- Scrapie, a disease of sheep
- Bovine spongiform encephalopathy (BSE)
- Feline spongiform encephalopathy (FSE)
- Chronic wasting disease of deer, mule and elk

Prion diseases in humans

- Sporadic: classic Creutzfeldt–Jakob disease (CJD)
- Inherited: CJD, Gerstmann–Sträussler–Scheinker syndrome, fatal familial insomnia (FFI)
- Acquired: kuru, variant CJD (vCJD)

There is evidence to suggest that in TSEs, of which vCJD is one, leucocytes (particularly lymphocytes) are the key cells in transportation of the putative infectious agent to the brain; therefore, as a risk reduction measure, leucodepletion of blood components was introduced in 1999 (Norfolk 2013). There were a total of 178 deaths in cases of definite or probable vCJD in the UK up to 31 December 2017. Analysis of the incidence of vCJD onsets and deaths from January 1994 to December 2011 indicates that a peak has passed (National CJD Research and Surveillance Unit 2017). While this is an encouraging finding, the incidence of vCJD may increase again, particularly if different genetic subgroups with longer incubation periods exist (National CJD Research and Surveillance Unit 2017).

Sepsis

Sepsis can occur as a result of bacteria entering the blood or blood component that is to be infused. The most common bacterial culprit is skin flora (Levy et al. 2018). The blood component that carries the largest risk of causing a bacterial infection is platelets (Bolton-Maggs 2018). Bacteria can enter at any point from the time of collection, during storage through to administration to the patient.

Complications: pulmonary

Transfusion-related acute lung injury (TRALI)

The current SHOT definition of transfusion-related acute lung injury (TRALI) is as follows:

> Transfusion-related acute lung injury (TRALI) is defined as acute dyspnoea with hypoxia and bilateral pulmonary infiltrates during or within 6 hours of transfusion, in the absence of circulatory overload or other likely causes, or in the presence of human leucocyte antigen (HLA) or human neutrophil antigen (HNA) antibodies cognate with the recipient. (Bolton-Maggs 2018, p.144)

The pathophysiology of TRALI is not completely understood and is thought to be complex (Bolton-Maggs 2018, Semple et al. 2019). The model that is proposed is a 'two-hit model' whereby an existing clinical pathophysiology has already caused neutrophils to sequest in the pulmonary capillaries and then a second hit is caused by the transfusion, whereupon a substance in the transfused component causes the neutrophils to activate (Semple et al. 2019, Skeate and Eastlund 2007). The 2017 SHOT report cited plans for a future workshop to address some of the gaps in knowledge regarding transfusion pulmonary complications (Bolton-Maggs 2018, p.142). A new consensus definition was published in 2019 with new terminology to define TRALI (Vlaar et al. 2019). The new consensus definition is dependent on the presence or absence of existing risk factors for acute respiratory distress syndrome (ARDS) in the patient prior to transfusion. In type 1 TRALI, the patient has no risk factors for ARDS but following transfusion develops acute-onset hypoxaemia with clear evidence of bilateral pulmonary oedema and no evidence of left anterior hemiblock, and this occurs within 6 hours of the end of the transfusion. Patients who have risk factors for ARDS or who have mild existing ARDS, but where the transfusion causes respiratory deterioration, are classified as type 2 TRALI (Vlaar et al. 2019).

TRALI is usually caused by anti-neutrophil antibodies reacting against donor leucocytes but there have been cases of TRALI that are antibody negative, and definitions of TRALI are shaped by the presence or absence of antibodies in serological testing (Bolton-Maggs 2018). In many cases, either HLA or neutrophil-specific antibodies were detected in the donors and most of the donors were multiparous (having been pregnant with one or more children) women. As the antibodies were mostly found in multiparous women and, as because SHOT reports demonstrate that in the majority of cases the donor is female, in 2003 NHSBT developed a strategy to use only the plasma from male donors for FFP and male plasma in pooled platelets (Bolton-Maggs 2018).

TRALI is usually treated the same way as any ARDS and therefore patients who develop TRALI may require ventilatory support (Tinegate et al. 2012) and should be treated as emergency cases. Diuretics should not be administered as patients are generally hypotensive and hypovolaemic. As TRALI is donor related, it is essential that cases are reported to the blood transfusion services so that donors can be contacted, investigated for antibodies to HLA and, if necessary, removed from the donor panel (Norfolk 2013). The consensus committee emphasized that clinicians should report all cases of post-transfusion pulmonary oedema to the transfusion service so that further investigation can take place (Vlaar et al. 2019).

Transfusion-associated circulatory overload (TACO)

Circulatory overload can occur when blood or any of its components is infused rapidly or administered to a patient with an increased plasma volume, causing hypervolaemia. Patients at risk are those with renal or cardiac deficiencies, the young and the elderly. Patients with signs of cardiac failure should receive their transfusion slowly with diuretic support (Norfolk 2013). A key recommendation of Narayan (2019) is that all patients must be risk assessed for TACO as part of the decision to transfuse. Patients at risk of TACO must be closely monitored and then reassessed after each pack of blood component.

Transfusion-associated dyspnoea (TAD)

"TAD is characterised by respiratory distress within 24 hours of transfusion that does not meet the criteria for TRALI, TACO or allergic reaction' (International Society of Blood Transfusion cited in Narayan 2019, p.147). In these cases, the patient's underlying condition should not provide an adequate explanation for their respiratory distress.

Complications: minor transfusion reactions

It should always be remembered that the symptoms of a 'minor' transfusion reaction may be the prelude to a major, life-threatening reaction. It is essential that staff take any transfusion reaction seriously. Symptomatic patients should have their vital signs monitored closely and they should be clearly observable. Patients with persistent or deteriorating symptoms should always be managed as a major reaction case, and urgent medical and specialist support should be sought (Norfolk 2013, Tinegate et al. 2012).

Symptoms of minor reactions include a temperature rise of up to 2°C, rash without systemic disturbance, and moderate tachycardia without hypotension but sometimes transient hypertension (Delaney et al. 2016). Such symptoms may be caused by an immunological reaction to components of the blood product. While it may be possible to manage such symptoms and continue with the transfusion, the actions listed in Box 12.11 should always be taken.

It may be possible to continue with the transfusion at a reduced rate once the patient's symptoms have been controlled; however, it may be necessary to increase the frequency of observations until the transfusion has been completed. Some patients who have regular transfusions may experience recurrent febrile reactions and may benefit from an antipyretic premedication. Aspirin and other non-steroidal anti-inflammatory drugs are contraindicated in patients with a thrombocytopenia or coagulopathy (BNF 2019).

Febrile non-haemolytic reactions

Febrile non-haemolytic reactions are caused by an immunological response to the transfusion of cellular components such as donor leucocytes. Specific patient groups are at risk of greater sensitization to leucocytes, for example critically ill patients, those receiving anti-cancer therapies and those who require multiple transfusion therapies (Bolton-Maggs 2018, Williamson et al. 1999). Such reactions present with a mild fever (up to 2°C from the baseline), rash without systemic disturbance and moderate tachycardia without hypotension (Norfolk 2013, Tinegate et al. 2012).

Urticaria

Urticaria is characterized by mild hives, rash or skin itching (Delaney et al. 2016). Symptoms can usually be treated with an antihistamine (Norfolk 2013) and patients require monitoring until their symptoms subside in case they develop into a severe reaction. If the reaction subsides then the transfusion can often be recommenced; however, if any other signs or symptoms develop, the transfusion must be discontinued completely (Norfolk 2013).

Complications: major transfusion reactions

Major transfusion reactions include anaphylaxis, haemolysis and sepsis and may present as a fever of over 38.5°C and tachycardia with or without hypertension. In such circumstances a severe reaction should always be considered and the transfusion should be stopped until a specialist assessment has been conducted (see Box 12.11).

Care should be taken when returning the blood components to the laboratory, to ensure that the components do not leak and that no needles remain attached. Any further components being held locally for the patient should also be returned to the hospital transfusion laboratory for assessment. The events surrounding the reaction should be clearly documented and reported in the following ways:

- Record the adverse event in the patient's clinical record.
- Complete a detailed incident report as per local policy.
- Follow local, regional and national criteria for reporting via SABRE and SHOT (this is usually done by the transfusion practitioner).

Acute haemolytic reactions

Acute haemolytic reactions are usually directly related to ABO incompatibilities due to either an IBCT or undetected antibody where antigen/antibody reactions occur when the recipient's antibodies react with surface antigens on the donor red cells. This reaction causes a cascade of events within the recipient, who can present with chills and/or rigors, facial flushing, pain and/or oozing at the cannula site, burning along the vein, chest pain, lumbar or flank pain, or shock. The BSH guideline (Tinegate et al. 2012) stresses that acute transfusion reactions can often present with an overlapping complex of signs and symptoms; the initial assessment should aim to identify patients with a serious or life-threatening reaction and then treatment should be targeted to the signs and symptoms (Tinegate et al. 2012).

Patients may express a feeling of anxiety or doom, which may be associated with cytokine activity. Haemolytic shock can occur after only a few millilitres of blood have been infused. Treatment is often vigorous to reverse hypotension, aid adequate renal perfusion and renal flow (to reduce potential damage to renal tubules), and start appropriate therapy for disseminated intravascular coagulation reactions (Norfolk 2013). It is important to remember that most acute haemolytic reactions are preventable as they are usually caused by human error when taking or labelling pre-transfusion

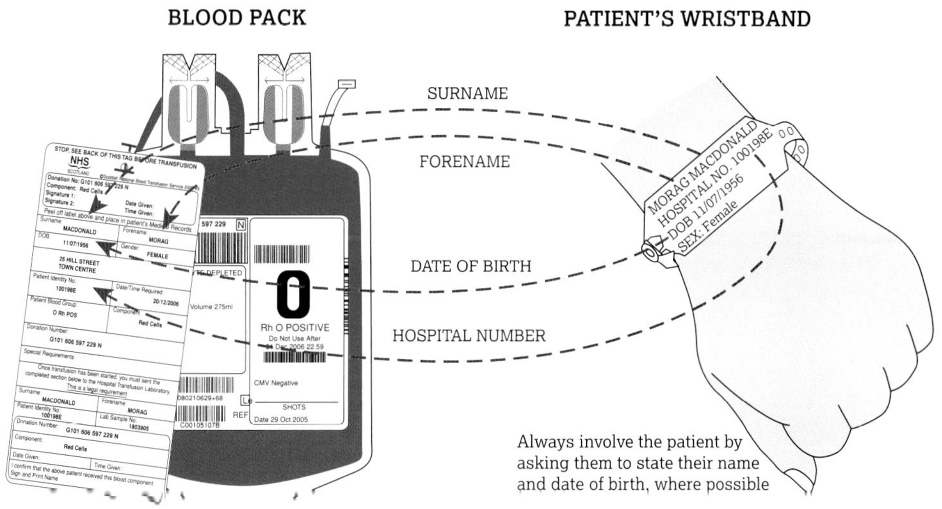

Figure 12.75 Checking the compatibility label or tie on tag against the patient's wristband.

samples or collecting blood components, and/or failing to perform a correct identity check of the blood pack and patient at the bedside (McClelland 2007, Norfolk 2013) (Figure 12.75).

Acute anaphylactic reactions

Allergic and anaphylactic reactions are most common with platelet transfusions but can occur with any blood component (Delaney et al. 2016). If a patient presents with shock and severe hypotension with accompanying wheeze or stridor, this is strongly suggestive of anaphylaxis (Tinegate et al. 2012). Urgent medical care should be sought immediately and Resuscitation Council guidelines followed (Norfolk 2013).

Hypothermia

Infusing large quantities of cold blood rapidly can cause hypothermia. Patients likely to experience this reaction are those who have suffered massive blood loss due to trauma, haemorrhage, clotting disorders or thrombocytopenia (Norfolk 2013). Such reactions present with alterations in vital signs and development of pallor and chills.

Complications: delayed transfusion reactions

Reactions may occur days, months or even years after transfusion. Delayed reactions can be haemolytic or serological with no signs of hemolysis (Delaney et al. 2016). Usually the reaction is seen in a patient who has already made an alloantibody and the antibody has fallen to an undetectable level so that it is not detected on a pre-transfusion antibody screen (Norfolk 2013). Re-exposure to the antigen in a subsequent transfusion causes the antibody level to rise again, usually within 24 hours but sometimes up to 28 days after the transfusion (Delaney et al. 2016). The most frequent signs and symptoms in delayed reactions include dark urine, jaundice, fever, back pain, dyspnoea, chills and hypertension (Delaney et al. 2016). When a delayed reaction is suspected, further laboratory testing is required; however, the treatment is usually supportive and may require further transfusions to maintain the desired level of haemoglobin (Delaney et al. 2016, Norfolk 2013).

Hyperkalaemia

Hyperkalaemia is a rare complication associated with haemorrhage and the subsequent infusion of large quantities of blood. Mortality is also associated with an increase rate of transfusion and stored blood, as potassium is known to leak out of red cells during storage, thereby increasing circulatory levels in recipients receiving blood products (Raza et al. 2015). The process is exacerbated if packed red cells are gamma irradiated as this changes the cell membrane's permeability and causes more potassium leakage into the extracellular space (Raza et al. 2015). A patient with hyperkalaemia requires urgent medical review.

Iron overload

Patients who are dependent on frequent transfusion, such as those with thalassaemic, sickle cell and other transfusion-dependent disorders, can become overloaded with iron (Norfolk 2013). A unit of red blood cells contains 250 mg iron, which the body is unable to excrete, and as a result patients receiving large volumes of blood are at risk of iron overload (Norfolk 2013). This can result in poor growth, pigment changes, hepatic cirrhosis, hypoparathyroidism, diabetes, arrhythmia, cardiac failure and death. Chelation therapy through the use of desferrioxamine, which induces iron excretion, minimizes the accumulation of iron (BNF 2019).

Websites

British Society for Haematology: Guidelines
https://b-s-h.org.uk/guidelines/?category=Transfusion&fromdate=&todate=

Joint UK Blood Transfusion and Tissue Transplantation Services Professional Advisory Committee
https://www.transfusionguidelines.org

NHS Blood and Transplant: Hospitals and Science
https://hospital.blood.co.uk

Serious Hazards of Transfusion
https://www.shotuk.org

TOXBASE
https://www.toxbase.org

References

AAGBI (Association of Anaesthetists of Great Britain and Ireland) (2016) AAGBI guidelines: The use of blood components and their alternatives 2016. *Anaesthesia*, 71(7), 829–842.

Academy of Medical Royal Colleges (2013) *Safe Sedation Practice for Healthcare Procedures: Standards and Guidelines*. Available at: www.aomrc.org.uk/wp-content/uploads/2016/05/Safe_Sedation_Practice_1213.pdf

Adam, S., Osborne, S. & Welch, J. (2017) *Critical Care Nursing*, 3rd edn. Oxford: Oxford University Press.

Adamson, R.T. (2015) The burden of hyperkalemia in patients with cardiovascular and renal disease. *American Journal of Managed Care*, 21, S307–S315.

[illegible]
L., Demoule, A., & Windlisch, W. (eds) *Pulmonary Emergencies*. Norwich: European Respiratory Society, pp.229–239.

Afacan, M.A., Colak, S., Gunes, H., et al. (2014) An unusual complication of cardiopulmonary resuscitation: Stomach perforation. *American Journal of Emergency Medicine*, 33(6), 1140.

Al Ashry, H.S. & Modrykamien, A.M. (2014) *Humidification during mechanical ventilation in the adult patient. BioMed Research International.* Available at: https://www.hindawi.com/journals/bmri/2014/715434

Alamdari, D.H., Asadi, M., Rahim, A.N., et al. (2018) Efficacy and safety of pleurodesis using platelet-rich plasma and fibrin glue in management of postoperative chylothorax after esophagectomy. *World Journal of Surgery*, 42(4), 1046–1055.

Al-Omari, A., Aljamaan, F., Alhazzani, W., et al. (2016) Cytomegalovirus infection in immunocompetent critically ill adults: Literature review. *Annals of Intensive Care*, 6(1), 110.

American Society of Anesthesiologists (2018) Practical guidelines for moderate procedural sedation and analgesia. *Anesthesiology*, 128(3), 437–479.

Ari, A., Harwood, R., Sheard, M., et al. (2016) Quantifying aerosol delivery in simulated spontaneously breathing patients with tracheostomy using different humidification systems with or without exhaled humidity. *Respiratory Care*, 61(5), 600–606.

Backhaus, R., Torka, E., Ertl, M., et al. (2017) Influence of positive end-expiratory pressure ventilation on cerebral perfusion and cardia haemodynamics. *Journal of Depression and Anxiety*, 6(4). DOI: 10.4172/2167-1044.1000285

Barbara, J.A. & Contreras, M. (2009) Infectious complications of blood transfusion: Bacteria and parasites. In: Contreras, M. (ed) *ABC of Transfusion*, 4th edn. Oxford: Blackwell, pp.69–73.

Barnett, M. (2012) Back to basics: Caring for people with a tracheostomy. *Nursing & Residential Care*, 14(8), 390–394.

Batuwitage, B., Webber, S. & Glossop, A. (2014) Percutaneous tracheostomy. *Continuing Education in Anaesthesia, Critical Care & Pain*, 14(6), 268–272.

BCSH (British Committee for Standards in Haematology) (2009) *Guideline on the Administration of Blood Components*. London: British Society of Haematology.

BCSH, Blood Transfusion Task Force, Boulton, F.E. & James, V. (2007) Guidelines for policies on alternatives to allogeneic blood transfusion. 1. Predeposit autologous blood donation and transfusion. *Transfusion Medicine*, 17(5), 354–365.

BCSH, Milkins, C., Berryman, J., et al. (2013) Guidelines for pre-transfusion compatibility procedures in blood transfusion laboratories. *Transfusion Medicine*, 23, 3–35.

Bein, T., Grasso, S., Moerer, O., et al. (2016) The standard of care of patients with ARDS: Ventilatory settings and rescue therapies for refractory hypoxemia. *Intensive Care Medicine*, 42(5), 699–711.

Beitler, J., Owen, R. & Malhotra, A. (2016) Unmasking a role for noninvasive ventilation in early acute respiratory distress syndrome. *JAMA*, 315(22), 2401–2403.

Bender, B., Murthy, V. & Chamberlain, R.S. (2016) The changing management of chylothorax in the modern era. *European Journal of Cardio-Thoracic Surgery*, 49(1), 18–24.

Bishop, E. (2008) Blood transfusion therapy. In: Dougherty, L. & Lamb, J. (eds) *Intravenous Therapy in Nursing Practice*, 2nd edn. Oxford: Blackwell, pp.377–394.

BMA (British Medical Association), Resuscitation Council UK (RCUK), & Royal College of Nursing (RCN) (2016) *Decisions Relating to Cardiopulmonary Resuscitation*, 3rd edn. London: British Medical Association.

BNF (British National Formulary) (2019) *British National Formulary*. National Institute for Health and Care Excellence. Available at: https://bnf.nice.org.uk

Bolton-Maggs, P.H.B. (ed) on behalf of the Serious Hazards of Transfusion (SHOT) Steering Group (2012) *The Annual SHOT Report 2011*. SHOT. Available at: https://www.shotuk.org/wp-content/uploads/myimages/SHOT ANNUAL REPORT_FinalWebVersionBookmarked_2012_06_22.pdf

Bolton-Maggs, P.H.B. (ed) on behalf of the Serious Hazards of Transfusion (SHOT) Steering Group (2014) *The Annual SHOT Report 2013*. SHOT. [illegible] 2013.pdf

Bolton-Maggs, P.H.B. (ed) on behalf of the Serious Hazards of Transfusion (SHOT) Steering Group (2018) *The Annual SHOT Report 2017*. SHOT. Available at: [illegible] SHOT Report 2017 WEB Final v4 25 9 18.pdf

Bonvento, B., Wallace, S., Lynch, J., et al. (2017) Role of the multidisciplinary team in the care of the tracheostomy patient. *Journal of Multidisciplinary Healthcare*, 10, 391–398.

Brady, D.R. (2018) Care of the patient with respiratory failure. In: Perrin, K.O. & Macleod, C.E. (eds) *Understanding the Essentials of Critical Care Nursing*. New York: Pearson, pp.51–80.

Brill, A. (2014) How to avoid interface problems in acute noninvasive ventilation. *Breathe*, 10(3), 231–242.

Brill, S.E. & Wedzicha, J.A. (2014) Oxygen therapy in acute exacerbations of chronic obstructive pulmonary disease. *International Journal of Chronic Obstructive Pulmonary Disease*, 9, 1241–1252.

British Heart Foundation (2018) *Cardiovascular Disease Statistics 2018*. Available at: https://www.bhf.org.uk/what-we-do/our-research/heart-statistics/heart-statistics-publications/cardiovascular-disease-statistics-2018

Bry, C., Jaffré, S., Guyomarc'h, B., et al. (2018) Noninvasive ventilation in obese subjects after acute respiratory failure. *Respiratory Care*, 63(1), 28–35.

BSQR (Blood Safety and Quality Regulations) (2005) Available at: www.opsi.gov.uk/si/si2005/20050050.htm

Cammarota, G., Vaschetto, G., Turucz, E., et al. (2011) Influence of lung collapse distribution on the physiologic response to recruitment maneuvers during noninvasive continuous positive airway pressure. *Intensive Care Medicine*, 37, 1095–1102.

Cardillo, G., Bintcliffe, O.J., Carleo, F., et al. (2016) Primary spontaneous pneumothorax: A cohort study of VATS with talc poudrage. *Thorax*, 71(9), 847–853.

Carless, P.A., Henry, D.A., Moxey, A.J., et al. (2010) Cell salvage for minimising perioperative allogeneic blood transfusion. *Cochrane Database of Systematic Reviews*, 4, CD001888.

Carson, J.L., Carless, P.A. & Hebert, P.C. (2012) Transfusion thresholds and other strategies for guiding allogeneic red blood cell transfusion. *Cochrane Database of Systematic Reviews*, 4, CD002042.

Ceachir, O., Hainarosie, R. & Zainea, V. (2014) Total laryngectomy: Past, present, future. *Maedica*, 9(2), 210–216.

Centers for Disease Control and Prevention (2019) *Variant Creutzfeldt-Jakob Disease (vCJD)*. Available at: https://www.cdc.gov/prions/vcjd/clinical-pathologic-characteristics.html

Cerfolio, R.J., Bryant, A.S., Skylizard, L. & Minnich, D.J. (2013) Optimal technique for the removal of chest tubes after pulmonary resection. *Journal of Thoracic and Cardiovascular Surgery*, 145(6), 1535–1539.

Chadwick, A.J., Halfyard, R. & Ali, M. (2015) Intercostal chest drains: Are you confident going on the pull? If not use the I-T-U approach. *Journal of Intensive Care Society*, 16(4), 312–325.

Cheng, H.M. & Jusof, F. (2018) Control of respiration. In: *Defining Physiology: Principles, Themes, Concepts*. Singapore: Springer, pp.117–124.

Cheung, N.H. & Napolitano, L.M. (2014) Tracheostomy: Epidemiology, indications, timing, technique, and outcomes. *Respiratory Care*, 59(6), 895–919.

Choi, W.I. (2014) Tuberculosis and respiratory diseases. *Pneumothorax*, 76(3), 99–104.

Chowdhury, O., Wedderburn, C., Duffy, D. & Greenough, A. (2012) CPAP review. *European Journal of Paediatrics*, 171, 1441–1448.

Cipriano, A., Mao, M.L., Hon, H.H., et al. (2015) An overview of complications associated with open and percutaneous tracheostomy procedures. *International Journal of Critical Illness and Injury Science*, 5(3), 179–188.

Clarke, P., Radford, K., Coffey, M. & Stewart, M. (2016) Speech and swallow rehabilitation in head and neck cancer: United Kingdom National Multidisciplinary Guidelines. *Journal of Laryngology & Otology*, 130(Suppl. 2), 176–180.

Collins, J.A., Rudenski, A., Gibson, J., et al. (2015) Relating oxygen partial pressure, saturation and content. The haemoglobin–oxygen dissociation curve. *Breathe*, 11(3), 194–201.

Corrêa, T.D., Sanches, P.R., de Morais, L.C., et al. (2015) Performance of noninvasive ventilation in acute respiratory failure in critically ill patients: A prospective, observational, cohort study. *BMC Pulmonary Medicine*, 15, 144.

Cortegiani, A., Russotto, V., Antonelli, M., et al. (2017) Ten important articles on noninvasive ventilation in critically ill patients and insights for the future: A report of expert opinions. *Anaesthesiology*, 17, 122.

Cosgrove, J.F. & Carrie, S. (2015) Indications for and management of tracheostomies. *Surgery*, 33(4), 172–179.

Cuquemelle, E., Pham, T., Papon, J.F., et al. (2012) Heated and humidified high-flow oxygen therapy reduces discomfort during hypoxemic respiratory failure. *Respiratory Care*, 57, 1571–1577.

Daniels, G. (2013) Human blood group systems. In: Murphy, M., Pamphilon, D. & Heddle, N. (eds) *Practical Transfusion Medicine*, 4th edn. Chichester: John Wiley & Sons, pp.21–30.

Davies, H.E., Davies, R.J.O. & Davies, C.W.H. (2010) Management of pleural infection in adults: British Thoracic Society pleural disease guideline 2010. *Thorax*, 65(Suppl. 2), i41–i53.

Davies, M., Allen, M., Bentley, A., et al. (2018) British Thoracic Society quality standards for acute non-invasive ventilation in adults. *BMJ*, 5, 1–13.

Davison, C., Banham, S., Elliott, M., et al. (2016) BTS/ICS guideline for the ventilatory management of acute hypercapnic respiratory failure in adults. *Thorax*, 71(Suppl. 2), i1–i35.

Dawson, D. (2014) Essential principles: Tracheostomy care in the adult patient. *British Association of Critical Care Nurses*, 19(2), 63–72.

Delaney, M., Wendel, S., Bercovitz, R.S., et al. (2016) Transfusion reactions: Prevention, diagnosis, and treatment. *Lancet*, 388(10061), 2825–2836.

Demoule, A., Hill, N. & Navalesi, P. (2016) Can we prevent intubation in patients with ARDS. *Intensive Care Medicine*, 42, 768–771.

DH (Department of Health) (2003) *Confidentiality: NHS Code of Practice*. Available at: https://assets.publishing.service.gov.uk/government/uploads/system/uploads/attachment_data/file/200146/Confidentiality_-_NHS_Code_of_Practice.pdf

DH (2007) *Better Blood Transfusion: Safe and Appropriate Use of Blood – HSC 2007/001*. Available at: https://webarchive.nationalarchives.gov.uk/20130105061013/www.dh.gov.uk/prod_consum_dh/groups/dh_digitalassets/documents/digitalasset/dh_080803.pdf

DH (2013) *Measures Currently in Place in the UK to Reduce the Potential Risk of vCJD Transmission via Blood*. Available at: https://www.gov.uk/government/news/measures-currently-in-place-in-the-uk-to-reduce-the-potential-risk-of-vcjd-transmission-via-blood

DH (2017) *Safe Transfusion Practice: Use a Bedside Checklist* [Alert Reference Number CEM/CMO/2017/005]. London: Department of Health.

Dhruve, H., Davey, C. & Pursell, J. (2015) Respiratory disease oxygen therapy: Emergency use and long term treatment. *Clinical Pharmacist*, 7(5). Available at: https://www.pharmaceutical-journal.com/learning/learning-article/oxygen-therapy-emergency-use-and-long-term-treatment/20068717.article

Dixon, C. & Jones, L. (2017) Oxygen prescription and safe administration on respiratory wards. *Journal of the Royal College of Physicians*, 17(Suppl. 3). DOI: 10.7861/clinmedicine.17-3-s2

Doctor, T.N., Foster, J.P., Stewart, A., et al. (2017) Heated and humidified inspired gas through heated humidifiers in comparison to non-heated and non-humidified gas in hospitalised neonates receiving respiratory support. *Cochrane Database of Systematic Reviews*, 2. DOI: 10.1002/14651858.CD012549

Dres, M. & Demoule, A. (2016) Noninvasive ventilation: Do not tolerate intolerance. *Respiratory Care*, 61(3), 393–394.

Dysart, K., Miller, T.L., Wolfson, M.R. & Shaffer, T.H. (2009) Research in high flow therapy: Mechanisms of action. *Respiratory Medicine*, 103, 1400–1405.

Egan, A.M., McPhillips, D., Sarkar, S. & Breen, D. P. (2014) Malignant pleural effusion. *QJM*, 107(3), 179–184.

Eldin, K.W. & Teruya, J. (2012) Blood components for hemostasis. *Laboratory Medicine*, 43(6), 237–244.

English, A.M. (2015). Physiotherapy in palliative care. In: Cherny, N., Fallon, M., Kaasa, S., et al. (eds) *Oxford Textbook of Palliative Medicine*, 5th edn. Oxford: Oxford University Press, pp.197–202.

ERC (European Resuscitation Council) (2015) *European Resuscitation Guidelines*. Available at: https://cprguidelines.eu

Estcourt, L.J., Birchall, J., Allard, S., et al. (2017) Guidelines for the use of platelet transfusions. *British Journal of Haematology*, 176(3), 365–394.

Everitt, E. (2016a) Caring for patients with a tracheostomy. *Nursing Times*, 112(9), 16–20.

Everitt, E. (2016b) Caring for patients with permanent tracheostomy. *Nursing Times*, 112(21), 20–22.

Everitt, E. (2016c) Supporting a patient following laryngectomy. *Nursing Times*, 112(1), 6–9.

Feller-Kopman, D.J. & Schwartzstein, R.M. (2017) The evaluation, diagnosis, and treatment of the adult patient with acute hypercapnic respiratory failure. *UpToDate*. Available at: https://www.uptodate.com/contents/the-evaluation-diagnosis-and-treatment-of-the-adult-patient-with-acute-hypercapnic-respiratory-failure

Fernandez, R., Compton, S., Jones, K.A. & Velilla, M.A. (2009) The presence of a family witness impacts physician performance during simulated medical codes. *Critical Care Medicine*, 37(6), 1956–1960.

Ferreira, J.C., Medeiros, P. Jr., Rego, F.M. & Caruso, P. (2015) Risk factors for noninvasive ventilation failure in cancer patients in the intensive care unit: A retrospective cohort study. *Journal of Critical Care*, 30(5), 1003–1007.

[illegible] failure. *Critical Care*, 21(1), 1–6.

Findlay, G.P., Shotton, H., Kelly, K. & Mason, M. (2012) *Time to Intervene? A Review of Patients who Underwent Cardiopulmonary Resuscitation as a Result of an In-Hospital Cardiorespiratory Arrest*. London: National Confidential Enquiry into Patient Outcome and Death.

Fisher & Paykel Healthcare (2013) *Airvo 2 User Manual*. Available at: https://www.fphcare.com/en-gb/hospital/adult-respiratory/optiflow/airvo-2-system/#downloads

Fitch, M.T., Nicks, B.A., Pariyadath, M., et al. (2012) Emergency pericardiocentesis. *New England Journal of Medicine*, 366(12), e17.

Frat, J.P., Thille, A.W., Mercat, A., et al. (2015) High-flow oxygen through nasal cannula in acute hypoxemic respiratory failure. *New England Journal of Medicine*, 372, 2185–2196.

Friedman, D. (2001) Hepatitis. In: Hillyer, C.D. (ed) *Handbook of Transfusion Medicine*. San Diego, CA: Academic Press, pp.275–284.

Gaffney, S. & Dalton, A. (2018) Humidification devices. *Anaesthesia & Intensive Care Medicine*, 19(8), 397–400.

[illegible] (2016) Advances in chest drain management in thoracic disease. *Journal of Thoracic Disease*, 8(Suppl. 1), S55–S64.

Global Tracheostomy Collaborative (2013) *Bite-Sized Training from the GTC*. Available at: https://members.globaltrach.org/wp-content/uploads/2014/02/2.9%20Decannulation.pdf

GMC (General Medical Council) (2008) *Consent: Patients and Doctors*. Available at: https://www.gmc-uk.org/ethical-guidance/ethical-guidance-for-doctors/consent/part-3-capacity-issues#paragraph-75

GOLD (Global Initiative of Chronic Obstructive Lung Disease) (2017) *A Guide to COPD Diagnosis, Management and Prevention: A Guide to Health Care Professionals*. Available at: https://goldcopd.org/wp-content/uploads/2016/12/wms-GOLD-2017-Pocket-Guide.pdf

Goldberger, Z.D., Nallamothu, B.K. & Nichol, G. (2015). Family presence during resuscitation and patterns of care during in-hospital cardiac arrest. *Circulation: Cardiovascular Quality and Outcomes*, 8(3), 226–234.

Green, J. & Pirie, L. (2009) *A Framework to Support Nurses and Midwives Making the Clinical Decision and Providing the Written Instruction for Blood Component Transfusion*. London: UK Blood Transfusion Services.

Green, L., Bolton-Maggs, P., Beattie, C., et al. (2018) British Society of Haematology guidelines on the spectrum of fresh frozen plasma and cryoprecipitate products: Their handling and use in various patient groups in the absence of major bleeding. *British Journal of Haematology*, 181(1), 54–67.

Greenwood, J.C. & Winters, M.E. (2014) Tracheostomy care. In: Roberts, J.R., Custalow, C.B., Thomsen, T.W. & Hedges, J.R. (eds) *Roberts and Hedges' Clinical Procedures in Emergency Medicine*, 6th edn. Philadelphia: Elsevier Saunders, pp.134–151.

Griffith, R. (2016) For the record: Keeping detailed notes. *British Journal of Nursing*, 25(7), 408–409.

Gulati, A., Oscroft, N., Chadwick, R., et al. (2015) The impact of changing people with sleep apnea using CPAP less than 4 h per night to a bi-level device. *Respiratory Medicine*, 109, 778–783.

Hafner, S., Beloncle, F., Koch, A., et al. (2015) Hyperoxia in intensive care, emergency, and peri-operative medicine: Dr. Jekyll or Mr. Hyde? A 2015 update. *Annals of Intensive Care*, 5(1), 42.

Hardinge, M., Annandale, J., Bourne, S., et al. (2015) British Thoracic Society guidelines for home oxygen use in adults. *Thorax*, 70(1), i1–i43.

Harper, R.J. (2010) Pericardiocentesis. In: Roberts, J.R. & Hedges, J.R. (eds) *Clinical Procedures in Emergency Medicine*, 5th edn. Philadelphia: Saunders Elsevier, pp.287–307.

Harrison, D.A., Patel, K., Nixon, E., et al. (2014) Development and validation of risk models to predict outcomes following in-hospital cardiac arrest attended by a hospital-based resuscitation team. *Resuscitation*, 85(8), 993–1000.

Hassan, M. & Shaarawy, H. (2018) Spontaneous pneumothorax: Time to depart from the 'chest tube underwater seal'? *Egyptian Journal of Bronchology*, 12(2), 137–142.

Havelock, T., Teoh, R., Laws, D. & Gleeson, F. (2010) Pleural procedures and thoracic ultrasound: British Thoracic Society pleural disease guideline 2010. *Thorax*, 65(Suppl. 2), ii61–ii76.

Henry, D.A., Carless, P.A., Moxey, A.J., et al. (2002) Pre-operative autologous donation for minimising perioperative allogeneic blood transfusion. *Cochrane Database of Systematic Reviews*, 2, CD003602.

Hernández, G., Vaguero, C., Gonzalez, P., et al. (2016) Effect of postextubation high-flow nasal cannula vs conventional oxygen therapy on reintubation in low-risk patients: A randomized clinical trial. *JAMA*, 315(13), 1354–1361.

Herren, T., Achermann, E., Hegi, T., et al. (2017) Carbon dioxide narcosis due to inappropriate oxygen delivery: A case report. *Journal of Medical Case Reports*, 11, 204.

Herring, N. & Paterson, D.J. (2018) *Levick's Introduction to Cardiovascular Physiology*, 6th edn. Boca Raton, FL: Taylor & Francis.

Hess, D.R. & Altobelli, N.P. (2014) Tracheostomy tubes. *Respiratory Care*, 59(6), 956–973.

Hilbert, G., Navalesi, P. & Girault, C. (2015) Is sedation safe and beneficial in patients receiving NIV? Yes. *Intensive Care Medicine*, 41, 1688–1691.

Holst, L.B., Petersen, M.W., Haase, N., et al. (2015) Restrictive versus liberal transfusion strategy for red blood cell transfusion: Systematic review of randomised trials with meta-analysis and trial sequential analysis. *BMJ*, 350, h1354.

Hooper, C., Lee, Y.C.G. & Maskell, N. (2010) Investigation of a unilateral pleural effusion in adults: British Thoracic Society pleural disease guideline 2010. *Thorax*, 65(Suppl. 2), ii4–ii17.

Huang, H., Xu, B., Liu, G., et al. (2017) Use of noninvasive ventilation in immunocompromised patients with acute respiratory failure: A systematic review and meta-analysis. *Critical Care*, 21(4), 1–9.

Human Rights Act (1998) Available at: www.legislation.gov.uk/ukpga/1998/42/contents

Hunt, B.J., Allard, S., Keeling, D., et al. (2015) A practical guideline for the haematological management of major haemorrhage. *British Journal of Haematology*, 170(6), 788–803.

Hyzy, R.C. & McSparron, J.I. (2018) Overview of tracheostomy. *UpToDate*. Available at: https://www.uptodate.com/contents/overview-of-tracheostomy

ICS (Intensive Care Society) (2014) *Standards for the Care of Adult Patients with a Temporary Tracheostomy*. London: Intensive Care Society.

Ireland, C., Chapman, T., Matthew, S., et al. (2014) Continuous positive airway pressure (CPAP) during the postoperative period for prevention of postoperative morbidity and mortality following major abdominal surgery (review). *Cochrane Database of Systematic Reviews*, 8, 1–55.

Jabre, P., Belpomme, V., Azoulay, E., et al. (2013) Family presence during cardiopulmonary resuscitation. *New England Journal of Medicine*, 368(11), 1008–1018.

Jeffries, M. (2017) Research for practice: Evidence to support the use of occlusive dry sterile dressings for chest tubes. *MEDSURG Nursing*, 26(3), 171–174.

Jones, R. & Berry, R. (2015) Mechanisms of hypoxaemia and the interpretation of arterial blood gases. *Surgery Journal*, 33(10), 461–466.

JPAC (Joint UK Blood Transfusion Society and National Institute for Biological Standards and Control Professional Advisory Committee) (2013) Care and selection of whole blood and component donors (including donors of pre-deposit autogous blood). In: *Guidelines for the Blood Transfusion Services in the United Kingdom*. London: The Stationery Office.

JPAC (2014) UK Cell Salvage Action Group. Available at: https://www.transfusionguidelines.org/transfusion-practice/uk-cell-salvage-action-group

Katz, L.M. & Dodd, R.Y. (2019) Transfusion-transmitted diseases. In: Shaz, B., Hillyer, C. & Gil, M.R. (eds) *Transfusion Medicine and Hemostasis: Clinical and Laboratory Aspects*, 3rd edn. Amsterdam: Elsevier Science, pp.437–453.

Kaufman, D.P. & Dhamoon, A.S. (2018) *Physiology, Oxyhemoglobin Dissociation Curve*. Treasure Island, FL: StatPearls.

Kaufman, R.M., Dinh, A., Cohn, C.S., et al. (2019) Electronic patient identification for sample labeling reduces wrong blood in tube errors. *Transfusion*, 59(3), 972–980.

Kayner, A.M. (2012) Respiratory failure. *Medscape*. Available at: http://emedicine.medscape.com/article/167981

Klein, H.G. & Anstee, D.J. (2014) *Mollison's Blood Transfusion in Clinical Medicine*, 12th edn. Chichester: Wiley Blackwell.

Konstantinides, S.V., Torbicki, A., Agnelli, G., et al. (2014) 2014 ESC guidelines on the diagnosis and management of acute pulmonary embolism. *European Heart Journal*, 35(43), 3033–3069.

Lautrette, A., Darmon, M., Megarbane, B., et al. (2007) A communication strategy and brochure for relatives of patients dying in the ICU. *New England Journal of Medicine*, 356, 469–478.

Laws, D., Neville, E. & Duffy, J. (2003) BTS guidelines for the insertion of a chest drain. *Thorax*, 58(Suppl. 2), ii53–ii59.

Lee, S.H., Kim, K.H. & Woo, S.H. (2015) The usefulness of the stay suture technique in tracheostomy. *Laryngoscope*, 125, 1356–1359.

Lenihan, C.R. & Cormac, T.T. (2013) The impact of hypoxia on cell death pathways: Regulation of metabolism in cancer and immune cells. *Biochemical Society Transactions*, 41(3), 657–663.

Levy, J.H., Neal, M.D. & Herman, J.H. (2018) Bacterial contamination of platelets for transfusion: Strategies for prevention. *Critical Care*, 22(1), 271.

Lewis, S.R., Pritchard, M.W., Evans, D.J., et al. (2018) Colloids versus crystalloids for fluid resuscitation in critically ill people. *Cochrane Database of Systematic Reviews*, 8. DOI: 10.1002/14651858.CD000567.pub7

Lin, C., Yu, H., Fan, H. & Li, Z. (2014) The efficacy of noninvasive ventilation in managing postextubation respiratory failure: A meta-analysis. *Heart & Lung*, 43(2), 99–104.

Liu, Q., Gao, Y., Chen, R. & Cheng, Z. (2016) Noninvasive ventilation with helmet versus control strategy in patients with acute respiratory failure: A systematic review and meta-analysis of controlled studies. *Critical Care*, 20(1), 265.

Loveday, H.P., Wilson, J.A., Pratt, R.J., et al. (2014) epic3: National evidence-based guidelines for preventing healthcare-associated infections in NHS hospitals in England. *Journal of Hospital Infection*, 86(Suppl. 1), S1–S70.

MacDuff, A., Arnold, A. & Harvey, J. (2010) Management of spontaneous pneumothorax: British Thoracic Society pleural disease guideline 2010. *Thorax*, 65(Suppl. 2), ii18–ii31.

Mach, W.J., Thimmesch, A.R., Pierce, J.T. & Pierce, J.D. (2011) Consequences of hyperoxia and the toxicity of oxygen in the lung. *Nursing Research and Practice*, 2011, 1–7.

MacIntyre, N.R. (2014) Tissue hypoxia: Implications for the respiratory clinician. *Journal of Respiratory Care*, 59(10), 1590–1596.

Mahmood, K. & Wahidi, M.M. (2013) Straightening out chest tubes. What size, what type, and when. *Clinics in Chest Medicine*, 34(1), 63–71.

Malhotra, S., Dhama, S.S., Kumar, M. & Jain, G. (2013) Improving neurological outcome after cardiac arrest: Therapeutic hypothermia the best treatment. *Anesthesia Essays and Researches*, 7(1), 18–24.

Mallet, J., Albarran, J.W. & Richardson, A. (2013) *Critical Care Manual of Clinical Procedures and Competencies*. Chichester: John Wiley & Sons.

Mao, M., Hughes, R., Papadimos, T.J. & Stawicki, S.P. (2015) Complications of chest tubes: A focused clinical synopsis. *Current Opinion in Pulmonary Medicine*, 21(4), 376–386.

Marhong, J. & Fan, E. (2014) Carbon dioxide in the critically ill: Too much or too little of a good thing? *Journal of Respiratory Care*, 59(10), 1597–1605.

Marieb, E.N. & Hoehn, K. (2016) *Human Anatomy & Physiology*, 10th edn. Harlow: Pearson.

Marieb, E.N. & Hoehn, K. (2018) *Human Anatomy & Physiology*, 11th edn. Harlow: Pearson.

Masa, J., Utrabo, I., Gomez de Terreros, J., et al. (2016) Noninvasive ventilation for severely acidotic patients in respiratory intermediate care units. *Pulmonary Medicine*, 16(97), 1–13.

Massey, E. (2016) *Clinical Guidelines for the Use of Granulocyte Transfusions.* Available at: https://nhsbtdbe.blob.core.windows.net/umbraco-assets-corp/14874/inf2764-clinical-guidelines-for-the-use-of-granulocyte-transfusions.pdf

McCauley, L. & Dean, N. (2015) Pneumonia and empyema: Causal, casual or unknown. *Journal of Thoracic Disease*, 7(6), 992–998.

McClelland, D.B. (2007) *Handbook of Transfusion Medicine.* London: The Stationery Office.

McCoy, R.W. (2013) Options for home oxygen therapy equipment: Storage and metering of oxygen in the home. *Respiratory Care Journal*, 58(1), 65–80.

McGrath, B.A., Bates, L., Atkinson, D. & Moore, J.A. (2012) Multidisciplinary guidelines for the management of tracheostomy and laryngectomy airway emergencies. *Anaesthesia*, 67, 1025–1041.

McNulty, G. & Eyre, L. (2015) Humidification in anaesthesia and critical care. *British Journal of Anaesthesia Education*, 15(3), 131–135.

Meaney, P.A., Nadkarni, V.M., Kern, K.B., et al. (2010) Rhythms and outcomes of adult in-hospital cardiac arrest. *Critical Care Medicine*, 38(1), 101–108.

Medicines Act (1968) Available at: www.legislation.gov.uk/ukpga/1968/67

Mental Capacity (Amended) Act (2019) Available at: https://www.legislation.gov.uk/ukpga/2019/18/contents/enacted

MHRA (Medicines and Healthcare products Regulatory Agency) (2010) *Medical Device Alert: All Chest Drains when Used with High-Flow, Low Vacuum Suction Systems (Wall Mounted) MDA/2010/040.* Available at: https://webarchive.nationalarchives.gov.uk/20150113080833/www.mhra.gov.uk/home/groups/dts-bs/documents/medicaldevicealert/con001090.pdf

MHRA (2013) *Top Tips on Care and Handling of Oxygen Cylinders and Their Regulators.* Available at: https://assets.publishing.service.gov.uk/government/uploads/system/uploads/attachment_data/file/428425/O2_cylinders_top_tips_2013.pdf

Mian, H., Foley, R. & O'Hoski, P. (2017) Haemopoietic stem cell processing and storage. In: Murphy, M. F., Roberts, D. J., & Yazer, M. H. (eds) *Practical Transfusion Medicine*, 5th edn. Chichester: John Wiley & Sons, pp.455–465.

Mitchell, R.B., Hussey, H.M., Setzen, G., et al. (2013) Clinical consensus statement: Tracheostomy care. *Otolaryngology: Head and Neck Surgery*, 148(1), 6–20.

Mollison, P.L., Engelfriet, C.P. & Contreras, M. (1997) *Blood Transfusion in Clinical Medicine*, 10th edn. Oxford: Blackwell Science.

Moffat, S., Skinner, J. & Fritz, Z. (2016) Does resuscitation status affect decision making in a deteriorating patient? Results from a randomised vignette study. *Journal of Evaluation in Clinical Practice*, 22(6), 921–927.

Mohammed, H.M. (2015) Chest tube care in critically ill patient: A comprehensive review. *Egyptian Journal of Chest Diseases and Tuberculosis*, 64(4), 849–855.

Möller, W., Celik, G., Feng, S., et al. (2015) Nasal high flow clears anatomical dead space in upper airway models. *American Journal of Physiology: Heart and Circulatory Physiology*, 18(12), 1525–1532.

Moore, J.E. (2016) The importance of the mundane: Nebuliser care and hygiene. *Journal of Cystic Fibrosis*, 15(1), 4–5.

Morris, L.L., Bedon, A.M., McIntosh, E. & Whitmer, A. (2015) Restoring speech to tracheostomy patients. *Critical Care Nurse*, 35, 13–28.

Mortimer, H. & Kubba, H. (2017) A retrospective case series of 318 tracheostomy-related adverse events over 6 years: A Scottish context. *Clinical Otolaryngology*, 42, 936–940.

Murdock, J., Watson, D., Doree, C.J., et al. (2009) Drugs and blood transfusions: Dogma- or evidence-based practice? *Transfusion Medicine*, 19(1), 6–15.

Murphy, M.F., Staves, J., Davies, A., et al. (2009) How do we approach a major change program using the example of the development, evaluation, and implementation of an electronic transfusion management system? *Transfusion*, 49(5), 829–837.

Na, M.J. (2014) Diagnostic tools of pleural effusion. *Tuberculosis and Respiratory Diseases*, 76(5), 199–210.

Narayan, S. (ed) on behalf of the Serious Hazards of Transfusion (SHOT) Steering Group (2019) *The Annual SHOT Report 2018.* Available at: https://www.shotuk.org/wp-content/uploads/myimages/SHOT-Report-2018_Web_Version.pdf

National Blood Transfusion Committee (2016a) *Indication Codes for Transfusion: An Audit Tool.* Available at: www.transfusionguidelines.org.uk/uk-transfusion-committees/national-blood-transfusion-committee/responses-and-recommendations

National Blood Transfusion Committee (2016b) *Requirements for Training and Assessment in Blood Transfusion.* Available at: www.transfusionguidelines.org/document-library/documents/nbtc-requirements-for-training-and-assessment-final

National CJD Research and Surveillance Unit (2017) *26th Annual Report 2017: Creutzfeldt-Jakob Disease Surveillance in the UK.* Edinburgh: National CJD Research and Surveillance Unit.

NBTC (National Blood Transfusion Committee) (2014) *Patient Blood Management: An Evidence Based Approach to Care.* Available at: https://www.transfusionguidelines.org/uk-transfusion-committees/national-blood-transfusion-committee/patient-blood-management

NBTC (2016) *Indication Codes for Transfusion.* Available at: https://www.transfusionguidelines.org/document-library/documents/nbtc-indication-codes-june-2016v2

NCEPOD (National Confidential Enquiry into Patient Outcome and Death) (2017) *Inspiring Change.* London: NCEPOD.

NHS England and NHSI (NHS Improvement) (2019) *Standard Infection Control Precautions: National Hand Hygiene and Personal Protective Equipment Policy.* Available at: https://improvement.nhs.uk/documents/4957/National_policy_on_hand_hygiene_and_PPE_2.pdf

NHS Improvement (2016) *Reducing the Risk of Oxygen Tubing Being Connected to Air Flowmeters.* Available at: https://improvement.nhs.uk/documents/408/Patient_Safety_Alert_-_Reducing_the_risk_of_oxygen_tubing_being_connected_to_a_bDUb3KY.pdf

NHS Improvement (2018a) *Patient Safety Alert: Risk of Death and Severe Harm from Failure to Obtain and Continue Flow from Oxygen Cylinders.* Available at: https://improvement.nhs.uk/documents/2206/Patient_Safety_Alert_-_Failure_to_open_oxygen_cylinders.pdf

NHS Improvement (2018b) *Patient Safety Alert: Safer Temporary Identification Criteria for Unknown or Unidentified Patients.* Available at: https://improvement.nhs.uk/documents/3535/Patient_Safety_Alert_-_unknown_or_unidentified_patients_FINAL.pdf

NHS Quality Improvement Scotland (2006) *Clinical Standards: Blood Transfusion.* Edinburgh: NHS Quality Improvement Scotland.

NHSBT (NHS Blood and Transplant) (2003) *National Comparative Audit of Blood Transfusion: Auditing the Administration of Blood at the Bedside.* Available at: https://hospital.blood.co.uk/audits/national-comparative-audit/blood-sampling-collection-and-administration-of-blood-components

NHSBT (2009) *National Comparative Audit of Blood Transfusion: 2008 Bedside Transfusion Re-audit.* Available at: https://nhsbtdbe.blob.core.windows.net/umbraco-assets-corp/14928/nca-2008_bedside_transfusion_audit_report_-_st_elsewheres.pdf

NHSBT (2011a) *National Comparative Audit of Blood Transfusion: 2011 Re-audit of Bedside Transfusion Practice.* Available at: https://hospital.blood.co.uk/audits/national-comparative-audit/blood-sampling-collection-and-administration-of-blood-components

NHSBT (2011b) *Strategic Plan 2011–14.* Available at: https://nhsbtdbe.blob.core.windows.net/umbraco-assets-corp/1854/nhsbt_strategic_plan_2011_14.pdf

NICE (National Institute for Health and Care Excellence) (2007) *Acutely Ill Adults in Hospital: Recognizing and Responding to Deterioration* [CG50]. Available at: www.nice.org.uk/guidance/cg50

NICE (2008) *Intraoperative Red Blood Cell Salvage during Radical Prostatectomy or Radical Cystectomy* [IPG258]. Available at: https://www.nice.org.uk/guidance/ipg258

NICE (2013) *Acute Illness in Adults in Hospital: Recognizing and Responding to Deterioration* [CG50]. Available at www.nice.org.uk/guidance/CG50

NICE (2015) *Blood Transfusion* [NG24]. Available at: https://www.nice.org.uk/guidance/NG24

NICE (2016) *Motor Neurone Disease: Assessment and Management* [NG42]. Available at: https://www.nice.org.uk/guidance/ng42

NICE (2017) *Healthcare-Associated Infections: Prevention and Control in Primary and Community Care* [CG139]. Available at: https://www.nice.org.uk/guidance/CG139

NICE (2018a) *Oxygen: Overview.* Available at: https://bnf.nice.org.uk/treatment-summary/oxygen.html

NICE (2018b) *Chronic Obstructive Pulmonary Disease in Over 16s: Diagnosis and Management* [NG115]. Available at: https://www.nice.org.uk/guidance/NG115

NICE (2018c) *Clinical Knowledge Summaries: Iron Deficiency Anaemia.* Available at: https://cks.nice.org.uk/anaemia-iron-deficiency#!scenario

Nishimura, M. (2015) High-flow nasal cannula oxygen therapy in adults. *Journal of Intensive Care*, 3(1), 15.

NMC (Nursing and Midwifery Council) (2018) *The Code: Professional Standards of Practice and Behaviour for Nurses, Midwives and Nursing Associates.* Available at: https://www.nmc.org.uk/standards/code

Noel, D., Fink, D.S., Kunduk, M., et al. (2016) Secondary tracheoesophageal puncture using transnasal esophagoscopy in gastric pull-up reconstruction after total laryngopharyngoesophagectomy. *Head Neck*, 38, E61–E63.

Nolan, J.P., Soar, J., Smith, G.B., et al. (2014) Incidence and outcome of in-hospital cardiac arrest in the United Kingdom National Cardiac Arrest Audit. *Resuscitation*, 85(8), 987–992.

Noorani, A. & Abu-Omar, Y. (2018) Chest drainage. In: Valchanov, K., Jones, N. & Hogue, C. (eds) *Core Topics in Cardiothoracic Critical Care.* Cambridge: Cambridge University Press, pp.70–76.

Norfolk, D. (2013) *Handbook of Transfusion Medicine*, 5th edn. London: The Stationery Office.

NPSA (National Patient Safety Agency) (2006) *Right Patient, Right Blood.* Available at: https://webarchive.nationalarchives.gov.uk/20171030131001/www.nrls.npsa.nhs.uk/resources/type/alerts/?entryid45=65838&p=4

NPSA (2007) *Standardising Wristbands Improves Patient Safety (Safer Practice Notice No. 24).* Available at: https://webarchive.nationalarchives.gov.uk/20171030124213/www.nrls.npsa.nhs.uk/resources/?entryid45=59824&p=14

NPSA (2010) *Rapid Response Report: The Transfusion of Blood and Blood Components in an Emergency.* Available at: https://www.transfusionguidelines.org/document-library/documents/npsa-rapid-response-report-the-transfusion-of-blood-and-blood-components-in-an-emergency-21-october-2010-pdf-100kb

NTSP (National Tracheostomy Safety Project) (2013) *Information Resource for Safer Management of Patients with Tracheostomies and Laryngectomies.* Available at: www.tracheostomy.org.uk/resources/documents

O'Connell, B., Lee, E.J. & Schiffer, C.A. (1988) The value of 10-minute post-transfusion platelet counts. *Transfusion*, 28(1), 66–67.

O'Connor, R. (2017) *Cardiac Arrest.* Available at: https://www.msdmanuals.com/en-gb/professional/critical-care-medicine/cardiac-arrest-and-cpr/cardiac-arrest

O'Driscoll, B.R., Howard, L.S., Earis, J., et al. (2017) British Thoracic Society Guideline for oxygen use in adults in healthcare and emergency settings. *Thorax*, 72(Suppl. 1), i1–i89.

Olivieri, C., Carenzo, L., Vignazia, G.L., et al. (2015) Does noninvasive ventilation delivery in the ward provide early effective ventilation? *Respiratory Care*, 60(1), 6–11.

Ozsancak Ugurlu, A., Sidhom, S., Khodabandeh, A., et al. (2016) Use and outcomes of noninvasive ventilation for acute respiratory failure in different age groups. *Respiratory Care*, 61(1), 36–43.

Papazian, L., Corley, A., Hess, D., et al. (2016) Use of high-flow nasal cannula oxygenation in ICU adults: A narrative review. *Intensive Care Medicine*, 42(9), 1336–1349.

Pasricha, S.R., Colman, K., Centeno-Tablante, E., et al. (2018) Revisiting WHO haemoglobin thresholds to define anaemia in clinical medicine and public health. *Lancet Haematology*, 5(2), e60–e62.

Patel, B.K., Wolfe, K.S., Pohlman, A.S., et al. (2016) Effect of noninvasive ventilation delivered by helmet vs face mask on the rate of endotracheal intubation in patients with acute respiratory distress syndrome. *JAMA*, 315(22), 2435–2441.

Patel, S. & Majmundar, S.H. (2020) *Physiology, Carbon Dioxide Retention.* StatPearls. Available at: https://www.ncbi.nlm.nih.gov/books/NBK482456

Pathmanathan, N., Beaumont, N. & Gratrix, A. (2014) Respiratory physiotherapy in the critical care unit. *Continuing Education in Anaesthesia, Critical Care & Pain*, 15(1), 20–25.

Patrini, D., Panagiotopoulos, N., Pararajasingham, J., et al. (2015) Etiology and management of spontaneous haemothorax. *Journal of Thoracic Disease*, 7(3), 520–526.

Perkins, G.D., Handley, A.J., Koster, R.W., et al. (2015) European Resuscitation Council Guidelines for resuscitation: Section 2 – Adult basic life support and automated external defibrillation. *Resuscitation*, 95, 81–99.

Pirie, E.S. & Gray, M.A. (2007) Exploring the assessors' and nurses' experience of formal assessment of clinical competency in the administration of blood components. *Nurse Education in Practice*, 7(4), 215–227.

Porcel, J.M. (2018a) Improving the management of spontaneous pneumothorax. *European Respiratory Journal*, 52(6), 1801918.

Porcel, J.M. (2018b) Chest tube drainage of the pleural space: A concise review for pulmonologists. *Tuberculosis and Respiratory Diseases*, 81(2), 106–115.

Porth, C. (2005) *Pathophysiology: Concepts of Altered Health States*, 7th edn. Philadelphia: Lippincott Williams & Wilkins.

Prasarn, M.L., Horodyski, M., Scott, N.E., et al. (2014) Motion generated in the unstable upper cervical spine during head tilt–chin lift and jaw thrust maneuvers. *Spine Journal*, 14(4), 609–614.

Provan, D., Baglin, T., Dokal, I. & de Vos, J. (2015) *Oxford Handbook of Clinical Haematology*, 4th edn. Oxford: Oxford University Press.

Ravi, C. & McKnight, C.L. (2018) *Chest Tube.* Treasure Island, FL: *Stat Pearls.*

Raza, S., Baig, M.A., Chang, C. et al. (2015) A prospective study on red blood cell transfusion related hyperkalemia in critically ill patients. *Journal of Clinical Medicine Research*, 7(6), 417–421.

RCN (Royal College of Nursing) (2005) *Right Blood, Right Patient, Right Time.* Available at: www.spitjudms.ro/_files/protocoale_terapeutice/anestezie/buna_practica_transfuzionala.pdf

RCN (2010) *Standards for Infusion Therapy*, 3rd edn. London: Royal College of Nursing.

RCN (2017) Principles of consent: Guidance for nursing staff. *British Journal of Healthcare Assistants*, 11(10), 498–502.

RCP (Royal College of Physicians) (2017) *National Early Warning Score 2 (NEWS2): Standardising the Assessment of Acute Illness Severity in the NHS.* Available at: https://www.rcplondon.ac.uk/projects/outputs/national-early-warning-score-news-2

RCS (Royal College of Surgeons) (2016) *Caring for Patients who Refuse Blood.* Available at: https://www.rcseng.ac.uk/-/media/files/rcs/library-and-publications/non-journal-publications/caring-for-patients-who-refuse-blood--a-guide-to-good-practice.pdf#targetText=For%20further%20information%20regarding%20doctors,Practice%20(GMC%2C%202013).&targetText=Consent%20refers%20to%20a%20patient's,must%20be%20confirmed%20in%20writing

RCUK (Resuscitation Council UK) (2015) *Advanced Life Support.* London: Resuscitation Council UK.

Retter, A., Wyncoll, D., Pearse, R., et al. (2013) Guidelines on the management of anaemia and red cell transfusion in adult critically ill patients. *British Journal of Haematology*, 160, 445–464.

Riou, M., Ball, S., Williams, T.A., et al. (2018) 'She's sort of breathing': What linguistic factors determine call-taker recognition of agonal breathing in emergency calls for cardiac arrest? *Resuscitation*, 122, 92–98.

Roberts, D.J., Leigh-Smith, S., Faris, P.D., et al. (2015) Clinical presentation of patients with tension pneumothorax: A systematic review. *Annals of Surgery*, 261(6), 1068–1078.

Robinson, S., Harris, A., Atkinson, S., et al. (2017) The administration of blood components: A British Society for Haematology guideline. *Transfusion Medicine*, 28(1), 3–21.

Rodriguez-Hortal, M., Nygren-Bonnier, M. & Hjelte, L. (2017) Non-invasive ventilation as airway clearance technique in cystic fibrosis. *Physiotherapy Research International*, 22(3), e1667.

Roth, D., Mayer, J., Schreiber, W., et al. (2018) Acute carbon monoxide poisoning treatment by non-invasive CPAP ventilation, and by face mask: Two simultaneous cases. *American Journal of Emergency Medicine*, 36(9), 1718e5–1718e6.

SaBTO (Advisory Committee on the Safety of Blood, Tissues and Organs) (2011) *Guidance for Clinical Staff to Support Patient Consent for Blood Transfusion*. Available at: www.transfusionguidelines.org.uk/transfusion-practice/consent-for-blood-transfusion-1

SaBTO (2012) *SaBTO Report of the Cytomegalovirus Steering Group*. Available at: www.dh.gov.uk/en/Publicationsandstatistics/Publications/PublicationsPolicyAndGuidance/DH_132965

Saguil, A., Wyrick, K. & Hallgren, J. (2014) Diagnostic approach to pleural effusion. *American Family Physician*, 90(2), 99–104.

Sarkar, M., Niranjan, N. & Banyal, P.K. (2017) Mechanisms of hypoxemia. *Lung India: Official Organ of Indian Chest Society*, 34(1), 47–60.

Schiavone, W.A. (2013) Cardiac tamponade: 12 pearls in diagnosis and management. *Cleveland Clinical Journal of Medicine*, 80(2), 109–116.

Schober, A., Sterz, F., Handler, C., et al. (2014) Cardiac arrest due to accidental hypothermia: A 20 year review of a rare condition in an urban area. *Resuscitation*, 85(6), 749–756.

Schnell, D., Timsit, J., Darmon, M., et al. (2014) Noninvasive mechanical ventilation in acute respiratory failure: Trends in use and outcomes. *Intensive Care Medicine*, 40, 582–591.

Scott, B. (2017) Skin integrity and the NIV patient. *AARC Times*, 2017, 5–8.

Seed, C.R., Hewitt, P.E., Dodd, R.Y., et al. (2018) Creutzfeldt–Jakob disease and blood transfusion safety. *Vox Sanguinis*, 113(3), 220–231.

Sekhon, M.S., Ainslie, P.N. & Griesdale, D.E. (2017) Clinical pathophysiology of hypoxic ischemic brain injury after cardiac arrest: A 'two-hit' model. *Critical Care*, 21(90), 30–33.

Semenza, G.L. (2012) Hypoxia-inducible factors in physiology and medicine. *Cell*, 148(3), 399–408.

Semple, J.W., Rebetz, J. & Kapur, R. (2019) Transfusion-associated circulatory overload and transfusion-related acute lung injury. *Blood*, 133(17), 1840–1853.

Shander, A., Gross, I., Hill, S., et al. (2013) A new perspective on best transfusion practices. *Blood Transfusion*, 11(2), 193–202.

Shander, A., Javidroozi, M., Perelman, S., et al. (2012) From bloodless surgery to patient blood management. *Mount Sinai Journal of Medicine*, 79(1), 56–65.

Sharma, D., Goswami, R., Arora, G., et al. (2016) Silicon airflow prosthetic device after laryngectomy: A clinical trial. *Karnataka Anaesthesia Journal*, 2(2), 59–61.

Shreeve, K. (2014) *SBAR: NPSA Safer Practice Notice 14, 'Right Patient, Right Blood'*. Pontyclun: Welsh Blood Service.

Sigurdson, C.J., Bartz, J.C. & Glatzel, M. (2019) Cellular and molecular mechanisms of prion disease. *Annual Review of Pathology: Mechanisms of Disease*, 14, 497–516.

Sikorski, R.A., Rizkalla, N.A., Yang, W.W. & Frank, S.M. (2017) Autologous blood salvage in the era of patient blood management. *Vox Sanguinis*, 112(6), 499–510.

Singh, R.K., Saran, S. & Baronia, A.K. (2017) The practice of tracheostomy decannulation: A systematic review. *Journal of Intensive Care*, 5, 38.

Sjoberg, F. & Singer, M. (2013) The medical use of oxygen: A time for critical reappraisal. *Journal of Internal Medicine*, 274(6), 505–528.

Skeate, R.C. & Eastlund, T. (2007) Distinguishing between transfusion related acute lung injury and transfusion associated circulatory overload. *Current Opinion in Hematology*, 14(6), 682–687.

Slichter, S.J., Kaufman, R.M., Assmann, S.F., et al. (2010) Dose of prophylactic platelet transfusions and prevention of hemorrhage. *New England Journal of Medicine*, 362(7), 600–613.

SNBTS (Scottish National Blood Transfusion Service) (2004) *Better Blood Transfusion Level 1: Safe Transfusion Practice: Self-Directed Learning Pack*. Available at: https://webarchive.nationalarchives.gov.uk/20130105054416/www.dh.gov.uk/en/Publicationsandstatistics/Lettersandcirculars/Healthservicecirculars/DH_080613

Soar, J., Nolan, J.P., Böttiger, B.W., et al. (2015) European Resuscitation Council guidelines for resuscitation 2015: Section 3 – Adult advanced life support. *Resuscitation*, 95, 100–147.

Spoletini, G. & Hill, N.S. (2016) High-flow nasal oxygen versus noninvasive ventilation for hypoxemic respiratory failure: Do we know enough? *Annals of Thoracic Medicine*, 11, 163–166.

Stickle, D. (2018) BiPAP noninvasive ventilation for COPD. *Journal for Respiratory Care Practitioners*, 2018, 15–16.

Sutt, A.L., Cornwell, P., Mullany, D., et al. (2015) The use of tracheostomy speaking valves in mechanically ventilated patients results in improved communication and does not prolong ventilation time in cardiothoracic intensive care unit patients. *Journal of Critical Care*, 30, 491–494.

Sztrymf, B., Messika, J., Bertrand, F., et al. (2011) Beneficial effects of humidified high flow nasal oxygen in critical care patients: A prospective pilot study. *Intensive Care Medicine*, 37(11), 1780–1786.

Tang, C.G. & Sinclair, C.F. (2015) Voice restoration after total laryngectomy. *Otolaryngologic Clinics of North America*, 48(4), 687–702.

Tekgündüz, S.A. & Özbek, N. (2016) ABO blood group mismatched hematopoietic stem cell transplantation. *Transfusion and Apheresis Science*, 54(1), 24–29.

Thomas, C. & Lumb, A. (2012) Physiology of haemaglobin. *Journal of Continuing Education in Anaesthesia, Critical Care & Pain*, 12(5), 251–256.

Tinegate, H., Birchall, J., Gray, A., et al. (2012) Guideline on the investigation and management of acute transfusion reactions: Prepared by the BCSH Blood Transfusion Task Force. *British Journal of Haematology*, 159, 143–153.

Tirkkonen, J., Huhtala, H. & Hoppu, S. (2018) In-hospital cardiac arrest after a rapid response team review: A matched case-control study. *Resuscitation*, 126, 98–103.

Tortora, G.J. & Derrickson, B.H. (2017) *Principles of Anatomy & Physiology*, 15th edn. Hoboken, NJ: John Wiley & Sons.

Treleaven, J., Gennery, A., Marsh, J., et al. (2011) Guidelines on the use of irradiated blood components prepared by the British Committee for Standards in Haematology blood transfusion task force. *British Journal of Haematology*, 152, 35–51.

Truhlar, A., Deakin, C.D., Soar, J., et al. (2015) European Resuscitation Council guidelines for resuscitation 2015: Section 4 – Cardiac arrest in special circumstances. *Resuscitation*, 95(10), 148–200.

Tschopp, J.M., Bintcliffe, O., Astoul, P., et al. (2015) ERS task force statement: Diagnosis and treatment of primary spontaneous pneumothorax. *European Respiratory Journal*, 46, 321–335.

UK Blood Services (2007) *Handbook of Transfusion Medicine*, 4th edn. Available at: www.transfusionguidelines.org.uk

Vadde, R. & Pastores, S. (2016) Management of acute respiratory failure in hematological malignancy patients. *Journal of Intensive Care Medicine*, 31(10), 627–641.

Vargas, M., Marra, A., Vivona, L., et al. (2018) Performances of CPAP devices with an oronasal mask. *Respiratory Care*, 63(8), 1033–1039.

Vlaar, A.P., Toy, P., Fung, M., et al. (2019) A consensus redefinition of transfusion-related acute lung injury. *Transfusion*, 59(7), 2465–2476.

Ward, E.C. & Van As-Brooks, C.J. (2014) *Head and Neck Cancer: Treatment, Rehabilitation and Outcomes*, 2nd edn. San Diego: Pleural.

Waugh, A. & Grant, A. (2014) *Ross & Wilson Anatomy and Physiology in Health and Illness*. Edinburgh: Churchill Livingstone.

Weil, I.A., Kumar, P., Seicean, S., et al. (2019) Platelet count abnormalities and peri-operative outcomes in adults undergoing elective, non-cardiac surgery. *PLOS ONE*, 14(2), e0212191.

WHO (World Health Organization) (2011) *Global Forum for Blood Safety: Patient Blood Management – 14–15 March 2011, Dubai, United Arab Emirates*. Available at: www.who.int/bloodsafety/events/gfbs_01_pbm_concept_paper.pdf

Wild, K. & Peate, I. (2012) Clinical observations 5/6: Breathing and respiratory rate. *British Journal of Healthcare Assistants*, 6(9), 438–441.

Wilkinson, I.B., Raine, T., Wiles, K., et al. (2017) *The Oxford Handbook of Clinical Medicine*, 10th edn. Oxford: Oxford University Press.

Wilkinson, K.A., Martin, I.C., Freeth, H., et al. (2014) *NCEPOD: On the Right Trach? A Review of the Care Received by Patients who Underwent a Tracheostomy*. National Confidential Enquiry into Patient Outcome and Death. Available at: https://www.ncepod.org.uk/2014report1/downloads/OnTheRightTrach_FullReport.pdf

Williamson, L.M., Lowe, S., Love, E., et al. (1999) *Serious Hazards of Transfusion*. Manchester: SHOT. Available at: https://www.shotuk.org/wp-content/uploads/myimages/2010/04/SHOT-Report-1997-98.pdf

Wittels, K.A. (2018) Basic airway management in adults. *UpToDate*. Available at: https://www.uptodate.com/contents/basic-airway-management-in-adults

Wong, C.Y.Y., Shakir, A.A., Farboud, A. & Whittet, H.B. (2016) Active versus passive humidification for self-ventilating tracheostomy and laryngectomy patients: A systematic review of the literature. *Clinical Otolaryngology*, 41(6), 646–651.

Woodrow, P. (2013) Intrapleural chest drainage. *Nursing Standard*, 27(40), 49–56.

Yeung, J., Couper, K., Ryan, E.G., et al. (2018) Non-invasive ventilation as a strategy for weaning from invasive mechanical ventilation: A systematic review and Bayesian meta-analysis. *Intensive Care Medicine*, 44(12), 2192–2204.

Yousuf, A. & Rahman, N.M. (2018) Chest drain insertion. In: Hunt, I., Rahman, N.M., Maskell, N.A. & Gleeson, F.V. (eds) *ABC of Pleural Diseases*. Oxford: John Wiley & Sons, pp.56–59.

Zaw, A.S., Bangalore Kantharajanna, S. & Kumar, N. (2017) Is autologous salvaged blood a viable option for patient blood management in oncologic surgery? *Transfusion Medicine Reviews*, 31(1), 56–61.

Zenga, J., Goldsmith, T., Bunting, G. & Deschler, D.G. (2018) State of the art: Rehabilitation of speech and swallowing after total laryngectomy. *Oral Oncology*, 86, 38–47.

Zisis, C., Tsirgogianni, K., Lazaridis, G., et al. (2015) Chest drainage systems in use. *Annals of Translational Medicine*, 3(3), 43.

Zwaginga, J.J. & van Ham, M. (2013) Essential immunology for transfusion medicine. In: Murphy, M., Pamphilon, D. & Heddle, N. (eds) *Practical Transfusion Medicine*, 4th edn. Oxford: John Wiley & Sons, pp.11–20.

Part Three

Supporting patients through the diagnostic process

Chapters

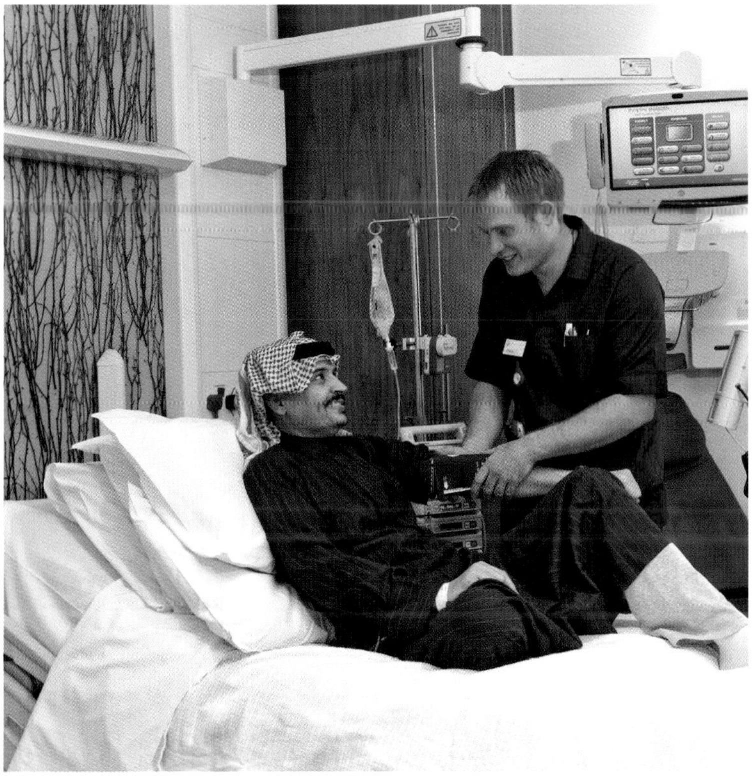

Chapter 13

Diagnostic tests

Andrew Dimech with Andreia Fernandes, Firza Gronthoud, Lilian Li and Barbara Witt

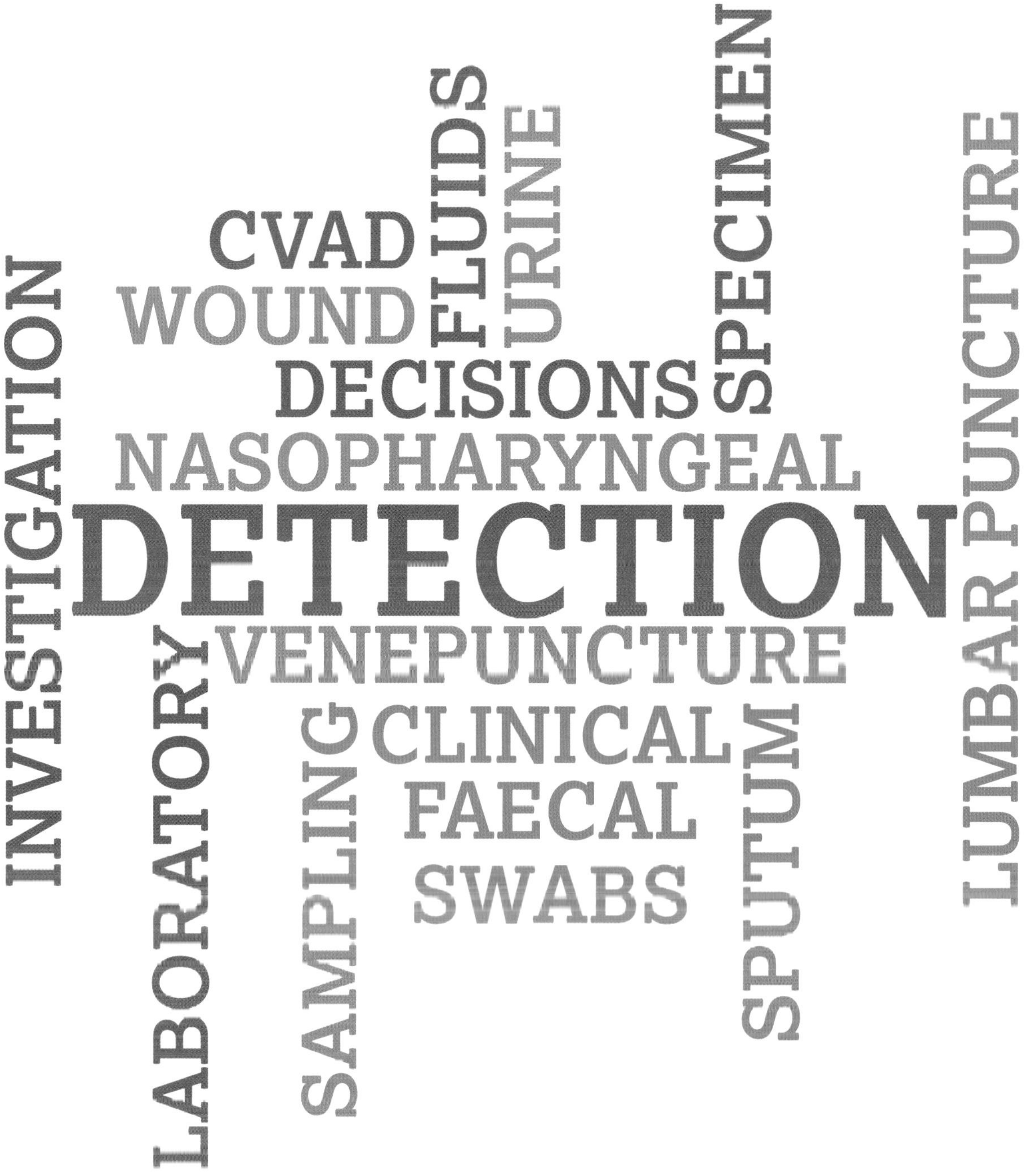

The Royal Marsden Manual of Clinical Nursing Procedures: Professional Edition, Tenth Edition. Edited by Sara Lister, Justine Hofland and Hayley Grafton.

Procedure guidelines

Being an accountable professional

At the point of registration, the nurse will:

2. Use evidence-based, best practice approaches to undertake the following procedures:

2.2 undertake venepuncture and cannulation and blood sampling, interpreting normal and common abnormal blood profiles and venous blood gases

2.9 collect and observe sputum, urine, stool and vomit specimens, undertaking routine analysis and interpreting findings

Future Nurse: Standards of Proficiency for Registered Nurses (NMC 2018)

Overview

In clinical practice, nursing staff are required to instigate, participate or assist in diagnostic tests and the collection of body fluids and/or specimens for various diagnostic purposes. This chapter discusses common diagnostic tests encountered in clinical practice that are used during the diagnostic process and to support ongoing treatment decisions.

Diagnostic tests

Definition

A diagnostic test is a procedure that is used to aid in the detection, confirmation, and elimination and/or monitoring of disease (Pagana and Pagana 2017).

Related theory

Diagnostic tests are undertaken to aid in the diagnosis and treatment of various conditions. The diagnostic tests are used to identify diseases from their characteristics, signs and symptoms and to identify changes or abnormalities. They may require the collection of body fluids and tissue samples using various techniques and medical devices. Depending on the clinical picture, radiological investigations – such as X-ray, computed tomography (CT) or magnetic resonance imaging (MRI) – may be required.

Evidence-based approaches

Rationale

Diagnostic tests are essential in the healthcare setting but their selection and use must be considered carefully. The overuse of or inefficient use of diagnostic tests is a contributor to needless healthcare costs. This leads to poor-quality services and continuing financial pressure on departments and organizations (Korenstein et al. 2012, Pagana and Pagana 2017). Hence, it is essential that healthcare providers and professionals ensure that the tests used are of adequate benefit to the patient's health (Pagana and Pagana 2017, Qaseem et al. 2012). For example, a faecal sample from a patient who has a history of recent travel would be investigated for organisms not normally looked for in a specimen from a patient without such a history. The sensitivity of the organism to a range of antimicrobials could then be tested to decide on the most appropriate and effective mode of treatment (Higgins 2013).

Successful laboratory diagnosis depends upon the collection of specimens at the appropriate time, using the correct technique and equipment, and transporting them to the designated laboratory safely and without delay (Box 13.1). For this to be achieved, it is essential that there is good liaison between medical, nursing, portering and laboratory staff. Diagnostic tests should not have to be repeated due to inadequate patient preparation, procedures or specimen collection techniques (Pagana and Pagana 2017).

Box 13.1 Good practice in specimen collection

- Appropriate to the patient's clinical presentation
- Collected at the right time
- Collected in a way that minimizes the risk of contamination
- Collected in a manner that minimizes the health and safety risk to all staff handling the sample
- Collected using the correct technique, with the correct equipment and in the correct container
- Documented clearly, informatively and accurately on the request forms
- Stored and transported appropriately

Source: Adapted from NHS Pathology (2014), Pagana and Pagana (2017), WHO (2015).

Indications

Conducting a diagnostic test is often the first crucial step in determining a diagnosis and subsequent mode of treatment for patients. In other contexts, the collection or diagnostic test may help to determine variation from normal values, such as in blood sampling or endoscopic findings.

Principles of care

Nursing staff play a key role within the diagnostic testing process because they often identify the need for diagnostic tests, initiate the collection of specimens, and assume responsibility for timely and safe transportation to the laboratory (Higgins 2013, Keogh 2017). The interpretation of findings or results is also a key role for nurses in various settings and facilitates timely and collaborative treatment plans (Pagana and Pagana 2017). Specimen collection is often the first crucial step in investigations that define the nature of the disease, determine a diagnosis and therefore decide the mode of treatment. Patient education is also a crucial component in ensuring accuracy and success of diagnostic tests. Patient understanding of all steps before, during and after the test or investigation is necessary and should form part of the nursing process (Pagana and Pagana 2017).

Methods of investigation

Various healthcare professionals, such as doctors, nurses, pharmacists and allied healthcare professionals, are able to identify the need for and request a variety of diagnostic tests. Those requesting a diagnostic test must also be able to interpret the findings. Each professional must have the ability to clinically assess the patient, and this assessment then informs the choice of diagnostic test. An understanding of the laboratory methods available is also important for those requesting a diagnostic test.

Initial examination and assessment

The initial examination and assessment of the patient will determine the potential diagnostic tests or samples that are required. Depending on how the patient progresses, their clinical history, a physical assessment and/or their symptom progression will subsequently determine the need for further diagnostic tests. The results of these tests will then form a treatment plan. The initial assessment is often undertaken by nurses and other healthcare professionals (Keogh 2017, Pagana and Pagana 2017).

Cytology

Cytology is the study of the cell, its structure, structural transformations, molecular biology and cell physiology. The specimen can be a fine-needle aspiration, a sample of body fluid or a scrape/brush. The specimen is placed onto a glass slide and examined for the presence of abnormal cells. These include benign, precancerous and cancer cells. The test can also be used to diagnose infective processes (Chernecky and Berger 2013).

Direct microscopy

The majority of specimens will then undergo direct microscopic investigation, which is valuable as an early indication of the causative organism. High magnification is required to visualize viruses, which are then identified according to their characteristic shapes (Gould and Brooker 2008). Certain parasitic protozoa, such as those causing malaria, are identified by direct microscopy, which necessitates the specimen being delivered to the laboratory as quickly as possible, while the protozoa are mobile and therefore visible (Higgins 2013). In combination with clinical presentations, this may be enough to initiate or change targeted treatments until a more definitive diagnosis is reached (Weston 2008).

Gram staining

Gram staining is a process for identifying bacterial species. A staining substance is added to a sample to differentiate the types of organism present. Cells with differing properties stain differently in relation to the structure of their cell wall. Gram staining allows for the differentiation of gram-positive bacteria (e.g. *Staphylococcus aureus*), which stain purple, and gram-negative bacteria (e.g. *Escherichia coli*), which stain pink when viewed under the microscope. The findings can be used to guide the choice of antimicrobial therapy until other investigation methods can provide a definitive identification of pathogenic micro-organisms. In blood cultures, gram staining is 67.9% sensitive for the detection of bacteria (Chernecky and Berger 2013).

Histology

Histology is the study of cells and tissues within the body. It also studies how the tissues are arranged to form organs. The histological focus is on the structure of individual cells and how they are arranged to form the individual organs. The types of tissues that are recognized are epithelial, connective, muscular and nervous (Kierszenbaum and Tres 2016, Mescher 2016).

The tissues are examined under a light microscope, where light passes through the tissue components after they have been stained. As most tissues are colourless, they are stained with dyes to enable visualization. An alternative is the electron microscope, in which cells and tissue can be viewed at magnifications of about 130,000 times (Kierszenbaum and Tres 2016, Mescher 2016).

Serology

A serological test looks for antibodies in a patient's blood. Serology is useful in identifying viral infections and bacterial infections with difficult culture organisms and is based upon the patient's immunological reaction. Detection of antigens or antibodies in serum, which are activated in response to infection, may suggest that the patient is, or has been, infected (Higgins 2013, Keogh 2017).

Clinical governance

An organization that provides any diagnostic services must have clear, identifiable policies and procedures. There must be open, bidirectional communication between the department, organizational board and national bodies such as the Medicines and Health products Regulatory Agency (MHRA) to ensure appropriate care is delivered. Internal monitoring processes must be in place to identify potential clinical or organizational risks, and there must be a clear reporting mechanism.

Competencies

In accordance with the Nursing and Midwifery Council's (NMC's) *The Code: Professional Standards of Practice and Behaviour for Nurses, Midwives and Nursing Associates* (NMC 2018), nurses must always practice using the best available evidence. This includes giving patients evidence-based information and advice, and maintaining their own skills and knowledge for safe and effective practice.

Consent

It is essential that healthcare professionals and healthcare support staff gain consent before beginning any treatment or care, or undertaking any diagnostic tests or procedures. Consent is continuous throughout any patient episode and the practitioner must ensure that the patient is kept informed at every stage (NMC 2018, RCN 2017a). For diagnostic tests and procedures, this may include:

- informing the patient of the reason for the diagnostic test or procedure
- telling the patient what the diagnostic test or procedure will involve
- ascertaining the patient's level of understanding (especially if they need to be directly involved in the preparation, sampling technique or positioning)
- telling the patient how long the results may take to be processed
- telling the patient how the results will be made available
- giving the patient information about the implications this may have for their care
- giving the patient information regarding any post-procedural considerations.

Risk management

New research and evidence continue to be produced. It is essential that any risk or change in practice is communicated to clinicians. Alerts from the MHRA – for example, concerning issues related to medical devices used in the diagnostic testing process and changes in practice – should be acted upon. Several agencies, such as the Health Protection Agency, also publish new guidance and best practice using the latest available evidence.

Accurate record keeping and documentation

Good record keeping is an integral part of nursing practice and it is essential to the provision of safe and effective care (NMC 2018). Accurate, specific and timely documentation of any diagnostic tests should be recorded in the patient's electronic or paper notes, care plan, or designated record charts or forms. This assists in the communication and dissemination of information between members of the inter-professional healthcare team.

Pre-procedural considerations

Specimen selection

Selecting a specimen that is representative of the disease process is critical to the ability of the laboratory to provide information that is accurate, significant and clinically relevant. The specimen may come from any part of the body and include blood, tissue or body fluids. Incorrect specimen selection or technique can be life threatening to patients (Chernecky and Berger 2013, Pagana and Pagana 2017). Specimens should only be taken when there are clinical indications – for example, signs of infection. Signs of infection, such as fever, should trigger a careful clinical assessment to ensure that unnecessary tests are avoided and the most useful laboratory samples are obtained to identify therapeutic options (Pagana and Pagana 2017).

The production of high-quality, accurate results that are clinically useful is very much dependent upon the quality of the specimen collection (Higgins 2013, Pagana and Pagana 2017). Additionally, the greater the quantity of material sent for laboratory examination, the greater the chance of isolating a causative organism.

Specimens should be taken as soon as possible after the manifestation of clinical signs and symptoms. The timing of specimen collection is especially important during the acute phase of viral infections. Many viral illnesses have a prodromal phase where multiplication and shedding of the virus are usually at their peak and when the patient is most infectious. This is often before the onset of clinical illness and has often ceased by about day 5 from the onset of symptoms. At this stage, the patient's immune response against the virus will already have been been mounted and may therefore affect organism isolation (Chernecky and Berger 2013, Keogh 2017, Pagana and Pagana 2017).

Specimens are readily contaminated by poor technique, and analysis of such specimens could lead to adverse outcomes such as misdiagnosis, misleading results, extended length of stay, inappropriate therapy or potentially disastrous consequences for the patient (Keogh 2017, Pagana and Pagana 2017). Therefore, a clean technique must be used to avoid inadvertent contamination of the site of the sample or the specimen itself. Specimens should also be collected in sterile containers with close-fitting lids.

Equipment selection

A variety of medical devices are used before, during and after diagnostic tests. For blood, body fluids and tissue specimens, various blood bottles, sterile pots, swabs and other receptacles are required (following local policy and guidelines) (Figures 13.1–13.4). It is essential that the specimen and its transport container are appropriate for the type of specimen or sample. Failure to use the correct collection method and equipment leads to inaccurate results and potentially incorrect or unnecessary treatments. Other medical devices, such as X-ray machines or endoscopes, may be used to undertake a diagnostic test or procedure. It is essential to ensure practitioners are aware of local variation in types and manufacturers of medical devices and have been trained in their use prior to undertaking a diagnostic test or procedure.

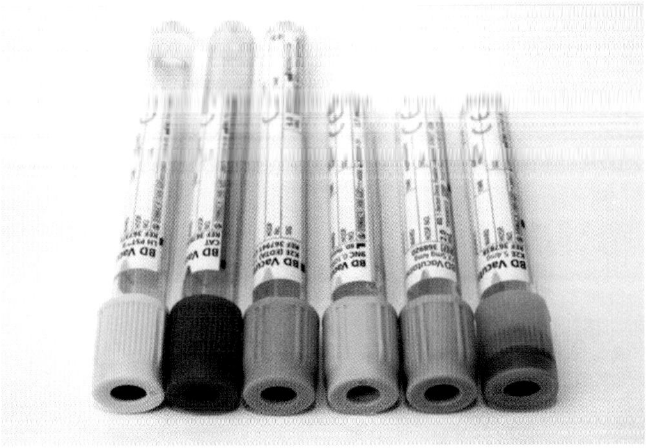

Figure 13.1 Various blood bottles. *Source*: Reproduced from Dougherty et al. (2019). © 2019 The Royal Marsden NHS Foundation Trust. Published 2019 by John Wiley & Sons, Ltd.

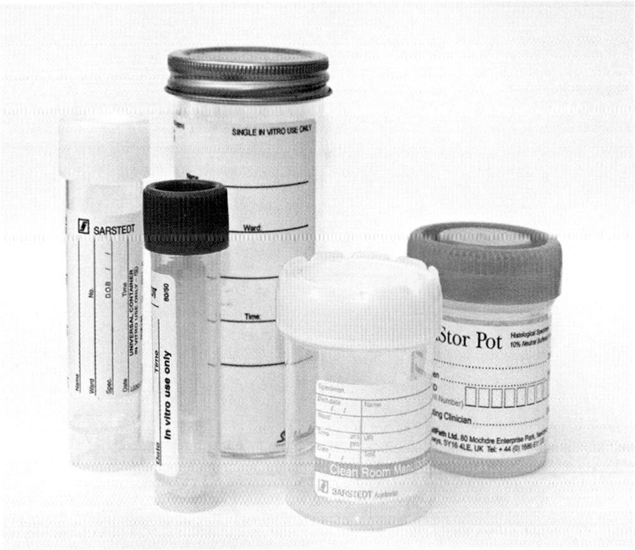

Figure 13.2 Various specimen pots. *Source*: Reproduced from Dougherty et al. (2019). © 2019 The Royal Marsden NHS Foundation Trust. Published 2019 by John Wiley & Sons, Ltd.

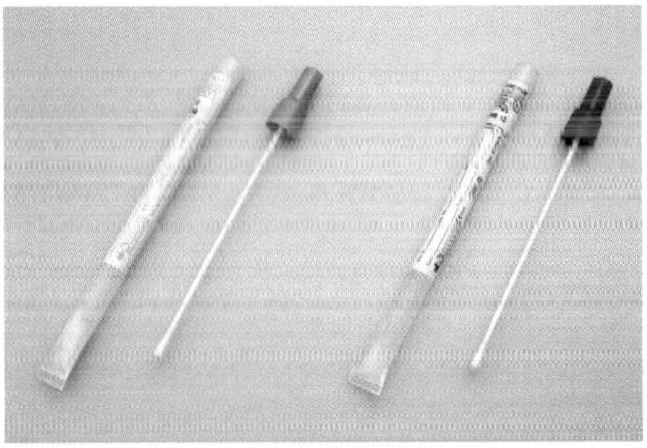

Figure 13.3 Two different swabs.

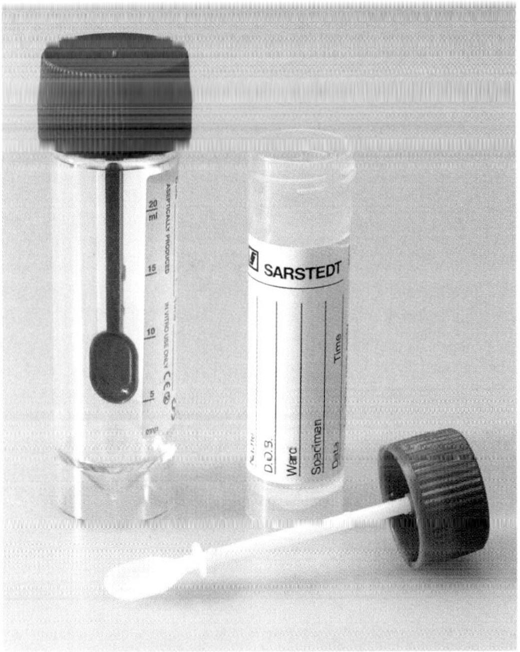

Figure 13.4 Two different stool pots.

Handling specimens

Specimens should be obtained using safe techniques and practices, and practitioners should be aware of the potential physical and infection hazards associated with the collection of diagnostic specimens within the healthcare environment. Standard (universal) infection control precautions should be adopted by healthcare workers who have direct contact or exposure to the blood, body fluids, secretions or excretions of patients (Gould and Brooker 2008). In addition to considering personal protection, the person collecting the specimen should be mindful of the collective health and safety of other people involved in the handling of samples. Every health authority must ensure that medical, nursing, phlebotomy, portering and any other staff involved in handling specimens are trained to do so (RCN 2017b, WHO 2015).

In relation to specimen collection, standard (universal) infection control precautions should include the following (RCN 2017b):

- hand hygiene
- the use of personal protection equipment
- safe sharps management
- safe handling, storage and transportation of specimens
- waste management
- clean environment management
- personal and collective management of exposure to body fluids and blood.

Selection of personal protection equipment should be based upon an assessment of risk of exposure to body fluids. As minimum precautions, gloves and aprons should be worn when handling all body fluids. Protective face wear (e.g. goggles, masks and visors) should be worn during any procedure where there is a risk of blood, body fluid, secretions or excretions splashing into the eyes or face (RCN 2017b).

Assessment and recording tools

The request form should include as much information as possible as this allows the laboratory or department conducting the diagnostic procedure or investigation to select the most appropriate equipment and/or media for examination (IBMS 2016). Request forms should include some or all of the following information, depending on the type of diagnostic test or procedure:

- patient's name, date of birth, ward and/or department
- hospital number

- test required
- date and time of diagnostic test, procedure or specimen collection
- type and site of specimen: this should specify the anatomical site, such as 'abdominal wound', as this allows the laboratory to differentiate the target and non-target pathogens and assess the significance of the results based upon the flora normally associated with that site (Wegerhoff 2006)
- diagnosis and relevant clinical information that could help in the interpretation of the sample (Higgins 2013)
- relevant signs and symptoms
- relevant history – for example, recent foreign travel
- present or recent antimicrobial therapy, if relevant
- whether the patient is immunocompromised, as these patients are highly susceptible to opportunistic infections and non-pathogenic organisms (Weston 2008)
- consultant's name
- name and contact details of the practitioner requesting the investigation, as it may be necessary to telephone the result before the report is dispatched
- 'danger of infection' label if the specimen is high risk (HSE 2003, WHO 2015).

Communication

For certain specimens that have specific collection techniques or require prompt processing, communication with the laboratory before the sample collection is essential. Providing specimen arrival time to the laboratory can improve efficiency of processing and accuracy of results. Where a diagnostic test is to be undertaken, it is essential that the patient is prepared appropriately with consideration of fasting times, the cessation of certain medications and post-procedural care. A patient information leaflet explaining the test can be given to prepare the patient for pre- and post-procedural care. Communication with the department where the test will be conducted is essential.

Post-procedural considerations

Handling specimens

Specimens should be placed in a double self-sealing bag with one compartment containing the specimen and the other containing the request form. The specimen container used should be appropriate for the purpose and the lid should be securely closed immediately to avoid spillage and contamination. The specimen should not be overfilled and not be externally contaminated by the contents. Any accidental spillages must be cleaned up immediately by staff wearing appropriate protective equipment (HSE 2003, RCN 2017b, WHO 2015) (see Chapter 4: Infection prevention and control). Standard precautions must be in place at all times when handling any body fluids or specimens irrespective of infectious status (Pagana and Pagana 2017).

Specimens from patients who have recently been treated with toxic therapy (such as gene therapy, cytotoxic drugs, radioactivity or active metabolites) need to be handled with particular caution. Local guidelines on the labelling, bagging and transportation of such samples to the laboratory should be followed. For example, in the case of gene therapy, the specimen must be labelled with a 'biohazard' label, double bagged and transported to the laboratory in a secure box with a secure lid (HSE 2003, WHO 2015).

Clinical waste

It is essential that all clinical waste is disposed of appropriately. This ensures that healthcare activities do not go on to pose further infection risks and that waste is securely managed. There are various regulatory regimes (e.g. concerning environment and waste, controlled drugs, infection control, health and safety, and transport) that pertain to the destruction of healthcare waste. Specialist disposal of cytotoxic and radioactive waste must also be considered. Due to variations in product availability and local waste arrangements, it is important to follow local policy and guidelines (DH 2013) (see Chapter 4: Infection prevention and control).

Documentation

Labelling specimens

Incorrectly labelled and unlabelled specimens will be discarded (HSE 2003, IBMS 2016). Samples should include the following information:

- patient's name, date of birth, ward and/or department
- hospital number
- date and time of specimen collection
- type and site of specimen: this should specify the anatomical site, such as 'abdominal wound', as this allows the laboratory to differentiate the target and non-target pathogens and assess the significance of the results based upon the flora normally associated with that site (Keogh 2017, Pagana and Pagana 2017).

Transporting specimens

An awareness of the type of specimen or organism being investigated gives the healthcare professional an insight into the correct storage and transportation methods. For example, most micro-organisms are extremely susceptible to environmental fluctuations, such as in pH, temperature, ultraviolet rays and oxidizing agents (Table 13.1) (Gould and Brooker 2008). Incorrect or prolonged storage or transportation may result in the organism not surviving before cultures can be made. Delays in transporting a specimen to the laboratory can compromise the specimen's integrity, leading to false-negative or false-positive results or a misdiagnosis because the sample is no longer representative of the disease process (Higgins 2013, Pagana and Pagana 2017).

The sooner a specimen arrives in the laboratory, the greater the chance of organisms or disease being identified. Some pathogens do not survive for very long once they have left the host, while normal body flora within the sample may proliferate and overgrow, inhibiting or killing the pathogen (Weston 2008).

If delays are anticipated, samples need to be stored appropriately, depending on the nature of the specimen, until they can be processed. This could be in an ambient temperature storage unit, specimen fridge or freezer (HSE 2003, WHO 2015). For example, blood cultures need to be incubated at 37°C, whereas swabs must be either refrigerated or kept at ambient temperature, depending on the site from which they were taken. Other specimens, such as tissue, may need to be stored in preservatives such as formaldehyde solution (WHO 2015).

Equipment used for transportation

Where a specimen is obtained within a healthcare setting, it should be transported either in a deep-sided tray that is not used for any other purpose and is disinfected after each use (HSE 2003, WHO 2015) or in a robust, leak-proof container that conforms to the regulation Biological Substances, Category B: UN3373 (HSE 2005, WHO 2015). Specimens that need to be moved outside the hospital or clinic must be transported using a triple-packaging

Table 13.1 Types of organism

Organism	Definition
Aerobic	Aerobic bacteria only grow in the presence of oxygen.
Anaerobic	Anaerobic bacteria prefer an atmosphere of reduced oxygen, such as deep in wound bed tissue, and facultative anaerobes can grow in either the presence or absence of oxygen.
Bacteria	Bacteria are unicellular organisms that multiply and die very rapidly, especially once they have been removed from their optimum environment.
Virus	Viruses are intracellular parasites that hijack the genetic material of the host cell and are therefore unable to multiply outside living cells.

Source: Adapted from Gould and Brooker (2008), Higgins (2013), Pagana and Pagana (2017).

system (HSE 2005, WHO 2015). This consists of a watertight, leak-proof, absorbent primary container; a durable, watertight, leak-proof secondary container; and an outer container that complies with Biological Substances, Category B: UN 3373 standards (HSE 2005, WHO 2015). A box for transportation is essential and should carry a warning label for hazardous material. It must be made of smooth, impervious material, such as plastic or metal, which will retain liquid and can be easily disinfected and cleaned in the event of a spillage (HSE 2003, WHO 2015).

Blood sampling

Definition

Blood sampling, or phlebotomy, is the collection of blood via various methods with the purpose of testing and analysing the components of the blood (Chernecky and Berger 2013, Keogh 2017, Pagana and Pagana 2017, WHO 2010a).

Evidence-based approaches

Rationale

Blood is the body fluid most frequently used for analysis. Blood sampling is undertaken to assess body processes and disorders and includes haematology, biochemistry and arterial blood gas analysis (Chernecky and Berger 2013, Keogh 2017, Pagana and Pagana 2017, WHO 2010a).

Indications

Indications for blood sampling include:

- defining baseline results
- establishing a diagnosis
- establishing a prognosis
- confirming or screening for disease
- ruling out a clinical problem
- monitoring disease
- regulating therapy or treatment

Methods of blood sampling

The methods of blood sampling vary depending on the blood sample required and include venepuncture, sampling via vascular access devices and arterial sampling. The samples obtained via these means will have different properties; for example, venous blood will be low in oxygen in comparison to an arterial sample (Pagana and Pagana 2017).

It is important that the correct blood tube is used for each test. Blood tubes contain special additives relevant to the type of test required, usually indicated by the colour of the tube top. The practitioner should ensure that the correct tube is selected by referring to local guidelines. Correct 'order of draw' should be followed to avoid transferring additive from one tube to another when filling (see Table 13.4) (Garza and Becan-McBride 2013, Pagana and Pagana 2017).

Methods of investigation

Numerous blood tests are available. Blood samples are sent to various departments within the laboratory, such as haematology, biochemistry or microbiology. Brief outlines of some routine tests are given below. Refer to specialist reference texts for more detail.

Haematology

The full blood count is the most commonly requested blood test (Higgins 2013). It involves monitoring the levels of red blood cells (erythrocytes), white blood cells (leucocytes) and platelets (thrombocytes). Variations to normal values can indicate anaemia, infection or thrombocytopenia (Table 13.2).

Table 13.2 Haematology

Test	Reference range	Functions and additional information
Red blood cells	Men: 4.5–6.5 × 10^{12}/L Women: 3.9–5.6 × 10^{12}/L	• The main function of the RBCs is the transport of oxygen and carbon dioxide using haemoglobin (Pagana and Pagana 2017).
Haemoglobin	Men: 135–175 g/L Women: 115–155 g/L	• Haemoglobin is a protein pigment found within the RBCs that carries oxygen. • Anaemia (deficiency in the number of RBCs or haemoglobin content) may occur for many reasons. Changes to cell production, deficient dietary intake or blood loss may be relevant and need to be investigated further.
White blood cells	Men: 3.7–9.5 × 10^9/L Women: 3.9–11.1 × 10^9/L	• The function of the WBCs is defence against infection. • There are different kinds of WBC: neutrophils, lymphocytes, monocytes, eosinophils and basophils. • Leucopenia is a WBC count lower than 3.7 × 10^9/L and is usually associated with the use of cytotoxic drugs. • Leucocytosis (high levels of neutrophils and lymphocytes) occurs as the body's normal response to infection and after surgery. • Leukaemia involves an increased WBC count caused by changes in cell production in the bone marrow. The leukaemic cells enter the blood in increased numbers in an immature state.
Platelets	Men: 150–400 × 10^9/L Women: 150–400 × 10^9/L	• Clot formation occurs when platelets and the blood protein fibrin combine. • A patient may be thrombocytopenic (low platelet count) due to drugs or poor production, or have a raised count (thrombocytosis) with infection or autoimmune disease.
Coagulation/INR	INR range 2–3 (in some cases a range of 3–4.5 is acceptable)	• Coagulation occurs to prevent excessive blood loss by the formation of a clot (thrombus). However, a clot that forms in an artery may block the vessel and cause an infarction or ischaemia, which can be fatal (Blann 2007). • Aspirin, warfarin and heparin are three drugs used for the prevention and/or treatment of thrombosis. • It is imperative that patients on warfarin therapy receive regular monitoring to ensure a balance of slowing the clot-forming process and maintaining the ability of the blood to clot (Blann 2007).

INR, international normalized ratio; RBC, red blood cell; WBC, white blood cell.

Group and save (blood transfusion)

All patients who require a blood transfusion need to have their blood type confirmed. It is essential that correct patient identification and accurate labelling are maintained. The sample will be screened to determine the blood type: A, B, O or Rh (Rhesus). All staff should receive formal documented training in blood transfusion practice (Robinson et al. 2017) (see Chapter 12: Respiratory care, CPR and blood transfusion).

Biochemistry

Urea and electrolytes are the most common biochemistry tests requested (Table 13.3).

Liver function tests

There are numerous tests that are used to assess liver function. These include alkaline phosphatase (AP), gamma-glutamyl transpeptidase (GGT), aspartate aminotransferase (AST) and alanine aminotransferase (ALT).

Microbiology

Various types of sample may be sent to the microbiology laboratory for screening, for example microbiological drug assays. Blood samples sent to microbiology may require screening for hepatitis B, hepatitis C and HIV.

Table 13.3 Biochemistry

Test	Reference range	Functions and additional information
Sodium	135–145 mmol/L	• The main function of sodium is to maintain extracellular volume (water stored outside the cells), acid-base balance and the transmitting of nerve impulses. • Hypernatraemia (serum sodium >145 mmol/L) may be an indication of dehydration due to fluid loss from diarrhoea, excessive sweating, increased urinary output or a poor oral intake of fluid. An increased salt intake may also cause an elevation. • Hyponatraemia (serum sodium <135 mmol/L) may be indicated in fluid retention (oedema).
Potassium	3.5–5.2 mmol/L	• Potassium plays a major role in nerve conduction, muscle function, acid-base balance and osmotic pressure. It has a direct effect on cardiac muscle, influencing cardiac output by helping to control the rate and force of each contraction. • The most common cause of hyperkalaemia (serum potassium >5.2 mmol/L) is chronic renal failure. The kidneys are unable to excrete potassium. The level may be elevated due to an increased intake of potassium supplements during treatment. Tissue cell destruction caused by trauma or cytotoxic therapy may cause a release of potassium from the cells and an elevation in the potassium plasma level. It may also be observed in untreated diabetic ketoacidosis. • Urgent treatment is required as hyperkalaemia may lead to changes in cardiac muscle contraction and cause subsequent cardiac arrest. • The main cause of hypokalaemia (serum potassium <3.5 mmol/L) is the loss of potassium via the kidneys during treatment with thiazide diuretics. Excessive or chronic diarrhoea may also cause a decreased potassium level.
Urea	[illegible]	• Urea is a waste product of metabolism that is transported to the kidneys and excreted as urine. Elevated levels of urea may indicate poor kidney function.
Creatinine	55–105 μmol/L	• Creatinine is a waste product of metabolism that is transported to the kidneys and excreted as urine. Elevated levels of creatinine may indicate poor kidney function.
Calcium	2.2–2.6 mmol/L	• Most of the calcium in the body is stored in the bone but ionized calcium, which circulates in the blood plasma, plays an important role in the transmission of nerve impulses and the functioning of cardiac and skeletal muscle. It is also vital for blood coagulation. • High calcium levels (hypercalcaemia >2.6 mmol/L) can be due to hyperthyroidism, hyperparathyroidism or malignancy. Elevation in calcium levels may cause cardiac arrhythmia, potentially leading to cardiac arrest (Chernecky and Berger 2013, Pagana and Pagana 2017). • Tumour cells can cause excessive production of a protein called parathormone-related polypeptide (PTHrP), which causes a loss of calcium from the bone and an increase in blood calcium levels. This is a major reason for hypercalcaemia in cancer patients (Higgins 2013). • Hypocalcaemia (<2.20 mmol/L) is often associated with vitamin D deficiency due to inadequate intake or increased loss due to gastrointestinal disease. Mild hypocalcaemia may be symptomless but severe hypocalcaemia may cause increased neuromuscular excitability and cardiac arrhythmias. It is also a common feature of chronic renal failure (Higgins 2013).
C-reactive protein (CRP)	<10 mg/L	• Elevation in the CRP level can be a useful indication of bacterial infection. CRP is monitored after surgery and for patients who have a high risk of infection. CRP level can help clinicians to monitor the severity of inflammation and assist in the diagnosis of conditions such as systemic lupus erythematosus, ulcerative colitis and Crohn's disease (Higgins 2013).
Albumin	35–50 g/L	• Albumin is a protein found in blood plasma that assists in the transport of water-soluble substances and the maintenance of blood plasma volume.
Bilirubin	(total) <17 μmol/L	• Bilirubin is produced from the breakdown of haemoglobin; it is transported to the liver for excretion in bile. Elevated levels of bilirubin may cause jaundice.

Pre-procedural considerations

Equipment

There are specific medical devices required for the various methods of blood sampling; however, blood tubes are common throughout the NHS. It is important that the correct blood tube is used for each test. Blood tubes contain special additives relevant to the type of test required, usually indicated by the colour of the tube top. The practitioner should ensure that the correct tube is selected by referring to local guidelines. Correct 'order of draw' should be followed to avoid transferring additive from one tube to another when filling (Garza and Becan-McBride 2018, Pagana and Pagana 2017).

Venepuncture: obtaining blood samples from a peripheral vein

Definition

Venepuncture is the procedure of entering a vein with a needle (McCall and Tankersley 2016).

Anatomy and physiology

The superficial veins of the upper limb are most commonly chosen for venepuncture. These veins are numerous and accessible, ensuring that the procedure can be performed safely and with minimum discomfort (McCall and Tankersley 2016). In adults, veins located on the dorsal portion of the foot may be selected but there is an increased risk of complications, especially if the patient has diabetes or a history of vascular or coagulation disorders (Hoeltke 2018). Therefore, veins in the lower limbs should be avoided where possible.

Veins

The veins commonly used for venepuncture are those found in the antecubital fossa because they are sizeable veins capable of providing copious and repeated blood specimens (Weinstein and Hagle 2014). However, the venous anatomy of individuals may differ. The main veins of choice are (Figure 13.5):

- median cubital veins
- cephalic vein
- basilic vein
- metacarpal veins (used only when the others are not accessible).

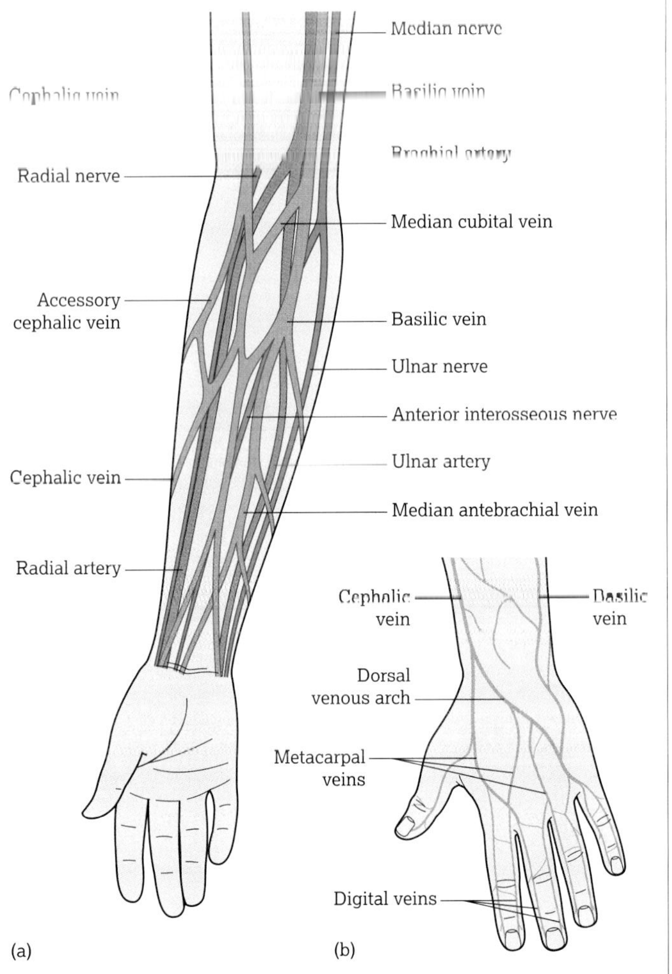

Figure 13.5 (a) Superficial veins of the forearm. (b) Superficial veins of the dorsal aspect of the hand. Green, nerves; red, arteries; blue, veins. *Source:* Reproduced with permission of Becton, Dickinson and Company.

Median cubital vein

The median cubital vein may not always be visible, but its size and location make it easy to palpate. It is also well supported by subcutaneous tissue, which prevents it from rolling under the needle (Hoeltke 2018).

Cephalic vein

On the lateral aspect of the wrist, the cephalic vein rises from the dorsal veins and flows upwards along the radial border of the forearm as the median cephalic vein and crossing the antecubital fossa as the median cubital vein. Care must be taken to avoid accidental arterial puncture, as this vein crosses the brachial artery. It is also in close proximity to the radial nerve (Dougherty 2008, Tortora and Derrickson 2017).

Basilic vein

The basilic vein, which has its origins in the ulnar border of the hand and forearm (Waugh and Grant 2018), is often overlooked as a site for venepuncture. It may well be prominent but it is not well supported by subcutaneous tissue, making it roll easily, which can result in difficult venepuncture. Owing to its position, a haematoma may occur if the patient flexes the arm on removal of the needle, as this squeezes blood from the vein into the surrounding tissues (McCall and Tankersley 2016). Care must also be taken to avoid accidental puncture of the median nerve and brachial artery (Hoeltke 2018).

Metacarpal veins

The metacarpal veins are easily visualized and palpated. However, the use of these veins may not be suitable in the elderly because skin turgor and subcutaneous tissue are diminished, which makes the veins more difficult to anchor (Hoeltke 2018).

Layers of the veins

Veins consist of three layers: the tunica intima, the tunica media and the tunica adventitia.

Tunica intima

The tunica intima is a smooth endothelial lining, which allows the passage of blood cells. If it becomes damaged, the lining may become roughened, leading to an increased risk of thrombus formation (Weinstein and Hagle 2014). Within this layer are folds of endothelium called valves, which keep blood moving towards the heart by preventing backflow. Valves are present in larger vessels and at points of branching and are seen as palpable bulges in the veins (Tortora and Derrickson 2017). However, when suction is applied during venepuncture, the valve can compress and close the lumen of the vein, preventing the withdrawal of blood (Weinstein and Hagle 2014). Therefore, if detected, venepuncture should be performed above the valve in order to facilitate collection of the sample (Weinstein and Hagle 2014).

Tunica media

The tunica media, the middle layer of the vein wall, is composed of muscular tissue and nerve fibres, both vasoconstrictors and vasodilators, which can stimulate the vein to contract or relax. This layer is not as strong or stiff as the equivalent layer in an artery and therefore veins can distend or collapse as the pressure rises or falls (Waugh and Grant 2018, Weinstein and Hagle 2014). Stimulation of this layer by a change in temperature, mechanical or chemical stimulation can produce venous spasm, which can make a venepuncture more difficult.

Tunica adventitia

The tunica adventitia is the outer layer and consists of connective tissue, which surrounds and supports the vessel (Waugh and Grant 2018).

Choosing a vein

The choice of vein must be that which is best for the individual patient. The most prominent vein is not necessarily the most suitable vein for venepuncture (Weinstein and Hagle 2014). There are two stages to locating a vein:

1 visual inspection
2 palpation.

Visual inspection

Visual inspection is the scrutiny of the veins in both arms and is essential prior to choosing a vein. Veins adjacent to foci of infection, bruising and phlebitis should not be considered, owing to the risk of causing more local tissue damage or systemic infection (Dougherty 2008). An oedematous limb should be avoided as there is danger of stasis of lymph, predisposing the patient to complications such as phlebitis and cellulitis, with increased risk of causing tissue damage from the tourniquet application (Hoeltke 2018). Areas of previous venepuncture should be avoided as a build-up of scar tissue can cause difficulty in accessing the vein and can result in pain due to repeated trauma (Hoeltke 2018).

Palpation

Palpation is an important assessment technique as it determines the location and condition of the vein, distinguishes veins from arteries and tendons, identifies the presence of valves and detects deeper veins (Dougherty 2008). The nurse should always use the same fingers for palpation as this will increase sensitivity and the ability of the nurse to know what they are feeling. The less dominant hand should be used for palpation so that in the event of a missed vein, the nurse can repalpate and realign the needle (Hoeltke 2018). The thumb should not be used as it is not as sensitive and has a pulse, which may lead to confusion in distinguishing veins from arteries in the patient (Hoeltke 2018).

Thrombosed veins feel hard and cord-like, and should be avoided along with tortuous, sclerosed, fibrosed, inflamed or fragile veins, which may be unable to accommodate the device to be used and will result in pain and repeated venepunctures (Dougherty 2008). Use of veins that cross over joints or bony prominences and those with little skin or subcutaneous cover (e.g. the inner aspect of the wrist) will also subject the patient to more discomfort (Dougherty 2008). Therefore, preference should be given to a vessel that is unused, easily detected by inspection and palpation, patent and healthy. These veins feel soft and bouncy and will refill when depressed (McCall and Tankersley 2016).

Arteries

Arteries tend to be placed more deeply than veins and can be distinguished by their thicker walls (which do not collapse), the presence of a pulse and the bright red blood they carry. It should be noted that aberrant arteries may be present; these are arteries located superficially in an unusual place (Weinstein and Hagle 2014).

Evidence-based approaches

Rationale

Indications

Venepuncture is carried out for two reasons:

- to obtain a blood sample for diagnostic purposes
- to monitor levels of blood components and a patient's condition (Garza and Becan-McBride 2018).

Contraindications

Contraindications to using certain veins or limbs include:

- previous surgery to an affected limb with axillary lymph node clearance
- lymphoedema on a particular limb
- amputation, fracture or cerebrovascular accident affecting a limb.

Methods of improving venous access

There are various ways of improving venous access:

- *Application of a tourniquet* promotes venous distension. The tourniquet should be tight enough to impede venous return but not restrict arterial flow. It should be placed about 7–8 cm above the venepuncture site. It may be more comfortable for the patient to position it over a sleeve or paper towel to prevent pinching the skin. The tourniquet should not be left on for longer than 1 minute as this may result in haemoconcentration (pooling of the blood) or haemolysis (rupturing of red blood cells), leading to inaccurate blood results (Hoeltke 2018).
- The patient may be asked to *clench their fist* to encourage venous distension but should avoid 'pumping' as this action may affect certain blood results (e.g. test for potassium levels, as cell damage releases potassium) (Garza and Becan-McBride 2018).
- *Lowering the arm* below heart level increases blood supply to the veins.
- *Light tapping of the vein* may be useful but can be painful and may result in the formation of a haematoma in patients with fragile veins, for example thrombocytopenic patients (Dougherty 2008).
- *The use of heat* in the form of a warm pack or by immersing the arm in a bowl of warm water for 10 minutes helps to encourage vasodilation and venous filling (Garza and Becan-McBride 2018).
- *Ointment or patches* containing small amounts of glyceryl trinitrate can be used to improve local vasodilation to aid venepuncture (Weinstein and Hagle 2014).

Methods of insertion

Asepsis is vital when performing a venepuncture as the skin is breached and a foreign device is introduced into a sterile circulatory system. The two major sources of microbial contamination are:

- cross-infection from practitioner to patient
- skin flora of the patient.

Good hand washing and drying techniques are essential and gloves should be changed between patients (see Chapter 4: Infection prevention and control).

To remove the risk presented by the patient's skin flora, firm and prolonged rubbing with an alcohol-based solution, such as chlorhexidine 2% in 70% alcohol, is advised (RCN 2017b). This cleaning should continue for a minimum of 30 seconds, although some authors state a minimum of 1 minute or longer (Weinstein and Hagle 2014). The area that has been cleaned should then be allowed to dry. This facilitates coagulation of the organisms, thus ensuring disinfection, and also prevents a stinging pain on insertion of the needle due to the alcohol being transferred onto the end of the needle. The skin must not be touched or the vein repalpated prior to venepuncture (McCall and Tankersley 2016).

Clinical governance

Venepuncture is one of the most commonly performed invasive procedures in the NHS and is now routinely undertaken by nurses. In order to perform venepuncture safely, the nurse must have basic knowledge of the following:

- the relevant anatomy and physiology
- the criteria for choosing both the vein and the device to use
- the problems that may be encountered, how to prevent them and necessary interventions
- the health and safety and the risk management of the procedure, as well as the correct disposal of equipment (RCN 2017b).

Certain principles, such as adherence to an aseptic technique, must be applied throughout (see Chapter 4: Infection prevention and control). The circulation is a closed, sterile system and a venepuncture, however quickly completed, is a breach of this system, providing a means of entry for bacteria.

Nurses must be aware of the physical and psychological comfort of the patient (Hoeltke 2018). They must appreciate the value of adequate explanation and simple measures to prevent the complications of venepuncture, such as haematoma formation, when it is neither a natural nor acceptable consequence of the procedure (Hoeltke 2018).

Risk management

The number of litigation cases within the healthcare environment has increased in recent years (Garza and Becan-McBride 2018). It is therefore vital that nurses receive accredited and appropriate training, supervision and assessment by an experienced member of staff (RCN 2017a). The nurse is then accountable and responsible for ensuring that skills and competence are maintained and knowledge is kept up to date, in order to fulfil the criteria set out in *The Code* (NMC 2018).

Pre-procedural considerations

Safety of the practitioner

It is recommended that well-fitting gloves are worn during any procedure that involves handling blood and body fluids, particularly venepuncture and cannulation (NHS England and NHSI 2019, RCN 2017b). This is to prevent contamination of the practitioner from potential blood spills. While it is recognized that gloves will not prevent a needle stick injury, the wiping effect of a glove on a needle may reduce the volume of blood to which the hand is exposed, thereby reducing the volume inoculated and the risk of infection (NHS Employers 2015). However, there is no substitute for good technique and practitioners must always work carefully when performing venepuncture.

A range of safety devices are now available for venepuncture that can reduce the risk of occupational percutaneous injuries among healthcare workers, in particular vacuum blood collection systems (see Figure 13.6) (Garza and Becan-McBride 2018). Regulations require the use of safer sharps systems that incorporate protective mechanisms such as safety shields or covers. Where practical, all conventional devices are to be replaced (HSE 2013). Used needles should always be discarded directly into an approved sharps container, without being resheathed (DH 2013, McCall and Tankersley 2016). The accompanying request forms should be kept separately from the specimen to avoid contamination (HSE 2003). All other non-sharp disposables should be placed in a universal clinical waste bag or discarded in accordance with local policy.

Equipment

Tourniquets

There are several types of tourniquet available. A good-quality, buckle-closure, single-hand-release type is most effective but the choice will depend on availability and operator. Consideration should be given to the type of material and the ability to decontaminate the tourniquet. Fabric tourniquets that cannot be cleaned are not recommended (RCN 2017b). Disposable tourniquets are recommended and are available for single use and should be discarded immediately after use, especially where there is potential for microbial cross-contamination (RCN 2017b). A blood pressure cuff can be applied instead of a tourniquet as it will apply pressure over a wider area and make the veins more prominent. The cuff should be inflated half way between the diastolic and systolic readings. The need for disposable cuffs should also be considered where cross-contamination may occur.

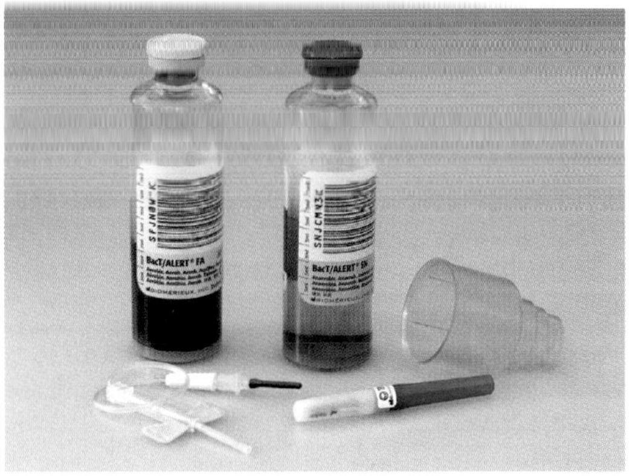

Figure 13.6 A vacuumed collection system: two blood culture bottles, a Vacutainer holder and a Vacutainer 'butterfly'.

Needles

The intravenous devices commonly used to perform a venepuncture for blood sampling are a straight steel needle and a steel winged infusion device. The optimum gauge to use is 21 swg (standard wire gauge), which measures internal diameter: the smaller the gauge size, the larger the diameter. This enables blood to be withdrawn at a reasonable speed without undue discomfort to the patient or possible damage to the blood cells (Garza and Becan-McBride 2018).

Vacuum systems

A vacuum system consists of a plastic holder that contains or is attached to a double-ended needle or adapter (Figure 13.6). It is important to use the correct Luer adapter to ensure a good connection and avoid blood leakage (Garza and Becan-McBride 2018). The blood tube is vacuumed in order to ensure that the exact amount of blood required is withdrawn when the tube is pushed into the holder. Filling ceases once the tube is full, which removes the need for decanting blood and also reduces blood wastage. The system can also be attached to winged infusion devices (WHO 2010a).

A number of vacuum systems can be used for taking blood samples. These are simple to use and cost-effective. The manufacturer's instructions should be followed. Vacuum systems reduce the risk of healthcare workers being contaminated, because they offer a completely closed system during the process of blood withdrawal. This makes them the safest method for collecting blood samples.

Blood collection tubes are available in various sizes and have different-coloured tops depending on the type of additive. The colour coding of the tops is generally universal but may vary depending on manufacturer. Local policy must be referred to in order to select the correct tubes for specific tests. Blood tubes should be used in a sequence referred to as the 'order of draw' to minimize the transferring of additives. The correct volume of blood should be collected into each tube to prevent erroneous results (Table 13.4). The expiry dates on the tubes should also be monitored regularly.

The equipment available will depend on local policy (Table 13.5). However, given increasing concerns about the possibility of contamination of practitioners, blood collection systems with integrated safety devices are now readily available and should be used for all procedures (HSE 2013, RCN 2017b). However, the nurse must always select the device after assessing the condition and accessibility of the vein.

Table 13.4 Blood collection tubes and draw order

Tube	Type	Determinations	Instructions
Blood culture	Blood cultures	Blood cultures	Aerobic followed by anaerobic – use aerobic bottle only if not enough blood for both bottles
Light blue	Sodium citrate	PT, PTT, INR, APTT, D-dimers, fibrinogen, clotting screen, factor assays, thrombophilia screen (four light blue tubes and one EDTA tube), lupus (three light blue tubes), anticoagulant	Fill tube completely and invert tube gently three or four times
Red	No additive	Antibiotic levels, steroid hormones, B_{12}	No need to invert tube
Gold	Clot activator and serum separator	Routine chemistry, lipids, thyroid (TFT), drug levels including lithium, proteins Supply additional tube for troponin I levels Does not do glucose, lactate or alcohol	Invert six times
Green	Lithium heparin	Chromosome studies	Invert 8–10 times
Lavender	EDTA	Haematology: FBC, sickle screen, haemoglobin, electrophoresis, red cell folate, malaria, lead, mercury, thalassaemia, PTH, ESR Biochemistry: cyclosporin and other drugs	Invert 8–10 times
Pink	EDTA Cross-match	Antibody and group screen	Invert 8–10 times
Grey	Fluoride oxalate	Alcohol, glucose, lactate	Invert 8–10 times
Black	ESR	ESR	Invert 8–10 times
Royal blue	Trace elements	Trace elements, manganese, zinc, whole blood	Invert 8–10 times

APTT, activated partial thromboplastin time; EDTA, ethylenediamine tetra-acetic acid; ESR, erythrocyte sedimentation rate; FBC, full blood count; INR, international normalized ratio; PT, prothrombin time; PTH, parathyroid hormone; PTT, partial thromboplastin time; TFT, thyroid function test.
Source: Adapted from Dojcinovska (2011) with permission of John Wiley & Sons, Ltd.

Table 13.5 Choice of [illegible] devices

Device	Gauge	Advantages	Disadvantages	Use
Needle	21	• Cheaper than winged infusion devices. • Easy to use with large veins.	• Rigid. • Difficult to manipulate with smaller veins in less conventional sites. • May cause more discomfort. • Venous access only confirmed when sample tube attached.	• In large, accessible veins in the antecubital fossa. • When small quantities of blood are to be drawn.
Winged infusion device with safety feature	21	• Flexible due to small needle shaft. • Easy to manipulate and insert at any site. • Increases the success rate of venepuncture and causes less discomfort (Garza and Becan-McBride 2018). • Usually shows a 'flashback' of blood to indicate a successful venepuncture.	• More expensive than steel needles. • The 12–30 cm length of tubing on the device may be caught and dislodge the needle.	• Veins in sites other than the antecubital fossa. • When quantities of blood greater than 20 mL are required from any site.
	23	• Flexible due to its small needle shaft. • Easy to manipulate and insert at any site. • Causes less discomfort than a needle. • Smaller swg and therefore useful with fragile veins.	• More expensive than steel needles, plus there can be damage to cells that can cause inaccurate measurements in certain blood samples, e.g. potassium.	• Small veins in more painful sites, e.g. inner aspect of the wrist, especially if measurements are related to plasma and not cellular components.

swg, standard wire gauge.

Pharmacological support

It is important to remember that patients may fear venepuncture and in some cases suffer from needle phobia. The use of topical local anaesthetic cream may be beneficial for anxious patients or children (Weinstein and Hagle 2014). Further information can be found in Chapter 17: Vascular access devices: insertion and management.

Non-pharmacological support

Patient anxiety about the procedure may result in vasoconstriction. The nurse's manner and approach will also have a direct bearing on the patient's experience (McCall and Tankersley 2016). Approaching the patient with a confident manner and giving an adequate explanation of the procedure may reduce anxiety. Careful preparation and an unhurried approach will help to relax the patient and this in turn will increase vasodilation (Dougherty 2008).

Specific patient preparation

There are various considerations in patient preparation for venepuncture:

- Injury, disease or treatment (e.g. amputation, fracture or cerebrovascular accident) may prevent the use of a limb for venepuncture, thereby reducing the venous access. Use of a limb may be contraindicated because of an operation on one side of the body (e.g. mastectomy and axillary node dissection) as this can lead to impairment of lymphatic drainage, which can influence venous flow regardless of whether there is obvious lymphoedema (Berreth 2010, McCall and Tankersley 2016).
- The age and weight of the patient will also influence choice. Young children have short, fine veins and the elderly have prominent but fragile veins. Care must be taken with fragile veins and the largest vein should be chosen along with the smallest-gauge device to reduce the amount of trauma to the vessel (Weinstein and Hagle 2014). Malnourished patients will often present with friable veins (Dougherty 2008).
- If the patient is in shock or dehydrated, there will be poor superficial peripheral access. It may be necessary to take blood after the patient is rehydrated as this will promote venous filling and blood will be obtained more easily (Dougherty 2008).
- Medications can influence the choice of vein in that patients on anticoagulants or steroids or those who are thrombocytopenic tend to have more fragile veins and will be at greater risk of bruising both during venepuncture and on removal of the needle. Therefore, choice may be limited by areas of bruising present or the inability to access the vessel without causing bruising (Dougherty 2008).
- The temperature of the environment will influence venous dilation. If the patient is cold, no veins may be evident on first inspection. Application of heat – for example, in the form of a warm compress or soaking the arm in warm water will increase the size and visibility of the veins, thus increasing the likelihood of a successful first attempt (Garza and Becan McBride 2018).
- Venepuncture itself may cause the vein to collapse or go into a spasm. This will produce discomfort and a reduction in blood flow. Careful preparation and choice of vein will reduce the likelihood of this, and stroking the vein or applying heat will help to resolve it (Dougherty 2008).
- Involving patients in the choice of vein, even if it is simply to choose the non-dominant arm, can increase a feeling of control, which in turn helps to relieve anxiety (Weinstein and Hagle 2014).
- The environment is also another important consideration. In the inpatient and outpatient settings, lighting, ventilation, privacy and position must be checked and optimized where possible. This will ensure that the patient and the operator are both comfortable. Having adequate lighting is also beneficial as it illuminates the procedure, ensuring the operator has a good view of the vein and equipment (Weinstein and Hagle 2014).

Procedure guideline 13.1 Venepuncture

Essential equipment

- Personal protective equipment
- Clean tray or receiver
- Disposable tourniquet or sphygmomanometer and cuff
- 21 swg multiple-sample safety needle or 21/23 swg winged safety infusion device and multiple-sample Luer adapter
- Plastic tube holder, standard
- Appropriate vacuumed specimen tubes
- Swab with chlorhexidine 2% in 70% alcohol, or isopropyl alcohol 70%
- Low-linting gauze swabs
- Sterile adhesive plaster or hypoallergenic tape
- Specimen request forms
- Sharps bin

Action	Rationale
Pre-procedure	
1 Introduce yourself to the patient, explain and discuss the procedure with them, and gain their consent to proceed.	To ensure that the patient feels at ease, understands the procedure and gives their valid consent (NMC 2018, **C**).
2 Check that the identity of the patient matches the details on the request form by asking for their full name and date of birth and checking their identification bracelet (where appropriate). If the patient is unable to communicate then check the identity band for full name, date of birth and hospital number.	To ensure the sample is taken from the correct patient (NPSA 2007a, **C**; RCN 2017a, **C**).
3 Allow the patient to ask questions and discuss any problems that have arisen previously.	Anxiety results in vasoconstriction; therefore, a patient who is relaxed will have dilated veins, making access easier. **E**

4 Consult the patient as to any preferences and problems that may have been experienced at previous venepunctures.	To involve the patient in the treatment, and to acquaint the nurse fully with the patient's previous venous history and identify any changes in clinical status (e.g. mastectomy), as both may influence vein choice (Dougherty 2008, **E**).
5 Check whether the patient has any allergies.	To prevent allergic reactions, for example to latex or chlorhexidine (McCall and Tankersley 2016, **E**; MHRA 2012, **C**).
6 Assemble the equipment necessary for venepuncture.	To ensure that time is not wasted and that the procedure goes smoothly without unnecessary interruptions. **E**
7 Wash hands using bactericidal soap and water or alcohol-based handrub, and dry before commencement.	To minimize risk of infection (NHS England and NHSI 2019, **C**).
8 Check own hands for any visibly broken skin, and cover any such areas with a waterproof dressing.	To minimize the risk of contamination to the practitioner (DH 2010, **C**; Fraise and Bradley 2009, **E**).
9 Check all packaging before opening and preparing the equipment on the chosen clean receptacle.	To maintain asepsis throughout and check that no equipment is damaged. **E**
Procedure	
10 Take all the equipment to the patient, exhibiting a confident manner.	To help the patient feel more at ease with the procedure. **E**
11 Support the chosen limb on a pillow.	To ensure the patient's comfort and facilitate venous access. **E**
12 Apply a tourniquet to the arm on the chosen side, making sure it does not obstruct arterial flow. If the radial pulse cannot be palpated then the tourniquet is too tight (Weinstein and Hagle 2014). The position of the tourniquet may be varied; for example, if a vein in the hand is to be used, the tourniquet may be placed on the forearm. A sphygmomanometer cuff may be used as an alternative.	To dilate the veins by obstructing the venous return (Dougherty 2008, **E**). To increase the prominence of the veins. **E** To slow down blood flow and therefore distend the veins (Garza and Becan-McBride 2018, **R**).
13 If the tourniquet does not improve venous access, the following methods can be used. If venous access appears possible, skip to step 19. *Either:* The arm may be placed in a dependent position. The patient may be asked to clench their fist. *Or:* The veins may be tapped gently or stroked. *Or:* Remove the tourniquet and apply moist heat (e.g. a warm compress), soak the limb in warm water or, with prescription, apply glyceryl trinitrate ointment/patch (Weinstein and Hagle 2014).	To improve venous access (Dougherty 2008, **E**).
14 Select the vein by careful palpation to determine size, depth and condition (**Action figure 14**).	To prevent inadvertent insertion of the needle into other anatomical structures (Witt 2011, **E**).
15 Release the tourniquet.	To ensure patient comfort. **E**
16 Select the device, based on vein size, site and volume of blood to be taken. Use a 23 swg winged infusion device for small veins, metacarpal or feet veins.	To reduce damage or trauma to the vein and prevent haemolysis (Dougherty 2008, **E**).
17 Wash hands with bactericidal soap and water or alcohol-based handrub and allow to dry.	To maintain asepsis and minimize the risk of infection (NHS England and NHSI 2019, **C**)
18 Reapply the tourniquet.	To dilate the veins by obstructing the venous return (Dougherty 2008, **E**).
19 Put on gloves.	To prevent possible contamination of the practitioner (NHS England and NHSI 2019, **C**).
20 Clean the patient's skin carefully for 30 seconds using an appropriate preparation, for example chlorhexidine 2% in 70% alcohol, and allow to dry. Do not repalpate or touch the skin (**Action figure 20**).	To maintain asepsis and minimize the risk of infection (DH 2010, **C**; Fraise and Bradley 2009, **E**; Loveday et al. 2014, **R**).
21 Remove the cover from the needle and inspect the device carefully.	To detect faulty equipment, for example bent or barbed needles. If these are present, place them in a safe container, record batch details and return to manufacturer (MHRA 2005, **C**).

(continued)

Procedure guideline 13.1 Venepuncture *(continued)*

Action	Rationale
22 Anchor the vein by applying manual traction on the skin a few centimetres below the proposed insertion site (**Action figure 22**).	To immobilize the vein and to provide counter tension to the vein, which will facilitate a smoother needle entry (Dougherty 2008, **E**).
23 Insert the needle smoothly at an angle of approximately 30°. However, the angle will depend on the size and depth of the vein (**Action figure 22**).	To facilitate a successful, pain-free venepuncture. **E**
24 Reduce the angle of descent of the needle as soon as a flashback of blood is seen in the tubing of a winged infusion device or when puncture of the vein wall is felt.	To prevent advancing too far through the vein wall and causing damage to the vessel (Dougherty 2008, **E**).
25 Slightly advance the needle into the vein, if possible.	To stabilize the device within the vein and prevent it becoming dislodged during withdrawal of blood. **E**
26 Do not exert any pressure on the needle.	To prevent a puncture occurring through the vein wall. **E**
27 Withdraw the required amount of blood using a vacuumed blood collection system (**Action figure 27**). Collect blood samples in the draw order shown in Table 13.4.	To minimize the risk of transferring additives from one tube to another and bacterial contamination of blood cultures (manufacturer's guidelines, **C**).
28 Release the tourniquet. This may be necessary at the beginning of sampling as inaccurate measurements may be caused by haemostasis, for example when taking blood to assess calcium levels.	To decrease the pressure within the vein. **E**
29 Remove the tube from the plastic tube holder.	To prevent blood spillage caused by vacuum in the tube (Hoeltke 2018, **E**).
30 Place a low-linting swab over the puncture point.	To apply pressure. **E**
31 Remove the needle, but do not apply pressure until the needle has been fully removed.	To prevent pain on removal and damage to the intima of the vein. **E**
32 Activate the safety device and then discard the needle immediately in a sharps bin.	To reduce the risk of accidental needle stick injury (HSE 2013, **C**).
33 Apply digital pressure directly over the puncture site. Pressure should be applied until bleeding has ceased; approximately 1 minute or longer may be required if the patient's current disease or treatment interferes with clotting mechanisms.	To stop leakage and haematoma formation. To preserve the vein by preventing bruising or haematoma formation. **E**
34 The patient may apply pressure with a finger but should be discouraged from bending the arm if a vein in the antecubital fossa is used.	To prevent leakage and haematoma formation (McCall and Tankersley 2016, **E**).
35 Gently invert as guided by the manufacturer's instructions.	To prevent damage to blood cells and to mix with additives (manufacturer's guidelines, **C**).
36 Label the bottles with the relevant details at the patient's side. Never pre-label bottles.	To ensure that the specimens from the right patient are delivered to the laboratory, the requested tests are performed and the results are returned to the correct patient's records (NMC 2018, **C**; NPSA 2007a, **C**).
Post-procedure	
37 Inspect the puncture point before applying a dressing.	To check that the puncture point has sealed. **E**
38 Confirm whether the patient is allergic to adhesive plaster.	To prevent an allergic skin reaction. **E**
39 Apply an adhesive plaster or alternative dressing.	To cover the puncture and prevent leakage or contamination. **E**
40 Ensure that the patient is comfortable.	To ascertain whether the patient wishes to rest before leaving (if an outpatient) or whether any other measures need to be taken. **E**
41 Remove gloves and discard waste and sharps according to local policy.	To ensure safe disposal and avoid laceration or other injury of staff (DH 2013, **C**; Fraise and Bradley 2009, **E**).
42 Follow hospital procedure for collection and transportation of specimens to the laboratory.	To make sure that specimens reach their intended destination. **E**
43 Document the procedure in the patient's records.	To ensure timely and accurate record keeping (NMC 2018, **C**).

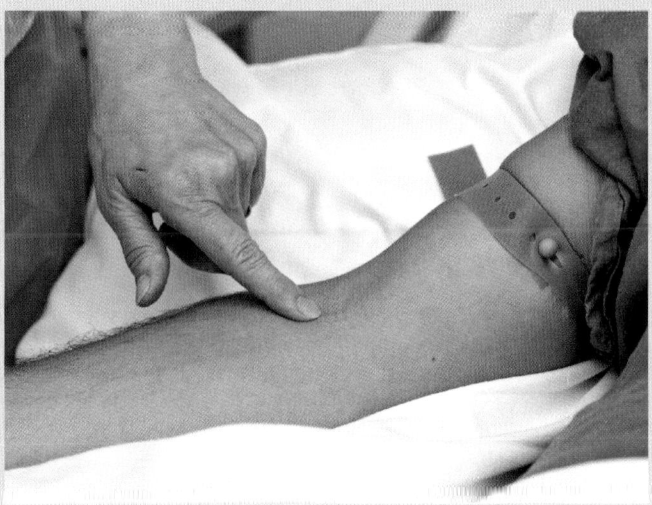

Action Figure 14 Palpating the vein.

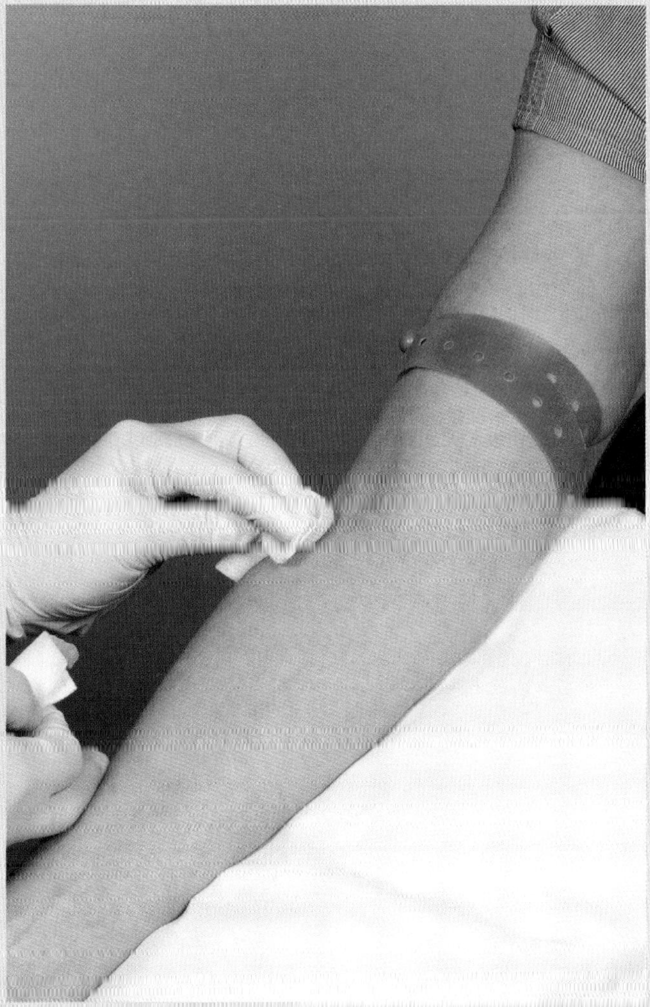

Action Figure 20 Cleaning the skin.

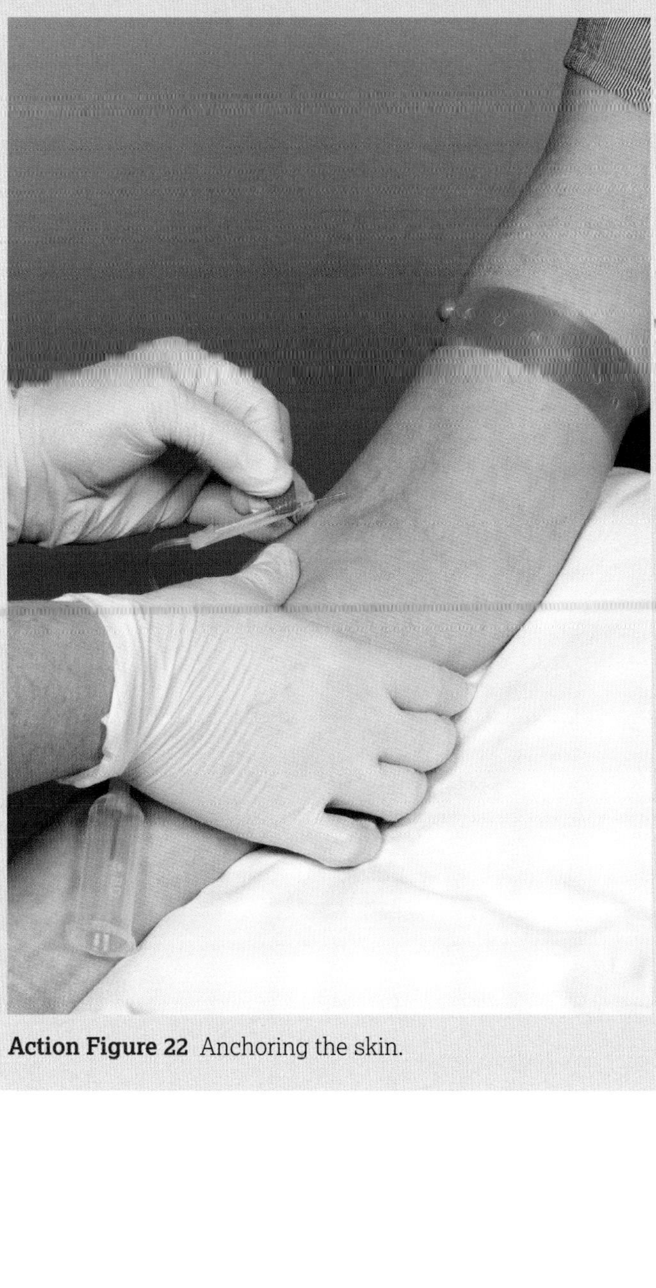

Action Figure 22 Anchoring the skin.

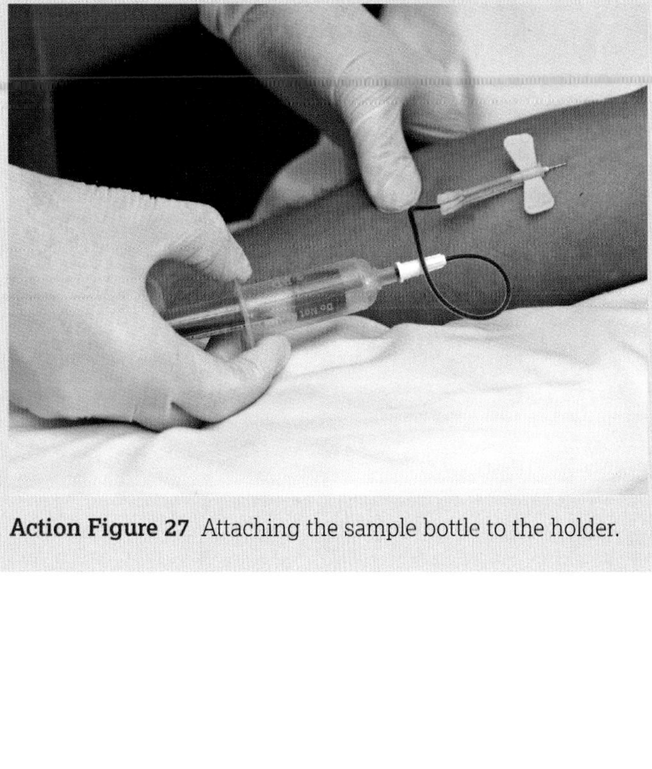

Action Figure 27 Attaching the sample bottle to the holder.

Problem solving table 13.1 Prevention and resolution (Procedure guideline 13.1)

Problem	Cause	Prevention	Action
Pain	Use of vein in sensitive area (e.g. wrist)	Avoid using veins in sensitive areas wherever possible. Use local anaesthetic cream	Complete the procedure as quickly as possible.
Anxiety	Previous trauma	Minimize the risk of a traumatic venepuncture. Use all methods available to ensure successful venepuncture.	Approach patient in a calm and confident manner. Listen to the patient's fears and explain what the procedure involves. Offer patient the opportunity to lie down. Suggest use of local anaesthetic cream (WHO 2010a).
	Fear of needles		All of the above and perhaps referral to a psychologist if fear is of phobic proportions.
Limited venous access	Repeated use of same veins Peripheral shutdown	Use alternative sites if possible. Ensure the room is not cold.	Do not attempt the procedure unless experienced.
	Dehydration	Ensure correct device and technique are used.	Put patient's arm in warm water. Apply glycerol trinitrate patch (as prescribed).
	Hardened veins (due to scarring and thrombosis)		May be necessary to rehydrate patient prior to venepuncture.
	Poor technique or poor choice of vein or device		Do not use these veins as venepuncture will be unsuccessful.
Needle inoculation of or contamination to practitioner	Unsafe practice Incorrect disposal of sharps	Maintain safe practice. Activate safety device. Ensure sharps are disposed of immediately and safely.	Follow accident procedure for sharps injury, for example make site bleed and apply a waterproof dressing. Report and document. An injection of hepatitis B immunoglobulin or triple therapy may be required.
Accidental blood spillage	Damaged/faulty equipment Reverse vacuum	Check equipment prior to use. Use vacuumed plastic blood collection system. Remove blood tube from plastic tube holder before removing needle.	Report within hospital and/or the Medicines and Healthcare products Regulatory Agency. Ensure blood is handled and transported correctly.
Missed vein	Inadequate anchoring Poor vein selection Wrong positioning Lack of concentration Poor lighting	Ensure that only properly trained staff perform venepuncture or that those who are training are supervised. Ensure the environment is well lit.	Repalpate, withdraw the needle slightly and realign it, providing the patient is not feeling discomfort. Ensure all learners are supervised. If the patient is feeling pain, then the needle should be removed immediately.
	Difficult venous access		Ask an experienced colleague to perform the procedure.
Spurt of blood on entry	Bevel tip of needle enters the vein before entire bevel is under the skin; usually occurs when the vein is very superficial		Reassure the patient. Wipe blood away on removal of needle.
Blood stops flowing	Through-puncture: needle inserted too far	Correct angle.	Draw back the needle, but if bruising is evident remove the needle immediately and apply pressure.
	Contact with valves	Palpate to locate.	Withdraw the needle slightly to move the tip away from the valve.
	Venous spasm	Results from mechanical irritation and cannot be prevented.	Gently massage above the vein or apply heat.
	Vein collapse	Use veins with large lumens. Use a smaller device.	Release tourniquet, allow veins to refill and retighten tourniquet.
	Small vein	Avoid use of small veins wherever possible.	May require another venepuncture.
	Poor blood flow	Use veins with large lumens.	Apply heat above vein.

Post-procedural considerations

Immediate care

It is important to ensure that the needle is removed correctly on completion of blood sampling and that the risk of haematoma formation is minimized. Pressure should be applied as the needle is removed from the skin. If pressure is applied too early, it causes the tip of the needle to drag along the intima of the vein, resulting in sharp pain and damage to the lining of the vessel (McCall and Tankersley 2016).

The practitioner should ensure that firm pressure is maintained until bleeding has stopped. The patient should also be instructed to keep their arm straight and not bend it as this increases the risk of bruising (McCall and Tankersley 2016). A longer period of pressure may be necessary where the patient's blood may take longer to clot, for example if the patient is receiving anticoagulants or is thrombocytopenic. The practitioner may choose to apply the tourniquet over the venepuncture site to ensure even and constant pressure on the area (Dougherty 2008). Alternatively, if safe and practical, they can elevate the arm slightly above the heart to decrease venous pressure (Weinstein and Hagle 2014).

The practitioner should inspect the site carefully for bleeding or bruising before applying a dressing and before the patient leaves the department. If bruising has occurred, the patient should be informed of why this has happened and given instructions for what to do to reduce the bruising and any associated pain.

Complications

Complications associated with venepuncture include arterial puncture, nerve injury, haematoma, fainting and infection. Careful assessment and preparation will minimize the risks but if any of these complications occur then appropriate action should be taken immediately.

Arterial puncture

To prevent an arterial puncture, careful assessment of vein selection is necessary. The nurse should palpate the vessel prior to needle insertion to confirm the absence of a pulse; the angle of insertion should be less than 30° and in the event of a missed vein, blind probing should be avoided (McCall and Tankersley 2016).

An arterial puncture can be identified by bright red blood, rapid blood flow and pain. The needle should be removed immediately and pressure applied for 5 minutes by the nurse. A pressure dressing should be applied and the patient should receive verbal and written advice to follow in the event of increased pain, swelling or loss of sensation. No tourniquet or blood pressure cuff should be reapplied to the arm for 24 hours. The incident should be documented in the patient's notes (NMC 2018, WHO 2010a, 2015).

Nerve injury

Careful vein selection and needle insertion should minimize the risk of nerve injury. The angle of insertion should be less than 30° and blind probing should be avoided (Hoeltke 2018). In the event of a nerve injury, the patient may complain of a sharp shooting pain, burning or electric shock sensation that radiates down the arm and they may experience numbness or tingling in their fingers. The needle should be removed immediately to prevent further nerve damage (Garza and Becan-McBride 2018). The patient should receive verbal and written advice to follow if the pain or numbness continues for more than a few hours. The incident should be documented in the patient's notes.

Haematoma

Haematoma formation is the most common complication of venepuncture (McCall and Tankersley 2016). A haematoma develops when blood leaks from the vein into the surrounding tissues. It may be caused by the needle penetrating completely through the vein wall, the needle only being partially inserted or insufficient pressure being placed on the site when the needle is removed. If a haematoma develops, the needle should be removed immediately and pressure applied. In the event of a large haematoma developing, the nurse can apply an ice pack to relieve pain and swelling. The application of a topical cream that is used for the treatment of superficial thrombophlebitis, bruising and/or haematoma may be beneficial (BNF 2019).

The patient should receive verbal and written advice as a haematoma may lead to a compression injury to the nerve (Hoeltke 2018). The incident should be documented in the patient's notes (NMC 2018, WHO 2015).

Fainting

Fainting may occur during or immediately following venepuncture. The patient may complain of feeling light-headed and appear pale and sweaty. Loss of consciousness may occur suddenly so the nurse should be vigilant throughout the procedure and routinely confirm with the patient that they do not feel unwell or faint. In the event of the patient feeling faint, the nurse should remove the device immediately, apply pressure to the site and encourage the patient to lower their head from upright or lie down and breathe deeply. The application of a cold compress to the forehead and increased ventilation (open a window if clinically acceptable) may help to make the patient more comfortable. If the patient suffers a loss of consciousness, the nurse should call for assistance and ensure the patient's safety until they recover. The patient should not be allowed to leave the department until fully recovered and should be advised not to drive for at least 30 minutes (McCall and Tankersley 2016). The incident should be documented in the patient's notes and the patient should be advised to inform staff on future occasions.

Infection

Infection at the venepuncture site is a rare occurrence and should be reported to a doctor or non-medical prescriber (McCall and Tankersley 2016). Aseptic technique should be maintained with careful attention to hand washing and skin preparation. The venepuncture site should not be repalpated after cleaning and the site should be covered for 15–20 minutes after the procedure.

CVAD sampling: sampling from a central venous access device

Definition

Sampling from a central venous access device (CVAD) involves the collection of blood from a CVAD, such as a central venous catheter (CVC) or peripherally inserted central catheter (PICC) (Hess and Decker 2017, Sousa et al. 2015).

Evidence-based approaches

Methods of taking blood samples from a central venous access device

Sampling from a CVAD has the advantage of using an existing line to obtain the sample, without the need of venepuncture, saving the patient potential pain and inconvenience. However, obtaining blood samples from a CVAD can lead to inaccurate results, if the correct method is not followed to ensure removal of any drug or intravenous fluid prior to sampling (Mendez 2012, WHO 2015). A number of methods may be used to withdraw samples and there appears to be no significant difference in laboratory results and no evidence that haemolysis or haemodilution can occur if the technique is undertaken appropriately (Mendez 2012, RCN 2010, WHO 2015).

Discard method

The discard method is the one most commonly used in the clinical setting (recommended by The Royal Marsden Hospital and demonstrated within Procedure guideline 13.2: Central venous access devices: taking a blood sample for vacuum sampling) where the first 5–10 mL of blood is withdrawn and discarded (Gorski et al. 2010, Mendez 2012). This ensures removal of any heparin, drugs or intravenous fluid. This may also result in an excessive blood removal in patients requiring multiple samples, for example for pharmacokinetic tests (Hess and Decker 2017, Mendez 2012).

Push–pull (mixing) method

In the push–pull (mixing) method, a syringe is attached to the catheter, the catheter is flushed with 0.9% sodium chloride, then 6 mL is withdrawn and pushed back without removing the syringe; this is repeated at least three times. This removes any residual solution and reduces exposure to blood, and there is no blood wastage (Adlard 2008, Mendez 2012). This method suggests that mixing of blood eliminates heparin, drugs or intravenous fluids from the CVAD lumen. However, it may be difficult to obtain enough blood to exchange three or four times.

Pre-procedural considerations

It is preferable to use the distal lumen of a multilumen catheter when obtaining a sample as it is normally the largest; where these catheters have different-sized lumens, the largest should be reserved for blood sampling (Gorski et al. 2010).

Post-procedural considerations

Whichever method is used, once the samples have been taken it is vital that the catheter is adequately flushed with 0.9% sodium chloride followed where appropriate with a heparin solution, to reduce the risk of clot formation and subsequent infection and/or occlusion (Goossens 2015, Gorski et al. 2010, RCN 2010, Sousa et al. 2015).

Procedure guideline 13.2 Central venous access devices: taking a blood sample for vacuum sampling

Essential equipment

- Personal protective equipment
- Sterile dressing pack
- Extra 10 mL blood bottle without heparin
- Vacuum system container holder (shell)
- Vacuum system adapter
- Clean tray or receiver
- Trolley
- Appropriate vacuumed blood bottles or needleless injection cap (as necessary)

Medicinal products

- 10 mL syringe containing 0.9% sodium chloride
- Flushing solution as per policy
- 10 mL syringe
- 2% chlorhexidine in 70% alcohol swab

Action	Rationale
Pre-procedure	
1 Introduce yourself to the patient, explain and discuss the procedure with them, and gain their consent to proceed. Check forms to ascertain sample bottles required and check patient's identity.	To ensure that the patient feels at ease, understands the procedure and gives their valid consent (NMC 2018, **C**). To ensure correct bottles are used and blood is taken from the correct patient (NPSA 2007a, **C**; RCN 2010, **C**).
Procedure	
2 Wash hands with bactericidal soap and water or alcohol-based handrub and allow to dry.	To reduce the risk of cross-infection (NHS England and NHSI 2019, **C**).
3 Prepare a tray or trolley and take it to the bedside. Clean hands as above. Open sterile pack and prepare equipment.	To reduce the risk of contamination of contents (DH 2010, **C**; RCN 2017b, **C**).
4 If intravenous fluid infusion is in progress, switch it off.	To prevent spillage of fluid following disconnection. **E**
5 Where required, disconnect the administration set from the catheter and cover the end of the set with a sterile cap.	To reduce the risk of contaminating the end of the administration set. **E**
6 Clean hands with an alcohol-based handrub.	To minimize the risk of introducing infection into the catheter. To enable the disinfection process to be completed (Loveday et al. 2014, **R**; RCN 2017b, **C**).
7 Put on non-sterile gloves.	To prevent possible contamination of the practitioner (NHS England and NHSI 2019, **C**).
8 Clean hub or needle-free cap thoroughly with a 2% chlorhexidine in 70% alcohol swab for at least 15 seconds and allow to dry before accessing the system.	To enable the disinfection process to be completed (Loveday et al. 2014, **R**).

9 Connect the vacuum container holder and adapter to the needleless injection cap and release the lumen clamp.	To maintain a closed system and prevent contamination of the practitioner or air entry. **E**
10 Attach the extra sample bottle; fill and discard.	To remove blood, heparin, drugs and intravenous fluids from the 'dead space' of the catheter. Samples from this dead space are likely to cause inaccuracies in blood tests. Using a spare bottle keeps the system closed (WHO 2010a, **C**).
11 Attach the required sample bottles in the correct order of draw (see Table 13.4) for the requested specimens.	To obtain the sample. It is not necessary to clamp the catheter when changing collection bottles, as the system is not open. **E**
12 Re-clamp the lumen/catheter and detach the vacuum container holder.	To prevent blood loss or air embolism. **E**
13 Flush with 10 mL 0.9% sodium chloride, using the push–pause method (i.e. 1 mL at a time).	To create turbulence, ensure removal of all blood in the catheter and prevent occlusion (Goossens 2015, **C**; Gorski 2011, **C**).
14 Reconnect the administration set, unclamp the catheter and recommence infusion or attach a new needle-free injection cap. Release the clamp and flush the catheter through the injection cap using the push–pause method and finishing with the positive pressure technique.	To prevent the catheter clotting between uses (Dougherty 2006, **E**; Goossens 2015 **C**; Gorski et al. 2010, **E**).
15 Ensure that the blood samples have been placed in the correct containers and invert as necessary (see Table 13.4) to prevent clotting.	To make certain that the specimens, correctly presented and identified, are delivered to the laboratory, enabling the requested tests to be performed and the results to be returned to the correct patient's records (NMC 2018, **C**; RCN 2010, **C**; WHO 2015, **C**).
16 Label the samples with the patient's name, number, date of birth, etc. at the patient's side and send them to the laboratory with the appropriate forms.	To prevent mislabelling when away from the patient. To maintain accurate records and provide accurate information for laboratory analysis (NMC 2018, **C**; Weston 2008, **E**; WHO 2015, **C**).
Post-procedure	
17 Remove gloves and discard waste, making sure it is placed in the correct containers (e.g. sharps into a designated receptacle).	To ensure correct clinical waste management and to reduce the risk of cross-infection (DH 2013, **C**).
18 Document the procedure in the patient's records.	To ensure timely and accurate record keeping (NMC 2018, **C**; WHO 2015, **C**).

673

Procedure guideline 13.3 Central venous access devices: taking a blood sample for syringe sampling

This may be necessary if the CVAD does not bleed when using a vacuum system, for example with silicone peripherally inserted central cannulas (PICCs).

Essential equipment

- Personal protective equipment
- Sterile dressing pack
- Extra 10 mL syringe
- Clean tray or receiver
- Appropriate blood bottles
- Sterile syringe of appropriate size for sample required
- Needleless injection cap (as necessary)
- Trolley

Medicinal products

- Flushing solution as per policy
- 10 mL syringe containing 0.9% sodium chloride
- 2% chlorhexidine in 70% alcohol swab

(continued)

Procedure guideline 13.3 Central venous access devices: taking a blood sample for syringe sampling *(continued)*

Action	Rationale
Pre-procedure	
1 Introduce yourself to the patient, explain and discuss the procedure with them, and gain their consent to proceed. Check forms to ascertain sample bottles required and check patient's identity.	To ensure that the patient feels at ease, understands the procedure and gives their valid consent (NMC 2018, **C**). To ensure correct bottles are used and blood is taken from the correct patient (NPSA 2007a, **C**; RCN 2010, **C**).
Procedure	
2 Wash hands with bactericidal soap and water or alcohol-based handrub and allow to dry.	To reduce the risk of cross-infection (NHS England and NHSI 2019, **C**)
3 Prepare a tray or trolley and take it to the bedside. Clean hands as above. Open sterile pack and prepare equipment.	To reduce the risk of contamination of contents (DH 2010, **C**; RCN 2017b, **C**).
4 If intravenous fluid infusion is in progress, switch it off.	To prevent spillage of fluid following disconnection. **E**
5 Where required, disconnect the administration set from the catheter and cover the end of the set with a sterile cap.	To reduce the risk of contaminating the end of the administration set. **E**
6 Clean hands with an alcohol based handrub and allow to dry.	To minimize the risk of introducing infection into the catheter. To enable the disinfection process to be completed (DH 2007, **C**; RCN 2017b, **C**).
7 Put on non sterile gloves.	To prevent possible contamination of the practitioner (WHO 2010a, **C**).
8 Clean the hub or needle-free cap thoroughly with a 2% chlorhexidine in 70% alcohol swab. Allow to dry.	To enable the disinfection process to be completed (DH 2007, **C**).
9 Attach a 10 mL syringe to the needleless injection cap. Release the clamp and withdraw 5–10 mL of blood.	To remove blood, heparin, drugs and intravenous fluids from the 'dead space' of the catheter. Samples from this dead space are likely to cause inaccuracies in blood tests (WHO 2010a, **C**).
10 Clamp and remove the syringe and discard.	To discard the contaminated sample and prevent mixing. **E**
11 Attach a new syringe of appropriate size. Unclamp and withdraw the required amount of blood.	To obtain the sample. **E**
12 Clamp and detach the syringe.	To prevent blood spillage or air entry. **E**
13 Decant blood into the sample bottles following the draw order shown in Table 13.4.	To ensure blood is placed into the sample bottles as soon as possible. **E**
14 Flush with 10 mL 0.9% sodium chloride, using the push–pause method (i.e. 1 mL at a time).	To create turbulence, ensure removal of all blood in the catheter and prevent occlusion (Goossens 2015, **C**).
15 Reconnect the administration set, unclamp the catheter and recommence infusion or attach a new needleless injection cap. Release the clamp and flush the catheter through the injection cap using the push–pause method and finishing with the positive pressure technique.	To prevent the catheter clotting between uses (Dougherty 2006, **E**; Goossens 2015, **C**; Gorski et al. 2010, **E**).
Post-procedure	
16 Remove gloves and discard waste, making sure it is placed in the correct containers (e.g. sharps into a designated receptacle).	To ensure correct clinical waste management and to reduce the risk of cross-infection (DH 2013, **C**).
17 Ensure that blood samples have been placed in the correct containers and agitated as necessary to prevent clotting.	To make certain that the specimens, correctly presented and identified, are delivered to the laboratory, enabling the requested tests to be performed and the results to be returned to the correct patient's records (NMC 2018, **C**; RCN 2010, **C**; WHO 2015, **C**).
18 Label the samples with the patient's name, number, date of birth, etc. at the patient's side and send them to the laboratory with the appropriate forms.	To prevent mislabelling when away from the patient. To maintain accurate records and provide accurate information for laboratory analysis (NMC 2018, **C**; Weston 2008, **E**; WHO 2015, **C**).
19 Document the procedure in the patient's records.	To ensure timely and accurate record keeping (NMC 2018, **C**; WHO 2015, **C**).

Problem-solving table 13.2 Prevention and resolution (Procedure guidelines 13.2 and 13.3)

Problem	Cause	Prevention	Action
Difficulty may be encountered when taking blood samples.	Difficulty is common when the central venous catheter is made of silicone and has been in place for a long time. One of the causes is that the tip of the soft catheter lies against the wall of the vessel and the suction required to draw blood brings this into close contact, leading to temporary occlusion. There could also be a collapse of the catheter walls when using the vacuum system, which may necessitate the use of syringes to obtain the blood.	Position the tip in the lower superior vena cava or right atrium.	Measures to use to try to dislodge the tip include asking the patient to: • cough and breathe deeply • roll from side to side • raise their arms • perform the Valsalva manoeuvre, if possible • increase their general activity, for example walk up and down stairs (Gorski et al. 2010).
	The tip of the catheter may be covered in a fibrin sheath, which may result in partial withdrawal occlusion (PWO).		This may be resolved with rapid flushing of the catheter with 0.9% sodium chloride or a dilute solution of heparin. If it is due to PWO then a fibrinolytic agent may be necessary to remove the fibrin (Goossens 2015, Goossens et al. 2013, Kumar et al. 2013).
	Pinch-off syndrome occurs when a CVAD inserted via the percutaneous subclavian site is compressed by the clavicle and first rib and aspirating blood becomes difficult (Mirza et al. 2004).		Ask the patient to lift their arm to the side. If blood aspiration improves and there is little resistance on flushing, suspect pinch-off and request a chest X-ray and cathetergram to check for catheter damage or embolism.

Arterial blood sampling

Definition

Arterial blood sampling is the collection of blood from an artery via an arterial puncture to measure arterial blood gases (ABGs) and other blood components (Kim 2013, Pagana and Pagana 2017).

ABGs are more difficult to undertake in comparison to venepuncture. The radial artery in the wrist is the artery most often used for intermittent or infrequent sampling. An ABG sample may also be drawn from the brachial or femoral artery provided the healthcare practitioner is trained to do so. The brachial and femoral arteries do not have adequate collateral supplies and are not routinely used for sampling. A pulse is felt by pressing on the area above an artery. If blood is drawn at the wrist, the healthcare provider will usually check the pulse to make sure blood is flowing into the hand from the radial and ulnar arteries in the forearm (Kim 2013, Pagana and Pagana 2017). If frequent sampling is required, an intra-arterial cannula is normally inserted (Keogh 2017, Osborne 2017, Pagana and Pagana 2017).

Anatomy and physiology

Arteries transport blood away from the heart and they vary in size. The arteries consist of three layers: tunica adventitia, tunica media and tunica intima. Arteries normally stretch easily or have high compliance with small increases in pressure due to the presence of elastic fibres (Tortora and Derrickson 2017). The brachial artery terminates as the radial and ulnar arteries, and an extensive collateral network of superficial and deep palmar arteries connects the radial and ulnar circulations. This normal pattern is present in 84% of patients. In 5% of cases, the radial artery is derived from the superficial brachial artery while the ulnar and interosseous arteries continue to originate from the brachial artery (Brzezinski et al. 2009).

Evidence-based approaches

Rationale

ABG sampling provides valuable information relating to a patient's respiratory, metabolic acid-base and electrolyte status (Table 13.6). It allows the partial pressure of oxygen (PaO_2), the partial pressure of carbon dioxide ($PaCO_2$) and the acid-base balance (pH) to be measured. It is also used to measure electrolytes and haemoglobin (for example) at a specific point in the course of a patient's illness (Keogh 2017, Pagana and Pagana 2017). The sample is often taken during a period of acute deterioration (Pagana and Pagana 2017, Welch and Black 2017).

There are two methods for sampling an ABG: arterial puncture and intra-arterial cannula. The latter method is usually used in the critical care unit, intensive care unit or high-dependency unit. In practice, interpreting the abnormalities in each value that may be compensated will help to determine the treatment plan. Compensation occurs when the body is able to respond to the acid-base imbalance to normalize the pH via the respiratory and/or metabolic systems (Table 13.7).

Indications

Indications for ABG sampling include the following:

- to enable the identification of respiratory, metabolic and mixed acid-base disorders, with or without physiological compensation, by means of pH (concentration of H^+ ions) and carbon dioxide (CO_2) levels (partial pressure of CO_2)
- to measure the partial pressures of respiratory gases involved in oxygenation and ventilation (PaO_2 and $PaCO_2$)
- to monitor acid-base status, as in a patient with diabetic ketoacidosis on insulin infusion; ABG and venous blood gas (VBG) could be obtained simultaneously for comparison, with VBG sampling subsequently used for further monitoring

Table 13.6 Arterial blood gas sampling

Test	Reference range	Functions and additional information
pH	7.35–7.45	The acidity of the blood is measured by the pH. The pH scale measures the number of hydrogen ions (H^+). A pH >7.45 is alkaline or basic and pH <7.35 is acidic
$PaCO_2$	4.6–6.0 kPa	The partial pressure of carbon dioxide is measured by the $PaCO_2$ and is a measure of ventilation or respiratory function
PaO_2	10.0–13.3 kPa	The PaO_2 measures the amount of oxygen carried by the blood.
HCO_3^-	22–26 mmol/L	The HCO_3^- is bicarbonate and measures the metabolic or renal part of the acid-base balance. The amount of HCO_3^- increases if the blood becomes too acidic.
Base excess/deficit	−2 to +2	A negative (deficit) base excess indicates a metabolic acidosis and a positive base excess a metabolic alkalosis or compensation.
O_2 saturation	>95%	The O_2 saturation is the percentage of haemoglobin saturated with O_2.

Source: Adapted from Keogh (2017), Pagana and Pagana (2017), Welch and Black (2017).

Table 13.7 Arterial blood gas abnormalities

Diagnosis	pH	$PaCO_2$	HCO_3^-
Acute respiratory acidosis	↓	↑	Normal
Acute respiratory alkalosis	↑	↓	Normal
Acute metabolic acidosis	↓	Normal or ↓	↓
Acute metabolic alkalosis	↑	Normal	↑
Compensated respiratory acidosis	Near normal	↑	↑
Compensated respiratory alkalosis	Normal	↓	↓
Compensated metabolic acidosis	Near normal	↓	↓
Compensated metabolic alkalosis	Near normal	↑	↑

Source: Adapted from Keogh (2017), Pagana and Pagana (2017), Welch and Black (2017).

- to assess the response to therapeutic interventions such as mechanical ventilation in a patient with respiratory failure
- to determine arterial respiratory gases during diagnostic evaluation (e.g. assessment of the need for home oxygen therapy in patients with advanced chronic pulmonary disease)
- to procure a blood sample in an acute emergency setting when venous sampling is not feasible (many blood chemistry tests can be performed from an arterial sample) (Danckers and Fried 2013, Keogh 2017, Pagana and Pagana 2017).

Contraindications

Absolute contraindications for ABG sampling include the following:

- an abnormal modified Allen test (Figure 13.7), in which case consideration should be given to attempting puncture at a different site
- local infection or distorted anatomy at the potential puncture site (e.g. from previous surgical interventions, congenital or acquired malformations, or burns)
- full-thickness burns
- Raynaud's syndrome
- the presence of arteriovenous fistulas or vascular grafts, in which case arterial vascular puncture should not be attempted
- known or suspected severe peripheral vascular disease of the limb involved.

Relative contraindications include the following:

- severe coagulopathy
- anticoagulation therapy with warfarin, heparin and derivatives, direct thrombin inhibitors or factor X inhibitors; aspirin is not a contraindication for arterial vascular sampling in most cases
- localized infection at the sampling site
- partial-thickness burns
- use of thrombolytic agents, such as streptokinase or tissue plasminogen activator (Danckers and Fried 2013, Keogh 2017, Pagana and Pagana 2017).

Arterial puncture

Arterial puncture may result in spasm, intraluminal clotting or bleeding, haematoma formation, or a transient obstruction of blood flow. These factors may decrease the arterial flow in distal tissues unless adequate collateral arterial vessels are available. Traditionally, palpation is the method used to locate the radial artery; however, Doppler ultrasound has also been used (Ueda et al. 2015). The radial artery at the wrist is the best site for obtaining an arterial sample because it is near the surface, is relatively easy to palpate and stabilize, and usually has good collateral supply from the ulnar arteries. This can be confirmed via a modified Allen test (Figure 13.7).

Multiple puncture attempts will increase the risk of patient discomfort, localized injury and haematoma, and delayed interventions, and

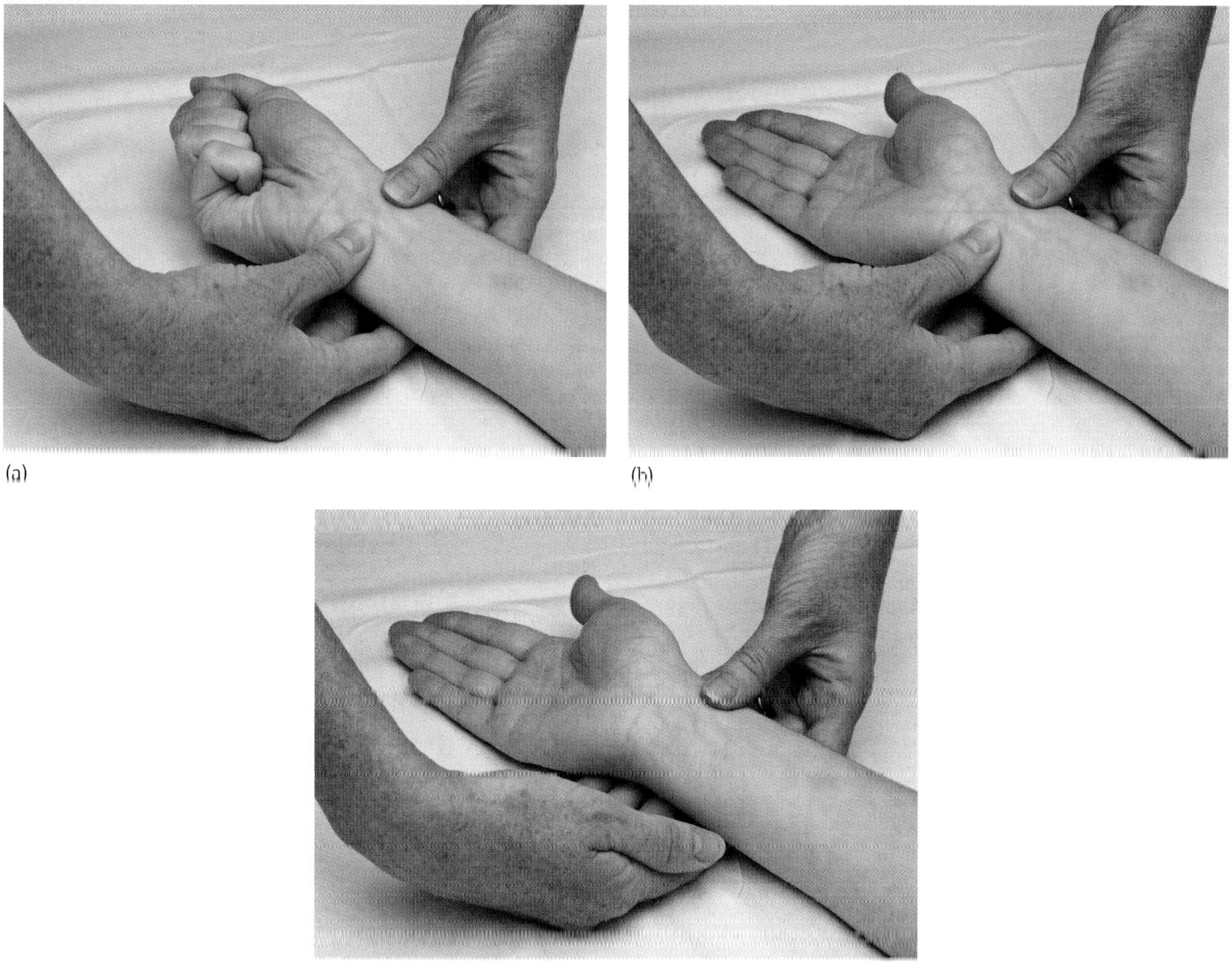

(a) (b) (c)

Figure 13.7 Modified Allen test. (a) Step 1: firmly compress the radial and ulnar arteries while the patient clenches their fist. (b) Step 2: ask the patient to open their hand, then release the arteries one at a time. (c) Step 3: the ulnar artery can be used for sampling if blood flow returns to the hand within 15 seconds of release of only the ulnar artery.

may also contribute to arterial spasm (Ueda et al. 2015). There are various factors that are associated with failed arterial puncture or cannulation and they include obesity, oedema, arterial scarring, hypotension and atherosclerosis (White et al. 2016). If the patient requires repetitive blood sampling, it may be more appropriate to admit them to a more clinically suitable area where intra-arterial cannulation is possible. This not only minimizes both the distress to the patient and the time taken by skilled personnel in obtaining each sample but also reduces the risks associated with multiple punctures (Brzezinski et al. 2009). It is worth noting that morbidity associated with arterial cannulation is less than that associated with five or more arterial punctures (Bersten et al. 2009; see also Chapter 17: Vascular access devices: insertion and management). Radial artery puncture and cannulation are relatively safe procedures with severe complications occurring rarely; however, there can be infections, thrombotic complications or mechanical complications in 1% of patients. Although the anatomy of the arteries in the forearm and hand is variable, adequate collateral flow in the event of radial artery thrombosis is present in most patients (Ueda et al. 2015, White et al. 2016).

Clinical governance

The practitioner must document their action in the patient's case notes and report the procedure, including assessment of the patient and any complications with the procedure itself. Any identified complications must be reported to a doctor as soon as practically possible. Practitioners are required to demonstrate knowledge of potential dangers and complications associated with the procedure. In addition, the practitioner must demonstrate knowledge of the signs and symptoms of associated complications, and be able to identify appropriate actions to safeguard the patient. Practitioners must undertake the role with due reference to the NMC *Code* (NMC 2018).

Competencies

Staff who undertake arterial puncture must be competent to do so. Each practitioner must be able to perform the relevant procedure in accordance with the trust policy or guidelines. Practitioners should not attempt arterial puncture more than twice on the same patient and must refer to a more experienced practitioner when practice limitations are recognized. See also Chapter 17: Vascular access devices: insertion and management.

Risk management

Sampling from arterial devices is risky and should only be done by competent, trained staff. Trusts should raise awareness of risks and review local guidelines. These should include criteria for requests for blood gas analyses, sampling technique, monitoring and interpretation of results (including unexpected results) (NPSA 2008a; see also Chapter 17: Vascular access devices: insertion and management).

Arterial infusion devices must be clearly identified. This means labelling or using specifically marked devices (O'Hare and Chilvers 2001, Osborne 2017). Any infusion (or additive) attached to an arterial device must be prescribed and checked before administration. Further checks should be made at regular intervals and key points (such as shift handover). Staff should use only sodium chloride 0.9% to keep devices open. Labels should clearly identify the contents of infusion bags, even when pressure bags are used (NPSA 2008a).

To minimize the risks, clinical staff should ask themselves the following questions (NPSA 2008a):

- Have I recorded the clinical reason for inserting this device?
- Is it clearly marked as an arterial device?
- Do I need to take this sample?
- Do I know how to do this safely (e.g. removing air from sample)?
- Have I picked the right infusion fluid bag? Did someone else check this?
- Can the label be seen, even if pressure bags are used?
- Is the reading from the sample within the expected range? Could it have been contaminated?

Pre-procedural considerations

Specific patient preparation

Ideally, prior to obtaining any ABG sample (Figure 13.8), the patient should be in a respiratory steady state for 15–20 minutes. The oxygen should not be reduced, and, if the patient is ventilated, suction should not be attempted and ventilation parameters should not be adjusted (Keogh 2017, Pagana and Pagana 2017). Arterial sampling and cannulation are associated with a considerable amount of pain due to adjacent nerves and the need for deeper puncture than venous sampling or cannulation. ABG sampling may be difficult to perform in patients who are unco-operative or in whom pulses cannot be easily identified (Danckers and Fried 2013).

Pain can be reduced by using local anaesthetic, which will also allow the healthcare professional to perform sampling without the patient moving their arm too much. In an emergency, there may be no time for local anaesthetic application. However, when it is feasible to wait for local anaesthetic to take effect before attempting arterial puncture, studies suggest higher success rates for arterial sampling (McSwain and Yeager 2015).

Despite its controversial value in predicting post-procedure ischaemia due to a radial arterial thrombosis, the modified Allen test (Figure 13.7) is still widely used and should be performed prior to accessing the radial artery to confirm patent collateral circulation to the hand. Adjuncts to the Allen test (e.g. pulse oximetry) have not been shown to increase the diagnostic power of the test (Pagana and Pagana 2017). The modified Allen test is performed by firmly compressing the radial and ulnar arteries while the patient clenches their

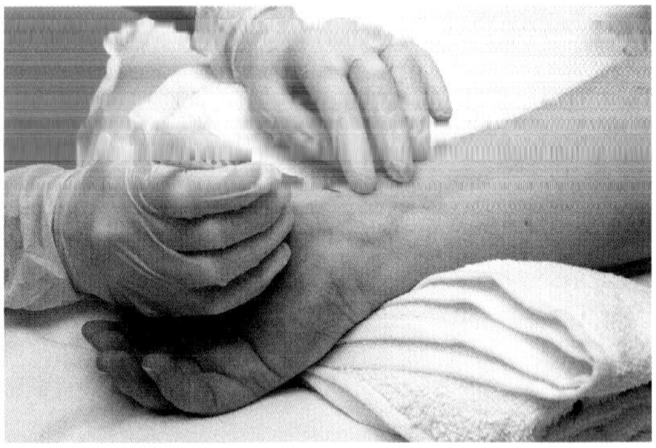

Figure 13.8 Arterial blood gas sampling.

fist (Step 1). The patient is then asked to open their hand (Step 2) and the arteries are released one at a time to check their ability to return blood flow to the hand, turning it pink or flushing again (Step 3) (Pagana and Pagana 2017). If blood flow to the hand returns within 15 seconds after release of only the ulnar artery (flushing), it is presumed the radial artery can be used for sampling. If after 15 seconds there is no blood flow returning to the hand (no flushing), the radial artery cannot be used (Pagana and Pagana 2017).

Where a sample is taken from an established arterial cannula, certain volumes of blood should be withdrawn and discarded. This is to ensure that any 0.9% sodium chloride, blood and small emboli from the dead space within the cannula and the three-way tap have been removed. Discarded volumes will vary according to arterial cannula placement due to the length of the arterial cannula:

- peripheral artery cannula: take 3 mL and discard
- femoral artery cannula: take 5 mL and discard (Danckers and Fried 2013).

When using a vacuum system, take one bottle and discard prior to obtaining requested samples.

ABG sampling may be difficult to perform in patients who are unco-operative or in whom pulses cannot be easily identified. Challenges arise when healthcare personnel are unable to position the patient properly for the procedure. This situation is commonly seen in patients with cognitive impairment, advanced degenerative joint disease or essential tremor. The amount of subcutaneous fat in overweight and obese patients may limit access to the vascular area and obscure anatomical landmarks. Arteriosclerosis of peripheral arteries, as seen in elderly patients and those with end-stage kidney disease, may cause increased rigidity in the vessel wall (Danckers and Fried 2013).

Procedure guideline 13.4 Arterial puncture: radial artery

Essential equipment

- Personal protective equipment
- Sterile dressing pack
- Trolley
- Clean tray or receiver
- Sterile adhesive plaster or hypoallergenic tape
- 2 mL syringe for local anaesthetic
- 20 swg needle for local infiltration
- 18 swg needle
- Sharps container
- Pre-heparinized ABG syringe (some syringes are vented or self-filling, whereas others require the user to draw back to fill – check manufacturer's instructions)
- 22 swg needle for sampling

Medicinal products

- 2% chlorhexidine in 70% alcohol
- Lidocaine 1%

Action	Rationale
Pre-procedure	
1 Introduce yourself to the patient, and explain and discuss the procedure with them. Obtain consent to proceed in all cases except in emergencies when the patient is unable to consent.	To ensure that the patient feels at ease, understands the procedure and gives their valid consent (NMC 2018, **C**). To minimize anxiety, which may distort analysis or exacerbate symptoms. **E** Consent may not be possible in certain clinical scenarios, such as where the patient is critically ill with rapid decompensation or has an altered level of consciousness (Danckers and Fried 2013, **E**).
2 Check the patient's identity and allergy status.	To ensure the procedure is undertaken with the correct patient and to minimize the risk of allergic reaction (NPSA 2007a, **C**; RCN 2017a, **C**).
3 Check the concentration of oxygen the patient is breathing and their body temperature at the time of sampling; document both on the sampling results.	Inspired oxygen concentration and temperature parameters are required to interpret arterial blood gases (ABGs) accurately (Adam et al. 2017, **E**).
4 Check the patient's current coagulation screen, platelet count, medical history and prescription chart for anticoagulation therapy.	To identify possible risk of bleeding and haematoma formation post procedure and, where appropriate, to prevent puncture until coagulation is corrected (Danckers and Fried 2013, **E**).
5 Prepare trolley and take to bedside.	To reduce the risk of cross-infection (DH 2010, **C**).
6 Wash hands with bactericidal soap and water or an alcohol-based handrub.	To reduce the risk of cross-infection (NHS England and NHSI 2019, **C**).
Procedure	
7 Assume a stable and comfortable position. If possible, sit down on a chair or stool near the patient.	To maximize the chance of successful sampling at the first attempt, thereby minimizing patient discomfort. To prevent back strain in the practitioner and minimize the risk of a needle stick injury. **E**
8 Inspect and assess the tissues and anatomical structures surrounding the intended sampling site.	To identify any areas of excoriation or infection, poor perfusion or other puncture sites. If any of these are present, the site should not be used (Pagana and Pagana 2017, **E**).
9 Locate and palpate the radial artery with the middle and index fingers of the non-dominant hand.	To assess maximum pulsation so as to ensure the radial artery is the optimum site for successful puncture. The dominant hand will be used to perform the puncture (Pagana and Pagana 2017, **E**; Weinstein and Plumer 2007, **E**).
10 Perform the modified Allen test (see Figure 13.7).	To confirm patency of ulnar artery circulation and adequate collateral circulation to the hand in the event of radial artery damage, for example thrombosis (Pagana and Pagana 2017, **E**).
11 Prepare the patient in a supine position: with forearm supinated at the wrist, gently extend the wrist at 40° over a rolled towel while avoiding overextension (ask for assistance if required) to bring the radial artery to a more superficial plane (Danckers and Fried 2013).	To reduce the risk of the patient moving unexpectedly, which could result in through-puncture (Hudson et al. 2006, **E**; Pagana and Pagana 2017, **E**). To flex the hand slightly to facilitate insertion. **E** Overextension of the wrist is discouraged, because interposition of flexor tendons may make the pulse difficult to detect (Danckers and Fried 2013, **E**).
12 Clean hands, open the pack and place the equipment onto it.	To ensure all equipment required is prepared. **E**
13 Withdraw the plunger of the ABG syringe 1–2 mL before the puncture. If using a vented sample syringe, withdraw fully.	To reduce blood haemolysis. Arterial pressure causes a brisk pulsatile reflux of blood into the syringe (unless the patient is severely hypotensive) (Weinstein and Plumer 2007, **E**).
14 Place a sterile field under the patient's wrist and maintain aseptic technique throughout the procedure.	To minimize the risk of infection (DH 2010, **C**).
15 Clean hands and then clean the site with chlorhexidine in 70% alcohol and allow to dry.	To minimize the risk of infection (DH 2010, **C**).
16 Prepare and administer subcutaneous local anaesthetic. Only inject 0.5–1 mL of the anaesthetic to create a small dermal papule at the site of puncture.	To minimize pain during the procedure. Local vasodilation effects of the local anaesthetic may reduce vasospasm, making for a successful puncture (Lipsitz 2004, **E**). Using larger amounts or injecting the anaesthetic into deeper planes may distort the anatomy and hinder identification of the vessel (Danckers and Fried 2013, **E**).
17 After the skin is punctured but just before the anaesthetic is injected, the clinician should pull back the plunger to confirm that the needle is not inside a blood vessel; intravascular placement will be indicated by blood filling up the anaesthetic syringe.	Injecting local anaesthetic directly intravascularly may cause cardiac arrhythmias (Danckers and Fried 2013, **E**).

(continued)

Procedure guideline 13.4 Arterial puncture: radial artery (continued)

Action	Rationale
18 Clean hands with bactericidal skin-cleaning solution or wash with soap and water.	To minimize the risk of infection (DH 2010, **C**).
19 Apply non-sterile gloves. Take care not to touch the puncture site after cleaning.	To minimize the risk of infection and prevent contamination of hands with blood (NHS England and NHSI 2019, **C**).
20 Uncap the ABG syringe, attach the 22 swg needle and hold it with two fingers of the dominant hand.	To guide the needle into position above the radial artery and aid successful puncture. **E**
21 Angle the needle at 30–45° for a radial artery, with the bevel of the needle up just distal to the planned puncture site. While palpating the radial pulse proximal to the planned puncture site, advance the needle slowly, aiming in the direction of the artery until a flashing pulsation is seen in the hub of the needle (see Figure 13.8).	To minimize trauma to the artery. **E** Rapid insertion may result in a through-puncture (Chernecky and Berger 2013, **E**). Take care not to touch the puncture site after cleaning, to minimize risk of infection (DH 2010, **C**; WHO 2010a, **C**). Pulsatile flow indicates access to radial artery. **E** Arterial pressure causes blood to pulsate spontaneously back into the syringe (Weinstein and Plumer 2007, **E**).
22 Slowly aspirate by gently pulling the plunger of the arterial gas syringe to a minimum of 0.6 mL of blood for the sample (check recommended amount of blood as directed by manufacturer's guidelines). If using a vented sample syringe, aspiration is not required as the syringe will fill automatically.	To minimize vasospasm. **E** To ensure the optimal volume is obtained in order to ensure an appropriate mix of blood with heparin (Chernecky and Berger 2013, **E**; see manufacturer's guidelines, **C**).
23 Withdraw the needle and immediately apply pressure using a low-linting swab.	To prevent haematoma formation and excessive bleeding. **E**
24 Discard the sharp into a sharps container. Promptly return the wrist to the neutral position following sampling.	To ensure correct clinical waste management and to reduce the risk of sharps injury (DH 2013, **C**). Prolonged hyperextension may be associated with changes in median nerve conduction (Chowet et al. 2004, **R**).
25 Apply pressure for a minimum of 5 minutes or until no signs of bleeding are observed. Ask for assistance from another nurse if necessary.	To minimize blood loss and to ensure pressure is exerted to prevent haematoma and blood loss (Pagana and Pagana 2017, **E**; RCN 2010, **C**).
Post-procedure	
26 Dispose of equipment safely.	To prevent contamination of others (DH 2013, **C**).
27 Expel any air bubbles from the syringe and cap the arterial syringe.	To keep the sample airtight and avoid inaccuracies (see manufacturer's guidelines, **C**).
28 Label the sample with the patient's name, number, date of birth, etc. at their bedside.	To prevent mislabelling when away from the patient. To maintain accurate records and provide accurate information for laboratory analysis (NMC 2018, **C**; Weston 2008, **E**).
29 Immediately send the sample to an area with ABG analysis machines, such as a laboratory, intensive care unit, high-dependency unit, theatre or A&E department.	ABG samples can be processed immediately and usually a result can be obtained within minutes. **E**
30 Check the puncture site and apply a clean, sterile, low-linting gauze dressing. Secure with tape.	To maintain pressure and prevent haematoma formation. **E**
31 Clearly document the rationale for the procedure in the patient's notes and verbally communicate the arterial analysis findings to relevant medical and nursing teams.	To acknowledge accountability for actions and ensure effective communication. To ensure prompt and appropriate treatment (NMC 2018, **C**).

Procedure guideline 13.5 Arterial blood gas sampling: arterial cannula

Essential equipment

- Personal protective equipment
- Sterile dressing pack
- 5 mL Luer-Lok syringe
- Sterile Luer-Lok cap
- 2% chlorhexidine in 70% alcohol
- Clean tray or receiver
- Trolley
- Pre-heparinized ABG syringe

Action	Rationale
Pre-procedure	
1 Introduce yourself to the patient, and explain and discuss the procedure with them. Obtain consent to proceed in all cases except in emergencies when the patient is unable to consent.	To ensure that the patient feels at ease, understands the procedure and gives their valid consent (NMC 2018, **C**).
2 Wash hands with bactericidal soap and water or an alcohol-based handrub.	To minimize the risk of cross-infection (NHS England and NHSI 2019, **C**).
3 Prepare trolley.	To minimize the risk of cross-infection (DH 2010, **C**).
4 Apply gloves and apron.	To prevent contamination of hands with blood (NHS England and NHSI 2019, **C**).
5 Check the three-way tap is closed to port (**Action figure 5**).	To prevent backflow of blood and blood spillage. **E**
6 If safe to do so, press the silence button on the arterial monitor for duration of sampling.	The continual alarm disturbs both the patient and others in the unit. Alarms of no clinical significance should be minimized. **E**
Procedure	
7 Remove the cap from the three-way tap and clean the port with a swab soaked in 2% chlorhexidine in 70% alcohol for 10 seconds and allow to dry.	To minimize the risk of infection (NHS England and NHSI 2019, **C**).
8 Attach a 5 mL Luer-Lok syringe.	To remove saline, old blood and small emboli from the dead space within the cannula (Danckers and Fried 2013, **E**).
9 Turn the three-way tap to the artery and port (**Action figure 9**).	To prevent contamination of blood with flush solution. **E**
10 Slowly withdraw 3–5 mL of blood.	To prevent the artery going into spasm and to withdraw the saline from the line to ensure the sample is fresh blood. **E**
11 Turn the three-way tap diagonally to close off both the artery and the flush (**Action figure 11**).	To enable the syringe to be removed without blood loss and to prevent saline from contaminating the sample. **E**
12 Remove the 5 mL syringe and discard.	To discard the contaminated sample. **E**
13 Connect the blood gas syringe to the three-port.	In order to withdraw the sample. **E**
14 Turn the three-way tap to the artery and port (**Action figure 9**).	To withdraw arterial blood. **E**
15 Slowly remove the recommended amount of blood (0.6–1 mL).	To prevent the artery going into spasm, ensuring the correct volume of blood mixes with the heparin in the gas syringe (Chernecky and Berger 2013, **E**; Lipsitz 2004, **R**).
16 Turn the three-way tap diagonally to close off both the artery and the flush (**Action figure 11**).	To prevent haemorrhage or blood spillage. **E**
17 Remove the gas syringe, gently rotating as you do so.	To ensure the blood and heparin contained within the syringe are mixed. **E**
Post-procedure	
18 Turn the three-way tap to the 'open to port' position; to flush the port, apply a sterile swab to the port and flush by squeezing the actuator (see manufacturer's instructions) (**Action figure 18**).	The swab will absorb the blood, preventing contamination. **E** Blood is cleared from the port, reducing the risk of thrombosis and microemboli. **E**
19 Turn the three-way tap to the 'open to artery' position and flush the cannula towards the artery by gently squeezing the actuator. As the cannula is flushed, observe the patient's digits for signs of blanching or discolouration, and listen for complaints of pain from the patient.	Blood is cleared from the cannula and arterial tubing. **E** To ensure early recognition of proximal or distal embolism. **E**
20 Clean the port with chlorhexidine in 70% alcohol swab and allow to dry.	To minimize the risk of infection (DH 2010, **C**).
21 Apply a new sterile Luer-Lok cap and check it is secure.	To minimize the risk of infection and prevent exsanguination. **E**
22 Remove gloves and wash hands.	To minimize the risk of infection (NHS England and NHSI 2019, **C**).
23 Check the pressure infuser cuff is inflated to 300 mmHg.	To prevent backflow of blood into the circuit. **E**
24 Analyse the sample or send it to the nearest blood gas analyser. Document the result and report abnormalities.	To obtain a result. **E** To ensure timely and accurate record keeping (NMC 2018, **C**; WHO 2015, **C**).

(continued)

Procedure guideline 13.5 Arterial blood gas sampling: arterial cannula *(continued)*

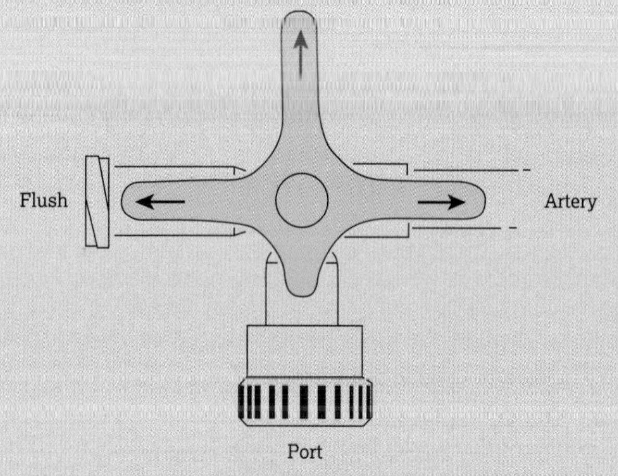

Action Figure 5 Three-way tap: closed to port.

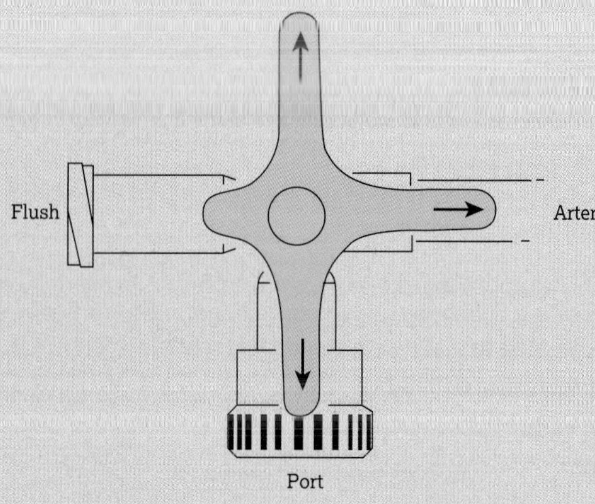

Action Figure 9 Three-way tap: turned to artery and port.

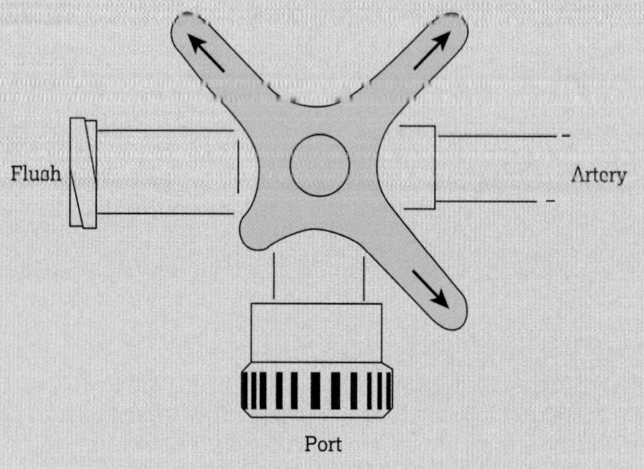

Action Figure 11 Three-way tap: turned diagonally to close off flush, artery and port.

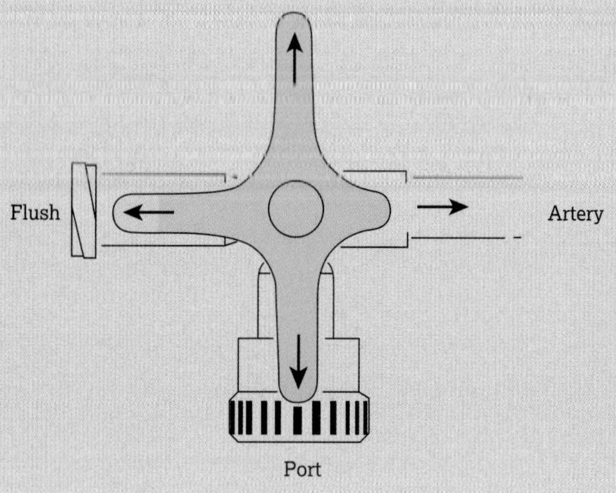

Action Figure 18 Three-way tap: turned to flush and port.

Equipment

Various types of blood gas syringe are available: some are pre-heparinized, whereas some are vented and self-fill on arterial blood sampling. If an intra-arterial cannula is inserted in a critical care environment then a sodium chloride 0.9% infusion is required to keep the cannula open (NPSA 2008a). If continuous arterial monitoring is done via a cannula, further equipment is required, including a transducer connected to a cardiac monitor and pressure bag set normally at 300 mmHg for arterial lines (Osborne 2017).

Post-procedural considerations

Monitoring and follow-up of the patient are essential. After the blood sampling procedure, nursing staff should monitor the patient for early and late signs and symptoms of potential complications. Active, profuse bleeding at the puncture site might raise suspicion of vessel laceration. Femoral artery bleeding carries an increased risk of circulatory compromise because of the large calibre and deep location of the vessel, which allow large amounts of blood to accumulate without initially giving rise to clinical findings (Chernecky and Berger 2013, Danckers and Fried 2013, Pagana and Pagana 2017).

A rapidly expanding haematoma may compromise regional circulation and increase the risk of compartment syndrome, especially in the forearm. This manifests as pain, paraesthesia, pallor and absence of pulses. Paresis and persistent pain may indicate a nerve lesion. Limb skin colour changes, absent pulses and distal coldness may be seen in ischaemic injury from artery occlusion caused by thrombus formation or vasospasm. Infection at the puncture site should be considered in the presence of regional erythema and fever (Chernecky and Berger 2013, Danckers and Fried 2013, Pagana and Pagana 2017).

Complications

Although patients with severe coagulopathy are at higher risk for bleeding complications, no clear evidence exists on the safety of arterial puncture in the setting of coagulopathy. In patients with coagulopathy, careful evaluation of the need for ABG sampling is recommended (Chernecky and Berger 2013, Danckers and Fried 2013, Pagana and Pagana 2017).

Complications of ABG sampling include the following:

- local haematoma
- artery vasospasm
- arterial occlusion
- air or thrombus embolism
- local anaesthetic anaphylactic reaction
- infection of the puncture site
- needle stick injury to healthcare personnel
- vessel laceration
- vasovagal response
- haemorrhage
- local pain (Chernecky and Berger 2013, Danckers and Fried 2013, Pagana and Pagana 2017).

Blood cultures

Definition

A blood culture is a specimen of blood obtained from a single venepuncture or central venous access device (CVAD) sample for the purpose of detecting blood-borne organisms (bacteria or fungi) and their associated infections (Lee et al. 2007, Pagana and Pagana 2017). Inoculation of an aerobic and an anaerobic sample of blood in two separate bottles comprises a set of blood cultures.

Related theory

Blood cultures are an essential part of the management of patients with serious blood-borne infections and are known as the gold standard investigation for such diseases (PHE 2018a), enabling the identification of the potential pathogens and antimicrobial susceptibility, and guiding treatment (Shore and Sandoe 2008). Bacteraemia (bacteria in the blood) and fungaemia (fungi in the blood) are associated with high morbidity and mortality among hospitalized patients, particularly those with compromised host defences (Panceri et al. 2004). The accurate and timely detection of the organism and susceptibilities has significant diagnostic and prognostic importance (PHE 2018a).

Micro-organisms may be present in the blood intermittently or continuously, depending upon the source of infection (PHE 2018a). In order to determine whether there is bacteraemia or fungemia, the bacteria or fungus must be 'grown' or 'cultured'. The blood sample needs to be inoculated into aerobic and anaerobic blood culture bottles and transported to the microbiology laboratory, where the blood culture bottles are incubated.

Most clinically significant bacteria are detected within the first 1 to 2 days of incubation. For fungi such as yeasts, it may take around 3 days. Blood culture bottles are usually incubated for up to 5 to 7 days before they are reported by the laboratory as having no growth. If there is evidence of bacterial growth, this will then be stained and examined under a microscope to carry out a gram stain (negative or positive) and to determine the morphology (shape – e.g. cocci or rods) before identifying the species and testing for antimicrobial drug susceptibility (Higgins 2013).

Evidence-based approaches

Rationale

Indications

There are many signs and symptoms in patients that may suggest bacteraemia, but clinical judgement is required. The following indicators should be taken into account when assessing a patient for signs of bacteraemia or sepsis, which would then indicate the need for blood culture sampling (HPA 2014a, Rhodes et al. 2017):

- altered mental state
- raised respiratory rate or new need for oxygen
- low blood pressure
- raised heart rate
- failure to pass urine (or less than 1 ml/kg of urine per hour for catheterized patients)
- core temperature out of normal range (>38°C or <36°C)
- changes in appearance of skin (mottled or ashen appearance; cyanosis of skin, lips or tongue; non-blanching rash of skin; signs of potential infection including redness, swelling or discharge at surgical site or breakdown of wound) (NICE 2017).

Coburn et al. (2012) suggest that an isolated fever or leucocytosis does not necessitate the collection of blood cultures, unless the patient is immunocompromised or endocarditis is suspected. Asai et al. (2012) recognize the limitations of blood culture sampling in terminally ill patients and do not recommend the routine use of this diagnostic tool for patients at the end of life. However, professional judgement will be required for each individual case.

Methods of blood culture specimen collection

In recognition of the importance of taking accurate blood cultures, there is now national guidance on procedure and policy to improve the quality of blood culture investigations and to reduce the risk of blood sample contamination (PHE 2018a). Contamination can come from a number of sources: the patient's skin, the equipment used to obtain the sample, the practitioner or the general environment (Murray and Masur 2012). Failure to use an aseptic technique or careful procedures when obtaining blood cultures can cause a false-positive result, which may lead to extensive diagnostic testing, excessive antibiotic use, prolonged hospitalization and artificially raised incidence rates (Rhodes et al. 2017).

Taking multiple blood cultures not only enhances the ability to detect bacteria but also helps to ascertain whether skin bacteria such as coagulase-negative staphylococci are clinically significant or contamination. Coagulase-negative staphylococci are frequent blood culture contaminants, but detection in a blood culture set from both the central line and the peripheral set increases the likelihood of it being a true pathogen. The initial samples should be obtained directly from a peripheral vein and not from existing peripheral cannulas or immediately above a cannula site, and the femoral vein should be avoided for venepuncture because it is difficult to ensure adequate skin cleansing and disinfection (DH 2010).

If the patient has an existing vascular access device (VAD) that has been *in situ* for more than 48 hours or is suspected to be a source of infection, a sample should also be taken from the device (Myers and Reyes 2011). Rhodes et al. (2017) suggest that, if feasible, a set of cultures should be taken from each lumen of the VAD.

It is suggested that the blood cultures should be taken when the temperature is rising or as soon as possible following a spike in temperature as this is when the serum concentration of the bacteria is at its highest (Higgins 2013). This is because organisms in the bloodstream elicit an immune response, causing symptoms such as fever and hypotension. However, in patients with a transient bacteraemia, organisms are immediately cleared from the blood by the immune system (Mahon et al. 2015). In such patients clinical symptoms, especially fever, may not occur until after the organisms are cleared from the bloodstream. Studies in the adult (Riedel et al. 2008) and paediatric (Kee et al. 2016) populations have shown that taking a blood culture when a patient spikes a temperature does not increase the sensitivity of the blood culture. In patients with a continuous bacteraemia (e.g. endocarditis), bacteria are constantly leaked into the blood vessels and are likely to grow from blood cultures taken at random times. The timing of taking blood cultures therefore is less important than the volume of blood taken (Miller et al. 2018).

Blood cultures should ideally be taken prior to commencing or changing antimicrobial therapy as antibiotics may delay or prevent bacterial growth, causing a falsely negative result (HPA 2014a). In accordance with the National Institute for Health and Care Excellence's sepsis guidelines (NICE 2017), antimicrobial therapy should be started within the first hour of recognition of severe sepsis and blood cultures should be taken before antimicrobial therapy is initiated. This is essential to confirm infection and the responsible pathogens while not causing significant delay in antibiotic administration (Rhodes et al. 2017). If antibiotic therapy has already been commenced, blood cultures should ideally be taken immediately prior to the next dose (DH 2010).

Clinical governance

Competencies

Blood cultures should be collected by practitioners who have been trained in the collection procedure and whose competence has been assessed (DH 2010). Practitioners must be competent and feel confident that they have the knowledge, skill and understanding to undertake blood culture sampling for microbiological analysis (NMC 2018).

Risk management

Contamination of a blood sample can lead to false positive results, which may in turn lead to inappropriate antibiotic therapy. This also has cost and resource implications (PHE 2018a). Contamination can be avoided by correctly decontaminating the patient's skin, ensuring adequate hand hygiene and decontaminating the bottle tops prior to obtaining a sample (Aziz 2011).

False-negative culture results can occur due to inadequate sample volumes, resulting in incorrect blood-to-media ratios and the administration of antimicrobials prior to taking the samples. False negatives result in present bacteria going undetected and therefore potentially being missed or untreated, which has clear consequences for the patient (PHE 2018a).

Pre-procedural considerations

Equipment

Most blood culture systems involve two collection bottles. Both bottles contain a particular medium that provides an optimal environment for bacterial growth. One bottle contains oxygen in the space above the medium for aerobic or oxygen-requiring bacteria and the other is suitable for anaerobic bacteria not requiring oxygen. The aerobic bottle should be filled first to avoid oxygen entering the anaerobic bottle (PHE 2018a).

The use of a needle to decant blood into the culture bottles is now largely redundant due to the wide use of closed, vacuumed blood collection systems (e.g. the Biomérieux BacT/ALERT system, which uses either a holder for venous access device sampling or a Luer adapter safety winged device for peripheral sampling) (see Figure 13.6). This reduces the health and safety risk to the healthcare professional and the risk of culture contamination. Needle-free or safety systems should be used where possible (HSE 2013).

Volume of blood culture specimen collection

The most important factor that determines the success of a blood culture is the volume of blood processed. A false-negative result could occur if an insufficient volume is introduced or if too much blood is introduced, due to the culture medium in the bottles being diluted (Higgins 2013). The liquid culture medium is a mixture of nutrients that supports microbial growth and inhibits phagocytosis and lysozyme activity (Shore and Sandoe 2008). This helps to determine whether there are pathogenic micro-organisms present in the blood. As there are a number of systems in use, the manufacturer's instructions should be followed as to the total volume required for each bottle. Adult patients with clinically significant bacteraemias often have a low number of colony-forming units per millilitre of blood and a minimum of 10 mL per culture bottle is recommended (Rhodes et al. 2017).

Pharmacological support

Skin preparation products

Poor aseptic technique and skin decontamination can cause contamination of a blood culture with the patient's own skin flora, such as coagulase-negative staphylococci (Weston 2008). A combination of 2% chlorhexidine gluconate in 70% isopropyl alcohol is recommended as being effective for skin antisepsis (DH 2010, Madeo and Barlow 2008, NHS England and NHSI 2019). Chlorhexidine gluconate maintains a persistent antimicrobial function by disrupting the cell membrane and precipitating the bacterial cell's contents, while the isopropyl alcohol quickly destroys micro-organisms by denaturing cell proteins (Inwood 2007). In order to achieve reduction and inhibition of the micro-organisms living on the skin, gentle friction is required for 30 seconds and the solution should be allowed to dry to achieve good skin antisepsis and to expose the cracks and fissures of the skin to the solution (NHS England and NHSI 2019). The top of each blood culture collection bottle should also be cleaned with 2% chlorhexidine gluconate in 70% isopropyl alcohol (DH 2010, Higgins 2013).

Infection related to central venous access devices (CVADs)

A CVAD presents a high risk of infection with an incidence of bacteraemia of between 4% and 8% (PHE 2018a). When it is suspected that the CVAD is the source of infection, a blood culture sample should ideally be obtained from each lumen of the vascular device as well as obtaining a peripherally drawn sample (DH 2010, Gabriel 2008, Rhodes et al. 2017). Adequate hub cleansing with 2% chlorhexidine in 70% isopropyl alcohol is essential in reducing cross-contamination of the sample (DH 2010).

Blood cultures from a CVAD can identify colonization from either the device itself or the bloodstream. To diagnose CVAD-related infections, comparison of the time it takes to achieve a positive result from both central and peripheral cultures is recommended (Catton et al. 2005). If a culture from the CVAD is positive much earlier than a culture from the peripheral culture (>2 hours earlier) then it can be assumed that the VAD is the source of the infection with up to 96% sensitivity and 92% specificity (Bouza et al. 2005). Results of such analyses can guide whether removal of the CVAD is indicated. Removal of the central venous catheter is indicated in cases of bacteraemia with a *Staphylococcus aureus* or *Pseudomonas aeruginosa* and fungemia.

Procedure guideline 13.6 Blood cultures: peripheral (winged device collection method)

Essential equipment

- Personal protective equipment
- Alcohol-based skin-cleaning preparation (2% chlorhexidine in 70% isopropyl alcohol)
- Two alcohol-based swabs for blood culture bottle decontamination (2% chlorhexidine in 70% isopropyl alcohol)
- A set of blood culture bottles (anaerobic and aerobic)
- Vacuum-assisted collection system (some include a winged device for peripheral cultures)
- Gauze swabs
- Appropriate document or form
- Clean tray or receiver
- Trolley

Action	Rationale
Pre-procedure	
1 Introduce yourself to the patient, explain and discuss the procedure with them, and gain their consent to proceed.	To ensure that the patient feels at ease, understands the procedure and gives their valid consent (NMC 2018, **C**).
2 Wash hands with bactericidal soap and water then dry, or decontaminate physically clean hands with alcohol-based handrub.	To reduce the risk of cross-infection and specimen contamination (NHS England and NHSI 2019, **C**).
3 Clean any visibly soiled skin on the patient with soap and water then dry.	To reduce the risk of contamination (DH 2010, **C**).
Procedure	
4 Apply a disposable tourniquet and palpate to identify vein. Release tourniquet.	To improve venous access and choose an appropriate vein (Witt 2011, **E**).
5 Clean skin with a 2% chlorhexidine in 70% isopropyl alcohol swab for 30 seconds and allow to dry for 30 seconds. Do not palpate site again after cleaning.	To enable adequate skin antisepsis and decontamination, and to prevent contamination from the practitioner's fingers (DH 2010, **C**; WHO 2010a, **C**).
6 Remove flip-off caps from culture bottles and clean with a second 2% chlorhexidine in 70% isopropyl alcohol swab and allow to dry.	To reduce the risk of environmental contamination causing false positive results (DH 2010, **C**).
7 Wash and dry hands again or use alcohol handrub and apply non-sterile gloves (sterile gloves are not essential).	To decontaminate hands having been in contact with the patient's skin to palpate vein and to prevent cross-infection. **E**
8 Attach winged blood collection set to the appropriate vacuum holder for taking blood cultures.	To reduce risk of contamination and health and safety risk to practitioner (DH 2010, **C**; WHO 2010a, **C**).
9 Reapply tourniquet.	To improve venous access. **E**
10 Remove sheath covering needle at wings and perform venepuncture.	To obtain blood samples. **E**
11 If blood is being taken for other tests, collect the blood culture first. Inoculate the aerobic culture first.	To reduce the risk of contamination of culture bottles after inoculating other blood bottles. **E**
12 Attach the aerobic bottle first, hold upright and use bottle graduation lines to accurately gauge sample volumes (at least 10 mL in each bottle or as recommended by manufacturer). Remove bottle and replace with anaerobic bottle, take same volume and remove bottle.	To ensure the anaerobic bottle does not become contaminated with oxygen from the sample (Myers and Reyes 2011, **E**).
13 Release tourniquet and remove winged device. Apply pressure to the venepuncture site.	To prevent bleeding at the site (de Verteuil 2011, **E**).
Post-procedure	
14 Activate safety feature and discard winged collection set in sharps container.	To reduce risk of sharps injury (HSE 2013, **C**).
15 Apply appropriate dressing.	To cover the puncture site after checking the patient has no allergy to the dressing (de Verteuil 2011, **E**).
16 Remove gloves, discard waste and wash or decontaminate hands.	To ensure correct clinical waste management and reduce risk of cross-infection (DH 2013, **C**).
17 Label bottles with appropriate patient details while in the presence of the patient, ensuring the bar codes on the bottles are not covered or removed.	To ensure that the specimens from the right patient are delivered to the laboratory, the requested tests are performed and the results are returned to the patient's records (NHSBT 2011, **C**; NHSBT 2012, **C**; NMC 2018, **C**; NPSA 2007a, **C**).
18 Complete microbiology request form (including relevant information such as indications, site and time of culture).	To maintain accurate records and provide accurate information for laboratory analysis (NMC 2018, **C**; Weston 2008, **E**; WHO 2015, **C**).
19 Arrange prompt delivery to the microbiology laboratory for immediate processing (or incubate at 37°C).	To increase the chance of accurate organism identification (Higgins 2013, **E**).
20 Document the procedure in the patient's records.	To ensure timely and accurate record keeping (NMC 2018, **C**).

Procedure guideline 13.7 Blood cultures: central venous access device

Essential equipment

- Personal protective equipment
- Alcohol-based skin-cleaning preparation (2% chlorhexidine in 70% isopropyl alcohol)
- Alcohol-based swab for blood culture bottle decontamination (2% chlorhexidine in 70% isopropyl alcohol)
- A set of blood culture bottles (anaerobic and aerobic)
- Vacuum-assisted collection system and tube holder for blood cultures
- Gauze swabs
- Microbiological request form
- 10 mL syringe
- 0.9% sodium chloride flushing solution as per hospital policy
- Clean tray or receiver
- Trolley

Action	Rationale
Pre-procedure	
1 Introduce yourself to the patient, explain and discuss the procedure with them, and gain their consent to proceed.	To ensure that the patient feels at ease, understands the procedure and gives their valid consent (NMC 2018, **C**).
2 Wash hands with bactericidal soap and water, or decontaminate physically clean hands with alcohol-based handrub. Apply gloves.	To reduce the risk of cross-infection and specimen contamination (DH 2010, **C**).
Procedure	
3 Prepare a cleaned trolley and sterile intravenous or dressing pack.	To ensure a clean and suitable workplace. **E**
4 Clean the end of each lumen with 2% chlorhexidine in 70% isopropyl alcohol swab and allow to dry for 15 seconds (if continuous life-sustaining infusions are running, this may not be possible from this lumen, so an alternative lumen must be used).	To enable adequate antisepsis and decontamination of each lumen (NHS England and NHSI 2019, **C**; Rhodes et al. 2017, **C**).
5 Remove flip-off caps from culture bottles and clean with a 2% chlorhexidine in 70% isopropyl alcohol swab and allow to dry.	To reduce the risk of environmental contamination causing false-positive results (DH 2010, **C**).
6 Using a 10 mL syringe, take and discard at least 10 mL of blood prior to attaching blood culture bottles.	To remove any 0.9% sodium chloride or other drug residue that may be present in the lumen (Danckers and Fried 2013, **E**).
7 If blood is being taken for other tests, collect the blood culture first. Inoculate the aerobic culture first.	To reduce the risk of contamination of culture bottles after inoculating other blood bottles. **E**
8 Attach adapter to holder and then attach vacuum-assisted collection system to hub of central venous access device (CVAD). Insert blood culture bottle and puncture septum.	To initiate vacuum collection. **E**
9 Attach aerobic bottle first, hold upright and use bottle graduation lines to accurately gauge sample volumes (at least 10 mL in each bottle or as recommended by manufacturer). Remove bottle and replace with anaerobic bottle.	To reduce the risk of a false-negative result due to insufficient volume or overdiluted culture medium (Higgins 2013, **E**).
10 Repeat steps 5–9 with each lumen if a multilumen device is *in situ*.	To accurately determine whether the CVAD is the source of infection (Rhodes et al. 2017, **C**).
11 Remove and discard the vacuumed collection holder in the sharps container.	To reduce risk of sharps injury and ensure correct waste management (DH 2013, **C**).
12 Flush with at least 10 mL 0.9% sodium chloride using the push–pause method (i.e. 1 mL at a time) and end with positive pressure.	To remove blood from the lumen and maintain patency (Dougherty 2008, **E**).
Post-procedure	
13 Remove and dispose of gloves and wash or decontaminate hands.	To ensure correct clinical waste management and reduce risk of cross-infection (DH 2013, **C**).
14 Label bottles with appropriate patient details, ensuring the bar codes on the bottles are not covered or removed.	To ensure correct patient and sample identity and to aid traceability within the laboratory. **E**
15 Complete microbiology request form (including relevant information such as indications, site and time of culture).	To maintain accurate records and provide accurate information for laboratory analysis (NMC 2018, **C**; Weston 2008, **E**).
16 Arrange prompt delivery to the microbiology laboratory for immediate processing (or incubate at 37°C).	To increase the chance of accurate organism identification (Higgins 2013, **E**)
17 Document the procedure in the patient's records.	To ensure timely and accurate record keeping (NMC 2018, **C**; WHO 2015, **C**).

Post-procedural considerations

Immediate care

Blood cultures should be dispatched to the laboratory for immediate processing. If cultures cannot be processed immediately, they should be incubated at 37°C in order for bacterial growth to begin and to prevent deterioration in pathogenic micro-organism yield (Higgins 2013).

Ongoing care

Decisions on commencing, changing or adding antimicrobial therapy may need to be considered depending upon the patient's condition and history. The increase in drug-resistant microorganisms has highlighted the need for prudent control of antibiotic prescribing and usage. It is estimated that up to 40% of patients with moderate-to-severe infections are given antibiotics that are unnecessary or inappropriate to treat the pathogen that is subsequently cultured *in vitro* (Johannes 2008).

The possibility of false results should also be considered before commencing any therapy. A false negative may be due to disproportionate blood volume to culture medium, inadequate incubation time and/or antibiotic administration prior to taking the sample. If the results are positive, the possibility of contamination should be considered, especially if the bacterium is one that commonly causes contamination (Higgins 2013). Occasionally a blood culture will provide a positive result for *Staphylococcus epidermidis*, which is normally present on the skin and therefore can contaminate the sample due to poor technique (Higgins 2013). Decisions regarding appropriate choice of empirical therapy as well as the duration and dosage should be made in conjunction with advice from the microbiology team (Tacconelli 2009).

Antimicrobial drug assay

Definition

Therapeutic drug monitoring of blood serum ensures that there are sufficient levels of particular antimicrobial drugs to be therapeutically effective while avoiding a potentially toxic excess that may lead to adverse effects (Thomson 2004, Walker and Whittlesea 2012).

Related theory

The majority of drugs used in clinical practice have a wide therapeutic window, meaning that quantitative analysis of serum levels is unnecessary. However, there are certain drugs that require monitoring of serum concentration levels due to their narrow therapeutic index where toxicity is associated with persistently high serum concentrations, while therapeutic failure can result from low concentrations (Egan et al. 2012, Thomson 2004).

Examples of drugs that need to be monitored in clinical practice include lithium, digoxin, theophylline, phenytoin, ciclosporin and certain antibiotics (Higgins 2013). This section focuses on aminoglycoside antibiotics, such as gentamicin and amikacin, and glycopeptide antibiotics, such as vancomycin, as these are the most commonly monitored via antimicrobial assays.

These drugs are excreted almost entirely by glomerular filtration and are potentially nephrotoxic and ototoxic:

- *Nephrotoxicity* involves the proximal tubules, which are capable of regeneration. Therefore, adverse effects may be reversible over time (Huth et al. 2011).
- *Ototoxicity* causes damage within the neuroepithelial cells of the inner ear, which can cause cochlear damage and/or vestibular impairment. These cells cannot be regenerated so the effects are irreversible (Huth et al. 2011). Ototoxicity occurs in 0.5–3% of patients and is usually associated with very high serum concentrations of the drugs (Pagkalis et al. 2011, Sha 2005).

When aminoglycosides or glycopeptides are used as single modes of treatment, rates of renal toxicity in patients are estimated to be 5–10%, although this can increase to as much as 30% if both are used synergistically (Pannu and Nadim 2008).

Aminoglycoside antibiotics

Aminoglycosides such as gentamicin and amikacin are antibiotics, which are mainly used against aerobic gram-negative bacteria. They can also be used synergistically with beta-lactam antibiotics against certain gram-positive organisms (Hammett-Stabler and Johns 1998). Traditional dosing follows standard 8-hour dosing regimens. Drug-level monitoring revolves around the determination of peak and trough drug concentrations. Subsequent changes to the doses, dose intervals or both are made with the aim of achieving a drug concentration within the accepted therapeutic range. The timing of serum sampling will be determined by the patient's clinical manifestations, particularly for renal function. For gentamicin, the trough level should be lower than 2 mg/L and that for amikacin should be <10 mg/L. The peak level for gentamicin should be 5–8 mg/L and that for amikacin should be 20–30 mg/L (Walker and Whittlesea 2012, Winter 2004).

Administering extended-interval dosing of aminoglycosides (high doses that are given less frequently) instead of traditional dosing has been found to be associated with fewer adverse events. The benefit of high doses results from their rapid 'concentration-dependent' action; the rate and extent of bacterial cell death are increased (Owens and Shorr 2009, Pagkalis et al. 2011). Extended-interval dosing also reduces the adaptive resistance of gram-negative bacilli to aminoglycosides and is known as the first exposure effect (Urban and Craig 1997). Even when the level of the drug falls below the minimum inhibitory concentration (MIC) of the organism, there is suppression of the regrowth of organisms that have been exposed to aminoglycosides; this is the post-antibiotic effect. Peak-level tests are not performed in extended interval dosing as such tests are designed to ensure a high peak level and a low trough level. Instead, a single drug-level test performed 6 to 14 hours after giving the dose is used to monitor therapy.

Glycopeptide antibiotics

Vancomycin is the glycopeptide antibiotic most widely used for the treatment of serious infections caused by gram-positive pathogens, such as those suspected to be meticillin resistant (Jones 2006). *In vitro* models suggest that vancomycin exhibits time-dependent effects on *Staphylococcus aureus* and coagulase-negative staphylococci. This means the effectiveness of vancomycin increases the longer the antibiotic serum concentration is above the MIC of susceptible pathogens (Lowdin et al. 1998). However, a study of 108 patients with *S. aureus* lower respiratory tract infections demonstrated highly significant associations between clinical cure and an AUC/MIC (area under the curve/minimum inhibitory concentration) over 400 and between bacteriological cure and an AUC/MIC over 850 (Moise-Broder et al. 2004). This suggests that there is time-dependent killing and that there are moderate to prolonged persistent effects, and that it is the amount of drug received that determines the ideal dosing regime.

The use and monitoring of vancomycin have increased due to the emergence of meticillin-resistant *S. aureus* (MRSA). However, the emergence of vancomycin-resistant *S. aureus* has further complicated this drug's clinical use (Roberts et al. 2011).

How often serum blood levels of vancomycin are determined depends on the frequency of administration. If it is given as an intermittent infusion (usually twice-daily doses), trough levels should be taken at set times, immediately before the administration of the next bolus dose (Jones 2006). The trough level should be between 10 and 20 mg/L (Rybak et al. 2009).

An alternative method of administration is the continuous infusion of vancomycin. This is as effective as intermittent administration and is associated with reduced nephrotoxicity (Cataldo et al. 2012). Continuous infusions aim to maintain serum concentrations at between 15 and 25 mg/L.

Evidence-based approaches

Rationale

The main criterion for monitoring serum drug concentration is to ensure that there is enough drug given for efficacy while avoiding concentrations associated with a significant risk of toxicity (Roberts et al. 2011).

Indications

Accurate and timely monitoring of antimicrobial assay levels is indicated in patients receiving intravenous aminoglycoside or glycopeptide antibiotics to ensure optimum therapeutic range and to minimize high serum levels, which may cause adverse side-effects of the drugs (particular caution should be exercised in patients who have renal impairment) (Roberts et al. 2011).

Contraindications

The samples should not be taken if there has been an insufficient time lapse since dose administration.

Principles of care

The initial dosage regimen should be appropriate for the clinical condition being treated, the patient's clinical characteristics (age, weight, renal function, etc.) and any concomitant drug therapy (Thomson 2004). The timing of the sample and interpretation of the results of analysis need consideration in relation to the dose given and the timing of previous dose administration.

Serum samples can be taken at two different times: the peak or the trough. A peak sample is collected at the drug's highest therapeutic concentration within the dosing period. The peak-level timing will vary depending on the drug; ordinarily this is 1 hour after the completion of an infusion of aminoglycoside (Tobin et al. 2002, Walker and Whittlesea 2012). The trough level can be taken 18–24 hours after the last dose.

Vancomycin trough levels are measured just prior to the administration of the next dose – that is, at the lowest concentration in the dosing period (Tobin et al. 2002). Therefore, trough levels are more commonly used than peak levels because the level is more representative of how the different variables (such as drug absorption and renal function) affect the concentration within a predetermined timeframe. The results can then be used to adjust dosages to achieve the optimal response with the minimal toxicity.

Abnormally elevated serum levels may be obtained if the samples are taken from a CVAD through which the drug has been administered. This is more likely when residual drugs remain in the catheter if it has not been flushed correctly following administration of the drug or when the first 5 to 10 mL of blood are not discarded (Himberger and Himberger 2001). If a multilumen CVAD is *in situ*, a different lumen from the one used to administer the drug should be used to obtain the blood specimen.

Procedure guideline 13.8 Blood sampling: antimicrobial drug assay

Essential equipment

- Personal protective equipment
- Sterile pack
- Appropriate blood sample bottles
- Vacuum-assisted blood collection system
- Clean tray or receiver
- Appropriate documentation/forms

Action	Rationale
Pre-procedure	
1 Introduce yourself to the patient, explain and discuss the procedure with them, and gain their consent to proceed.	To ensure that the patient feels at ease, understands the procedure and gives their valid consent (NMC 2018, **C**).
2 Wash hands with bactericidal soap and water, or decontaminate physically clean hands with alcohol-based handrub. Apply gloves.	To reduce the risk of cross-infection and specimen contamination (Fraise and Bradley 2009, **E**).
3 Establish whether a trough, random or peak drug level is required. Then: • If trough, take sample immediately prior to next due dose. • If peak, the timing is drug dependent; discuss with the prescriber or pharmacist. • If random, take sample when convenient.	To ensure the correct test is undertaken.
Procedure	
4 *If venepuncture is required to obtain the sample*: following venepuncture (see Procedure guideline 13.1: Venepuncture), withdraw the volume of blood appropriate to the blood sample bottle using the vacuum-assisted collection system.	To ensure the correct volume of blood is obtained and to reduce the safety risk to the practitioner (DH 2010, 2013, **C**).
5 *If a CVAD is available from which to obtain the sample*: follow Procedure guideline 13.2: Central venous access devices: taking a blood sample for vacuum sampling or 13.3: Central venous access devices: taking a blood sample for syringe sampling, remembering the following: • The device must be flushed thoroughly before taking the blood sample. • Take and discard enough blood to clear the device of any residual flush solution or medications (usually 5–10 mL is sufficient), then attach the vacuum-assisted collection system to take the drug-level sample. • Indicate on the blood sample bottle and appropriate form that the sample is from a CVAD.	To reduce contamination by previously administered therapeutic agents and to allow appropriate interpretation of the results (NPSA 2007b, **C**; RCN 2010, **C**).

6 Clearly label the blood sample bottle and appropriate form with request details (trough, peak or random) and note the time of the last administered dose.	To ensure there is no confusion between the peak and trough drug serum level specimens (WHO 2015, **C**).
Post-procedure	
7 Ensure microbiology or biochemistry request forms are completed correctly, including date, exact time and dosage of previously administered dose.	To maintain accurate records and provide accurate information for laboratory analysis (NMC 2018, **C**; Weston 2008, **E**).
8 Arrange prompt delivery to pathology.	To allow for prompt analysis and timely adjustments to patient's drug therapy regimen if indicated. **E**
9 Document the procedure in the patient's records.	To ensure timely and accurate record keeping (NMC 2018, **C**; WHO 2015, **C**).

Post-procedural considerations

Ongoing care

Changes in dosage regimens will depend upon interpretation of the results by the microbiology, pharmacy, medical and nursing teams. A low drug serum level would instigate an increase in the dosage of the drug (Roberts et al. 2011). A high drug serum level would potentially instigate omitting the subsequent dose, and adjusting the dose and/or time interval. Any changes to the drug regimen should be clearly documented on the patient's prescription.

Documentation

In accordance with the principles of good record keeping, the date and time when a trough and/or peak drug assay level is sent to the laboratory should be documented clearly and promptly in the patient's notes, care plan and/or drug chart (or antimicrobial flow charts as provided by the pharmacy department) (NMC 2018, WHO 2015). This assists in communication and the dissemination of information between members of the inter-professional healthcare team.

Cerebrospinal fluid obtained by lumbar puncture

Definition

Lumbar puncture is a technique used to sample cerebrospinal fluid (CSF). It involves inserting a hollow spinal needle into the lumbar subarachnoid space and is a technique first described by Quincke (1891). It may be used for either diagnostic or therapeutic procedures (Doherty and Forbes 2014, Engelborghs et al. 2017, Pagana and Pagana 2017).

Anatomy and physiology

The spinal cord lies within the spinal column, extending from the medulla oblongata to the level of the second lumbar vertebra. The adult spinal cord is 2 cm wide at the midthoracic region and 42–45 cm long (Figure 13.9). Like the brain, the spinal cord is enclosed and protected by the meninges – that is, the dura mater, arachnoid mater and pia mater. The dura and arachnoid mater are separated by a potential space known as the subdural space. The arachnoid mater and pia mater are separated by the subarachnoid space, where the CSF continually circulates. Below the termination of the spinal cord, the subarachnoid space contains CSF, the filum terminale and the cauda equina (the anterior and posterior roots of the lumbar and sacral nerves) (Doherty and Forbes 2014, Pagana and Pagana 2017, Tortora and Derrickson 2017). So as to avoid damage to the spinal cord, it is imperative that lumbar puncture is performed at the lowest palpable intervertebral space (Figure 13.10). The higher the space, the greater the risk of spinal cord injury.

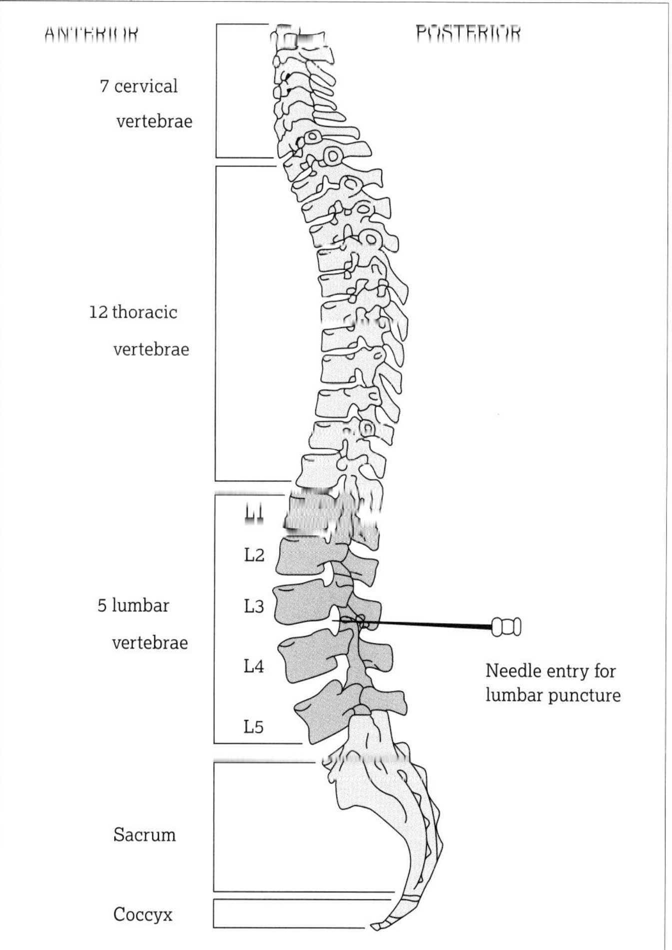

Figure 13.9 Lateral view of the spinal column and vertebrae, showing the needle entry site for a lumbar puncture.

The spinal needle has to pass through the following structures: skin, subcutaneous tissue, supraspinal ligament, interspinous ligament, ligamentum flavum, epidural space, dura mater and arachnoid mater.

CSF is formed primarily by filtration and secretion from networks of capillaries, called choroid plexuses, located in the ventricles of the brain. Eventually, absorption takes place through the arachnoid villi, which are finger-like projections of the arachnoid mater that push into the dural venous sinuses. CSF is a clear, colourless liquid with various functions and properties. In an adult, the total volume of CSF

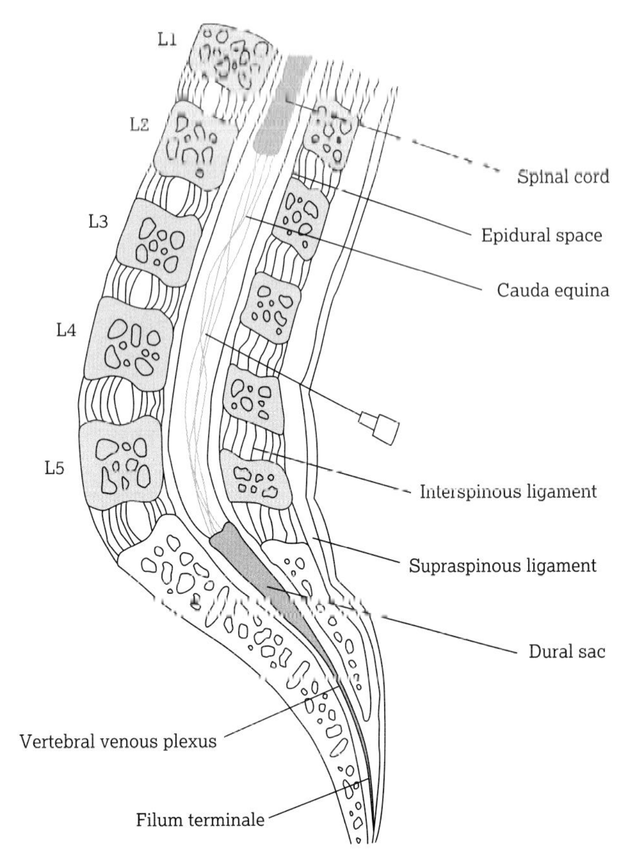

Figure 13.10 Lumbar puncture. Sagittal section through the lumbosacral spine. The most common sites for lumbar puncture are between L3 and L4 and between L4 and L5 as the spinal cord terminates at L1.

is 80–150 mL; it is reabsorbed at a rate of 20 mL/hour or 480 mL/day (Tortora and Derrickson 2017). CSF's constituents include:

- mineral salts
- glucose
- lactic acid
- protein (16–45 mg/dL)
- urea
- cations (Na^+, K^+, Ca^{2+}, Mg^{2+})
- anions (Cl^-, HCO_3^-)
- white blood cells (Tortora and Derrickson 2017).

There are three basic functions of CSF:

- *Mechanical protection*: acts as a shock absorber and buoys the brain, enabling it to 'float' in the cranial cavity.
- *Chemical protection*: ensures an optimal chemical and ionic environment.
- *Circulation*: enables the exchange of nutrients and waste products between adjacent nervous tissue and blood (Tortora and Derrickson 2017).

Related theory

Abnormalities of cerebrospinal fluid

Blood

Red discolouration of the CSF is indicative of the presence of blood. If the presence of blood is caused by a traumatic spinal tap, the blood will usually clot and the fluid will clear as the procedure continues. If the presence of blood is due to subarachnoid haemorrhage, no clotting will occur (Lindsay et al. 2010, Pagana and Pagana 2017).

Colour

Hyperbilirubinaemia, hypercarotenaemia, melanoma and elevated protein levels can each cause a change in the colour of the CSF. A cloudy CSF is indicative of the presence of a large number of white cells or protein.

Cells

The presence of different types of blood cells in the CSF can be diagnostic of a variety of neurological disorders:

- Erythrocytes are indicative of haemorrhage.
- Neutrophils (polymorphonuclear leukocytes) are indicative of bacterial meningitis, a cerebral abscess.
- Neutrophils (mononuclear leukocytes) are indicative of viral or tubercular meningitis or encephalitis.
- Monocytes are indicative of a viral or tubercular meningitis or encephalitis.
- Lymphocytes present in larger numbers are indicative of viral, tubercular, fungal or syphilitic meningitis or infiltration of the meninges by malignant disease.
- The presence of leukaemic blast cells is indicative of infiltration of the meninges by leukaemia.
- Viral, bacterial and fungal cultures from the CSF sample are indicative of infection (Barker and Laia 2008, Pagana and Pagana 2017)

Pressure

Normal CSF pressure falls within a range of 10–15 cmH_2O (Lindsay et al. 2010). Spinal pressure may be raised in the presence of cerebrovascular accident, a space-occupying lesion or bacterial meningitis (Barker and Laia 2008, Pagana and Pagana 2017).

Evidence-based approaches

Rationale

A number of tests can be performed on CSF to aid diagnosis (Tortora and Derrickson 2017):

- *Culture and sensitivity*: identifying the presence of micro-organisms confirms the diagnosis of bacterial or fungal meningitis or a cerebral abscess. Organisms may include atypical bacteria, *Mycobacterium tuberculosis* or fungi. The isolation of the causative organism enables the initiation of appropriate antibiotic or antifungal therapy (Pagana and Pagana 2017).
- *Virology screening*: isolation of a causative virus enables appropriate therapy to be initiated promptly.
- *Serology for syphilis*: tests include the Wassermann Reaction (WR), Venereal Disease Research Laboratory (VDRL) and *Treponema pallidum* Immobilization (TPI) tests.
- *Cytology*: central nervous system tumours and secondary meningeal disease tend to shed cells into the CSF, where they float freely. Examination of these cells morphologically after lumbar puncture determines whether the tumour is malignant or benign (Pagana and Pagana 2017).

Indications

A lumbar puncture and withdrawal of CSF, with or without the introduction of therapeutic agents, is performed for the following purposes:

- It can be used to exclude subarachnoid haemorrhage.
- It can be used to investigate neurological disorders such as multiple sclerosis and to exclude or investigate meningitis (Doherty and Forbes 2014, Pagana and Pagana 2017).
- It can be used to manage disorders of intracranial pressure (ICP) such as spontaneous intracranial hypotension and idiopathic intracranial hypertension (Doherty and Forbes 2014, Lee and Lueck 2014).
- It can be used to administer therapeutic and diagnostic agents. A number of drugs do not cross the blood–brain barrier, so in the treatment and prophylaxis of some malignant diseases (such as leukaemia and lymphoma) a lumbar puncture is used to insert the drugs. Cytarabine, methotrexate and corticosteroids are the drugs most commonly administered intrathecally. Other drugs

include intrathecal antibiotics to treat infection, radiopaque contrast to provide myelograms of the spinal cord and the administration of a local anaesthetic agent (such as bupivacaine) into the CSF to enable lower body surgery and/or to provide pain relief (Bottros and Christo 2014, Doherty and Forbes 2014, Gilbar 2014, Tortora and Derrickson 2017).

Contraindications

The procedure should not be undertaken in the following circumstances:

- In patients in whom raised ICP is suspected or present due to the risk of brain herniation (Lindsay et al. 2010, Pagana and Pagana 2017).
- In patients with papilloedema, bacterial meningitis or deteriorating neurological symptoms in whom raised ICP or an intracranial mass is suspected. In this situation, neuroimaging (CT or MRI scan) should be undertaken prior to lumbar puncture in order to avoid resultant potentially fatal brainstem compression, herniation or coning (Engelborghs et al. 2017). However, a normal CT scan does not always ensure that it is safe to perform a lumbar puncture so, until better non-invasive procedures to monitor ICP become available and are routinely used, the decision to proceed must be left to clinical expertise and judgement (Engelborghs et al. 2017).
- Local skin infection may result in meningitis by passage of the bacteria from the skin to the CSF during the procedure. Cutaneous or osseous infection at the site of the lumbar puncture may be considered an absolute contraindication (Chernecky and Berger 2013, Pagana and Pagana 2017).
- In patients who are unable to co-operate or who are too drowsy to give a history. Patient co-operation is essential to carry out a baseline neurological examination and to minimize the potential risk of trauma associated with this procedure (Chernecky and Berger 2013, Pagana and Pagana 2017).
- In patients who have severe degenerative spinal joint disease. In such cases, difficulty will be experienced both in positioning the patient and in accessing the spaces between the vertebrae (Chernecky and Berger 2013, Pagana and Pagana 2017).
- In those patients undergoing anticoagulant therapy or who have coagulopathies or thrombocytopenia (less than 50×10^9/L). These patients are at increased risk of bleeding and therefore coagulopathies and thrombocytopenia must be corrected prior to undertaking lumbar puncture (Lindsay et al. 2010, Pagana and Pagana 2017).

Principles of care

The principles of lumbar puncture are to gain access to the CSF of the patient while maintaining sterility and patient comfort throughout the procedure. For patients receiving intrathecal medication, it is essential that the correct agent is given. For diagnostic procedures, it is imperative that accurate measurements are taken and that the sample is handled and labelled correctly. The role of the nurse in caring for a patient undergoing a lumbar puncture procedure may include helping to explain the procedure to the patient, preparing the patient, supporting both the patient and the doctor or practitioner during the procedure, and close follow-up monitoring (Doherty and Forbes 2014, Pagana and Pagana 2017).

Clinical governance

Competencies

If a lumbar puncture is being undertaken to administer medication (e.g. for intrathecal chemotherapy administration), the practitioner performing the procedure must comply with the national guidance (DH 2008). Organizations must ensure that only appropriately trained staff are conducting lumbar punctures.

Risk management

In order to minimize risk to patients, the equipment used in the procedure was modified by the manufacturers to reduce the risk of incorrect drug administration and/or technique (DH 2012, NPSA 2011). Wrong route administration of intravenous or other chemotherapy into the intrathecal space is a Department of Health 'Never Event' and is therefore considered unacceptable and eminently preventable (DH 2012). All needles, syringes and connectors utilized in intrathecal (spinal) boluses or lumbar puncture samples must not be able to connect to any other intravenous device. This must also include any epidural, spinal and regional anaesthesia boluses or infusions (NPSA 2011).

Pre-procedural considerations

Equipment

Enhancements to the design of lumbar puncture needles can confer benefits to patients in terms of reducing complications and can also contribute to reducing drug errors. The newer 'non-cutting' needles, such as the Sprotte and Whitacre types, cause fewer post-lumbar puncture headaches (PLPHs) than the older 'cutting' needles, such as the Quincke type (Doherty and Forbes 2014, Engelborghs et al. 2017). This is because the vertically aligned dural fibres are split and parted instead of being cut, thus allowing some degree of dural self-sealing. In the same manner, thinner-gauge needles create less of a CSF leak and further reduce the occurrence of PLPHs (Engelborghs et al. 2017, NPSA 2011). It is important to be aware of alerts in relation to equipment problems, such as an incorrect needle size supplied in certain packs (MHRA 2013).

Assessment and recording tools

Depending on the patient's condition and the reason for the lumbar puncture, various observations and recording tools should be used. As a baseline, the patient's vital signs must be recorded before and after the procedure and documented on an observation chart. If the patient is being investigated for a neurological problem, then the inclusion of pre-procedural Glasgow Coma Scale (GCS) assessment is advised. In all cases, neurological observations, including GCS and pupillary response, should be recorded on a neurological observation chart following the procedure. The patient should be monitored for headache and backache and the puncture site should be inspected, particularly if there have been fluctuations in the neurological observations (Chernecky and Berger 2013, Doherty and Forbes 2014, Pagana and Pagana 2017).

Specific patient preparation

Preparation includes advising the patient to empty their bowels and bladder to ensure comfort during the correct flexed (knee-to-chest) position that the patient must assume during the procedure. This position is required to increase the space between adjacent vertebral spines to allow for the passage of the needle (Chernecky and Berger 2013, Doherty and Forbes 2014, Lindsay et al. 2010, Pagana and Pagana 2017).

Skin disinfection is of extreme importance to prevent serious spinal infection. A chlorhexidine or equivalent antiseptic is the most effective solution in this regard, but it must be allowed to air dry completely to prevent the neurotoxic chlorhexidine from coming into contact with neural tissue (Doherty and Forbes 2014).

Post-procedural considerations

Immediate care

Patients will usually be nursed flat for a period of up to 4 hours in order to reduce the risk of post-spinal headache. There is no evidence that longer periods are useful (Doherty and Forbes 2014). Follow-up care will include neurological observations, monitoring for issues such as difficulties with voiding, raised temperature, headache and discomfort. Analgesia and reassurance may be required (Chernecky and Berger 2013, Pagana and Pagana 2017).

Ongoing care

If the procedure has been performed in an outpatient setting, the patient may be discharged home after 1–2 hours but with clear instructions to lie flat in transport and at home, and to report any of the following: leakage from the site, headaches, backaches and neurological symptoms. Backache with leg weakness and bladder disturbance may be caused by a spinal haematoma (cauda equina syndrome) and is (usually) a surgical emergency (Chernecky and Berger 2013, Doherty and Forbes 2014, Pikis et al. 2013).

Procedure guideline 13.9 Lumbar puncture

Essential equipment

- Personal protective equipment
- Antiseptic skin-cleaning agents, for example chlorhexidine in 70% alcohol or isopropyl alcohol
- Selection of needles and syringes
- Sterile gloves
- Sterile dressing pack
- Lumbar puncture needles of assorted sizes
- Disposable manometer
- Three sterile specimen bottles; these should be labelled 1, 2 and 3
- Plaster dressing

Medicinal products

- Local anaesthetic, for example lidocaine 1%

Action	Rationale
Pre-procedure	
1 Introduce yourself to the patient, explain and discuss the procedure with them, and gain their consent to proceed.	To ensure that the patient feels at ease, understands the procedure and gives their valid consent (NMC 2018, **C**).
2 Patient should empty their bladder and bowels before the procedure.	To ensure comfort (Doherty and Forbes 2014, **E**; Pagana and Pagana 2017, **E**).
3 Assist patient into the required position on a firm surface. *Either lying* (**Action figure 3**): • one pillow under the patient's head • on side with knees drawn up to the abdomen and clasped by the hands • support patient to maintain this position.	To ensure maximum widening of the intervertebral spaces and thus easier access to the subarachnoid space (Lindsay et al. 2010, **E**). To avoid sudden movement by the patient, which would produce trauma (Barker and Laia 2008, **E**).
Or sitting: • patient straddles a straight-backed chair so that their back is facing the doctor • patient folds arms on the back of the chair and rests head on them.	Either sitting or lying may be used, depending on what the patient can tolerate. The sitting position allows more accurate identification of the spinous processes and thus the intervertebral spaces (Barker and Laia 2008, **E**; Doherty and Forbes 2014, **E**).
4 Continue to support and observe the patient throughout the procedure, and explain the procedure.	To facilitate psychological and physical wellbeing (Barker and Laia 2008, **E**).
Procedure	
5 Wash hands with antibacterial detergent. Put on gloves and apron.	To reduce the risk of contamination and cross-infection (Fraise and Bradley 2009, **E**).
6 Assist doctor/practitioner as required; doctor/practitioner will proceed to put on a hat and mask, clean hands with antiseptic solution, and put on a sterile apron and gloves.	To minimize the risk of cross-contamination (Gemmell et al. 2008, **E**).
7 Clean the skin with the antiseptic cleaning agent.	To ensure the removal of skin flora to minimize the risk of infection (Lindsay et al. 2010, **E**).
8 Identify the area to be punctured and infiltrate the skin and subcutaneous layers with local anaesthetic.	To minimize discomfort from the procedure (Barker and Laia 2008, **E**).
9 Introduce a spinal puncture needle below the second lumbar vertebra and into the subarachnoid space.	This is below the level of the spinal cord but still within the subarachnoid space (Lindsay et al. 2010, **E**).
10 Ensure that the subarachnoid space has been entered and attach the manometer to the spinal needle, if required.	To obtain a cerebrospinal fluid (CSF) pressure reading (normal pressure is 10–15 cmH_2O). This can only be measured if the patient is in a lateral position (Doherty and Forbes 2014, **E**; Lindsay et al. 2010, **E**).
11 Obtain the appropriate specimens of CSF (approx. 10 mL) for analysis. Cell count and gram stain can be performed using 1 mL of fluid.	To establish a diagnosis (Pagana and Pagana 2017, **E**). The first specimen, which may be blood-stained due to needle trauma, should go into bottle 1. This will assist the laboratory to differentiate between blood due to procedure trauma and blood due to subarachnoid haemorrhage (Chernecky and Berger 2013, **E**).
12 Ensure the specimens are labelled appropriately (as 1, 2 and 3) and sent with the correct forms to the laboratory.	To maintain accurate records and provide accurate information for laboratory analysis (NMC 2018, **C**; Weston 2008, **E**).
13 If intrathecal medication is to be instilled, the drug and dose must be checked and administered safely according to national guidelines.	To ensure the correct drug and dosage of drug are safely administered (Coward and Cooley 2006, **E**; DH 2008, **C**).

14 Withdraw the spinal needle once specimens have been obtained, appropriate pressure measurements have been taken and intrathecal medication has been administered.	To minimize the risks of the procedure (Barker and Laia 2008, **E**).
15 When the needle has been withdrawn, apply pressure over the lumbar puncture site using a sterile topical swab.	To maintain asepsis and to stop blood and CSF flow (Doherty and Forbes 2014, **E**).
16 When all leakage from the puncture site has ceased, apply a plaster dressing.	To prevent secondary infection (Barker and Laia 2008, **E**).

Post-procedure

17 Make the patient comfortable. They should lie flat or the head should be tilted slightly downwards. Time to lie flat varies from hospital to hospital, but it is usually around 4 hours if there is no headache.	To avoid headache and decrease the possibility of brainstem herniation (coning) due to a reduction in CSF pressure (Barker and Laia 2008, **E**; Doherty and Forbes 2014, **E**).
18 Remove equipment and dispose of it as appropriate.	To prevent the spread of infection and reduce the risk of needle stick injury (DH 2013, **C**).
19 Document the procedure in the patient's records.	To ensure timely and accurate record keeping (NMC 2018, **C**).
20 Patient should be monitored for the next 24 hours with careful observation of the following: • leakage from the puncture site • headache • backache • neurological observations and vital signs.	Clear fluid may be a cerebrospinal leak (Barker and Laia 2008, **E**). Headache and backache are not unusual following lumbar puncture and may be due to loss of CSF. **E** Neurological observations and vital signs may indicate signs of change in intracranial pressure (Doherty and Forbes 2014, **E**). For further information see Chapter 14: Observations.
21 Encourage fluid intake.	To replace lost fluid. The patient may have difficulty micturating due to the procedure and the supine position (Doherty and Forbes 2014, **E**; Pagana and Pagana 2017, **E**).

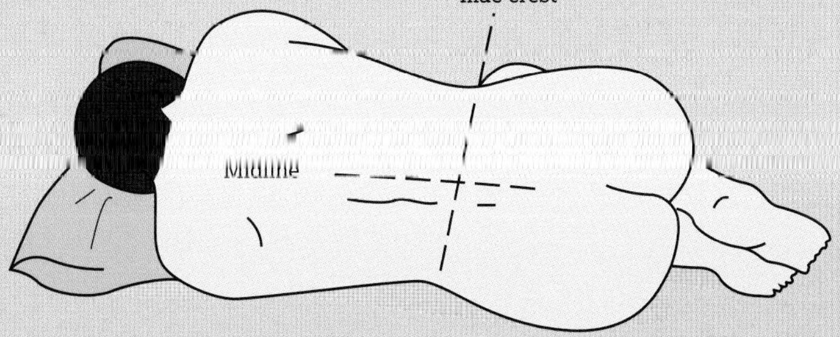

Action Figure 3 Position for lumbar puncture: head is flexed onto chest and knees are drawn up.

Problem-solving table 13.3 Prevention and resolution (Procedure guideline 13.9)

Problem	Cause	Prevention	Action
Pain down one leg during the procedure	A dorsal nerve root may have been touched by the spinal needle.	Make sure the spinal needle is in the midline. Advance the needle slowly and stop as soon as CSF is obtained.	Inform the doctor or practitioner, who will probably move the needle. Reassure the patient.
Fluctuation of neurological observations: level of consciousness, pulse, respirations, blood pressure or pupillary reaction	Herniation (coning) of the brainstem due to the decrease of ICP. Raised ICP is a contraindication to lumbar puncture.	Check that relevant neuroimaging has been reviewed prior to the procedure.	Observe the patient constantly for signs of alteration in ICP. The frequency may be decreased as the patient's condition allows. Report any fluctuations in these observations to a doctor immediately (Barker and Laia 2008).

ICP, intracranial pressure.

Documentation

The procedure should be documented in the patient's notes along with a record of informed consent. Any problems or immediate complications should be noted along with any treatment required. The sample bottles must be labelled correctly and sent to the laboratory.

Education of the patient and relevant others

Patients should be informed about relevant signs of complications and be given verbal and written information prior to discharge. Clear instructions should be given about side-effects and information on whom to call if side-effects occur.

Complications

Infection

Infection may be inadvertently introduced during the procedure. It may be superficial or deep and may be caused by either skin commensals surviving on the patient or respiratory flora from the person performing the lumbar puncture. Deep infection includes the serious complications of meningitis and spinal abscess and will need urgent intravenous antibiotics after discussion with a microbiologist. Spinal abscess causing nerve root compression may need urgent neurosurgical decompression. Adequate disinfection of the skin and the use of surgical face-masks will reduce the risk to the patient (Chernecky and Berger 2013, Doherty and Forbes 2014, Schneider 2013).

Haemorrhage

Haemorrhage or localized bruising may be caused by a traumatic procedure or in the presence of thrombocytopenia or a coagulopathy (Barker and Laia 2008, Lindsay et al. 2010). Haematoma formation may become a surgical emergency if there is nerve root compression.

Herniation

Transtentorial or tonsillar herniation is possible if lumbar puncture is carried out in the presence of raised ICP (Doherty and Forbes 2014). This is a serious and life-threatening complication and so brain imaging studies should be done if raised ICP is suspected. Consultation with a neurologist may also be warranted.

Headache

Frequency of PLPH varies among studies and between diagnostic and therapeutic procedures. Most symptoms develop within 24 hours. The following risk factors have been identified: young age, female gender and the presence of headache before or at the time of the lumbar puncture (Chernecky and Berger 2013, Doherty and Forbes 2014, Engelborghs et al. 2017). In more than 85% of cases, PLPH will resolve without any treatment. Rehydration, pain relief and antiemetic medications can help in milder cases (Doherty and Forbes 2014). If severe or prolonged, the headache may be treated with an epidural blood patch, usually after referral to an anaesthetist (Engelborghs et al. 2017, Gruener and Biller 2008).

Backache

Backache after lumbar puncture may be due to either local bruising from the lumbar puncture needle or excessive spinal flexion for prolonged periods of time (i.e. during difficult procedures). It does not seem to be affected by different needle sizes or by repeated attempts to gain CSF (Engelborghs et al. 2017, Pagana and Pagana 2017). In rare cases, backache may be suggestive of spinal haematoma or abscess, particularly if associated with leg weakness or bladder/bowel disturbance.

Leakage from puncture site

There may be a small amount of blood-stained oozing (Doherty and Forbes 2014, Pagana and Pagana 2017). The presence of clear fluid should be reported immediately to the doctor, especially if it is accompanied by fluctuation of other symptoms (e.g. level of consciousness, motor changes, problems voiding), as it may indicate a CSF leak (Barker and Laia 2008).

Semen collection and analysis

Definition

Semen collection is the collection of human male semen. Semen analysis may be called sperm count, sperm examination, seminal cytology or semen examination (Keogh 2017, Pagana and Pagana 2017).

Anatomy and physiology

Two of the three key functions of the male reproductive system are to produce and deliver sperm to the female ova for fertilization; the third is to produce and secrete male sex hormones in order to maintain the male reproductive system (Tortora and Derrickson 2017).

Spermatogenesis takes place in the testes in a constant and continuous cycle throughout an adult human male's life. On average, 300 million sperm complete spermatogenesis each day. Primary male germ cells are initially created in the outer wall of the germinal epithelium of the seminiferous tubules (Tortora and Derrickson 2017). As the sperm cells mature, they move into the lumen of the tubule to begin a circuitous journey through the male reproductive system. On this journey, sperm cells are augmented with nutritional and biochemical supplements, resulting in a greyish-white viscous fluid (semen). Semen not only helps sperm to survive but also eases the transfer of sperm into the female reproductive tract and facilitates successful fertilization (Tortora and Derrickson 2017).

Components of normal semen

The volume of semen released per ejaculate varies between 2 and 5 mL. The average ejaculate is 3.4 mL. Semen contains:

- fructose-rich fluid from the seminal vesicles (65–70%)
- secretions from the prostate gland containing enzymes, citric acid, lipids and acid phosphatase (25–30%)
- 200–500 million sperm (2–5%)
- secretions produced by the bulbourethral glands that aid the mobility of sperm in the vagina and cervix (1%) (Mandal 2010).

Semen is released during the two-phase process of ejaculation. It is controlled by the central nervous system; ejaculation occurs when there is friction on the genitalia or other forms of sexual stimulation occur, leading to impulses that are sent via the spinal cord to the brain. Phase 1 occurs when the vas deferens contracts to squeeze the sperm towards the base of the penis through the prostate gland and into the urethra. The seminal vesicles release their part of the semen, which combines with the sperm (Mulhall 2013, Tortora and Derrickson 2017).

Phase 2 is when the muscles at the base of the penis and urethra contract. This forces the semen out of the penis. During this phase, the bladder neck contracts to prevent the backflow of the semen into the urinary tract (if this occurs, it is called retrograde ejaculation). The final components of the semen join together in the posterior urethra and mix only after ejaculation (Mulhall 2013, Tortora and Derrickson 2017).

Evidence-based approaches

Rationale

Semen collection may be required for diagnostic and/or therapeutic purposes (Keogh 2017, Pagana and Pagana 2017). Common reasons to collect semen include:

- to evaluate the quality of the sperm
- to investigate and evaluate the cause of infertility
- to assess the success of vasectomy or vasectomy reversal (Pagana and Pagana 2017)
- cryopreservation of semen prior to treatments that may affect fertility, such as treatments for cancer (NICE 2013, RCP, RCR and RCOG 2007)
- prior to artificial insemination (Hammarberg et al. 2010)
- for sperm donation (Van den Broek et al. 2013).

Principles of care

Studies have shown that male infertility can cause extreme loss of self-esteem and impaired gender identity (Schmidt et al. 2005). There exists evidence on the importance of the relationship between body and mind in self-identity and perception (Greil et al. 2010) and on the idea that male infertility threatens the perception of masculinity (Gannon et al. 2004).

However, much of the infertility literature suggests that the focus has previously been on the female rather than male partner so best practice is now that couples (opposite sex or same sex) having difficulty conceiving should be seen together as decisions made in relation to investigations and treatment affect both partners (HFEA 2017). Evidence-based information should be made available to ensure informed decisions are made. Information can be given verbally and supplemented with written and/or audio-visual information (NICE 2013).

For men and teenage young adults with cancer, semen collection is common as a means of fertility preservation. Education and information should be given to inform donors' consent for cryopreservation. It is essential for patients to consider practical issues regarding how sperm is collected, stored and managed in the event of death prior to any cancer treatment (Pacey and Fiser 2011). Clinical judgement should be employed in the timing of this consultation, but doing so at the earliest opportunity is encouraged.

Whatever the reason for collecting semen, the donor should have adequate verbal and written information. They should also have time and counselling to consider the decision, reflect on the consequences of donation and fully understand the process of how their semen will be collected.

Methods of semen collection

Masturbation

Collecting semen for sperm cryopreservation is generally obtained by masturbation. For many men, this may be an embarrassing or uncomfortable process (Williams 2010). It is critical that men understand how to collect semen and that they are offered a private and relaxing environment in which to do so.

For adolescent males, careful counselling as well as careful and age-appropriate instructions are necessary, as these patients are at risk for emotional distress from this process (Crawshaw and Hale 2005). Parents should be included in discussions, although separate sessions with the adolescent are often useful. Unfortunately, no guidelines exist on the best approach to semen cryopreservation in adolescent males, but individual institutional strategies are available.

Electroejaculation

In some patients who have suffered a spinal cord injury, ejaculation by masturbation is not an option for sperm collection. In this case, the ejaculatory nerves can be electrically stimulated using a low-voltage rectal probe. This is usually sufficient to produce a semen ejaculate, although the quality of the ejaculate is often less using this method compared to masturbation (Brackett et al. 2010).

Microepididymal sperm aspiration

Microepididymal sperm aspiration (MESA) is a surgical procedure for collection of sperm when the ejaculatory tubes are blocked or have been interrupted by previous vasectomy (Bernie et al. 2013). A surgical incision is made into the outer covering of the testis and the epididymis is exposed; expanded areas of the epididymis likely to contain sperm are incised and the sperm is extracted (Bernie et al. 2013).

Percutaneous epididymal sperm aspiration

Percutaneous epididymal sperm aspiration (PESA) is a variant of MESA; rather than an incision, needle aspiration is used to extract sperm from the epididymis. PESA can be performed under local anaesthesia, but it is often the case that less sperm is collected using this approach (Esteves et al. 2013). Both MESA and PESA yield enough sperm for use with assisted reproductive techniques (ARTs) but not enough for a standard insemination (Bernie et al. 2013, Esteves et al. 2013).

Testicular sperm extraction

For men who have a low sperm count, recovery of sperm from the epididymis may not be successful (Dabaja and Schlegel 2012). Testicular sperm extraction (TESE) and possibly tissue biopsy may be the best option for collecting sperm suitable for ARTs. The outer covering of the testicle is pulled back so that the seminiferous tubules can be visualized. An enlarged tubule is cut to permit sperm to flow from the tubule, where it can be aspirated (Schlegel 1999). Testicular tissue can be dissected in a culture dish and the released sperm collected for ARTs (Dabaja and Schlegel 2012). Some men with permanent azoospermia after chemotherapy can be successfully treated by TESE and intracytoplasmic sperm injection (ICSI) (Meseguer et al. 2003).

Anticipated patient outcomes

Usually, a diagnosis and/or analysis of results in relation to fertility treatments is made available to patients after semen collection has taken place. Cryopreservation of semen gives patients the opportunity to conceive after fertility-damaging treatment such as chemotherapy and/or radiotherapy.

Clinical governance

The Human Fertilisation and Embryology Act 1990 provided for the establishment of the Human Fertilisation and Embryology Authority (HFEA), the first statutory body of its type in the world. With the creation of the HFEA, the 1990 Act ensured the regulation, through licensing, of:

- the creation of human embryos outside the body and their use in treatment and research
- the use of donated gametes and embryos
- the storage of gametes and embryos.

The Act was radically amended in 2008 (Human Fertilisation and Embryology Act 2008) to ensure that the legislative framework was in line with major technological, social and medical changes that had taken place since its original publication. Amendments included:

- extending regulation to the creation and use of all embryos outside the human body, regardless of the processes used in their creation
- increasing the scope of legitimate embryo research activities, i.e. allowing hybrid embryos to be created for research purposes
- banning sex selection of offspring for non-medical reasons
- retention of a duty, when providing fertility treatment, to take account of the welfare of the child, but removal of the reference to 'the need for a father'
- recognizing same-sex couples as legal parents of children conceived through the use of donated sperm, eggs or embryos (Birk 2009).

Human Fertilisation and Embryology Authority

The HFEA is the independent regulator of the licensing and monitoring of fertility clinics and research involving human embryos in the UK. In accordance with the Human Fertilisation and Embryology Acts (1990 and 2008), the Human Fertilisation and Embryology (Quality and Safety) Regulations (2017) and the European Union Tissues and Cells Directive (European Parliament and European Council 2004), the HFEA provides authoritative information for the public, in particular for people seeking treatment, donor-conceived people and donors. The HFEA also determines the policy framework for fertility issues, which are sometimes ethically and clinically complex.

European Union Tissues and Cells Directives

The European Union Tissues and Cells Directive, published in 2004 (European Parliament and European Council 2004), introduced common safety and quality standards for human tissues and cells across the European Union. The purpose of the directive is to facilitate a safer and easier exchange of tissues and cells (including human eggs and sperm) between member states of the European Union and to improve safety standards for European citizens.

Ethical considerations

Beyond the scientific processes in ARTs and cryopreservation, there are ethical considerations to keep in mind in the collection, storage and use of semen (Gong et al. 2009). The legal ownership of sperm as unfertilized gametes varies from country to country. However, ethical principles must respect the interests and welfare of those who will be born as a result of semen collection as well as the health and welfare of the donor (Gong et al. 2009).

Consent

Counselling and gaining informed consent are integral parts of all patient activities. Prior to the collection of semen for any reason, it is essential that practitioners gain fully informed consent (RCN 2017a). Consent is a continuous process throughout any patient episode and the practitioner must ensure that the patient is kept informed at every stage (Stuart and White 2012). For semen collection, this includes:

- informing the patient of the rationale for specimen collection
- telling the patient what the procedure will involve
- ascertaining the patient's level of understanding (especially if they need to be directly involved in the sampling technique)
- telling the patient how long the results may take to be processed
- telling the patient how the results will be made available
- giving the patient information on how this may affect their care.

In the UK, if the donor is a child (i.e. under the age of 18 years), then the normal rules for gaining consent in this age group apply (Shaw 2001):

- When obtaining consent, the person gaining consent must establish whether the child is legally competent (has capacity) to give consent.
- All people aged 16 and over are presumed in law to have capacity unless there is evidence to the contrary.
- However, as with adults, this does not mean that all 16-year-olds have capacity, and competence must be assessed along the following lines:
  - Are they able to understand and retain the information pertinent to the decision about their care, i.e. the nature, purpose and possible consequences of undergoing or not undergoing the proposed investigations or treatment?
  - Are they able to use this information to consider whether or not they should consent to the intervention offered?
  - Are they able to communicate their wishes?

If a child is deemed not legally competent, consent will need to be obtained from someone with parental responsibility (Shaw 2001).

Pre-procedural considerations

Equipment

A sterile specimen container from the laboratory is required. Container lids must not be waxed cardboard or have plastic or rubber liners to maintain the quality of the sample. Contraceptive condoms are not suitable as the lubricants are spermicidal. Men who are unable to provide a sample on religious or moral grounds may use silastic condoms such as the seminal collection device (Brinsden 2005).

Recording tools

Specimens must be accurately labelled. Prompt specimen analysis is only possible if specimens and their accompanying request forms are sent with specific, accurate and complete patient information. Incorrectly labelled and unlabelled specimens will be discarded (HSE 2003). The form should include as much information as possible as this allows the laboratory to select the most appropriate media inoculation for examination and interpretation of results (Weston 2008). General labelling should be conducted accurately, as discussed at the beginning of this chapter.

Specific patient preparation

It takes between 3 and 4 days for the sperm count to return to normal after ejaculation so patients should be advised that neither sexual intercourse nor masturbation should have taken place for 2 days prior to semen collection. This will ensure that the semen will have an optimum count and motility (NICE 2013, Tortora and Derrickson 2017). The patient should have ejaculated at least once between 2 and 7 days before collection. The patient should also be screened for the use of medicines and/or herbal remedies that may have an impact on sperm production or motility, such as St John's wort, which has a mutagenic effect on sperm cells (Chernecky and Berger 2013).

Education

Patients who are to be treated with ICSI should undergo appropriate investigations to determine the diagnosis and enable informed discussion prior to the procedure. This will prepare the patient or couple for the potential implications of treatment. Genetic counselling and testing should be offered to men who have a specific or suspected genetic defect in relation to their infertility (NICE 2013).

Patients who are undergoing treatments that may lead to infertility should be offered independent counselling to prepare them to cope with the possible physical and psychological implications of the treatment and its side-effects prior to commencing treatment (NICE 2013, Wo and Viswanathan 2009).

Procedure guideline 13.10 Semen collection

Essential equipment

- Private room
- Sterile specimen collection container for assisted reproduction or microbiological analysis (WHO 2010b)
- Clean specimen collection container for diagnostic or research purposes (WHO 2010b)
- Tissues

Action	Rationale
Pre-procedure	
1 Introduce yourself to the patient, explain and discuss the procedure with them, and gain their consent to proceed. Give clear, comprehensive written and verbal instructions.	To ensure that the patient feels at ease, understands the procedure and gives their valid consent (NMC 2018, **C**).

2 Instruct the patient not to ejaculate for 2 to 3 days prior to the procedure.	To ensure the sperm count will be at maximum levels (Keogh 2017, **E**; Pagana and Pagana 2017, **E**).
3 Discourage abstinence for no more than 7 days prior to specimen collection.	To ensure the sperm count and quality will be at maximum levels (WHO 2010b, **C**; Keogh 2017, Pagana and Pagana 2017, **E**).
4 Instruct the patient to report any loss of any part of the sample during collection	To ensure accurate results are obtained (WHO 2010b, **C**).
5 Ensure the patient has a private room near to the laboratory.	To ensure privacy for the patient. **E** To limit fluctuations in temperature of the semen (WHO 2010b, **C**).
6 Give the patient a specimen container.	To ensure the specimen is not contaminated and can be transported to the laboratory (Chernecky and Berger 2013, **E**).
Procedure	
7 Instruct the patient to only open the lid prior to ejaculation and replace it immediately after collection.	To minimize microbiological contamination (Brinsden 2005, **E**).
8 A fresh masturbated specimen must be collected in a sterile container.	To ensure the optimum sample is obtained (Chernecky and Berger 2013, **E**).
Post-procedure	
9 Complete the specimen form and label the specimen container (including relevant information such as date and time of collection and date of previous semen emission).	To maintain accurate records and provide accurate information for laboratory analysis (NMC 2018, **C**; Pagana and Pagana 2017, **E**).
10 Specimens must be transported to the laboratory as quickly as possible (within 1 hour of collection) and analysed within 3 hours.	To ensure a sample of optimum quality is obtained (Chernecky and Berger 2013, **E**; Pagana and Pagana 2017, **E**).
11 Keep the specimen between 25°C and 37°C in a laboratory incubator.	To ensure a sample of optimum quality is obtained (Brinsden 2005, **E**).
12 Document the procedure in the patient's records.	To ensure timely and accurate record keeping (NMC 2018, **C**).

Post-procedural considerations

Immediate care

It is important that the patient has information to take away and has a contact number in case further questions arise. The patient should be informed of when the results are likely to be available and how they will be communicated.

Ongoing care

Patients who are undergoing treatments that may lead to infertility should be offered independent counselling to help them cope with the possible physical and psychological implications of the treatment and its side-effects.

Cervical screening

Definition

Cervical screening (previously known as a smear test) is a test used to detect abnormalities in the cervix; it involves a specimen of cellular material being scraped from the cervix. The specimen is then stained and examined under a microscope by a cytologist to identify early cellular changes (Kumar and Clark 2016). As human papillomavirus (HPV) of the high-risk type is the cause of 99.7% of all cervical cancers, HPV testing is now routinely offered in many countries as part of cervical screening (RCN 2017b). While women may test positive to high-risk HPV, this does not necessarily mean that they will develop cervical cancer. It means that they are at greater risk than those who test negative (RCN 2018).

Anatomy and physiology

The cervix is the narrow neck of the uterus and is located between the vagina and the uterus. It projects into the vagina and the cavity of the cervix is known as the cervical canal. The cervical canal's glands secrete a mucus that blocks the entry of sperm except in the midcycle, when a reduction in viscosity allows sperm to pass (Marieb and Hoehn 2015) (Figure 13.11).

Related theory

The intention of a cervical screening test is to collect squamous epithelial cells and some endocervical cells from the transformation zone and squamocolumnar junction of the cervix (Figure 13.11). The sampling technique must take into consideration that the position of the squamocolumnar junction changes with age, contraception and parity (Higgins 2013, WHO 2014).

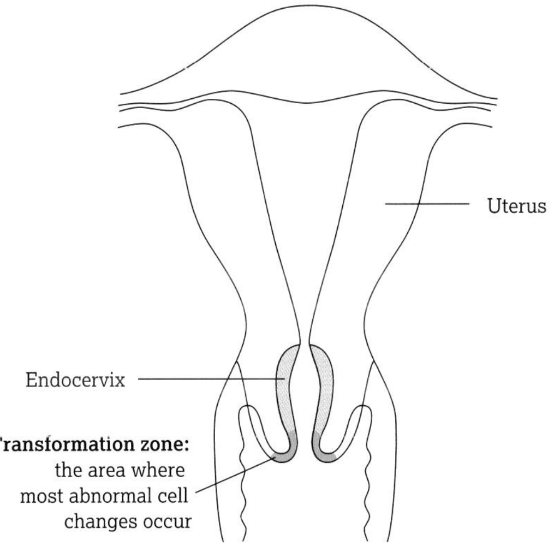

Figure 13.11 The cervix

Evidence-based approaches

Rationale

The ideal time for obtaining a cervical smear is midcycle if the woman is premenopausal; this prevents contamination from menstrual flow and allows for accuracy of results (Higgins 2013, WHO 2014). It is not ideal to take a cervical smear if a woman is pregnant or immediately post-partum as the results obtained can be misleading. The World Health Organization suggests that if a woman is in the target age group and there are concerns about access to screening post-partum, then a cervical smear should be taken following childbirth after consent is obtained (WHO 2014).

In the UK, 80% of cervical smears are taken in the primary care setting and most are taken by practice nurses. Screening is recommended in the UK for all women between the ages of 25 and 64 years and is an investigation to confirm that the cervix is healthy and there are no abnormal changes to the cells; it is not a test for diagnosing cervical cancer (Higgins 2013, NHSCSP 2016b). HPV testing was introduced into the NHS cervical screening programme in April 2011. HPV testing does not require any other additional procedures in addition to the regular smear test. In practice, the residual smear sample is used to test for HPV and this is conducted in a laboratory (NHSCSP 2013).

Indications

Women between the ages of 25 and 64 are indicated for cervical screening.

Contraindications

Women should not normally be offered a cervical screen:

- during menstruation
- during pregnancy
- immediately post-partum.

Method for cervical smears: liquid-based cytology

Liquid-based cytology (LBC) is the established method for cervical smears in Europe and the USA. Other countries may still use the conventional cytology methods, depending on their human, infrastructure and financial resources. The sample used to test for HPV DNA can also be used to test for sexually transmitted diseases such as chlamydia and gonorrhoea (Schuiling and Likis 2013).

Clinical governance

Healthcare professionals conducting cervical smears should be familiar with national guidance (NHSCSP 2016a). Women should be offered the option of having a chaperone present and their decision should be documented (GMC 2013, NMC 2018). The chaperone may be a person of the patient's choice who will accompany them throughout the procedure.

When attending for cervical screening, women can raise a number of other issues and these might be private in nature. Healthcare professionals must be prepared to listen and provide support, including details of other sources of information local to them. The concerns raised should be recorded (RCN 2018). Women may also have questions regarding HPV, cervical cancer and the HPV vaccine, vaginal discharge or abnormal bleeding, menopausal symptoms, and sexual difficulties (RCN 2018).

Governance

Smear tests are often performed by doctors and nurses. Training for cervical sample takers is designed to support the education and training of competent practitioners (NHSCSP 2016a). Training should reflect current trends, developments and understanding of the cervical screening process in light of new recommendations (RCN 2013).

Risk management

It is essential that women are informed that the likelihood of an inadequate test is about 1–2% for LBC and 9% for conventional cytology (NHSCSP 2016a).

Pre-procedural considerations

Equipment

There are several devices that are used in sampling the uterine cervix (Figure 13.12).

Vaginal speculum

The vaginal speculum is an instrument used during gynaecological examination to facilitate the visualization of the vagina and cervix. The speculum is introduced via the vagina and its cylinder (with a rounded end) allows easy passage. Once *in situ*, the speculum is opened, holding the vagina open and allowing the health professional to have access to the cervix and perform the cervical smear. Most speculums are now made of plastic and are single use, replacing those formerly made of metal and requiring sterilization after use. There are two categories of speculum: virgin and non-virgin. The latter is available in four sizes: small, medium, large and long. Special attention should be paid when selecting a speculum for use in women previously treated with pelvic radiotherapy or who are postmenopausal (Singh et al. 2013).

Cervical broom

The cervical broom is a plastic broom-shaped tool with a pyramidal arrangement of flexible flat 'teeth'. The longer 'central' tuft fits into the cervical os and must be rotated clockwise through a full circle five times. When used to take a conventional smear, this brush is an adequate and effective sampling device (NHSCSP 2016a). The brush should be inserted into the cervical os with the lower bristles remaining visible and rotated between a half and a whole turn to reduce trauma (NHSCSP 2016b).

The brush should be inserted into the cervical os with the lower bristles remaining visible and rotated between half and a whole turn to minimise trauma (Insinga et al. 2004).

Storage

LBC is the current standard method of screening in the NHS cervical screening programme (NHSCSP 2016a). The National Institute for Health and Care Excellence (2003) has recommended that LBC is used as the primary means of processing samples in the cervical screening program in England and Wales. It achieves 'cleaner' preparations, which are generally easier to read. Its advantage is a reduction in inadequate samples and there may be gains in reducing borderline results and increasing sensitivity (PHE 2019).

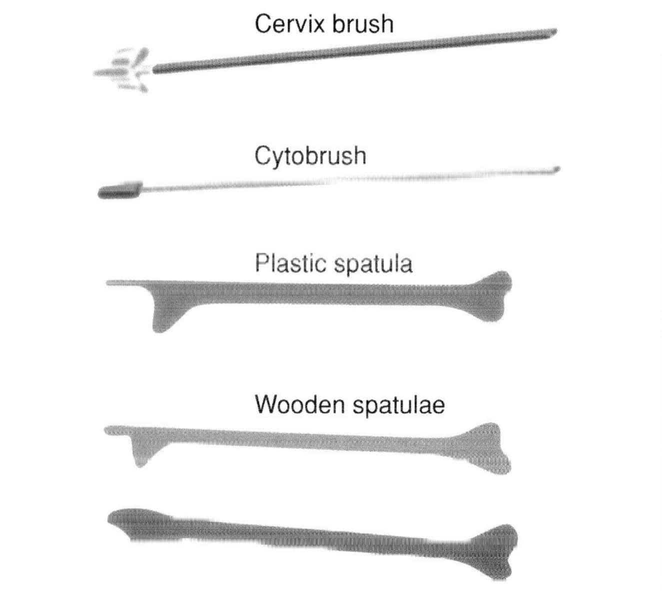

Figure 13.12 Types of device used for sampling the cervix.

Once the sample has been taken, it is vital that the cells collected are transferred onto a glass slide and preserved immediately or placed into the correct vial containing liquid preservative and fixative. Slides must not be placed in a refrigerator (Higgins 2013, NHSCSP 2016b).

Environment

The environment is also important, with the following equipment required:

- height-adjustable couch
- angle-positioned light source that is ideally free-standing for manoeuvrability (RCN 2013).

Specific patient preparation

The examination must be undertaken in a private room that cannot be entered during the procedure. Adequate private changing facilities should also be available that are warm and comfortable, and, if possible, there should be a separate waiting and recovery area (NHSCSP 2016a). Where possible, face the examination couch away from the door to enhance privacy and dignity for the patient (RCN 2013). Privacy can be achieved by locking the door after informing the woman. Having to attend for cervical screening can be perceived as embarrassing. For some women, this feeling of embarrassment prevents them from attending cervical screening.

The patient should be given the opportunity to empty her bladder prior to the examination. Ask the patient to remove her underwear and explain the position required on the couch. The most common position is supine or alternatively left lateral as it is comfortable and aids in the visualization of the cervix. Once the patient is ready, she should inform the practitioner. A modesty towel or covering should be supplied to enable the patient to partially cover herself (RCN 2013).

Education

Explain the procedure to the patient prior to commencing. It is good practice to offer the patient a demonstration of the speculum and to explain what part will be inserted into the vagina. Possible side-effects, such as spotting post-examination, should also be discussed prior to commencing the examination (RCN 2013).

Procedure guideline 13.11 Cervical uterine smear using liquid-based cytology

Essential equipment

- Personal protective equipment
- Light source
- Examination couch
- Disposable clean paper couch covers
- Variously sized specula (disposable or reusable)
- Cervix brush
- Liquid based cytology (LBC) container
- Black pen for labelling LBC container
- Specimen form and plastic specimen bag
- Container of warm water
- Box of tissue paper
- Clinical waste container
- Trolley
- Lubricant

Optional equipment

- A collecting container for central sterile services (CSS) if reusable instruments are used

Action	Rationale
Pre-procedure	
1 Introduce yourself to the patient, explain and discuss the procedure with them, and gain their consent to proceed. Discuss the benefits and limitations of screening and the significance of smear results. Explain the purpose of the procedure and what will occur at each step.	To ensure that the patient feels at ease, understands the procedure and gives her valid consent. To ensure that she understands that the procedure involves removing underwear and that the speculum will be inserted into her vagina (NHSCSP 2016b, **C**; NMC 2018, **C**). To allow the patient time to ask any questions. **E**
2 Document the woman's clinical and screening history, specifically: • date of last menstruation • any abnormal bleeding • any unusual vaginal discharge • contraception • date of last cervical smear • any abnormal smear results • any treatment to the cervix.	To ensure a relevant history is recorded (NHSCSP 2016b, **C**).
3 Place all the equipment required for the procedure on the trolley.	To facilitate the efficient taking of the sample. **E**
4 Close the room door and/or curtains and ask the woman to remove her underwear.	To provide privacy and comfort for the woman. **E**
Procedure	
5 Turn the light source on and position it at the end of the examination table.	To provide illumination of the cervix and increase the accuracy of the smear taking (NHSCSP 2016b, **C**; RCN 2013, **C**).

(continued)

Procedure guideline 13.11 Cervical uterine smear using liquid-based cytology (continued)

Action	Rationale
6 Assist the patient into a supine position on the couch, with knees drawn up and legs parted. Keep her as covered as possible.	To facilitate easy access of the vaginal speculum and the taking of the cervical smear (NHSCSP 2016b, WHO 2014, **C**).
7 Wash hands with antibacterial detergent and running hand-hot water. Ensure hands are dried with disposable paper hand towels.	To reduce the risk of contamination and cross-infection (NHS England and NHSI 2019, **C**, **E**; RCN 2012, **C**).
8 Apply gloves and apron.	To reduce the risk of contamination and cross-infection (NHS England and NHSI 2019, **C**; RCN 2012, **C**).
9 Select the appropriate size of speculum, from small, medium and large, or a long-bladed narrow speculum if the vagina is long or the cervix is lying posterior. The sterilized speculum can be warmed or cooled using clean tap water.	To promote patient comfort and reduce anxiety (NHSCSP 2016b, **C**). If removed from a sterilizer, the speculum may need to be cooled down; if cold, it may need to be warmed up to reduce patient discomfort. It must be explained to the patient that the speculum has been sterilized but that the water will not contaminate it. **E**
10 Apply lubricant to the speculum. Part the labia and, holding the speculum blades together sideways, slip the speculum into the vagina.	To insert the speculum and reduce patient discomfort (Fraise and Bradley 2009, **E**; RCN 2013, **C**; WHO 2014, **C**).
11 When the speculum is half way into the vagina, turn it so that the handle is facing down.	To promote patient comfort and reduce contamination of the cervix with lubricants (NHSCSP 2016b, **C**).
12 Gently open the blades of the speculum and look for the cervix. It may be necessary to move the speculum up or down until the entire cervix is visible.	To reduce patient discomfort and visualize the cervix (WHO 2014, **C**).
13 Using the cervix brush, insert the central bristles into the endocervical canal so that the shorter, outer bristles fully contact the ectocervix.	To ensure accuracy of the site sampled (NHSCSP 2016b, **C**; Singh et al. 2013, **R**).
14 Using pencil pressure, rotate the brush in a clockwise direction five times. *Note*: the plastic fronds of the brush are bevelled for rotation in a clockwise direction only.	To ensure good contact with the ectocervix and gather a high cellular yield (NHSCSP 2016b, **C**). Firm pressure is required to ensure the cells cling to the brush (NHSCSP 2016b, **C**).
Either:	
If using ThinPrep, using a swirling motion, rinse the brush into the fixative vial; then push the brush into the base of the vial at least 10 times, forcing the bristles apart.	To ensure a usable amount of cellular material is collected (NHSCSP 2016b, **C**).
Inspect the brush for any residual material and remove any remaining material by passing the brush over the edge of the fixative vial.	To ensure the cellular material reaches the preservative solution (NHSCSP 2016b, **C**).
Ensure that the material reaches the liquid. Then tighten the cap so that the material passes the torque line on the vial and give the vial a shake.	To ensure that the cells do not cling to the device (NHSCSP 2016b, **C**).
Or:	
If using SurePath, remove the head of the brush from the stem and place into the vial of fixative. Then screw the lid on tightly and shake the vial. *Note*: it is essential that the sample is placed into the vial immediately in order to achieve fixation.	To ensure accurate preservation of cervical material (NHSCSP 2016b, **C**).
15 Gently pull the speculum out until the blades are clear of the cervix, then close the blades and remove the speculum, placing it in a clinical waste bin if disposable or into a CSS container if reusable.	To prevent pinching the cervix or vaginal walls and to ensure safe disposal of contaminated equipment (NHSCSP 2016b, **C**).
16 Cover the patient and offer tissue paper to wipe away any excess vaginal discharge.	To ensure dignity and privacy while promoting hygiene and comfort. **E**
Post-procedure	
17 Remove gloves and dispose of waste in clinical waste receiver.	To safely dispose of clinical waste (DH 2013, **C**).
18 Assist the patient off the examination table and allow her to dress.	To ensure safety and promote dignity and privacy. **E**
19 Using a black ballpoint pen, label the vial with the patient's name, clinic number and date of birth.	To ensure the patient's details are documented correctly. **E**
20 Place the vial into a plastic specimen bag with the correctly labelled specimen form and send it to the laboratory.	To ensure safe handling and transportation of a biohazard (DH 2013, **C**; HSE 2003, **C**; WHO 2015, **C**).
21 Document the procedure in the patient's records.	To ensure timely and accurate record keeping (NMC 2018, **C**).

Problem-solving table 13.4 Prevention and resolution (Procedure guideline 13.11)

Problem	Cause	Prevention	Action
Inadequate sample	Cervix has not been scraped firmly enough to obtain adequate epithelial cells (WHO 2014).	Ensure adequate pressure to obtain sample.	Repeat cervical smear.
	Brush not rinsed immediately, allowing the sample to dry and causing the cells to become misshapen.	Ensure brush is rinsed immediately after scraping the cervix.	Repeat cervical smear.
	Sample contaminated with lubricants, spermicide or blood (Higgins 2013).	Ensure sample is not contaminated by educating the patient not to use lubricants or spermicide 24 hours prior to the test.	Repeat cervical smear.
Unable to visualize the cervix	Position of the patient or anatomical position of the cervix.	Adequate positioning of the patient.	Reposition the patient from the prone to the lateral position. Place a pillow under the buttocks or turn the speculum. Consider requesting assistance from another sample taker or refer to colposcopy clinic if unable to visualize.

Post-procedural considerations

Immediate care
Ensure patient modesty is maintained throughout and directly after the examination. To maintain privacy and dignity, the nurse should leave the room while the patient gets undressed and dressed, and advise her to call when ready (RCN 2013).

Ongoing care
The nurse should explain when and how the results will be communicated to the woman, and in the event of abnormal results how her care will progress (RCN 2018). It is important that the nurse considers how the patient may react if abnormal results are to be delivered and ensures necessary support (RCN 2013).

Documentation
The nurse should ensure that the request form has been adequately completed and that the samples are also labelled correctly and accurately. If other microbiological tests are conducted, ensure that the correct forms are completed and that the samples are labelled, and document any findings and resulting actions (RCN 2018).

Education of the patient and relevant others
It is not unusual for a patient to experience some spotting after a cervical smear. This must be explained to the patient to ensure she is aware and knows not to worry. The nurse should promote health education programmes and encourage screening to those who are eligible, such as by providing accurate information and advice on the prevention of cervical cancer. Information leaflets should be offered to patients to ensure they have the appropriate information (RCN 2018).

Specimen collection: swab sampling

Definition
Sterile swabs are commonly used in clinical practice to obtain samples of material from skin and mucous membranes. They are utilized to identify micro-organisms in suspected infection or as part of a screening programme to identify patients who may be carrying pathogens without displaying clinical signs or symptoms. Swab cultures provide useful data that can be used to augment diagnostic and therapeutic decision making (Bonham 2009, Panpradist et al. 2014).

Related theory
Swabbing is aimed at collection of body fluid or cutaneous material for the purpose of obtaining a specimen for microbiological analysis; when properly performed, a swab is a simple, non-invasive and cost-effective method of culturing in clinical practice (Bonham 2009, Panpradist et al. 2014). Samples of infected material can be obtained from any accessible part of the body by using a sterile swab tipped with cotton wool or synthetic material (Chernecky and Berger 2013, Huddleston Cross 2014, Pagana and Pagana 2017).

Evidence-based approaches

Rationale

Indications
Taking a swab is indicated:

- if there are clinical signs of infection, which may manifest as symptoms such as pain, redness, inflammation, heat, pus or odour
- if a patient shows signs of systemic infection or has a pyrexia of unknown origin
- as part of a screening programme.

Contraindications
Taking a swab is not indicated:

- as routine use (unless part of a screening regimen)
- on chronic wounds, which will be colonized with skin flora.

Principles of care
Although swabs are relatively simple to use, absorbency of infected material is variable and adequate material collection that is representative of pathogenic changes, for example to wounds, is often dependent upon correct sampling technique (Gould and Brooker 2008, Panpradist et al. 2014). Swab specimens should be collected using an aseptic technique with sterile swabs, with the principal aim of gathering as much material as possible from the site of infection or inflammation. Care should be taken to avoid contamination with anything other than the sample material, such as surrounding tissue, which will be contaminated with other pathogens such as skin flora (Weston 2008).

If an infected area is producing copious amounts of pus or exudate, a specimen should be aspirated using a sterile syringe because swabs tend to absorb excess overlying exudate, resulting in an inadequate specimen (Huddleston Cross 2014). If the area to be swabbed is relatively dry (e.g. in nasal or skin swabs), the tip of the swab can be moistened with sterile 0.9% sodium chloride, which makes it more absorbent and increases the survival of pathogens (Weston 2008).

Obtaining a swab should be considered in conjunction with a comprehensive nursing assessment. This could include observation of localized infection, such as inflammation or discharge from a wound during a dressing change.

Practitioners should know what type of pathogenic micro-organism they are testing (e.g. whether a bacterial or viral infection is suspected), as this will determine which swab is the most appropriate. Advice should be sought from the microbiology laboratory prior to taking a swab to ensure appropriate and resource-effective sampling or specimen collection. For example, while viruses cause the majority of throat infections, group A streptococcus is the main bacterial cause of sore throats and therefore, if suspected, a swab with bacterial transport medium would need to be used rather than one containing viral transport medium (PHE 2015a).

Clinical governance

Competencies

Obtaining specimens for microbiological analysis is a key component in the patient's assessment and subsequent nursing care. Therefore, practitioners must be competent and feel confident that they have the knowledge, skill and understanding to obtain and correctly process samples for specimen collection (NMC 2018).

Pre-procedural considerations

Equipment

Commercially available transport media offer a cheap and effective method to enable the culture of both aerobic and anaerobic micro-organisms. Wound swabbing most frequently involves the use of a cotton- or alginate-tipped swab, although these have been found to inhibit the detection of certain bacteria (Faoagali 2010). Despite being more expensive, flocked nylon swabs now provide a sensitive collection method for culture, rapid and near-patient testing, and molecular detection of a variety of bacteria and viruses. This is because of their ability to absorb cells and then release them effectively to increase the sensitivity of detection of infecting microbes (Faoagali 2010). If unsure, the practitioner should liaise with the microbiology laboratory to clarify which is the most suitable swab for a particular investigation or type of specimen.

Specific patient preparation

It may be necessary to position the patient in order to obtain the required sample.

Procedure guideline 13.12 Swab sampling: ear

Essential equipment

- Personal protective equipment
- Sterile swab (with transport medium)
- Appropriate documentation/form

Action	Rationale
Pre-procedure	
1 Introduce yourself to the patient, explain and discuss the procedure with them, and gain their consent to proceed.	To ensure that the patient feels at ease, understands the procedure and gives their valid consent (NMC 2018, **C**).
2 Wash hands with bactericidal soap and water, or decontaminate physically clean hands with an alcohol-based handrub. Put on apron and gloves.	To reduce the risk of cross-infection and specimen contamination (NHS England and NHSI 2019, **C**).
3 Ensure no antibiotics or other therapeutic drops have been used in the aural region within the 3 hours before taking the swab.	To prevent collection of such therapeutic agents, which may mask pathogenic organisms and invalidate the specimen. **E**
Procedure	
4 Remove the swab from outer packaging and place at the entrance of the auditory meatus, as shown in **Action figure 4**. Rotate gently once.	To avoid trauma to the ear and to collect secretions and/or suitable specimen material. **E**
Post-procedure	
5 Remove cap from plastic transport tube.	To avoid contamination of the swab and to maintain the viability of the sampled material during transportation. **E**
6 Carefully place swab into plastic transport tube, ensuring it is fully immersed in the transport medium. Ensure cap is firmly secured.	To avoid contamination of the swab and to maintain the viability of the sampled material during transportation. See manufacturer's guidance. **E**
7 Remove gloves and apron, and wash and/or decontaminate hands.	To reduce the risk of cross-infection (NHS England and NHSI 2019, **C**).
8 Label swab immediately.	To maintain accurate records and provide accurate information for laboratory analysis (NMC 2018, **C**; Weston 2008, **E**).
9 Complete microbiology request form (including relevant information, such as exact site, nature of specimen and investigation required).	To maintain accurate records and provide accurate information for laboratory analysis (NMC 2018, **C**; Weston 2008, **E**).

10 Arrange prompt delivery to the microbiology laboratory or refrigerate at 4–8°C.	To achieve optimal conditions for analysis (PHE 2018b, **C**).
11 Document the procedure in the patient's records.	To ensure timely and accurate record keeping (NMC 2018, **C**).

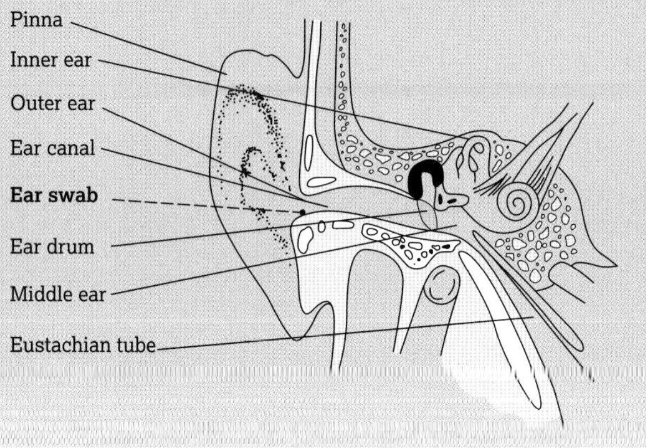

Action Figure 4 Area to be swabbed when sampling the outer ear

Procedure guideline 13.13 Swab sampling: eye

Essential equipment

- Personal protective equipment
- Appropriate documentation/form
- Sterile bacterial or viral swab (with transport medium)

Action	Rationale
Pre-procedure	
1 Introduce yourself to the patient, explain and discuss the procedure with them, and gain their consent to proceed.	To ensure that the patient feels at ease, understands the procedure and gives their valid consent (NMC 2018, **C**).
2 Seek advice from the microbiology laboratory as to the correct culture medium and swab required.	Different culture media and swabs are required for bacteria, viruses and chlamydia (Shaw et al. 2010, **E**).
3 Wash hands with bactericidal soap and water, or decontaminate physically clean hands with an alcohol-based handrub. Put on apron and gloves.	To reduce the risk of cross-infection and specimen contamination (NHS England and NHSI 2019, **C**).
Procedure	
4 Remove swab from outer packaging.	To ensure collection of specimen material. **E**
5 Ask patient to look upwards.	To prevent corneal damage (Shaw et al. 2010, **E**).
6 Hold the swab parallel to the cornea and gently rub the conjunctiva in the lower eyelids from nasal side outwards.	To ensure that a swab of the correct site is taken and to avoid contamination by touching the eyelid (Shaw et al. 2010, **E**).
7 *If for chlamydia specimen*: apply slightly more pressure when swabbing.	To obtain as many organisms as possible from the follicles and to sweep organisms away from the lower punctum (Shaw et al. 2010, **E**).
8 If both eyes are to be swabbed, label swabs 'right' and 'left' accordingly.	To prevent the wrong swab being placed in the wrong culture medium (Shaw et al. 2010, **E**).
Post-procedure	
9 Remove cap from plastic transport tube.	To avoid contamination of the swab. **E**
10 Carefully place swab into plastic transport tube, ensuring it is fully immersed in the transport medium. Ensure cap is firmly secured.	To avoid contamination of the swab and to maintain the viability of the sampled material during transportation. See manufacturer's guidance. **E**
11 Remove gloves and apron, and wash and/or decontaminate hands.	To reduce the risk of cross-infection (NHS England and NHSI 2019, **C**).
12 Label swab immediately.	To maintain accurate records and provide accurate information for laboratory analysis (NMC 2018, **C**; Weston 2008, **E**).
13 Complete microbiology request form (including relevant information such as exact site, nature of specimen and investigation required).	To maintain accurate records and provide accurate information for laboratory analysis (NMC 2018, **C**; Weston 2008, **E**).
14 Arrange prompt delivery to the microbiology laboratory.	To achieve optimal conditions for analysis (PHE 2018b, **C**).
15 Document the procedure in the patient's records.	To ensure timely and accurate record keeping (NMC 2018, **C**).

Procedure guideline 13.14 Swab sampling: nose

Essential equipment

- Personal protective equipment
- Sterile bacterial or viral swab (with transport medium)

Optional equipment

- 0.9% sodium chloride
- Appropriate documentation/form

Action	Rationale
Pre-procedure	
1 Introduce yourself to the patient, explain and discuss the procedure with them, and gain their consent to proceed.	To ensure that the patient feels at ease, understands the procedure and gives their valid consent (NMC 2018, **C**).
2 Wash hands with bactericidal soap and water, or decontaminate physically clean hands with an alcohol-based handrub. Put on apron and gloves.	To reduce the risk of cross-infection and specimen contamination (NHS England and NHSI 2019, **C**).
Procedure	
3 Remove swab from outer packaging.	To ensure collection of specimen material. **E**
4 Ask patient to tilt head backwards.	To optimize visualization of the area to be swabbed (Gould and Brooker 2008, **E**).
5 Moisten swab with sterile saline.	To prevent discomfort to the patient as the nasal mucosa is normally dry and organisms will adhere more easily to a moist swab. **E**
6 Insert swab inside the anterior nares with the tip directed upwards and gently rotate (**Action figure 6**).	To ensure that an adequate specimen from the correct site is obtained and to avoid damage to the epithelium, which is delicate (Gould and Brooker 2008, **E**).
7 Repeat the procedure with the same swab in the other nostril.	To optimize organism collection. **E**
Post-procedure	
8 Remove cap from plastic transport tube.	To avoid contamination of the swab. **E**
9 Carefully place swab into plastic transport tube, ensuring it is fully immersed in the transport medium. Ensure cap is firmly secured.	To avoid contamination of the swab and to maintain the viability of the sampled material during transportation. See manufacturer's guidance. **E**
10 Provide the patient with a tissue if required.	For patient comfort (Higgins 2013, **E**).
11 Remove gloves and apron, and wash and/or decontaminate hands.	To reduce the risk of cross-infection (NHS England and NHSI 2019, **C**).
12 Label swab immediately	To maintain accurate records and provide accurate information for laboratory analysis (NMC 2018, **C**; Weston 2008, **E**).
13 Complete microbiology request form (including relevant information such as exact site, nature of specimen and investigation required).	To maintain accurate records and provide accurate information for laboratory analysis (NMC 2018, **C**; Weston 2008, **E**).
14 *If sample taken for screening*: state clearly on the microbiology request form, for example for MRSA screening.	To ensure only these organisms are being analysed, so the result will only indicate their presence or absence, and sensitivities (Weston 2008, **E**).
15 Arrange prompt delivery to the microbiology laboratory.	To achieve optimal conditions for analysis (PHE 2015b, **C**).
16 Document the procedure in the patient's records.	To ensure timely and accurate record keeping (NMC 2018, **C**).

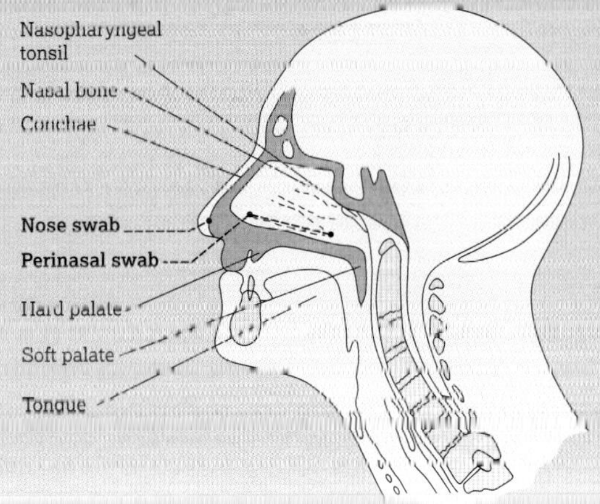

Action Figure 6 Area to be swabbed when sampling the nose.

Procedure guideline 13.15 Swab sampling: penis

Essential equipment

- Personal protective equipment
- Sterile bacterial or viral swab (with transport medium)
- Appropriate documentation/form

Action	Rationale
Pre-procedure	
1 Introduce yourself to the patient, explain and discuss the procedure with them, and gain their consent to proceed.	To ensure that the patient feels at ease, understands the procedure and gives their valid consent (NMC 2018, **C**).
2 Wash hands with bactericidal soap and water, or decontaminate physically clean hands with an alcohol-based handrub. Put on apron and gloves.	To reduce the risk of cross-infection and specimen contamination (NHS England and NHSI 2019, **C**).
Procedure	
3 The patient should not have passed urine for at least 1 hour.	To ensure a representative sample of the area being swabbed (PHE 2017, **C**).
4 Remove swab from outer packaging.	To ensure collection of specimen material. **E**
5 Retract the prepuce.	To obtain maximum visibility of the area to be swabbed (PHE 2017, **C**).
6 Pass the swab gently through the urethral meatus and rotate gently.	To collect a specimen of discharge or secretions (HPA 2014b, **C**).
Post-procedure	
7 Remove cap from plastic transport tube.	To avoid contamination of the swab (PHE 2017, **C**).
8 Label swab immediately.	To maintain accurate records and provide accurate information for laboratory analysis (NMC 2018, **C**; Weston 2008, **E**).
9 Carefully place swab into plastic transport tube, ensuring it is fully immersed in the transport medium. Ensure cap is firmly secured.	To avoid contamination of the swab and to maintain viability of the sampled material during transportation. See manufacturer's guidance. **E**
10 Remove gloves and apron, and wash and/or decontaminate hands.	To reduce the risk of cross-infection (NHS England and NHSI 2019, **C**).
11 Complete microbiology request form (including relevant information such as exact site, nature of specimen and investigation required).	To maintain accurate records and provide accurate information for laboratory analysis (NMC 2018, **C**; Weston 2008, **E**).
12 Arrange prompt delivery to the microbiology laboratory (within 4 hours).	To increase the chance of accurate organism identification and to ensure the best possible conditions for laboratory analysis (PHE 2017, **C**).
13 Document the procedure in the patient's records.	To ensure timely and accurate record keeping (NMC 2018, **C**).

Procedure guideline 13.16 Swab sampling: rectum

Essential equipment

- Personal protective equipment
- Appropriate documentation/form
- Sterile bacterial or viral swab (with transport medium)

Action	Rationale
Pre-procedure	
1 Introduce yourself to the patient, explain and discuss the procedure with them, and gain their consent to proceed.	To ensure that the patient feels at ease, understands the procedure and gives their valid consent (NMC 2018, **C**).
2 Ensure a suitable location in which to carry out the procedure.	To maintain patient privacy and dignity. **E**
3 Wash hands with bactericidal soap and water, or decontaminate physically clean hands with an alcohol-based handrub. Put on apron and gloves.	To reduce the risk of cross-infection and specimen contamination (NHS England and NHSI 2019, **C**).

(continued)

Procedure guideline 13.16 Swab sampling: rectum *(continued)*

Action	Rationale
Procedure	
4 Remove swab from outer packaging.	To ensure collection of specimen material. **E**
5 Pass the swab, with care, through the anus into the rectum and rotate gently.	To avoid trauma and to ensure that a rectal, not an anal, sample is obtained. **E**
6 *If specimen is for suspected threadworm*: take swab from the perianal area.	Threadworms lay their ova on the perianal skin. **E**
Post-procedure	
7 Remove cap from plastic transport tube.	To avoid contamination of the swab. **E**
8 Carefully place swab into plastic transport tube, ensuring it is fully immersed in the transport medium. Ensure cap is firmly secured.	To avoid contamination of the swab and to maintain viability of the sampled material during transportation. See manufacturer's guidance. **E**
9 Remove gloves and apron, and wash and/or decontaminate hands.	To reduce the risk of cross-infection (NHS England and NHSI 2019, **C**).
10 Label swab immediately.	To maintain accurate records and provide accurate information for laboratory analysis (NMC 2018, **C**; Weston 2008, **E**).
11 Complete microbiology request form (including relevant information such as exact site, nature of specimen and investigation required).	To maintain accurate records and provide accurate information for laboratory analysis (NMC 2018, **C**; Weston 2008, **E**).
12 Arrange prompt delivery to the microbiology laboratory.	To achieve optimal conditions for analysis (PHE 2018b, **C**).
13 Document the procedure in the patient's records.	To ensure timely and accurate record keeping (NMC 2018, **C**).

Procedure guideline 13.17 Swab sampling: skin

Essential equipment

- Personal protective equipment
- Appropriate documentation/form
- Sterile bacterial or viral swab (with transport medium)

Optional equipment

- Scalpel blade or U blade (for trained practitioners only)

Action	Rationale
Pre-procedure	
1 Introduce yourself to the patient, explain and discuss the procedure with them, and gain their consent to proceed.	To ensure that the patient feels at ease, understands the procedure and gives their valid consent (NMC 2018, **C**).
2 Wash hands with bactericidal soap and water, or decontaminate physically clean hands with an alcohol-based handrub. Put on apron and gloves.	To reduce the risk of cross-infection and specimen contamination (NHS England and NHSI 2019, **C**).
Procedure	
3 Remove swab from outer packaging.	To ensure collection of specimen material. **E**
4 *For cutaneous sampling (for screening, e.g. groin)*: moisten swab with sterile saline and roll one swab along the area of skin along the inside of the thighs close to the genitalia.	Organisms adhere more easily to a moist swab (Hampson 2006, **C**).
5 *For suspected fungal infection*: skin scrapings should be obtained. Take a scalpel blade and, with the affected area of skin stretched taut between two fingers, gently scrape the skin with a piece of dark paper underneath. Do not cause bleeding.	To identify superficial fungi that inhabit the outer layer of the skin (MacKie 2003, **E**). To visualize the amount of sample and to allow easier transfer. **E**
Post-procedure	
6 *Either:* *For swab specimen:* • Remove cap from plastic transport tube. • Carefully place swab into plastic transport tube, ensuring it is fully immersed in the transport medium. Ensure cap is firmly secured.	To avoid contamination of the swab and to maintain the viability of the sampled material during transportation. See manufacturer's guidance. **E**

Or: *For skin scrapings:* • Transfer scrapings into sterile container.	To allow samples to be processed appropriately in the laboratory. **E**
7 Remove gloves and apron, and wash and/or decontaminate hands.	To reduce the risk of cross-infection (NHS England and NHSI 2019, **C**).
8 Label swabs immediately.	To maintain accurate records and provide accurate information for laboratory analysis (NMC 2018, **C**; Weston 2008, **E**).
9 Complete microbiology request form (including relevant information such as exact site, nature of specimen and investigation required).	To maintain accurate records and provide accurate information for laboratory analysis (NMC 2018, **C**; Weston 2008, **E**).
10 Arrange prompt delivery to the microbiology laboratory (keep at room temperature).	To achieve optimal conditions for analysis (PHE 2018b, **C**).
11 Document the procedure in the patient's records.	To ensure timely and accurate record keeping (NMC 2018, **C**).

Procedure guideline 13.18 Swab sampling: throat

Essential equipment

- Personal protective equipment
- Sterile bacterial or viral swab (with transport medium)
- Light source
- Tongue spatula
- Appropriate documentation/form

Action	Rationale
Pre-procedure	
1 Introduce yourself to the patient, explain and discuss the procedure with them, and gain their consent to proceed.	To ensure that the patient feels at ease, understands the procedure and gives their valid consent (NMC 2018, **C**).
2 Wash hands with bactericidal soap and water, or decontaminate physically clean hands with an alcohol-based handrub. Put on apron and gloves.	To reduce the risk of cross-infection and specimen contamination (NHS England and NHSI 2019, **C**).
Procedure	
3 Remove swab from outer packaging.	To ensure collection of specimen material. **E**
4 Ask patient to sit upright facing a strong light, tilt head backwards, open mouth and stick out tongue.	To ensure maximum visibility of the area to be swabbed and avoid contact with the oral mucosa (Gould and Brooker 2008, **E**).
5 Depress tongue with a spatula.	The procedure may cause the patient to gag. The spatula prevents the tongue moving to the roof of the mouth, which would contaminate the specimen. **E**
6 Ask patient to say 'Ah'.	Assists with depression of the tongue and prevents the patient from feeling the gag reflex. **E**
7 Quickly but gently roll the swab over any area of exudate or inflammation or over the tonsils and the posterior pharynx (**Action figure 7**).	To obtain the required sample (Weston 2008, **E**).
8 Carefully withdraw the swab, avoiding touching any other area of the mouth or tongue.	To prevent contamination of the specimen with the resident flora of the oropharynx (Weston 2008, **E**).
Post-procedure	
9 Remove cap from plastic transport tube.	To avoid contamination of the swab. **E**
10 Carefully place swab into plastic transport tube, ensuring it is fully immersed in the transport medium. Ensure cap is firmly secured.	To avoid contamination of the swab and maintain the viability of the sampled material during transportation. See manufacturer's guidance. **E**
11 Remove gloves and apron, and wash and/or decontaminate hands.	To reduce the risk of cross-infection (NHS England and NHSI 2019, **C**).
12 Label swab immediately.	To maintain accurate records and provide accurate information for laboratory analysis (NMC 2018, **C**; Weston 2008, **E**).

(continued)

Procedure guideline 13.18 Swab sampling: throat (continued)

Action	Rationale
13 Complete microbiology request form (including relevant information such as exact site, nature of specimen and investigation required).	To maintain accurate records and provide accurate information for laboratory analysis (NMC 2018, **C**; Weston 2008, **E**).
14 Arrange prompt delivery to the microbiology laboratory.	To achieve optimal conditions for analysis (PHE 2018b **C**).
15 Document the procedure in the patient's records.	To ensure timely and accurate record keeping (NMC 2018, **C**).

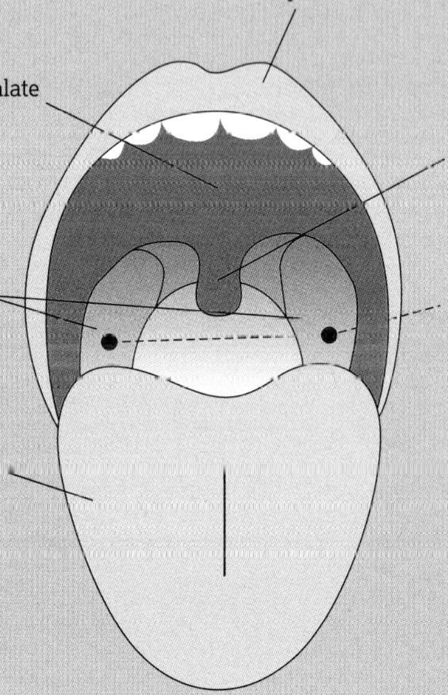

Action Figure 7 Area to be swabbed when sampling the throat.

Procedure guideline 13.19 Swab sampling: vagina

Essential equipment

- Personal protective equipment
- Sterile bacterial or viral swab (with transport medium)
- Appropriate documentation/form
- Light source
- Sterile speculum

Action	Rationale
Pre-procedure	
1 Introduce yourself to the patient, explain and discuss the procedure with them, and gain their consent to proceed.	To ensure that the patient feels at ease, understands the procedure and gives their valid consent (NMC 2018, **C**).
2 Ensure a suitable location in which to carry out the procedure.	To maintain patient privacy and dignity and to help her to relax and be comfortable during the procedure. **E**
3 Wash hands with bactericidal soap and water, or decontaminate physically clean hands with an alcohol-based handrub. Put on apron and gloves.	To reduce the risk of cross-infection and specimen contamination (NHS England and NHSI 2019, **C**).
4 Position the patient with her knees bent and legs apart. Adjust the light.	To be able to visualize the vulva and cervix. **E**
Procedure	
5 Remove swab from outer packaging.	To ensure collection of specimen material. **E**
6 *Either:*	
For low vaginal swab: Insert the swab into the lower part of the vagina and rotate gently but firmly.	To obtain appropriate sample. **E**

Or:	
For high vaginal swab: moisten the speculum with warm water and insert into the vagina to separate the vaginal walls. Wipe away any excess cervical mucus with a cotton swab. Using a sterile swab, sample as high as possible in the vaginal vault. Remove the speculum and wipe the vagina and vulval area with a tissue.	To ensure maximum visibility of the area to be swabbed and to obtain the appropriate sample. **E**
7 Allow the patient to resume a comfortable position.	To aid patient comfort. **E**
Post-procedure	
8 Remove cap from plastic transport tube.	To avoid contamination of the swab. **E**
9 Carefully place swab into plastic transport tube, ensuring it is fully immersed in the transport medium. Ensure cap is firmly secured.	To avoid contamination of the swab and to maintain the viability of the sampled material during transportation. See manufacturer's guidance. **E**
10 Remove gloves and apron, and wash and/or decontaminate hands.	To reduce the risk of cross-infection (NHS England and NHSI 2019, **C**).
11 Label swab immediately.	To maintain accurate records and provide accurate information for laboratory analysis (NMC 2018, **C**; Weston 2008, **E**).
12 Complete microbiology request form (including relevant information such as exact site, nature of specimen and investigation required).	To maintain accurate records and provide accurate information for laboratory analysis (NMC 2018, **C**; Weston 2008, **E**).
13 Arrange prompt delivery to the microbiology laboratory (within 4 hours).	To achieve optimal conditions for analysis (PHE 2018b, **C**).
14 Document the procedure in the patient's records.	To ensure timely and accurate record keeping (NMC 2018, **C**).

Procedure guideline 13.20 Swab sampling: wound

Essential equipment

- Personal protective equipment
- Sterile bacterial or viral swab (with transport medium)
- Appropriate documentation/form
- Dressing pack containing sterile gloves, cleansing solution and dressing (post-sampling procedure)

Optional equipment

- 0.9% sodium chloride

Action	Rationale
Pre-procedure	
1 Introduce yourself to the patient, explain and discuss the procedure with them, and gain their consent to proceed.	To ensure that the patient feels at ease, understands the procedure and gives their valid consent (NMC 2018, **C**).
2 Wash hands with bactericidal soap and water, or decontaminate physically clean hands with an alcohol-based handrub. Put on apron and gloves.	To reduce the risk of cross-infection and specimen contamination (NHS England and NHSI 2019, **C**).
3 Remove current dressing, if applicable.	To expose the wound in preparation for swabbing. **E**
4 Remove gloves and decontaminate hands. Open sterile dressing pack, decant sterile swab and put on sterile gloves.	To reduce the risk of cross-infection (RCN 2012, **E**) and prepare equipment for sampling (NHS England and NHSI 2019, **C**).
Procedure	
5 Remove swab from outer packaging.	To ensure collection of specimen material. **E**
6 Rotate the swab tip over a 1 cm^2 area of viable tissue, at or near the centre of the wound, for 5 seconds, applying enough pressure to express tissue fluid from the wound bed.	Expressed tissue fluids are likely to contain the true infecting organisms and less likely to contain surface contaminants (Huddleston Cross 2014, **E**).
7 If the wound is dry, the tip of the swab should be moistened with 0.9% sodium chloride.	To make the swab more absorbent and to increase the survival of pathogens present prior to culture (Huddleston Cross 2014, **E**).
8 If pus is present, it should be aspirated using a sterile syringe and decanted into a sterile specimen pot.	To yield the optimum number of micro-organisms present within the wound (Weston 2008, **E**).

(continued)

Procedure guideline [illegible] Swab sampling: wound (continued)

Action	Rationale
Post-procedure	
9 Remove cap from plastic transport tube.	To avoid contamination of the swab. **E**
10 Carefully place swab into plastic transport tube, ensuring it is fully immersed in the transport medium. Ensure cap is firmly secured.	To avoid contamination of the swab and to maintain the viability of the sampled material during transportation. See manufacturer's guidance. **E**
11 Redress the wound, if applicable, as per patient care plan.	To redress the wound. **E**
12 Remove gloves and apron, discard all clinical waste and wash and/or decontaminate hands.	To reduce the risk of cross-infection (NHS England and NHSI 2019, **C**).
13 Label swab immediately.	To maintain accurate records and provide accurate information for laboratory analysis (NMC 2018, **C**; Weston 2008, **E**).
14 Complete microbiology request form (including relevant information such as exact site, nature of specimen and investigation required).	To maintain accurate records and provide accurate information for laboratory analysis (NMC 2018, **C**; Weston 2008, **E**).
15 Arrange prompt delivery to the microbiology laboratory (keep at room temperature).	To achieve optimal conditions for analysis (PHE 2018b, **C**).
16 Document the procedure in the patient's records.	To ensure timely and accurate record keeping (NMC 2018, **C**).

Post-procedural considerations

Immediate care

Specimens should be sent to the laboratory immediately or no later than 2 hours following collection (Bonham 2009). For specimens that cannot be transferred to the laboratory within 2 hours, storage at room temperature is considered to be appropriate for the maintenance of aerobic and anaerobic micro-organisms. Advice should be sought from the microbiology laboratory if practitioners are unsure of the storage requirements for the sample.

Documentation

Relevant and detailed information – such as clinical presentation, signs and symptoms of infection, and the site and nature of the swab – should be indicated on the sample and microbiology request form. This allows the microbiology laboratory to select the most appropriate processing technique and assist in differentiating organisms that would normally be expected at a particular site from those causing infection (Weston 2008).

In accordance with the principles of good record keeping, the date and time when a swab is sent to the laboratory should be documented clearly and promptly in the patient's notes and care plan (NMC 2018). This should be done alongside documentation of the clinical nursing assessment, particularly in relation to significant findings that have prompted the collection of the sample, such as observation of inflammation or discharge at the site. This assists in the communication and dissemination of information between members of the inter-professional healthcare team.

Specimen collection: urine sampling

Definition

Urine samples are intended to identify any organisms causing infection within the urinary tract. Urinalysis encompasses the tests that involve microbiological, chemical, microscopical and physical examination of the urine (Higgins 2013, Pagana and Pagana 2017). Urinary tract infections (UTIs) result from the presence and multiplication of bacteria in one or more structures of the urinary tract with associated tissue invasion (Keogh 2017, Pagana and Pagana 2017, PHE 2018c).

Related theory

Protection against infection is normally given by the constant flow of urine and regular bladder emptying, which prevent the colonization of micro-organisms (PHE 2018c). The urethra is colonized with naturally occurring flora but urine proximal to the distal urethra is normally sterile. As urine passes through the urethra, some of these micro-organisms are flushed through and normal urine will naturally contain a small number of bacteria. Therefore, the presence of bacteriuria is insignificant in the absence of clinical symptoms of an infection (Keogh 2017, Pagana and Pagana 2017, Weston 2008).

UTIs account for up to 20% of all hospital-acquired infections overall. This is the second largest group of infections in the healthcare setting (PHE 2018c). The majority of the 20% are generally catheter-related infections with only 2–6% actual UTIs (PHE 2018c). UTIs in adults are common, particularly in women due to the short female urethra and its close proximity to the perineum, but age, sex and predisposing factors are other important considerations (PHE 2018c).

Evidence-based approaches

Rationale

Urine sample requests for microscopy, culture and sensitivity constitute the largest single category of specimens examined in microbiological laboratories. The main value of urine culture is to identify bacteria and their sensitivity to antibiotics (Higgins 2013).

Urine sampling should be considered in combination with clinical assessment and urinalysis to avoid unnecessary sample processing, which has time and cost implications for the microbiology laboratory (Pagana and Pagana 2017; Thomas 2008). A clinical assessment involves examining the odour, turbidity and colour; determining whether there are obvious signs of haematuria; and ascertaining whether there is pain, particularly around the suprapubic area. Urinalysis may reveal a high pH, the presence of blood, or positivity to leucocyte esterase (an enzyme released by white blood cells) or nitrite, all of which indicate a high probability of bacteriuria (Higgins 2013, Pagana and Pagana 2017).

Indications

Obtaining a urine specimen is indicated:

- when there are clinical signs and symptoms to indicate a UTI
- if there are signs of a systemic infection or in patients with a pyrexia of unknown origin

- on development of new patient confusion as toxicity from infection can cause alterations in mental status or impairments in cognitive ability (Pagana and Pagana 2017; Pellowe 2009).

Principles of care

Urine may be collected using a midstream urine (MSU) clean-catch technique or from a catheter using a sterile syringe to access the sample port (PHE 2018c). To minimize the contamination of a specimen by bacteria (which may be present on the skin, the perianal region or the external genital tract), good hand and genital hygiene should be encouraged. Therefore, patients should be encouraged to wash their hands prior to collecting a clean-catch MSU specimen and to clean around the urethral meatus prior to sample collection (Higgins 2013).

The principle for obtaining a midstream collection of urine is that any bacteria present in the urethra are washed away in the first portion of urine voided and therefore the specimen collected more accurately represents the urine in the bladder. A study conducted by Jackson et al. (2005) using a urinary collection device showed a reduction in contamination compared with other MSU techniques. However, a study in pregnant women found that there was no difference between MSU, clean-catch samples and morning samples with regard to potential contamination (Schneeberger et al. 2013).

Catheter-associated urinary tract infections

The presence of a urinary catheter and the amount of time *in situ* are contributory factors in the development of a UTI. For every day the catheter remains *in situ*, the risk of bacteriuria is 5%, such that 50% of patients catheterised for longer than 7–10 days will have bacteriuria (Pellowe 2009). Although often asymptomatic, up to 30% of patients with bacteriuria will develop symptoms of catheter-associated UTIs (CAUTIs), with 1–4% of those subsequently developing bacteraemia or sepsis, with an obvious impact on patient morbidity and increased hospital length of stay.

In order to minimize CAUTIs, catheters should only be inserted where absolutely necessary and should not be placed for the management of urinary incontinence except in exceptional circumstances when all other management methods have been unsuccessful. Additional techniques – such as closed catheter systems, antimicrobial coated catheters and carrying out drainage bag changes according to the manufacturer's guidance – can reduce the risk of a CAUTI (Hooton et al. 2010, Loveday et al. 2014).

Pre-procedural considerations

Equipment

Specimen jars for urine collection must be sterile to ensure no contamination occurs, as this may lead to an incorrect diagnosis and inappropriate treatment. The jar must close securely to prevent leakage of the sample and have a CE marking (PHE 2018c) (see Figure 13.2).

Specific patient preparation

When collecting an MSU, the patient must pass a small amount of urine before collecting the specimen. This reduces the risk of contamination of the specimen with naturally occurring micro-organisms and/or flora within the urethra. Periurethral cleansing is recommended although the need for this has been questioned in both men and women as its effectiveness has been debated (PHE 2018c, Saint and Lipsky 1999).

Procedure guideline 13.21 Urine sampling: midstream specimen of urine: male

Essential equipment

- Personal protective equipment
- Cleaning solution (e.g. soap and water, 0.9% sodium chloride or disinfectant-free solution)
- Sterile specimen container with wide opening (CE marked)
- Appropriate documentation/forms

Action	Rationale
Pre-procedure	
1 Introduce yourself to the patient, explain and discuss the procedure with them, and gain their consent to proceed.	To ensure that the patient feels at ease, understands the procedure and gives their valid consent (NMC 2018, **C**).
2 Fully explain the steps of the procedure.	The patient needs to fully understand the procedure in order to avoid inadvertent contamination of the specimen and optimize the quality of the sample (Higgins 2008a, **E**).
3 Ensure a suitable private location.	To maintain patient privacy and dignity. **E**
Procedure	
4 Ask patient to wash hands with soap and water.	To reduce the risk of cross-infection (NHS England and NHSI 2019, **C**).
5 *If practitioner's assistance is required*: wash hands with bactericidal soap or decontaminate physically clean hands with alcohol rub and put on apron.	To prevent cross-contamination (NHS England and NHSI 2019, **C**).
6 Ask patient to retract the foreskin and clean the skin surrounding the urethral meatus with soap and water, 0.9% sodium chloride or a disinfectant-free solution.	To optimize general cleansing and minimize contamination of the specimen with other organisms. **E** Disinfectant solutions may irritate the urethral mucous membrane (Higgins 2013, **E**).
7 Ask patient to begin voiding first stream of urine (approx. 15–30 mL) into a urinal, toilet or bedpan.	To commence the flow of urine and avoid contamination of the specimen with naturally occurring micro-organisms and/or flora within the urethra (PHE 2018c, **C**).
8 Place the wide-necked sterile container into the urine stream without interrupting the flow.	To prevent contamination of the specimen and ensure the collection of the midstream urine, which most accurately represents the urine in the bladder (PHE 2018c, **C**).

(continued)

Procedure guideline 13.21 Urine sampling: midstream specimen of urine: male (continued)

Action	Rationale
9 Ask the patient to void his remaining urine into the urinal, toilet or bedpan.	For patient to comfortably continue passing urine (PHE 2018c, **C**).
10 Allow patient to wash hands.	To maintain personal hygiene. **E**
Post-procedure	
11 Label sample immediately and complete microbiological request form (including relevant clinical information, such as signs and symptoms of infection, and antibiotic therapy).	To maintain accurate records and provide accurate information for laboratory analysis (NMC 2018, **C**; Weston 2008, **E**).
12 Dispatch sample to laboratory immediately (within 4 hours) or refrigerate at 4°C.	To ensure the best possible conditions for microbiological analysis and to prevent micro-organism proliferation (PHE 2018c, **C**).
13 Document the procedure in the patient's records.	To ensure timely and accurate record keeping (NMC 2018, **C**).

Procedure guideline 13.22 Urine sampling: midstream specimen of urine: female

Essential equipment

- Personal protective equipment
- Cleaning solution (e.g. soap and water, 0.9% sodium chloride or disinfectant-free solution)
- Sterile specimen container with wide opening (CE marked)
- Appropriate documentation/forms

Action	Rationale
Pre-procedure	
1 Introduce yourself to the patient, explain and discuss the procedure with them, and gain their consent to proceed.	To ensure that the patient feels at ease, understands the procedure and gives their valid consent (NMC 2018, **C**).
2 Fully explain the steps of the procedure.	The patient needs to fully understand the procedure in order to avoid inadvertent contamination of the specimen and optimize the quality of the sample (Higgins 2008a, **E**).
3 Ensure a suitable private location.	To maintain patient privacy and dignity. **E**
Procedure	
4 Ask patient to wash hands with soap and water.	To reduce the risk of cross-infection (NHS England and NHSI 2019, **C**).
5 *If practitioner's assistance is required*: wash hands with bactericidal soap or decontaminate physically clean hands with alcohol rub and put on apron.	To prevent cross-contamination (NHS England and NHSI 2019, **C**).
6 Ask the patient to part the labia and clean the urethral meatus with soap and water, 0.9% sodium chloride or a disinfectant-free solution.	To optimize general cleansing and minimize contamination of the specimen with other organisms. **E** Disinfectant solutions may irritate the urethral mucous membrane (Higgins 2013, **E**).
7 Use a separate swab for each wipe and wipe downwards from front to back.	To prevent cross-infection and perianal contamination (Weston 2008, **E**).
8 Ask the patient to begin voiding first stream of urine (approx. 15–30 mL) into a toilet or bedpan while separating the labia.	To commence the flow of urine and avoid contamination of the specimen with naturally occurring micro-organisms and/or flora within the urethra (PHE 2018c, **C**).
9 Place the wide-necked sterile container into the urine stream without interrupting the flow.	To prevent contamination of the specimen and to ensure the collection of the midstream urine, which most accurately represents the urine in the bladder (PHE 2018c, **C**).
10 Ask the patient to void her remaining urine into the toilet or bedpan.	For patient to comfortably continue passing urine (PHE 2018c, **C**).
11 Allow patient to wash hands.	To maintain personal hygiene. **E**
Post-procedure	
12 Label sample immediately and complete microbiological request form (including relevant clinical information, such as signs and symptoms of infection, and antibiotic therapy).	To maintain accurate records and provide accurate information for laboratory analysis (NMC 2018, **C**; Weston 2008, **E**).
13 Dispatch sample to laboratory immediately (within 4 hours) or refrigerate at 4°C.	To ensure the best possible conditions for microbiological analysis and to prevent micro organism proliferation (PHE 2018c, **C**).
14 Document the procedure in the patient's records.	To ensure timely and accurate record keeping (NMC 2018, **C**).

Procedure guideline 13.23 Urine sampling: catheter specimen of urine

Essential equipment

- Personal protective equipment
- Sterile gloves
- Syringe
- Non-traumatic clamps
- Appropriate documentation/forms
- Universal specimen container
- Alcohol-based swab

Action	Rationale
Pre-procedure	
1 Introduce yourself to the patient, explain and discuss the procedure with them, and gain their consent to proceed.	To ensure that the patient feels at ease, understands the procedure and gives their valid consent (NMC 2018, **C**).
2 Ensure a suitable private location.	To maintain patient privacy and dignity. **E**
3 Prepare equipment and place on sterile trolley.	To prepare equipment for use. **E**
Procedure	
4 *If no urine is visible in catheter tubing:* wash and/or decontaminate physically clean hands with alcohol rub, put on apron and apply non-sterile gloves prior to manipulating the catheter tubing.	To minimize the risk of cross-infection (NHS England and NHSI 2019, **C**).
5 Apply non-traumatic clamp a few centimetres distal to the sampling port.	To ensure sufficient sample has collected to allow for accurate sampling (Higgins 2013, **E**).
6 Wash hands with bactericidal soap and water, or decontaminate physically clean hands with alcohol rub and put on gloves.	To prevent cross-contamination (NHS England and NHSI 2019, **C**).
7 Wipe sampling port with 2% chlorhexidine in 70% isopropyl alcohol and allow to dry for 30 seconds.	To decontaminate sampling port and prevent false-positive results (NHS England and NHSI 2019, **C**).
8 In a needleless system: insert syringe firmly into centre sampling port (according to manufacturer's guidelines), aspirate the required amount of urine and remove syringe.	To reduce the risk of sharps injury (European Biosafety Network 2010, **C**).
9 Transfer an adequate volume of the urine specimen (approx. 10 mL) into a sterile container immediately.	To avoid contamination and to allow for accurate microbiological processing (PHE 2018c, **C**).
10 Discard needle and syringe into sharps container.	To reduce the risk of needle stick injury. **E**
11 Wipe the sampling port with an alcohol wipe and allow to dry for 15 seconds.	To reduce contamination of access port and reduce the risk of cross-infection (DH 2007, **C**).
Post-procedure	
12 Unclamp catheter tubing.	To allow drainage to continue. **E**
13 Dispose of waste, remove apron and gloves, and wash hands.	To ensure correct clinical waste management and reduce the risk of cross-infection (DH 2013, **C**).
14 Label sample immediately and complete microbiological request form (including relevant clinical information, such as signs and symptoms of infection, and antibiotic therapy).	To maintain accurate records and provide accurate information for laboratory analysis (NMC 2018, **C**; Weston 2008, **E**).
15 Dispatch sample to laboratory immediately (within 4 hours) or refrigerate at 4°C.	To ensure the best possible conditions for microbiological analysis and to prevent micro-organism proliferation (PHE 2018c, **C**).
16 Document the procedure in the patient's records.	To ensure timely and accurate record keeping (NMC 2018, **C**).

Procedure guideline 13.24 Urine sampling: sampling from an ileal conduit

Essential equipment

- Personal protective equipment
- Sterile trolley
- Sterile dressing pack (with gloves)
- Urinary catheter (not larger than 14 Fr)
- Universal specimen container
- Clean stoma appliance
- Appropriate documentation/forms
- Sterile water or 0.9% sodium chloride

(continued)

Procedure guideline 13.24 Urine sampling: sampling from an ileal conduit *(continued)*

Action	Rationale
Pre-procedure	
1 Introduce yourself to the patient, explain and discuss the procedure with them, and gain their consent to proceed.	To ensure that the patient feels at ease, understands the procedure and gives their valid consent (NMC 2018, **C**).
2 Ensure a suitable private location.	To maintain patient privacy and dignity. **E**
3 Ensure the patient is in a comfortable position (sitting up, supported by pillows) and that the stoma is easily accessible.	For patient comfort and to allow access to the stoma. **E**
4 Prepare equipment and place on sterile trolley.	To prepare equipment for use. **E**
Procedure	
5 Wash hands with bactericidal soap and water and dry, or decontaminate physically clean hands with alcohol rub. Put on non-sterile gloves.	To prevent cross-contamination (NHS England and NHSI 2019, **C**).
6 Remove the appliance from stoma. Decontaminate hands, apply gloves and place sterile towel/pad under stoma.	To absorb any spillage from the stoma. **E**
7 Clean around the stoma with sterile water or 0.9% sodium chloride from the centre outwards.	Cleaning of the area reduces the risk of introducing surface pathogens into the ileal conduit. **E**
8 Apply gentle skin traction to make the stoma opening more visible.	To avoid the catheter coming into contact with the external surface of the stoma. **E**
9 Insert the catheter tip gently into the stoma to a depth of 2.5–5 cm only.	Gentle handling reduces the risk of ileal perforation and is more comfortable for the patient. **E**
10 Allow approximately 10 mL of drain through into a sterile specimen container.	To avoid contamination and to allow for accurate microbiological processing (PHE 2018c, **C**).
11 Remove the catheter and discard.	As catheter is no longer required. **E**
12 Change gloves, attend to stoma and apply new stoma appliance.	To ensure patient comfort. **E**
Post-procedure	
13 Dispose of waste, remove apron and gloves, and wash and/or decontaminate hands.	To ensure correct clinical waste management and reduce the risk of cross-infection (DH 2013, **C**).
14 Label sample immediately and complete microbiological request form (including relevant clinical information, such as signs and symptoms of infection, and antibiotic therapy).	To maintain accurate records and provide accurate information for laboratory analysis (NMC 2018, **C**; Weston 2008, **E**).
15 Dispatch sample to laboratory immediately (within 4 hours) or refrigerate at 4°C.	To ensure the best possible conditions for microbiological analysis and to prevent micro-organism proliferation (PHE 2018c, **C**).
16 Document the procedure in the patient's records.	To ensure timely and accurate record keeping (NMC 2018, **C**).

Procedure guideline 13.25 Urine sampling: 24-hour urine collection

Essential equipment

- Personal protective equipment
- Clean urine collection containers (e.g. wide-necked pot)
- Large urine containers with label attached for patient details
- Appropriate documentation/forms

Optional equipment

- Written patient instruction sheet

Action	Rationale
Pre-procedure	
1 Introduce yourself to the patient, explain and discuss the procedure with them, and gain their consent to proceed.	To ensure that the patient feels at ease, understands the procedure and gives their valid consent (NMC 2018, **C**).
2 Fully explain the steps of the procedure, emphasizing the importance of not discarding any urine within the 24-hour period (provide written information if needed).	The patient needs to fully understand the procedure in order to avoid inadvertent contamination of the specimen and optimize the quality of the sample. **E**

Procedure	
3 Ask patient to void urine and discard this specimen.	To establish the exact start time of the 24-hour period. **E**
4 All urine passed in the 24 hours after this appointed time should be collected in a clean urine collection container.	To ensure the specimen is representative of the variables of altering body chemistry within the 24 hours (Pagana and Pagana 2017, **E**).
5 *If catheter in situ*: completely empty catheter bag and hourly chamber (if applicable) or attach new catheter bag. Attach label indicating start time of 24-hour urine collection.	To clearly indicate to all practitioners the 24-hour collection period. **E**
6 If applicable, transfer urine from collection container into large specimen container.	To ensure specimen is collected in a suitable container for safe transportation to the laboratory. **E**
Post-procedure	
7 Label sample and complete request form.	To maintain accurate records and provide accurate information for laboratory analysis (NMC 2018, **C**; Weston 2008, **E**).
8 Dispatch sample to laboratory as soon as possible after completion of the 24-hour period.	To allow accurate laboratory processing and analysis (Higgins 2013, **E**).
9 Document the procedure in the patient's records.	To ensure timely and accurate record keeping (NMC 2018, **C**).

Post-procedural considerations

Immediate care

Urine is a very good culture medium so any bacteria present at the time of collection will continue to multiply in the specimen container. Rapid transport or special measures to ensure preservation of the sample are essential for laboratory diagnosis. The specimens should be transported and processed within 4 hours (PHE 2018c). Therefore, specimens should be processed immediately as delays of more than 2 hours at room temperature between collection and examination will yield unreliable results, suggesting falsely raised bacteriuria. If a delay occurs, the sample should be stored in a designated sample refrigerator (Higgins 2013).

Where delays in processing are unavoidable, specimens should be refrigerated at 4°C; alternatively, a boric acid preservative, which holds the bacterial population steady for 48–96 hours, should be utilized. Facilities with semi-automated urine analysers should ensure that they have been validated and follow the manufacturer's and local guidance (PHE 2018c).

Specimen collection: faecal sampling

Definition

Faecal specimens are primarily obtained for microbiological analysis to isolate and identify pathogenic bacterial, viral or parasitic organisms suspected of causing gastrointestinal (GI) infections or in patients with diarrhoea of potentially infectious aetiology (Pagana and Pagana 2017). Faecal specimens may also be obtained for other non-microbiological testing to detect the presence of other substances, such as occult blood, or as part of the national screening programme for colorectal cancer (NHS BCSP 2018).

Related theory

There are a number of enteric pathogens normally present within the GI tract, along with resident flora, that play an important role in digestion and in forming a protective, structural and metabolic barrier against the growth of potentially pathogenic bacteria (Chernecky and Berger 2013, Tortora and Derrickson 2017). Pathogenic agents that disrupt the balance within the GI tract manifest in symptoms such as prolonged diarrhoea, bloody diarrhoea, nausea, vomiting, abdominal pain and/or fever. Bacteria in faeces are representative of the bacteria present in the GI tract, so the culture of a faecal sample is necessary for identification of GI tract colonization (Chernecky and Berger 2013, Keogh 2017, Pagana and Pagana 2017).

Laboratory investigations are requested for bacterial infections such as *Salmonella spp.*, *Campylobacter spp.*, *Helicobacter spp.*, *Shigella spp.*, *Escherichia coli* and *Clostridioides difficile*; viral infections such as norovirus and rotavirus; and parasitic pathogens such as protozoa, tapeworms and amoebiasis (HPA 2014c, Weston 2008).

Diarrhoea can be defined as an unusual frequency of bowel actions with the passage of loose, unformed faeces and may be associated with other symptoms such as nausea, abdominal cramping, fever and malaise. It may be attributable to a variety of bacterial, viral or parasitic pathogens and may be associated with antibiotic use, food or travel related agents (HPA 2014c, 2016). Prompt collection of a faecal sample for microbiological investigation is essential in determining the presence and identification of such agents.

Evidence-based approaches

Rationale

Timely and accurate identification of patients with infective diarrhoea is crucial in individual management of colonization and within the context of effective infection control management. Obtaining the specimen provides important diagnostic information that can be used to decide how to manage the patient's condition and the mode of treatment (PHE 2014). Prompt diagnosis can influence aspects of care such as isolation and cohort nursing of infected patients, infection control procedures, environmental decontamination and antibiotic prescribing (Loveday et al. 2014, PHE 2014).

Indications

Collection of a faecal specimen is indicated:

- to identify an infective agent in the presence of chronic, persistent or extended periods of diarrhoea
- if patients are systemically unwell with symptoms of diarrhoea, nausea and vomiting, pain, abdominal cramps, weight loss and/or fever
- to investigate diarrhoea occurring after foreign travel
- to identify parasites, such as tapeworms
- to identify occult (hidden) blood if rectal bleeding is suspected in the presence of diarrhoea associated with prolonged antibiotic administration

- for symptomatic contacts of individuals with certain organisms where an infection can have serious clinical sequelae (PHE 2014)
- for bowel cancer screening.

Contraindications

Collection of a faecal specimen is not indicated:

- as routine testing
- in the absence of diarrhoea in suspected infective colonization.

Principles of care

A sample should be obtained as soon as possible after the onset of symptoms, ideally within the first 48 hours of illness, as the chance of successfully identifying a pathogen diminishes once the acute stage of the illness passes (Weston 2008).

Pre-procedural considerations

Assessment and recording tools

Collecting a faecal sample should be considered in conjunction with a comprehensive nursing assessment. This includes the observation of faeces for colour, presence of blood, consistency and odour (Chernecky and Berger 2013, Pagana and Pagana 2017). The most widely used assessment tool is the Bristol Stool Chart (see Figure 6.3), which categorizes faeces into seven classifications (types) based upon appearance and consistency. Samples sent to the microbiology laboratory for analysis of suspected *C. difficile* should be classified as type 6/7 on the Bristol Stool Chart.

In addition to covering other associated symptomatology (such as vomiting, fever, myalgia or abdominal pain), an accurate history should include the onset, frequency and duration of diarrhoea, and other information such as history of foreign travel or potential food poisoning.

Procedure guideline 13.26 Faecal sampling

Essential equipment

- Personal protective equipment
- Clinically clean bedpan or disposable receiver
- Sterile specimen container (CE marked) (with integrated spoon) (see Figure 13.2)
- Appropriate documentation/forms

Action	Rationale
Pre-procedure	
1 Introduce yourself to the patient, explain and discuss the procedure with them, and gain their consent to proceed.	To ensure that the patient feels at ease, understands the procedure and gives their valid consent (NMC 2018, **C**).
2 Wash hands with bactericidal soap and water, or decontaminate physically clean hands with an alcohol-based handrub. Put on apron and gloves.	To reduce the risk of cross-infection and specimen contamination (NHS England and NHSI 2019, **C**).
Procedure	
3 Ask the patient to defaecate into a clinically clean bedpan or receiver.	To avoid unnecessary contamination from other organisms. **E**
4 *If the patient has been incontinent*: a sample may be obtained from bedlinen or pads; try to avoid contamination with urine.	Urine would cause contamination of the sample (Higgins 2008b, **E**).
5 Using the integrated spoon, scoop enough faecal material to fill a third of the specimen container (or 10–15 mL of liquid stool).	To obtain a suitable amount of specimen for laboratory analysis. **E**
6 Apply specimen container lid securely.	To prevent risk of spillage. **E**
Post-procedure	
7 Dispose of waste, remove apron and gloves, and wash hands with soap and water.	To reduce the risk of cross-infection (DH 2013, **C**). Soap and water must be used as alcohol-based handrub is ineffective for *C. difficile* (DH 2010, **C**).
8 Examine the specimen for features such as colour, consistency and odour. Record observations in nursing notes and/or care plans.	To complete a comprehensive nursing assessment (NMC 2018, **C**; WHO 2015, **C**).
9 *In cases of suspected tapeworm*: segments of tapeworm are easily seen in faeces and should be sent to the laboratory for identification.	Unless the head is dislodged, the tapeworm will continue to grow. Laboratory confirmation of the presence of the head is essential (Gould and Brooker 2008, **E**).
10 Label the sample and complete the microbiology request form (including relevant information such as onset and duration of diarrhoea, fever or recent foreign travel).	To maintain accurate records and provide accurate information for laboratory analysis (NMC 2018, **C**; Weston 2008, **E**).
11 Dispatch sample to the laboratory as soon as possible or refrigerate at 4–8°C and dispatch within 12 hours.	To increase the chance of accurate organism identification and to ensure the best possible conditions for laboratory analysis (Higgins 2013, **E**).
12 *In cases of suspected amoebic dysentery*: dispatch the sample to the laboratory immediately.	The parasite causing amoebiasis must be identified when mobile and survives for a short period only. Therefore, faeces should remain fresh and warm (Kyle 2007, **E**).
13 *In cases of prolonged diarrhoea, especially in the presence of a fever*: dispatch the sample to the laboratory immediately.	Due to the risk of *C. difficile* and to ensure prompt diagnosis and initiation of appropriate infection control measures (DH 2010, **C**)
14 Document the procedure in the patient's records.	To ensure timely and accurate record keeping (NMC 2018, **C**)

Post-procedural considerations

Immediate care

A faecal sample should be transported to the laboratory and processed as soon as possible because a number of important pathogens, such as *Shigella spp.*, may not survive changes in pH and temperature once outside the body (PHE 2014). If there is an anticipated delay in dispatching the sample to the laboratory, it should be refrigerated at 4–8°C and processed within 12 hours (PHE 2014).

Ongoing care

The result of specimen analysis will determine the patient's ongoing care. The involvement of the microbiology and infection control teams is essential to ensure prudent and safe treatment and nursing care. This should include:

- effective hand-washing techniques to minimize the transmission of organisms
- implementation of standard precautions (gloves and aprons)
- nursing of patients with unexpected or unexplained diarrhoea in isolation or cohorted with other infected patients
- thorough environmental decontamination
- prudent antibiotic prescribing (NHS England and NHSI 2019).

Education of the patient and relevant others

Patients should be provided with information and involved in their care as much as they choose to be (NMC 2018). Confirmation of an infection diagnosis should be relayed to patients and their families alongside information on management strategies (such as antibiotic therapy, the use of personal protective equipment, reasons for isolation and visiting restrictions). The provision of written information, such as leaflets, may also be useful.

Specimen collection: respiratory tract secretion sampling

Definition

Obtaining a specimen from the respiratory tract is important in diagnosing various illnesses, infections and conditions, such as tuberculosis and lung cancer (Chernecky and Berger 2013, Guest 2008, Pagana and Pagana 2017). A sample can be obtained invasively or non-invasively and the correct technique will enable a representative sample to identify respiratory tract pathology and to guide treatment.

Related theory

Excessive respiratory secretions may be due to increased mucus production in cases of infection, impaired mucociliary transport or a weak cough reflex. Lower airway secretions that are not cleared provide an ideal medium for bacterial growth. Suitable microbiological analysis in diagnosing infection will depend upon (PHE 2018d):

- adequacy of lower respiratory tract specimens
- avoidance of contamination by upper respiratory tract and oral flora
- use of microscopic techniques and culture methods
- current and recent antimicrobial therapy.

Sputum is a combination of mucus, inflammatory and epithelial cells, and degradation products from the lower respiratory tract. It is never free from organisms since material originating from the lower respiratory tract has to pass through the pharynx and the mouth, which have commensal populations of bacteria (Keogh 2017, Pagana and Pagana 2017, PHE 2018d). However, it is important to ensure that material sent to the microbiology laboratory is sputum rather than a saliva sample, which will contain squamous epithelial cells and be unrepresentative of the underlying pulmonary pathology.

Evidence-based approaches

Rationale

The main aim of sputum or secretion collection is to provide reliable information on the causative agent of bacterial, viral or fungal infection within the respiratory tract and its susceptibility to antibiotics, in order to guide treatment (Chernecky and Berger 2013, Pagana and Pagana 2017, PHE 2018d).

Indications

A respiratory tract secretion specimen is indicated:

- when there are clinical signs and symptoms of a respiratory tract infection, such as a productive cough, particularly with purulent secretions
- if there are signs of systemic infection or in patients with a pyrexia (Pagana and Pagana 2017, PHE 2018d).

The presence of sputum, especially when discoloured, is commonly interpreted to represent the presence of bacterial infection and seen as an indication for antibiotic therapy. However, purulence primarily occurs when inflammatory cells or sloughed mucosal epithelial cells are present, and can result from either viral or bacterial infection (Chernecky and Berger 2013, PHE 2018d). One strategy for limiting or targeting antimicrobial prescribing is to send a respiratory tract specimen for microbiological analysis to either demonstrate that a substantial infection is not present or identify an organism for which antimicrobial treatment is deemed necessary.

The accuracy of microbiological analysis can depend on the quality of the specimen obtained as well as the time taken for transportation and the method by which it is stored and transported (Pagana and Pagana 2017, PHE 2018d).

Methods of non-invasive and semi-invasive sampling

There are various methods of non-invasive and invasive sampling methods, from self-expectoration to a bronchoalveolar lavage. A sufficient quality of sputum will yield a representative sample; early morning sputum samples are preferred as they contain pooled overnight secretions in which pathogenic bacteria are more likely to be concentrated (PHE 2018d, Philomina 2009).

Self-expectoration

For patients who are self-ventilating, co-operative and able to cough, expectorate and follow commands, a sputum sample is a suitable collection method. Sputum produced as a result of infection is usually purulent and a good sample can yield a high bacterial load. Ideally at least 1 ml of sputum should be collected (PHE 2018d). In cases of suspected *Mycobacterium tuberculosis*, three sputum specimens collected on at least three consecutive days are required (as the release of the organism is intermittent) before the pathogenic organisms can be isolated (Damani 2012, PHE 2018d). See Procedure guideline 13.27: Sputum sampling.

Nasopharyngeal samples

Nasopharyngeal suctioning is a viable alternative for patients who are obtunded or whose cough is weak (Chernecky and Berger 2013, PHE 2018d). Sampling techniques to obtain specimens from the nasopharynx are semi-invasive but can be used on patients who are self-ventilating. They are indicated in suspected viral infections such as respiratory syncytial virus (RSV), influenza and parainfluenza. The main aim is to collect epithelial cells from the posterior nasopharynx and a sample can be obtained using nasal washing or vacuum-assisted aspiration (see Procedure guideline 13.28: Nasopharyngeal wash: syringe method). This method can yield a more reliable sample because the normal flora present in the oropharynx are bypassed (Philomina 2009).

Methods of invasive sampling

Intubated patients who are unable to clear secretions independently or who require more accurate specimen collection may need a more invasive technique to obtain a sample. Invasive techniques

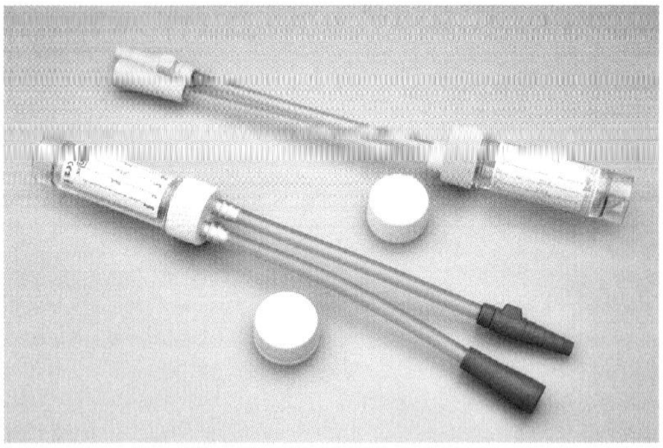

Figure 13.13 Types of vacuum-assisted sputum trap.

obtain secretions directly from the lower airway and are designed to avoid contamination by upper airway colonization, which may lead to misinterpretation of cultures (PHE 2018d).

Vacuum-assisted aspirate via endotracheal tube

Endotracheal suctioning is frequently used as a diagnostic method and to obtain specimens in intubated patients with suspected pulmonary infection. This technique bypasses the upper respiratory airways and provides an accurate microbiological result. Suctioning aids the clearance of secretions by the application of negative pressure through a sterile flexible suction catheter or a closed suction system. A sterile sputum trap is attached to the suction catheter at one end, while the other end is attached to the suction tubing to collect the sample (Figure 13.13).

Bronchoalveolar lavage

Bronchoalveolar lavage (BAL) is a reliable and accurate technique that provides a good diagnostic yield in cases of pulmonary infection, particularly invasive fungal infections and malignancies (PHE 2018d). BAL specimens are particularly useful in immunocompromised patients with diffuse pneumonia (Brooks et al. 2010). This method is used to clear secretions and to obtain washings for the retrieval of cellular and non-cellular components of the epithelial surface of the lower respiratory tract (PHE 2018d). Endotracheal aspiration can eliminate some of the contamination problems of expectoration in the sampling of sputum.

Flexible fibreoptic bronchoscopy is a relatively safe and well-tolerated means by which to obtain BAL fluid (Chernecky and Berger 2013, PHE 2018d). A flexible bronchoscope is inserted through the endotracheal tube and advanced distally into a subsegmental bronchus. The area selected for sampling is based upon a correspondent area of infiltration on a chest X-ray or by visualization of a subsegment containing purulent secretions. A volume of sterile 0.9% sodium chloride (normally 20–30 mL) is then instilled through a port on the bronchoscope and suctioned back through another port into a sterile sputum trap. The procedure is repeated three to five times and the samples are then dispatched to the laboratory for microscopy and microbiological analysis (Chernecky and Berger 2013, Keogh 2017, Pagana and Pagana 2017, PHE 2018d).

Clinical governance

Competencies

Practitioners must be competent and feel confident that they have the knowledge, skill and understanding to undertake respiratory tract secretion sampling for microbiological analysis (NMC 2018). For more advanced skills of specimen collection, such as suctioning, the practitioner should receive training and be assessed on their knowledge and understanding of the technique and potential adverse effects that may occur, such as hypoxia, cardiovascular instability and mucosal trauma (NMC 2018). BAL is normally performed by a member of the medical team who has received specialist training and has been deemed competent in the skill.

Pre-procedural considerations

Equipment

The use of vacuum-assisted and invasive suctioning techniques requires a comprehensive assessment of clinical indication and safety considerations. These include the following:

- the use of an appropriately sized, single-use, multi-eyed suction catheter, which causes less tracheal mucosal trauma; if suctioning through an endotracheal tube, the suction catheter diameter should be half the diameter or less, which prevents occlusion of the airway and avoids generation of large negative intrathoracic pressures (Russian et al. 2014) (Table 13.8)
- the use of the lowest effective suction pressure that is high enough to clear secretions while avoiding trauma to the bronchial mucosa
- the use of a suction duration time of 15 seconds to decrease the risk of adverse side-effects such as desaturation (Welch and Black 2017).

Procedures that involve suctioning present a risk of suction-induced hypoxaemia, hypertension, cardiac arrhythmias and other problems that warrant patient monitoring, in particular oxygen saturation and cardiac monitoring (Welch and Black 2017).

Pharmacological support

Adequate analgesia is a key consideration in ensuring that an effective sputum expectoration technique can be achieved. For example, pre-procedural analgesia should be given time to be effective, and wounds need to be supported to maximize inhalation and minimize pain (Guest 2008).

Nebulization of 0.9% sodium chloride and/or mucolytic agents, such as N-acetylcysteine, may need to be administered to help loosen tenacious secretions and to elicit an effective cough. However, there is no clear consensus on the effectiveness of N-acetylcysteine when compared to 0.9% sodium chloride in mechanically ventilated patients (Masoompour et al. 2015).

Non-pharmacological support

Collaboration with the physiotherapy team may assist in obtaining a good-quality sample (Welch and Black 2017). For sputum sampling, physiotherapeutic modalities may include appropriate positioning, active cycle of breathing, deep breathing and effective coughing techniques (PHE 2018d).

Specific patient preparation

Patient position is important in optimizing secretion sampling. Patients should be sat upright or on the edge of the bed, if able, or in a high semi-Fowler position (head elevated to 30–45°) in bed supported by pillows (Chernecky and Berger 2013).

The quality and quantity of secretion production and mucociliary clearance depend on systemic hydration. Patient hydration can boost sputum production and thereby enable a good sample. This can be further enhanced with sufficient airway humidity and nebulization (Chernecky and Berger 2013, Keogh 2017, Welch and Black 2017).

Table 13.8 Catheter sizes and suction pressures

Patient age	Catheter size (Fr)	Suction pressure (mmHg)
Premature infant	6	80–100
Infant	8	80–100
Toddler/preschooler	10	100–120
School age	12	100–120
Adolescent/adult	14	120–150

Procedure guideline 13.27 Sputum sampling

Essential equipment

- Personal protective equipment
- Universal container
- Appropriate documentation/form
- Eye protection (e.g. goggles/visor)

Optional equipment

- Nebulizer

Action	Rationale
Pre-procedure	
1 Introduce yourself to the patient, explain and discuss the procedure with them, and gain their consent to proceed.	To ensure that the patient feels at ease, understands the procedure and gives their valid consent (NMC 2018, **C**).
2 Fully explain the steps of the procedure.	The procedure requires the patient to fully understand and co-operate in order to optimize the quality of the sample (NMC 2018, **C**).
3 Position the patient upright in a chair or in a high semi-Fowler position, supported as necessary with pillows.	For comfort and to facilitate optimum chest and lung expansion. **E**
4 *If secretions are thick or tenacious, or are difficult to clear:* administer nebulization therapy and/or enlist the help of a physiotherapist.	To loosen secretions and assist in techniques that will optimize sputum sample collection (Welch and Black 2017, **E**).
5 Wash hands with bactericidal soap, or decontaminate physically clean hands with alcohol rub. Put on apron, gloves and eye protection.	To reduce the risk of cross-infection and splash injury to the practitioner (NHS England and NHSI 2019, **C**).
Procedure	
6 Ask the patient to take three deep breaths in through their nose, exhale through pursed lips and then force a deep cough.	Deep breathing helps to loosen secretions and a deep cough will ensure a lower respiratory tract sample is obtained. **E**
7 Ask the patient to expectorate into a clean container. Secure the lid.	To prevent contamination. **E**
Post-procedure	
8 Dispose of waste; remove apron, gloves and eye protection; and wash and/or decontaminate hands.	To ensure correct clinical waste management and reduce the risk of cross-infection (DH 2013, **C**).
9 Label the sample immediately and complete the microbiology request form (including relevant information such as indication for sample and current or recent antimicrobial therapy).	To maintain accurate records and provide accurate information for laboratory analysis (NMC 2018, **C**; Weston 2008, **E**).
10 Dispatch the sample to the laboratory as soon as possible (within 4 hours).	To increase the chance of accurate organism identification (Higgins 2013, **E**).
11 Document the procedure in the patient's records.	To ensure timely and accurate record keeping (NMC 2018, **C**).

Procedure guideline 13.28 Nasopharyngeal wash: syringe method

Essential equipment

- Personal protective equipment
- Universal container
- 5 mL syringe or wide-bore bladder syringe
- Sterile tubing cut to approximately 5–8 cm (e.g. size 8 Fr nasogastric tube or cut-off tip from a suction catheter if using a 5 mL syringe)
- 3–5 mL 0.9% sodium chloride
- Viral transport medium (if required by laboratory)
- Eye protection (e.g. goggles, visor)
- Appropriate documentation/form
- Sterile water-soluble lubricant

Action	Rationale
Pre-procedure	
1 Introduce yourself to the patient, explain and discuss the procedure with them, and gain their consent to proceed.	To ensure that the patient feels at ease, understands the procedure and gives their valid consent (NMC 2018, **C**).
2 Position the patient upright in a chair or in a high semi-Fowler position, supported as necessary with pillows.	For comfort and to facilitate optimum specimen collection. **E**

(continued)

Procedure guideline 13.28 Nasopharyngeal wash: syringe method *(continued)*

Action	Rationale
3 Wash hands with bactericidal soap, or decontaminate physically clean hands with alcohol rub. Put on apron, gloves and eye protection.	To reduce the risk of cross-infection and splash injury to the practitioner (NHS England and NHSI 2019, **C**).
Procedure	
4 Fill syringe with 3–5 mL of 0.9% sodium chloride and attach tubing to syringe tip.	To facilitate instillation of 0.9% sodium chloride high into the patient's nostril. **E**
5 Ask the patient to tilt their head backwards slightly while sitting upright.	To promote the flow of 0.9% sodium chloride into the nostril. **E**
6 Dip the end of the catheter into the water-soluble lubricant.	To facilitate comfortable passing of the catheter. **E**
7 Carefully insert the tubing into the nostril and quickly instil 0.9% sodium chloride into one nostril while holding the second nostril closed.	To facilitate optimal recovery of epithelial cells. **E**
8 Aspirate the fluid while withdrawing and rotating the tube to dislodge cells and secretions. *Note*: recovery must occur rapidly or instilled fluid will drain down the throat.	To obtain the desired nasopharyngeal specimen. **E**
9 *Either:*	
Where appropriate, the patient may tilt their head forward and gently push the fluid out of the nostril into a sterile container.	Patients may find this method more comfortable. **E**
Or:	
If aspirated: inject aspirated specimen from the syringe into suitable dry, sterile container or one containing viral transport medium, according to virology laboratory requirements.	To ensure a good-quality specimen and to prevent cross-contamination. **E**
10 Repeat procedure with the other nostril and inject the specimen into the same container (**Action figure 10**).	A combined specimen will promote optimal yield of micro-organisms. **E**
Post-procedure	
11 Dispose of waste; remove apron, gloves and eye protection; and wash and/or decontaminate hands.	To ensure correct clinical waste management and reduce the risk of cross-infection (DH 2013, **C**).
12 Label the sample immediately and complete the microbiology request form (including relevant information such as indication for sample and current or recent antimicrobial therapy).	To maintain accurate records and provide accurate information for laboratory analysis (NMC 2018, **C**; Weston 2008, **E**).
13 Dispatch the sample to the laboratory as soon as possible (within 4 hours).	To increase the chance of accurate organism identification (Higgins 2013, **E**).
14 Document the procedure in the patient's records.	To ensure timely and accurate record keeping (NMC 2018, **C**).

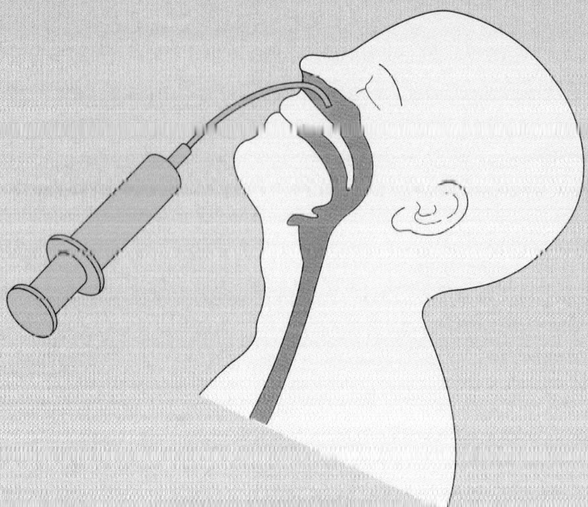

Action Figure 10 Nasopharyngeal wash: syringe method.

Procedure guideline 13.29 Nasopharyngeal wash: vacuum-assisted aspirate method

Essential equipment

- Personal protective equipment
- Suction pump (wall or portable)
- Sterile suction catheter (see Table 13.8 for appropriate size)
- Sterile sputum trap
- Viral transport medium (if required by laboratory)
- Sterile gloves
- Eye protection (e.g. goggles, visor)
- Appropriate documentation/form
- Sterile water-soluble lubricant

Action	Rationale
Pre-procedure	
1 Introduce yourself to the patient, explain and discuss the procedure with them, and gain their consent to proceed.	To ensure that the patient feels at ease, understands the procedure and gives their valid consent (NMC 2018, **C**).
2 Position the patient upright in a chair or in a high semi-Fowler position, supported as necessary with pillows.	For comfort and to facilitate optimum specimen collection. **E**
3 Wash hands with bactericidal soap, or decontaminate physically clean hands with alcohol rub. Put on apron and eye protection.	To reduce the risk of cross-infection and splash injury to the practitioner (NHS England and NHSI 2019, **C**).
Procedure	
4 Attach suction tubing to the male adapter of the specimen trap and attach the rubber tubing on the trap to the end of the suction catheter, leaving the packaging on.	To enable correct set-up and to ensure the suction catheter remains sterile. **E**
5 Turn suction on and adjust to correct pressure (see Table 13.8).	To ensure suction pressure is high enough to clear secretions while avoiding trauma. **E**
6 Put on sterile gloves and remove the suction catheter from the packaging aseptically.	To prevent cross-contamination of the specimen. **E**
7 Ask the patient to tilt their head backwards slightly while sitting upright.	To optimize recovery of specimen collection. **E**
8 Dip the end of the catheter into the water-soluble lubricant.	To facilitate comfortable passing of the catheter. **E**
9 Without applying suction, carefully insert the catheter into the nostril and direct it posteriorly towards the external ear (**Action figure 9**). *Note*: the depth of insertion necessary to reach the posterior pharynx is equivalent to the distance between the anterior naris and the external ear.	To prevent damage to the nasopharynx and to minimize patient discomfort. **E**
10 Apply suction. Using a rotating movement, slowly withdraw the catheter. *Note*: the catheter should remain in the nasopharynx for no longer than 10 seconds.	To prevent damage to the nasopharynx and to obtain the desired nasopharyngeal specimen. **E** To reduce the risk of hypoxaemia, mucosal damage and atelectasis. **E**
11 Hold the trap upright to prevent secretions being suctioned into the suction pump.	To prevent loss of the specimen. **E**

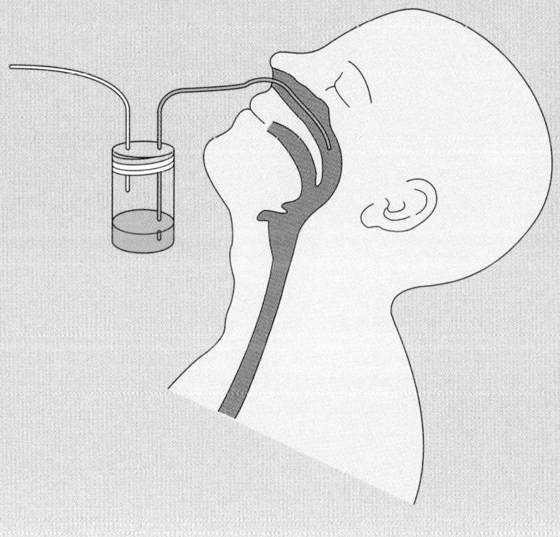

Action Figure 9 Nasopharyngeal wash: vacuum-assisted aspirate method.

(continued)

Procedure guideline 13.29 Nasopharyngeal wash: vacuum-assisted aspirate method *(continued)*

Action	Rationale
12 Rinse the catheter (if necessary) with approximately 10–20 mL of viral transport medium.	To ensure maximum recovery of epithelial cells and to prevent cross-contamination (Higgins 2013, **E**).
13 Disconnect suction. Depending on the sputum trap type, connect the tubing to the arm of the sputum trap to seal, or detach and apply the sealable lid.	To ensure the specimen container is securely sealed and to prevent cross-contamination. **E**
Post-procedure	
14 Dispose of waste; remove apron, gloves and eye protection; and wash and/or decontaminate hands.	To ensure correct clinical waste management and to reduce the risk of cross-infection (DH 2013, **C**).
15 Label the sample immediately and complete the microbiology request form (including relevant information such as indication for sample and current or recent antimicrobial therapy).	To maintain accurate records and provide accurate information for laboratory analysis (NMC 2018, **C**; Weston 2008, **E**).
16 Dispatch the sample to the laboratory as soon as possible (within 4 hours).	To increase the chance of accurate organism identification (Higgins 2013, **E**).
17 Document the procedure in the patient's records.	To ensure timely and accurate record keeping (NMC 2018, **C**).

Post-procedural considerations

Immediate care

Many organisms responsible for infection of the lower respiratory tract do not survive well outside the host, so specimens should be dispatched to the laboratory immediately and processed within 2 hours. If there is an anticipated delay in dispatching the sample to the laboratory, it should be refrigerated at 4–8°C and sent as soon as possible (PHE 2018d).

Documentation

The date and time when a sputum sample is sent to the laboratory should be documented clearly and promptly in the patient's notes and care plan (NMC 2018). This should be done alongside documentation in relation to significant findings that have prompted the collection of the sample (such as a description of the type and colour of the sputum and/or secretions) and the method used to obtain the sample.

Specimen collection: pleural fluid

Definition

Specimens of pleural fluid for microbiological analysis are obtained via thoracocentesis to assist in the diagnosis of infection in fluid that has accumulated within the inner and outer (visceral and parietal) layers of the pleural cavity; such infections can include parapneumonia, empyema and tuberculosis (Chernecky and Berger 2013, Pagana and Pagana 2017). In the context of microbiological analysis, thoracocentesis is the insertion of a needle into the pleural space to obtain a fluid sample for diagnostic testing (Pagana and Pagana 2017).

Anatomy and physiology

See Chapter 12: Respiratory care, CPR and blood transfusion.

Related theory

Pleural fluid is generated from pleural vessels as a result of negative intrapleural pressure. It exits via the parietal pleural lymphatic system. Pleural effusions occur when there is an accumulation of fluid within the pleural cavity, which implies an increased production of fluid that exceeds the capacity of lymphatic removal and/or obstruction of drainage of the pleural space (Chernecky and Berger 2013, Pagana and Pagana 2017, PHE 2018e).

Analysis of pleural effusion fluid is obtained via thoracocentesis, which determines the cause of the effusion. Effusion occurs when factors that influence the formation and absorption of fluid are altered either systematically, for example in cirrhosis or congestive heart failure (transudate effusions), or locally, for example in infection or malignancy (exudate effusions). Pleural fluid in a patient with undiagnosed exudative effusions should be cultured for bacteria (aerobic and anaerobic), mycobacteria and fungi (Chernecky and Berger 2013, PHE 2018e).

Infection of pleural fluid caused by bacteria, viruses or fungi may originate in the pleura or translocate from another site. Micro-organisms can infiltrate the pleural space by various routes: directly in cases of empyema or a primary tuberculous focus rupturing into the pleural cavity; from an adjacent area of pneumonia, thoracic surgery or drainage; from chest trauma; or from transdiaphragmatic spread from intra-abdominal infection (PHE 2018e).

Pleural fluid is clear and straw-coloured, and contains a small number of white blood cells but no red blood cells or micro-organisms (PHE 2018e). In cases of suspected infection, it appears cloudy due to the presence of micro-organisms and/or increased white blood cells (Chernecky and Berger 2013, Pagana and Pagana 2017). Differential white blood cell counts assist further in the diagnosis of infection because increased numbers of neutrophils indicate bacterial infection. Other changes include decreased glucose levels, increased protein or albumin levels, and disturbances in lactate level.

Evidence-based approaches

Rationale

Detection of micro-organisms in fluids that are normally sterile indicates significant infection (PHE 2018e). Pleural fluid may be sent to the microbiology laboratory for bacterial culture to identify the cause of an effusion, isolate pathogenic micro-organisms and establish susceptibility to antimicrobial therapy.

Indications

Obtaining a specimen of pleural fluid is indicated in patients with:

- bacterial pneumonia with radiological suggestion of significant pleural effusions
- systemic infection with pyrexia, severe pleuritic pain and leucocytosis
- suspected tuberculous focus with clinical signs or radiological evidence of significant pleural effusions (PHE 2018e).

Methods of pleural fluid collection

Diagnosis of infection is established via the microbiological analysis of pleural fluid obtained by thoracocentesis using a strict aseptic technique, including meticulous skin antisepsis (Chernecky and Berger 2013, Pagana and Pagana 2017).

Following clinical assessment and possibly radiological guidance, local anaesthetic is infiltrated into the area of intended thoracocentesis. A needle is advanced superiorly to the ribs to avoid neuromuscular bundle damage and to reduce the risk of causing a pneumothorax (Pendharkar and Tremblay 2007). Between 50 and 100 mL of fluid is drawn, transferred into a sterile container and sent to the laboratory for analysis.

The samples can initially be observed for characteristics such as colour and turbidity, and gram stains allow for direct observation of bacteria under a microscope. When bacterial infection of pleural fluid is suspected, a specimen should be drawn and inoculated directly into aerobic and anaerobic blood culture bottles (Pendharkar and Tremblay 2007).

Specimens should be dispatched to the laboratory immediately and liaison with the laboratory is essential to enable efficient processing of the sample. If there are any delays, the sample should be refrigerated at 4°C (PHE 2018e).

Endoscopic investigations

Definition

Occasionally, patients will be required to undergo further invasive diagnostic procedures such as an endoscopy. An endoscopy is the direct visual examination of the GI tract (Figure 13.14) and it may include gastroscopy or colonoscopy. Endoscopy allows the practitioner to evaluate the appearance of the visualized mucosa for the purpose of diagnosis and therapeutic procedures (Chernecky and Berger 2013, Pagana and Pagana 2017).

Gastroscopy

Definition

A gastroscopy, or oesophagogastroduodenoscopy, is a procedure in which a long, flexible endoscope is passed through the mouth, allowing the doctor or nurse endoscopist to look directly at the mucosal lining of the oesophagus, stomach and proximal duodenum. The endoscope is generally less than 10 mm in diameter but a larger scope may be required for therapeutic procedures where suction channels are required (Chernecky and Berger 2013, Pagana and Pagana 2017) (Figure 13.14).

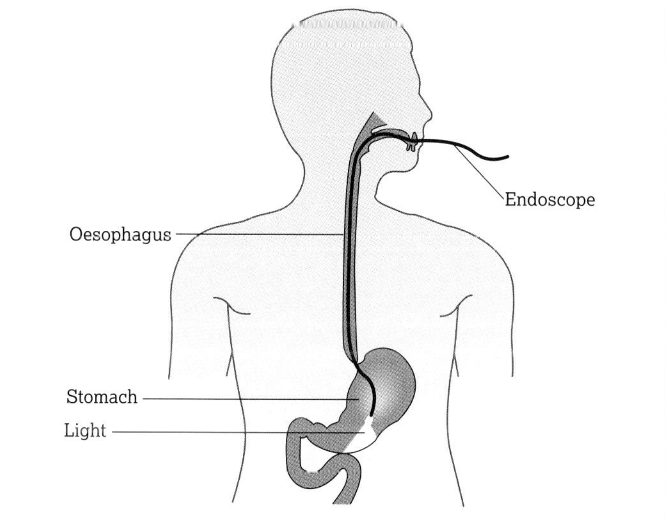

Figure 13.14 Endoscopy. *Source*: Reproduced with permission of the patient information website of Cancer Research UK (www.cancerresearchuk.org/cancerhelp).

Anatomy and physiology

See Figure 13.15.

Oesophagus

The oesophagus is a muscular thin-walled tube approximately 25 cm long and about 2 cm in diameter. It is located behind the trachea and in front of the vertebral column. It begins at the inferior end of the laryngopharynx and ends at the stomach. There are two sphincters within the oesophagus: the upper or hypopharyngeal sphincter and the lower gastro-oesophageal or cardiac sphincter. The upper moves food from the pharynx to the oesophagus and the lower enables the food to pass into the stomach. The oesophagus has three layers – the mucosa, submucosa and muscularis – with the innermost layer consisting of stratified squamous epithelium (Tortora and Derrickson 2017).

Stomach

The stomach connects the oesophagus to the small intestine or duodenum. It is a J-shaped dilated portion of the alimentary tract and one of its functions is as a holding reservoir and mixing chamber. It is located between the epigastric, umbilical and left hypochondriac regions of the abdomen. It is divided into four regions: the cardia, fundus, body and pyloric part. Distally, the pyloric sphincter is located between the stomach and the duodenum. The stomach has three muscle layers to allow for gastric motility to move the contents adequately whereas other parts of the alimentary tract only have two muscle layers (Tortora and Derrickson 2017).

Duodenum

The duodenum is part of the small intestine. It is approximately 25 cm long and 3.5 cm in diameter and is the shortest region. It begins at the pyloric sphincter of the stomach and joins the jejunum.

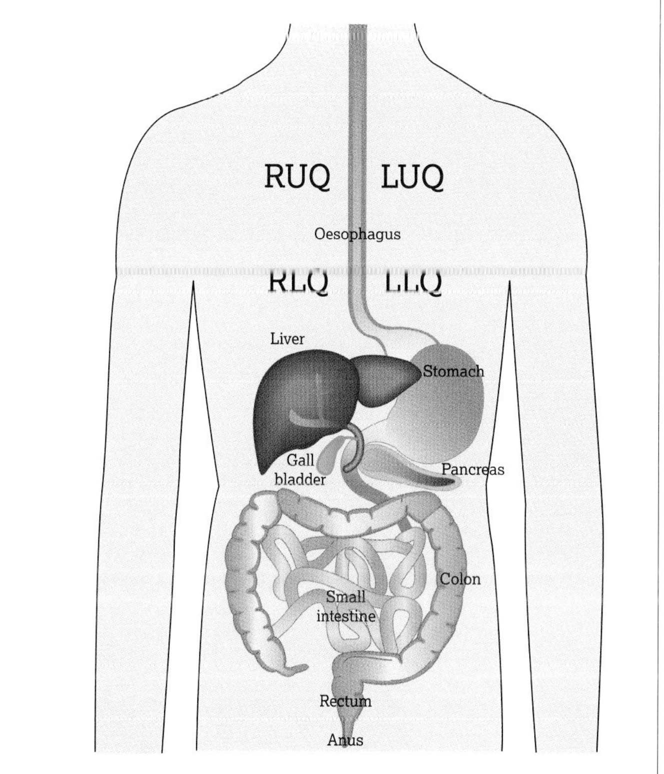

Figure 13.15 Anatomy of the lower gastrointestinal tract. RUQ, right upper quadrant; LUQ, left upper quadrant; RLQ, right lower quadrant; LLQ, left lower quadrant.

Both the pancreas and the gallbladder release secretions into the duodenum (Tortora and Derrickson 2017).

Evidence-based approaches

Rationale

A gastroscopy is undertaken to investigate symptoms originating from the upper GI tract, such as reflux and dysphagia. The doctor or nurse endoscopist uses direct vision to diagnose, sample and document changes in the upper GI tract.

Indications

Indications for gastroscopy include:

- dysphagia
- odynophagia
- achalasia
- unresponsive reflux disease
- gastric and peptic ulcers
- haematemesis and melaena
- suspected carcinoma
- oesophageal or gastric varices
- monitoring Barrett's oesophagus disease.

Contraindications

Contraindications for gastroscopy include:

- fractured base of skull
- metastatic adenocarcinoma
- some head and neck tumours
- thrombocytopenia
- symptoms that are functional in origin.

Clinical governance

Nurse endoscopists

In some centres, nurse endoscopists work alongside medical endoscopists to undertake endoscopy. In 1995, the British Society of Gastroenterology began to support the development of non-medical endoscopists. The nurse endoscopist must work within their own professional boundaries and complement the medical endoscopist teams (BSG 2005, Smith and Watson 2005). Studies have shown that nurse endoscopists perform procedures at a high standard and adhere to international standards, and most patients had no specific preference for a doctor or nurse endoscopist and expressed high satisfaction (Tursi 2013, Van Putten et al. 2012). It is essential that all practitioners are adequately trained in the administration of conscious sedation and are aware of its side-effects and reversal agents. Conscious sedation is used to relax the patient, minimize pain during the procedure and improve procedural efficiency (Choi 2012). Clinical units must also limit the possibility of overdose, particularly with midazolam, as highlighted by the National Patient Safety Agency (NPSA) (2008b).

Consent

It is essential that valid consent is obtained prior to any investigation, as previously discussed in this chapter. This is important as conscious sedation may be utilized during this procedure.

Governance

It is a priority that an organization providing endoscopic services has clear, identifiable policies and procedures. There must be open, bidirectional communication between the department, organizational board and national bodies to ensure that appropriate care is delivered. Monitoring processes must be in place to identify potential clinical or organizational risks, and there must be a clear reporting mechanism.

Risk management

The organization must ensure that relevant policies and procedures are in place to reduce risk. Responding to national alerts and guidance is essential, as is implementing relevant evidence. In 2008, the NPSA (2008b) issued an alert regarding the use of midazolam during conscious sedation. It had been found that some patients were receiving an overdose of midazolam with a subsequent over-reliance on the use of flumazenil as a reversal agent.

Pre-procedural considerations

Equipment

To conduct a gastroscopy, a flexible side- or end-viewing endoscope is required. The endoscope allows visualization of the oesophagus, stomach and proximal duodenum (Chernecky and Berger 2013, MacKay et al. 2010, Pagana and Pagana 2017, Smith and Watson 2005). Access to resuscitation equipment is also essential if conscious sedation is going to be administered (BSG 2007).

Assessment and recording tools

A medical and nursing history and assessment must be undertaken to identify any care needs or concerns that may be significant, in particular the patient's current drug therapy, drug reactions and allergies, any organ dysfunctions (such as cardiac and/or respiratory disease), and previous and current illnesses. It is also important to be aware of any coagulopathies, as samples of tissue or biopsy may need to be taken during the procedure. This can be pre-empted by reviewing blood results prior to the gastroscopy. A set of observations (including temperature, pulse, blood pressure, respiration rate and oxygen saturations) should also be taken to identify any pre-procedural abnormalities and provide a baseline. If the patient has diabetes, their blood glucose level should be checked (BSG 2003, 2007, MacKay et al. 2010, Pagana and Pagana 2017, Smith and Watson 2005).

Pharmacological support

Prior to the procedure, a local anaesthetic spray may be used on the back of the throat. In some cases, conscious sedation may be administered. This technique involves the administration of a benzodiazepine such as midazolam in small doses. Doses must be titrated for elderly patients or those with co-morbidities such as cardiac or renal failure (BNF 2019). Oxygen therapy should also be administered for patients at risk of hypoxia and those requiring sedation. Generally, 2 L per minute is adequate for most circumstances to maintain oxygen saturation levels and prevent hypoxaemia (BSG 2003, 2007).

Specific patient preparation

The patient must fast for at least 4–8 hours prior to the gastroscopy to ensure that the stomach is relatively empty. Clear fluids may be taken up to 2 hours before, but local guidelines must be followed. This increases the visual field for the endoscopist and also minimizes the risk of aspiration if the patient vomits (Kang and Hyun 2013, Saied et al. 2012). If the patient has undergone previous gastric surgery, this fasting time may be longer, depending on the type of surgery, to ensure gastric emptying (Ahn et al. 2013).

The nurse can assist by getting the patient to lie on their left side on the trolley (Chernecky and Berger 2013, Pagana and Pagana 2017, Smith and Watson 2005). If a sedative is used, it is essential that the patient is monitored with pulse oximetry and observed for any respiratory depression. Nursing staff can observe and record oxygen saturations and respiratory rate. ECG (electrocardiography) monitoring may only be required if a patient is at risk of cardiac instability during the procedure (BSG 2003).

Post-procedural considerations

Immediate care

Physiological monitoring must continue in the immediate recovery period. Supplemental oxygen and oxygen saturations may be required, especially if a sedative has been used. The patient should avoid drinking or eating for an hour after the use of the throat spray to minimize the risk of aspiration. Once stable, awake and reviewed by the team, the patient may be discharged or transferred to another department (BSG 2003, 2007).

Ongoing care

It is recommended that patients who have been sedated with an intravenous benzodiazepine do not drive a car, operate machinery, sign legal documents or drink alcohol for 24 hours (BSG 2003). This is irrespective of whether their sedation has been reversed with flumazenil. The patient must be accompanied home if they have been given a sedative. The accompanying adult should stay with the patient for 12 hours at home if they live alone. It is important to remember that aspiration pneumonia may develop hours or days later and the patient should be informed to report any symptoms such as temperature or breathing difficulty (BSG 2003, 2007, Smith and Watson 2005).

Documentation

Any samples should be clearly documented with the appropriate forms, as previously discussed in this chapter. All drugs administered, complications and/or findings should be documented.

Complications

Respiratory depression

If oversedation occurs, respiratory function will be affected. It is essential that close monitoring occurs during and after the procedure. A reversal agent may be required, such as flumazenil for midazolam (BSG 2003, NPSA 2008b, Pagana and Pagana 2017, Smith and Watson 2005).

Perforation

Although rare, it is possible that perforation of the oesophagus, stomach or duodenum may occur. Further medical and/or surgical intervention will be required to manage this potential complication (Borgaonkar et al. 2012, Pagana and Pagana 2017, Smith and Watson 2005).

Haemorrhage

Where biopsy samples have been taken, this may increase the risk of post-procedural bleeding. Further intervention may be required to stop the bleeding. Patients should be advised to seek medical assistance if, following discharge, there are signs of bleeding that include the presence of fresh blood in the sputum and melaena (Chernecky and Berger 2013).

This will be dependent on the specific aetiology of the bleed; for example, if it is from varices, variceal band ligation may be required (Borgaonkar et al. 2012, Pagana and Pagana 2017, SIGN 2008, Smith and Watson 2005).

Colonoscopy

Definition

A colonoscopy is conducted by inserting a colonoscope through the anus into the colon. It provides information regarding the lower GI tract and allows a complete examination of the colon. The colonoscope is similar to the endoscope used in gastroscopy. Its length ranges from 1.2 to 1.8 m. It is the most effective method of diagnosing rectal polyps and carcinoma (MacKay et al. 2010, Pagana and Pagana 2017, Smith and Watson 2005, Swan 2005, Taylor et al. 2009).

Anatomy and physiology

The large intestine is about 1.5 m long. It begins at the ileum and ends at the anus. The four major structures are the caecum, colon, rectum and anal canal (Tortora and Derrickson 2017) (see Figure 13.15).

Caecum

The caecum is about 6 cm long and opens from the ileum and ileocaecal valve (Tortora and Derrickson 2017).

Colon

The colon consists of three parts. The ascending colon runs from the caecum and joins the transverse colon and the hepatic flexure. The transverse colon is in front of the duodenum, where it joins the descending colon at the splenic flexure. The descending colon travels down towards the middle of the abdomen, where it joins the sigmoid colon, which is S-shaped and becomes the rectum (Tortora and Derrickson 2017).

Rectum and anal canal

The rectum is approximately 20 cm long and is a dilated section of the colon. It joins the anal canal, which is approximately 2–3 cm long (Tortora and Derrickson 2017).

Evidence-based approaches

Rationale

A colonoscopy is performed to investigate specific symptoms originating from the lower GI tract, such as bleeding. The endoscopist uses direct vision to diagnose, sample and document changes in the lower GI tract (MacKay et al. 2010, Pagana and Pagana 2017, Taylor et al. 2009).

Indications

Colonoscopy is indicated in the following circumstances:

- screening of patients with a family history of colon cancer, which is a serious but highly curable malignancy
- determining the presence of suspected polyps
- monitoring ulcerative colitis
- monitoring diverticulosis and diverticulitis
- active or occult lower GI bleeding
- unexplained bleeding or faecal occult blood specifically in patients aged 50 years or over
- abdominal symptoms, such as pain or discomfort, particularly if associated with weight loss or anaemia
- chronic diarrhoea, constipation or a change in bowel habits
- surveillance of inflammatory bowel disease
- population screening for colorectal carcinoma
- palliative supportive treatments, such as stent insertion.

Contraindications

Colonoscopy is contraindicated in the following circumstances:

- upper GI bleeding
- acute diarrhoea
- recent colon anastomosis
- toxic megacolon
- pregnancy (Chernecky and Berger 2013, Pagana and Pagana 2017).

Clinical governance

Competencies and consent

Competencies and consent are the same as those discussed in the section on gastroscopy, above.

Risk management

The NPSA (2009) has highlighted the risks in relation to bowel preparation and actions required to minimize these. Harm to patients has occurred where oral bowel preparations were prescribed to those with definite contraindications; however, the majority of the incidents (56%) were related to the administration of the bowel preparations (Connor et al. 2012). The NPSA (2009) identified that one death and 218 patient safety incidents resulting in moderate harm were related to the use of oral bowel preparations where contraindications were not considered or assessed.

Pre-procedural considerations

Equipment

A colonoscope is a flexible endoscope that generally uses fibreoptics to allow direct visualization of the rectum and colon (Chernecky and Berger 2013, MacKay et al. 2010, Pagana and Pagana 2017, Smith and Watson 2005).

Pharmacological support

Bowel preparation agents, such as senna tablets and Citramag, are given to the patient to take 1 day before the colonoscopy to clear the bowel and minimize faecal contamination (Connor et al. 2012). A sedative and possibly an analgesic are usually administered before the procedure. This involves the administration of a benzodiazepine such as midazolam and an opioid such as fentanyl or pethidine. Doses must be titrated for elderly patients and those with co-morbidities such as cardiac or renal failure. An antispasmodic may also be given. Oxygen therapy should also be administered during sedation. Generally, 2 litres per minute is adequate for most circumstances to maintain oxygen saturation levels and prevent hypoxaemia (BSG 2007, Connor et al. 2012, MacKay et al. 2010, Riley 2008).

Specific patient preparation

A medical and nursing history and assessment must be undertaken to identify any care needs or concerns that may be significant. In particular, this should cover the patient's current drug therapy, drug reactions and allergies, any organ dysfunctions (such as cardiac and/or respiratory disease), and previous and current illnesses. It is also important to be aware of any coagulopathies, as samples of tissue or biopsy may need to be taken during the procedure. This can be pre-empted by reviewing blood results prior to the colonoscopy (Chernecky and Berger 2013, Pagana and Pagana 2017).

To complete a successful colonoscopy, the bowel must be clean so that the physician can clearly view the colon. Most patients will require a bowel preparation. It is very important that the patient is given clear written instructions for bowel preparation well in advance of the procedure. Without proper preparation, the colonoscopy will not be successful and the test may have to be repeated. The patient must be individually assessed before being supplied with the bowel preparation and the potential contraindications, considered below.

The choice of bowel preparation must consider the advantages and disadvantages of each product, the tolerability, efficacy and possible side-effects. If the patient feels nauseated or vomits while taking the bowel preparation, they are advised to wait 30 minutes before drinking more fluid and start with small sips of solution. Some activity such as walking or a few cream crackers may help decrease the nausea (Connor et al. 2012, Smith and Watson 2005, Swan 2005).

Two days prior to the colonoscopy, specific light foods may be eaten, such as steamed white fish, and others avoided, such as high-fibre foods. On the day before the colonoscopy, breakfast from the approved food groups may be eaten while drinking plenty of clear fluids. The period of bowel cleansing generally should not be longer than 24 hours. On the day of the procedure, patients can drink tea or coffee with no milk 4 hours before and water up to 2 hours before. Some patients who are at risk of hypovolaemia and dehydration may need to be admitted to hospital for pre-hydration (Connor et al. 2012, MacKay et al. 2010, Smith and Watson 2005, Swan 2005).

A set of observations (including temperature, pulse, blood pressure, respiration rate and oxygen saturations) should also be taken to identify any pre-procedural abnormalities and provide a baseline. If the patient has diabetes, their blood glucose level should be checked (BSG 2003, 2007, Connor et al. 2012, Smith and Watson 2005).

Contraindications to bowel preparation

Bowel preparation is contraindicated in the following circumstances:

- GI obstruction, perforation, ileus or gastric retention
- severe acute inflammatory bowel disease
- toxic megacolon
- a reduction in consciousness level
- allergies or hypersensitivity to bowel preparation
- the inability to swallow
- ileostomy (Connor et al. 2012).

Post-procedural considerations

Immediate care

Physiological monitoring and care post-sedation should be the same as those for gastroscopy. However, larger doses of sedative and opioids may have been used so further observation is required. The patient may feel some cramping or a sensation of having gas, but this quickly passes on eating and drinking. Bloating and distension typically occur for about an hour after the examination until air in the bowel that developed during the procedure is expelled. Unless otherwise instructed, the patient may immediately resume a normal diet, but it is generally recommended that the patient waits until the day after the procedure to resume normal activities (BSG 2007, MacKay et al. 2010).

Ongoing care

If a biopsy was taken or a polyp was removed, the patient may notice light rectal bleeding for 1–2 days after the procedure. Large amounts of bleeding, the passage of clots or abdominal pain should be reported immediately.

Complications

Polypectomy syndrome

When an endoscopic mucosal resection (EMR) or an endoscopic submucosal dissection (ESD) is conducted, a thermal injury to the bowel wall may occur. The patient may present with localized tenderness and pyrexia. Generally, conservative management is adequate, but it is essential to monitor the patient's condition as they may go on to develop a perforation (MacKay et al. 2010).

Perforation

During the procedure, the greatest risk or possible complication is bowel perforation; this may be apparent during the procedure but it can present 3–4 days after the procedure. It occurs in 1 in 1000 cases (MacKay et al. 2010, Pagana and Pagana 2017). If a snare polypectomy was conducted, the incidence of perforation is 0.1–0.3%. The incidence rises to 5% following an EMR (MacKay et al. 2010, Smith and Watson 2005). The nurse monitoring the patient after colonoscopy should be familiar with potential signs and symptoms, such as unresolved abdominal pain, rigidity and/or bleeding. If a perforation occurs, surgical intervention is likely to be required (MacKay et al. 2010, Pagana and Pagana 2017, Smith and Watson 2005, Suissa et al. 2012).

Haemorrhage

On average, haemorrhage occurs in 3 in 1000 procedures but the incidence and complication rates may be higher where a procedure involves a polypectomy. MacKay et al. (2010) state that the incidence post-polypectomy should be less than 1%, and it should be 0.5–6.0% following EMR. Post-procedure monitoring by the nurse again includes observing for signs and symptoms of bleeding (MacKay et al. 2010, Smith and Watson 2005). Depending on the severity of the bleed, it may be managed conservatively, but embolization may be required in haemodynamically unstable patients (MacKay et al. 2010, Pagana and Pagana 2017, Suissa et al. 2012).

Cystoscopy

Definition

A flexible cystoscopy is a camera examination used to visualize the lower urinary tract, including the urethra (or prostatic urethra), sphincter, bladder and ureteric orifices. Cystoscopy can assist in identifying problems with the urinary tract, such as early signs of bladder cancer, infection, strictures, obstruction, bleeding and other abnormalities; it is also used for surveillance of bladder cancer. Furthermore, it is an effective method for removing ureteric stents when they are no longer therapeutically indicated and in some cases treating bladder abnormalities. The procedure is performed under local anaesthetic with the patient awake in a dedicated outpatient facility (Kumar and Clark 2016, Tortora and Derrickson 2017).

Anatomy and physiology

Urethra

The urethra extends from the external urethral orifice to the bladder (Tortora and Derrickson 2017).

Male urethra

The male urethra is approximately 20 cm long and provides a common pathway for urine, semen and reproductive organ secretions. The three parts of the male urethra are the prostatic urethra, the membranous urethra and the spongy or penile urethra. Originating at the urethral orifice of the bladder, the prostatic urethra passes through the prostate gland (Figure 13.16). The narrowest and shortest part of the urethra is the membranous urethra, originating at the prostate gland and extending to the bulb of the penis. The penile urethra ends at the urethral orifice (Tortora and Derrickson 2017).

Female urethra

The female urethra is located behind the symphysis pubis and opens at the external urethral orifice (Figure 13.17). It is approximately 4 cm long (Tortora and Derrickson 2017).

Evidence-based approaches

Rationale

A cystoscopy is undertaken to gain direct visualization of the urethra and the bladder to aid diagnosis of urological complications and diseases such as bladder cancer (British Association of Urological Surgeons 2013, Pagana and Pagana 2017).

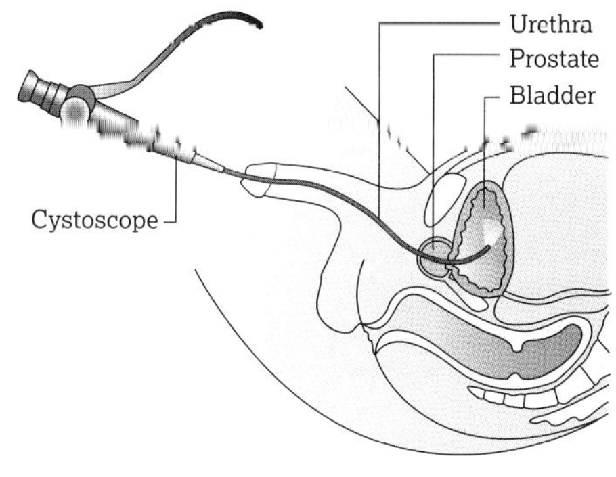

Figure 13.16 Cystoscopy for a man. *Source*: Reproduced with permission of the patient information website of Cancer Research UK (www.cancerresearchuk.org/cancerhelp).

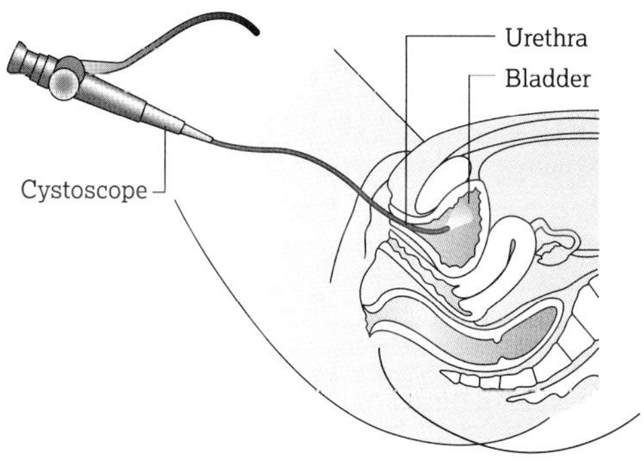

Figure 13.17 Cystoscopy for a woman. *Source*: Reproduced with permission of the patient information website of Cancer Research UK (www.cancerresearchuk.org/cancerhelp).

Indications

Indications for cystoscopy include:

- bladder dysfunction
- unexplained haematuria
- diagnosis of bladder cancer
- staging of bladder cancer
- obstruction or strictures
- dysuria.

Contraindications

Confirmed urinary tract infection (UTI) is a contraindication for cystoscopy.

Pre-procedural considerations

Equipment

A cystoscope may be flexible or rigid. A rigid cystoscope is utilized in the operating theatre, where the patient is anaesthetized. The flexible cystoscope (Figure 13.18) is used with a video stack (Figure 13.19) and can be used in the outpatient setting with local anaesthesia. The flexible cystoscope is useful for patients who require more regular examinations for follow-up after bladder cancer treatment (Chernecky and Berger 2013, Fillingham and Douglas 2004, Pagana and Pagana 2017).

Specific patient preparation

It is essential that the patient does not have a UTI as the organism responsible for the infection may be spread into the bloodstream during the procedure. A dipstick and/or midstream urine test should be performed at least one week prior to a flexible cystoscopy to exclude a UTI. If the patient is having a general anaesthetic, they will have to fast prior to the procedure, depending on anaesthetic instruction. Prior to the procedure, patients undergoing a local anaesthetic can usually eat and drink as normal and should empty their bladder prior to the procedure. It may be necessary for some patients to be treated with antibiotics before the procedure to reduce the risk of infection (American Urological Association 2012, Pagana and Pagana 2017).

Post-procedural considerations

Immediate care

Depending on the type of procedure, recovery will vary. After a general anaesthetic, the patient will recover under the care of dedicated nursing staff. In the outpatient setting, physiological observations may be required. Nursing staff should monitor the patient for signs of haematuria, infection, urinary retention and excessive pain in the abdomen or urethral area. It is also possible that the patient may experience bladder spasms, which can be minimized

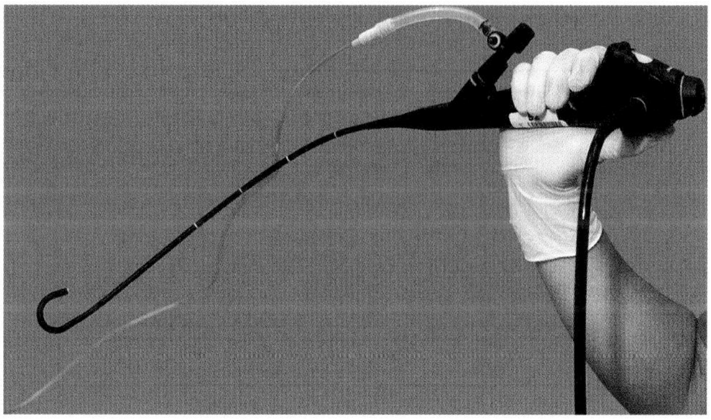

Figure 13.18 A flexible cystoscope. *Source*: Reproduced from Dougherty et al. (2019). © 2019 The Royal Marsden NHS Foundation Trust. Published 2019 by John Wiley & Sons, Ltd.

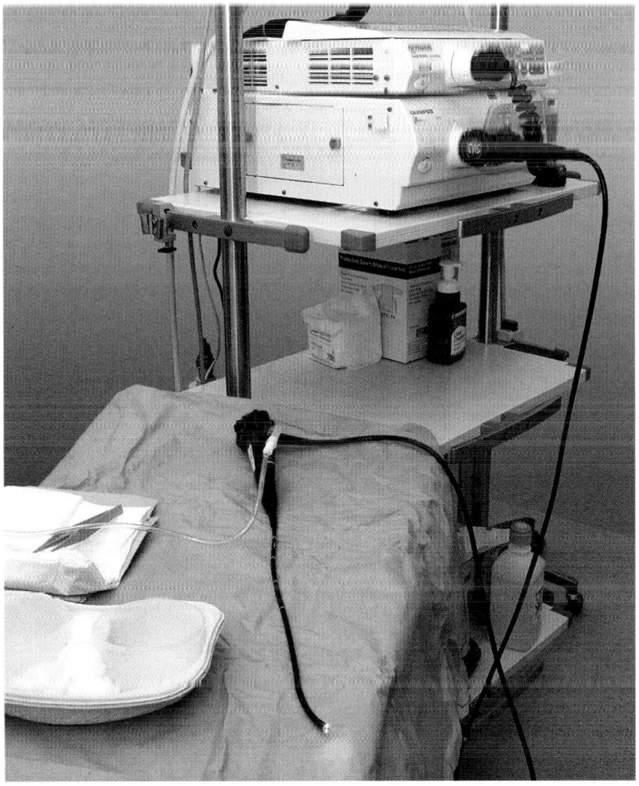

Figure 13.19 A video stack.

with prescribed analgesics. Oral fluids should be encouraged (Chernecky and Berger 2013, Pagana and Pagana 2017).

Ongoing care

It is common for patients to experience some burning sensations while passing urine for a few days. It is advised that patients drink plenty of water post-procedure to flush the bladder and reduce the risk of infection. Any signs of excessive bleeding should be reported to the medical team (Chernecky and Berger 2013, Pagana and Pagana 2017).

Complications

There are various potential complications associated with a flexible cystoscopy. These include infection, bleeding, urinary retention and pain. If any of these symptoms arise, the patient should be reviewed by a clinician (Chernecky and Berger 2013, Pagana and Pagana 2017).

Liver biopsy

Definition

Liver biopsy involves percutaneous puncture using a biopsy needle and removal of a small piece of the liver to diagnose pathological liver conditions (Al Knawy and Shiffman 2007, Pagana and Pagana 2017).

Anatomy and physiology

The liver is the heaviest organ in the body. It weighs approximately 1.4 kg and is highly vascular. It is incompletely covered by a layer of peritoneum and enclosed in a thin inelastic capsule. There are two main lobes in the liver: the large right lobe and the smaller left lobe, which is wedge shaped. The caudate and quadrate lobes are on the posterior surface and are continuations of the left lobe (Tortora and Derrickson 2017).

Functions of the liver

The liver has many functions, including:

- carbohydrate metabolism and contributing to maintenance of blood glucose levels
- lipid metabolism
- protein metabolism: converting ammonia into urea
- drug and hormone processing: detoxifying the body
- activation of vitamin D
- excretion of bilirubin
- phagocytosis of some bacteria and aged blood cells
- storage of some vitamins, iron, copper and glycogen (Tortora and Derrickson 2017).

Evidence-based approaches

Rationale

A liver biopsy is an invaluable tool for diagnosing or monitoring conditions affecting the liver, such as cirrhosis, inflammation or hepatitis of various causes, and some metabolic liver disorders. The risks, although small, must be weighed against the potential benefits (Pagana and Pagana 2017, Tannapfel et al. 2012).

Indications

Liver biopsy is indicated in the following circumstances:

- diagnosis of cirrhosis
- diagnosis of cancer, both primary and secondary
- miliary tuberculosis
- amyloidosis
- viral hepatitis for grading, staging and exclusion of co-morbidities
- diagnosis of autoimmune diseases affecting the liver
- grading and staging of chronic hepatitis B or C.

Contraindications

Liver biopsy is contraindicated in the following circumstances:

- an unco-operative or confused patient
- severe purpura
- coagulation defects
- prolonged clotting time
- increased bleeding time
- severe jaundice
- patient under 3 years of age
- current right lower lobe pneumonia
- current pleuritis (Pagana and Pagana 2017, Tannapfel et al. 2012).

Methods of liver biopsy

There are a variety of methods for conducting a liver biopsy. The ultrasound-guided technique is considered the standard (Tannapfel et al. 2012).

Percussion palpation approach

The percussion palpation approach is also known as the 'blind approach'. The liver is palpated in order to determine the position required for the liver biopsy.

Image-guided approach

Image guidance may be conducted using ultrasound, CT or MRI, but the preferred method is ultrasound. The ultrasound method utilizes continuous ultrasound or site marking immediately prior to the procedure (Al Knawy and Shiffman 2007, Pagana and Pagana 2017).

Ultrasound-assisted approach

The ultrasound is utilized immediately prior to the procedure and a mark is left on the skin indicating the puncture site. It is also known as the 'X marks the spot' technique. This technique has been shown to yield larger tissue samples, require fewer needle passes and have a decreased biopsy failure rate than the non-ultrasound-assisted approach (Di Teodoro et al. 2013).

Ultrasound-guided approach

The ultrasound is utilized throughout the procedure with the liver and biopsy needle viewed in real time. This method is simple, reasonably fast, inexpensive and safer than other methods. In 1% of cases, significant complications have been reported with a mortality of 0.1% (Tannapfel et al. 2012).

Transjugular liver biopsy

When the percutaneous approach is contraindicated due to coagulopathy, vascular tumours, ascites or failed percutaneous attempts, the transjugular technique is indicated and is a safer approach (BSG 2004). The biopsy needle is inserted via the hepatic vein and this approach avoids the peritoneum and liver capsule (Keshava et al. 2008).

Pre-procedural considerations

Equipment

Aspiration- or suction-type needle

There are a few varieties of aspiration- or suction-type needles, such as the Jamshidi needle, Klatskin needle and Menghini needle (Figure 13.20). The Menghini needle has a retaining device to minimize the risk of the sample being aspirated into the syringe and is the most commonly used. It is 6 cm long and approximately 1.4 mm wide.

Cutting-type needles

The Tru-Cut and Vim-Silverman needles utilize a cutting sheath to obtain the specimen. They are advanced approximately 2–3 cm into the liver and a sample of 1–2 cm with a diameter of 1 mm is collected. These needles are associated with low failure rates but they also have higher complication rates (Karamshi 2008).

Automated spring-loaded needle biopsy guns

Automated spring-loaded needle biopsy guns automatically trigger and insert the needle. These generally only require one hand to operate, allowing the clinician to use the other hand for visual guidance, such as the use of ultrasound (Karamshi 2008).

Pharmacological support

Medications should be reviewed by medical and nursing staff and arrangements made by the medical team for alternative anticoagulant and diabetic medication if necessary. A local anaesthetic, such as lidocaine 2%, is infiltrated into the area where the biopsy is to be taken. In some cases, where the patient is extremely anxious, conscious sedation may be considered (Al Knawy and Shiffman 2007).

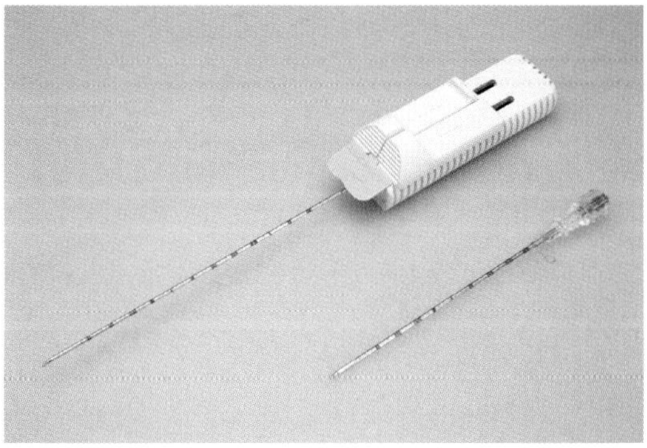

Figure 13.20 Liver biopsy needles. *Source*: Reproduced from Dougherty et al. (2019). © 2019 The Royal Marsden NHS Foundation Trust. Published 2019 by John Wiley & Sons, Ltd.

Specific patient preparation

Nursing staff should take a nursing history, reviewing social and medical history and determining allergy status. Up to 7 days prior to the procedure, the referring medical team must ensure that a full blood count, clotting screen and biochemistry have been taken. Nursing staff should review bloods as part of their pre-procedure assessment. If a patient is currently taking an anticoagulant such as warfarin, a clotting sample must be taken within 24 hours of the procedure.

A baseline set of physiological observations must be undertaken. If conscious sedation is used, the patient must be nil by mouth and they must have patent intravenous access (Academy of Medical Royal Colleges 2013, Australian and New Zealand College of Anaesthetists 2014). The patient is usually in the supine position with the right side as close to the edge of the bed as possible. The left side may be supported by a pillow. The patient's right hand is positioned under their head and their head turned to the left. Oxygen therapy may be required if there are pre-existing conditions or when conscious sedation is used. The patient may be asked to hold their breath at the end of expiration so nursing staff should explain this prior to the procedure (Karamshi 2008, Pagana and Pagana 2017).

Post-procedural considerations

Immediate care

Immediately following the procedure, the patient must lie on their right side for 3 hours and remain on bedrest for a total of 6 hours. They may be able to go to the toilet after 3 hours. Physiological observations are required every 15 minutes for the first hour and every 30 minutes for the following 2 hours; the frequency can then be reviewed by the registered nurse (Chernecky and Berger 2013, Karamshi 2008, Pagana and Pagana 2017). Any abnormality must be reported to the medical team immediately. The nurse should also observe the puncture site and abdomen for signs of bleeding and ensure that pain is adequately controlled. Pain is the most common problem reported by patients and can develop within 3 hours of the procedure, so it may be necessary to record the patient's pain scores and provide analgesia. Severe pain must always be reported to the medical team as it may be an indicator of a bleed or bile leak (Karamshi 2008, Pagana and Pagana 2017). The patient may also require emotional care throughout and after the procedure (Karamshi 2008).

Ongoing care and education

A post-procedure information sheet should be given to the patient identifying possible complications and instructions on what to do if any symptoms occur (Chernecky and Berger 2013, Pagana and Pagana 2017).

Complications

Haemorrhage

An inadvertent puncture of an intrahepatic or extrahepatic blood vessel can lead to haemorrhage manifesting within 4 hours. However, it is normal to lose approximately 5–10 mL of blood from the surface of the liver after the biopsy. Conservative management with blood products may be appropriate but surgical intervention may also be required to treat haemorrhage (Chernecky and Berger 2013, Karamshi 2008).

Peritonitis

An inadvertent puncture of the bile duct that consequently results in bile leaking into the peritoneal cavity can lead to peritonitis. Treatment may range from antimicrobial therapy to surgical and/or critical care intervention depending on the severity (Chernecky and Berger 2013, Karamshi 2008, Pagana and Pagana 2017).

Pneumothorax

An inadvertent puncture of the pleura can lead to a pneumothorax. If this occurs, urgent medical intervention is required. A formal chest drain may be necessary to relieve the pneumothorax (Chernecky and Berger 2013, Denzer et al. 2007, Pagana and Pagana 2017).

Radiological investigations: X-ray

Definition

An X-ray is a short-wavelength dose of electromagnetic radiation that passes through matter and is used in diagnostic radiology and radiotherapy (Martin 2010).

Evidence-based approaches

Rationale

The general X-ray department performs a wide range of examinations, many of which require no patient preparation in advance and can often be performed on the day of the request. In accordance with the Ionizing Radiation (Medical Exposure) Regulations (2017), known as IR(ME)R, to ensure radiation safety, there is a requirement for radiologists to justify and radiographers to authorize and optimize radiation exposure of a patient.

Indications

Diagnostic X-rays are performed to diagnose medical conditions such as damage to the skeletal structures and organ dysfunction, for example chest X-rays for respiratory complications.

Contraindications

IR(ME)R prohibits any medical exposure from being carried out that has not been justified and authorized, and provides an optimization process to ensure that doses arising from exposures are kept 'as low as reasonably practicable' (ALARP), consistent with the diagnostic task.

It is also necessary to be aware of the Protection of Pregnant Patients during Diagnostic Medical Exposures to Ionizing Radiation guidelines, issued by the Royal College of Radiologists, the Health Protection Agency and the College of Radiographers (2009). For women known or likely to be pregnant, where the examination has been justified on the basis of clinical urgency and involves irradiation of the abdomen, operators must optimize the technique to minimize irradiation of the foetus. Radiography of areas remote from the foetus, for example the chest, skull or hand, may be carried out safely at any time during pregnancy as long as good beam collimation and proper shielding equipment are used.

Clinical governance

IR(ME)R sets out the legal roles and responsibilities of all duty holders related to medical exposures to X-rays. In accordance with IR(ME)R, the completed request form for a medical exposure must be clear and legible and the following information must be supplied:

- unique patient identification, to include at least three identifiers from name, date of birth, hospital number and NHS number
- sufficient details of the clinical problem to allow the IR(ME)R practitioner to justify the medical exposure or the IR(ME)R operator to authorize it, and indication of examination thought to be appropriate
- if applicable, information on the patient's possible pregnancy status
- signature uniquely identifying the referrer as it is important that the referrer is qualified to order an X-ray.

Blank request cards, pre-signed by a referrer, are a breach of the regulations. Any entries on the request form made by others should be checked and initialled by the referrer prior to signing the form.

Competencies

IR(ME)R requires employers to only accept requests for X-ray or nuclear medicine investigations from approved and authorized 'referrers'. When the referrer is not a trained medical doctor or dentist, they must have received appropriate information, instruction and training in clinical assessment and radiation protection of the patient, and the scope and range of investigations for which they are authorized to request must be documented. All 'referrers' must be made aware of the appropriate referral criteria for such investigations, as set down by each individual's organization in its IR(ME)R procedures and protocols.

Risk management

Radiation protection is based on the three principles of justification, optimization and limitation:

- The procedure must be *justified* and be of net benefit to the patient.
- *Optimization* ensures that exposure to the patient, staff and public must be as low as reasonably practicable (ALARP).
- *Limitation* is essential to ensure that radiation doses to staff and members of the public do not exceed the dose limits (IR(ME)R 2017).

Note that there are no dose limits for patient exposures.

Pre-procedural considerations

Pharmacological support

For some types of X-ray, such as the barium swallow or enema, the patient is usually required to drink the contrast or have it administered via an enema, and a series of X-ray pictures is taken at various intervals. Afterwards, the patient must be advised to drink plenty of fluids to clear their system of the contrast as quickly as possible (Chernecky and Berger 2013).

Specific patient preparation

The radiology department should inform the patient of any requirements prior to the booked procedure, such as being nil by mouth. For most examinations, the patient will be asked to remove some of their clothing and change into a hospital gown, to ensure that no artefacts (any feature in an image that misrepresents the object in the field of view) are caused in the area of clinical interest on the X-ray image (McRobbie 2007). It is advisable for the patient not to wear jewellery at the time of the appointment as in most cases this will have to be removed, again to prevent the presence of artefacts on the image. For all X-rays, the patient will be required to keep still to prevent any blurring of the images. Some procedures are performed on inspiration or expiration, and the patient will be given the appropriate breathing instructions by the operator performing the procedure (Chernecky and Berger 2013).

Magnetic resonance imaging (MRI)

Definition

Magnetic resonance imaging is a non-invasive diagnostic scanning technique that provides cross-sectional images of the body. The patient lies inside the bore of a very strong magnet, typically 1.5 tesla, although 3 tesla scanners are becoming increasingly prevalent. Protons in the body's water molecules spin or 'precess' when exposed to such a strong magnetic field. Radio waves are transmitted into the patient at the same frequency at which the protons are precessing and the patient transmits a signal, which is detected by a receiver coil (Chernecky and Berger 2013, Pagana and Pagana 2017).

Evidence-based approaches

Rationale

Soft tissue structures (such as the brain, spinal cord, musculoskeletal system, liver and pelvic structures) are particularly well demonstrated using MRI. Although MRI is often targeted to particular areas of the body, it is also possible to scan the whole body with scan times ranging from 20 to 60 minutes. MRI is increasingly being used as a tool in radiotherapy treatment planning (Prestwich et al. 2012) and can be used to guide interventional procedures, for example breast biopsies (O'Flynn et al. 2010, Pagana and Pagana 2017). MRI does *not* use ionizing radiation and can therefore be used for repeated examinations, which is useful for the evaluation of radiotherapy and chemotherapy response during cancer treatments. The magnetic field is always present so strict safety procedures are necessary to protect staff and patients (Pagana and Pagana 2017; Shellock and Spinazzi 2008).

An MRI may be used instead of a computed tomography (CT) scan as the contrast between normal and pathological tissue is better and there are no obscuring bone artefacts. Blood vessels also appear dark from the fast-moving blood; therefore, this results in a natural contrast between the blood vessels and the surrounding tissues (Pagana and Pagana 2017).

Indications

There are various indications for an MRI, which include:

- scanning of the brain to assess for stroke, tumour or meningeal disease
- evaluation of the central nervous system, neck, back and heart
- evaluation of the back, bones, soft tissues and joints
- spinal pathology, including intervertebral disc pathology, tumour, infarction, spinal dysraphism, infection and degenerative diseases (spinal pathology is particularly well demonstrated)
- differentiation and characterization of benign versus malignant pathology in the liver
- imaging of the breast (MRI is particularly sensitive for this area)
- assessment of pelvic malignancy and pelvic anatomy (MRI is the gold standard for this area) (Keogh 2017, Pagana and Pagana 2017, Royal College of Radiologists 2012).

MRI scans (Table 13.9) can also be used to identify and quantify various conditions.

Contraindications

Patients with non-MRI-compatible implanted devices, such as cardiac pacemakers and cochlear implants, must not be scanned. Other implanted devices, for example stents, must be confirmed as MRI-safe prior to scanning. Other contraindications are confused or agitated patients and patients weighing more than 140 kg, unless specified by the manufacturer. If a patient is claustrophobic and an enclosed scanner is used, a medical review is required and antianxiety medications may be prescribed (Pagana and Pagana 2017).

Magnetic resonance imaging tends not to be used for acute trauma, for which CT is usually the preferred imaging modality. Nor is it generally used for primary whole-body staging of malignancies, although a role for whole-body MRI is increasingly being proposed in some areas for non-oncological and oncological diagnostic purposes (Lambregts et al. 2011, Lin et al. 2013).

Pre-procedural considerations

Assessment and recording tools

A pre-MRI checklist must undertaken for all patients to identify risks from implanted devices that may be harmful to the patient or that may severely degrade the image quality (Chernecky and Berger 2013, Pagana and Pagana 2017, Shellock and Spinazzi 2008).

Pharmacological support

The patient may require intravenous access for contrast injection, most often of a gadolinium-based contrast agent. This is used to enhance areas of suspected pathology, to define tumour bulk or to improve the efficacy of the scan by delineation or characterization of a pathological process. It is important to be aware of potential allergies and that gadolinium-based contrasts have been linked to nephrogenic fibrosing dermopathy (NFD) and nephrogenic systemic fibrosis (NSF) (Pagana and Pagana 2017; Runge et al. 2009). These contrast agents may be contraindicated in patients with poor renal function and therefore recent blood tests – such as for creatinine,

Table 13.9 Common MRI scans

Scan area	Potential findings
MRI of brain and meninges	Benign and malignant neoplasms Brain oedema Intracranial haemorrhage
Magnetic resonance spectroscopy (MRS)	Enhanced image of high-grade malignancy Chemical abnormalities of the brain related to the human immunodeficiency virus (HIV)
Magnetic resonance angiography (MRA)	Possible arterial blockages Cardiac abnormalities Aortic aneurysm
MRI of breast	Localized staging of breast cancer Surgical staging Fracture of a breast implant
MRI of heart	Evaluation of pericardial disease Congenital heart disease
Magnetic resonance cholangiopancreatography (MRCP)	Images of pancreas, pancreatic duct, gall bladder and biliary tree Pancreatobiliary stones, infection and tumours Underlying cause of pancreatitis
MRI of liver	Liver and biliary tumours
Magnetic resonance enterography (MRE)	Inflammatory bowel disease
MRI of cervical or lumbar spine	Herniated disc

Source: Adapted from Keogh (2017), Pagana and Pagana (2017).

glomerular filtration rate (GFR) and/or blood urea nitrogen (BUN) – may be required to demonstrate adequate renal function (Pagana and Pagana 2017). It is also routine practice in some centres to administer antispasmodic agents prior to abdominal or pelvic scans to reduce bowel peristalsis and improve image quality.

Claustrophobia can also be an issue and in some cases patients may require an oral sedative to relax them during the procedure. In severe claustrophobia or when scanning young children or individuals with learning difficulties, sedation or a general anaesthetic may be necessary. This will require specialist nursing and anaesthetic support with continuous vital sign monitoring and predominantly support by the emergency or critical care teams.

Non-pharmacological support

The scanner is very noisy so it is mandatory that patients are given ear protection during the scan. If the patient feels mildly claustrophobic but not enough to consider pharmacological support, there are strategies to manage this, such as:

- adapting the patient's position
- changing the scanning technique
- using blindfolds or mirrors
- relaxation therapy (Chernecky and Berger 2013).

Specific patient preparation

Apart from safety checking, for most scans there is no preparation. However, for certain body scans the patient may have to abstain from food but may drink clear (non-caffeine) fluids to ensure their bladder does not fill too quickly, resulting in movement artefacts (Chernecky and Berger 2013).

Patients must be able to lie very still, usually on their back, for significant time periods. Patient comfort is paramount so patients requiring pain relief should continue with pain medication as normal.

Procedure

The patient lies on the MRI table and is positioned as required. If needed, the contrast medium is administered and then the radiographer moves the patient into the scanner.

Post-procedural considerations

Immediate care

It is important to ensure that any intravenous cannula used to administer a contrast medium is removed post procedure. If the patient required sedation, cannula removal, post-sedation monitoring and observations will be required. Patients who have had a sedation or anaesthetic will need to be accompanied home by a relative or other responsible adult (Chernecky and Berger 2013).

Computed tomography (CT)

Definition

Computed tomography is also known as a CT or CAT scan. The CT images are created when radiation passes through the patient and is absorbed in varying degrees by the body tissue. A three-dimensional and cross-sectional view of the structures is then produced (Keogh 2017, Pagana and Pagana 2017).

Evidence-based approaches

Rationale

Multi slice CT has an excellent image resolution and is used for diagnosis, staging and monitoring treatment as well as being a research tool. The scan produces detailed images of the structures within the body. Soft tissues, bone and other anatomy (such as the lungs) are all seen well on CT scans. Patients can be given an intravenous iodine-containing contrast medium, which perfuses the body tissues and enhances the images (Husband and Reznek 2010, Pagana and Pagana 2017).

A CT scan uses radiation, but protocols are optimized to give the best image with the lowest dose. Additionally, the number of body areas scanned and the intervals between scans are closely monitored in accordance with IR(ME)R (2017) regulations.

Indications

CT can image all parts of the body and is used for:

- diagnosis
- pre-treatment cancer staging
- interval scans to monitor treatment
- follow-up post-treatment
- diagnosis and assessment of complications:
  - bowel obstructions and perforation
  - pulmonary embolism
  - stroke and cerebral bleeds
- perfusion CT
- guidance during procedures such as biopsies (Chernecky and Berger 2013, Keogh 2017).

CT scans (Table 13.10) can also be used to identify and quantify various conditions.

Table 13.10 Common CT scans

Scan area	Potential findings
Brain/head	Tumours Infarction Bleeding Haematoma Degenerative abnormalities such as multiple sclerosis and Alzheimer's disease
Chest	Chest wall: fracture of ribs or thoracic spine, tumour Diaphragm: hernia Heart: pericarditis, pericardial effusion Lungs: tumours, pneumonia, pleural effusion, tuberculosis Mediastinum: enlarged lymph nodes
Abdomen and pelvis	Adrenal gland: cancer, adenoma, haemorrhage Gallbladder and biliary system: gallstones, tumours Gastrointestinal system: appendicitis, inflammatory bowel disease, perforation, tumours, diverticulitis Kidneys: calculi, cysts, obstruction, tumours Liver: abscess, bile duct dilation, tumours Pancreas: bleeding, inflammation, tumours, pseudocysts Peritoneum: abscess, ascites Prostate: tumours Retroperitoneum: lymphadenopathy, abdominal aneurism, tumours Spleen: laceration, haematoma, tumours, thrombus (venous) Uterus, ovaries and fallopian tubes: cysts, fibroids, infection, tumours, abscess
Full body	All of the above Obstructions Tumours Fluid collection Bleeding Foreign objects Inflammation or infection

Source: Adapted from Keogh (2017), Pagana and Pagana (2017).

Contraindications

CT is contraindicated in the following circumstances:

- pregnancy: CT is not recommended unless the clinical benefit outweighs the radiation risk
- patient has poor renal function (or patients having iodine therapy may have CT without intravenous contrast)
- patient is allergic to iodine or shellfish
- patient had a previous CT within a short timeframe (unless the new CT is clinically urgent)
- patient is unable to lie down in order to pass through the machine (Royal College of Radiologists 2010).

Pre-procedural considerations

Assessment and recording tools

Patients must complete a questionnaire prior to CT in order to assess their suitability for CT and IV contrast. IV contrast contains iodine, so patients with an iodine allergy, an allergy to shellfish or a previous history of reaction to IV contrast should have a [illegible]

Equipment

Emergency equipment must be available if IV contrast or a general anaesthetic is used (Chernecky and Berger 2013).

Pharmacological support

The patient will be cannulated for the intravenous injection of iodine-based contrast medium to enhance the blood vessels and bodily organs. During the injection, it is normal for the patient to transiently feel warm over their whole body and to experience a metallic taste at the back of the throat, and some patients feel nauseous. Some CT examinations, such as CT pulmonary angiograms, demand contrast to flow at a fast rate and therefore a large gauge cannula (20 G) is required. CT compatible ports and peripherally inserted central cannulas (PICCs) may also be used (Thomsen et al. 2009). Antihistamines and steroids may be required to treat a reaction (Pagana and Pagana 2017).

Non-pharmacological support

Although CT is a fast imaging technique (5–20 seconds), some patients are very concerned about feeling claustrophobic during scanning. However, with kind, careful explanations, most manage to be scanned. For more information, see the advice on claustrophobia above in the section on MRI.

Specific patient preparation

Patients are prepared for CT by drinking an oral contrast, usually water, which shows the digestive tract. This serves to hydrate the patient, which is beneficial post-IV contrast, and also acts as a negative contrast agent in the digestive tract. Patients must refrain from eating for 2 hours prior to CT in order to allow them to drink easily and to reduce nausea after the IV contrast medium (Keogh 2017; Thomsen et al. 2009). IV access must be established prior to the CT scan to facilitate injection of the IV contrast. Radiopaque objects, such as jewellery, must be removed (Chernecky and Berger 2013).

Procedure

Patients lie on the CT scan couch and pass through the doughnut-shaped machine. The examination is painless and the majority of patients tolerate the examination well (Chernecky and Berger 2013, Pagana and Pagana 2017, Thomsen et al. 2009).

Post-procedural considerations

Immediate care

If any monitoring leads were moved prior to the CT, they should be replaced immediately. Some patients may experience side-effects, which should be observed for after the administration of a contrast. These may include headache, nausea and vomiting. If an allergic reaction occurs, this must be treated and the allergy status of the patient amended. The patient must then be informed that they have had an allergic reaction (Chernecky and Berger 2013).

Websites

British Infertility Counselling Association
www.bica.net

Cancer Research UK
www.cancerresearchuk.org/about-cancer

Diagnostic tests
www.library.wmuh.nhs.uk/pil/diagnostictests.htm

Human Fertilisation and Embryology Authority
www.hfea.gov.uk

Macmillan Cancer Support
www.macmillan.org.uk

NHS Cancer Screening Programme publications related to cervical screening
www.cancerscreening.nhs.uk/cervical

NHS Information Centre
www.ic.nhs.uk

References

Academy of Medical Royal Colleges (2013) *Safe Sedation Practice for Healthcare Procedures: Standards and Guidance*. Available at: https://www.rcoa.ac.uk/system/files/PUB-SafeSedPrac2013.pdf

Adam, S., Osborne, S. & Welch, J. (eds) (2017) *Critical Care Nursing*, 3rd edn. Oxford: Oxford University Press.

Adlard, K. (2000) Examining the push–pull method of blood sampling from central venous access devices. *Journal of Pediatric Oncology Nursing*, 25(4), 200–208.

Ahn, J.I., Jung, H.Y., Bae, S.E., et al. (2013) Proper preparation to reduce endoscopic reexamniation due to food residue after distal gastrectomy for gastric cancer. *Surgical Endoscopy*, 27(3), 910–917.

Al Knawy, B. & Shiffman, M. (2007) Percutaneous liver biopsy in clinical practice. *Liver International*, 27(9), 1166–1173.

American Urological Association (2012) *Best Practice Policy Statement on Urological Surgery Antimicrobial Prophylaxis*. American Urological Association. Available at: https://www.auanet.org/guidelines/antimicrobial-prophylaxis-(2008-reviewed-and-validity-confirmed-2011-amended-2012)

Asai, A., Aoshima, M., Ohkui, Y., et al. (2012) Should blood cultures be performed in terminally ill cancer patients? *Indian Journal of Palliative Care*, 18(1), 40–44.

Australian and New Zealand College of Anaesthetists (2014) *Guidelines on Sedation and/or Analgesia for Diagnostic and Interventional Medical, Dental or Surgical Procedures*. Available at: https://www.anzca.edu.au/documents/ps09–2014-guidelines-on-sedation-and-or-analgesia

Aziz, A.M. (2011) Audit of blood culture technique and documentation to improve practice. *British Journal of Nursing*, 20(8), 26–34.

Barker, E. & Laia, A. (2008) Neurodiagnostic studies. In: Barker, E.M. (ed) *Neuroscience Nursing: A Spectrum of Care*, 3rd edn. St Louis, MO: Mosby, pp.99–129.

Bernie, A.M., Ramasamy, R., Stember, D.S. & Stahl, P.J. (2013) Microsurgical epididymal sperm aspiration: Indications, techniques and outcomes. *Asian Journal of Andrology*, 15(1), 40–43.

Berreth, M. (2010) Minimising the risk of lymphoedema: Implications for the infusion nurse. *INS Newsline*, 32(3), 6–7.

Bersten, A.D., Soni, N. & Oh, T.E. (2009) *Oh's Intensive Care Manual*, 6th edn. Oxford: Butterworth-Heinemann.

Birk, D. (2009) *Human Fertilization and Embryology: The New Law*. London: Jordan Publishing.

Blann, A.D. (2007) *Routine Blood Results Explained*, 2nd edn. Keswick, UK: M&K Update.

BNF (British National Formulary) (2019) *British National Formulary.* National Institute for Health and Care Excellence. Available at: https://bnf.nice.org.uk

Bonham, P.A. (2009) Swab cultures for diagnosing wound infections: A literature review and clinical guideline. *Journal of Wound, Ostomy and Continence Nursing*, 36(4), 389–395.

Borgaonkar, M.R., Hookey, L., Hollingworth, R., et al. (2012) Indicators of safety compromise in gastrointestinal endoscopy. *Canadian Journal of Gastroenterology*, 26(2), 71–78.

Bottros, M.M. & Christo, P.J. (2014) Current perspectives on intrathecal drug delivery. *Journal of Pain Research*, 7, 615–626.

Bouza, E., Munoz, P., Burillo, A., et al. (2005) The challenge of anticipating catheter tip colonization in major heart surgery patients in the intensive care unit: Are surface cultures useful? *Critical Care Medicine*, 33(9), 1953–1960.

Brackett, N., Lynne, C., Ibrahim, E., et al. (2010) Treatment of infertility in men with spinal cord injury. *Nature Reviews: Urology*, 7(3), 162–172.

Brinsden, P.R. (2005) *Textbook of* In Vitro *Fertilization and Assisted Reproduction: The Bourn Hall Guide to Clinical and Laboratory Practice*, 3rd edn. London: Taylor & Francis.

British Association of Urological Surgeons (2013) *Multi-disciplinary Team (MDT) Guidance for Managing Bladder Cancer*, 2nd edn. London: BAUS.

Brooks, G.F., Carroll, K.C., Butel, J.S., et al. (2010) *Jawetz, Melnick & Adelberg's Medical Microbiology*, 25th edn. Philadelphia: McGraw-Hill.

Brzezinski, M., Luisetti, T. & London, M.J. (2009) Radial artery cannulation: A comprehensive review of recent anatomic and physiologic investigations. *Anesthesia & Analgesia*, 109(6), 1763–1781.

BSG (British Society of Gastroenterology) (2003) *Guidelines on Safety and Sedation during Endoscopic Procedures.* Available at: https://www.bsg.org.uk/resource/guidelines-on-safety-and-sedation-for-endoscopic-procedures.html

BSG (2004) *Guidelines on the Use of Liver Biopsy in Clinical Practice.* Available at: https://www.bsg.org.uk/resource/bsg-guidelines-on-the-use-of-liver-biopsy-in-clinical-practice.html

BSG (2005) *Non-medical Endoscopists.* Available at: https://www.bsg.org.uk/resource/non-medical-endoscopists.html

BSG (2007) *BSG Quality and Safety Indicators for Endoscopy.* Available at: https://www.thejag.org.uk/Downloads/Accreditation/Guidance%20-%20BSG%20Quality%20and%20Safety%20Indicators.pdf

Cataldo, M.A., Tacconelli, E., Grilli, E., et al. (2012) Continuous versus intermittent infusion of vancomycin for the treatment of gram-positive infections: Systematic review and meta-analysis. *Journal of Antimicrobial Chemotherapy*, 67, 17–24.

Cotton, J.A., Dobbins, B.M., Kite, P., et al. (2005) In situ diagnosis of intravascular catheter-related bloodstream infection: A comparison of quantitative culture, differential time to positivity, and endoluminal brushing. *Critical Care Medicine*, 33(4), 787–791.

Chernecky, C.C. & Berger, B.J. (2013) *Laboratory Tests and Diagnostic Procedures*, 6th edn. St Louis, MO: Elsevier.

Choi, C.H. (2012) Safety and prevention of complications in endoscopic sedation. *Digestive Diseases and Sciences*, 57, 1745–1747.

Chowet, A.L., Lopez, J.R., Brock-Utne, J.G. & Jaffe, R.A. (2004) Wrist hyperextension leads to median nerve conduction block: Implications for intra-arterial catheter placement. *Anesthesiology*, 100 (2), 287–291.

Coburn, B., Morris, A.M., Tomlinson, G. & Detsky, A.S. (2012) Does this adult with suspected bacteremia require blood cultures? *JAMA*, 308(5), 502–511.

Connor, A., Tolan, D., Hughes, S., et al. (2012) *Consensus Guidelines for the Safe Prescription and Administration of Oral Bowel-Cleansing Agents.* Available at: https://www.rcr.ac.uk/docs/radiology/pdf/obca_12.pdf

Coward, M. & Cooley, H.M. (2006) Chemotherapy. In: Kearney, N. & Richardson, A. (eds) *Nursing Patients with Cancer: Principles and Practice.* Edinburgh: Elsevier Churchill Livingstone, pp.283–302.

Crawshaw, M. & Hale, J. (2005) Sperm storage and the adolescent male: A multi-disciplinary approach. *Human Fertility*, 8(3), 175–176.

Dabaja, A. & Schlegel, P. (2012) Microdissection testicular sperm extraction: An update. *Asian Journal of Andrology*, 15, 35–39.

Damani, N. (2012) *Manual of Infection Prevention and Control*, 3rd edn. Oxford: Oxford University Press.

Danckers, M. & Fried, E.D. (2013) *Arterial Blood Gas Sampling.* Available at: http://emedicine.medscape.com/article/1902703-overview

de Verteuil, A. (2011) Procedures for venepuncture and cannulation. In: Phillips, S., Collins, M. & Dougherty, L. (eds) *Venepuncture and Cannulation.* Oxford: John Wiley & Sons, pp.131–174.

Denzer, U., Arnoldy, A., Kanzler, S., et al. (2007) Prospective randomised comparison of minilaparoscopy and percutaneous liver biopsy: Diagnosis of cirrhosis and complications. *Journal of Clinical Gastroenterology*, 41(1), 103–110.

DH (Department of Health) (2007) *Saving Lives: Reducing Infection, Delivering Clean and Safe Health Care – High Impact Intervention No.6: Urinary Catheter Care Bundle.* Available at: https://webarchive.nationalarchives.gov.uk/+/www.dh.gov.uk/en/Publicationsandstatistics/Publications/PublicationsPolicyAndGuidance/DH_078134

DH (2008) *Updated National Guidance on the Safe Administration of Intrathecal Chemotherapy.* London: Department of Health.

DH (2010) *Clean Safe Care: High Impact Intervention – Taking Blood Cultures: A Summary of Best Practice.* London: Department of Health.

DH (2012) *The 'Never Events' List 2012/13.* London: Department of Health.

DH (2013) *Environment and Sustainability: Health Technical Memorandum 07–01 – Safe Management of Healthcare Waste.* London: Department of Health.

Di Teodoro, L.I., Pudhota, S.G., Vega K.J., et al. (2013) Ultrasound marking by gastroenterologists prior to percutaneous liver biopsy removes the need for a separate radiological evaluation. *Hepato-Gastroenterology*, 60, 821–824.

Doherty, C.M. & Forbes, R.B. (2014) Diagnostic lumbar puncture. *Ulster Medical Journal*, 83(2), 93–102.

Dojcinovska, M. (2011) Selection of equipment. In: Phillips, S., Collins, M. & Dougherty, L. (eds) *Venepuncture and Cannulation.* Oxford: John Wiley & Sons, pp.68–90.

Dougherty, L. (2006) *Central Venous Access Devices: Care and Management.* Oxford: Blackwell.

Dougherty, L. (2008) Obtaining peripheral venous access. In: Dougherty, L. & Lamb, J. (eds) *Intravenous Therapy in Nursing Practice*, 2nd edn. Oxford: Blackwell Publishing, pp.225–270.

Dougherty, L., Lister, S. & McNamara, L. (eds) (2019) *The Royal Marsden Manual of Cancer Nursing Procedures.* Chichester: Wiley Blackwell.

Egan, S., Murphy, P.G., Fennell, J.P., et al. (2012) Using Six Sigma to improve once daily gentamicin dosing and therapeutic drug monitoring performance. *BMJ Quality & Safety*, 21, 1042–1051.

Engelborghs, S., Niemantsverdriet, E., Struyfs, H., et al. (2017) Consensus guidelines for lumbar puncture in patients with neurological diseases. *Alzheimer's & Dementia: Diagnosis, Assessment & Disease Monitoring*, 8, 111–126.

Esteves, S., Lee, W., David, B., et al. (2013) Reproductive potential of men with obstructive azoospermia undergoing percutaneous sperm retrieval and intracytoplasmic sperm injection according to the cause of obstruction. *Journal of Urology*, 189(1), 232–237.

European Biosafety Network (2010) *Prevention of Sharps Injuries in the Hospital and Healthcare Sector.* Available at: https://www.europeanbiosafetynetwork.eu/wp-content/uploads/2017/01/EU-Sharps-Injuries-Implementation-Guidance.pdf

European Parliament and European Council (2004) *Directive 2004/23/EC of the European Parliament and the Council of 31 March 2004 on Setting Standards of Quality and Safety for the Donation, Procurement, Testing, Processing, Preservation, Storage and Distribution of Human Tissues and Cells* [European Union Tissues and Cells Directive]. Brussels: European Parliament.

Faoagali, J. (2010) 'Swabs' then and now: Cotton to flocked nylon. *Microbiology Australia*, September, 133–136.

Fillingham, S. & Douglas, J. (2004) *Urological Nursing*, 3rd edn. Edinburgh: Baillière Tindall.

Fraise, A.P. & Bradley, T. (2009) *Ayliffe's Control of Healthcare-Associated Infection: A Practical Handbook*, 5th edn. London: Hodder Arnold.

Gabriel, J. (2008) Long-term central venous access. In: Dougherty, L. & Lamb, J. (eds) *Intravenous Therapy in Nursing Practice*, 2nd edn. Oxford: Blackwell, pp.321–351.

Gannon, K., Glover, L. & Abel, P. (2004) Masculinity, infertility, stigma and media reports. *Social Science & Medicine*, 59(6), 1169–1175.

Garza, D. & Becan-McBride, K. (2013) *Phlebotomy Simplified*, 2nd edn. Hoboken, NJ: Pearson Education.

Garza, D. & Becan-McBride, K. (2018) *Phlebotomy Handbook: Blood Specimen Collection from Basic to Advanced*, 10th edn. Hoboken, NJ: Pearson Education.

Gemmell, L., Birks, R., Radford, P., et al. (2008) AAGBI safety guideline: Infection control in anaesthesia. *Anaesthesia*, 63, 1027–1036.

Gilbar, P.J. (2014) Intrathecal chemotherapy: Potential for medical error. *Cancer Nursing*, 37(4), 299–309.

GMC (General Medical Council) (2013) *Intimate Examinations and Chaperones*. Available at: https://www.gmc-uk.org/-/media/documents/maintaining-boundaries-intimate-examinations-and-chaperones_pdf-58835231.pdf?la=en

Gong, D., Liu, Y.L., Zheng, Z., et al. (2009) An overview on ethical issues about sperm donation. *Asian Journal of Andrology*, 11, 645–652.

Goossens, G.A. (2015) Flushing and locking of venous catheters: Available evidence and evidence deficit. *Nursing Research and Practice*, 2015, 1–12.

Goossens, G.A., Jérôme, M., Janssens, C., et al. (2013) Comparing normal saline versus diluted heparin to lock non-valved totally implantable venous access devices in cancer patients: A randomised, non-inferiority, open trial. *Annals of Oncology*, 24(7), 1892–1899.

Gorski, L. (2011) Infusion nursing standards of practice. *Journal of Infusion Nursing*, 34, S3–S3.

Gorski, L., Perucca, R. & Hunter, M. (2010) Central venous access devices: Care, maintenance, and potential problems. In: Alexander, M., Corrigan, A., Gorski, L., et al. (eds) *Infusion Nursing: An Evidence-Based Approach*, 3rd edn. St Louis, MO: Saunders Elsevier, pp.495–515.

Gould, D. & Brooker, C. (2008) *Infection Prevention and Control: Applied Microbiology for Healthcare*, 2nd edn. Basingstoke: Palgrave Macmillan.

Greil, A., Slausen-Blevens, K. & McQuillan, J. (2010) The experience of infertility: A review of recent literature. *Sociology of Health & Illness*, 32(1), 140–162.

Gruener, G. & Biller, J. (2008) Spinal cord anatomy, localization, and overview of spinal cord syndromes. *Continuum*, 14(3), 11–35.

Guest, J. (2008) Specimen collection: Part 5 – Obtaining a sputum sample. *Nursing Times*, 104(21), 26–27.

Hammarberg, K., Baker, H. & Fisher, J. (2010) Men's experiences of infertility and infertility treatment 5 years after diagnosis of male factor infertility: A retrospective cohort study. *Human Reproduction*, 25(11), 2815–2820.

Hammett-Stabler, C.A. & Johns, T. (1998) Laboratory guidelines for monitoring of antimicrobial drugs: National Academy of Clinical Biochemistry. *Clinical Chemistry*, 44(5), 1129–1140.

Hampson, G.D. (2006) *Practice Nurse Handbook*, 5th edn. Oxford: Blackwell.

Hess, S. & Decker, M. (2017) Comparison of the single-syringe push–pull technique with the discard technique for obtaining blood samples from pediatric central venous access devices. *Journal of Pediatric Oncology Nursing*, 34(6), 381–386.

HFEA (Human Fertilisation and Embryology Authority) (2017) *Code of Practice*, 8th edn. Available at: https://www.hfea.gov.uk/media/2062/2017-10-02-code-of-practice-8th-edition-full-version-11th-revision-final-clean.pdf

Higgins, C. (2013) *Understanding Laboratory Investigations for Nurses and Health Professionals*, 3rd edn. Oxford: Blackwell.

Higgins, D. (2008a) Specimen collection: Obtaining a midstream specimen of urine. *Nursing Times*, 104(17), 26–27.

Higgins, D. (2008b) Specimen collection: Part 3 – Collecting a stool specimen. *Nursing Times*, 104(19), 22–23.

Himberger, J.R. & Himberger, L.C. (2001) Accuracy of drawing blood through infusing intravenous lines. *Heart & Lung*, 30(1), 66–73.

Hoeltke, L.B. (2018) *The Complete Textbook of Phlebotomy*, 5th edn. Boston: Delmar Cengage Learning.

Hooton, T.M., Bradley, S.F., Cardens, D.D., et al. (2010) Diagnosis, prevention, and treatment of catheter-associated urinary tract infection in adults: 2009 International Clinical Practice Guidelines from the Infectious Diseases Society of America. *Clinical Infectious Diseases*, 50(5), 625–663.

HPA (Health Protection Agency) (2014a) *UK Standards for Microbiology Investigations: Investigation of Blood Cultures (for Organisms other than Mycobacterium Species)*. London: Health Protection Agency.

HPA (2014b) *UK Standards for Microbiology Investigations: Investigation of Genital Tract and Associated Specimens*. Available at: www.hpa.org.uk/webc/hpawebfile/hpaweb_c/1317132861109

HPA (2014c) *UK Standards for Microbiology Investigations: Investigation of Faecal Specimens for Enteric Pathogens*. Available at: www.hpa.org.uk/webc/hpawebfile/hpaweb_c/1317132856754

HPA (2018) *UK Standards for Microbiology Investigations: Processing of Faeces for* Clostridium difficile. Available at: https://assets.publishing.service.gov.uk/government/uploads/system/uploads/attachment_data/file/758284/B_10i1.7.pdf

HSE (Health and Safety Executive) (2003) *Safe Working and the Prevention of Infection in Clinical Laboratories and Similar Facilities*, 2nd edn. Sudbury, UK: HSE Books.

HSE (2005) *Biological Agents: Managing the Risks in Laboratories and Healthcare Premises*. Sudbury: HSE Books.

HSE (2013) *Health and Safety (Sharp Instruments in Healthcare) Regulations 2013*. London: Health and Safety Executive.

Huddleston Cross, H. (2014) Obtaining a wound swab culture specimen. *Nursing*, 44(7), 68–69.

Hudson, T.L., Dukes, S.F. & Reilly, K. (2006) Use of local anesthesia for arterial punctures. *American Journal of Critical Care*, 15, 595–599.

Human Fertilisation and Embryology Act (1990) Available at: https://www.legislation.gov.uk/ukpga/1990/37/contents

Human Fertilisation and Embryology Act (2008) Available at: https://www.legislation.gov.uk/ukpga/2008/22/contents

Human Fertilisation and Embryology (Quality and Safety) Regulations (2017) Department of Health. Available at: https://assets.publishing.service.gov.uk/government/uploads/system/uploads/attachment_data/file/598616/HFE_Act_consultation_document_A.pdf

Husband, J.E. & Reznek, R.H. (2010) *Husband & Reznek's Imaging in Oncology*, 3rd edn. London: Informa Healthcare.

Huth, M.E., Ricci, A.J. & Cheng, A.G. (2011) Mechanisms of aminoglycoside ototoxicity and targets of hair cell protection. *International Journal of Otolaryngology*, 2011, 1–19.

IBMS (Institute of Biomedical Science) (2016) *Patient Sample and Request Form Identification Criteria*. Available at: https://www.ibms.org/resources/documents/patient-sample-and-request-form-identification-criteria

Insinga, R.P., Glass, A.G. & Rush, B.B. (2004) Diagnoses and outcomes in cervical cancer screening: A population based study. *American Journal of Obstetrics & Gynecology*, 191, 105–113.

Inwood, S. (2007) Skin antisepsis: Using 2% chlorhexidine gluconate in 70% isopropyl alcohol. *British Journal of Nursing*, 16(22), 1390, 1392–1394.

Ionizing Radiation (Medical Exposure) Regulations (2017) Available at: www.legislation.gov.uk/uksi/2017/1322/made

Jackson, S.R., Dryden, M., Gillett, P. et al. (2005) A novel midstream urine-collection device reduces the contamination rates in urine cultures amongst women. *BJU International*, 96, 360–364.

Johannes, R.S. (2008) Epidemiology of early-onset bloodstream infection and implications for treatment. *American Journal of Infection Control*, 36(10), S171.e13–S171.e17.

Jones, R.N. (2006) Microbiological features of vancomycin in the 21st century: Minimum inhibitory concentration creep, bactericidal/static activity, and applied breakpoints to predict clinical outcomes or detect resistant strains. *Clinical Infectious Diseases*, 42(Suppl. 1), S13–S24.

Kang, H. & Hyun, J.J. (2013) Preparation and patient evaluation for safe gastrointestinal endoscopy. *Clinical Endoscopy*, 46(3), 212–218.

Karamshi, M. (2008) Performing a percutaneous liver biopsy in parenchymal liver diseases. *British Journal of Nursing*, 9(17), 746–752.

Kee, P.P., Chinnappan, M., Nair, A., et al. (2016) Diagnostic yield of timing blood culture collection relative to fever. *Pediatric Infectious Disease Journal*, 35(8), 846–850.

Keogh, J. (2017) *Nursing, Laboratory & Diagnostic Tests*, 2nd edn. New York: McGraw-Hill.

Keshava, S., Mammen, T., Surendrababu, N.R.S. & Moses, V. (2008) Transjugular liver biopsy: What to do and what not to do. *Interventional Radiology Symposium*, 18(3), 245–248.

Kierszenbaum, A.L. & Tres, L.L. (2016) *Histology and Cell Biology: An Introduction to Pathology*, 4th edn. Philadelphia: Elsevier.

Kim, H.T. (2013) Arterial puncture and cannulation. In: Roberts, J.R. & Hedges, J.R. (eds) *Clinical Procedures in Emergency Medicine*, 6th edn. Philadelphia: Elsevier Saunders, pp.368–384.

Korenstein, D., Falk, R., Howell, E.A., et al. (2012) Overuse of health care services in the United States: An understudied problem. *Archives of Internal Medicine*, 172(2), 171–178.

Kumar, A.H.D., Srinivasan, N.M., Thakkar, J.M. & Mathew, S. (2013) A prospective observational study of the outcome of central venous catheterization in 100 patients. *Anesthesia Essays and Researches*, 7(1), 71–75.

Kumar, P.J. & Clark, M.L. (2016) *Kumar & Clark's Clinical Medicine*, 9th edn. Edinburgh: Saunders/Elsevier.

Kyle, G. (2007) Bowel care: Part 3 – Obtaining a stool sample. *Nursing Times*, 103(44), 24–25.

Lambregts, D.M., Maas, M., Cappendijk, V.C., et al. (2011) Whole-body diffusion-weighted magnetic resonance imaging: Current evidence in oncology and potential role in colorectal cancer staging. *European Journal of Cancer*, 47(14), 2107–2116.

Lee, A., Mirrett, S., Reller, L.B. & Weinstein, M.P. (2007) Detection of bloodstream infections in adults: How many blood cultures are needed? *Journal of Clinical Microbiology*, 45(11), 3546–3548.

Lee, S.C.M. & Lueck, C.J. (2014) Cerebrospinal fluid pressure in adults. *Journal of Neuro-Opthalmology*, 34, 278–283.

Lin, C., Luciani, A., Itti, E., et al. (2012) Whole-body diffusion magnetic resonance imaging in the assessment of lymphoma. *Cancer Imaging*, 12(2), 403–408.

Lindsay, K.W., Bone, I. & Fuller, G. (2010) *Neurology and Neurosurgery Illustrated*, 5th edn. Edinburgh: Churchill Livingstone.

Lipsitz, E.C. (2004) Cannulation injuries of the radial artery. *American Journal of Critical Care*, 13(4), 314, 319.

Loveday, H.P., Wilson, J.A., Pratt, R.J., et al. (2014) epic3: National evidence-based guidelines for preventing healthcare-associated infections in NHS hospitals in England. *Journal of Hospital Infection*, 86(Suppl. 1), S1–S70.

Lowdin, E., Odenholt, I. & Cars, O. (1998) *In vitro* studies of pharmacodynamic properties of vancomycin against *Staphylococcus aureus* and *Staphylococcus epidermidis*. *Antimicrobial Agents and Chemotherapy*, 42, 2739–2744.

MacKay, G.J., Dorrance, H.R., Molloy, R.G. & O'Dwyer, P.J. (2010) *Colorectal Surgery*. Oxford: Oxford University Press.

MacKie, R.M. (2003) *Clinical Dermatology*, 5th edn. Oxford: Oxford University Press.

Madeo, M. & Barlow, G. (2008) Reducing blood-culture contamination rates by the use of a 2% chlorhexidine solution applicator in acute admission units. *Journal of Hospital Infection*, 69(3), 307–309.

Mahon, C.R., Lehman, D.C. & Manuselis, G. (2015) *Textbook of Diagnostic Microbiology*, 5th edn. Philadelphia: Saunders.

Mandal, A. (2010) *Semen Physiology*. Medical Life Sciences. Available at: www.news-medical.net/health/Semen-Physiology.aspx

Marieb, E.N. & Hoehn, K. (2015) *Human Anatomy and Physiology*, 10th edn. San Francisco: Pearson.

Martin, E.A. (2010) *Concise Colour Medical Dictionary*, 5th edn. Oxford: Oxford University Press.

Masoompour, S.M., Anushiravani, A. & Norouz, A.T. (2015) Evaluation of the effect of nebulized N-acetylcysteine on respiratory secretions in mechanically ventilated patients: Randomized clinical trial. *Iranian Journal of Medical Sciences*, 40(4), 309–315.

McCall, R.E. & Tankersley, C.M. (2016) *Phlebotomy Essentials*, 6th edn. Philadelphia: Wolters Kluwer.

McRobbie, D.W. (2007) *MRI from Picture to Proton*, 2nd edn. Cambridge: Cambridge University Press.

McSwain, S.D. & Yeager, B.E. (2015) Reducing pain of arterial punctures. *Respiratory Care*, 60(1), 141–143.

Mendez, S.J. (2012) Evidence-based practice for obtaining blood specimens from a central venous access device. *Oncology Nursing Forum*, 39(3), 247–251.

Mescher, A.L. (2016) *Basic Histology: Text and Atlas*, 14th edn. London: McGraw-Hill Medical.

Meseguer, M., Garrido, N., Remohí, J., et al. (2003) Testicular sperm extraction (TESE) and ICSI in patients with permanent azoospermia after chemotherapy. *Human Reproduction*, 18(6), 1281–1285.

MHRA (Medicines and Healthcare products Regulatory Agency) (2005) *Reporting Adverse Incidents and Disseminating Medical Device Alerts*. London: Medicines and Healthcare products Regulatory Agency.

MHRA (2010) *All Medical Devices and Medicinal Products Containing Chlorhexidine*. London: Medicines and Healthcare products Regulatory Agency.

MHRA (2013) *Custom Portex® Epidural and Spinal Kits*. Available at: www.mhra.gov.uk/home/groups/fsn/documents/fieldsafetynotice/con[illegible].pdf

Miller, J.M., Binnicker, M.J., Campbell, S., et al. (2018) A guide to utilization of the microbiology laboratory for diagnosis of infectious diseases: 2018 update by the Infectious Diseases Society of America and the American Society for Microbiology. *Clinical Infectious Diseases*, 67(6), e1–e94.

Mirza, B., Vanek, V. & Kupensky, D.T. (2004) Pinch-off syndrome: Case report and collective review of the literature. *American Journal of Surgery*, 70, 635–644.

Moise-Broder, P.A., Forrest, A., Birmingham, M.C., et al. (2004) Pharmacodynamics of vancomycin and other antimicrobials in patients with *Staphylococcus aureus* lower respiratory tract infections. *Clinical Pharmacokinetics*, 43, 925–942.

Mulhall, J. (2013) Physiology of ejaculation. In: Mulhall, J., Applegarth, L., Oates, R. & Schlegel, P. (eds) *Fertility Preservation in Male Cancer Patients*. Cambridge: Cambridge University Press, pp.35–38.

Murray, P.R. & Masur, H. (2012) Current approaches to the diagnosis of bacterial fungal bloodstream infections in the ITU. *Critical Care Medicine*, 40(12), 3277–3282.

Myers, F.E. & Reyes, C. (2011) Blood cultures: 5 steps to doing it right. *Nursing*, 41(3), 62–63.

NHS BCSP (Bowel Cancer Screening Programme) (2018) *Bowel Cancer Screening: Programme Overview*. Available at: https://www.gov.uk/guidance/bowel-cancer-screening-programme-overview

NHS Employers (2015) *Managing the Risk of Sharps Injuries*. London: NHS Employers.

NHS England and NHSI (NHS Improvement) (2019) *Standard Infection Control Precautions: National Hand Hygiene and Personal Protective Equipment Policy*. Available at: https://improvement.nhs.uk/documents/4957/National_policy_on_hand_hygiene_and_PPE_2.pdf

NHS Pathology (2014) *Samples and Request Forms*. Previously available at: www.nhspathology.fph.nhs.uk/Core-Service/TestDirectory/General_Information_Samples_and _Request_Forms.aspx

NHSBT (NHS Blood and Transplant) (2011) *Blood and Transplant Matters*. Watford: NHS Blood and Transplant.

NHSBT (2012) *Blood and Transplant Matters*. Watford: NHS Blood and Transplant.

NHSCSP (NHS Cancer Screening Programmes) (2013) *Achievable Standards, Benchmarks for Reporting, and Criteria for Evaluating Cervical Cytopathology*, 3rd edn. Sheffield: NHS Cancer Screening Programmes.

NHSCSP (2016a) *NHS Cervical Screening Programme: Colposcopy and Programme Managment*. Available at: https://www.bsccp.org.uk/assets/file/uploads/resources/NHSCSP_20_Colposcopy_and_Programme_Management_(3rd_Edition)_(2).pdf

NHSCSP (2016b) *NHS Cervical Screening Programme Guidance for the Training of Cervical Sample Takers*. Available at: https://assets.publishing.service.gov.uk/government/uploads/system/uploads/attachment_data/file/577158/NHS_Cervical_Screening_Progamme_-_guidance_for_cervical_sample_takers.pdf

NICE (National Institute for Health and Care Excellence) (2003) *Guidance on the Use of Liquid-Based Cytology for Cervical Screening*. London: National Institute for Health and Care Excellence.

NICE (2013) *Fertility Problems: Assessment and Treatment*. Available at: https://www.nice.org.uk/guidance/cg156/resources/fertility-problems-assessment-and-treatment-pdf-35109634660549

NICE (2017) *Sepsis: Recognition, Diagnosis and Early Management*. Available at: https://www.nice.org.uk/guidance/ng51/resources/sepsis-recognition-diagnosis-and-early-management-pdf-1837508256709

NMC (Nursing and Midwifery Council) (2018) *The Code: Professional Standards of Practice and Behaviour for Nurses, Midwives and Nursing Associates*. Available at: https://www.nmc.org.uk/standards/code

NPSA (National Patient Safety Agency) (2007a) *Standardising Wristbands Improves Patient Safety*. London: National Patient Safety Agency.

NPSA (2007b) *Promoting the Safer Use of Injectable Medicines*. London: National Patient Safety Agency.

NPSA (2008a) *Infusions and Sampling from Arterial Lines*. London: National Patient Safety Agency.

NPSA (2008b) *Reducing Risk of Overdose with Midazolam Injection in Adults*. London: National Patient Safety Agency.

NPSA (2009) *Reducing Risk of Harm from Oral Bowel Cleansing Solutions*. London: National Patient Safety Agency.

NPSA (2011) *Safer Spinal (Intrathecal), Epidural and Regional Devices*. London: National Patient Safety Agency.

O'Flynn, E.A.M., Wilson, A.R.M. & Michell, M.J. (2010) Image-guided breast biopsy: State-of-the-art. *Clinical Radiology*, 65(4), 259–270.

O'Hare, D. & Chilvers, R.J. (2001) Arterial blood sampling practices in intensive care units in England and Wales. *Anaesthesia*, 56, 568–584.

Osborne, S. (2017) Cardiovascular problems. In: Adam, S., Osborne, S. & Welch, J. (eds) *Critical Care Nursing*, 3rd edn. Oxford: Oxford University Press, pp.143–226.

Owens, R.C. Jr. & Shorr, A.F. (2009) Rational dosing of antimicrobial agents: Pharmacokinetic and pharmacodynamic strategies. *American Journal of Health-System Pharmacy*, 66(12 Suppl. 4), S23–S30.

Pacey, A. & Eiser, C. (2011) Banking sperm is only the first of many decisions for men: What healthcare professionals and men need to know. *Human Fertility*, 14(4), 208–217.

Pagana, K.D. & Pagana, T.J. (2017) *Mosby's Manual of Diagnostic and Laboratory Tests*, 6th edn. St Louis, MO: Elsevier.

Pagkalis, S., Mantadakis, E., Mavros, M.N., et al. (2011) Pharmacological considerations for the proper clinical use of aminoglycosides. *Drugs*, 71(17), 2277–2294.

Panceri, M.L., Vegni, F.E., Goglio, A., et al. (2004) Aetiology and prognosis of bacteraemia in Italy. *Epidemiology & Infection*, 132(4), 647–654.

Pannu, N. & Nadim, M.K. (2008) An overview of drug-induced acute kidney injury. *Critical Care Medicine*, 36(4 Suppl.), S216–S223.

Panpradist, N., Toley, B.J., Zhang, X., et al. (2014) Swab sample transfer for point-of-care diagnostics: Characterization of swab types and manual agitation methods. *PLOS ONE*, 9(9), e105786.

Pellowe, C. (2009) Using evidence-based guidelines to reduce catheter related urinary tract infections in England. *Journal of Infection Prevention*, 10(2), 44–49.

Pendharkar, S.R. & Tremblay, A.T. (2007) A diagnostic approach to pleural effusion: Guidance on how to identify the cause. *Journal of Respiratory Diseases*, 28(12), 565–572.

PHE (Public Health England) (2014) *UK Standards for Microbiology Investigations: Investigation of Faecal Specimens for Enteric Pathogens*. Available at: https://www.gov.uk/government/publications/smi-b-30-investigation-of-faecal-specimens-for-enteric-pathogens

PHE (2015a) *UK Standards for Microbiology Investigations: Investigation of Throat Related Specimens*. Available at: https://assets.publishing.service.gov.uk/government/uploads/system/uploads/attachment_data/file/423204/B_9i9.pdf

PHE (2015b) *UK Standards for Microbiology Investigations: Investigation of Nasal Samples*. Available at: https://assets.publishing.service.gov.uk/government/uploads/system/uploads/attachment_data/file/394716/B_5i7.1.pdf

PHE (2017) *UK Standards for Microbiology Investigations: Investigation of Genital Tract and Associated Specimens*. Available at: https://assets.publishing.service.gov.uk/government/uploads/system/uploads/attachment_data/file/611011/B_28i4.6.pdf

PHE (2018a) *UK Standards for Microbiology Investigations: Investigation of Blood Cultures (for Organisms other than Mycobacterium Species)*. https://www.gov.uk/government/uploads/system/uploads/attachment_data/file/732278/B37i8.1.odt

PHE (2018b) *UK Standards for Microbiology Investigations: Investigation of Specimens for Screening for MRSA*. https://assets.publishing.service.gov.uk/government/uploads/system/uploads/attachment_data/file/674688/B_29i6_under_review.pdf

PHE (2018c) *Investigation of Urine: BSOP 41 – Issue 7*. Available at: https://www.gov.uk/government/publications/smi-b-41-investigation-of-urine

PHE (2018d) *Investigation for Bronchovascular Lavage, Sputum and Associated Specimens: BSOP57 – Issue 2.3*. Available at: https://www.gov.uk/government/publications/smi-b-57-investigation-of-bronchoal veolar-lavage-sputum-and-associated-specimens

PHE (2018e) *Investigation of Fluids from Normally Sterile Sites*. Available at: https://www.gov.uk/government/publications/smi-b-26-investigation-of-fluids-from-normally-sterile-sites

PHE (2019) *NHS Cervical Screening: Cytology Reporting Failsafe (Primary HPV)*. Available at: https://www.gov.uk/government/publications/cervical-screening-cytology-reporting-failsafe/cervical-screening-failsafe-guidance

Philomina, B. (2009) Role of respiratory samples in the diagnosis of lower respiratory tract infections. *Pulmonology*, 11(1), 12–14.

Pikis, S., Cohen, J.E., Gomori, J., et al. (2013) Cauda equina syndrome after spinal epidural steroid injection into an unrecognized paraganglioma. *Clinical Journal of Pain*, 29(12), e39–e41.

Prestwich, R.J., Sykes, J., Carey, B., et al. (2012) Improving target definition for head and neck radiotherapy: A place for magnetic resonance imaging and 18-fluoride fluorodeoxyglucose positron emission tomography? *Clinical Oncology*, 24(8), 577–589.

Qaseem, A., Alguire, P., Dallas, P., et al. (2012) Appropriate use of screening and diagnostic tests to foster high-value, cost-conscious care. *Annals of Internal Medicine*, 156(2), 147–149.

Quincke, H. (1891) Verhandlungen des Congresses für Innere Medizin, Zehnter Congress. *Wiesbaden*, 10, 321–331.

RCN (Royal College of Nursing) (2010) *Standards for Infusion Therapy*, 3rd edn. London: Royal College of Nursing.

RCN (2012) *Wipe It Out: Essential Practice for Infection Prevention and Control: Guidance for Nursing Staff*. London: Royal College of Nursing.

RCN (2013) *Cervical Screening: RCN Guidance for Good Practice*. London: Royal College of Nursing.

RCN (2017a) *Principles of Consent: Guidance for Nursing Staff*. Available at: https://www.rcn.org.uk/professional-development/publications/pub-006047

RCN (2017b) *Essential Practice for Infection Prevention and Control: Guidance for Nursing Staff*. Available at: https://www.rcn.org.uk/professional-development/publications/pub-005940

RCN (2018) *Human Papillomavirus (HPV), Cervical Screening and Cervical Cancer*. London: Royal College of Nursing.

RCP, RCR & RCOG (Royal College of Physicians, Royal College of Radiologists & Royal College of Obstetricians and Gynaecologists) (2007) *The Effects of Cancer Treatment on Reproductive Functions: Guidance on Management*. Available at: https://www.rcr.ac.uk/system/files/publication/field_publication_files/Cancer_fertility_effects_Jan08.pdf

Rhodes, A., Evan, L.E., Alhazzani, W., et al. (2017) Surviving sepsis campaign: International guidelines for management of sepsis and septic shock: 2016. *Intensive Care Medicine*, 43(3), 304–377.

Riedel, S., Bourbeau, P., Swartz, B., et al. (2008) Timing of specimen collection for blood cultures from febrile patients with bacteremia. *Journal of Clinical Microbiology*, 46(4), 1381–1385.

Riley, S.A. (2008) *Colonocopic Polypectomy and Endoscopic Mucosal Resection: A Practical Guide*. British Society of Gastroenterology. Available at: https://www.bsg.org.uk/resource/colonoscopic-polypectomy-and-endoscopic-mucosal-resection--a-practical-guide.html

Roberts, J., Norris, R., Paterson, D.L. & Martin, J.H. (2011) Therapeutic drug monitoring of antimicrobials. *British Journal of Clinical Pharmacology*, 73(1), 27–36.

Robinson, S., Harris, A., Atkinson, S., et al. (2017) The administration of blood components: A British Society for Haematology guideline. *Transfusion Medicine*, 28(1), 3–21.

Royal College of Radiologists (2010) *Standards for Intravascular Contrast Agent Administration to Adult Patients*. London: Royal College of Radiologists.

Royal College of Radiologists (2012) *iRefer: Making the Best Use of Clinical Radiology*. London: Royal College of Radiologists.

Royal College of Radiologists, Health Protection Agency & College of Radiographers (2009) *Protection of Pregnant Patients during Diagnostic Medical Exposures to Ionizing Radiation*. Available at: https://www.rcr.ac.uk/system/files/publication/field_publication_files/HPA_preg_2nd.pdf

Runge, V.M., Nitz, W.R. & Schmeets, S.H. (2009) *The Physics of Clinical MR Taught through Images*, 2nd edn. New York: Thieme.

Russian, C.J., Gonzales, J.F. & Henry, N.R.H. (2014) Suction catheter size: An assessment and comparison of 3 different calculation methods. *Respiratory Care*, 59(1), 32–38.

Rybak, M., Lomaestro, B., Rotschafer, J.C., et al. (2009) Therapeutic monitoring of vancomycin in adult patients: A consensus review of the

American Society of Health-System Pharmacists, the Infectious Diseases Society of America, and the Society of Infectious Diseases Pharmacists. *American Journal of Health-System Pharmacy*, 66, 82–98.

Saied, N., Chopra, A. & Agarwal, B. (2012) Parenteral erythromycin for potential use to empty retained gastric contents encountered during upper gastrointestinal endoscopic procedures. *Open Journal of Gastroenterology*, 2, 119–123.

Saint, S. & Lipsky, B.A. (1999) Preventing catheter-related bacteriuria. *Archives of Internal Medicine*, 159, 800–808.

Schlegel, P. (1999) Testicular sperm extraction: Microdissection improves sperm yield with minimal tissue excision. *Human Reproduction*, 14(1), 131–135.

Schmidt, L., Christensen, U. & Holstein, B.E. (2005) The social epidemiology of coping with infertility. *Human Reproduction*, 20(4), 1044–1052.

Schneeberger, C., van den Heuvel, E.R., Erwich, J.J., et al. (2013) Contamination rates of three urine-sampling methods to assess bacteriuria in pregnant women. *Obstetrics & Gynecology*, 121, 299–305.

Schneider, V.F. (2013) Lumbar puncture. In: Dehn, R. & Asprey, D.P. (eds) *Essential Clinical Procedures*, 3rd edn. Philadelphia: Elsevier Saunders, pp.146–155.

Schuiling, K.D. & Likis, F.E. (2013) *Women's Gynecological Health*, 2nd edn. Sudbury, MA: Jones & Bartlett Learning.

Sha, S. (2005) Physiological and molecular pathology of aminoglycoside ototoxicity. *Volta Review*, 105(3), 325–335.

Shaw, M. (2001) Competence and consent to treatment in children and adolescents. *Advances in Psychiatric Treatment*, 7, 150–159.

Shaw, M., Lee, A. & Stollery, A. (2010) *Ophthalmic Nursing*, 4th edn. Oxford: Blackwell.

Shellock, F.G. & Spinazzi, A. (2008) MRI safety update 2008: Part 2 – Screening patients for MRI. *American Journal of Roentgenology*, 191(4), 1140–1149.

Shore, A. & Sandoe, J. (2008) Blood cultures. *BMJ*, 16(4), 324–325.

SIGN (2008) *Management of Acute Upper and Lower Gastrointestinal Bleeding: A National Guideline*. Edinburgh: NHS Quality Improvement Scotland. Available at: https://pdfs.semanticscholar.org/646b/ed5610e7030ea0fccad8d8d5897137682962.pdf

Singh, S., van Herwijnen, I. & Phillips, C. (2013) The management of lower urogenital changes in the menopause. *Menopause International*, 19(2), 77–81.

Smith, G.D. & Watson, R. (2005) *Gastrointestinal Nursing*. Oxford: Blackwell.

Sousa, B., Furlanetto, J., Hutka, M., et al. (2015) Central venous access in oncology: ESMO clinical practice guidelines. *Annals of Oncology*, 26(5), 152–168.

Stuart, M. & White, M. (2012) Consent. *Anaesthesia and Intensive Care Medicine*, 13(4), 141–144.

Suissa, A., Bentur, S., Lachter, J., et al. (2012) Outcome and complications of colonoscopy: A prospective multicenter study in northern Israel. *Diagnostic and Therapeutic Endoscopy*, 2012, 612542.

Swan, E. (2005) *Colorectal Cancer*. London: Whurr.

Tacconelli, E. (2009) Antimicrobial use: Risk driver of multidrug resistant microorganisms in healthcare settings. *Current Opinion in Infectious Diseases*, 22(4), 352–358.

Tannapfel, A., Dienes, H.P. & Lohse, A.W. (2012) The indications for liver biopsy. *Deutsches Ärzteblatt International*, 109(27/28), 477–483.

Taylor, I., van Cutsem, E. & Garcia-Aguilar, J. (2009) *Colorectal Disease*, 3rd edn. Abingdon, UK: Health Press.

Thomas, N. (2008) *Renal Nursing*, 3rd edn. Edinburgh: Baillière Tindall Elsevier.

Thomsen, H.S., Webb, J.A.W. & Aspelin, P. (eds) (2009) *Contrast Media: Safety Issues and ESUR Guidelines*, 2nd rev. edn. Berlin: Springer.

Thomson, A. (2004) Why do therapeutic drug monitoring? *Pharmaceutical Journal*, 273(7310), 153–155.

Tobin, C.M., Darville, J.M., Thomson, A.H., et al. (2002) Vancomycin therapeutic drug monitoring: Is there a consensus view? The results of a UK National External Quality Assessment Scheme (UK NEQAS) for Antibiotic Assays questionnaire. *Journal of Antimicrobial Chemotherapy*, 50(5), 713–718.

Tortora, G.J. & Derrickson, B.H. (2017) *Principles of Anatomy & Physiology*, 15th edn. Hoboken, NJ: John Wiley & Sons.

Tursi, A. (2013) Colonoscopy by nurse endoscopists: The right answer for the growing demand for colonoscopy in clinical practice? *Endoscopy*, 45(5), 408.

Ueda, K., Bayman, E.O., Johnson, C., et al. (2015) A randomized controlled trial of radial artery cannulation guided by Doppler vs palpation vs ultrasound. *Anaesthesia*, 70, 1039–1044.

Urban, A.W. & Craig, W.A. (1997) Daily dosage of aminoglycosides. *Current Clinical Topics in Infectious Disease*, 17, 236–255.

Van den Broek, U., Vandermeeren, M., Vanderschueren, D., et al. (2013) A systematic review of sperm donors: Demographic characteristics, attitudes, motives and experiences of the process of sperm donation. *Human Reproduction Update*, 19(1), 37–51.

Van Putten, P.G., ter Borg, F., Adang, R.P., et al. (2012) Nurse endoscopists perform colonoscopies according to the international standard and with high patient satisfaction. *Endoscopy*, 44(12), 1127–1132.

Walker, R. & Whittlesea, C. (2012) *Clinical Pharmacy and Therapeutics*, 5th edn. London: Churchill Livingstone.

Waugh, A. & Grant, A. (2018) *Ross and Wilson Anatomy and Physiology in Health and Illness*, 13th edn. Edinburgh: Elsevier.

Wegerhoff, F. (2006) It's a bug's life: Specimen collection, transport, and viability. *Microbe*, 1, 180–184.

Weinstein, S. & Hagle M.E. (2014) *Plumer's Principles & Practice of Intravenous Therapy*, 9th edn. Philadelphia: Lippincott Williams & Wilkins.

Weinstein, S. & Plumer, A.L. (2007) *Plumer's Principles & Practice of Intravenous Therapy*, 8th edn. Philadelphia: Lippincott Williams & Wilkins.

Welch, J. & Black, C. (2017) Respiratory problems. In: Adam, S., Osborne, S. & Welch, J. (eds) *Critical Care Nursing*, 3rd edn. Oxford: Oxford University Press, pp.83–142.

Weston, D. (2008) *Infection Prevention and Control: Theory and Clinical Practice for Healthcare Professionals*. Oxford: John Wiley & Sons.

White, L., Halpin, A., Turner, M. & Wallace, L. (2016) Ultrasound-guided radial artery cannulation in adult and paediatric populations: A systematic review and meta-analysis. *British Journal of Anaesthesia*, 116(5), 610–617.

WHO (World Health Organization) (2010a) *WHO Guidelines on Drawing Blood: Best Practices in Phlebotomy*. Geneva: World Health Organization.

WHO (2010b) *WHO Laboratory Manual for the Examination and Processing of Human Semen*, 5th edn. Geneva: World Health Organization.

WHO (2014) *Comprehensive Cervical Cancer Control: A Guide to Essential Practice*. Geneva: World Health Organization.

WHO (2015) *Guidance on Regulations for the Transport of Infectious Substances 2015–2016*. Geneva: World Health Organization.

Williams, D. (2010) Sperm banking and the cancer patient. *Therapeutic Advances in Urology*, 2(1), 19–34.

Winter, M.E. (2004) *Basic Clinical Pharmacokinetics*, 4th edn. Philadelphia: Lippincott Williams & Wilkins.

Witt, B. (2011) Vein selection. In: Phillips, S., Collins, M. & Dougherty, L. (eds) *Venepuncture and Cannulation*. Oxford: John Wiley & Sons, pp.91–107.

Wo, J.Y. & Viswanathan, A.N. (2009) Impact of radiotherapy on fertility, pregnancy, and neonatal outcomes in female cancer patients. *International Journal of Radiation Oncology, Biology, Physics*, 73(5), 1304–1312.

Chapter 14

Observations

Filipe Carvalho with Emma-Claire Breen, Zoë Bullock, Sonya Hussein, Elodie Malard, Yara Osman De Oliveira, Marie Parsons and Heather Thexton

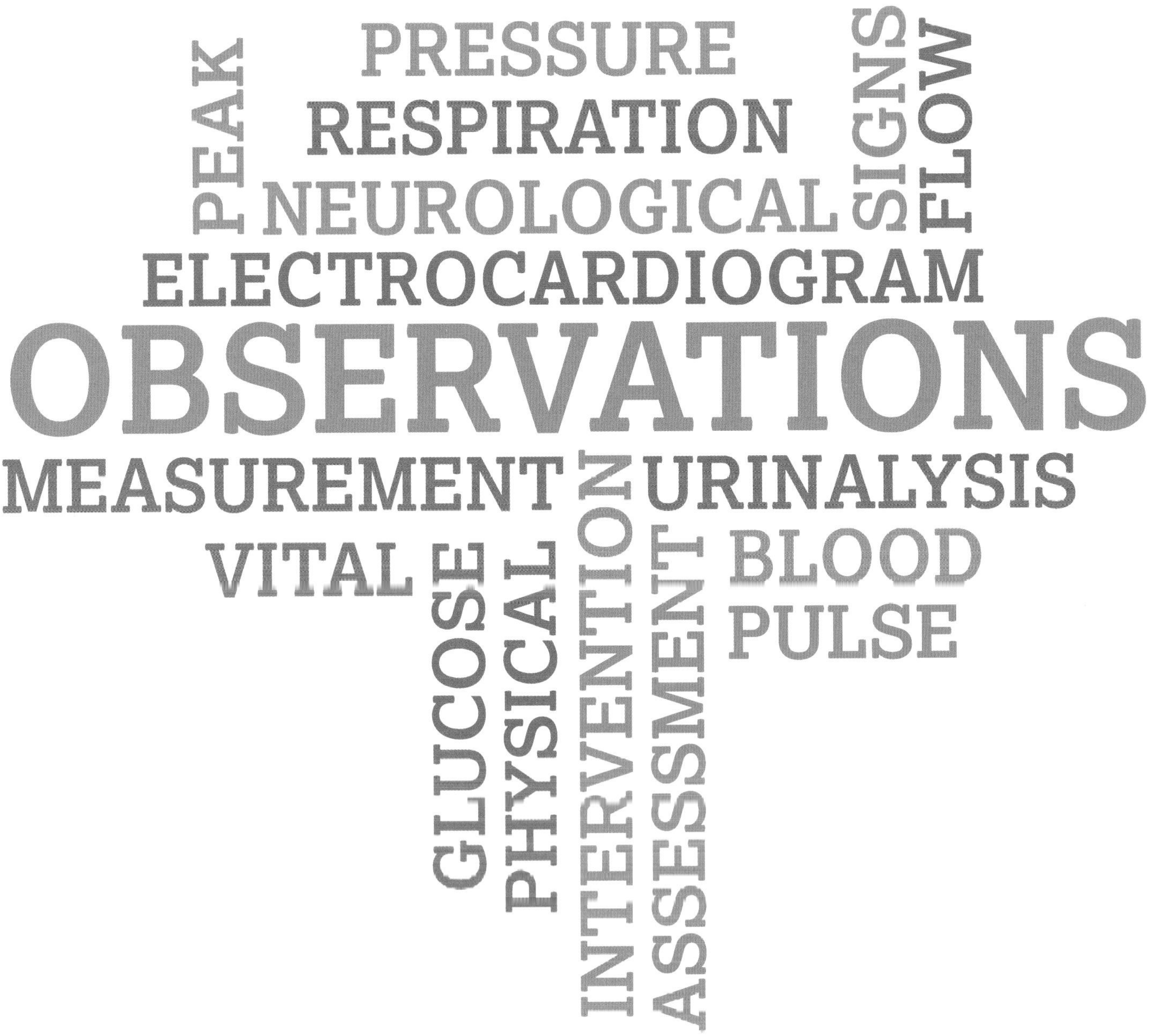

The Royal Marsden Manual of Clinical Nursing Procedures: Professional Edition, Tenth Edition. Edited by [illegible]

Procedure guidelines

Being an accountable professional

At the point of registration, the nurse will:

2. Use evidence-based, best practice approaches to undertake the following procedures:
- **2.1** take, record and interpret vital signs manually and via technological devices
- **2.3** set up and manage routine electrocardiogram (ECG) investigations and interpret normal and commonly encountered abnormal traces
- **2.5** manage and interpret cardiac monitors, infusion pumps, blood glucose monitors and other monitoring devices
- **2.7** undertake a whole body systems assessment including respiratory, circulatory, neurological, musculoskeletal, cardiovascular and skin status
- **2.10** measure and interpret blood glucose levels
- **2.12** undertake, respond to and interpret neurological observations and assessments
- **2.13** identify and respond to signs of deterioration and sepsis

Future Nurse: Standards of Proficiency for Registered Nurses (NMC 2018)

Overview

This chapter discusses the following observations: pulse, electrocardiogram (ECG), blood pressure, respiration, pulse oximetry, peak flow, temperature, urinalysis, blood glucose and neurological observations. For each observation discussed, the chapter provides a definition, a rationale, a summary of governance and professional issues, a procedure guideline and a guide to problem solving.

Observations

Definition

The term 'observation' refers to the physical assessment of a patient, which in addition to vital signs and specialized assessments (such as neurological observations) includes a review of wounds, intravenous therapy, wound drains and pain (Adam et al. 2017, Sprigings and Chambers 2017) (note that the latter topics are discussed elsewhere in this manual). The term 'vital signs' is traditionally used in the context of the collection of a cluster of physical measurements, such as pulse, respiration rate, temperature, blood pressure, pulse oximetry and more recently level of consciousness (Jarvis et al. 2015).

Evidence-based approaches

Rationale

The taking of patient observations forms a fundamental part of the assessment process (Churpek et al. 2017; see also Chapter 2: Admissions and assessment). The findings and results will help to determine the level of care a patient requires and to establish whether an intervention is needed to prevent the patient deteriorating (Uppanisakorn et al. 2018).

Indications

Observations are usually undertaken:

- to act as a baseline and to help determine a patient's usual range (Bickley 2016)
- to assist in recognizing whether a patient's condition is deteriorating or improving (Keep et al. 2016)
- to assess the effectiveness of interventions (Hodgson et al. 2017).

Principles of care

Adult patients in acute hospital settings should have:

- observations taken when they are admitted or initially assessed (including on transfer from one ward or area to another)
- a clearly documented plan that identifies which observations should be taken and how frequently, taking into consideration the diagnosis, the patient's treatment plan and any co-morbidities
- observations taken at least once every 12 hours, unless specified otherwise by senior staff or the patient's medical team (NICE 2018).

National Early Warning Score and standardizing communication

Caring for acutely unwell patients can be daunting and challenging; however, early detection of changes in observations helps to identify patients who are at risk of clinical deterioration. Early detection may provide an opportunity to intervene and avoid further deterioration (Adam et al. 2017, Tait et al. 2015). Various early warning scores have been created and used across UK hospitals to assist with the identification of critically ill patients and improve patient safety (Farenden et al. 2017). However, in 2012, and with the view of facilitating a standardized approach, the Royal College of Physicians (RCP) introduced a physiological scoring system called the National Early Warning Score (NEWS). This simple scoring system relies on healthcare staff performing patient observations (respiratory rate, heart rate, blood pressure, peripheral oxygen saturation, temperature and fluid balance) and informing medical staff and/or critical outreach teams of deviations from the norm (Keep et al. 2016). The total score helps to identify not just patients who are at risk and require immediate assessment but also those who are being safely managed, supporting clinical decision making and improving patient outcomes (NICE 2018).

More recently, in December 2017, the RCP updated its 2012 NEWS and published NEWS 2 (Figure 14.1) with the aim of improving the recognition of clinical deterioration in adults due to sepsis and hypercapnic respiratory failure (NICE 2018). The updated version now includes a new oxygen saturation scoring system for such patients and recognizes the patient's level of consciousness as an important sign of clinical deterioration (RCP 2017a). A final score of 5 or more identifies patients who require further assessment and early intervention, and this can help to prevent further clinical deterioration and potentially death (NICE 2018). Once a patient 'triggers', they are usually referred to critical care outreach teams or medical emergency teams, who are available in most hospitals to provide support to staff, assess the patient, initiate any required interventions, and avert or assist in critical care admissions (NICE 2018, RCP 2017a).

Initially, the implementation of NEWS in 2012 was targeted at UK hospital wards and emergency departments; however, since then, other clinical settings, such as ambulance services and general practices, have also embraced its use. In addition, NEWS is currently used across the world to assist health services to identify acutely unwell patients, improve patient outcomes and ultimately save lives (Blows 2018, Lee et al. 2018, NICE 2018, RCP 2017a, Wilkinson et al. 2017).

The use of NEWS has been shown to help nurses improve and focus their recognition of patients who may need further support and monitoring; therefore, it is important that time is taken to accurately calculate the score and act accordingly (Adam et al. 2017, Peate and Wild 2018). Obtaining an accurate measure of a patient's condition relies not just on an early warning score but also on clinical judgement and a holistic assessment (Farenden et al. 2017, NICE 2018).

A tool that assists with structuring and standardizing communication when reporting concerns is the Situation-Background-Assessment-Recommendation (SBAR) tool (Figure 14.2). SBAR is an easy-to-remember mechanism that is useful for framing any conversation, especially critical ones. It aims to focus the clinician's immediate attention on the presenting problem (Adam et al. 2017, Wilkinson et al. 2017), and it allows the person raising the concern to communicate key, succinct points and to highlight expected actions. It provides an easy and focused way to communicate key points and enables the person raising the concern to express what action is expected to result from the conversation (Müller et al. 2018).

Anticipated patient outcomes

Physiological observations will be assessed and recorded appropriately. Any actual or potential deterioration will be recognized early and communicated to the necessary teams (RCP 2017a).

Clinical governance

Nurses are accountable and responsible for providing optimum care for their patients (NMC 2018). The Nursing and Midwifery Council's *The Code* provides a framework of professional accountability for nurses and nursing associates (NMC 2018). It is essential that nursing staff objectively examine the information gathered from assessments and observations, including the patient's baseline as well as any information previously recorded (NICE 2018).

For nurses' own professional accountability and in order to achieve safe, effective and proficient care of patients, it is essential that nurses are able to discuss (using physiological rationale) the potential cause of any changes in the patient's observations (Farenden et al. 2017, Jackson 2016). Professional accountability demands more than just recording observations; it requires knowledge of underlying pathophysiology, the ability to interpret results, an understanding of clinical relevance and the ability to take appropriate action (Adam et al. 2017, NICE 2018).

NEWS key	FULL NAME	
0 1 2 3	DATE OF BIRTH	DATE OF ADMISSION

Parameter	Range	Score	Range
	DATE		DATE
	TIME		TIME
A+B Respirations Breaths/min	≥25	3	≥25
	21–24	2	21–24
	18–20		18–20
	15–17		15–17
	12–14		12–14
	9–11	1	9–11
	≤8	3	≤8
A+B SpO_2 Scale 1 Oxygen saturation (%)	≥96		≥96
	94–95	1	94–95
	92–93	2	92–93
	≤91	3	≤91
SpO_2 Scale 2† Oxygen saturation (%) Use Scale 2 if target range is 88–92%, eg in hypercapnic respiratory failure	≥97 on O_2	3	≥97 on O_2
	95–96 on O_2	2	95–96 on O_2
	93–94 on O_2	1	93–94 on O_2
	≥93 on air		≥93 on air
	88–92		88–92
	86–87	1	86–87
†ONLY use Scale 2 under the direction of a qualified clinician	84–85	2	84–85
	≤83%	3	≤83%
Air or oxygen?	A=Air		A=Air
	O_2 L/min	2	O_2 L/min
	Device		Device
C Blood pressure mmHg Score uses systolic BP only	≥220	3	≥220
	201–219		201–219
	181–200		181–200
	161–180		161–180
	141–160		141–160
	121–140		121–140
	111–120		111–120
	101–110	1	101–110
	91–100	2	91–100
	81–90	3	81–90
	71–80		71–80
	61–70		61–70
	51–60		51–60
	≤50		≤50
C Pulse Beats/min	≥131	3	≥131
	121–130	2	121–130
	111–120		111–120
	101–110	1	101–110
	91–100		91–100
	81–90		81–90
	71–80		71–80
	61–70		61–70
	51–60		51–60
	41–50	1	41–50
	31–40	3	31–40
	≤30		≤30
D Consciousness Score for NEW onset of confusion (no score if chronic)	Alert		Alert
	Confusion	3	Confusion
	V		V
	P		P
	U		U
E Temperature °C	≥39.1°	2	≥39.1°
	38.1–39.0°	1	38.1–39.0°
	37.1–38.0°		37.1–38.0°
	36.1–37.0°		36.1–37.0°
	35.1–36.0°	1	35.1–36.0°
	≤35.0°	3	≤35.0°
NEWS TOTAL			TOTAL
	Monitoring frequency		Monitoring
	Escalation of care Y/N		Escalation
	Initials		Initials

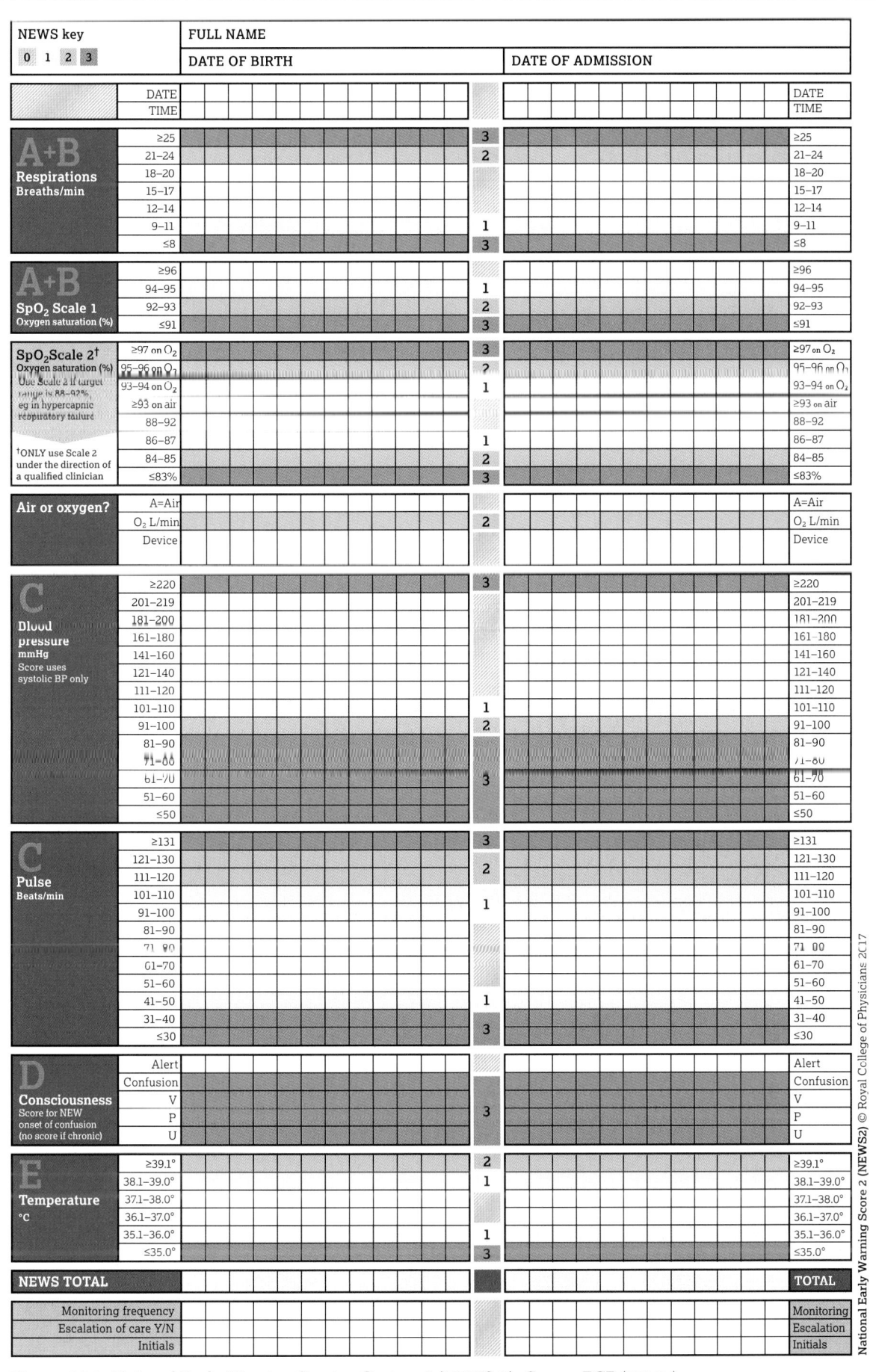

Figure 14.1 National Early Warning Scoring System 2 (NEWS 2). *Source:* RCP (2017a).

The ROYAL MARSDEN
NHS Foundation Trust

SBAR – Sepsis Tool

Scan onto EPR under SEPSIS or SBAR

S – Situation

Date	Time :	Ward
Referrer's name and designation		
Patient's name		
Hospital no		
Reason for referral		

B – Background

Diagnosis
Reason for admission

A – Assessment

RR	SpO_2	FiO_2	Temp
BP	HR	AVPU / New confusion *(circle)*	
PEW/NEW score			
Referrer's clinical impression			
Assessment/Action taken			

R – Recommendation

I would like you to: **Attend / Be aware**
Agreed plan and timescale
Name of person receiving referral

SEPSIS

1. Suspicion of an infection *(please tick all that apply)*:

Chest ☐	Urine ☐	Abdomen ☐	Skin/wound ☐
CVAD ☐	Meningitis ☐	Other ☐	Source unclear ☐

+ Red flags Time identified .... / .... hrs

RR ≥ 25bpm ☐	Needs Oxygen to keep SpO2 ≥ 92% (88% if COPD) ☐	HR > 130bpm ☐	Systolic BP ≤ 90mmHg (or drop of 40 from normal) ☐
Temp < 36°C or > 38°C and recent anticancer treatment (last 6 weeks) ☐		Responds only to voice, pain or unresponsive ☐	Non blanching rash, mottled, ashen, cyanotic ☐
Lactate > 2mmol/L ☐		New onset of confusion ☐	
Not passed urine in last 18 h/ UO <0.5 ml/kg/hr ☐			

or Amber flags Time identified .... / .... hrs

RR > 21-24bpm ☐	HR 91-130bpm ☐ New onset arrhythmia ☐	Systolic BP 91-100mmHg ☐	Acute deterioration in functional ability or mental status ☐
Clinic signs of wound, device or skin infection ☐		Not passed urine in last 12-18 hours ☐	

2. Time sepsis suspected .... / .... hrs

3. Sepsis 6

1. IV Antibiotics Time administered ...... /...... hrs **Please ensure time is filled in**	Tazocin ☐ Amikacin ☐ Ceftazidime ☐ Ciprofloxacin ☐ Teicoplanin ☐ Other	Was this a new or change in IVAB therapy? Y ☐ or N ☐	If Neutropenic Sepsis was suspected were IVAB's given before Neutrophil count known? Y ☐ or N ☐ Neutrophil count ....
2. Oxygen ☐	3. VBG ☐ Lactate result	4. Blood cultures: Peripheral ☐ CVAD ☐	Urine ☐ Sputum ☐ Wound swab ☐ Other ....
5. IV fluid bolus ☐	6. Monitor urine output ☐	If any of the above not done, please document why:	

NR570 V4 February 2019

Figure 14.2 Situation-Background-Assessment-Recommendation (SBAR) tool.

Observations should only be taken by staff who have undergone the appropriate training and assessment to ensure their competence in the use of the relevant equipment, the accurate recording and documentation of the observations, and the ability to interpret and act on results (MHRA 2013b, NICE 2018).

Pre-procedural considerations

Equipment

All practitioners need to be aware of the strengths and limitations of the devices they are using and need to have adequate training in the use of all equipment. In addition, they must ensure that the devices are validated, checked, maintained and recalibrated regularly according to the manufacturer's instructions in order to be used effectively and safely (MHRA 2013a, 2013b).

Pulse (heart rate)

Definition

The pulse is a pressure wave that is transmitted through the arterial tree with each heart beat following the alternating expansion and recoil of arteries during each cardiac cycle (Marieb and Hoehn 2018). The pulse is strongest in the arteries closest to the heart, becomes weaker in the arterioles and disappears altogether in the capillaries (Tortora and Derrickson 2017). It can be palpated in any artery that lies close to the surface of the body (Peate and Wild 2018). The portion of the radial artery at the wrist is easily accessible and therefore the radial pulse is frequently used (Figure 14.3), but there are several other clinically important arterial pulse points, such as the carotid artery, femoral artery and brachial plexus (Marieb and Hoehn 2018, Tortora and Derrickson 2017) (Figure 14.4).

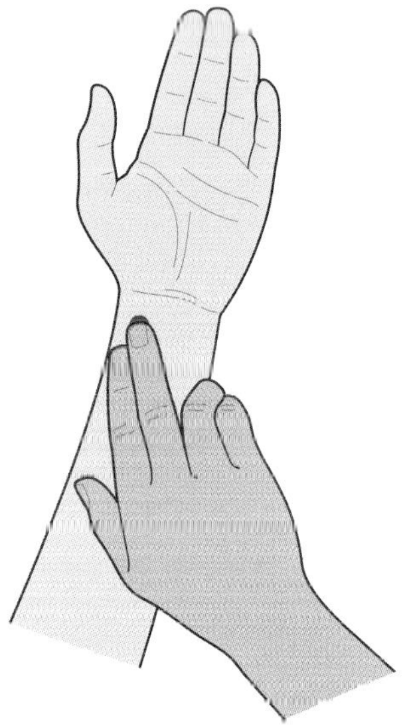

Figure 14.3 Taking a radial pulse. *Source:* Reproduced from Peate and Wild (2018) with permission of John Wiley & Sons.

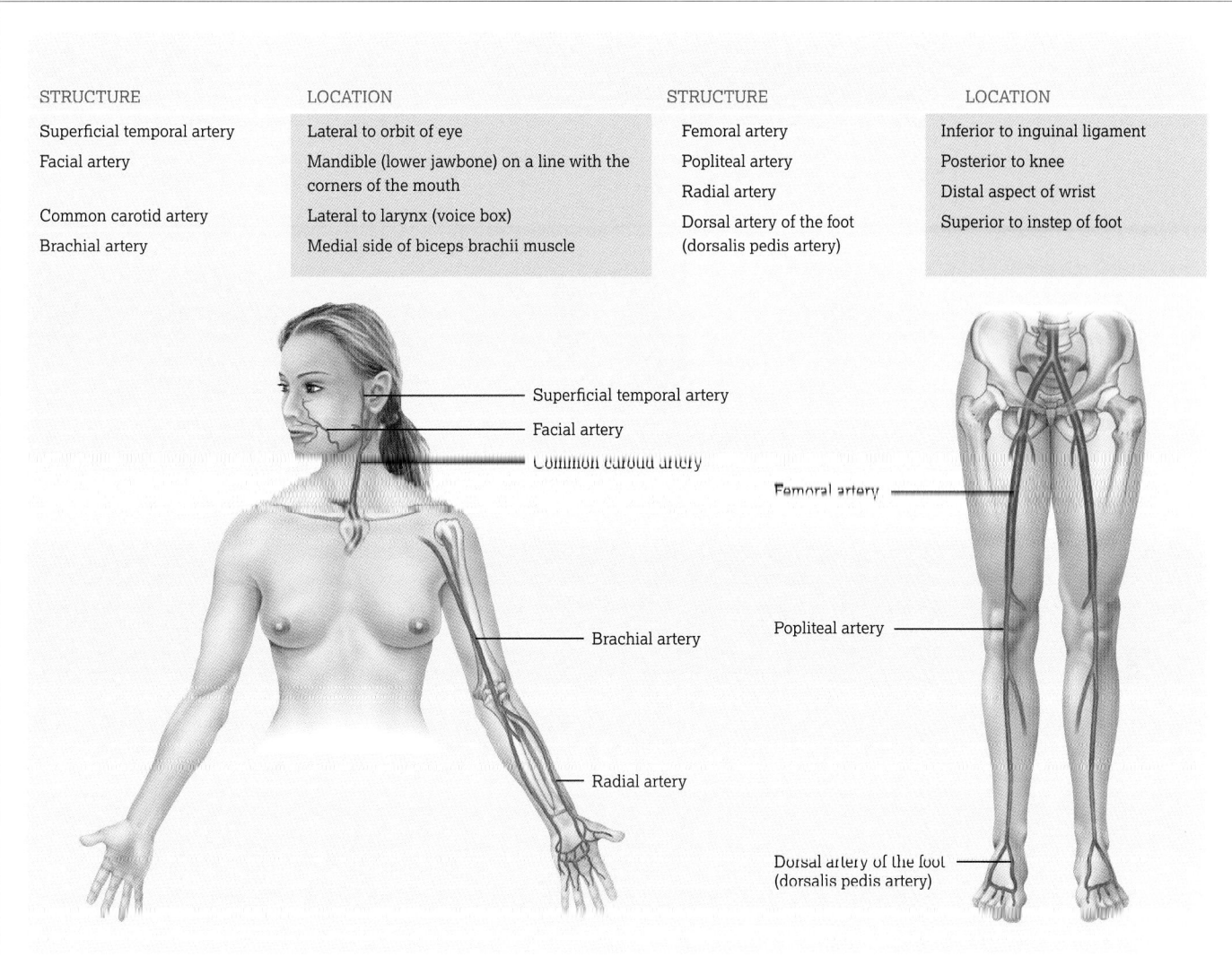

STRUCTURE	LOCATION	STRUCTURE	LOCATION
Superficial temporal artery	Lateral to orbit of eye	Femoral artery	Inferior to inguinal ligament
Facial artery	Mandible (lower jawbone) on a line with the corners of the mouth	Popliteal artery	Posterior to knee
Common carotid artery	Lateral to larynx (voice box)	Radial artery	Distal aspect of wrist
Brachial artery	Medial side of biceps brachii muscle	Dorsal artery of the foot (dorsalis pedis artery)	Superior to instep of foot

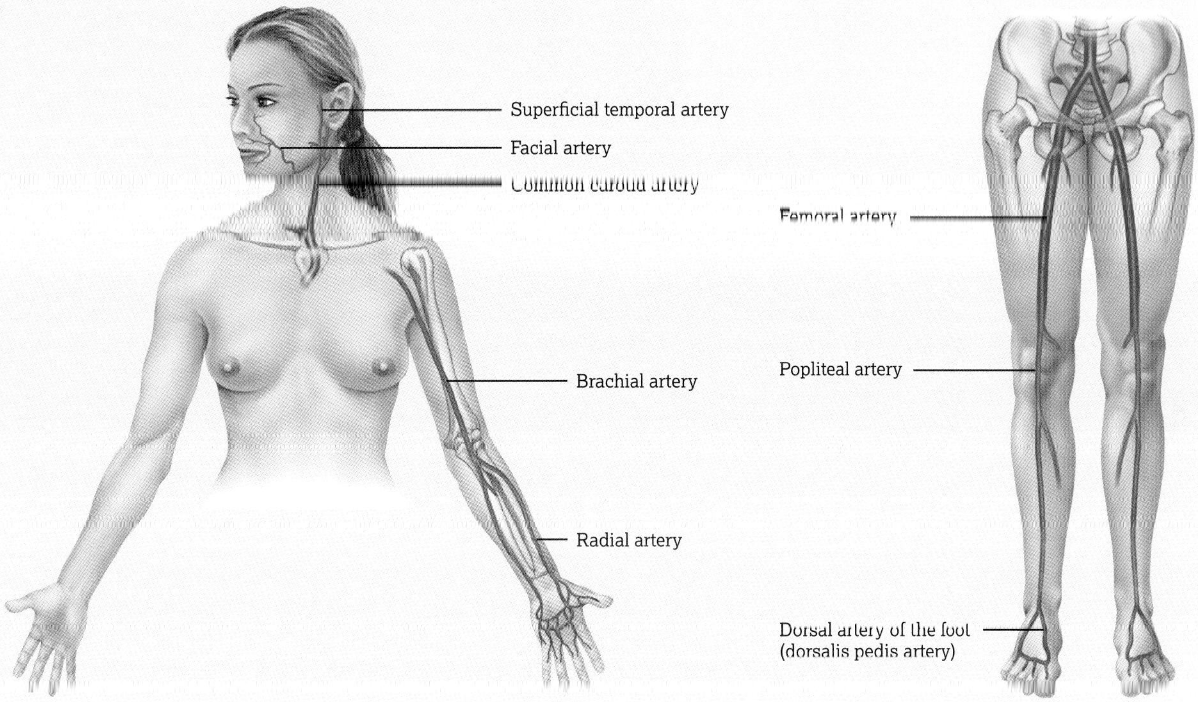

Figure 14.4 Pulse points. *Source*: Reproduced from Tortora and Derrickson (2011) with permission of John Wiley & Sons.

Anatomy and physiology

In health, the arterial pulse is commonly used to assess the effects of activity, postural changes and emotions, such as anxiety, on heart rate (Marieb and Hoehn 2018). In ill health, pulse measurement can be used to assess the effects of disease, treatments and response to therapy (Blows 2018). Each time the heart beats, it pushes blood through the arteries and the pumping action causes the walls of the arteries to expand and distend, creating a wave-like sensation that can then be felt as the pulse (Marieb and Hoehn 2018).

The pulse can be measured manually by lightly compressing an artery against firm tissue and counting the number of beats in a minute (Peate and Wild 2018). The pulse is palpated to note the following:

- rate
- rhythm
- amplitude (Bickley 2016).

Rate

A person's pulse rate can be influenced by several factors, including age, the person's sex, exercise, temperature, medications, intravascular volume, stress, positioning, pathology, hormones and electrolytes (Marini and Dries 2016, Wilkinson et al. 2017). The approximate usual ranges are illustrated in Table 14.1.

Table 14.1 Normal resting pulse rates per minute at various ages

Age	Approximate range
1 week to 3 months	100–160
3 months to 2 years	80–150
2–10 years	70–110
10 years to adulthood	55–90

The pulse may also vary depending on posture. For example, the pulse of a healthy man may be around 66 beats per minute when he is lying down, but it may increase to 70 beats per minute when he is sitting up and 80 beats per minute when he suddenly stands; in women, the pulse is slightly faster (Marieb and Hoehn 2018).

The pulse rate of an individual with a healthy heart tends to be relatively constant; however, when blood volume drops suddenly or when the heart has been weakened by disease, the stroke volume declines and cardiac output is maintained only by increasing the rate of the heart beat (Tortora and Derrickson 2017).

Cardiac output (CO) is the amount of blood pumped out by each ventricle in 1 minute (Lin 2016). It is the product of heart rate (HR) and stroke volume (SV) (Box 14.1). Stroke volume is defined as the volume of blood pumped out by one ventricle with each beat (Lin 2016, Mehta and Arora 2014).

Box 14.1 Cardiac output equation

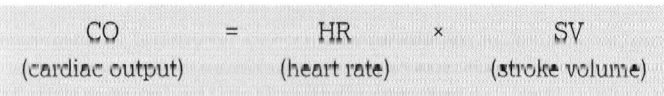

CO	=	HR	×	SV
(cardiac output)		(heart rate)		(stroke volume)

Using normal resting values for HR (75 beats per minute) and SV (70 mL per beat), the average adult cardiac output can be calculated as (Tortora and Derrickson 2017):

$$CO = 75\,\text{beats/min} \times 70\,\text{mL/beat} = 5250\,\text{mL/min} = 5.25\,\text{L/min}$$

The heart rate and therefore pulse rate are influenced by various factors acting through neural, chemical and physically induced homeostatic mechanisms (see Figure 14.5 for factors that increase cardiac output):

- Neural changes in heart rate are caused by activation of the sympathetic nervous system, which increases heart rate, while parasympathetic activation decreases heart rate (Patton 2018).
- Chemical regulation of the heart is affected by hormones (adrenaline and thyroxine) and electrolytes (sodium, potassium and calcium) (Patton 2018). High or low levels of electrolytes, particularly potassium, magnesium and calcium, can cause alterations in the heart's rhythm and rate (Blows 2018).
- Other factors that influence heart rate are age, gender, exercise and body temperature; hyperthermia and hypothermia cause the metabolism to increase or slow down, depending on the tissues' demand for oxygen (Marieb and Hoehn 2018, Tortora and Derrickson 2017).

Tachycardia

Tachycardia is an abnormally fast heart rate, over 100 beats per minute in adults (Wilkinson et al. 2017). It may result from exercise or exertion, an elevated body temperature, stress, certain drugs or heart disease (Marieb and Hoehn 2018). Persistent tachycardia (even at rest) is considered pathological because tachycardia can lead to fibrillation (Marieb and Hoehn 2018).

Bradycardia

Bradycardia is a heart rate slower than 60 beats per minute, which can result from low body temperature, certain drugs or parasympathetic nervous system activation (Marieb and Hoehn 2018, Patton 2018). It can also occur in fit athletes as physical and cardiovascular conditioning leads to hypertrophy of the heart, increasing stroke volume and leading to a lower resting heart rate but with the same cardiac output (Marieb and Hoehn 2018). If persistent bradycardia occurs in an individual as a result of illness, then blood circulation to body tissues may be inadequate. After head trauma, bradycardia can be a warning of brain oedema and is one of the indications of raised intracranial pressure (Marieb and Hoehn 2018).

Rhythm

The pulse rhythm is the sequence of beats, which in health should be regular (Wilkinson et al. 2017). The co-ordinated action of the muscles of the heart in producing a regular heart rhythm is caused

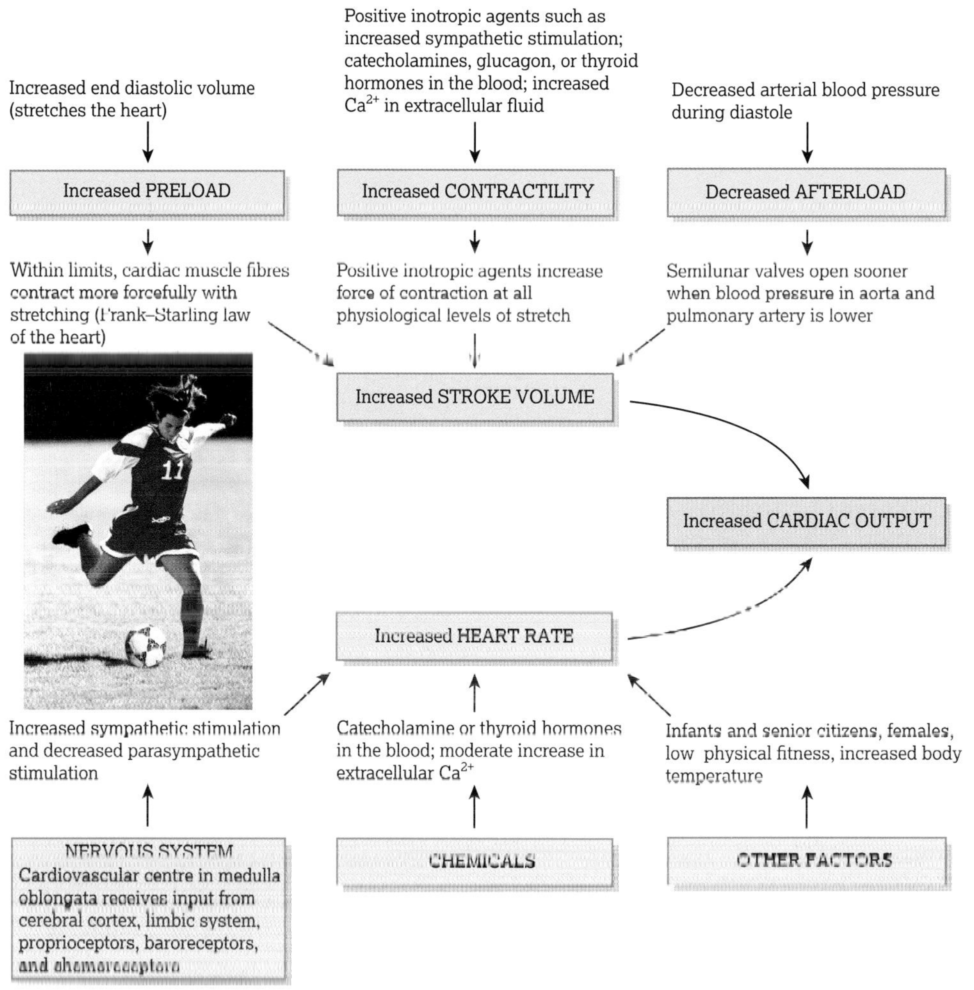

Figure 14.5 Factors that increase cardiac output. *Source*: Reproduced from Tortora and Derrickson (2011) with permission of John Wiley & Sons.

by the ability of cardiac muscle to contract inherently without nervous control (Marieb and Hoehn 2018). The co-ordinated action of the muscles in the heart results from two physiological factors:

- Gap junctions in the cardiac muscles form interconnections between adjacent cardiac muscles and allow transmission of nerve impulses from cell to cell.
- Specialized nerve-like cardiac cells form the nodal system, which initiates and distributes impulses throughout the heart so that the heart beats as one unit (Marieb and Hoehn 2018).

The nodal or conduction system is composed of the sinoatrial node, the atrioventricular node, the atrioventricular bundle and the Purkinje fibres (Marieb and Keller 2017). The sinoatrial node is the pacemaker and initiates each impulse, which leads to a wave of contraction, setting the rhythm for the heart as a whole (Figure 14.6) (Waugh and Grant 2018). A rhythm that is initiated at the sinoatrial node is called 'sinus rhythm' (Waugh and Grant 2018).

In patients younger than 40 years, irregularities may be linked to breathing when the heart rate increases on inspiration and decreases on expiration (Blows 2018). Although this is rarely noticeable in adults, it is normal and is known as sinus arrhythmia (Tortora and Derrickson 2017). Defects in the conduction system of the heart can cause irregular heart rhythms, or arrhythmias, which result in unco-ordinated contraction of the heart (Marieb and Keller 2017). These can be felt when palpating the pulse and can be seen on an ECG tracing.

Amplitude

Amplitude is a reflection of pulse strength and the elasticity of the arterial wall, which varies with alternating strong and weak ventricular contractions (Bickley 2016). In patients with arteriosclerosis, the arteries feel hard and different, in terms of flexibility, when compared to those of young, healthy adults (Tortora and Derrickson 2017). It takes some clinical experience to be able to identify these differences in amplitude; however, it is important to be able to recognize major changes, such as the faint flickering pulse of the severely hypovolaemic patient or the irregular pulse of cardiac arrhythmias (Adam et al. 2017).

Abnormal heart rhythms

Irregular heart rhythms can be present in patients of all age groups regardless of previous medical history or co-morbidities (Brown and Cadogan 2016). Among all of the different types, atrial fibrillation is the most common, especially in the older population, and it can lead to heart failure and potentially death (Sprigings and Chambers 2017). It starts with a disruption of rhythm in the atrial areas of the heart, occurring at extremely rapid and unco-ordinated intervals (Wilkinson et al. 2017). The rapid impulses result in the ventricles not being able to respond to every atrial beat and, therefore, the ventricles contract irregularly (Adam et al. 2017). Among the possible causes of atrial fibrillation, some of the most common are ischaemic heart disease, acute illness, electrolyte imbalance and thyrotoxicosis (Mann and Dries 2016). If poorly managed, patients with atrial fibrillation are at increased risk of arterial thromboembolism and stroke (Phang and Manning 2019).

Assessing and detecting abnormalities in the ventricular rate by checking the radial pulse is considered an unreliable method as some contractions may not be strong enough to transmit a pulse wave that is detectable at the radial artery (Sprigings and Chambers 2017). Hence, monitoring of the apex beat and radial pulse is advisable in patients with atrial fibrillation, because it will determine the ventricular rate more reliably and identify whether there is an apex beat–radial pulse deficit (Sprigings and Chambers 2017). This procedure requires

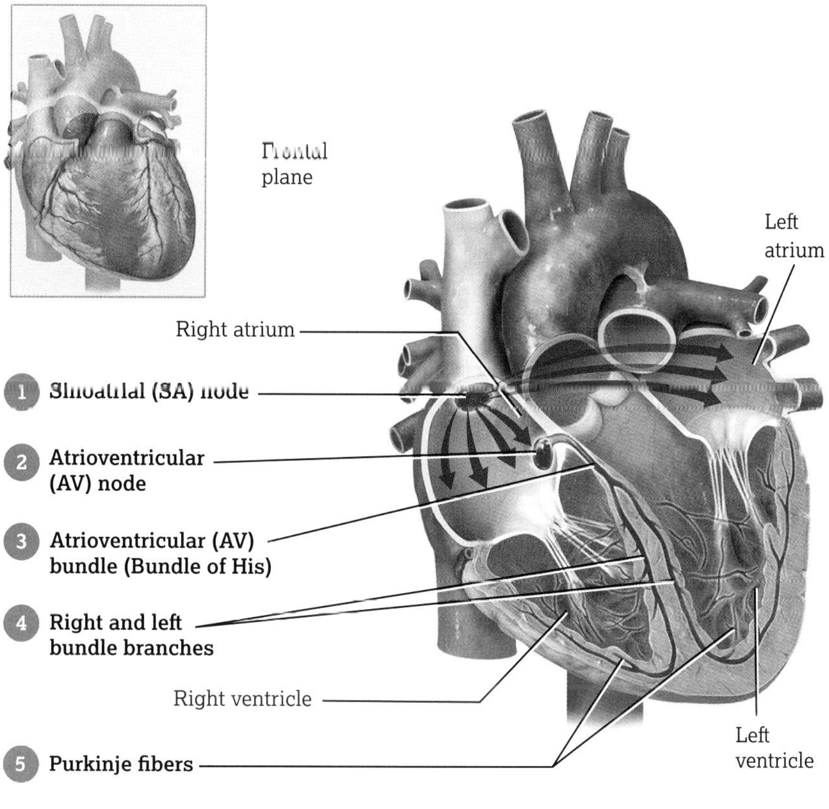

Figure 14.6 Conduction system of the heart. Auto-rhythmic fibres in the SA node, located in the right atrial wall, act as the heart's pacemaker, initiating cardiac action potentials that cause contraction of the heart's chambers. The conduction system ensures that the chambers of the heart contract in a co-ordinated manner. *Source:* Reproduced from Tortora and Derrickson (2017) with permission of John Wiley & Sons.

two nurses and is described below in the section on assessing gross pulse irregularity. In addition, a 12-lead ECG should be taken to confirm any arrhythmias (see the section on ECG below).

Assessing gross pulse irregularity

A paradoxical pulse is a pulse that markedly decreases in amplitude during inspiration (Swanevelder 2016). On inspiration, blood is pooled in the lungs, decreasing the amount of blood that is returned to the left side of the heart; this affects the consequent stroke volume (Marieb and Keller 2017). A paradoxical pulse is usually regarded as normal, although, in conjunction with features such as hypotension and dyspnoea, it may indicate cardiac tamponade, hypovolaemia, severe airway obstruction or tension pneumothorax (Bickley 2016).

When there is a gross pulse irregularity, a stethoscope may be used to assess the apical heartbeat by placing the diaphragm of the stethoscope over the apex of the heart and counting the beats for 60 seconds (Bickley 2016). A second nurse should record the radial pulse at the same time and the deficit between the two should be noted using, for example, different colours on the patient's chart to indicate the apex and radial rates (Jackson 2016).

Assessing lower limb perfusion

Co-morbidities such as atherosclerosis, diabetes, heart failure, and peripheral arterial or vascular disease can affect the blood circulation in the lower limbs (Wilkinson et al. 2017). Palpating the dorsalis pedis pulse (Figure 14.7), which is on the dorsal surface of the foot; the posterior tibial pulse (Figure 14.8), which is located near the Achilles tendon; and the popliteal pulse (Figure 14.9), which is felt at the back of the knee, can provide an insight into the amount of circulatory compromise, if any (Bickley 2016). Where indicated, feeling for the femoral pulses is also of value for an accurate clinical assessment (Bickley 2016).

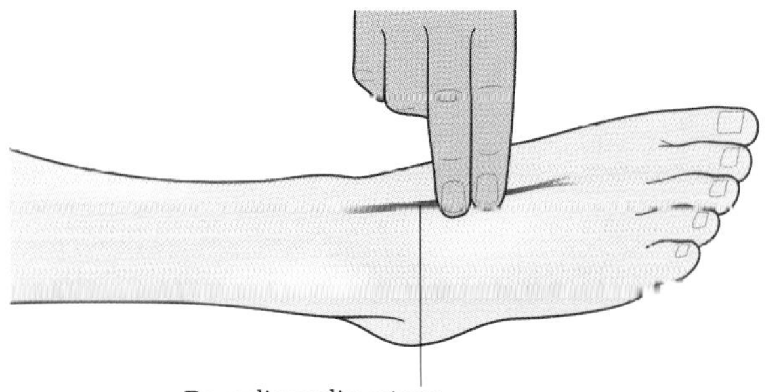

Figure 14.7 Dorsalis pedis pulse. *Source*: Reproduced from Peate and Wild (2018) with permission of John Wiley & Sons.

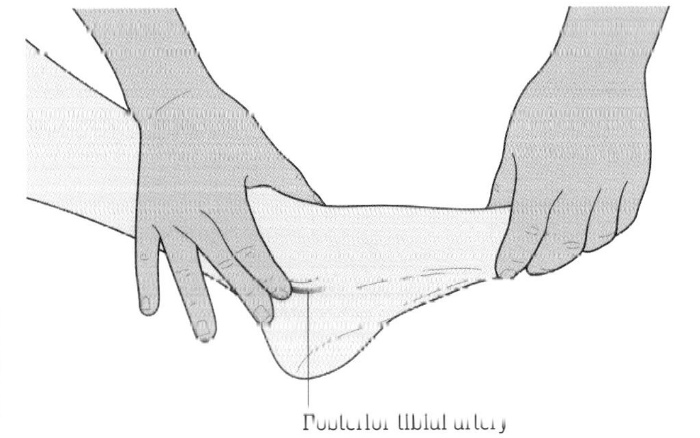

Figure 14.8 Posterior tibial pulse. *Source*: Reproduced from Peate and Wild (2018) with permission of John Wiley & Sons.

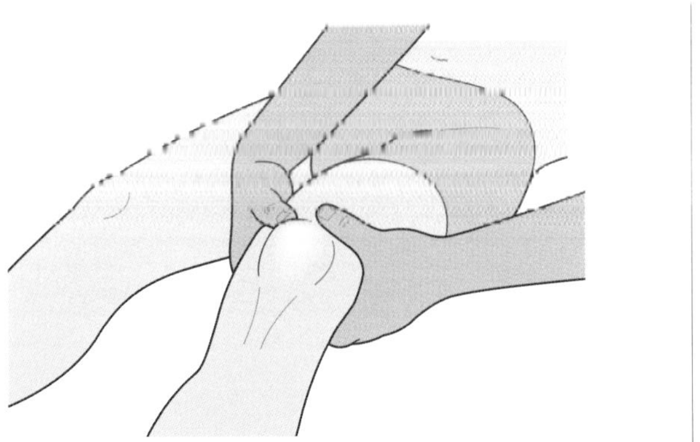

Figure 14.9 Popliteal pulse. *Source*: Reproduced from Peate and Wild (2018) with permission of John Wiley & Sons.

Inspection is another form of assessment as ischaemia, deep vein thrombosis and any other compromising vascularity illness may cause changes in the warmth and colour of the lower limbs, including in the capillary refill (Bajwa et al. 2014). Patients with certain types of cancer or who have previously had vascular interventions, such as coronary artery bypass, are more prone to circulatory changes in the lower limbs and therefore a precise assessment will prevent complications that may lead to, for example, amputation (Bailey et al. 2014).

Evidence-based approaches

Rationale

The pulse is taken for the following reasons:

- to gather information on the heart rate, pattern of beats (rhythm) and amplitude (strength) of the pulse (RCN 2017b)
- to determine the individual's pulse on admission as a base for comparison with future measurements (NHS Health Check 2017)
- to monitor changes in pulse (Marieb and Hoehn 2018)
- to monitor the efficiency of the individual's circulatory system (Peate and Wild 2018)
- to ensure the perfusion of peripheries (Bickley 2016).

Indications

Conditions in which a patient's pulse may need careful monitoring, as part of an overall assessment and in conjunction with other vital signs, are as follows:

- Post-operative and critically ill patients require monitoring of the pulse to assess cardiovascular stability (the patient's pulse should be recorded pre-operatively in order to establish a baseline and to make comparisons) (Adam et al. 2017, Peate and Wild 2018).
- Hypovolaemic shock can occur post-surgery due to the loss of plasma or blood from the circulatory blood volume (RCUK 2015). The resulting acceleration in heart rate causes a tachycardia that can be felt in the pulse; the greater the loss in volume, the threadier the pulse is likely to feel (Swanevelder 2016).
- Blood transfusions require careful monitoring of the pulse as an incompatible blood transfusion may lead to a rise in pulse rate early in the transfusion (Robinson et al. 2017) (see Chapter 12: Respiratory care, CPR and blood transfusion).
- Patients with local or systemic infections or inflammatory reactions require monitoring of their pulse to detect sepsis or severe sepsis (Blows 2018). This is characterized by a decrease in the mean arterial pressure and a rise in pulse rate (Marieb and Hoehn 2018).
- Patients with cardiovascular conditions require regular assessment of the pulse to monitor their condition and the efficacy of medications (Wilkinson et al. 2017).

- It is necessary to monitor the pulse of any patient at risk of deterioration, as a change in heart rate is often a response to other pathophysiology and can be a compensatory mechanism (Adam et al. 2017).
- Any patient with compromised circulation or perfusion to a limb, for example post-surgery or trauma or with vascular disease, requires their pulse to be monitored (Bajwa et al. 2014).

Methods of pulse measurement

Manual

The pulse is measured by lightly compressing the appropriate artery against firm tissue and counting the number of beats in a minute and/or by auscultation the apex of the heart with a stethoscope (Bickley 2016).

Electronic

Automated electronic equipment – such as a pulse oximeter, blood pressure recording devices, 12-lead ECG or continuous cardiac monitoring – may be used to determine a patient's pulse (Marini and Dries 2016). However, even when a patient has continuous ECG monitoring, it is still essential to manually feel for a pulse to determine amplitude and volume and whether the pulse is irregular (Jackson 2016). In the specific case of pulseless electrical activity, the monitor shows a heart rhythm; however, a pulse is not palpable due to insufficient cardiac output (Coviello 2015).

Pre-procedural considerations

Equipment

Monitoring a pulse may require a stethoscope (if it is necessary to count the apical beat along with palpating the pulse). Alternatively, an electronic pulse measurement device (pulse oximeter) may be used; this is a small electronic device consisting of a probe that is placed onto the end of a finger to record pulse rate and peripheral oxygen saturations.

Specific patient preparation

Ideally a patient should be at rest for 20 minutes before any attempt to obtain an accurate pulse, as strenuous activity can result in falsely elevated readings (Blows 2018).

Procedure guideline 14.1 Pulse measurement

Essential equipment

- Personal protective equipment
- A watch that has a second hand
- Observations chart
- Black pen
- A stethoscope (if counting the apical beat)
- Electronic pulse measurement device, for example pulse oximeter, blood pressure measuring device or cardiac monitor

Action	Rationale
Pre-procedure	
1 Introduce yourself to the patient, explain and discuss the procedure with them, and gain their consent to proceed.	To ensure that the patient feels at ease, understands the procedure and gives their valid consent (NMC 2018, **C**).
2 Decontaminate hands with soap and water and/or an alcohol-based handrub, and apply personal protective equipment.	To prevent cross-infection (NHS England and NHSI 2019, **C**).
3 Where possible, measure the pulse under the same conditions each time.	To ensure continuity and consistency in recording (Tait et al. 2015, **E**).
4 Ensure that the patient is comfortable and relaxed. Ideally the patient should refrain from physical activity for 20 minutes before their pulse is measured.	To ensure that the patient is comfortable. **E** Strenuous activity will result in falsely elevated readings (Bickley 2016, **E**).
Procedure	
5 Place the first and second fingers, and optionally also the third finger, along the appropriate artery and apply light pressure until the pulse is felt (**Action figure 5**).	The fingertips are sensitive to touch. Practitioners should be aware that the thumb and forefinger have pulses of their own and therefore these may be mistaken for the patient's pulse (Peate and Wild 2018, **E**).
6 For apical heart rate, place a stethoscope on the fourth or fifth intercostal space on the left mid-clavicular line (typically under the breast area) and listen to the heart beat.	The apical heart rate is usually recorded if the heart rate is irregular; this ensures a more accurate count (Bickley 2016, **E**).
7 Count the pulse for 60 seconds.	Sufficient time is required to detect irregularities in rhythm or volume; however, if the pulse is regular and of good volume, subsequent readings may be taken for 30 seconds and then doubled to give beats per minute (Blows 2018, **E**). If the rhythm or volume changes on subsequent readings, the pulse must be taken for 60 seconds (Bickley 2016, **E**).
8 Accurately document the result; additional factors, such as the rhythm, volume and skin condition (dry, sweaty or clammy), may be described in the patient's nursing notes.	To monitor differences and detect trends; any irregularities should be brought to the attention of the appropriate senior nursing and medical teams (NMC 2018, **C**). Additional qualitative characteristics of the pulse may aid diagnosis of the patient's condition (Brown and Cadogan 2016, **E**).

(continued)

Procedure guideline 14.1 Pulse measurement *(continued)*

Action	Rationale
Post-procedure	
9 Discuss the result and any further action with the patient.	To involve the patient in their care and provide assurance of a normal result or explain the actions to be undertaken in the event of an abnormal result (NMC 2018, **C**).
10 Wash and dry or decontaminate hands with an alcohol-based handrub. Decontaminate any equipment used as per local policy.	To prevent cross-infection (NHS England and NHSI 2019, **C**; NICE 2014, **C**).

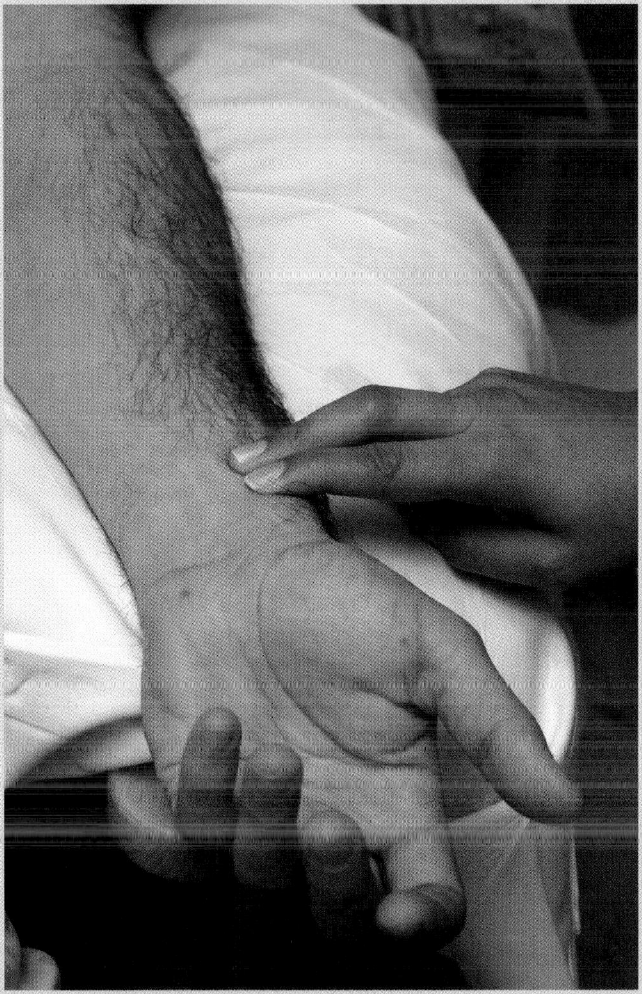

Action Figure 5 Taking a radial pulse.

Problem-solving table 14.1 Prevention and resolution (Procedure guideline 14.1)

Problem	Cause	Prevention	Action
No pulse palpable	Incorrect positioning of fingers	Refer to Figure 14.4 for palpation sites.	Place two or three fingers over the appropriate artery and lightly depress against the tissue or bone. Try alternative sites such as the brachial or carotid artery.
Absent or faint pulse	Poor perfusion	Assess the patient's existing co-morbidities for further information and identify any possible causes of hypovolaemia (Lin 2010).	Inform the medical team if the patient is cardiovascularly compromised (RCUK 2015).

Problem	Cause	Prevention	Action
	Obstruction to flow, for example clot, swelling or trauma	Perform a venous thromboembolism risk assessment on admission and ensure appropriate preventative measures are in place, for example anti-embolism stockings, mechanical devices applying intermittent pneumatic compression, or pharmacological prophylaxis such as injections of low-molecular-weight heparin preparations (NICE 2018). Monitor lower lib circulation.	Perform a neurovascular assessment, assessing all pulse sites to determine the compromised area (Sprigings and Chambers 2017). Also feel for warmth and sensation and capillary refill to provide further information on the degree of vascular sufficiency (Bickley 2016). Evaluate the vascularity of the lower limbs (see the section above on assessing lower limb perfusion).
Pulse too fast and irregular to palpate manually	Patient may be in an abnormal rhythm	Conduct a haemodynamic assessment, and monitoring and maintenance of electrolyte balance (Jackson 2016).	Irregular rhythms should prompt a full set of observations, and it is essential to perform a 12-lead ECG and have this reviewed by a practitioner competent in ECG interpretation (Adam et al. 2017).

ECG, electrocardiogram.

Post-procedural considerations

Documentation

The pulse should be recorded in the patient's notes on the institution's approved observation chart. The recording should be dated and timed so that the pulse trend may be viewed easily as part of ongoing patient monitoring (Peate and Wild 2018).

Electrocardiogram (ECG)

Definition

Muscle contraction is associated with electrical activity in the heart called depolarization, which can be monitored, amplified and recorded with a simple test called an electrocardiogram (ECG) (Marieb and Hoehn 2018). An ECG provides a graphical representation of the myocardium's electrical conduction and excitation (Marieb and Hoehn 2018), and illustrates a three-dimensional event in a two-dimensional graph recorded over a period of time (Blows 2018). It is a non-invasive, routine clinical examination that can be performed by a range of healthcare professionals by applying electrodes on the surface of the patient's body (Peate and Wild 2018).

When used correctly and in the context of the patient's clinical history, it is a valuable tool that can be used to ascertain information about the electrophysiology of the heart and provide guidance relevant to diagnosis, prognosis and treatment (Marieb and Hoehn 2018, Marini and Dries 2016).

Types of ECG monitoring

12-lead ECG

A 12-lead ECG provides 12 different views of the heart from 10 electrodes placed on the patient's chest and limbs (Aehlert 2017, Wesley 2016) (Figure 14.10). Electrical changes take place as the cardiac muscle depolarizes and repolarizes, and the 12 views show the three-dimensional electrical activity occurring in the heart (Aehlert 2017). A 12-lead ECG provides a snapshot of myocardial activity and is used for diagnostic purposes (Wesley 2016).

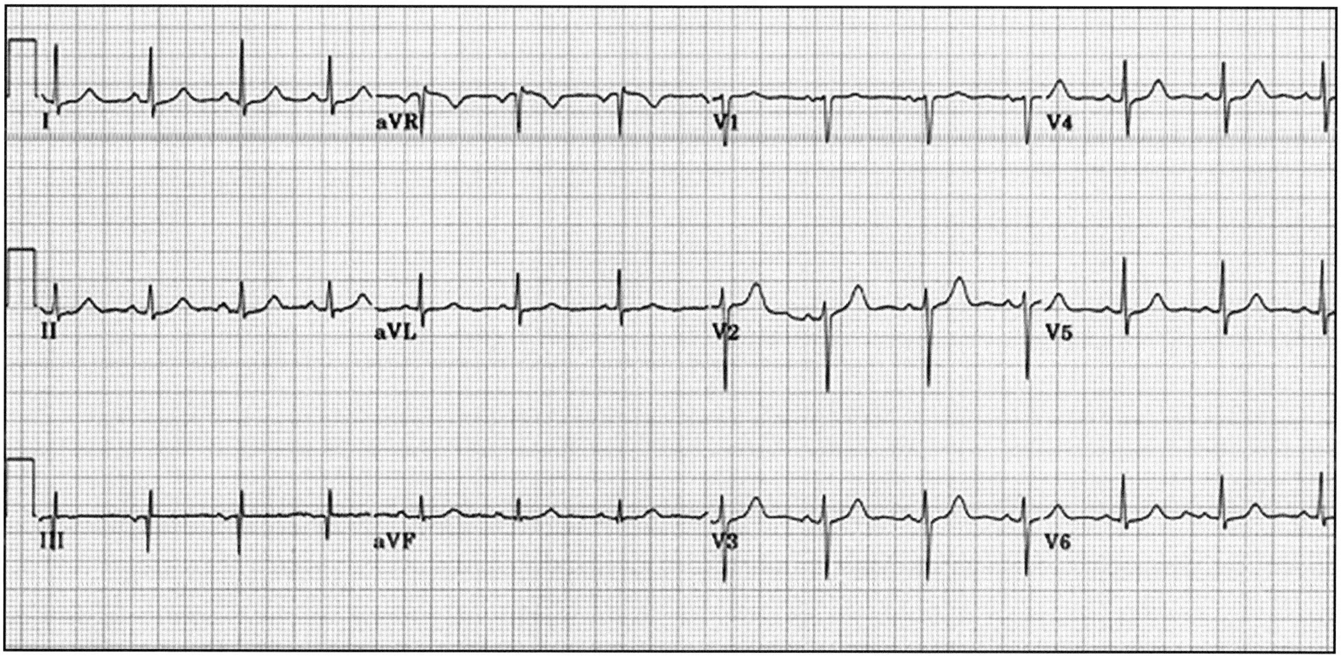

Figure 14.10 A 12-lead electrocardiogram (ECG). *Source*: Reproduced from https://meds.queensu.ca/central/assets/modules/ECG/the_12_lead_ecg.html.

Three- and five-lead ECG

Three-lead ECG monitoring is most commonly used for cardiac rhythm assessment and continuous cardiac monitoring (Coviello 2015). Three leads are placed on the torso: one on each shoulder and one on the lower left chest (Figure 14.11). A five-lead ECG is used for similar purposes but has the addition of an extra two leads/views, which gives a more detailed picture of the activity in the heart; it is commonly used in critical care settings (Bunce and Ray 2016, Wesley 2016).

Anatomy and physiology

All myocardial cells are able to spontaneously generate impulses and initiate the cardiac electrical cycle without the need for external stimulation; this is known as automaticity (Patton 2018). Cardiac conduction normally begins in the sinoatrial (SA) node (see Figure 14.6), located in the wall of the right atrium. Considered the heart's natural pacemaker, the SA node normally initiates impulses at a faster rate than other myocardial cells, generating impulses at a rate of 60–100 beats per minute (Waugh and Grant 2018). The impulse generated by the SA node spreads through the atrial muscle fibres (depolarization) to the atrioventricular (AV) node, causing atrial contraction as it spreads (Aehlert 2017).

The AV node acts as a gateway into the ventricular conduction system, delaying impulses for approximately 0.1–0.2 seconds and creating a short period of electrical standstill before the depolarization spreads through the AV node into the ventricles, allowing the atria to finish contracting before ventricular contraction commences (Waugh and Grant 2018, Wesley 2016). From the AV node, the impulse travels rapidly through specialized conduction tissues in the ventricles, firstly through the bundle of His, along the left and right bundle branches, and then more slowly through the mass of ventricular muscle along the Purkinje fibres, resulting in a powerful ventricular contraction (Tortora and Derrickson 2017). See Figure 14.6 for the conduction pathway of the heart.

The normal ECG waveform depicts five deflections or waves known as P, Q, R, S and T waves (Figure 14.12). The P wave (which is small) reflects atrial depolarization, the QRS waves (which are large) reflect the rapid spread of depolarization from the AV node to the Purkinje fibres through the ventricles, and the T wave reflects ventricular repolarization – the return of the ventricular muscle to its resting state (Aehlert 2017, SCST 2017). Atrial repolarization is not graphically represented on the ECG as it is hidden in the QRS complex (Wesley 2016).

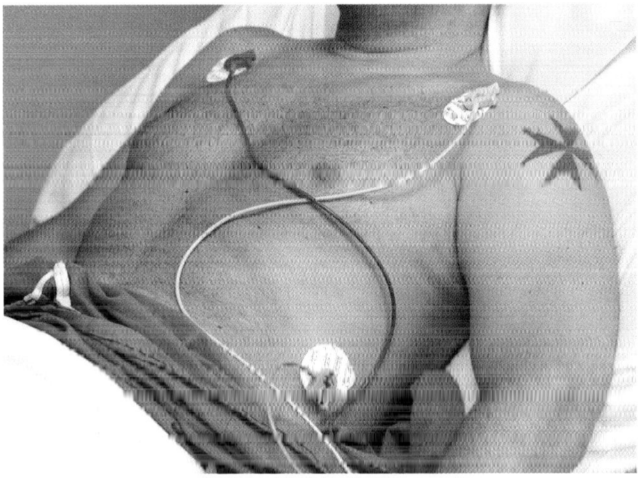

Figure 14.11 Three-lead electrocardiogram (ECG) electrode placement.

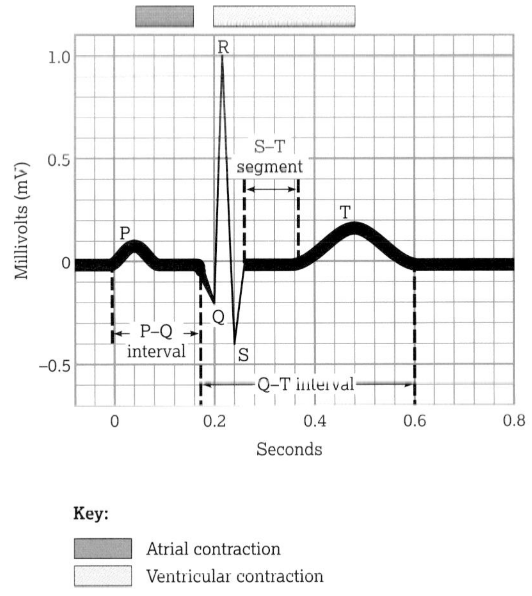

Figure 14.12 A normal electrocardiogram (ECG) (lead II). P wave, arterial depolarization; QRS complex, onset of ventricular depolarization; T wave, ventricular repolarization. *Source*: Reproduced from Tortora and Derrickson (2017) with permission of John Wiley & Sons.

Evidence-based approaches

12-lead ECG

A 12-lead ECG (see Figure 14.10) provides 12 views (also termed 'leads') of the electrical current of the heart. It consists of the following:

- Three bipolar leads (I, II and III) are also called 'standard limb leads' because they are obtained from the electrodes placed on the right arm, left arm and left foot. They measure the electric potential between a positive and a negative electrode and create a triangle around the heart called the Einthoven triangle (Figure 14.13) (Wesley 2016).
- Three augmented unipolar leads (aVR, aVL and aVF) and six unipolar chest leads or precordial leads (V1–V6). Contrary to the bipolar leads, the unipolar leads have only one positive electrode (Wesley 2016).
- One neutral lead is connected to an electrode placed on the right leg; this reduces interference (Aehlert 2017).

Electrode placement

Table 14.2 describes the anatomical locations of each chest electrode and Figure 14.14 shows the standard positions of the six chest electrodes. The limb electrodes should be placed just proximally to the wrist and ankle bones unless there is a clinical reason, such as amputation, burns or surgical wounds, to do otherwise; ECGs recorded using any other limb position must be clearly labelled as such to account for any changes that might affect interpretation (SCST 2017). It does not matter if the electrode is positioned on the inside or outside of the limb – position the patient comfortably and use the most accessible aspect for electrode placement (Blows 2018).

The 12 leads (or viewpoints) look at the heart from different directions. Each lead records a positive or negative wave depending on which direction the impulse is travelling in relation to the observing lead; a positive wave will be recorded if the impulse is travelling towards the observing lead, whereas a negative wave will be recorded if the impulse is travelling away from the observing lead (SCST 2017). Correct electrode placement is essential to ensure an accurate ECG recording is obtained. Incorrect electrode

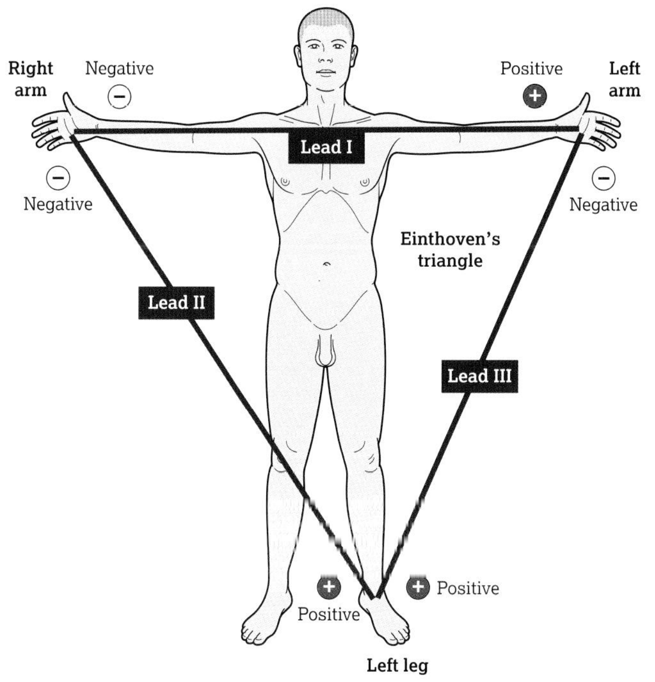

Figure 14.13 Einthoven triangle.

Table 14.2 Three- and five-lead ECG positioning

Electrode	Position
Three-lead placement	
Right arm limb lead (RA, red)	Right clavicle proximal to right shoulder
Left arm limb lead (LA, yellow)	Left clavicle proximal to left shoulder
Left leg limb lead (LL, green)	Lower edge of left ribcage, below pectoral muscles
Five-lead placement	
Right arm limb lead (RA, red)	Right clavicle proximal to right shoulder
Left arm limb lead (LA, yellow)	Left clavicle proximal to left shoulder
Left leg limb lead (LL, green)	Lower edge of left ribcage, below pectoral muscles
V (white electrode)	Fourth intercostal space at the right sternal edge
RL (black electrode)	Lower edge of the right ribcage, on a non-muscular area.

placement can lead to morphology changes or alter the amplitude of waves, meaning that ECG changes may be caused by artefacts rather than physiological abnormalities, which may lead to misdiagnosis (Aehlert 2017, Wesley 2016).

An alternative positioning of the limb electrodes on the torso, known as the Mason–Likar 12-lead ECG system (Figure 14.15), can be used when continuous 12-lead ECG monitoring is required, as it enables the waveforms to be easily viewed without interference from limb movement (Khan 2015). However, it should be noted that the QRS complexes are slightly different in amplitude and axis when repositioned on the torso in the Mason–Likar position and so any deviation from the standard 12-lead electrode placement should be clearly documented on the ECG trace (SCST 2017, Wesley 2016).

Three-lead and five-lead ECGs

The three-lead ECG is mostly used in acute clinical areas where continuous cardiac monitoring is required (Adam et al. 2017). The three limb electrodes can be placed according to Figure 14.11 and Table 14.2. The monitor should be set to display lead II as this

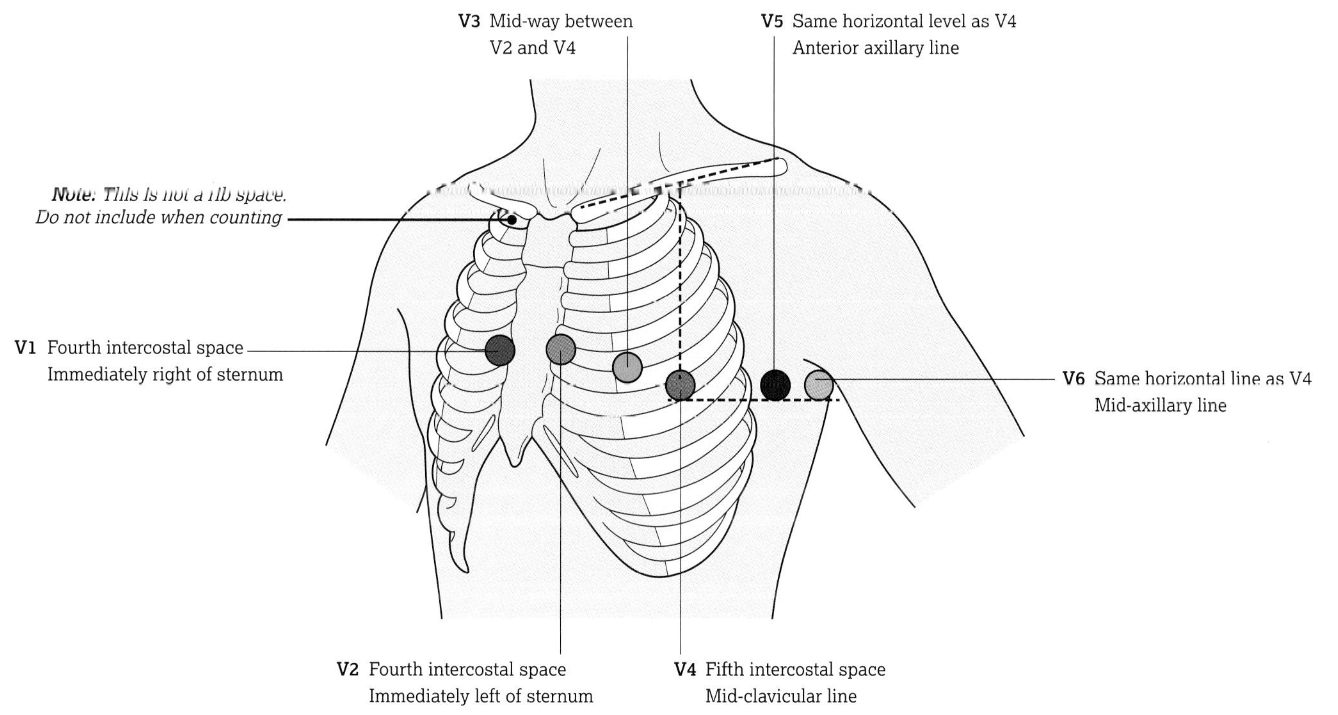

Figure 14.14 Position of chest electrodes for a 12-lead electrocardiogram (ECG). *Source*: SCST (2017) – The Society for Cardiological Science and Technology (www.scst.org.uk).

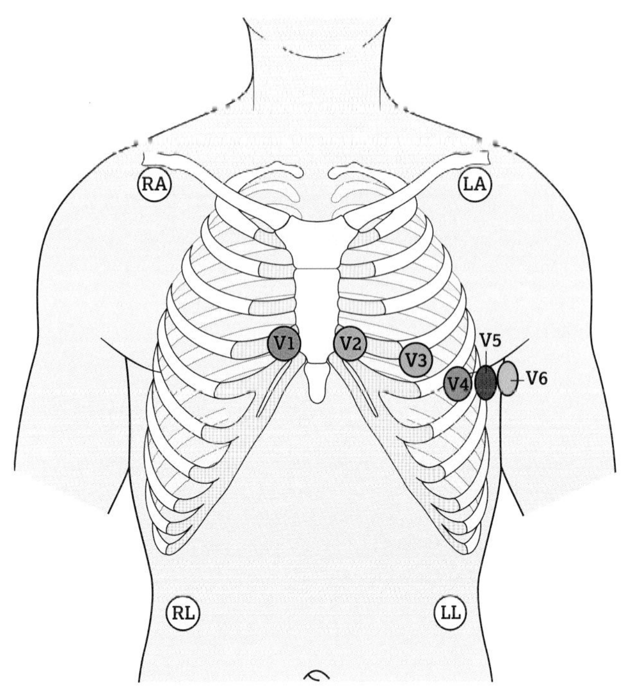

Figure 14.15 Mason–Likar 12-lead electrocardiogram (ECG) system.

runs from the right arm to the left foot and so is normally positive, showing the greatest deflection of all the limb leads in a normal heart (Marini and Dries 2016).

A five-lead ECG offers the features of a three-lead ECG with the addition of two extra leads, offering more detailed views of the heart.

The 12-lead ECG is, however, the gold standard for diagnostic purposes and is described in Procedure guideline 14.2: Electrocardiogram (ECG).

Rationale

Indications

A 12-lead ECG may be performed electively or to aid diagnosis following any acute deterioration or after any cardiac event. For example, it may be performed in the following circumstances:

- to provide a baseline prior to surgery or a course of medical treatment
- sudden onset of chest pain
- shortness of breath
- haemodynamic disturbance
- cardiac rhythm or rate changes
- suspected acute coronary syndrome
- suspected or confirmed myocardial infarction
- cardiac surgery
- percutaneous coronary intervention
- after successful cardiopulmonary resuscitation (RCUK 2015).

Serial 12-lead ECGs may be required in patients known to have cardiac toxicity, developing myocardial ischaemia or infarction (Bunce and Ray 2016).

Ambulatory ECG monitoring, also known as a '24-hour tape', may be used to record and analyse a patient's heart rhythm during normal daily activities (Wesley 2016). Usually applied and interpreted by specialist cardiac services, it is useful to capture abnormalities that might be missed with a standard 12-lead ECG. It is typically recorded continuously over a period of 24–48 hours (Aehlert 2017).

Contraindications

There are no absolute contraindications to performing a 12-lead ECG, but obtaining the ECG should not compromise or delay immediate care – for example, if a patient presents with an arrhythmia requiring immediate shock or in cardiac arrest (RCUK 2015).

Clinical governance

Competencies

Any healthcare professional who has been trained and assessed as competent can perform a 12-lead ECG in line with local hospital policy. However, its analysis and diagnosis are usually undertaken by medical staff or specialist nurses (SCST 2017).

Pre-procedural considerations

Equipment

12-lead ECG machine

A 12-lead ECG machine has 10 cables, which are connected to electrodes fixed to the body. The machine detects and amplifies the electrical impulses that occur at each heart beat and record the waveforms onto graphed paper (using a stylus) or onto a computer. All ECG machines should be tested to ensure accurate data are recorded. Calibration is usually undertaken by qualified engineers; however, this should be verified in the clinical setting to confirm that when a voltage of (usually) 1 mV over 0.2 seconds is put through the machine, the machine produces the expected deflection of 10 mm and the paper moves at the correct speed: 25 mm per second (Aehlert 2017, SCST 2017). This calibration verification should be printed at the beginning or end of each line of the ECG as a box shape with a 5 mm width and a 10 mm height (Figure 14.16) (Wesley 2016).

Electrodes

The 10 electrodes are attached to the patient's body in the positions described above and in Procedure guideline 14.2: Electrocardiogram (ECG). The cables clip onto these electrodes and record 12 views of the heart using different combinations of electrodes to measure various signals from the heart.

ECG paper

ECG graph paper is divided into small squares of 1 mm each, and five small squares make up a large square. The horizontal axis of the ECG paper represents time and the vertical axis represents amplitude. Standard ECG paper speed is 25 mm per second; each small square equals 0.04 seconds and one large square equals 0.2 seconds, so five large squares equal 1 second. ECG machines are calibrated so that the deflection amplitude of cardiac conduction is measured in mm/mV; 10 small squares or two large squares

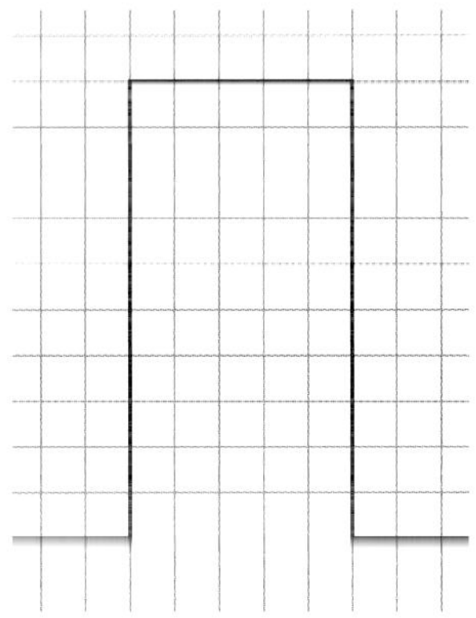

Figure 14.16 Electrocardiogram (ECG) calibration verification signal. *Source*: Reproduced from Crawford and Doherty (2010) with permission of MA Healthcare.

show a deflection of 1 mV (10 mm/mV) (see Figure 14.16) (Aehlert 2017, Wesley 2016).

Filter

Filters are electronic devices that remove artefacts from the ECG, improving the tracing obtained. ECG machines have internal pre-programmed filters set by the manufacturer or clinical engineers, which cannot be altered by clinical staff, and also control panel filters, which can be deployed by clinical staff. However, these can distort the ECG waveform, and therefore are not recommended for routine use, but they may be required if all other actions to reduce artefacts have been unsuccessful. If a filter is used, this must be clearly documented on the ECG (SCST 2017, Wesley 2016).

Maintenance and storage

All ECG machines should be used and maintained in accordance with the manufacturer's instructions. In addition, as they are often used in emergency situations, they should always be available and in good working order (SCST 2017). After use, the ECG machine should be cleaned, returned to its storage location and plugged into a mains electrical supply to charge the internal battery ready for use in an emergency (SCST 2017). Any malfunctioning machine should be taken out of clinical use until repair or service can be undertaken by the relevant department, in accordance with local policy (Wesley 2016).

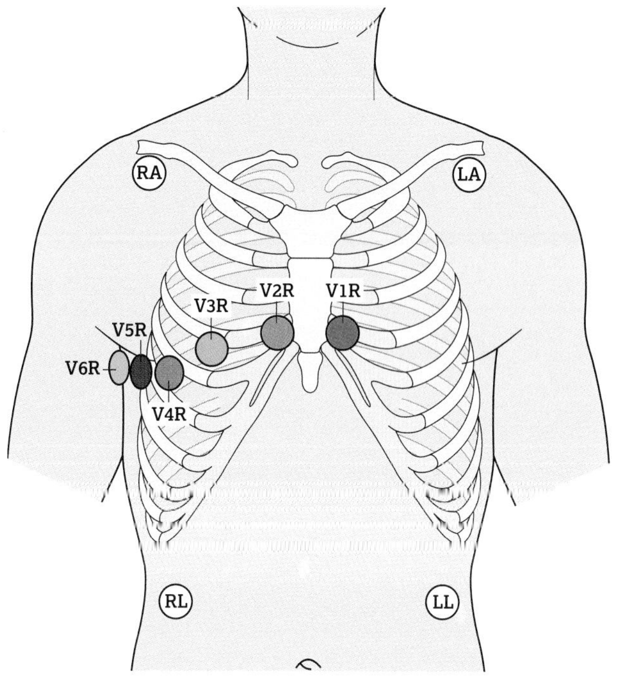

Figure 14.17 Right-sided chest lead positioning for an electrocardiogram (ECG).

Specific patient preparation

Female patients

The conventional placement of the lateral chest leads (V4, V5 and V6) is beneath the left breast. While there is emerging evidence to support the positioning of these over the breast, it is insufficient to suggest a change of procedure (SCST 2017). It is also worth noting that the fifth intercostal space can only be found by lifting the breast and therefore it is logical to position the electrodes here (SCST 2017).

Dextrocardia

Dextrocardia is any situation where the heart is located within the right side of the chest rather than the left. This may be associated with the condition situs inversus, believed to occur in 1 out of 8000 people, where all of the patient's organs are in mirror-image positions (Sharma et al. 2015).

The SCST (2017) suggests the following approach to ECG recording for patients with suspected or known dextrocardia:

- Dextrocardia should be suspected if the ECG shows an inverted P wave in lead I (P-axis >90°) together with poor R wave progression across the chest leads. In this case a second ECG should be recorded with the chest electrodes positioned on the right side of the chest using the same intercostal spacing and anatomical landmarks to provide a true ECG representation (Figure 14.17). The limb lead complexes will continue to appear inverted, demonstrating the abnormal location of the heart, but the repositioned chest leads will now show the appropriate R wave progression. The revised electrode positions should be clearly documented on the second ECG, and both ECGs should be retained for inclusion in the patient's notes.
- Patients who are known to have dextrocardia should have the ECG recorded with the limb electrodes in the usual positions and the chest electrodes placed across the right side of the chest, as described above. Note that swapping of the right- and left-limb electrodes will normalize the appearance of the limb leads; therefore, when repositioning electrodes, it is imperative that the ECG is clearly annotated to describe the new positions of the electrodes (V3R, V4R, etc.) to prevent the possibility of dextrocardia being overlooked.

Education

The patient must give their consent for the ECG to be performed, after appropriate explanation of what the procedure consists of, the rationale and the intent (NMC 2018, Peate and Wild 2018). The patient's privacy and dignity should be ensured and reassurance should be provided, along with an explanation that an ECG is not a painful procedure (NMC 2018, SCST 2017). The patient should be positioned comfortably either lying or sitting, preferably in a semi-recumbent position (at an angle of 45°) with their head supported (SCST 2017, Wesley 2016). It is important that the patient is relaxed and keeps still during the procedure to reduce interference and artefacts and to facilitate recording of a clear and stable ECG trace (Aehlert 2017, SCST 2017).

Procedure guideline 14.2 Electrocardiogram (ECG)

Essential equipment

- Personal protective equipment
- ECG machine with chest and limb leads labelled respectively, for example LA to left arm and V1 to first chest lead
- Disposable electrodes (check that these are in date and not dry prior to use)

Action	Rationale
Pre-procedure	
1 Introduce yourself to the patient, explain and discuss the procedure with them, and gain their consent to proceed.	To ensure that the patient feels at ease, understands the procedure and gives their valid consent (NMC 2018, **C**).

(continued)

Procedure guideline 14.2 Electrocardiogram (ECG) *(continued)*

Action	Rationale
2 Wash and dry hands and/or use an alcohol-based handrub.	To prevent cross-infection (NHS England and NHSI 2019, **C**).
3 Ensure that the patient is comfortably positioned in a semi-recumbent position with their chest exposed. Any variations to the standard recording techniques must be highlighted on the ECG recording (e.g. 'ECG recorded while patient in wheelchair').	To ensure optimal recording and comfort of the patient (SCST 2017, **E**). The ECG may vary depending on the patient's position so it is important to note this on the ECG (Wesley 2016, **C**).
4 If necessary, prepare skin by cleaning with soap and water and/or shaving using a single-use razor.	To ensure a good grip and therefore good contact between the skin and electrodes, which results in fewer electrical artefacts (SCST 2017). Shaving should be avoided due to the risk of infection if the skin is grazed or bleeding if the patient is on anticoagulation therapy. **E**
Procedure	
5 Apply the limb and chest electrodes as described in Table 14.2 or as shown in Figure 14.14. For advice on placement in females and patients with known cardiac abnormalities see the section on specific patient preparation above.	To obtain a three-dimensional view of the electrical activity of the heart (Wesley 2016, **E**). Following a standard arrangement ensures consistency between recordings and prevents invalid recordings and misdiagnosis (SCST 2017, **C**).
6 Attach the cables from the ECG machine to the electrodes, checking that the cables are connected correctly and to the relevant electrodes.	To obtain the ECG recording and to ensure the correct polarity (Blows 2018, **E**).
7 Ensure that the cables are not pulling on the electrodes or lying over each other. Offer the patient a gown or sheet to place over their exposed chest.	To reduce the number of electrical artefacts and to obtain a clear ECG recording (Aehlert 2017, **E**). To ensure patient dignity and reduce shivering (SCST 2017, **C**).
8 Ask the patient to relax and refrain from movement.	To obtain the optimal recording via the reduction of artefacts from muscular movement (SCST 2017, **C**).
9 Encourage the patient to breathe normally and not to speak while the recording is being taken.	Speaking can alter the recording (Blows 2018, **E**).
10 Switch the machine on and enter the patient's details.	To ensure that it is clear which patient the ECG was taken from (NMC 2018, **C**).
11 Check that the machine is functioning correctly and that calibration is 10 mm/mV.	To ensure standard recording and to aid interpretation (SCST 2017, **C**).
12 Commence the recording by pressing 'Start', 'Go' or 'Capture' (according to the specific machine).	To obtain the ECG. **E**
13 In the case of artefacts or poor recording, check the electrodes and connections.	To ensure optimal recording (Wesley 2016, **E**).
14 During the procedure, give reassurance to the patient.	To ensure the patient is informed and reassured (SCST 2017, **E**).
15 Detach the ECG print-out and ensure the recording contains the patient's name and hospital number, and the date and time of the procedure. Also include any diagnostic information (i.e. if the patient had chest pain during the recording) and deviations from the standard electrode placement.	To ensure that the ECG forms part of the correct patient's medical record (NMC 2018, **C**). To help with diagnosis and interpretation (SCST 2017, **C**).
Post-procedure	
16 Inform the patient that the procedure is completed, remove the electrodes and help the patient to re-dress if required.	To ensure that the patient can relax and that the electrodes are removed to prevent them drying out and causing skin irritation. **E**
17 Wash and dry hands and/or use an alcohol-based handrub.	To prevent cross-infection (NHS England and NHSI 2019, **C**).
18 Inform the relevant nursing and medical staff that the ECG has been completed. Show the recording to the person who will analyse it.	To enable relevant nursing and medical staff to use the ECG data in their care planning and treatment (NMC 2018, SCST 2017, **C**).
19 File the ECG recording in the appropriate documentation.	To ensure appropriate record keeping and aid continuity of care (NMC 2018, **C**).
20 Clean the ECG machine in accordance with the manufacturer's recommendations. Return it to its storage place and plug it in to mains electricity to keep the battery fully charged.	The ECG machine forms part of a department's emergency equipment and should always be available and in good working order with a charged battery for use in an emergency (SCST 2017, **E**).

Problem-solving table 14.2 Prevention and resolution (Procedure guideline 14.2)

Problem	Cause	Prevention	Action
Unable to turn on the ECG machine	Low battery	Ensure the ECG is left on continuous charge when not in use.	Connect the ECG machine to mains electricity. It should function once it has been connected to a power supply.
The ECG machine is working but the rhythm display is blank	Loose connection	Carefully store the cables after use to prevent damage.	Check that each lead is connected to the electrode clip and that the base of the cable is connected to the ECG machine.
	Electrode stickers peel off from the patient's skin	Prepare the patient's skin prior to electrode application (see step 4 of Procedure guideline 14.2: Electrocardiogram (ECG)).	Cleanse the electrode sites with soap and water to remove any lotion or reduce skin moisture, and allow to dry. Reapply new electrode stickers. If the patient has a lot of chest hair, try to push the hair out of the way when applying stickers to make a better contact; reinforcement with tape may be required. If this is unsuccessful, ask the patient for permission to clip or shave the hair at the electrode sites, cleanse to remove loose hair, allow to dry and apply new electrode stickers.
	The electrode stickers may be intact but there is still no rhythm – the patient's skin may be excessively dry and flaky	Identify underlying causes and severity of dry skin and address them with the multidisciplinary team as appropriate.	With the patient's consent, perform vigorous but gentle rubbing with soap and water to remove the superficial dead skin cells. The skin should be allowed to dry and new electrode stickers applied.
The ECG is printing but some of the views are missing	A loose connection	Ensure good skin preparation and maintenance of the ECG machine.	Check that the electrode stickers are intact and follow the above suggestions for skin preparation. Check that the cables are all securely connected.
The ECG is printing but there is interference, making it difficult to interpret accurately	Patient movement	Ask the patient to remain still and not to speak, but to breathe normally.	Ensure the patient is not moving or talking and repeat the ECG once the displayed rhythm has stabilized.
	The patient is cold and therefore involuntarily shivering	If at all possible and not clinically dangerous, wait for the patient to warm up.	Once the electrodes are connected, place a gown, sheet or blanket over the patient to warm them.
	Peripheral interference	As above – ask the patient to remain still and ensure they are warm.	Place the limb electrodes more centrally, as shown in the Mason–Likar system (see Figure 14.15), to reduce interference from limb movement.
	General interference or a wandering baseline	Ensure there is good skin contact with the electrodes and good electrode placement, and ask the patient to avoid thoracic movement.	Ensure good skin preparation. Ask the patient to lie still and breathe normally. Check that the electrodes are properly placed. If necessary, record an additional ECG with the 'filter' function on to limit interference. Write on the ECG that the filter function was used.
	Electrical interference from nearby devices (such as infusion pumps, other monitoring devices or haemodialysis machines)	It may be necessary to temporarily remove or suspend electrical devices if safe and appropriate to do so.	Repeat the ECG once the displayed rhythm has stabilized. If necessary, record an additional ECG with the 'filter' function on to limit interference. Write on the ECG that the filter function was used.
The ECG is working and displays a rhythm but the print-out is blank	A different manufacturer's ECG paper has been loaded	Only use the manufacturer's recommended paper for the ECG machine.	Reload the machine using the correct paper and repeat the recording.
	Internal fault	Ensure the manufacturer's recommendations on maintenance and servicing are followed.	Contact the in-house engineer, medical device technician or manufacturer for advice in accordance with local policy.

Post-procedural considerations

Immediate care

Once the ECG is complete, it must be interpreted by a competent and trained healthcare professional so that any changes that might require urgent medical attention are identified and appropriate action taken (Peate and Wild 2018, SCST 2017). If the patient had any cardiac symptoms at the time of the recording, such as chest pain or palpitations, this should be noted on the tracing and brought to the immediate attention of a senior member of the nursing or medical staff (SCST 2017). Examples of a normal 12-lead ECG and some important types of abnormal ECG tracing are shown in Figure 14.18.

Documentation

It is good practice for the reviewer, who may be a doctor or senior nurse, to document their interpretation of the ECG directly onto the ECG and to sign and date it or the equivalent if using electronic documentation. Once reviewed, the ECG should be filed in the patient's medical notes. Nurses should document in the nursing notes when the ECG was recorded, who was asked to review it and the time the ECG was reviewed; they should also indicate whether it was normal or, if abnormal, what further action was taken (Adam et al. 2017, Blows 2018, SCST 2017).

Blood pressure

Definition

Blood pressure may be defined as the force of blood inside the blood vessels against the vessel walls (Marieb and Hoehn 2018). Systolic pressure is the peak pressure caused by the left ventricle contracting and blood entering the aorta, which causes the aorta to stretch; therefore, systolic pressure in part reflects the function of the left ventricle (Waugh and Grant 2018). Diastolic pressure is caused by the aortic valve closing, blood flowing from the aorta into the smaller vessels and the aorta recoiling back (Marieb and Keller 2017). This is when the aortic pressure is at its lowest and tends to reflect the resistance of the blood vessels (Marieb and Hoehn 2018).

Related theory

Blood pressure is determined by cardiac output and vascular resistance and can be described as shown in the equation in Box 14.2. If that equation is combined with the equation for cardiac output (see Box 14.1), which uses heart rate (HR) and stroke volume (SV), blood pressure (BP) could be seen as (Blows 2018):

$$BP = SV \times HR \times SVR$$

In theory, anything that alters one of the above components (stroke volume, heart rate or systemic vascular resistance) will therefore produce a change in blood pressure (Tortora and Derrickson 2017). However, this is not always the case as a drop in one may be compensated for by an increase in either of the others (Patton 2018).

Normal blood pressure

Normal blood pressure ranges between 100 and 140 mmHg systolic and 60 and 90 mmHg diastolic at rest (Lough 2015). However, it varies depending on age (increasing with age), activity, sleep, emotion, positioning, physical condition and fitness (Tortora and Derrickson 2017). It also varies depending on the time of day, being at its lowest during sleep (Blows 2018). Blood pressure

Box 14.2 Blood pressure equation

BP	=	*CO*	×	*SVR*
(blood pressure)		(cardiac output)		(systemic vascular resistance)

Source: Marini and Dries (2016).

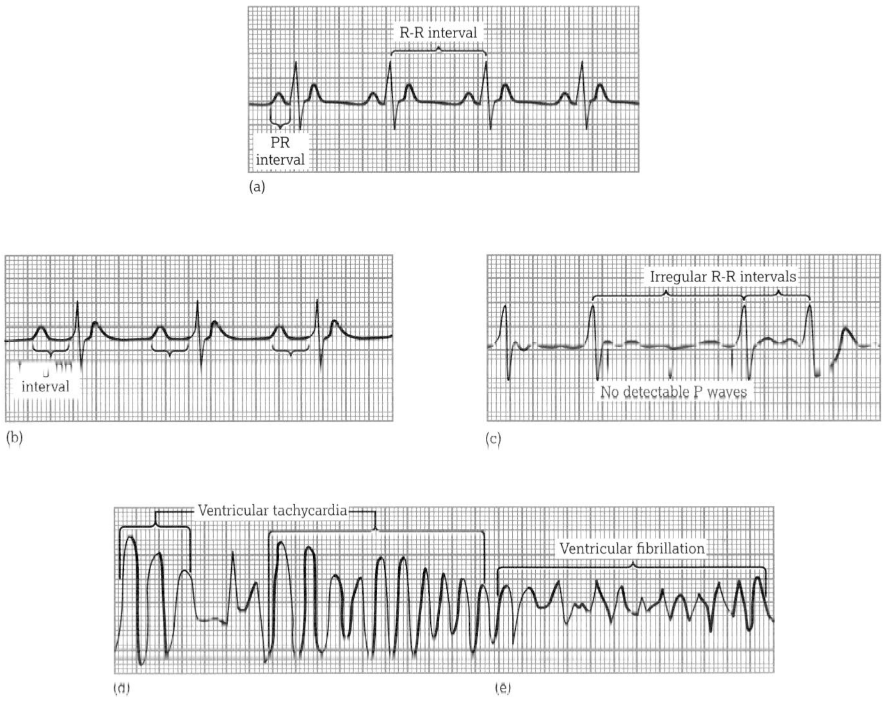

Figure 14.18 (a) Normal electrocardiogram tracing. Abnormal electrocardiogram tracings: (b) first-degree AV block, (c) atrial fibrillation, (d) ventricular tachycardia and (e) ventricular fibrillation. *Source*: Reproduced from Tortora and Derrickson (2011) with permission of John Wiley & Sons.

therefore reflects individual variations but an abnormal blood pressure should not be assumed to be the individual's norm; rather, it should be assessed in relation to their previous results, general condition and other observations (Bunce and Ray 2016).

Hypotension

Hypotension is generally defined in adults as a systolic blood pressure below 100 mmHg (Marieb and Hoehn 2018). A low blood pressure may indicate orthostatic hypotension – that is, a sudden drop in blood pressure when the patient rises from a supine or sitting position (Brown and Cadogan 2016). This is usually compensated for by the baroreceptor reflex and the sympathetic nervous system but, especially in older people, this compensatory mechanism may not work as efficiently (Marieb and Hoehn 2018). Hypotension can also be a symptom of many other conditions, including shock, haemorrhage and malnutrition, all of which can result in reduced tissue perfusion and lead to hypoxia and an accumulation of waste products (Sprigings and Chambers 2017).

Hypertension

Hypertension is defined as blood pressure of 140/90 mmHg or greater and can be either *primary* hypertension, with no single known cause, or *secondary* hypertension, which means it is related to another factor such as kidney disease (NICE 2016b).

Factors leading to hypertension include sex, genetic factors and age, alongside risk factors such as obesity, lack of exercise, smoking, and high caffeine and/or alcohol intake (Patton 2018). If hypertension is sustained, the heart will have an increased workload to maintain circulation; greater stress will be placed on the blood vessel walls and cardiac ischaemia can occur (Wilkinson et al. 2017).

There are many illnesses and factors that can lead to changes in blood pressure (Figure 14.19), and hypertension is one of the most important preventable causes of premature morbidity and mortality in the UK (NICE 2016b). It has been suggested that a patient's knowledge of their own 'goal blood pressure' is associated with improved blood pressure control (NICE 2016b). Interventions to improve knowledge of specific blood pressure targets may have an important role in optimizing blood pressure management (NICE 2016b).

Mean arterial pressure

The mean arterial pressure (MAP) is the average pressure of blood throughout the pulse cycle and thus is a reliable indication of perfusion (Lin 2016). Mathematically, the MAP is derived from the diastolic pressure and the pulse pressure (which is the difference between the systolic and diastolic blood pressures) (Marieb and Hoehn 2015):

$$MAP = diastolic\ pressure + (pulse\ pressure \div 3)$$

Therefore, a patient with a blood pressure of 123/90 mmHg has a MAP of 101 mmHg. An adequate MAP is usually deemed to be between 65 and 70 mmHg (Marini and Dries 2016).

Resistance

Resistance is effectively the opposition to blood flow and is created by friction between the walls of blood vessels and the blood itself (Patton 2018). It is termed 'peripheral' or 'systemic' vascular resistance because most of the resistance occurs in the vessels away from the heart (Marieb and Hoehn 2018). Systemic vascular resistance varies depending on the degree of vasoconstriction or vasodilation, the viscosity of blood and the length of the vessels, although the last two factors generally remain relatively static (Marieb and Hoehn 2018). Arterioles can dilate or constrict; when they are constricted, systemic vascular resistance increases and blood flow to the tissues decreases, increasing the arterial blood pressure (Patton 2018). The blood pressures in the vessels of the cardiovascular system can be seen in Figure 14.20.

Blood pressure control

Hormonal control

Many hormones help to regulate blood pressure, including adrenaline and noradrenaline, which are released from the adrenal medulla in response to a drop in blood pressure; these hormones increase cardiac contractility and vasoconstriction, and thus increase cardiac output (Patton 2018). Atrial natriuretic peptide is a hormone that is produced from the atria of the heart in response to hypertension. It works by inhibiting the renin–angiotensin system, raising the glomerular filtration rate by causing vasodilation in the afferent arteriole, inhibiting sodium reabsorption and causing fluid transfer into the interstitial space (Waugh and Grant 2018) in an attempt to lower blood pressure.

Neural control

When blood pressure increases, the baroreceptors, or stretch receptors, are stimulated and in turn stimulate the cardiac inhibitory centre, reducing sympathetic nerve impulses and increasing

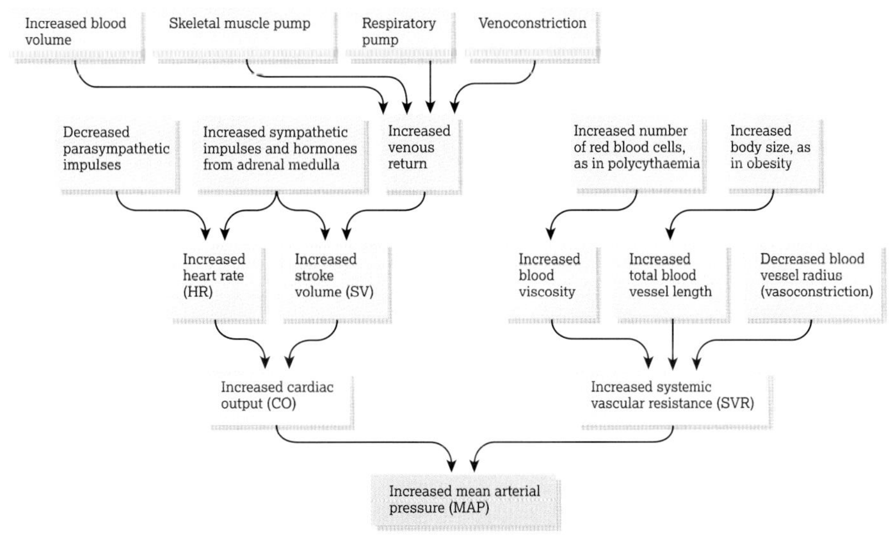

Figure 14.19 Factors that lead to an increase in blood pressure. Changes noted within green boxes increase cardiac output, whereas changes noted within blue boxes increase systemic vascular resistance. *Source*: Reproduced from Tortora and Derrickson (2017) with permission of John Wiley & Sons.

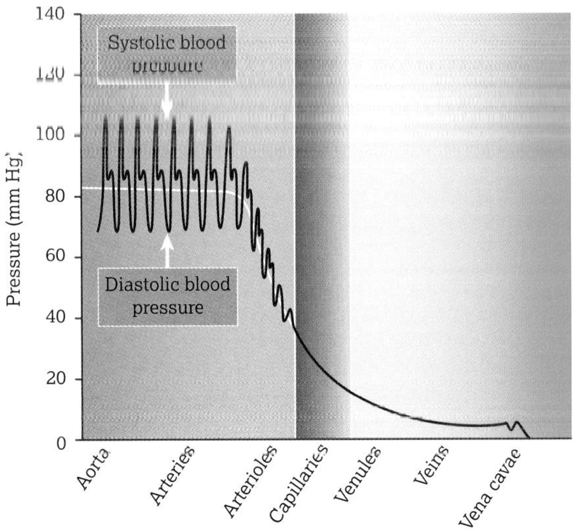

Figure 14.20 Blood pressures in various parts of the cardiovascular system. The white line is the mean (average) blood pressure in the aorta, arteries and arterioles. *Source*: Reproduced from Peate and Wild (2018) with permission of John Wiley & Sons.

parasympathetic nerve impulses (Marieb and Keller 2017). This causes vasodilation and a decrease in cardiac output, thereby reducing blood pressure (Blows 2018). When blood pressure is low, the opposite occurs. This response is termed a 'reflex arc', and it continually maintains homeostasis (Marieb and Hoehn 2018). Baroreceptors are located in the aortic arch, the carotid sinuses and the walls of most of the large arteries in the thorax and neck (Marieb and Hoehn 2018). Close to these are chemoreceptors, which are stimulated when the pH of the blood drops or when carbon dioxide rises, and when oxygen levels drop significantly; this causes an increase in cardiac output and vasoconstriction, leading to an increase in blood pressure (Marieb and Hoehn 2018).

Renal control

The juxtaglomerular cells within the kidneys are stimulated to release renin when blood volume or pressure falls (Tortora and Derrickson 2017). This leads to the production of angiotensin I, which is converted to angiotensin II (with the aid of angiotensin-converting enzyme) (Patton 2018). Angiotensin II has a potent effect on blood pressure, increasing cardiac output and vasoconstriction and stimulating the production of aldosterone. Aldosterone increases reabsorption of water and sodium and stimulates the thirst receptors (Patton 2018) in an attempt to increase the circulatory volume of fluid and thereby blood pressure (Blows 2018). These mechanisms are known collectively as the renin–angiotensin–aldosterone system (Figure 14.21). Anti-diuretic hormone is produced in the hypothalamus in response to low blood pressure or volume and increases vasoconstriction and water reabsorption in the kidneys. These mechanisms are inhibited when fluid volume in the circulatory system is high (Marieb and Keller 2017).

Other mechanisms that influence blood pressure

Skeletal muscle contractions and the mechanism of respiration promote venous return of blood to the heart and therefore assist in maintaining cardiac output (Lin 2016). Skeletal muscles contract on movement, compressing the veins and pushing the blood towards the heart, and respiration causes a change in thoracic and abdominal pressure, which acts to pump venous blood (Patton 2018). Starling's law states that the force of the contraction of the heart is directly related to how much blood volume is in the heart (Patton 2018). The more stretched the muscle fibres are prior to contraction, the stronger the contraction and the greater volume the heart will pump (Marieb and Keller 2017).

Evidence-based approaches

Rationale

Indications

Blood pressure measurements should be taken as follows:

- on admission or during initial assessment (NICE 2007)
- when a patient is transferred to a ward setting from intensive or high-dependency care (NICE 2018)
- regularly for inpatients, as per local policy (RCP 2017b)
- in patients at risk of, or with known, infections (NICE 2017e)
- to assess response to interventions intended to correct a patient's blood pressure (Peate and Wild 2018)
- pre-operatively to establish a baseline, and post-operatively to assess cardiovascular stability (Tait et al. 2015)
- in critically or acutely ill patients, or those who are at risk of rapid deterioration and who might require close and potentially continuous monitoring (Goulden 2016)
- in patients who are being transfused blood or blood products, to establish a baseline and also during and after the transfusion (NICE 2015b)
- in any patient who is receiving medications that could alter their blood pressure, such as epidurals or anaesthetics, antiarrhythmics, anti-hypertensives, nitrates or vasopressors (Lin 2016).

Contraindications

There are times when certain methods of blood pressure measurement should be used with caution:

- Oscillometric blood pressure devices may not be accurate in patients with weak or thready pulse or those with pre-eclampsia (Chen et al. 2018).
- The brachial artery should not be used to measure blood pressure in patients with arteriovenous fistulas (Adam et al. 2017).
- Patients with atrial fibrillation should have auscultatory blood pressure measurements taken, rather than oscillometric, and may require multiple readings (Marini and Dries 2016).
- Korotkoff sounds (see the section on indirect methods of measuring blood pressure below) are not dependably audible in children under the age of 1 year and many children under 5 years; therefore, ultrasound, doppler or oscillometric devices are recommended in these patients (Duncombe et al. 2017).
- Patients who have had trauma to the upper arm, a mastectomy or a forearm amputation should not have their blood pressure measured on the affected side at the brachial artery (Lin 2016).
- Oscillometric devices should be used with caution in patients with atherosclerosis and/or high or low blood pressure, as they may not measure accurately (Chen et al. 2018).
- Blood pressure should not be measured on an arm that has had brachial artery surgery or is at risk of lymphoedema (Bickley 2016).

In all cases, the manufacturer's guidance should be sought for contraindications specific to the device used (NICE 2016b).

Methods of measuring blood pressure

There are two main methods of measuring blood pressure: direct and indirect.

Direct

The direct method enables continuous monitoring of the blood pressure and so is commonly used for critically ill patients, for example in intensive care units and theatres (Adam et al. 2017). To do this, a cannula is inserted into an artery, most commonly the radial artery, as it is easy to access and monitor (Lin 2016). The cannula has a transducer attached to it that is connected to a

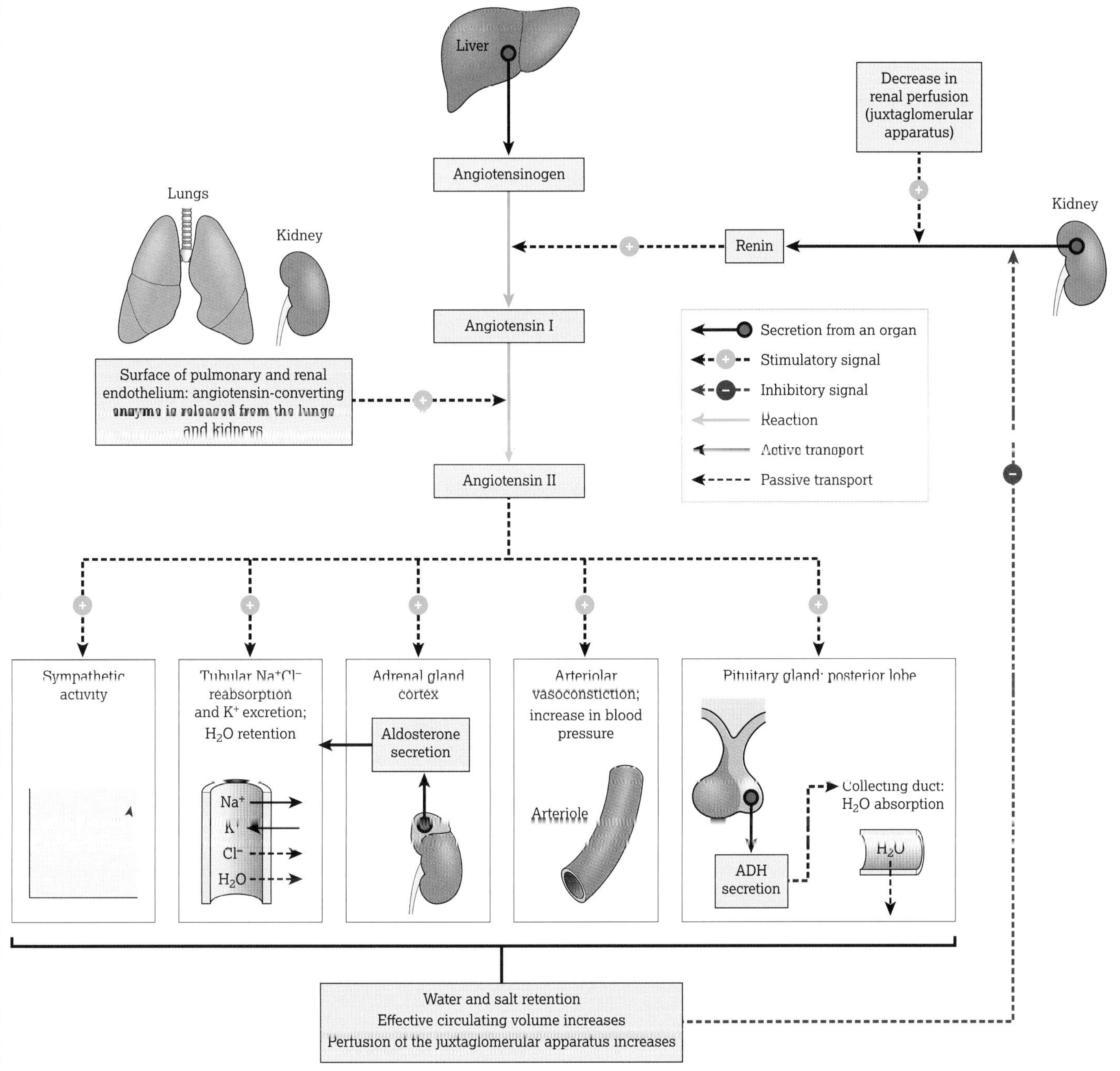

Figure 14.21 The renin–angiotensin–aldosterone system. *Source*: Reproduced with permission of Soupvector – Own work, CC BY-SA 4.0 https://commons.wikimedia.org/w/index.php?curid=66583851.

cardiac monitor, where the blood pressure is shown as a waveform; the cannula is also attached to a pressurized flush of solution to prevent blood backflow (Figure 14.22) (Tait et al. 2015). This method has risks of severe haemorrhage, thrombosis and air embolism; therefore, it must only be used where patients can be continuously observed (Adam et al. 2017).

Indirect

For indirect blood pressure measurement, either manual auscultatory sphygmomanometers or automated oscillometric devices are used (Duncombe et al. 2017). Oscillometric devices electronically measure blood pressure by measuring the oscillation of air pressure in the cuff, so when the artery begins to pulse it causes a corresponding oscillation of cuff pressure (Babbs 2015). Manual auscultatory blood pressure involves occluding the artery by use of a pressurized cuff and then gradually releasing the pressure; when the systolic blood pressure exceeds the cuff pressure, blood re-enters the arteries, producing vibrations in the artery during systole, enabling a pulse to be auscultated (Benmira et al. 2016). As the cuff pressure descends, the sounds cease as the artery remains open throughout the pulse wave (Chen et al. 2017). These sounds are called the Korotkoff sounds (Figure 14.23). Box 14.3 outlines which sounds relate to which phases of blood pressure.

Systolic blood pressure is usually defined as being phase 1 of the Korotkoff sounds, and diastolic is usually defined as being phase 5 (Marieb and Hoehn 2018, Patton 2018). However, in some patients the Korotkoff sounds may continue until the cuff is completely deflated; in such cases, phase 4 will represent the diastolic blood pressure (Pan et al. 2017). Some patients may present with an 'auscultatory gap'; this is evident as a silence between the Korotkoff sounds, in that phase 1 may be audible but

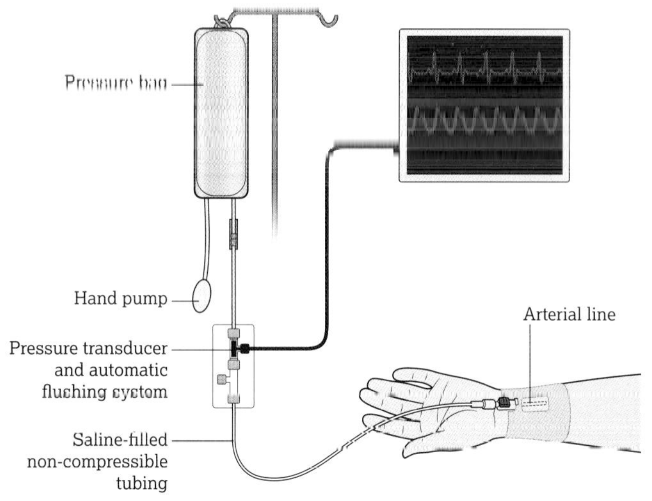

Figure 14.22 Arterial line and transducer set.

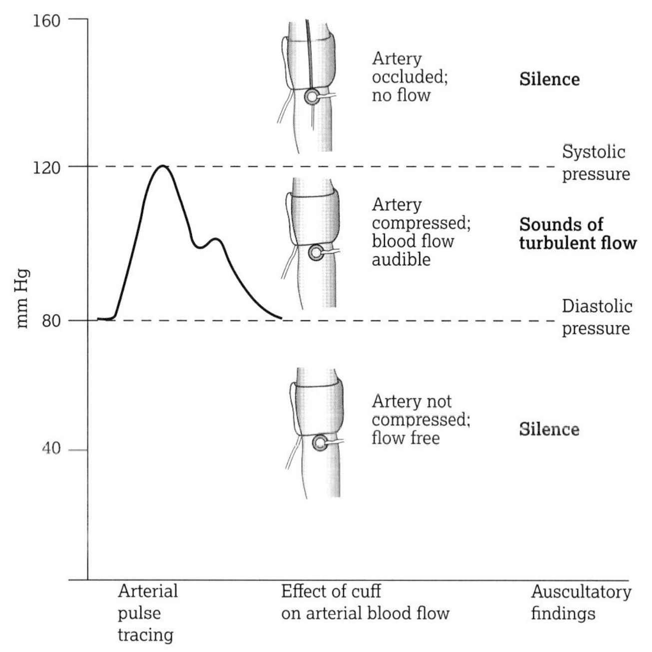

Figure 14.23 Korotkoff sounds.

Box 14.3 The five phases of the Korotkoff sounds

The sounds heard are called the Korotkoff sounds and have five phases.

1 The first phase is clear tapping, repetitive sounds, which increase in intensity and indicate the systolic pressure.
2 The second phase is murmuring or swishing sounds heard between systolic and diastolic pressures. Some people may have an auscultatory gap – a disappearance of sounds between the second and third phases.
3 The third phase is sharper and crisper sounds.
4 The fourth phase is the distinct muffling of sounds, which may be heard as soft and blowing noises.
5 The fifth phase is silence as the cuff pressure drops below the diastolic blood pressure. This disappearance is considered to be the diastolic blood pressure.

Source: NICE (2016b), O'Brien et al. (2003).

then a gap follows before the sounds of phase 3 are audible again. It is vital to establish whether the patient has an auscultatory gap as the blood pressure may be misread (missing phase 1 all together). Having an auscultatory gap is often associated with arterial stiffness.

Blood pressure measurement sites

The brachial artery is usually the favoured site for blood pressure measurement; however, in some patients this is inappropriate and so alternative sites have to be considered (Adam et al. 2017), such as the thigh, calf or wrist (Bickley 2016). However, local guidelines should be followed, as specific cuffs and different sizes of cuff can be advised, according to the blood pressure measurement site, in order to give an equal pressure to that in the brachial artery (Bickley 2016).

Measurement of orthostatic blood pressure

Orthostatic blood pressure measurement may be indicated if the patient has a history of dizziness or syncope on changing position (Brown and Cadogan 2016). The patient should rest on a bed in the supine position for at least 5 minutes prior to the initial blood pressure measurement, and the measurement should be taken in this position. The patient should then stand upright and have their blood pressure taken again in the first minute (RCP 2017b). A third blood pressure reading should be taken after the patient has been standing for 3 minutes (RCP 2017b). While the patient is in the standing position, the practitioner should support the patient's arm at the elbow to maintain it parallel to the hips and ensure accuracy (Chen et al. 2018). Orthostatic (postural) hypotension is defined by a drop in arterial blood pressure of at least 20 mmHg for systolic and 10 mmHg for diastolic blood pressure, with symptoms (RCP 2017b).

Pre-procedural considerations

Equipment

Sphygmomanometer

The device used to measure blood pressure is called a sphygmomanometer. It consists of a rubber cuff connected to a rubber bulb that is used to inflate the cuff and a meter that registers the pressure in the cuff (Tortora and Derrickson 2017). Sphygmomanometers that are uncalibrated or not working accurately can cause blood pressure measurement error (Benmira et al. 2016). If using a manual sphygmomanometer, check that the dial is set at zero prior to commencing (Chen et al. 2018). In addition, follow the manufacturer's recommendations and local policies regarding servicing and care of the device (NICE 2016b).

Manual mercury sphygmomanometers have gradually been phased out of mainstream clinical practice and replaced with dial or electronic manometers (Environment Agency 2015). This is primarily due to potential mercury leaks, which are hazardous to both the environment and humans, and secondly because since April 2009 they have no longer been available to either members of the public or healthcare professionals (Environment Agency 2015).

Cuff

The cuff is made of an inelastic material that encloses an inflatable bladder and encircles the arm. It is important that the correct cuff size is selected for the individual patient as cuffs that are too small yield a reading that is falsely high and large cuffs give a falsely low reading (British Hypertension Society 2017, MHRA 2013b). With the correct size of cuff, the bladder should encircle 80% of the patient's arm (British Hypertension Society 2017).

Inflatable bladder, valve, pump and tubing

In a manual sphygmomanometer, the system used to inflate and deflate the bladder consists of a bulb attached to the bladder with rubber tubing. When the bulb is compressed, air is forced into the bladder; to deflate the bladder, there is a release valve. The rubber tubes have conventionally been placed so they are inferior to the cuff; however, it is now recommended that they are placed superiorly to prevent them impeding auscultation (British Hypertension Society 2017).

Stethoscope

It is recommended that the stethoscope, which should be of high quality with well-fitting earpieces, should be placed over the brachial artery at the antecubital fossa (Bickley 2016, Pan et al. 2014). The bell part of the stethoscope may capture the low pitch of the Korotkoff sounds better than the diaphragm but the diaphragm has a larger surface area and is easier to manipulate with one hand (Pan et al. 2014, 2017).

Specific patient preparation

It is important to maintain a standardized environment in which to take the patient's blood pressure (NICE 2016b). The patient should empty their bladder and be seated (unless thigh or orthostatic blood pressure measurements are required) in a relaxed, quiet and comfortable setting (BHS 2017b). Their arm should be outstretched and supported (an unsupported arm may result in an increase of diastolic blood pressure by 10%) (NICE 2016b). The brachial artery at the antecubital fossa should be positioned level with the heart, approximately level with where the fourth intercostal space meets the sternum (Bickley 2016, Waugh and Grant 2018).

The patient's back should be supported and if they are in a chair their feet should be on the floor as systolic blood pressure can increase in people with their legs crossed (Privšek et al. 2018). Correct patient positioning can be seen in Figure 14.24.

Blood pressure should initially be measured in both arms as often people have a significant difference in blood pressure measurement between their arms (NICE 2016b). Patients who have a large and persistent disparity may have underlying conditions such as occlusive artery disease (Bickley 2016). Differences of up to 10 mmHg can be due to random variation (RCP 2017b). The arm with the highest reading should be the one used for subsequent measurements (NICE 2016b).

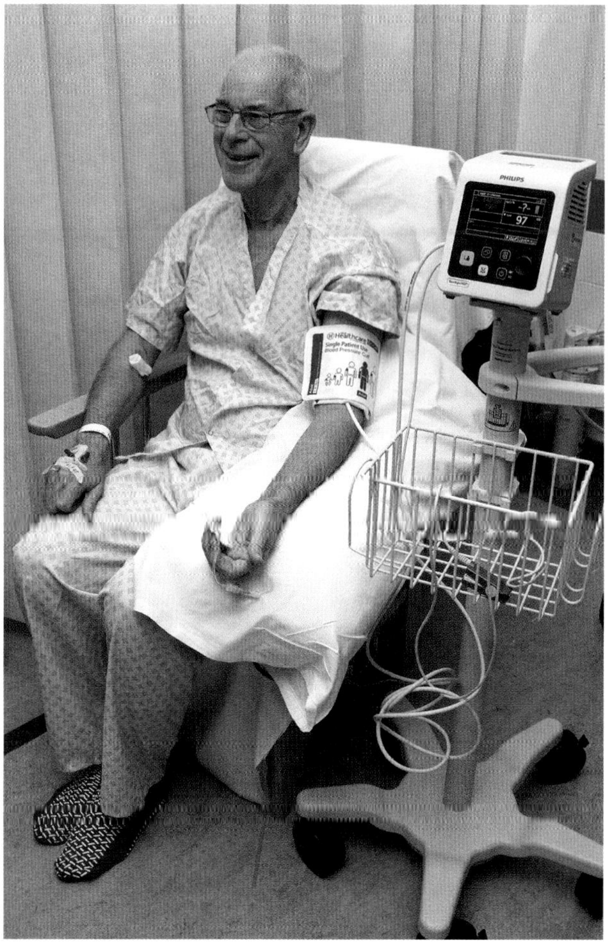

Figure 14.24 Correct blood pressure reading technique.

Procedure guideline 14.3 Blood pressure measurement (manual)

Essential equipment

- Personal protective equipment
- A range of cuffs
- Documentation chart
- Sphygmomanometer (working and calibrated)
- Stethoscope
- Cleaning wipes

Optional equipment

- Pillow if required to provide extra arm support
- Bed or examination bench, so the patient can have their blood pressure measured lying down if necessary

Action	Rationale
Pre-procedure	
1 Introduce yourself to the patient, explain and discuss the procedure with them, and gain their consent to proceed.	To ensure that the patient feels at ease, understands the procedure and gives their valid consent (NMC 2018, **C**).
2 Wash and dry hands and/or use an alcohol-based handrub.	To prevent cross-infection (NHS England and NHSI 2019, **C**).
3 Assess whether the patient has any of the following: • lymphoedema or risk of lymphoedema • arteriovenous fistula • trauma or surgery to the arm or axilla • previous brachial artery surgery • intravenous (IV) infusion in progress. If there is a contraindication, use the other arm, or, if the condition is bilateral, a lower extremity.	To ensure there are no contraindications to using a particular arm (Bickley 2016, **E**). Taking a blood pressure measurement is not recommended on a limb with an IV infusion in progress because the pressure could damage the vein, placing the patient at risk of extravasation or infiltration (Jackson 2016, **E**). If there is no other choice, blood pressure can be taken on a limb with an IV catheter *in situ* although the infusion must be temporarily stopped if clinically safe to do so (Tait et al. 2015, **C**).

(continued)

Procedure guideline 14.3 Blood pressure measurement (manual) *(continued)*

Action	Rationale
4 Provide a relaxed and comfortable environment. The patient should be seated in a chair with back support or supine in bed for at least 5 minutes prior to measuring their blood pressure.	To enable comparisons to be drawn with prior blood pressure results (NICE 2016b, E). Variations in temperature and emotions can alter blood pressure readings (RCP 2017b, **E**). Resting for 5 minutes will ensure an optimum reading (RCP 2017b, **E**).
5 Ensure the cuff is the correct size for the arm.	To prevent falsely high readings, which may occur if small cuffs are used, or falsely low readings, which may occur if large cuffs are used (NICE 2016b, **E**; RCP 2017b, **C**).
6 Check the patient's arm is free from clothing, supported (e.g. with a pillow, whether the patient is sitting or standing) and placed at heart level (midsternal level). The patient's bladder should have been emptied recently. Their legs should be uncrossed with their feet flat on the floor (if they are positioned in a chair) and ankles uncrossed (if they are in a bed). See Figure 14.24.	Taking measurements over clothing or with tight clothing pushed up on the arm can cause a tourniquet effect and also produce significant artefacts (Sprigings and Chambers 2017, **E**). If the arm is lower than the heart, it can lead to falsely high readings, and vice versa (NICE 2016b, **E**). Obtaining a measurement before bladder emptying can increase blood pressure, as can having the legs crossed (Blows 2018, **E**).
Procedure	
7 Wrap the cuff of the sphygmomanometer around the bare arm with the artery marking centred over the brachial artery and superior to the elbow. The lower edge of the cuff should be 2–3 cm above the brachial artery pulsation.	To obtain an accurate reading and so that the artery can easily be palpated (NICE 2016b, **C**).
8 Ask the patient to stop talking and eating during the procedure.	Activity can cause a falsely high blood pressure (RCP 2017b, **C**).
9 Palpate the brachial artery while pumping air into the cuff using the bulb. Once the pulse can no longer be felt, rapidly inflate the cuff a further 20–30 mmHg.	Palpation of the artery prior to obtaining a blood pressure is recommended as it locates the correct position for stethoscope placement (NICE 2016b, **E**). Although the radial artery is also available for palpating, the brachial artery is selected due to its proximity to the most common cuff position (superior to the elbow). **C** Inflating the cuff to only 20–30 mmHg above the predicted systolic level prevents undue discomfort (Bickley 2016, **E**).
10 Slowly deflate the cuff and note the point at which the pulse becomes detectable again. This approximates the systolic blood pressure.	This provides an indication of systolic pressure and can ensure accurate results in patients who have an auscultatory gap (see Box 14.3) (Tortora and Derrickson 2017, **E**).
11 Deflate the cuff completely and wait 15–30 seconds.	To allow venous congestion to resolve (Bickley 2016, **E**).
12 The diaphragm of the stethoscope should be firmly, but without too much pressure, placed on bare skin over the brachial artery where the pulse was palpable.	The bell of the stethoscope may hear the tone of the Korotkoff sounds better; however, the diaphragm has a larger surface area and is easier to hold in place (Tait et al. 2015, **E**). If the stethoscope is in contact with material, it may distort the Korotkoff sounds. In addition, applying pressure may partially occlude the artery (Babbs 2015, Bickley 2016, **E**).
13 Inflate the cuff again to 20–30 mmHg above the predicted systolic blood pressure.	To ensure an accurate measurement (Bickley 2016, **C**).
14 Release the air in the cuff slowly (at an approximate rate of 2–3 mmHg per pulsation) until the first tapping sounds are heard (first Korotkoff sound). This is the systolic blood pressure.	The cuff should not be deflated too quickly as this may result in [illegible] 2017, **E**).
15 Continue to deflate the cuff slowly, listening to the Korotkoff sounds; the point at which the sound completely disappears is the best representation of the diastolic blood pressure.	To ensure an accurate diastolic blood pressure measurement (Bickley 2016, **E**).
16 Once sounds can no longer be heard, rapidly deflate the cuff.	To prevent venous congestion to the arm (Chen et al. 2018, **E**).
17 If it is necessary to recheck the blood pressure, wait 1–2 minutes before proceeding (RCP 2017b).	Venous congestion may make the Korotkoff sounds less audible (Bickley 2016, **E**).

Post-procedure

18 Inform the patient that the procedure is now finished.	To reassure the patient (NMC 2018, **C**).
19 Wash hands using bactericidal soap and water and/or an alcohol-based handrub. Clean the bell and diaphragm of the stethoscope and cuff with cleaning wipes.	To minimize the risk of infection (Loveday et al. 2014, **R**; NHS England and NHSI 2019, **C**).
20 Document as soon as the measurement has been taken and compare it with previous results. Take action as appropriate and document the action.	Any interruption in the process may result in the measurement being incorrectly remembered (RCP 2017b, **E**). Records should identify any risks or problems that have arisen and show the action taken to deal with them (NMC 2018, **C**).

Problem-solving table 14.3 Prevention and resolution (Procedure guideline 14.3)

Problem	Cause	Prevention	Action
The result is unexpectedly low or high	Poor technique, incorrect cuff size or faulty equipment Patient incorrectly positioned or recently having exercised	Check the sphygmomanometer prior to use to see when it was last serviced. Check all the components for signs of damage. Choose the correct size of cuff. Ensure the patient is correctly positioned and has rested prior to the procedure.	Wait 1–2 minutes before repeating the blood pressure measurement (NICE 2016b). If the measurement is still unexpected, consider changing devices or asking a colleague to repeat the procedure. If it remains abnormal, notify the medical team of the result.
On auscultation, the Korotkoff sounds disappear after the initial sound, then reappear and then disappear again	This is called the auscultatory gap – it may mislead the practitioner into obtaining an incorrect result (Pan et al. 2017)	Palpate the pulse as the cuff is being deflated to gain an approximation of the systolic blood pressure (NICE 2016b).	Document that the patient has an auscultatory gap and ensure other practitioners are aware to prevent future errors. Recheck using the correct procedure.
On auscultation, the Korotkoff sounds are inaudible or very weak	Poor placement of the stethoscope A noisy environment Venous congestion The patient may be in shock (Bickley 2016)	Find a quiet environment in which to measure the patient's blood pressure; listen with the bell of the stethoscope rather than the diaphragm; wait for venous congestion to resolve (Bickley 2016).	If still inaudible, ask the patient to elevate their arm overhead for 30 seconds, then bring it back to the correct height to inflate the cuff and measure their blood pressure; this increases the loudness of the sounds (Bickley 2016).

Post-procedural considerations

Immediate care

Abnormal blood pressure results should be notified to medical or senior nursing staff (NICE 2018). As the treatment will depend on what is causing the abnormality, and its severity, it is important that practitioners try to ascertain any possible causes of the physiological change in blood pressure (Brown and Cadogan 2016). Hypovolaemia will require fluid replacement and, if persistent, inotropes or vasopressors and other cardiovascular drugs may be necessary (Bunce and Ray 2016). If hypertension is evident it may be transient, for example related to anxiety or pain, in which case it is important to address that issue and monitor the blood pressure until it resolves (Bickley 2016). However, if the patient is diagnosed as having hypertension, they might require medication to control their condition (NICE 2016b). To determine the cause of the altered blood pressure, more information will be required, including:

- a comprehensive medical history from the patient
- a full set of observations
- an ECG
- urinalysis including protein, leucocytes, blood and the osmolality of the urine
- blood tests for full blood count, urea, creatinine and electrolytes and fasting blood tests for glucose and lipids
- a chest X-ray or further radiological investigations (if required)
- a septic screen including blood cultures, sputum specimen, and swabs of any wounds or potential sites of infection (if required)
- current fluid balance (Adam et al. 2017, Bickley 2016, Blows 2018, Sprigings and Chambers 2017, Wilkinson et al. 2017).

Ongoing care

If the patient is hypertensive and in primary care, they will require at least monthly blood pressure measurements and more frequent measurement if it is accelerated hypertension or there are any further concerns (NICE 2016b). Additionally, it will be necessary to give lifestyle advice on eating healthily and smoking cessation, if relevant (NICE 2016b).

If the patient has orthostatic hypotension, they should be advised to change position slowly so their baroreceptors and sympathetic nervous system have time to adapt their blood pressure to each stage (Marieb and Hoehn 2018).

Documentation

As well as accurately recording the blood pressure measurement, it is important to record:

- the position the patient was in
- the arm used – and, if both arms were used initially, the pressure of each
- arm circumference and cuff size used

- whether there is an auscultatory gap
- whether there were any difficulties in obtaining a reading, such as the absence of stage 5 of the Korotkoff sounds
- the state of the patient, for example whether they were in pain, frightened and so on
- any medication they are on and when they last took it (Bickley 2016, NICE 2016b, RCP 2017b).

When documenting what medication the patient is taking, it is important to include not only cardiovascular medication but also other medication that might affect their blood pressure, including tricyclic antidepressants, neuroleptic agents, contraceptives, decongestants and non-steroidal anti-inflammatory drugs (Bickley 2016, Bunce and Ray 2016, Wilkinson et al. 2017).

Respiration and pulse oximetry

Definitions

Respiration

The major function of the respiratory system is to supply the cells of the human body with oxygen and to remove carbon dioxide, to ensure the cells can function effectively (Tortora and Derrickson 2017). Respiration is composed of four processes:

- *pulmonary ventilation*: movement of air into and out of the lungs to continually refresh the gases there, commonly called 'breathing'
- *external respiration*: movement of oxygen from the lungs into the blood, and carbon dioxide from the blood into the lungs, commonly called 'gaseous exchange'
- *transport of respiratory gases*: transport of oxygen from the lungs to the cells, and of carbon dioxide from the cells to the lungs, accomplished by the cardiovascular system
- *internal respiration*: movement of oxygen from blood into the cells, and of carbon dioxide from the cells to the blood (Marieb and Hoehn 2018).

Pulse oximetry

Pulse oximetry provides continuous and non-invasive monitoring of the oxygen saturation from haemoglobin in arterial blood (Peate and Wild 2018). Pulse oximetry is an effective method of monitoring for hypoxaemia and detecting a fall in arterial oxygen saturation, often even before any obvious symptoms are displayed (Marini and Dries 2016). It also provides useful information about heart rate (Tait et al. 2015).

Anatomy and physiology

The organs and structures of the respiratory system can be split into two zones: the conducting zone and the respiratory zone (Marieb and Hoehn 2018). The conducting zone consists of a number of interconnecting passageways, both outside and within the lungs, through which air passes to get to the area of gaseous exchange, such as the nasal cavity, trachea and bronchi (Marieb and Keller 2017). The function of this area is to provide conduits through which air can pass, and it can also filter, cleanse, warm and humidify the air while conducting it to the lungs (Tortora and Derrickson 2017). The respiratory zone consists of the bronchioles, alveolar ducts and alveoli, which are the main sites where gaseous exchange occurs (Marieb and Hoehn 2018).

A variety of efficient inter-relationships exist between the different body systems in order for effective respiration to occur; these include the cardiovascular system, nervous system and musculoskeletal system (Patton 2018). The respiratory muscles (the diaphragm and intercostal muscles) promote ventilation by causing volume and pressure changes within the respiratory system (Marieb and Hoehn 2018).

The mechanism of breathing

The key mechanism of pulmonary ventilation is that changes of volume within the respiratory system lead to changes in pressure, and these in turn lead to a flow of gases to equalize the pressure (Marieb and Hoehn 2018). The relationship between the pressure and volume of a gas is called Boyle's law, whereby at a constant temperature the pressure of a gas varies inversely with its volume; in a larger container, the pressure of a gas is less than in a smaller one (Marieb and Hoehn 2018). As air will flow from an area of high pressure to an area of lower pressure, air moves into the lungs when the air pressure inside the lungs is lower than the air pressure in the atmosphere, and out of the lungs when the air pressure outside the lungs is greater than the air pressure in the atmosphere (Tortora and Derrickson 2017).

Inspiration

For inspiration to occur, the pressure in the alveoli must be lower than the air pressure in the atmosphere; this is achieved by increasing the size (volume) of the lungs through the contraction of the muscles of inhalation – the diaphragm and the intercostal muscles (Marieb and Keller 2017). The diaphragm flattens and descends and the intercostal muscles lift the ribcage and sternum, causing the ribs to broaden outwards and increasing the diameter of the thoracic cavity, both from side to side and from front to back (Patton 2018). During normal inspiration, the pressure between the two pleural layers in the pleural cavity (intrapleural pressure) is always just lower than atmospheric pressure (756 mmHg at an atmospheric pressure of 760 mmHg) (Marieb and Hoehn 2018). As the volume of the lungs and pleural cavity increases, the intrapleural pressure drops to 754 mmHg (Marieb and Hoehn 2018). At the same time, the pressure within the lungs (alveolar or intrapulmonary pressure) drops from 760 mmHg to 758 mmHg, and so a pressure difference between the atmosphere and the alveoli is established and air flows into the lungs (Tortora and Derrickson 2017). The relationship between these pressures can be seen in Figure 14.25.

Expiration

Expiration also occurs due to a pressure gradient but in the opposite direction, such that the pressure within the lungs is greater than the pressure of the atmosphere (Patton 2018). In normal gentle breathing, the process of expiration is largely passive, not involving any muscular contractions but resulting from elastic recoil of the chest wall and lungs (Tortora and Derrickson 2017).

Expiration begins when the inspiratory muscles relax, causing the diaphragm to move superiorly and the ribs to depress, which decreases the diameter of the thoracic cavity and returns it to its normal size (Marieb and Keller 2017). This results in a decrease in lung volume and compression of the alveoli, causing an increase in alveolar (intrapulmonary) pressure to 762 mmHg (Tortora and Derrickson 2017). This forces gases to flow out from the area of higher pressure in the lungs to the area of lower pressure in the atmosphere (Tortora and Derrickson 2017). A summary of the events that occur during inspiration and expiration can be seen in Figure 14.26.

The accessory muscles

The accessory muscles of inspiration further increase the volume of the thoracic cavity and, therefore, increase the volume of breathing. These muscles include the sternocleidomastoid muscles, which elevate the sternum, and the scalene muscles and the pectoralis minor muscles, which elevate the first to the fifth ribs (Tortora and Derrickson 2017). These muscles may be used during exercise or in situations where the individual is in respiratory distress (Marieb and Hoehn 2018).

The accessory muscles of expiration are used only during forceful breathing, such as when playing a wind instrument or during exercise (Tortora and Derrickson 2017). Contraction of the abdominal wall muscles, primarily the oblique and transversus muscles, increases intra-abdominal pressure, forcing the abdominal organs upwards against the diaphragm, and also depresses the ribcage

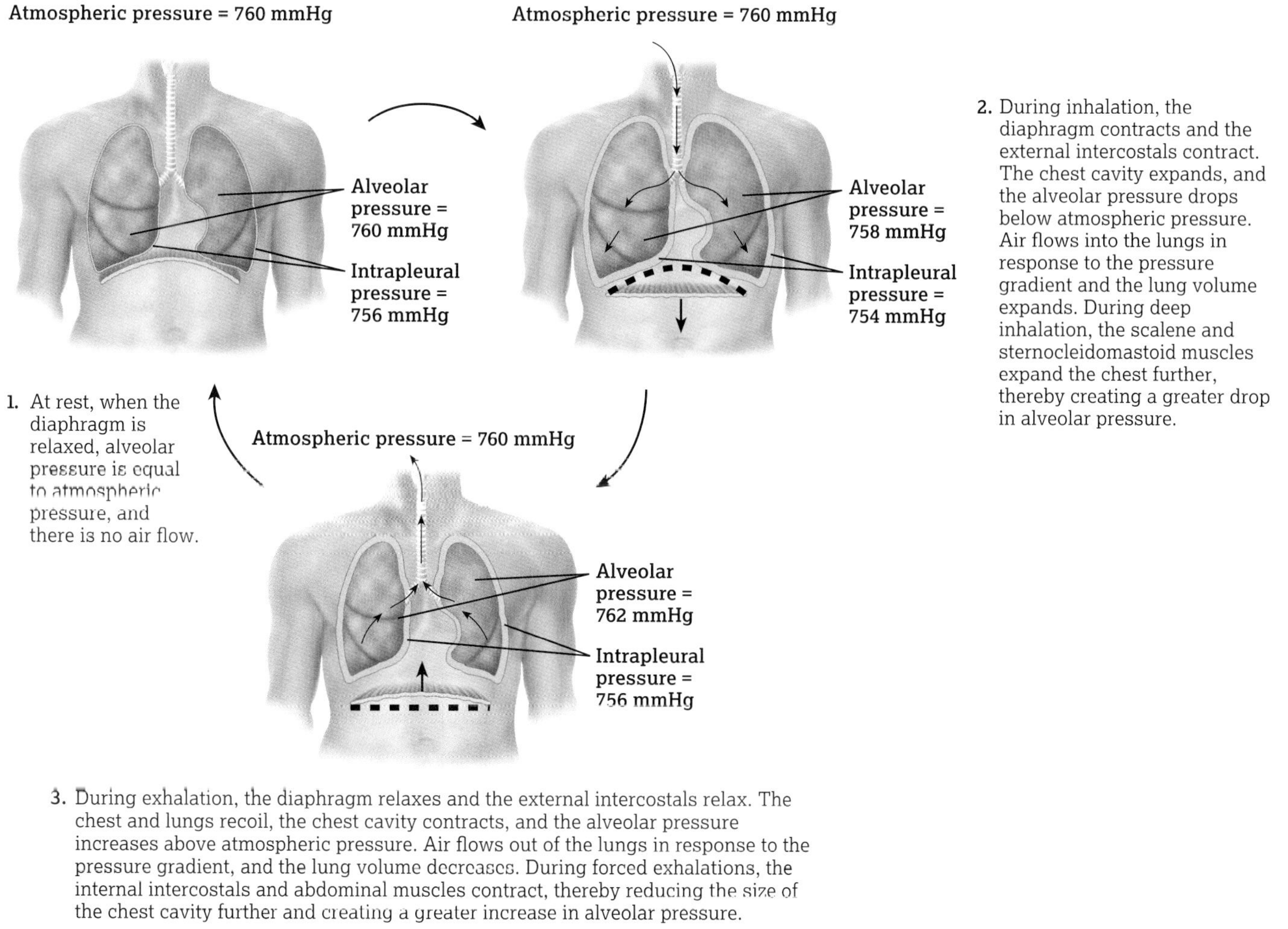
Atmospheric pressure = 760 mmHg
Atmospheric pressure = 760 mmHg
Alveolar pressure = 760 mmHg
Intrapleural pressure = 756 mmHg
Alveolar pressure = 758 mmHg
Intrapleural pressure = 754 mmHg
2. During inhalation, the diaphragm contracts and the external intercostals contract. The chest cavity expands, and the alveolar pressure drops below atmospheric pressure. Air flows into the lungs in response to the pressure gradient and the lung volume expands. During deep inhalation, the scalene and sternocleidomastoid muscles expand the chest further, thereby creating a greater drop in alveolar pressure.
1. At rest, when the diaphragm is relaxed, alveolar pressure is equal to atmospheric pressure, and there is no air flow.
Atmospheric pressure = 760 mmHg
Alveolar pressure = 762 mmHg
Intrapleural pressure = 756 mmHg
3. During exhalation, the diaphragm relaxes and the external intercostals relax. The chest and lungs recoil, the chest cavity contracts, and the alveolar pressure increases above atmospheric pressure. Air flows out of the lungs in response to the pressure gradient, and the lung volume decreases. During forced exhalations, the internal intercostals and abdominal muscles contract, thereby reducing the size of the chest cavity further and creating a greater increase in alveolar pressure.

Figure 14.25 Pressure changes in pulmonary ventilation. *Source*: Reproduced from Tortora and Derrickson (2017) with permission of John Wiley & Sons.

(Waugh and Grant 2018). The internal intercostal muscles also depress the ribcage and decrease thoracic volume, forcing air out of the lungs (Marieb and Hoehn 2018).

Control of respiration

Oxygen consumption increases exponentially during periods of strenuous exercise; several mechanisms help to match respiratory effort to the metabolic demand of the cells (Tortora and Derrickson 2017). Higher brain centres, chemoreceptors and other reflexes modify the basic respiratory rhythms generated in the brainstem (Marieb and Keller 2017). Control of respiration primarily involves neurons in the medulla and pons (Marieb and Hoehn 2018).

The respiratory centres

Within the medulla are two clusters of neurones that are critically important in the co-ordination of the respiratory system: the dorsal respiratory group (DRG) and the ventral respiratory group (VRG) (Marieb and Hoehn 2018).

The DRG contains neurones that generate impulses; they stimulate the diaphragm and the external intercostal muscles to contract, via the phrenic and intercostal nerves, and contraction of these muscles leads to inspiration. Generation of the impulses is then paused, allowing the diaphragm and intercostal muscles to relax, leading to passive expiration (Marieb and Hoehn 2018). The VRG contains neurones that act as 'pacemakers' and control the rhythm of breathing (Marieb and Hoehn 2018). It is also from the VRG that active or forceful breathing is controlled (Tortora and Derrickson 2017).

The DRG co-ordinates input from the peripheral baroreceptors (or stretch receptors) and chemoreceptors and relays this to the VRG to alter respiratory rate as required (Marieb and Hoehn 2018). Baroreceptors monitor the stretch of the bronchi and bronchioles during overinflation of the lungs (Tortora and Derrickson 2017). Chemoreceptors monitor the arterial blood for changes in the partial pressure of carbon dioxide ($PaCO_2$) and pH, but also, to a lesser extent, the partial pressure of oxygen (PaO_2) (Patton 2018). For more information on the chemical factors that affect respiration, see Chapter 12: Respiratory care, CPR and blood transfusion.

Additionally, pontine respiratory centres relay impulses to the VRG to modify breathing rhythms so that there is a smooth transition from inspiration to expiration and so that breathing can be modified to allow for speech, exercise and sleep (Marieb and Hoehn 2018).

Carbon dioxide

Although oxygen is essential for every cell in the body, the body's need to rid itself of carbon dioxide is the most influential stimulus to respiration in a healthy person (Marieb and Hoehn 2018). Arterial $PaCO_2$ is closely monitored and acceptable levels maintained by a sensitive homeostatic mechanism mediated mainly by the effect that increased carbon dioxide levels have on the central chemoreceptors of the brainstem (Tortora and Derrickson 2017). Carbon dioxide passes easily from the blood into the cerebrospinal fluid, where it forms carbonic acid, releasing hydrogen ions (H^+) (Marieb and Keller 2017). This increase of H^+ causes the pH to drop, stimulating the central chemoreceptors in the brainstem to

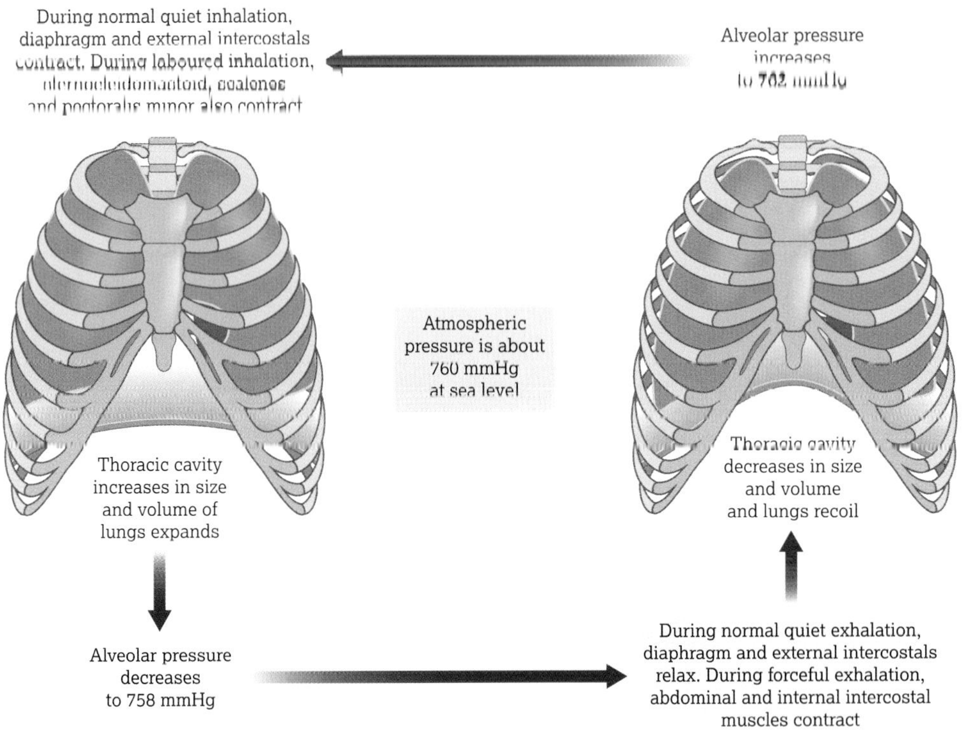
During normal quiet inhalation,
diaphragm and external intercostals
contract. During laboured inhalation,
sternocleidomastoid, scalenes
and pectoralis minor also contract
Alveolar pressure
increases
to 762 mmHg
Atmospheric
pressure is about
760 mmHg
at sea level
Thoracic cavity
increases in size
and volume of
lungs expands
Thoracic cavity
decreases in size
and volume
and lungs recoil
Alveolar pressure
decreases
to 758 mmHg
During normal quiet exhalation,
diaphragm and external intercostals
relax. During forceful exhalation,
abdominal and internal intercostal
muscles contract

Figure 14.26 Summary of events of inhalation and exhalation. *Source*: Reproduced from Peate and Wild (2018) with permission of John Wiley & Sons.

increase the rate and depth of breathing and so increase the amount of carbon dioxide exhaled (Marieb and Hoehn 2018). Similarly, should a metabolic acidosis or acidaemia (low pH) exist (such as a build-up of lactic acid), a change in respiration will ensue in an attempt to compensate for this (Marieb and Hoehn 2018). See Figure 14.27 for negative feedback mechanisms by which changes in $PaCO_2$ and blood pH regulate ventilation. Abnormally low $PaCO_2$ levels cause inhibition of respiration, with breathing becoming slow and shallow, and periods of apnoea may occur until arterial $PaCO_2$ rises again and stimulates respiration (Marieb and Hoehn 2018).

Oxygen

The peripheral chemoreceptors, found in the aortic arch and carotid arteries, are responsible for sensing the arterial PaO_2 (Marieb and Hoehn 2015). Normally, decreasing levels of oxygen only affect respiratory rate by causing the peripheral chemoreceptors to have an increased sensitivity to carbon dioxide (Marieb and Hoehn 2018). A normal arterial PaO_2, regardless of age, should be greater than 10.6 kPa (80 mmHg); a significant drop will cause the central receptors to become suppressed and at the same time the peripheral receptors will stimulate the respiratory centres to increase ventilation even if $PaCO_2$ is normal (Marieb and Hoehn 2018).

Other ways in which respiration is controlled

There are a number of receptors in the lungs that respond to a variety of irritants (Marieb and Keller 2017). Accumulated mucus or inhaled debris stimulates receptors in the bronchioles that cause reflex constriction of those air passages (Tortora and Derrickson 2017). When these receptors are stimulated in the bronchi or trachea, a cough is initiated, whereas when they are stimulated in the nasal cavity, a sneeze is triggered (Marieb and Hoehn 2018). These irritant receptors have a protective mechanism to prevent obstruction or aspiration of food or liquids (Patton 2018). There are also stretch receptors present in the conducting passages and the visceral pleura that are stimulated when the lungs inflate; these then signal the respiratory centres to end inspiration (Marieb and Hoehn 2018). These receptors are thought to act more as a protective response to prevent excessive stretching of the lungs than as a normal regulatory mechanism (Marieb and Hoehn 2018).

Respiration can also be altered in the higher cortical centres in response to factors such as strong emotions, pain and alteration of temperature (Tortora and Derrickson 2017). The cerebral motor cortex yields a degree of voluntary control over breathing; however, this can be overridden by the other mechanisms (Patton 2018).

Some of the mechanisms through which breathing is controlled are summarized in Figure 14.28.

Related theory

Respiratory volumes

The volume of air that is breathed in and out of the lungs varies depending on the conditions of inspiration and expiration (Marieb and Hoehn 2018). As such, several respiratory volumes can be described, combinations of which (termed 'respiratory capacities') are measured to gain information about a person's respiratory status (Marieb and Hoehn 2018). A summary of these volumes can be seen in Figure 14.29. See Table 14.3 for a summary of respiratory volumes and capacities for males and females.

Gaseous exchange

Gaseous exchange occurs during *external respiration* where oxygen diffuses from the air in the alveoli of the lungs into blood in the pulmonary capillaries, and carbon dioxide diffuses from the blood into the alveolar air (Patton 2018). This occurs as there is a flow of gases from areas of higher pressure to areas of lower pressure; oxygen diffuses from alveolar air, where the partial pressure is higher than that in the capillary blood, and carbon dioxide diffuses from the blood, where the partial pressure is higher than that in the alveolar air (Tortora and Derrickson 2017).

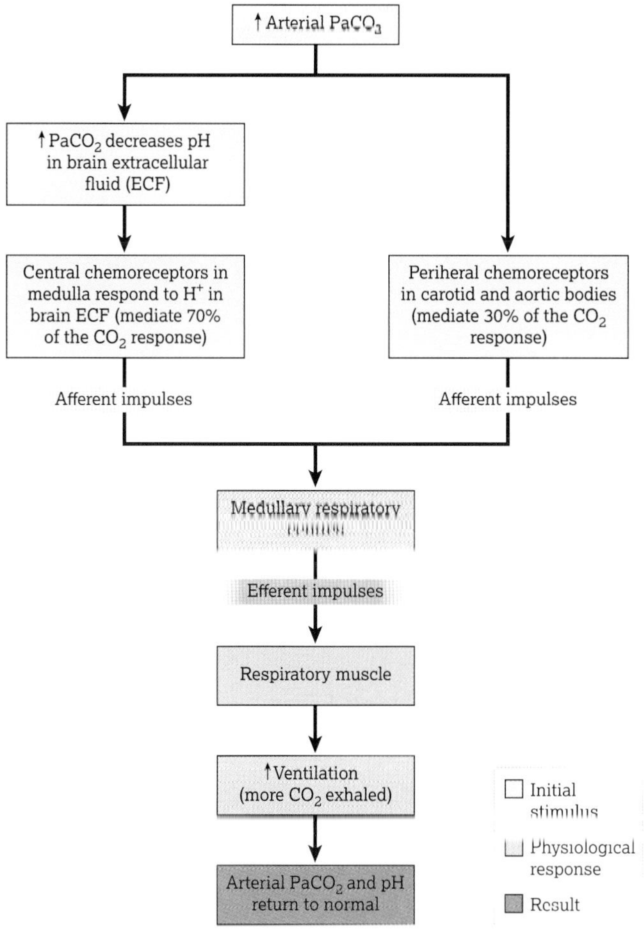

Figure 14.27 Negative feedback mechanisms by which changes in $PaCO_2$ and blood pH regulate ventilation. *Source*: Marieb and Hoehn (2016).

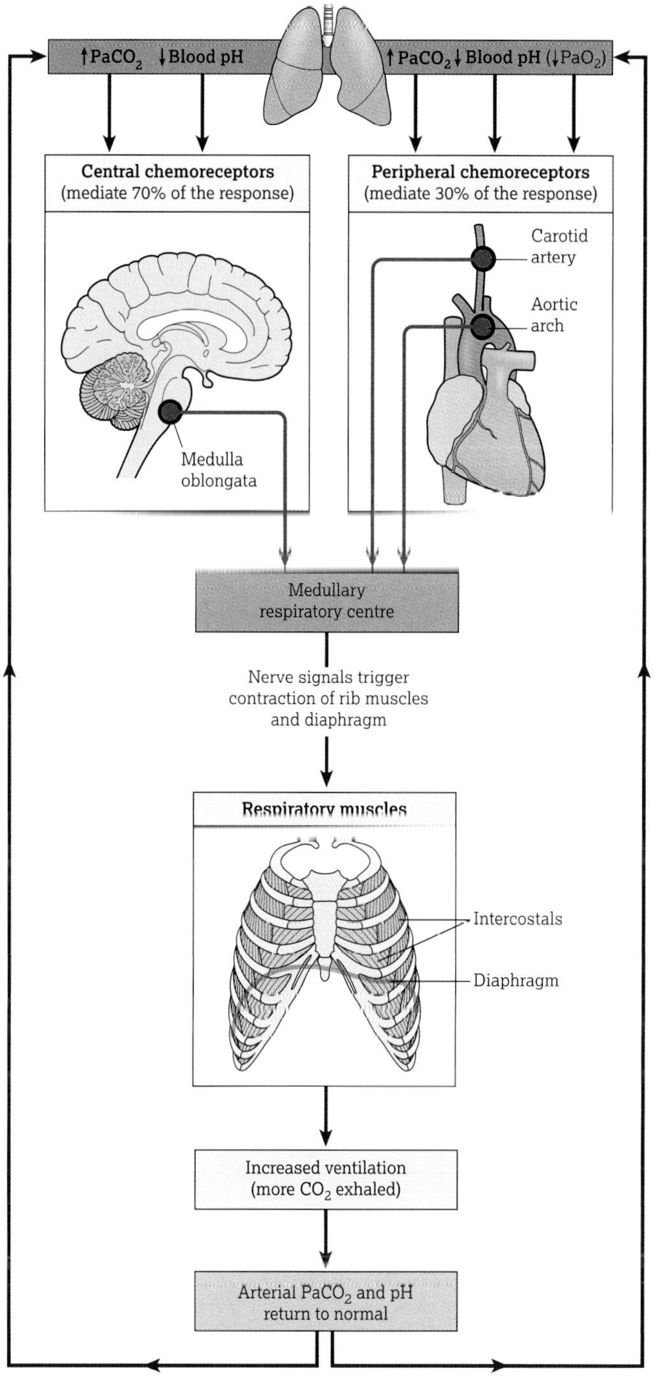

Figure 14.28 Factors that influence rate and depth of breathing. *Source*: Marieb and Hoehn (2016).

Internal respiration, or systemic gas exchange, takes place where the same gases move into or out of the cells of the body by diffusion, so oxygen moves into the tissues and carbon dioxide moves out of them (Tortora and Derrickson 2017). See Figure 14.30 for the changes that occur in the partial pressures of oxygen and carbon dioxide during internal and external respiration. See Chapter 12: Respiratory care, CPR and blood transfusion for further information.

Transport through the blood

Oxygen does not dissolve easily in water and therefore only 1.5% of the oxygen is transported in the blood by being dissolved in the plasma; the other 98.5% is bound to haemoglobin in the red blood cells, forming oxyhaemoglobin (Hb–O_2) (Tortora and Derrickson 2017). The majority of carbon dioxide is transported in the blood as bicarbonate ions (HCO_3^-) within the plasma (70%); approximately 20–23% is bound to haemoglobin, forming carbaminohaemoglobin (Hb–CO_2); and the remaining 7–10% is dissolved in the plasma (Marieb and Hoehn 2018). This process is summarized in Figure 14.31; see also Chapter 12: Respiratory care, CPR and blood transfusion.

Hypoxia

Hypoxia is defined as inadequate oxygen delivery to the tissues, which can have various causes. Based on these causes, it can be classified into four types (Marieb and Hoehn 2018, Tortora and Derrickson 2017):

- *Hypoxaemic hypoxia*: caused by a low PaO_2 in arterial blood as a result of breathing air with inadequate oxygen (such as at high altitude) or abnormal ventilation/perfusion matching in the lungs (due to airway obstruction or fluid in the lungs); carbon monoxide poisoning can also cause this.
- *Anaemic hypoxia*: caused by too little functioning haemoglobin being present in the blood (e.g. due to haemorrhage or anaemia), which reduces the transport of oxygen to the cells.
- *Ischaemic hypoxia*: caused when blood flow to a specific area is inadequate to supply enough oxygen (due to embolism or thrombosis), even though PaO_2 and Hb–O_2 levels are normal.
- *Histotoxic hypoxia*: caused by the cells being unable to use the oxygen that has been delivered; this can occur as a result of poisons such as cyanide.

Signs of hypoxia include tachypnoea, dyspnoea, tachycardia, restlessness and confusion, headache, mild hypertension and pallor.

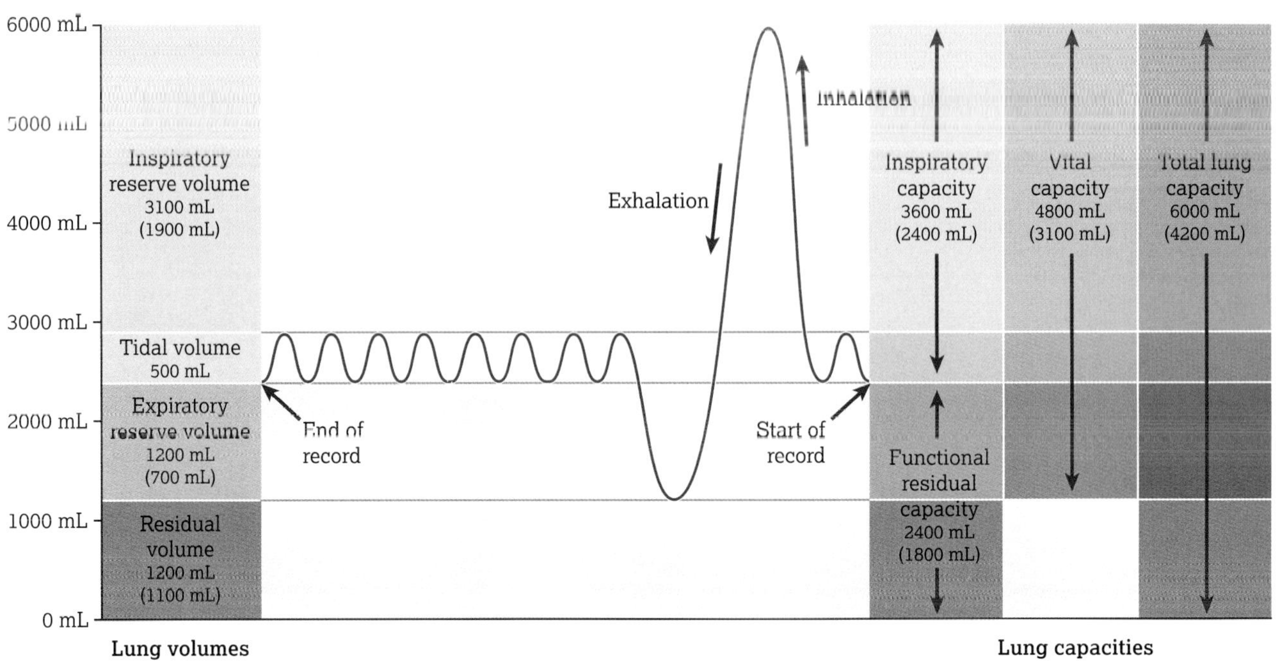

Figure 14.29 Spirogram of lung volumes and capacities. The average values for a healthy average male and female are indicated, with the values for a female in parentheses. Note that the spirogram is read from right (start of record) to left (end of record). *Source*: Reproduced from Peate and Wild (2018) with permission of John Wiley & Sons.

Table 14.3 Respiratory volumes and capacities

Respiratory volumes and capacities	Adult male average value (mL)	Adult female average value (mL)	Description
Tidal volume (V_T)	500	500	The volume of air inhaled or exhaled in one breath
Minute volume (MV)	6000	6000	The total volume of air inhaled or exhaled each minute: = 12 breaths per minute × 500 mL/breath = 6000 mL/minute
Inspiratory reserve volume (IRV)	3100	1900	The volume of air that can be forcibly inhaled after a normal tidal volume inhalation
Expiratory reserve volume (ERV)	1200	700	The volume of air that can be forcibly exhaled after a normal tidal volume exhalation
Residual volume (RV)	1200	1100	The volume of air left in the lungs after a forced exhalation
Inspiratory capacity (IC)	3600	2400	The sum of the tidal volume and inspiratory reserve volume
Functional residual capacity (FRC)	2400	1800	The sum of the residual volume and expiratory reserve volume
Vital capacity (VC)	4800	3100	The sum of the tidal volume, inspiratory reserve volume and expiratory reserve volume
Total lung capacity (TLC)	6000	4200	The sum of the vital capacity and residual volume

Source: Adapted from Tortora and Derrickson (2017).

In its severe stages, the symptoms will worsen, leading to slow, irregular breathing, cyanosis, hypotension, altered level of consciousness, blurred vision and eventually respiratory arrest (Sprigings and Chambers 2017).

Hypercapnia

Hypercapnia is an elevated level of carbon dioxide in the blood. Signs include tachypnoea (eventually becoming bradypnoea as it worsens), dyspnoea, tachycardia, hypertension, headaches, vasodilation, drowsiness, sweating and a red coloration (Sprigings and Chambers 2017). Patients with hypercapnia require urgent medical attention and close monitoring as hypercapnia causes respiratory acidosis (Cleave 2016). Patients with chronic hypercapnia, such as those who have chronic obstructive pulmonary disease, will have at least partially adapted to the chronically high levels of carbon dioxide, which means their primary respiratory drive will be a low PaO_2 rather than a high PaCO2. Oxygen therapy therefore needs to be administered with caution in these

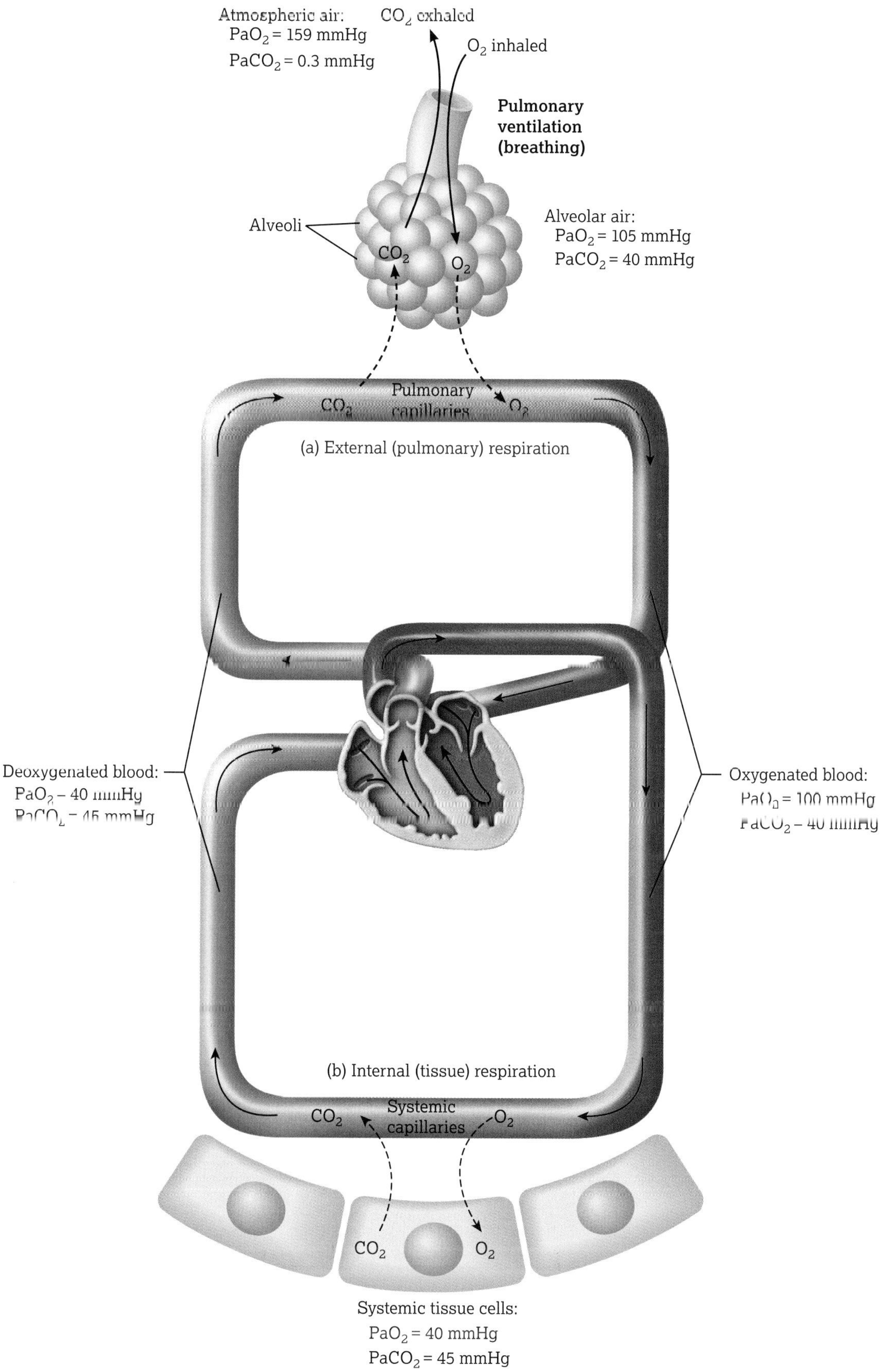

Figure 14.30 Changes to partial pressures of oxygen and carbon dioxide (in mmHg) during internal and external respiration. *Source*: Reproduced from Tortora and Derrickson (2011) with permission of John Wiley & Sons.

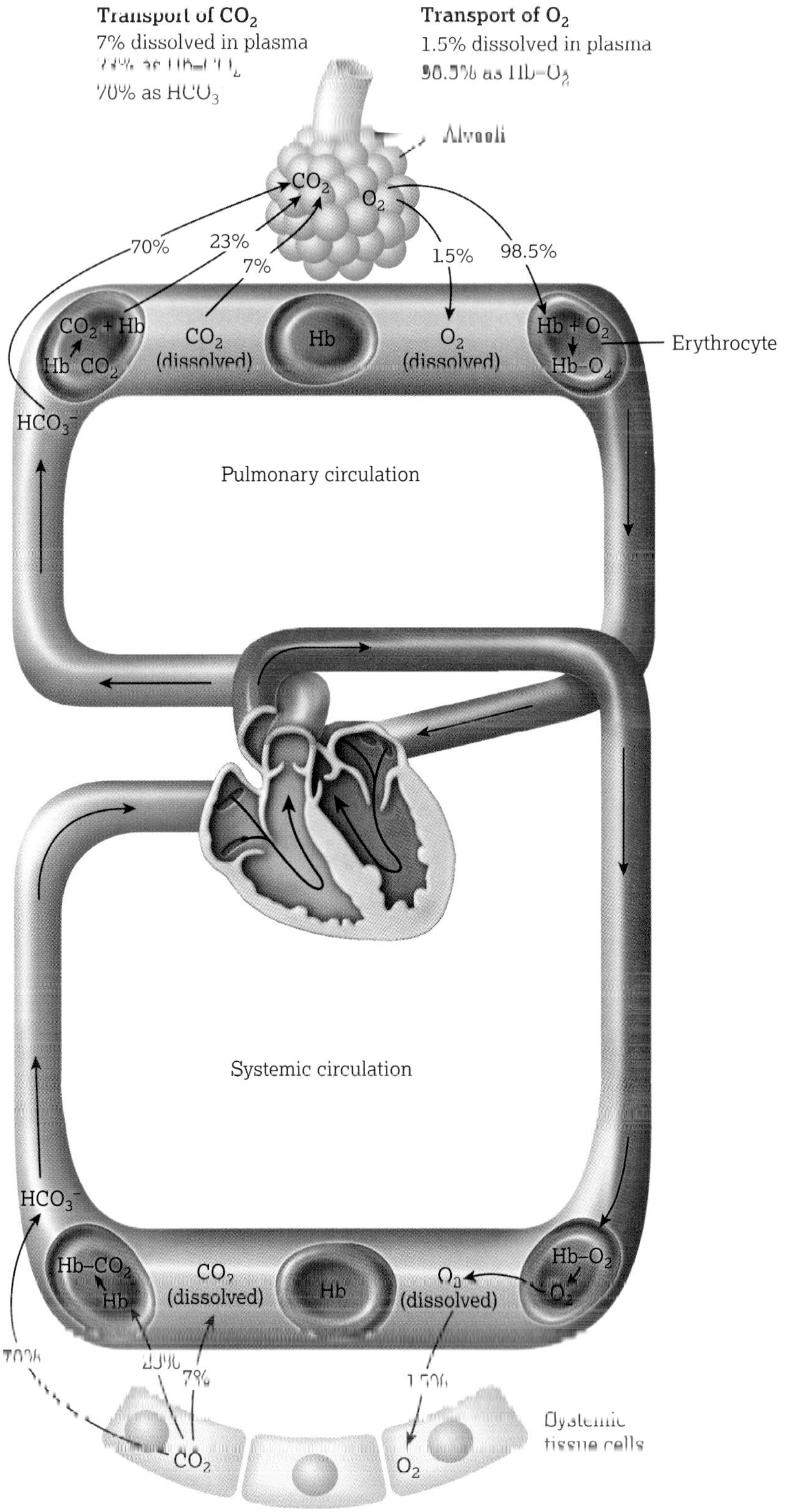

Figure 14.31 Transport of oxygen (O_2) and carbon dioxide (CO_2) in the blood. *Source*: Reproduced from Tortora and Derrickson (2011) with permission of John Wiley & Sons.

patients, often aiming for lower than usual peripheral oxygen saturations (90–92%) (O'Driscoll et al. 2017).

Pulse oximetry

Normal oxygen saturation sits at 96% or above; however, patients with chronic respiratory conditions may have adjusted to lower oxygen saturation levels, hence oxygen saturations should be targeted to be as near to the patient's normal range as possible (O'Driscoll et al. 2017). In general terms, [illegible] 91% is of concern, but the trend of oxygen saturations may be of more importance than individual readings as this gives an indication of whether the patient is responding to therapy or deteriorating (O'Driscoll et al. 2017). Supplementary oxygen may be required to achieve saturations of 94–98% in an acutely ill adult or 88–92% in patients with a chronic respiratory disease and those at risk of hypercapnic respiratory failure (O'Driscoll et al. 2017). Oxygen therapy should be regarded as a drug and be prescribed in line with local policy (BNF 2019). In addition, a sudden drop of greater than 3% in oxygen saturation suggests a thorough clinical assessment should be performed (O'Driscoll et al. 2017).

Evidence-based approaches

Rationale

The purpose of respiratory assessment is to determine the respiratory status of the patient (Bickley 2016). A thorough respiratory assessment is vital to:

- identify patients who are at risk of deterioration
- commence treatment that may stabilize and improve the patient's condition and outcomes
- help prevent unnecessary admission to critical care units (Sprigings and Chambers 2017).

Derangement of respiratory observations may indicate difficulties in a range of body systems, not simply the respiratory system, so it is a vital indicator of morbidity. Changes to the respiratory system are a known precursor to adverse events, with an associated increase in mortality (Cleave 2016). Breathing, and more specifically respiratory rate, is one of the most sensitive indicators of critical illness and is usually the first vital sign to alter in a deteriorating patient; therefore, timely, accurate observations, with early, effective and appropriate interventions, may vastly improve patient outcomes (Adam et al. 2017).

Indications

Patients who are in hospital should have observations, including respiratory observations, taken and recorded regularly, as follows:

- during and following surgery, investigative procedures, trauma, infections and emergency situations in order to identify any changes from baseline observations and compare different sets of observations
- for monitoring before and during blood or blood product transfusions or intravenous fluids
- to monitor response to medications, including opiates and bronchodilators (Blows 2018).

If the patient is acutely ill or at risk of respiratory deterioration, they will require continuous pulse oximetry and frequent respiratory assessment (Tait et al. 2015). Similarly, if the patient is receiving oxygen therapy, they will need to be closely monitored to ensure its efficacy (Marini and Dries 2016). Any patient who has, or is at risk of, chronic hypercapnia should have close monitoring of their respiratory function, with observations performed accordingly (O'Driscoll et al. 2017).

Any healthcare professional who has been trained and assessed as competent can perform a respiratory assessment and pulse oximetry in accordance with local hospital policy.

Contraindications for pulse oximetry

Although pulse oximetry is a useful tool in the assessment of respiratory status, its limitations should be recognized. One of the main limitations is its inability to reliably detect hypoventilation (particularly in patients receiving supplemental oxygen) and carbon dioxide retention (Lough 2015); the latter is usually confirmed by measurement of $PaCO_2$ via arterial blood gas analysis (Brown and Cadogan 2016). Likewise, pulse oximetry does not give an indication of haemoglobin, so if the patient is profoundly anaemic then their oxygen saturation may be normal but they may still be hypoxic (Adam et al. 2017). Other factors that may affect pulse oximetry readings include the following:

- *Nail polish*: dark colours in particular will affect the accuracy of readings (Peate and Wild 2018).
- *Intravenous dyes*: pulse oximetry may be inaccurate in patients who have received dye treatment, such as methylene blue, indocyanine green or indigo carmine (Blows 2018).
- *Poor peripheral perfusion*: to work effectively, an adequate peripheral blood flow is required, but this can be impaired by factors such as hypovolaemia, hypotension, hypothermia, vasoconstriction or heart failure, and may result in falsely low readings (Tait et al. 2015).
- *Cardiac arrhythmias, e.g. atrial fibrillation*: these can cause inadequate or irregular perfusion, resulting in falsely low readings (Blows 2018).
- *Recording blood pressure*: inflation of the blood pressure cuff will cause the readings to be inaccurate; the probe should be positioned on a finger of the opposite arm to where blood pressure is being taken (Peate and Wild 2018).
- *Carbon monoxide poisoning*: pulse oximetry should not be used on patients with suspected or confirmed carbon monoxide poisoning as the sensor cannot differentiate between oxyhaemoglobin and carboxyhaemoglobin and will therefore provide falsely elevated oxygen saturation readings; arterial blood gas analysis should be undertaken instead (Sprigings and Chambers 2017). 773
- *Methaemoglobinaemia*: changes in the structure of haemoglobin, caused by lignocaine, nitrates, metoclopramide and local anaesthetics, can inhibit oxygen release from the haemoglobin, resulting in tissue hypoxia and unreliable oxygen saturation measurements (Appadu and Lin 2016).
- *Bright external light*: fluorescent lighting or light interference from surgical lamps, infra-red warming lamps or direct sunlight can give falsely high readings (Adam et al. 2017).
- *Movement*: sudden movement, due to shivering, seizures or restlessness, may dislodge the sensor or cause motion artefact, affecting the ability of light to travel from the light-emitting diode to the detector in the probe (Adam et al. 2017).

Methods of assessing respiration

Airway assessment

In a conscious patient, a quick way to check airway patency is to ask them a question; a normal verbal response confirms that the patient's airway is clear (this also indicates that they are breathing and that their brain is being perfused) (Goulden and Clarke 2016; see also Chapter 12: Respiratory care, CPR and blood transfusion).

Airway obstruction can have a subtle presentation, with signs and symptoms that depend on the type of obstruction; regardless, it is usually a medical emergency (Brown and Cadogan 2016). A partial airway obstruction, where some air is allowed through, is generally associated with noises such as choking, snoring, hoarseness (harsh, deep voice) or stridor (harsh, high-pitched sound occurring usually on inspiration) (Wilkinson et al. 2017). In this case, the person may be agitated and panicked. It is important to assess whether there is any obstruction to the patient's airway as a result of vomit, blood, foreign bodies or the patient's tongue (Sprigings and Chambers 2017).

In contrast, in a complete airway obstruction, where there is no air getting through, there will be no breath sounds and the chest will not move (Sprigings and Chambers 2017); the patient will be extremely distressed and, if left untreated, they will lose consciousness quickly. In both cases, the presence of hypoxia implies a medical emergency due to impending respiratory arrest, irrespective of the location of the obstruction (upper or lower airway) (Adam et al. 2017). Its management can include the Heimlich manoeuvre (a technique used to release foreign objects from a person's airway), epinephrine injection (used to reverse airway swelling caused by an allergic reaction) and CPR (Brown and Cadogan 2016).

Breathing assessment

Breathing assessment is required to assess the patient's ability to adequately ventilate; it starts by observing the patient and how they breathe (Bickley 2016). It is important that the following aspects are observed:

- colour of the patient's skin and mucous membranes
- use of accessory muscles or other respiratory signs
- rhythm, rate and depth of respiration
- shape and expansion of the chest (Bickley 2016).

Skin colour

Cyanosis is a blue tone to the skin and mucous membranes, which may occur when high levels of unsaturated haemoglobin are present in the blood; it may be detectable when oxygen saturation of arterial blood drops below 90% (Peate and Wild 2018). Cyanosis is, however, often considered a late sign of respiratory deterioration and may be difficult to detect, particularly in artificial lighting (Brown and Cadogan 2016). There are two types of cyanosis: central, affecting the lips and oral mucosa, usually indicating cardiorespiratory insufficiency, and peripheral, observed in the skin and nail beds, usually indicating poor peripheral circulation if seen in isolation (Wilkinson et al. 2017). Patients who are anaemic may not be cyanotic as there is insufficient haemoglobin to generate the blue tone (Adam et al. 2017). Similarly, a pale skin tone may indicate that the patient is anaemic or in shock (Bickley 2016).

Use of accessory muscles

The use of accessory muscles (such as the sternocleidomastoid, scalene, trapezius and abdominals) to increase inspiration may suggest that the patient has difficulty breathing and is in respiratory distress (Bickley 2016). Observe the patient's neck during inspiration to see whether there is any contraction of the sternomastoid or other accessory muscles (Cleave 2016). In addition, some patients may breathe through pursed lips in an attempt to increase resistance on expiration, which helps to keep the alveoli open, or have nasal flaring as they attempt to force more air into their lungs (Bickley 2016).

Rhythm, rate and depth of respiration

The normal respiratory rate in adults is 12–18 breaths per minute with expiration lasting approximately twice as long as inspiration (Peate and Wild 2018). The rate should be counted for one full minute to fully assess both the rate and the rhythm (Bickley 2016). An increase from the patient's normal respiratory rate by as little as 3–5 breaths per minute is an early and important sign of respiratory distress or acute illness (Blows 2018). Patients with a respiratory rate greater than 21 breaths per minute should have frequent observations and be closely monitored; if they also have other physiological alterations, they should receive prompt medical attention, as should all patients with a respiratory rate greater than 25 breaths per minute (RCP 2017a). Respiratory rates of 9 or less also require urgent medical care (RCP 2017a). Respiratory rate can be classified as follows.

- *Eupnoea*: unconscious, gentle respiration. This is the normal respiratory rate and rhythm, usually between 12 and 18 breaths per minute (Patton 2018).
- *Bradypnoea*: a respiratory rate that is slower than the normal range – less than 12 breaths per minute. This may signify depression of the respiratory centre, opioid overdose, increased intracranial pressure or a diabetic coma. Regardless of the cause, it may indicate a severe deterioration in the patient's condition (Blows 2018).
- *Tachypnoea*: a respiratory rate that is faster than the normal range and shallow – greater than 21 breaths per minute. This may indicate a number of conditions, including anxiety, pain, restrictive lung disease, cardiac or circulatory problems, or pyrexia. It is the first indication of respiratory distress (Peate and Wild 2018).
- *Dyspnoea*: breathing where the individual is conscious of the effort to breathe and finds it increasingly difficult. When dyspnoea occurs when the patient lies flat, it is termed 'orthopnoea' (Patton 2018).
- *Apnoea*: a temporary cessation of breathing (Wilkinson et al. 2017).
- *Biot's breathing*: irregular respiratory rate and depth, alternating periods of deep gasping with periods of apnoea. This is seen in patients with increased intracranial pressure, head trauma, brain abscess, spinal meningitis and encephalitis (Waugh and Grant 2018).
- *Cheyne–Stokes breathing*: regular pattern of alternating periods of deep breathing with periods of apnoea. This may have many causes, including heart failure, renal failure, brain damage, drug overdose or increased intracranial pressure, and may also be present at the end of life (Marini and Dries 2016).
- *Kussmaul breathing*: rapid deep breathing resulting from stimulation of the respiratory centre caused by metabolic acidosis, such as in the case of diabetic ketoacidosis (Sprigings and Chambers 2017).
- *Hyperventilation*: increase in respiratory rate and depth, which can be caused by anxiety, exercise, metabolic acidosis, diabetic ketoacidosis or alteration in blood gas concentrations (Brown and Cadogan 2016).
- *Hypoventilation*: shallow and irregular breathing, which can be caused by an overdose of certain drugs, such as anaesthetic agents or opiates. It may also occur with prolonged bedrest or conscious splinting of the chest to avoid respiratory or abdominal pain (Bickley 2016).

Shape and expansion of the chest

The respiratory assessment should also consider the shape and expansion of the chest (Bickley 2016). The anteroposterior diameter of the chest wall may give an indication of underlying respiratory conditions or other problems (Brown and Cadogan 2016); it may change with age or increase in chronic pulmonary disease (Bickley 2016). It is also important to view the way the chest expands with each breath; when normal, it should be equal and bilateral (Sprigings and Chambers 2017). Any paradoxical movements – such as only one side of the chest moving, greater movement on one side, or one side moving up and the other moving down – should be noted as they can indicate a particular problem with one side of the chest (Adam et al. 2017). Asymmetrical chest expansion is abnormal and may indicate pleural disease, pulmonary fibrosis, collapse of upper lobes or bronchial obstruction; spinal deformities such as kyphosis also influence lung expansion (Wilkinson et al. 2017).

Further assessment

Following the above – and if a more thorough assessment is required in order to assess the patient's ability to adequately ventilate – percussion, palpation and auscultation of the chest should be performed (Adam et al. 2017). These assessment techniques will enable the identification of any added or absent breath sounds that may indicate lung abnormalities (such as an infection or pneumothorax).

In addition, respiratory assessment involves assessing the entire patient for other signs or symptoms, such as high temperature (which may be suggestive of pneumonia), increased pulse (which may indicate cardiovascular disease) and low blood pressure (which may indicate sepsis) (Bickley 2016). The patient's level of consciousness should also be assessed, including how alert and orientated they are and whether they appear to be distressed (Peate and Wild 2018). If the patient can only speak in very short sentences or can only say a few words without needing to stop to breathe, then they are in respiratory distress (Bickley 2016).

Methods of assessing oxygen saturation (pulse oximetry)

Arterial blood gas analysis has been the gold standard for monitoring arterial oxygen saturation, but it is invasive, time consuming and costly, and involves repeated arterial blood sampling, which only provides intermittent information (Sprigings and Chambers 2017; Tait et al. 2015). Therefore, the use of pulse oximetry should be considered in order to reduce the need for arterial samples to be taken (Clarke and Beaumont 2016).

Pre-procedural considerations

Equipment

Pulse oximeter

A pulse oximeter is a device that measures the amount of haemoglobin saturation in the tissue capillaries (Blows 2018). The probe consists of two light-emitting diodes (one red and one infra-red) on one side of the probe and a photodetector on the other side (Appadu and Lin 2016). The device projects light through the tissue to the detector and measures absorption in pulsatile blood by saturated haemoglobin (visible red) and desaturated haemoglobin (infra-red wavelength) (Appadu and Lin 2016). This is translated by the receiver into a percentage of oxygen saturation of the blood, symbolized as SpO_2.

In order to achieve a successful reading, the sensor of the pulse oximeter should be placed on an appropriate site with an adequate pulsating vascular bed (the probe must be designed for use on the chosen site) (Blows 2018). Therefore, the sensor may be attached to the patient's fingers (most common), ears, toes or nose (Goodell 2012, Johnson et al. 2012).

Pulse oximeters are vital in all areas where oxygen is administered and form part of any acute medical department's essential equipment (O'Driscoll et al. 2017). They should be checked, calibrated, maintained and stored as per the manufacturer's recommendations to ensure accurate and reliable results (Peate and Wild 2018).

Specific patient preparation

Appropriate positioning of the patient can help to ease any respiratory distress and facilitate the assessment and observation of their breathing (Cleave 2016). The patient should have rested and not have engaged in any strenuous physical activity prior to the assessment (Bickley 2016). If this is not contraindicated, the patient should be positioned upright or lying in bed with the head section elevated to an angle of 45–60° to allow good lung expansion; pillows can help to support the patient in this position (Peate and Wild 2018). With the patient's consent (RCN 2017a), it may be useful to remove clothing from their thorax to aid with observation of breathing (Bickley 2016). Positioning can also help to relax the patient and therefore potentially reduce the distress resulting from breathlessness (Adam et al. 2017).

The patient should give their consent to the assessment and remain still while pulse oximetry is being performed so that an accurate result can be obtained (Blows 2018). As mentioned previously, non-invasive blood pressure measurement should not be performed while pulse oximetry recording is underway, and nail polish should be removed from the probe site (Peate and Wild 2018).

Procedure guideline 14.4 Respiratory assessment and pulse oximetry

Essential equipment

- Personal protective equipment
- Pulse oximeter
- Cleaning materials (according to the manufacturer's recommendations and local policy)
- Sensor (probe) applicable to the chosen site
- A watch with a second hand
- Appropriate method of documentation and a pen

Optional equipment

- Variety of sensors (probes) available for different sites

Action	Rationale
Pre-procedure	
1 Introduce yourself to the patient, explain and discuss the procedure with them, and gain their consent to proceed.	To ensure that the patient feels at ease, understands the procedure and gives their valid consent (NMC 2018, **C**).
2 Wash and dry hands and/or use an alcohol-based handrub.	To prevent cross-infection (NHS England and NHSI 2019, **C**).
3 Ask the patient to remain as still as possible during the procedure and ensure that a constant temperature is maintained in the patient's environment.	Artefacts from movement, such as shivering, may adversely affect the accuracy of the measurement (Blows 2018, **E**).
4 While talking to the patient, assess their respiratory status, including their ability to talk in full sentences, the colour of their skin, whether they appear to be in distress or not, and whether they are alert and orientated.	This initial assessment can give important information about the patient's respiratory function and any potential problems (Bickley 2016, **E**).
5 Determine the site to be used to perform pulse oximetry. The site should have a good blood supply, determined by checking it is warm, with a proximal pulse and brisk capillary refill.	To ensure the sensor will receive strong enough signals to produce a result by being located in a well-perfused area (Adam et al. 2017, **E**).
6 Ensure that the area to be used is clean and free from dirt, and that the sensor is clean. If using the patient's fingers, ensure that all nail polish and any artificial nails have been removed.	Dirt, nail polish and artificial nails may interfere with the transmission of the light signals, causing inaccurate results (Peate and Wild 2018, **E**).
7 Select the correct pulse oximeter sensor for the site that is most appropriate for your patient, depending on their circulation and the manufacturer's instructions.	The correct sensor should be used for each site to ensure that the contact is good, that excessive pressure is not applied and that an accurate reading from the chosen site is obtained (Appadu and Lin 2016, **E**; Johnson et al. 2012, **E**).

(continued)

Procedure guideline 14.4 Respiratory assessment and pulse oximetry *(continued)*

Action	Rationale
Procedure	
8 Position the sensor securely but do not fix it with tape (unless specifically recommended by the manufacturer) (**Action figure 8**). If the pulse oximetry is to be continuous then the site should be changed at least every 4 hours.	If the probe is too tight, it may impede blood flow, leading to inaccurate results and the potential for pressure ulcer formation on the site, particularly in patients with compromised skin integrity (Appadu and Lin 2016, **E**).
9 Turn the pulse oximeter on and, if using it continuously, set the alarms on the device depending on the patient's condition and within locally agreed limits.	To ensure that the pulse oximeter is ready to use (Adam et al. 2017, **E**).
10 Ask the patient not to talk while you palpate their pulse. Check that the pulse reading on the device corresponds with the patient's actual pulse.	Any large deviations in pulse may show that the device is not measuring accurately or is being affected by movement (Blows 2018, **E**).
11 Assess respiration by keeping your fingers on the patient's wrist once the pulse rate has been obtained. Count their respiratory rate for a full minute – one breath is equal to one inspiration and expiration and is obtained by watching the abdomen or chest wall move in and out (Peate and Wild 2018). Assess the regularity and depth of breathing and the shape and expansion of the chest, and look for any use of accessory muscles. If possible, do not tell the patient you are counting their breathing.	To determine the patient's respiration rate, depth and rhythm. **E** The patient should ideally not be aware that their breathing is being counted as this may produce inaccurate results (Brown and Cadogan 2016, **E**).
Post-procedure	
12 Document the results clearly, including the time and date of the reading.	Records must be kept of all assessments made and care provided (NMC 2018, **C**).
13 Clean the pulse oximeter according to the manufacturer's recommendations and local policy.	The pulse oximeter may become colonized and be a source of infection to another patient (NICE 2014, **E**).
14 Wash and dry hands and/or use an alcohol-based handrub.	To prevent cross-infection (NHS England and NHSI 2019, **C**).

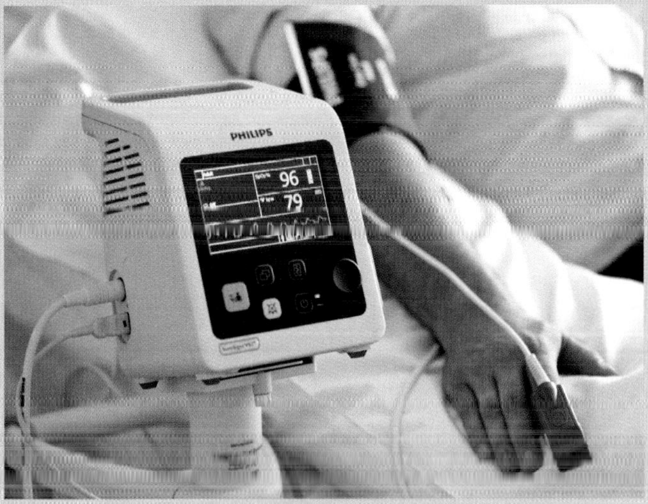

Action Figure 8 Position of an oxygen saturation probe.

Problem-solving table 14.4 Prevention and resolution (Procedure guideline 14.4)

Problem	Cause	Prevention	Action
Unable to turn on the pulse oximeter	Low battery	Ensure the pulse oximeter is left on continuous charge when not in use.	Connect the pulse oximeter to mains electricity. It should function once it is connected to a power supply.
The pulse oximeter is working but the heart rate and saturations display is blank	Loose connection	Carefully store the cables after use to prevent damage.	Check that the probe is securely connected to the machine.

Problem	Cause	Prevention	Action
Poor trace or inconsistent reading	Movement from shivering, seizures or tremors can affect the accuracy of the reading (Blows 2018)	Encourage the patient to keep as still as possible. If still unable to obtain an accurate reading, try to use a site that is less affected by movement, for example an ear lobe.	If the finger has been used, compare the pulse rate as given by the oximeter with the palpated radial pulse. If there is a difference then the oxygen saturation reading will not be accurate and arterial blood gases may be required to monitor the patient's oxygen saturation, if accurate pulse oximetry cannot be obtained from an alternative site (Adam et al. 2017).
Unexpectedly low result that does not correlate with the patient's clinical condition	The site chosen may not have an adequate blood supply	Check for perfusion by palpating for a pulse and checking the area is warm, with good capillary refill.	Reposition the sensor on a new site. If the result remains low, arterial blood gases may need to be considered (Adam et al. 2017).
Pulse oximetry heart rate does not correlate with palpated pulse	Not all pulsations are being detected	Check for perfusion by palpating for a pulse and checking the area is warm, with good capillary refill.	Obtain a replacement probe and/or monitor (Peate and Wild 2018).

Post-procedural considerations

Immediate care

Any abnormalities discovered during the respiratory assessment should prompt rapid action; early intervention is essential to improve patient outcomes (Sprigings and Chambers 2017). If there is a risk of a compromised airway or respiratory insufficiency or failure, then in-house emergency or outreach teams (e.g. cardiac arrest team) should be sought, and senior nursing and medical teams should be made aware (Clarke and Deaumont 2016). Further information will be needed, including obtaining:

- a full set of observations, including temperature, blood pressure and heart rate (Adam et al. 2017)
- a history of the patient's current condition and any past medical history, including a list of the medications they are taking (Brown and Cadogan 2016).

Other tests may also be required depending on the condition of the patient. These may include the following:

- arterial blood gases to check for carbon dioxide level, oxygen level, pH and acid/base balance (Adam et al. 2017)
- sputum collection to assess for infection and/or specific diseases such as tuberculosis (Marini and Dries 2016)
- chest X-ray or CT (computed tomography) scan (Wilkinson et al. 2017)
- blood tests, including a full blood count, urea and electrolytes, clotting screen and cross-match (Marini and Dries 2016)
- fluid balance to monitor for signs of fluid overload or dehydration (Tait et al. 2015).

Airway management and administration of oxygen

If a patient's condition necessitates the administration of oxygen, this should be provided as quickly and efficiently as possible. Although oxygen should be prescribed, in an emergency situation the absence of a prescription should not delay its administration (O'Driscoll et al. 2017). For further information see Chapter 12: Respiratory care, CPR and blood transfusion.

Ongoing care

As well as involving senior nurses, the medical team and potentially anaesthetists in the care of the patient, it may be useful to refer the patient to the physiotherapy team for further support and appropriate interventions, such as deep breathing exercises (Cleave 2016).

Documentation

Documentation should state the oxygen saturation result and whether the patient was breathing room air or supplementary oxygen; the flow of oxygen and method of administration should also be noted (O'Driscoll et al. 2017). If the oxygen is given in an emergency situation without a prescription, then subsequent documentation must state the rationale for the administration (O'Driscoll et al. 2017).

Education of the patient and relevant others

One of the key focuses of education for patients with respiratory conditions concerns smoking cessation. Ascertaining whether the patient smokes (both regular and e-cigarettes), including how much and how often, and offering advice on how to stop, is an essential part of nursing health promotion. Discussions should focus on explaining the impact of smoking and how stopping may improve the patient's condition and prognosis; advice on how to stop should then be offered (Patel and Steinberg 2016).

Complications

It is recommended that to prevent any tissue damage, the pulse oximeter sensor is not taped in place (unless recommended by the manufacturer) and that the sensor should be re-sited routinely every 4 hours or more frequently if necessary, depending on the patient's condition and the manufacturer's recommendation. Assessment of tissue integrity before siting the probe is essential to avoid placement on existing damaged tissue (Adam et al. 2017).

Peak flow

Definition

Peak expiratory flow (PEF) is the highest flow achieved on forced expiration from a position of maximum lung inflation expressed in litres per minute (L/min) (Hill and Winter 2017). PEF is a simple test of lung function, commonly used to help detect and monitor moderate and severe respiratory disease. It is particularly useful in the diagnosis and monitoring of patients with asthma to assess the degree of airway obstruction, the severity of an asthma attack and response to treatment (Dakin et al. 2016, NICE 2017b).

Anatomy and physiology

In healthy individuals without any pathological conditions of the airways, factors that determine PEF include:

- the quality of the large airways
- the volume of the lungs (a function of thoracic dimensions and the individual's stature)
- the elastic properties of the lungs (the degree of stretch the lungs have been subjected to previously and the recoil ability of the lungs)

the power and co-ordination of the expiratory muscles, primarily the abdominal muscles (related to lung inflation and the speed with which maximum alveolar pressure is reached)

- the resistance of the instrument used to measure PEF (Cavill and Kerr 2016, Chapman et al. 2014).

Any condition that alters any of the above factors could affect PEF. However, a reduction in one of these factors may be compensated for by an increase in one of the others, meaning that PEF may not alter, resulting in staff potentially underestimating the severity of the patient's condition (Dakin et al. 2016, Hill and Winter 2017).

Related theory

PEF reflects a range of physiological characteristics of the lungs, airways and neuromusculature; the most common disorders that affect PEF are those that increase the resistance to air flow in the large conducting intrathoracic airways, such as asthma (NICE 2016e, West and Luks 2015). However, PEF may also be impaired by:

- disorders that limit chest movement
- respiratory musculoskeletal problems
- obstruction of the extrathoracic airways
- impairment of the nerves that supply the respiratory system (Dakin et al. 2016, Hill and Winter 2017).

PEF readings are subject to individual variation depending on the patient's age, sex, ethnic origin and stature (British Thoracic Society 2016). Therefore, the patient's results should be compared against normal reference values for people of the same age, sex and height (Figure 14.32) and, more importantly, against previous results for that individual (Dakin et al. 2016, NICE 2017b).

Measuring PEF is similar to measuring forced expired volume in 1 second (FEV_1) but the two are not interchangeable and each measure different aspects of lung function (Cavill and Kerr 2016). FEV_1 measures the volume of air exhaled during the first second of forced vital capacity (FVC), which occurs when an individual exhales forcefully to their maximum capacity following a deep inspiration (Marieb and Hoehn 2018). FEV_1 is usually 80% of FVC in healthy participants and is felt to be more sensitive than PEF in detecting mild airway obstruction as PEF is effort dependent and so can have a greater degree of intra-subject variability (Marieb and Hoehn 2018). However, FEV_1 and PEF can have similar predictive

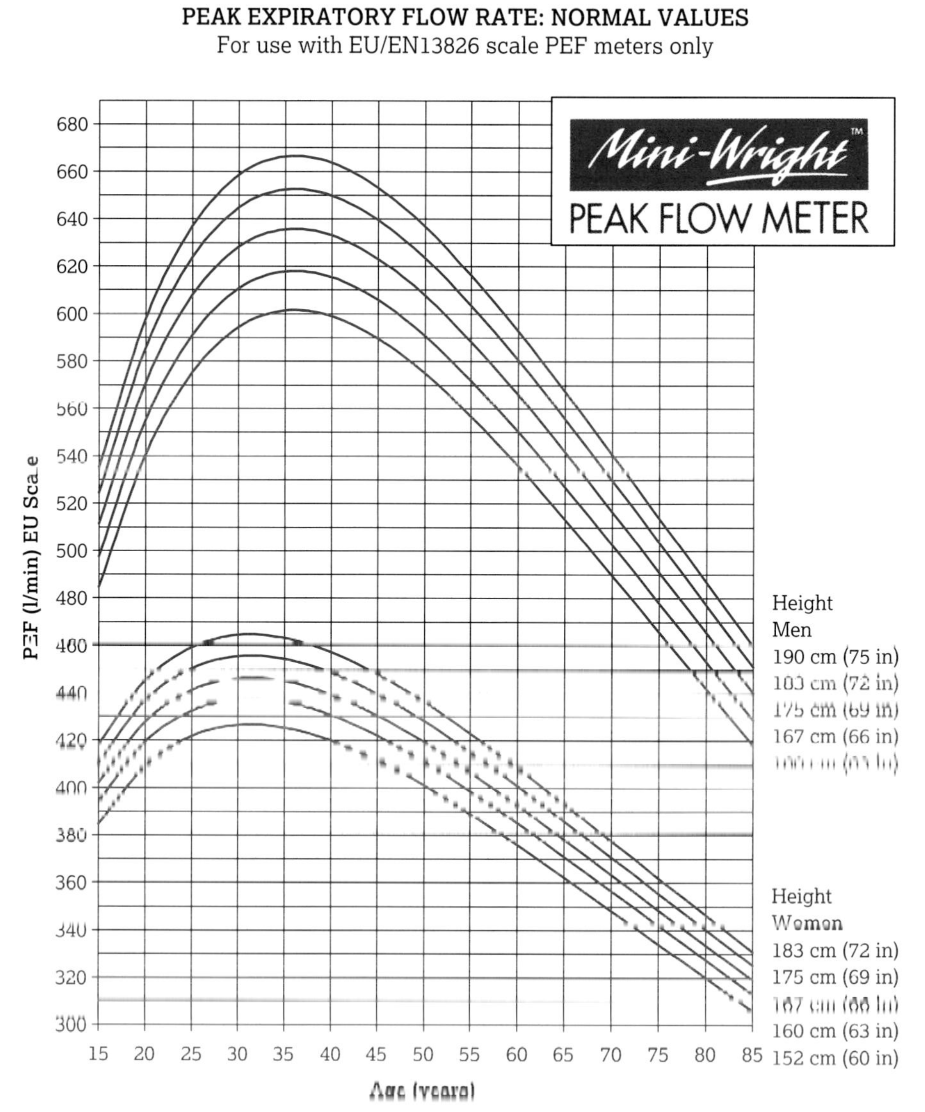

Figure 14.32 Normal peak expiratory flow rate measurements. *Source*: Reproduced with permission of Clement Clarke International, Ltd (www.peakflow.com).

ability in relation to mortality in patients with chronic obstructive pulmonary disease, although FEV_1 is considered to be a better predictor in patients with asthma (Chapman et al. 2014, NICE 2017b).

Evidence-based approaches

Rationale

PEF is a simple, objective procedure that can be used to measure the degree of air flow limitation. Although it may not give a full representation of lung function, it can monitor efficacy of treatment and progression of a condition (Cavill and Kerr 2016).

Indications

PEF can be used to:

- confirm a diagnosis of asthma
- determine the severity of an asthma exacerbation
- monitor the severity of the condition in patients with chronic severe asthma
- identify exacerbating factors
- monitor the progression of respiratory disease
- evaluate the effectiveness of treatment (Dakin et al. 2016, West and Luks 2015).

Contraindications

There are no absolute contraindications to PEF measurement, but PEF should be used and interpreted with caution in the following situations:

- patients who are acutely breathless, as the procedure requires physical effort
- patients with severe air flow obstruction, as included in the measurement may be air coming from the collapsing airway, which would yield an erroneously high result
- patients unable to take a full inspiration, for example if they have a persistent cough, as the results will be inaccurate
- where consecutive results could produce a reduction in scoring – the procedure itself may cause an exacerbation of the air flow limitation
- young children or anyone with learning difficulties may not understand or be able to comply with the procedure correctly (Cavill and Kerr 2016, Hill and Winter 2017).

Methods of measuring peak flow

Treatment is often based on PEF measurements and so it is vital that these are as accurate as possible (Wilkinson et al. 2017). Patients should be advised to perform PEF measurements in accordance with their monitoring regimen even if symptom free (NICE 2016e) as trends can be more important than isolated results (unless the isolated results reflect an exacerbation) (Dakin et al. 2016). Patients should repeat the procedure three times with the best result of the three being documented (Chapman et al. 2014). Unless the procedure induces an exacerbation, there should be consistency between the three results; if the top two results have a greater disparity than 40 L/min then, as long as the patient is not fatigued, a further two attempts can be made to reach a greater level of consistency (Cavill and Kerr 2016).

Timing of peak flow readings

While an isolated PEF measurement can indicate a restriction in air flow, in general sequential measurements are of more value, as they display trends, which are essential to understanding the severity and progression of the disease (Hill and Winter 2017). However, there may be significant diurnal variations, with higher values obtained in the evenings and the lowest measurements occurring during the night and first thing in the morning (Dakin et al. 2016). Therefore, it is recommended that measurements should be taken and documented on waking, in the afternoon and prior to going to bed (Frew et al. 2016). If it is suspected that the patient may have restricted air flow due to occupational causes, the patient should take measurements for a minimum of 2 weeks while at work and 2 weeks while not at work to enable a comparison (Frew et al. 2016).

Clinical governance

Competencies

All healthcare professionals who measure PEF must have received appropriate approved training and undertaken supervised practice, and this role should be undertaken in accordance with local hospital policy (Hill and Morgan 2016, Hill and Winter 2017).

Pre-procedural considerations

Equipment

The mini-Wright peak flow meter

Peak flow is measured by the patient exhaling as quickly and as forcefully as possible following maximal inspiration; the maximum expiratory flow is measured using a PEF meter and usually occurs early in expiration (West and Luks 2015). The mini-Wright peak flow meter, which is commonly used today, uses EU scales of measurement ranging from 60 L/min to 800 L/min, which are thought to increase the accuracy of the assessment (Hill and Winter 2017, West and Luks 2015).

Patients with their own meter should be encouraged to bring it with them to appointments (NICE 2016e). If a patient does not have their own meter then most hospitals and clinics have multiple patient-use PEF meters that are valved and have disposable single-use mouthpieces to prevent cross-infection (British Thoracic Society 2016). Most hand-held PEF meters do not need day-to-day calibration but all PEF meters should be replaced annually as with regular use the spring becomes slack and so the meter becomes inaccurate (NICE 2017b).

All PEF meters should be used and maintained in accordance with the manufacturer's instructions. In settings where meters are used between patients, a log should be kept of cleaning and disinfection procedures, and disposable one-way mouthpieces that prevent patients inhaling through the meter should be used (Hill and Winter 2017).

Spirometers

Spirometers can produce a reading for PEF alongside other lung function measurements such as FVC. However, to enable comparison with previous results, the patient should use the same equipment and technique each time (Dakin et al. 2016).

Assessment and recording tools

Recording peak flow measurements on individualized action plans or booklets gives patients a greater degree of control and awareness about when they need to access medical care; therefore, their use is strongly advocated (British Thoracic Society 2016).

Specific patient preparation

The procedure should be performed when the patient is at rest (unless otherwise specified) and may be performed with them sitting upright or standing as long as their neck is not flexed (NICE 2017b). To increase reliability and enable comparisons to be drawn, it is advisable that the patient uses the same posture each time (Hill and Winter 2017).

Education

The practitioner must ensure that the patient is fully informed about how to perform the procedure and performs it accurately, as even small alterations in technique may produce inaccurate results (Bickley 2016). If the patient has not performed the procedure previously then they will need a full explanation of what PEF is, what it measures, and how they should interpret and act on the results (Hill and Winter 2017). Patients should have the opportunity to have the procedure demonstrated to them and have their own practice attempts (Peate and Wild 2018).

Procedure guideline 14.5 Peak flow reading using a manual peak flow meter

Essential equipment

- Personal protective equipment
- Peak flow meter
- Disposable mouthpiece
- Peak flow chart and pen to document results

Action	Rationale
Pre-procedure	
1 Introduce yourself to the patient, explain and discuss the procedure with them, and gain their consent to proceed.	To ensure that the patient feels at ease, understands the procedure and gives their valid consent (NMC 2018, **C**).
2 Ask the patient what their best peak flow measurements have been and what their current peak flow readings are.	To enable a comparison to be drawn between their current and previous results (British Thoracic Society 2016, **C**).
3 Wash and dry hands or use alcohol-based handrub.	To minimize the risk of cross-infection (NHS England and NHSI 2019, **C**).
4 Assemble the equipment. Ask the patient to use their own meter if it is in good working order and less than 1 year old. If using a multiple-patient device, ensure that it is valved and has a disposable single-use mouthpiece.	Different equipment can have slight variations in results; therefore, using the same equipment will allow a reliable comparison (Dakin et al. 2016, **E**). However, regular use causes the spring to become slack and so the meter may become inaccurate if it older than 1 year (Hill and Winter 2017, **E**). To prevent cross-infection (NICE 2014, Weston 2013, **E**).
5 Ask the patient to adopt the position in which they normally undertake the procedure; this can be either standing or sitting. They should be advised not to flex their neck.	In order that their maximal lung volume can be reached and so that there is no positional obstruction that could affect the results, and to enable comparisons between results (Peate and Wild 2018, **E**).
6 Push the needle on the gauge down to zero.	To ensure the results are accurate (Hill and Winter 2017, **E**).
Procedure	
7 Ask the patient to hold the peak flow meter horizontally, ensuring their fingers do not impede the gauge.	So that the movement of the needle is not obstructed (Hill and Winter 2017, **E**).
8 Ask the patient to take a deep breath in through their mouth to full inspiration.	To ensure they achieve the greatest measurement (NICE 2016e, **E**).
9 Ask the patient to immediately place their lips tightly around the mouthpiece. The inspiration should be held for no longer than 2 seconds at total lung capacity.	To ensure a good seal around the mouthpiece and to prevent the patient's tongue and teeth from obstructing it (NICE 2017b, **E**). To ensure the full, total lung capacity is held. **E**
10 Ask the patient to blow out through the meter in a short, sharp 'huff' as forcefully as they can. See **Action figure 10**.	This can be very quick and need only take about 1 second, to enable accuracy of results (British Thoracic Society 2016, **E**).
11 Take a note of the reading and return the needle on the gauge to zero. Ask the patient to take a moment to rest and then repeat the procedure twice, noting the reading each time. Ideally there should be less than 20 L/min difference between the three readings. If there is more than 40 L/min difference, two additional blows can be performed. Document the highest of the three acceptable readings.	To ensure that the best possible result is achieved (Hill and Winter 2017, **E**).

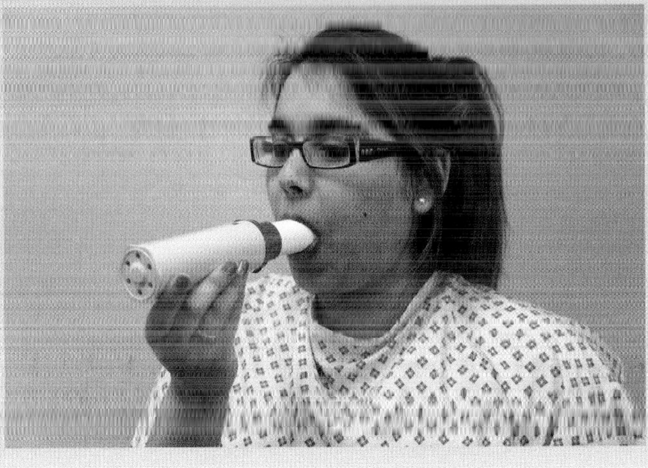

Action Figure 10 Manual peak flow meter technique.

Post-procedure	
12 Document the readings on the patient's record chart, comparing measured values against predicted values or patient trends. Report any abnormalities to medical or senior nursing staff.	Records must be kept of all assessments, treatment and care, and the outcomes of these (NMC 2018, **C**).
13 Dispose of the mouthpiece (unless using the patient's own) and clean the meter in line with local policies and the manufacturer's recommendation.	To prevent the risk of cross-infection (NICE 2014, Weston 2013, **E**).
14 Wash and dry hands and/or use an alcohol-based handrub.	To minimize the risk of cross-infection (NHS England and NHSI 2019, **C**).

Problem-solving table 14.5 Prevention and resolution (Procedure guideline 14.5)

Problem	Cause	Prevention	Action
Result is higher than expected	Needle was not being pushed back to zero prior to commencement Poor technique leading to 'explosive decompression' where there is sudden opening of the glottis, or release of the tongue occluding the mouthpiece; alternatively, the patient may be coughing or spitting into the mouthpiece (Dakin et al. 2016)	Allow practice runs prior to the procedure and ensure that the patient is educated on the correct technique.	Reset the needle back to zero. Educate the patient on the correct technique and, if they appear fatigued, allow them to rest prior to repeating the procedure.
Result is lower than expected	Failing to take a maximal inhalation Holding breath at maximal inhalation and delaying blowing into the meter Failure to make maximum effort Mouthpiece leaks due to blowing out cheeks, loose-fitting dentures or facial palsy (Hill and Winter 2017)	As above.	As above.

Post-procedural considerations

Immediate care

A reduction in peak flow may indicate a life-threatening situation and so should receive urgent medical attention (Wilkinson et al. 2017). For example, a PEF below 50% of the reference value indicates acute severe asthma and a PEF below 33% indicates acute life-threatening asthma (Dakin et al. 2016). The treatment provided will be aimed at increasing air flow and oxygenation (Frew et al. 2016). Oxygen therapy is usually given with the aim of keeping oxygen saturations at a target saturation range (Sprigings and Chambers 2017). In patients who are known, or suspected, to have hypercapnia, oxygen therapy should target saturations of 88–92% (see Chapter 12: Respiratory care, CPR and blood transfusion for methods of oxygen administration).

Patients will require arterial blood gas samples to be taken at the earliest opportunity to enable their condition to be more thoroughly assessed (Adam et al. 2017, O'Driscoll et al. 2017). Medication can be used to try to improve air flow and will usually include a combination of inhaled bronchodilators and steroids (British Thoracic Society 2016, NICE 2017b).

Ongoing care

It should be noted whether the patient has experienced or been in contact with any of the following prior to the exacerbation:

- cold air
- heightened levels of emotion
- exposure to allergens
- viral infection
- inhaled irritants such as pollution or dust
- medication or drugs, including anti-inflammatories and beta-adrenoreceptor blocking agents
- occupational sensitizers (Hill and Winter 2017, NICE 2017b).

The patient may require additional investigations, such as a chest X-ray and blood and sputum tests (Frew et al. 2016, West and Luks 2015).

Education of the patient and relevant others

Patient education is vital so that patients can manage their own condition (NICE 2017b). This will include information on exacerbating factors, smoking cessation and when to access medical help (NICE 2016e). Written personalized action plans used as part of self-management education have been shown to improve health outcomes for people with asthma, with particularly good evidence for those with moderate to severe disease; patients report improved outcomes such as self-efficacy, knowledge and confidence (British Thoracic Society 2016).

Temperature

Definition

Body temperature represents the balance between heat production (metabolism) and heat loss (Marieb and Hoehn 2018). If the rate of heat generated equates to the rate of heat lost, the core body temperature will be stable (Tortora and Derrickson 2017). All body tissues produce heat depending on how metabolically active they are (Marieb and Keller 2017). When the body is resting, most heat is generated by the heart, liver, brain and endocrine organs (Marieb and Hoehn 2018).

Anatomy and physiology

The core body temperature is set and closely regulated by the thermoregulatory centre of the hypothalamus in the brain. The normal range of 36.0–37.5°C is optimal for cell metabolic activity (Tortora and Derrickson 2017).

All tissues produce heat as a result of cell metabolism, and this is increased by exercise and activity (Marieb and Hoehn 2018). Humans have the ability through homeostasis to maintain a constant core temperature despite environmental changes (Tortora and Derrickson 2017). The body's core (arterial blood) generally has the highest temperature while the skin has the coolest (Marieb and Hoehn 2018, Marieb and Keller 2017).

The hypothalamus contains a group of neurones in the anterior and posterior portions, referred to as the 'preoptic area', that work as a thermostat (Figure 14.33) (Tortora and Derrickson 2017). The body requires stability of its temperature to produce an optimum environment for biochemical and enzymic reactions to maintain cellular function (Tortora and Derrickson 2017). Body temperature above or below the normal range affects total body function (Marieb and Hoehn 2018). A temperature above 41°C can cause convulsions and a temperature of 43°C renders life unsustainable (Wilkinson et al. 2017).

Heat is a by-product of the metabolic reactions of all cells in the body, especially those of the muscles and liver (Waugh and Grant 2018). Heat loss is achieved through the skin by the processes of radiation, convection, conduction and evaporation (Marieb and Hoehn 2018). Various factors cause fluctuations of temperature:

- The body's *circadian rhythms* cause daily fluctuations; however, body temperature is usually higher in the evening than in the morning (Marieb and Hoehn 2018). Differences can reach 1.5°C.
- *Ovulation* can elevate the body's temperature as it influences the basal metabolic rate (Tortora and Derrickson 2017).
- *Exercise and eating* cause elevations in temperature (Marieb and Hoehn 2018).
- *Age* affects a person's response to environmental change as the core temperature of healthy people over 65 years is lower than that of younger people, resulting in limitations to their tolerance of thermal extremes (Waugh and Grant 2018). This is due to the deterioration of thermoregulatory functions with advancing age (Blatteis 2012, Greaney et al. 2016). However, thermoregulation is also inadequate in newborns, and especially in low-birth-weight babies and those delivered by caesarean section (Vilinsky and Sheridan 2014).

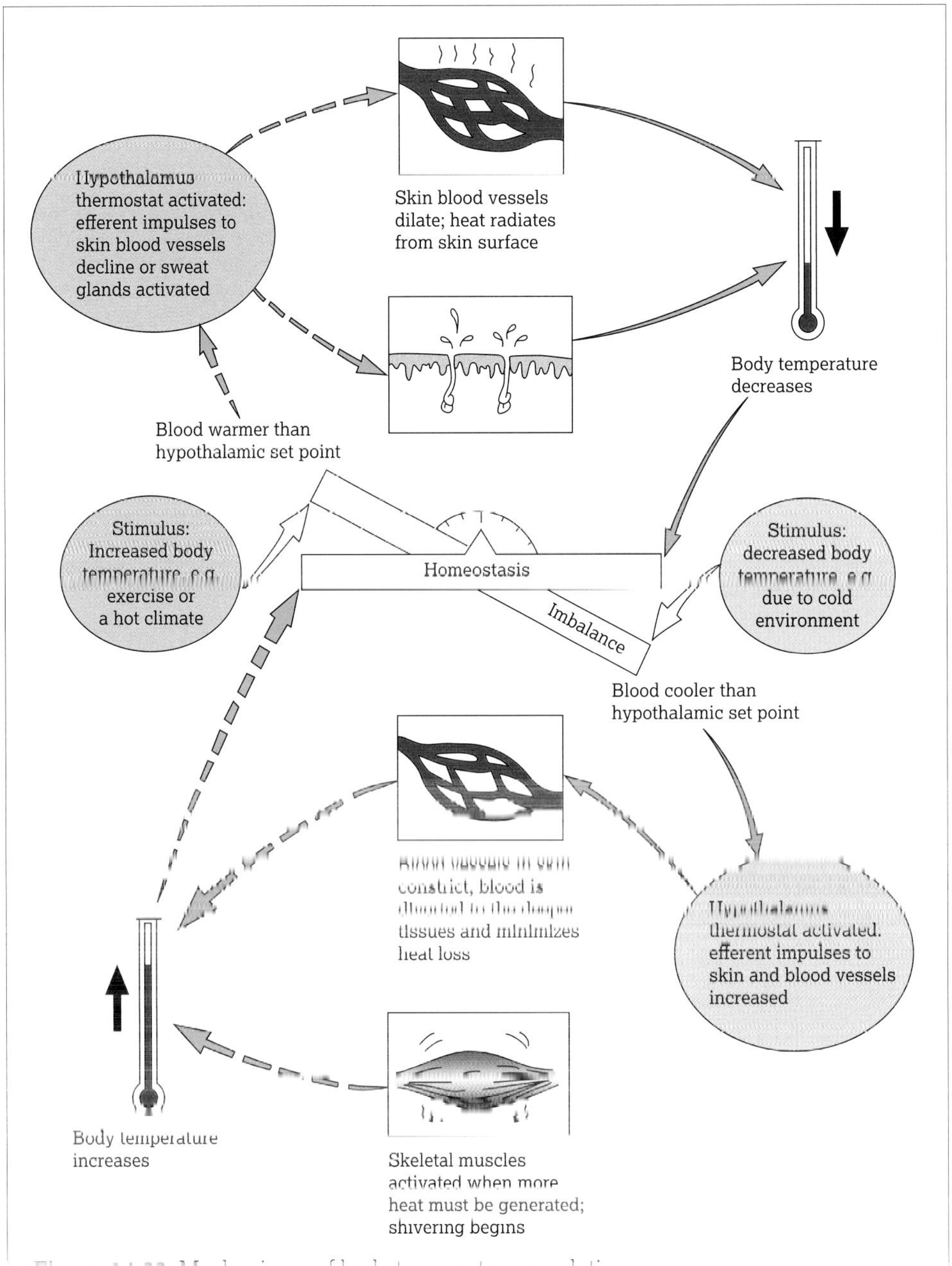

Figure 14.33 Mechanisms of body temperature regulation.

Related theory

Hypothermia

Hypothermia (low body temperature) is defined as a core temperature of 35°C or below (Sequeira et al. 2017), which causes the metabolic rate to decrease (Cobas and Vera-Arroyo 2017). Hypothermia may be classified as mild (32–35°C), moderate (30–32°C) and severe (below 30°C) (Malhotra et al. 2013). Hypothermia occurs when the body loses heat and is subsequently unable to maintain homeostasis (Grainger 2013, Marieb and Keller 2017). In contrast to a raised temperature, during hypothermia cellular metabolism slows, and the need for oxygen is reduced as more oxygen remains bound to haemoglobin, leading to a reduction in respiratory rate (Tortora and Derrickson 2017).

If a patient's temperature falls below 35°C, they can start to shiver severely (O'Donnell and Waskett 2016). However, hypothermia can cause non-specific symptoms, and ascertaining the exact temperature is challenging; for example, when using an oral thermometer, hypothermia frequently escapes detection (Bodkin et al. 2014, Marini and Dries 2016). It can occur in all ages, although the elderly are at particular risk, and it is often multifactorial in origin with other risk factors, including a low body mass index or an ambient temperature lower than 20°C (Breathett et al. 2016, Chambers and Burlingame 2016, Torossian et al. 2015).

Hypothermia can arise as a result of:

- environmental exposure
- medications and other substances that can alter the perception of cold, increase heat loss through vasodilation or inhibit heat generation, for example paracetamol or alcohol
- metabolic conditions, for example hypoglycaemia and adrenal insufficiency
- the exposure of the body and internal organs during surgery
- the use of drugs that dampen the vasoconstrictor response (Marini and Dries 2016).

Acute hypothermia occurs when the body is accidentally exposed to cold environmental temperatures, for example following cold water immersion or cold weather exposure, while chronic hypothermia can arise due to endogenous factors including ageing and diseases such as diabetes (Peiris et al. 2018). Induced hypothermia is based on the theorized protective effects on apoptosis and post-traumatic immune response (RCUK 2015). Therapeutic hypothermia was previously common practice following cardiac arrest (Cobas and Vera-Arroyo 2017). However, clinicians are now electing to use 36°C as the preferred target temperature following the recent large Target Temperature Management trial, which found no difference in mortality between target temperatures of 36°C and lower ones (Nielsen et al. 2013, RCUK 2015). The use of therapeutic hypothermia in traumatic brain injury also remains controversial (Andrews et al. 2015, Cobas and Vera-Arroyo 2017), mainly due to a lack of robust evidence (Carney et al. 2017, Cobas and Vera-Arroyo 2017); hence, it has not been incorporated into the Brain Trauma Foundation guidelines (Carney et al. 2017).

Endogenous hypothermia results from a metabolic dysfunction with decreased heat production (e.g. hypothyroidism, hypoglycaemia and hypoadrenalism) or disturbed thermoregulation (e.g. intracranial tumour or degenerative neurological disorders) (Marieb and Keller 2017). Finally, accidental hypothermia is characterized by an unintentional decrease of the core temperature due to exposure to a cold environment without a thermoregulative dysfunction (Waugh and Grant 2018).

Surgical patients having procedures longer than 1 hour have increased disruption to normal homeostatic mechanisms, and this results in a drop in temperature (Marini and Dries 2016). Complications can include cardiovascular ischaemia, delayed wound healing, increased risk of wound infections and increase in post-operative recovery time (Bashaw 2016). To prevent unplanned perioperative hypothermia, aggressive use of convective and conductive warming measures and an increased ambient temperature are recommended (Bashaw 2016), especially for the following patients:

- those undergoing major surgery
- those with compromised thermoregulatory systems (such as older adults)
- those with conditions that affect their general health, such as hypertension or diabetes
- those needing anaesthesia for longer than 2 hours or a combination of general and regional anaesthesia (Horn et al. 2017, NICE 2016c).

Hyperthermia

Sudden temperature elevations usually indicate inflammation or infection, making it prudent to perform a physical examination and, if indicated, obtain appropriate cultures and institute antibiotics. However, although infection is the most common explanation, several life-threatening, non-infectious causes of fever are frequently overlooked (Marini and Dries 2016) (Table 14.4).

Fever caused by pyrexia (elevated body temperature) is the result of the internal thermostat resetting to a higher level (Tait et al. 2015). This is the result of the action of pyrogens, which are chemical substances now known to be cytokines (Tortora and Derrickson 2017). Cytokines are chemical mediators that are involved in cellular immunity; they enhance the immune response by being released from white blood cells, injured tissues and macrophages (Marieb and Hoehn 2018). This causes the hypothalamus to release prostaglandins, which in turn reset the hypothalamic thermostat (Zampronio et al. 2015). The body then promotes heat-producing mechanisms such as vasoconstriction and, as a result, heat loss from the body surface declines, the skin cools and shivering begins to generate heat (Marieb and Keller 2017). These 'chills' are a sign that body temperature is rising and are often referred to as 'rigors' (Marieb and Hoehn 2018). A full list of the physiological changes that occur following a quick temperature rise is as follows:

- thermoreceptors in the skin are stimulated, resulting in vasoconstriction (this decreases heat loss through conduction and convection)
- sweat gland activity is reduced to minimize evaporation
- shivering occurs: muscles contract and relax out of sequence with each other, generating heat
- the body increases catecholamine and thyroxine levels, elevating the metabolic rate in an attempt to increase temperature (Grainger 2013, Marieb and Hoehn 2018, Waugh and Grant 2018).

All of these changes contribute to a rise in metabolism and a faster rate of diffusion, with increases in carbon dioxide excretion and the need for oxygen, leading to an increased respiratory rate (Tortora and Derrickson 2017). When the body temperature reaches its new 'set point', the patient no longer complains of feeling cold, shivering ceases and sweating commences (Marieb and Keller 2017).

There are several grades of pyrexia, and these are described in Table 14.5. However, the intensity of a pyrexia is not an indicator of the severity of infection (DeFronzo et al. 2015, NICE 2017e), as this varies from person to person (Wilkinson et al. 2017).

Table 14.4 Non-infectious causes of hyperthermia

Agonist drugs	Malignancy
Alcohol withdrawal	Malignant hyperthermia
Anticholinergic drugs	Neuroleptic malignant syndrome
Allergic drug or transfusion reaction	Phaeochromocytoma
	Salicylate intoxication
Autonomic insufficiency	Status epilepticus
Crystalline arthritis (gout)	Stroke or central nervous system damage
Drug allergy	
Heat stroke	Vasculitis hyperthyroidism

Table 14.5 Grades of pyrexia

Level of pyrexia	Temperature	Remarks
Low-grade pyrexia	37–38°C	Indicative of an inflammatory response due to a mild infection, allergy, disturbance of body tissue by trauma, surgery, malignancy or thrombosis
Moderate to high-grade pyrexia	38–40°C	May be caused by wound, respiratory or urinary tract infections
Hyperpyrexia	40°C and above	May arise because of bacteraemia, damage to the hypothalamus or high environmental temperatures

Evidence-based approaches

Rationale

Core body temperature measurements are taken to assess for deviation from the normal range. These may indicate disease, deterioration in condition, infection or reaction to treatment (Tait et al. 2015).

Body temperature measurement is part of routine observations in clinical practice and can influence important decisions regarding tests, diagnosis and treatment (Morrow-Barnes 2014). Temperature needs to be measured accurately and monitored effectively to enable changes to be detected quickly and any necessary interventions commenced (NICE 2017e). Temperature assessment accuracy depends on several factors, such as measurement technique, device type, body site and the healthcare professional's training (Sund-Levander and Grodzinsky 2013). Temperature recording is a core assessment (and reassessment) in nursing practice, but it may lead to mismanagement of the patient if not performed appropriately (El-Radhi 2013).

Indications

Circumstances in which a patient's temperature requires careful monitoring include the following:

- Conditions that affect basal metabolic rate, such as disorders of the thyroid gland, including hyperthyroidism or hypothyroidism (Wilkinson et al. 2017). Hypothyroidism is a condition where inadequate secretion of hormones from the thyroid gland results in slowing of physical and metabolic activity; thus, the individual has a decrease in body temperature (Obermeyer et al. 2017). Hyperthyroidism is a hypermetabolic condition that causes an increase in all metabolic processes as a result of excessive activity of the thyroid gland (Wilkinson et al. 2017). The individual complains of low heat tolerance, and, if thyrotoxic crisis develops (i.e. a sudden increase in thyroid hormones), hyperpyrexia occurs (Chiha et al. 2015).
- Post-operative and critically ill patients, as hyperthermia or hypothermia could indicate a reaction to surgical or medical treatments (NICE 2016c).
- Immunosuppression, conditions that cause a lower than normal white blood cell count (<1 10^9/L) and treatments (such as radiotherapy, chemotherapy or steroids) that make patients more susceptible to infections and less able to mount a normal response to infection (Annane 2018).
- Systemic or local infections, to assess development or improvement of the infection (Greaney et al. 2016, Rhodes et al. 2016).
- Blood transfusions: pyrexia can occur as a result of a severe transfusion reaction, usually within the first 15 minutes (Robinson et al. 2017).

Methods of recording temperature

All metabolizing body cells manufacture heat in varying amounts; therefore, temperature is not evenly distributed across the body (Marini and Dries 2016). True core temperature readings can only be measured by invasive means, such as placing a temperature probe into the oesophagus, pulmonary artery or urinary bladder (Sund-Levander and Grodzinsky 2013), and are therefore used most in the critical care setting (Tait et al. 2015). This must be undertaken by specialists or nurses who have received additional training that incorporates anatomical imaging technology (Marini and Dries 2016).

Traditionally, the mouth, axilla, rectum and external auditory canal have been the preferred sites for obtaining temperature readings, due to their accessibility (Bijur et al. 2016). More recently, infra-red thermometers have been developed to detect the temperature of the temporal lobe and these have been widely adopted in practice (Bijur et al. 2016). As the temperatures between these sites can vary, ideally the same site should be used continuously throughout patient assessment to allow for comparison, and the location of the site must be recorded on the observation chart (Grainger 2013). Unfortunately, an accurate, non-invasive method of measuring core temperature has yet to be established, and the current instruments produce wide variations in results (Bijur et al. 2016).

Oral

Oral temperature measurement continues to be used in practice as a quick and easy method of obtaining an estimate of the core body temperature (Bijur et al. 2016). When taking an oral temperature, the thermometer is placed in the posterior sublingual pocket of tissue at the base of the tongue (Sund-Levander and Grodzinsky 2013). The temperature difference between the anterior and posterior sublingual regions can be up to 1.6°C in febrile patients (Sund-Levander and Grodzinsky 2013). This area is in close proximity to the thermoreceptors, which respond rapidly to changes in the core temperature, hence changes in core temperature are reflected quickly here (Sund-Levander and Grodzinsky 2013). Oral temperatures are thought to be affected by ingested foods and fluids, smoking, the muscular activity of chewing, and rapid breathing (Sund-Levander and Grodzinsky 2013).

Rectal

Rectal temperatures have been demonstrated in clinical trials to be more accurate than oral or axillary; however, due to its invasive nature, assessing temperature via this route is not advocated, and aspects relating to privacy, dignity and patient choice need to be considered (Bijur et al. 2016, Hernandez and Upadhye 2016).

The rectal temperature is often higher than the peripheral one and offers greater precision in terms of obtaining the core temperature as it is more sheltered from the external environment (Sund-Levander and Grodzinsky 2013); however, false readings can occur in the presence of stool (Tait et al. 2015). In adults, the rectal thermometer should be inserted at least 4 cm into the rectum for an accurate reading (Adam et al. 2017). However, use of a rectal thermometer is contraindicated in immunosuppressed patients and in children under 5 years old as it carries a risk of rectal ulceration or perforation (NICE 2017c).

Axillary

The axilla is considered less desirable than the other sites because of the difficulty in achieving accurate and reliable readings (Asadian et al. 2016) as it is not close to major vessels, and skin surface temperatures vary more with changes in the temperature of the environment (Marui et al. 2017). However, axillary temperature measurement, using an electronic or chemical dot thermometer, is recommended in children aged 4 weeks to 5 years to detect fevers (NICE 2017c). In the clinical setting, it is mainly used in neonatal or paediatric units, where ambient temperatures are stable and patients are unsuitable for, or cannot tolerate, rectal thermometers (El-Radhi 2013, NICE 2017c).

To take an axillary temperature reading, the thermometer should be placed in the centre of the armpit, with the patient's arm firmly against the side of the chest (Barry et al. 2016). It is important that the same arm is used for each measurement, as there is often variation in temperature between left and right (Barry et al. 2016).

Tympanic

Measuring temperature using the tympanic membrane has become increasingly popular as it is less invasive than other methods, reduces the risk of cross-contamination and provides rapid results (<1 minute) (El-Radhi 2013). A tympanic thermometer uses infra-red light to detect thermal radiation; it is designed for intermittent use and provides a digital reading (Barry et al. 2016). It has been suggested by some that tympanic membrane thermometers give an accurate representation of actual body temperature (Kiekkas et al. 2016). This is because the tympanic membrane lies close to the temperature regulation centre in the hypothalamus, shares the same artery and is therefore considered to directly reflect core temperature in adults (Basak et al. 2013).

However, some limitations to this method of temperature measurement have been identified. In 2003, the Medicines and Healthcare products Regulatory Agency (MHRA) published a medical device alert following reports of tympanic thermometers providing low temperature readings, which were attributed to dirty probes and probe covers and user error (MHRA 2003). A soiled probe or probe cover would record a low temperature because the infra-red emissions from the tympanic membrane would be affected (Basak et al. 2013). In addition, this method is not suitable for patients who have undergone ear surgery or who use a hearing aid. Occlusion and otitis media resulting from ear wax can also lead to inaccurate values (Basak et al. 2013).

The accuracy of these devices is still subject to much debate within the literature. For example, their use is not yet recommended by the National Institute for Health and Care Excellence (NICE) for measuring temperature perioperatively as they do not provide a direct estimate of core body temperature (devices used in this setting should be accurate to within 0.5°C) (NICE 2016c). However, their use is recommended in children aged 4 weeks to 5 years when screening for fever (NICE 2017c).

Temporal artery

Temperature from the temporal region can be measured using an infra-red temporal artery thermometer (El-Radhi 2013). However, readings can be inaccurate due to the presence of perspiration, make-up and hair (Geijer et al. 2016). Thickness of tissue and bone, local blood flow, device placement and ambient temperature can also affect accuracy (Sund-Levander and Grodzinsky 2013). This is especially the case during rapid changes in body temperature, for example during episodes of pyrexia (Sund-Levander and Grodzinsky 2013).

Use of non-touch infra-red devices on the temporal artery site produces an indirect estimate of the true temperature using a correction factor to account for the difference in temperature between the outer surface of the head and the arterial blood flow (NICE 2016c). Temporal artery thermometers produce rapid readings and do not require any skin contact (Basak et al. 2013, Gasim et al. 2013), which reduces the risk of infection and discomfort. They are also cost-effective and easy to use (Basak et al. 2013). Measurements from this area are considered accurate because it shares the same blood flow as the hypothalamus, originating from the carotid artery, and is therefore considered to reflect the body's core temperature (Gasim et al. 2013). However, studies disagree on the precision and accuracy of this temperature measurement method: some say that the existing evidence does not support its use and that it cannot replace ordinary invasive and non-invasive methods in adult patients (Geijer et al. 2016, Kiekkas et al. 2016), while others support the use of these devices as an alternative to invasive temperature measurement (Barry et al. 2016, Reynolds 2014, Smith et al. 2018) but on paediatric patients only (Morgensen et al. 2018).

Anticipated patient outcomes

The patient's temperature will be determined on admission as a baseline for comparison with future measurements and to monitor fluctuations in temperature.

Pre-procedural considerations

Temperature can be measured at a number of different sites, using different tools for measurement (see above). However, whichever route is used for temperature measurement, it is important that this is then used consistently, as switching between sites can produce a record that is misleading or difficult to interpret (El-Radhi 2013).

It is also vital to control any factors that could affect the precision of the device used, in order to ensure accuracy. Such factors should be addressed when educating staff on the use of different temperature measurement methods. Therapeutic decisions should not be made on the basis of a single vital sign (Grainger 2013).

It should also be considered that the average person experiences circadian rhythms that result in fluctuations in body temperature. Body temperature is generally highest in the late afternoon (around 5pm) and falls to its lowest point in the early hours of the morning (around 4am) (Bracci et al. 2016, Taylor et al. 2014).

Equipment

There are a number of devices on the market, including electronic contact thermometers, chemical thermometers and infra-red-sensing thermometers, each of which obtains temperature in a different time frame and in a different way. If a device can be used on multiple sites, its programming will need to be altered to reflect the chosen site per the manufacturer's guidelines. Clinical thermometry is governed by International Standard BS EN ISO 80601-2-56:2017 (British Standards Institution 2017), which stipulates the need for regular calibration and maintenance.

In the UK, it is no longer advised that mercury thermometers are used in healthcare practice due to the high risk of toxicity to humans (Environment Agency 2015, Marini and Dries 2016). Devices currently available for recording body temperature are:

- single-use plastic-coated strips with heat-sensitive recorders (dots) that change colour to indicate the temperature (record from 35.5°C to 40.4°C)
- digital analogue probe thermometers with plastic disposable sheets (record from 32°C to 42°C)
- invasive thermometers attached to a pulmonary artery catheter (record from 0°C to 50°C)
- tympanic probe thermometers with disposable covers
- temporal infra-red non-contact devices (Launey et al. 2016).

Tympanic membrane thermometer

Measuring tympanic temperature (see Procedure guideline 14.6: Tympanic temperature measurement) requires a tympanic membrane thermometer. This is a small hand-held device that has a disposable probe cover that is inserted into the patient's ear canal. The sensor at the end of the probe records the infra-red radiation that is emitted by the tympanic membrane, as a result of its warmth, and converts this into a temperature reading presented on a digital screen (El-Radhi 2013). The probe is protected by a disposable cover, which is changed between patients to prevent cross-infection (Grainger 2013). Advantages of tympanic membrane thermometry are speed (temperature reading available within seconds), safety and ease of use (Gasim et al. 2013).

A common problem with using tympanic thermometers is poor technique leading to inaccurate temperature measurements (Bijur et al. 2016, Jevon and Ewens 2012). The placement of the probe to fit snugly within the ear canal (Figure 14.34) is crucial

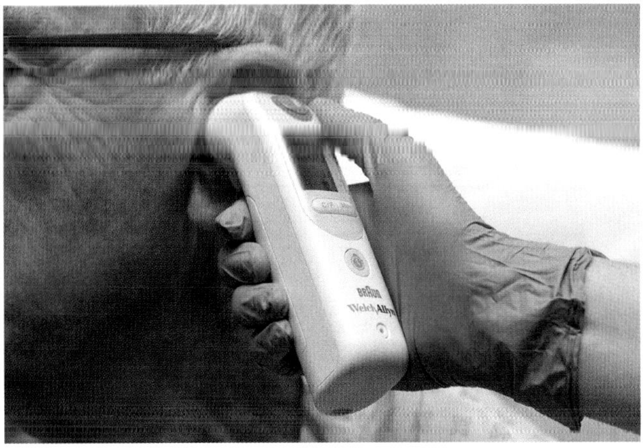

Figure 14.34 Tympanic membrane thermometer.

as the difference in temperature between the opening of the ear canal and the tympanic membrane can be as high as 2°C (Lewis 2013). Other causes of false readings include a dirty or cracked probe lens and incorrect installation of the probe cover (WelchAllyn 2015). Ear infections and wax are reported to influence the true temperature of the tympanum (Basak et al. 2013); therefore, the ear should be inspected prior to obtaining a reading, and, if wax or evidence of an infection is present, an alternative route for obtaining the temperature should be sought (Grainger 2013). For infection prevention and control purposes, the appropriate disposable probe cover should be used and the healthcare professional should inspect the cover to ensure that it has been fitted correctly and that there are no wrinkles over the tip end. This will ensure an accurate reading is achieved (Grainger 2013).

Specific patient preparation

Ask the patient when they last ate, smoked or had anything to drink as these activities may influence their temperature.

Procedure guideline 14.6 Tympanic temperature measurement

Essential equipment

- Personal protective equipment
- Tympanic membrane thermometer
- Disposable probe covers
- Lint-free swab

Action	Rationale
Pre-procedure	
1 Introduce yourself to the patient, explain and discuss the procedure with them, and gain their consent to proceed.	To ensure that the patient feels at ease, understands the procedure and gives their valid consent (NMC 2018, **C**).
2 If the patient is wearing a hearing aid, ask the patient to remove the device from the ear (or remove it for them if appropriate) and wait 10 minutes before taking a reading.	To allow the temperature within the ear canal to normalize. **E**
3 Wash and dry hands and/or use an alcohol-based handrub.	To minimize the risk of cross-infection and contamination (NHS England and NHSI 2019, **C**).
Procedure	
4 Inspect the ear canal for the presence of ear drainage, blood, cerebrospinal fluid, vernix, cerumen (compacted ear wax) or foreign bodies.	The presence of these substances can affect the accuracy of the reading (Basak et al. 2013, **C**). Ear wax does not affect accuracy but cerumen plugs and impactions containing debris can lower the temperature measurement by several tenths of a degree (Basak et al. 2013, **C**).
5 Remove the thermometer from the base unit and ensure the lens is clean and not cracked, and that the probe lens is free of smudges and debris. Use a dry lint-free swab to wipe it clean if required and calibrate it according to the manufacturer's guidelines.	Alcohol-based wipes should not be used as this can lead to a false low temperature measurement (WelchAllyn 2015, **E**).
6 Verify the mode setting on the display to show the route (ear) by which the temperature is due to be measured.	To ensure accuracy when interpreting the result (Grainger 2013, **C**).
7 Place a disposable probe cover on the probe tip, ensuring the manufacturer's instructions are followed, e.g. ensuring the cover is flush with the thermometer end and not touching the plastic film on the distal tip of the probe cover.	The probe cover protects the tip of the probe and is necessary for the functioning of the instrument (WelchAllyn 2015, **E**)
8 Ensure the patient has not been lying on either ear in the 20-minute interval immediately preceding temperature measurement. If the patient is lying on their side, always take the temperature in the exposed ear.	Lying on an ear causes significant changes in tympanic temperature (Arslan et al. 2011, **C**).
9 Align the probe tip with the ear canal and gently advance it into the ear canal until the probe lightly seals the opening, ensuring a snug fit (see Figure 14.34).	To prevent air at the opening of the ear from entering it, causing a false low temperature measurement (Covidien 2011, **C**; Jevon and Ewens 2013, **E**).
10 Press and release the 'scan' button (the name of the button may vary between models).	To commence the scanning (Covidien 2011, **C**).

11	Remove the probe tip from the ear as soon as the thermometer display reads 'done' (or equivalent) or displays the temperature reading, usually indicated by beeps. Read the temperature display and document in the patient's records (along with the ear used).	To ensure the procedure is carried out for the necessary amount of time. Measurement is usually complete within seconds (Gasim et al. 2013, **E**). Any interruption in the process may result in the measurement being incorrectly remembered (Fuller et al. 2018, **E**).
12	Obtain a reading from both ears and take the greater of the readings. A new probe cover must be used for each reading to ensure the highest degree of accuracy and to prevent cross-contamination between the ears.	Recent evidence suggests that any anatomical differences between the two ears are irrelevant with the newest generation of infra-red tympanic thermometers (Haugan et al. 2013, **E**; Salota et al. 2016, **E**).
13	Compare the result with previous results. Take action as appropriate.	Deviations from normal temperature ranges may require urgent medical/clinical attention (NMC 2018, **C**).
Post-procedure		
14	Press the 'release' or 'eject' button (or equivalent) to discard the probe cover into a waste bin per local infection control guidelines.	Probe covers are for single use only (Grainger 2013, **E**).
15	Wipe the thermometer clean as per the manufacturer's guidelines and return it to the base unit for storage.	To reduce the risk of cross-infection (NICE 2014, **E**).

Problem-solving table 14.6 Prevention and resolution (Procedure guideline 14.6)

Problem	Cause	Prevention	Action
Thermometer is not working properly, for example 'error' is showing	Battery is low (note that in most devices, the low battery indicator appears when around 100 more temperatures can be taken) Device is dirty	Clean thermometer device, including probe, after each use.	Replace the battery. Clean the thermometer as per the manufacturer's guidelines.
The 'wait' indicator is on	'Wait' indicator appears when the practitioner attempts to take successive temperatures in too short a period of time	Pause briefly between taking temperatures until the 'wait' indicator disappears.	Retry; if still instructed to 'wait', send for repair.
'Use new cover' showing even though probe cover has been installed	Probe cover replaced too quickly	Ensure that the probe cover has been fitted correctly.	Press the 'release' or 'eject' button (or equivalent) and reinstall the probe cover.

Post-procedural considerations

Immediate care

Hyperthermia

A rise in temperature can be regarded as a normal response, in that it is part of the autonomic response to create an environment inhospitable for bacteria and organisms, and it is also a favourable environment for antibiotics (Fletcher et al. 2017). A postoperative fever is often a normal inflammatory response to surgery; however, it can also be a manifestation of a serious underlying infectious or non-infectious aetiology (Annane 2018). If a temperature rises above 40°C (hyperthermia), it is dangerous and may indicate that the patient's regulatory systems have failed (Kiekkas et al. 2013).

It is common practice to try to reduce fever with medications (such as antipyretics) and physical cooling methods (O'Donnell and Waskett 2016). Antipyretics, including paracetamol and ibuprofen, can mask the function of the hypothalamus by reducing temperature while hiding the underlying signs of disease (Chiumello et al. 2017). It is thought that these drugs inhibit the inflammatory action of prostaglandins, affecting the hypothalamus by temporarily resetting the thermostat to a normal level (Marieb and Keller 2017). Currently the evidence on how to reduce fever in practice is weak and does not support the routine administration of antipyretic therapies (Drewry et al. 2017). Therefore, nurses should assess patients individually, using antipyretic therapies selectively and with caution (Tait et al. 2015).

It is recommended by many studies that antipyretic treatment should begin with drug administration and proceed with external cooling, but the adverse effects of both methods should be considered (Kiekkas et al. 2013). A large multi-centre trial looking at the effects of external cooling alone in septic patients did, however, find that this method was beneficial and safe (Schortgen et al. 2012). Various surface and endovascular automatic cooling devices allowing tight temperature control are available, such as air and water circulating blankets (Doyle and Schortgen 2016). There is little evidence to support fanning for temperature control, and this is usually only considered for patient comfort. Fanning can actually increase body temperature as it can stimulate a compensatory response by the hypothalamus, initiating heat-gaining activities such as shivering and peripheral vasoconstriction, which could compromise unstable patients by depleting their metabolic reserve (Gardner 2012, Young et al. 2018). Shivering not only impedes thermal control but also increases oxygen consumption (Doyle and Schortgen 2016).

Healthcare professionals should be aware of the side-effects associated with cooling techniques, such as:

- arrhythmias and bradycardia
- coagulation pathway impairment
- electrolyte disorders from intracellular shifts and renal excretion (calcium, magnesium, phosphate and potassium levels can be affected)

- insulin resistance with hyperglycaemia
- patient discomfort from shivering and skin breakdown (Knowlton 2013).

Comfort measures, in addition to reassurance, may include:

- providing dry clothing and bed linen
- offering oral hygiene to keep the mouth moist
- limiting patient exertion to minimize heat production
- offering sufficient nutrition and fluids (2.5–3 L daily) to meet the patient's higher metabolic demands and to avoid dehydration
- providing extra blankets when the patient feels cold, but removing surplus blankets when the patient complains of too much warmth (Knowlton 2013, Kozier et al. 2008).

Hypothermia

A low temperature can lead to complications such as cardiac arrhythmias and hypotension, as well as fluid and electrolyte shifts (Wilkinson et al. 2017). Therefore, immediate management should address these aspects and focus on preventing further heat loss and rewarming the body in order to increase core temperature. There is an increased risk of mortality and morbidity with a body temperature below 32°C (Perlman et al. 2016).

There are three basic types of hypothermia treatment: passive external rewarming, active external rewarming and active internal rewarming (Perlman et al. 2016). Passive external rewarming involves removing wet clothing and providing more insulation for patients with mild hypothermia (32–35°C), who are neither neurologically nor cardiovascularly compromised and are still able to generate heat (Sequeira et al. 2017). Active external methods are advised for moderate (28–32°C) accidental hypothermia and patients with no cardiac co-morbidities; they include forced-air blankets, warm blankets and heating pads (Perlman et al. 2016). Active internal methods are reserved for patients who have severe hypothermia (<28°C) and are haemodynamically unstable (Sequeira et al. 2017). Internal rewarming restores temperature to normal levels at a faster rate than surface methods and is associated with rapid normalization of cardiac output (Perlman et al. 2016). Active internal methods include the use of warmed intravenous fluids, such as saline or blood. The fluids must be warmed because a 2 L crystalloid bag administered at the usual temperature of 18°C will decrease a patient's core temperature by about 0.6°C (Zaman et al. 2016). Other active internal techniques include warmed oxygen administration and bladder, peritoneal or thoracic lavage (Perlman et al. 2016).

During any rewarming process, attention must be paid to speediness, as rewarming can cause vasodilation and the patient's metabolic rate can change rapidly (RCUK 2015). Rebound hyperthermia is associated with increased mortality and neurological morbidity (Winters et al. 2013). The optimal rate is unknown but 0.25–0.5°C per hour is recommended (RCUK 2015). For both active external and internal treatment types, specific training and knowledge of the associated devices and products are necessary (Perlman et al. 2016).

Documentation

Recordings of body temperature are an index of biological function and a valuable indicator of a patient's health.

Urinalysis

Definition

Urinalysis is the analysis of the volume and the physical, chemical and microscopic properties of urine (Tortora and Derrickson 2017). It can provide valuable information about a patient's condition, allowing detection of systemic disease and infection (Wilkinson et al. 2017).

Anatomy and physiology

The kidneys process approximately 180 L of blood-derived fluid a day (Tortora and Derrickson 2017); approximately 1% of this total leaves the body as urine, whereas the rest returns to the circulation (Marieb and Hoehn 2018). Urine formation and the simultaneous adjustment of blood composition occur within the kidneys and involve three processes (Figure 14.35):

- glomerular filtration
- tubular reabsorption
- tubular secretion (Marieb and Hoehn 2018).

Glomerular filtration

Glomerular filtration occurs in the glomeruli of the kidney, which act as non-selective filters. Filtration occurs as a result of glomerular blood pressure, which is determined by the difference in diameter between afferent and efferent arterioles (Tortora and Derrickson 2017). The effect is a simple mechanical filter that permits substances smaller than plasma proteins to pass from the glomeruli to the glomerular capsule (Marieb and Hoehn 2018).

Tubular reabsorption

Tubular reabsorption then occurs, where substances such as sodium ions and water are reabsorbed, primarily in the proximal convoluted tubules but also in the distal tubules and collecting ducts (Marieb and Hoehn 2018). Necessary substances are removed from the filtrate and returned to the peritubular capillaries, where they go back into the circulation (Waugh and Grant 2018). Others, such as creatinine and drug metabolites, are not reabsorbed because of their size, insolubility or a lack of carriers (Marieb and Keller 2017).

Tubular reabsorption is hormonally controlled as aldosterone increases the reabsorption of sodium, and antidiuretic hormone (ADH) enhances water reabsorption by the collecting ducts (Marieb and Hoehn 2018).

Tubular secretion

Tubular secretion is an active process that is important in eliminating drugs, certain wastes and excess ions and in maintaining the acid/base balance of blood (Marieb and Hoehn 2018).

Regulation of urine concentration and volume occurs in the loop of Henle, where the osmolarity (concentration) of the filtrate is controlled (Tortora and Derrickson 2017). As the filtrate flows through the tubules, the permeability of the walls controls how diluted or concentrated the resulting urine will be (Waugh and Grant 2018). In the absence of ADH, diluted urine is formed because the filtrate is not reabsorbed as it passes through the kidneys (Marieb and Keller 2017). As levels of ADH increase, the collecting ducts become more permeable to water, and water moves out of the filtrate back into the blood; consequently, more concentrated urine is produced, and in smaller amounts, as a response to the physiological need for increased intravascular volume and/or maintaining electrolyte balance (Marieb and Hoehn 2018).

The composition, smell and colour of urine can change dramatically as a result of disease processes (Eyer et al. 2016). An unusual colour, such as pink or brown, may result from eating certain foods (beetroot or rhubarb), it or may be due to the presence of bile products or blood (Marieb and Hoehn 2018). A turbid (cloudy) colour can mean an infection of the urinary tract, which is one of the most common sites of bacterial infection (Wilkinson et al. 2017). Risk factors for urinary tract infections (UTIs) include the presence of a urinary catheter, female sex, diabetes and advanced age (Sheerin 2015). See Figure 14.36 for other predisposing factors. A fruity smell, instead of the natural slightly aromatic smell, can indicate the presence of ketones, a result of disease processes such as diabetes mellitus (Marieb and Hoehn 2018).

Urinalysis allows the assessment of the composition of urine, giving an indication of renal function and the effectiveness of the mechanisms described above.

RENAL CORPUSCLE

Glomerular filtration rate: 105–125 mL/min of fluid that is isotonic to blood

Filtered substances: water and all solutes present in blood (except proteins) including ions, glucose, amino acids, creatinine, uric acid

PROXIMAL CONVOLUTED TUBULE

Reabsorption (into blood) of filtered:

Water	65% (osmosis)
Na^+	65% (sodium–potassium pumps, symporters, antiporters)
K^+	65% (diffusion)
Glucose	100% (symporters and facilitated diffusion)
Amino acids	100% (symporters and facilitated diffusion)
Cl^-	50% (diffusion)
HCO_3^-	80–90% (facilitated diffusion)
Urea	50% (diffusion)
Ca^{2+}, Mg^{2+}	variable (diffusion)

Secretion (into urine) of:

H^+	variable (antiporters)
NH^{4+}	variable, increases in acidosis (antiporters)
Urea	variable (diffusion)
Creatinine	small amount

At end of PCT, tubular fluid is still isotonic to blood (300 mOsm/liter).

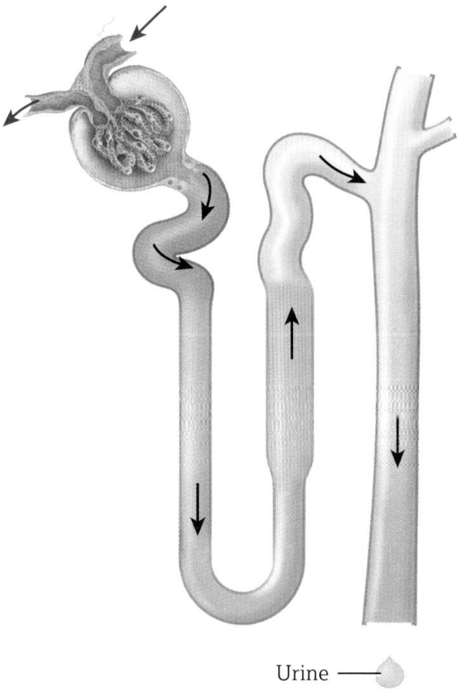

EARLY DISTAL CONVOLUTED TUBULE

Reabsorption (into blood) of:

Water	10–15% (osmosis)
Na^+	5% (symporters)
Cl^-	5% (symporters)
Ca^{2+}	variable (stimulated by parathyroid hormone)

LATE DISTAL CONVOLUTED TUBULE AND COLLECTING DUCT

Reabsorption (into blood) of:

Water	5–9% (insertion of water channels stimulated by ADH)
Na^+	1–4% (sodium–potassium pumps and sodium channels stimulated by aldosterone)
HCO_3^-	variable amount, depends on H^+ secretion (antiporters)
Urea	variable (recycling to nephron loop)

Secretion (into urine) of:

K^+	variable amount to adjust for dietary intake (leakage channels)
H^+	variable amounts to maintain acid–base homeostasis (H^+ pumps)

Tubular fluid leaving the collecting duct is dilute when ADH level is low and concentrated when ADH level is high.

NEPHRON LOOP

Reabsorption (into blood) of:

Water	15% (osmosis in descending limb)
Na^+	20–30% (symporters in ascending limb)
K^+	20–30% (symporters in ascending limb)
Cl^-	35% (symporters in ascending limb)
HCO_3^-	10–20% (facilitated diffusion)
Ca^{2+}, Mg^{2+}	variable (diffusion)

Secretion (into urine) of:

Urea	variable (recycling from collecting duct)

At end of nephron loop, tubular fluid is hypotonic (100–150 mOsm/liter).

Figure 14.35 Summary of filtration, reabsorption and secretion in the nephron and collecting duct. *Source*: Reproduced from Tortora and Derrickson (2011) with permission of John Wiley & Sons.

Evidence-based approaches

Rationale

Urinalysis (urine testing) is commonly undertaken in clinical practice as a non-invasive means of:

- measuring response to certain treatments
- assessing particular symptoms
- assisting in the diagnosis of medical conditions
- undertaking routine health assessments (Marini and Dries 2016).

Interpretation of urinalysis is generally based on reviewing all of the test's components and correlating them with the results of a physical examination and the patient's clinical signs and symptoms (Bickley 2016).

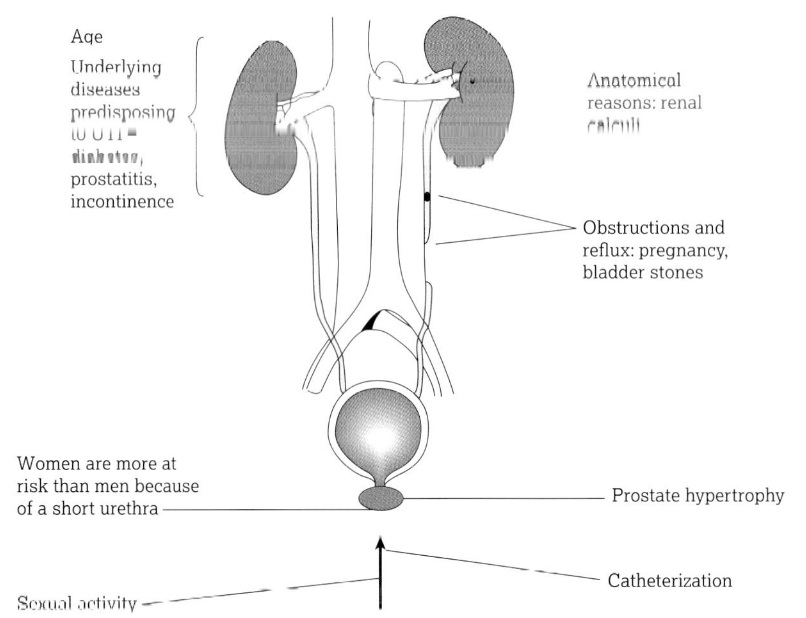

Figure 14.36 Reasons for predisposition to urinary tract infections (UTIs).

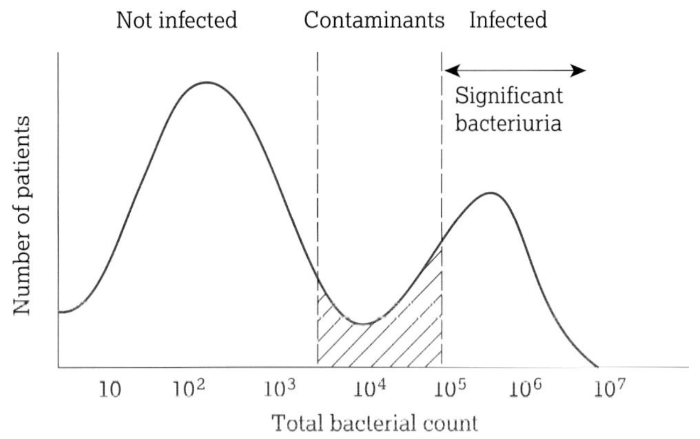

Figure 14.37 Significant bacteriuria. Specimens of urine are rarely sterile. A cut-off point is identified to distinguish true infection (significant bacteriuria) from the effects of contamination from surrounding tissues.

Carrying out a urinalysis can identify the level of ketones (and many other substances, such as proteins) in the urine; it can also identify bacteriuria (the presence of bacteria in the urine) (D[illegible] 2015). However, urine specimens are rarely sterile, as a result of contamination with periurethral flora during collection (Weston 2013). Therefore, significant bacteriuria is defined as the presence of more than 10^5 organisms per millilitre of urine and the presence of clinical symptoms (Sheerin 2015). See Figure 14.37 for an illustration of significant bacteriuria.

A clean-catch urine sample should ideally be obtained to try to avoid contamination; however, if this is not practical, for example in infants, other methods should be used (NICE 2017f). These include use of a pad, a catheter specimen of urine or a suprapubic aspirate collected via the rubber specimen side port (Herreros et al. 2018, NICE 2017f). An initial urine investigation with a dipstick, from a fresh spontaneous urine sample, is sufficient in most clinical situations; however, in other circumstances, a clean-catch midstream urinalysis (MSU) will be required due to the risk of contamination in 'spontaneous' urine collected without any special hygiene precautions (Dolan and Cornish 2013). This is especially the case in women, where urine contains leucocytes in the presence of vaginal discharge and erythrocytes in the presence of the products of menstruation (Provan 2018). In addition, dipstick testing is not effective in catheterized patients as the presence of a catheter causes elevated pyuria without the presence of infection (NICE 2015c).

When collecting an MSU, it is necessary to clean the genitals to ensure the culture specimen is processed with as little contamination as possible and to minimize the presence of contaminating elements, such as bacteria, analytes and formed particles (Adam et al. 2017, Weston 2013).

Consideration must be given to whether a urine sample should be obtained randomly (at any time) or at the first void. This will be guided by referring to local guidelines and liaising with the requesting party. Random voids have been proven worthwhile for most test purposes (Delanghe and Speeckaert 2016). However, there are some clinical circumstances where using the first morning void may be essential, including testing for microalbuminuria and spot urine testing to evaluate daily salt intake. This is because the urine has been in the bladder for a reasonably long period, so its composition is independent of daily variations in food and fluid intake and physical activity (Delanghe and Speeckaert 2016).

Indications

Urinalysis is performed for several reasons:

- for screening, prevention and diagnosis of systemic diseases, for example diabetes mellitus, haemolytic disorders, or renal and liver diseases
- for diagnosis of suspected conditions, such as UTIs
- for management and planning, with the aim of ascertaining a baseline and then monitoring the progress of an existing condition and treatment efficacy
- to assess for pregnancy
- to detect the presence of drug metabolites or alcohol
- to assess hydration status (Bickley 2016, Provan 2018, Wilkinson et al. 2017).

Midstream urine specimens are indicated in adults and children who are continent and can empty their bladder on request (Holm and Aabenhus 2016).

Methods of urinalysis

There are three main methods by which urinalysis is performed:

- urine reagent test strips (dipstick)
- light microscopy
- timed collection (Provan 2018).

Reagent test strips

Before using a reagent strip to analyse a sample of urine, the following observations should be made to support the overall assessment:

- colour
- clarity/debris
- odour (Provan 2018).

See Table 14.6 for further information on visual observations of urine.

The main advantages of using a urine dipstick are that it is convenient, quick and non-invasive, with results usually determined in a few minutes (Provan 2018). The main disadvantages are in terms of accuracy, which can be affected by the following factors:

- Bilirubin and urobilinogen are relatively unstable when subjected to light and at room temperature, so it is important to use fresh urine to obtain the most accurate result (Provan 2018).
- Exposure of unpreserved urine at room temperature for a considerable period of time (>4 hours) may result in an increase in micro-organisms in the urine and a change in pH (Shapiro and Yaney 2015).
- Bacterial growth of contaminated organisms in urine may produce a positive blood reaction (Delanghe and Speeckaert 2016).
- Urine that is highly alkaline may show false-positive results for the presence of protein (Delanghe and Speeckaert 2016).
- The presence of glucose in urine may reduce its pH as a result of the metabolism of glucose by organisms present in the urine (Delanghe and Speeckaert 2016).
- The presence of urea-splitting organisms, which convert urea to ammonia, may cause urine to become more alkaline (Trimarchi et al. 2015).
- Certain drugs and chemicals (e.g. meropenem, imipenem, clavulanic acid and nitrofurantoin) can cause false positives due to their influence on the leucocyte reading (Delanghe and Speeckaert 2016). See Table 14.7.

Table 14.6 Visual observations of urine and possible indications

Observation	Possible indications
Colour	
Green	*Pseudomonas* infection, presence of bilirubin Excretion of cytotoxic agents (e.g. mitomycin) or substances (e.g. methylene blue)
Pink/red	Blood
	Excretion of cytotoxic agents (e.g. doxorubicin)
Orange	Excess urobiliogen or rifampicin
Yellow	Presence of bilirubin
Brown	Presence of bilirubin
Odour	
Fishy	Infection
Sweet-smelling	Ketones
Debris	
Cloudy	Infection, stale urine
Sediment	Infection, contamination

Source: Reproduced from Rigby and Gray (2005) with permission of EMAP Publishing, Ltd.

Light microscopy

[illegible] necessary under laboratory conditions. This may include culture and sensitivity testing to identify organisms responsible for infection and to determine the most effective treatment (Provan 2018).

Optical or light microscopy involves passing visible light transmitted through or reflected from the sample through single or multiple lenses to allow for a magnified view of the sample (Provan 2018). The image generated can then be read and interpreted by the eye, imaged on a photographic plate or captured digitally (Provan 2018). Light microscopy examines the number and types of cells and/or material in the urine and can yield a great deal of information and suggest a more specific diagnosis (Provan 2018). For light microscopy, an MSU should be used as opposed to a fresh spontaneous sample so that any contaminating bacteria in the urethra are flushed out first and thus the sample represents the bladder's contents (Weston 2013). This reduces the chance of contamination of the specimen with epithelial cells, especially vaginal flora (Provan 2018).

In the microbiology laboratory, urine samples constitute a large proportion of the total workload and most of these samples show no infection (Paattiniemi et al. 2017). Therefore, it is vital to only send samples where a urine dipstick has indicated cause for concern (Lelli et al. 2018).

Timed urinalysis

Timed urine collection is typically undertaken over an 8-, 12- or 24-hour period. It simply requires a person to collect their urine in a special container over the set period (Provan 2018). This test typically focuses on renal creatinine clearance, sodium and protein (Provan 2018). Renal clearance refers to the volume of plasma that is cleared of a particular substance in a given time, usually 1 minute, and is tested to determine the glomerular filtration rate, which allows detection of glomerular damage and the examination

Table 14.7 How drugs may influence the results of reagent stick testing

Drug	Reagent test	Effect on the results
Ascorbic acid	Glucose, blood, nitrite	High concentrations may diminish colour
L-dopa	Glucose	High concentrations may give a false-negative reaction
	Ketones	Atypical colour
Nalidixic acid	Urobilinogen	Atypical colour
Phenazopyridine	Protein	May give atypical colour
	Ketones	Coloured metabolites may mask a small reaction
	Urobilinogen, bilirubin	May mimic a positive reaction
	Nitrite	May cause a false-positive result
Rifampicin	Bilirubin	Coloured metabolites may mask a small reaction
Salicylates (aspirin)	Glucose	High doses may give a false-negative reaction

of the progress of renal disease (Mareb and Hoehn 2018). Timed urinalysis may also examine hormone levels and measure substances such as steroids, white cells and electrolytes; it can also determine urine osmolarity, which makes it a vital test in illnesses such as hyponatraemia and diabetes ([illegible]).

Pre-procedural considerations

Equipment

Dipstick (reagent) tests

Dipstick reagents are primarily used as screening tools for components in the urine such as protein, blood, bilirubin, glucose, ketones, nitrites and leucocyte esterase, which can be indicators of bacterial infection; it is also used to check the urine's pH (Provan 2018).

A urine dipstick is usually a narrow plastic strip that has several different coloured squares on it, each representing the components described above, impregnated with chemicals (Provan 2018). When dipped in urine, the chemicals react with abnormal substances and change colour (Marini and Dries 2016). Once the strip has been quickly dipped into the urine sample and the necessary time has lapsed for the colour changes to take place, the strip is compared to a standardized colour chart that displays results in terms of parameters (Tait et al. 2015). It is essential to use the strips according to the manufacturer's instructions and be aware of factors that may affect their results, including specific drugs (see Table 14.7), the quality of the urine specimen itself and the possibility of false negative results (Marini and Dries 2016).

Specific patient preparation

Education

Most patients need advice on hygiene and technique before collecting a urine sample to prevent contamination from hands or the genital area and to ensure that the midstream sample is collected correctly (Holm and Aabenhus 2016).

Post-procedural considerations

Documentation

When sending a urine specimen to the laboratory, check that the laboratory form has been completed and that all relevant

Procedure guideline 14.7 Urinalysis: reagent strip

Essential equipment

- Personal protective equipment
- Urine dipsticks that are in date and have been stored according to the manufacturer's recommendations
- Appropriate urine specimen pot

Action	Rationale
Pre-procedure	
1 Introduce yourself to the patient, explain and discuss the procedure with them, and gain their consent to proceed.	To ensure that the patient feels at ease, understands the procedure and gives their valid consent (NMC 2018, **C**).
2 Wash and dry hands and/or use an alcohol-based handrub and put on gloves and apron.	To maintain infection control and prevent cross-infection (NHS England and NHSI 2019, **C**).
Procedure	
3 Check the reagent sticks have been stored in accordance with the manufacturer's instructions. This is usually a dark, dry place in an airtight container.	To ensure reliable results. Tests may depend on enzymic reaction, so expired, contaminated or improperly stored strips can give false-positive results (e.g. in leucocyte and blood readings) (Delanghe and Speeckaert 2016, **C**).
4 Prepare the sample area. • If taking the specimen from a urinary catheter, it should be collected using an aseptic technique via the catheter side port. • For women, the labia should be separated with cotton wool or a sponge moistened with water, and the vulva should be wiped from the front to the back, although disinfectant must never be used. • Men should clean the glans penis with soap and water.	To reduce sample contamination (Adam et al. 2017, **C**).
5 Instruct the patient that, to obtain a clean, midstream specimen of fresh urine, they should allow a few millilitres of urine to pass into the toilet (not collected), then introduce a container or sterile receptacle into the urine stream. Once a sufficient sample has been collected, the remaining urine can pass into the toilet.	To ensure that any contaminating bacteria in the urethra are flushed out first and the sample represents the bladder contents (Adam et al. 2017, **C**).
6 Dip the reagent strip into the urine. The time that the dipstick remains in the urine should be governed by the manufacturer's recommendations. The strip should be completely immersed in the urine and then removed. Run the edge of the strip along the container to remove excess urine.	To ensure accuracy and to remove any excess urine, preventing mixing of chemicals from adjacent reagent areas (Provan 2018, **C**).
7 Hold the stick sideways in a horizontal position.	Urine reagent strips should not be held upright when reading them because urine may run from square to square, mixing the different reagents (Provan 2018, **C**).
8 Wait the required time, as per the manufacturer's instructions, before reading each test on the strip against the colour chart.	The strips must be read at exactly the time interval specified or the reagents will not have had time to react or may display an inaccurate result (Provan 2018, **C**).

Post-procedure	
9 If an abnormality is found (Table 14.8), the urine sample should be sent to the laboratory for a more detailed analysis; otherwise, dispose of the sample appropriately in either the sluice or a toilet. Dispose of the urinalysis stick and gloves in the correct wastage bin. Ensure the cap on the package of urine reagent strips is replaced immediately and closed tightly.	To prevent misdiagnosis and to ensure strips are stored in an airtight container according to storage guidelines (Bardsley 2015, **C**).
10 Wash and dry hands and/or use an alcohol-based handrub.	To maintain infection control and prevent cross-infection (NHS England and NHSI 2019, **C**).
11 Document urinalysis readings and inform medical staff of any abnormal readings.	To allow prompt action if a change of treatment plan is required (NMC 2018, **C**).

Table 14.8 Interpretation of the results (interpretation should always be made with consideration of the whole clinical picture)

Parameter	Interpretation
Specific gravity (relative density)	Usual range: 1.001–1.035; this is a measure of the concentration of the urine and indicates hydration status
pH	Usual range: 6.4–6.8 Urine is usually slightly acidic, but elevated acidity may suggest kidney stones whereas an alkaline result may suggest an infection Many other factors, such as diet, can also affect pH
Leucocytes (white blood cells)	Usually absent and therefore negative Present in infection or inflammation of the urinary tract
Nitrates	Usually absent and therefore negative Present in a bacterial infective process (as produced by bacteria)
Protein	Usually present in small amounts If the reading is '+++' or more and there is associated haematuria, may indicate infection or damage to renal glomerulus Proteinuria in the absence of haematuria may indicate high serum albumin levels or tubular damage
Glucose	Usually absent in normal urine and therefore negative Present in hyperglycaemia (if serum glucose >10–11 mmol/L) If present without high serum glucose, may indicate renal tubular dysfunction
Ketones	Usually absent and therefore negative Present in 'starvation' states (where the body breaks down fat rather than using glucose for energy) Ketoacidosis (diabetic/alcoholic) Poor carbohydrate intake
Urobilinogen	Usually present in urine; however, excessive amounts may indicate liver disease
Bilirubin	Usually absent and therefore negative Positive result may indicate liver disease or an obstructive liver process
Blood	Usually absent or present in very small amounts Significant presence indicates damage or disease in the urinary tract

Source: Adapted from Yates (2016).

information is included, taking care not to contaminate the outside of the container or the request forms (Bardsley 2015).

Education of the patient and relevant others

Patients should be made aware that further tests and investigations may be required following the urine dipstick test (Bardsley 2015).

Blood glucose

Definition

Blood glucose is the amount of glucose in the blood (Whitmore 2012). Table 14.9 outlines the normal target ranges, which are expressed as millimoles per litre (mmol/L). Normally, blood glucose levels stay within narrow limits (4–8 mmol/L) throughout the day. However, some fluctuations can occur throughout the day: readings are usually slightly higher after meals and lowest in the morning (Whitmore 2012).

Anatomy and physiology

Blood glucose is regulated by insulin and glucagon. Insulin is synthesized and secreted from the beta cells within the islets of Langerhans, which are found in the pancreas (Marieb and Hoehn 2018). It is produced in response to high blood glucose levels, usually after food is consumed, and promotes the uptake and storage of sugar by fat and muscle tissue as glycogen (Wallymahmed 2013). Glucagon is secreted by the alpha cells in response to low blood glucose levels and results in the release of stored sugar back into the blood (Marieb and Hoehn 2018), allowing blood sugar levels to rise (glycogenolysis). Both processes are controlled by a negative feedback system; this is shown in Figure 14.38. In health,

Table 14.9 Normal target blood glucose ranges

Target levels by type	Upon waking (mmol/L)	Before meals (pre-prandial) (mmol/L)	At least 90 minutes after meals (post-prandial) (mmol/L)
[illegible]	4.0–5.9	4.0–5.9	under 7.8
Type 2 diabetes	5.0–7.0	4.0–7.0	under 8.5
Type 1 diabetes	5.0–7.0	4.0–7.0	5.0–9.0
Children with type 1 diabetes	4.0–7.0	4.0–7.0	5.0–9.0

Source: Adapted from Diabetes.co.uk.

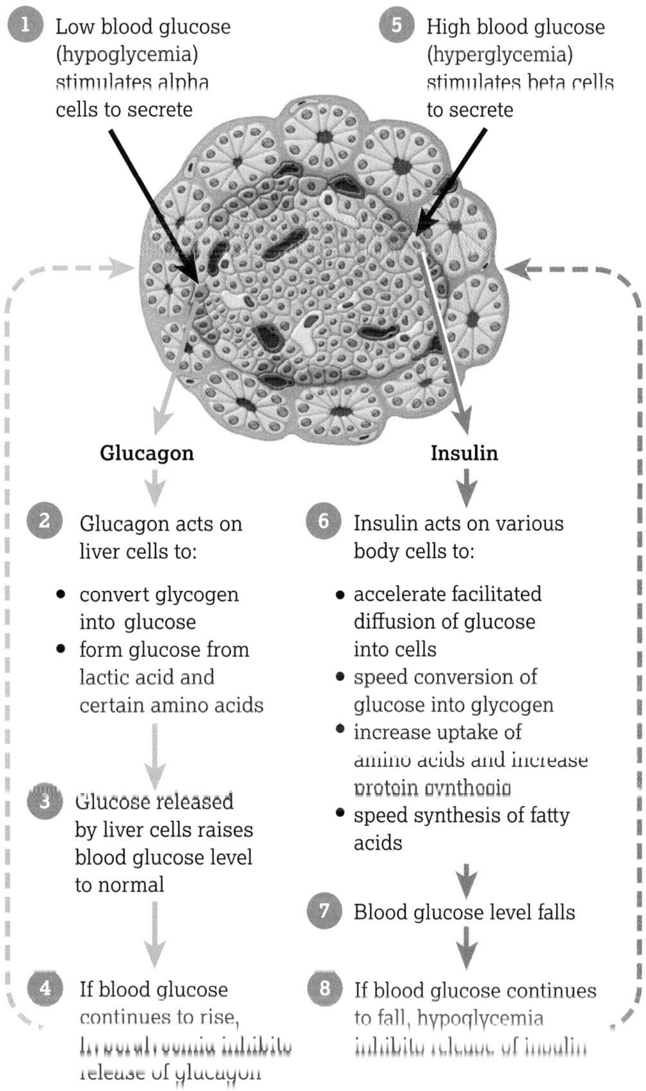
1 Low blood glucose (hypoglycemia) stimulates alpha cells to secrete
5 High blood glucose (hyperglycemia) stimulates beta cells to secrete
Glucagon
Insulin
2 Glucagon acts on liver cells to:
• convert glycogen into glucose
• form glucose from lactic acid and certain amino acids
3 Glucose released by liver cells raises blood glucose level to normal
4 If blood glucose continues to rise, hyperglycemia inhibits release of glucagon
6 Insulin acts on various body cells to:
• accelerate facilitated diffusion of glucose into cells
• speed conversion of glucose into glycogen
• increase uptake of amino acids and increase protein synthesis
• speed synthesis of fatty acids
7 Blood glucose level falls
8 If blood glucose continues to fall, hypoglycemia inhibits release of insulin

Figure 14.38 Negative feedback regulation of the secretion of glucagon and insulin *Source*: Reproduced from Tortora and Derrickson (2017) with permission of John Wiley & Sons.

these processes maintain blood glucose's stability within the body (homeostasis) (DeFronzo et al. 2015).

Diabetes mellitus

Diabetes mellitus (DM) is a heterogeneous disorder characterized by chronic hyperglycaemia due to complete insulin deficiency, increased insulin resistance or production of insulin that is inadequate to meet the individual's need (ADA 2019). It is estimated that in 2015, 3.8 million deaths were directly caused worldwide by diabetes and higher-than-optimal blood glucose (WHO 2016). This rate is thought to be related to the global increase in the prevalence of people living with diabetes, currently estimated at 422 million and expected to increase to around 629 million by 2045 (WHO 2016).

There are two main types of DM: type 1 and type 2. Type 1 is an autoimmune condition that causes destruction of the beta cells in the pancreas, leading to a complete loss of insulin production (ADA 2019) with known genetic, epidemiological and environmental factors (Phillips 2016a). Age was previously believed to be a factor but this is now known not to be the case (NICE 2016d). Type 2 is a multifactorial disease characterized by a resistance to insulin that is frequently triggered by poor diet, lifestyle and obesity; however, genetic predisposition has been recognized as a key factor in its development (Phillips 2016b). Insulin resistance commences prior to the development of type 2 diabetes (Casey 2018), with the hypersecretion of insulin occurring concurrently (Phillips 2016b). This contributes to beta cell exhaustion and lack of insulin production (Casey 2018), which leads to hyperglycaemia (high blood glucose) (Phillips 2016b). As the process is frequently much slower than seen in type 1 diabetes, the period of sustained low-level hyperglycaemia is longer, in some cases years, which allows long-term complications to occur, such as cardiovascular disease and degenerative changes affecting the kidneys, nerves (neuropathy) and eyes (blindness) (Patel et al. 2016, Wilkinson et al. 2017). Further complications of uncontrolled blood glucose include coronary artery and peripheral vascular disease, stroke, and central and peripheral nerve damage, possibly resulting in the need for amputations (NICE 2016a).

A diagnosis of diabetes can primarily be based on a fasting blood glucose level of more than or equal to 7 mmol/L or a random plasma glucose of more than or equal to 11.1 mmol/L accompanied by symptoms associated with diabetes such as polydipsia, polyuria and weight loss (NICE 2017a). These features of diabetes do not appear until 80% of beta cells are lost; therefore, with increasing insulin resistance being a major driver of type 2 diabetes, changes to lifestyle, diet and exercise have the potential to reverse its development if it is picked up early enough (Van Ommen et al. 2018). However, it must be acknowledged that sustained lifestyle changes require multifactorial components including diet, physical activity, stress management, self-empowerment and active participation by the individual supported by an appropriate healthcare professional (Van Ommen et al. 2018).

Furthermore, during infection, major surgery or critical illness (such as sepsis, pancreatitis or respiratory distress), counter-regulatory or stress hormones (adrenaline, noradrenaline, cortisol, growth hormone and glucagon) are released, causing significant metabolic alterations (Rau et al. 2017). These hormones increase insulin resistance, which decreases peripheral uptake of glucose and also promotes glycogenolysis by stimulating glycogen and fat breakdown, causing further hyperglycaemia, also known as stress hyperglycaemia (Palermo et al. 2016). For this reason, patients with diabetes may need additional treatment with insulin or anti-diabetic medication during acute illness, in order to replicate this homeostasis or improve the body's ability to produce or use insulin (Kotagal et al. 2015).

Hyperglycaemia

Hyperglycaemia can lead to poor clinical outcomes, increased mortality and extended hospital length of stay (Mabrey and Setji 2015). It is defined as random blood glucose of more than

11.1 mmol/L; however, in the absence of symptoms, diagnosis should be established using plasma blood levels and not a random glucose test (NICE 2017a). When insulin is deficient or absent, as in type 1 or 2 diabetes, blood glucose levels will remain high after a meal and be raised in times of illness or stress because glucose is unable to enter most cells (Rau et al. 2017). In this way, cells are starved of glucose and the body reacts inappropriately by producing stress hormones that cause glycogenolysis (the breakdown of glycogen to release glucose), lipolysis (the breakdown of stored fat into glycerol and fatty acids) and gluconeogenesis (the conversion of glycerol and amino acids into glucose) (Marieb and Keller 2017).

This causes blood glucose to increase further, which results in a number of signs and symptoms (Kotagal et al. 2015). Water reabsorption in the kidneys becomes inhibited, resulting in frequent, large volumes of urine (polyuria) (Wilkinson et al. 2017). This will cause the person to feel excessive thirst (polydipsia) and may also result in extreme hunger (polyphagia) (NICE 2016d). Polyuria and polydipsia will cause dehydration, a fall in blood pressure and electrolyte imbalance (Marieb and Keller 2017, Marini and Dries 2016). Moreover, the subsequent loss of sodium (hyponatraemia) and potassium (hypokalaemia) leads to muscle cramps, nausea, vomiting and diarrhoea, confusion, blurred vision, lethargy, cardiac events, coma and eventually death (Wilkinson et al. 2017).

Despite the excessive level of glucose in the body, due to the lack of insulin, the body cannot utilize it effectively, so the body starts to break down its fat and protein stores for energy, which leads to high levels of fatty acids in the blood (lipidaemia) (Marieb and Keller 2017). This can also cause sudden and dramatic weight loss (Tortora and Derrickson 2017). These fatty acids are converted to ketones, which accumulate in the blood more quickly than they can be excreted or used and so cause the blood's pH to fall, resulting in ketoacidosis (Marieb and Keller 2017). Ketones will also be present in the urine. If ketoacidosis is allowed to continue, it can become life threatening, disrupting all physiological processes, including oxygen transportation and heart activity, and causes depression of the nervous system, leading to coma and death (Marieb and Keller 2017). Potential reasons for hyperglycaemia are described in Table 14.10.

It has been found that enteral and parenteral feeding contribute to hyperglycaemia both in patients with a diagnosis of diabetes and in those without (Gosmanov and Umpierrez 2013). This is particularly true of patients receiving parenteral nutrition, as it bypasses the gut and therefore the incretin hormones, which help to maintain glucose homeostasis (Gosmanov and Umpierrez 2013). Hyperglycaemia in response to steroids, for example dexamethasone, is another consideration and some researchers believe that steroids' hypermetabolic action decreases glucose uptake, increases hepatic glucose production and may directly inhibit insulin release (Marieb and Keller 2017). For this reason, these patients will need blood glucose monitoring and may require changes to their insulin treatment or temporary insulin (Wilkinson et al. 2017).

Hypoglycaemia

Hypoglycaemia is a blood glucose level that is unable to meet the metabolic needs of the body (Marini and Dries 2016), normally lower than 4 mmol/L (Adam et al. 2017). It is an acute complication of diabetes that increases morbidity, mortality and the economic cost of diabetes (Kreider et al. 2017).

In healthy individuals, the glucoregulatory system rapidly reduces insulin production and mobilizes energy reserves from the fat and liver to counter hypoglycaemia (Tortora and Derrickson 2017). However, when it does not act promptly, the increasing levels of insulin in the blood cause an abrupt drop of glucose levels (Wilkinson et al. 2017). Often young, healthy individuals can be asymptomatic during episodes of hypoglycaemia, but early symptoms can include sweating, tremor, weakness, nervousness, tachycardia and hypertension (Wilkinson et al. 2017), although these depend not only on the absolute blood glucose but also on its rate of decline (Tortora and Derrickson 2017). Severe hypoglycaemia can lead to mental disorientation, convulsions, unconsciousness and death (Marini and Dries 2016). In addition, research is now suggesting that frequency and severity of hypoglycaemia episodes can cause an increase in diabetic individuals developing dementia in later life (Rhee 2017). Potential reasons for hypoglycaemia are described in Table 14.10.

Table 14.10 Possible causes of hyperglycaemia and hypoglycaemia

Hyperglycaemia	Inadequate doses of insulin Stress Infection/sepsis Surgery Medications (e.g. steroids) Variability in oral or nutritional intake Nutritional support, for example parenteral nutrition or enteral nutrition Critical illness
Hypoglycaemia	Missed or delayed meals Not eating enough Exercise without carbohydrate compensation Too much glucose-lowering medication (e.g. insulin) Excessive alcohol intake Infection Muscle and fat depletion (e.g. anorexia) Diarrhoea and vomiting Hepatic failure due to tumour or cirrhosis Adrenal insufficiency Salicylate poisoning Insulin-secreting tumours Congestive heart failure Cerebral vascular accident Concurrent medications (beta blockers, adrenaline) Surgery

Source: Adapted from Marieb and Keller (2017), Marini and Dries (2016), Wilkinson et al. (2017).

There are several ways to reduce the risk of hypoglycaemia, including frequent monitoring of blood sugars with home blood glucose tests and occasionally continuous glucose monitoring (Adam et al. 2017). Treatment should ideally consist of the administration of glucose, and the route of administration will depend on the consciousness level of the patient, their treatment and their ability to take oral substances (Marini and Dries 2016). If they can tolerate oral or enteral intake, they should be given a fast-acting carbohydrate such as 4–5 glucose tablets, 60 mL of glucose juice, 150–200 mL of pure fruit juice or 3–4 teaspoons of sugar dissolved in water (Walden et al. 2018). Drinks such as Lucozade or Ribena are no longer recommended following the 'sugar tax' implementation in 2016. Alternatively, give two tubes of 40% glucose gel (e.g. Glucogel) squeezed into the mouth between the teeth and gums (Walden et al. 2018). If the patient is unconscious or the enteral route is inappropriate, give 1 mg of glucagon intramuscularly and repeat capillary blood glucose levels after 10–15 minutes. If the level of blood glucose remains below 4 mmol/L, 10% glucose intravenous administration should be considered, or treatment should be provided as per local policies (Walden et al. 2018). Once blood glucose is above 4 mmol/L and the patient is alert and able to swallow, a long-acting carbohydrate food should be offered to the patient, such as biscuits, bread or milk (Walden et al. 2018).

Management of type 1 diabetes usually involves administration of multiple doses of insulin through subcutaneous injections. A single episode of hypoglycaemia does not always necessitate omitting insulin; however, if it remains a consistent problem, the treatment should be reviewed and tailored to the patient's current needs (Walden et al. 2018). For optimal control, patients should have access to continuous subcutaneous insulin infusion (CSII) pump therapy (NICE 2015a, Phillips 2016a).

Evidence-based approaches

Rationale

Blood glucose monitoring provides an accurate indication of how the body is controlling glucose metabolism. It enables clinicians and patients to adjust their treatment accordingly to achieve optimal glucose control (Kreider et al. 2017). In the short term it can prevent hypoglycaemia and hyperglycaemia, and in the long term it can significantly reduce the risk of prolonged, life-threatening vascular complications (NICE 2016d, Walden et al. 2018).

Capillary blood glucose monitoring provides immediate results and shows whether blood sugar is high or low, whereas urine testing indicates instances of high blood sugar and the presence of ketones (Adam et al. 2017, Marini and Dries 2016).

Indications

Conditions in which blood glucose monitoring will need to take place include the following:

- to make a diagnosis of diabetes
- to monitor and manage the day-to-day treatment of known type 1 and type 2 diabetes (NICE 2016a)
- in acute management of unstable diabetes – that is, where there is evidence of hyperglycaemia, hypoglycaemia, diabetic ketoacidosis or hyperosmolar non-ketotic coma (once severe dehydration has been corrected) (Walden et al. 2018)
- in hospitalized patients with diabetes, who may require sliding-scale treatments and/or nutritional support (Walden et al. 2018)
- for initial parenteral and enteral nutritional support of all patients (Gosmanov and Umpierrez 2013)
- in patients taking steroids and other drugs that cause raised blood glucose (Wilkinson et al. 2017).

Contraindications

The following conditions can affect the accuracy of capillary blood glucose monitoring, meaning that it may be necessary to obtain a blood plasma sample for more reliable results, especially where treatment (e.g. insulin) is due to be initiated on the basis of the acquired result:

- peripheral circulatory failure and severe dehydration, for example diabetic ketoacidosis, peripheral vascular disease, shock, hypotension, vomiting or diarrhoea, and the use of diuretics (these conditions cause peripheral shutdown, which can cause artificially low capillary readings)
- extreme values of haematocrit, which may lead to inaccurate levels, such as in the case of neonatal blood samples or in pregnancy
- intravenous infusion of ascorbic acid, which can lead to false increases in glucose levels
- some dialysis treatments, as the fluids used may contain maltose, which can interfere with some blood glucose tests
- hyperlipidaemia and/or parenteral and enteral nutrition, which may lead to artificially raised capillary blood glucose readings (MHRA 2013a).

Principles of care

Although capillary blood glucose monitoring is an essential part of diabetic management, it can have severe consequences if not done correctly; therefore, it is imperative that on initial diagnosis the individual is shown the correct basic technique (NICE 2016d). In addition, appropriate healthcare staff should undergo formal training and any equipment used should be subjected to strict quality control (MHRA 2013a).

Blood glucose monitoring needs to be performed regularly enough for patterns to be established on which treatment changes (e.g. to insulin regimes) can be based (Phillips 2016a). What constitutes 'regularly' will vary in different circumstances; for example, illness, change of daily routine and hospitalization may affect diabetes control and therefore require more frequent testing (Walden et al. 2018). Generally, people with type 1 diabetes will need to test their blood glucose several times a day or more depending on their treatment regime, while those with type 2 diabetes will require less testing due to the lower risk of large fluctuations in blood glucose levels (Meetoo et al. 2018). There is variation in the literature surrounding the frequency of blood glucose monitoring for type 2 diabetes, however, for patients with type 1 diabetes it is suggested that monitoring four or more times daily is a minimal requirement, with measurement being imperative on waking and prior to going to bed (NICE 2015a). Closer monitoring has been proven to have a positive impact on the control of blood glucose levels (Elgart et al. 2016).

Testing regularly will permit the individual to be aware of their blood sugar levels, allowing them to have better control and thus better stabilize their glycaemic variability. This will in turn reduce the likelihood of long-term complications, in particular vascular complications such as retinopathy, nephropathy and cardiac autonomic neuropathy (Virk et al. 2016).

Blood glucose monitoring should be individualized depending on the type of treatment (diet versus oral medication versus insulin), level of haemoglobin A1c (HbA1c) (see below for further information) and treatment goals (WHO 2016). These should be evaluated frequently and reassessed with the support of a healthcare professional (NICE 2015a). HbA1c measurement provides information relevant to overall glucose control as it measures the amount of glucose surrounding a haemoglobin molecule (Peate and Bennet-Long 2016); it is a vital component of overall diabetic control (NICE 2017a). It is typically lower than 6% in a normal healthy person (NICE 2015a). As the body's glucose levels increase, more haemoglobin becomes glycosylated (glucose binds with haemoglobin), and, in a person with diabetes, further glucose molecules attach to the haemoglobin molecules, which can remain for around 3 months – that is, the life of the blood cell (Marieb and Keller 2017). Guidelines suggest that diabetic patients should aim for an HbA1c of 6.5% or lower; however, individual targets may be given by the healthcare team depending on the individual and type of treatment (NICE 2015a).

Within the hospital setting, self-monitoring of blood glucose may be appropriate for competent adult patients who are medically stable and successfully self-managing their diabetes at home (Mabrey and Setji 2015). This would need to be supported by local policy, adequate patient assessment and the necessary documentation.

Methods of blood glucose testing

Blood glucose testing involves obtaining a drop of capillary blood and adding it to a testing strip, which is then analysed by a blood glucose meter (Marini and Dries 2016). Previously, most glucometers offered the option of using blood from the palm of the hand or the side of the hand; however, it is now routinely recommended that blood is only used from fingertips as the blood from this area responds rapidly to changes in blood glucose level and provides more reliable results (NICE 2015a). The fingertips contain nerve endings, which can become painful and less sensitive with frequent testing; therefore, the outer parts of the finger, the thumb and the forefinger should be used sparingly due to their continual use in apposition and because these tend to be more painful (Adam et al. 2017). It is important to rotate the areas used for blood glucose testing to avoid infection from multiple stabbings, to avoid areas becoming toughened and to reduce pain (Walden et al. 2018).

Anticipated patient outcomes

The patient will have their blood sugar levels kept as near normal as possible via blood glucose testing and control (Meetoo et al. 2018). Trials have shown the benefits of tight glycaemic control at near normal levels, which resulted in reductions in length of hospital stay, sepsis, dialysis, and hospital mortality and morbidity (Preiser et al. 2016, Wise 2014). Improved glycaemic control positively impacts patients' quality of life and reduces the risk of further complications (Penning et al. 2015).

Clinical governance

The MHRA (2013a) has highlighted the need for standardization in training (including regular updates) and for reliability and quality control of blood glucose testing. In order to achieve these, careful and systematic selection of appropriate equipment must occur. The following aspects must be considered when selecting monitoring devices:

- The equipment must be designed for use by non-laboratory staff.
- The equipment must be suitable for use in the intended setting (e.g. in a critical care unit or in an ambulance).
- It must be clear whether the meter or lancing device is for single patient use or can be used on multiple patients.
- The design must suit the needs and requirements of the patient or user.
- The equipment must be CE marked under the IVD directive (MHRA 2017).
- Support and advice must be provided by the hospital laboratory on device purchase, interpretation of results, troubleshooting, quality control, and health and safety.
- The equipment should be easy to use and an appropriate service co-ordinator should be identified.
- Written standard operating procedures should be available and kept with the device.
- Training must be given to the operators of the equipment and refreshed appropriately. The training should include:
  - basic principles of measurement
  - expected results in normal and pathological states
  - demonstration of the proper use of the equipment in accordance with the manufacturer's specification
  - demonstration of the consequences of improper use
  - knowledge of operator-dependent steps
  - instruction in the collection of appropriate blood samples
  - health and safety aspects
  - instruction in the importance of complete documentation of all data produced
  - appropriate calibration and quality control techniques
  - practical experience of the relevant procedures, including a series of analyses to satisfy the instructor that the trainee is competent
  - information regarding contraindications
  - information on basic troubleshooting, error messages and potential sources of error (MHRA 2013a).

It is recommended to keep records of training and quality testing results. The frequency of these quality control tests may vary according to manufacturer or hospital policy (MHRA 2013a).

Pre-procedural considerations

Equipment

Errors can occur during any phase of the testing process. Common sources of error include patient or operator method, environmental exposure and device malfunction (Sudhakaran and Surani 2015). All equipment should be checked for expiry dates (according to individual hospital trust policy), and it should be calibrated and stored according to the manufacturer's guidelines (MHRA 2013a).

Equipment selection should include:

- *Blood glucose monitor*: a medical device that measures the concentration of glucose in a human blood sample using a blood glucose test strip.
- *Testing strip*: a strip with a small window used to collect a sample of the patient's blood to be inserted into the blood glucose monitor. The strips must be calibrated with the monitor prior to use.
- *Disposable lancet*: a device used to draw out a small amount of blood from the patient for testing of glucose level. Single-use lancets are used to minimize the risk of cross-infection and accidental needle stick injury; they must be set to the correct depth according to the skin's turgor (Roche Diagnostics 2017).

The accuracy of glucose meters is a factor for consideration when purchasing or renting glucose meters (MHRA 2013a). Home glucose meters, which have been adopted for use in some hospitals without additional testing, may not give the high level of accuracy required (Karon et al. 2017).

Specific patient preparation

Patients should be advised to wash their hands prior to testing. Alternatively, the test area should be cleaned with soap and water and then dried, and the use of alcohol based handrub should be avoided to ensure non-contamination of the result (Adam et al. 2017). The patient should be encouraged to warm their hands before sampling to promote blood flow and increase the chance of obtaining an adequate sample of blood to cover the test strip (Wallymahmed 2013).

Procedure guideline 14.8 Blood glucose monitoring

Essential equipment

- Personal protective equipment
- Blood glucose monitor
- Test strips
- Control solution
- Single-use safety lancets
- Cotton wool or low-linting gauze
- Sharps box

Action	Rationale
Pre-procedure	
1 Turn the machine on and ensure the correct date and time are presented on screen, and that there is adequate battery life. Where applicable, enter or scan operator number and/or password.	To ensure accuracy in the record and patient safety (Roche Diagnostics 2017, **C**).
2 Ensure that the device is reading in mmol/L prior to each use.	Units of measure may change from mmol/L to mg/dL, which could result in an incorrect result (MHRA 2013a, **C**).

(continued)

Procedure guideline 14.8 Blood glucose monitoring *(continued)*

Action	Rationale
3 Before taking the device to the patient, calibrate the monitor and test strips (where applicable) using the relevant steps below (always follow the manufacturer's instructions in case of any difference): • Ensure the testing strips are in date and have not been left exposed to air. • Calibrate the monitor and test strips together. • Carry out a quality control test using both high and low or level 1 and 2 solutions (in accordance with trust and manufacturer's guidelines). Ensure the LOT number is recorded, either manually or via a bar code scanning system. • Record the result (pass or fail) in the equipment log book and sign it. • Where an automated device is used, ensure the device is docked in its base unit to enable the centrally held electronic records to be updated. • Ensure the meter has been decontaminated per local guidelines and is fit for use. • Ensure the meter service record is in date according to local policy. • Ensure the screen or display is intact and the 'screen safety check' has been completed in accordance with the manufacturer's guidelines (Roche Diagnostics 2017).	To ensure the device can be used under safe conditions (MHRA 2013a, E). Some machines will self calibrate: check the manufacturer's instructions.
4 Identify the patient, introduce yourself, explain and discuss the procedure with them, and gain their consent to proceed.	To ensure that the patient feels at ease, understands the procedure and gives their valid consent (NMC 2018, **C**).
5 Select a site that is warm, well perfused and free of any skin damage. The ideal site for lancing is the palmar surface of the distal segment of the third or fourth finger (**Action figure 5**) of the non-dominant hand, avoiding the thumb and the index finger. Also avoid sites that have recently been punctured.	Fingers on the non-dominant hand are generally less callused and the index finger is potentially more sensitive to pain due to additional nerve endings (Marini and Dries 2016, **C**). The thumb also may be callused and has a pulse, indicating arterial presence, and the distance between the skin surface and the bone in the fifth finger makes it unsuitable for puncture (WHO 2010, **C**). Tips and pads of fingers should be avoided as they have a denser nerve supply and can be more painful (WHO 2010, **C**). Rotating puncture sites avoids fingertip soreness and reduces callus formation (WHO 2010, **C**).
Procedure	
6 Ask the patient to wash their hands with soap and water and dry them thoroughly.	To avoid sample contamination (Adam et al. 2017, **C**). Not washing hands can lead to inaccurate results, especially with fingers exposed to fruit or a sugar-containing product (Pickering and Marsden 2014, **R**).
7 Ask patient to sit or lie down.	To ensure the patient's safety and minimize the risks if they feel faint when blood is taken (Roche Diagnostics 2017, **C**).
8 Wash and dry hands and/or use an alcohol-based handrub and apply personal protective equipment.	To minimize the risk of cross-infection and contamination (NHS England and NHSI 2019, **C**).
9 Turn on the device (where applicable and if not automated) and insert a testing strip.	Some devices will turn on automatically once the strip has been inserted. The manufacturer's guidelines should be followed to ensure accurate results (MHRA 2013a, **C**).
10 Take a single-use lancet and set the appropriate depth (if applicable).	To minimize the risk of cross-infection and accidental needle stick injury (NICE 2015a, **C**; Pickering and Marsden 2014, **E**; Weston 2013, **E**). The correct depth setting will minimise patient pain (Roche Diagnostics 2017, **C**).
11 Using the lancet, puncture the chosen site (see step 5). If necessary, 'milk' the fingertip from the palm of the hand towards the finger to gain a large enough droplet of blood.	Reusable lancet devices may be used in the patient's own environment; they should never be used for more than one person due to the risk of blood-borne viruses (Weston 2013, **C**). Milking the finger only (and not from the palm) can cause tissue fluid contamination and a false low reading (WHO 2010, **R**).
12 Dispose of the lancet in a sharps container.	To minimize the risk of cross-infection and accidental needle stick injury (Pickering and Marsden 2014, **E**; Weston 2013, **E**).
13 Apply the drop of blood to the testing strip (some strips are hydrophilic and are dosed/filled from the side, whereas others require a drop of blood to be placed directly onto the strip). Ensure that the window on the test strip is entirely covered with blood (**Action figure 13**).	To ensure the result is accurate, the window on the test strip needs to be adequately filled as per the manufacturer's guidelines (Roche Diagnostics 2017, **C**).

14 Immediately read and make note of the result on the display screen (**Action figure 14**). Document the result.	To interpret the results of the test. Some devices will turn off automatically after the result has been displayed for a short while. **E** To ensure accuracy in record keeping (NMC 2018, **C**).
15 Dispose of the testing strip in a sharps container.	To minimize the risk of sharps injury and cross-infection (Weston 2013, **E**).
16 Place gauze over the puncture site, apply firm pressure and monitor for excess bleeding.	To ensure patient safety (Walden et al. 2018, **E**) and to stop the bleeding (WHO 2010, **C**).
17 Once the bleeding has subsided, the site can be left exposed. It is not necessary to dress the site unless bleeding persists.	To allow the site to heal effectively. **E**
18 Remove gloves, place them in the clinical waste and perform hand hygiene again.	To prevent cross-infection (NHS England and NHSI 2019, **C**).
Post-procedure	
19 Where applicable, dock the machine.	To ensure centralized records are maintained and the machine is charged (Roche 2017, **C**).
20 Report and/or act on any unexpected results.	To ensure appropriate treatment and obtain an optimal blood glucose range (Adam et al. 2017, **E**).

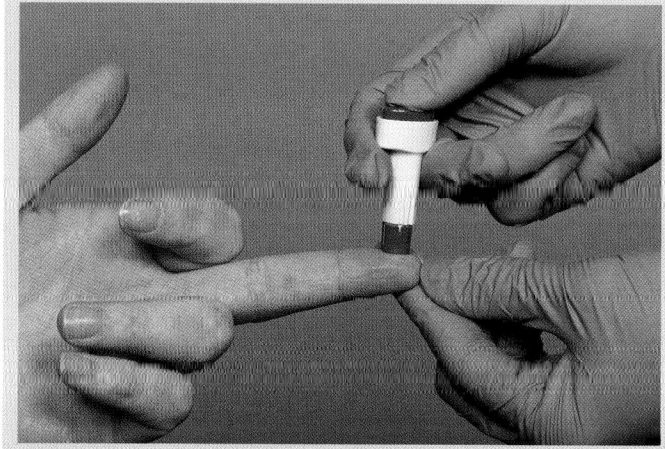

Action Figure 5 Take a blood sample from the side of the finger using a lancet, ensuring that the site of piercing is rotated.

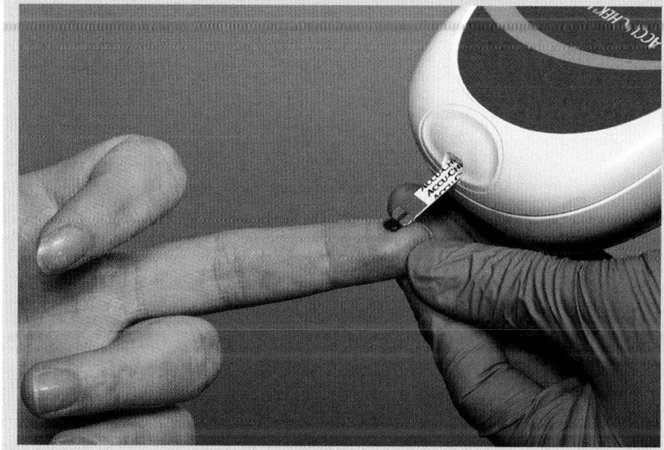

Action Figure 13 Insert the test strip into the blood glucose monitor and apply the blood to the test strip. Ensure that the window on the test strip is entirely covered with blood.

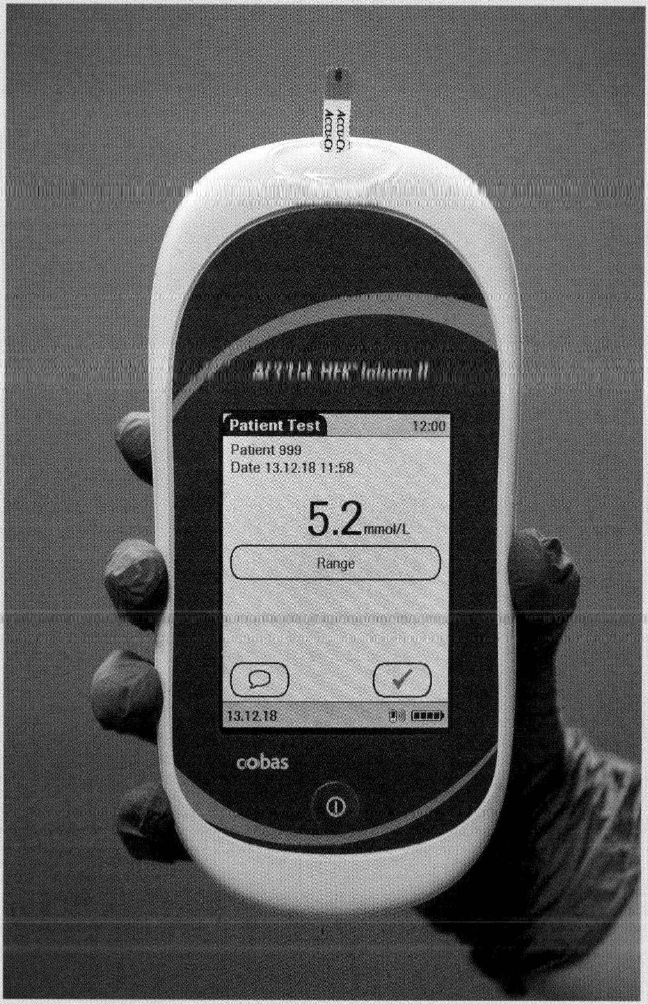

Action Figure 14 Read the result.

Problem-solving table 14.7 Prevention and resolution (Procedure guideline 14.8)

Problem	Cause	Prevention	Action
Inaccurate results	Device maintenance issues: • inadequate meter calibration • failure to code correctly • poor meter maintenance • out-of-date test strips	Ensure staff receive adequate training and clear instructions on how to calibrate the device (MHRA 2013a, Walden et al. 2018).	Repeat steps 1, 2 and 3 of Procedure guideline 14.8: Blood glucose monitoring appropriately and according to the manufacturer's instructions and/or local guidelines.
	Inadequate amount of blood on the test strip	Ensure staff receive adequate training. Ensure there is an adequate amount of blood available to apply to the testing strip.	Repeat the blood sugar measurement, ensuring that the window on the test strip is entirely covered with blood. If the error persists, ask a colleague to repeat the test. If the error still persists, report glucose meter to a technician and use another machine.

Post-procedural considerations

Immediate care

If a true abnormal blood glucose result is detected then the appropriate action should be taken according to medical advice and hospital policy.

Education of the patient and relevant others

Diabetes mellitus is a long-term, often lifelong condition affecting all aspects of a person's life (Preiser et al. 2016). Diabetes care primarily consists of self-care, and all people with diabetes should have access to self-monitoring (WHO 2016). Research has found that diabetes self-management education improves quality of life (Meetoo et al. 2018). Nurses have a role in educating patients and promoting self-management of diabetes. Advising patients on the type and frequency of monitoring based on individual clinical need will enable them to monitor and adjust their own treatment (Walden et al. 2018). Furthermore, a specialist nurse can be equipped to provide essential support in guiding patients' day-to-day management of their disease (Hamilton et al. 2017). People with diabetes should be given annual updates to ensure they are still able to perform tests accurately and inform them of any new developments, and it is important to ensure that key assessments are completed, such as retinal eye screening and foot checks (NICE 2016d). Healthcare professionals should advocate a healthy lifestyle for patients with diabetes, including regulating blood pressure, a low-sugar diet and exercise; these may be invaluable to patients and allow them to have a full, unrestricted life (NICE 2016d).

Neurological observations

Definition

Neurological observation is the collection of information about a patient's central nervous system (Wilkinson et al. 2017). Despite advances in neuromonitoring, clinical observation of patients remains the most sensitive measure of neurological function (Adam et al. 2017).

Anatomy and physiology

The nervous system is the most complex of the body's systems and is responsible for the co-ordination of all body functions and for adapting to changes in internal and external environments. The activities of the nervous system can be grouped into three basic functions (Tortora and Derrickson 2017):

- *sensory (input)*: detection of internal or external stimuli; this information is carried to the spinal cord and the brain through the cranial and spinal nerves
- *integrative (process)*: analysis of sensory information and initiating appropriate responses
- *motor (output)*: eliciting an appropriate motor response by activating effectors (muscles and glands) through the cranial and spinal nerves.

The intricate network of neurones and neuroglia that comprise the nervous system are divided into two main subdivisions: the central nervous system and the peripheral nervous system.

The central nervous system

The central nervous system consists of the brain and spinal cord (Tortora and Derrickson 2017).

The brain

Located within the skull, the brain is the control centre for registering sensations, correlating them with one another and stored information, making decisions and taking actions; it is also the centre for intellect, emotions, behaviour and memories (Tortora and Derrickson 2017). The adult brain consists of four regions: the brainstem, the cerebellum, the diencephalon and the cerebrum (Figure 14.39).

The cerebrum is the largest part of the brain and provides us with the ability to read, write and speak; to make calculations; and to remember the past, plan for the future and imagine things (Wilkinson et al. 2017).

The cerebral hemispheres contain the greatest mass of brain tissue. Each hemisphere is subdivided into several lobes named after the bones that cover them: frontal, parietal, temporal and occipital (Figure 14.40). Each of these lobes has a particular function:

- The *frontal lobe* is located at the front of the brain and is associated with cognitive function (orientation, memory, insight, judgement, calculation and abstraction), expressive language (verbal and written) and voluntary motor function (through skeletal muscle).
- The *parietal lobe* is located in the middle section of the brain and is associated with sensory function, including integration of sensory information; awareness of body parts; interpretation of touch, pressure and pain; and recognition of object size, shape and texture.
- The *occipital lobe* is located at the back of the brain; it is associated with interpreting visual stimuli and receives impulses from the optic nerve.
- The *temporal lobe* is located in the bottom section of the brain and is primarily associated with hearing, speech, behaviour and memory (Adam et al. 2017).

The spinal cord

The spinal cord is a cylindrical mass of nerve tissue encased within the vertical canal of the vertebral column; it extends

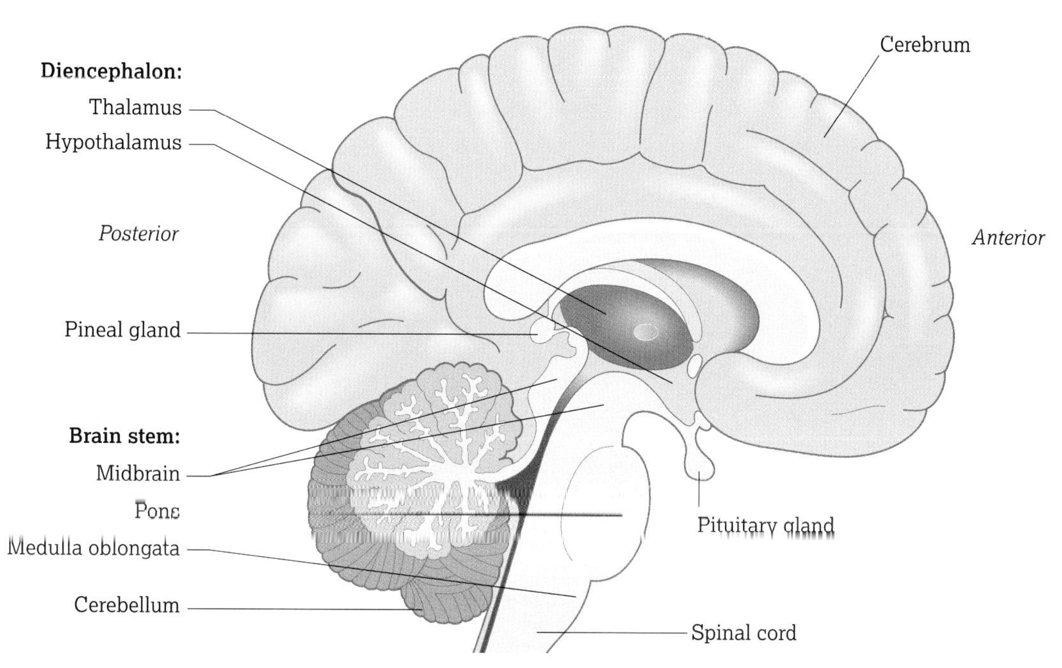

Figure 14.39 The brain. *Source*: Reproduced from Peate and Wild (2018) with permission of John Wiley & Sons.

from the medulla oblongata of the brainstem to the superior border of the second lumbar vertebra (Tortora and Derrickson 2017). It contains important motor and sensory nerve pathways that exit and enter the cord through anterior and posterior nerve roots and spinal and peripheral nerves, and it also mediates reflex activity of the deep tendons from the spinal nerves (Bickley 2016). The spinal cord is divided into five segments: cervical, from C1 to C8; thoracic, from T1 to T12; lumbar, from L1 to L5; sacral, from S1 to S5; and coccygeal (Bickley 2016) (Figure 14.41).

The peripheral nervous system

The cranial nerves

There are 12 pairs of cranial nerves that emerge from the brain. They are named according to their distribution and are numbered I to XII in order of their attachment to the brain (Tortora and Derrickson 2017). Cranial nerves II–XII arise from the diencephalon and the brainstem (Table 14.11). Cranial nerves I and II are actually fibre tracts emerging from the brain (Tortora and Derrickson 2017). Some cranial nerves are limited to general motor or sensory functions whereas others are specialized, enabling smell, vision or hearing (I, II and VIII) (Bickley 2016).

The peripheral nerves

In addition to the cranial nerves, the peripheral nervous system includes spinal and peripheral nerves that carry impulses to and from the spinal cord. The 31 pairs of spinal nerves are named and numbered in accordance with the region and level of the spinal cord from which they emerge: eight cervical, twelve thoracic, five lumbar, five sacral and one coccygeal. The spinal nerves are typically connected to the spinal cord by a posterior root (containing sensory fibres) and an anterior root (containing motor fibres) (Tortora and Derrickson 2017).

Related theory

Changes in neurological status can be rapid and dramatic or subtle, developing over minutes, hours, days, weeks or even longer (Wilkinson et al. 2017). The frequency of neurological observations will depend upon the patient's condition and the rapidity with which changes are occurring or expected to occur, and should include:

- assessment of level of consciousness
- pupil size and reaction to light
- limb assessments (including both motor and sensory function)
- vital signs (Adam et al. 2017).

Assessment of level of consciousness

Level of consciousness is the most sensitive indicator of neurological deterioration and is therefore the most important aspect of any neurological assessment (Brain Trauma Foundation 2016). Consciousness is a state of awareness of self and the environment and is dependent on two components: arousal and awareness (Baumann 2017). These correspond to two brain structures: the reticular activating system (RAS) and the cerebral cortex (Tortora and Derrickson 2017). Consciousness depends on the interaction between the neurones in the RAS in the brainstem and the neurones in the cerebral cortex (Adam et al. 2017).

Arousal

Arousal is a primitive state managed by the RAS. The core of nuclei that make up the RAS extends from the brainstem with projections upwards to the cortex and downwards to the spinal cord (Tortora and Derrickson 2017). The RAS receives auditory, visual and sensory impulses (such as pain, touch, movement of limbs, bright light or noise), and because of its connections is ideal for governing arousal of the brain as a whole (Adam et al. 2017). Unless inhibited by other areas of the brain, the reticular neurones send a continuous stream of impulses to the cerebral cortex, maintaining the cortex in an alert, conscious state; the RAS is selective, however, forwarding only essential information to the cortex and filtering out unnecessary information (Tortora and Derrickson 2017). Certain drugs have a direct effect on the RAS; alcohol, sleep-inducing drugs and tranquillizers depress the RAS and drugs such as lysergic acid diethylamide (LSD) remove the RAS's filter system, leading to heightened sensory arousal (Adam et al. 2017).

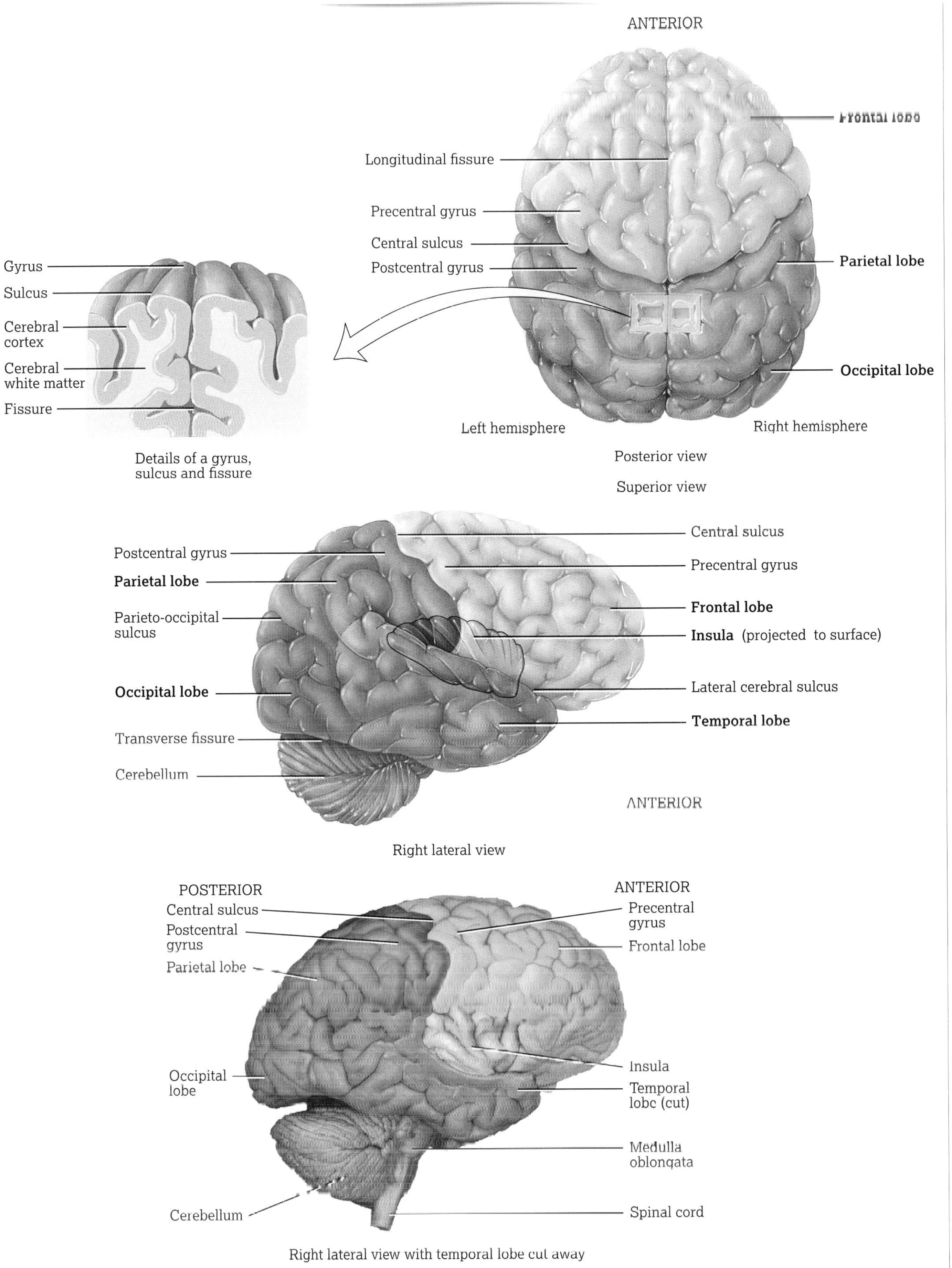

Figure 14.40 The cerebrum. *Source:* Reproduced from Tortora and Derrickson (2017) with permission of John Wiley & Sons.

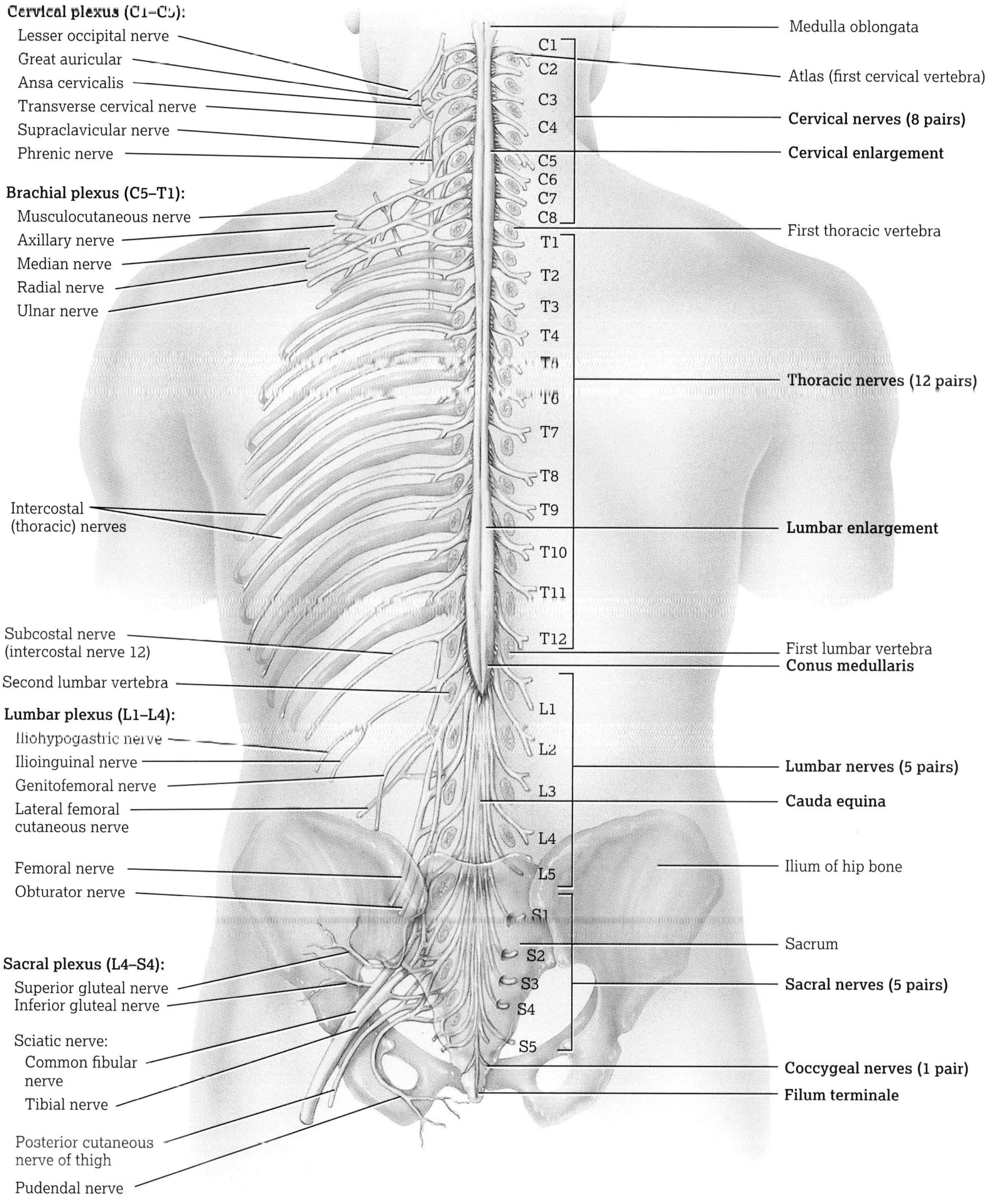

Figure 14.41 External anatomy of the spinal cord and the spinal nerves (posterior view). *Source*: Reproduced from Tortora and Derrickson (2017) with permission of John Wiley & Sons.

Table 14.11 Summary of cranial nerves

Cranial nerve	Components	Principal functions
Olfactory (I)	**Special sensory**	Olfaction (smell)
Optic (II)	**Special sensory**	Vision (sight)
Oculomotor (III)	**Motor**	
	Somatic	Movement of eyeballs and upper eyelid
	Motor (autonomic)	Adjusts lens for near vision (accommodation)
		Constriction of pupil
Trochlear (IV)	**Motor**	
	Somatic	Movement of eyeballs
Trigeminal (V)	**Mixed**	
	Sensory	Touch, pain, and thermal sensations from scalp, face, and oral cavity (including teeth and anterior two-thirds of tongue)
	Motor (branchial)	Chewing and controls middle ear muscle
Abducens (VI)	**Motor**	
	Somatic	Movement of eyeballs
Facial (VII)	**Mixed**	
	Sensory	Taste from anterior two-thirds of tongue
		Touch, pain, and thermal sensations from skin in external ear canal
	Motor (branchial)	Control of muscles of facial expression and middle ear muscle
	Motor (autonomic)	Secretion of tears and saliva
Vestibulocochlear (VIII)	**Special sensory**	Hearing and equilibrium
Glossopharyngeal (IX)	**Mixed**	
	Sensory	Taste from posterior one-third of tongue
		Proprioception in some swallowing muscles
		Monitors blood pressure and oxygen and carbon dioxide levels in blood
		Touch, pain, and thermal sensations from skin of external ear and upper pharynx
	Motor (branchial)	Assists in swallowing
	Motor (autonomic)	Secretion of saliva
Vagus (X)	**Mixed**	
	Sensory	Taste from epiglottis
		Proprioception from throat and voice box muscles
		Monitors blood pressure and oxygen and carbon dioxide levels in blood
		Touch, pain, and thermal sensations from skin of external ear
		Sensations from thoracic and abdominal organs
	Motor (branchial)	Swallowing, vocalisation, and coughing
	Motor (autonomic)	Motility and secretion of gastrointestinal organs
		Constriction of respiratory passageways
		Decreases heart rate
Accessory (XI)	**Motor**	
	Branchial	Movement of head and pectoral girdle
Hypoglossal (XII)	**Motor**	
	Somatic	Speech, manipulation of food, and swallowing

Source: Reproduced from Tortora and Derrickson (2017) with permission of John Wiley & Sons.

Awareness

Awareness is the more sophisticated part of consciousness and requires an intact cerebral cortex to interpret sensory input and respond accordingly (Adam et al. 2017).

Assessing consciousness

Consciousness cannot be measured directly but is assessed by observing behaviour in response to different stimuli. The response indicates the level at which the sensory information has been translated within the central nervous system (Adam et al. 2017).

Assessment of arousal focuses on the patient's ability to respond appropriately to verbal and non-verbal stimuli. It begins with verbal stimuli in a normal tone; if there is no response, the stimulus is progressively increased, initially by raising the voice, then by gently shaking the patient and finally by applying noxious (painful) stimuli (see section on application of painful stimuli below).

Assessment of awareness is concerned with the patient's orientation to person, place and time. Changes in this may be the first sign of neurological deterioration leading to confusion and disorientation (Baumann 2017).

Previous and/or co-existing problems should be considered when assessing levels of consciousness, for example deafness, hemiparesis or hemiplegia, as a manifestation of altered consciousness implies an underlying brain dysfunction (Adam et al. 2017). Its onset may be sudden, for example following an acute head injury, or it may occur more gradually, such as in hypoglycaemia (Wilkinson et al. 2017). Similarly, alterations in level of consciousness can vary from slight to severe, indicating the degree of brain dysfunction (Adam et al. 2017). For a full assessment, it is essential to take a detailed history and to involve family and/or friends to describe the patient's usual function (Adam et al. 2017).

Consciousness ranges across a continuum from alert wakefulness to deep coma with no apparent responsiveness (Baumann 2017). Level of consciousness can be measured using the Glasgow Coma Scale (GCS) or, during a rapid assessment of an acutely unwell patient, the AVPU (alert, verbal, pain, unresponsive) scale (see the section below on assessment and recording tools) (Adam et al. 2017, Brain Trauma Foundation 2016, Braine and Cook 2017).

Application of painful stimuli

Painful stimuli should be employed only if the patient does not respond to firm and clear commands (Braine and Cook 2017). The stimulus should be applied in a standard way, increasing from light pressure and being maintained until a response is elicited, for a maximum of 10 seconds, to avoid soft tissue injury and unnecessary pain (Adam et al. 2017, Brain Trauma Foundation 2016, Braine and Cook 2017).

As the ability to localize pain is lost, various responses may be observed when painful stimuli are applied (Baumann 2017). It is important to note, when applying a painful stimulus peripherally, that it may only elicit a spinal reflex that does not involve cerebral function; therefore, evaluation of cerebral function requires the application of central stimuli (Braine and Cook 2017).

Central stimuli include the trapezium squeeze (Figure 14.42), supraorbital pressure and the sternal rub (Baumann 2017), which are described below (although the sternal rub is no longer advocated). Local policies and guidelines should be followed as some practices are not recommended in some organizations.

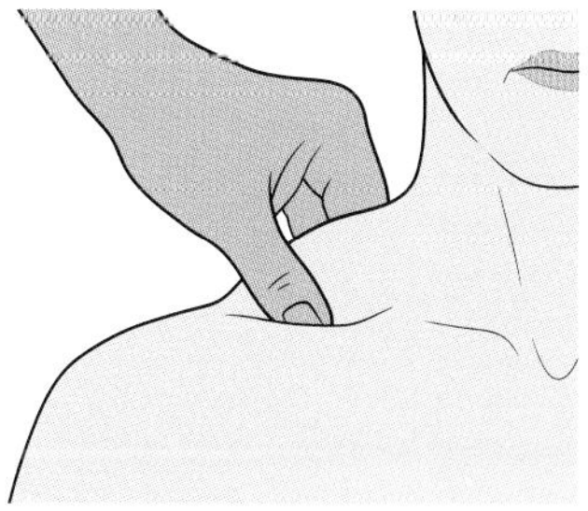

Figure 14.42 Trapezium squeeze.

- *Trapezium squeeze*: using the thumb and two fingers, hold 5 cm of the trapezius muscle where the neck meets the shoulder and twist the muscle.
- *Supraorbital pressure*: run a finger along the supraorbital margin (the bony ridge along the top of the eye) to feel a notch. Apply pressure to the notch to stimulate the supraorbital nerve and cause an ipsilateral (on that side) sinus headache-type pain. This method should not be used if the facial or cranial bones are unstable, if facial fractures are suspected or after facial surgery. Using supraorbital pressure as a painful stimulus may also make the patient grimace and lead to them closing the eye rather than opening it (Fairley et al. 2005).
- *Sternal rub*: the use of a sternal rub is no longer recommended as it has been shown to cause excessive bruising and discomfort to the patient (Dawes and Durham 2007, Naalla et al. 2014).

If there is no response to central stimuli (e.g. flexion, eye movement or verbal response) then a peripheral stimulus should be applied (Adam et al. 2017). One technique is to place the patient's finger between the assessor's thumb and a pencil or pen, apply pressure gradually and increase it over a few seconds or until the slightest response is seen (Braine and Cook 2017). Due to the risk of bruising, pressure should not be applied to the nail bed and, again, local policies and guidelines should be followed.

Assessment of pupillary activity

Careful examination of the reactions of the pupils to light is an important part of the neurological assessment and can lead to important findings, as listed in Table 14.12 (Fuller 2013). The size (Figure 14.43), shape, equality, reaction to light (in both the eye directly exposed to light (direct) and the eye not directly exposed to it (consensual)) and position of the eyes should be noted as well as whether the eyes are deviated upwards or downwards, and whether the eyes are conjugate (moving together) or dysconjugate (not moving together) (Bickley 2016). Pupillary response to light relies on unimpaired afferent and efferent function (which

Table 14.12 Examination of pupils

Observation	Pupil size	Pupil reactiveness	Possible indication
Pupils equal	Pinpoint	–	Opiates or pontine lesion
	Small	Reactive	Metabolic encephalopathy
	Mid-sized	Fixed	Midbrain lesion
		Reactive	Metabolic lesion
Pupils unequal	Dilated	Unreactive	Third nerve palsy
	Small	Reactive	Horner's syndrome

Source: Reproduced from Fuller (2013) with permission of Elsevier.

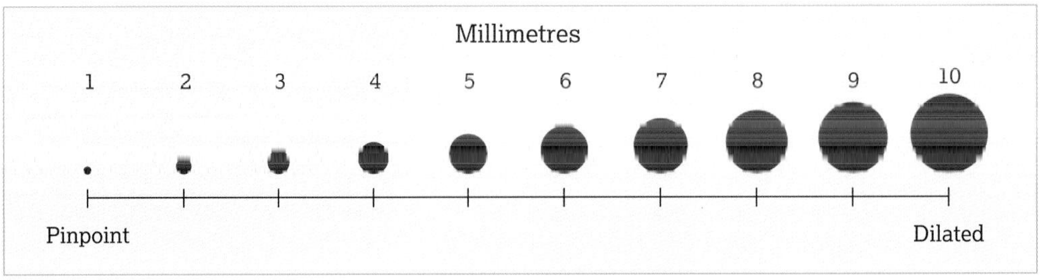

Figure 14.43 Pupil size guide.

respectively rely on the optic and oculomotor nerves), which allow the retina to communicate the light impulse to the pupillary musculature and to the midbrain (Adam et al. 2017). Due to its resistance to metabolic changes, the pupillary pathway reaction to light aids in the differentiation of a metabolic coma from a structural one (Wilkinson et al. 2017). When a brain mass is suspected, compromised pupillary response to light is likely due to the midbrain being under pressure; in these cases, changes in the constriction and dilation of the pupils may reflect pressure on the oculomotor nerve (cranial nerve III) or brainstem damage (Adam et al. 2017).

Assessment of limb function

Motor function

Damage to any part of the motor nervous system can affect the ability to move (Baumann 2017). After assessing motor function on one side of the body, the contralateral muscle group should also be evaluated to detect asymmetry (Adam et al. 2017). Motor function assessment involves evaluation of the following:

- muscle strength
- muscle tone
- muscle co-ordination
- reflexes
- abnormal movements (Bickley 2016).

Muscle strength

This involves testing the patient's muscle strength against the pull of gravity and then against resistance applied by another person. Changes in motor strength, especially between the right and left sides, may indicate imminent or existing neurological failure (Baumann 2017).

Muscle tone

This involves flexing and extending the patient's limbs on both sides and noting how well such movements are resisted. Increased resistance (compared to normal tone) denotes increased muscle tone and decreased resistance denotes decreased tone (Baumann 2017, Bickley 2016).

Muscle co-ordination

Any disease or injury that involves the cerebellum or basal ganglia will affect co-ordination (Bickley 2016). Assessment of hand and leg co-ordination can be achieved by testing the rapidity and rhythm of alternating movements and point-to-point movements (Baumann 2017).

Reflexes

Among the most important reflexes are blink, gag and swallow, oculocephalic and plantar:

- *Blink (corneal)*: this is a protective reflex and can be affected by damage to the fifth cranial nerve (trigeminal) and the seventh cranial nerve (facial). Facial weakness (seventh cranial nerve) will affect eye closure, and absence of the corneal reflex may result in corneal damage (Fuller 2013).
- *Gag and swallow*: damage to the ninth cranial nerve (glossopharyngeal) and 10th cranial nerve (vagus) may impair protective reflexes. These two cranial nerves are always assessed together as their functions overlap. Muscle innervation of the palate is from the vagus, while sensation is supplied by the glossopharyngeal nerves (Wilkinson et al. 2017).
- *Oculocephalic*: this reflex is an eye movement that occurs only in patients with a severely decreased level of consciousness (in conscious patients this reflex is not present). When the reflex is present, the patient's eyes will move in the opposite direction from the side to which the head is turned. However, in patients with absent brainstem reflexes, the eyes will appear to remain stationary in the centre. This reflex should not be assessed if there is suspected instability of the cervical spine as the necessary head movement could exacerbate any spinal injury (Baumann 2017).
- *Plantar*: abnormalities of the plantar reflex will help to locate the anatomical site of the lesion. The upgoing plantar (extension) reflex is termed 'positive Babinski' (dorsiflexion of the big toe and fanning of the other toes) and indicates an upper motor neurone lesion. Note that the upgoing plantar reflex is normal in children of less than 1 year of age (Baumann 2017, Bickley 2016).

Abnormal movements

When carrying out neurological observations, any abnormal movements (such as seizures, tics and tremors) must be noted (Bickley 2016).

Sensory function

Constant sensory input enables individuals to alter their responses and behaviour to suit the environment. When disease or injury damages the sensory pathways, the sensory responses are always affected. Any assessment of sensory function should include an evaluation of the following:

- central and peripheral vision
- hearing and ability to understand verbal communication
- superficial sensations (light touch, pain) and deep sensations (muscle and joint pain, muscle and joint position) (Baumann 2017, Fuller 2013).

Visual acuity

Clarity or clearness of vision may be tested with a Snellen chart, which uses decreasing letter sizes or newspaper prints. If the patient wears glasses, they should be worn during the test (Bickley 2016).

Visual fields

Lesions at various points in the visual pathways affect vision. It should be noted that loss of vision is always described with reference to the visual fields rather than the retinal fields (Bickley 2016).

Vital signs

It is recommended that assessment of vital signs should include respiration rate, oxygen saturation, temperature, and blood pressure and pulse.

Respiration and oxygen saturation

Respiratory patterns can give a clear indication of how the brain is functioning as the complex process of respiration is controlled by more than one area of the brain: the cerebral hemispheres, the cerebellum and the brainstem (Adam et al. 2017). Any disease or injury that affects these areas may produce respiratory changes (Wilkinson et al. 2017). The rate, character and pattern of a patient's respiration must be noted. Abnormal respiratory patterns are listed in Table 14.13 (Adam et al. 2017, Wilkinson et al. 2017). Any change in respiration may lead to a change in oxygen saturation; this should therefore also be assessed.

Constant re-evaluation of the patient's ability to maintain and protect their airway is essential when there is evidence of reduced consciousness or coma (i.e. when the GCS score is less than 8) (Baumann 2017). At this stage, muscles often become flaccid and use of the recovery position may need to be considered (Adam et al. 2017). Patients whose neurological function has deteriorated may require adjuncts to protect the airway and possibly artificial ventilation (RCUK 2015). Close liaison with physiotherapists and speech and language therapists is important to minimize the danger of chest infections (due to the patient's inability to clear secretions) and the risk of aspiration (Adam et al. 2017).

Temperature

Damage to the hypothalamus (the temperature-regulating centre) may result in grossly fluctuating temperatures (Adam et al. 2017).

Blood pressure and pulse

Hypertension with a widening pulse pressure, bradycardia and a fall in respiratory rate may be indicative of rising intracranial pressure and is part of the Cushing reflex (Adam et al. 2017). Abnormalities of blood pressure and pulse usually occur late (and may not appear at all in some patients); usually, the patient's level of consciousness will have begun to deteriorate before there is any alteration in their vital signs (Adam et al. 2017).

Evidence-based approaches

Rationale

Neurological observations are carried out to assess a patient's level of consciousness and neurological function. It is appropriate to carry out these observations in any clinical scenario where the level of consciousness has changed or normal neurological function is in question.

Indications

An accurate neurological assessment is essential in planning appropriate patient care (Bickley 2016). The information gained from a neurological assessment can be used in the following ways:

- to aid diagnosis (Braine and Cook 2017)
- as a baseline for observations (Braine and Cook 2017)
- to determine both subtle and rapid changes in an individual's condition (Summers and McLeod 2017)
- to monitor neurological status following a neurological procedure or trauma (Summers and McLeod 2017)
- to observe for deterioration and establish the extent of a traumatic head injury (Braine and Cook 2017)
- to detect life-threatening situations (Braine and Cook 2017)
- to monitor the effectiveness of interventions (Braine and Cook 2017).

Frequency of observations

It is impossible to be prescriptive with regard to the frequency of neurological observations as these will depend on the patient's presenting condition, medical diagnosis and underlying pathology, and the possible consequences (Braine and Cook 2017). Clinical knowledge and judgement will dictate the necessary timing interval for the assessment (Adam et al. 2017) and local guidelines should be followed. If the patient's condition is deteriorating, observations may need to be carried out as frequently as every 10–15 minutes for the first few hours and then every 1–2 hours for a further 48 hours (Adam et al. 2017).

The nurse must be competent to take appropriate action if changes in the patient's neurological status occur, and they must report any subtle signs that may indicate deterioration (Braine and Cook 2017). For example, patients will often become increasingly restless, or a previously restless patient may become atypically quiet (Adam et al. 2017). It should never be assumed that difficulty to rouse a patient is due to night-time sleep as even a deeply asleep patient with no focal deficit should respond to pain (Baumann 2017). If the patient requires an increased amount of stimulus to achieve the same response as before, this may be an indication of subtle deterioration (Fuller 2013).

Pre-procedural considerations

Equipment

The following equipment may be used as part of a neurological assessment:

- *Pen torch*: used to assess the reaction of the pupils to light and the consensual light reflex (Bickley 2016).
- *Tongue depressor*: a device used to depress the tongue to allow for examination of the mouth and throat (Fuller 2013).

Table 14.13 Abnormal respiratory patterns

Type	Pattern	Significance
Apneustic breathing	Prolonged inspiration with a pause at full inspiration; there may also be expiratory pauses.	May indicate a lesion of the lower pons or upper medulla, hypoglycaemia or drug-induced respiratory depression.
Ataxic breathing	A completely irregular pattern with random deep and shallow respirations; irregular pauses may also appear.	May indicate a lesion of the medulla.
Central neurogenic hyperventilation	Sustained, regular, rapid respirations, with forced inspiration and expiration.	May indicate a lesion of the low midbrain or upper pons areas of the brainstem.
Cheyne–Stokes breathing	Rhythmic waxing and waning of both rate and depth of respirations, alternating regularly with briefer periods of apnoea. Greater than normal rate of respiration (i.e. 16–24 breaths per minute).	May indicate deep cerebral or cerebellar lesions, usually bilateral; may occur with upper brainstem involvement.
Cluster breathing	Clusters of irregular respirations alternating with longer periods of apnoea.	May indicate a lesion of the lower pons or upper medulla.

- *Patella hammer*: a tendon hammer used to strike the patella tendon below the knee to assess the deep knee-jerk/reflex (Fuller 2013).
- *Neuro tips*: a sharp instrument (such as a safety pin or other suitable sharp object) used to apply pressure and test for superficial sensations to pain (Fuller 2013).
- *Snellen chart*: a letter chart used to measure visual acuity (Bickley 2016).

Assessment and recording tools

The initial assessment of a patient should include a history (taken from relatives or friends if necessary) that notes changes in mood, intellect, memory and personality, since these may be indicators of a long-standing problem (Baumann 2017).

Assessment of level of consciousness can be carried out using the GCS or the AVPU scale (Adam et al. 2017).

Glasgow Coma Scale

The GCS, first published by Teasdale and Jennett (1974), is a widely used tool for assessing level of consciousness and should be employed to assess all patients with head injuries (NICE 2017d). It forms a quick, objective and easily interpreted mode of neurological assessment (Braine and Cook 2017). The GCS measures arousal and awareness by assessing three areas of the patient's behaviour: eye opening, verbal response and motor response (Wilkinson et al. 2017). Each area is allocated a score, enabling objectivity, ease of recording and comparison between recordings (Baumann 2017). The sum provides a score out of 15, where a score of 15 indicates a fully alert and responsive patient and a score of 3 (the lowest possible score) indicates unconsciousness (Adam et al. 2017). When used consistently, the GCS provides a graphical representation that shows any improvement or deterioration of the patient's consciousness level at a glance (Figure 14.44; Table 14.14) (Adam et al. 2017, Brain Trauma Foundation 2016, Braine and Cook 2017). However, a thoughtful, educated approach is essential to enhance its coherency and practicality (Braine and Cook 2017).

A limitation in the use of the GCS is that most healthcare professions will require the scale to be available for review in order to score a patient's consciousness level (as very few healthcare professions have memorized the scores for each area of assessment) (Reith et al. 2016). In an urgent or highly acute situation, this may not be possible, in which case the AVPU method may be more appropriate (see below) (RCUK 2015).

Assessment using the GCS involves three phases (Baumann 2017):

- evaluation of eye opening
- evaluation of verbal response
- evaluation of motor response.

Evaluation of eye opening

Eye opening indicates that the arousal mechanism in the brain is active (Fuller 2013). Eye opening may occur spontaneously, in response to speech, in response to a painful stimulus or not at all (Baumann 2017). Arousal (eye opening) is always the first measurement undertaken when performing the GCS, as without arousal, cognition cannot occur (Baumann 2017, Brunker and Harris 2015). Eye opening is scored as follows.

- *Spontaneous*: the patient is observed to be awake, with their eyes open, without any speech or touch (allocated a score of 4).
- *To speech*: the patient opens their eyes to loud and clear commands (allocated a score of 3).
- *To pain*: the patient opens their eyes to a painful stimulus (allocated a score of 2).
- *None*: the patient does not open their eyes to a painful stimulus (allocated a score of 1) (Baumann 2017, Brunker and Harris 2015, Fuller 2013).

A patient with flaccid ocular muscles may lie with their eyes open all the time; this is not a true arousal response and should be recorded as 'none' (Fuller 2013). If a patient's eyes are closed as a result of swelling or facial fractures, eye opening cannot be used to determine a falling consciousness level; this should be recorded as a 'C' (closed) on the chart (Brunker and Harris 2015, Fuller 2013).

Evaluation of verbal response

Verbal response is scored as follows.

- *Orientated*: the patient can correctly identify who they are (person), where they are (place) and the current year (time) (allocated a score of 5).
- *Confused*: the patient's responses to the above questions are incorrect and they are unaware of person, place or time (allocated a score of 4).
- *Inappropriate words*: the patient responds using intelligible words that are unsuitable as conversational responses; swearing is common, as are single-word responses (allocated a score of 3).
- *Incomprehensible*: the patient may mumble, moan or groan without recognizable words (allocated a score of 2).
- *Absent*: the patient does not speak or make sounds at all (allocated a score of 1) (Baumann 2017, Brunker and Harris 2015, Fuller 2013).

The absence of speech may not always indicate a falling level of consciousness; for example, the patient may not speak English but may still be able to speak. A patient with a tracheostomy or endotracheal tube should be recorded as 'T' on the chart under no response and allocated a score of 1 (Baumann 2017). Likewise, if the patient is dysphasic, the best verbal response cannot be determined accurately. The patient may have a motor (expressive) dysphasia and therefore be able to understand but be unable to find the right word, or a sensory (receptive) dysphasia, which means they will be unable to comprehend what is being said to them (Fuller 2013). At times, patients with expressive dysphasia may also have receptive problems; therefore, it is important to make an early referral to a speech and language therapist. This should be recorded as a 'D' on the chart under no response and allocated a score of 1 (Baumann 2017).

If a patient cannot follow an instruction due to a language barrier or unconsciousness, observe their spontaneous movements and note how strong they appear to be (Adam et al. 2017). Then, if necessary, apply painful stimuli (Fuller 2013). The nurse should also consider that some patients may need a lot of stimulation to maintain their concentration to answer questions, even though they can answer them correctly (Brunker and Harris 2015). It is therefore important to note the amount of stimulation that the patient required as part of the baseline assessment (Baumann 2017).

Evaluation of motor response

Motor response is the most important prognostic aspect of the GCS after traumatic brain injury (Adam et al. 2017). To obtain an accurate picture of brain function, motor response is tested by using the upper limbs because responses in the lower limbs reflect spinal function (Adam et al. 2017). The patient should be asked to obey a couple of simple commands; for example, they can be asked to squeeze the nurses hands (both sides). The nurse should note the power in the hands and the patient's ability to release the grip in order to discount a reflex action (Brain Trauma Foundation 2016). In addition, the patient should be asked to raise their eyebrows or stick out their tongue, and the best motor response should be recorded (Bickley 2016). If movement is spontaneous, the nurse should note which limbs move and whether the movement is purposeful (Fuller 2013). If the patient is able to obey commands, they should be allocated a score of 6 (Baumann 2017).

If the patient is unresponsive to simple commands, their response to painful stimuli should be assessed. This may be:

- *Localized*: the patient moves their hand to the site of the stimulus, either up beyond the chin or across the midline of the body (allocated a score of 5).

The ROYAL MARSDEN
NHS Foundation Trust

Name: ....
Hospital No: .... NHS No: ....

Adult Neurological Observations

			Key
		Date	
		Time	
Glasgow Coma Scale	Eyes open	Eyes open spontaneously 4	C = Eyes closed by swelling
		Eye opening to speech 3	
		Eye opening to pain 2	
		No eye opening 1	
	Best verbal response	Orientated 5	T = Endotracheal tube or Tracheostomy D = Dysphasia LB = Language barrier
		Confused 4	
		Inappropriate words 3	
		Incomprehensible sounds 2	
		No verbal response 1	
	Best motor response (Record best arm)	Obeys commands 6	M = Muscle relaxant P = Paralysed
		Localises pain 5	
		Normal flexion to pain 4	
		Abnormal flexion to pain 3	
		Extension to pain 2	
		No motor response 1	
		Total GCS Score out of 15 *	

* See overleaf for guidance (Clinical Response)

			Key
Pupils	Left	Size	+ = Reacts – = No reaction SL = Sluggish C = Eye closed
		Reaction	
	Right	Size	
		Reaction	
Limb movement	Arms	Normal power	Record right (R) and left (L) separately if there is a difference between the two sides P = Paralysed
		Mild weakness	
		Severe weakness	
		Flexion	
		Extension	
		No response	
	Legs	Normal power	
		Mild weakness	
		Severe weakness	
		Flexion	
		Extension	
		No response	

Temperature°C

Pupil scale (mm): 1, 2, 3, 4, 5, 6, 7, 8

Blood pressure ∧ ∨

Pulse rate •

230
220
210
200
190
180
170
160
150
140
130
120
110
100
90
80
70
60
50
40
35
30
25
20
15
10
5

Respiration (write number)

O_2 Sats
Inspired O_2%
Monitoring Frequency
Initials

Figure 14.44 Glasgow Coma Scale and neurological observations chart.

Scoring the Activities of the Glasgow Coma Scale

Eye Opening Scored 1–4		
Spontaneously	4	Eyes open without need of stimulus
To speech	3	Eyes open to verbal stimulation (normal, raised or repeated)
To pain	2	Eyes open to central pain only
No eye opening	1	No eye opening to verbal or painful stimuli

Note
Normal pupils are spherical, usually at mid position and have a diameter ranging from 1.5 to 6mm.
Look at both pupils together: size, equality and shape – monitor reaction to light.

Verbal Response Scored 1–5		
Orientated	5	Able to accurately describe details of time, person and place
Confused	4	Can speak in sentences but does not answer orientation questions correctly
Inappropriate words	3	Speaking incomprehensible, inappropriate words only
Incomprehensible sounds	2	Incomprehensible sounds following both verbal and painful stimuli
No verbal response	1	No verbal response following verbal and painful stimuli

Note
The absence of speech may not always indicate a falling level of consciousness. The patient may not speak English (though he/she can still speak), may have a tracheostomy or may be dysphasic. Some patients may need a lot of stimulation to maintain their concentration to answer questions, even though they can answer correctly.

Motor Response Scored 1–6		
Obeys commands	6	Follows and acts out commands, e.g. Lift up right arm
Localises pain	5	Purposeful movement to remove noxious stimulus
Normal flexion to pain	4	Flexes arm at elbow without wrist rotation in response to central painful stimulus
Abnormal flexion to pain (Withdrawal from pain)	3	Flexes arm at elbow with accompanying rotation of the wrist into spastic posturing in response to central pain
Extension to pain	2	Extends arm at elbow with some inward rotation in response to central pain
No motor response	1	No response to central painful stimulus

Motor response

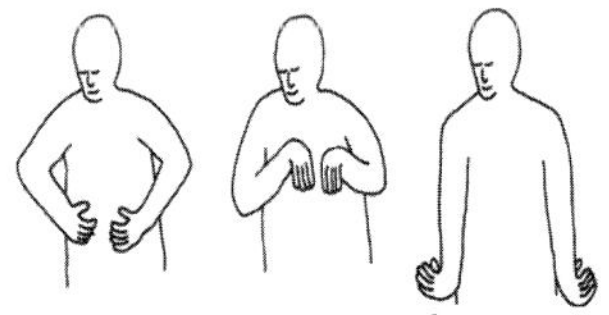

Motor response is tested using the upper limbs since responses to the lower limbs may reflect spinal function.

Evaluation of Painful Stimuli
Painful stimulus should be employed only if the patient does not respond to firm and clear commands. It is always important that the least amount of pressure to elicit a response is applied so as to avoid bruising the patient.

1. Trapezium squeeze – using the thumb and two fingers, hold 5 cms of the trapezius muscle where the neck meets the shoulder and twist the muscle. If the trapezius muscle is pinched the hand should move above the nipple line.
2. Supra-orbital pressure – to be performed only by health care professional competent in this method.
3. Sternal rub – not recommended for repeated assessment.

Clinical Response
If Glasgow Coma Score drops by 2 points or more or is <13 seek urgent assessment by medical team/critical care outreach and an anaesthetist, as this may indicate a neurological emergency. A drop of 1 point must also be considered as a significant change/deterioration and review sought from the nurse in charge/medical team. Any change, and action, should be documented in the patients notes.

Figure 14.44 *Continued*

- *Normal flexion*: no localization is seen; instead, the patient bends their arms at the elbow in response to painful stimuli. This is a rapid response associated with abduction of the shoulder (allocated a score of 4).
- *Abnormal flexion*: internal rotation, adduction of the shoulder and flexion of the elbow in response to painful stimuli. This is much slower than normal flexion and may be accompanied by spastic flexion of the wrist (allocated a score of 3) (Figure 14.45).
- *Extension*: no abnormal flexion is seen. The patient has straightening of the elbow joint, adduction and internal rotation of the shoulder, and inward rotation and spastic flexion of the wrist limb in response to painful stimuli (allocated a score of 2) (Figure 14.45).
- *Flaccid/none*: no motor response is seen at all in response to painful stimuli (allocated a score of 1) (Brain Trauma Foundation 2016).

The AVPU scale

The AVPU scale is a simple, rapid and effective method for assessing consciousness and forms part of the National Early Warning Score 2 (NEWS2) (RCP 2017b). It is particularly useful during the rapid assessment of an acutely unwell patient (RCUK 2015).

AVPU is a mnemonic for a neurological scoring system that quantifies the patient's response to stimulation and assesses their level of consciousness (Brunker and Harris 2015). It stands for Alert, response to Voice, response to Pain or Unresponsive. Assessment using the AVPU method is done in sequence and only one outcome

Table 14.14 Scoring activities of the GCS; the scores are summed, with the highest score (15) indicating full consciousness

Category	Score	Response
Eye opening		
Spontaneous	4	Eyes open spontaneously without stimulation
To speech	3	Eyes open to verbal stimulation (normal, raised or repeated)
To pain	2	Eyes open with painful/noxious stimuli
None	1	No eye opening regardless of level of stimulation
Verbal response		
Orientated	5	Able to give accurate information regarding time, person and place
Confused	4	Able to answer in sentences using correct language but cannot answer orientation questions appropriately
Inappropriate words	3	Uses incomprehensible words in a random or disorganized fashion
Incomprehensible sounds	2	Makes unintelligible sounds, for example moans and groans
None	1	No verbal response despite verbal or other stimuli
Best motor response		
Obeys commands	6	Obeys and can repeat simple commands, for example arm raise
Localizes to pain	5	Purposeful movement to remove painful stimuli
Normal flexion	4	Withdraws extremity from source of pain, for example flexes arm at elbow without wrist rotation in response to painful stimuli
Abnormal flexion	3	Decorticate posturing (flexion of arms, hyperextension of legs) spontaneously or in response to noxious stimuli
Extension	2	Decerebrate posturing (limbs extended and internally rotated) spontaneously or in response to noxious stimuli
None	1	No response to noxious stimuli; flaccid limbs

Source: Adapted from Baumann (2017).

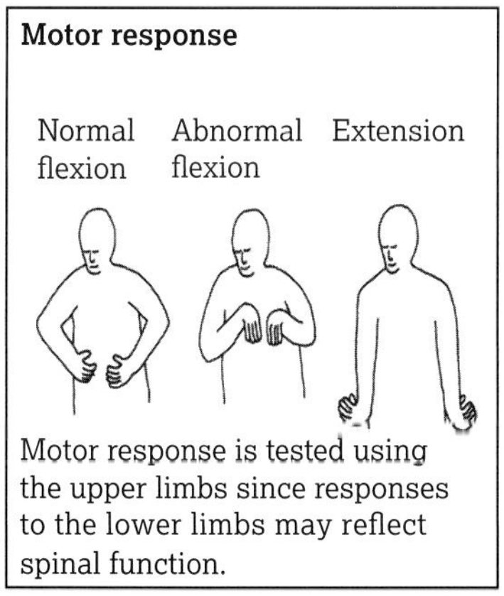
Motor response
Normal flexion
Abnormal flexion
Extension
Motor response is tested using the upper limbs since responses to the lower limbs may reflect spinal function.

Figure 14.45 Normal and abnormal flexion and extension.

is recorded; for example, if the patient responds to voice, it is not necessary to assess the response to pain (Wilkinson et al. 2017):

- *Alert*: a fully awake (although not necessarily orientated) patient. The patient has spontaneous opening of the eyes, responds to voice (although they may be confused) and has motor function.
- *Voice*: the patient makes some kind of response when the assessor talks to them. The response can be in any of the three component measures of eyes, voice or motor. For example, the patient's eyes might open on being asked, 'Are you OK?'. The response can be as small as a grunt, moan or slight movement of a limb when prompted by voice.
- *Pain*: the patient makes a response to a pain stimulus. A patient who is not alert and who has not responded to voice is likely to exhibit only withdrawal from pain, or even involuntary flexion or extension of the limbs from the pain stimulus.
- *Unresponsive*: commonly referred to as 'unconscious'. This outcome is recorded if the patient does not give any eye, voice or motor response to voice or pain (RCP 2017a).

Procedure guideline 14.9 Neurological observations and assessment

Essential equipment

- Personal protective equipment
- Pen torch
- Thermometer
- Sphygmomanometer
- Tongue depressor
- Patella hammer
- Neuro tips
- Glasgow Coma Scale

(continued)

Procedure guideline 14.9 Neurological observations and assessment *(continued)*

Optional equipment
- Low-linting swabs
- Snellen chart
- Ophthalmoscope

Action	Rationale
Pre-procedure	
1 Whether or not the patient is conscious, introduce yourself to the patient, and explain and discuss the procedure with them. If possible, gain their consent to proceed.	Sense of hearing is frequently unimpaired even in unconscious patients. To ensure that the patient feels at ease, understands the procedure and gives their valid consent as far as possible (NMC 2018, **C**).
Procedure	
2 Wash and dry hands and/or use an alcohol-based handrub.	To minimize the risk of cross-contamination (NHS England and NHSI 2019, **C**).
Assessment using the Glasgow Coma Scale (GCS) and AVPU	
3 Observe the patient without speech or touch.	To assess eye opening as part of the GCS and level of consciousness as part of the AVPU (RCP 2017a, **C**).
4 Talk to the patient. Note whether they are alert and giving their full attention, restless, or lethargic and drowsy. Ask the patient who they are, where they are and what day, month and year it is. Also ask them to give details about their family.	To establish whether the patient's level of consciousness is deteriorating. If the patient is becoming disorientated, changes will occur in this order: a disorientation as to time b disorientation as to place c disorientation as to person (Bickley 2016, **E**).
5 Ask the patient to squeeze and release your fingers (both sides should be assessed) and then to stick out their tongue or raise their eyebrows.	To assess the patient's ability to follow commands, to evaluate their motor responses and to ensure that the responses are equal and not reflexive (Baumann 2017, **E**).
6 If the patient does not respond, apply painful stimuli, such as the trapezium squeeze (see the section above on application of painful stimuli).	Responses grow less purposeful as the patient's level of consciousness deteriorates. As their condition worsens, the patient may no longer localize to pain (Baumann 2017, **E**).
7 Extend both hands and ask the patient to squeeze your fingers as hard as possible. Compare grip and strength.	To test grip and ascertain strength. Record the best arm in the GCS chart to reflect the best outcome (Baumann 2017, **E**).
Pupil assessment	
8 Reduce any external bright light by darkening the room, if necessary, or shield the patient's eyes with your hands.	To allow accurate monitoring of pupil reaction and enable a better view of the eye (Bickley 2016, **E**).
9 Ask the patient to open their eyes. If the patient cannot do so, hold their eyelids open and note the size and shape of both pupils simultaneously, and whether they are equal.	To assess the size, shape and equality of the pupils as an indication of brain damage (Kerr et al. 2016, **E**). Normal pupils are round and equal in size with a diameter ranging from 2 to 5 mm (Wilkinson et al. 2017, **E**). See Figure 14.43.
10 Hold each eyelid open in turn. Shine a bright light into the eye, moving from the outer corner towards the pupil. This should cause the pupil to constrict immediately, and there should be an immediate and brisk dilation of the pupil once the light is withdrawn.	To assess the direct light reflex of the pupils (Kerr et al. 2016, **E**).
11 Hold both eyelids open but shine the light into one eye only. Both pupils should constrict immediately and then briskly dilate once the light is withdrawn.	To assess the consensual light reflex (Baumann 2017, **E**).
12 Record pupillary size (in mm) and reactions on the observation chart. Brisk reaction is documented as '+', no reaction as '–', and sluggish response of one pupil compared to the other as 'S'.	Accurate recording will enable continuity of assessment and comply with Nursing and Midwifery Council (NMC) guidelines (NMC 2018, **C**).
13 Record unusual eye movements, such as nystagmus or deviation to the side.	To assess cranial nerve damage (Kerr et al. 2016, **E**).
Vital signs in relation to neurological assessment	
14 Note the rate, character and pattern of the patient's respirations.	Respirations are controlled by different areas of the brain. When disease or injury affects these areas, respiratory changes may occur (Adam et al. 2017, **E**, Baumann 2017, **E**).

15 Take and record the patient's temperature at specified intervals.	Damage to the hypothalamus (the temperature-regulating centre in the brain) will be reflected in grossly abnormal temperatures (Adam et al. 2017, **E**).
16 Take and record the patient's blood pressure and pulse at specified intervals.	To monitor for signs of increased intracranial pressure. Hypertension and bradycardia usually occur late, after the patient's level of consciousness has begun to deteriorate. Call for medical assistance as soon as it is evident that there is deterioration in the patient's level of consciousness (Adam et al. 2017, **E**; Tortora and Derrickson 2017, **E**).
Assessment of strength and co-ordination	
17 Ask the patient to close their eyes and hold their arms straight out in front, with palms upwards, for 20–30 seconds. Observe for any sign of weakness or drift.	To detect any weakness and/or difference of strength in limbs (Baumann 2017, **E**; Bickley 2016, **E**).
18 Stand in front of the patient and extend your hands. Ask the patient to push and pull against your hands. Ask the patient to lie on their back in bed. Place the patient's leg with knee flexed and foot resting on the bed. Instruct the patient to keep the foot down as you attempt to extend the leg. Then instruct the patient to straighten the leg while you offer resistance.	To test arm strength. If one arm drifts downwards or turns inwards, it may indicate hemiparesis. To test flexion and extension strength in the patient's extremities by having the patient push and pull against resistance (Baumann 2017, **E**).
19 Flex and extend all the patient's limbs in turn. Note how well the movements are resisted.	To test muscle tone (Baumann 2017, **E**).
20 Ask the patient to pat their thigh as quickly as possible. Note whether the movements seem slow or clumsy. Ask the patient to turn their hand over and back several times in succession. Evaluate co-ordination. Ask the patient to touch the back of their fingers with the thumb of the same hand in sequence rapidly.	To assess hand and arm co-ordination. The dominant hand should perform better (Baumann 2017, **E**; Bickley 2016, **E**).
21 Extend one of your hands towards the patient. Ask the patient to touch your index finger, then their nose, several times in succession. Repeat the test with the patient's eyes closed.	To assess hand and arm co-ordination and cerebellar function (Baumann 2017, **E**).
22 Ask the patient to place a heel on the opposite knee and slide it down the shin to the foot. Check each leg separately.	To assess leg co-ordination (Bickley 2016, **E**).
Assessment of reflexes	
23 Ask the patient to look up, or hold their eyelid open. With your hand, approach the eye unexpectedly or touch the eyelashes.	To test the corneal (blink) reflex – only if indicated (Bickley 2016, **E**; Fuller 2013, **E**).
24 Ask the patient to open their mouth and hold down the tongue with a tongue depressor. Touch the back of the pharynx, on each side, with a low-linting swab.	To test the gag reflex – only if indicated (Bickley 2016, **E**; Fuller 2013, **E**).
25 Ask the patient to lie on their back in bed. Place your hand under the knee, and raise and flex the leg. Tap the patellar tendon. Note whether the leg responds.	To assess the deep tendon knee-jerk reflex (Bickley 2016, **E**; Fuller 2013, **E**).
26 Stroke the lateral aspect of the sole of the patient's foot. If the response is abnormal (Babinski's response), the big toe will dorsiflex and the remaining toes will fan out.	To assess for upper motor neurone lesions (Baumann 2017, **E**; Bickley 2016, **E**; Fuller 2013, **E**).
27 Ask the patient to read something aloud. Check each eye separately. If their vision is so poor that they are unable to read, ask the patient to count your upraised fingers or distinguish light from dark.	To test for visual acuity (Fuller 2013, **E**).
28 Occlude one ear with a low-linting swab. Stand a short way away from the patient. Whisper numbers into the open ear. Ask for feedback. Repeat for the other ear.	To test hearing and comprehension (Fuller 2013, **E**).
29 Ask the patient to close their eyes. Using the point of a neuro tip (a sharp instrument for applying pressure), stroke the skin. Use the blunt end occasionally. Ask the patient to tell you what is felt. See whether the patient can distinguish between sharp and dull sensations.	To test superficial sensations to pain (Bickley 2016, **E**; Fuller 2013, **E**).
30 Stroke a low-linting swab lightly over the patient's skin. Ask the patient to say what they feel.	To test superficial sensations to touch (Fuller 2013, **E**).

(continued)

Procedure guideline 14.9 Neurological observations and assessment *(continued)*

Action	Rationale
31 Ask the patient to close their eyes. Hold the tip of one of the patient's fingers between your thumb and index finger. Move it up and down and ask the patient to say in which direction it is moving. Repeat with the other hand. For the legs, hold the big toe.	To test proprioception (Bickley 2016, **E**). Proprioception is the receipt of information from muscles and tendons in the labyrinth, which enables the brain to determine movements and position of the body (Tortora and Derrickson 2017, **E**).
Post-procedure	
32 Record the findings precisely in the appropriate sections, noting the patient's best responses. Write exactly what stimulus was used, where it was applied, how much pressure was needed to elicit the response and how the patient responded. Do not be influenced by previous observations.	Vague terms can easily be misinterpreted. Accurate recording will enable continuity of assessment and comply with NMC guidelines (NMC 2018, **C**).
33 Report any abnormal findings to medical staff.	To prevent further deterioration and allow timely intervention (Adam et al. 2017, **E**).
34 Wash and dry hands and/or use an alcohol-based handrub.	To minimize the spread of cross-infection (NHS England and NHSI 2019, **C**).
35 Clean the equipment after use.	To prevent cross-infection (NICE 2014, **E**).

Problem-solving table 14.8 Prevention and resolution (Procedure guideline 14.9)

Problem	Cause	Prevention	Action
Patient's speech difficulties or a language barrier make it difficult to conduct the assessment	Language barrier or dysphasia	Ensure adequate knowledge of methods of interacting with patients speech difficulties. Be aware of translation resources available.	Use an interpreter if there is a language barrier. Use other communication tools (such as picture boards, signalling or allowing the patient to write) as necessary.
Patient not compliant with instructions	Patient is scared or frustrated or does not have a clear understanding of what is being asked	Tell the patient what you are doing and explain the procedure, whether they are conscious or not.	Give details to the patient of what you will be asking, including examples of commands. Explain that some of these might seem unusual but are essential assessments of specific brain functions. If the patient's family are present, ask them not to answer any questions directed at the patient.
Unable to assess strength or movement of limbs due to spinal cord compression, fracture, cast, etc.	Injuries	Ensure thorough knowledge of the patient's previous medical history and current clinical condition.	If at all possible, assess the best response of each limb individually; otherwise chart N/A (not applicable) and record the reasons in the patient's medical notes.
Eyelids closed due to oedema	Fluid overload, trauma, allergic reaction, clinical situation, etc.	Knowledge of patient's previous medical history and current clinical condition.	Attempt to open the patient's eyelids gently but do not force the eyelids open; otherwise record a 'C' for closed.

Post-procedural considerations

Documentation

A validated observation chart (see Figure 14.44) is the most common method of monitoring and recording neurological observations (Adam et al. 2017). Although the layout may differ from chart to chart, in essence all neurological observation charts measure and record the same clinical information, including the level of consciousness, pupil size and response, motor and sensory response, and vital signs (Goulden and Clarke 2016).

Observation charts ensure a systematic approach to collecting and analysing essential information regarding a patient's condition (RCP 2017a). Such charts also act as a means of communication between nurses and other healthcare professionals (Müller et al. 2018).

References

ADA (American Diabetes Association) (2019) Classification and diagnosis of diabetes: Standards of medical care in diabetes – 2019. *Diabetes Care*, 42(Suppl. 1), S13–S28.

Adam, S., Osborne, S. & Welch, J. (2017) *Critical Care Nursing: Science and Practice*, 3rd edn. Oxford: Oxford University Press.

Aehlert, B. (2017) *ECGs Made Easy*, 6th edn. St Louis, MO: Elsevier.

Andrews, P.J.D., Sinclair, L., Rodriguez, A., et al. (2015) Hypothermia for intracranial hypertension after traumatic brain injury. *New England Journal of Medicine*, 373(25), 2403–2412.

Annane, D. (2018) Body temperature in sepsis: A hot topic. *Lancet Respiratory Medicine*, 6(3), 162–163.

Appadu, B. & Lin, T. (2016) Respiratory physiology. In: Lin, T., Smith, T. & Pinnock, C. (eds) *Fundamentals of Anaesthesia*, 4th edn. Cambridge: Cambridge University Press, pp.371–404.

Arslan, G., Eser, I. & Khorshid, L. (2011) Analysis of the effect of lying on the ear on body temperature measurement using a tympanic thermometer. *Journal of Pakistan Medical Association*, 61(11), 1065–1068.

Asadian, S., Khatony, A., Moradi, G., et al. (2016) Accuracy and precision of four common peripheral temperature measurement methods in intensive care patients. *Medical Devices*, 9, 301–308.

Babbs, F. (2015) The origin of Korotkoff sounds and the accuracy of auscultatory blood pressure measurements. *Journal of the American Society of Hypertension*, 9(12), 935–950.

Bailey, M., Griffin, K. & Scott, D. (2014) Clinical assessment of patients with peripheral arterial disease. *Seminars in Interventional Radiology*, 31(4), 292–299.

Bajwa, A., Wesolowski, R., Patel, A., et al. (2014) Assessment of tissue perfusion in the lower limb: Current methods and techniques under development. *Circulation: Cardiovascular Imaging*, 7(5), 836–843.

Bardsley, A. (2015) How to perform a urinalysis. *Nursing Standard*, 30(2), 34–36.

Barry, L., Branco, J., Kargbo, N., et al. (2016) The impact of user technique on temporal artery thermometer measurements. *Nursing Critical Care*, 11(5), 13–14.

Dabuli, T., Acikgoz, O., Tosun, D., et al. (2013) Comparison of three different thermometers in evaluating the body temperature of healthy young adult individuals. *International Journal of Nursing Practice*, 19(5), 471–478.

Bashaw, M.A. (2016) Guideline implementation: Preventing hypothermia. *AORN Journal*, 103(3), 304–313.

Baumann, J. (2017) Neurologic clinical assessment and diagnostic procedures. In: Urden, L., Stacy, K.M. & Lough, M.E. (eds) *Critical Care Nursing: Diagnosis and Management*, 8th edn. St Louis, MO: Elsevier, pp.550–575.

Benmira, A., Perez-Martin, A., Schuster, I., et al. (2016) From Korotkoff and Marey to automatic non-invasive oscillometric blood pressure measurement. Does easiness come with reliability? *Expert Review of Medical Devices*, 13(2), 179–189.

Bickley, L. (2016) *Bates' Guide to Physical Examination and History Taking*, 12th edn. Philadelphia: Wolters Kluwer.

Bijur, P., Shah, P.D. & Esses, D. (2016) Temperature measurement in the adult emergency department: Oral, tympanic membrane and temporal artery temperatures versus rectal temperature. *Emergency Medicine Journal*, 33(12), 843–847.

Blatteis, C. (2012) Age-dependent changes in temperature regulation: A mini review. *Gerontology*, 58(4), 289–295.

Blows, W. (2018) *The Biological Basis of Clinical Observations*, 3rd edn. New York: Routledge.

BNF (British National Formulary) (2019) *British National Formulary*. National Institute for Health and Care Excellence. Available at: https://bnf.nice.org.uk

Bodkin, R., Acquisto, N.M., Zwart, J.M. & Toussaint, S.P. (2014) Differences in noninvasive thermometer measurements in the adult emergency department. *American Journal of Emergency Medicine*, 32(9), 987–989.

Bracci, M., Ciarapica, V., Copertaro, A., et al. (2016) Peripheral skin temperature and circadian biological clock in shift nurses after a day off. *International Journal of Molecular Sciences*, 17(5), E623.

Brain Trauma Foundation (2016) *Guideline for the Management of Severe Traumatic Brain Injury*. Available at: https://braintrauma.org/uploads/03/12/Guidelines_for_Management_of_Severe_TBI_4th_Edition.pdf

Braine, M. & Cook, N. (2017) The Glasgow Coma Scale and evidence informed practice: A critical review of where we are and where we need to be. *Journal of Clinical Nursing*, 26(1/2), 280–290.

Breathett, K., Mehta, N., Yildiz, V., et al. (2016) The impact of body mass index on patient survival after therapeutic hypothermia after resuscitation. *American Journal of Emergency Medicine*, 34(4), 722–725.

British Hypertension Society (2017) *Home Blood Pressure Monitoring Protocol*. Available at https://bihsoc.org/wp-content/uploads/2017/09/Protocol.pdf

British Standards Institution (2017) *Medical Electrical Equipment: Particular Requirements for Basic Safety and Essential Performance of Clinical Thermometers for Body Temperature Measurement*. London: British Standards Institution.

British Thoracic Society (2016) *British Guideline on the Management of Asthma*. Available at: https://www.sign.ac.uk/sign-153-british-guideline-on-the-management-of-asthma.html

Brown, A. & Cadogan, M. (2016) *Emergency Medicine: Diagnosis and Management*, 7th edn. Boca Raton, FL: CRC Press.

Brunker, C. & Harris, R. (2015) How accurate is the AVPU scale in detecting neurological impairment when used by general ward nurses? An evaluation study using simulation and a questionnaire. *Intensive and Critical Care Nursing*, 31(2), 69–75.

Bunce, N. & Ray, R. (2016) Cardiovascular disease. In: Kumar, P. & Clark, M. (eds) *Clinical Medicine*, 9th edn. London: Elsevier, pp.931–1056.

Carney, A., Totten, A.M., O'Reilly, C., et al. (2017) Guidelines for the management of severe traumatic brain injury. *Neurosurgery*, 80(1), 6–15.

Casey, G. (2018) Type 2 diabetes mellitus. *Kai Taiki Nursing New Zealand*, 24(4), 20–24.

Cavill, G. & Kerr, K. (2016) Preoperative management. In: Lin, T., Smith, T. & Pinnock, C. (eds) *Fundamentals of Anaesthesia*, 4th edn. Cambridge: Cambridge University Press, pp.1–28.

Chambers, K. & Burlingame, B. (2016) Clinical issues. *AORN Journal*, 103(3), 338–345.

Chapman, S., Robinson, G., Stradling, J., et al. (2014) *Oxford Handbook of Respiratory Medicine*, 3rd edn. Oxford: Oxford University Press.

Chen, W., Chen, F., Feng, Y., et al. (2017) Quantitative assessment of blood pressure measurement accuracy and variability from visual auscultation method by observers without receiving medical training. *BioMed Research International*, 2017, 1–8.

Chen, Y., Lei, L. & Wang, J.-G. (2018) Methods of blood pressure assessment used in milestone hypertension trials. *Pulse*, 6(1/2), 112–123.

Chiha, M., Samarasinghe, S. & Kabaker, A.S. (2015) Thyroid storm: An updated review. *Journal of Intensive Care Medicine*, 30(3), 131–140.

Chiumello, D., Gotti, M. & Vergani, G. (2017) Paracetamol in fever in critically ill patients: An update. *Journal of Critical Care*, 38, 245–252.

Churpek, M., Snyder, A., Han, X., et al. (2017) Quick sepsis-related organ failure assessment, systemic inflammatory response syndrome, and early warning scores for detecting clinical deterioration in infected patients outside the intensive care unit. *American Journal of Respiratory and Critical Care Medicine*, 195(7), 906–911.

Clarke, D. & Beaumont, P. (2016) Traumatic brain injury. In: Clarke, D. & Ketchell, A. (eds) *Nursing the Acutely Ill Adult*, 2nd edn. London: Palgrave, pp.88–111.

Cleave, L. (2016) Chronic obstructive pulmonary disease. In: Clarke, D. & Ketchell, A. (eds) *Nursing the Acutely Ill Adult*, 2nd edn. London: Palgrave, pp.185–215.

Cobas, M. & Vera-Arroyo, A. (2017) Hypothermia update on risks and therapeutic and prophylactic applications. *Advances in Anaesthesia*, 35(1), 25–45.

Covidien (2011) *Genius™ 2 Tympanic Thermometer and Base Operating Manual*. Mansfield, MA: Covidien.

Coviello, J. (2015) *ECG Interpretation Made Incredibly Easy*, 6th edn. London: Lippincott Williams & Wilkins.

Crawford, J. & Doherty, L. (2010) Ten steps to recording a 12-lead ECG. *Practice Nursing*, 21(12), 622–630.

Dakin, J., Mottershaw, M. & Kourteli, E. (2016) *Making Sense of Lung Function Tests*, 2nd edn. Boca Raton, FL: CRC Press.

Dawes, E. & Durham, L. (2007) Monitoring and recording patients' neurological observations. *Nursing Standard*, 22(10), 40–45.

DeFronzo, R.A., Ferrannini, E., Groop, L., et al. (2015) Type 2 diabetes mellitus. *Nature Reviews: Disease Primers*, 1, 15019.

Delanghe, J. & Speeckaert, M. (2016) Preanalytics in urinalysis. *Clinical Biochemistry*, 49(18), 1346–1350.

Dolan, V. & Cornish, N. (2013) Urine specimen collection: How a multidisciplinary team improved patient outcomes using best practices. *Urologic Nursing*, 33(5), 249–256.

Doyle, J. & Schortgen, F. (2016) Should we treat pyrexia? And how do we do it? *Critical Care*, 20(1), 303.

Drewry, M.A., Ablordeppey, E.A., Murray, E.T., et al. (2017) Antipyretic therapy in critically ill septic patients: A systematic review and meta-analysis. *Critical Care Medicine*, 45(5), 806–813.

Duncombe, S.L., Voss, C. & Harris, K.C. (2017) Oscillometric and auscultatory blood pressure measurement methods in children: A systematic review and meta-analysis. *Journal of Hypertension*, 35(2), 213–224.

Elgart, J.F., Gonzalez, L., Prestes, M., et al. (2016) Frequency of self-monitoring blood glucose and attainment of HbA1c target values. *Acta Diabetologica*, 53(1), 57–62.

El-Radhi, A. (2013) Temperature measurement: The right thermometer and site. *British Journal of Nursing*, 22(4), 208–211.

Environment Agency (2015) *Mercury in Medical Devices Guidance Note*. Available at: https://assets.publishing.service.gov.uk/government/uploads/system/uploads/attachment_data/file/481116/LIT_7108.pdf

Eyer, M.M., Lang, M., Aujesky, D. & Marschall, J. (2016) Overtreatment of asymptomatic bacteriuria: A qualitative study. *Journal of Hospital Infection*, 93(3), 297–230.

Fairley, D., Timothy, J., Donaldson-Hugh, M., et al. (2005) Using a coma scale to assess patient consciousness levels. *Nursing Times*, 101(25), 38–41.

Farenden, S., Gamble, D. & Welch, J. (2017) Impact of implementation of the National Early Warning Score on patients and staff. *British Journal of Hospital Medicine*, 78(3), 132–136.

Fletcher, T., Bleeker-Rovers, C.P., Beeching, N.J. (2017) Fever. *Medicine*, 45(3), 177–183.

Frew, A., Doffman, S.R., Hurt, K. & Buxton-Thomas, R. (2016) Respiratory disease. In: Kumar, P. & Clark, M. (eds) *Clinical Medicine*, 9th edn. London: Elsevier, pp. 1057–1138.

Fuller, G. (2013) *Neurological Examination Made Easy*, 5th edn. Edinburgh: Churchill Livingstone.

Fuller, T., Fox, B., Lake, D. & Crawford, K. (2018) Improving real-time vital sign documentation. *Nursing Management*, 49(1), 28–33.

Gardner, J. (2012) Is fever after infection part of the illness or the cure? *Emergency Nurse*, 19(10), 20–25.

Gasim, G.I., Musa, I.R., Abdien, M.T. & Adam, I. (2013) Accuracy of tympanic temperature measurement using an infrared tympanic membrane thermometer. *BMC Research Notes*, 6(1), 194.

Geijer, H., Udumyan, R., Lohse, G. & Nilsagard, Y. (2016) Temperature measurements with a temporal scanner: Systematic review and meta-analysis. *BMJ Open*, 6(3), e009509.

Goodell, T. (2012) An in vitro quantification of pressures exerted by earlobe pulse oximeter probes following reports of device-related pressure ulcers in ICU patients. *Ostomy Wound Management*, 58(11), 30–34.

Gosmanov, A.R. & Umpierrez, G.E. (2013) Management of hyperglycaemia during enteral and parenteral nutrition therapy. *Current Diabetes Reports*, 13(1), 155–162.

Goulden, I. (2016) Shock presentation. In: Clarke, D. & Ketchell, A. (eds) *Nursing the Acutely Ill Adult*, 2nd edn. London: Palgrave, pp.45–70.

Goulden, I. & Clarke, D. (2016) Acute stroke. In: Clarke, D. & Ketchell, A. (eds) *Nursing the Acutely Ill Adult*, 2nd edn. London: Palgrave, pp.112–139.

Grainger, A. (2013) Principles of temperature monitoring. *Nursing Standard*, 27(50), 48–55.

Greaney J.L., Kenney, W.L. & Alexander, L.M. (2016) Sympathetic regulation during thermal stress in human ageing and disease. *Autonomic Neuroscience: Basic and Clinical*, 196, 81–90.

Hamilton, H., Knudsen, G., Vania, C.L., et al. (2017) Children and young people with diabetes: Recognition and management. *British Journal of Nursing*, 26(6), 340–347.

Haugan, B., Langerud, A.K., Kalvoy, H., et al. (2013) Can we trust the new generation of infrared tympanic thermometers in clinical practice? *Journal of Clinical Nursing*, 22(5/6), 698–709.

Hernandez, J. & Upadhye, S. (2016) Do peripheral thermometers accurately correlate to core body temperature? *Annals of Emergency Medicine*, 68(5), 562–563.

Herreros, M.L., Tagarro, A., García-Pose, A., et al. (2018) Performing a urine dipstick test with a clean-catch urine sample is an accurate screening method for urinary tract infections in young infants. *Acta Paediatrica*, 107(1), 145–150.

Hill, S. & Morgan, M. (2016) *Improving the Quality of Diagnostic Spirometry in Adults: The National Register of Certified Professionals and Operators*. Available at: https://www.pcc-cic.org.uk/sites/default/files/articles/attachments/improving_the_quality_of_diagnostic_spirometry_in_adults_the national register of certified professionals and operators.pdf

Hill, S. & Winter, R. (2017) *A Guide to Performing Quality Assured Diagnostic Spirometry*. Available at: https://www.pcc-cic.org.uk/sites/default/files/articles/attachments/spirometry_e-guide_1-5-13_0.pdf

Hodgson, L.E., Dimitrov, B.D., Congleton, J., et al. (2017) A validation of the National Early Warning Score to predict outcome in patients with COPD exacerbation. *Thorax*, 72(1), 23–30.

Holm, A. & Aabenhus, R. (2016) Urine sampling techniques in symptomatic primary-care patients: A diagnostic accuracy review. *BMC Family Practice*, 17, 72.

Horn, E., Klar, E., Höcker, J., et al. (2017) Prevention of perioperative hypothermia: Implementation of the S3 guideline [in German]. *Chirurg*, 88(5), 422–428.

Jackson, J. (2016) Principles of assessment. In: Clarke, D. & Ketchell, A. (eds) *Nursing the Acutely Ill Adult*, 2nd edn. London: Palgrave, pp.17–44.

Jarvis, S., Kovacs, C., Briggs, J., et al. (2015) Aggregate National Early Warning Score (NEWS) values are more important than high scores for a single vital signs parameter for discriminating the risk of adverse outcomes. *Resuscitation*, 87, 75–80.

Jevon, P. & Ewens, B. (2012) *Monitoring the Critically Ill Patient*, 3rd edn. Chichester: John Wiley & Sons.

Johnson, C., Anderson, M.A. & Hill, P.D. (2012) Comparison of pulse oximetry measures in a healthy population. *MEDSURG Nursing*, 21(2), 70–75.

Karon, B.S., Donato, L.J., Larsen, C.M., et al. (2017) Accuracy of capillary and arterial whole blood glucose measurements using a glucose meter in patients under general anesthesia in the operating room. *Anesthesiology*, 127(3), 466–474.

Keep, J.W., Messmer, A.S., Sladden, R., et al. (2016) National early warning score at emergency department triage may allow earlier identification of patients with severe sepsis and septic shock: A retrospective observational study. *Emergency Medicine Journal*, 33(1), 37–41.

Kerr, R.G., Bacon, A.M., Baker, L.L., et al. (2016) Underestimation of pupil size by critical care and neurosurgical nurses. *American Journal of Critical Care*, 25(3), 213–219.

Khan, G. (2015) A new electrode placement method for obtaining 12-lead ECGs. *Open Heart*, 2(1), e000226.

Kiekkas, P., Aretha, D., Bakalis, N., et al. (2013) Fever effects and treatment in critical care: Literature review. *Australian Critical Care*, 26(3), 130–135.

Kiekkas, P., Stefanopoulos, N., Bakalis, N., et al. (2016) Agreement of infrared temporal artery thermometry with other thermometry methods in adults: Systematic review. *Journal of Clinical Nursing*, 25(7/8), 894–905.

Knowlton, C. (2013) Nurses know how to manage fever, but what about the shivering? *Nursing*, 43(11), 49–51.

Kotagal, M., Symons, R.G., Hirsch, I.B., et al. (2015) Perioperative hyperglycemia and risk of adverse events among patients with and without diabetes. *Annals of Surgery*, 261(1), 97–103.

Kozier, B., Erb, G., Berman, A. & Snyder, S. (2008) *Fundamentals of Nursing: Concepts, Process and Practice*, 8th edn. Harlow: Pearson.

Kreider, K.E., Pereira, K. & Padilla, B.I. (2017) Practical approaches to diagnosing, treating and preventing hypoglycaemia in diabetes. *Diabetes Therapy*, 8(6), 1427–1435.

Launey, Y., Larmet, R., Nesseler, N., et al. (2016) The accuracy of temperature measurements provided by the Edwards Lifesciences pulmonary artery catheter. *Anesthesia & Analgesia*, 122(5), 1480–1483.

Lee, Y.S., Choi, J.W., Park, Y.H., et al. (2018) Evaluation of the efficacy of the National Early Warning Score in predicting in-hospital mortality via the risk stratification. *Journal of Critical Care*, 47, 222–226.

Lelli, D., Pedone, C., Alemanno, P., et al. (2018) Voltammetric analysis for fast and inexpensive diagnosis of urinary tract infection: A diagnostic study. *Journal of Translational Medicine*, 16(1), 17.

Lewis, R. (2013) Too hot … or too cold? *Nursing Standard*, 27(51), 72.

Lin, T. (2016) Physiology of the circulation. In: Lin, T., Smith, T., Pinnock, C. & Mowatt, C. (eds) *Fundamentals of Anaesthesia*, 4th edn. Cambridge: Cambridge University Press, pp.315–344.

Lough, M. (2015) *Hemodynamic Monitoring: Evolving Technologies and Clinical Practice*. St Louis, MO: Elsevier.

Loveday, H.P., Wilson, J.A., Pratt, R.J., et al. (2014) epic3: National evidence-based guidelines for preventing healthcare-associated infections in NHS hospitals in England. *Journal of Hospital Infection*, 86(Suppl. 1), S1–S70.

Mabrey, M. & Setji, T. (2015) Patient self-management of diabetes care in the inpatient setting: Pro. *Journal of Diabetes Science and Technology*, 9(5), 1152–1154.

Malhotra, S., Dhama, S.S., Kumar, M. & Jain, G. (2013) Improving neurological outcome after cardiac arrest: Therapeutic hypothermia the best treatment. *Anesthesia Essays and Researches*, 7(1), 18–24.

Marieb, E. & Hoehn, K. (2016) *Human Anatomy & Physiology*, 10th edn. Harlow: Pearson.

Marieb, E.N. & Hoehn, K. (2018) *Human Anatomy & Physiology*, 11th edn. Harlow: Pearson.

Marieb, E. & Keller, S. (2017) *Essentials of Human Anatomy & Physiology*, 12th edn. Harlow: Pearson.

Marini, J. & Dries, D. (2016) *Critical Care Medicine: The Essentials and More*, 5th edn. Philadelphia: Wolters Kluwer.

Marui, S., Misawa, A., Tanaka, Y. & Nagashima, K. (2017) Assessment of axillary temperature for the evaluation of normal body temperature of healthy young adults at rest in a thermoneutral environment. *Journal of Physiological Anthropology*, 36(1), 18.

Meetoo, D., Wong, L. & Fatani, T. (2018) Knowing where I am: Self-monitoring of blood glucose in diabetes. *British Journal of Nursing*, 27(10), 537–541.

Mehta, Y. & Arora, D. (2014) Newer methods of cardiac output monitoring. *World Journal of Cardiology*, 6(9), 1022–1029.

MHRA (Medicines and Healthcare products Regulatory Agency) (2003) *Infra-red Ear Thermometer: Home Use*. London: Medicines and Healthcare products Regulatory Agency.

MHRA (2013a) *Blood Glucose Meters: Point of Care Testing*. Available at: https://www.gov.uk/government/publications/point-of-care-testing-with-blood-glucose-meters-leaflet

MHRA (2013b) *Blood Pressure Measurement Devices*. Available at: https://www.gov.uk/government/publications/blood-pressure-measurement-devices

MHRA (2017) *IVD Directive: Agency*. Available at: https://www.gov.uk/guidance/medical-devices-eu-regulations-for-mdr-and-ivdr

Morgensen, C.B., Wittenhoff, L., Fruerhoj, G. & Hansen, S. (2018) Forehead or ear temperature measurement cannot replace rectal measurements, except for screening purposes. *BMC Pediatrics*, 18(1), 15.

Morrow-Barnes, A. (2014) Temperature monitoring. *Nursing Standard*, 28(37), 61.

Müller, M., Jürgens, J., Redaèlli, M., et al. (2018) Impact of the communication and patient hand-off tool SBAR on patient safety: A systematic review. *BMJ Open*, 8(8), e022202.

Naalla, R., Chitriala, P., Chittarulu, P. & Atreyapuropua, V. (2014) Sternal rub causing presternal abrasion in a patient with capsuloganglionic haemorrhage. Available at: https://casereports.bmj.com/content/2014/bcr-2014-204028.full

NHS England and NHSI (NHS Improvement) (2019) *Standard Infection Control Precautions: National Hand Hygiene and Personal Protective Equipment Policy*. Available at: https://improvement.nhs.uk/documents/4957/National_policy_on_hand_hygiene_and_PPE_2.pdf

NHS Health Check (2017) *Best Practice Guidance*. London: Public Health England.

NICE (National Institute for Health and Care Excellence) (2007) *Acutely Ill Adults in Hospital: Recognising and Responding to Deterioration* [CG50]. Available at https://www.nice.org.uk/guidance/cg50

NICE (2014) *Infection Prevention and Control Quality Standard* [QS61]. Available at: https://www.nice.org.uk/guidance/qs61

NICE (2015a) *Diabetes (Type 1 and 2) in Children and Young People: Diagnosis and Management* [NG18]. Available at: https://www.nice.org.uk/guidance/ng18

NICE (2015b) *Blood Transfusion* [NG24]. Available at: https://www.nice.org.uk/guidance/ng24

NICE (2015c) *Urinary Tract Infections in Adults* [QS90]. Available at: https://www.nice.org.uk/guidance/qs90

NICE (2016a) *Diabetes in Adults* [QS6]. Available at: https://www.nice.org.uk/guidance/qs6

NICE (2016b) *Hypertension in Adults: Diagnosis and Management* [CG127]. Available at: https://www.nice.org.uk/guidance/cg127

NICE (2016c) *Hypothermia: Prevention and Management in Adults Having Surgery* [CG65]. Available at: https://www.nice.org.uk/guidance/cg65

NICE (2016d) *Type 1 Diabetes in Adults: Diagnosis and Management* [NG17]. Available at: https://www.nice.org.uk/guidance/ng17

NICE (2016e) *Chronic Obstructive Pulmonary Disease in Adults* [QS10]. Available at: https://www.nice.org.uk/guidance/qs10

NICE (2017a) *Type 2 Diabetes in Adults: Management* [NG28]. Available at: https://www.nice.org.uk/guidance/ng28

NICE (2017b) *Asthma: Diagnosis, Monitoring and Chronic Asthma Management* [NG80]. Available at: https://www.nice.org.uk/guidance/ng80

NICE (2017c) *Fever in Under 5s: Assessment and Initial Management* [CG160]. Available at: https://www.nice.org.uk/guidance/cg160

NICE (2017d) *Head Injury: Assessment and Early Management* [CG176]. Available at: https://www.nice.org.uk/guidance/cg176

NICE (2017e) *Sepsis: Recognition, Diagnosis and Early Management* [NG51]. Available at: https://www.nice.org.uk/guidance/ng51

NICE (2017f) *Urinary Tract Infection in Under 16s: Diagnosis and Management* [CG54]. Available at: https://www.nice.org.uk/guidance/cg54

NICE (2018) *Emergency and Acute Medical Care in Over 16s: Service Delivery and Organisation* [NG94]. Available at: https://www.nice.org.uk/guidance/ng94

Nielsen, N., Wetterslev, J., Cronberg, T., et al. (2013) Targeted temperature management at 33°C versus 36°C after cardiac arrest. *New England Journal of Medicine*, 369(23), 2197–2206.

NMC (Nursing and Midwifery Council) (2018) *The Code: Professional Standards of Practice and Behaviour for Nurses, Midwives and Nursing Associates*. Available at: https://www.nmc.org.uk/standards/code

O'Brien, E., Asmar, R., Beilin, L., et al. (2003) European Society of Hypertension recommendations for conventional, ambulatory and home blood pressure measurement. *Journal of Hypertension*, 21(5), 821–848.

O'Donnell, P. & Waskett, C. (2016) Understanding sepsis. In: Clarke, D. & Ketchell, A. (eds) *Nursing the Acutely Ill Adult*, 2nd edn. London: Palgrave, pp.71–87.

O'Driscoll, B.R., Howard, L.S., Earis, J. & Mak, V. (2017) BTS guideline for oxygen use in adults in healthcare and emergency settings. *Thorax*, 72(1), ii1–ii90.

Obermeyer, Z., Samra, J.K. & Mullainathan, S. (2017) Individual differences in normal body temperature: Longitudinal big data analysis of patient records. *BMJ*, 359, j5468.

Paattiniemi, E.-L., Karumaa, S., Viita, A.-M., et al. (2017) Analysis of the costs for the laboratory of flow cytometry screening of urine samples before culture. *Infectious Diseases*, 49(3), 217–222.

Palermo, N.E., Gianchandani, R.Y., McDonnell, M.E. & Alexanian, S.M. (2016) Stress hyperglycemia during surgery and anesthesia: Pathogenesis and clinical implications. *Current Diabetes Report*, 16(3), 33.

Pan, F., He, P., Lui, C., et al. (2017) Variation of the Korotkoff stethoscope sounds during blood pressure measurement: Analysis using a convolutional neural network. *Journal of Biomedical and Health Informatics*, 21(6), 1593–1598.

Pan, F., Zheng, D., He, P. & Murray, A. (2014) Does the position or contact pressure of the stethoscope make any difference to clinical blood pressure measurements: An observational study. *Medicine (Baltimore)*, 93(29), e301.

Patel, M. & Steinberg, M. (2016) In the clinic: Smoking cessation. *Annals of Internal Medicine*, 164(5), ITC33.

Patel, T.P., Rawal, K., Bagchi, A.K., et al. (2016) Insulin resistance: An additional risk factor in the pathogenesis of cardiovascular disease in type 2 diabetes. *Heart Failure Reviews*, 21(1), 11–23.

Patton, K. (2018) *Anatomy & Physiology*, 10th edn. St Louis, MO: Elsevier.

Peate, I. & Bennet-Long, L. (2016) Tests, scans and investigations, 3: Blood HbcA1. *British Journal of Healthcare Assistants*, 10(10), 476–479.

Peate, I. & Wild, K. (2018) *Nursing Practice: Knowledge and Care*, 2nd edn. Oxford: Wiley Blackwell.

Peiris, A.N., Jaroudi, S. & Gavin, M. (2018) Hypothermia. *JAMA*, 319(12), 1290.

Penning, S., Pretty, C., Presier, J.-C., et al. (2015) Glucose control positively influences patient outcome: A retrospective study. *Journal of Critical Care*, 30(3), 445–459.

Perlman, R., Callum, J., Laflamme, C., et al. (2016) A recommended early goal directed management guideline for the prevention of hypothermia-related transfusion, morbidity and mortality in severely injured trauma patients. *Critical Care*, 20(1), 107.

Phang, R. & Manning, W.J. (2019) Prevention of embolization prior to and after restoration of sinus rhythm in atrial fibrillation. *UpToDate*. Available at: https://www.uptodate.com/contents/prevention-of-embolization-prior-to-and-after-restoration-of-sinus-rhythm-in-atrial-fibrillation?search=atrial%20fibrit&topicRef=908&source=see_link

Phillips, A. (2016a) Supporting patients with type 1 diabetes. *British Journal of Nursing*, 25(6), 330–334.

Phillips, A. (2016b) Optimising the person-centred management of type 2 diabetes. *British Journal of Nursing*, 25(10), 535–538.

Pickering, D. & Marsden, J. (2014) How to measure blood glucose. *Community Eye Health*, 27(87), 56–57.

Preiser, J.-C., Chase, J.G., Hovorka, R., et al. (2016) Glucose control in the ICU: A continuing story. *Journal of Diabetes Science and Technology*, 10(6), 1372–1381.

Privšek, E., Hellgren, M., Råstam, L., et al. (2018) Epidemiological and clinical implications of blood pressure measured in seated versus supine position. *Medicine (Baltimore)*, 97(31), e11603.

Provan, A. (2018) *Oxford Handbook of Clinical and Laboratory Investigation*, 3rd edn. Oxford: Oxford University Press.

Rau, C.-S., Wu, S.-C., Chen, Y.-C., et al. (2017) Stress-induced hyperglycemia in diabetes: A cross-sectional analysis to explore the definition based on the trauma registry data. *International Journal of Environmental Research and Public Health*, 14(12), 1527.

RCN (Royal College of Nursing) (2017a) *Principles of Consent: Guidance for Nursing Staff*. London: Royal College of Nursing.

RCN (2017b) *Standards for Assessing, Measuring and Monitoring Vital Signs in Infants, Children and Young People*. London: Royal College of Nursing.

RCP (Royal College of Physicians) (2017a) *National Early Warning Score (NEWS) 2: Standardising the Assessment of Acute-Illness Severity in the NHS*. London: Royal College of Physicians.

RCP (2017b) *Measurement of Lying and Standing Blood Pressure: A Brief Guide for Clinical Staff*. London: Royal College of Physicians.

RCUK (Resuscitation Council UK) (2015) *Resuscitation Guidelines*. London: Resuscitation Council UK.

Reith, F., Brennan, P., Maas, A. & Teasdale, G. (2016) Lack of standardization in the use of the Glasgow Coma Scale: Results of international surveys. *Journal of Neurotrauma*, 33(1), 89–94.

Reynolds, M. (2014) Are temporal artery temperatures accurate enough to replace rectal temperature measurement in pediatric ED patients? *Journal of Emergency Nursing*, 40(1), 46–50.

Rhee, S. (2017) Hypoglycemia and dementia. *Endocrinology and Metabolism*, 32(2), 195–199.

Rhodes, A., Evans, L.E., Alhazzani, E., et al. (2016) Surviving sepsis campaign: International guidelines for management of sepsis and septic shock. *Intensive Care Medicine*, 43(3), 304–377.

Rigby, D. & Gray, K. (2005) Understanding urine testing. *Nursing Times*, 101(12), 60–62.

Robinson, S., Harris, A., Atkinson, S., et al. (2017) The administration of blood components: A British Society for Haematology guideline. *Transfusion Medicine*, 28(1), 3–21.

Roche Diagnostics (2017) *ACCU-CHEK® Safe-T-Pro Plus Lancet*. Available at: https://usdiagnostics.roche.com/en/document/Safety-Pro-Plus-72975.pdf

Salota, V., Slovakova, Z., Panes, C., et al. (2016) Is postoperative tympanic membrane temperature measurement effective? *British Journal of Nursing*, 25(9), 490–493.

Schortgen, F., Clabault, K., Kastahian, S., et al. (2012) Fever control using external cooling in septic shock: A randomized controlled trial. *American Journal of Respiratory and Critical Care Medicine*, 185(10), 1088–1095.

SCST (Society for Cardiology Science and Technology) (2017) *Clinical Guidelines by Consensus: Recording a Standard 12-Lead Electrocardiogram – An Approved Methodology by the Society for Cardiology Science and Technology*. London: Society for Cardiology Science and Technology.

Sequeira, H.R., Mohamed, H.E., Wakefield, D.B. & Fine, J. (2017) A guideline-based policy to decrease intensive care unit admission rates for accidental hypothermia. *Journal of Intensive Care Medicine*. DOI: 10.1177/0885066617731337.

Shapiro, R. & Yaney, E. (2015) Analysis of urinalysis and urine culture methods: Preventing false positive urine specimens. *American Journal of Infection Control*, 43(6), 32.

Sharma, P., Nagarajan, V. & Underwood, D.A. (2015) Heart on the right may [illegible]

Sheerin, N. (2015) Urinary tract infection. *Medicine*, 43(8), 435–439.

Smith, S., Keltner, C., Sikes, R., et al. (2018) Comparison of axillary and temporal artery thermometry in preterm neonates. *Journal of Obstetric, Gynecologic & Neonatal Nursing*, 47(3), 352–361.

Sprigings, D. & Chambers, J. (2017) *Acute Medicine: A Practical Guide to the Management of Medical Emergencies*, 5th edn. Oxford: Wiley Blackwell.

Sudhakaran, S. & Surani, S. (2015) Guidelines for perioperative management of the diabetic patient. *Surgery Research and Practice*, 2015, 1–8.

Summers, C. & McLeod, A. (2017) What influences nurses to undertake accurate assessment of the Glasgow Coma Scale? *British Journal of Neuroscience Nursing*, 13(1), 216–224.

Sund Levander, M. & Grodzinsky, E. (2013) Assessment of body temperature measurement options. *British Journal of Nursing*, 22(15), 882–888.

Swanevelder, J. (2016) Cardiac physiology. In: Lin, T., Smith, T. & Pinnock, C. (eds) *Fundamentals of Anaesthesia*, 4th edn. Cambridge: Cambridge University Press, pp.282–314.

Tait, D., James, J., Williams, C. & Barton, D. (2015) *Acute and Critical Care in Adult Nursing*, 2nd edn. London: Sage.

Taylor, N.S., Michael, J. & Kenny, G.P. (2014) Considerations for the measurement of core, skin and mean body temperatures. *Journal of Thermal Biology*, 46, [illegible]101.

Teasdale, G. & Jennett, B. (1974) Assessment of coma and impaired consciousness: A practical scale. *Lancet*, 2(7872), 81–84.

Torossian, A., Bräuer, A., Höcker, J., et al. (2015) Preventing inadvertent perioperative hypothermia. *Deutsches Ärzteblatt International*, 112(10), 166–172.

Tortora, G. & Derrickson, B. (2011) *Principles of Anatomy & Physiology*, 13th edn. Hoboken, NJ: John Wiley & Sons.

Tortora, G. & Derrickson, B. (2017) *Principles of Anatomy & Physiology*, 15th edn. Hoboken, NJ: John Wiley & Sons.

Trimarchi, H., Young, P. & Lombi, F. (2015) Milky urine and struvite crystals. *Kidney International*, 88(1), 205.

Uppanisakorn, S., Bhurayanotachai, R., Boonyarat, J. & Kaewpradit, J. (2018) National Early Warning Score (NEWS) at ICU discharge can predict early clinical deterioration after ICU transfer. *Journal of Critical Care*, 43, 225–229.

Van Ommen, B., Wopereis, S., van Empelen, P., et al. (2018) From diabetes care to diabetes cure: The integration of systems biology. *Frontiers in Endocrinology*, 8, 381.

Vilinsky, A. & Sheridan, A. (2014) Hypothermia in the newborn: An exploration of its cause, effect and prevention. *British Journal of Midwifery*, 22(8), 557–562.

Virk, S., Donaghue, K.C., Cho, Y.H., et al. (2016) Association between HbA1c variability and risk of microvascular complications in adolescents with type 1 diabetes. *Journal of Clinical Endocrinology & Metabolism*, 101(9), 3257–3263.

Walden, E., Stanisstreet, D. & Graveling, A. (2018) *The Hospital Management of Hypoglycaemia in Adults with Diabetes Mellitus*, 3rd edn. London: Royal College of Nursing.

Wallymahmed, M. (2013) Encouraging people with diabetes to get the most from blood glucose monitoring: Observing and acting upon blood glucose patterns. *Journal of Diabetes Nursing*, 17(1), 6–13.

Waugh, A. & Grant, A. (2018) *Ross & Wilson Anatomy and Physiology in Health and Illness*, 13th edn. London: Elsevier.

WelchAllyn (2015) *Braun ThermoScan Pro6000 Ear Thermometer: User Manual*. Available at: https://www.welchallyn.com/content/dam/welchallyn/documents/sap-documents/LIT/80020/80020802LITPDF.pdf

Wesley, K. (2016) *Huszar's ECG and 12-Lead Interpretation*, 5th edn. St Louis, MO: Elsevier.

West, J. & Luks, A. (2015) *West's Respiratory Physiology: The Essentials*, 10th edn. Philadelphia: Wolters Kluwer.

Weston, D. (2013) *Fundamentals of Infection Prevention and Control: Theory and Practice*, 2nd edn. Oxford: John Wiley & Sons.

Whitmore, C. (2012) Blood glucose monitoring: An overview. *British Journal of Nursing*, 21(10), 583–587.

WHO (World Health Organization) (2010) *WHO Guidelines on Drawing Blood: Best Practices in Phlebotomy*. Geneva: World Health Organization.

WHO (2016) *Global Report on Diabetes*. Geneva: World Health Organization.

Wilkinson, I.B., Raine, T., Wiles, K., et al. (2017) *Oxford Handbook of Clinical Medicine*, 10th edn. Oxford: Oxford University Press.

Winters, S.A., Wolf, K.H., Kettinger, S.A., et al. (2013) Assessment of risk factors for post-rewarming 'rebound hyperthermia' in cardiac arrest patients undergoing therapeutic hypothermia. *Resuscitation*, 84(9), 1245–1249.

Wise, J. (2014) Tight glycaemic control in critically ill children could shorten hospital stays, finds trial. *BMJ*, 38, g137

Yates, A. (2016) Urinalysis: How to interpret results. *Nursing Times*, 7 June. Available at: https://www.nursingtimes.net/clinical-archive/continence/urinalysis-how-to-interpret-results-07-06-2016

Young, P.J., Nielsen, N. & Saxena, M. (2018) Fever control. *Intensive Care Medicine*, 44(2), 227–230.

Zaman, S.S., Rahmani, F., Majedi, M.A., et al. (2016) A clinical trial of the effect of warm intravenous fluids on core temperature and shivering in patients undergoing abdominal surgery. *Journal of PeriAnesthesia Nursing*, [illegible].

Zampronio, A.R., Soares, D.M. & Souza, G.E.P. (2015) Central mediators involved in the febrile response: Effects of antipyretic drugs. *Temperature*, 2(4), 506–521.

Part Four

Supporting patients through treatment

Chapters

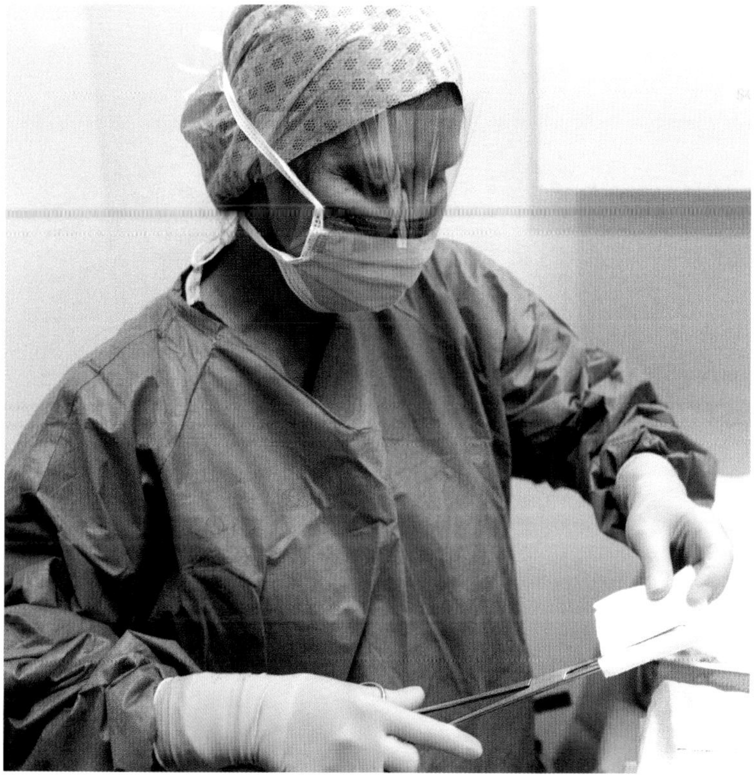

Chapter 15

Medicines optimization: ensuring quality and safety

Lisa Barrott, Emma Foreman and Jatinder Harchowal with Kulpna Daya, Lisa Dougherty and Suraya Quadir

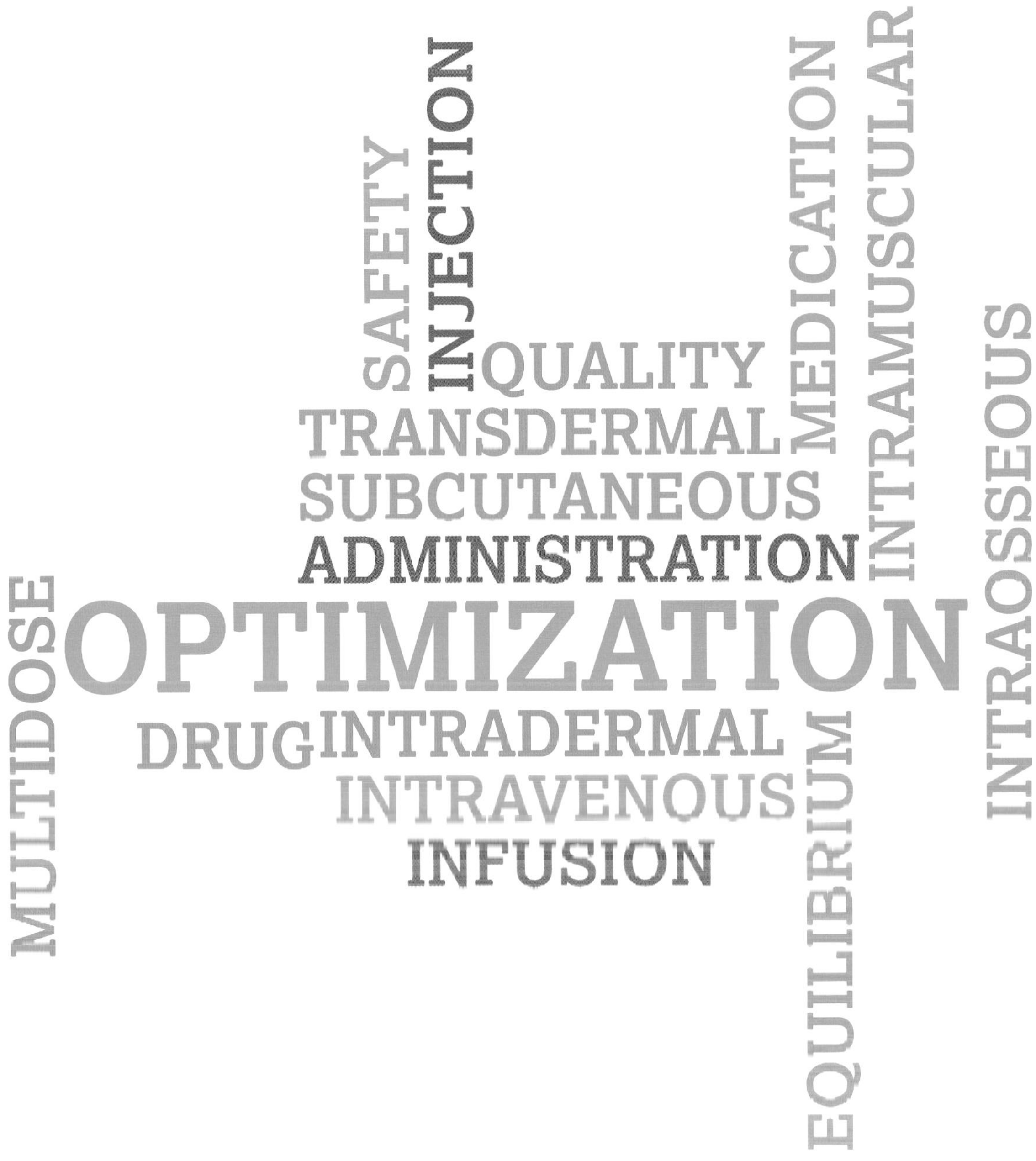
INJECTION
SAFETY
MEDICATION
INTRAMUSCULAR
QUALITY
TRANSDERMAL
SUBCUTANEOUS
ADMINISTRATION
INTRAOSSEOUS
MULTIDOSE
OPTIMIZATION
DRUG
INTRADERMAL
INTRAVENOUS
INFUSION
EQUILIBRIUM

The Royal Marsden Manual of Clinical Nursing Procedures, Professional Edition, Tenth Edition. Edited by Sara Lister, Justine Hofland and Hayley Grafton.

Procedure guidelines

Being an accountable professional

At the point of registration, the nurse will have:

11. Procedural competencies required for best practice, evidence-based medicines administration and optimization.

Future Nurse: Standards of Proficiency for Registered Nurses (NMC 2018)

Overview

This chapter discusses the optimization of medicines. Medicines optimization is about ensuring that the right patients get the right choice of medicine at the right time. By focusing on patients and their experiences, the goal is to help patients to:

- improve their outcomes
- take their medicines correctly
- avoid taking unnecessary medicines
- reduce wastage of medicines
- improve medicines safety.

Ultimately, medicines optimization can help to encourage patients to take ownership of their treatment. However, the medicines optimization approach requires multidisciplinary team working to an extent that has not been seen previously. Healthcare professionals need to work together to individualize care, monitor outcomes more carefully, review medicines more frequently and support patients when needed (NICE 2015c, RPS 2013b). Figure 15.1 shows how this works.

Medicines management

Definitions

Medicinal products and medical devices

The definition of a *medicine* is:

- any substance or combination of substances presented as having properties for treating or preventing disease in human beings; or
- any substance or combination of substances that may be used in or administered to human beings with a view to either (a) restoring, correcting or modifying physiological functions by exerting a pharmacological, immunological or metabolic action, or (b) making a medical diagnosis (Human Medicines Regulations 2012).

The definition of a *medical device* is any instrument, apparatus, appliance, material or other article, whether used alone or in combination, including the software necessary for its proper application, intended by the manufacturer to be used for human beings for the purpose of:

- diagnosis, prevention, monitoring, treatment or alleviation of disease
- diagnosis, monitoring, treatment, alleviation of or compensation for an injury or handicap
- investigation, replacement or modification of the anatomy or of a physiological process.

Additionally, such devices must not achieve their principal intended action in or on the human body by pharmacological, immunological or metabolic means, but may be assisted in their function by such means.

There are three main types of medical device that incorporate or are used to administer a medicinal product:

- devices that are used to administer medicinal products (e.g. medicine spoons, oral syringes or droppers)
- devices for administering medicinal products where the device and the medicinal product form a single integral product designed to be used exclusively in the given combination and that are not reusable or refillable (e.g. pre-filled syringes or eye drop containers)

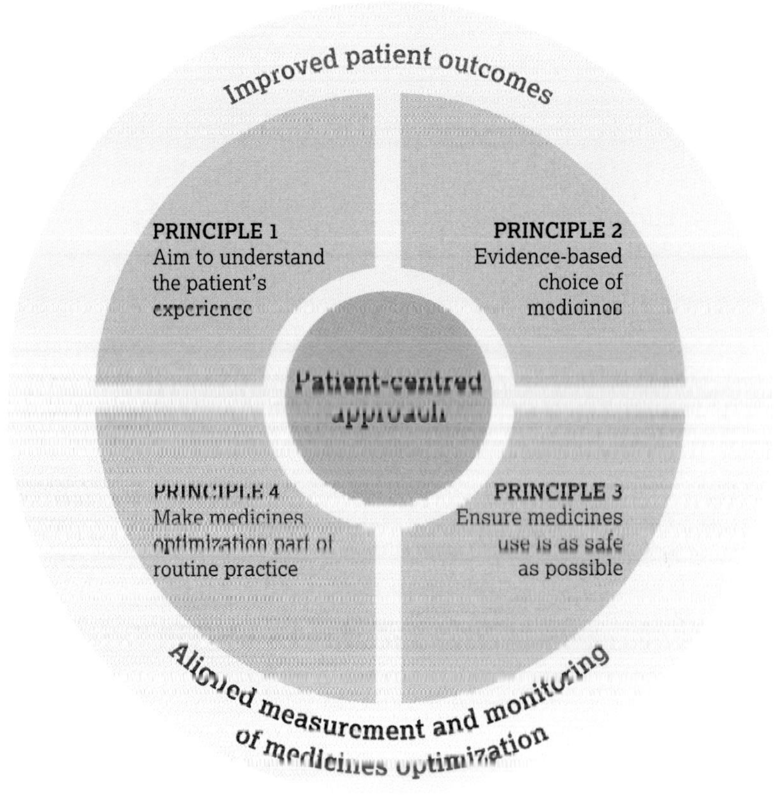

Figure 15.1 A patient-centred approach.

- devices incorporating, as an integral part, a substance that, if used separately, may be considered to be a medicinal product and that is such that the substance is liable to act upon the body with action ancillary to that of the device (e.g. wound dressings with antimicrobial agents) (Council of the European Communities 1993).

Pharmacology

Several terms are relevant to pharmacology:

- *Pharmacology* can be defined as the study of the effects of drugs on the function of living systems. Its purpose is to understand what drugs do to living organisms and, more practically, how their effects can be applied to the treatment of diseases (Rang et al. 2015).
- *Pharmacokinetics* looks at the absorption, distribution, metabolism and excretion of drugs within the body (i.e. what the body does to the drugs). When these four factors are considered alongside the dose of the drug given, the concentration of the drug in the body over a period of time can be determined. Pharmacokinetics is most useful when considered with *pharmacodynamics*, which is the study of the mechanisms of action of drugs and other biochemical and physiological effects (i.e. what the drug does to the body) (Rang et al. 2015).
- The *indication* for a drug refers to the use of that drug for treating a particular disease. Drugs often have more than one indication, which means that there is more than one disease for which they can be used. Indications may be diagnostic, prophylactic or for therapeutic purposes. The licensed indication(s) for a medicinal product are the indication(s) that have been approved by the medicines regulator, which in the UK is the Medicines and Healthcare products Regulatory Agency (MHRA). This means the product has a current marketing authorization – that is, it can be marketed, advertised and supplied for that/those indications.
- A *contraindication* to a medicine is a specific situation in which a medicine should not be used, because it may be harmful to the patient. This could be due to the patient's allergy status, co-morbidities, current disease state or other medicines they are taking.
- A *drug interaction* occurs when a substance (e.g. another medicine or food) affects the activity of a drug when both are administered together. This action can be synergistic (when the drug's effect is increased) or antagonistic (when the drug's effect is decreased) or a new effect can be produced that neither substance produces on its own. Interactions between drugs are termed 'drug–drug interactions' and interactions between drugs and foods are known as 'drug–food interactions' (Medicines Complete 2018). It is important not to forget over-the-counter, herbal and complementary medicines when considering potential interactions.
- *Side-effects* of a medicine are defined by Aronson (2016) as any effects that are in addition to its intended primary effect that can be harmful, unpleasant or in some cases beneficial to the patient. Harmful or unpleasant side-effects are more commonly described as 'adverse drug reactions' (Aronson 2016).

Legislation relating to medicines

Legislative frameworks, government guidelines and professional regulations govern medicines management in the UK. The primary pieces of legislation are the Human Medicines Regulations (2012) and the Misuse of Drugs Act (1971) (see the section below on controlled drugs (CDs) for information on the Misuse of Drugs Act).

The Human Medicines Regulations (2012)

The Human Medicines Regulations (2012) set out a comprehensive regimen for:

- the authorization of medicinal products for human use
- the manufacturing, importing, distribution, sale and supply of those products
- the products' labelling and advertising
- pharmacovigilance.

The regulations were the result of a review of UK medicines legislation by the MHRA and a subsequent consolidation of changes in the law pertaining to medicines for humans since the enactment of the Medicines Act (1968). The regulations replaced nearly all UK medicines legislation, including most of the Medicines Act (1968) and over 200 other statutory instruments.

A number of policy changes were introduced through the regulations to help ensure that medicines legislation is currently fit for purpose. Relevant changes included:

- Medicines legislation allows health professionals and others to sell, supply and/or administer medicines by way of exemptions from the usual restrictions. The regulations removed a number of obsolete exemptions, amended or extended some current exemptions, and introduced some new exemptions in order to reflect modern clinical practice.
- There were updates to the process by which independent hospitals, clinics and agencies are able to continue using patient group directions to ensure processes reflect changes to the registration requirements for these organizations.
- The regulations consolidated provisions enabling a pharmacist, if in the exercise of their professional skill and judgement they believe it is appropriate to do so, to make changes to a prescription relating to the name of the product or its common name; directions for use of the product; and precautions relating to the use of the product. The regulations removed the requirement for the pharmacist to attempt to contact the prescriber before making such changes. 823

The regulations are comprehensive but in terms of medicines optimization they lay out the legal framework for the prescribing, sale and supply of medicines. In addition, they lay out the requirements for labelling of medicines, patient information leaflets and packaging. They also regulate the licensed status of medicines. Apart from some exemptions of specific categories of persons and situations when a prescription-only medicine may be administered without a prescription, there is no reference in the regulations to administration of medicines. The regulations state that a person may not parenterally administer (other than to themselves) a prescription-only medicine unless they are an appropriate practitioner other than a European Economic Area (EEA) health professional or are acting in accordance with the directions of such an appropriate practitioner. There are no regulations relating to medicines administered by the oral or other routes if there is a prescription.

Medicine administration is regulated primarily through professional regulation and governmental guidance, as well as the application of good clinical governance.

Independent prescribers, supplementary prescribers and patient group directions

The Human Medicines Regulations (2012) and subsequent amendments (in 2013 and 2018) state that in addition to medical practitioners and dentists, a number of other healthcare professionals can train to become independent prescribers (IPs) and/or supplementary prescribers (SPs). Furthermore, patient group directions (PGDs) allow specified medicines to be given without a prescription.

Independent prescribers

Independent prescribing allows nurses, pharmacists and other healthcare professionals (as outlined below) who have successfully completed an accredited prescribing course and are registered as IPs to prescribe any medicine including unlicensed medicines (DH 2009) for any medical condition. This includes CDs (Human Medicines Regulations 2012) but only within the healthcare professional's own level of experience and competence, and in accordance with the relevant professional codes. For nurses this is the Nursing and Midwifery Council's (NMC) *Code* (NMC 2018, Public Health England 2006), while other professions have equivalent ethical codes and requirements. Prescribing must also be considered to be part of that nurse's role.

The full list of healthcare professionals who can become IPs is as follows:

- nurses
- optometrists
- paramedics (since 2018)
- pharmacists
- physiotherapists
- podiatrists
- therapeutic radiographers.

IPs, except optometrist IPs, can prescribe medicines for any medical condition within their competence. Optometrist IPs are restricted to prescribing for ocular conditions affecting the eye and surrounding tissue only. Nurse and pharmacist IPs can prescribe any controlled drugs (CDs) except cocaine, dipipanone or diamorphine for the control of addiction. They can prescribe these drugs for other conditions. Physiotherapist and podiatrist IPs can prescribe a restricted list of CDs (see Table 15.1) while optometrist IPs are not permitted to prescribe CDs. There are proposed changes to the legislation that would permit therapeutic radiographer and paramedic IPs to prescribe a range of CDs.

All IPs with the exception of optometrist IPs can authorize an emergency supply of medicines but not for Schedule 1, 2 or 3 CDs, with the exception of phenobarbital for the treatment of epilepsy. Nurse and pharmacist IPs can prescribe unlicensed medicines, subject to accepted good clinical practice, while physiotherapists, podiatrists, optometrists and therapeutic radiographers are limited to 'off label' medicines (i.e. licensed medicines used outside their marketing authorization, again subject to accepted good clinical practice). Presently, paramedic IPs cannot prescribe any unlicensed medicines or prescribe off label.

Supplementary prescribers

Supplementary prescribing has been defined as 'a voluntary prescribing partnership between an IP and an SP to implement an agreed patient specific clinical management plan with the patient's agreement' (DH 2003a). Amendments to the Prescription Only Medicines (Human Use) Order (1997) and the NHS regulations allowed supplementary prescribing by suitably trained nurses from April 2003. SPs prescribe in partnership with a doctor or dentist (the IP) and are able to prescribe any medicine, including CDs and unlicensed medicines, that are listed in an agreed clinical management plan. The plan is drawn up with the patient's agreement, following diagnosis of the patient by an IP and following consultation and agreement between the independent and SPs (DH 2003a, pp.6–7). A range of other professions can be SPs, including some that currently are not permitted to be IPs (Human Medicines Regulations 2012). Practitioners who are SPs have to successfully complete a course of accredited training and be annotated on their professional register as such.

The following professions can be SPs:

- chiropodists
- dietitians
- midwives
- nurses
- optometrists
- paramedics
- pharmacists
- physiotherapists
- radiographers.

All prescribing carried out by an SP must be subject to the practitioner's clinical competence and within an agreed clinical management plan with the patient and IP partner. SPs can prescribe CDs (with the exception of cocaine, dipipanone and diamorphine for the treatment of addiction) and unlicensed medicines, subject to accepted good clinical practice, if they are included in the clinical management plan. Community nurse prescribers can prescribe a range of dressings, appliances and licensed medicines that are listed in the *Nurse Prescribers' Formulary* (BNF 2019a).

The key principles that underpin supplementary prescribing are:

- the importance of communication between the prescribing partners
- the need for access to shared patient records
- the need for the patient to be treated as a partner in their care and to be involved at all stages in decision making, including regarding whether part of their care is delivered via supplementary prescribing (NPC 2003).

Independent and supplementary non-medical prescribers must demonstrate the competencies outlined in the Royal Pharmaceutical Society's Prescribing Competency Framework. This framework is supported by all prescribing professions and accredited by the National Institute for Health and Care Excellence (NICE) (RPS 2019b). The competency framework was developed to set out what good prescribing looks like. It has 10 competencies divided into two domains: 'The Consultation' and 'Prescribing Governance'.

Table 15.1 Controlled drug (CD) prescribing by independent prescribers

Profession	CDs permitted	Notes
Nurse	All CDs with the exception of cocaine, dipipanone and diamorphine for the treatment of addiction.	
Optometrist	Not permitted.	
Paramedic	Proposed changes to legislation still to be considered by the Home Office.	Likely to be a list of CDs for use in emergency situations. No date presently known – check current legislation.
Pharmacist	All CDs with the exception of cocaine, dipipanone and diamorphine for the treatment of addiction.	
Physiotherapist	Restricted to: • diazepam, dihydrocodeine, lorazepam, oxycodone and temazepam for oral administration only • morphine for oral administration or injection • fentanyl for transdermal administration.	
Podiatrist	Restricted to diazepam, dihydrocodeine, lorazepam and temazepam for oral administration only.	
Therapeutic radiographer	Proposed changes to legislation still to be considered by the Home Office.	No date presently known. Check current legislation.

Table 15.2 Royal Pharmaceutical Society's Prescribing Competency Framework

Domain	Competency	Example statements
The Consultation	Assess the patient	1.1 Takes an appropriate medical, social and medication history including allergies and intolerances 1.2 Undertakes an appropriate clinical assessment 1.6 Understands the condition(s) being treated, their natural progression and how to assess their severity, deterioration and anticipated response to treatment
	Consider the options	2.1 Considers both non-pharmacological (including no treatment) and pharmacological approaches to modifying disease and promoting health 2.2 Considers all pharmacological treatment options including optimizing doses as well as stopping treatment (appropriate polypharmacy, de-prescribing) 2.6 Takes into account any relevant patient factors (e.g. ability to swallow, religion) and the potential impact on route of administration and formulation of medicines
	Reach a shared decision	3.1 Works with the patient/carer in partnership to make informed choices, agreeing a plan that respects patient preferences including their right to refuse or limit treatment 3.3 Explains the rationale behind and the potential risks and benefits of management options in a way the patient/carer understands 3.6 Explores the patient's/carer's understanding of a consultation and aims for a satisfactory outcome for the patient/carer and prescriber
	Prescribe	4.1 Prescribes a medicine only with adequate, up-to-date awareness of its actions, indications, dose, contraindications, interactions, cautions and unwanted effects 4.3 Prescribes within relevant frameworks for medicines use as appropriate (e.g. local formularies, care pathways, protocols and guidelines)
	Provide information	5.2 Gives the patient/carer clear, understandable and accessible information about their medicines (e.g. what it is for, how to use it, possible unwanted effects and how to report them, and expected duration of treatment) 5.4 Ensures that the patient/carer knows what to do if there are any concerns about the management of their condition, if the condition deteriorates or if there is no improvement in a specific time frame
	Monitor and review	6.1 Establishes and maintains a plan for reviewing the patient's treatment 6.4 Adapts the management plan in response to ongoing monitoring and review of the patient's condition and preferences
Prescribing Governance	Prescribe safely	7.1 Prescribes within own scope of practice and recognizes the limits of own knowledge and skill 7.6 Reports prescribing errors, near misses and critical incidents, and reviews practice to prevent recurrence
	Prescribe professionally	8.2 Accepts personal responsibility for prescribing and understands the legal and ethical implications 8.4 Makes prescribing decisions based on the needs of patients and not the prescriber's personal considerations
	Improve prescribing practice	9.1 Reflects on own and others' prescribing practice, and acts upon feedback and discussion 9.3 Understands and uses available tools to improve prescribing (e.g. patient and peer review feedback, prescribing data analysis and audit)
	Prescribe as part of a team	10.1 Acts as part of a multidisciplinary team to ensure that continuity of care across care settings is developed and not compromised 10.4 Provides support and advice to other prescribers or those involved in administration of medicines where appropriate

Source: Adapted from RPS (2019b).

Within each competency there are a number of statements that describe the activities or outcomes the prescriber should be able to demonstrate. The domains and competencies, along with some example statements, are outlined in Table 15.2.

Patient group directions

Patient group directions (PGDs) allow healthcare professionals to supply and administer specified medicines to predefined groups of patients without a prescription (NICE 2017b). PGDs were defined in Health Service Circular 2000/026 as 'written instructions for the supply or administration of medicines to groups of patients who may not be individually identified before presentation for treatment' (DH 2000b). Both the NICE guidance and original legislation identify that the preferred method of providing clinical care involving supplying and/or administering medicines should be on an individual, patient-specific basis, usually involving a prescriber. However, it is recognized that there may be situations where PGDs offer an advantage for patient care, without compromising patient safety, and there are clear arrangements for governance and accountability in place. A tool is available (SPS 2018) to help organizations and potential authors and signatories of PGDs to think about and follow necessary procedures before and during the stages of developing and authorizing PGDs, including determining whether the use of a PGD is appropriate.

PGDs must be used only by named and authorized registered health professionals who can legally supply and/or administer medicines using a PGD in line with the Human Medicines Regulations (2012). Healthcare professionals who may supply or administer medicines using a PGD are:

- pharmacists
- registered chiropodists and podiatrists
- registered dental hygienists
- registered dental therapists
- registered dietitians
- registered midwives
- registered nurses
- registered occupational therapists
- registered optometrists
- registered orthoptists
- registered orthotists and prosthetists
- registered paramedics
- registered physiotherapists
- registered radiographers
- registered speech and language therapists.

PGDs must only include medicines with a UK marketing authorization (i.e. licensed medicines), although off-label use of a licensed medicine can be included in a PGD when it is clearly justified by best clinical practice. It is a requirement that the PGD states that the medicine is being used outside the terms of the marketing authorization. 'Black triangle medicines' (i.e. those subject to close adverse drug reaction monitoring and reporting) can also be included when clearly justified by best clinical practice and when the black triangle status is stated on the PGD. If antimicrobials are included on a PGD, care should be taken not to jeopardize local and national strategies to combat antimicrobial resistance and healthcare-associated infections, and a local specialist in microbiology must agree that a PGD is needed.

Schedule 4 and 5 CDs can be included in a PGD, while nurses and pharmacists can supply and/or administer diamorphine or morphine for the immediate necessary treatment of sick or injured persons.

The contents of a PGD are laid out in the legislation (Human Medicines Regulations 2012, NICE 2017b) A PGD should be developed by a multidisciplinary PGD working group with a named lead author. The group must include a doctor (or dentist), a pharmacist and a representative of any other professional group using the PGD. Institutions should have a multidisciplinary PGD approval group, and the group may be an existing local medicines decision-making group, such as a drug and therapeutics committee or medicines management committee.

Similar guidance is available for Scotland (NES 2018).

Unlicensed and off-label medicines

The MHRA states:

> A marketing authorisation or product licence defines a medicine's terms of use: its summary of product characteristics outlines, among other things, the indication(s), recommended dose(s), contraindications, and special warnings and precautions for use on which the licence is based, and it is in line with such use that the benefits of the medicine have been judged to outweigh the potential risks. Furthermore, a licensed medicine: has been assessed for efficacy, safety, and quality; has been manufactured to appropriate quality standards, and when placed on the market is accompanied by appropriate product information and labelling. (MHRA 2014b)

However, there are clinical situations when the use of unlicensed medicines or use of medicines outside the terms of the licence (i.e. 'off label') may be judged by the prescriber to be in the best interest of the patient on the basis of available evidence. Such practice is particularly common in certain areas of medicine, for instance in paediatrics, where difficulties in the development of age-appropriate formulations mean that many medicines prescribed for children are used off label or are unlicensed (MHRA 2014b).

At present, the following healthcare professionals can prescribe unlicensed medicines:

- doctors
- dentists
- independent nurse and pharmacist prescribers
- in some circumstances, SPs (who can be pharmacists, nurses, midwives, community nurses, optometrists, physiotherapists, radiographers, or chiropodists or podiatrists).

In addition to these health professional groups, the following can prescribe a licensed medicine off label:

- nurse IPs
- pharmacist IPs
- optometrist IPs.

However, all healthcare professionals who can prescribe as outlined above are subject to their individual clinical competence, the professional codes and ethics of their statutory bodies, and the prescribing policies of their employers (MHRA 2014b).

The responsibility that falls on healthcare professionals when prescribing an unlicensed medicine or an off-label medicine may be greater than when prescribing a licensed medicine within the terms of its licence. Prescribers should pay particular attention to the risks associated with using unlicensed medicines or using a licensed medicine off label. These risks may include adverse reactions, product quality issues, and discrepant product information or labelling (e.g. absence of information for some unlicensed medicines, information in a foreign language for unlicensed imports, and potential confusion for patients or carers when the patient information leaflet is inconsistent with a medicine's off-label use) (MHRA 2014b).

Supply of medicines

Medicines reconciliation

NICE (2015c) highlights medicines reconciliation as an important component of medicines optimization. NICE uses the Institute for Healthcare Improvement's definition:

> Medicines reconciliation ... is the process of identifying an accurate list of a person's current medicines and comparing them with the current list in use, recognising any discrepancies, and documenting any changes, thereby resulting in a complete list of medicines, accurately communicated. The term 'medicines' also includes over-the-counter or complementary medicines, and any discrepancies should be resolved. The medicines reconciliation process will vary depending on the care setting that the person has just moved into – for example, from primary care into hospital, or from hospital to a care home. (NICE 2015c, p.18)

Medicines reconciliation is the process of determining an accurate list of medicines currently being taken by a patient. The process of medicines reconciliation has five steps (Aronson 2017):

1. list the patient's current medications
2. list the medications currently needed
3. compare the lists
4. make a new list based on the comparison
5. communicate the new list to the patient and caregivers.

NICE (2015c) recommends that in acute settings, an accurate list of all of the person's medicines (including prescribed, over-the-counter and complementary medicines) should be assembled and a medicines reconciliation carried out within 24 hours or sooner if clinically necessary, when the person moves from one care setting to another, typically if they are admitted to hospital. It is also important to recognize that a medicines reconciliation may need to be carried out on more than one occasion during a hospital stay (e.g. when the person is admitted, transferred between wards and discharged).

In primary care, NICE (2015c) recommends that medicines reconciliation is carried out for all people who have been discharged from hospital or another care setting. This should happen as soon as is practically possible, before a prescription or new supply of medicines is issued and within 1 week of the GP practice receiving the information.

Irrespective of the care setting, organizations should ensure that a designated healthcare professional has overall organizational responsibility for the medicines reconciliation process, including:

- organizational responsibilities
- responsibilities of health and social care practitioners involved in the process (including who they are accountable to)
- individual training and competency needs.

Medicines reconciliation should be carried out by a trained and competent healthcare professional, ideally a pharmacist, pharmacy technician, nurse or doctor, who has the necessary knowledge, skills and expertise. In most UK hospitals, medicines reconciliation is performed by a member of the pharmacy team who has completed the necessary local accreditation processes deemed essential to perform this role safely and accurately. NICE (2015c) also recommends that patients and their family members or carers, where appropriate, should be involved in the medicines reconciliation process.

The NICE pathway on medicines optimization highlights the place and role of medicines reconciliation in the overall medicines optimization process (NICE 2015b).

Use of patients' own drugs

Currently, the use of patients' own drugs falls under guidance from the Royal Pharmaceutical Society (RPS 2018). Patients are encouraged to bring their medications into hospital with them to facilitate a comprehensive medicines reconciliation process. Patients' own medicines that are brought into hospital to be used to continue their treatment should be checked for quality and accuracy of labelling. This is frequently done during the medicines reconciliation procedures. Patients' own drugs should be stored at the same security standards as other medicine stock on the ward. They should be used solely for that patient and returned to them on discharge as they remain the patient's property (RPS 2018). They should not be destroyed without prior consent from the patient or, if appropriate, their representative. If the patient agrees to the destruction of the medicines, they must be sent to the pharmacy for destruction. If the patient does not want the medicines to be stored in the hospital or sent to the pharmacy for destruction, they must be sent home with the patient's representative.

Safe storage of medicines

Professional guidance on the safe and secure handling of medicines (RPS 2018) recommends that the overall responsibility for establishing and maintaining a system for the security of medicines should be that of the chief pharmacist in the hospital. They should do this in consultation with senior nursing staff and appropriate medical staff. The appointed nurse in charge of the area will have the responsibility of ensuring that this system is followed and that the security of medicines is maintained. The nurse in charge may delegate some of these duties but always remains responsible for this task. The safe and secure handling of medicines on the ward is governed by a number of principles, as follows.

Security

All medicines (including intravenous fluids) should be stored in a locked cupboard that complies with British Standard (BS) 2881 and/or a locked room with separate storage for internal medicines, external medicines, and medicines needing refrigeration or storage in a freezer. Locks for cupboards (except for patients' own lockers) must comply with BS 3621 as a minimum. All medicines, including intravenous infusion fluids and small-volume injection ampoules, must be securely stored in their original packaging and not loose or decanted (RPS 2018).

A separate cupboard should be provided for CDs; this cupboard must comply with the specifications set out by the Misuse of Drugs (Safe Custody) Regulations (1973) as a minimum. The cupboard must be locked with a key and locking mechanism that complies with BS 3621. Intravenous infusion fluids should also be securely stored in a locked facility.

Diagnostic reagents, including for urine testing, should have a separate cupboard, and there should be separate areas for flammable fluids and gases. Bulk flammable solutions must be stored in a metal cabinet, and a risk assessment must be carried out to determine whether a fire-resistant cabinet is required (RPS 2018).

Where computer-controlled cabinets are used for medicines, they should provide at least the same level of security as traditional lockable cupboards (RPS 2018).

Finally, medicine trolleys should be lockable and immobilized when not in use.

Stability

No medicinal preparation should be stored where it may be subject to substantial variations in temperature (e.g. it should not be stored in direct sunlight). The normal temperature ranges for storage are as follows.

- *Cold storage*: for products that need to be stored between 2°C and 8°C. Refrigerators should be placed in an area where the ambient temperature does not affect the temperature control within them. Refrigerators should have minimum and maximum thermometers fitted; these should be read and reset daily, including at weekends.
- *Cool storage*: for products that need to be stored in a cool place or between 8°C and 15°C. If these temperatures cannot be achieved, these products should be stored in a fridge provided that temperatures below 8°C do not affect the stability of the product.
- *Room temperature*: for products that need to be stored at room temperature or not above 25°C. Temperatures must be monitored on a daily basis and action taken in accordance with local procedures if maximum temperature limits are exceeded (RPS 2018).

Containers

The type of container used may have been chosen for specific reasons. Therefore, all medicines should be stored in the containers in which they were supplied by the pharmacy. Medicinal preparations should never be decanted or transferred from one container to another except in the pharmacy.

Stock control

A system of stock rotation must be operated (e.g. first in, first out) to ensure that there is no accumulation of old stock. Only one pack or container of a named medicine should be in use at any one time. A list of stock medicines to be kept on the ward should be regularly reviewed according to usage figures. The medicines to be held on the ward should be discussed between the nurse in charge and a pharmacist with relevant medical staff (RPS 2018).

Storage requirements for specific preparations

Certain preparations have specific storage requirements:

- *Flammables* must be stored in a separate metal cupboard. If large quantities are required to be stored, then a specific flammables cupboard should be used.
- *Aerosol containers* should not be stored in direct sunlight or over radiators: there is a risk of explosion if they are heated. They must also not be punctured.
- *External creams* may deteriorate rapidly if subjected to extremes of temperature, while *ointments* can become liquid if stored at excessively high temperatures.
- *Eye drops and eye ointments* may become contaminated with micro-organisms during use and thus pose a danger to the recipient. Therefore, in hospitals, eye preparations should be discarded 7 days after they are first opened, unless local policies extend this limit. Eye preparations prescribed for use at home should be discarded after 28 days unless otherwise advised by the manufacturer (BNF 2019a).

- *Reconstituted liquid preparations* have a limited shelf life and therefore will have a short expiry date once reconstituted. If they have been prepared by a pharmacy, the expiry date will be clearly written on the label. In the unusual situation of the product having to be reconstituted by ward staff or the patient/carer, the packaging should be consulted and the expiry date clearly written on the label of the bottle.
- *Liquids* must be used within 6 months of opening unless stated otherwise by the manufacturer.
- *Tablets and capsules* are relatively stable but are susceptible to moisture unless correctly packed. They should be stored only in the containers in which they were supplied by the pharmacy. It is important to ensure that if a bottle contains a desiccant this remains in the pack until it is empty, and it is essential that the desiccant is never inadvertently administered to a patient.
- *Vaccines and similar preparations* usually require refrigerated storage and may deteriorate rapidly if exposed to heat.
- *Medical gases* should be securely stored in a separate area. The health and safety issues associated with medical gas cylinders must also be adhered to (see Chapter 12: Respiratory care, CPR and blood transfusion).

Safe and secure handling of medicines

Handling of medicines is a frequent, everyday nursing activity that carries great responsibility. Nursing associates were added to the NMC register as a separate role in January 2019, and this task has been extended to them, as they are able supply, dispense and administer medicines (but not prescribe them) (NMC 2018).

The effective and safe prescribing, dispensing and administration of medicines to patients demands a partnership between the various healthcare professionals concerned – that is, doctors, pharmacists, nurses and nursing associates. *Professional Guidance on the Administration of Medicines in Healthcare Settings* (RPS 2019a) details how the key principles of compliance with legislation, adherence to guidance, and safety of patients and staff should be applied to the management and handling of medicines. In order to achieve this, organizations should have in place standard operating procedures for each activity in the medicines trail; these should indicate clear responsibilities, training, competencies and performance standards for each member of staff. Processes for validation, audit and risk assessment of the activities also need to be included.

Safe administration of medicines

All nurses and other staff who administer medicines must be familiar with the professional guidance on administration of medicines included in *Professional Guidance on the Administration of Medicines in Healthcare Settings* (RPS 2019a). Nurses are accountable for the safe administration of medicines, which is arguably one of the most common clinical procedures that they will undertake. This can be regarded as the greatest area of risk in nursing practice. To achieve safe administration, nurses must have a sound knowledge of the therapeutic use, usual dose, side-effects, precautions and contraindications of the drug being administered. If nurses lack knowledge of a particular medicine, they must not administer it and must seek advice from a senior colleague.

Institutional policies and procedures will assist nurses to administer drugs safely, and a sound working knowledge of these is essential. Medicines administration requires thought and the exercise of professional judgement. There are a number of 'rights' associated with medicines administration; publications refer respectively to five rights (Federico 2011, MacDonald 2010), six rights (Perry 2015), eight rights (Bonsell 2011) and nine rights (Elliot and Liu 2010) (Table 15.3).

Key principles for administration of medicines

Patient identification

When administering a medicine, the nurse must be certain of the identity of the patient to whom the medicine is to be administered (RPS 2019a), and it is recommended that at least two patient identifiers should be used (e.g. check name, hospital number and date of birth) (Joint Commission 2019). To avoid misidentification of patients, staff should check the patient's identity using an identification wristband, which should meet the nationally required standards for wristbands (NPSA 2007b).

Electronic prescribing and medicines administration (EPMA) systems provide further safeguards when both the patient's identity and the medicine to be administered are confirmed through the use of a bar code reader or similar. If available, these should be used according to local policies and procedures.

Patient misidentification can occur at any stage of a patient's journey (Joint Commission 2018), with incidents relating to medication administration not always captured as they may not always be recognized (Paparella 2012). Not identifying the patient correctly can result in the administration of the wrong drug or dose, and can sometimes be fatal (Schulmeister 2008). The patient's prescription chart should be taken to the bedside to ensure verification against two patient identifiers (e.g. patient name, date of birth and/or hospital number) (Gunningberg et al. 2014, Joint Commission 2018).

Allergy status

Accurate and up-to-date allergy information is important in reducing medicine-related harm to patients. The patient's allergy status must be current at all times. This should include identifying positively where a patient does not have an allergy. If it is not possible to determine whether a patient has an allergy, this should be documented as 'unable to ascertain', and the actual allergy status should be documented as soon as the information is available (NICE 2014). It is the responsibility of all healthcare professionals involved in the patient's care to update and document any identified allergies, hypersensitivities, anaphylaxis or drug intolerances (Jevon 2008, Shelton and Shivnan 2011).

Allergic reactions are immune mediated and can be classified as in Table 15.4. There are many risk factors that increase the likelihood of an allergic reaction. These can be split into those that are specific to the patient and those that are specific to the drug. The patient-related factors and drug-related factors are listed in Boxes 15.1 and 15.2 respectively.

Although the incidence of true allergic drug reactions is low, the potential morbidity and mortality related to these reactions can be high, so it is important that drug allergies are accurately diagnosed and treated. The first step towards an accurate diagnosis is a detailed history (Mirakian et al. 2009). Guidance on what information should be collated and accurately recorded is detailed in the British Society for Allergy and Clinical Immunology's drug allergy guidelines (Mirakian et al. 2009) and in NICE (2014) guidance, and include the following:

- Detailed description of reaction:
  - symptom sequence and duration
  - treatment provided
  - outcome.
- Timing of symptoms in relation to drug administration.
- Has the patient had the suspected drug before this course of treatment?
  - How long had the drug(s) been taken before onset of reaction?
  - When was/were the drug(s) stopped?
  - What was the effect?
- Witness description (from patient, relative or doctor).
- Is there a photograph of the reaction?
- Illness for which suspected drug was being taken – that is, underlying illness (this may be the cause of the symptoms, rather than the drug).
- List of all drugs taken at the time of the reaction (including regular medication, over-the-counter medications and 'alternative' remedies).
- Previous history
  - other drug reactions
  - other allergies
  - other illnesses.

Table 15.3 The rights associated with medicines administration

	Five rights	Six rights	Eight rights	Nine rights
Patient • Check name on prescription • Use at least two identifiers (e.g. name and date of birth) • Ask patient to identify themselves • Use technology when available (bar codes)	✓	✓	✓	✓
Medicine • Check the prescription • Check the medication label	✓	✓	✓	✓
Route • Check the prescription and appropriateness • Confirm the patient can take or receive the medication by the prescribed route	✓	✓	✓	✓
Time • Check the frequency on the prescription • Check the medication is being given at the right time • Confirm when the last dose was given	✓	✓	✓	✓
Dose • Check name on prescription • Check appropriateness • Calculate dose if necessary	✓	✓	✓	✓
Documentation • Document *after* giving the prescribed medication • Chart the time and route, your signature and any other specific information as necessary		✓	✓	✓
Reason/Action • Confirm the rationale for the prescribed medication			✓	✓
Response/Form • Has the drug had the desired effect? • Document monitoring			✓	✓
Education/Consent • Check whether the patient understands what the medication is for Make the patient aware that they should contact their healthcare professional if they experience side-effects or reactions • Ensure you have patient consent to administer medication, and be aware that patients have the right to refuse medication if they have capacity to do so				✓

Source: Adapted from Bonsell (2011), Elliot and Lui (2010), Federico (2011), MacDonald (2010), Perry (2015).

Table 15.4 Types of allergic reactions

Type of reaction	Result of reaction	Example of reaction
Type I: IgE-mediated reactions	Urticaria, angio-oedema, anaphylaxis and bronchospasm	Anaphylaxis from beta-lactam antibiotic
Type II: IgG/M-mediated cytotoxic reactions	Anaemia, cytopenia and thrombocytopenia	Haemolytic anaemia from penicillin
Type III: IgG/M-mediated immune complexes (also known as 'serum sickness')	Vasculitis, lymphadenopathy, fever, arthropathy and rashes	Serum sickness from antithymocyte globulin
Type IV: Delayed hypersensitivity reactions	Dermatitis, bullous exanthema, maculopapular and pustular xanthemata	Contact dermatitis from topical antihistamine

IgE, immunoglobulin type E; IgG/M, immunoglobulin type G/M.

Source: Adapted from Beijnen and Schellens (2004), Riedl and Casillas (2003).

Advice on the management of a drug reaction is provided in Box 15.3. In some cases desensitization may be considered, but this is rarely indicated.

Following an allergic reaction, it is extremely important that the patient is given information regarding what substances they should avoid. This information must be recorded clearly in the patient's medical records, including paper and electronic records. All inpatients with an allergy should have this indicated by wearing a red-coloured identity band (NHSI 2018b). The allergic drug reaction should also be reported using the Yellow Card Scheme (Mirakian et al. 2009) (see 'Adverse drug reactions' below).

Prior to administering any medication, the nurse must confirm the patient's allergy status and where necessary document any changes.

Box 15.1 Allergic reactions: patient-related risk factors

- *Immune status*: previous reaction to the same or related compound.
- *Age*: younger adults are more likely to have an allergic reaction than infants or the elderly.
- *Gender*: women are more likely than men to suffer skin reactions.
- *Genetic*: atopic predisposition is more likely to result in a severe reaction, and genetic polymorphisms (e.g. G6PD deficiency, slow acetylators) may predispose a person to drug hypersensitivity.
- *Concomitant disease*: viral infections such as HIV and herpes are associated with an increased risk of allergic reactions. Cystic fibrosis is associated with an increased risk of allergic reactions to antibiotics, which is thought to be due to prolonged use in this group of patients.

Source: Adapted from Mirakian et al. (2009) with permission of John Wiley & Sons.

Box 15.2 Allergic reactions: drug-related risk factors

- *Drug chemistry*: some drugs are more likely to cause drug reactions than others. These are high-molecular-weight compounds, such as insulin. Additionally, drugs that bind to proteins called haptens (e.g. beta-lactam antibiotics) form complexes that can cause an immune response.
- *Route of administration*: the topical route is most likely to cause an allergic reaction, with the oral route being the least likely. The intramuscular route is more likely to cause an allergic reaction than the intravenous route.
- *Dose*: a large single dose is less likely to cause a reaction than prolonged or frequent doses.

Source: Adapted from Mirakian et al. (2009) with permission of John Wiley & Sons.

Box 15.3 Treatment of acute drug reactions

An acute drug reaction must be treated promptly and appropriately:

1 Stop the suspected drug.
2 Treat the reaction.
3 Identify and avoid potential cross-reacting drugs.
4 Record precise details of the reaction and its treatment.
5 Identify a safe alternative. In some cases this may not be possible so, where the case is less severe, it may be decided to continue with the medication with suppression of the symptoms with, for example, a corticosteroid and an antihistamine.

See also 'Complications' within 'Intravenous injections and infusions' below.

Source: Adapted from Mirakian et al. (2009) with permission of John Wiley & Sons.

Medication checks

The nurse must know the therapeutic uses of the medicine to be administered as well as its normal dosage, side-effects, precautions and contraindications. If the nurse has concerns regarding the prescription or the prescription is not clear, the prescriber or pharmacist must be contacted. If weight and/or height are required for calculation of the dose, a recent height and weight must have been used.

Calculating the required dose is vital as any miscalculation of medication dosage represents a potential threat to both patient safety and clinical effectiveness (Hayes et al. 2009). It is important for nurses to acquire and maintain mathematical competency in practice in order to prevent medication errors (Brady et al. 2009), although there is insufficient evidence to conclude that medication errors can be linked to nurses' poor calculation skills (Sherriff et al. 2011, Wright 2010). Incorporating computer-based competency within practice and practice simulation assessments has been shown to be highly effective in medication calculation training for nurses (Sabin et al. 2013), but more research is required (Stolic 2014).

To ensure the patient receives the intended treatment, the following checks must be performed:

- correct medicine and formulation selected
- correct dose prepared
- medicine within expiry date
- correct route, administration time and rate (if applicable).

If a delivery device is required, the correct device must be used (e.g. a vascular access device for intravenous therapy or an epidural catheter for epidural drug administration).

Record of administration

The nurse must document a clear, accurate and immediate record of all medicines administered, intentionally withheld or refused by the patient, ensuring all written entries and signatures are clear and legible. If any medication is withheld or refused by a patient, the reasons must be documented, and, where appropriate, the prescriber and/or multiprofessional team must be informed (RPS 2019a).

Single or double checking of medicines

Medicines can be prepared and administered by a single qualified nurse or by two nurses (known as double checking). There are certain times when double or second checking is required. It is recommended that for the administration of CDs, a secondary signature is required. Additionally, where the administration of a medicine requires complex calculations, it is deemed good practice for a second practitioner (a registered professional) to check the calculation independently in order to minimize the risk of error (RPS 2019a).

Single checking can ensure greater accountability, increase attentiveness to procedures, encourage updating of drug knowledge and better use nursing time (Cross et al. 2017). In contrast, double checking can dilute individual responsibility and contribute to increased medication errors (Armitage 2009). More research is required, however, especially in paediatric management (Conroy et al. 2012).

An alternative is the use of independent double checking. This is when two nurses check a drug independently of each other. In the setting up of ambulatory chemotherapy pumps, a study showed that the use of independent double checking showed no significantly statistical difference in dose, rate or documentation errors when compared with traditional double checking, but it did show a reduction in errors related to patient identification (Savage and Tripp 2008).

Those nurses who wish or need to have their administration supervised should retain the right to do so until such a time as all parties agree that the requested level of proficiency has been achieved. The nurse checking the medicine must be able to justify any action taken and be accountable for the action taken. This is in keeping with the principles of *The Code* (NMC 2018).

Delegation of medicines administration

If a registered nurse or nursing associate delegates any aspect of the administration of a medicinal product to a patient, their carer or a care assistant, they remain accountable for the delegatee's actions and non-actions and any omissions that occur (NMC 2018). As a registered professional, they are accountable for all aspects of their practice, which includes delegating a task or accepting a task delegated to them. When delegating, the registered nurse or nursing associate must ensure that the task is within the individual's scope of competence, that the individual fully understands the instructions, and that they are adequately supervised and supported (NMC 2018). Student nurses must never administer or supply medicinal products without direct supervision, and both the student and the registered nurse must sign the medication chart or document the administration in the notes (NMC 2018).

Additional factors to consider

Drug interactions

Consideration should also be given to potential interactions between concomitant drugs and/or food. These interactions can result in an increased effect (causing toxicity) or a decreased effect (resulting in decreased efficacy of the drug). Drug interactions can be divided into pharmacokinetic (Table 15.5) and pharmacodynamic (Table 15.6) interactions.

Herbal and complementary medicines have increasingly been used in the UK over recent years and as a result there has been an increase in the reporting of interactions between these agents and conventional drugs. Some of the most common herbal interactions are those containing St John's wort, a popular herbal product used as an antidepressant. Concomitant use should be avoided with, for example, antiepileptics, antivirals and warfarin.

Interactions can also occur between drugs and food. Food can have an effect on drugs by changing gastrointestinal motility or by binding to drugs while in transit in the gastrointestinal tract. An example of interactions between food and a drug can be seen with monoamine oxidase inhibitors (MAOIs) and tyramine-containing foods (such as mature and aged cheeses, yeast or meat extracts, pickled fish, salami, broad bean pods and heavy red wines). Tyramine is a chemical present in certain foods that are rich in protein and can interact with MAOIs. As procarbazine has mild MAOI properties, taking both together can result in a hypertensive reaction, which can cause symptoms of raised blood pressure, headache, pounding heart, neck stiffness, sweating, flushing and vomiting. Patients taking MAOIs should therefore be advised to avoid tyramine-rich foods (Medicines Complete 2018). The *British National Formulary* has a comprehensive list of drug interactions and the potential clinical consequences (BNF 2019a). Concerns over actual drug interactions and their management should be discussed with a pharmacist.

Adverse drug reactions

Although drugs are used to diagnose, prevent or treat disease, no drug is administered without risk. It is important when choosing a drug treatment that consideration is given to the balance between clinical effect and undesired effects.

The World Health Organization's (WHO) definition of adverse drug reactions (ADRs) is 'harmful, unintended reactions to medicines that occur at doses normally used for treatment' (WHO 2008, p.1). ADRs can be classified as type A or type B reactions. Type A ('augmented') reactions are considered to be exaggerations of the medicine's normal effect when given at the usual dose. This category includes unwanted reactions that are predictable from the drug's pharmacology and are usually dose dependent (e.g. respiratory depression with opioids and bleeding with warfarin). In many instances this type of unwanted effect is reversible and the problem can often be dealt with by reducing the dose (Rang et al. 2015).

Type B ('bizarre or idiosyncratic') reactions are effects that are not pharmacologically predictable and can include hypersensitivity reactions (e.g. anaphylaxis with beta-lactam antibiotics). These are not related to the pharmacological action of the drug and are not dose related, and therefore cannot be controlled by dose reduction. Type A reactions are more common than type B but type B reactions tend to cause higher rates of serious illness and mortality.

Table 15.5 Types of pharmacokinetic interaction

Type of interaction	Interaction caused by	Example of when to consider in clinical practice
Drug absorption interactions	• Changes in the gastrointestinal (GI) pH • Adsorption or chelation in the GI tract • Changes in GI motility • Induction or inhibition of transporter proteins or malabsorption	In cases of tetracycline absorption interaction with milk, bisphosphonate use, etc. (Medicines Complete 2018)
Drug distribution interactions	• Protein binding or inhibition or induction of drug transporter proteins	Therapeutic drug monitoring, as drugs that can be displaced in this way (e.g. phenytoin) can appear subtherapeutic when monitored but doses would not need to be increased (Medicines Complete 2018)
Drug metabolism interactions	• Changes in first pass metabolism, enzyme induction, enzyme inhibition and genetic factors • The hepatic cytochrome P450 enzyme system is the major site of drug metabolism and most drug–drug interactions occur at this site	Grapefruit juice can inhibit the cytochrome P450 isoenzyme CYP3A4, thus reducing the metabolism of calcium channel blockers (Medicines Complete 2018)
Drug excretion interactions	• Changes in urinary pH, active renal tubular excretion, renal blood flow and biliary excretion, or the enterohepatic shunt	Probenecid and penicillin compete for the same active transport systems in the renal tubules; as a result, probenecid reduces the excretion of penicillin, which can lead to penicillin toxicity (Medicines Complete 2018)

Table 15.6 Types of pharmacodynamic interaction

Type of interaction	Interaction caused by	Example of when to Consider in Clinical practice
Additive or synergistic interactions	• Two drugs can have the same pharmacological effect and therefore the results can be additive	Opioids with benzodiazepines can cause increased drowsiness (Medicines Complete 2018)
Antagonistic or opposing interactions	• Two drugs can have opposing activities	Vitamin K and warfarin result in the effects of the anticoagulant being opposed (Medicines Complete 2018)

The WHO (2008) states that 'ADRs are among the leading causes of death in many countries'. Drug-related adverse events, including ADRs, have been reported to be among the leading causes of morbidity and mortality (de Vries 2008, Lazarou et al. 1998). ADRs occur in both outpatients and inpatients (Kongkaew et al. 2008, Krähenbühl-Melcher et al. 2007, Leendertse et al. 2010). In a meta-analysis conducted in 2002, an average of 4.9% of hospital admissions were associated with ADRs, with the rate ranging between 0.2% and 41.3% in individual studies (Beijer and de Blaey 2002). This meta-analysis considered that 28.9% of the ADR-related hospitalizations were preventable. Of inpatients, 10.9% are estimated to experience an ADR during hospitalization (Lazarou et al. 1998). A more recent meta-analysis has shown that among adult outpatients, 2% had ADRs, of which 52% were preventable. Among inpatients, 1.6% had ADRs, of which 45% were preventable (Hakkarainen et al. 2012).

According to the WHO (2008), the cost of ADRs, including hospitalizations, surgery and lost productivity, exceeds the cost of medicines in some countries. Work in the US a number of years ago (Rodriguez-Monguio et al. 2003) showed that significant costs may be avoided if drug-related adverse events, including ADRs, are prevented.

Although the effect of a drug cannot always be predicted, it is important that when a drug is given to a patient, the risk of harm is minimized by ensuring that the prescribed medicine is of good quality, safe, effective and used by the right patient in the right dose at the right time. Consideration should always be given to predisposing factors that drugs or a patient may have that could increase the risk of ADRs, including:

- polypharmacy
- age of the patient
- gender
- co-morbidities (e.g. renal disease)
- race
- genetic factors
- allergies
- drug–drug interactions (Medicines Complete 2018, Whittlesea and Hodson 2018, Zeind and Carvalho 2018).

Preventing and detecting adverse effects from medicines is termed 'pharmacovigilance'. It is an important factor for all healthcare professionals to consider in order to identify potential new hazards relating to medicines and prevent harm to patients (MHRA 2010a).

Although medicines are widely tested within clinical trials before they become commercially available, trials do not provide information about how different patient populations may respond to the medicines. The only way for this information to be collected is through careful patient monitoring and further collection of data through post-marketing surveillance. In the UK this information is collected through the Yellow Card Scheme, which is run by the MHRA and the Commission on Human Medicines. The scheme is used to collect information from both healthcare professionals and patients about suspected ADRs with prescribed medicines, over-the-counter medicines and herbal medicines. Yellow Cards can be completed via the MHRA website (https://yellowcard.mhra.gov.uk) or by completing the paper card found in the *British National Formulary*.

Medication errors: definition and causes

A medication error is a failure in treatment procedures that leads to, or has the potential to lead to, patient harm (Aronson 2009). Medication administration errors occur frequently and are more likely to result in serious harm and death than other types of medication error (Westbrook et al. 2011). Direct observational studies in hospitals estimate that errors occur in 19–27% of instances when drugs are administered to patients (Westbrook et al. 2011). Studies have demonstrated that interruptions are common and that these and other distractions can increase error and accident rates relating to drug administration (Relihan et al. 2010, Westbrook et al. 2010) (Box 15.4).

Box 15.4 Key areas of risk for medication error

- Wrong drug or diluent
- Calculation errors
- Level of knowledge
- Administration to wrong patient
- Administration via wrong route
- Unsafe handling or poor aseptic technique

Clinical governance

Medicines safety, governance and risk management

Medication is the most common intervention in medicine and is a critical component of modern healthcare. Medication has huge potential to do good, but errors can occur at many points in the medication cycle; these can have a significant impact on patients and be a considerable burden on the NHS.

In 2000, the report *An Organisation with a Memory* (DH 2000a) recognized that preventable harms were occurring frequently in the NHS. Following this report, the National Patient Safety Agency (NPSA) and the National Reporting and Learning System (NRLS), a single, national reporting system for patient safety incidents in England and Wales, were set up in 2001 and 2003 respectively. Another national initiative, the Yellow Card Scheme, for the reporting of side-effects of medicines, was set up in 1964 and is now run by the MHRA.

In 2014, NHS England and the MHRA issued a joint alert *Improving Medication Error Incident Reporting and Learning* (NHS England 2014), which aimed to improve the quality of data reported by providers and introduce national networks to maximize learning and provide guidance on minimizing harm relating to medication error reporting. In 2016, NHSI became the central body responsible for overseeing patient safety in England and in 2019 it merged with NHS England to form one central body. The WHO Global Patient Safety Challenge was launched in 2017 to reduce the level of severe, avoidable harm related to medications by 50% over 5 years globally. Its three early priority actions focus on polypharmacy, high-risk situations and transfers of care. These sit within an overarching strategic framework of four domains:

- patients and the public
- medicines
- healthcare professionals
- systems and practices of medication.

Reduction in medication errors will be achieved by encouraging countries and key stakeholders to focus on early action priorities as well as developmental programmes to improve practice and health systems.

Medication errors can include prescribing, dispensing, administration and monitoring errors. Medication errors can result in ADRs, drug–drug interactions, lack of efficacy, suboptimal patient adherence, and poor quality of life and patient experience. It has been reported that:

- an estimated 237 million medication errors occur in the NHS in England every year
- 28% of this total cause moderate or serious harm, and 72% cause little or no harm
- the estimated costs to the NHS of definitely avoidable ADRs are £98.5 million per year; ADRs also consume 181,626 bed days, cause 712 deaths and contribute to 1708 deaths (Elliott et al. 2018).

A review of all medication safety incidents reported to the NRLS between 2005 to 2010 highlighted that incidents involving administration (50%) and prescribing (18%) followed by dispensing or preparation of medicines (16%) caused the highest number of reports. Omitted and delayed medication (16%) and wrong dose (15%) represented the largest error categories (Cousins et al. 2012).

Organizations should have clinical governance structures in place to ensure that medication reporting systems are operating effectively and that important medication safety incidents are addressed locally. Organizations should have defined medication safety roles, such as a medicines optimization lead, a controlled drugs accountable officer and a medication safety officer. Procedures for reporting and investigating near misses and patient safety incidents should aim to support active learning and ensure that the positive lessons learned from these events are embedded into the organization's culture and practices. Learning from incidents and near misses is an essential part of integrated governance and risk management.

Never Events

'Never Events' are defined as serious patient safety incidents that are 'wholly preventable because guidance or safety recommendations that provide strong systemic protective barriers are available at a national level and should have been implemented by all healthcare providers' (NHSI 2018c, p.4).

Each Never Event type has the potential to cause serious patient harm or death. However, serious harm or death does not need to have happened as a result of a specific incident for that incident to be categorized as a Never Event. For each Never Event type, there is evidence that the Never Event has occurred in the past and that the risk remains. Occurrence of a Never Event indicates that an organization may not have put the right systems and processes in place to prevent incidents from happening. It is important that when a Never Event happens, the problem is identified and analysed through a comprehensive investigation to understand how and why it occurred, as described in the Serious Incident framework. This will ensure that effective action can be taken to prevent incident recurrence (NHSI 2018c).

There are currently five Never Events that are associated with medicines use (NHSI 2018c):

- *Mis-selection of a strong potassium solution*: this refers to when a patient is intravenously given a strong (greater or equal to 10%, 1 g/mL or 1.3 mmol/mL of potassium chloride) potassium solution rather than the intended medication. There is clear guidance on supply, storage and preparation of potassium containing injectable products as well as prescribing advice. Wherever possible, ready-mixed intravenous infusions must be used. Note that in addition to potassium chloride solutions for injection, this alert applies to some other potassium-containing products, such as potassium acid tartrate injection (NPSA 2002).
- *Administration of medication by the wrong route*: this occurs when a patient is given one of the following (NPSA 2007c, 2007e):
  - intravenous chemotherapy by the intrathecal route
  - oral/enteral medication or feed/flush by any parenteral route
  - intravenous administration of an epidural medication that was not intended to be administered by the intravenous route.
- *Overdose of insulin due to abbreviations or incorrect device*: 'overdose' refers to when (NHSI 2016, NICE 2017c, NPSA 2010b):
  - a patient is given a 10-fold overdose of insulin because the words 'unit' or 'international unit' are abbreviated
  - such an overdose was given in a care setting with an electronic prescribing system
  - a healthcare professional fails to use a specific insulin administration device, that is, an insulin syringe or pen is not used to measure the insulin
  - a healthcare professional withdraws insulin from an insulin pen or pen refill and then administers this using a syringe and needle.
- *Overdose of methotrexate for non-cancer treatment*: this refers to when a patient is given a dose of methotrexate, by any route, for non-cancer treatment that is more than the intended weekly dose. It is important to note that such an overdose has been given in a care setting with an electronic prescribing system (NPSA 2006b).
- *Mis-selection of high-strength midazolam during conscious sedation*:
  - This occurs when a patient is given an overdose of midazolam due to the selection of a high-strength preparation (2 or 5 mg/mL) instead of a 1 mg/mL preparation, in a clinical area that performs conscious sedation.
  - The guidance does exclude clinical areas where the use of high-strength midazolam is appropriate: these are generally only those performing general anaesthesia, intensive care or palliative care, and areas where the drug's use has been formally risk assessed in the organization (NPSA 2008b).

Patient Safety Alerts are identified using the National Reporting and Learning System to spot emerging patterns at a national level, so that appropriate guidance can be developed and issued to protect patients from harm. Patient Safety Alerts are issued via the Central Alerting System (CAS), a web-based cascading system for issuing alerts, important public health messages, and other critical safety information and guidance to the NHS and other organizations including independent providers of health and social care.

All Patient Safety Alerts issued since 2012 can be found on the NHS Improvement website (https://improvement.nhs.uk). Alerts issued prior to April 2012 are available through the archived National Patient Safety website (available via https://improvement.nhs.uk/resources/patient-safety-alerts). These older alerts should be used with caution as they were only updated to reflect changes in current safety knowledge until their 'action complete' date was reached and some are now over 15 years old. No National Patient Safety Agency (NPSA) publications have been updated since the closure of the agency in 2012, with the exception of key actions still relevant to the Never Events policy and framework. New alerts are released frequently, and all staff are responsible for ensuring that they are followed.

Self-administration of medicines

Definition

'Self-administration' is when a person in a care setting can look after and take their own medicines (CQC 2018b). The Royal Pharmaceutical Society (RPS 2016) states that this preserves independence regardless of the social care environment and is an important feature of intermediate care because it prepares people to look after their own medicines when they return home.

Related theory

Organizations should have a policy for self-administration of medicines. This should set out any exclusion criteria for self-administration and the responsibilities and accountabilities of the staff for the care of patients who have assumed responsibility for the self-administration of their medicines (RPS 2005).

Self-administration is not an all-or-nothing process. Patients may retain or assume responsibility for some or all of their own medicines during their stay in hospital, including any items dispensed by the pharmacy for the patient during their inpatient stay, as part of a 'one-stop' dispensing process. The patient's ability to manage the tasks involved in self-administration of medicines must be assessed, with the patient's agreement (Figure 15.2), by the nursing staff to determine the patient's level of responsibility. The assessment must be completed daily as an ongoing process to document how the patient manages their medicines. All records must be retained in the patient's notes.

To aid self-administration, patients' medicines must be stored at the required temperatures. Each medication should be checked to ensure it is fit for use by the pharmacy team or nursing staff, and it should be stored in the patient's own locked cupboard or

SELF-ADMINISTRATION OF MEDICINES (SAM) NURSING ASSESSMENT CHART

Name:
DOB:
Hospital no:
Ward:
Or use patient's ID sticker
Sheet no:

	Yes	No	Comments
1. Has the patient read and understood the Patient information leaflet?			If no then give leaflet before progressing from level 0.
2. Does the patient wish to be included in the self-administration scheme?			If no, then patient is not suitable for SAM, continue at level 0.
3. Does the patient have capacity to consent?			If no, then patient is not suitable for SAM, continue at level 0.
4. Has the patient been consented?			Do not proceed without written consent.
5. Does the patient usually self-administer their medication?			If no, then patient is not suitable for SAM, continue at level 0.
6. Does the patient understand the following about their medication? - the dosage and frequency - what to do if a dose is missed			If no, then patient should remain at level 0 until re-educated by nursing/pharmacy staff.
7. Is the medication regime stable? Has the patient been admitted due to poor compliance?			Frequent dose changes will make SAM difficult – consider level 0 until patient stabilised.
8. Is the patient's clinical condition likely to deteriorate, e.g. sedation post-operatively, which may result in temporary exclusion from the scheme?			If yes, then patient to be changed to level 0 prior to surgery and reassessed daily after until stabilised.
9. Does the patient have any history of self-harm?			If yes, then patient is not suitable for SAM, continue at level 0.
10. Does the patient understand the principles of safe storage of medicines, including their responsibility for safekeeping of locker keys?			If no, then patient not suitable for SAM, do not give patient custody of medicines.

Based on the patient's knowledge of their drug treatment plus the assessment as above, please circle the level of supervision that you recommend for this patient.

Level of Supervision after Initial Assessment (please circle):

Level 0   Level 1

Date & Time initiated:	Signature: *(Nursing Staff)*	Print Name: *Job Title:*

Figure 15.2 Self-administration nursing assessment chart. *Source:* The Royal Marsden NHS Foundation Trust.

Level	Description
Level 0	**Nurse administration, no self-administration activity** - Nurse administers medicines from cabinet - Key locked in cabinet and nurse uses master key - Nurse signs administration chart
Level 1	**Self-administration of medication** - Self administration sticker placed on front of drug chart - Patient self-administers own medication - Medicines locked in cupboard and the key kept by patient - Nurse will check within 2 hours of the ward's regular drug round that the appropriate medicine was taken and endorse the chart with number 5 and initial
Level S	**Supported self-administration for parents of patients within paediatric units only** - Nurse prepares the medication for administration and labels - Nurse confirms with parent: drug, dose route and time of medication and allergy status - Nurse confirms parent remains willing to administer to their child - Nurse will check within 2 hours of the ward's regular drug round that the appropriate medicine was taken and endorse the chart with number 5 and initial

Figure 15.2 *Continued*

cabinet (by the patient's bedside) to enable easy accessibility. Each lockable cupboard or cabinet should have an individual key for that patient's use only (where appropriate), to ensure medicines cannot be accessed by unauthorized individuals (e.g. other patients) (RPS 2005).

Controlled drugs

Definition

Drugs that are subject to control are listed as controlled drugs (CDs) in Schedule 2 to the Misuse of Drugs Act (1971). The term 'controlled drug' means any substance or product listed in Schedule 2 or in a temporary class drug order as a drug subject to temporary control (Police Reform and Social Responsibility Act 2011).

Clinical governance

Legislation

Medicines Act (1968)

The Medicines Act (1968) and the regulations made under the act set out the requirements for the legal sale, supply and administration of medicines. They also allow certain exemptions from the general restrictions on the sale, supply and administration of medicines; for example, these enable midwives to supply and/or administer diamorphine, morphine, pethidine and pentazocine.

A number of healthcare professionals are permitted to supply and/or administer medicines generally in accordance with a patient group direction (PGD) (see 'Patient group directions' above). Some of these professional groups, but not all, are permitted to possess, supply or administer CDs in accordance with a PGD under the misuse of drugs legislation.

Misuse of Drugs Act (1971)

The Misuse of Drugs Act (1971) controls certain classes of dangerous drugs (e.g. diamorphine, morphine, amphetamines and benzodiazepines), which are listed in Schedule 2 and are subject to the controls stipulated in the act. The use of CDs in medicine is permitted by the Misuse of Drugs Regulations (2001) (see below) and related regulations. The regulations' main purpose is to prevent the misuse of these drugs by imposing a total ban on the possession, supply, manufacture or importation of CDs, except as allowed by regulations.

Drugs controlled under the Misuse of Drugs Act (1971) are divided into three classes (A, B and C) for the purposes of establishing the maximum penalties that can be imposed. The act also controls the manufacture of CDs. Other regulations of the act govern safe storage, destruction and supply to known addicts.

Practitioners responsible for ordering, administering, prescribing or safe custody of CDs should familiarize themselves with the Misuse of Drugs Act (1971) and the regulations (as summarized in BNF 2019a).

Misuse of Drugs (Safe Custody) Regulations (1973)

The Misuse of Drugs (Safe Custody) Regulations (1973) control the storage of CDs. The level of control of storage depends on the premises in which the drugs are being stored and the schedule of the drug.

Misuse of Drugs Regulations (2001)

The use of CDs in medicine is regulated by the Misuse of Drugs Regulations (2001). The regulations define the classes of person who are authorized to supply and possess CDs while undertaking their professional duties and stipulates the conditions in which they must undertake these tasks. The requirements of the regulations as they apply to nurses working in a hospital with a pharmacy department are described in Table 15.7.

Under these regulations, CDs are classified into five schedules, each representing a different level of control for each task, including prescribing and recording keeping (Table 15.8). The schedule in which a CD is placed depends on its medicinal or therapeutic benefit balanced against its harm when misused:

- *Schedule 1 CDs* are subject to the highest level of control: hallucinogenic drugs. They include LSD and cannabis (non-medicinal use), which may only be possessed or used by persons with a Home Office licence for research or other special purposes, although some cannabis-based products for medicinal use in humans, pregabalin and gabapentin have recently been moved to Schedule 2 (DH 2018).
- *Schedule 2 CDs* include opiates (e.g. diamorphine, morphine, methadone, nabilone, remifentanil and pethidine) and major stimulants (e.g. amphetamine, quinalbarbitone and ketamine).
- *Schedule 3 CDs* include temazepam, the barbiturates (including phenobarbital), buprenorphine, pentazocine, flunitrazepam, midazolam, diethyl propion, tramadol and Sativex.

Table 15.7 Legal requirements for the schedules of controlled drugs (CDs)

	Schedule 2 *Includes opioids and major stimulants, e.g. amphetamines*	Schedule 3 *Includes pregabalin, gabapentin, temazepam, barbiturates, tramadol and minor stimulants*	Schedule 4 Part I *Includes benzodiazepines (except temazepam and midazolam), zopiclone and Sativex*	Schedule 4 Part II *Includes anabolic steroids and growth hormones*	Schedule 5 *Includes low-dose opioids*
Designation	CD	CDs with no register entry requirements	CDs (benzodiazepines)	CDs (anabolic steroids)	CDs (needing invoice retention)
Safe custody	Yes, except quinalbarbitone	Yes, except certain exemptions listed in *Medicines, Ethics and Practices* (RPS 2012), including phenobarbitone, gabapentin and pregabalin	No	No	No
Prescription requirements	Yes	Yes, except temazepam	No	No	No
Requisitions necessary	Yes	Yes	No	No	No
Records to be kept in CD register	Yes	No (but retention of invoices is required for 2 years)	No, except for Sativex	No	No
Pharmacist must ascertain the identity of the person collecting the CD	Yes	No	No	No	No
Emergency supplies allowed	No	No, except phenobarbitone for epilepsy	Yes	Yes	Yes
Validity of prescription	28 days	28 days	28 days	28 days	6 months
Maximum duration that can be prescribed	30 days as good practice	30 days as good practice	30 days as good practice	30 days as good practice	30 days as good practice

For further details see the Misuse of Drugs and Misuse of Drugs (Safe Custody) (Amendment) (England and Wales and Scotland) Regulations (2018)

Source: Adapted from DH (2007). © Crown copyright. Reproduced under the Open Government Licence v3.0.

836

- *Schedule 4 CDs* include most of the benzodiazepines (zaleplon, zolpidem and zopiclone) and anabolic and androgenic steroids.
- *Schedule 5 CDs* are subject to a much lower level of control and include certain preparations of CDs that are exempt from full control when present in medical products of low strength (e.g. codeine in co-dydramol or co-codamol).

This list is not exhaustive and as updates to legislation occur, they will inform practice. A comprehensive list of drugs included within the schedules is given in the Misuse of Drugs Regulations (2001) and can be accessed at https://tinyurl.com/hdvm9uh.

Controlled Drugs (Supervision of Management and Use) Regulations (2006)

The Controlled Drugs (Supervision of Management and Use) Regulations (2006) were introduced as part of the government's response to the Shipman Inquiry's fourth report (Shipman Enquiry 2004). The aim of these regulations was to strengthen the governance arrangements for the use and management of CDs, which are essential to modern clinical care. As such, it is essential that the NHS enforces robust arrangements for the management and use of CDs to minimize patient harm, misuse and criminality. As a consequence of the passage of the Health and Social Care Act (2012), the 2006 regulations have been revised to reflect the new architecture in the NHS in England. The Controlled Drugs (Supervision of Management and Use) Regulations (2013) came into force in England on 1 April 2013.

There is a statutory requirement for NHS bodies to appoint an accountable officer for CDs within their organization, responsible for the safe management of CDs. The duties and responsibilities of the accountable officer are to improve the management and use of CDs. These regulations also allow for the periodic inspection of premises

Misuse of Drugs and Misuse of Drugs (Safe Custody) (Amendment) Regulations (2007)

The Misuse of Drugs and Misuse of Drugs (Safe Custody) (Amendment) Regulations (2007) give accountable officers authority to nominate persons to witness the destruction of Schedules 1 and 2 CDs. Accountable officers must be independent of the day-to-day management of CDs and therefore are not authorized to witness destructions, but they must be able to ensure there are adequate witnesses within their organization to prevent build-up of expired or surplus stock, which can lead to associated risk of diversion or misuse.

The 2007 regulations removed the descriptive term 'sister' (which was considered obsolete), replacing it with 'senior registered

Table 15.8 Summary of legal requirements for handling of controlled drugs (CDs) as they apply to nurses in hospitals with a pharmacy

	Schedule 1: CDs requiring a Home Office licence	Schedule 2: CDs subject to full controls	Schedule 3: CDs with no register entry	Schedule 4: anabolic steroids and benzodiazepines	Schedule 5: CDs needing invoice retention
Drugs in the schedule	Cannabis (non-medicinal use) and derivatives but excluding nabilone and LSD (lysergic acid diethylamide)	Most opioids in common use, including cannabis-based product for medicinal use, alfentanyl, amphetamines, cocaine, diamorphine, methadone, morphine papaveretum, fentanyl phenoperidine, pethidine, codeine, dihydrocodeine injections and pentazocine	Minor stimulants; barbiturates (excluding hexobarbitone and thiopentone); diethylpropion; buprenorphine; midazolam; temazepam;* tramadol; gabapentin and pregabalin	Part I: anabolic steroids and zopiclone Part II: benzodiazepines	Some preparations containing very low strengths of cocaine; codeine morphine; pholcodine and some other opioids
Ordering	Possession and supply permitted only by special licence from the Secretary of State issued (to a doctor only) for scientific or research purposes	A requisition must be signed in duplicate by the nurse in charge; the requisition must be endorsed to indicate that the drugs have been supplied copies should be kept for 2 years	As Schedule 2	No requirement (except Sativex)**	No requirement**
Storage	Must be kept in a locked steel cabinet that complies with British Standard 2881:1989 and the Misuse of Drugs (Safe Custody) Regulations (1973) and where access is restricted	As Schedule 1	Yes, except there are certain exemptions listed in *Medicines, Ethics and Practices* (RPS 2012), including phenobarbitone, gabapentin and pregabalin	No requirement**	No requirement**
Record keeping	Controlled drug register must be used	As Schedule 1	No requirement**	No requirement**	No requirement**
Prescription	Prescription must include: • the name and address of the patient • the drug, dose, form of preparation and strength (if more than one strength) • the total quantity of drug or the total number of dosage units to be supplied (this quantity must be stated in words and figures) • the words 'for dental treatment only' if prescribed by a dentist All prescription requirements must be indelible and signed by the prescriber with the date of prescribing Dental prescriptions must be endorsed	As Schedule 1	As Schedule 1 except for phenobarbitone (this includes all preparations of phenobarbitone and phenobarbitone sodium); because of its use as an antiepileptic, it does not need to comply with prescription requirements	No requirement**	No requirement**

* Temazepam preparations are exempt from record keeping and prescription requirements but are subject to storage requirements.

** 'No requirement' indicates that the Misuse of Drugs Act (1971) imposes no legal requirements additional to those imposed by the Medicines Act (1968).

Source: Misuse of Drugs and Misuse of Drugs (Safe Custody) (Amendment) (England and Wales and Scotland) Regulations (2018). © Crown copyright. Reproduced under the Open Government Licence v3.0.

nurse' to reflect current terminology. The 2007 regulations also allow operating department practitioners to order, possess and supply CDs.

In addition, the 2007 regulations set out changes to the requirements around record keeping and CDs; for example, each strength and form of CD is recorded on a separate page. Other mandatory fields of information included are the person collecting the Schedule 2 CD (the patient, the patient's representative or a healthcare professional). If it is a healthcare professional, there is a requirement for the name and address of that person to be recorded. Records need to be kept regarding whether proof of identity was requested of the patient or the patient's representative and whether this proof of identity was provided.

The amendment rescheduled midazolam from Schedule 4 to Schedule 3 to ensure there were tighter controls in respect of the prescribing, requisition and record keeping of this CD.

Implications of the legislation for nursing practice

Accountability and responsibility

The nurse in charge of an area is responsible for the safe and appropriate management of CDs in that area. Certain tasks, such as holding keys, can be delegated to a registered nurse but the overall responsibility remains with the nurse in charge.

To ensure CDs are managed appropriately and safely, most hospitals will store Schedule 3 CDs (e.g. tramadol, temazepam, midazolam, pregabalin and gabapentin) in a lockable cupboard, as for Schedule 2 CDs.

A witness is required for the administration of a CD; this may be a registered healthcare professional or another competent health or social care practitioner, depending on the setting and local procedures (NICE 2016a). The witness should observe the whole administration process, from access of medications from the CD cupboard to administration at the patient's bedside.

Requisition

The nurse in charge of an area is responsible for the requisition of CDs for that area. This task can be delegated to a registered nurse but the overall responsibility remains with the nurse in charge. Orders should be written on suitable stationery and must be signed by an authorized signatory. All those who are authorized to order CDs should have a copy of their signatures in the front of the order book, which must be countersigned by the senior registered nurse for validation. All stationery that is used to order, record, supply and return CDs must be stored securely in a locked cupboard and access to it should be restricted.

Receipt

When CDs are delivered to the ward, they must be delivered in a tamper-evident bag or locked box and must be handed to a registered nurse and not left unattended. The registered nurse receiving the CD order should then check (in the presence of a second registered nurse) the contents of the tamper-evident bag against the requisition order, including the quantity ordered and received. If the items supplied are correct, the nurse should sign the 'received by' section of the order book (Figure 15.3).

The CD should then be entered in the CD record book with the following information:

- date of receipt
- requisition number
- quantity
- name of the CD
- formulation and strength of drug
- name and signature of the person making the entry
- name and signature of the witness
- total balance of stock.

The updated balance should be checked against the CD physical stock to ensure these are the same. The CDs should then be placed in the CD cupboard.

Storage and equipment

CDs should be stored in a locked cupboard reserved solely for the storage of CDs that is fixed permanently to the wall. The CD cupboard must conform to British Standard BS2881. Cupboards should be locked when not in use. The lock must not be common to any other lock in the hospital.

Key holding and access

The nurse in charge of the ward or clinical area is responsible for the CD keys and is responsible for controlling access to the CD cupboard. To prevent delays in access to medication, the responsibility can be delegated to another registered nurse if the registered nurse in charge is occupied for a length of time, but overall responsibility lies with the registered nurse in charge.

For the purpose of stock checking, the key may be handed to an authorized member of pharmacy staff. If keys are lost, the senior nurse, the pharmacy manager and the accountable officer must be contacted. Appropriate actions must be taken to replace the lock to ensure that patient care is not impeded.

Record keeping

Each ward that holds CDs should keep a record of received and administered CDs in a CD record book. The nurse in charge is

Drug Name *morphine sulphate solution* **Form** *liquid* **Strength** *10 mg/5 mL*

Amount	Req No.	AMOUNT(S) ADMINISTERED							
		Date	Time	Patient's Name	Dose & Volume		Given By (Signature)	Witnessed By (Signature)	Balance Remaining
					Amount Given	Amount Destroyed			
				Balance Carried Forward From Page No................................					
		1/1/20	12:00	Balance Transferred			S SMITH *S Smith*	Jones *Jones*	335 mL
300 mL	25	2/1/20	11.40	Received from Pharmacy			S SMITH *S Smith*	Jones *Jones*	635 mL
		[illegible]	[illegible]	Joe Bloggs	25 mg/12.5 mL		S SMITH *S Smith*	Jones *Jones*	[illegible] mL

Figure 15.3 An example of recording the receipt from pharmacy and the supply to a patient of controlled drugs in a controlled drugs register.

responsible for keeping the CD record book up to date and available for inspection at any time. The record book should not be used for any other purpose and should be kept for a minimum of 2 years after the date of the last entry or the last use of the book. A computerized CD record may also be used, subject to it meeting the requirements of the relevant regulations (see DH 2006, paras. 9 and 10).

The CD record book should have sequentially numbered pages and a separate page for each drug and strength. Entries should be in chronological order and in ink. The entries in the CD record book should be signed by a registered nurse and then witnessed by a second registered nurse. If a second nurse is unavailable, the transaction can be witnessed by another registered practitioner such as a doctor, pharmacist or pharmacy technician.

To avoid staff using patients' own CDs, most organizations stipulate that if patients bring their CDs into hospital with them, they must be segregated from ward CD stock and recorded in separate CD record books.

When the end of a page is reached, the balance should be transferred to another page. The new number should be written on the bottom of the finished page and as a matter of good practice the transfer should be witnessed.

If a mistake is made in the record book, for audit purposes the mistake should be bracketed and 'error' written with the amended details written adjacent to the entry (Figure 15.4). This must be signed, dated and witnessed by a second registered nurse, who must also sign the amendment.

Stock checks and discrepancies

The registered nurse in charge is responsible for ensuring the stock balance of CDs is checked at least once every 24 hours. However, it is good practice to check the stock balance once per shift.

The stock balance entered in the CD record book should be checked against the physical amount in the cupboard, and any CDs not accounted for in the record book must be reported to the nurse. In addition, quarterly stock checks should be carried out by the pharmacy. The stock checks should be carried out by two registered nurses. When checking the balance:

- Packs with unopened tamper-evident seals do not need to be opened.
- Stock balances of liquid medicines may be checked by visual inspection but the balance must be confirmed to be correct on completion of a bottle.

A record should be made in the record book of the date and time that the stock was checked, with words such as 'CD stock level checked' together with the signature of the registered nurse and the witness. Any discrepancy must be reported to the nurse in charge immediately. In the event of a discrepancy in a CD's stock balance or the loss of CDs, the matter should be investigated immediately.

The registered nurse in charge of investigating the discrepancy should check that:

- all requisitions have been entered
- all drugs administered have been entered
- items have not been recorded in the wrong place in the record book
- the drugs have not been placed in the wrong cupboard
- the balances have been added up correctly.

If an error is found, the nurse in charge should make an entry to correct the balance, and this should be witnessed. If an error is identified but its source cannot be found, the chief pharmacist and the accountable officer should be contacted immediately.

Archiving

CD record books, order books and returns book must be stored for a minimum of 2 years from the date the last entry was made or the date of use.

Administration

Any registered practitioner can administer any drug specified as Schedule 2, 3 or 4, provided they are acting in accordance with the directions of an appropriately qualified prescriber (see 'Prescribing' below). CDs must usually be administered at the specified time; if they are not, the reason should be documented on the patient's drug chart. CDs must not be administered if the prescription is unclear, illegible or ambiguous or if there is any reason for doubt.

Two practitioners must be involved in the administration of CDs, and both practitioners should be present during the whole administration procedure (NICE 2016a). The two practitioners should have clearly defined roles. One should be the checker and the other should take responsibility for taking the drug out of the cupboard, preparing it and administering it. These roles should not be interchangeable during the procedure as this can result in errors. Both practitioners should witness the preparation, the CD being administered and the destruction of any surplus drug. An entry should be made in the CD record book recording the following information:

- the date and time the dose was administered
- the name of the patient
- the name of the CD
- the formulation
- the dose and volume being administered
- the dose and volume being wasted (e.g. if only a part vial is required)
- the name and signature of the person administering the dose
- the name and signature of the witness
- the remaining stock balance, which must be manually checked every time a drug is administered.

Drug Name *fentanyl* **Form** *patches* **Strength** *25 μg/hr*

AMOUNT(S) ADMINISTERED									
Amount	Req No.	Date	Time	Patient's Name	Dose & Volume		Given By (Signature)	Witnessed By (Signature)	Balance Remaining
					Amount Given	Amount Destroyed			
		Balance Carried Forward From Page No................................							
		1/1/20	12:00	Balance Transferred			S SMITH *S Smith*	Jones *Jones*	2
5	15	2/1/20	11.40	Received from Pharmacy			S SMITH *S Smith*	Jones *Jones*	[3] * 7 error 2/1/20 *JJ*

Figure 15.4 An example of the incorrect recording of the receipt of a supply of controlled drugs from pharmacy in a controlled drugs register.

Return and disposal, including of part vials

Unused CD stock should be returned to the pharmacy. CDs that have expired should also be returned to the pharmacy for safe destruction. All returns to the pharmacy should be completed with a pharmacist or pharmacy technician. An entry of the CD being returned should be made in the CD returns book and in the relevant page of the record book recording the following information:

- date
- reason for return
- returns requisition number (from the returns book)
- name and signature of registered nurse
- name and signature of witness
- quantity removed
- name, form and strength
- the balance remaining.

Disposal of CDs can take place on the ward if a part vial is administered to the patient or if individual doses of CDs were prepared and not administered. If a part vial is being destroyed, the registered nurse should record the amount given and the amount wasted under the administration entry in the record book. For example, if a patient is prescribed diamorphine 2.5 mg and only a 5 mg preparation is available, the record should show '2.5 mg given and 2.5 mg wasted'.

The entry and destruction should be witnessed by a registered nurse or other registered professional. If an unused prepared CD is being destroyed, this should also be recorded in the record book and the entry and destruction witnessed by another registered professional. Destructions must be disposed of in a yellow sharps bin. Solid preparations should be crushed and mixed with a small amount of water prior to disposal, liquids should be directly emptied into the sharps bin, and patches should have their backing removed and then be folded over.

Stationery

CD record books, patients' own CD record books, CD order books and CD returns books are controlled stationery and must be obtained from the pharmacy. CD stationery is issued by the pharmacy against a written requisition signed by an appropriate member of staff. Only one requisition order book should be in use by a ward. CD stationery should not be stored in the CD cupboard but should be stored in a locked cupboard or drawer.

Transport

CDs should be transferred in a secure, locked or sealed, tamper-evident container. A person collecting CDs should be aware of safe storage and security requirements, and of the importance of handing over to an authorized person to obtain a signature. They must also have a valid identification badge.

Supply under patient group directions

Nurses, when acting in their capacity as such under a PGD, are authorized to supply or offer to supply diamorphine and morphine where administration of such drugs is required for the immediate, necessary treatment of sick or injured persons (excluding the treatment of addiction) in any setting. They can also supply or administer any Schedule 3 or 4 CD in accordance with a PGD (except anabolic steroids in Schedule 4 Part II and injectable formulations for the purpose of treating a person who is addicted to a drug).

Prescribing

CDs must be prescribed in accordance with the British National Formulary (BNF 2019a), NICE guidance (NICE 2016a) and the Misuse of Drugs Regulations (2001).

Schedules 1–3 of the Misuse of Drugs Act (1971) require prescriptions to be written legibly and indelibly on an FP10 or the organization's CD prescription, stating:

- *Name and address of patient*: patient details can be in the form of a tamper-evident sticky label as long as the prescriber signs or part signs that label.
- *Patient's unique identifier or hospital number.*
- *Name and form of the preparation*: form of preparation should include modified release or immediate release where appropriate.
- *Strength of the preparation*: this may be different from the dose if the total dose is a combination of strengths – for example, the dose 'morphine M/R capsules 30 mg twice daily' would require two strengths: 10 mg MR capsules and 20 mg MR capsules. Both should be specified.
- *Dose instructions.*
- *Total quantity or number of dose units in both words and figures*: for liquids, this should be the total volume in millilitres (in both words and figures) of the preparation to be supplied; for dosage units, this should be the number (in both words and figures) of dosage units to be supplied; in any other case, this should be the total quantity (in both words and figures) of the CD to be supplied. This requirement applies to outpatient and discharge prescriptions but not to inpatient prescriptions.
- *Name (in capitals), contact number and signature of the prescriber.*
- *Date.*

When prescribing opioid medicines, the practitioner should:

- obtain a full drug history
- confirm any recent opioid dose, the formulation, the frequency of administration and any other analgesic medicines prescribed for the patient
- ensure that, where a dose increase is intended, the calculated dose is safe for the patient
- ensure they are familiar with the following characteristics of the medicine and formulation: usual starting dose, frequency of administration, standard dosing increments, symptoms of overdose and common side-effects
- use a recognized opioid dose conversion guide when prescribing, reviewing or changing opioid prescriptions to ensure that the total opioid load is considered
- inform the person's GP of all prescribing decisions and record this information in the person's discharge letter so the GP has access to it.

When prescribing strong opioids, practitioners should be aware of the relevant guidance issued by NICE (2012) and ensure that patient counselling is documented in the patient's record.

Prescriptions for all CDs, including temazepam, are valid for 28 days from the date of prescribing or from the 'start date' specified by the prescriber.

In hospital, FP10(HNC) prescriptions may be used to prescribe CDs for outpatients in exceptional circumstances. *These prescriptions are for NHS patients only.*

FP10 prescriptions can be used in the community to prescribe CDs for patients under the care of the medical or non-medical independent prescriber (IP). In the case of non-medical IPs, individuals must ensure that the CD is within their scope of practice and that they are competent to prescribe the CD. Prescribers must not prescribe or administer CDs for themselves, close family or friends except in exceptional circumstances.

A supplementary prescriber (SP), when acting in accordance with a clinical management plan, can prescribe a CD provided the CD is included in the clinical management plan. Nurse IPs may prescribe any CD listed in Schedules 2–5 for any medical condition, except diamorphine, cocaine and dipipanone for the treatment of addiction (other CDs can be prescribed by nurse IPs for the treatment of addiction). The authority to prescribe any CD is given on the basis that nurses must only prescribe within their competence.

In response to seven case reports published between 2000 and 2005 regarding deaths caused by the administration of high-dose

Box 15.5 High-dose opiate guidance

- High-strength preparations of morphine or diamorphine (30 mg or above) should be stored in a location separate from lower strength preparations (10 mg) within the controlled drug cupboard.
- Awareness should be raised of similarities in drug packaging, and use should be considered of alert stickers attached to high-strength preparations by the pharmacy.
- A review of stock levels should be undertaken in all clinical areas where morphine and diamorphine are stored to assess whether high-strength preparations need to be kept on a permanent basis or whether they could be ordered according to specific patient requirements.
- Clear guidance should be provided to ensure that doses of diamorphine and morphine are prepared in a manner that is appropriate to the clinical situation. For example, diamorphine 5 mg and 10 mg ampoules could be used for both bolus administration and patients newly commenced on diamorphine infusions; diamorphine 30 mg ampoules could be reserved for patients already receiving diamorphine infusions and who require higher daily doses.
- Patients should be observed for the first hour after receiving their first dose of diamorphine or morphine injection.
- Naloxone injections should be available in all clinical areas where morphine and diamorphine are stored.

Source: Adapted from NPSA (2006a). © Crown copyright. Reproduced under the Open Government Licence v2.0. For updates see www.england.nhs.uk.

(30 mg or greater) morphine or diamorphine to patients who had not previously received doses of opiates, the NPSA released a Safer Practice Notice titled *Ensuring Safer Practice with High Dose Ampoules of Morphine and Diamorphine* (NPSA 2006a). In line with this Safer Practice Notice, the guidance in Box 15.5 should be adhered to.

Between 2005 and 2008, 4223 incidents were reported to the NRLS involving opioid medicines and the 'wrong/unclear dose or strength' or 'wrong frequency' of medication. As a result, the NPSA released a Rapid Response Report in July 2008 containing the guidance shown in Box 15.6.

The NPSA was notified of 498 midazolam patient safety incidents between November 2004 and November 2008 where the dose prescribed or administered to the patient was inappropriate. Three midazolam-related incidents resulted in death. As a result, the NPSA released a Rapid Response Report in 2008 containing the guidance in Box 15.7.

Box 15.6 Opioid dose and strength guidance

- Confirm any recent opioid dose, the formulation, the frequency of administration and any other analgesic medicines prescribed for the patient. This may be done, for example, through discussion with the patient or their representative (although not in the case of treatment for addiction), through discussion with the prescriber or through medication records.
- Where a dose increase is intended, ensure that the calculated dose is safe for the patient (e.g. for oral morphine or oxycodone in adult patients, not normally more than 50% higher than the previous dose).
- Ensure familiarity with the following characteristics of the medicine and formulation: usual starting dose, frequency of administration, standard dosing increments, symptoms of overdose and common side-effects.

Source: Adapted from NPSA (2008a). © Crown copyright. Reproduced under the Open Government Licence v2.0. For updates see www.england.nhs.uk.

Box 15.7 Midazolam guidance

- Ensure that the storage and use of high-strength midazolam (5 mg/mL in 2 mL and 10 mL ampoules, or 2 mg/mL in 5 mL ampoules) are restricted to general anaesthesia, intensive care, palliative medicine, and clinical areas and situations where the drug's use has been formally risk assessed, for example where syringe drivers are used.
- Ensure that in other clinical areas, high-strength midazolam is replaced with low-strength midazolam (1 mg/mL in 2 mL or 5 mL ampoules).
- Review therapeutic protocols to ensure that the guidance on the use of midazolam is clear and that the risks, particularly for the elderly and frail, are fully assessed.
- Ensure that all healthcare practitioners involved directly or participating in sedation techniques have the necessary knowledge, skills and competencies.
- Ensure that stocks of flumazenil are available where midazolam is used and that the use of flumazenil is regularly audited as a marker of excessive dosing of midazolam.
- Ensure that sedation is covered by organizational policy and that overall responsibility is assigned to a senior clinician, who in most cases will be an anaesthetist.

Source: Adapted from NPSA (2008b). © Crown copyright. Reproduced under the Open Government Licence v2.0. For updates see www.england.nhs.uk.

Procedure guideline 15.1 Medication: controlled drug administration

Essential equipment

- Prescription chart
- Controlled drug record book
- Appropriate medication container, for example medicine pot or syringe

Action	Rationale
Pre-procedure	
1 Introduce yourself to the patient, explain and discuss the procedure with them, and gain their consent to proceed.	To ensure that the patient feels at ease, understands the procedure and gives their valid consent (NMC 2018, **C**).
2 Before administering any prescribed drug, look at the patient's prescription chart and check the following:	To ensure that the patient is given the correct drug, in the correct formulation, in the prescribed dose using the appropriate diluent and by the correct route (DH 2003b, **C**).

(continued)

Procedure guideline 15.1 Medication: controlled drug administration *(continued)*

Action	Rationale
• drug name (generic) • dose • date and time of administration • frequency • route and method of administration	
• formulation of oral preparation, e.g. modified release or immediate release	To ensure the correct formulation is given as many different formulations are available for the same drug. **R**
• diluent as appropriate	
• validity of prescription	To ensure the prescription is legal (DH 2003b, **C**).
• legible signature and contact details of prescriber	To ensure the prescription is legal and complies with hospital policy (DH 2003b, **C**).
• when the drug was last administered.	To ensure the patient requires the drug at this time. **E**
If any of these pieces of information are missing, unclear or illegible, do not proceed with the administration. Consult with the prescriber.	To prevent any errors occurring. **E**
Procedure	
3 With the second registered nurse or registered healthcare professional, take the keys and open the controlled drug (CD) cupboard. Take the ward CD record book that contains the prescribed CD, consult the contents page, and turn to the relevant page headed with the name and strength of the CD.	To check the stock and enter the details into the CD record book (DH 2003b, **C**; NICE 2016a, **C**).
4 With the second registered nurse or registered healthcare professional, take the correct drug out of the CD cupboard.	To comply with hospital policy and to ensure the patient receives the correct medicine (DH 2003b, **C**; NPSA 2006a, **C**).
5 With the second registered nurse or registered healthcare professional, check the stock level against the last entry in the ward record book.	To comply with hospital policy (DH 2003b, **C**; NPSA 2006a, **C**).
6 With the second registered nurse or registered healthcare professional, check the appropriate dose and concentration/ strength (e.g. 10 mg in 1 mL or 5 mg in 5 mL) and formulation against the prescription chart. Remove the dose from the box/bottle and place it into an appropriate container, e.g. medicine pot or syringe.	To comply with hospital policy and to ensure the patient receives the correct dose and strength of medicine (DH 2003b, **C**; NPSA 2006a, **C**).
7 Return the remaining stock to the cupboard and lock the cupboard.	To comply with hospital policy (DH 2003b, **C**; NPSA 2006a, **C**).
8 Enter the date, dose, new stock level and patient's name in the ward record book, ensuring that both you and the second registered nurse sign the entry. *Note*: it may be necessary to make the entry in different sections if the dose is to be made up of different doses (e.g. 70 mg = 1 × 50 mg and 2 × 10 mg). If any is wasted then ensure it is documented correctly (e.g. '5 mg given and 5 mg wasted').	To comply with hospital policy (DH 2003b, **C**; NICE 2016a, **C**; NPSA 2006a, **C**).
9 a With the second registered nurse or registered healthcare professional, take the prepared dose to the patient and check the patient's identity by asking them to verbally identify themselves (where possible). Check the information the patient gives against the identification wristband they are wearing.	To prevent error and confirm the patient's identity (NPSA 2005, **C**; NPSA 2007b, **C**).
b Tell the patient the name and dose of the drug where possible; advise them on the different methods of administration and check their understanding (NICE 2016a).	
c Ask the patient whether they have any allergies, checking their response against the prescription chart.	
d Check when the patient last had the medication against the prescription chart.	To ensure that the patient has not already received the medication. **E**
10 Administer the drug. If given orally, wait until the patient has swallowed the medication.	To ensure the patient receives the medication (DH 2003b, **C**).

Post-procedure	
11 Once the drug has been administered, ensure the prescription chart is signed by the nurse responsible for administering the medication and the registered nurse or registered healthcare professional who witnessed the administration.	To prevent duplication of treatment and to comply with hospital policy (DH 2003b, **C**; NICE 2016a, **C**; NPSA 2006a, **C**). To maintain accurate records, provide a point of reference in the event of any queries and prevent any duplication of treatment (NICE 2016a, **C**).
12 Check the patient after administration for effectiveness and/or toxicity.	To ensure that the drug has been effective and to administer a breakthrough dose if necessary. To check that the patient has not experienced any toxicity that may require interventions. **E**
13 If the drug was given via a syringe pump, return to check the infusion (for rate) and site (for signs of any local complications) and document in the appropriate records.	To ensure that the infusion is infusing at the correct rate and the site is suitable. **E**

Post-procedural considerations

Ongoing care

Patients should be monitored for signs of adverse effects from opioids and signs of toxicity. The most common side-effects are constipation, nausea and vomiting, and drowsiness. All patients who are prescribed an opioid regularly should be prescribed laxatives concurrently to prevent constipation. Nausea and vomiting should subside after a few days but patients should be prescribed antiemetics and given reassurance. Drowsiness due to opioids should also subside after a few days; therefore, if patients experience this symptom, they should be given reassurance that it will pass in time (Regnard and Hockley 2004).

The warning signs of toxicity due to opioids are:

- pinpoint pupils
- confusion
- myoclonus
- hallucinations and nightmares
- respiratory depression.

If patients are showing signs of toxicity, the opioid dose should be reduced or stopped and as-required opioid pain relief given (Regnard and Hockley 2004). Changing to an alternative opioid can also be considered (Regnard and Hockley 2004).

Naloxone, a specific opioid antagonist, has a high affinity for opioid receptors and reverses the effect of opioid analgesics. It is rarely needed but may be required in the case of opioid-induced respiratory depression (a respiration rate of eight breaths per minute or below).

Care must be taken not to give naloxone to patients who have non-life-threatening opioid-induced drowsiness, confusion or hallucinations, as this may risk reversing the opioid analgesic effect (Twycross et al. 2007). Naloxone should be used with care, especially in patients with opioid dependence; there have been Patient Safety Alerts whose guidance should be followed (NHS England 2014, 2015b).

Naloxone should be given in doses of 400 μg every 2 minutes until respiratory function is satisfactory, and doses should be titrated against respiratory function and not the level of consciousness of the patient in order to avoid total reversal of the analgesic effect (Twycross et al. 2007). Registered nurses administering opioids should be aware of local policy, procedures and protocols. Flumazenil is used for reversal of the effects of benzodiazepine toxicity.

Routes of administration

The five basic routes of administration are enteral, parenteral, pulmonary, transdermal and topical (Tables 15.9 and 15.10). The enteral route uses the gastrointestinal (GI) tract for absorption of drugs. The parenteral route bypasses the GI tract and is associated with all forms of injections. The pulmonary route is used to administer drugs to the lungs and bronchi, usually for local activity. Transdermal, also known as percutaneous, administration of medicines is used to deliver drugs systemically through the skin, usually for a systemic effect, although some preparations are designed for local action. The topical route is used to administer drugs to the skin and mucous membranes, including the eyes, ears, nasal cavity and sublingually, usually for a local action.

Enteral (oral) administration

Definition

Enteral (oral) medication is taken by mouth – that is, it is swallowed by the patient (e.g. liquid, tablets or capsules; Merck 2011) or administered via a feeding tube (e.g. nasogastric tube or percutaneous endoscopic gastrostomy) (Potter and Perry 2016) (Figure 15.5).

Oral administration is the most convenient route for medicine administration and may result in high levels of compliance (Kelly and Wright 2009). It is usually the safest and least expensive route. Due to the widespread use of oral drugs, they are prepared in a variety of dosage forms.

Related theory

Solid dosage forms

Tablets

Tablets come in a great variety of shapes, sizes, colours and types. The formulation may be very simple (a plain white uncoated tablet) or complex (designed with specific therapeutic aims, e.g. sustained-release preparations). Sugar coatings are used to improve appearance and palatability. In cases where the drug is a gastric irritant or is broken down by gastric acid, an enteric coating may be used; this is designed to allow the tablet to remain intact in the stomach and to pass unchanged into the small bowel, where the coating dissolves and the drug is released and absorbed.

Tablets may be formulated specifically to control the rate of release of the drug from the tablet as it passes through the GI tract.

Table 15.9 Advantages and disadvantages of the routes of administration

Route	Advantages	Disadvantages
Enteral (oral)	Convenient Easy to administer Least expensive Easy for patients to use	Compliance Some drugs not suitable for oral route Patient may not be able to swallow or take oral medications Subject to first-pass metabolism
Topical	Easy to apply Local effects	Can stain clothing Local irritation Risk of burns from paraffin preparations
Parenteral (injections and infusions)	Absorbed quickly Rapid action when required Avoids gastrointestinal tract Valuable when fine control of action required	Invasive Pain Potentially toxic if used inappropriately Complications such as infection May be difficult to self-administer
Pulmonary	Local effects Minimize side-effects Rapid onset of action	Complexity of devices Requires patient dexterity and ability
Transdermal (percutaneous)	Controlled long-term release Drug reaches systemic circulation, avoiding first-pass mechanism Patches can be removed easily and quickly in cases where an adverse drug reaction occurs Patient adherence is relatively high Easy to apply	Potential toxicity if not used correctly Limited number of drugs available
Site specific, e.g. eye, ear, nasal, vaginal or rectal	Often for local effects Minimal systemic adverse effects	Discomfort and embarrassment May be difficult to self-administer Occasional unwanted systemic effects

Table 15.10 Considerations for specific types of administration

Consideration	Rationale
Administer drugs that may irritate the gastrointestinal tract with meals or snacks.	To minimize their effect on the gastric mucosa (Jordan et al. 2003, Shepherd 2002).
Administer drugs that interact with food, that are destroyed in significant proportions by digestive enzymes, or that have their absorption significantly affected by food between meals or on an empty stomach (usually 1 hour before or 2 hours after food).	To prevent interference with the absorption of the drug (Jordan et al. 2003, Shepherd 2002).
Do not break a tablet unless it is scored and appropriate to do so. Break scored tablets with a file or a tablet cutter. Wash the file or cutter after use.	Breaking may cause incorrect dosage, gastrointestinal irritation or destruction of a drug in an incompatible pH. To reduce risk of contamination between tablets (DH 2007, Jordan et al. 2003, Shepherd 2002).
Do not interfere with time-release capsules and enteric coated tablets. Ask patients to swallow these whole and not to chew them.	The absorption rate of the drug will be altered (Harrison 2015, Jordan et al. 2003).
Dissolve effervescent and soluble tablets in water, and allow to disperse fully before administration.	The absorption rate of the drug will be altered (Harrison 2015, Jordan et al. 2003).
Sublingual tablets must be placed under the tongue and buccal tablets between gum and cheek.	To allow for correct absorption (Harrison 2015).
When administering liquids to babies and young children, or when an accurately measured dose in multiples of 1 mL is needed for an adult, an oral syringe should be used in preference to a medicine spoon or measure.	An oral syringe is much more accurate than a measure or a 5 mL spoon. Use of a syringe makes administration of the correct dose much easier in an unco-operative child. Oral syringes are available and are designed to be washable and reused for the same patient. However, in immunocompromised patients, single-use only is recommended. Oral syringes must be clearly labelled for oral or enteral use only (DH 2007, NPSA 2007c).

Consideration	Rationale
In babies and children especially, correct use of the syringe is very important. The tip should be gently pushed into and towards the side of the mouth. The contents are then *slowly* discharged towards the inside of the cheek, pausing if necessary to allow the liquid to be swallowed.	To prevent injury to the mouth and eliminate the danger of choking the patient (Watt 2003).
If children are unco-operative, it may help to place the end of the barrel between the teeth.	To get the dose in and to prevent the patient spitting it out (Watt 2003).
When administering gargling medication, throat irrigations should not be warmer than body temperature.	Liquid warmer than body temperature may cause discomfort or damage tissue.

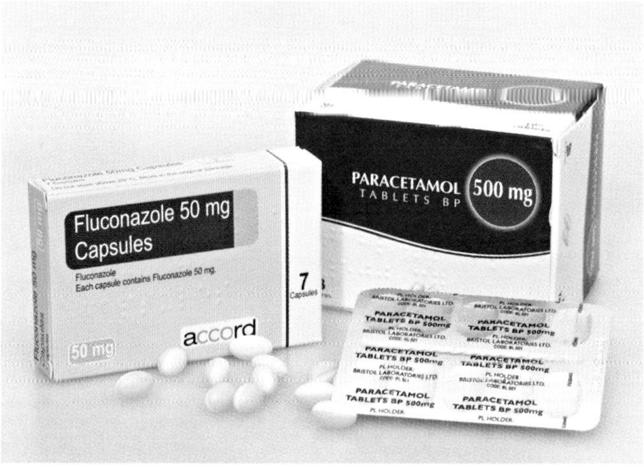

Figure 15.5 Examples of oral medication.

Terms such as 'sustained release', 'controlled release' and 'modified release' are used by manufacturers to describe these preparations. Care should be taken with these as different formulations of modified-release preparations may not be bioequivalent (BNF 2019a). These preparations may be prescribed by brand name to ensure the patient gets the same formulation each time (BNF 2019a). Tablets may also be formulated specifically to dissolve or disperse readily in water before administration ('soluble' or 'effervescent'). Other tablets are formulated to disperse in the mouth ('oro-dispersible'), while others must be chewed. The contents of these are swallowed by the patient after the contents have dispersed. Other tablets are designed to be placed and held under the tongue ('sublingual') or placed between the gum and inside of the mouth ('buccal'). On release, the drug from these formulations is absorbed through the sublingual or buccal mucosa. Unscored or coated tablets should not be crushed or broken, nor should most modified-release tablets, since this can affect the pharmacokinetic profile of the drug and may result in excessive peak plasma concentrations and side-effects (Smyth 2006). Advice on whether modified-release preparations can be split should be sought from a pharmacist.

Capsules

Capsules offer a useful method of formulating drugs that are difficult to make into a tablet or that are particularly unpalatable. Capsules can also be easier for some patients to swallow.

Medicines are formulated in both hard and soft capsule shells. Capsule shells are usually made of gelatine and this may pose a problem for patients who are vegetarian or vegan, as well as some with religious beliefs with regard to products of animal origin. Capsule contents may be solid, liquid or of a paste-like consistency. The contents do not cause deterioration of the shell. The shell, however, is dissolved by the digestive fluids and the contents are then released. Delayed-release capsule formulations also exist. Gastro-resistant capsules are delayed-release capsules that are intended to resist the gastric fluid and to release their active substance or substances in the intestinal fluid (British Pharmacopoeia 2019).

If for any reason a capsule is unpalatable or the patient is unable to take it, the contents should not routinely be removed from the shell without first seeking advice from a pharmacist. Removing the contents from the capsule could destroy its properties and cause gastric irritation or premature release of the drug into an incompatible pH (Downie et al. 2003).

Lozenges and pastilles

Lozenges and pastilles are solid, single-dose preparations intended to be sucked to obtain a local or systemic effect to the mouth and/or throat (British Pharmacopoeia 2019).

Oral liquid dosage forms

There are a variety of liquid oral dosage forms, including solutions, suspensions, mixtures, syrups, linctuses, elixirs and emulsions. The nature of the liquid dosage form will depend on the nature of the drug, particularly its solubility and stability (Aulton and Taylor 2018). The nature of the condition being treated will also have some bearing in some circumstances – for example, the use of linctuses for the management of coughs.

Solutions

Oral solutions are swallowed and the drug may exert a local effect on the GI tract or be absorbed into the blood to exert a systemic effect. Solutions can be relatively simple aqueous solutions but to be acceptable they must be palatable to patients and must be of an appropriate viscosity for pouring and palatability. Solutions can contain flavourings, colourings and sweeteners to improve taste; agents to increase viscosity; and preservatives. These are known as 'excipients'. Some solutions are complex and may require the use of excipients to improve solubility (co-solvents and surfactants) and/or stability (Aulton and Taylor 2018).

Patients may be allergic to excipients and details of excipients can be found in the summary of product characteristics for the medicine. These are readily available online at https://www.medicines.org.uk/emc.

A few medicines are formulated in non-aqueous solutions and these may pose adherence challenges due to their palatability.

Suspensions

Suspensions are used where a drug is not water-soluble but remains as solid particles dispersed throughout a liquid. A suspension will be formulated to ensure that the drug is optimally dispersed (Aulton and Taylor 2018) but this is challenging to achieve and most suspensions settle. It is essential, therefore, to thoroughly shake a suspension to disperse the drug before each use.

Mixtures

Mixtures are usually aqueous preparations, frequently containing more than one active ingredient. They can be in the form of either a solution or a suspension.

Syrups

Syrups are formulations where the active ingredients are dissolved or suspended in an aqueous liquid containing a high proportion of dissolved sugar to form a syrup. The high sugar content acts as a preservative as well as making the medicine more palatable. The sugar content can contribute to dental caries (especially with long-term medication), and patients should be advised on good dental hygiene (Roberts and Roberts 1979).

Due to long-term stability problems in water, some liquid medicines are presented as powders or granules for reconstitution before use. The correct amount of water should be added and the medicine discarded after its expiry date. This will frequently be a relatively short period, typically 1–2 weeks.

Linctuses

These are viscous oral liquids that may contain one or more active ingredients; the solution usually contains a high proportion of sucrose. Linctuses are intended for use in the treatment or relief of coughs.

Elixirs

Traditionally elixirs are liquid medicines that contain alcohol as a cosolvent to dissolve the active ingredient. However, not all medicines that contain alcohol are designated as elixirs (Aulton and Taylor 2018)

Emulsions

Emulsions are formulations of two or more liquids that do not normally mix, with the drug usually dissolved in one of the liquids. They contain an emulsifier to produce either small water droplets in oil (water in oil emulsion) or small droplets of oil in water (oil in water emulsion). Like suspensions, oral emulsions must be shaken thoroughly to ensure even dispersion of the active ingredient. Although there some oral emulsions available, the majority of commercially available emulsions are currently for topical or injectable products (Aulton and Taylor 2018).

Evidence-based approaches

Older observational studies suggest that medication administration errors for oral medicine range from 3% to 8% (Ho et al. 1997, Taxis et al. 1999) but the rate has been found to be twice as high in mental health patients who have swallowing difficulties (Haw et al. 2007). However, more recent work suggests the rate of error may be higher; a systematic review of 91 research studies found that the median error rate for medication administration errors (MAEs) was 19.6% (8.6–28.3%) of the total opportunities for error including wrong-time errors, and 8.0% (5.1–10.9%) without timing errors (Keers et al. 2013). A higher median MAE rate was observed for the intravenous route (53.3% excluding timing errors; 26.6–57.9%) compared to when all administration routes were studied (20.1%; 9.0–24.6%). There was consistency in the types of error reported: wrong time, omission and wrong dosage were among the three most common MAEs. Common medication groups associated with MAEs were those affecting nutrition and blood, the GI system, the cardiovascular system and the central nervous system, and antimicrobials. The MAE rates varied greatly as the research studies used a variety of medication error definitions, data collection methods and settings.

Another review looking primarily at the effects of methodological variations and their effects on MAE rates (McLeod et al. 2013) reviewed 16 studies. Overall, adult MAE rates were 5.6% out of a total of 31 533 non intravenous (IV) opportunities for error and 35% of a total of 1164 IV opportunities for error. As in the review by Keers et al. (2013), MAEs were more prevalent in IV compared to non-IV doses, this time by a factor of five. Including timing errors of ±30 minutes increased the MAE rate from 27% to 69% of 320 IV doses in one study. Five studies were unclear as to whether the denominator included dose omissions; omissions accounted for 0–13% of IV doses and 1.8–5.1% of non-IV doses.

Swallowing difficulties

Problems occur when patients have an aversion to swallowing tablets, or difficulties in swallowing (Kelly and Wright 2009). When giving medicines to patients with dysphagia, both the patient and the medicine should be reviewed on a regular basis. Guidance has been published by a working group that advocates a multidisciplinary approach (Wright et al. 2017). If patients cannot swallow tablets then licensed liquid or dispersible medications should be considered next (NEWT 2018). If the oral route is not patent then alternative routes should be used.

Advice is available on tailoring medication for patients with swallowing difficulties (Barnett and Parmar 2018). The NEWT (2018) guidelines provide guidance on the administration of medication to patients with enteral feeding tubes or swallowing difficulties.

Covert drug administration

Medicines should only be administered covertly (e.g. by disguising them in food or drink) as part of an agreed management plan, to people who refuse their medication and who are considered to lack mental capacity (RPS 2019b); this should be in exceptional circumstances only (CQC 2018a, Griffith 2016). A pharmacist must be involved in these decisions as adding medication to food or drink can alter its pharmacological properties and thereby affect its performance.

It is vital to meet the requirements of the Mental Capacity Act (2005) when considering covert drug administration:

- All the relevant circumstances should be considered.
- Is it likely the patient will regain capacity and can treatment be delayed until then?
- As far as is reasonably possible, the patient should be encouraged and assisted in participating in any decision making.
- Decisions regarding life-sustaining treatments must not be motivated by a desire to hasten death.
- The patient's past and current wishes must be taken into account where available (particularly those written at a time when the patient had capacity).
- The patient's beliefs and values that might have influenced their decision (if they had capacity) should be considered.
- Other factors that might have influenced their decision if they had capacity should be taken into account.
- Where practical, the views of the following should be considered: any person named by the patient to be consulted on such decisions, carers and other people with an interest in the patient's welfare, and any person with lasting power of attorney for the patient.
- What is deemed to be in the patient's best interests must be taken into account.

NICE (2015a) provides guidance on covert administration of medicines in care homes:

> The covert administration of medicines should only be used in exceptional circumstances when such a means of administration is judged necessary, in accordance with the Mental Capacity Act 2005. However, once a decision has been made to covertly administer a particular medicine (following an assessment of the capacity of the resident to make a decision regarding their medicines and a best interests meeting), it is also important to consider and plan how the medicine can be covertly administered, whether it is safe to do so and to ensure that need for continued covert administration is regularly reviewed (as capacity can fluctuate over time). Medicines should not be administered covertly until after a best interests meeting has been held. If the situation is urgent, it is acceptable for a less formal discussion to occur between the care home staff, prescriber and family or advocate to make an urgent decision. However, a formal meeting should be arranged as soon as possible. (p.29)

Pre-procedural considerations

Equipment

Medicine pots

Medicine pots (Figure 15.6) allow a dosage form to be taken from its original container for immediate administration to a patient. The person who removes medication from its original container and places it into a medicine pot must oversee the administration of this medication. This responsibility cannot be transferred to someone else.

Tablet splitters

The practices of crushing, opening and splitting tablets should be avoided wherever possible due to a number of potential factors (RPS 2011):

- risks to healthcare workers and carers due to exposure of toxic or irritant materials
- drug instability, although in most circumstances this is less of an issue if the dosage form is crushed, opened or split immediately before administration
- changes in the pharmacokinetics and/or bioavailability of the drug
- irritation to the patient's GI tract from the drug
- unmasking unpleasant taste.

If the practice is necessary, then commercially available tablet splitters (Figure 15.7) may increase the accuracy of tablet splitting (Verrue et al. 2010). Tablets that are unscored, unusually thick or oddly shaped, sugar coated, enteric coated or modified release are not suitable for splitting. Areas for consideration when using a tablet splitter include the following:

- Can the tablet be split? This must always be discussed with the pharmacy department.
- Does the patient have the manual dexterity to use a tablet splitter when at home?
- Will splitting the tablets affect patient adherence when they are at home? Will the patient skip or double dose rather than split tablets?
- How will the storage of split tablets affect the stability of the tablets? What about the effect of light and air (Marriott and Nation 2002)?

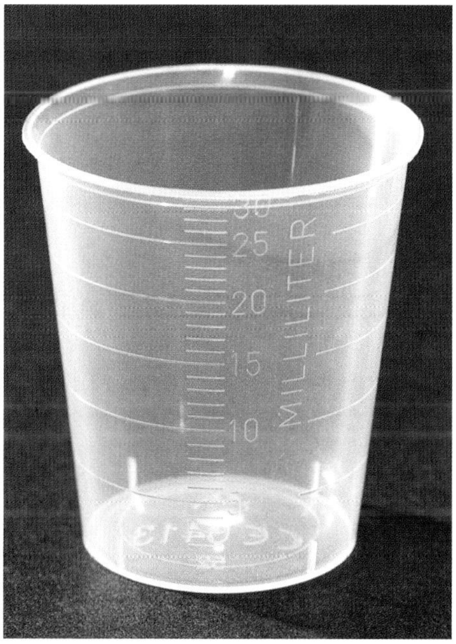

Figure 15.6 Medicine pot.

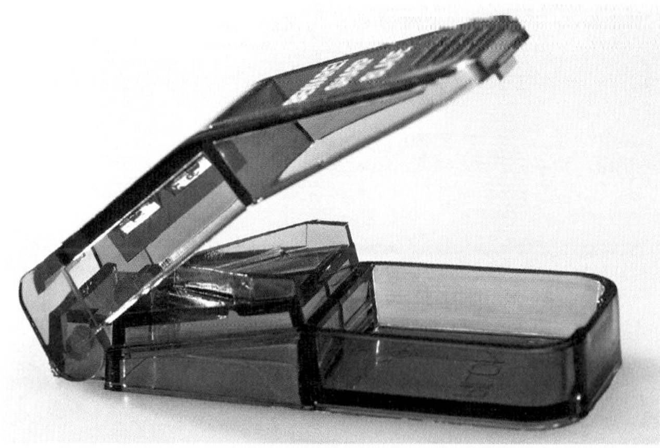

Figure 15.7 Tablet splitter.

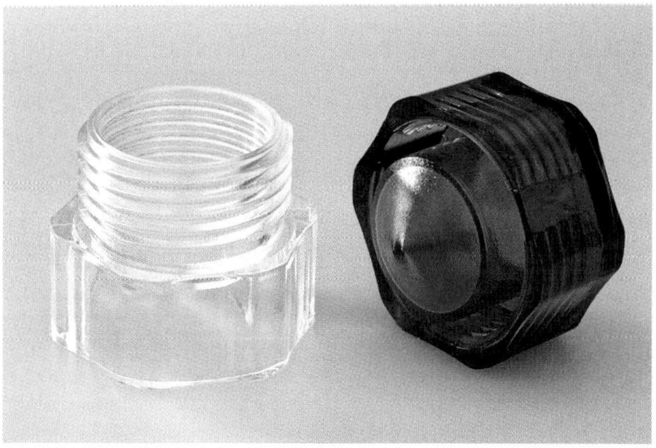

Figure 15.8 Tablet crusher.

Tablet crushers

Tablet crushers (Figure 15.8) can be used when a patient has swallowing difficulties and no alternative dosage form exists. The crushing or splitting of dosage forms will be an unlicensed use of the medicine (unless this form of manipulation is covered by the product's marketing authorization). The Human Medicines Regulations (2012) state that unlicensed medicines can only be authorized by a prescriber, so if tablets are going to be crushed, there should be discussion and agreement between the prescriber and the person who will administer the medicine. Discussion should also take place with a pharmacist to check that the tablet is suitable for crushing and that the efficacy of the medication will not be changed as a result. Tablets that are enteric coated, sustained release or chewable cannot be crushed. Areas for consideration when crushing a tablet include the following (RPS 2011):

- Can the tablet be crushed? This must always be discussed with the pharmacy department.
- Will crushing make the tablet unpalatable?
- Will crushing the tablet cause any adverse effects for the patient, for example burning of the oral mucosa?
- Will crushing the tablet result in inaccurate dosing (Kelly and Wright 2009)?

When a tablet crusher is used, water should be added to the crushed tablet and the resulting solution drawn up using an oral syringe. The crusher should then be rinsed and the process repeated if necessary. Tablet crushers should be rinsed before and after use to prevent cross-contamination with other medicines (Fair and Proctor 2007, Smyth 2006). When a tablet crusher has been used, it should be opened and washed under running water, dried with a tissue and left to air dry on a tissue or paper towel.

Monitored dosage systems and compliance aids

Monitored dosage systems and compliance aids, for example dosette boxes (Figure 15.9), are designed to help patients remember when to take their medication. They can also let carers know whether patients have taken their medication. However, the default approach should be to dispense medicines in their standard packaging, on the assumption that patients can manage their medicines unless indicated otherwise. This is in line with NICE (2009) guidance stating that monitored dosage systems should be considered as an option to improve adherence on a case-by-case basis, and only if there is a specific need to overcome practical problems. This should follow a discussion with the patient to explore possible reasons for nonadherence and the options available to improve adherence, if that is their wish. More recent guidance from NICE (2017a) on managing medicines for adults receiving social care reinforces this with the following recommendation:

> Consider using a monitored dosage system only when an assessment by a health professional (for example, a pharmacist) has been carried out, in line with the Equality Act 2010, and a specific need has been identified to support medicines adherence. Take account of the person's needs and preferences, and involve the person and/or their family members or carers and the social care provider in decision-making. (p.19)

NICE has also produced a quality and productivity case study (NICE 2016b), which outlines actions intended to reduce the inappropriate use of monitored dosage systems by ensuring they are only issued on a case-by-case basis to address specific practical problems with medicines adherence. The inappropriate use of monitored dosage systems can make patients and carers less familiar with their medicines. The preparation and checking of unnecessary monitored dosage systems creates significant additional workload for hospital pharmacies, which can be reduced.

Therefore, monitored dosage systems should only be initiated in patients where there is a likely benefit and full assessment and consultation have been carried out. The RPS (2013a) reinforces these principles as well as providing guidance for pharmacists and their staff on filling and dispensing these devices.

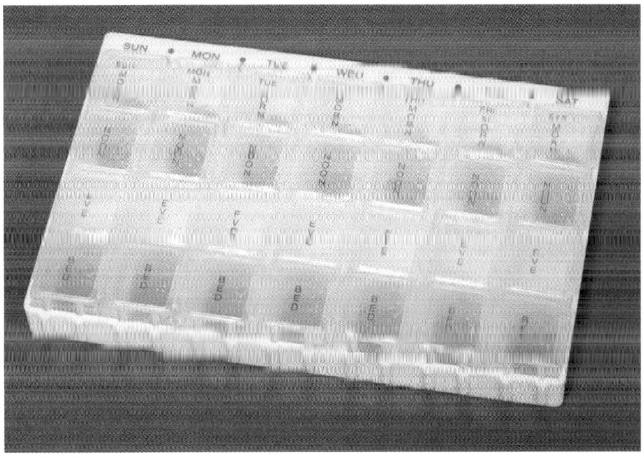

Figure 15.9 Dosette box.

The following should be considered when using these systems (RPS 2013a):

- They can only be used for tablets and capsules.
- Medicines that are susceptible to moisture should not be put in these systems.
- Light sensitive medicines should not be put in these systems.
- Medicines that are harmful when handled should not be put in these systems.
- If the patient is on medications that cannot be stored in these systems, precautions should be put in place to ensure that they can cope with two systems.
- If the patient's drug regimen is not stable, consideration should be given to how easy it will be to make changes to the system.
- As-required medication cannot be placed in these systems.
- These systems are subject to labelling and leaflet legislation so they must always be dispensed by a pharmacy department.

Oral syringes

The BNF for children (BNF 2019b) recommends that an oral syringe should be used for accurate measurement and controlled administration of an oral liquid medicine to a child. For adults, the BNF (2019a) recommends that an oral syringe is supplied when oral liquid medicines are prescribed in doses other than multiples of 5 mL. The oral syringe should be marked in 0.5 mL divisions from 1 to 5 mL to measure doses of less than 5 mL (other sizes of oral syringe may also be available). It should be provided with an adaptor and an instruction leaflet. Otherwise, a 5 mL medicine spoon must be used for doses of 5 mL (or multiples thereof).

If a syringe is needed to measure and administer an oral dose, an oral syringe (Figure 15.10) that cannot be attached to intravenous catheters or ports should be used. These syringes are purple in colour. All oral syringes containing oral liquid medicines must usually be labelled by the person who prepared the syringe with the name and strength of the medicine, the time it was prepared and the patient's name. However, labelling is unnecessary if the preparation and administration is one uninterrupted process and the labelled syringe does not leave the hands of the person who prepared it. Only one unlabelled syringe should be handled at any one time (NHS England 2015a, NPSA 2007c).

Specific patient preparation

Before administering oral medication, the nurse should assess for:

- the patient's ability to understand the purpose of the medication being administered

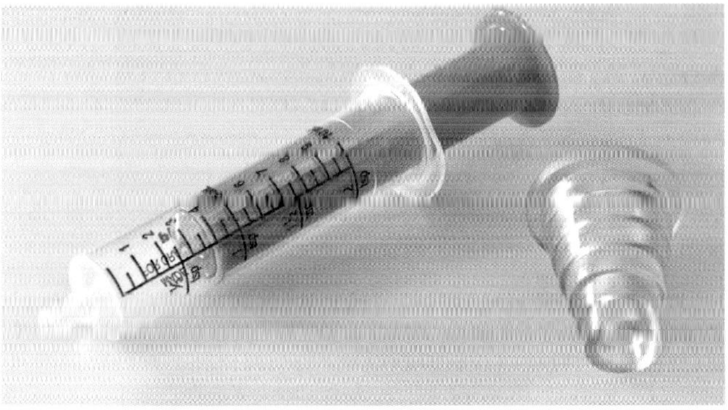

Figure 15.10 Oral syringe (compliant with NHS Improvement guidance).

- any medication allergies and hypersensitivities
- nil-by-mouth status
- the patient's ability to swallow the form of medication
- the patient's cough and gag reflexes
- any contraindications to oral medications including nausea and vomiting, absence of bowel sounds or reduced peristalsis, nasogastric suctioning, or any circumstance affecting bowel motility or absorption of medication, for example general anaesthesia, GI surgery or inflammatory bowel disease
- any possibility of drug–drug or drug–food interactions
- any pre-administration assessment for specific medications, for example pulse or blood pressure (Chernecky et al. 2005, Perry 2015).

Procedure guideline 15.2 Medication: oral drug administration

Essential equipment

- Personal protective equipment
- Medicine(s) to be administered
- Recording sheet or book as required by law or hospital policy
- Patient's prescription chart, to check dose, route, etc.
- Electronic identity check equipment, where relevant
- Glass of water
- Medicine container (disposable if possible)

Action	Rationale
Pre-procedure	
1 Introduce yourself to the patient, explain and discuss the procedure with them, and gain their consent to proceed.	To ensure that the patient feels at ease, understands the procedure and gives their valid consent (NMC 2018, **C**).
2 Wash hands with bactericidal soap and water or an alcohol-based handrub.	To minimize the risk of cross-infection (DH 2007, **C**; Fraise and Bradley 2009, **E**).
3 Before administering any prescribed drug, check that it is due and has not already been given. Carry out any required assessments, such as pulse, blood pressure and respiration. Check that the information contained in the prescription chart is complete, correct and legible.	To protect the patient from harm (DH 2003b, **C**; NMC 2018, **C**). Assessments are required to ensure the patient is fit enough to receive medication, for example blood pressure check before antihypertensives (Chernecky et al. 2005, **E**).
4 Before administering any prescribed drug, look at the patient's prescription chart and check the following: a the correct patient is being given the drug b drug c dose d date and time of administration e route and method of administration f diluent as appropriate g validity of prescription h signature of prescriber i the prescription is legible.	To ensure that the correct patient is given the correct drug in the prescribed dose using the appropriate diluent and by the correct route (DH 2003b, **C**; RPS 2019a, **C**). To protect the patient from harm (DH 2003b, **C**; NMC 2018, **C**).
If any of these pieces of information are missing, unclear or illegible, do not proceed with the administration. Consult with the prescriber.	To prevent any errors occurring. **E**
Procedure	
5 Select the required medication and check the expiry date.	Treatment with medication that is outside the expiry date is dangerous. Drugs deteriorate with storage. The expiry date indicates when a particular drug is no longer pharmacologically efficacious (DH 2003b, **C**; RPS 2019a **C**).
6 Empty the required dose into a medicine container. Avoid touching the preparation.	To minimize the risk of cross-infection. To minimize the risk of harm to the nurse (DH 2007, **C**; Fraise and Bradley 2009, **E**).
7 Take the medication and the prescription chart to the patient. Check the patient's identity by asking them to state their full name and date of birth. If the patient is unable to confirm these details, then check the patient identity band against the prescription chart. If an electronic identity check system for the patient and/or medicine identification is in place, then use it in accordance with hospital policy and procedures. Check the patient's allergy status by asking them or by checking the name band.	To ensure that the medication is administered to the correct patient and prevent any errors related to drug allergies (NPSA 2005, **C**).

(continued)

Procedure guideline 15.2 Medication: oral drug administration *(continued)*

Action	Rationale
8 Evaluate the patient's knowledge of the medication being offered by asking them to tell you what the medication is for and what side-effects to expect. If this knowledge appears to be faulty or incorrect, offer an explanation of the use, action, dose and potential side-effects of the drug or drugs involved.	Patients have a right to information about treatment (NMC 2018, **C**). To ensure that the patient understands the procedure and gives their valid consent (Griffith and Jordan 2003, **E**; NMC 2018, **C**).
9 Assist the patient into a sitting position where possible. A side-lying position may also be used if the patient is unable to sit.	To ease swallowing and prevent aspiration (Chernecky et al. 2005, **E**).
10 Administer the drug as prescribed.	To meet legal requirements and adhere to hospital policy (DH 2003b, **C**; NMC 2018, **C**; RPS 2019a, **C**).
11 Offer a glass of water, if allowed, assisting the patient where necessary.	To facilitate swallowing of the medication (Chernecky et al. 2005, **E**; Jordan et al. 2003, **E**).
12 Stay with the patient until they have swallowed all the medication.	To ensure that the medication is taken on time (Chernecky et al. 2005, **E**).
Post-procedure	
13 Record the dose given and sign the prescription chart. Also sign in any other place made necessary by legal requirement or hospital policy.	To meet legal requirements and adhere to hospital policy (DH 2003b, **C**; NMC 2018, **C**; RPS 2019a **C**).

Problem-solving table 15.1 Prevention and resolution (Procedure guideline 15.2)

Problem	Cause	Prevention	Action
Patient vomits when taking or after taking tablets	Patient suffering from nausea	Administer antiemetics prior to administration of tablets. These may need to be given via the rectal, intramuscular or intravenous routes.	If the patient vomits immediately after swallowing the tablet then it may be given again (potentially after antiemetics). If the patient vomits some time after the tablet is taken, it may depend on the type and frequency of medication as to whether it can be retaken. Ensure that the patient retakes the medication if they can see a whole tablet in the vomit.
Patient unable to swallow tablets	Patient suffering from dysphagia or has issues swallowing tablets	Ask the pharmacy whether the medication is available in liquid, sublingual, buccal or percutaneous forms (Barnett and Parmar 2018).	Discuss with the prescriber as to administering the medicine in another form or route.

Topical administration

Definition

Topical administration involves medication applied onto the skin and mucous membranes primarily for its local effects, for example creams, ointments and lotions (Perry 2015).

Related theory

Creams

Creams are emulsions of oil in water and are generally well absorbed into the skin. They are usually more cosmetically acceptable than ointments because they are less greasy and easier to apply (Aulton and Taylor 2018, BNF 2019a). They may be used as a 'base' in which a variety of drugs may be applied for local therapy (BNF 2019a).

Ointments

Ointments are greasy and/or oily preparations that are normally anhydrous and insoluble in water, and are more occlusive than creams (BNF 2019a). They are absorbed more slowly into the skin and leave a greasy residue. They have similar uses to creams and are particularly suitable for dry, scaly lesions (BNF 2019a). Care should be taken with extensive use of ointments as they pose a risk to the patient of their clothes or skin catching fire (NPSA 2007a).

Lotions

Lotions have a cooling effect and may be preferred to ointments or creams for application over a hairy area (BNF 2019a). Lotions are more liquid than ointments and creams and spread easily; they can become a slip hazard if spilt on the floor.

Pastes

Pastes are stiff preparations containing a high proportion of finely powdered solids, such as zinc oxide suspended in ointment. They are less occlusive than ointments and can be used to protect inflamed or excoriated skin (BNF 2019a, Perry 2015).

Wound products

See Chapter 18: Wound management.

Evidence-based approaches

The risk of serious effects from topical administration is generally low, but systemic effects can occur if the skin is thin, if the drug concentration is high or if contact is prolonged (Perry 2015). This is a particular problem with topical corticosteroids, as systemic absorption can occur. Mild and moderately potent corticosteroids are associated with few side-effects but particular care is required when treating neonates and babies and when using potent and very potent corticosteroids. Absorption through the skin can sometimes (rarely) cause adrenal suppression and even Cushing's syndrome (BNF 2019a). Central serous chorioretinopathy is a retinal disorder that has been reported after local administration of corticosteroids. Patients should be advised to report any blurred vision or other visual disturbances (MHRA 2017).

Pre-procedural considerations

Specific patient preparation

The condition of the affected site should be assessed for altered skin integrity as applying medicines to broken skin can cause them to be absorbed too rapidly, resulting in systemic effects (Chernecky et al. 2005, Perry 2015). The affected area must be washed and dried before applying the topical medicines where appropriate, unless the prescription directs otherwise.

Procedure guideline 15.3 Medication: topical applications

Essential equipment

- Personal protective equipment
- Medicine(s) to be applied
- Recording sheet or book as required by law or hospital policy
- Patient's prescription chart, to check dose, route, etc.
- Electronic identity check equipment, where relevant
- Sterile topical swabs
- Applicators

Action	Rationale
Pre-procedure	
1 Introduce yourself to the patient, explain and discuss the procedure with them, and gain their consent to proceed.	To ensure that the patient feels at ease, understands the procedure and gives their valid consent (Griffith and Jordan 2003, **E**; NMC 2018, **C**).
2 Wash hands with bactericidal soap and water or an alcohol-based handrub.	To minimize the risk of cross-infection (DH 2007, **C**; Fraise and Bradley 2009, **E**).
3 Before administering any prescribed drug, look at the patient's prescription chart and check the following: a the correct patient is being given the drug b drug c dose d date and time of administration e route and method of administration f diluent as appropriate g validity of prescription h signature of prescriber i the prescription is legible j the patient's allergy status.	To ensure that the correct patient is given the correct drug in the prescribed dose using the appropriate diluent and by the correct route (DH 2003b, **C**; RPS 2019a, **C**). To protect the patient from harm (DH 2003b, **C**; RPS 2019a, **C**).
If any of these pieces of information are missing, unclear or illegible, do not proceed with the administration. Consult with the prescriber.	To prevent any errors occurring. **E**
Procedure	
4 Put on a plastic apron and assist the patient into the required position.	To protect the patient from infection and the nurse from the topical agent as well as to allow access to the affected area of skin. **E**
5 Close the room door or curtains if appropriate.	To ensure patient privacy and dignity. **E**
6 Take the medication and the prescription chart to the patient. Check the patient's identity by asking them to state their full name and date of birth. If the patient is unable to confirm these details, then check the patient identity band against the prescription chart. If an electronic identity check system for the patient and/or medicine identification is in place, then use it in accordance with hospital policy and procedures. Check the patient's allergy status by asking them or by checking the name band.	To ensure that the medication is administered to the correct patient and prevent any errors related to drug allergies (NPSA 2005, **C**).
7 Expose the area that requires the medication and where necessary cover the patient with a towel or sheet.	To gain access to the affected area and to ensure patient dignity. **E**
8 Apply gloves and assess the condition of the skin, using aseptic technique if the skin is broken.	To prevent local or systemic infection (DH 2007, **C**; Fraise and Bradley 2009, **E**).
9 If the medication is to be rubbed into the skin, the preparation should be placed on a sterile topical swab.	To minimize the risk of cross-infection. To protect the nurse (DH 2007, **C**; Fraise and Bradley 2009, **E**).

(continued)

Procedure guideline 15.3 Medication: topical applications *(continued)*

Action	Rationale
10 If the preparation causes staining, advise the patient of this.	To ensure that adequate precautions are taken beforehand such as removal of clothing and to prevent stains (NMC 2018, **C**).
11 Apply the medication.	[illegible]
12 Apply a sterile dressing if required.	To ensure the ointment remains in place (Chernecky et al. 2005, **E**).
Post-procedure	
13 Remove gloves and apron and dispose of waste appropriately.	To ensure safe disposal and prevent reuse of equipment (HWR 2005, **C**; MHRA 2004, **C**).
14 Record the administration on the appropriate charts.	To maintain accurate records, provide a point of reference in the event of any queries and prevent any duplication of treatment (RPS 2019a, **C**).

Post-procedural considerations

Ask the patient to report any itching, skin colour change or signs of a rash following application.

Complications

Local skin reaction

The skin site may appear inflamed, and oedema with blistering indicates that subacute inflammation or eczema has developed from worsening of skin lesions. Patients may also complain of pruritus and tenderness, which could indicate slow or impaired healing and should be referred to the prescriber; alternative therapies may be required (Perry 2015).

Transdermal (percutaneous) administration

Definition

Transdermal drug delivery is the application of a formulation to the skin for absorption into the systemic circulation (Aulton and Taylor 2018). Medication is applied to the outermost layer of the skin (the stratum corneum) as a patch, ointment, cream or paste. Most transdermal products are designed for a systemic effect but some are designed for a local effect, such as non-steroidal anti-inflammatory drug (NSAID) creams designed to act within a joint.

Related theory

Transdermal ointments, creams and pastes

Transdermal ointments, creams and pastes consist of a semisolid medicine such as a paste or ointment where a quantity, usually specified in terms of length, is measured and rubbed into the skin. It can be rubbed into any non-hairy area of skin. However, where a local effect is required (e.g. for NSAID gels) then the quantity should be rubbed over the affected area(s). Drugs that can be delivered in this way include glyceryl trinitrate and oestradiol. Disadvantages of transdermal preparations in these forms include that they can be messy for patients and can also result in variations of the dose delivered due to the amount applied, the amount of rubbing in of the product and the amount of product transferred onto clothing.

Transdermal patches

Numerous types of transdermal patch exist and their properties differ, so it is important to use them as directed. A transdermal patch (Figure 15.11) contains a certain amount of drug and delivers it in a controlled manner over a specific period of time that is sufficient to cause the desired pharmacological effect when the drug passes through the skin and systemically into the body. A major advantage of all transdermal patch systems is to deliver a drug at a constant rate over a prolonged period of time (Aulton and Taylor 2018). Drugs that can be delivered via a transdermal system include fentanyl, hyoscine, nicotine, rivastigmine, rotigotine and oestradiol (Aulton and Taylor 2018).

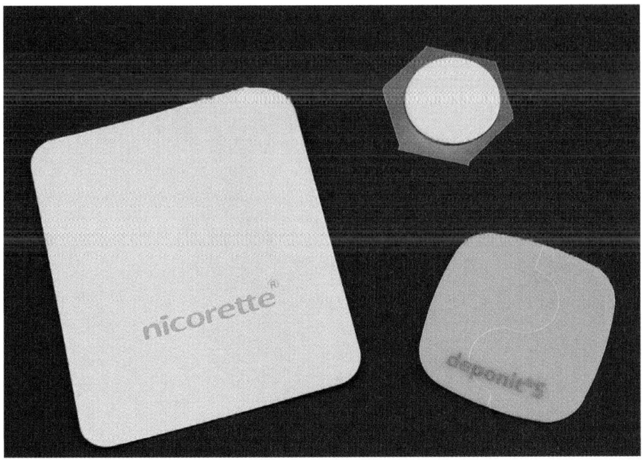

Figure 15.11 Transdermal patches.

Three types of transdermal patch are available: drug in adhesive patches, drug in matrix patches and rate-limiting membrane-type patches.

Drug in adhesive patches

These are simply designed patches that consist of a drug-containing adhesive and a backing material. They are widely used to deliver nicotine, oestradiol and glyceryl trinitrate. They tend to be thinner and more flexible than other patches and this may aid patient comfort and hence adherence. Various daily doses can be delivered, and the patches can be designed to deliver their drug over different periods of time, such as up to 1 day for nicotine patches and up to 7 days for buprenorphine, granisetron and oestradiol (Aulton and Taylor 2018).

Drug in matrix patches

In these patches, the drug is contained within a separate matrix that can be designed to either increase the drug content or control the drug release (Aulton and Taylor 2018). These patches consist of a drug-containing matrix, an adhesive layer and a backing material. The drug-containing matrix controls the release of the drug from the system (Aulton and Taylor 2018).

Rate-limiting membrane-type patches

These are more complex patches where the drug is contained within a reservoir and the release of the drug is controlled through a semi-permeable membrane. The reservoir may be liquid or a gel. A characteristic of this type of patch is that it can be designed to contain a high drug load.

Evidence-based approaches

The advantages of transdermal systems include the following.

- avoidance of drug loss due to first-pass metabolism
- the drug's effects can be maintained within the therapeutic window for longer, which reduces side-effects and maintains constant dosing
- potentially improved patient compliance
- the drug's effects can be stopped with the withdrawal of the patch and avoidance of first-pass metabolism (Aulton and Taylor 2018).

First-pass metabolism occurs when a drug is absorbed from the GI tract and enters the hepatic portal system and thus the liver before it reaches the rest of the body. The liver metabolizes many drugs, thus reducing their bioavailability before they reach the rest of the circulatory system (Hardman et al. 1996).

A disadvantage of transdermal systems is the limited number of drugs for which the system is suitable; for example, drugs have to have suitable physical and chemical properties to allow them to be absorbed through the skin and exert their effect. Tolerance-inducing drugs need a period during which they are not administered, which is not always possible with transdermal systems. In addition, drugs to be used in transdermal systems cannot be irritating to the skin otherwise they will not be tolerated by patients (Hillery et al. 2001).

Pre-procedural considerations

Specific patient preparation

The condition of the affected site should be assessed for altered skin integrity as applying medicines to broken skin can cause too-rapid absorption, resulting in systemic effects (Perry 2015). The affected area must be washed and dried before applying the patch or ointment. Both patches and ointments should be applied to a hairless area of skin. The upper chest, upper arms and upper back are recommended sites and the distal areas of the extremities should be avoided (Chernecky et al. 2005). For local use (e.g. NSAID ointment) they should be applied to the relevant area of the body. Patches should not be trimmed or cut. It is important to remove previously applied patches as they will have residual drugs, which will continue to be absorbed and may lead to adverse effects.

Procedure guideline 15.4 Medication: transdermal applications

Essential equipment

- Personal protective equipment
- Medicine(s) to be applied
- Recording sheet or book as required by law or hospital policy
- Patient's prescription chart, to check dose, route, etc.
- Electronic identity check equipment, where relevant

Action	Rationale
Pre-procedure	
1 Introduce yourself to the patient, explain and discuss the procedure with them, and gain their consent to proceed.	To ensure that the patient feels at ease, understands the procedure and gives their valid consent (Griffith and Jordan 2003, **E**; NMC 2018, **C**).
2 Wash hands with bactericidal soap and water or an alcohol-based handrub.	To minimize the risk of cross-infection (DH 2007, **C**; Fraise and Bradley 2009, **E**).
3 Before administering any prescribed drug, look at the patient's prescription chart and check the following: a the correct patient is being given the drug b drug c dose d date and time of administration e route and method of administration f diluent as appropriate g validity of prescription h signature of prescriber i the prescription is legible.	To ensure that the correct patient is given the correct drug in the prescribed dose using the appropriate diluent and by the correct route (DH 2003b, **C**; RPS 2019a, **C**). To protect the patient from harm (DH 2003b, **C**; NMC 2018, **C**).
If any of these pieces of information are missing, unclear or illegible, do not proceed with the administration. Consult with the prescriber.	To prevent any errors occurring. **E**
Procedure	
4 Put on a plastic apron and assist the patient into the required position.	To allow access to the affected area of skin. **E**
5 Close the room door or curtains if appropriate.	To ensure patient privacy and dignity. **E**
6 Take the medication and the prescription chart to the patient. Check the patient's identity by asking them to state their full name and date of birth. If the patient is unable to confirm these details, then check the patient identity band against the prescription chart. If an electronic identity check system for the patient and/or medicine identification is in place, then use it in accordance with hospital policy and procedures. Check the patient's allergy status by asking them or by checking the name band.	To ensure that the medication is administered to the correct patient and prevent any errors related to drug allergies (NPSA 2005, **C**).
7 Expose the area where the patch, ointment, cream or paste will be applied. Where necessary, cover the patient with a towel or sheet.	To gain access to the affected area and to ensure patient privacy and dignity. **E**

(continued)

Procedure guideline 15.4 Medication: transdermal applications *(continued)*

Action	Rationale
8 Apply gloves and assess the condition of the skin. Do not apply to skin that is oily, burnt, cut or irritated in any way.	To prevent local or systemic infection (DH 2007, **C**; Fraise and Bradley 2009, **E**). To prevent local or systemic effects and to ensure the patch will remain in place (DH 2007, **C**; Perry 2015, **E**).
9 Where necessary, remove any used patch and fold it in half, adhesive side inwards. Place it in the original sachet (if still available) and dispose of it into clinical waste.	To ensure that the release membrane is not exposed. **E**
10 Remove any drug residue from the former site before placing the next patch.	To avoid any skin irritation (Chernecky et al. 2005, **E**).
11 Carefully remove the patch from its protective cover and hold it by the edge without touching the adhesive edges (or touching the adhesive edges as little as possible).	To ensure the patch will adhere and the medication dose will not be affected (Perry 2015, **E**).
12 Apply the patch immediately, pressing firmly with the palm of the hand for up to 10 seconds, making sure the patch sticks well around the edges.	To ensure adequate adhesion and prevent loss of the patch, which would result in reduced dose and effectiveness (Perry 2015, **E**).
13 Date and initial the patch.	To ensure all staff know when it must be changed (Perry 2015, **E**).
14 For ointment, creams and pastes, apply the prescribed quantity and gently rub until absorbed.	To ensure the medication is applied. **E**
Post-procedure	
15 Remove and dispose of waste in appropriate waste bags.	To ensure safe disposal and prevent reuse of equipment. **E**
16 Record the administration on the appropriate charts.	To maintain accurate records, provide a point of reference in the event of any queries and prevent any duplication of treatment (RPS 2019a, **C**).

Post-procedural considerations

Ongoing care
A different skin site should be used each time to avoid skin irritation (Chernecky et al. 2005). After use, the patch still contains substantial quantities of active ingredients, which may have harmful effects if they reach the aquatic environment. Hence, after removal, the used patch should be folded in half (adhesive side inwards so that the release membrane is not exposed), placed in the original sachet (if still available) and then discarded safely out of reach of children. Any used or unused patches should be discarded according to local policy or returned to the pharmacy. Used patches should not be flushed down the toilet or placed in liquid waste disposal systems.

Complications
See 'Topical applications' above.

Rectal administration

Definition
These preparations are administered via the rectum, which may exert a local effect on the GI mucosa (e.g. an anti-inflammatory effect in ulcerative colitis) or have systemic effects (e.g. analgesics or to relieve vomiting) (Potter and Perry 2016).

Related theory

Suppositories
Suppositories are solid preparations that may contain one or more drugs. The drugs are normally ground or sieved and then dissolved or dispersed into a glyceride-type fatty acid or water-soluble base. These suppositories will either melt after insertion into the body or dissolve and mix with the available volume of rectal fluid (Aulton and Taylor 2018).

Enemas
Enemas are solutions or dispersions of a drug in a small volume of water or oil. These preparations are presented in a small plastic container in the shape of a bulb, which contains the drug and an application tube. The bulb can be compressed when the tube has been inserted in the rectum to deliver the drug. Retention enemas are often in larger volumes, up to 100 mL, while some rectal preparations come in the form of foams. Enemas can be difficult for patients to use by themselves compared to suppositories and therefore their use is not as widespread (Aulton and Taylor 2018).

Evidence-based approaches
The advantages of rectal administration include the following (Chernecky et al. 2005, Perry 2015):

- The drug can be administered when the patient cannot use the oral route, for example if the patient is vomiting or is post-operative and therefore either unconscious or unable to ingest anything via the oral route.
- In some categories of patient (e.g. children and the elderly), it may be easier to use the rectal route than the oral one as it does not require swallowing.
- The drug may be less suited to the oral route; for example, the oral route can cause severe local GI side-effects.
- The drug may not be stable after GI administration or it may have an unacceptable taste that makes it unpalatable via the oral route.
- Rectal administration rarely causes local irritation or side-effects.

The disadvantages of the rectal route include the following (Chernecky et al. 2005, Downie et al. 2003, Perry 2015):

- Some patients have strong feelings against the rectal route, and some have feelings of discomfort and embarrassment.
- There can be slow and incomplete absorption.
- The development of proctitis has been reported with rectal drug administration.
- It is contraindicated in patients who have had rectal surgery or have active rectal bleeding.

After a suppository has been inserted into the rectum, body temperature melts the suppository so the medication can be distributed. Proper placement is important to promote retention of the medication until it dissolves and is absorbed into the mucosa (Perry 2015).

For further information about the administration of rectal medication, see Procedure guideline 6.22: Suppository administration.

Vaginal administration

Definition

Medications are inserted into the vaginal canal usually for local effects such as treatment of infections (e.g. *Trichomonas* and *Candida* infections) and contraceptive purposes. They can also be used for systemic effects (e.g. administration of oestrogens and progesterones) but this is less common (Chernecky et al. 2005, Perry 2015).

Related theory

Vaginal preparations can be delivered in a wide variety of dosage forms including pessaries, creams, aerosol foams, gels and tablets (Chernecky et al. 2005, Perry 2015).

Evidence-based approaches

The advantages of the vaginal route include the following (Hillery et al. 2001).

- The vagina offers a large surface area for drug absorption.
- A rich blood supply ensures rapid absorption of the drug.
- This route can act as an alternative for drugs that cannot be delivered via the oral route (as for suppositories).
- The vaginal route can deliver a drug over a controlled period of time, thus avoiding peaks and troughs, which can result in toxicity and risk ineffectiveness.

The disadvantages of the vaginal route include the following (Hillery et al. 2001).

- The route is limited to drugs that are potent molecules and are therefore easily absorbed.
- The vagina can easily be irritated by the use of devices or locally irritating drugs.
- Care must be taken with the use of vaginal devices to ensure they are sterilized and do not act as a growth medium for bacteria.
- Vaginal bioavailability can be affected by hormone levels and can therefore change during menstrual cycles, with age and during pregnancy.
- Leakage can occur with vaginal preparations. This can be alleviated by using the preparation at night.
- This route may not be acceptable to some patients.

Pre-procedural considerations

Specific patient preparation

Check the patient's allergy status and also ascertain whether they have recently given birth or undergone vaginal surgery, as this may alter tissue integrity and the level of discomfort. Additionally, review the patient's willingness and ability to self-administer the medication (Chernecky et al. 2005, Perry 2015).

Procedure guideline 15.5 Medication: vaginal administration

Essential equipment

- Personal protective equipment
- Medicine(s) to be administered
- Recording sheet or book as required by law or hospital policy
- Patient's prescription chart, to check dose, route, etc.
- Electronic identity check equipment, where relevant
- Topical swabs
- Disposable sanitary pad
- Lubricating jelly
- Warm water

Optional equipment

- Light source (e.g. lamp or torch)

Medicinal products

- Pessary

Action	Rationale
Pre-procedure	
1 Introduce yourself to the patient, explain and discuss the procedure with them, and gain their consent to proceed.	To ensure that the patient feels at ease, understands the procedure and gives their valid consent (NMC 2018, **C**).
2 Wash hands with bactericidal soap and water or an alcohol-based handrub.	To minimize the risk of cross-infection (DH 2007, **C**; Fraise and Bradley 2009, **E**).
3 Before administering any prescribed drug, look at the patient's prescription chart and check the following: a the correct patient is being given the drug b drug c dose d date and time of administration e route and method of administration f diluent as appropriate g validity of prescription h signature of prescriber i the prescription is legible.	To ensure that the correct patient is given the correct drug in the prescribed dose using the appropriate diluent and by the correct route (DH 2003b, **C**; RPS 2019a, **C**). To protect the patient from harm (DH 2003b, **C**; NMC 2018, **C**).
If any of these pieces of information are missing, unclear or illegible, do not proceed with the administration. Consult with the prescriber.	To prevent any errors occurring. **E**

(continued)

Procedure guideline 15.5 Medication: vaginal administration *(continued)*

Action	Rationale
4 Select the appropriate pessary and check it against the prescription chart.	To ensure that the correct medication is given to the correct patient at the appropriate time (RPS 2019a, **C**).
Procedure	
5 Close the room door or curtains, keeping the patient covered as much as possible.	To ensure patient privacy and dignity. **E**
6 Take the medication and the prescription chart to the patient. Check the patient's identity by asking them to state their full name and date of birth. If the patient is unable to confirm these details, then check the patient identity band against the prescription chart. If an electronic identity check system for the patient and/or medicine identification is in place, then use it in accordance with hospital policy and procedures. Check the patient's allergy status by asking them or by checking the name band.	To ensure that the medication is administered to the correct patient and prevent any errors related to drug allergies (NPSA 2005, **C**).
7 Apply an apron and assist the patient into the appropriate position, either left lateral with buttocks to the edge of the bed or supine with the knees drawn up and legs parted. A light source (e.g. lamp or torch) may be needed.	To facilitate easy access to the vaginal canal, visualize the external genitalia and vaginal canal, and facilitate correct insertion of the pessary (Chernecky et al. 2005, **E**; Perry 2015, **E**).
8 Wash hands with bactericidal soap and water or an alcohol-based handrub, and put on gloves.	To minimize the risk of cross-infection (DH 2007, **C**; Fraise and Bradley 2009, **E**).
9 Clean the area with warm water if necessary.	To remove any previously applied creams (Downie et al. 2003, **E**).
10 Remove the pessary from the wrapper and apply lubricating jelly to a topical swab and from the swab onto the pessary. Lubricate the gloved index finger of the dominant hand.	To facilitate insertion of the pessary and ensure the patient's comfort. **C**
11 With the non-dominant gloved hand, gently retract the labial folds to expose the vaginal orifice.	To enable insertion of the pessary into the correct orifice (Perry 2015, **E**).
12 Insert the rounded end of the pessary along the posterior vaginal wall and into the top of the vagina (entire length of finger).	To make sure the pessary is inserted in the correct position to ensure equal distribution of the medication (Perry 2015, **E**). To ensure that the pessary is retained and that the medication can reach its maximum efficiency (Chernecky et al. 2005, **E**).
13 Wipe away any excess lubricating jelly from the patient's vulval and/or perineal area with a topical swab.	To promote patient comfort (Potter and Perry 2016, **E**).
14 Make the patient comfortable and explain that there may be a small amount of discharge. Apply a clean sanitary pad.	To absorb any excess discharge (Potter and Perry 2016, **E**).
Post-procedure	
15 Remove and dispose of gloves and apron safely and in accordance with locally approved procedures.	To ensure safe disposal (HWR 2005, **C**; MHRA 2004, **C**).
16 Record the administration on appropriate charts.	To maintain accurate records, provide a point of reference in the event of any queries and prevent any duplication of treatment (RPS 2019a, **C**).

Post-procedural considerations

The patient needs to retain the medication so it is recommended that the medication is administered prior to the patient going to bed, or the patient should remain supine for 5–10 minutes after the pessary is instilled (Chernecky et al. 2005, Perry 2015). Explain to the patient that they may also notice discharge following administration and that it is nothing to be concerned about.

Pulmonary administration

Definition

Pulmonary administration involves dosage forms that enter the body via the lungs in aerosol form with the aim of achieving local effects, such as improving bronchodilation or improving clearance of pulmonary secretions (Chernecky et al. 2005, Perry 2015). Systemic effects can also be achieved through the pulmonary route, for example via volatile anaesthetics (Hillery et al. 2001). Doses are inhaled via the mouth, some via the nose, and some via the nose and mouth (Downie et al. 2003).

Related theory

In order for drugs to reach the lungs, they must be delivered in an aerosol form. The aerosol penetrates the lung airways, the deeper passages of the respiratory tract provide a large surface area for drug absorption, and the alveolar–capillary network absorbs medication rapidly (Potter and Perry 2016).

There are three ways in which an aerosol form can be produced: by nebulizer, by pressurized metered dose inhalers and by drug powder inhalers:

- *Nebulization* involves the passage of air or oxygen driven through a solution of a drug. The resulting fine mist is then inhaled via a face-mask (Trounce and Gould 2000). Some antibiotics and bronchodilators may be given in this way (Figure 15.12).
- *Metered dose inhalers* (MDIs) involve a drug being suspended in a propellant in a small hand-held aerosol can in the form of a spray, mist or fine powder. Metered doses can then be delivered from the aerosol by the use of a metering valve within the device, which is designed to release a fixed volume, for example of salbutamol.

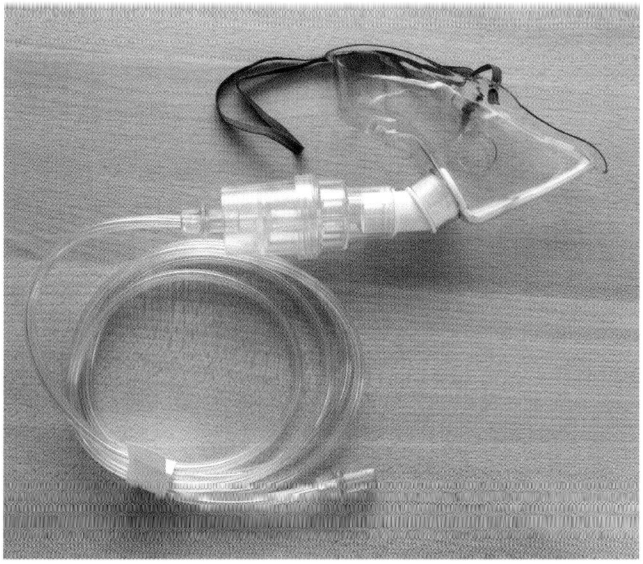

Figure 15.12 Nebulizer.

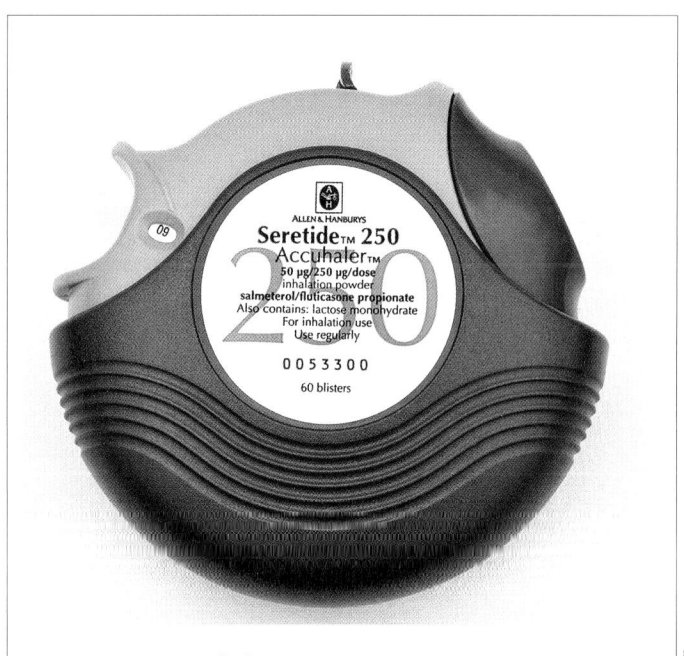

Figure 15.14 Accuhaler.

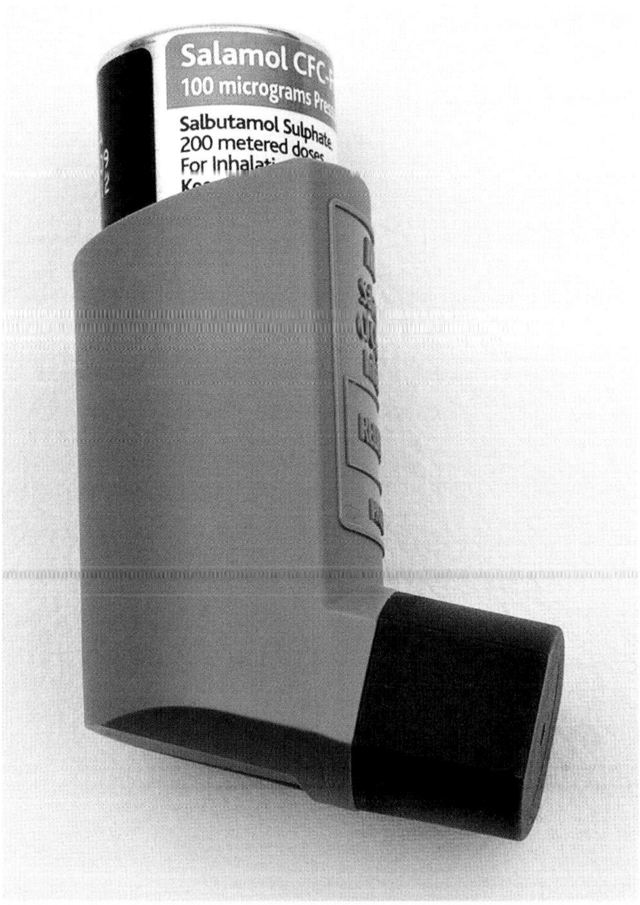

Figure 15.13 Metered dose inhaler (MDI).

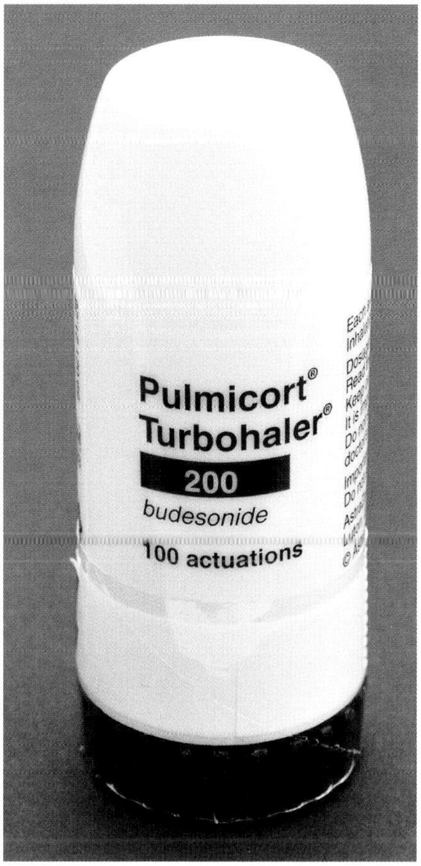

Figure 15.15 Turbohaler.

Steroid medications are often administered by MDI to treat long-term reactive airway disease (Chernecky et al. 2005, Perry 2015) (Figure 15.13).

- *Dry powder inhalers* involve a powder being delivered to the lungs via a breath-actuated device. Examples of inhalers in this group are the Accuhaler (Figure 15.14) and the Turbohaler (Figure 15.15).

Pre-procedural considerations

Equipment

Nebulizer

The advantage of nebulizers is that they can deliver drugs to the lungs consistently with better deposition in greater amounts, if necessary, than standard inhalers because of the smaller particles that are generated. They also do not require any co-ordination in order to deliver the drug to the lungs. Nebulization can also be used to deliver drugs where the dose is large or needs to be dispersed in a large volume. The disadvantages are that they are expensive, they are not easily portable and the delivery of the drug can be difficult to control, for example due to loss in the tubing and mouthpiece.

Solutions and suspensions for nebulization may be available in single-dose units or multiple-dose containers. Careful measurement is required in the case of the latter. Some products are presented as dry powders that require reconstitution, while some solutions require dilution before administration. The manufacturer's instructions should be followed to ensure that the drug is properly dispersed and at the appropriate concentration for nebulization.

Metered dose inhaler

The advantages of MDIs are that they are convenient, can deliver a fixed dose and are inexpensive. The disadvantage can be the co-ordination needed to use one. In order for the MDI to be effective, the patient needs to trigger it during a deep, slow inhalation and then hold their breath for around 10 seconds. This need for co-ordination between actuation of the dose and inhalation can be removed by using a spacer device (Figure 15.16). The spacer device reduces the speed with which the dose is delivered and the resulting 'cold freon' effect that can occur, which can prevent a patient from continuing to inhale after actuation of the MDI. Spacers are also useful for patients on high-dose inhaled steroids in order to prevent oral candidiasis, for children and patients requiring higher doses, and can improve dose delivery to 15% (Downie et al. 2003). Spacer devices are designed to be compatible with specific inhalers and therefore care should be taken to ensure the correct spacer device is used.

Medication in MDIs is under pressure and so they should not be punctured or stored near heat or in hot conditions (e.g. patients must be informed not to leave their MDI in a hot car) (Chernecky et al. 2005).

Dry powder inhalers

Dry powder inhalers are also useful when there are problems with co-ordination. However, they can initiate a cough reflex and patients need to have sufficient breath inhalation to activate the device. It is also important to remember that because these medications are absorbed rapidly through the pulmonary circulation, most create systemic side-effects (Chernecky et al. 2005, Perry 2015).

There are multiple types and brands of device available, including a number of combination products. Care must be taken in product selection, and the current recommendation is to keep patients on inhaler devices from the same range (BTS and SIGN 2016).

Specific patient preparation

Patients who suffer from chronic respiratory disease and require airway management frequently receive inhalation medications. Maximum benefit is obtained only when the correct technique of inhalation is used so it is vital that patients are taught how to use these devices correctly and safely. Placebo inhalers and devices are available for educating patients on the use of their inhalers. Periodic checks should be carried out to ensure that efficiency is being maintained.

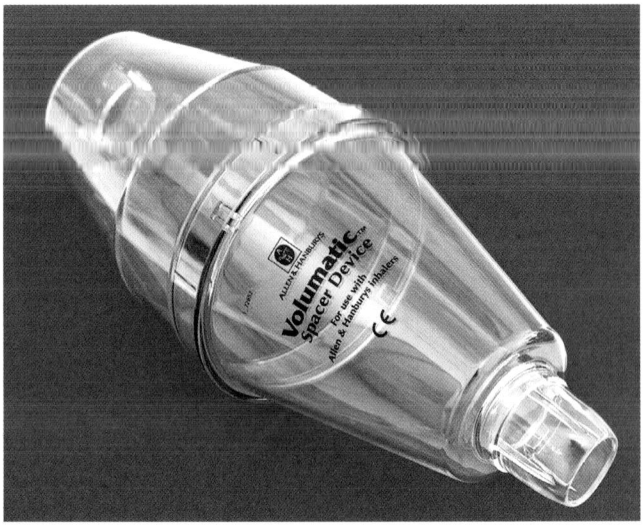

Figure 15.16 Spacer device.

Use of an MDI requires co-ordination during the breathing cycle, and impairment of grasp or presence of tremors of the hands interferes with patients' ability to depress the canister within the inhaler (Chernecky et al. 2005, Perry 2015). Studies have shown that both adults and children have difficulties with aerosol inhalers; problems include co-ordinating activation and inhalation, too rapid inhalation and too short breaths after inspiration (Hilton 1990). Baseline observations of pulse, respirations and breath sounds should be performed before beginning treatment to use as a comparison during and after treatment (Potter and Perry 2016). Patients who are to receive nebulized medicines should be in a sitting position either in bed or in a chair (Downie et al. 2003).

Education

Compliance is more likely to be achieved if the patient is well informed. It is the responsibility of the nurse, doctor and pharmacist to ensure that patients have adequate teaching and demonstration and are monitored at intervals. The patient should know the following:

- about the disease, the purpose of the therapy, and how to recognize and report deterioration in their condition
- how to use and care for the inhaler
- the dose to be taken
- the time interval
- the maximum number of inhalations that should be taken in 24 hours (Downie et al. 2003).

Procedure guideline 15.6 Medication: administration by inhalation using a metered dose or dry powder inhaler

Essential equipment

- Personal protective equipment
- Inhaler(s) to be used
- Spacer device if appropriate
- Recording sheet or book as required by law or hospital policy
- Patient's prescription chart, to check dose, route, etc.
- Electronic identity check equipment, where relevant

Action	Rationale
Pre-procedure	
1 Introduce yourself to the patient, explain and discuss the procedure with them, and gain their consent to proceed.	To ensure that the patient feels at ease, understands the procedure and gives their valid consent (Griffith and Jordan 2003, **E**; NMC 2018, **C**).
2 Wash hands with bactericidal soap and water or an alcohol-based handrub.	To minimize the risk of cross-infection (DH 2007, **C**; Fraise and Bradley 2009, **E**).
3 Carefully explain and demonstrate the inhaler to the patient. If further advice is required, contact the hospital pharmacist.	Correct use of inhalers is essential (see the manufacturer's information leaflet). Incorrect use may result in most of the dose remaining in the mouth and/or being expelled almost immediately. This renders treatment ineffective (Watt 2003, **E**).
Procedure	
4 Assist the patient into an upright position, if possible in the bed or a chair.	To permit full expansion of the diaphragm. **E**
5 Before administering any prescribed drug, look at the patient's prescription chart and check the following: a the correct patient is being given the drug b drug c dose d date and time of administration e route and method of administration f diluent as appropriate g validity of prescription h signature of prescriber i the prescription is legible.	To ensure that the correct patient is given the correct drug in the prescribed dose using the appropriate diluent and by the correct route (DH 2003b, **C**; RPS 2019a, **C**). To protect the patient from harm (DH 2003b, **C**).
If any of these pieces of information are missing, unclear or illegible, do not proceed with the administration. Consult with the prescriber.	To prevent any errors occurring. **E**
6 Take the medication and the prescription chart to the patient. Check the patient's identity by asking them to state their full name and date of birth. If the patient is unable to confirm these details, then check the patient identity band against the prescription chart. If an electronic identity check system for the patient and/or medicine identification is in place, then use it in accordance with hospital policy and procedures. Check the patient's allergy status by asking them or by checking the name band.	To ensure that the medication is administered to the correct patient and prevent any errors related to drug allergies (NPSA 2005, **C**).
7 Remove the mouthpiece cover from the inhaler.	To expose the area for use. **E**
8 Shake the inhaler well for 2–5 seconds.	To ensure mixing of medication in the canister (Potter and Perry 2016, **E**).
9 • *Without a spacer device*: ask the patient to take a deep breath and exhale completely, open their lips and place the inhaler mouthpiece in their mouth with the opening towards the back of the throat, then close their lips tightly around it.	To prepare the airway to receive medication and direct the aerosol towards the airway (Potter and Perry 2016, **E**).
• *With a spacer device*: insert the metered dose inhaler (MDI) into the end of the spacer device. Ask the patient to exhale and then grasp the spacer mouthpiece with teeth and lips while holding inhaler.	To enable the medication to reach the airways instead of hitting the back of the throat. The spacer improves delivery of correct dose of inhaled medication. **E**
10 Ask the patient to tip their head back slightly then inhale slowly and deeply through their mouth while depressing the canister fully.	To allow the medication to be distributed to the airways during inhalation. **E**
11 Instruct the patient to breathe in slowly for 2–3 seconds and hold their breath for approximately 10 seconds, then remove the MDI from their mouth (if not using a spacer) before exhaling slowly through pursed lips.	To enable the aerosol spray to reach the deep branches of the airways (Chernecky et al. 2005, **E**).
12 Instruct the patient to wait 20–30 seconds between inhalations (if same medication) or 2–5 minutes between inhalations (if different medication). Always administer bronchodilators before steroids.	To ensure that the medication has the optimum effect and minimal side-effects. **E**
13 If steroid medication is administered, ask the patient to rinse their mouth with water approximately 2 minutes after inhaling the dose.	To remove any medication residue from the oral cavity. Steroids may alter the normal flora of the oral mucosa and lead to development of fungal infection (Lilley et al. 2007, **E**).

(continued)

Procedure guideline 15.6 Medication: administration by inhalation using a metered dose or dry powder inhaler *(continued)*

Action	Rationale
Post-procedure	
14 Clean any equipment used and discard all disposable equipment in appropriate containers.	To minimize the risk of infection (Fraise and Bradley 2009, **E**).
15 Record the administration on the appropriate charts.	To maintain accurate records, provide a point of reference in the event of any queries and prevent any duplication of treatment (NPSA 2007c, **C**; RPS 2019a, **C**).

Procedure guideline 15.7 Medication: administration by inhalation using a nebulizer

Essential equipment

- Personal protective equipment
- Recording sheet or book as required by law or hospital policy
- Patient's prescription chart, to check dose, route, etc.
- Electronic identity check equipment, where relevant
- Face-mask or mouthpiece
- Nebulizer and tubing
- Measuring equipment, e.g. needles and syringes (if relevant)

Medicinal products

- Medication required
- Materials and equipment for reconstitution and/or dilution (if relevant)

Action	Rationale
Pre-procedure	
1 Introduce yourself to the patient, explain and discuss the procedure with them, and gain their consent to proceed.	To ensure that the patient feels at ease, understands the procedure and gives their valid consent (Griffith and Jordan 2003, **E**; NMC 2018, **C**).
2 Wash hands with bactericidal soap and water or an alcohol-based handrub.	To minimize the risk of cross-infection (DH 2007, **C**; Fraise and Bradley 2009, **E**).
3 Assist the patient into an upright position, if possible in bed or a chair.	To permit full expansion of the diaphragm and facilitate effective inhalation (Jevon et al. 2010, **E**).
4 Before administering any prescribed drug, look at the patient's prescription chart and check the following: a the correct patient is being given the drug b drug c dose d date and time of administration e route and method of administration f diluent as appropriate g validity of prescription h signature of prescriber i the prescription is legible.	To ensure that the correct patient is given the correct drug in the prescribed dose using the appropriate diluent and by the correct route (DH 2003b, **C**; RPS 2019a, **C**). To protect the patient from harm (DH 2003b, **C**).
If any of these pieces of information are missing, unclear or illegible, do not proceed with the administration. Consult with the prescriber.	To prevent any errors occurring. **E**
Procedure	
5 Take the medication and the prescription chart to the patient. Check the patient's identity by asking them to state their full name and date of birth. If the patient is unable to confirm these details, then check the patient identity band against the prescription chart. If an electronic identity check system for the patient and/or medicine identification is in place, then use it in accordance with hospital policy and procedures. Check the patient's allergy status by asking them or by checking the name band.	To ensure that the medication is administered to the correct patient and prevent any errors related to drug allergies (NPSA 2005, **C**).
6 Administer only one drug at a time unless specifically instructed to the contrary.	Several drugs used together may cause undesirable reactions or may inactivate each other (Jordan et al. 2003, **E**).

7 Assemble the nebulizer equipment as per the manufacturer's instructions.	To ensure correct administration. **C**
8 Measure any liquid medication with a syringe. Add the prescribed medication and diluent (if needed) to the nebulizer.	To ensure the correct dose is given (DH 2007, **C**).
9 Attach the mouthpiece or face-mask via the tubing to medical piped air or oxygen as prescribed.	To ensure it is ready to use when switched on. **E**
a If the patient has a clinical need for supplementary oxygen therapy, oxygen therapy must *not* be discontinued while the nebulizer is in progress. In this situation the drug should be nebulized with oxygen therapy. The patient should receive continuous pulse oximetry for at least the duration of the nebulizer treatment.	To ensure the patient maintains their target saturation (Jevon et al. 2010, **E**).
b If the patient is hypercapnic or acidotic (e.g. chronic obstructive pulmonary disease), the nebulizer should be driven by medical air, not oxygen.	To avoid worsening hypercapnia (NICE 2010, **C**).
10 Ask the patient to hold the mouthpiece between their lips or apply the face mask and take a slow, deep breath.	To promote greater deposition of medication in the airways (Potter and Perry 2016, **E**).
11 After inspiration, ask the patient to pause briefly and then exhale.	To improve the effectiveness of the medication. **E**
12 Turn on the piped air or oxygen and ensure a sufficient mist is formed. A minimum flow rate of 6–8 L per minute is required.	To ensure effective nebulization of the medication (Downie et al. 2003, **E**; Jevon et al. 2010, **E**).
13 Ask the patient to continue to breathe as above until all the nebulized medication has been used (0.5 mL will remain in the chamber). Optimal nebulization of 4 mL takes approximately 10 minutes.	To ensure all medication has been received. **E** To ensure the medication is effective. **E**
Post-procedure	
14 If appropriate and prescribed, recommence oxygen therapy at the appropriate dose.	To continue the patient's required therapy (Jevon et al. 2010, **E**).
15 Clean any equipment used and/or discard all single-use disposable equipment in appropriate containers.	To minimize the risk of infection (DH 2007, **C**; Fraise and Bradley 2009, **E**; Jevon et al. 2010, **E**).
16 Record the administration on the appropriate charts.	To maintain accurate records, provide a point of reference in the event of any queries and prevent any duplication of treatment (RPS 2019a, **C**).

Post-procedural considerations

If the nebulizer is marked as single use then it must be discarded after use. However, nebulizers should not be treated as single use unless clearly indicated by the manufacturer. If they can be reused, then the nebulizer chamber and mask should be washed in hot soapy water, rinsed thoroughly and dried with paper towels to reduce bacterial contamination and also to prevent any build-up of crystallized medication in the nebulizer (Downie et al. 2003). Spacer devices should be washed, rinsed and allowed to dry naturally on a weekly basis and replaced after 6–12 months (Downie et al. 2003).

Complications

There is a risk of patients developing oral candidiasis when using a corticosteroid MDI or dry powder inhaler. This can be reduced by using a spacer device for an MDI and encouraging the patient to rinse their mouth after administration.

Overuse of some inhalers can result in cardiac dysrhythmias and patients may suffer from tachycardia, palpitations, headache, restlessness and insomnia. The doctor should be informed and observations commenced (Potter and Perry 2016).

Ophthalmic administration

Definition

Ophthalmic administration involves dosage forms introduced into the eye for local effects (e.g. to treat infections), to dilate or constrict the pupil, or to treat eye conditions such as glaucoma (Potter and Perry 2016).

Related theory

The topical route is the most popular way to introduce drugs into the eye in the form of eye drops or eye ointment. Most types of drop are instilled into the inferior fornix (the pocket formed by gently pulling on the lower eyelid), as the conjunctiva in this area is less sensitive than that overlying the cornea and will aid the retention of the medication (Jevon et al. 2010).

There are many factors that affect how much of an effect the instilled drug will have on the eye. The eye has a highly selective corneal barrier, which can prevent absorption of drugs. It also has a tear film, which provides an effective clearance mechanism. When an excess volume of fluid is present in the eye, this fluid either will be spilled onto the cheeks and eyelashes or will enter the nasolacrimal drainage system, with the potential for systemic absorption of the drug. Drugs also need to be introduced to the eye at a neutral pH, as acidic or alkaline preparations will result in reflex lachrymation, which will remove the drug from the eye.

Evidence-based approaches

In order to optimize the effects of topical eye preparations, attempts should be made to ensure that there is proper placement of eye drops and ointments and that the volume applied is kept to a minimum. The number of drops instilled depends on the type of solution used and its purpose. Usually one drop only is required into the affected eye(s) and will be sufficient if it is instilled in the correct manner. The exceptions to the 'one drop' rule are as follows:

- *Oil-based solutions*: these are used to lubricate the eyeball. Usually one drop is instilled, with further drops given as required.
- *Anaesthetic drops*: these are used to anaesthetize the eye; one drop should be instilled at a time. This is repeated until the drop cannot be felt on the eye.

The tip of the dropper bottle should be held as close to the eye as possible without touching the lids or the cornea. This will avoid corneal damage and reduce the risk of cross-infection. If the drop falls from too great a height, it is difficult to control and will be uncomfortable for the patient. The eye should be closed for as long as possible after application, preferably for 1–2 minutes.

It is important to remember that systemic effects may arise from absorption of drugs into the body's circulation; this absorption is highly variable but can be minimized by applying pressure to the lacrimal punctum for at least 1 minute after applying eye drops. Some eye drops are contraindicated or have special precautions in some patients due to the risk of adverse effects (e.g. beta blockers, such as timolol, in patients with asthma or chronic obstructive pulmonary disease) (EMC 2019).

If patients need to use more than one eye drop preparation at the same time of the day, they may experience overflow and dilution when one immediately follows the other, so they should be advised to leave an interval of at least 5 minutes between the two. If eye drops have an extended contact time (e.g. gels and suspensions), then this interval should be extended (BNF 2019a). If both drops and ointments are prescribed, the drops should be applied before the ointment, as the ointment will leave a film on the eye and hamper the absorption of the medication in drop form (Aldridge 2010).

Useful properties of eye ointments include:

- longer duration of action than eye drops
- a soothing emollient action
- easy to apply
- long shelf life (Downie et al. 2003).

Ointments are applied to the upper rim of the inferior fornix using a similar technique to eye drops (Figures 15.17 and Figure 15.18). A 2 cm line of ointment should be applied from the nasal canthus outwards. Similarly to the instillation of eye drops, the nozzle should be held as close to the eye as possible to avoid contact with the cornea and eyelids (Aldridge 2010, Alexander et al. 2007).

Pre-procedural considerations

Equipment

A variety of droppers and bottles are available for the instillation of eye preparations. These include glass bottles incorporating droppers, plastic bottles with an integral dropper and single-dose forms, such as Minims. The vast majority of eye drops are supplied in plastic bottles with an integrated dropper. Droppers from glass bottles expose the drops to potential contamination and can become contaminated themselves. Plastic bottles are squeezed between the fingers, so avoiding the need for a separate dropper. They are also less expensive than glass bottles with a dropper. Single-dose units usually consist of small plastic dropper tubes that are squeezed and discarded after a single use.

Due to the risk of eye drops introducing infection into the eye and between individual patients and eyes, the BNF (2019a) provides extensive guidelines to minimize the risk of microbial contamination. Preparations for use in the eye should be sterile on issue.

Eye drops in multiple-application containers used at home (domiciliary use) should not be used for more than 4 weeks after first opening (unless otherwise stated by the manufacturer). Multiple-application eye drops for use on hospital wards are normally discarded 1 week after first opening, although different hospitals have different policies so practice may vary. Individual containers should be supplied for each patient. Separate containers for each eye should only be used if there are concerns about contamination. The BNF (2019a) advises that a fresh supply should be provided on discharge from hospital, although local policies may vary.

There is specific advice for patients undergoing eye operations and in specialist ophthalmic units, and the current BNF and/or local guidance should be consulted (BNF 2019a).

In clinics, single-application containers should be used. If there is a need to use multiple-application containers, they should be discarded after single patient use within one clinical session.

A number of patients (particularly the elderly and patients with arthritic symptoms, visual impairments or Parkinson's disease) may experience problems instilling eye medication. This may be due to co-ordination and/or dexterity difficulties, or difficulties squeezing the bottle. Aids are available to assist patients with these problems. Some manufacturers supply devices specific to their drug containers (see individual manufacturer guidance for further information). Patients will need guidance in how to use aids (Downie et al. 2003).

Preservatives and sensitizers

Apart from preservative-free eye drops, all multiple-application eye drops contain a preservative. These and other contents of eye drops may act as sensitizers in some patients. Preservative-free eye drops may be required instead. Preservatives also cause problems in contact lens wearers (see below).

Contact lenses

Many people wear contact lenses in preference to spectacles. In addition, contact lenses are sometimes used to treat medical conditions. Special care is required when using eye medication in patients using contact lenses. Some drugs and preservatives in

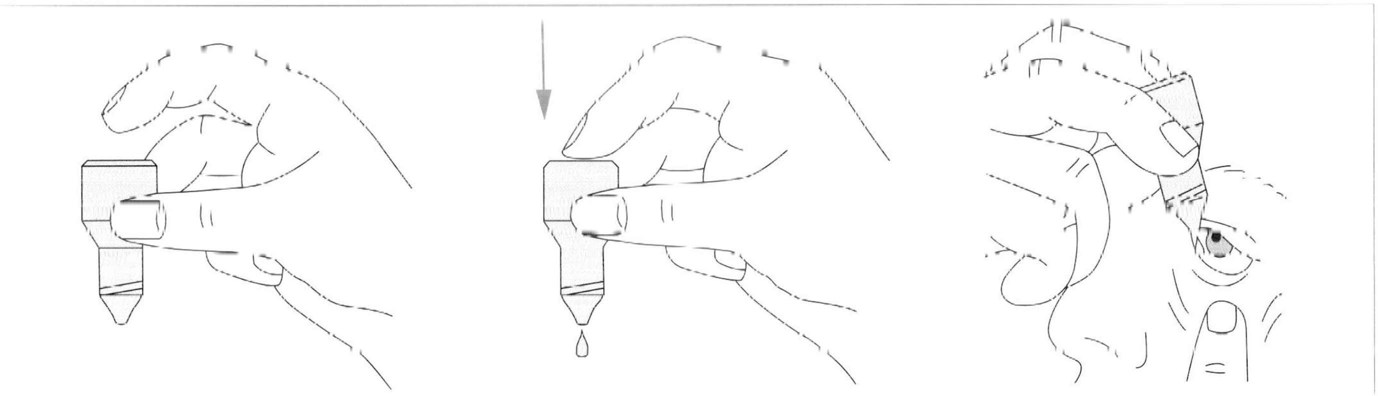

Figure 15.17 How to instil eye drops.

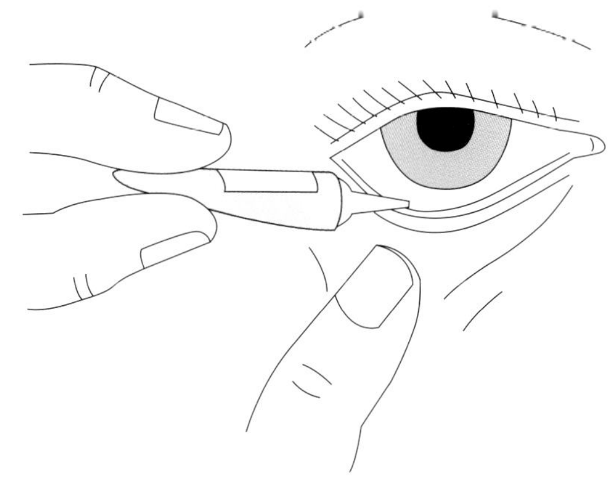

Figure 15.18 How to instil eye ointment.

eye preparations can accumulate in hydrogel lenses (soft contact lenses). Therefore, unless medically indicated, lenses should be removed before instillation of the eye preparation and not worn during the period of treatment. Alternatively, preservative-free drops can be used. Eye drops can be instilled in patients with rigid corneal lenses (hard or gas permeable). Eye ointments should never be used in conjunction with contact lenses and oily eye drops should also be avoided (BNF 2019a).

Eye drop storage

Some eye drops need to be kept in refrigerator storage, and it is customary practice in many institutions for in-use eye preparations to be stored in the fridge to minimize the risk of contamination. Products should be removed from the fridge and allowed to come to room temperature before administration to minimize patient discomfort.

Pharmacological support

Drugs may be given either systemically or topically to exert an effect on the eye (BNF 2019a). However, if they are given systemically, the prescribing doctor needs to take account of the blood–aqueous barrier that which exists within the eye. This barrier is selective in allowing drugs to pass into the intraocular fluids. The permeability of this barrier may increase during inflammatory conditions or following paracentesis (the removal of excess fluid with a needle or cannula) (Andrew 2006).

Medications applied topically meet some resistance at the barrier presented by the lacrimal system (tear film barrier). A further barrier is the cornea, which is selectively permeable and only allows the passage of water and not drugs. However, corneal resistance may alter if there is damage to the corneal epithelium (Kirkwood 2006). Many drugs will produce similar effects in healthy and diseased eyes.

Drugs for use in the eye are usually classified according to their action.

Anti-inflammatories and drugs for allergic conditions

Anti-inflammatory drugs include steroids, antihistamines, lodoxamide and sodium cromoglycate. The most commonly used steroid preparations are dexamethasone, prednisolone and beta-methasone (BNF 2019a).

Corticosteroid eye drops should be used with caution as they can cause cataract formation or a gradual rise in intraocular pressure in a small percentage of people, particularly if the individual has a history of glaucoma (Forrester et al. 2002).

Antibacterials, antivirals and antifungals

Antibacterials and antivirals can be used for the active treatment of eye infections or as prophylactic treatment for eye surgery, after removal of a foreign body or following an eye injury. Antibiotic preparations in common use are chloramphenicol, fusidic acid and gentamicin. Aciclovir is the most commonly used antiviral eye preparation and is licensed for local treatment of herpes simplex infections (BNF 2019a).

Artificial tears and ocular lubricants

Artificial tears and ocular tears are used when there is a deficiency in natural tear production. This can be due to a disease process or radiotherapy treatment, can occur as a side-effect of certain drugs, or result when the eye-blink reflex is absent. These artificial lubricants commonly contain hypromellose or hydroxyethylcellulose (BNF 2019a). These eye drops may have to be instilled frequently (e.g. hourly). Carbomer-containing eye drops may help to reduce application to four times a day. The severity of the problem and the patient's choice will determine the treatment.

Treatment of glaucoma

A range of drugs available in ophthalmic preparations are used in the treatment of glaucomas. These include beta-adrenoreceptor blockers, carbonic anhydrous inhibitors, prostaglandin inhibitors, prostamides and sympathomimetics, and pilocarpine. Many patients are on combination therapy and a range of combination products are available (BNF 2019a). It should be noted that although the action of eye drops is local, a number of them can also have systemic effects.

Local anaesthetics

Local anaesthetics render the eye and the inner surfaces of the lids insensitive. They are used before minor surgery, removal of foreign bodies and tonometry (measurement of intraocular pressure). The most widely used eye anaesthetics are oxybuprocaine and tetracaine (BNF 2019a).

Mydriatics and cycloplegics

Mydriatics and cycloplegics cause pupil dilation and produce their effects by paralysing the ciliary muscle, stimulating the dilator muscle of the pupil (Figure 15.19) or a combination of both. They are used mainly for diagnostic purposes and most have an anticholinergic action. The most commonly used preparations are cyclopentolate hydrochloride, tropicamide and atropine (BNF 2019a).

Miotics

Miotics produce their effects by contracting the ciliary muscle and constricting the pupil (Figure 15.20). They open the inefficient drainage channels in the trabecular meshwork (BNF 2019a). Miotics help in the drainage of aqueous humour and are used mainly in the treatment of primary angle-closure glaucoma. An example is pilocarpine (BNF 2019a). However, in the treatment of glaucoma, they have mainly been superseded by other drug groups.

Specific patient preparation

The eye to be treated must be ascertained and the unaffected eye should not be dosed. Ascertain whether the patient is wearing contact lenses as contact of the medication with the lens can lead to increased drug absorption, visual distortion and discoloration of the lens (Chernecky et al. 2005). It may be necessary for the patient to remove the lenses and replace them with glasses for the duration of their treatment.

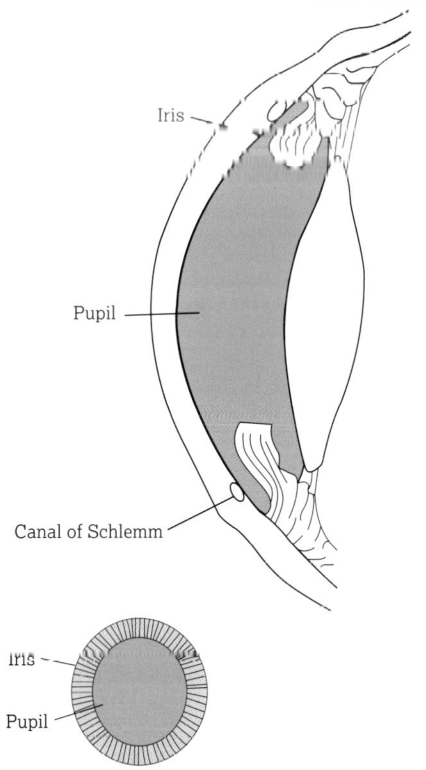

Figure 15.19 Effects of mydriatics.

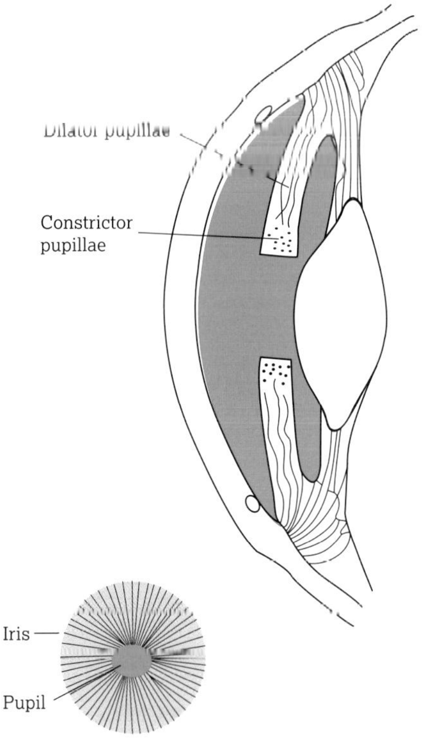

Figure 15.20 Effect of miotics.

Procedure guideline 15.8 Medication: eye administration

Essential equipment

- Personal protective equipment
- Non-sterile powder-free gloves
- Eye preparation to be administered
- Recording sheet or book as required by law or hospital policy
- Patient's prescription chart, to check dose, route, etc.
- Electronic identity check equipment, where relevant
- Low-linting swabs
- Sterile 0.9% sodium chloride or warm water
- Eye drops at room temperature or eye ointment

Optional equipment

- Eye swab

Action	Rationale
Pre-procedure	
1 Introduce yourself to the patient, explain and discuss the procedure with them, and gain their consent to proceed.	To ensure that the patient feels at ease, understands the procedure and gives their valid consent (NMC 2018, **C**).
2 Ask the patient to explain how their eyes feel, if they are able to.	To gain a baseline understanding of current problems or changes the patient is experiencing. **E**
3 Before administering any prescribed drug, look at the patient's prescription chart and check the following: a the correct patient is being given the drug b drug c dose d date and time of administration e route and method of administration f diluent as appropriate g validity of prescription h signature of prescriber i the prescription is legible.	To ensure that the correct patient is given the correct drug in the prescribed dose using the appropriate diluent and by the correct route (DH 2003b, **C**; RPS 2019a **C**). To protect the patient from harm (DH 2003b, **C**).

	Action	Rationale
	If any of these pieces of information are missing, unclear or illegible, do not proceed with the administration. Consult with the prescriber.	To prevent any errors occurring. **E**
4	Wash hands and apply gloves.	To reduce the risk of cross-infection (DH 2007, **C**; Fraise and Bradley 2009, **E**).
	Procedure	
5	Take the medication and the prescription chart to the patient. Check the patient's identity by asking them to state their full name and date of birth. If the patient is unable to confirm these details, then check the patient identity band against the prescription chart. If an electronic identity check system for the patient and/or medicine identification is in place, then use it in accordance with hospital policy and procedures. Check the patient's allergy status by asking them or by checking the name band.	To ensure that the medication is administered to the correct patient and prevent any errors related to drug allergies (NPSA 2005, **C**).
6	Ask the patient to sit back with their neck slightly hyperextended or lie down.	To ensure a position that allows easy access for medication instillation and to avoid excess running down the patient's cheek (Stollery et al. 2005, **E**). Correct positioning minimizes drainage of eye medication into the tear duct (Potter and Perry 2016, **E**).
7	If there is any discharge, proceed as for eye swabbing (see Chapter 13: Diagnostic tests). If any crusting or drainage is present around the eye, gently wash it away with warm water or 0.9% sodium chloride and a swab. Always wipe from the inner to the outer canthus.	To prevent the introduction of micro-organisms into the lacrimal ducts (Potter and Perry 2016, **E**).
8	Ask the patient to look at the ceiling and carefully pull the skin below the affected eye using a wet swab to expose the conjunctival sac.	To move the sensitive cornea up and away from the conjunctival sac and reduce stimulation of the blink reflex (Potter and Perry 2016, **E**).
9	If administering both drops and ointment, administer drops first.	Ointment will leave a film in the eye, which may hamper the absorption of medication in drop form (Jevon et al. 2010, **E**).
10	*Either:*	
	Administer the prescribed number of drops, holding the eye dropper 1–2 cm above the eye. If the patient blinks or closes their eye, repeat the procedure.	To provide even distribution of medication across the eye. The therapeutic effect of drugs is obtained only when drops enter the conjunctival sac (Potter and Perry 2016, **E**).
	Or:	
	Apply a thin stream of ointment evenly along the inner edge of the lower eyelid on the conjunctiva from the nasal corner outwards. If there is excess medication on the eyelid, gently wipe it from the inner to the outer canthus.	To provide even distribution of medication across the eye and lid margin and reduce the risk of cross-infection, contamination of the tube and trauma to the eye (Fraise and Bradley 2009, **E**; Perry 2015, **E**; Stollery et al. 2005, **E**). To avoid excess ointment irritating the surrounding skin (Stollery et al. 2005, **E**).
11	Ask the patient to close their eyes and keep them closed for 1–2 minutes.	To help distribute the medication (Aldridge 2010, **E**; Potter and Perry 2016, **E**).
12	Explain to the patient that they may have blurred vision for a few minutes after application. Explain that they should refrain from driving or operating machinery until their vision returns to normal.	To ensure the patient understands why they have blurred vision (Aldridge 2010, **E**).
	Post-procedure	
13	Clean any equipment used and discard all disposable equipment in appropriate containers.	To minimize the risk of infection (DH 2007, **C**; Fraise and Bradley 2009, **E**).
14	Record the administration on the appropriate charts.	To maintain accurate records, provide a point of reference in the event of any queries and prevent any duplication of treatment (RPS 2019a, **C**).

Post-procedural considerations

Immediate care

After using any eye medications, any excess medication should be wiped off from the inner to the outer canthus. If an eye patch is to be worn, it should be secured without putting any pressure on the eye. Patients should be warned not to drive for 1–2 hours, until their vision is clear, after instillation of mydriatics (which dilate the pupil and paralyse the ciliary muscle) (BNF 2019a). Patients should be taught how to instil eye medication. If it is difficult for them to do so then it may be necessary for a community nurse to attend and administer the eye medication (Chernecky et al. 2005).

Nasal administration

Definition

Nasal administration involves introducing medication into the cavity of the nose for local or systemic effects (Aldridge 2010).

Related theory

The nasal passages are lined with highly vascular mucous membranes covered with ciliated epithelium, which warms and moistens air and traps dust. Medication can be delivered directly to the nasal cavity to relieve local symptoms, such as allergic rhinitis, in the form of nasal drops or nasal sprays (Aldridge 2010). Nasal ointments are used to treat and prevent infections in the nasal cavity.

The nasal cavity can also be used to allow the delivery of drugs systemically. Examples include sumatriptan for migraine, desmopressin for the treatment of diabetes insipidus, and nocturia and fentanyl for the treatment of breakthrough pain.

Evidence-based approaches

The advantages of the delivery of drugs using the nasal route include:

- the large vascular surface of the nasal cavity, which allows rapid absorption
- the avoidance of first-pass metabolism
- the accessibility of the nose
- the ease of administration
- the fact that this route can be used when patients are unable to swallow.

There are some disadvantages to the nasal route, including:

- the presence of mucus, which acts as a barrier to absorption
- mucociliary clearance, which reduces the time that drugs are held in the nasal cavity
- colds can affect absorption from the nasal cavity
- some drugs may irritate the nasal cavity.

Pre-procedural considerations

Specific patient preparation

The patient should be encouraged to clear their nostrils by blowing or manually cleaning with a tissue or damp cotton bud to ensure that the drug has access to the nasal mucosa (Aldridge 2010).

Procedure guideline 15.9 Medication: nasal drop administration

Essential equipment

- Personal protective equipment
- Recording sheet or book as required by law or hospital policy
- Patient's prescription chart, to check dose, route, etc.
- Electronic identity check equipment, where relevant
- Tissues

Medicinal product

- Nasal spray, drops, ointment or cream

Optional equipment

- Cotton bud

Action	Rationale
Pre-procedure	
1 Introduce yourself to the patient, explain and discuss the procedure with them, and gain their consent to proceed.	To ensure that the patient feels at ease, understands the procedure and gives their valid consent (NMC 2018, **C**).
2 Wash hands with bactericidal soap and water or an alcohol-based handrub.	To minimize the risk of cross-infection (DH 2007, **C**; Fraise and Bradley 2009, **E**).
3 Before administering any prescribed drug, look at the patient's prescription chart and check the following: a the correct patient is being given the drug b drug c dose d date and time of administration e route and method of administration f diluent as appropriate g validity of prescription h signature of prescriber i the prescription is legible.	To ensure that the correct patient is given the correct drug in the prescribed dose using the appropriate diluent and by the correct route (DH 2003b, **C**; RPS 2019a **C**). To protect the patient from harm (DH 2003b, **C**).
If any of these pieces of information are missing, unclear or illegible, do not proceed with the administration. Consult with the prescriber.	To prevent any errors occurring. **E**
4 Have paper tissues available.	To wipe away secretions and/or medication. **E**

Procedure	
5 Take the medication and the prescription chart to the patient. Check the patient's identity by asking them to state their full name and date of birth. If the patient is unable to confirm these details, then check the patient identity band against the prescription chart. If an electronic identity check system for the patient and/or medicine identification is in place, then use it in accordance with hospital policy and procedures. Check the patient's allergy status by asking them or by checking the name band.	To ensure that the medication is administered to the correct patient and prevent any errors related to drug allergies (NPSA 2005, **C**).
6 Ask the patient to blow their nose to clear the nasal passages, if appropriate.	To ensure maximum penetration of the medication (Chernecky et al. 2005, **E**).
7 Assist the patient into a supine position and hyperextend the neck (unless clinically contraindicated, e.g. due to cervical spondylosis).	To obtain the safest optimum position for insertion of the medication. **E**
8 Wash hands and put on gloves.	To reduce the risk of cross-infection (DH 2007, **C**; Fraise and Bradley 2009, **E**).
9 With the non-dominant hand, gently push upward on the end of the patient's nose.	To aid in opening the nostrils. **E**
10 Avoid touching the external nares with the dropper and instil the drops just inside the nostril of the affected side.	To prevent the patient from sneezing. **E**
11 Ask the patient to sniff any liquid into the back of the nose or to maintain their position for 2–3 minutes.	To ensure full absorption of the medication. **E**
12 Discard any remaining medication in the dropper into a sink before returning the dropper to the container.	To minimize the risk of cross-infection (Chernecky et al. 2005, **E**; DH 2007, **C**; Fraise and Bradley 2009, **E**).
13 Instruct the patient not to blow their nose for several minutes.	To keep the medication in contact with the nasal passages. **E**
14 Each patient should have their own medication and dropper.	To minimize the risk of cross-infection (DH 2007, **C**; Fraise and Bradley 2009, **E**).
Post-procedure	
15 Record the administration on the appropriate charts.	To maintain accurate records, provide a point of reference in the event of any queries and prevent any duplication of treatment (RPS 2019a, **C**).

Post-procedural considerations

The patient should be discouraged from sniffing too vigorously post-administration as this can cause 'run-off' of the medication down the nasopharynx. This can cause an unpleasant taste in the throat and affect absorption of the medication (Aldridge 2010).

Otic administration

Definition

Otic administration involves introducing medication into the ear for local effects, such as treatment of ear infections and softening of ear wax (cerumen) prior to ear syringing (Aldridge 2010, Chernecky et al. 2005, Nichols and O'Brien 2012).

Related theory

Drugs administered via this route are intended to have a localized effect and act within the anatomy of the ear and auditory canal (Aldridge 2010). Ear preparations can be presented in the form of drops, sprays, ointments or solutions. Certain factors can affect the absorption or action of drugs in the ear, including ear wax and the acidic environment around the ear skin's surface.

Evidence-based approaches

The internal structures of the ear are very sensitive to temperature extremes and so solutions should be administered at room temperature. When drops are instilled cold, patients may experience vertigo, ataxia or nausea (Chernecky et al. 2005, Perry 2015). Solutions should never be forced into the ear canal as medication administered under pressure can injure the eardrum. The ear drop solution should be labelled to indicate the ear it is intended to treat.

The dropper should be held as close to the ear as possible without touching to reduce the risk of cross-infection. Some ear drops are highly coloured and can stain skin and the patient's clothing. Care should be taken to minimize excess liquid running out of the ear and causing staining. The use of a tissue to catch excess liquid is usually sufficient. In addition, although ototoxic drugs such as gentamicin are safe to use in ears with an intact tympanic membrane, they should not be used if the membrane is perforated (BNF 2019a).

Pre-procedural considerations

Specific patient preparation

The ear should be examined, taking note of any discharge, redness or swelling, and the amount and texture of any ear wax present, as these will give an indication of the general health of the ear (Rotherham NHS Foundation Trust 2019). The patient's current level of hearing should also be ascertained. It should be explained to the patient that they must lie still during the procedure as sudden movements could cause injury from the ear dropper.

Procedure guideline 15.10 Medication: ear drop administration

Essential equipment

- Personal protective equipment
- Recording sheet or book as required by law or hospital policy
- Patient's prescription chart, to check dose, route, etc.
- Electronic identity check equipment, where relevant
- Tissues

Medicinal products

- Ear drops

Action	Rationale
Pre-procedure	
1 Introduce yourself to the patient, explain and discuss the procedure with them, and gain their consent to proceed.	To ensure that the patient feels at ease, understands the procedure and gives their valid consent (NMC 2018, **C**).
2 Wash hands with bactericidal soap and water or an alcohol-based handrub.	To minimize the risk of cross-infection (DH 2007, **C**; Fraise and Bradley 2009, **E**).
3 Before administering any prescribed drug, look at the patient's prescription chart and check the following: a the correct patient is being given the drug b drug c dose d date and time of administration e route and method of administration f diluent as appropriate g validity of prescription h signature of prescriber i the prescription is legible.	To ensure that the correct patient is given the correct drug in the prescribed dose using the appropriate diluent and by the correct route (DH 2003b, **C**; RPS 2019a, **C**). To protect the patient from harm (DH 2003b, **C**).
If any of these pieces of information are missing, unclear or illegible, do not proceed with the administration. Consult with the prescriber.	To prevent any errors occurring. **E**
Procedure	
4 Take the medication and the prescription chart to the patient. Check the patient's identity by asking them to state their full name and date of birth. If the patient is unable to confirm these details, then check the patient identity band against the prescription chart. If an electronic identity check system for the patient and/or medicine identification is in place, then use it in accordance with hospital policy and procedures. Check the patient's allergy status by asking them or by checking the name band.	To ensure that the medication is administered to the correct patient and prevent any errors related to drug allergies (NPSA 2005, **C**).
5 Ask the patient to lie on their side with the ear to be treated uppermost.	To ensure the best position for insertion of the drops. **E**
6 Warm the drops to near body temperature by holding the container in the palm of the hand for a few minutes.	To prevent trauma to the patient (ASHP 1982, **C**; Rotherham NHS Foundation Trust 2019, **E**; Perry 2015, **E**).
7 Wash hands and apply gloves.	To reduce the risk of cross-infection (DH 2007, **C**; Fraise and Bradley 2009, **E**).
8 Pull the cartilaginous part of the pinna backwards and upwards (**Action figure 8**).	To prepare the auditory meatus for instillation of the drops (Rotherham NHS Foundation Trust 2019, **E**).
9 If cerumen (ear wax) or drainage occludes the outermost portion of the ear canal, wipe it out gently with a cotton-tipped applicator.	To enable the medication to enter the ear. **E**
10 Allow the drop(s) to fall in the direction of the external canal. The dropper should not touch the ear.	To ensure that the medication reaches the area requiring therapy. **E**
11 Gently massage over the tragus to help work in the drops.	To aid the passage of medication into the ear and prevent the escape of medication. **E**
12 If necessary, temporarily place a gauze swab over the ear canal.	To prevent escape of the medication (Chernecky et al. 2006, **E**).
13 Request the patient to remain in their current position for 2–3 minutes.	To allow the medication to reach the eardrum and be absorbed. To prevent escape of the medication (Aldridge, 2010, **E**; Perry 2015, **E**).
Post-procedure	
14 Record the administration on the appropriate charts.	To maintain accurate records, provide a point of reference in the event of any queries and prevent any duplication of treatment (RPS 2019a, **C**).

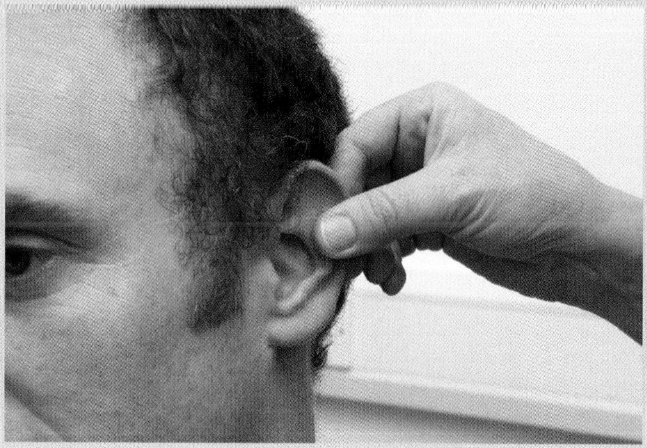

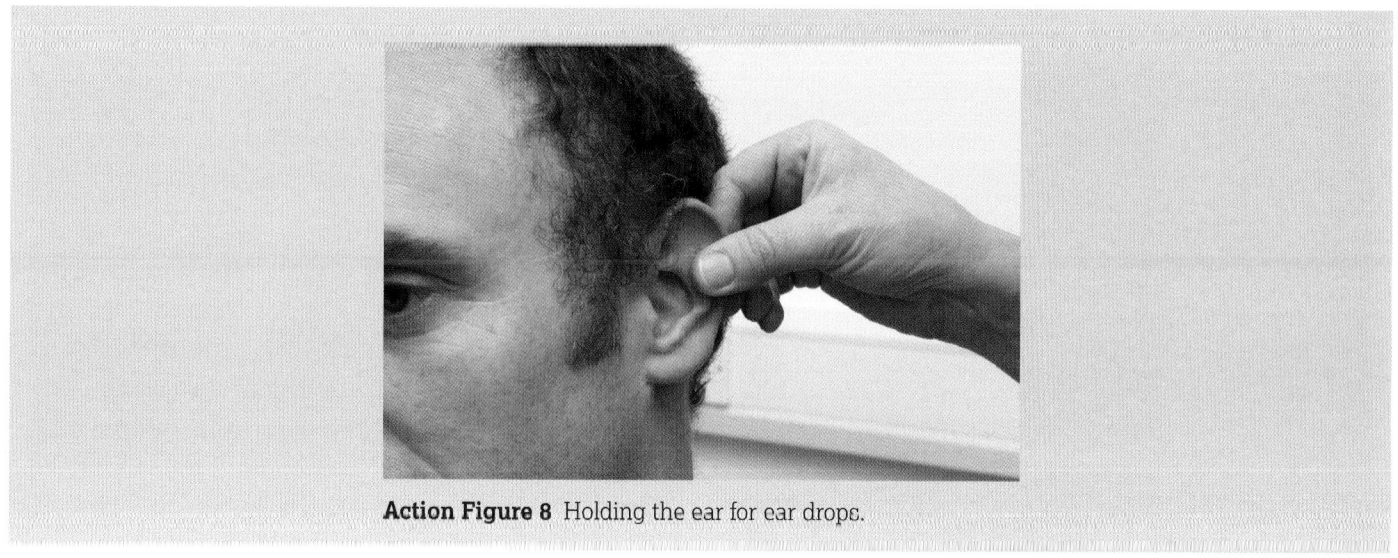

Action Figure 8 Holding the ear for ear drops.

Post-procedural considerations

Ask the patient to report any changes in order to monitor the effectiveness of the intervention. Consideration should also be given to the patient's hearing aids (where relevant) and assistance should be given to help clean these. Check for any irritation and/or pain of the meatus.

Parenteral administration (injections and infusions)

Definitions

An injection can be described as the act of giving medication by use of a syringe and needle. An infusion can be defined as a drug or fluid given over a prolonged period. This may be due to the volume of the preparation, the risk of toxicity if the drug is given too rapidly or the need to maintain activity over a long period. Many medications are given in relatively small volumes (50–100 mL) or over a short period of time (30–60 minutes) (Weinstein and Hagle 2014).

Injections and infusions consist of sterile solutions, emulsions or suspensions. They are prepared by dissolving, emulsifying or suspending the active ingredient and any added substances in water (for injections), a suitable non-aqueous liquid or a mixture of these vehicles (British Pharmacopoeia 2019). Box 15.8 lists the types of injections and infusions.

Anatomy and physiology

The skin is made up of two layers: the dermis and the epidermis. Within the dermis there is the papillary layer (upper dermal region), which contains capillaries as well as pain and touch receptors. The reticular layer contains blood vessels as well as sweat and oil glands. Both collagen and elastic fibres are found throughout the dermis. Collagen fibres are responsible for the toughness of the dermis. The skin also has a rich nerve supply (Marieb and Hoehn 2018).

There are three types of muscle: skeletal, cardiac and smooth. Skeletal muscles are attached to the body's skeleton and are also known as striated muscle because the fibres appear to be striped (Marieb and Hoehn 2018).

Box 15.8 Types of injections and infusions

- Intra-arterial injection
- Intra-articular injection
- Intrathecal injection and infusion
- Intradermal injection
- Subcutaneous injection and infusion
- Intramuscular injection
- Intraosseous injection
- Intravenous injection and infusion:
  - bolus injection
  - intermittent and continuous infusion

Evidence-based approaches

Medicines should only be administered by injection when no other route is suitable or available, or administration by injection is clinically indicated. As injections avoid the GI tract, this is described as parenteral administration. Injections are administered when:

- the medication might be destroyed by the stomach
- rapid first-pass metabolism may be extensive
- the drug is not absorbed if given orally
- precise control over dosage is required
- the drug cannot be given by mouth
- there is a need to achieve high drug plasma levels (Downie et al. 2003, Ostendorf 2015).

There are disadvantages as injections are invasive, cause pain and discomfort, and can put patients at risk of infection and (in the case of intravenous injections) infiltration and extravasation.

Methods for injection or infusion

There are a number of routes for injection or infusion (see Box 15.8). The selection may be predetermined, for example in the cases of intra-arterial or intra-articular injections. The choice of other routes will normally depend on the desired therapeutic effect and the patient's safety and comfort.

Pre-procedural considerations

Dosage forms

Ampoules

Ampoules (Figure 15.21) are traditionally single-dose glass containers although increasingly plastic ampoules are used for a number of products (Downie et al. 2003). They are sealed by heat fusion to exclude any contamination. They have a thin wall that allows rupture of the glass to expose the contents of the liquid or powder. There is a narrow constriction leading to the neck, which

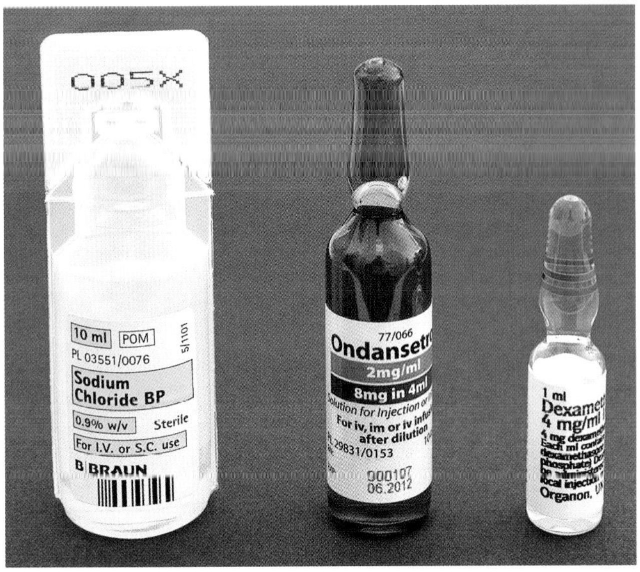

Figure 15.21 Ampoules.

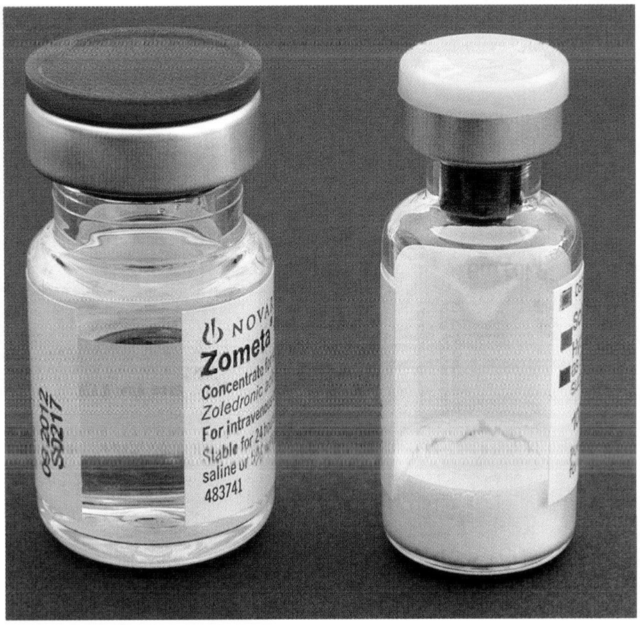

Figure 15.22 Vials.

is often marked with a white ring, which indicates the place where the neck can be snapped off (Downie et al. 2003). Ampoule opening devices of various designs are available. Ampoules are available in several sizes, from 1 to 20 mL (Ostendorf 2015).

Vials

Vials (Figure 15.22) are glass containers with a rubber closure that can be penetrated to allow the addition of a diluent to dissolve powder contents and withdrawal of a dose via the needle. The exposed rubber surface is usually covered by a protective pull-off metal or plastic cap, which prevents tampering or damage but does not provide sterility (Downie et al. 2003, Ostendorf 2015). A vial may be packaged with a specific transfer needle, and it is important to follow the manufacturer's instructions in these instances. Most vials are intended for single use but a small number are multidose containers.

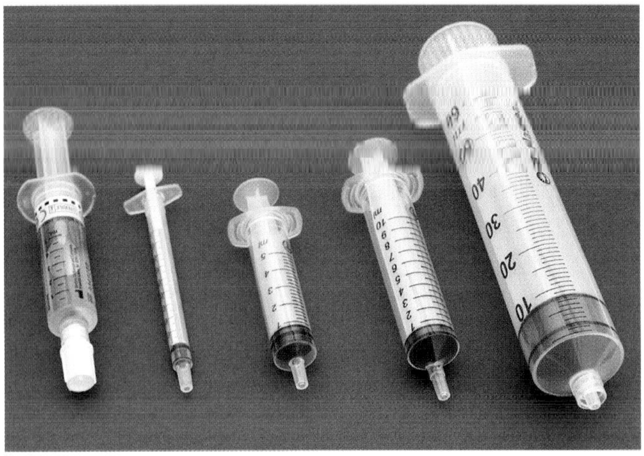

Figure 15.23 Syringes: Luer-Lok (far left and far right) and Luer-Slip (middle three).

Pre-filled syringes

A number of drugs (e.g. insulin and low-molecular-weight heparins) are presented in pre-filled syringes with a needle attached. There are various designs and the nurse must ensure that they are familiar with the device being used. Drugs should never be transferred from these specialist dosage forms into other containers or syringes for administration due to the danger of error (NHS England 2016, NPSA 2010a). In addition, there are a number of pre-prepared syringes that contain 0.9% sodium chloride specifically for flushing or ready-to-administer medicines for use in emergency situations.

Equipment

Syringes

Syringes are commonly plastic and disposable, although occasionally a medicine must be administered via a glass syringe (e.g. adenosine). They consist of a graduated barrel and a plunger and a tip. It is the tip that classifies the type of syringe as either Luer-Lok or Luer-Slip (Figure 15.23).

Syringes come in various sizes, from 1 to 60 mL. The choice of syringe is made according to the volume of medication to be administered so it is important to choose the smallest syringe possible to ensure accuracy (Downie et al. 2003, Ostendorf 2015). For Luer-Lok syringes, the needle must be twisted onto the tip and 'locked' into position. This provides security and these syringes are recommended for use with intravenous medicines, especially cytotoxic medications and any medicines administered via a syringe pump. Luer-Slip syringes tend to be used for intramuscular and subcutaneous injections. Insulin syringes are low dose syringes often calibrated in units and are only used for insulin administration (Downie et al. 2003, NICE 2017d, Ostendorf 2015). They should be stored and distinguished from intravenous syringes (MHRA 2008a, Reid 2012). Injection pens are pre-filled syringes that contain a disposable cartridge. They provide a convenient delivery method and allow patients to self-administer their medications subcutaneously (e.g. insulin and adrenaline) (Ostendorf 2015).

Following intrathecal incidents, the NPSA (2009) issued a safety alert stating that all spinal (intrathecal) bolus doses and lumbar puncture samples (part A) and all epidural, spinal (intrathecal) and regional anaesthesia infusions and bolus doses (part B) should be performed using syringes, needles and other devices with connectors that *will not* also connect with intravenous equipment.

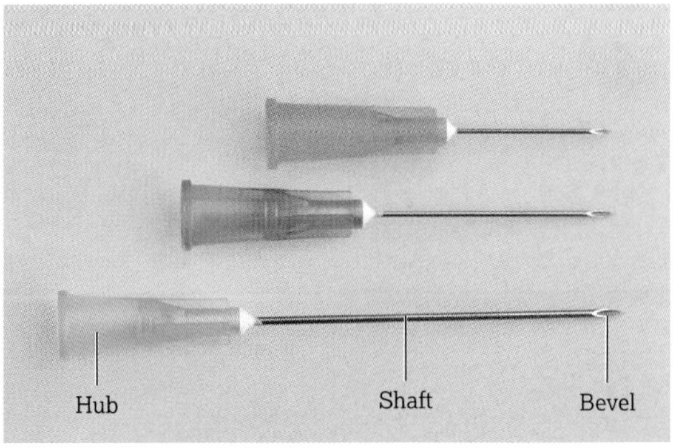

Figure 15.24 Needles.

Needles

A hypodermic needle is composed of three parts (Figure 15.24):

- the *hub*, which fits onto the tip of the syringe
- the *shaft*, which connects to the hub
- the *bevel* or slanted tip or eye of the needle (different bevels are required depending on the use of the needle).

Needle sizes are known as 'gauges' – for example 19 G (used for intravenous injections), 21 G (used for intramuscular injections), 23 G (used for subcutaneous injections) and 25 G (used for intradermal injections). This indicates their diameter. The higher the gauge, the finer the needle, and selection is made depending on the viscosity of the liquid to be injected (Downie et al. 2003, Ostendorf 2015). Needles vary in length from 10 to 16 mm, and selection of length will depend on the size and weight of the patient, and the type of tissue into which the drug is to be injected (e.g. longer for intramuscular injections and shorter for subcutaneous injections). Each needle is enclosed in a removable plastic guard and then sealed in a sterile pack. Filter needles may be used to prevent drawing up glass and rubber particles into the syringe (Downie et al. 2003, Ostendorf 2015).

There are now a variety of safety needles available to prevent needle stick injury, where a plastic guard or sheath slips over the needle after an injection (EASHW 2010) (Figure 15.25) or the needle retracts into the barrel.

Three categories of needle bevel are available:

- *regular*: for all intramuscular and subcutaneous injections
- *intradermal*: for diagnostic injections and other injections into the epidermis
- *short*: rarely used.

Spinal needles

Spinal needles are used for lumbar punctures, spinal anaesthesia and the administration of intrathecal therapy. Spinal needles are classified according to their needle tip (De Leon and Wong 2017):

- *Cutting-tip needles*: Quincke spinal needles have sharp cutting tips, with the hole at the end of the needle.
- *Pencil-point needles*: Whitacre and Sprotte needles have a closed tip shaped like a pencil, with the hole on the side of the needle near the tip. These needles are designed to minimize the leak of cerebrospinal fluid after puncture and reduce the risk of post-dural puncture headache.

Non-Luer-Lok connectors (NRFit) are required for all neuraxial devices, including spinal needles. This is to prevent the delivery of intravenous drugs into the neuraxial space and also prevent

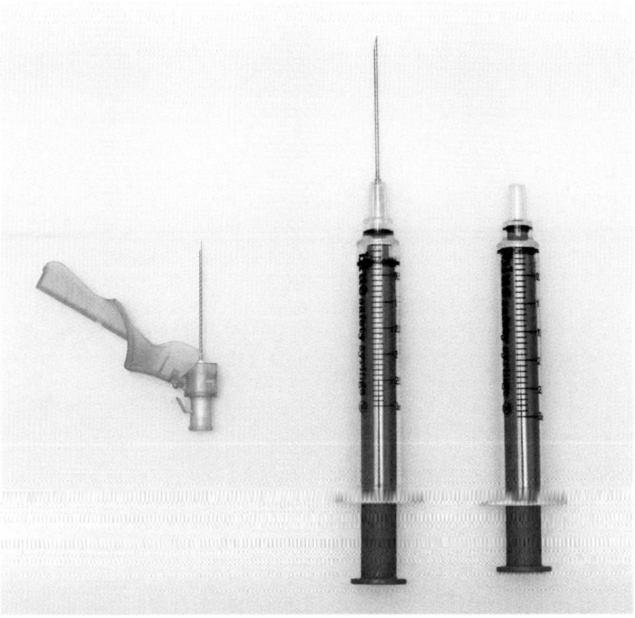

Figure 15.25 Safety needles.

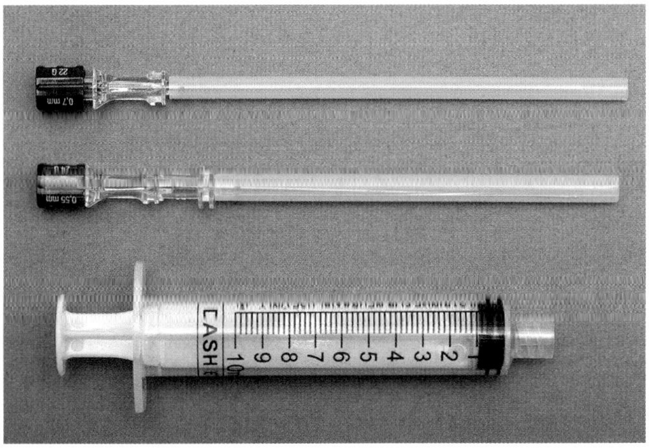

Figure 15.26 Lumbar puncture needles and intrathecal syringe.

wrong-route delivery of neuraxial medicines (e.g. bupivacaine) (NHSI 2017) (Figure 15.26).

Medication preparation

Medicines presented as liquids can be drawn up directly from the vial or ampoule. If the medicine has been presented in a powder form, it will need to be reconstituted. This is usually done using water for injections but some medications will require special diluents, which are often supplied with the medication. When adding a diluent to a powder, for example 2 mL to a 100 mg vial, the final volume will exceed 2 mL although this is usually not of any consequence if the total dose is to be administered (Downie et al. 2003). In order to ensure that the correct volume is withdrawn, it is necessary to perform a calculation.

Medication calculations

Following is how to calculate the drug volume required from the stock strength:

$$\frac{strength\ required}{stock\ strength} \times volume\ of\ stock\ solution = volume\ required$$

Another way of expressing this is to start with the strength you want, divide it by the strength of the stock you have, and then multiply the result by the volume of stock solution.

Displacement values

Displacement values are relevant when a drug is dissolved in a solution (e.g. water). The resulting solution will have a greater volume than before. Displacement values can vary from drug to drug and may be so small that the increased volume is not considered in calculating doses (Lapham and Agar 2003). However, the total volume may be increased significantly and, if this is not taken into account when calculating a dose, errors in dosage may occur, particularly when small doses are involved (e.g. for neonates) (Lapham and Agar 2003). Displacement volumes may be stated in the relevant drug information sheet.

To calculate dose using displacement volumes, use the following equation:

$$\textit{volume to be added} = \textit{diluent volume} - \textit{displacement volume}$$

Single-dose preparations

The volume of the injection in a single-dose container is sufficient to permit the withdrawal and administration of the required dose using a normal technique.

Multidose preparations

Multidose aqueous injections contain a suitable antimicrobial preservative at an appropriate concentration except when the preparation itself has adequate antimicrobial properties. When it is necessary to present a preparation for parenteral use in a multidose container, the precautions to be taken for the preparation's administration and more particularly for its storage between successive withdrawals will be provided.

Parenteral infusions

Parenteral infusions are sterile, aqueous solutions or emulsions with water; they are free from pyrogens and are usually made isotonic with blood. They are principally intended for administration in large volumes. Parenteral infusions do not contain any added antimicrobial preservative (British Pharmacopoeia 2018, Hillery et al. 2001).

Pre-procedural considerations

Specific patient preparation

Patients are often afraid of receiving injections because they believe the injection will be painful (Downie et al. 2003). Torrance (1989) listed a number of factors that can cause pain:

- the needle
- the chemical composition of the drug or solution
- the technique
- the speed of the injection
- the volume of drug.

Applying manual pressure to an injection site before performing the injection can be an effective means of reducing pain intensity (Chung et al. 2002). A small study carried out by Chan (2001) showed that administering subcutaneous heparin slowly (over 30 seconds rather than 10) can reduce site pain intensity as well as bruising. Pain may also be reduced when using retractable needles (Lamblet et al. 2011). Other ways of reducing pain during injections are covered in Box 15.9.

Box 15.9 Reducing the pain of injections

- Use correct length and gauge of needle (use smallest possible)
- Use correct site
- Use correct angle (90° for intramuscular injections)
- Use correct volume (no more than 3 mL at a site for intramuscular injections)
- Rotate sites to prevent formation of indurations or abscesses
- Consider using ice, freezing spray or topical local anaesthetic to numb the skin
- Listen to the views of experienced patients
- Explain the benefits of the injection
- Position the patient so that the muscles are relaxed
- Use distraction
- If appropriate, ask the patient to turn their foot inwards (for intramuscular injections into the upper leg)
- Insert and remove the needle smoothly and quickly
- Hold the syringe steady once the needle is in the tissue to prevent tissue damage
- Inject the medication slowly but smoothly

Source: Adapted from Dickerson (1992), Downie et al. (2003), Perry (2015).

Procedure guideline 15.11 Medication: single-dose ampoule: solution preparation

Essential equipment

- Personal protective equipment
- Medication ampoule
- Needle
- Syringe
- Sterile topical swab
- Sharps container
- Ampoule opening aid

Action	Rationale
Pre-procedure	
1 Wash hands with bactericidal soap and water or an alcohol based handrub.	To prevent contamination of medication and equipment (DH 2007, **C**).
2 Inspect the solution for cloudiness or particulate matter. If present, discard and follow hospital guidelines on action to take; for example, return drug to pharmacy.	To prevent the patient from receiving an unstable or contaminated drug (NPSA 2007d, **C**).

Procedure	
3 Tap the neck of the ampoule gently.	To ensure that all the solution is in the bottom of the ampoule (NPSA 2007d, **C**).
4 Cover the neck of the ampoule with a sterile topical swab and snap it open. If there is any difficulty, a file or ampoule opening aid may be required.	To minimize the risk of contamination. To prevent aerosol formation or contact with the drug, which could lead to a sensitivity reaction. To reduce the risk of injury to the nurse (NPSA 2007d, **C**).
5 Inspect the solution for glass fragments; if present, discard.	To minimize the risk of injection of foreign matter into the patient (NPSA 2007d, **C**).
6 Open the packaging and attach the needle onto the syringe.	To assemble the equipment. **E**
7 Withdraw the required amount of solution, tilting the ampoule if necessary.	To avoid drawing in any air (NPSA 2007d, **C**).
8 Tap the syringe to dislodge any air bubbles. Expel air. *Or:* An alternative to expelling the air with the needle sheath in place is to use the ampoule or vial to receive any air and/or drug.	To prevent needle stick injury and aerosol formation (NPSA 2007d, **C**). To ensure that the correct amount of drug is in the syringe (NPSA 2007d, **C**).
9 Attach a new needle if required (and discard the used needle into the appropriate sharps container) or attach a plastic end cap or insert the syringe into the syringe packet.	To reduce the risk of contamination of the syringe tip. To avoid tracking medications through superficial tissues and to ensure that the correct size of needle is used for intramuscular or subcutaneous injection. To reduce the risk of injury to the nurse (NPSA 2007d, **C**).
10 Attach a label to the syringe.	To ensure the practitioner can identify the medication in the syringe (NPSA 2007d, **C**).
11 Keep all ampoules/vials and diluents in the tray with the syringe.	To enable checking at the bedside. **E**

873

Procedure guideline 15.12 Medication: single-dose ampoule: powder preparation

Essential equipment

- Personal protective equipment
- Medication ampoule
- Diluent
- Needle
- Syringe
- Sharps container
- Swab

Action	Rationale
Pre procedure	
1 Wash hands with bactericidal soap and water or an alcohol-based handrub.	To prevent contamination of medication and equipment (DH 2007, **C**).
2 Open the packaging and attach the needle to the syringe.	To assemble the equipment. **E**
Procedure	
3 Open the diluent and draw up the required volume.	To ensure the correct volume of diluent. **E**
4 Tap the neck of the ampoule gently.	To ensure that any powder lodged here falls to the bottom of the ampoule (NPSA 2007d, **C**).
5 Cover the neck of the ampoule with a sterile topical swab and snap it open. If there is any difficulty, an ampoule opening device may be required.	To minimize the risk of contamination. To prevent contact with the drug, which could cause a sensitivity reaction. To prevent injury to the nurse (NPSA 2007d, **C**).
6 Inject the correct diluent slowly into the powder within the ampoule.	To ensure that the powder is thoroughly wet before agitation and is not released into the atmosphere (NPSA 2007d, **C**).
7 Agitate the ampoule.	To dissolve the drug (NPSA 2007d, **C**).
8 Inspect the contents.	To detect any glass fragments or any other particulate matter. If present, continue agitation or discard as appropriate (NPSA 2007d, **C**).

(continued)

Procedure guideline 15.12 Medication: single-dose ampoule: powder preparation *(continued)*

Action	Rationale
9 When the solution is clear, withdraw the prescribed amount, tilting the ampoule if necessary.	To ensure the powder is dissolved and has formed a solution with the diluent. To avoid drawing in air (NPSA 2007d, **C**)
10 Tap the syringe to dislodge any air bubbles. Expel air.	To prevent aerosol formation. To ensure that the correct amount of drug is in the syringe (NPSA 2007d, **C**).
11 Attach a new needle if required (and discard the used needle into the appropriate sharps container) or attach a plastic end cap or insert the syringe into the syringe packet.	To reduce the risk of contamination of the syringe tip. To avoid possible trauma to the patient if the needle has barbed (become bent or hooked), to avoid tracking medications through superficial tissues and to ensure that the correct size of needle is used for intramuscular or subcutaneous injection. To reduce the risk of injury to the nurse (NPSA 2007d, **C**).
12 Attach a label to the syringe.	To ensure the practitioner can identify the medication in the syringe (NPSA 2007d, **C**).
13 Keep all ampoules/vials and diluents in the tray with the syringe.	To enable checking at the bedside. **E**

Procedure guideline 15.13 Medication: multidose vial: powder preparation using a venting needle

Essential equipment

- Personal protective equipment
- Medication ampoule
- Diluent
- Needles × 2
- Syringe
- Alcohol swab

Action	Rationale
Pre-procedure	
1 Wash hands with bactericidal soap and water or an alcohol-based handrub.	To prevent contamination of medication and equipment (DH 2007, **C**).
2 Open the packaging and attach the needle to the syringe.	To assemble the equipment. **E**
Procedure	
3 Open the diluent and draw up the required volume.	To ensure the correct volume of diluent. **E**
4 Remove the tamper-evident seal on the vial. Clean the rubber septum with an alcohol swab and let it air dry for at least 30 seconds.	To prevent bacterial contamination of the drug, as the plastic lid prevents damage but does not ensure sterility (NPSA 2007d, **C**).
5 Insert a 21 G needle into the cap to vent the bottle (**Action figure 5a**).	To prevent pressure differentials, which can cause separation of needle and syringe (NPSA 2007d, **C**).
6 Insert the needle bevel up, at an angle of 45–60°. Before completing the insertion of the needle tip, lift the needle to 90° and proceed (**Action figure 6**).	To minimize the risk of coring when inserting the needle into the cap. **E**
7 Inject the correct diluent slowly into the powder within the vial.	To ensure that the powder is thoroughly wet before it is mixed and is not released into the atmosphere (NPSA 2007d, **C**).
8 Remove the needle and the syringe.	To enable adequate mixing of the solution. **E**
9 Place a sterile topical swab over the venting needle (**Action figure 5b**) and gently swirl to dissolve the powder.	To prevent contamination of the drug or the atmosphere. To mix the diluent with the powder and dissolve the drug (NPSA 2007d, **C**).
10 Inspect the solution for cloudiness or particulate matter. If this is present, discard. Follow hospital guidelines on what action to take: for example, return drug to pharmacy.	To prevent the patient from receiving an unstable or contaminated drug (NPSA 2007d, **C**).
11 Withdraw the prescribed amount of solution. Inspect for pieces of rubber, which may have been 'cored out' of the cap (**Action figure 5c**).	To ensure that the correct amount of drug is in the syringe (NPSA 2007d, **C**). To prevent the injection of foreign matter into the patient (NPSA 2007d, **C**).

12 Remove air from the syringe without spraying into the atmosphere by injecting air back into the vial (**Action figure 5d**) and tap the syringe to dislodge any air bubbles. Expel air.	To reduce the risk of contamination of the practitioner. To prevent aerosol formation (NPSA 2007d, **C**).
13 Attach a new needle if required (and discard the used needle into the appropriate sharps container) or attach a plastic end cap or insert the syringe into the syringe packet.	To reduce the risk of contamination of the syringe tip. To avoid possible trauma to the patient if the needle has barbed (become bent or hooked), to avoid tracking medications through superficial tissues and to ensure that the correct size of needle is used for intramuscular or subcutaneous injection. To reduce the risk of injury to the nurse (NPSA 2007d, **C**).
14 Attach a label to the syringe.	To ensure the practitioner can identify the medication in the syringe (NPSA 2007d, **C**).
15 Keep all ampoules/vials and diluents in the tray with the syringe.	To enable checking at the bedside. **E**

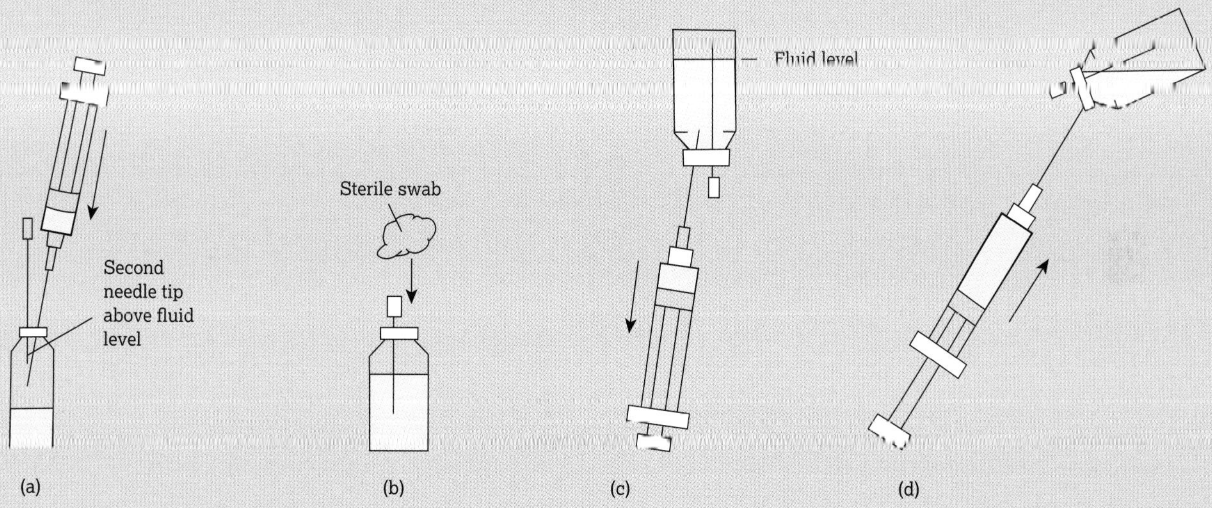

Action Figure 5 Suggested method of vial reconstitution to avoid environmental exposure. (a) When reconstituting the vial, insert a second needle to allow air to escape when adding diluent for injection. (b) When gently swirling the vial to dissolve the powder, push in a second needle up to the Luer connection and cover with a sterile swab. (c) To remove the reconstituted solution, insert the syringe needle and then invert the vial. Ensuring that the tip of the second needle is above the fluid, withdraw the solution. (d) Remove the air from the syringe without spraying into the atmosphere by injecting air back into the vial.

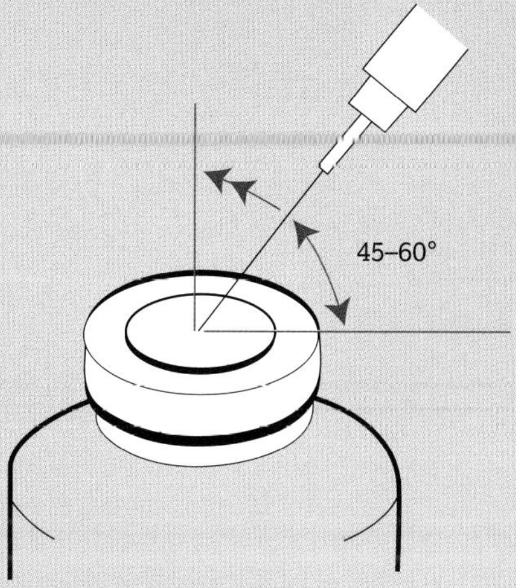

Action Figure 6 Method to minimize coring.

Procedure guideline 15.14 Medication: multidose vial: powder preparation using the equilibrium method

Essential equipment

- Personal protective equipment
- Medication vial
- Diluent
- Needle
- Syringe
- Alcohol swab

Action	Rationale
Pre-procedure	
1 Wash hands with bactericidal soap and water or an alcohol-based handrub.	To prevent contamination of medication and equipment (DH 2007, **C**).
2 Open the packaging and attach the needle to the syringe.	To assemble the equipment. **E**
Procedure	
3 Open the diluent and draw up the required volume.	To ensure the correct volume of diluent. **E**
4 Remove the tamper evident seal on the vial. Clean the rubber septum with an alcohol swab and let it air dry for at least 30 seconds.	To prevent bacterial contamination of the drug, as the plastic lid prevents damage but does not ensure sterility (NPSA 2007d, **C**).
5 Inject the diluent into the vial. Keeping the tip of the needle above the level of the solution in the vial, release the plunger. The syringe will fill with air that has been displaced by the solution.	To prevent bacterial contamination of the drug (NPSA 2007d, **C**).
6 With the syringe and needle still in place, gently swirl the vial to dissolve all the powder.	To mix the diluent with the powder and dissolve the drug (NPSA 2007d, **C**).
7 Inspect the solution for cloudiness or particulate matter. If this is present, discard. Follow hospital guidelines on what action to take; for example, return drug to pharmacy.	To prevent the patient from receiving an unstable or contaminated drug (NPSA 2007d, **C**).
8 Invert the vial. Keep the needle in the solution and slowly depress the plunger to push the air into the vial.	To create equilibrium in the vial (NPSA 2007d, **C**).
9 Release the plunger so that the solution flows back into the syringe (if a large volume of solution is to be withdrawn, use a push–pull technique).	To create equilibrium in the vial (NPSA 2007d, **C**).
10 Re-inject the diluent into the vial. Keeping the tip of the needle above the level of the solution in the vial, release the plunger. The syringe will fill with the air that has been displaced by the solution.	This 'equilibrium method' helps to minimize the build-up of pressure in the vial (NPSA 2007d, **C**).
11 Withdraw the prescribed amount of solution and inspect for pieces of rubber, which may have been 'cored out' of the cap (see **Action figure 5c** in Procedure guideline 15.13).	To ensure that the correct amount of drug is in the syringe (NPSA 2007d, **C**). To prevent the injection of foreign matter into the patient (NPSA 2007d, **C**).
12 Remove air from the syringe without spraying into the atmosphere by injecting air back into the vial (see **Action figure 5d** in Procedure guideline 15.13) and tap the syringe to dislodge any air bubbles.	To reduce the risk of contamination of the practitioner. To prevent aerosol formation (NPSA 2007d, **C**).
13 Attach a new needle if required (and discard the used needle into the appropriate sharps container) or attach a plastic end cap or insert the syringe into the syringe packet.	To reduce the risk of contamination of the syringe tip. To avoid possible trauma to the patient if the needle has barbed (become bent or hooked), to avoid tracking medications through superficial tissues and to ensure that the correct size of needle is used for intramuscular or subcutaneous injection. To reduce the risk of injury to the nurse (NPSA 2007d, **C**).
14 Attach a label to the syringe.	To ensure the practitioner can identify the medication in the syringe (NPSA 2007d, **C**).
15 Keep all ampoules/vials and diluents in the tray with the syringe.	To enable checking at the bedside. **E**

Procedure guideline 15.15 Medication: injection administration

Essential equipment

- Personal protective equipment
- Clean tray or receiver in which to place the drug and equipment
- 21 G needle(s) to ease reconstitution and drawing up; 23 G if from a glass ampoule
- 21, 23 or 25 G needle, size dependent on route of administration
- Syringe(s) of appropriate size for the amount of drug to be given
- Swabs saturated with isopropyl alcohol 70%
- Sterile topical swab, if the drug is presented in ampoule form
- Drug(s) to be administered
- Patient's prescription chart, to check dose, route and so on
- Recording sheet or book as required by law or hospital policy
- Electronic identity check equipment, where relevant

Action	Rationale
Pre-procedure	
1 Introduce yourself to the patient, explain and discuss the procedure with them, and gain their consent to proceed.	To ensure that the patient feels at ease, understands the procedure and gives their valid consent (Griffith and Jordan 2003, **E**; NMC 2018, **C**).
2 Collect and check all equipment.	To prevent delays and enable full concentration on the procedure. **E**.
3 Check that the packaging of all equipment is intact.	To ensure sterility. If any seal is damaged, discard (NPSA 2007d, **C**).
4 Wash hands with bactericidal soap and water or an alcohol-based handrub.	To prevent contamination of medication and equipment (DH 2007, **C**).
Procedure	
5 Prepare needle(s), syringe(s) and other necessary materials, placing them on a tray or receiver.	To contain all items in a clean area. **E**
6 Inspect all equipment.	To check that none is damaged; if so, discard or report to the MHRA. **C**
7 Before administering any prescribed drug, look at the patient's prescription chart and check the following: a the correct patient is being given the drug b drug c dose d date and time of administration e route and method of administration f diluent as appropriate g validity of prescription h signature of prescriber i the prescription is legible.	To ensure that the patient is given the correct drug in the prescribed dose using the appropriate diluent and by the correct route (DH 2003b, **C**; RPS 2019a, **C**). To protect the patient from harm (DH 2003b, **C**).
If any of these pieces of information are missing, unclear or illegible, do not proceed with the administration. Consult with the prescriber.	To prevent any errors occurring. **E**
8 Check the patient's allergy status with the patient and the patient's records.	To prevent an adverse allergic reaction. **C**
9 Check all details with another nurse if required by hospital policy.	To minimize any risk of error (RPS 2019a, **C**).
10 Select the drug in the appropriate volume, dilution or dosage and check the expiry date.	To reduce wastage. Treatment with medication that is outside the expiry date is dangerous. Drugs deteriorate with storage. The expiry date indicates when a particular drug is no longer pharmacologically efficacious (NPSA 2007d, **C**).
11 Proceed with the preparation of the drug, using protective clothing if advisable.	To protect the practitioner during preparation (NPSA 2007d, **C**).
12 Take the prepared dose to the patient and close the door or curtains as appropriate.	To ensure patient privacy and dignity. **E**
13 Check the patient's identity. If an electronic identity check system for patient and/or medicine identification is in place, then use in accordance with hospital policy and procedures.	To prevent error and confirm the patient's identity (NPSA 2005, **C**).

(continued)

Procedure guideline 15.15 Medication: injection administration *(continued)*

Action	Rationale
14 Evaluate the patient's knowledge of the medication being offered. If this knowledge appears to be faulty or incorrect, offer an explanation of the use, action, dose and potential side-effects of the drug or drugs involved.	Patients have a right to information about treatment (NMC 2018, **C**).
15 Administer the drug as prescribed.	To ensure the patient receives treatment. **E**
Post-procedure	
16 Dispose of all equipment in the appropriate waste containers and sharps bins.	To ensure safe disposal of all equipment. **C**
17 Record the administration on the appropriate charts.	To maintain accurate records, provide a point of reference in the event of any queries and prevent any duplication of treatment (NPSA 2007d, **C**; RPS 2019a, **C**).

Intra-arterial injections and infusions

Definition

This special technique allows the delivery of a high concentration of drug to the tissues or organ supplied by a particular artery; it is used when the medications required are rapidly metabolized or systemically toxic (Downie et al. 2003). This route can be used for the administration of chemotherapy and vasodilators and for diagnostic purposes. Injection of drugs into an artery is a rare and hazardous procedure. The introduction of the cannula or catheter must be performed with care as the vessel may go into spasm, causing pain and occlusion. This can result in necrosis of an organ or part of a limb.

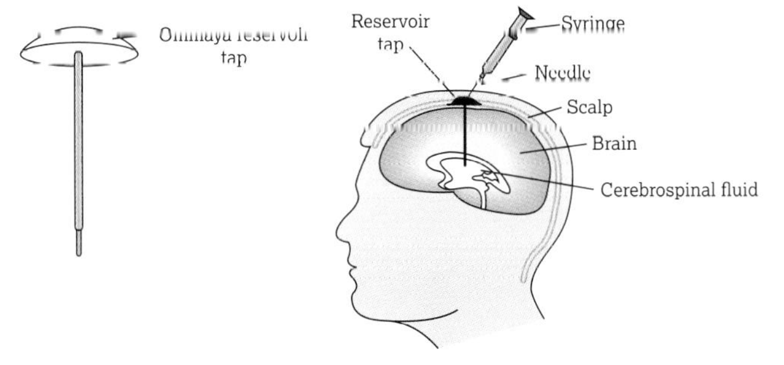

Figure 15.27 Ommaya reservoir.

Intra-articular injections and infusions

Definition

In inflammatory conditions of the joints, corticosteroids are given by intra-articular injection to relieve inflammation and increase joint mobility (Downie et al. 2003).

Intrathecal administration of medication

Definition

Intrathecal administration is the administration of drugs into the central nervous system (CNS) via the cerebrospinal fluid. This is usually achieved using a lumbar puncture (Polovich et al. 2014, Stanley 2002, Wilkes 2018).

Related theory

Medications can be administered intrathecally if they have poor lipid solubility and therefore do not pass the blood–brain barrier (Downie et al. 2003). Only medication specially prepared for the intrathecal route should be used; doses should be carefully calculated and are usually much smaller than would be given by intramuscular or intravenous injection. Water-soluble antibiotics are administered by the intrathecal route to achieve adequate concentrations in the cerebrospinal fluid in the treatment of meningitis. Other medicines administered via this route include antifungal agents, opioids, cytotoxic therapy and radio-opaque substances (used in the diagnosis of spinal lesions) (Downie et al. 2003).

The advantage of this route is that it allows direct access to the CNS by drugs that do not normally cross the blood–brain barrier in sufficient amounts; it thus ensures constant levels of the drug in this area. The main disadvantage is that it requires a standard lumbar puncture before the drug can be injected, and this may need to be performed on a daily to weekly basis (Wilkes and Barton-Burke 2018). Although this can be quick and easy to perform, it can be distressing for the patient, and can even result in CNS trauma and infection. It may also only reach the epidural or subdural spaces and therefore the concentrations in the ventricles may not be therapeutic (Wilkes and Barton-Burke 2018). However, central instillation of the drug into the ventricle can be achieved via an Ommaya reservoir (Figure 15.27), which is surgically implanted through the cranium (Weinstein and Hagle 2014, Wilkes and Barton-Burke 2018). It carries more risk but provides permanent access and can be inserted under local or general anaesthetic (Wilkes and Barton-Burke 2018). Doses of intraventricular drugs tend to be lower than those given intrathecally.

Evidence-based approaches

Rationale

Indications

Intrathecal administration has proved to be of benefit in prophylactic treatment in cases of leukaemias and some lymphomas, where the CNS may provide a sanctuary site for tumour cells not reached during systemic chemotherapy (Wilkes and Barton-Burke 2018). It has no place in the treatment of CNS metastases of solid tumours (Wilkes and Barton-Burke 2018). Water-soluble antibiotics are administered by the intrathecal route in the treatment of meningitis, and radio-opaque substances are administered for the diagnosis of spinal lesions (Downie et al. 2003).

Principles of care

Preparation of the drug must be performed using aseptic technique to reduce the risk of infection. The drug should be free from preservatives to reduce neurotoxicity. Cerebrospinal fluid removal and volumes of medication should not exceed 2 mL/min.

Clinical governance

Chemotherapy administered using this route has the potential to cause great harm and it was associated with the deaths of at least

13 patients between 1985 and 2002 (Sewell et al. 2002). The risks of intrathecal chemotherapy were well documented in *An Organisation with a Memory* (DH 2000a) and the government set a target to eliminate the incidents of patients dying or being paralysed by maladministered intrathecal injections by the end of 2001 (DH 2000a). Two reports on injection errors (see Toft 2001) gave rise to the publication of national guidance on the safe administration of intrathecal chemotherapy.

Following the publication of the guidance, all UK trusts that undertake to administer intrathecal cytotoxic chemotherapy must ensure safe practice guidelines have been introduced and that they are fully compliant with the *Updated National Guidance on the Safe Administration of Intrathecal Chemotherapy* (DH 2008). The key requirements of the guidance are noted in Box 15.10.

The hospital's chief executive must identify a 'designated lead', who in turn must ensure the appropriate induction, training and continuing professional development of designated personnel authorized to administer intrathecal chemotherapy. A register of these personnel must be kept along with details of certain competency based tasks such as prescribing, dispensing, issuing, checking and administration. It is important to keep up to date with relevant safety alerts concerning intrathecal therapy; these may be issued by Department of Health agencies such as the Medicines and Healthcare products Regulatory Agency (MHRA), previously known as the National Patient Safety Agency (NPSA), whose function was taken over by the NHS Commissioning Board in 2012. Such reports have highlighted concerns over the risk of neurological injury due to implantable drug pumps for intrathecal therapy (MHRA 2008b) and the storage of vinca alkaloid minibags (NPSA 2008c). More recently, the NPSA published two alerts to ensure that all needles, syringes and other devices used for intrathecal administration of medication cannot be attached to any intravenous equipment to prevent maladministered injections (NPSA 2011). Injection of a drug intended for intravenous use into the intrathecal space is considered a 'Never Event' (NHSI 2018a).

Box 15.10 Summary: requirements of intrathecal guidance

- Only trained, designated personnel whose names are recorded on the appropriate intrathecal register are authorized to prescribe, dispense, check or administer intrathecal chemotherapy.
- All staff involved in the intrathecal chemotherapy process must undertake a formal competency-based induction programme that is appropriate to their role, and annual training must be provided for all professional staff for them to remain on the register.
- Staff involved with intrathecal chemotherapy must follow policy in conjunction with DH (2008) and NPSA (2008c), the latter of which relates to intravenous vinca alkaloid administration.
- Staff should be given an annual date-expiring certificate on satisfactory completion of their training.
- Intrathecal chemotherapy must be prescribed by a consultant, associate specialist, specialist registrar, staff grade or ST3 grade doctor only, and they must be on the appropriate intrathecal register.
- Intrathecal chemotherapy drugs must be issued and received by designated staff only. Any such products not used must be returned to the pharmacy at the end of the intrathecal chemotherapy session.
- In adults, intravenous drugs must be administered *before* intrathecal drugs are issued (or once intravenous continuous infusions have been started).
- Children receiving intrathecal therapy under general anaesthetic will have their intrathecal treatment first, in theatre. Intravenous drugs (excluding vinca alkaloids) may be given later in day care or on the ward, but never in theatre.
- Intrathecal chemotherapy should always be administered in a designated area, within normal working hours; out-of-hours administration must only occur in exceptional circumstances.
- Checks must be made by medical, nursing and pharmacy staff at relevant stages throughout the prescribing, preparation and administration process.
- This guidance predominantly relates to treatment given intrathecally, by lumbar puncture (i.e. via spinal injection), but is also relevant to intraventricular chemotherapy (i.e. via injection into the ventricles of the brain).

Source: Adapted from DH (2008).

879

Intradermal injection

Definition

An intradermal injection is given into the dermis of the skin just below the epidermis, where the blood supply is reduced and drug absorption can occur slowly (Chernecky et al. 2005). The intradermal route provides a local rather than systemic effect and is used primarily for administering small amounts of local anaesthetic and skin testing, for example allergy or tuberculin testing (Perry 2015).

Evidence-based approaches

Observation of the skin for an inflammatory reaction is a priority, so the best sites are those that are lowly pigmented, thinly keratinized and hairless. The inner forearms and the scapulae are commonly chosen. The injection site most commonly used for skin testing is the medial forearm area, as this allows for easy inspection (Downie et al. 2003). Volumes of 0.5 mL or less should be used (Chernecky et al. 2005).

Pre-procedural considerations

Equipment

These injections are best performed using a 25 or 27 G needle inserted at a 10–15° angle, bevel up, just under the epidermis. Usually a tuberculosis or 1 mL syringe is used to ensure accuracy of the dose.

Procedure guideline 15.16 Medication: intradermal injection

Essential equipment

- Personal protective equipment
- Medication to be injected
- Recording sheet or book as required by law or hospital policy
- Patient's prescription chart, to check dose, route, etc.
- Electronic identity check equipment, where relevant
- Needle (25 or 27 G)
- 1 mL syringe containing medication
- Alcohol swab
- Clinically clean receiver or tray containing the prepared drug (prepare as described in Procedure guidelines 15.11, 15.12, 15.13 or 15.14)

(*continued*)

Procedure guideline 15.16 Medication: intradermal injection *(continued)*

Action	Rationale
Pre-procedure	
1 Introduce yourself to the patient, explain and discuss the procedure with them, and gain their consent to proceed.	To ensure that the patient feels at ease, understands the procedure and gives their valid consent (NMC 2018, **C**).
2 Before administering any prescribed drug, look at the patient's prescription chart and check the following: a the correct patient is being given the drug b drug c dose d date and time of administration e route and method of administration f diluent as appropriate g validity of prescription h signature of prescriber i the prescription is legible.	To ensure that the patient is given the correct drug in the prescribed dose using the appropriate diluent and by the correct route (DH 2003b, **C**; RPS 2019a, **C**). To protect the patient from harm (DH 2003b, **C**).
If any of these pieces of information are missing, unclear or illegible, do not proceed with the administration. Consult with the prescriber.	To prevent any errors occurring. **E**
Procedure	
3 Apply apron, close the curtains or door, and assist the patient into the required position. Wash hands.	To ensure patient privacy and dignity. **E** To allow access to the appropriate injection site (Workman 1999, **E**).
4 Take the medication and the prescription chart to the patient. Check the patient's identity by asking them to state their full name and date of birth. If the patient is unable to confirm these details, then check the patient identity band against the prescription chart. If an electronic identity check system for the patient and/or medicine identification is in place, then use it in accordance with hospital policy and procedures. Check the patient's allergy status by asking them or by checking the name band.	To ensure that the medication is administered to the correct patient and prevent any errors related to drug allergies (NPSA 2005, **C**).
5 Assist the patient to remove the appropriate garments to expose the injection site.	To gain access for the injection (Workman 1999, **E**).
6 Assess the injection site for signs of inflammation, oedema, infection and skin lesions.	To promote the effectiveness of the administration (Workman 1999, **E**). To reduce the risk of infection (Fraise and Bradley 2009, **E**; Workman 1999, **E**). To avoid skin lesions and possible trauma to the patient (Workman 1999, **E**).
7 Choose the correct needle size and attach the needle.	To minimize the risk of missing the subcutaneous tissue and any ensuing pain (Workman 1999, **E**).
8 Apply gloves and clean the injection site with a swab saturated with isopropyl alcohol 70%.	To reduce the number of pathogens introduced into the skin by the needle at the time of insertion. **E** (For further information on this action see 'Skin preparation' below.)
9 Remove the needle sheath and hold the syringe with the dominant hand with the bevel of the needle pointing up.	To facilitate needle placement (Ostendorf 2015, **E**).
10 With the non-dominant hand, stretch the skin over the site with forefinger and thumb.	To facilitate the needle piercing the skin more easily (Ostendorf 2015, **E**).
11 With the needle almost against the patient's skin, insert the needle into the skin at an angle of 10–15° and advance through the epidermis so the needle tip can be seen through the skin.	To ensure the needle tip is in the dermis (Ostendorf 2015, **E**).
12 Inject the medication slowly. It is not necessary to aspirate as the dermis is relatively avascular.	To minimize discomfort at the site (Ostendorf 2015, **E**).
13 While injecting the medication, a bleb (resembling a mosquito bite) will form (**Action figure 13**).	To indicate the medication is in the dermis (Ostendorf 2015, **E**).
14 Withdraw the needle rapidly and apply pressure gently. Do not massage the site.	To prevent dispersing the medication into underlying tissue layers and altering test results (Chernecky et al. 2005, **E**; Ostendorf 2015, **E**).

Post-procedure

15 Where appropriate, activate safety devices. Ensure that all sharps and non-sharp waste are disposed of safely and in accordance with locally approved procedures – for example, sharps into sharps bin and syringes into an orange clinical waste bag.	To ensure safe disposal and to avoid laceration or other injury to staff (EASHW 2010, **C**; HWR 2005, **C**; MHRA 2004, **C**).
16 Record the administration on the appropriate charts.	To maintain accurate records, provide a point of reference in the event of any queries and prevent any duplication of treatment (NPSA 2007d, **C**; RPS 2019a, **C**).

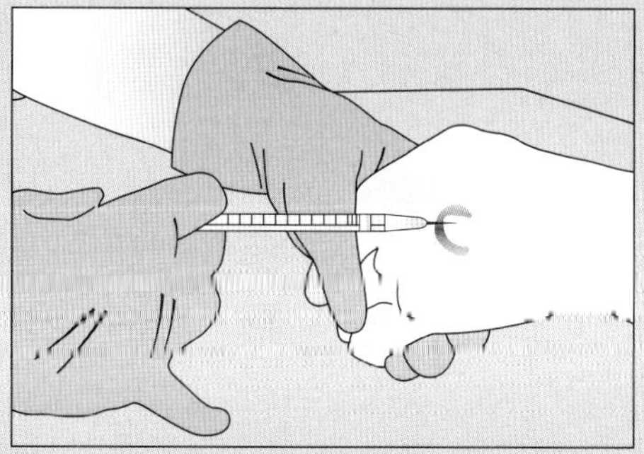

Action Figure 13 Intradermal bleb. *Source*: Adapted from Springhouse (2009) with permission of Wolters Kluwer.

Subcutaneous injection

Definition

Subcutaneous injections are given beneath the epidermis into the loose fat and connective tissue underlying the dermis and are used for administering small doses of non-irritating water-soluble substances such as insulin or heparin (Downie et al. 2003).

Related theory

Subcutaneous tissue is not richly supplied with blood vessels and so medication is absorbed more slowly here than when given intramuscularly. The rate of absorption is influenced by factors that affect blood flow to tissues, such as physical exercise and local application of hot or cold compresses (Ostendorf 2015). Other conditions can prevent or delay absorption due to impaired blood flow, so subcutaneous injections are contraindicated in conditions such as circulatory shock and occlusive vascular disease (Ostendorf 2015).

Evidence-based approaches

Injection sites recommended are the abdomen (in the umbilical region), the lateral or posterior aspect of the lower part of the upper arm, the thighs (under the greater trochanter rather than midthigh) and the buttocks (Downie et al. 2003) (Figure 15.28). It has been found that the amount of subcutaneous tissue varies more than was previously thought; this is particularly significant for administration of insulin, as inadvertent intramuscular administration can result in rapid absorption and hypoglycaemic episodes (King 2003). Rotation of sites can decrease the likelihood of irritation and ensure improved absorption. If using the abdominal area, try to inject each subsequent injection 2.5 cm from the previous one (Chernecky et al. 2005). Injection sites should be free of infection, skin lesions, scars, birthmarks, bony prominences, and large underlying muscles or nerves (Ostendorf 2015).

The skin should be gently pinched into a fold to elevate the subcutaneous tissue, which lifts the adipose tissue away from the underlying muscle (FIT 2016). The practice of aspirating to ensure a blood vessel has not been pierced is no longer recommended as it has been shown that this is unlikely to occur (Ostendorf 2015,

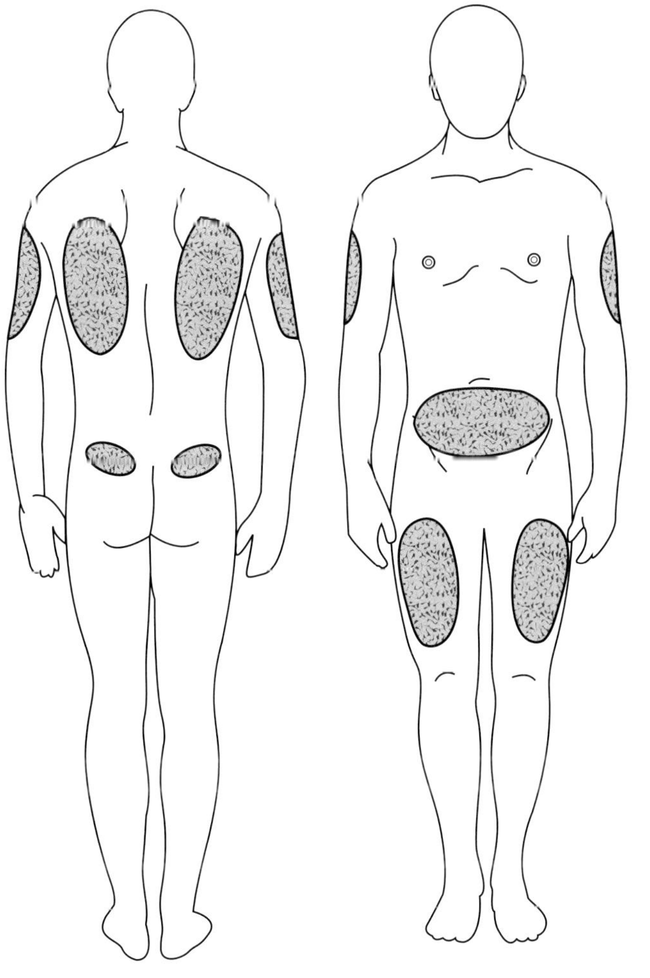

Figure 15.28 Sites recommended for subcutaneous injection. *Source*: Adapted from Perry et al. (2015) with permission of Elsevier.

Peragallo-Dittko 1997). The maximum volume tolerable using this route for injection is 2 mL and drugs should be highly soluble to prevent irritation (Downie et al. 2003).

Pre-procedural considerations

Equipment

Subcutaneous injections are usually given using a 25 G needle. There is no clinical reason to recommend needles longer than 8 mm in adults (FIT 2016). Where a needle is 6mm or shorter, it may not be necessary to lift a skin fold, unless injecting into slim limbs or the abdomen (FIT 2016). When using a needle of 6 mm length or less, insulin injections should be given at an angle of 90° in adults (FIT 2016). Needles of 6 mm or less should be used in children and adolescents; a skin fold should be lifted, unless a smaller needle (4 mm) is being used, in which case this is not usually required. An angle of 90° is recommended for most insulin injections when using a 4 mm needle (FIT 2016). If the medication is presented in a pre-filled syringe, do not transfer it into another container or delivery system.

Specific patient preparation

Skin preparation

There are differences of opinion regarding skin cleaning prior to subcutaneous or intramuscular injections. It has been stated that it is not necessary to use an alcohol swab to clean the skin prior to administration of injections providing the skin is socially clean (FIT 2016). Further studies have suggested that cleaning with an alcohol swab is not always necessary, as not cleaning the site does not result in infections and may predispose the skin to hardening (Dann 1969, Koivistov and Felig 1978, Workman 1999).

In a study over a period of 5 years involving more than 5000 injections, Dann (1969) found no single case of local and/or systemic infection. Koivistov and Felig (1978) concluded that while skin preparations do reduce skin bacterial count, they are not necessary to prevent infections at the injection site. Some hospitals accept that if the patient is physically clean and the nurse maintains a high standard of hand hygiene and asepsis during the procedure, skin disinfection is not necessary (Workman 1999). There is no recent research currently available on what is appropriate skin preparation prior to a simple intramuscular or subcutaneous injection (Wolf et al. 2005).

In immunosuppressed patients, consideration may be given to skin preparation as such patients may become infected by inoculation of a relatively small number of pathogens (Downie et al. 2003); however, advice on this subject will vary between healthcare providers as there is minimal evidence available. The practice at the Royal Marsden Hospital is to clean the skin prior to injection in order to reduce the risk of contamination from the patient's skin flora. The skin is cleaned using an alcohol swab (containing 70% isopropyl alcohol) for 30 seconds and then allowed to dry. If the skin is not dry before proceeding, skin cleaning is ineffective and the antiseptic may cause irritation by being injected into the tissues (Downie et al. 2003).

Procedure guideline 15.17 Medication: subcutaneous injection

Essential equipment

- Personal protective equipment
- Recording sheet or book as required by law or hospital policy
- Patient's prescription chart, to check dose, route, etc.
- Electronic identity check equipment, where relevant
- Alcohol swab
- Needle
- Syringe containing prepared medication
- Sterile gauze
- Clinically clean receiver or tray containing the prepared drug (prepare as described in Procedure guidelines 15.11, 15.12, 15.13 or 15.14)

Action	Rationale
Pre-procedure	
1 Introduce yourself to the patient, explain and discuss the procedure with them, and gain their consent to proceed.	To ensure that the patient feels at ease, understands the procedure and gives their valid consent (NMC 2018, **C**).
2 Before administering any prescribed drug, look at the patient's prescription chart and check the following: a the correct patient is being given the drug b drug c dose d date and time of administration e route and method of administration f diluent as appropriate g validity of prescription h signature of prescriber i the prescription is legible.	To ensure that the correct patient is given the correct drug in the prescribed dose using the appropriate diluent and by the correct route (DH 2003b, **C**; NMC 2018, **C**; RPS 2019a, **C**). To protect the patient from harm (DH 2003b, **C**).
If any of these pieces of information are missing, unclear or illegible, do not proceed with the administration. Consult with the prescriber.	To prevent any errors occurring. **E**
3 Wash hands and apply an apron.	To prevent contamination of medication and equipment (DH 2007, **C**). To prevent cross-contamination (Fraise and Bradley 2009, **E**).

Procedure	
4 Close the curtains or door and assist the patient into the required position.	To ensure the patient's privacy and dignity. **E** To allow access to the appropriate injection site (Ostendorf 2015, **E**).
5 Take the medication and the prescription chart to the patient. Check the patient's identity by asking them to state their full name and date of birth. If the patient is unable to confirm these details, then check the patient identity band against the prescription chart. If an electronic identity check system for the patient and/or medicine identification is in place, then use it in accordance with hospital policy and procedures. Check the patient's allergy status by asking them or by checking the name band.	To ensure that the medication is administered to the correct patient and prevent any errors related to drug allergies (NPSA 2005, **C**).
6 Assist the patient to remove the appropriate garments to expose the injection site.	To gain access for the injection. **E**
7 Assess the injection site for signs of inflammation, oedema, infection and skin lesions.	To promote the effectiveness of the administration (Ostendorf 2015, **E**). To reduce the risk of infection (Fraise and Bradley 2009, **E**; Workman 1999, **E**). To avoid skin lesions and possible trauma to the patient (Ostendorf 2015, **E**).
8 Wash and dry hands and apply non-sterile gloves.	To prevent contamination of medication and equipment (DH 2007, **C**). To prevent possible cross-contamination (Fraise and Bradley 2009, **E**).
9 Select the appropriate needle size.	To minimize the risk of missing the subcutaneous tissue and any ensuing pain (FIT 2016, **C**; Ostendorf 2015, **E**).
10 Where appropriate, clean the injection site with a swab saturated with isopropyl alcohol 70%.	To reduce the number of pathogens introduced into the skin by the needle at the time of insertion (FIT 2016, **C**). (For further information on this action see 'Skin preparation' below.)
11 Remove the needle sheath.	To prepare the syringe for use. **E**
12 Consider whether pinching a skin fold is required.	To elevate the subcutaneous tissue and lift the adipose tissue away from the underlying muscle (FIT 2016, **C**; Ostendorf 2015, **E**).
13 Hold the syringe between thumb and forefinger of the dominant hand as if grasping a dart.	To enable a quick, smooth injection (Ostendorf 2015, **E**).
14 Insert the needle into the skin at an angle of 45° and release the grasped skin (unless administering insulin, when an angle of 90° should usually be used). Inject the drug slowly over 10–30 seconds.	Injecting medication into compressed tissue irritates nerve fibres and causes discomfort (Ostendorf 2015, **E**). The introduction of shorter insulin needles makes 90° the more appropriate angle (FIT 2016, **C**; Trounce and Gould 2000, **E**).
15 Withdraw the needle rapidly. Apply gentle pressure with sterile gauze. Do not massage the area.	To aid absorption. Massage can injure the underlying tissue (Ostendorf 2015, **E**).
Post-procedure	
16 Ensure that all sharps and non-sharp waste are disposed of safely and in accordance with locally approved procedures.	To ensure safe disposal and to avoid laceration or other injury to staff (HWR 2005, **C**; MHRA 2004, **C**).
17 Record the administration on the appropriate charts.	To maintain accurate records, provide a point of reference in the event of any queries and prevent any duplication of treatment (NPSA 2007d, **C**; RPS 2019a, **C**).

Post-procedural considerations

Education of the patient and relevant others

Patients often have to administer their own subcutaneous injections, for example insulin for diabetics. The nurse must teach the patient how to prepare and administer self-injection, including aspects such as equipment, storage, hand washing, injection technique, rotation of sites, and safe disposal of equipment and sharps (FIT 2016, Ostendorf 2015).

Complications

If medications collect within the tissues, this can cause sterile abscesses, which appear as hardened, painful lumps (Ostendorf 2015). In rare cases, lipohypertrophy (wasting of the subcutaneous tissue at injection sites) can develop (FIT 2016). The nurse must monitor and report these, and avoid using these areas for further injections (FIT 2016).

Subcutaneous infusion

Definition

A subcutaneous infusion is a continuous infusion of fluids or medication into the subcutaneous tissues (Ostendorf 2015).

Evidence-based approaches

Methods for subcutaneous infusions of fluids (hypodermoclysis)

Hypodermoclysis is a method of infusing fluid into subcutaneous tissue that is an alternative to administering intravenous fluids

(Sasson and Shvartzman 2001). Subcutaneous fluids can be given to maintain adequate hydration in patients with mild or moderate dehydration (Scales 2011, Walsh 2005) and have been shown to be as effective as the intravenous route for replacing fluid and electrolytes (Barton et al. 2004, Barua and Bhowmick 2005, Luk et al. 2008). The use of this route is generally limited to palliative care and elderly patients (Scales 2011, Walsh 2005). It is not recommended for patients needing rapid administration of fluids, and is also contraindicated in patients with clotting disorders or who have problems with fluid overload (such as those with cardiac failure) (Mei and Auerhahn 2009, Walsh 2005).

A volume of 1000–2000 mL can be given over 24 hours; this can be given as a continuous infusion, over a number of hours (such as overnight) or as intermittent boluses (Moriarty and Hudson 2001, Scales 2011, Walsh 2005). More than one site can be used if greater volumes are required. It is recommended that electrolyte-containing fluids such as 0.9% sodium chloride or dextrose saline be used, although 5% glucose has also been used (Hypodermoclysis Working Group 1998, Sasson and Shvartzman 2001).

Advantages of this route include the following:

- side-effects are few and not generally significant
- it is a relatively easy procedure that can be carried out at home, reducing the need for hospitalization
- it may be set up and administered by nurses in almost any setting
- it has a low cost
- it is less likely than intravenous infusion to cause fluid overload
- intravenous access can be problematic in elderly or debilitated patients; avoidance of this issue can reduce anxiety and distress (Mei and Auerhahn 2009, Scales 2011).

Side-effects of subcutaneous fluid administration include pain, bruising, local oedema, erythema and local inflammation, which can be reduced by changing the site of the infusion (Mei and Auerhahn 2009, Scales 2011).

Hyaluronidase is an enzyme that temporarily increases the permeability of subcutaneous connective tissue by degrading hyaluronic acid and has been shown to increase the dispersion and absorption of co-administered molecules (Thomas et al. 2009). It can be given as a subcutaneous injection before commencing fluids or added to infusion bags (Sasson and Shvartzman 2001). A randomized study compared absorption and the side-effects of administration of subcutaneous fluids with and without hyaluronidase. No significant differences were found although patients not receiving hyaluronidase showed an increase in the size of the limb in which the fluid had been administered, but no differences in pain or local discomfort were found so no clear benefit to the use of hyaluronidase was demonstrated (Constans et al. 1991). Most agree that it is not necessary to use hyaluronidase if the infusion rate is 1 mL/min or less (Mei and Auerhahn 2009).

Methods for subcutaneous infusions of drugs

Subcutaneous infusion may be the route of choice in patients with problems such as vomiting, diarrhoea or dysphagia, and in those who are unable to tolerate drugs by the oral route. Some patients with bowel obstruction whose gut absorption may be impaired may also benefit. Subcutaneous infusion is also commonly used for patients who are dying and no longer able to manage medication orally (Dickman et al. 2016, Dychter et al. 2012, Menahem and Shvartzman 2010, Ostendorf 2015). Continuous subcutaneous infusion of insulin is used in a small number of diabetic patients, particularly when adequate control cannot be achieved with multiple daily insulin doses. Such patients need to be under the care of a multidisciplinary team familiar with the use of such infusions (NICE 2003).

Infusions of a single drug, such as an antiemetic or analgesic, do not generally cause problems with drug stability. The drug should be diluted with a suitable diluent (sodium chloride is recommended for most drugs) and given over 12–24 hours (Dickman et al. 2016). The use of a combination of drugs can be problematic; there is anecdotal evidence regarding combinations of drugs but not many pharmaceutical studies have confirmed compatibility. Combinations of up to four drugs have been reported; however, if compatibility is uncertain, it may be best to use a second syringe pump. It is also important to ensure that the diluent used is compatible with all the drugs in the infusion. It is recommended that infusions are not exposed to direct sunlight or to increased temperatures as drug instability may result (Dickman et al. 2016). Hyaluronidase may be used to enhance the pharmacokinetics of drugs such as subcutaneous morphine (Menahem and Shvartzman 2010, Thomas et al. 2009).

The subcutaneous route can be used in the palliative care setting for parenteral hydration. The decision to commence subcutaneous fluids is individual and the decision process should involve the patient (if possible), their family and/or carers, and the multiprofessional team (Bruera et al. 2015). The overall comfort and wellbeing of the patient should be central to the decision (Gabriel 2012), as the evidence to support the use of the subcutaneous route for this purpose is limited (Bruera et al. 2015).

Pre-procedural considerations

Equipment

Access devices

Research has shown that the use of peripheral cannulas rather than steel winged infusion devices results in sites remaining viable for longer (Torre 2002). Incidence of needle stick injuries may also be reduced (Dawkins et al. 2000). It is now recommended that subcutaneous infusion be given via a plastic cannula. Administration of infusions of drugs or fluids requires the insertion of a 25 G winged infusion set or a 24 G cannula (RCN 2016, Scales 2011). These should be inserted at an angle of 45° and secured with a transparent dressing to enable inspection of the site. This may also be appropriate for patients not receiving a continuous infusion but requiring frequent subcutaneous injections; this is common practice in palliative care in order to reduce the number of needles inserted into the patient and the subsequent trauma caused.

Syringe pump

A syringe pump is a portable battery-operated infusion device. It is used to deliver drugs at a predetermined rate via the appropriate parenteral route (e.g. subcutaneous) and is suitable for symptom management and palliative care (Bailey and Harman 2018, Dickman et al. 2016). It should be used for patients who are unable to tolerate oral medication, for example in nausea and vomiting, dysphagia, intestinal obstruction, local disease or sometimes in intractable pain that is unrelieved by oral medications and where rapid-dose titration is required. Drugs administered by subcutaneous infusion include opioid analgesics, antiemetics, anxiolytic sedatives, corticosteroids, non-steroidal anti-inflammatory drugs and anticholinergic drugs (Dickman et al. 2016, Dychter et al. 2012).

There are various types of syringe pump available; they must meet the standards required by the MHRA, and nurses should consult the manufacturer's instruction manual for details on their use. One type used widely in the UK is CME Medical's T34 syringe pump (previously the McKinley T34 syringe pump)

Most sizes and brands of plastic syringe can be used with these devices; however, it is recommended to use Luer-Lok syringes to avoid leakage or accidental disconnection.

The advantages of syringe drivers are as follows (Dickman et al. 2016):

- They avoid the necessity of intermittent injections.
- Mixtures of drugs may be administered.
- Infusion timing is accurate, which is particularly advantageous in the community, where it is not possible to constantly monitor the rate.
- The devices are lightweight and compact, allowing mobility and independence.

- Rate can be increased.
- Simple calculations of dosage are required over a 12 or 24 hour period.
- They allow patients to spend more time at home with their symptoms managed effectively.

The disadvantages are as follows (Dickman et al. 2016):

- The patient may become psychologically dependent on the device.
- Inflammation or infection may occur at the insertion site of the subcutaneous cannula.
- They should be used with caution in patients with peripheral oedema.
- Close proximity to a mobile phone may interfere with their action.

Specific patient preparation

Choice of infusion site should be based on both thickness of subcutaneous tissue and patient convenience. Sites recommended for subcutaneous infusion of drugs or fluids are the lateral aspects of the upper arms and thighs, the abdomen, the chest and the scapulae (Walsh 2005). If the patient is ambulant then the chest or abdomen are the preferred sites, but the patient should be included in the decision-making process wherever possible (Dickman et al. 2016). The following areas should not be used:

- lymphoedematous areas, as absorption may be impaired and infection may be introduced
- sites over bony prominences, as there may be insufficient subcutaneous tissue
- previously irradiated skin areas, as absorption may be impaired
- sites near a joint, as movement may cause the cannula to become dislodged
- skin folds or breast tissue (Dickman et al. 2016)
- areas directly over a tumour (Dickman et al. 2016)
- any areas of inflamed, infected or broken skin (Dickman et al. 2016, Ostendorf 2015).

In general, an infusion site need not be changed for at least 72 hours, unless there is a local reaction to the infusion (Dickman et al. 2016).

Procedure guideline 15.18 Medication: subcutaneous infusion of fluids

Essential equipment

- Personal protective equipment
- Recording sheet or book as required by law or hospital policy
- Patient's prescription chart, to check dose, route, etc.
- Electronic identity check equipment, where relevant
- Clinically clean receiver or tray
- Sharps box
- Isopropyl alcohol 70% swab
- Transparent adhesive dressing
- Winged infusion set or 24 G cannula
- Infusion fluid
- Administration set

Action	Rationale
Pre-procedure	
1 Introduce yourself to the patient, explain and discuss the procedure with them, and gain their consent to proceed.	To ensure that the patient feels at ease, understands the procedure and gives their valid consent (NMC 2018, **C**).
2 Before administering any prescribed fluid, check that it is due and has not already been given.	To protect the patient from harm (NPSA 2007d, **C**).
3 Before administering any prescribed fluid, look at the patient's prescription chart and check the following: a the correct patient is being given the drug b drug/fluid c dose d date and time of administration e route and method of administration f diluent as appropriate g validity of prescription h signature of prescriber i the prescription is legible.	To ensure that the correct patient is given the correct fluid in the prescribed dose using the appropriate diluent and by the correct route (DH 2003b, **C**; RPS 2019a, **C**). To protect the patient from harm (DH 2003b, **C**; NMC 2018, **C**).
If any of these pieces of information are missing, unclear or illegible, do not proceed with the administration. Consult with the prescriber.	To prevent any errors occurring. **E**
4 Wash hands with bactericidal soap and water or an alcohol-based handrub, and assemble the necessary equipment.	To minimize the risk of infection (Fraise and Bradley 2009, **E**; NHS England and NHSI 2019, **C**).
Procedure	
5 Check the name and volume of the infusion fluid against the prescription chart.	To ensure that the correct type and quantity of fluid are administered (NPSA 2007d, **C**; RPS 2019a, **C**).
6 Check the expiry date of the infusion bag.	To prevent an ineffective or toxic compound being administered to the patient (NPSA 2007d, **C**).

(continued)

Procedure guideline 15.18 Medication: subcutaneous infusion of fluids *(continued)*

Action	Rationale
7 Check that the packaging is intact and inspect the container and contents in good light for cracks, punctures and air bubbles.	To check that no contamination of the infusion container has occurred (NPSA 2007d, **C**).
8 Inspect the fluid for discoloration, haziness, and crystalline or particulate matter. If this is found, discard.	To prevent any toxic or foreign matter being infused into the patient (NPSA 2007d, **C**). To detect any incompatibility or degradation (NPSA 2007d, **C**).
9 Establish the correct drip rate setting using the correct calculation.	To monitor rate and ensure fluid is infused safely (Pickstone 1999, **E**).
10 Place the infusion bag and administration set in a clean receptacle. Wash hands and proceed to the patient.	To minimize the risk of contamination (Loveday et al. 2014, **C**; NHS England and NHSI 2019, **C**).
11 Check the identity of the patient against the prescription chart, and with the patient. If an electronic identity check system for patient and/or medicine identification is in place, then use in accordance with hospital policy and procedures.	To minimize the risk of error and ensure the correct fluid is administered to the correct patient (NPSA 2007d, **C**).
12 Place the infusion bag on a flat surface, remove the seal and insert the spike of the administration set fully into the infusion bag port.	To prevent puncturing the side of the infusion bag and to reduce the risk of contamination (DH 2007, **C**).
13 Hang the infusion bag from a drip stand.	To allow flow due to gravity. **E**
14 Open the roller clamp and allow the fluid through the set to prime it. Close the clamp.	To remove air from the set. **E**
15 Apply an apron and assist the patient into a comfortable position.	To ensure patient comfort during the procedure. **E**
16 Expose the chosen site for infusion.	To expose the area. **E**
17 Apply gloves and clean the chosen site with a swab saturated with 70% isopropyl alcohol. Wait until the alcohol evaporates.	To reduce the risk of infection and prevent a stinging sensation on insertion of the needle (Fraise and Bradley 2009, **E**; Loveday et al. 2014, **C**).
18 Pinch a fold of skin firmly.	To elevate the subcutaneous tissue. **E**
19 Insert the infusion needle into the skin at an angle of 45°, bevel up, and release the grasped skin. (If using a cannula, remove the stylet.)	To gain access to the subcutaneous tissue (Walsh 2005, **E**).
20 Connect the administration set to the device.	To commence the infusion. **E**
21 Apply a transparent dressing to secure the infusion device.	To prevent movement and reduce the risk of mechanical phlebitis and infection (Fraise and Bradley 2009, **E**; Loveday et al. 2014, **C**; Weinstein and Hagle 2014, **E**).
22 Open the roller clamp and adjust until the flow rate is achieved. The rate is usually 1 mL/min per site by gravity.	To ensure the correct rate is set. **E**
Post-procedure	
23 Complete the patient's prescription chart and other hospital and/or legally required documents.	To comply with local drug administration policies and provide a record in the event of any queries, and to prevent any duplication of treatment (RPS 2019a, **C**).
24 Monitor the patient for any infusion- or site-related complications and document these in the patient's notes.	To detect complications promptly (Sasson and Shvartzman 2001, **E**).
25 Ask the patient to report any pain or tenderness at the infusion site.	To ascertain whether there are any problems that may require nursing care and to enable referral to medical staff where appropriate. **E**
26 Discard waste, making sure that it is placed in the correct containers, for example sharps into a designated receptacle.	To ensure safe disposal and avoid injury to staff, and to prevent reuse of equipment (HWR 2005, **C**; MHRA 2004, **C**).

Procedure guideline 15.19 Medication: subcutaneous administration using a CME Medical T34 syringe pump (previously McKinley)

Essential equipment

- Personal protective equipment
- Clinically clean receiver or tray containing the prepared drug
- Syringe pump
- Battery (PP3 size, 9 volt alkaline)
- Plastic peripheral cannulas (e.g. 24 G) and microbore extension set (100 cm) with needle-free Y connector injection site (or 100 cm winged infusion set)

- Luer-Lok syringe of a suitable size (minimum size 20 mL)
- Swab saturated with isopropyl alcohol 70%
- Transparent adhesive dressing
- Drugs and diluent
- Needle (to draw up drug)
- Drug additive label
- Patient's prescription chart
- Recording chart or book as required by law or hospital policy
- Electronic identity check equipment, where relevant
- Sharps box

Action	Rationale
Pre-procedure	
1 Introduce yourself to the patient, explain and discuss the procedure with them, and gain their consent to proceed.	To ensure that the patient feels at ease, understands the procedure and gives their valid consent (NMC 2018, **C**).
2 Before administering any prescribed drug, check that it is due and has not already been given.	To protect the patient from harm (NPSA 2007d, **C**).
3 Before administering any prescribed drug, look at the patient's prescription chart and check the following: a the correct patient is being given the drug b drug c dose d date and time of administration e route and method of administration f diluent as appropriate g validity of prescription h signature of prescriber i the prescription is legible.	To ensure that the correct patient is given the correct drug in the prescribed dose using the appropriate diluent and by the correct route (DH 2003b, **C**; NMC 2018, **C**). To protect the patient from harm (DH 2003b, **C**; RPS 2019a, **C**).
If any of these pieces of information are missing, unclear or illegible, do not proceed with the administration. Consult with the prescriber.	To prevent any errors occurring. **E**
4 Calculate and check the dosage of the drugs required over a 24-hour period.	To establish the correct doses of drugs (Pickstone 1999, **E**).
5 Wash hands with bactericidal soap and water or an alcohol-based handrub, and assemble the necessary equipment.	To minimize the risk of infection (Fraise and Bradley 2009, **E**; NHS England and NHSI 2019, **C**).
Procedure	
6 Check the name, strength and volume of the subcutaneous drug(s) against the prescription chart.	To ensure that the correct type and quantity of fluid are administered (NPSA 2007d, **C**; RPS 2019a, **C**).
7 Check the expiry date of the drug(s).	To prevent an ineffective or toxic compound being administered to the patient (NPSA 2007d, **C**).
8 Check that the packaging is intact and inspect the container and contents in good light for cracks, punctures and air bubbles.	To check that no contamination of the infusion container has occurred (NPSA 2007d, **C**).
9 Check the identity and amount of drug to be prepared. If an electronic identity check system for patient and/or medicine identification is in place, then use in accordance with hospital policy and procedures.	To minimize any risk of error, and to ensure safe and effective administration of the drug (NPSA 2007d, **C**).
Consider: a compatibility of drugs b stability of mixture over the prescription time c any special directions for dilution, for example pH or optimum concentration d sensitivity to external factors such as light e any anticipated allergic reaction. If any doubts exist about the listed points, consult a pharmacist or appropriate reference works.	To enable anticipation of toxicities and the nursing implications of these (NPSA 2007d, **C**).
10 Prepare the medication as described in Procedure guidelines 15.11, 15.12, 15.13 or 15.14. Using a Luer-Lok syringe, draw up the drugs required with diluent to measure the total volume (this will depend on the type of syringe pump used). See Box 15.11 for CME Medical T34 recommended volumes and **Action figure 10** for a CME Medical T34 syringe pump.	To ensure accuracy and avoid any infusion errors. To ensure the drug is prepared correctly (NPSA 2007d, **C**).

(continued)

Procedure guideline 15.19 Medication: subcutaneous administration using a CME Medical T34 syringe pump (previously McKinley) *(continued)*

Action	Rationale
11 Inspect the fluid for discoloration, haziness, and crystalline or particulate matter. If this is found, discard and re-evaluate drug compatibility. *Note*: this can occur even if the mixture is theoretically compatible, thus making vigilance essential.	To prevent any toxic or foreign matter being infused into the patient (NPSA 2007d, **C**). To detect any incompatibility or degradation (NPSA 2007d, **C**).
12 Establish the correct rate setting of the pump using the correct calculation.	To monitor rate and ensure the drug is infused safely (Dickman et al. 2016, **E**; Pickstone 1999, **E**).
13 Complete the drug additive label and fix it onto the syringe without obscuring the markings.	To identify which drug has been added, when and by whom, and to be able to visually inspect the amount in the syringe (NPSA 2007d, **C**).
14 Wash hands with bactericidal soap and water or an alcohol-based handrub.	To minimize the risk of infection (Fraise and Bradley 2009, **E**; NHS England and NHSI 2019, **C**).
15 Connect the prepared syringe to a 100 cm microbore driver set with needle-free Y connector injection site.	This length of tubing allows the patient greater freedom of movement. **E**
16 Prime the infusion by gently depressing the plunger of the syringe until the fluid is visible at the end of the infusion set. Priming the infusion set after calculation will reduce the delivery time by approximately half an hour for the first infusion. Do not alter previously the calculated rate setting despite the volume reduction in the barrel of the syringe.	To remove extraneous air from the system. **E** To ensure the patient receives the drugs immediately and accurately. **E**
17 Place the syringe and infusion set in a clean receptacle. Wash hands and proceed to the patient.	To minimize the risk of contamination (Loveday et al. 2014, **C**; NHS England and NHSI 2019, **C**).
18 Check the identity of the patient against the prescription chart, syringe drug additive label and with the patient if possible. If an electronic identity check system for patient and/or medicine identification is in place, then use in accordance with hospital policy and procedures.	To minimize the risk of error and ensure the correct drug is administered to the correct patient (NPSA 2007d, **C**; RPS 2019a, **C**).
19 Apply an apron and assist the patient into a comfortable position.	To aid patient comfort. **E**
20 Expose the chosen site for infusion.	To gain access to the site. **E**
21 Apply gloves and clean the chosen site with a swab saturated with 70% isopropyl alcohol. Wait until the alcohol evaporates.	To reduce the risk of infection and prevent a stinging sensation on insertion of the needle (Fraise and Bradley 2009, **E**; Loveday et al. 2014, **C**).
22 Pinch a fold of skin firmly.	To elevate the subcutaneous tissue. **E**
23 Insert the infusion needle into the skin at an angle of 45° and release the grasped skin. (If using a cannula, remove the stylet and connect the extension set.)	Positioning shallower than 45° may shorten the life of the infusion site. **E**
24 Apply a transparent dressing to secure the infusion device.	To prevent movement and reduce the risk of mechanical phlebitis and infection (Fraise and Bradley 2009, **E**; Loveday et al. 2014, **C**; Weinstein and Hagle 2014, **E**).
25 Check that the infusion set and syringe are securely connected.	To ensure that there is no disconnection so that the drug(s) are administered correctly. **E**
26 Connect the syringe to the syringe pump.	To ensure the syringe is correctly connected to the syringe pump. **E**
27 Press the 'Back' key to adjust the actuator to accommodate the syringe. Lift the barrel arm and ensure the syringe is loaded correctly. If the syringe is not loaded into the barrel, collar and plunger correctly, this will be identified on the LED screen.	To ensure the syringe is in the correct position. **C**
28 The pump will detect the size and brand of syringe. Check and confirm by pressing the 'YES' key.	To enable the pump mechanism to operate correctly (manufacturer's instructions, **C**).
29 Set a new programme for each syringe.	To clear the previous programme and reduce the risk of error (manufacturer's instructions, **C**).
30 Set pump measurements for the deliverable volume in the syringe.	To check the volume is as required. **E**
31 Press 'YES' to confirm the volume to be infused. Press 'YES' to confirm the infusion duration. The pump will display the rate calculated for the volume and duration set by the user. Then press 'YES' to confirm.	To complete set-up of the device (manufacturer's instructions, **C**).

32	Secure the syringe in the clear Perspex lock box (for syringes of 30 mL or larger only).	To ensure extra security and minimize the risk of errors in infusion rates. **E**
	Post-procedure	
33	Discard waste, making sure that it is placed in the correct containers, for example sharps into a designated receptacle.	To ensure safe disposal and avoid injury to staff. To prevent reuse of equipment (HWR 2005, **C**; MHRA 2004, **C**).
34	Complete the patient's prescription chart and other hospital and/or legally required documents. This should include infusion device serial number and infusion device and site checks.	To comply with local drug administration policies and ensure the safe administration and monitoring of the infused drug and accurate records. To provide a record in the event of any queries (RPS 2019a, **C**). To prevent any duplication of treatment (RPS 2019a, **C**).
35	Monitor the patient for any infusion-related complications.	To detect complications promptly (Dickman et al. 2016, **E**; Dougherty 2002, **E**; MHRA 2010b, **C**; Pickstone 1999, **E**; Quinn 2000, **E**).
36	Ask the patient to report any pain or tenderness at the infusion site and if they experience any change in their symptoms or have new symptoms.	To ascertain whether there are any problems that may require nursing care and to enable referral to medical staff where appropriate. **E**

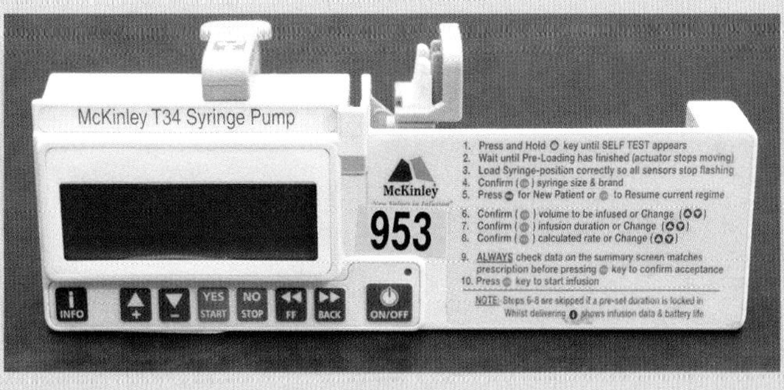

Action Figure 10 A CME MediCal (previously McKinley) T34 syringe pump.

Problem-solving table 15.2 Prevention and resolution (Procedure guideline 15.19)

Problem	Cause	Prevention	Action
Precipitation or cloudiness in the syringe.	Incompatibility	Check compatibility prior to mixing. See http://book.pallcare.info for up-to-date advice.	Remove syringe, dispose of contents and prepare a new syringe.

Box 15.11 Volumes for syringe pumps

- 10 mL syringe must be drawn up to 10 mL (approx. rate = 0.42 mL per 24 hours)
- 20 mL syringe must be drawn up to 17 mL (approx. rate = 0.71 mL per 24 hours)
- 30 mL syringe must be drawn up to 22 mL (approx. rate = 0.92 mL per 24 hours)
- 60 mL syringe must be drawn up to 32 mL (approx. rate = 1.33 mL per 24 hours)

Post-procedural considerations

Ongoing care

Accurate documentation of the site, rate, flow, start time and drugs used is imperative in order to avoid confusion and errors among staff (Dickman et al. 2016, Dougherty 2002, MHRA 2010b, Quinn 2000, Sasson and Shvartzman 2001). Sites and tubing will need to be changed every 1–4 days.

At the start of the infusion, record the date, time, start volume, infusion rate setting and name of the person setting up the infusion. Checks should subsequently be carried out at a frequency determined by the type of infusion and the patient's condition; however, at minimum, checks should be carried out 15 minutes and 1 hour after the initial set-up and thereafter a minimum of every 4 hours. Additionally, the device must be checked at the start of each shift and when setting up an infusion.

The following should be taken into account when performing a check:

- Check and record the date, time, rate and volume remaining, and that the battery and syringe pump are working.
- Record any reasons for changing the drug, dose, rate setting of the syringe pump, or site.
- Check the subcutaneous site for:
  - pain or discomfort
  - swelling or induration
  - erythema
  - leakage of fluid
  - bleeding.

Complications

Some drugs are particularly likely to cause skin irritation and may need to be diluted in a greater volume of diluent; cyclizine and levomepromazine are among these. Skin irritation may result in skin sites that break down rapidly or site reactions. The following methods can help to prevent this:

- Check the compatibility of drugs and diluents, and consider changing the drug combination.
- Dilute the solution as much as possible or change the diluent.
- Rotate the site at least every 72 hours.
- Use a non-metal cannula.
- Use a different site cleanser.
- Change the dressing used.
- Consider adding dexamethasone 1 mg to the pump; this may be helpful but is not currently recommended for routine use; care should also be taken as dexamethasone is incompatible with a number of drug combinations (Dickman et al. 2016).

Intramuscular injections

Definition

An intramuscular injection deposits medication into deep muscle tissue under the subcutaneous tissue (Chernecky et al. 2005). The vascularity of muscle aids the rapid absorption of medication (Ostendorf 2015).

Evidence-based approaches

Site and volume of injection

Selecting the site requires correct identification of the muscle groups by using landmarks to identify the relevant anatomical features (Hunter 2008). Choice will be influenced by the patient's physical condition and age. Intramuscular injections should be given into the densest part of the muscle (Pope 2002). Active patients will probably have greater muscle mass than older or emaciated patients (Hunter 2008).

The choice of muscle bed depends on the volume of medication to be injected; however, it appears that it is the medicine rather than just the volume that affects how a patient tolerates an injection. Malkin (2008) uses Botox injections as an example where a volume of 1–3 mL can be injected into facial muscle groups, supporting the view that tolerance of the drug is more important than the volume.

Current research evidence suggests that there are five sites that can be used for the administration of intramuscular injections (Rodger and King 2000, Tortora and Derrickson 2011). There is debate over which site to use. The two recommended are the vastus lateralis site and the ventrogluteal site, but most nurses tend to use the dorsogluteal site as it is more familiar (Greenway 2004).

Ventrogluteal site

The ventrogluteal site (Figure 15.29a) is relatively free of major nerves and blood vessels, and the muscle is large and well defined, making it easy to locate (Greenway 2004). It is located by placing the palm of the hand on the patient's opposite greater trochanter (right hand on left hip). The index finger is then extended to the anterior superior iliac spine to make a V. Injection in the centre of the V will ensure the injection is given into the gluteus medius muscle (Hunter 2008). This is the site of choice for intramuscular injections (Cocoman and Murray 2010) and is used for antibiotics, antiemetics, deep intramuscular and Z-track injections in oil, narcotics and sedatives. Up to 2.5 mL can be safely injected into the ventrogluteal site (Rodger and King 2000).

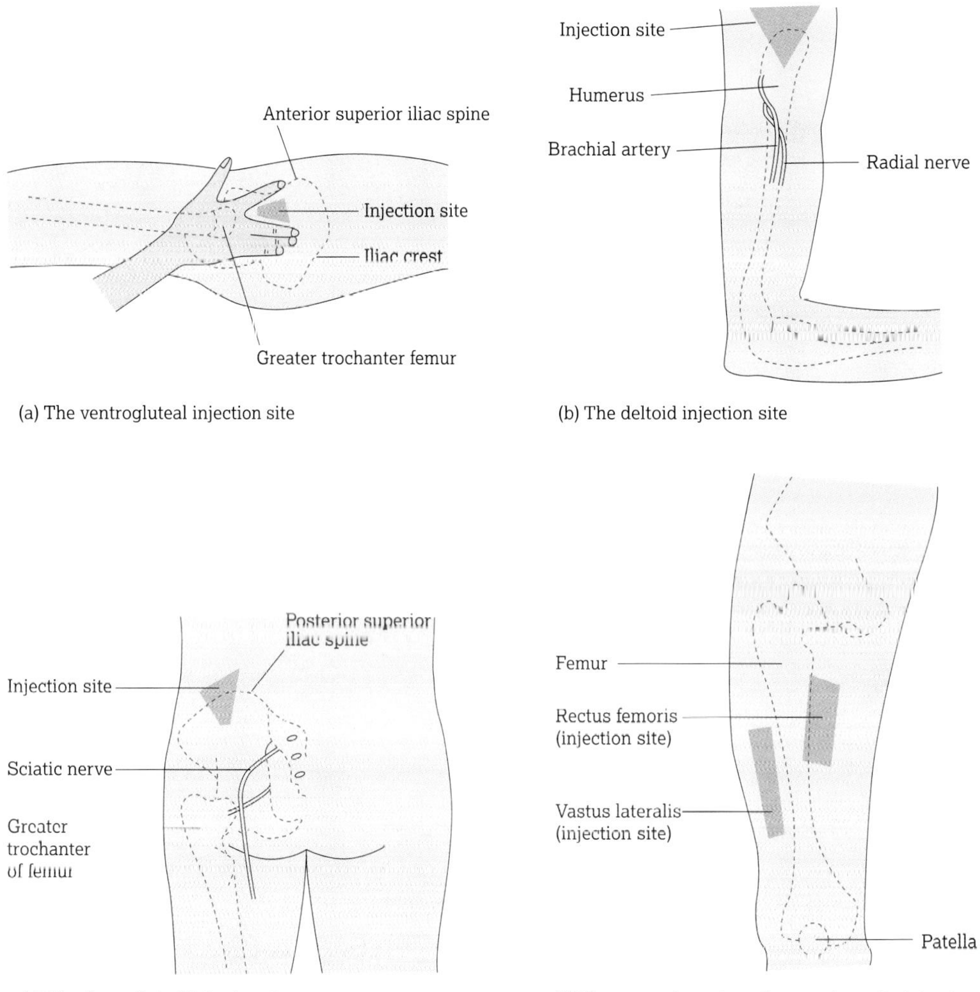

(a) The ventrogluteal injection site

(b) The deltoid injection site

(c) The dorsogluteal injection site

(d) The rectus femoris and vastus lateralis injection sites

Figure 15.29 Intramuscular injection sites. *Source*: Adapted from Rodger and King (2000) with permission of John Wiley & Sons.

Deltoid site

The deltoid site (Figure 15.29b) has the advantage of being easily accessible whether the patient is standing, sitting or lying down. It is found by visualizing a triangle where the horizontal line is located 2.5–5.0 cm below the acromial process and the mid-point of the lateral aspect of the arm, in line with the axilla, to form the apex (Hunter 2008). The injection is then given 2.5 cm down from the acromial process, avoiding the radial and brachial nerves. Owing to the small area of this site, the number and volume of injections that can be given into it are limited. Only small-volume, non-irritating medications, such as vaccines, antiemetics and narcotics, should be administered into this muscle. Rodger and King (2000) state that the maximum volume that should be administered at this site is 1 mL.

Dorsogluteal site

The dorsogluteal site (Figure 15.29c), or upper outer quadrant, is the traditional site of choice and is used for deep intramuscular and Z-track injections. It is located by using imaginary lines to divide the buttocks into four quarters. However, this site carries the danger of the needle hitting the sciatic nerve and the superior gluteal arteries (Small 2004). The gluteus muscle has the lowest drug absorption rate and this can result in a build-up in the tissues, increasing the risk of overdose (Malkin 2008). The muscle mass is also likely to have atrophied in elderly, non-ambulant and emaciated patients. Finally, it appears that there is a risk that the medication will not reach the muscle due to the amount of subcutaneous tissue in this area (Greenway 2004) and so it is not recommended for routine immunizations due to the poor absorption and risk of nerve injury (Public Health England 2006, WHO 2004). In adults, up to 4 mL can be safely injected into this site (Rodger and King 2000).

Rectus femoris site

The rectus femoris site (Figure 15.29d) is a well-defined muscle found by measuring a hand's breadth from the greater trochanter and the knee joint, which identifies the middle third of the quadriceps muscle (Hunter 2008). It is used for antiemetics, narcotics, sedatives, injections in oil, deep intramuscular injections and Z-track injections. It is rarely used by nurses, but is easily accessed for self-administration of injections or for infants (Workman 1999). At this site, 1–5 mL can be injected (1–3 mL in children).

Vastus lateralis site

The vastus lateralis site (Figure 15.29d) is used for deep intramuscular and Z-track injections. One of the advantages of this site is its ease of access and, more importantly, there are no major blood vessels or significant nerve structures associated with this site. It is the best option in obese patients (Nisbet 2006). Up to 5 mL can be safely injected (Rodger and King 2000).

Rate of administration

It is recommended that the plunger is depressed at a rate of 10 seconds per millilitre.

Technique

The syringe should be held like a pen so it can be inserted with a dart-like motion. The nurse should assess whether aspiration is appropriate; if there is a risk that the medication, dose, administration rate, complications of injections associated with the patient's condition, or accidental administration via the intravenous route would be harmful to the patient, then aspiration should be undertaken (Thomas et al. 2016). If aspiration is indicated, this should be over 5–10 seconds to ensure effectiveness and to reduce the risk of patient harm (Mraz et al. 2018).

The Z-track method reduces the leakage of medication through the subcutaneous tissue, decreases the chance of skin lesions forming at the injection site and may hurt less. It involves pulling the skin of the injection site downwards or laterally, which moves the cutaneous and subcutaneous tissues by approximately 2–3 cm, and inserting the needle at a 90° angle to the skin (Antipuesto 2010, Take 5 2006). The injection is given and the needle withdrawn, releasing the retracted skin at the same time. This manoeuvre seals off the puncture track.

Pre-procedural considerations

Equipment

The most commonly used size of needle for intramuscular injections is 21 G (23 G may also be used in a thin patient) but it does depend on the viscosity of the medication. The more important aspect of the needle is the length. The correct choice of needle length will result in fewer adverse events and reduce complications relating to abscess, pain and bruising (Malkin 2008). Needles should be long enough to penetrate the muscle and still allow a quarter of the needle to remain external to the skin (Workman 1999). Lenz (1983) states that when choosing the correct needle length for intramuscular injections, it is important to assess the muscle mass of the injection site, the amount of subcutaneous fat and the weight of the patient. Without such an assessment, most injections intended for gluteal muscle are deposited in the gluteal fat.

For the deltoid and vastus lateralis muscles, to determine the most suitable size of needle to use, the muscle should be grasped between the thumb and forefinger to determine the depth of the muscle mass or the amount of subcutaneous fat at the injection site. For the gluteal muscles, the layer of fat and skin above the muscle should be gently lifted with the thumb and forefinger for the same reasons as before.

The patient's weight indicates the length of needle to use:

- children: 16 mm needle
- 31.5–90.0 kg: 25 mm needle
- above 90 kg: 38 mm needle.

Women have more subcutaneous tissue than men so a longer needle will be needed (Pope 2002).

Procedure guideline 15.20 Medication: intramuscular injection

Essential equipment

- Personal protective equipment
- Recording sheet or book as required by law or hospital policy
- Patient's prescription chart, to check dose, route, etc.
- Electronic identity check equipment, where relevant
- 70% alcohol swab
- Needle
- Syringe containing prepared intramuscular medication
- Clinically clean receiver or tray containing the prepared drug (prepare as described in Procedure guidelines 15.11, 15.12, 15.13 or 15.14)

(continued)

Procedure guideline 15.20 Medication: intramuscular injection *(continued)*

Action	Rationale
Pre-procedure	
1 Introduce yourself to the patient, explain and discuss the procedure with them, and gain their consent to proceed.	To ensure that the patient feels at ease, understands the procedure and gives their valid consent (NMC 2018, **C**).
2 Before administering any prescribed drug, look at the patient's prescription chart and check the following: a the correct patient is being given the drug b drug c dose d date and time of administration e route and method of administration f diluent as appropriate g validity of prescription h signature of prescriber i the prescription is legible.	To ensure that the correct patient is given the correct drug in the prescribed dose using the appropriate diluent and by the correct route (DH 2003b, **C**; RPS 2019a, **C**). To protect the patient from harm (DH 2003b, **C**; NMC 2018, **C**).
If any of these pieces of information are missing, unclear or illegible, do not proceed with the administration. Consult with the prescriber.	To prevent any errors occurring. **E**
Procedure	
3 Apply apron, close the curtains or door, and assist the patient into the required position. Wash hands.	To ensure patient privacy and dignity. **E** To allow access to the injection site and to ensure the designated muscle group is relaxed (Workman 1999, **E**).
4 Take the medication and the prescription chart to the patient. Check the patient's identity by asking them to state their full name and date of birth. If the patient is unable to confirm these details, then check the patient identity band against the prescription chart. If an electronic identity check system for the patient and/or medicine identification is in place, then use it in accordance with hospital policy and procedures. Check the patient's allergy status by asking them or by checking the name band.	To ensure that the medication is administered to the correct patient and prevent any errors related to drug allergies (NPSA 2005, **C**).
5 Assist the patient to remove the appropriate garment(s) to expose the injection site.	To gain access for the injection (Workman 1999, **E**).
6 Apply gloves and assess the injection site for signs of inflammation, oedema, infection and skin lesions.	To promote the effectiveness of the administration (Workman 1999, **E**). To reduce the risk of infection (Fraise and Bradley 2009, **E**; Workman 1999, **E**). To avoid skin lesions and possible trauma to the patient (Ostendorf 2015, **E**; Workman 1999, **E**).
7 Clean the injection site with a swab saturated with isopropyl alcohol 70% for 30 seconds and allow to dry for 30 seconds (Workman 1999).	To reduce the number of pathogens introduced into the skin by the needle at the time of insertion and to prevent a stinging sensation if the alcohol is taken into the tissues upon needle entry (Antipuesto 2010, **E**; Hunter 2008, **E**). (For further information on this action see 'Skin preparation' above.)
8 With the non-dominant hand, stretch the skin slightly around the injection site.	To displace the underlying subcutaneous tissues, facilitate the insertion of the needle and reduce the sensitivity of nerve endings (Antipuesto 2010, **E**; Hunter 2008, **E**).
9 Holding the syringe in the dominant hand like a dart, inform the patient and quickly plunge the needle into the skin at an angle of 90° until about 1 cm of the needle is left showing.	To ensure that the needle penetrates the muscle (Hunter 2008, **E**; Workman 1999, **E**).
10 Pull back the plunger. If no blood is aspirated, depress the plunger at approximately 1 mL every 10 seconds to slowly inject the drug. If blood appears, withdraw the needle completely, replace it and begin again. Explain to the patient what has occurred.	The plunger is pulled back to confirm that the needle is in the correct position and not in a vein (Antipuesto 2010, **E**). Slow injection allows time for the muscle fibres to expand and absorb the solution (Hunter 2008, **E**; Workman 1999, **E**). To prevent pain and ensure even distribution of the drug (Ostendorf 2015, **E**)
11 Wait 10 seconds before withdrawing the needle.	To allow the medication to diffuse into the tissue (Ostendorf 2015, **E**; Workman 1999, **E**).

12 Withdraw the needle rapidly. Apply gentle pressure to any bleeding point but do not massage the site.	To ensure that the injected medication is not forced out of the tissues (Antipuesto 2010, **E**).
13 Apply a small plaster over the puncture site.	To prevent tissue injury and haematoma formation (Ostendorf 2015, **E**).
Post-procedure	
14 Where appropriate, activate any safety device. Ensure that all sharps and non-sharp waste are disposed of safely and in accordance with locally approved procedures, for example put sharps into sharps bin and syringes into orange clinical waste bag.	To ensure safe disposal and to avoid laceration or other injury to staff (EASHW 2010, **C**; HWR 2005, **C**; MHRA 2004, **C**).
15 Record the administration on the appropriate charts.	To maintain accurate records, provide a point of reference in the event of any queries and prevent any duplication of treatment (NPSA 2007d, **C**; RPS 2019a, **C**).

Intraosseous administration

Definition

Intraosseous administration of medications generally involves delivery via the medullary cavity of a long bone and has been used for decades (Vizcarra and Clum 2010).

Related theory

This route can be used for emergency or short-term treatment when access by the vascular route is difficult or impossible and the patient's condition is considered life threatening (Resuscitation Council 2015). It provides rapid systemic action of medications and fluids, while being more rapidly and easily achieved than other forms of central venous access. Unlike the peripheral vessels, the medullary cavity does not collapse in the presence of hypovolaemia or circulatory failure. It acts like a rigid vein, making it an ideal site in a situation where circulatory access is urgently required (e.g. clinical shock or cardiac arrest). The onset of action of medications administered via the intraosseous route is almost as rapid as conventional central venous delivery and considerably quicker than those given by the peripheral vessels. Medications can be delivered as a bolus injection or continuous infusion. The intraosseous route can also be used to obtain bone marrow samples for some emergency testing (e.g. cross-match).

There are several insertion sites that may be considered, including the humerus, the proximal or distal tibia, and the sternum, and a range of intraosseous devices are available (Resuscitation Council 2015). Decisions concerning which site or device to use should be made locally, and staff should be adequately trained in the devices' use before undertaking this procedure (Resuscitation Council 2015).

Any drug administered intravenously can be administered via the intraosseous route. Common indications for use of intraosseous devices are cardiac arrest, circulatory collapse, hypovolaemic shock, respiratory arrest, major trauma and emergency clinical situations (all advocated after two attempts at intravenous access or after 2 minutes of trying). However, this list is not exhaustive and administration may be based on the clinical judgement of a competent practitioner (Vizcarra and Clum 2010).

Contraindications include (Vizcarra and Clum 2010):

- suspected fracture of the tibia, femur or humeral head
- known previous orthopaedic procedure on the selected limb
- an extremity that is significantly compromised due to a pre-existing medical condition
- inability to locate anatomical landmarks
- previous intraosseous administration at the same site within the previous 48 hours
- local infection at the proposed insertion site
- prosthesis
- known thrombocytopenia (ideally the patient's platelet count should be at least 50, but in an emergency intraosseous access may be required irrespective of platelet count).

Fluids and blood products can also be given via the intraosseous route but need the application of pressure to achieve reasonable flow rates, ideally using a pressure bag.

Clinical governance

Any attempt at intraosseous access must be undertaken by a clinical practitioner who has undergone appropriate education, training and assessment. Intraosseous access is usually carried out by a resuscitation officer.

Pre-procedural considerations

Equipment

There are three types of device:

- *Manual* (hollow needle with removable trocar): manually inserted into the medullary space using pressure and twisting of the device.
- *Impact driven* (spring-loaded device with hollow needle and removable trocar): a spring-loaded device that triggers penetration when the safety catch is removed and the spring-loaded device is pressed; it triggers penetration into the sternum or the medullary space of the tibia.
- *Powered drill* (battery-operated drill with a hollow needle and removable stylet): the device drills the needle to the appropriate depth in the intraosseous space (Vizcarra and Clum 2010).

Vizcarra and Clum (2010) report success rates of 55–93% for sternal access (although rates increase with experience) whereas the drill device has a success rate of 97%.

Intraosseous needles are available in three sizes. The size of the needle to use is dependent on the weight of the patient and clinical judgement.

Specific patient preparation

As this method of administration is often used in an emergency, there may not be time to prepare the patient. However, the clinician inserting the intraosseous device must select the most appropriate site; it is suggested that the proximal tibia is the preferred insertion site.

Procedure guideline 15.21 Inserting an intraosseous needle

Essential equipment

- Personal protective equipment
- Sterile gloves
- Intraosseous needle
- Power driver
- Connector (e.g. EZ-Connect)
- Dressing pack (e.g. EZ-Stabilizer)
- Intraosseous needle (e.g. EZ-IO)
- Syringe (10 mL)

Optional equipment

- Intravenous administration set

Medicinal products

- 0.9% sodium chloride
- Lidocaine 2%
- Chlorhexidine 2% in 70% alcohol sponge

Action	Rationale
Pre-procedure	
1 Introduce yourself to the patient or their family, explain and discuss the procedure with them, and gain their consent to proceed.	To ensure that the patient feels at ease, understands the procedure and gives their valid consent (NMC 2018, **C**). In a cardiac arrest, it may not be possible to gain consent. **E**
2 Wash hands with bactericidal soap and water or an alcohol-based handrub, apply an apron and assemble the necessary equipment.	To minimize the risk of infection (DH 2007, **C**; Fraise and Bradley 2009, **E**).
3 Assess the patient and the chosen limb to determine what size of intraosseous needle is required (**Action figure 3**).	To ensure that the correct needle is selected (Vizcarra and Clum 2010, **E**).
4 Obtain assistance as required.	To maintain safety. **E**
Procedure	
5 Wash hands with bactericidal soap and water or an alcohol-based handrub, and apply gloves.	To minimize the risk of infection (DH 2007, **C**; Fraise and Bradley 2009, **E**).
6 Take the medication and the prescription chart to the patient. Check the patient's identity by asking them to state their full name and date of birth. If the patient is unable to confirm these details, then check the patient identity band against the prescription chart. If an electronic identity check system for the patient and/or medicine identification is in place, then use it in accordance with hospital policy and procedures. Check the patient's allergy status by asking them or by checking the name band. *Note*: in an emergency setting, it may not be possible to follow all of these steps.	To ensure that the medication is administered to the correct patient and prevent any errors related to drug allergies (NPSA 2005, **C**).
7 Inspect the needle set packaging to ensure sterility and then open the sterile pack and all packaging.	To ensure the device is safe to use and reduce the risk of complications. **E**
8 Draw up a syringe of 0.9% sodium chloride (10 mL).	To prepare for priming. **E**
9 Connect the 10 mL syringe to the connector (e.g. EZ-Connect) and prime with 0.9% sodium chloride. If lidocaine 2% is indicated, prime the set with the lidocaine.	To prepare for administration and remove air from the set. **E**
10 Leave the syringe connected to the connector.	To prepare for administration once sited. **E**
11 Connect the needle set to the driver, leaving the needle cap on until ready to insert.	To prepare for insertion. **E**
12 Palpate the site to locate the appropriate anatomical landmarks for the needle set placement (**Action figure 12**).	To ensure the intraosseous needle is placed in the correct position for optimal drug administration and minimization of tissue damage (Vizcarra and Clum 2010, **E**).
13 Select the insertion site. For the proximal tibia, it is approximately 2 cm below the patella and approximately 2 cm (depending on the patient's anatomy) medial to the tibial tuberosity along the flat aspect of the tibia.	To ensure the optimal site is used for insertion. **E**
14 Wash hands and apply gloves.	To minimize the risk of infection (Fraise and Bradley 2009, **E**).
15 Clean the site using 2% chlorhexidine in 70% alcohol and allow the site to air dry (**Action figure 15**).	To minimize the risk of infection (DH 2007, **C**; Fraise and Bradley 2009, **E**).

16 Stabilize the insertion site, keeping hand and fingers away from the needle.	To guard against unexpected patient movement and avoid a sharps injury. **E**
17 Remove the needle cap (**Action figure 17**).	To prepare for insertion. **E**
18 Identify the two markings on the needle. The distal mark should be visible once the needle is inserted into the skin. The proximal mark is the maximum insertion point.	To ensure that the insertion landmarks are identified. **E**
19 Insert the intraosseous needle (e.g. EZ-IO) through the skin at a 90° angle to the bone until the bone is reached (**Action figure 19**). The distal mark on the needle should be visible. If not, consider using another size of needle or site.	To ensure that the needle reaches the medullary space. **E**
20 Press the driver trigger while applying minimal pressure, driving through the bone until a give is heard or felt. Allow the driver to do the work.	To ensure that no excess pressure is applied and that the needle is inserted within the bone. **E**
21 Release the driver trigger when the proximal mark on the needle at the hub end is level with the skin.	To ensure that the needle reaches the medullary space. **E**
22 Remove the intraosseous needle's power driver from the needle set while stabilizing the needle hub.	To prepare for drug or fluid administration. **E**
23 Hold the base of the needle hub with one hand while turning the upper part of the needle anticlockwise.	To remove the stylet and prepare for fluid or drug administration. **E**
24 Remove the stylet from the needle (**Action figure 24**).	To prepare the needle for drug or fluid administration. **E**
25 Dispose of the stylet into a sharps container immediately.	To ensure safe disposal and avoid injury to staff (HWR 2005, **C**; MHRA 2004, **C**; NHS Employers 2007, **E**; NHS Employers 2015, **C**).
26 Confirm placement by: a ensuring the catheter is firmly seated and does not move b observing blood at the catheter hub c aspirating marrow from the catheter.	To ensure the needle is in the correct position. **E**
27 Apply a suitable dressing (e.g. EZ-Stabilizer).	To secure the intraosseous port and prevent dislodgement. **E**
28 Connect the primed connector to the exposed Luer-Lok hub and flush with the designated solution (**Action figure 28**).	To ensure patency of the intraosseous needle. **E**
29 Disconnect the 10 mL syringe from the connector.	To prepare for drug and/or fluid administration. **E**
30 Connect a primed intravenous administration set or administer bolus drugs.	To deliver the prescribed medication or fluids. **E**
Post-procedure	
31 Remove gloves and discard waste, placing it in the correct containers, for example sharps into a designated container.	To ensure safe disposal and avoid injury to staff (EASHW 2010, **C**; HWR 2005, **C**; MHRA 2004, **C**).
32 Document the time and date of insertion, the size and length of needle, the number of attempts, the location of the device, and the name of the practitioner who inserted the device.	To maintain accurate records, provide a point of reference in the event of any queries and prevent any duplication of treatment (NMC 2018, **C**).
	To ensure staff are aware of the insertion date as an intraosseous device should not remain in place for longer than 24 hours (NMC 2018, **C**).
33 Assess the site for potential complications or extravasation.	To minimize the risk of complications and to treat any complications promptly. **E**

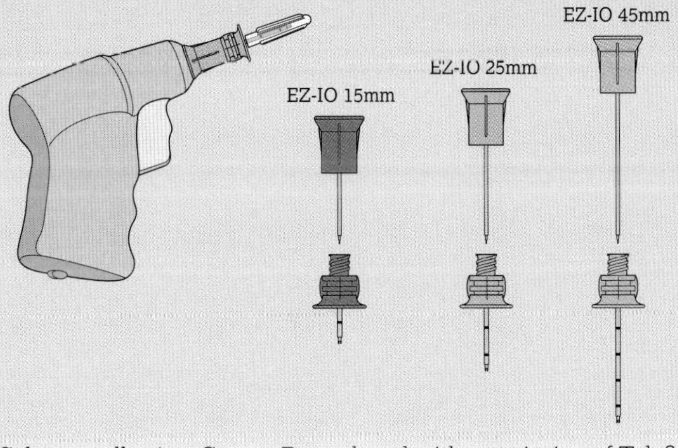

Action Figure 3 Select needle size. *Source:* Reproduced with permission of Teleflex Group UK, Ltd.

(continued)

Procedure guideline 15.21 Inserting an intraosseous needle *(continued)*

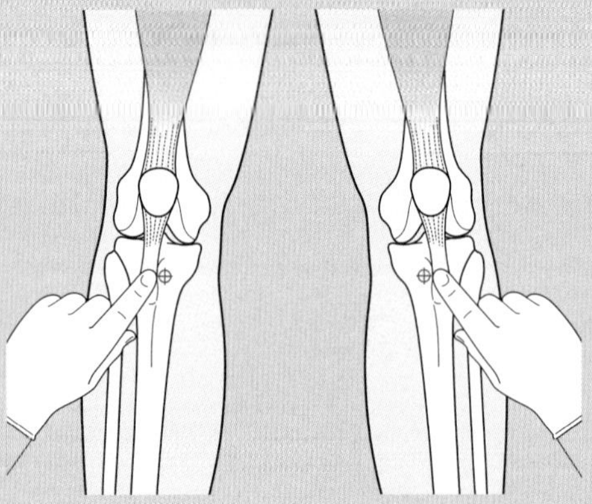

Action Figure 12 palpate the site to locate anatomical landmarks. *Source*: Reproduced with permission of Teleflex Group UK, Ltd.

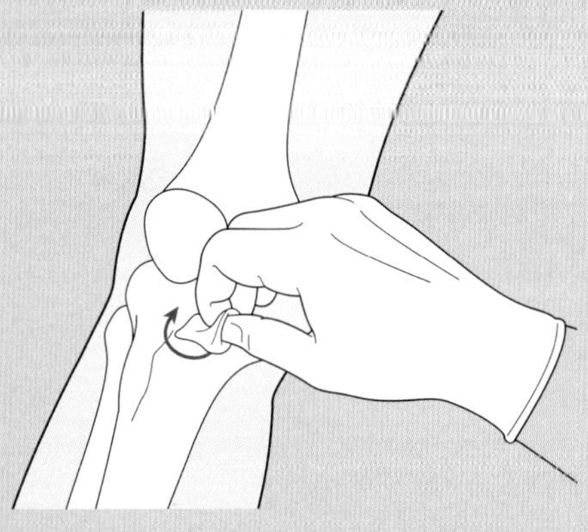

Action Figure 15 Clean the site. *Source*: reproduced with permission of Teleflex Group UK, Ltd.

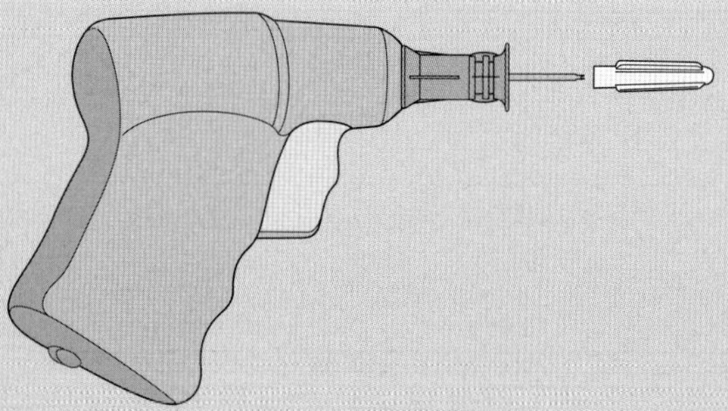

Action Figure 17 Remove the needle cap. *Source*: Reproduced with permission of Teleflex Group UK, Ltd.

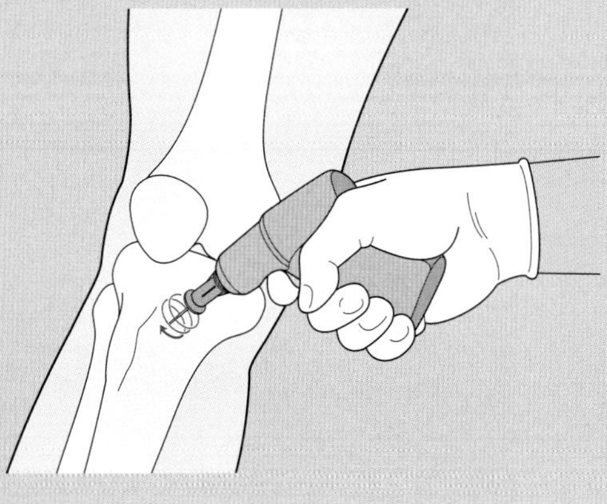

Action Figure 19 Insert the needle. *Source*: Reproduced with permission of Teleflex Group UK, Ltd.

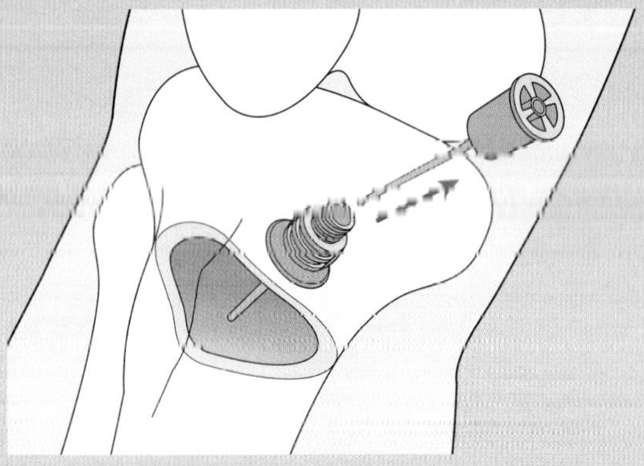

Action Figure 24 Remove the stylet. *Source*: Reproduced with permission of Teleflex Group UK, Ltd.

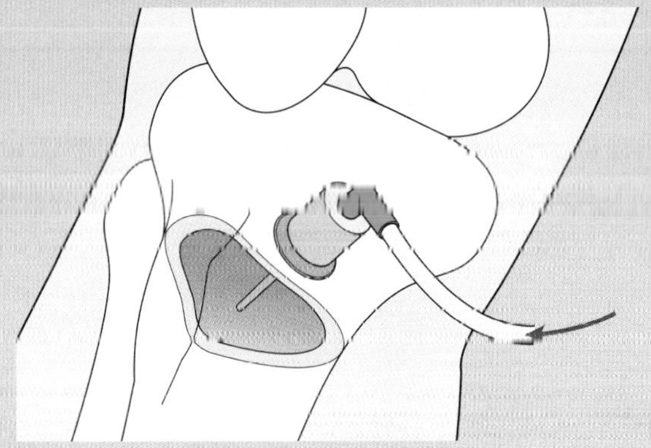

Action Figure 28 Connect EZ-Connect and flush. *Source*: Reproduced with permission of Teleflex Group UK, Ltd.

Procedure guideline 15.33 Removing an intraosseous needle

Essential equipment

- Personal protective equipment
- Sterile gloves
- Dressing pack
- Syringe (10 mL)
- Dressing

Action	Rationale
Pre-procedure	
1 Introduce yourself to the patient or their family, explain and discuss the procedure with them, and gain their consent to proceed.	To ensure that the patient feels at ease, understands the procedure and gives their valid consent (NMC 2018, **C**). In a cardiac arrest, it may not be possible to gain consent. **E**
2 Wash hands with bactericidal soap and water or an alcohol-based handrub, apply an apron and sterile gloves, and assemble and open the necessary equipment.	To minimize the risk of infection (DH 2007, **C**; Fraise and Bradley 2009, **E**). To prepare the equipment for use. **E**
Procedure	
3 Remove the extension set from the needle hub.	To facilitate the removal of the needle. **E**
4 Carefully remove the dressing.	To allow the safe removal of the needle. **E**
5 Attach a 10 mL sterile syringe with a Luer-Lok fitting.	To act as a handle and cap the open port. **E**
6 Grasp the syringe and continuously rotate it clockwise while gently pulling the catheter out, maintaining a 90° angle to the bone. *Do not rock or bend during removal.*	To enable the catheter to be removed easily without damaging the bone. **E**
7 Dispose of the intraosseous catheter into a sharps container.	To ensure safe disposal and avoid injury to staff (HWR 2005, **C**; MHRA 2004, **C**; NHS Employers 2007, **C**; NHS Employers 2015, **C**).
8 Apply pressure to the site with sterile gauze until bleeding has stopped.	To ensure bleeding has stopped. **E**
9 Apply an adhesive dressing.	To protect the puncture site from infection. **E**
Post-procedure	
10 Dispose of waste in the correct containers.	To ensure safe disposal (HWR 2005, **C**).
11 Document the time and date of removal.	To maintain accurate records, provide a point of reference in the event of any queries and prevent any duplication of treatment (NMC 2018, **C**).

Post-procedural considerations

Manufacturers recommend that the maximum length of time all intraosseous needles should stay *in situ* is 24 hours. It is good practice to document the time and location of insertion in the patient's medical and nursing notes (Resuscitation Council 2015).

Complications

Complications associated with the use of intraosseous devices are rare, but care must be taken during the insertion and use of such devices. Possible complications include:

- infection
- extravasation
- embolism
- compartment syndrome
- fracture of the selected limb
- skin necrosis (Resuscitation Council 2015).

Intravenous injections and infusions

Definition

Intravenous injections and infusions involve the introduction of medication or solutions into the circulatory system via a peripheral or central vein (Chernecky et al. 2005).

Anatomy and physiology

See Chapter 17: Vascular access devices: insertion and management for anatomy and physiology related to the venous system.

Related theory

Intravenous therapy is now an integral part of the majority of nurses' professional practice (RCN 2016). The nurse's role has progressed considerably from being able to add drugs to infusion bags (DHSS 1976) to now assessing patients and inserting the appropriate vascular access device (VAD) prior to drug administration (Gabriel et al. 2005).

Any nurse administering intravenous drugs must be competent in all aspects of intravenous therapy and act in accordance with *The Code* (NMC 2018) – that is, they must maintain their knowledge and skills (Hyde 2008, RCN 2016). Training and assessment should comprise both theoretical and practical components and include legal and professional issues, fluid balance, pharmacology, drug administration, local and systemic complications, infection control issues, use of equipment and risk management (Hyde 2008, RCN 2016).

The nurse's responsibilities in relation to intravenous drug administration include the following:

- knowing the therapeutic use of the drug or solution as well as its normal dosage, side-effects, precautions and contraindications

- preparing the drug aseptically and safely, checking the container and drug for faults, using the correct diluent and only preparing the drug immediately prior to administration
- identifying the patient and checking their allergy status
- checking the prescription chart
- checking and maintaining the patency of the VAD
- inspecting the site of the VAD and managing or reporting complications where appropriate
- controlling the flow rate of the infusion and/or the speed of the injection
- monitoring the condition of the patient and reporting changes
- clearly and immediately making records of all drugs administered (Finlay 2008, RCN 2016, RPS 2019a).

Evidence-based approaches

Methods of administering intravenous drugs

There are three methods of administering intravenous drugs: continuous infusion, intermittent infusion and direct intermittent injection.

Continuous infusion

Continuous infusion may be defined as the intravenous delivery of a medication or fluid at a constant rate over a prescribed time period, ranging from several hours to several days, to achieve a controlled therapeutic response (Turner and Hankins 2010). The greater dilution also helps to reduce venous irritation (Weinstein and Hagle 2014, Whittington 2008).

A continuous infusion may be used when:

- the drugs to be administered must be highly diluted
- maintenance of steady blood levels of the drug is required (Turner and Hankins 2010).

Pre-prepared infusion fluids with additives (such as potassium chloride) should be used whenever possible. This reduces the risk of extrinsic contamination, which can occur during the mixing of drugs (Weinstein and Hagle 2014). Only one addition should be made to each bottle or bag of fluid after the compatibility has been ascertained. More additions can increase the risk of incompatibility occurring, for example precipitation (Weinstein and Hagle 2014, Whittington 2008). The additive and fluid must be mixed well to prevent a layering effect, which can occur with some drugs (Whittington 2008). The danger is that a bolus injection of the drug may be delivered. To safeguard against this, any additions should be made to the infusion fluid and the container inverted a number of times to ensure mixing of the drug, before the fluid is hung on the infusion stand (NPSA 2007d). The infusion container should be labelled clearly after the addition has been made. The infusion fluid mixture should constantly be monitored for cloudiness or the presence of particles (Weinstein and Hagle 2014, Whittington 2008), and the patient's condition and the intravenous site should be checked for patency, extravasation or infiltration (Loveday et al. 2014).

Intermittent infusion

Intermittent infusion is the administration of a small-volume infusion (25–250 mL) over a period of between 15 minutes and 2 hours (Turner and Hankins 2010). This may be given as a specific dose at one time or at repeated intervals during 24 hours (Pickstone 1999).

An intermittent infusion may be used when:

- a peak plasma level is required therapeutically
- the pharmacology of the drug dictates this specific dilution
- the drug will not remain stable for the time required to administer a more dilute volume
- the patient is on a restricted intake of fluids (Whittington 2008).

Delivery of the drug by intermittent infusion can be piggy-backed (via a needle-free injection port) if the primary infusion is of a compatible fluid, using a system such as a 'Y' set or a burette set with a chamber capacity of 100 or 150 mL (Turner and Hankins 2010). This technique involves adding the drug to the burette and infusing it while the primary infusion is switched off. A small-volume infusion may also be connected to a cannula specifically to keep the vein open and maintain patency.

All of the points to be considered when preparing for a continuous infusion should be taken into account here, for example pre-preparing fluids, only adding one drug, and adequate mixing, labelling and monitoring.

After completion of an intermittent infusion, an appropriate diluent solution should be administered via the administration set. This is to ensure the full dose of medication has been administered to the patient.

The National Infusion and Vascular Access Society has published guidance on appropriate line flushing after infusion. This was prompted by concerns about the theoretical risk of underdosing in intravenous infusions, when some of the drug is left in the tubing of the giving set at the end of the administration (NIVAS 2019). As this guidance is new and under regular review, it is advised that it be accessed online for the most up-to-date advice (https://nivas.org.uk). All organizations should ensure that their policies and procedures reflect the current guidance.

Direct intermittent injection

Direct intermittent injection (also known as intravenous push or bolus) involves the injection of a drug from a syringe into the injection port of an administration set or directly into a VAD (Dougherty and Lamb 2008, Turner and Hankins 2010). Most are administered over a time span of anywhere from 3 to 10 minutes depending upon the drug (Weinstein and Hagle 2014, Whittington 2008).

A direct injection may be used when:

- the vital organs require the maximum concentration of the drug – this is a 'bolus' injection, which is given rapidly over seconds, often in an emergency (e.g. adrenaline)
- the drug cannot be further diluted for pharmacological or therapeutic reasons or does not require dilution – this is given as a controlled 'push' injection over a few minutes
- a peak blood level is required and cannot be achieved by small-volume infusion (Turner and Hankins 2010).

Rapid administration can result in toxic levels and an anaphylactic-type reaction. Manufacturers' recommendations on rates of administration (i.e. millilitres or milligrams per minute) should be adhered to. In the absence of such recommendations, administration should proceed slowly, over 5–10 minutes (Dougherty 2002).

Delivery of a drug by direct injection may be achieved via a cannula through a resealable needleless injection cap, an extension set or the injection site of an administration set. If a peripheral device is *in situ*, the bandage and dressing must be removed to inspect the insertion of the cannula, unless a transparent dressing is in place (Finlay 2008). Patency of the vein must be confirmed prior to administration and the vein's ability to accept an extra flow of fluid or irritant chemical must also be checked (Dougherty 2008a).

Administration into the injection site of a fast-running drip may be advised if the infusion in progress is compatible, in order to dilute the drug further and reduce local chemical irritation (Dougherty 2002). Alternatively, a stop–start procedure may be employed if there is doubt about venous patency. This allows the nurse to constantly check the patency of the vein and detect early signs of extravasation. If the infusion fluid is incompatible with the drug, the administration set may be switched off and a compatible solution may be used as a flush (NPSA 2007d).

If a number of drugs are being administered, 0.9% sodium chloride must be used to flush the device between each drug to prevent interactions. In addition, 0.9% sodium chloride should be used at the end of the administration to ensure that all of the drug has been delivered. The device should then be flushed to ensure patency is maintained (see Chapter 17: Vascular access devices: insertion and management) (Dougherty 2008a).

Principles to be followed when administering intravenous drugs

The following principles should be applied throughout preparation and administration of intravenous drugs.

Asepsis and reducing the risk of infection

Microbes on the hands of healthcare personnel contribute to healthcare-associated infection (Weinstein and Hagle 2014). Therefore, aseptic technique must be adhered to throughout all intravenous procedures (see Chapter 17: Vascular access devices: insertion and management). The nurse must employ good hand washing and drying techniques using a bactericidal soap or an alcohol-based handrub. If asepsis is not maintained, local infection, septic phlebitis or septicaemia may result (Hart 2008, Loveday et al. 2014, RCN 2016).

The insertion site should be inspected at least once per day for complications such as infiltration, phlebitis or any indication of infection, for example redness at the insertion site or pyrexia (RCN 2016). These problems may necessitate the removal of the device and/or further investigation (Finlay 2008).

It is desirable that a closed system of infusion is maintained wherever possible, with as few connections as are necessary (Finlay 2008, Hart 2008). This reduces the risk of bacterial contamination. Any extra connections within the administration system increase the risk of infection. Three-way taps have been shown to encourage the growth of micro-organisms. They are difficult to clean due to their design, as micro-organisms can become lodged and are then able to multiply in the warm, moist environment (Finlay 2008, Hart 2008). This reservoir of micro-organisms may then be released into the patient's circulation.

The injection sites on administration sets or injection caps should be cleaned using a 2% chlorhexidine alcohol-based antiseptic, allowing time for it to dry (Loveday et al. 2014). Connections should be cleaned before changing administration sets and manipulations kept to a minimum. Administration sets should be changed according to use (intermittent or continuous therapy), type of device and type of solution, and the set must be labelled with the date and time of the change (NPSA 2007d, RCN 2016).

To ensure safe delivery of intravenous fluids and medication:

- Replace all tubing when the VAD is replaced (Loveday et al. 2014).
- Replace solution administration sets and stopcocks used for continuous infusions every 96 hours unless clinically indicated, for example if drug stability data indicate otherwise (Loveday et al. 2014, RCN 2016). A Cochrane review of 13 randomized controlled trials found no evidence that changing intravenous administration sets more often than every 96 hours reduces the incidence of bloodstream infection (Loveday et al. 2014).
- Replace solution administration sets used for lipid emulsions and parenteral nutrition at the end of the infusion or within 24 hours of initiating the infusion (Loveday et al. 2014, RCN 2016).
- Replace blood administration sets at least every 12 hours and after every second unit of blood (Loveday et al. 2014, McClelland 2007, RCN 2016).
- All solution sets used for intermittent infusions (e.g. of antibiotics) should be discarded immediately after use and not be allowed to hang for reuse (RCN 2016).
- If administering more than one infusion via a multilumen extension set or multiple ports, be aware of the risk of backtracking of medication and consider using sets with one-way, non-return or anti-reflux valves (MHRA 2010a).

Inspection of fluids, drugs, equipment and their packaging must be undertaken to detect any points where contamination may have occurred during manufacture and/or transport. Such intrinsic contamination may be detected as cloudiness, discoloration or the presence of particles (BNF 2019a, RCN 2016, Weinstein and Hagle 2014). Infusion bags should not be left hanging for longer than 24 hours. In the case of blood and blood products, this limit is reduced to 5 hours (McClelland 2007, RCN 2016).

Safety

All details of the prescription and all calculations must be checked carefully in accordance with hospital policy in order to ensure safe preparation and administration of the drug(s). Accurate labelling of additives and records of administration are essential (NPSA 2007d, RCN 2016).

The nurse must also check the compatibility of the drug with the diluent or infusion fluid. The nurse should be aware of the types of incompatibilities and the factors that could influence them. These include pH, concentration, time, temperature, light and the brand of the drug. If insufficient information is available, a reference book (e.g. the *British National Formulary*; BNF 2019a) or the product data sheet must be consulted (NPSA 2007d, Whittington 2008). If the nurse is unsure about any aspect of the preparation and/or administration of a drug, they should not proceed and should consult with a senior member of staff (NMC 2018). Constant monitoring of both the mixture and the patient is important. The preferred method and rate of intravenous administration must be determined.

Drugs should never be added to the following:

- blood
- blood products – i.e. plasma or platelet concentrate (see Chapter 8: Nutrition and fluid balance and Chapter 12: Respiratory care, CPR and blood transfusion)
- mannitol solutions
- sodium bicarbonate solution.

Only specially prepared additives should be used with fat emulsions or amino acid preparations (Downie et al. 2003).

Any protective clothing that is advised should be worn, and vinyl gloves should be used to reduce the risk of latex allergy (Hart 2008). Healthcare professionals who use gloves frequently or for long periods face a high risk of allergy from latex products. All healthcare facilities should develop policies and procedures that determine measures to protect staff and patients from latex exposure and outline a treatment plan for latex reactions (RCN 2016).

Preventing needle stick injuries should be key in any health and safety programme, and organizations should introduce safety devices and needle-free systems wherever possible (EASHW 2010). Basic rules of safety include not resheathing needles, disposal of needles into a recognized sharps bin immediately after use, and convenient location of sharps bins in all areas where needles and sharps are used (Hart 2008, MHRA 2004, RCN 2016).

Comfort

Both the physical and the psychological comfort of the patient must be considered. Comprehensive explanation of the practical aspects of the procedure together with information about the effects of the treatment will contribute to reducing anxiety, although the provision of such information must be tailored to each patient's individual needs.

Clinical governance

At least one patient will experience a potentially serious intravenous drug error every day in an 'average' hospital. Intravenous drug errors have been estimated to account for a third of all drug errors. According to the NPSA (2004), 'fifteen million infusions are performed in the NHS every year and 700 unsafe incidents are reported each year with 19% attributed to user error' (p.1). Between 2005 and 2010, the MHRA investigated 1085 reports involving infusion pumps (MHRA 2011). In 69% of incidents, no cause was established. However, of the remaining incidents, 20% were attributed to user error (e.g. misloading the administration set or syringe, setting the wrong rate or confusing the pump type) and 11% to device-related issues (e.g. poor maintenance or inadequate cleaning) (MHRA 2011). Syringe pumps have given rise to the most significant problems in terms of patient mortality and morbidity (Fox 2000, MHRA 2010b, NPSA 2003).

The high frequency of human error in the intravenous administration of drugs has highlighted the need for more formalized,

Box 15.12 Checklist: how safe is your practice?

- Have I been trained in the use of the infusion device?
- Was the training formalized and recorded or did I just pick it up as I went along?
- How was my competency in relation to the infusion device assessed?
- Have I read the user instructions on how to use the infusion device and am I familiar with any warning labels?
- When was the infusion device last serviced?
- Are there any signs of wear, damage or faults?
- Do I know how to set up and use the infusion device?
- Is the infusion device and any additional equipment in good working order?
- Do I know how the infusion device should perform and the monitoring that needs to be done to check its performance?
- Am I using the correct additional equipment, for example the appropriate disposable administration set for the infusion pump?
- Do I know how to recognize whether the infusion device has failed?
- Do I know what to do if the infusion device fails?
- Do I know how and to whom to report an infusion device-related adverse incident?
- Does checking the infusion device indicate it is functioning correctly and to the manufacturer's specification?
- What action should be taken if the infusion device is not functioning properly?
- Is there up-to-date documentation to record regular checking of the infusion device?
- What are the details (name and serial number) of the infusion device being used?
- What is the cleaning and/or decontamination procedure for the infusion device and what are my responsibilities in this process?
- Do I know how to report an adverse incident?
- Do I have access to MHRA device bulletins of relevance to my area of practice and do I read and take note of hazard and safety notices?

Source: Reproduced with permission of the Medical Devices Agency. © Crown copyright. Reproduced under the Open Government Licence v2.0.

validated and competency-based training and assessment (MHRA 2010b, NPSA 2003, 2004, Pickstone 2000, Quinn 2000). Nurses must be familiar with the device they are using and not attempt to operate any device that they have not been fully trained to use (MHRA 2011, Murray and Glenister 2001, NPSA 2003). As a minimum, the training should cover the device, relevant drugs and solutions, and the practical procedures related to setting up the device and problem solving (MHRA 2010b, MHRA 2011, 2014a). Staff should also be made aware of the mechanisms for reporting faults with devices and procedures for adverse incident reporting within their trust and to the MHRA (MHRA 2006b, MHRA 2011).

A useful checklist (Box 15.12) has been produced by the Medical Devices Agency for staff to follow prior to using a medical device to ensure safe practice (see also MHRA 2010b, 2014a).

Nurses must have knowledge of the relevant solutions, their effects, rates of administration, factors that affect the flow of infusions, and the complications that can occur when flow is not controlled (Weinstein and Hagle 2014). They should also have an understanding of which groups require accurate flow control in order to prevent complications (Box 15.13) and how to select the most appropriate device for accuracy of delivery to best meet the patient's flow control needs (according to age, condition, setting and prescribed therapy) (Weinstein and Hagle 2014).

The identification of risks is crucial. Risks include the potential for error in complex calculations, prescription errors (Dougherty 2002, Weinstein and Hagle 2014), and risks specifically associated with infusions, such as neonatal risk infusions, high-risk infusions, low-risk infusions and ambulatory infusions (MHRA 2010b, Quinn 2000). Early detection of errors and infusion-related complications, for example overinfusion or underinfusion (Box 15.14), is imperative in order to instigate the appropriate interventions in response to an error or to manage any complications, as serious errors or complications can result in patient death (Dougherty 2002, NPSA 2003, Quinn 2008). Overinfusion accounts for about half of the reported errors involving infusion pumps, with 80% due to user error rather than a fault with the device (MHRA 2014a). The use of infusion devices, both mechanical and electronic, has increased the level of safety of intravenous therapy. However, it is recommended that a clearly defined structure for management of infusion systems should exist within a hospital (Department of Health (Northern Ireland) 2006, MHRA 2010b, 2011, NPSA 2004) (Box 15.15)

Strategies must be developed for the replacement of old, obsolete or inappropriate devices (MHRA 2015). Healthcare professionals are personally accountable for their use of infusion devices and they must therefore ensure they have appropriate training before using any pump (MHRA 2015). Records of training must also be maintained.

Box 15.13 Groups at risk of complications associated with flow control

- Infants and young children
- The elderly
- Patients with compromised cardiovascular status
- Patients with impairment or failure of organs, for example kidneys
- Patients with major sepsis
- Patients suffering from shock, whatever the cause
- Post-operative or post-trauma patients
- Stressed patients, whose endocrine homeostatic controls may be affected
- Patients receiving multiple medications, whose clinical status may change rapidly

Source: Reproduced from Quinn (2008) with permission of John Wiley & Sons.

Box 15.14 Complications of inadequate flow control

Complications associated with overinfusion

- Fluid overload with accompanying electrolyte imbalance
- Metabolic disturbances during parenteral nutrition, mainly related to serum glucose levels
- Toxic concentrations of medications, which may result in a shock-like syndrome ('speed shock')
- Air embolism, due to containers running dry before expected
- An increase in venous complications, for example chemical phlebitis, caused by reduced dilution of irritant substances (Weinstein and Hagle 2014)

Complications associated with underinfusion

- Dehydration
- Metabolic disturbances
- A delayed response to medications or below therapeutic dose
- Occlusion of a cannula/catheter due to slow flow or cessation of flow

Source: Reproduced from Quinn (2008) with permission of John Wiley & Sons.

Box 15.15 Criteria for selection of an infusion device

- Rationalization of devices
- Clinical requirement
- Education
- Compatibility with other equipment
- Disposable components
- Product support
- Costs
- Service and maintenance
- Regulatory issues

Source: Adapted from Department of Health (Northern Ireland) (2006), Health Care Standards Unit (2007a, 2007b), MHRA (2010b), Quinn (2000).

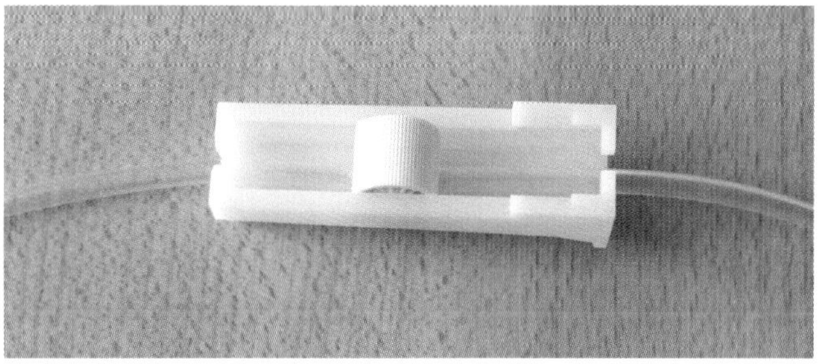

Figure 15.31 Roller clamp.

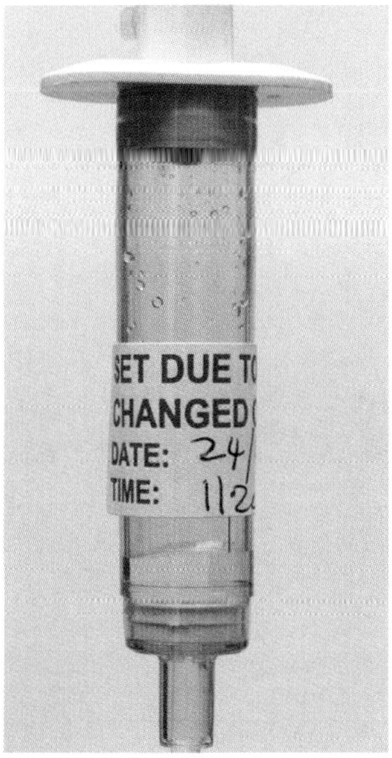

Figure 15.32 Labelled administration set.

Improving infusion device safety

As mentioned, a high frequency of human error is reported in the use of infusion device systems, so competence-based training is advocated for users of these systems (MHRA 2010b, NPSA 2004). By rationalizing the range of infusion device types within organizations and establishing a centralized equipment library, the number of patient safety incidents will be reduced (MHRA 2010b, NPSA 2004). Smart infusion pumps reduce pump programming errors by setting pre-programmed upper and lower dose limits for specific drugs. The pump will alert the nurse if it has been set outside the pre-determined dose limits (Keohane et al. 2005, MHRA 2011, Weinstein and Hagle 2014, Wilson and Sullivan 2004). Whatever infusion device is used, the need to monitor the patient and the device remains paramount for patient safety (Quinn 2008, RCN 2016).

Pre-procedural considerations

Equipment

Vascular access devices

For VADs see Chapter 17: Vascular access devices: insertion and management.

Administration sets

An administration set is used to administer fluids, blood or medications via an infusion bag into a VAD. The set comprises a number of components (see Figures 15.30, 15.31 and 15.32). At the top is a spike, which is inserted into the infusion container via an entry port. The spike is covered by a sterile plastic lid, which is removed just prior to insertion into the container (Downie et al. 2003). The plastic tubing continues from the spike to a drip chamber, which may contain a filter. This is filled by squeezing it when the tubing is attached to the fluid and waiting for the chamber to fill half way, thus allowing the practitioner to observe the drops. Along the tubing is a roller clamp, which allows the tubing to be incrementally occluded as the clamp can be tightened to pinch the tubing; this is used to adjust the rate of flow (Hadaway 2010). The clamp is usually positioned on the upper third of the administration set but should be repositioned along the set at intervals as the tubing can develop a 'memory' and not regain its shape, making it difficult to regulate (Hadaway 2010). The clamp is opened to allow the fluid along the tubing so as to remove the air, and then closed until the set has been attached to the patient's VAD. Finally, the Luer-Lok end is covered with a plastic cap to maintain sterility until it is attached (Downie et al. 2003).

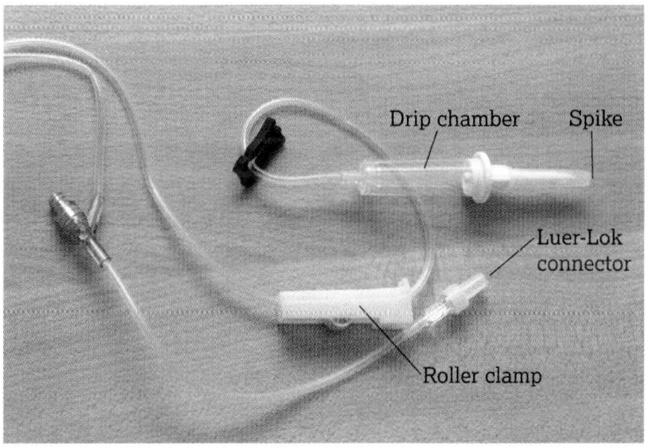

Figure 15.30 Fluid administration set.

There is a variety of sets. A solution set is used to administer crystalloid solutions (it can be used as a primary or secondary set and is also available as a Y-set to allow for dual administration of compatible solutions). Parenteral nutrition is also administered via solution sets. Solution sets may have needle-free injection ports, which allow for the administration of bolus injections or the connection of secondary infusions. Sets may also have back-check valves, which allow solutions to flow in one direction only and are especially used when a secondary set is needed (Hadaway 2010).

Blood and blood products are administered via a blood administration set (Figure 15.33), which has a special filter. Platelets can be administered via blood administration sets (check the manufacturer's guidance) or specialist platelet administration sets. Some medications, such as taxanes, must be administered via special taxane administration sets, which have a 0.22 μm filter.

Extension sets

Extension sets are used to add length (Hadaway 2010). Short (under 50 cm) extension sets tend to have a needle-free connector (Figure 15.34) and are attached directly to the VAD to provide a closed system; other equipment is then attached via the needle-free

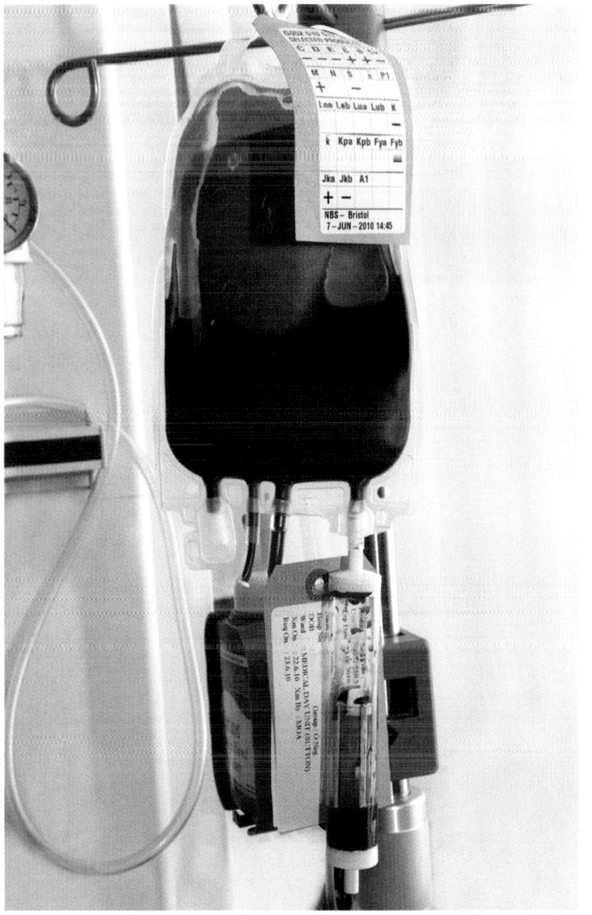

Figure 15.33 Blood administration set.

connector. Long (50–200 cm) extension sets are used to connect syringe pumps to a VAD and usually have a back-check or anti-siphon valve. They can be single, double or triple and may contain a slide or pinch clamp but do not regulate flow (Hadaway 2010).

Needleless connectors and injection caps

These are caps that are attached to the end of a VAD or extension set (see Figure 15.34) to provide a closed system and remove the need for needles when administering medications, thus removing the risk of needle stick injury. There are various types available, categorized by the internal mechanisms (split septum or mechanical valve) (Hadaway 2010) and how they function (i.e. the presence of fluid displacement inside the device). There are three main types:

- *negative*: blood is pulled back into the catheter lumen; for example, this occurs when an empty fluid container is left connected, which can lead to occlusion
- *positive*: these caps have a valve with a reservoir that holds a small amount of fluid, upon disconnection, this fluid is pushed out to the catheter lumen to overcome the reflux of blood that has occurred
- *neutral*: these caps contain valves that prevent blood reflux upon connection and disconnection (Hadaway 2010).

Others are coated with antimicrobial or antibacterial solutions on their external or internal parts to reduce the risk of infection (Hadaway 2010). These require regular changing in accordance with the manufacturer's instructions as well as cleaning before and after each use (MHRA 2007, 2008b).

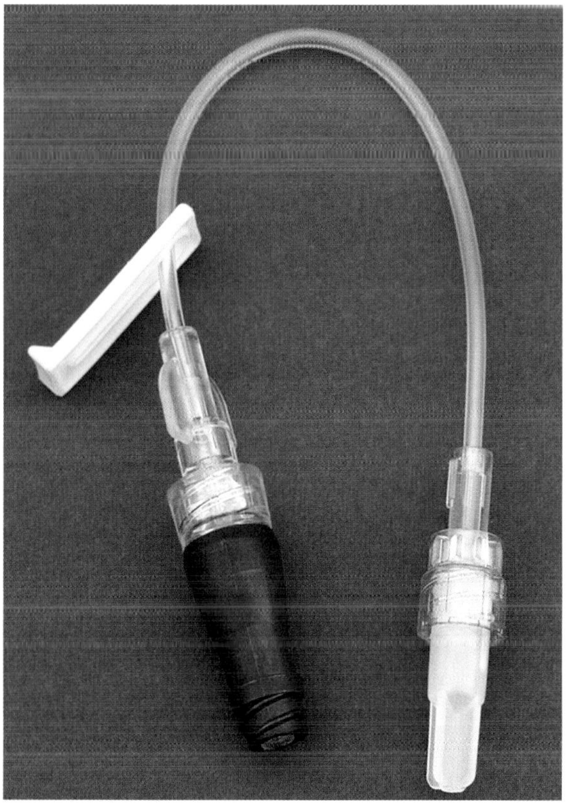

Figure 15.34 Extension set with needle-free injection cap.

It has been suggested that needle-free systems can increase the risk of bloodstream infections (Danzig et al. 1995). However, most studies have found no differences in rates of microbial contamination when comparing conventional and needle free systems (Brown et al. 1997, Luebke et al. 1998, Mendelson et al. 1998). It appears that an increased risk is only likely where there is lack of compliance with cleaning protocols or changing of equipment (Loveday et al. 2014).

Other equipment

Other intravenous equipment includes stopcocks (used to direct flow), which are usually three- or four-way devices. These tend to be used in critical care but their use is discouraged in the general setting due to misuse and contamination issues. If used, they should be capped off (Hadaway 2010).

Infusion devices

An infusion device is designed to accurately deliver measured amounts of fluid or drugs via a number of routes (intravenous, subcutaneous or epidural) over a period of time. The infusion device is set at an appropriate rate to achieve the desired therapeutic response and prevent complications (Dougherty 2002, MHRA 2010b, 2011).

Gravity infusion devices

Gravity infusion devices depend entirely on gravity to deliver the infusion. The system consists of an administration set containing a drip chamber and a roller clamp to control the flow, which is usually measured by counting drops (Pickstone 1999). The indications for their use are:

- delivery of fluids without additives
- administration of drugs or fluids where adverse effects are not anticipated and absolute precision is not required

- administration of drugs or fluids where the patient's condition does not give cause for concern and no complication is predicted (Quinn 2008).

The flow rate is calculated using a formula that requires the following information:

- the volume to be infused
- the number of hours the infusion will run for
- the drop rate of the administration set (which will differ depending on type of set).

The number of drops per millilitre is dependent on the type of administration set used and the viscosity of the infusion fluid. Increased viscosity causes the size of the drop to increase. For example, crystalloid fluid administered via a solution set is delivered at the rate of 20 drops/mL, whereas the rate of packed red cells given via a blood set will be calculated at 15 drops/mL (Quinn 2008).

The rate of administration of a continuous or intermittent infusion may be calculated from the following equation (Pickstone 1999)

$$\frac{\textit{volume to be infused}}{\textit{time in hours}} \times \frac{\textit{drop rate}}{60} = \textit{drops per minute}$$

In this equation, 60 is a factor for the conversion of the number of hours to the number of minutes.

Factors influencing flow rates are as follows.

Type of fluid

The composition, viscosity and concentration of the fluid affect flow (Pickstone 1999, Quinn 2000, Springhouse 2009, Weinstein and Hagle 2014). Irritating solutions may result in venospasm and impede the flow rate, but this may be resolved by the use of a warm pack over the cannula site and the limb (Springhouse 2009, Weinstein and Hagle 2014).

Height of the infusion container

Intravenous fluids run by gravity and so any changes in the height of the container will alter the flow rate. The container can be hung up to 1.5 m above the infusion site, which will provide a hydrostatic pressure of 110 mmHg (MHRA 2010b, Springhouse 2009). One metre above the infusion site would create 70 mmHg of pressure, which is adequate to overcome venous pressure (the normal range in an adult is 25–80 mmHg) (Pickstone 1999). If it is hung too high then it can create too great a pressure within the vein, leading to infiltration of the medication (MHRA 2006a). Therefore, any alterations in the patient's position may alter the flow rate and necessitate a change in the speed of the infusion to maintain the appropriate rate of flow (Hadaway 2010, MHRA 2011, Weinstein and Hagle 2014). Positioning of the patient will affect flow; patients should be instructed to keep the arm that is receiving the infusion lower than the container, if the infusion is reliant on gravity (Quinn 2008).

Administration set

The flow rate of the infusion may be affected in several ways:

- Roller clamps (see Figure 15.31) or screw clamps, used to adjust and maintain rates of flow on gravity infusions, vary considerably in their efficiency and accuracy. This variability is often dependent on a number of factors, such as patient movement and height of the infusion container (Hadaway 2010). The roller clamp should be used as the primary means of occluding the tubing even if there is an anti free flow device (MHRA 2010b).
- The inner diameter of the lumen and the length of tubing will also affect flow. Microbore sets have a narrow lumen, so flow is restricted to some degree. However, these sets may be used as a safeguard against 'runaway' or bolus infusions by either an integrated anti-siphon valve or an anti-free-flow device (Hadaway 2010, Quinn 2000, Weinstein and Hagle 2014).
- Inclusion of other in-line devices, for example filters, may also affect the flow rate (Hadaway 2010, MHRA 2010b).

Vascular access device

The flow rate may be affected by any of the following.

- *The condition and size of the vein*: for example, phlebitis can reduce the lumen size and decrease flow (Quinn 2008, Weinstein and Hagle 2014).
- *The gauge of the cannula or catheter* (MHRA 2010b, Springhouse 2009, Weinstein and Hagle 2014).
- *The position of the device within the vein*: that is, whether it is up against the vein wall (Quinn 2008).
- *The site of the VAD*: for example, the flow may be affected by changes in the position of a limb, such as a decrease in flow when a patient bends their arm if a cannula is sited over the elbow joint (Springhouse 2009).
- *Kinking, pinching or compression* of the cannula/catheter or tubing of the administration set may cause variation in the set rate (MHRA 2010b, Springhouse 2009).
- *Restricted venous circulation*: for example, a blood pressure cuff or the patient lying on the limb increases the risk of occlusion and may result in clot formation (Quinn 2008).

The patient

Patients occasionally adjust the control clamp or other parts of the delivery system (e.g. changing the height of the container), thereby making flow unreliable. Some pumps have tamper-proof features to minimize the risk of accidental manipulation of the infusion device (Hadaway 2010) or unauthorized changing of infusion device controls (Amoore and Adamson 2003).

Advantages and disadvantages of gravity infusion devices

A gravity flow system is simple to set up. It is low cost and the infusion of air is less likely than with electronic devices (Pickstone 1999). However, the system does require frequent observation and adjustment due to:

- the tubing changing shape over time
- creep or distortion of tubing made of polyvinyl chloride (PVC)
- fluctuations of venous pressure, which can affect the flow of the solution
- the roller clamp can be unreliable, leading to inconsistent flow rates.

There can also be variability of drop size and, if the roller clamp is inadvertently left open, free flow will occur. Infusion rates with viscous fluids can be reduced (particularly if administered via small cannulas) and there is a limitation on the type of infusion as these devices are not suitable for arterial infusions: this is because viscosity and arterial flow offer a high resistance to flow that cannot be overcome by gravity (Pickstone 1999, Quinn 2008). If more than one infusion is infusing and one is slower than the other or there is no flow in the second set, then there is a risk of backtracking, which leads to underinfusion or bolus delivery of medicines. The MHRA (2007) recommends that in these systems, the sets should include anti-reflux valves.

Gravity drip rate controllers

A gravity drip rate controller is a mechanical device that operates by gravity. These devices use standard solution sets and, although they look much like a pump, they have no pumping mechanism. The desired flow rate is set in drops per minute and controlled by battery- or mains-powered occlusion valves (MHRA 2010b).

Advantages and disadvantages of gravity drip rate controllers

Although they can maintain a drip rate within 1% of the target rate, volumetric accuracy is not guaranteed and many of the disadvantages associated with gravity flow still remain. The main advantages are that they are relatively inexpensive and can usually be used with standard gravity sets. They also incorporate some audible and visual alarm systems (MHRA 2010b).

Infusion pumps

These devices use pressure to overcome resistance from many causes along the fluid pathway, for example length and bore of tubing or particulate matter in the tubing (Hadaway 2010). There are a number of general features required of infusion pumps.

Accuracy of delivery

In order to meet requirements for high-risk and neonatal infusions, pumps must be accurate to within ±5% of the set rate when measured over a 60-minute period, although some may be as accurate as ±2% (Hadaway 2010, MHRA 2010b). They also have to satisfy short-term, minute-to-minute accuracy requirements, which demand smoothness and consistency of output (MHRA 2010b).

Occlusion response and pressure

Flow will occur if the pressure at the tip of an intravascular device is just fractionally above the pressure in the vein; the pressure does not need to be excessive. In an adult peripheral vein, the pressure is approximately 25 mmHg, while in a neonate it is 5 mmHg (Quinn 2000). Most pumps have a variable pressure setting that allows the user to employ their own judgement about the pressure needed to deliver therapy safely. The normal pumping pressure is only slightly lower than the occlusion pressure (Hadaway 2010). Flow is dependent upon pressure divided by resistance. If long extension sets of small internal bore are used, the resistance to flow will increase (Pickstone 1999, Quinn 2000).

If an administration set occludes, the resistance increases and the infusion will not flow into the vein. The longer the occlusion lasts, the greater the pressure, and the pump will continue to pump until an occlusion alarm is activated. There are two types of occlusion: upstream (between the pump and the container) and downstream (between the pump and the patient). An upstream occlusion alarm will be triggered when a vacuum is created in the upstream tubing or full reservoir, due to a collapsed or empty plastic fluid container or due to clamped or kinking tubing. A downstream occlusion occurs when the pressure required by the pump exceeds a certain limit of pounds per square inch (psi) to overcome the pressure created by the occlusion. Downstream occlusion pressures range from 1.5 to 15.0 psi (Hadaway 2010).

Pump alarms are triggered at 'occlusion alarm pressure', and many pumps allow the user to set the pressure within a range (MHRA 2010b). Therefore, the time it takes for an alarm to sound depends on the rate of flow: high rates activate the alarm more quickly. When the alarm is activated, a certain amount of stored medication will be present and it is important that what could be a potentially large bolus is not released into the vein. The release of the stored bolus could lead to rupture of the vein or constitute overinfusion, which may be detrimental to the patient, particularly if it is a critical medication (Amoore and Adamson 2003, MHRA 2010b). With a syringe pump, to prevent a bolus being delivered to the patient, the clamp should not be opened as this will release the bolus; the first action is to remove the pressure by opening the syringe plunger clamp, following which the occlusion can be dealt with.

A pump's downstream occlusion alarm must not be relied upon to detect infiltration or extravasation (Huber and Augustine 2009, Marders 2012, MHRA 2011) and routine assessment of intravenous sites is still vital to prevent these complications. Single-unit variable pressure pump settings that allow an earlier alarm alert are used in neonatal and paediatric units (Quinn 2008).

Air in line

Air-in-line detectors are designed to detect only visible or microscopic 'champagne' bubbles. They should not create anxiety over small particles of air but alert the nurse to the integrity of the system (MHRA 2011). Most air bubbles detected are too small to have a harmful effect but the nurse should clarify the cause of any alarms (MHRA 2010b).

Anti-siphonage

Uncontrolled flow from a syringe is called 'siphonage'; this is a result of gravity or leakage of air into the syringe and administration set. Siphonage can occur whether or not the syringe is fixed into an infusion device (Quinn 2008). It has been reported that 'in practice, a 50 mL syringe attached to a length of administration set with an internal diameter of 3 mm has been shown to empty by siphonage in less than 1 minute' (Pickstone 1999, p.57).

To minimize the risk of siphonage, the following safe practices should be undertaken:

- The syringe (plunger and barrel) should be correctly located and secured (MHRA 2011).
- Intravenous administration extension sets should always be micro or narrow bore in diameter to increase the resistance to flow; wide-bore extension sets should be avoided.
- The syringe pump should always be positioned at the same level as the infusion site (MHRA 2011).
- Extension sets with an integral anti-siphonage or anti-reflux valve should be used (MHRA 2007, 2010b, Quinn 2008).

Safety software: smart pumps

Smart pump technology incorporates safeguards such as a list of high-alert medications, soft and hard dosage limits, and a drug library that can be tailored to specific patient care areas (Agius 2012, Harding 2012, Hertzel and Sousa 2009). It has provided an important step in improving patient safety (Breland 2010), and the use of pumps that incorporate this technology is increasingly widespread. A number of studies have evaluated the effectiveness of using smart pumps to prevent medication errors, showing the success of these systems (Dennison 2007, Fields and Peterson 2005, Larson et al. 2005, Manrique-Rodriguez et al. 2013, Rothschild et al. 2005). It is now recommended that nurses use this technology when administering intravenous fluids and medications (Harding 2011), but careful device selection and training are vital for compliance and to ensure safety outcomes (Longshore et al. 2010). Additionally, organizations that provide acute care in the UK have been recommended to minimize the range of device types available and to introduce centralized equipment libraries in order to reduce the chances of user error and improve patient safety (Lacovides et al. 2015, NPSA 2004).

Advantages and disadvantages of smart pumps

Smart pumps incorporate technology to improve their 'intelligence' when compared to standard volumetric pumps, supporting improved patient safety. Whereas volumetric pumps are predominantly reliant on individual users' vigilance, smart pumps are able to monitor infusion rates, alert the user if defined dosing limits are exceeded, and generate reports on organizational infusion practices (Breland 2010). The drug library can usually be adapted to individual clinical areas within hospitals, reflecting different dosing requirements across specialities (Heron 2017). Evidence suggests that these features are improving the recognition of user errors, specifically in relation to the programming of doses and infusion rates (Manrique-Rodriguez et al. 2013).

Smart pumps' disadvantages are that staff may struggle to introduce these new-style pumps due to existing device contracts, the infrastructure and resources required to use them fully (such as their wireless features), and financial constraints (Iacovides et al. 2015).

Volumetric pumps

Volumetric pumps (Figure 15.35) pump fluid from an infusion bag or bottle via an administration set and work by calculating the volume delivered (Quinn 2008). This is achieved when the pump measures the volume displaced in a 'reservoir'. The reservoir is an integral component of the administration set (Hadaway 2010). The mechanism of action may be piston or peristaltic (Hadaway 2010). The indications for use are all large-volume infusions, both venous and arterial.

All volumetric pumps are mains and battery powered, with the rate selected in millilitres per hour. The accuracy of flow is usually within ±5% when measured over a period of time, which is more than adequate for most clinical applications (MHRA 2010b, Pickstone 1999).

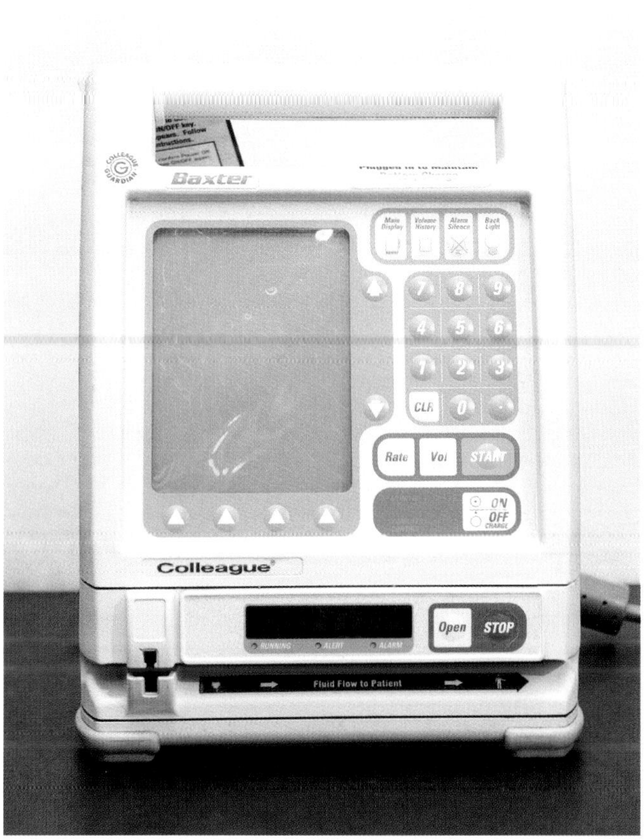

Figure 15.35 Volumetric pump.

Advantages and disadvantages of volumetric pumps

These pumps are able to overcome resistance to flow by increased delivery pressure and do not rely on gravity. This generally makes the performance of these pumps predictable, and they are capable of accurate delivery over a wide range of flow rates (MHRA 2010b).

Volumetric pumps also incorporate a wide range of features, including air-in-line detectors, variable pressure settings and comprehensive alarms, such as 'end of infusion', 'keep vein open' (where the pump switches to a low flow rate, e.g. 5 mL/h, in order to continue flow to prevent occlusion of the device) and 'low battery'. Many have a secondary infusion facility, which allows for intermittent therapy, for example antibiotics. The pump is programmed to switch to a secondary set and, when completed, it reverts back to the primary infusion at the previously set rate. The changing hospital environment has led to increased demand on volumetric pumps, which in turn has resulted in the development of multichannel and dual-channel infusion pumps. These may consist of two devices with an attached housing or of several infusion channels within a single device (Hadaway 2010).

The disadvantages of volumetric pumps are that they are usually relatively expensive, and often dedicated administration sets are required. The use of the wrong set could result in error even if the pump appears to work. Some are complicated to set up, which can also lead to errors (MHRA 2010b).

Syringe pumps

Syringe pumps (Figure 15.36) are low-volume, high-accuracy devices designed to infuse at low flow rates. The plunger of a syringe containing the substance to be infused is driven forward by the syringe pump at a controlled rate to deliver the substance to the patient (MHRA 2010b).

Syringe pumps are useful where small volumes of highly concentrated drugs need to be infused at low flow rates (Quinn 2008). The volume for infusion is limited to the size of the syringe used in the device, which is usually 60 mL, but most pumps will accept different sizes and brands of syringe.

These devices are calibrated for delivery in millilitres per hour (Weinstein and Hagle 2014).

Advantages and disadvantages of syringe pumps

Syringe pumps are mains and/or battery powered, are usually easy to operate, and tend to cost less than volumetric pumps. The alarm systems have become more comprehensive and include 'low

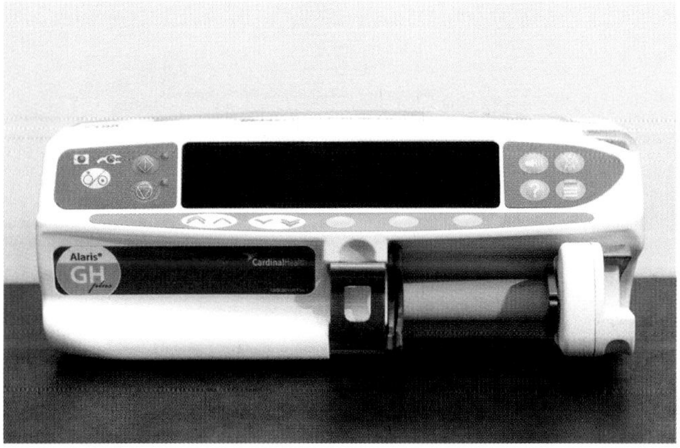

Figure 15.36 Syringe pump.

battery', 'end of infusion' and 'syringe clamp open' alarms. Most of the problems associated with the older models – for example, free flow, mechanical backlash (slackness that delays the start-up time of the infusion) and incorrect fitting of the syringe – have been eliminated in the newer models (MHRA 2010b, Quinn 2008). The risk of free flow is minimized by the use of an anti-siphonage valve, which may be integral to the administration set (Pickstone 1999). Despite the use of an anti-siphonage valve, the clamp of the administration set must still be used (MHRA 2010b). Where mechanical backlash is an issue and there is a prime (also called purge) option, this should be used at the start of the infusion to take up the mechanical slack (Amoore et al. 2001).

Specialist pumps

Patient-controlled analgesia pumps

Patient-controlled analgesia (PCA) devices are typically syringe pumps (although some are based on volumetric designs) (MHRA 2010b) (Figure 15.37). The syringe pump forces down the syringe piston, collapsing the syringe at a pre-set rate, but the distinguishing feature is the ability of the pump to deliver doses on demand, which occurs when the patient pushes a button (Schug et al. 2015). Whether or not the dose is delivered is determined by pre-set parameters in the pump. That is, if the maximum amount of drug over a given period of time has already been delivered, a further dose cannot be delivered.

PCA pumps are useful for patients who require pain control. They are used most commonly in the acute setting but are also useful in ambulatory situations (Schug et al. 2015).

The infusion options of a PCA pump are usually categorized into three types:

- *PCA demand mode only*: drug delivered by intermittent infusion when a button is pushed. Doses can be limited to a designated maximum amount (Macintyre and Schug 2015).
- *Continuous*: designed for patients who need maximum pain relief without the option of demand dosing (e.g. epidural).
- *A combination of PCA demand mode with a continuous infusion (background)*: a small dose of opioid is delivered in the background in addition to PCA demand dosing. This option may be useful if patients are on high-dose opiates or have high pain levels (Schug et al. 2015).

PCA pumps can dispense a bolus dose, with an initial bolus being called a 'loading dose'. This may benefit patients as the one-time dose is significantly higher than a demand dose in order to achieve immediate pain relief (see Chapter 9: Patient comfort and supporting personal hygiene and Chapter 11: Symptom control and care towards the end of life).

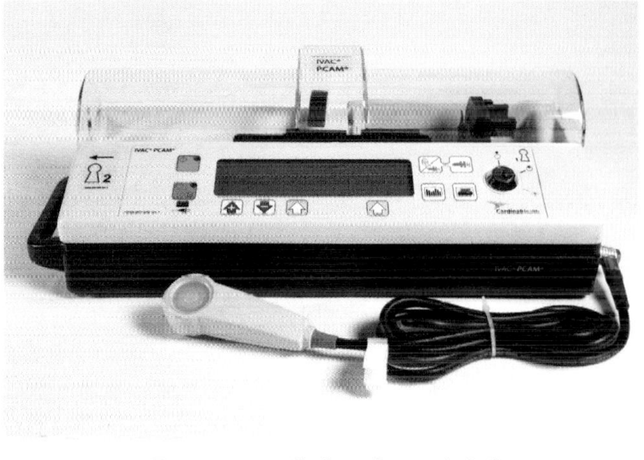

Figure 15.37 Patient-controlled analgesia (PCA) pump, generally used in acute hospital settings.

Advantages and disadvantages of patient-controlled analgesia pumps

To ensure patient safety, a key or software code is needed to access control of the pump. In addition, these devices offer a 'clinician override' feature with a predetermined key code to enable authorized personnel to modify running programmes in specific clinical situations. They have an extensive memory capability, which can be accessed through the display via a printer or computer (MHRA 2010b). This facility is critical for the pumps' effective use in pain management (Hadaway 2010), as it enables clinicians to determine when and how often demand is made by a patient and what total volume has been infused (Hadaway 2010). It has also been shown that PCA pumps increase patient satisfaction and also reduce their anxiety, their nursing needs and their time in hospital (McNicol et al. 2015).

While PCA pumps have advantages in relation to safety and efficacy, there is still a risk of adverse events, such as respiratory depression, with a continuous background infusion (Schug et al. 2015).

Anaesthesia pumps

Anaesthesia pumps are syringe pumps designed for delivery of anaesthesia or sedation and must only ever be used for those purposes. They should be restricted to operating theatres and critical care units, and should be clearly labelled. They are designed to allow rapid changes in flow rate and bolus to be made while the pump is infusing (Quinn 2008). Total intravenous anaesthesia (TIVA) and target-controlled infusion (TCI) pumps are available, designed to control the induction, maintenance and reversal phases of anaesthesia (Absalom and Struys 2006).

Epidural pumps

Epidural pumps (Figure 15.38) provide analgesia (most commonly a combination of opioids and anaesthetic agents) via a fine catheter inserted directly into the epidural space. As a form of analgesia delivery, the efficacy of the epidural route has been well documented (Block et al. 2003, Werawatganon and Charuluxanun 2005, Wheatley et al. 2001) and it is used effectively in several specialities, across medical and surgical settings (Gizzo et al. 2014, Janaki et al. 2008). See also Chapter 9: Patient comfort and supporting personal hygiene and Chapter 11: Symptom control and care towards the end of life.

Ambulatory infusion devices

Ambulatory infusion devices were developed to allow patients more freedom and to enable patients to continue with normal activities or to move unencumbered by a large infusion device (Hadaway 2010). Ambulatory devices range in size and weight. They are used for small volumes of drugs and are mainly designed for patients to wear and use when ambulant. The solution containers are often more cumbersome than the actual pump itself. Due to their size, the number of alarms may be limited. Considerations for selection of an ambulatory device include the following:

- type of therapy
- patient's ability to understand how to manage the infusion device
- drug stability
- frequency of doses
- reservoir volumes required
- control of flow and flow rate
- type of access

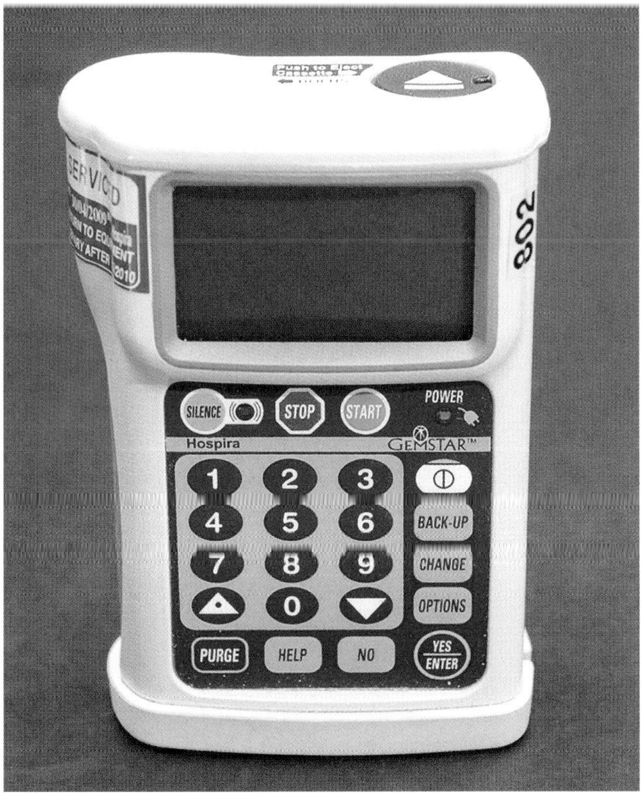

Figure 15.38 Epidural pump.

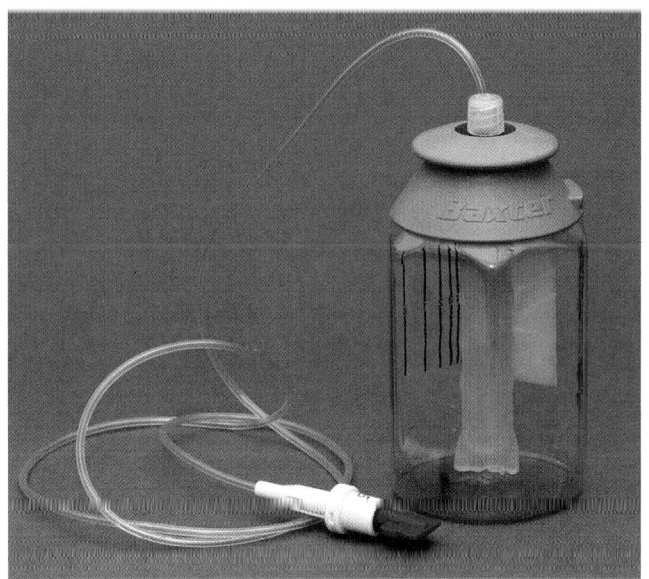

Figure 15.39 Elastomeric device.

- cost-effectiveness
- portability
- convenience.

Ambulatory pumps fall into two categories: mechanical and battery-operated infusion devices.

Mechanical infusion devices

These are simple and compact but may not necessarily be cost-effective as they are usually disposable. The mechanism for delivery is by balloon or simple spring, or they may be gas powered. They are usually very user friendly as they require minimal input from the patient and no battery. They can also be purchased pre-filled (Quinn 2008). Their flow rates are influenced by pressure gradient, viscosity and temperature, which can lead to inaccuracies (Ackermann et al. 2007, HWR 2005, Skryabina and Dunn 2006).

Mechanical infusion devices have two types:

- *Elastomeric balloon devices*: these are made of a soft rubberized material capable of being inflated to a predetermined volume, and the drug is then administered over a very specific infusion time. The balloon is encapsulated inside a rigid transparent container, which may be round or cylindrical. The rate of infusion is not controlled by the balloon but by the diameter of the restricting outlet, located in the pre-attached tubing (Quinn 2008). These devices are designed to supply a patient's need for a single-dose infusion of drugs (e.g. intermittent small-volume parenteral therapies, such as antibiotics). Their small size causes little disruption to the patient's daily activities and they tend to be well tolerated (Broadhurst 2012, Hadaway 2010). Figure 15.39 shows an elastomeric device.
- *Spring mechanism*: spring coil piston syringes have a spring that powers the plunger of a syringe in the absence of manual pressure. The volume is restricted by the size of the syringe, which is usually pre-filled. The spring coil container tends to be a multidose, small-volume administration device and is a combination of a spring coil in a collapsible flattened disc. Its shape can accommodate many therapies and volumes (Hadaway 2010).

Battery-operated infusion devices

Battery-operated pumps are small and light enough to be carried around by the patient without interfering with most everyday activities. They are operated using rechargeable or alkaline batteries but, owing to their size, the available battery capacity tends to be low. The length of time the battery lasts is often dependent on the rate at which the pump is set. Most give an output in the form of a small bolus delivered every few minutes, and most have an integral case or pouch that allows the pump and the reservoir or syringe to be worn with discretion by the patient.

There are two types: ambulatory volumetric infusion pumps and syringe drivers. Both are infusion devices that pump in the same way as a large volumetric pump; however, by nature of their size, they are portable and useful in the ambulatory setting (hospital or home care) (MHRA 2011).

These pumps are suitable for patients who have been prescribed continuous infusional treatment for a period of time, for example from 4 days to 6 months. They enable patients, where appropriate, to receive treatment at home, because they are small and portable.

Advantages and disadvantages of ambulatory infusion devices

The advantages of ambulatory pumps are as follows:

- They are able to deliver drugs continuously or intermittently.
- They can be used with a variety of infusion routes: central, peripheral venous, epidural, intra-arterial, intrathecal and subcutaneous.
- They deliver drugs accurately over a set period of time.
- They can improve the outcomes of treatment by delivering treatment continuously.

- They heighten the patient's independence and control by allowing them to be at home and participate in their own care.
- They are compact, light and easy to use.
- They have audible alarm systems.

The disadvantages of ambulatory pumps are as follows:

- They may require the insertion of a central venous access device, which has associated complications and problems.
- They may malfunction at home, which could be distressing and dangerous for the patient.
- In spite of their ease of use, some patients may not be able to cope with them at home.
- Patients may have to adapt their lifestyle to cope with living with a pump continuously (MHRA 2011).

Specific patient preparation

Selecting the appropriate infusion device for the patient

The nurse has a responsibility to determine when and how to use an infusion device to deliver hydration, drugs, transfusions and nutritional support, and how to select the most appropriate device to manage the needs of the patient. The following factors should be considered when selecting an infusion delivery system (Quinn 2008):

- Risk to the patient of:
  - overinfusion
  - underinfusion
  - uneven flow
  - inadvertent bolus
  - high-pressure delivery
  - extravascular infusion.
- Delivery parameters:
  - infusion rate and volume required
  - accuracy required (over a long or short period of time)
  - alarms required
  - ability to infuse into site chosen (venous, arterial or subcutaneous)
  - suitability of the device for infusing the required drug (e.g. ability to infuse viscous drugs).
- Environmental features:
  - ease of operation
  - frequency of observation and adjustment
  - type of patient (e.g. neonate, child or critically ill)
  - mobility of patient.

Paediatric considerations

The MHRA (2014a) classifies infusions into categories of risk. Neonatal infusions are the highest risk category, and infusion of fluids in children carries the next highest level of risk, as accuracy in the flow rate is essential. Infusion therapy within the paediatric setting requires very specific skills (Frey and Pettit 2010). It is paramount for practitioners to be competent in calculating paediatric doses, maintaining a stringent fluid balance, using paediatric-specific devices and managing complications.

The MHRA (2010b) has published recommendations on the safety and performance of infusion devices in order to enable users to make the appropriate choice of equipment to suit most applications. These recommendations include a classification system that is divided into three major categories according to the potential risks involved. These are shown in Table 15.11. A pump suited to the most risky category of therapy (A) can safely be used for the other categories (B and C). A pump suited to category B can be used for B and C, whereas a pump with the lowest specification (C) is suited only to category C therapies (MHRA 2010b) (Figure 15.40). Hospitals are required to label each infusion pump with its category, and it is necessary to know the category of the proposed therapy and match it with a pump of the same or a better category. A locally produced list of drugs and fluids along with their categories will need to be provided to all device users (MHRA 2010b).

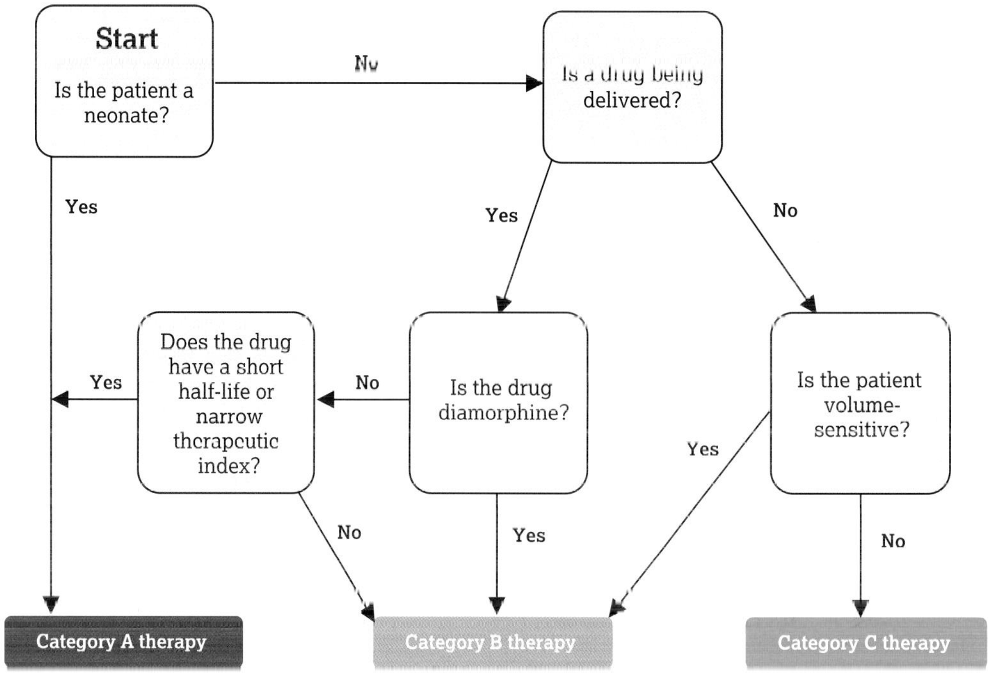

Figure 15.40 Decision tree for selection of an infusion device. *Source*: Adapted from MHRA (2010b). © Crown copyright. Reproduced under the Open Government Licence v2.0.

Table 15.11 Therapy categories and performance parameters

Therapy category	Therapy description	Patient group	Critical performance parameters
A	Drugs with a narrow therapeutic margin	Any	Good long-term accuracy Good short-term accuracy
	Drugs with a short half-life	Any	Rapid alarm after occlusion
	Any infusion given to neonates	Neonates	Small occlusion bolus Able to detect very small air embolus (volumetric pumps only) Small flow rate increments Good bolus accuracy Rapid start-up time (syringe pumps only)
B	Drugs other than those with a short half-life	Any except neonates	Good long-term accuracy Alarm after occlusion
	Parenteral nutrition	Volume sensitive except neonates	Small occlusion bolus
	Fluid maintenance	Volume sensitive except neonates	Able to detect small air embolus (volumetric pumps only)
	Transfusions	Volume sensitive except neonates	Small flow rate increments
C	Diamorphine	Any except neonates	Bolus accuracy
	Parenteral nutrition	Any except volume sensitive or neonates	Long-term accuracy
	Fluid maintenance	Any except volume sensitive or neonates	Alarm after occlusion
	Transfusions	Any except volume sensitive or neonates	Small occlusion bolus Able to detect air embolus (volumetric pumps only) Incremental flow rates

Procedure guideline 15.23 Medication: continuous infusion of intravenous drugs

This procedure may be carried out for the infusion of drugs from a bag, bottle or burette.

Essential equipment

- Personal protective equipment
- Clinically clean tray
- Patient's prescription chart
- Recording chart or book as required by law or hospital policy
- Electronic identity check equipment, where relevant
- Protective clothing as required by hospital policy for the administration of specific drugs
- Container of appropriate intravenous infusion fluid
- 2% chlorhexidine skin preparation
- Drug additive label
- Sterile needle

Action	Rationale
Pre-procedure	
1 Introduce yourself to the patient, explain and discuss the procedure with them, and gain their consent to proceed.	To ensure that the patient feels at ease, understands the procedure and gives their valid consent (NMC 2018, **C**).
2 Inspect the infusion in progress.	To check the correct infusion is being administered at the correct rate and that the contents are due to be delivered on time in order for the next prepared infusion bag to be connected. To check whether the patient is experiencing any discomfort at the site of insertion, which might indicate the peripheral device needs to be re-sited (NPSA 2007d, **C**).
3 Before administering any prescribed drug, check that it is due and has not already been given.	To protect the patient from harm (NPSA 2007d, **C**).

(continued)

Procedure guideline 15.23 Medication: continuous infusion of intravenous drugs *(continued)*

Action	Rationale
4 Before administering any prescribed drug, look at the patient's prescription chart and check the following: a the correct patient is being given the drug b drug c dose d date and time of administration e route and method of administration f diluent as appropriate g validity of prescription h signature of prescriber i the prescription is legible.	To ensure that the correct patient is given the correct drug in the prescribed dose using the appropriate diluent and by the correct route (DH 2003b, **C**; RPS 2019a, **C**). To protect the patient from harm (DH 2003b, **C**).
If any of these pieces of information are missing, unclear or illegible, do not proceed with the administration. Consult with the prescriber.	To prevent any errors occurring. **E**
5 Wash hands with bactericidal soap and water or an alcohol-based handrub, and assemble the necessary equipment.	To minimize the risk of infection (DH 2007, **C**; Fraise and Bradley 2009, **E**).
6 Prepare the drug for injection as described in Procedure guidelines 15.11, 15.12, 15.13 or 15.14.	To ensure the drug is prepared (NPSA 2007d, **C**).
7 Check the name, strength and volume of intravenous fluid against the prescription chart.	To ensure that the correct type and quantity of fluid are administered (NMC 2018, **C**; NPSA 2007d, **C**).
8 Check the expiry date of the fluid.	To prevent an ineffective or toxic compound being administered to the patient (NPSA 2007d, **C**).
9 Check that the packaging is intact and inspect the container and contents in good light for cracks, punctures and air bubbles.	To check that no contamination of the infusion container has occurred (NPSA 2007d, **C**).
10 Inspect the fluid for discoloration, haziness, and crystalline or particulate matter.	To prevent any toxic or foreign matter being infused into the patient (NPSA 2007d, **C**).
11 Check the identity and amount of drug to be added. Consider: a compatibility of fluid and additive b stability of mixture over the prescribed duration of the infusion c any special directions for dilution, for example pH or optimum concentration d sensitivity to external factors, such as light e any anticipated allergic reaction. If any doubts exist about the listed points, consult the pharmacist or appropriate reference works.	To minimize the risk of error. To ensure safe and effective administration of the drug. To enable anticipation of toxicities and the nursing implications of these (NPSA 2007d, **C**).
12 Any additions must be made immediately before use.	To prevent any possible microbial growth or degradation (NPSA 2007d, **C**).
13 Wash hands thoroughly using bactericidal soap and water or an alcohol-based handrub.	To minimize the risk of cross-infection (DH 2007, **C**; Fraise and Bradley 2009, **E**).
14 Place the infusion bag on a flat surface.	To prevent puncturing the side of the infusion bag when making additions (NPSA 2007d, **C**).
15 Remove any seal present.	To expose the injection site on the container. **E**
Procedure	
16 Clean the site with a swab and allow it to dry.	To reduce the risk of contamination (NPSA 2007d, **C**).
17 Inject the drug (using a new sterile needle) into the bag, bottle or burette. A 23 or 25 G needle should be used. If the addition is made into a burette at the bedside: a avoid contamination of the needle and inlet port b check that the correct quantity of fluid is in the chamber c switch the infusion off briefly d add the drug.	To minimize the risk of contamination. To enable resealing of the latex or rubber injection site (NPSA 2007d, **C**). To minimize the risk of contamination (NPSA 2007d, **C**). To ensure the correct dilution (NPSA 2007d, **C**). To ensure a bolus injection is not given (NPSA 2007d, **C**).
18 Invert the container a number of times, especially if adding to a flexible infusion bag.	To ensure adequate mixing of the drug (NPSA 2007d, **C**).
19 Check again for haziness, discoloration and particles. This can occur even if the mixture is theoretically compatible, thus making vigilance essential.	To detect any incompatibility or degradation (NPSA 2007d, **C**).

20 Complete the drug additive label and fix it on the bag, bottle or burette.	To identify which drug has been added, when and by whom (NPSA 2007d, **C**).
21 Place the container in a clean receptacle. Wash hands and proceed to the patient.	To minimize the risk of contamination (DH 2007, **C**).
22 Check the identity of the patient against the prescription chart and infusion bag. If an electronic identity check system for patient and/or medicine identification is in place, then use in accordance with hospital policy and procedures.	To minimize the risk of error and ensure the correct infusion is administered to the correct patient (NPSA 2007d, **C**).
23 Check that the contents of the previous container have been fully delivered.	To ensure that the preceding prescription has been administered (NPSA 2007d, **C**).
24 Switch off the infusion. Apply gloves. Place the new infusion bag on a flat surface and then disconnect the empty infusion bag.	To ensure that the administration set spike will not puncture the side wall of the infusion bag (Finlay 2008, **E**; NPSA 2007d, **C**).
25 Push the spike in fully without touching it and hang the new infusion bag on the infusion stand. Insert tubing into the infusion pump where appropriate.	To reduce the risk of contamination (DH 2007, **C**). To ensure accuracy of delivery (Quinn 2008, **E**).
26 For gravity infusion, restart the infusion and adjust the rate of flow as prescribed. If using an infusion pump, start the pump and set the rate.	To ensure that the infusion will be delivered at the correct rate over the correct period of time (NPSA 2007d, **C**).
27 If the addition is made into a burette, the infusion can be restarted immediately following mixing and recording, with the infusion rate adjusted accordingly.	To ensure that the infusion will be delivered correctly (NPSA 2007d, **C**).
28 Ask the patient to report any abnormal sensations.	To ascertain whether there are any problems that may require nursing care and to enable referral to medical staff where appropriate. **E**.
Post-procedure	
29 Discard waste, making sure that it is placed in the correct containers, for example sharps into a designated receptacle.	To ensure safe disposal and avoid injury to staff. To prevent reuse of equipment (EASHW 2010, **C**; HWR 2005, **C**; MHRA 2004, **C**).
30 Complete the patient's recording chart and other hospital and/or legally required documents.	To maintain accurate records. To provide a point of reference in the event of any queries. To prevent any duplication of treatment (NMC 2018, **C**; RPS 2019a, **C**).

Procedure guideline 15.24 Medication: intermittent infusion of intravenous drugs

Essential equipment

- Personal protective equipment
- Patient's prescription chart
- Recording chart
- Electronic identity check equipment, where relevant
- Container of appropriate intravenous infusion fluid
- Drug additive label
- Intravenous administration set
- Intravenous infusion stand
- Clean dressing trolley
- Clinically clean tray
- Sterile needles and syringes
- 10 mL of a compatible flush solution (for injection), for example 0.9% sodium chloride or 5% dextrose
- Flushing solution to maintain patency plus sterile injection cap
- 2% chlorhexidine skin preparation
- Sterile dressing pack
- Hypoallergenic tape
- Bandage
- Sharps bin

Action	Rationale
Pre-procedure	
1 Introduce yourself to the patient, explain and discuss the procedure with them, and gain their consent to proceed.	To ensure that the patient feels at ease, understands the procedure and gives their valid consent (NMC 2018, **C**).

(continued)

Procedure guideline 15.24 Medication: intermittent infusion of intravenous drugs *(continued)*

Action	Rationale
2 Before administering any prescribed drug, check that it is due and has not been given already.	To protect the patient from harm (NPSA 2007d, **C**; RPS 2019a, **C**).
3 Before administering any prescribed drug, look at the patient's prescription chart and check the following:	To ensure that the correct patient is given the correct drug in the prescribed dose using the appropriate diluent and by the correct route (DH 2003b, **C**; RPS 2019a, **C**). To protect the patient from harm (DH 2003b, **C**).
a the correct patient is being given the drug b drug c dose d date and time of administration e route and method of administration f diluent as appropriate g validity of prescription h signature of prescriber i the prescription is legible.	To protect the patient from harm. **E** To comply with RPS (2019a). **E** To comply with RPS (2019a). **E**
If any of these pieces of information are missing, unclear or illegible, do not proceed with the administration. Consult with the prescriber.	To prevent any errors occurring. **E**
4 Wash hands with bactericidal soap and water or an alcohol based handrub.	To prevent contamination of medication and equipment (DH 2007, **C**).
5 Prepare the intravenous infusion and additive as described in Procedure guidelines 15.11, 15.12, 15.13 or 15.14.	To ensure the drug is prepared correctly (NPSA 2007d, **C**).
6 Prime the intravenous administration set with infusion fluid mixture and hang it on the infusion stand.	To ensure removal of air from the set and check that the tubing is patent. To prepare for administration (NPSA 2007d, **C**).
7 Draw up 10 mL of compatible flush solution for injection using an aseptic technique.	To ensure sufficient flushing solution is available. **E**
8 Draw up solution (as advised by hospital policy) to be used to maintain patency, for example 0.9% sodium chloride. Add the additive drug label to the bag/syringe.	To prepare for administration. **E**
9 Place the syringes in a clinically clean tray on the bottom shelf of the dressing trolley.	To ensure the top shelf is used for the sterile dressing pack in order to minimize the risk of contamination. **E**
10 Collect the other equipment and place it on the bottom shelf of the dressing trolley.	To ensure all equipment is available to commence the procedure. **E**
11 Place the sterile dressing pack on top of the trolley.	To minimize the risk of contamination. **E**
12 Check that all necessary equipment is present.	To prevent delays and interruption of the procedure. **E**
13 Wash hands thoroughly using bactericidal soap and water or an alcohol-based handrub.	To minimize the risk of cross-infection (DH 2007, **C**; Fraise and Bradley 2009, **E**).
14 Proceed to the patient. Check the patient's identity against the prescription chart and prepared drugs. If an electronic identity check system for patient and/or medicine identification is in place, then use in accordance with hospital policy and procedures.	To minimize the risk of error and ensure the correct drug is given to the correct patient (NPSA 2007d, **C**; RPS 2019a, **C**).
Procedure	
15 Open the sterile dressing pack.	To minimize the risk of cross infection (DH 2007, **C**; Fraise and Bradley 2009, **E**).
16 Open the 2% chlorhexidine skin preparation packet and empty it onto the pack.	To ensure the correct cleaning swab is available (DH 2007, **E**).
17 Wash hands with bactericidal soap and water or an alcohol-based handrub.	To minimize the risk of cross-infection. (DH 2007, **C**; Fraise and Bradley 2009, **E**).
18 If a peripheral device is *in situ*, remove the patient's bandage.	To observe the insertion site (Dougherty 2008a, **E**).
19 Inspect the insertion site of the device.	To detect any signs of inflammation, infiltration and so on. If present, take appropriate action (see Problem-solving table 15.3) (DH 2003c, **C**).
20 Wash and dry hands.	To minimize the risk of contamination (DH 2007, **C**).

21 Put on gloves.	To protect against contamination with hazardous substances, for example cytotoxic drugs (NPSA 2007d, **C**).
22 Place a sterile towel under the patient's arm.	To create a sterile area on which to work. **E**
23 Clean the needle-free cap with the 2% chlorhexidine skin preparation.	To minimize the risk of contamination and maintain a closed system (Loveday et al. 2014, **C**).
24 Gently inject 10 mL of 0.9% sodium chloride for injection.	To confirm the patency of the device. **E**
25 Check that no resistance is met, no pain or discomfort is felt by the patient, no swelling is evident, no leakage occurs around the device and there is a good backflow of blood on aspiration.	To ensure the device is patent (Dougherty 2008a, **E**).
26 Connect the infusion to the device.	To commence treatment. **E**
27 Open the roller clamp and/or insert the tubing into an infusion pump and start the pump.	To check the infusion is flowing freely. **E**
28 Check the insertion site and ask the patient whether they are comfortable.	To confirm that the vein can accommodate the extra fluid flow and that the patient experiences no pain. **E**
29 Adjust the flow rate as prescribed.	To ensure that the correct speed of administration is established (NPSA 2007d, **C**).
30 Tape the administration set in a way that places no strain on the device, which could in turn damage the vein.	To reduce the risk of mechanical phlebitis or infiltration (Dougherty 2008a, **E**).
31 Remove gloves.	To ensure disposal. **E**
32 If the infusion is to be completed within 30 minutes, bandaging is unnecessary and the patient may be instructed to keep the arm resting on the sterile towel. Otherwise apply a new bandage.	To reduce the risk of dislodging the device. **E**
33 The equipment must be cleared away and new equipment only prepared when required at the end of the infusion.	To ensure that the equipment used is sterile prior to use. **E**
34 Monitor flow rate and device site frequently.	To ensure the flow rate is correct and the patient is comfortable, and to check for signs of infiltration (NPSA 2007d, **C**).
35 When the infusion is complete, wash hands using bactericidal soap and water or an alcohol-based handrub, and recheck that all the equipment required is present.	To maintain asepsis and ensure that the procedure runs smoothly (DH 2007 **C**; Finlay 2008, **E**).
36 Stop the infusion when all of the fluid has been delivered.	To ensure that all of the prescribed mixture has been delivered and prevent air infusing into the patient (NPSA 2007d, **C**).
37 Put on non-sterile gloves.	To protect against contamination with hazardous substances. **E**
38 Disconnect the infusion set and flush the device with 10 mL of 0.9% sodium chloride or another compatible solution for injection. (A 'minibag' may be used to flush the drug through the tubing but the cost implications of this as well as the risk to patients on restricted intake should be considered before this is adopted routinely.)	To flush any remaining irritating solution away from the cannula. **E**
39 Attach a new sterile injection cap if necessary.	To maintain a closed system (Hart 2008, **E**).
40 Flush the device.	To maintain the patency of the device (Dougherty 2008a, **E**).
41 Clean the injection site of the cap with 2% chlorhexidine skin preparation.	To minimize the risk of contamination (Hart 2008, **E**).
42 Administer flushing solution using the push–pause technique and ending with positive pressure.	To maintain the patency of the device and, if a needle was used, to enable resealing of the injection site (Dougherty 2008a, **E**).
43 Reapply bandage.	To reduce the risk of dislodging the cannula. **E**
44 Remove gloves.	To ensure disposal. **E**
45 Assist the patient into a comfortable position.	To ensure the patient is comfortable. **E**
Post-procedure	
46 Discard waste, placing it in the correct containers, for example sharps into a designated container.	To ensure safe disposal and avoid injury to staff (EASHW 2010, **C**; HWR 2005, **C**; MHRA 2004, **C**; NHS Employers 2007, **C**).
47 Record the administration on the appropriate charts.	To maintain accurate records, provide a point of reference in the event of any queries and prevent any duplication of treatment (NMC 2018, **C**; RPS 2019a, **C**).

Procedure guideline 15.25 Medication: injection (bolus or push) of intravenous drugs

Essential equipment

- Personal protective equipment
- Clinically clean tray
- Patient's prescription chart
- Recording sheet or book as required by law or hospital policy
- Electronic identity check equipment, where relevant
- Clean dressing trolley
- Sterile needles and syringes
- 0.9% sodium chloride or another compatible solution (20 mL for injection)
- Flushing solution, in accordance with hospital policy
- 2% chlorhexidine skin preparation
- Sterile dressing pack
- Hypoallergenic tape
- Sharps container

Action	Rationale
Pre-procedure	
1 Introduce yourself to the patient, explain and discuss the procedure with them, and gain their consent to proceed.	To ensure that the patient feels at ease, understands the procedure and gives their valid consent (NMC 2018, **C**).
2 Before administering any prescribed drug, check that it is due and has not been given already.	To protect the patient from harm (RPS 2019a, **C**).
3 Before administering any prescribed drug, look at the patient's prescription chart and check the following:	To ensure that the correct patient is given the correct drug in the prescribed dose using the appropriate diluent and by the correct route (DH 2003b, **C**; RPS 2019, **C**). To protect the patient from harm (DH 2003b, **C**).
a the correct patient is being given the drug	
b drug	
c dose	
d date and time of administration	To protect the patient from harm. **E**
e route and method of administration	To comply with RPS (2019a). **E**
f diluent as appropriate	To comply with RPS (2019a). **E**
g validity of prescription	
h signature of prescriber	
i the prescription is legible.	
If any of these pieces of information are missing, unclear or illegible, do not proceed with the administration. Consult with the prescriber.	To prevent any errors occurring. **E**
4 Select the required medication and check the expiry date.	Treatment with medication that is outside the expiry date is dangerous. Drugs deteriorate with storage. The expiry date indicates when a particular drug is no longer pharmacologically efficacious (NPSA 2007d, **C**).
5 Wash hands with bactericidal soap and water or an alcohol-based handrub, and assemble the necessary equipment.	To minimize the risk of infection (DH 2007, **C**; Fraise and Bradley 2009, **E**).
6 Prepare the drug for injection as described in Procedure guidelines 15.11, 15.12, 15.13 or 15.14.	To prepare the drug correctly. **E**
7 Prepare a 20 mL syringe of 0.9% sodium chloride (or another compatible solution) for injection using aseptic technique.	To use for flushing between each drug (NPSA 2007d, **C**).
8 Draw up the flushing solution, as indicated by local hospital policy.	To prepare for administration. **E**
9 Place the syringes in a clinically clean receptacle on the bottom shelf of the dressing trolley, along with the receptacle containing any drug(s) to be administered.	To ensure the top shelf is used for the sterile dressing pack in order to minimize the risk of contamination. **E**
10 Collect the other equipment and place it on the bottom of the trolley.	To ensure all equipment is available to commence the procedure. **E**
11 Place a sterile dressing pack on top of the trolley.	To minimize the risk of contamination. **E**
12 Check that all necessary equipment is present.	To prevent delays and interruption of the procedure. **E**

13 Wash hands thoroughly.	To minimize the risk of infection (DH 2007, **C**; Fraise and Bradley 2009, **E**).
14 Proceed to the patient and check their identity and the prepared drug against the prescription chart. If an electronic identity check system for patient and/or medicine identification is in place, then use in accordance with hospital policy and procedures.	To minimize the risk of error and ensure the drug is given to the correct patient (NPSA 2007d, **C**).
Procedure	
15 Open the sterile dressing pack, and open the 2% chlorhexidine skin preparation and empty it onto the pack.	To gain access to the necessary equipment and to ensure there is a cleaning swab available (DH 2007, **C**).
16 Wash hands with bactericidal soap and water or an alcohol-based handrub.	To reduce the risk of infection (DH 2007, **C**; Fraise and Bradley 2009, **E**).
17 If a peripheral device is *in situ*, remove the bandage.	To observe the insertion site. **E**
18 Inspect the insertion site of the device.	To detect any signs of inflammation, infiltration and so on. If present, take appropriate action (see Problem-solving table 15.3) (DH 2003c, **C**).
19 Observe the infusion, if in progress.	To confirm that it is infusing as desired (NPSA 2007d, **C**).
20 Check whether the infusion fluid and the drugs are compatible. If not, change the infusion fluid to 0.9% sodium chloride to flush between the drugs if necessary.	To prevent drug interaction. Some manufacturers recommend that the drug is given into the injection site of a rapidly running infusion (NPSA 2007d, **C**). A compatible fluid must be used to remove the medication and prevent precipitation or drug incompatibility if medications mix in the tubing (Whittington 2008, **E**).
21 Wash hands with bactericidal soap and water or an alcohol-based handrub.	To minimize the risk of infection (DH 2007, **C**; Fraise and Bradley 2009, **E**).
22 Place a sterile towel under the patient's arm.	To create a sterile field. **E**
23 Apply gloves. Clean the injection site with a 2% chlorhexidine skin preparation and allow to dry.	To reduce the number of pathogens introduced by the needle at the time of the insertion. To ensure complete disinfection has occurred (Loveday et al. 2014, **C**).
24 Switch off the infusion.	To prevent excessive pressure within the vein. To prevent contact with an incompatible infusion fluid. To allow the nurse to concentrate on the site of insertion and injection (NPSA 2007d, **C**).
25 If a peripheral device is *in situ*, gently inject 0.9% sodium chloride. This may not be necessary if the patient has a 0.9% sodium chloride infusion in progress.	To confirm patency of the vein. To prevent contact with an incompatible infusion solution (NPSA 2007d, **C**).
26 Open the roller clamp of the administration set fully. Inject the drug at a speed sufficient to slow but not stop the infusion and inject the drug smoothly in the direction of flow at the specified rate.	To prevent backflow of drug up the tubing. To prevent excessive pressure within the vein. To prevent speed shock (NPSA 2007d, **C**).
27 Ensure the needles and syringes are disposed of immediately into appropriate sharps containers (or are returned to the tray). Do not leave any sharps on the opened sterile pack.	To reduce the risk of needle stick injury and to prevent contamination of the pack (RCN 2016, **C**).
28 Observe the insertion site of the device throughout.	To detect any complications at an early stage, for example extravasation or local allergic reaction (Dougherty 2008b, **E**).
29 Frequently check for blood return and/or 'flashback' throughout the injection (i.e. every 3–5 mL), but other signs and symptoms must be taken into consideration too.	To confirm that the device is correctly placed and that the vein remains patent (Weinstein and Hagle 2014, **E**). Flashback alone is not an indicator that the vein is patent (Dougherty 2008a, **E**).
30 Consult the patient during the injection about any discomfort.	To detect any complications at an early stage and ensure patient comfort (Dougherty 2008a, **E**).
31 If more than one drug is to be administered, flush with 0.9% sodium chloride between administrations by restarting the infusion or changing syringes.	To prevent drug interactions (NPSA 2007d, **C**).
32 At the end of the injection, flush with 0.9% sodium chloride by restarting the infusion or attaching a syringe containing 0.9% sodium chloride.	To flush any remaining irritant solution away from the device site (NPSA 2007d, **C**).
33 After the final flush of 0.9% sodium chloride, adjust the infusion rate as prescribed, open the fluid path of the tap/stopcock, or administer the flushing solution using pulsatile flush and ending with positive pressure.	To continue delivery of therapy. To maintain the patency of the cannula (Finlay 2008, **E**).

(continued)

Procedure guideline 15.25 Medication: injection (bolus or push) of intravenous drugs *(continued)*

Action	Rationale
34 Apply a bandage.	To reduce the risk of dislodging the cannula. **E**
35 Assist the patient into a comfortable position.	To ensure the patient is comfortable. **E**
Post-procedure	
36 Dispose of used syringes (with the needle unsheathed) directly into a sharps container during the procedure, or place them back onto the plastic tray and then dispose of them in a sharps container as soon as possible. *Do not* disconnect needles from syringes prior to disposal. Other waste should be placed into the appropriate plastic bags.	To avoid needle stick injury (EASHW 2010, **C**; MHRA 2004, **C**; NHS Employers 2007, **C**).
37 Record the administration on the appropriate charts.	To maintain accurate records, provide a point of reference in the event of any queries and prevent any duplication of treatment (NMC 2018, **C**; RPS 2019a, **C**).

Problem-solving table 15.3 Prevention and resolution (Procedure guidelines 15.23, 15.24 and 15.25)

Problem	Cause	Prevention	Action
Infusion slows or stops due to a change in position of the patient or any equipment	Patient has changed position	Check the height of the fluid container if the patient is active and receiving an infusion using gravity flow.	Adjust the height of the container accordingly. The infusion should not hang higher than 1 m above the patient as the increased height will result in increased pressure and possible rupture of the vessel or device (Quinn 2008).
	Limb has changed position	Avoid inserting peripheral devices at joints of limbs. Instruct the patient on the amount of movement permitted. Continued movement could result in mechanical phlebitis (Lamb and Dougherty 2008).	Move the arm or hand until the infusion starts again. Secure the device, then bandage or splint the limb again carefully in the desired position. Take care not to cause damage to the limb.
	Administration set has moved	Tape the administration set so that it cannot become kinked or occluded.	Check for kinks and/or compression if the patient is active or restless, and correct accordingly.
	Cannula has moved	Secure the cannula firmly to prevent movement. It may come into contact with the vein wall or a valve. Infusions sited in small veins are prone to this problem.	Remove the bandage and dressing and manoeuvre the peripheral device gently, without pulling it out of the vein, until the infusion starts again. Secure adequately.
Infusion slows or stops due to technical problems	Negative pressure prevents flow of fluid	Ensure that the container is vented using an air inlet.	Vent if necessary, using a venting needle.
	Empty container	Check fluid levels regularly.	Replace the fluid container before it runs dry.
	Venous spasm due to chemical irritation or cold fluids/drugs	Dilute drugs as recommended. Remove solutions from the refrigerator a short time before use.	Apply a warm compress to soothe and dilate the vein, increase the blood flow and dilute the infusion mixture.
	Injury to the vein	Detect any injury early as it is likely to progress and cause more serious conditions.	Stop the infusion and re-site the cannula.

Problem	Cause	Prevention	Action
	Occlusion of the device due to fibrin formation	Maintain a continuous, regular fluid flow or ensure that patency is maintained by flushing. Instruct the patient to keep their arm below the level of the heart if ambulant and attached to a gravity flow infusion.	*If peripheral device*: remove extension set/injection cap and attempt to flush the cannula gently using a 10 mL syringe of 0.9% sodium chloride. If resistance is met, stop and re-site the peripheral device (see Chapter 17: Vascular access devices: insertion and management). *If central venous access device*: remove injection cap and attempt to flush the cannula gently using a 10 mL syringe of 0.9% sodium chloride. If resistance is met, attempt to instil a fibrinolytic agent such as urokinase (see Chapter 17: Vascular access devices: insertion and management).
	The cannula has become displaced either completely or partially; that is, fluid or drug has leaked into the surrounding tissues ('infiltration'; if the drugs were vesicant in nature, this would then be called 'extravasation')	Secure the cannula and tape the administration set to prevent pulling and dislodgement. Instruct the patient on the amount of movement permitted regarding the limb that has the device *in situ* (Fabian 2000).	Confirm that infiltration of drugs has or has not occurred by: • inspecting the site for leakage, swelling, and so on • testing the temperature of the skin: it will be cooler if infiltration has occurred • comparing the size of the limb with the opposite limb. If infiltration is confirmed, stop the infusion and request a re-siting of the device. If the infusion is allowed to progress, discomfort and tissue damage will result. Apply cold or warm compresses (whichever provides the most comfort for the patient) to provide symptomatic relief. Reassure the patient by explaining what is happening. Document the incident in the care plan and monitor the site (Lamb and Dougherty 2008). If extravasation occurs, follow hospital policy and procedure.
Infusion pump alarm: air detected	Air bubbles in administration set	Ensure all air is removed from all equipment prior to use.	Remove all air from the administration set and restart the infusion.
Infusion pump alarm: tube misload	Administration set has been incorrectly loaded	Ensure the set is loaded correctly.	Check that the set is loaded correctly and reload if necessary.
Infusion pump alarm: upstream occlusion	Closed clamp, obstruction or kink in the administration set is preventing fluid flow	Ensure the container/fluid bag has been adequately pierced by the administration spike.	Inspect the administration set and restart the infusion.
		Ensure the tubing is taped to prevent kinking.	If tubing is kinked, reposition, tape and restart infusion.
		Ensure the regulating (roller) clamp is open.	Check the administration set and open the clamp; restart the infusion.
Infusion pump alarm: downstream occlusion	Phlebitis/ infiltration or extravasation	Observe the site regularly for signs of swelling, pain or erythema.	Remove the peripheral device, provide symptomatic relief where appropriate. Initiate extravasation procedure. Re-site as appropriate.
	Closed distal clamp	Ensure clamps are open.	Locate distal occlusion and restart infusion.

(continued)

Problem-solving table 15.3 Prevention and resolution (Procedure guidelines 15.23, 15.24 and 15.25) (*continued*)

Problem	Cause	Prevention	Action
Infusion pump alarm: KVO (keep vein open) alert	The volume infused is complete and the device is infusing at the KVO rate	Programme in a new volume as appropriate.	Do not turn the device off. Allow KVO mode to run to maintain the patency of the device. Prepare a new infusion or discontinue as appropriate.
Infusion device malfunctioning (electrical/mechanical)	Not charging at mains	Ensure that the device is kept plugged in where appropriate.	Change device and remove device from use until fully charged. Send to clinical engineering to check plug.
	Low battery	Push lead in adequately.	Check lead is pushed in adequately. Contact clinical engineering if fault persists.
	Batteries keep requiring replacement	Do not use small rechargeable batteries in ambulatory devices.	Ensure non-rechargeable batteries have been used. Contact clinical engineering if fault persists.
	Technical fault	Ensure all infusion devices are serviced regularly.	Remove infusion device from use and contact clinical engineering department or relevant personnel.
	Device soiled inside mechanism	Maintain equipment and keep clean and free from contamination.	Remove administration set, wipe pump and reload. Do not use alcohol-based solutions on internal mechanisms.
Unstable infusion device.	Mounted on an old, poorly maintained stand	Ensure that stands are maintained and kept clean. Replace old stands.	Remove device from stand. Remove stand and send to clinical engineering for repair.
	Mounted on an incorrect stand	Ensure the correct stands are used.	Check the stand and change to an appropriate stand.
	Equipment not balanced on stand	Ensure that all equipment is balanced around the stand.	Remove the devices and attach them to two stands if necessary. Balance the equipment.

Post-procedural considerations

Ongoing care

Monitoring of the infusion while in progress includes monitoring the patient's condition and response to therapy, the VAD site, the rate and the volume infused. It may also include monitoring the battery life and occlusion pressure. The frequency of monitoring is often based on the type of therapy and the patient's condition; for example, the rate of infusion and the infusion site may be checked 15 minutes after setting up the infusion, then again after 1 hour and then 4-hourly (or more frequently depending on the medication). The check must be documented on the patient's fluid balance chart or in their notes. The type and make of pump along with the serial number should also be documented (this is useful if any errors occur) (MHRA 2008a).

Complications

In cases of phlebitis, thrombosis, septicaemia or embolism, see Chapter 17: Vascular access devices: insertion and management.

Infiltration and extravasation

Definitions

There is variation in the definitions attached to 'infiltration' and 'extravasation', and the terms are often used interchangeably (Reynolds et al. 2014), which can make reviewing the literature around them problematic. For the purposes of this manual, the following definitions are used.

Infiltration

Infiltration tends to refer to the leakage of non-vesicant solutions or medications into the surrounding tissues (INS 2016). It generally does not cause tissue necrosis but can result in long term injury due to local inflammatory reactions or compression of the surrounding tissues (if a large volume infiltrates), which is known as 'compartment syndrome' (Doellman et al. 2009, RCN 2016, Schulmeister 2009).

Extravasation

Extravasation literally means 'leaking into the tissues' but it has been linked with vesicants to describe a process that requires immediate action if local tissue damage is to be prevented (INS 2016, Polovich et al. 2014, Schulmeister 2009). A vesicant is any solution or medication that causes the formation of blisters with subsequent tissue necrosis and may be DNA-binding or non-DNA-binding (INS 2016, Polovich et al. 2014). The most well-known group of vesicants is cytotoxic chemotherapy agents, but several non-antineoplastic drugs also have these properties (Buter et al. 2019).

Related theory

It is important to recognize and distinguish extravasation and infiltration from flare reaction. Flare reaction is a not uncommon transient painless skin-streaking erythema that looks like urticaria with skin elevation; it may occur with anthracycline administration (Kreidieh et al. 2016, Polovich et al. 2014). It is caused by a venous inflammatory response to histamine release. It can involve itching, burning and potentially pain, which usually resolve in 1–2 hours (Kreidieh et al. 2016). Slowing infusion rates may be helpful, but flare reaction responds well within a few minutes to the application of a topical steroid (Schulmeister 2009, Weinstein and Hagle 2014).

The extent of tissue damage following extravasation of vesicant drugs depends on a number of factors:

- Whether the drugs bind to DNA or not:
  - DNA-binding vesicants (e.g. doxorubicin and epirubicin) bind to nucleic acids in the DNA of healthy cells, resulting in cell death. There is then cellular uptake of extracellular substances and this sets up a continuing cycle of tissue damage as the DNA-binding vesicant is retained and recirculated in the tissue, sometimes for a prolonged period of time (Goolsby and Lombardo 2006, Polovich et al. 2014, Schulmeister 2009).
  - Non-DNA-binding vesicants (e.g. paclitaxel and vinca alkaloids) have an indirect rather than a direct effect on the cells. They are eventually metabolized in the tissue and then neutralized (more easily than DNA-binding vesicants) (Polovich et al. 2014).
- The concentration and amount of vesicant drug in the tissue.
- The location of the extravasation, for example hand or arm.
- Patient factors: certain patient groups are more susceptible, such as neonates, the elderly, those with malnourishment, those with several co-morbidities and those with cancer (Doornaert et al. 2013, Polovich et al. 2014, Schulmeister 2009).

Evidence-based approaches

Extravasation is a well-recognized complication of intravenous chemotherapy administration, but in general is a condition that is often underdiagnosed, undertreated and under-reported (Stanley 2002). Estimates of the incidence of extravasation vary between 0.5% and 6% of all cytotoxic drug administrations (Goolsby and Lombardo 2006, Kassner 2000, Khan and Holmes 2002, Lawson 2003, Masoorli 2003), but some estimates of the incidence of peripheral extravasation are between 23% and 25% (Roth 2003). Compilation of such figures is problematic, however, due to the lack of any centralized reporting or nationally or internationally agreed parameters, rendering it difficult to obtain true figures (Pérez Fidalgo 2012). There are no available figures for the incidence of non-neoplastic vesicant extravasations (Buter et al. 2019).

There appears to have been a reduction in the incidence of extravasation with the increased use of central venous access devices (CVADs) in chemotherapy administration (Buter et al. 2019), although the incidence is estimated to still be up to 6% with ports (Masoorli 2003). However, when extravasation does occur alongside the use of a CVAD, the severity of the injuries can be greater than with the use of a port due to delayed detection (Kassner 2000, Polovich et al. 2014, Stanley 2002) and the site of the CVAD (Pérez Fidalgo et al. 2012).

Even when practitioners have many years of experience, extravasation of vesicant agents can occur and is an extremely stressful event for both patient and practitioner. However, it is not in itself an act of negligence by the practitioner (Weinstein and Hagle 2014).

Early detection and treatment are crucial if the consequences of an untreated or poorly managed extravasation are to be avoided (Box 15.16 and Figure 15.41). However, the initial signs and symptoms of an extravasation may be subtle, and, while they usually occur immediately, there can be a delay of up to 1–2 weeks before they appear (Susser et al. 1999). Signs and symptoms may include (Polovich et al. 2014):

- blistering (typically occurs 1–2 weeks post-extravasation)
- peeling and sloughing of the skin (about 2 weeks post-extravasation)
- tissue necrosis (2–3 weeks post-extravasation) with resulting pain
- damage to tendons, nerves and joints
- functional and sensory impairment of affected area, such as limb disfigurement (Polovich et al. 2014).

These can all result in hospitalization and plastic surgery, delay in the treatment of disease, lifelong disability and psychological distress for the patient.

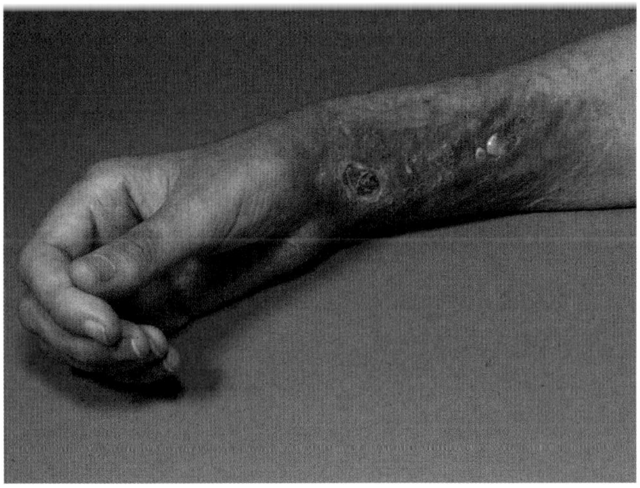

Figure 15.41 Extravasation.

Box 15.16 Considerations for the prevention of extravasation

- Monitoring the site
- Location of the device
- Identification of patients at risk
- Sequence of drugs
- Types of devices
- Method of administration
- Skill of practitioner
- Informing the patient of early signs and risks

Before administration of any vesicant drugs, the nurse should know which agents are capable of producing tissue necrosis; damage is usually caused by the ability to bind to DNA, or the pH, osmolarity or vasoconstrictive nature of the drugs (Table 15.12). Drugs should not be reconstituted to give solutions that are higher in concentration than is recommended by the manufacturer, and the method of administration (e.g. infusion or injection) should be checked. If in any doubt, the drug data sheet should be consulted; if this information is insufficient, the pharmacy department should be contacted regarding the action to take if a vesicant drug extravasates. Consideration should be given to the management of mixed vesicant drug extravasation in terms of which drug to treat with which antidote. For example, if drug A and drug B were in the same infusion and they required different antidotes, but drug A would cause more damage than drug B, the correct action would be to use the antidote for drug A (How and Brown 1998). Possible causes of extravasation are shown in Table 15.13.

Methods of preventing infiltration and extravasation

The nurse's focus should be on safe intravenous technique and implementing strategies to minimize risk (Weinstein and Hagle 2014). These include the following considerations.

Patients at risk

Patients who are at increased risk of extravasation (Box 15.17) should be observed particularly closely and cared for with extra caution.

Types of device

The use of steel needles is associated with a greater risk of extravasation and should be discouraged; a plastic cannula should be used instead (INS 2016, Polovich et al. 2014, Rodrigues et al. 2012, Sauerland et al. 2006). Vesicants should be given via a newly established cannula wherever possible (Dougherty 2010, Goolsby and Lombardo 2006) and consideration should be given to changing the cannula site after 24 hours (Wilkes 2018).

Table 15.12 Examples of vesicant cytotoxic and non-cytotoxic drugs in common use

Group A drugs	Group B drugs
Vinblastine	Amsacrine
Vindesine	Carmustine (concentrated solution)
Vinorelbine	Dacarbazine (concentrated solution)
Vincristine	Dactinomycin
Vinflunine	Daunorubicin
Paclitaxel	Doxorubicin
Calcium chloride	Epirubicin
Calcium gluconate	Amrubicin
Phenytoin	Actinomycin D
Hypertonic solutions (e.g. sodium chloride >0.9%)	Mitomycin C
Sodium bicarbonate (>5%)	Idarubicin
Glucose 50%	Mechlorethamine
	Streptozocin
	Aciclovir
	Amphotericin
	Cefotaxime
	Diazepam
	Ganciclovir
	Mannitol
	Potssium chloride (>40 mmol/L)
	Potassium phosphate
	Thiopental

Table 15.13 Possible causes of extravasation

Peripheral devices	Central venous access devices
• Vein wall puncture or trauma • Dislodgement of the cannula from the vein • Administration of a vesicant in a vein below a recent venepuncture or cannulation site (<24 hours)	• Perforation of the vein • Catheter leakage, rupture or fracture • Separation of the catheter from the portal body of an implanted port • Incomplete insertion of needle into an implanted port • Needle dislodgement from an implanted port • Fibrin sheath – leading to backflow of drug along the catheter from the insertion site

Source: Adapted from Mayo (1998), Polovich et al. (2014), Schulmeister (1998).

However, if the fluid runs freely, there is good blood return, and there are no signs of erythema, pain or swelling at the site, there is no reason to inflict a second cannulation on the patient (Weinstein and Hagle 2014). Consideration should be given to use of a CVAD if peripheral access is difficult; a decision-making tool can assist with this, for example the Vessel Health and Preservation tool (Hallam et al. 2016) – see Chapter 17: Vascular access devices: insertion and management.

Location of the device

The most appropriate site for a peripheral cannula is considered to be the forearm (Pérez Fidalgo et al. 2012, Polovich et al. 2014, Weinstein and Hagle 2014). However, a large, straight vein on the dorsum of the hand is preferable to a smaller vein in the forearm (Weinstein and Hagle 2014). Siting over joints should be avoided as tissue damage in this area may limit joint movement in the future. It is also recommended that the antecubital fossa should never be used for the administration of vesicants because of the risk of damage to local structures such as nerves and tendons (Gabriel 2008, Weinstein and Hagle 2014). Avoid venepuncture sites in limbs with impaired circulation, sclerosis, thrombosis or scar formation. Also avoid cannulation below a recent venepuncture site (Goolsby and Lombardo 2006). Use of the ipsilateral limb in women post-mastectomy is controversial, but it can be considered where lymphoedema is absent (Pérez Fidalgo et al. 2012).

Box 15.17 Patients at risk of extravasation

- Infants and young children
- Elderly patients
- Patients who are unable to communicate, due to sedation, unconsciousness, confusion or language issues
- Patients with chronic diseases, for example cancer, peripheral vascular disease, superior vena cava syndrome or lymphoedema
- Patients on anticoagulants or steroids
- Patients who have undergone repeated intravenous cannulation or venepuncture
- Patients with fragile veins or who are thrombocytopenic
- Obese patients, due to increased difficulty in locating and palpating a vein, and reduced ability to observe any swelling
- Malnourished patients
- Patients with skin disorders such as eczema or psoriasis
- Restless patients

Source: Adapted from Goolsby and Lombardo (2006), Polovich et al. (2014), Sauerland et al. (2006), Wilkes and Barton-Burke (2011).

Table 15.14 Drug sequencing: rationales for administering vesicant drugs first or last

Vesicants first	Vesicants last
• Vascular integrity decreases over time • Vein is most stable and least irritated at start of treatment • Initial assessment of vein patency is most accurate • Patient's awareness of changes will be more acute at the start of treatment	• Vesicants are irritating and increase vein fragility • Venous spasm may occur and mask signs of extravasation

Source: Adapted from Weinstein and Hagle (2014), Wilkes (2018).

Sequence of drugs

While there is some variation in opinion on the optimal order of administration (Table 15.14), vesicants should be administered first (Goolsby and Lombardo 2006, Wilkes 2018).

Methods of administration

Many vesicants must be given as a slow bolus injection, often via the side arm of a fast-running intravenous infusion of a compatible solution, for example doxorubicin or epirubicin via an infusion of 0.9% sodium chloride. If repeated infusions are to be given then use of a CVAD may be appropriate (Stanley 2002, Weinstein and Hagle 2014).

Monitoring the site and early recognition of extravasation

Confirm venous patency by flushing with 0.9% sodium chloride solution with at least 5–10 mL prior to administration of vesicants and monitor frequently thereafter (Goolsby and Lombardo 2006, Weinstein and Hagle 2014). Checking blood return after every 2–5 mL is recommended but cannot be relied upon as the key sign when giving a bolus injection; monitor the site every 5–10 minutes for any swelling (Weinstein and Hagle 2014).

It is important that the nurse does not rely on infusion pumps to raise an alarm about downstream occlusion and alert them to an infiltration or extravasation (Huber and Augustine 2009, INS 2016, Marders 2012) (Table 15.15 and Box 15.18).

Table 15.16 Nursing assessment of extravasation

Assessment parameter	Flare reaction	Venous irritation	Immediate manifestations of extravasation, i.e. during drug administration	Delayed manifestations, i.e. from 24 hours after extravasation
Pain	None	Aching, throbbing sensation along vein and in the limb	Severe stinging or burning pain (not always present); this can last from minutes to hours and will eventually subside; occurs during drug administration at the device site and surrounding areas	Can continue following extravasation or start within 48 hours; pain may intensify over time
Redness	Immediate blotches or tracking along the vein; this will subside within 30–45 minutes with or without treatment (usually steroid cream)	Vein may become red or darkened	Not always present immediately; more likely to see blanching of the skin; as the area becomes inflamed, redness will appear around the device site	Later occurrence
Swelling	Unlikely	Unlikely	May occur immediately but may not always be easy to identify immediately	Usually within 48 hours
Blood return	Usually present	Usually present and may require application of heat to improve blood return	Inability to obtain blood return (peripheral or central) but blood return may be present throughout	None
Ulceration	Unlikely	Unlikely	Unlikely	Can occur within 48–96 hours but may take 3–4 weeks to develop
Others	Urticaria	None	Change in quality of the infusion or pressure on the syringe	Local tingling and sensory deficits

Box 15.18 Signs and symptoms of extravasation

- The patient complains of *burning, stinging pain or any other acute change at the injection site*, although this is not always present (Polovich et al. 2014, Wilkes 2018). This should be distinguished from a feeling of cold (which may occur with some drugs) or venous spasm (which can be caused by irritation and is usually accompanied by pain described as an achiness or tightness) (Wilkes 2018). Any change of sensation warrants further investigation (Goolsby and Lombardo 2006).
- *Swelling* is a common symptom (Polovich et al. 2014). Induration or leakage may also occur at the injection site. Swelling may not always be immediately obvious if the patient has the cannula sited in an area of deep subcutaneous fat or in a deep vein, or if the leak is via the posterior vein wall (Dougherty 2008b).
- *Blanching of the skin* occurs (Terry 2017). Erythema can occur around the injection site but this is not usually present immediately (Wilkes 2018). It is important that this is distinguished from a flare reaction (Polovich et al. 2014).
- *Blood return* is one of the most misleading of all signs, particularly related to peripheral devices. In peripheral devices, if blood return is sluggish or absent, this may indicate lack of patency or incorrect position of the device. However, if no other signs are apparent, this should not be regarded as an indication of a non-patent vein, as a vein may not bleed back for a number of reasons and extravasation may occur even in the event of good blood return as the device may still be in the vein but the leak may be in the posterior vein wall (Wilkes 2018). Any change in blood flow should be investigated (Weinstein and Hagle 2014, Wilkes 2018). In central venous access devices, there should always be blood return; if this is absent, steps should be followed to verify correct tip and needle position or resolve a fibrin sheath (see Chapter 17: Vascular access devices: insertion and management and Figure 17.4).
- A *resistance* is felt on the plunger of the syringe if drugs are given by bolus (Stanley 2002).
- There is *absence of free flow* when administration is by infusion, once other reasons have been excluded, for example position (Polovich et al. 2014, Stanley 2002).
- There is *leaking* around the intravenous cannula or implanted port needle (Polovich et al. 2014).

Note: one or more of the above may be present. If extravasation is suspected or confirmed, the injection or infusion must be stopped immediately and action must be taken (INS 2016, Polovich et al. 2014, Weinstein and Hagle 2014).

Clinical governance

Competencies

Nurses are now being named in malpractice allegations, and infiltration and extravasation injuries are an area for concern (Dougherty 2003, Masoorli 2003, Roth 2003, Weinstein and Hagle 2014). Therefore, it is vital that nurses have the necessary level of knowledge and skills in order to:

- correctly choose the device and location
- understand the medication and whether it is a vesicant
- use the most appropriate vasodilation techniques

- recognize infiltration and extravasation early, and take prompt action (Dougherty 2008b, Goolsby and Lombardo 2006, Sauerland et al. 2006, Schrijvers 2003).

Successful cannulation at the first attempt is ideal, as vesicants have been known to seep into tissues at a vein entry site of a previous cannulation (Cault and Challands 1997). This also includes accessing a port as it is vital that the correct needle is selected and that the device is secured adequately (Camp-Sorrell and Cope 2011).

Consent

Patients should be informed of the potential problems when administering vesicants and the possible consequences of extravasation (Polovich et al. 2014, Sauerland et al. 2006, Stanley 2002, Weinstein and Hagle 2014). Giving adequate information to patients will help to ensure early recognition and co-operation as patients are the first to notice pain. Patients should be urged to report any change in sensation, such as burning or stinging, immediately (Goolsby and Lombardo 2006).

Pre-procedural considerations

Equipment

The use of extravasation kits is widely recommended in order to provide immediate management (Doornaert et al. 2013, Pérez Fidalgo et al. 2012). Kits should be assembled according to the particular needs of individual institutions. They should be kept in all areas where staff are regularly administering vesicant drugs, so that staff have immediate access to equipment (Gabriel 2008, Pérez Fidalgo et al. 2012). Kits should be simple, to avoid confusion, but comprehensive enough to meet all reasonable needs (Wilkes 2018) (see Procedure guideline 15.26: Extravasation management: peripheral cannula). Instructions should be clear and easy to follow, and the use of a flowchart enables staff to follow the management procedure in easy steps (Figure 15.42).

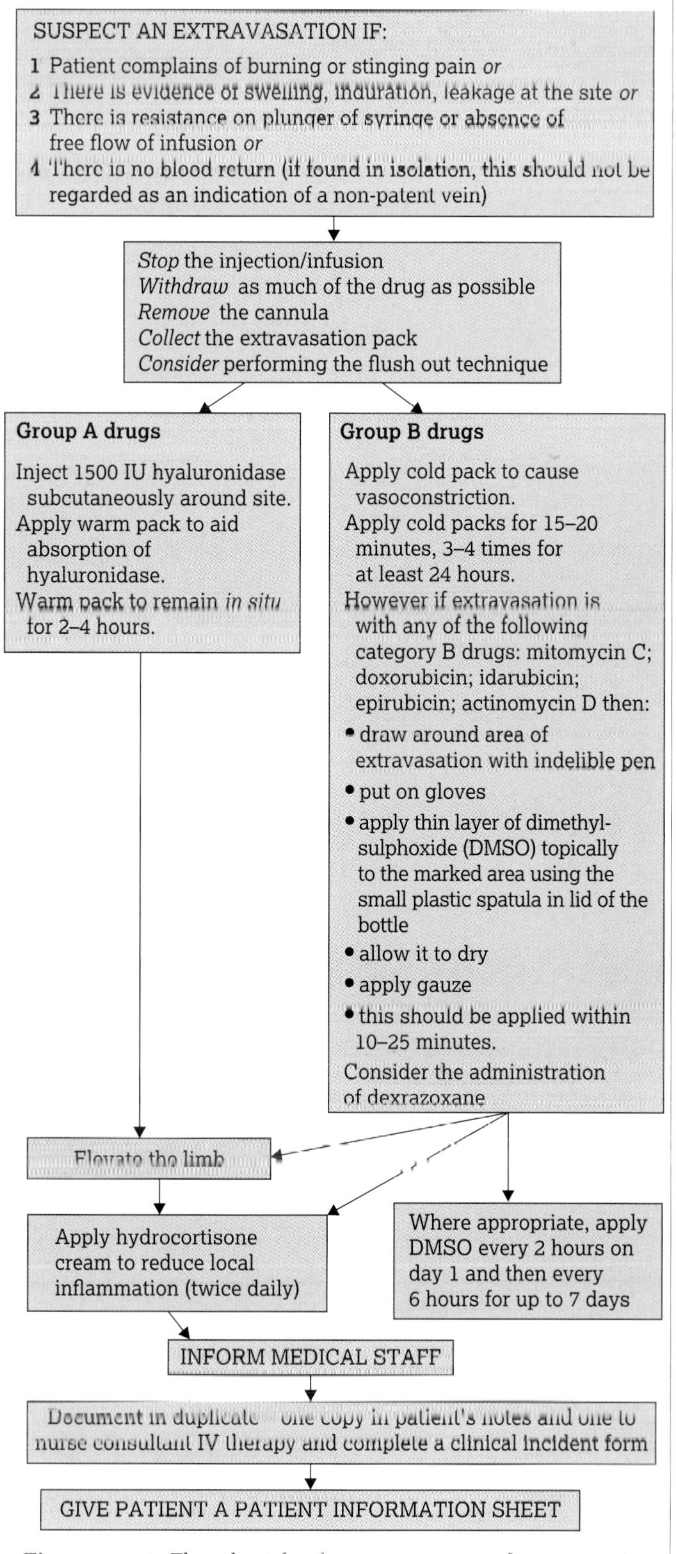

Figure 15.42 Flowchart for the management of extravasation.

Assessment and recording tools

Decision-making tools have been developed both nationally and locally to address issues related to selecting the correct vascular access device (Hallam et al. 2016) and to help with grading infiltration (INS 2016). See Figure 15.43 for an example and also consult the Vessel Health and Preservation tool (Hallam et al. 2016) in Chapter 17: Vascular access devices: insertion and management.

Pharmacological support

A number of 'antidotes' are available, but there is a lack of scientific evidence to demonstrate their value, with no randomized controlled trials establishing the role of any of the agents currently available, meaning their role is unclear (Polovich et al. 2014). There is therefore variation in what individual institutions recommend. There appear to be two main methods by which 'antidotes' work:

- localize and neutralize
- spread and dilute (Stanley 2002).

Administration of injectable antidotes (if not via cannula) is carried out using the pincushion technique – that is, instilling small volumes around and over the areas affected using a small-gauge (25 G) needle, as if moving towards the centre of a clock face. The procedure causes considerable discomfort to patients and if large areas are to be tackled, analgesia should be considered (Stanley 2002).

The following are the most widely accepted pharmacological treatments for extravasation

Hyaluronidase

Hyaluronidase is an enzyme that breaks down hyaluronic acid, a normal component of tissue 'cement', and helps to reduce or prevent tissue damage by allowing rapid (within 10 minutes) diffusion of the extravasated drug (Pérez Fidalgo et al. 2012) and restoration of tissue permeability within 24–48 hours (Doellman et al. 2009, INS 2016). The usual dose is 1500 international units (BNF 2019a). It should be injected within 1 hour of extravasation, ideally through the intravenous device delivering the enzyme to the same tissue (Pérez Fidalgo et al. 2012, Weinstein and Hagle 2014). Hyaluronidase is recommended for use with specific chemotherapy agents, specifically vinca alkaloids (Pérez Fidalgo et al. 2012; Polovich et al. 2014) and also taxanes (Pérez Fidalgo et al. 2012).

Any drug to be delivered by a continuous ambulatory drug delivery system or TPN must be administered via central venous access.

Patient Identification label		Date	
	Regimen		
	Planned length of treatment		

Vein assessment	Yes	No	
Absence of larger palpable veins			*Does the patient have accessible peripheral veins of sufficient quality suitable to provide the required level of venous access? Does your team have the necessary skill level to establish peripheral venous access for the patient at every visit?*
Extensive oedema/adipose tissue over forearms			
Inadequate venous fill of target veins			
Significant vein wall rigidity			
Significant cellulitis of forearm and/or upper arms			

Vein availability	Yes	No	
Axillary lymph node clearance			*Will the patient have accessible peripheral veins available for the proposed term of treatment (accounting for vein rotation and deterioration)?*
Upper limb/axilla/SVC venous thrombosis			
Extensive skin lesions – forearms			
Previous CVA			
Thrombo-phlebitis present			

VAD insertion & patency factors	Yes	No	
Fragile skin quality			*Is there an increased risk of cannula dislodgement, haematoma formation or thrombo-phlebitis for the patient with peripheral venous access? Is there an increased risk of infection for this patient? e.g. long-term steroid therapy*
Decreased platelets $<50 \times 10^9$/L			
Anticoagulant therapy i.e warfarin, aspirin, LMW heparin			
Anxiety/needle phobia			

Factors affecting long-term venous access patency			
Vesicant and/or irritant therapy for >6 cycles			*Will the patient be receiving therapy where intensive fluid management will be required (such as concentrated electrolytes)? Is there an increased risk of vein deterioration and thrombo phlebitis in the patient? Would a skin tunnelled catheter or implanted port offer a lower risk of site infection for the patient?*
Anticipated intensive IV therapy, i.e. blood products, electrolyte support, fluid support, multiple antimicrobial therapy			
Expected periods of sustained neutropenia ($<0.5 \times 10^9$/L for >7 days)			

Co-morbidities that may affect peripheral venous access	Yes	No	
Diabetes			*The effects of co-morbidities individual to the patient must be accounted when undertaking a venous access assessment. Would the patient be able to cope with the presence of a CVAD and notify the team appropriately to report adverse events?*
Peripheral vascular disease			
Raynaud's phenomenon			
Hypotension			
Other (please state):			
Other (please state):			

Practitioner recommended venous access device:	
Comments:	
Patient & practitioner agreed venous access device:	
Comments:	

Figure 15.43 Vascular access device decision tool. CVA, cerebrovascular accident; CVAD, central venous access device; IV, intravenous; LMW, low molecular weight; SVC, superior vena cava; TPN, total parenteral nutrition.

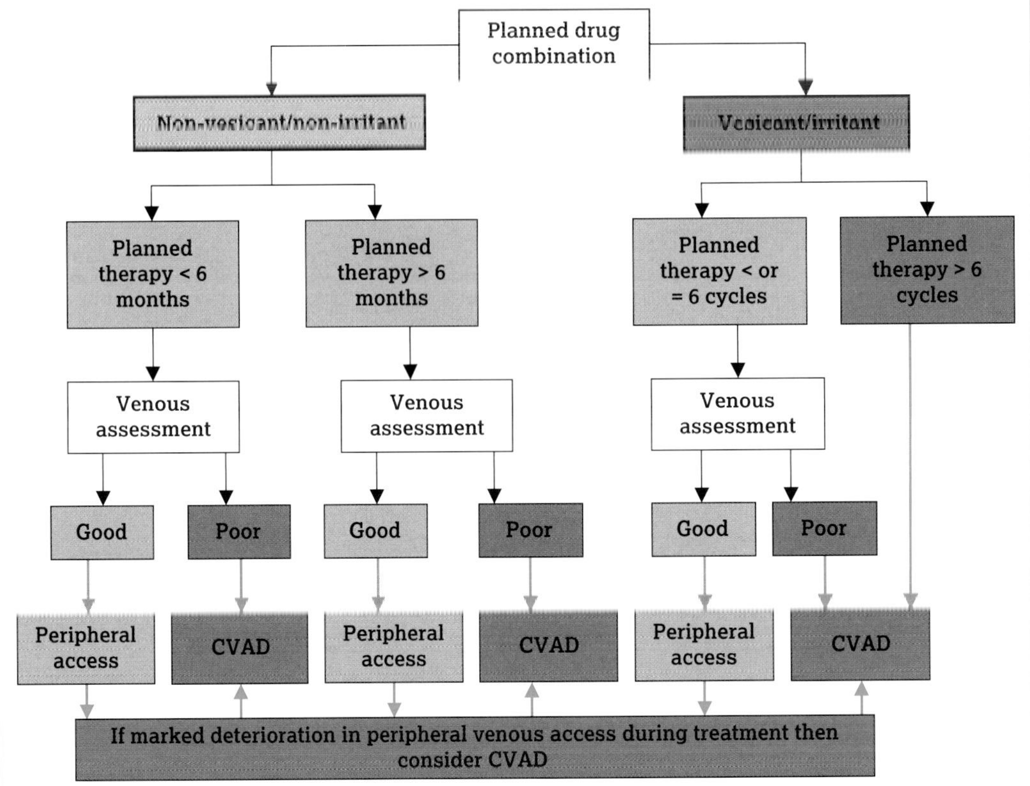

Figure 15.43 *Continued*

Note that hyaluronidase increases the absorption of local anaesthetic. Therefore, if local anaesthetic has been applied to the area (e.g. Ametop gel prior to cannulation) within 6 hours of extravasation, the patient should be monitored for signs and symptoms of systemic anaesthesia, such as increased pulse rate and decreased respirations, and the doctor should be informed immediately (BNF 2019a).

Corticosteroids

While corticosteroids were advocated as a treatment for anthracycline extravasation in the past, due to their action on inflammatory processes, there is no evidence that tissue damage in extravasation is secondary to inflammation (Buter et al. 2019). As a result, they are not usually recommended, except in large-volume extravasations of oxaliplatin (Pérez Fidalgo et al. 2012, Polovich et al. 2014). However, given as a cream, they can help to reduce local trauma and irritation (Stanley 2002) and are often recommended in this form.

Dimethylsulphoxide (DMSO)

DMSO is a topically applied solvent that may improve systematic absorption of vesicants. It acts as a potent free radical scavanger that rapidly penetrates tissues and prevents DNA damage (Doellman et al. 2009, Pérez Fidalgo et al. 2012). Reports on the clinical use of topical DMSO show it is effective and well tolerated in extravasation (Bertelli 1995, Pérez Fidalgo et al. 2012). However, this is based on the use of a high-dose (99%) solution, which is not always available (Pérez Fidalgo et al. 2012). Side-effects of DMSO include itching, erythema, mild burning and a characteristic breath odour (Bertelli 1995).

Dexrazoxane (Savene)

Dexrazoxane (more specifically, the branded drug Savene) is a topoisomerase II catalytic inhibitor traditionally used clinically to minimize the cardiotoxicity of doxorubicin. It was first tested in animals (Langer et al. 2000) and then in a small number of patients for its use in extravasation (Doroshow 2012). It is given intravenously as soon as possible after extravasation and it appears to reduce the wound size and duration of tissue damage with anthracyclines. Triple dosage appears to be more effective than a single dose (El-Saghir et al. 2004, Langer et al. 2000). In two multicentre studies, it was shown that the administration of dexrazoxane reduced the need for surgical interventions, and late sequelae (such as pain, fibrosis, atrophy and sensory disturbance) were judged as mild (Doroshow 2012, Mouridsen et al. 2007).

A consensus group (Jackson 2006) has developed recommendations for the use of dexrazoxane, and these have been further adapted by the European Oncology Nursing Society (2007), which recommends that for anthracycline extravasations resulting from peripheral administration, the site expert or team should be consulted in order to determine whether the use of dexrazoxane is indicated. Absolute indications are if the peripherally extravasated volume exceeds 3–5 mL and in the event of a CVAD extravasation (Langer 2008). Dexrazoxane is now included in many treatment algorithms for anthracycline extravasations (Gonzalez 2013, INS 2016, Pérez Fidalgo et al. 2012, Roe 2011, Vidall et al. 2013).

Granulocyte-macrophage colony-stimulating factor

Granulocyte-macrophage colony-stimulating factor (GM-CSF) is a growth factor. It is effective in accelerating wound healing and inducing formation of granulation tissue (El-Saghir et al. 2004, Ulutin et al. 2000).

Non-pharmacological support

Stopping infusion or injection and aspirating the drug

It appears that most authors agree that aspirating as much of the drug as possible, as soon as extravasation is suspected, is beneficial (Polovich et al. 2014, Rudolph and Larson 1987, Weinstein and Hagle 2014) and can help to lower the concentration of the drug in the area (Goolsby and Lombardo 2006). However, withdrawal is only possible immediately during bolus injections, because if the drug were being delivered via an infusion, this would need to be stopped and a syringe attached in an attempt to aspirate. Aspiration may be successful if extravasation presents as a raised blister, but it may be unsuccessful if the tissue is soft and soggy (Stanley 2002). In practice, it may achieve little and often distresses the patient (Gault and Challands 1997). The likelihood of withdrawing blood, as suggested by Ignoffo and Friedman (1980), is small and the practitioner may waste valuable time attempting this, which could lead to delay in the rest of the management procedure.

Removing the device

Some clinicians advocate that the peripheral vascular access device be left *in situ* in order to instil the antidote into the affected tissues via the device (Kassner 2000, Stanley 2002, Weinstein and Hagle 2014). However, others recommend that the peripheral device should be removed to prevent any injected solution increasing the size of the affected area (Rudolph and Larson 1987). There appears to be no research evidence to support either practice. It is therefore important to adhere to local institutional policies.

Application of hot or cold packs

Cooling appears to be a better choice, with the exception of the vinca alkaloids and some non-cytotoxic drugs, than warming (Bertelli 1995, Buter et al. 2019). Cold causes vasoconstriction, localizing the extravasation and perhaps allowing time for the local vascular and lymphatic systems to contain the drug (INS 2016). It should be applied for 15–20 minutes, 3–4 times a day for up to 3 days (Polovich et al. 2014, Wilkes 2018). Heat promotes healing after the first 24 hours by increasing the blood supply (Polovich et al. 2014, Weinstein and Hagle 2014). It also decreases local drug concentration, increasing the blood flow, which results in enhanced resolution of pain and reabsorption of any localized swelling.

Elevation of limb

Elevation of the limb is widely recommended as it minimizes swelling (Buter et al. 2019). This can be achieved by use of a Bradford sling, but this is usually recommended when the extravasation has occurred in the hand. Gentle movement should be encouraged to prevent adhesion of damaged areas to underlying tissue (Gabriel 2008, INS 2016).

Surgical techniques

It is now recognized that a plastic surgery consultation should form part of the management procedure in order to consider debridement of the affected area, although there are no standard procedures for surgical management (Boulanger et al. 2015). Surgical intervention should be considered, especially if the lesion is larger than 2 cm, if there is significant residual pain 1–2 weeks after extravasation or if there is minimal healing 2–3 weeks after injury despite local therapeutic measures (Goolsby and Lombardo 2006, Pérez Fidalgo et al. 2012). A liposuction cannula can be used to aspirate extravasated material, and subcutaneous fat or a flush-out technique can remove the extravasated drug without resorting to excision and skin grafting.

Flush-out technique

If there is little subcutaneous fat, then the saline flush-out technique is recommended, particularly if it is done within the first 24 hours (Dionyssiou et al. 2011, Gault 1993). It has been suggested as a less traumatic and cheaper procedure than surgery. Only appropriately trained doctors and nurses may perform the flush-out technique, and it may only be used for superficial peripheral extravasations where there is no visible skin damage or extensive swelling (Dougherty and Oakley 2011). A number of small stab incisions are made and large volumes of 0.9% sodium chloride are administered, which flush out the extravasated drug (Dougherty and Oakley 2011, Gault and Challands 1997) (see Procedure guideline 15.27: Extravasation: performing flush-out following an extravasation).

Management of infiltration

Treatment is often dependent upon the severity of the infiltration. There should be ongoing observation and assessment of the infiltrated site. The presence and severity of the infiltration should be documented. Infiltration statistics should include frequency, severity and type of infusate. The infiltration rate should be calculated according to a standard formula (INS 2016, RCN 2016).

Procedure guideline 15.26 Extravasation management: peripheral cannula

This procedure relates specifically to the management of extravasation of a drug from a peripheral cannula.

Essential equipment

- Personal protective equipment
- Gel packs × 2: one to be kept in the fridge and one available for heating (an electric heating blanket can be used while the pack is heating)
- 2 mL syringe
- 25 G needle
- 23 G needle
- Alcohol swabs
- Documentation forms
- Copy of extravasation management procedure
- Patient information leaflet
- Prescription chart

Medicinal products

- Hyaluronidase (1500 international units) and 2 mL sterile water for injection
- Hydrocortisone cream 1% (15 g tube)
- Savene (dexrazoxane) (optional)
- DMSO (dimethylsulphoxide) topical solution (99%)

Action	Rationale
Pre-procedure	
1 Introduce yourself to the patient, explain and discuss the procedure with them, and gain their consent to proceed.	To ensure that the patient feels at ease, understands the procedure and gives their valid consent (NMC 2018, **C**).

(continued)

Procedure guideline 15.26 Extravasation management: peripheral cannula *(continued)*

Action	Rationale
2 Wash hands with bactericidal soap and water or an alcohol-based handrub.	To minimize the risk of infection (DH 2007, **C**; Fraise and Bradley 2009, **E**).
Procedure	
3 Stop the injection or infusion *immediately*, leaving the cannula in place.	To minimize local injury. To allow aspiration of the drug to be attempted (Polovich et al. 2014, **C**; RCN 2016, **C**).
4 Aspirate any residual drug from the device and suspected extravasation site.	To minimize local injury by removing as much drug as possible (but only attempt if appropriate). Subsequent damage is related to the volume of the extravasation, in addition to other factors (Polovich et al. 2014, **C**; RCN 2016, **C**).
5 Consider removing the cannula.	Some sources recommend doing this to prevent the device from being used for antidote administration (Rudolph and Larson 1987, **E**). Others state that the cannula may be used to instil antidote to the affected tissue (Kassner 2000, **E**; Stanley 2002, **E**; Weinstein and Hagle 2014, **E**).
6 Consider contacting the extravasation team and whether the flush-out technique would be appropriate (see Figure 15.42).	Flush-out is most effective if undertaken as soon as extravasation is suspected (Dionyssiou et al. 2011, **E**).
7 Collect an extravasation pack and take it to the patient.	It contains all the equipment necessary for managing extravasation (Dougherty 2010, **E**; Stanley 2002, **E**).
8 *Either:*	
For Group A drugs (see Table 15.12):	
• Draw up 1500 international units of hyaluronidase in 1 mL sterile water for injection and inject volumes of 0.1–0.2 mL subcutaneously at points of the clock around the circumference of the area of extravasation. • Apply warm pack.	This is the recommended agent for Group A drugs. The warm pack speeds up absorption of the drug by the tissues (Polovich et al. 2014, Weinstein and Hagle 2014, **E**).
Or:	
For Group B drugs (see Table 15.12) (except those listed below):	
• Apply cold pack or ice instantly.	To localize the area of extravasation, slow cell metabolism and decrease the area of tissue destruction. To reduce local pain (Polovich et al. 2014, **C**).
Or:	
If extravasation is with any of the following category B drugs: mitomycin C, doxorubicin, idarubicin, epirubicin, actinomycin D:	
• Draw around the area of extravasation with an indelible pen. • Put on gloves. • Apply a thin layer of DMSO topically to the marked area using the small plastic spatula in the lid of the bottle. Allow it to dry. • Apply gauze. • This should be applied within 10–25 minutes.	DMSO is the recommended agent for these anthracyclines and helps to reduce local tissue damage (Bertelli 1995, **E**, Pérez Fidalgo et al. 2012, **C**).
Or:	
If extravasation of doxorubicin, epirubicin, idarubicin or daunorubicin occurs (i.e. 5 mL or more peripherally or any volume from a central venous access device) then stop use of the cold pack, do not apply DMSO and contact a member of the extravasation team to advise on use of dexrazoxane.	Cooling and DMSO interfere with the efficacy of dexrazaxone and it should be administered as soon as possible after extravasation of these drugs (El-Saghir et al. 2004, **E**; Langer et al. 2000, **E**).
9 Where possible, elevate the extremity and/or encourage movement.	To minimize swelling and prevent adhesion of the damaged area to underlying tissue, which could result in restriction of movement (Buter et al. 2019, **E**).
Post-procedure	
10 Inform a member of the medical staff at the earliest opportunity and administer any other prescribed antidotes, for example dexrazoxane.	To enable actions differing from agreed policy to be taken if considered in the best interests of the patient. To notify the doctor of the need to prescribe any other drugs. **E**

11	Apply hydrocortisone cream 1% twice daily, and instruct the patient on how to do this. Continue as long as erythema persists.	To reduce local inflammation and promote patient comfort (Stanley 2002, **E**).
12	Where appropriate, apply DMSO every 2 hours on day 1 and then every 6 hours for up to 7 days (patients will need to have this prescribed as a 'to take out' (TTO) and continue treatment at home where necessary).	To help reduce local tissue damage (Bertelli 1995, **E**).
13	Heat packs (for Group A drugs) should be reapplied after initial management for 2–4 hours. Cold packs (for Group B drugs) should be applied for 15–20 minutes, 3–4 times a day for up to 3 days.	To localize the steroid effect in the area of extravasation. To reduce local pain and promote patient comfort (Bertelli 1995, **E**).
14	Provide analgesia as required.	To promote patient comfort. To encourage movement of the limb as advised. **E**
15	Dispose of waste in appropriate containers.	To ensure safe disposal and avoid laceration or injury to other staff (EASHW 2010, **C**; HWR 2005, **C**).
16	Document the following details, in duplicate, on the form provided: a patient's name/number b ward/unit c date and time d signs and symptoms e cannulation site (on diagram) f drug sequence g drug administration technique, i.e. bolus or infusion h approximate amount of the drug extravasated i diameter, length and width of extravasation area j appearance of the area k step-by-step management with date and time of each step performed and medical officer notification l patient's complaints, comments and statements m indication that the patient information sheet has been given to the patient n follow-up actions required over subsequent days o whether photograph was taken p if required, when patient referred to plastic surgeon q signature of the nurse.	To provide an immediate and full record of all details of the incident that may be referred to if necessary. To provide a baseline for future observation and monitoring of the patient's condition. To comply with professional guidelines (RCN 2016, **C**; RPS 2019a, **C**; Schulmeister 2009, **E**; Weinstein and Hagle 2014, **E**).
17	Explain to the patient that the site may remain sore for several days.	To reduce anxiety and ensure continued co-operation. **E**
18	As part of the follow-up, all patients should receive written information explaining what has occurred, what management has been carried out, what they need to look for at the site and when to report any changes. For example, increased discomfort, peeling or blistering of the skin should be reported immediately.	To detect any changes as early as possible and allow for a review of future management. This may include referral to a plastic surgeon (Gault and Challands 1997, **E**; Polovich et al. 2014, **C**; RCN 2016, **C**).
19	Observe the area regularly for erythema, induration, blistering or necrosis. Where appropriate, take photographs. *Inpatients*: monitor daily.	To detect any changes at the earliest possible moment (RCN 2016, **C**).
20	If blistering or tissue breakdown occurs, begin dressing techniques and seek advice regarding wound management.	To minimize the risk of a superimposed infection and increase healing (Naylor 2005, **E**).
21	Depending on size of lesion, degree of pain and type of drug, consider referral to plastic surgeon.	To prevent further pain and other complications, as chemically induced ulcers rarely heal spontaneously (Dougherty 2010, **E**; Polovich et al. 2014, **C**).

Procedure guideline 15.27 Extravasation: performing flush-out following an extravasation

This procedure would begin once the immediate management of extravasation (i.e. stop the infusion or injection, aspirate any drug if possible, apply appropriate pack and elevate limb) has been performed.

Essential equipment

- Personal protective equipment
- Sterile gloves
- Eye protection
- Disposable gown
- 20 mL Luer-Lok syringe
- 10 mL Luer-Lok syringe
- 5 mL Luer-Lok syringe
- 25 G needle
- 23 G needle × 2
- Disposable scalpel (size 11)
- Bandage
- Sterile pack (containing gauze, drapes/towels and gallipot)
- Cleaning solution (2% chlorhexidine Chloraprep 3 mL)
- Blunt needle, or 18 G or 20 G cannula × 4
- Three-way tap with extension set
- Blank labels for syringes
- Solution administration set
- Sterile marker pen
- Plastic-backed towel (e.g. incontinence pad)
- Transparent dressing (large)
- Sterile scissors
- Extra gauze swabs

Medicinal products

- 1% lidocaine (10 mL) (kept at room temperature)
- Hyaluronidase (1500 international units) and 2 mL sterile water for injection
- Mepitel dressing
- 500 mL 0.9% sodium chloride infusion bag

Action	Rationale
Pre-procedure	
1 Introduce yourself to the patient, explain and discuss the procedure with them, and gain their consent to proceed.	To ensure that the patient feels at ease, understands the procedure and gives their valid consent (NMC 2018, **C**).
2 Ascertain what emergency treatment has been carried out. For example, was hyaluronidase administered?	To ensure that only required treatment is carried out; for example, if hyaluronidase has been given, no further dose would be administered as this could result in a sensitivity reaction. **E**
3 Assemble all of the equipment necessary for the procedure.	To ensure that time is not wasted and the procedure goes smoothly without any unnecessary interruptions. **E**
4 Check all packaging before opening and preparing the equipment to be used.	To maintain asepsis throughout and check that no equipment is damaged or out of date (Fraise and Bradley 2009, **E**).
5 Wash hands using bactericidal soap and water or an alcohol-based handrub and dry.	To minimize the risk of infection (DH 2007, **C**).
6 Place the patient's arm on a plastic-backed towel.	To prevent leakage of the flushed-out solution and possible contamination of the area with cytotoxic drugs. **E**
7 Apply a disposable gown and eye protection.	To prevent contamination of the practitioner with cytotoxic drugs. **E**
8 Open a pack, empty all equipment onto the pack and place a sterile dressing towel under the patient's arm.	To create a sterile working area. **E**
9 Wash hands using bactericidal soap and water.	To minimize the risk of infection (DH 2007, **C**; Fraise and Bradley 2009, **E**).
10 Apply sterile gloves.	To minimize the risk of infection and prevent contamination of the nurse (DH 2007, **C**; Fraise and Bradley 2009, **E**).
11 Clean the skin with 2% chlorhexidine and allow the area to dry.	To maintain asepsis and remove skin flora (DH 2007, **C**; Fraise and Bradley 2009, **E**).
Procedure	
12 Draw up 1% lidocaine in a 10 mL syringe.	To prepare for infiltration of the area. **E**
13 Mix the hyaluronidase with sterile water in a separate 5 mL syringe.	To ensure the drug is reconstituted correctly (BNF 2019a, **C**).

14 Mark the area of extravasation with a sterile marker; this is where incisions will be made.	To ensure the correct area is treated. **E**
15 Using a 25 G needle, make a small bleb by inserting the needle intradermally and administering 0.1–2 mL of lidocaine slowly as if towards the points of a clock face. Allow it to take effect.	To reduce any discomfort to the patient. **E**
16 Then, using a 23 G needle, infiltrate the marked area with lidocaine subdermally as if towards the points of a clock face. Check with the patient what kind of sensation they can feel (e.g. sharp or dull) before proceeding.	To ensure administration of anaesthetic to the area and to ensure the anaesthetic has taken effect. **E**
17 Attach a 23 G needle to the syringe of hyaluronidase and infiltrate the anaesthetized area towards the points of a clock face.	To facilitate the flush-out by loosening the tissues. **E**
18 Cut an opening in a transparent dressing that matches the size of the infiltrated area and apply it to the patient's skin.	To protect the skin from the flushed-out vesicant drugs. **E**
19 Attach the administration set, three-way tap and extension set to the bag of 0.9% sodium chloride and withdraw 20 mL via the tap.	To prepare the syringe and to enable continued access without having to open the system. **E**
20 Make at least four incisions around a clock face using a size 11 scalpel by inserting the blade straight down to a depth of no more than 0.5 cm. Make one further small incision to use for insertion of the cannula.	To prepare the area for flushing. The number of incisions will depend on the size of the area to be treated. To reduce risk of damage to tendons and other anatomical structures (Gault 1993, **E**).
21 Gently press on the area.	This alone may allow the fluid to escape (Gault 1993, **E**).
22 Insert the cannula through one of the incisions and push along tissues within the marked area.	To free up tissues from the skin and to aid advancement of the cannula and flush (Gault 1993, **E**).
23 Remove the stylet and attach the extension set to the cannula.	To facilitate the flushing. **E**
24 Flush the 0.9% sodium chloride through – it will exit out of the other incision holes. Pat with a sterile gauze swab, massaging and milking the area at the same time. The area will become puffy and swollen – this is normal.	To commence the flushing procedure. To assist with removal of saline (Gault 1993, **E**).
25 Draw up more 0.9% sodium chloride and repeat the procedure using a minimum of 100 mL (up to 500 mL) of 0.9% sodium chloride.	To facilitate the flushing of the drug from the area (Gault 1993, **E**).
26 If saline does not flow out of one incision, it may be necessary to remove the cannula from the original incision and insert a new cannula into another one.	To ensure all areas are flushed. **E**
Post-procedure	
27 Remove the transparent dressing and clean and dry the area, although it will continue to leak.	To promote patient comfort. **E**
28 Apply a Mepitel dressing and a loose bandage (do not wrap tightly).	To reduce the risk of infection and to prevent compression of the skin. **E**
29 Elevate the limb so that the hand is level with the head whenever the patient is at rest.	To aid reduction of oedema. **E**
30 Discard waste in appropriate containers.	To ensure safe disposal in the correct containers and avoid laceration or injury of other staff (EASHW 2010, **C**; HWR 2005, **C**).
31 Document the procedure in the patient's medical and nursing notes and on the flush-out technique form.	To ensure adequate records are kept and enable continued care of the patient (NMC 2018, **C**).
32 Discuss with medical colleagues the prescribing of oral antibiotics (flucloxacillin is recommended to reduce skin pathogens) and if necessary analgesia.	If the patient is neutropenic, they may be more at risk of infection. To minimize pain and discomfort. **E**
33 Refer to a plastic surgeon if there are any problems during the procedure or if there are any skin problems.	To ensure rapid access for further management. **E**
34 Monitor and review within the first 24 hours. Have photographs taken if possible.	To observe and document for any skin changes or infection and provide immediate treatment. **E**
35 Change the dressing every 48 hours and ensure that it remains *in situ* for up to a week. The skin incisions will heal within 1–2 weeks.	To reduce the risk of infection. **E**
36 Ensure the patient knows when and how to make contact if they have any problems once at home. Arrange for the patient to return for dressing changes at the hospital or with the community nurse. Inform the patient to contact the hospital if: • the swelling does not reduce • they have ongoing severe pain • there is any tingling or numbness in the fingers or arm.	To ensure the patient receives immediate treatment should there be any problems post-procedure. **E**

Post-procedural considerations

Ongoing care

Follow-up will be dependent on the patient's needs and the degree of damage. Assessment should be carried out using a standardized tool (INS 2016) and include inspection and management of the area of extravasation, skin integrity, the presence of pain and other symptoms (such as impaired mobility or sensation in the limb) (Table 15.16). If damage has occurred, it will be affected by the site, the amount of drug, the concentration of the agent and whether the drug binds to DNA or not (Polovich et al. 2014). Blistering may occur within 24 hours (e.g. with vinorelbine) or ulceration may occur over a period of days to weeks (e.g. with epirubicin), and extravasation wounds may be complicated by tissue ischaemia related to endothelial damage (Naylor 2005). The type of injury will dictate the type of dressing. Assessment of the wound should include the position and size of the wound, the amount and type of tissue present, the amount and type of exudate, and the extent and spread of erythema (Naylor 2005). If the flush-out technique has been undertaken then the incisions should be dressed using a dressing that allows the fluid to continue to leak from the site, for example Mepitel. It is also important to recognize the impact on the patient's psychological and situational dynamics, which may diminish their quality of life (Gonzalez 2013).

Documentation

An extravasation must be reported and fully documented as it is an adverse incident and the patient may require follow-up care (RCN 2016). The Oncology Nursing Society lists the key elements of vesicant extravasation documentation (Polovich et al. 2014) (Box 15.19). Statistics on the incidence, degree, causes and corrective action should be monitored and analysed (Gonzalez 2013, INS 2016, Pérez Fidalgo et al. 2012). Finally, records may be required in the case of litigation, which is now on the increase (Doellman et al. 2009, Dougherty 2003, Masoorli 2003).

Education of the patient and relevant others

Patients should always be informed when an extravasation has occurred and be given an explanation of what has happened and what management has been carried out (INS 2016, McCaffrey Boyle and Engelking 1995). An information sheet should be given to patients with instructions on what symptoms to look out for and when to contact the hospital during the follow-up period (Gabriel 2008).

Complications

If the extravasation is not managed correctly then an injury will result. In certain circumstances, in spite of managing an extravasation, an injury can still result and must be dealt with on an individual basis. Following the flush-out technique, it may be necessary to administer prophylactic antibiotics to prevent local infection (although this is rare).

Allergic reaction

Allergic reaction is a complication associated with any medication administration. However, because it happens more rapidly when intravenous medication is administered, it is often considered more of an issue in this context.

An allergic reaction is a response to a medication or solution to which the patient is sensitive and may be immediate or delayed (Lamb and Dougherty 2008, Perucca 2010). Clinical features may start with chills and fever, with or without urticaria, erythema and itching. The patient may then go on to experience shortness of breath with or without wheezing, then angioneurotic oedema and in severe cases anaphylactic shock (Lamb and Dougherty 2008). Prevention is achieved by assessing and recording patient allergies (drug, food and products) and applying allergy identification wristbands (NPSA 2008a, Perucca 2010). In the event of an allergic reaction, the infusion should be stopped immediately, the tubing and container changed, and the vein kept patent. The doctor should be notified and any required interventions undertaken (Lamb and Dougherty 2008).

Circulatory overload (isotonic fluid expansion)

A critical and common complication of intravenous therapy is circulatory overload, or 'isotonic fluid expansion'. It is caused by infusion of fluids of the same tonicity as plasma into the vascular circulation, for example 0.9% sodium chloride. As isotonic solutions do not affect osmolarity, water does not flow from the extracellular to the intracellular compartment. The result is that the extracellular compartment expands in proportion to the fluid infused (Weinstein and Hagle 2014). Because of the electrolyte concentration, no extra water is available to enable the kidneys to selectively excrete and restore the balance. Circulatory overload can also occur due to:

- infusing excessive amounts of sodium chloride solutions
- large-volume infusions running over multiple days
- rapid fluid infusion into patients with compromised cardiac, liver or renal status (Lamb and Dougherty 2008, Macklin and Chernecky 2004).

Prevention includes thorough assessment of the patient before commencing intravenous therapy, close monitoring of the patient, maintaining infusion rates as prescribed and the use of infusion devices where required (Lamb and Dougherty 2008). If circulatory overload is detected early, the patient should be sat upright (Macklin and Chernecky 2004). Treatment consists of withholding all fluids until excess water and electrolytes have been eliminated by the body and/or administration of diuretics to promote rapid diuresis (Weinstein and Hagle 2014). However, careful monitoring should be continued to prevent the occurrence of isotonic contraction (where there is loss of fluid and electrolytes isotonic to the extracellular fluid, such as blood and large volumes of fluid from

Table 15.16 Grading scale for monitoring extravasation

Grade	1	2	3	4	5
Skin colour	Normal	Pink	Red	Blanched area surrounded by red	Blackened
Skin integrity	Unbroken	Blistered	Superficial skin loss	Tissue loss and exposed subcutaneous tissue	Tissue loss and exposed bone/muscle with necrosis/crater
Skin temperature	Normal	Warm	Hot		
Oedema	Absent	Non-pitting	Pitting		
Mobility	Full	Slightly limited	Very limited	Immobile	
Pain	Grade using a scale of 0–10 where 0 = no pain and 10 = worst pain				
Temperature	Normal	Elevated (indicate actual temperature)			

Box 15.12 Key elements of vesicant extravasation documentation

- Date and time the extravasation occurred
- Type and size of vascular access device
- Length and gauge of needle (ports only)
- Location of device
- Details of how patency was established before and during administration (description and quality of blood return)
- Number and location of all cannulation attempts
- Vesicant administration method (e.g. bolus or infusion)
- Estimated amount of extravasated drug
- Symptoms reported by the patient
- Description of device site (e.g. swelling or redness)
- Assessment of limb (where applicable) for range of movement
- Immediate nursing interventions
- Follow-up interventions
- Patient information

diarrhoea and vomiting) (Weinstein and Hagle 2014). If fluid administration is allowed to continue unchecked, it can result in left-sided heart failure, circulatory collapse and cardiac arrest (Dougherty 2002).

Dehydration

Dehydration may be categorized as either hypertonic or hypotonic contraction and may be caused by underinfusion. Hypertonic contraction occurs when water is lost without corresponding loss of salts (Weinstein and Hagle 2014) and occurs in patients unable to take sufficient fluids (the elderly, unconscious patients and incontinent patients) or who have excessive insensible water loss via skin and lungs or as a result of certain drugs in excess. Hypotonic contraction occurs when fluids containing more salt than water are lost; this results in a decrease in osmolarity of the extracellular compartment (Weinstein and Hagle 2014).

It is important that nurses recognize the symptoms of overinfusion or underinfusion; certain factors should be considered when monitoring patients (Weinstein and Hagle 2014) (Table 15.17).

Speed shock

Speed shock is a systemic reaction that occurs when a substance foreign to the body is rapidly introduced into the circulation (Perucca 2010, Weinstein and Hagle 2014). This complication can manifest following administration of intravenous bolus injections or when large volumes of fluid are given too rapidly (Perucca 2010). It should not be confused with pulmonary oedema, which relates to the volume of fluid infused into the patient. Rapid, uncontrolled administration of drugs will result in toxic concentrations reaching vital organs (Lamb and Dougherty 2008). Toxicity may be manifested via an exaggeration of the usual pharmacological actions of the drug or via signs and symptoms specific to that drug or class of drugs. The most extreme toxic response that can occur if a drug is given at a dose or rate exceeding that recommended is termed the 'lethal response'.

Signs of speed shock include:

- flushed face
- headache and dizziness
- congestion of the chest
- tachycardia and fall in blood pressure
- syncope
- shock
- cardiovascular collapse (Perucca 2010, Weinstein and Hagle 2014).

Table 15.17 Monitoring overinfusion and underinfusion

Type of fluid or electrolyte imbalance	Patients at risk	Signs and symptoms	Treatment
Circulatory overload (isotonic fluid expansion)	Early post-operative or post-trauma patients, older people, those with impaired renal and cardiac function, and children	• Weight gain • A relative increase in fluid intake compared to output • A high bounding pulse pressure, indicating a high cardiac output • Raised central venous pressure measurements • Peripheral hand vein emptying time longer than normal (peripheral veins will usually empty in 3–5 seconds when the hand is elevated and will fill in the same length of time when the hand is lowered to a dependent position) • Peripheral oedema • Hoarseness • Dyspnoea, cyanosis and coughing due to pulmonary oedema and neck vein engorgement	If detected early: withhold all fluids until excess water and electrolytes have been eliminated by the body and/or administer diuretics to promote rapid diuresis
Dehydration (hypertonic contraction or hypotonic contraction)	*Hypertonic*: elderly, unconscious or incontinent patients *Hypotonic*: • Infants are at greatest risk, especially if they have diarrhoea • Patients with loss of salt from various sources: excess diuresis, fistula drainage, burns, vomiting or sweating	*Hyper/hypotonic contraction*: weight loss *Hypercontraction*: • Thirst (although this may be absent in the elderly) • Irritability and restlessness, and possible confusion • Diminished skin turgor • Dry mouth and furred tongue *Hypocontraction*: • Negative fluid balance • Weak, thready, rapid pulse rate • Increased 'hand filling time' • Increased skin turgor	Replace fluids and electrolytes

Prevention of speed shock involves the nurse having knowledge of the drug and the recommended rate of administration. When commencing an infusion using gravity flow, check that the solution is flowing freely before adjusting the rate and monitoring regularly (Perucca 2010). Movement of the patient or the device within the vessel can cause the infusion to flow more or less freely after a few minutes of setting the rate (Weinstein and Hagle 2014). For high-risk medications, an electronic flow-control device is recommended (RCN 2016). Although most pumps have an anti-free-flow mechanism, always close the roller clamp prior to removing the set from the pump (MHRA 2006a, Pickstone 1999).

If speed shock occurs, the infusion must be slowed down or discontinued. Medical staff should be notified immediately and the patient's condition treated as clinically indicated (Perucca 2010).

Monoclonal antibodies

Definition

Monoclonal antibodies (mAbs) were introduced to clinical practice in the 1980s and play a vital role in a variety of treatments and clinical interventions including cancer, inflammatory disease, organ transplantation, cardiovascular disease, infection, respiratory disease and ophthalmological disease (Suzuki et al. 2015).

Related theory

The efficacy of mAbs stems from the various natural functions of antibodies, which include neutralization, antibody-dependent cell-mediated cytotoxic (ADCC) activity, and complement-dependent cytotoxic (CDC) activity, or the antibody can be used as a drug delivery carrier (Suzuki et al. 2015). However, the possible consequences of their actions at a molecular level are not fully understood (Halsen & Kramer 2010).

Evidence-based approaches

Minimal data is available on the possible long-term risks to health professionals of handling these drugs (King et al. 2014; NHS PQAC 2015), but there is some research to show that staff are at risk of 'internalization' while handling them; this may occur via inhalation or via mucosal, oral or dermal contact (Alexander et al. 2014; Halsen & Kramer 2010; Langford et al. 2008), particularly during the preparation process (King et al. 2014). It is possible that low-level occupational exposure may produce neutralizing antibodies against mAbs proteins, which may mean the drug would be less effective should the staff member require it therapeutically in the future (Alexander et al. 2014; Langford et al. 2008), although the evidence for this is limited. Also, as they are proteinaceous products, usually of animal origin, they have the potential to cause sensitization of healthcare staff, potentially leading to allergic reactions.

While there is limited evidence that there is a risk of toxicity from low-grade occupational exposure to mAbs (Alexander et al. 2014; Langford et al. 2008), the lack of substantial research or evidence leads many staff to have significant concerns about what is a safe level of exposure, especially given mAbs' increasing availability and use (Meade 2015).

Unfortunately, there is a paucity of guidance on best practice (Meade 2015), in part as mAbs either do not fulfil hazardous drugs criteria or lack sufficient agent-specific information to be classified appropriately (NHS PQAC 2015). This has led to inconsistencies in the management of mAbs at national and international levels. There is, however, widespread agreement that every effort should be made by healthcare organizations to minimize staff exposure (Meade 2015).

Clinical governance

Risk assessment

It is vital that any mAb that is introduced into clinical practice should undergo an appropriate risk assessment to ensure the area and method of preparation are appropriate for that particular mAb (NHS Pharmaceutical Quality Assurance Committee 2015). Two factors must be considered during this process (NHS PQAC 2015):

1 What risk does the mAb pose to staff handling the product due to the agent's nature or mode of action?
2 What is the risk of a calculation error being made or of damage or contamination of the product occurring during preparation, leading to risk to the patient?

It is recommended that the National Patient Safety Agency 20 methodology is used to undertake this risk assessment (NHS PQAC 2015). However, this does not provide information specific to staff exposure risks and instead focuses only on the risk of error and product contamination. A modified version of this risk assessment is therefore recommended, which takes into account the level of staff exposure. An example of such an assessment is provided in Figure 15.44.

The risk assessment should stratify the mAb into a low, medium or high risk category. High-risk mAbs should be prepared in pharmacy aseptic units only, medium-risk mAbs require suitable risk controls to be put in place, and low-risk mAbs require standard ward-based aseptic techniques only (NHS PQAC 2015).

Where a medium-risk mAb is deemed appropriate for preparation in the clinical area, appropriate personal protective equipment (PPE) – including gowns, protective eyewear, masks and respiratory masks – should be provided (NHS PQAC 2015). While the use of closed system reconstitution devices (CSRDs) is not seen as essential for mAb preparation (NHS PQAC 2015), they do provide an additional level of safety in terms of operator protection and can reduce the risk of product contamination in clinical areas (NHS PQAC 2015). They are recommended for use alongside PPE by many organizations (Alexander et al. 2014; King et al. 2014; Meade 2015).

Pre-procedural condiderations

The area for preparation should have been assessed for its suitability for mAb preparation. It should meet the following criteria (NHS PQAC 2015):

- It should be a clearly defined, well-ventilated preparation area of a suitable size to accommodate the expected level of activity.
- Adequate bench space should be available to allow segregation of activities during preparation.
- It should be a separate clinical room rather than a thoroughfare.
- Surfaces must be easily cleaned and resistant to any cleaning products used.

Adequate information should be provided to staff, usually in the form of standard operating procedures and an organizational policy, on the appropriate risk assessment of mAbs, cleaning of clinical areas, management of spillages, and preparation, management and labelling of mAbs. Adequate training on mAb preparation should also be provided by expert staff, such as aseptic teams in pharmacy departments where these are available (NHS PQAC 2015).

Part 1 Health and safety score		(please circle)
Origin (O)	≥ 75% humanised (suffix -zumab or -mumab)	1
	Partially humanised (chimeric; suffix -ximab)	2
	Completely murine (mouse or hamster protein; suffix -momab)	3
Toxicities arising from therapeutic use(T)	Low risk of harm to the operator	1
	Theoretical risk of immunological, cutaneous or haematological adverse effects to the operator with prolonged low-dose exposure	2
	Known risk of immunological, cutaneous, haematological or other adverse effects to the operator with prolonged low-dose exposure	3
	Known or potential teratogenic or embryotoxic properties	4
	Known cytotoxic, radioactive or risk of initiating a cancer	5
Health and safety score (O+T)	**1–3 = low risk,** **4–5 = moderate** **6+ = high**	

Part 2 NPSA 20 risk assessment		
Risk factors	Description	✓
Therapeutic risk	Where there is a significant risk of patient harm if the injectable medicine is not used as intended.	
Use of a concentrate	Where further dilution (after reconstitution) is required before use, i.e. slow IV bolus not appropriate.	
Complex calculation	Any calculation with more than one step required for preparation and/or administration, e.g. microgram/kg/hour, dose unit conversion (such as mg to mmol or % to mg).	
Complex method	More than five non-touch manipulations involved or others including syringe-to-syringe transfer, preparation of a burette, use of a filter.	
Reconstitution of powder in a vial	Where a dry powder has to be reconstituted with a liquid.	
Use of a part vial or ampoule, or use of more than one vial or ampoule	Examples: 5 mL required from a 10 mL vial or four 5 mL ampoules required for a single dose.	
Use of a pump or syringe driver	All pumps and syringe drivers require some element of calculation and therefore have potential for error and should be included in the risk factors. However it is important to note that this potential risk is considered less significant than the risks associated with not using a pump when indicated.	
Use of non-standard giving set/device required	Examples: light protected, low adsorption, in-line filter or air inlet.	
Total number of product risk factors	Six or more risk factors = high-risk product (Red). Three to five risk factors = moderate-risk product (Amber). One or two risk factors = lower-risk product (Green).	

Risk Assessment Summary **Product:**

Health and Safety Score	NPSA Score	Preparation details
Low	Green	Nurse
Low	Amber	Nurse
Low	Red	Nurse
Moderate	Green	Aseptics/closed system
Moderate	Amber	Aseptics/closed system
Moderate	Red	Aseptics
High	Green	Aseptics
High	Amber	Aseptics
High	Red	Aseptics

This product has been assessed as ....risk and will therefore be prepared by ....

Risk assessment completed by: Date: Position:

Agreed by Consultant Chemotherapy Nurse Date:

Agreed by Senior Pharmacist: Date: Position:

Approved by: Date: Committee:

Figure 15.44 Monoclonal antibodies risk assessment form. *Source*: adapted from Langford et al. (2008).

Websites

EMC (Electronic Medicines Compendium)
https://www.medicines.org.uk/emc

Institute for Healthcare Improvement
www.ihi.org/explore/adesmedicationreconciliation/Pages/default.aspx

List of Most Commonly Encountered Drugs Currently Controlled under the Misuse of Drugs Legislation
https://tinyurl.com/hdvm9uh

MHRA
www.mhra.gov.uk
www.yellowcard.gov

NHS Improvement
https://improvement.nhs.uk

Stockley's Drug Interactions
www.medicinescomplete.com

References

Absalom, A. & Struys, M. (2006) *An Overview of TCI & TIVA*. Ghent, Belgium: Academia Press.

Ackermann, M., Maier, S., Ing, H. & Bonnabry, P. (2007) Evaluation of the design and reliability of three elastomeric and one mechanical infusers. *Journal of Oncology Pharmacy Practice*, 13(2), 77–84.

Agius, C.R. (2012) Intelligent infusion technologies: Integration of a smart system to enhance patient care. *Journal of Infusion Nursing*, 35(6), 364–368.

Aldridge, M. (2010) Miscellaneous routes of medication administration. In: Jevon, P., Payne, L., Higgins, D. & Endecott, R. (eds) *Medicines Management: A Guide for Nurses*. Hoboken, NJ: John Wiley & Sons, pp.239–261.

Alexander, M., Fawcett, J. & Runciman P. (2007) *Nursing Practice: Hospital and Home*, 3rd edn. London: Churchill Livingstone.

Alexander, M., King, J., Lingaratnam, S., et al. (2014) A survey of manufacturing and handling practices for monoclonal antibodies (MABs) by pharmacy, nursing and medical personnel. *Journal of Oncology Pharmacy Practice*, 22(2), 219–227.

Amoore, J. & Adamson, L. (2003) Infusion devices: Characteristics, limitations and risk management. *Nursing Standard*, 17(28), 45–52.

Amoore, J., Dewar, D., Ingram, P. & Lowe, D. (2001) Syringe pumps and start up time: Ensuring safe practice. *Nursing Standard*, 15(17), 43–45.

Andrew, S. (2006) Pharmacology. In: Marsden, J. (ed) *Ophthalmic Care*. Chichester: Whurr, pp.42–65.

Antipuesto, D.J. (2010) Z-Track Method. *Nursing Crib*, 13 October. Available at: https://nursingcrib.com/nursing-notes-reviewer/fundamentals-of-nursing/z-track-method

Armitage, G. (2009) The risks of double checking. *Nursing Times* 16(2), 30–35.

Aronson, J. (2009) Medication errors: Definitions and classification. *British Journal of Clinical Pharmacology*, 67(6), 599–604.

Aronson, J. (ed) (2016) *Meyler's Side Effects of Drugs: The International Encyclopedia of Adverse Drug Reactions and Interactions*, 16th edn. Philadelphia: Elsevier Science.

Aronson, J. (2017) Medicines reconciliation. *BMJ*, 356, i5336.

ASHP (American Society of Hospital Pharmacists) (1982) ASHP standard definition of a medication error. *American Journal of Hospital Pharmacy*, 3(2), 321.

Aulton, M.E. & Taylor, K.M.G. (eds) (2018) *Aulton's Pharmaceutics: The Design and Manufacture of Medicines*. Edinburgh: Elsevier.

Bailey, F. & Harman, S. (2018) Palliative care: The last hours and days of life. *UpToDate*. Available at: https://www.uptodate.com/contents/palliative-care-the-last-hours-and-days-of-life

Barnett, N. & Parmar, P. (2018) How to tailor medication formulations for patients with dysphagia. *Pharmaceutical Journal*, 297(7892). DOI: 10.1211/PJ.2016.20201498

Barton, A., Fuller, R. & Dudley, N. (2004) Using subcutaneous fluids to rehydrate older people: Current practices and future challenges. *Quarterly Journal of Medicine*, 97(11), 765–768.

Barua, P. & Bhowmick, B. (2005) Hypodermoclysis: A victim of historical prejudice. *Age and Ageing*, 34(3), 215–217.

Beijer, H.J. & de Blaey, C.J. (2002) Hospitalisations caused by adverse drug reactions (ADR): A meta-analysis of observational studies. *Pharmacy World & Science*, 24(2), 46–54.

Beijnen, J.H. & Schellens, J.H.M. (2004) Drug interactions in oncology. *Lancet Oncology*, 5, 489–496.

Bertelli, G. (1995) Prevention and management of extravasation of cytotoxic drugs. *Drug Safety*, 12(4), 245–255.

Block, B.M., Liu, S., Rowlingson, A., et al. (2003) Efficacy of postoperative analgesia: A meta-analysis. *JAMA*, 290, 2455–2463.

BNF (British National Formulary) (2019a) *British National Formulary*. National Institute for Health and Care Excellence. Available at: https://bnf.nice.org.uk

BNF (2019b) *British National Formulary for Children*. National Institute for Health and Care Excellence. Available at: https://bnfc.nice.org.uk

Bonsell, L. (2011) *8 Rights of Medication Administration*. Available at: www.nursingcenter.com/Blog/post/2011/05/27/8-rights-of-medication-administration.aspx

Boulanger, J., Ducharme, A., Dufour, A., et al. (2015) Management of extravasation of anti-neoplastic agents. *Support Cancer Care*, 23, 1459–1471.

Brady, A.M., Malone, A.M. & Fleming, S. (2009) A literature review of the individual and systems factors that contribute to medication errors in nursing practice. *Journal of Nursing Management*, 17(6), 679–697.

Breland, B. (2010) Continuous quality improvement using intelligent infusion pump data analysis. *American Journal of Health-System Pharmacy*, 67, 1446–1455.

British Pharmacopoeia (2019) *British Pharmacopoeia*. Medicines and Healthcare products Regulatory Agency. Available at: https://www.pharmacopoeia.com/BP2019

Broadhurst, D. (2012) Transition to an elastomeric infusion pump in home care: An evidence-based approach. *Journal of Infusion Nursing*, 35(3), 143–151.

Brown, J., Moss, H. & Elliot, T. (1997) The potential for catheter microbial contamination from a needleless connector. *Journal of Hospital Infection*, 36(3), 181–189.

Bruera, E., Higginson, I., von Gunten, C.F. & Morita, T. (eds) (2015) *Textbook of Palliative Medicine and Supportive Care*, 2nd edn. Boca Raton, FL: CRC Press.

BTS (British Thoracic Society) & SIGN (Scottish Intercollegiate Guidelines Network) (2016) *British Guideline for the Management of Asthma*. Edinburgh: Scottish Intercollegiate Guidelines Network.

Buter, J., Steele, K.T., Chung, K.C. & Elzinga, K. (2019) Extravasation injury from chemotherapy and other non-antineoplastic vesicants. *UpToDate*. Available at: https://www.uptodate.com/contents/extravasation-injury-from-chemotherapy-and-other-non-antineoplastic-vesicants/print

Camp-Sorrell, D. & Cope, D. (2011) *Oncology Nursing Society Access Device Guidelines: Recommendations for Nursing Practice and Education*. Pittsburgh: Oncology Nursing Society.

Chan, H. (2001) Effects of injection duration on site-pain intensity and bruising associated with subcutaneous heparin. *Journal of Advanced Nursing*, 35(6), 882–892.

Chernecky, C., Infortuna, H. & Macklin, D. (2005) *Saunders Nursing Survival Guide: Drug Calculations and Drug Administration*, 2nd edn. Philadelphia: W.B. Saunders.

Chung, J.W., Ng, W.M. & Wong, T.K. (2002) An experimental study on the use of manual pressure to reduce pain in intramuscular injection. *Journal of Clinical Nursing*, 11, 457–461.

Cocoman, A. & Murray, J. (2010) Recognizing the evidence and changing practice on injection sites. *British Journal of Nursing*, 19(18), 1170–1174.

Conroy, S., Davar, Z. & Jones, S. (2012) Use of checking systems in medicines administration with children and young people. *Nursing Children & Young People*, 24(3), 20–24.

Constans, T., Dutertre, J. & Froge, E. (1991) Hypodermoclysis in dehydrated elderly patients: Local effects with and without hyaluronidase. *Journal of Palliative Care*, 7(2), 10–12.

Controlled Drugs (Supervision of Management and Use) Regulations (2006) Available at: www.legislation.gov.uk/uksi/2006/3148/contents/made

Controlled Drugs (Supervision of Management and Use) Regulations (2013) Available at: https://www.legislation.gov.uk/uksi/2013/373/contents/made

Council of the European Communities (1993) *Council Directive 93/42/EEC of 14 June 1993 concerning Medical Devices.* Available at: https://eur-lex.europa.eu/legal-content/EN/TXT/?uri=CELEX%3A31993L0042

Cousins, D.H., Gerrett, D. & Warner, B. (2012) A review of medication incidents reported to the National Reporting and Learning System in England and Wales over 6 years (2005–2010). *British Journal of Clinical Pharmacology*, 74(4), 597–604.

CQC (Care Quality Commission) (2018a) *Administering Medicines Covertly.* Available at: https://www.cqc.org.uk/guidance-providers/adult-social-care/administering-medicines-covertly

CQC (2018b) *Self-Administered Medicines in Care Homes.* Available at: https://www.cqc.org.uk/guidance-providers/adult-social-care/self-administered-medicines-care-homes

Cross, R., Bennett, P.N., Ockerby, C., et al. (2017) Nurses' attitudes toward the single checking of medications. *Worldviews on Evidence-Based Nursing*, 14(4), 274–281.

Dann, T.C. (1969) Routine skin preparation before injection: An unnecessary procedure. *Lancet*, 294(7611), 96–97.

Danzig, L.E., Short, L., Collins, K., et al. (1995) Bloodstream infections associated with a needleless intravenous infusion system in patients receiving home infusion therapy. *JAMA*, 273(23), 1862–1864.

Dawkins, L., Britton, D., Johnson, I., et al. (2000) A randomised trial of winged Vialon cannulae and metal butterfly needles. *International Journal of Palliative Nursing*, 6(3), 110–116.

De Leon, A. & Wong, C. (2017) Spinal anesthesia: Technique. *UpToDate.* https://www.uptodate.com/contents/spinal-anesthesia-technique

de Vries, E.N., Ramrattan, M.A., Smorenburg, S.M., et al. (2008) The incidence and nature of in-hospital adverse events: A systematic review. *Quality & Safety in Health Care*, 17(3), 216–223.

Dennison, R.D. (2007) A medication safety education program to reduce the risk of harm caused by medication errors. *Journal of Continuing Education in Nursing*, 38(4), 176–184.

Department of Health (Northern Ireland) (2006) *Controls Assurance Standards: Medical Devices and Equipment Management.* Previously available at: www.dhsspsni.gov.uk/medical_device_and_equipment_management_-_version_2008_-_pdf.pdf

DH (Department of Health) (2000a) *An Organisation with a Memory.* London: Department of Health.

DH (2000b) *Patient Group Directions* [HSC 2000/026]. London: Health and Safety Commission.

DH (2003a) *Supplementary Prescribing by Nurses and Pharmacists within the NHS in England: A Guide for Implementation.* London: NHS.

DH (2003b) *Building a Safer NHS for Patients: Improving Medication Safety.* London: Department of Health.

DH (2003c) *Winning Ways: Working Together to Reduce Healthcare-Associated Infection in England.* London: Department of Health.

DH (2006) *Safer Management of Controlled Drugs (CDs): Changes to Record Keeping Requirements Guidance for Implementation.* London: Department of Health.

DH (2007) *Safer Management of Controlled Drugs: A Guide to Good Practice in Secondary Care (England).* London: Department of Health.

DH (2008) *Updated National Guidance on the Safe Administration of Intrathecal Chemotherapy* [HSC 2008/001]. Available at: https://webarchive.nationalarchives.gov.uk/20130104235816/http:/www.dh.gov.uk/prod_consum_dh/groups/dh_digitalassets/documents/digitalasset/dh_086844.pdf

DH (2009) *Changes to Medicines Legislation to Enable Mixing of Medicines Prior to Administration in Clinical Practice.* London: Department of Health.

DH (2018) *Cannabis Scheduling Review Part 1: The Therapeutic and Medicinal Benefits of Cannabis-Based Products.* Available at: https://www.gov.uk/government/publications/cannabis-scheduling-review-part-1

DHSS (Department of Health and Social Security) (1976) *Health Services Development: Addition of Drugs to Intravenous Fluids* [HC(76)9; Breckenridge Report]. Available at: https://www.sps.nhs.uk/wp-content/uploads/2019/04/HC769-Health-Services-Development-Additon-of-Drugs-to-IV-Fluids-The-Breckenridge-Report-DH-1976-1.pdf

Dickerson, R.J. (1992) 10 tips for easing the pain of intramuscular injections. *Nursing*, 22(8), 55.

Dickman, A., Schneider, J. & Varga, J. (2016) *The Syringe Driver: Continuous Subcutaneous Infusions in Palliative Care*, 4th edn. Oxford: Oxford University Press.

Dionyssiou, D., Chantes, A., Gravvanis, A., et al. (2011) The wash-out technique in the management of delayed presentations of extravasation injuries. *Journal of Hand Surgery*, 36(1), 66–69.

Doellman, D., Hadaway, L., Bowe-Geddes, L.A., et al. (2009) Infiltration and extravasation: Update on prevention and management. *Journal of Infusion Nursing*, 32(4), 203–211.

Doornaert, M., Monstrey, S. & Roche, N. (2013) Extravasation injuries: Current medical and surgical treatment. *Acta Chirurgica Belgica*, 113, 1–7.

Doroshow, J.H. (2012) Dexrazoxane for the prevention of cardiac toxicity and treatment of extravasation injury from the anthracycline antibiotics. *Current Pharmaceutical Biotechnology*, 13(10), 1949–1956.

Dougherty, L. (2002) Delivery of intravenous therapy. *Nursing Standard*, 16(16), 45–56.

Dougherty, L. (2003) The expert witness: Working within the legal system of the United Kingdom. *Journal of Vascular Access Devices*, 8(2), 29–35.

Dougherty, L. (2008a) Obtaining peripheral access. In: Dougherty, L. & Lamb, J. (eds) *Intravenous Therapy in Nursing Practice*, 2nd edn. Oxford: Blackwell, pp.225–270.

Dougherty, L. (2008b) IV therapy: Recognizing the differences between infiltration and extravasation. *British Journal of Nursing*, 17(14), 896, 898–901.

Dougherty, L. (2010) Extravasation: Prevention, recognition and management. *Nursing Standard*, 24(52), 48–55.

Dougherty, L. & Lamb, J. (eds) (2008) *Intravenous Therapy in Nursing Practice*, 2nd edn. Oxford: Blackwell.

Dougherty, L. & Oakley, C. (2011) Advanced practice in the management of extravasation. *Cancer Nursing Practice*, 10(5), 16–18.

Downie, G., MacKenzie, J. & Williams, A. (2003) Medicine management. In: Downie, G., MacKenzie, J. & Williams, A. (eds) *Pharmacology and Medicines Management for Nurses*, 3rd edn. London: Churchill Livingstone, pp.49–91.

Dychter, S.S., Gold, D.A. & Haller, M.F. (2012) Subcutaneous drug delivery: A route to increased safety, patient satisfaction, and reduced costs. *Journal of Infusion Nursing*, 35(3), 154–160.

EASHW (European Agency for Safety and Health at Work) (2010) *Directive 2010/32/EU: Prevention from Sharp Injuries in the Hospital and Healthcare Sector.* Available at: www.osha.europa.eu/en/legislation/directives/sector-specific-and-worker-related-provisions/osh-directives/council-directive-2010-32-eu-prevention-from-sharp-injuries-in-the-hospital-and-healthcare-sector

Elliott, M. & Liu, Y. (2010) The nine rights of medication administration: An overview. *British Journal of Nursing*, 19(5), 300–305.

Elliott, R.A., Camacho, E., Campbell, F., et al. (2018) *Prevalence and Economic Burden of Medication Errors in the NHS in England.* Policy Research Unit in Economic Evaluation of Health & Care Interventions. Available at: www.eepru.org.uk/wp-content/uploads/2018/02/eepru-report-medication-error-feb-2018.pdf

El-Saghir, N., Otrock, Z., Mufarrij, A., et al. (2004) Dexrazoxane for anthracycline extravasation and GM-CSF for skin ulceration and wound healing. *Lancet Oncology*, 5(5), 320–321.

EMC (Electronic Medicines Compendium) (2019) Timoptol 0.25% and 0.5% w/v eye drops solution summary of product characteristics. Available at: https://www.medicines.org.uk/emc/product/5110/smpc

European Oncology Nursing Society (2007) *Extravasation Guidelines: Guidelines Implementation Toolkit.* Brussels: European Oncology Nursing Society.

Fabian, B. (2000) IV complications: Infiltration. *Journal of Intravenous Nursing*, 23(4), 229–231.

Fair, R. & Proctor, B. (2007) *Administering Medicines through Enteral Feeding Tubes*, 2nd edn. Belfast: Royal Hospitals.

Federico, F. (2011) *The Five Rights of Medication Administration.* Institute for Healthcare Improvement. Available at: www.ihi.org/resources/Pages/ImprovementStories/FiveRightsofMedicationAdministration.aspx

Fields, M. & Peterson, J. (2005) Intravenous medication safety system averts high risk medication errors and provides actionable data. *Nursing Administration Quarterly*, 29(1), 78–87.

Finlay, T. (2008) Safe administration and management of peripheral intravenous therapy. In: Dougherty, L. & Lamb, J. (eds) *Intravenous Therapy in Nursing Practice*, 2nd edn. Oxford: Blackwell, pp.143–166.

FIT (Forum for Injection Technique) (2010) *The First Injection Technique Recommendations*, 4th edn. Available at: www.fit4diabetes.com/files/4514/7946/3482/FIT_UK_Recommendations_4th_Edition.pdf

Forrester, J., Dick, A.D., McMenamin, P.G. & Lee, W.R. (2002) *The Eye: Basic Science in Practice*, 2nd edn. Edinburgh: Saunders.

Fox, N. (2000) Armed and dangerous. *Nursing Times*, 96(44), 24–26.

Fraise, A.P. & Bradley, T. (eds) (2009) *Ayliffe's Control of Healthcare-Associated Infection: A Practical Handbook*, 5th edn. London: Hodder Arnold.

Frey, A.M. & Pettit, J. (2010) Infusion therapy in children. In: Alexander, M., Corrigan, A., Gorski, L., et al. (eds) *Infusion Nursing: An Evidence-Based Approach*, 3rd edn. St Louis, MO: Saunders Elsevier, pp.550–568.

Gabriel, J. (2008) Safe administration of intravenous cytotoxic drugs. In: Dougherty, L. & Lamb, J. (eds) *Intravenous Therapy in Nursing Practice*, 2nd edn. Oxford: Blackwell, pp.461–494.

Gabriel, J. (2012) Subcutaneous infusion in palliative care: The neria soft infusion set. *International Journal of Palliative Care*, 18(11), 526–530.

Gabriel, J., Bravery, K., Dougherty, L., et al. (2005) Vascular access: Indications and implications for patient care. *Nursing Standard*, 19(26), 45–52.

Gault, D. (1993) Extravasation injuries. *British Journal of Plastic Surgery*, 46(2), 91–96.

Gault, D. & Challands, J. (1997) Extravasation of drugs. *Anaesthesia Review*, 13, 223–241.

Gizzo, S., Noventa, M., Fagherazzi, S., et al. (2014) Update on best available options in obstetrics anaesthesia: Perinatal outcomes, side effects and maternal satisfaction – Fifteen years systematic literature review. *Archives of Gynaecology and Obstetrics*, 290(1), 21–34.

Gonzalez, T. (2013) Chemotherapy extravasations: Prevention, identification, management, and documentation. *Clinical Journal of Oncology Nursing*, 17(1), 61–66.

Goolsby, T.V. & Lombardo F.A. (2006) Extravasation of chemotherapeutic agents: Prevention and treatment. *Seminars in Oncology*, 33(1), 139–143.

Greenway, K. (2004) Using the ventrogluteal site for intramuscular injection. *Nursing Standard*, 18(25), 39–42.

Griffith, R. (2016) Can covert administration of medicines be in a patient's best interests? *British Journal of Nursing*, 25(15), 872–873.

Griffith, R. & Jordan, S. (2003) Administration of medicines part 1: The law and nursing. *Nursing Standard*, 18(2), 47–53.

Gunningberg, L., Pöder, U., Donaldson, N. & Leo Swenne, C. (2014) Medication administration accuracy: Using clinical observation and review of patient records to assess safety and guide performance improvement. *Journal of Evaluation in Clinical Practice*, 20(4), 411–416.

Hadaway, L.C. (2010) Anatomy and physiology related to infusion therapy. In: Alexander, M., Corrigan, A., Gorski, L., et al. (eds) *Infusion Nursing: An Evidence-Based Approach*, 3rd edn. St Louis, MO: Saunders Elsevier, pp.139–177.

Hakkarainen, K.M., Hedna, K., Petzold, M. & Haegg, S. (2012) Percentage of patients with preventable adverse drug reactions and preventability of adverse drug reactions: A meta-analysis. *PLOS ONE*, 7(3), e33236.

Hallam, C., Weston, V., Denton, A., et al. (2016) Development of the UK Vessel Health and Preservation (VHP) framework: A multi-organisational collaborative. *Journal of Infection Prevention*, 17(2), 65–72.

Halsen, G. & Kramer, I. (2010) Assessing the risk to health care staff from long-term exposure to anticancer drugs: The case of monoclonal antibodies. *Journal of Oncology Pharmacy Practice*, 17(1), 68–80.

Harding, A.D. (2011) Use of intravenous smart pumps for patient safety. *Journal of Emergency Nursing*, 37(1), 71–72.

Harding, A.D. (2012) Increasing the use of 'smart' pump drug libraries by nurses: A continuous quality improvement project. *American Journal of Nursing*, 112(1), 26–35.

Hardman, J.G., Limbird, L.E., Molinoff, P.B., et al. (eds) (1996) *Goodman and Gilman's The Pharmacological Basis of Therapeutics*, 9th edn. New York: McGraw-Hill.

Harrison, R.J. (2015) Preparation for safe medication administration. In: Perry, A.G., Potter, P.A. & Ostendorf, W. (eds) *Nursing Interventions & Clinical Skills*, 6th edn. St Louis, MO: Elsevier, pp.537–554.

Hart, S. (2008) Infection control in intravenous therapy. In: Dougherty, L. & Lamb, J. (eds) *Intravenous Therapy in Nursing Practice*, 2nd edn. Oxford: Blackwell, pp.87–116.

Harvey, S., Murphy, F., Lake, R., et al. (2009) Diagnosing a problem: Using a tool to identify pre-registration nursing students' mathematical ability. *Nurse Education in Practice*, 10(3), 119–125.

Haw, C., Stubbs, J. & Dickens, G. (2007) An observational study of medication administration: Errors in old age psychiatric inpatients. *International Journal of Quality in Health Care*, 19(4), 210–216.

Health Care Standards Unit (2007a) *First Domain: Safety (Info Bank) C4b*. Previously available at: www.hcsu.org.uk/index.php?option=com_content&task=view&id=197&Itemid=109

Health Care Standards Unit (2007b) *Updated Signpost C4b*. Previously available at: www.hcsu.org.uk/index.php?option=com_content&task=view&id=309 &Itemid=111

Health and Social Care Act (2012) Available at: www.legislation.gov.uk/ukpga/2012/7/contents/enacted

Heron, C. (2017) Implementing smart infusion pumps with dose-error reduction software: Real-world experiences. *British Journal of Nursing*, 26(8), 13–16.

Hertzel, C. & Sousa, V.D. (2009) The use of smart pumps for preventing medication errors. *Journal of Infusion Nursing*, 32(5), 257–267.

Hillery, A., Lloyd, A. & Swarbrick, J. (eds) (2001) *Drug Delivery and Targeting for Pharmacists and Pharmaceutical Scientists*. Boca Raton, FL: CRC Press.

Hilton, S. (1990) An audit of inhaler technique among patients of 34 general practitioners. *British Journal of General Practice*, 40(341), 505–506.

Ho, C.Y., Dean, B.S. & Barber, N. (1997) When do medication administration errors happen to hospital in-patients? *International Journal of Pharmacy Practice*, 5, 91–96.

How, C. & Brown, J. (1998) Extravasation of cytotoxic chemotherapy from peripheral veins. *European Journal of Oncology Nursing*, 2(1), 51–59.

Huber, C. & Augustine, A. (2009) IV infusion alarms: Don't wait for the beep. *American Journal of Nursing*, 109(4), 32–33.

Human Medicines Regulations, The (2012) Available at: www.legislation.gov.uk/uksi/2012/1916/contents

Human Medicines (Amendment) Regulations, The (2013) Available at: www.legislation.gov.uk/uksi/2013/1855/made

Human Medicines (Amendment) Regulations, The (2018) Available at: www.legislation.gov.uk/uksi/2018/199/made

Hunter, J. (2008) Intramuscular injection techniques. *Nursing Standard*, 22(24), 35–40.

HWR (Hazardous Waste (England and Wales) Regulations) (2005) Available at: https://www.legislation.gov.uk/uksi/2005/894/contents/made

Hyde, L. (2008) Legal and professional aspects of intravenous therapy. In: Dougherty, L. & Lamb, J. (eds) *Intravenous Therapy in Nursing Practice*, 2nd edn. Oxford: Blackwell, pp. 3–20.

Hypodermoclysis Working Group (1998) *Hypodermoclysis: Guidelines on the Technique*. Wrexham, UK: CP Pharmaceuticals.

Iacovides, I., Blandford, A., Cox, A., et al. (2015) Infusion device standardisation and dose error reduction software. *British Journal of Healthcare Management*, 21(2), 68–76.

Ignoffo, R.J. & Friedman, M.A. (1980) Therapy of local toxicities caused by extravasation of cancer chemotherapeutic drugs. *Cancer Treatment Reviews*, 7(1), 17–27.

INS (Infusion Nurses Society) (2016) Infusion therapy standards of practice. *Journal of Infusion Nursing*, 39(Suppl. 1), S1–S159.

Jackson, G. (2006) *Consensus Opinion on the Use of Dexrazoxane (Savene) in the Treatment of Anthracycline Extravasation*. UK: Topotarget.

Janaki, M., Nirmala, S., Kadam, A.R., et al. (2008) Epidural analgesia during brachytherapy for cervical cancer patients. *Journal of Cancer Research and Therapeutics*, 4(2), 60–63.

Jevon, P. (2008) Severe allergic reaction: Management of anaphylaxis in hospital. *British Journal of Nursing*, 17(2), 104–108.

Jevon, P., Payne, L., Higgins, D. & Endecott, R. (eds) (2010) *Medicines Management: A Guide for Nurses*. Hoboken, NJ: John Wiley & Sons.

Joint Commission (2018) *National Patient Safety Goals Effective January 2018*. Available at: https://www.jointcommission.org/assets/1/6/2018_HAP_NPSG_goals_final.pdf

Joint Commission (2019) *Joint Commission Accreditation Standards*. Washington, DC: Joint Commission.

Jordan, S., Griffiths, H. & Griffith, R. (2003) Administration of medicines part 2: Pharmacology. *Nursing Standard*, 18(3), 45–54.

Kassner, E. (2000) Evaluation and treatment of chemotherapy extravasation injuries. *Journal of Pediatric Oncology Nursing*, 17(3), 135–148.

Keers, R.N., Williams, S.D., Cooke, J., et al. (2013) Prevalence and nature of medication administration errors in health care settings: A systematic review of direct observational evidence. *Annals of Pharmacotherapy*, 47(2), 237–256.

Kelly, J. & Wright, D. (2009) Administering medication to adult patients with dysphagia. *Nursing Standard*, 23(29), 61–68.

Keohane, C.A., Hayes, J., Saniuk, C., et al. (2005) Intravenous medication safety and smart infusion systems. *Journal of Infusion Nursing*, 28(5), 321–328.

Khan, M.S. & Holmes, J.D. (2002) Reducing the morbidity from extravasation injuries. *Annals of Plastic Surgery*, 48(6), 628–632, discussion 632.

King, J., Alexander, M., Byrne, J., et al. (2014) A review of the evidence for occupational exposure risks to novel anticancer agents: A focus on monoclonal antibodies. *Journal of Oncology Pharmacy Practice*, 22(1), 121–134.

King, L. (2003) Subcutaneous insulin injection technique. *Nursing Standard*, 17(34), 45–52.

Kirkwood, B. (2006) The cornea. In: Marsden, J. (ed) *Ophthalmic Care*. Chichester: Whurr, pp.339–369.

Kongkaew, C., Noyce, P.R. & Ashcroft, D.M. (2008) Hospital admissions associated with adverse drug reactions: A systematic review of prospective observational studies. *Annals of Pharmacotherapy*, 42(7), 1017–1025.

Koivistov, V.A. & Felig, P. (1978) Is skin preparation necessary before insulin injection? *Lancet*, 1(8073), 1072–1073.

Krähenbühl-Melcher, A., Schlienger, R., Lampert, M., et al. (2007) Drug-related problems in hospitals: A review of the recent literature. *Drug Safety*, 30(5), 379–407.

Kreidieh, F.Y., Moukadem, H.A. & El Saghir, N.S. (2016) Overview, prevention and management of chemotherapy extravasation. *World Journal of Clinical Oncology*, 7(1), 87–97.

Lamb, J. & Dougherty, L. (2008) Local and systemic complications of intravenous therapy. In: Dougherty, L. & Lamb, J. (eds) *Intravenous Therapy in Nursing Practice*, 2nd edn. Oxford: Blackwell, pp.167–196.

Lamblet, L.C.R., Meira, E.S.A., Torres, S., et al. (2011) Randomized clinical trial to assess pain and bruising in medicines administered by means of subcutaneous and intramuscular needle injection: Is it necessary to have needles changed? *Revista Latino-Americana de Enfermagem*, 19(5), 1063–1071.

Langer, S. (2008) Treatment of anthracycline extravasation from centrally inserted venous catheters. *Oncology Reviews*, 2(2), 114–116.

Langer, S.W., Sehested, M. & Jensen, P.B. (2000) Treatment of anthracycline extravasation with dexrazoxane. *Clinical Cancer Research*, 6(9), 3680–3686.

Langer, S.W., Thougaard, A.V., Sehested, M. & Jensen, P.B. (2006) Treatment of anthracycline extravasation in mice with dexrazoxane with or without DMSO and hydrocortisone. *Cancer Chemotherapy and Pharmacology*, 57(1), 125–128.

Langford, S., Fradgley, S., Evans, M. & Blanks, C. (2008) Assessing the risk of handling monoclonal antibodies. *Hospital Pharmacist*, 15, 60–64.

Lapham, R. & Agar, H. (2003) *Drug Calculations for Nurses: A Step-by-Step Approach*, 2nd edn. London: Arnold.

Larson, G.Y., Parker, H., Cash, J., et al. (2005) Standard drug concentrations and smart pump technology reduce continuous medication infusion errors in pediatric patients. *Pediatrics*, 116(1), 21–25.

Lawson, T. (2003) A legal perspective on CVC-related extravasation. *Journal of Vascular Access Devices*, 8(1), 25–27.

Lazarou, J., Pomeranz, B.H. & Corey, P.N. (1998) Incidence of adverse drug reactions in hospitalized patients: A meta-analysis of prospective studies. *JAMA*, 279(15), 1200–1205.

Leendertse, A.J., Visser, D., Egberts, A.C. & van den Bemt, P.M. (2010) The relationship between study characteristics and the prevalence of medication-related hospitalizations: A literature review and novel analysis. *Drug Safety*, 33(3), 233–244.

Lenz, C.L. (1983) Make your needle selection right to the point. *Nursing*, 13(2), 50–51.

Lilley, L.L., Collins, S.R. & Snyder, J.S. (2007) *Pharmacology and the Nursing Process*, 5th edn. St Louis, MO: Elsevier Health Sciences.

Longshore, L., Smith, T. & Weist, M. (2010) Successful implementation of intelligent infusion technology in a multihospital setting: Nursing perspective. *Journal of Infusion Nursing*, 33(1), 38–47.

Loveday, H., Wilson, J., Pratt, R., et al. (2014) epic3: National evidence-based guidelines for preventing healthcare-associated infections in NHS hospitals in England. *Journal of Hospital Infection*, 86(Suppl. 1), S1–S70.

Luebke, M.A., Arduino, M., Duda, D., et al. (1998) Comparison of the microbial barrier properties of a needleless and conventional needle based intravenous access system. *American Journal of Infection Control*, 26, 437–441.

Luk, J., Chan, F. & Chu, L. (2008) Is hypodermoclysis suitable for frail Chinese elderly? *Asian Journal of Gerontology & Geriatrics*, 3(1), 49–50.

MacDonald, M. (2010) Patient safety: Examining the adequacy of the 5 rights of medication administration. *Clinical Nurse Specialist*, 24(4), 196–201.

Macintyre, P.E. & Schug, S.A. (2015) *Acute Pain Management: A Practical Guide*, 4th edn. Boca Raton, FL: CRC Press.

Macklin, D. & Chernecky, C.C. (2004) *IV Therapy*. St Louis, MO: Saunders.

Malkin, B. (2008) Are techniques used for intramuscular injection based on research evidence? *Nursing Times*, 104(50/51), 48–51.

Manrique-Rodriguez, S., Sanchez-Galindo, A., Lopez-Herce, J., et al. (2013) Impact of implementing smart infusion pumps in a pediatric intensive care unit. *American Journal of Health-System Pharmacy*, 70, 1897–1906.

Marders, J. (2012) Sounding the alarm for IV infiltration. *Nursing*, 35(4), [illegible]

Marieb, E.N. & Hoehn, K. (2018) *Human Anatomy & Physiology*, 11th edn. Harlow: Pearson.

Marriott, J.L. & Nation, R.L. (2002) Splitting tablets. *Australian Prescriber*, 25(6), 133–135.

Masoorli, S. (2003) Extravasation injuries associated with the use of central vascular access devices. *Journal of Vascular Access Devices*, 8(1), 21–23.

Mayo, D.J. (1998) Fibrin sheath formation and chemotherapy extravasation: A case report. *Supportive Care in Cancer*, 6(1), 51–56.

McCaffrey Boyle, D. & Engelking, C. (1995) Vesicant extravasation: Myths and realities. *Oncology Nursing Forum*, 22(1), 57–67.

McClelland, B. (2007) *Handbook of Transfusion Medicine*, 3rd edn. London: The Stationery Office.

McLeod, M.C., Barber, N. & Franklin, B.D. (2013) Methodological variations and their effects on reported medication administration error rates. *BMJ Quality & Safety*, 22(4), 278–89.

McNicol, E.D., Ferguson, M.C. & Hudcova, J. (2015) Patient controlled opioid analgesia versus non-patient controlled opioid analgesia for postoperative pain. *Cochrane Database of Systematic Reviews*, 2(6), CD003348.

Meade, E. (2015) Use of closed-system drug transfer devices in the handling and administration of MABs. *British Journal of Nursing*, 24(16 Suppl. 1), S21–S27.

Medicines Act (1968) Available at: www.legislation.gov.uk/ukpga/1968/67

Medicines Complete (2018) *Stockley's Drug Interactions*. Available at: https://about.medicinescomplete.com/publication/stockleys-drug-interactions

Mei, A. & Auerhahn, C. (2009) Hypodermoclysis. Maintaining hydration in the frail older adult. *Annals of Long-Term Care*, 17(5), 28–30.

Menahem, S. & Shvartzman, P. (2010) Continuous subcutaneous delivery of medications for home care palliative patients: Using an infusion set or a pump? *Supportive Care in Cancer*, 18(9), 1165–1170.

Mendelson, M.H., Short, L., Schechter, C., et al. (1998) Study of a needleless intermittent intravenous access system for peripheral infusions: Analysis of staff, patient and institutional outcomes. *Infection Control & Hospital Epidemiology*, 19(6), 401–406.

Mental Capacity Act (2005) Available at: www.legislation.gov.uk/ukpga/2005/9/contents

Merck (2011) *Merck Manual for Professionals*, 19th edn. White House Station, NJ: Merck Sharp & Dohme.

MHRA (Medicines and Healthcare products Regulatory Agency) (2004) *Reducing Needlestick and Sharps Injuries*. London: Medicines and Healthcare products Regulatory Agency.

MHRA (2006a) *Free-Flow Situations*. London: Medicines and Healthcare products Regulatory Agency.

MHRA (2006b) *Reporting Adverse Incidents and Disseminating Medical Device Alerts* [DB2006(01)]. Available at: http:/www.mhra.gov.uk/Publications/Safetyguidance/DeviceBulletins/CON2030705https://webarchive.nationalarchives.gov.uk/20110505000131/www.mhra.gov.uk/Publications/Safetyguidance/DeviceBulletins/CON2030705

MHRA (2007) *Medical Device Alert 2007/080. Intravenous (IV) Infusion Lines All Brands*. London: Medicines and Healthcare products Regulatory Agency.

MHRA (2008a) *Devices in Practice: A Guide for Professionals in Health and Social Care*. London: Medicines and Healthcare products Regulatory Agency.

MHRA (2008b) *Medical Device Alert [illegible] Needle Free Intravascular Connectors – All Brands*. London: Medicines and Healthcare products Regulatory Agency.

MHRA (2010a) *Good Pharmacovigilance Practice*. London: Medicines and Healthcare products Regulatory Agency.

MHRA (2010b) *Device Bulletin Infusion Systems* [DB 2003 (02) v2.0 November]. London: Medicines and Healthcare products Regulatory Agency.

MHRA (2011) *Report on Devices Adverse Incidents in 2010* [DB2011(02)]. Available at: https://webarchive.nationalarchives.gov.uk/20140713225354/www.mhra.gov.uk/home/groups/dts-bs/documents/publication/con129234.pdf

MHRA (2014a) *Devices in Practice: Checklist for Using Medical Devices*. London: Medicine and Healthcare products Regulatory Agency.

MHRA (2014b) *Off-Label or Unlicensed Use of Medicines: Prescribers' Responsibilities*. Available at: https://www.gov.uk/drug-safety-update/off-label-or-unlicensed-use-of-medicines-prescribers-responsibilities

MHRA (2015) *Managing Medical Devices: Guidance for Healthcare and Social Services Organisations*. Available at: https://assets.publishing.service.gov.uk/government/uploads/system/uploads/attachment_data/file/421028/Managing_medical_devices_-_Apr_2015.pdf

MHRA (2017) *Corticosteroids: Rare Risk of Central Serous Chorioretinopathy with Local as well as Systemic Administration*. London: Medicine and Healthcare products Regulatory Agency.

Mirakian, R., Ewan, P.W., Durham, S.R., et al. (2009) BSACI guidelines for the management of drug allergy. *Clinical & Experimental Allergy*, 39, 43–61.

Misuse of Drugs Act (1971) Available at: www.legislation.gov.uk/ukpga/1971/38/contents

Misuse of Drugs and Misuse of Drugs (Safe Custody) (Amendment) (England and Wales and Scotland) Regulations (2018) Available at: www.legislation.gov.uk/uksi/2018/1383/contents/made

Misuse of Drugs and Misuse of Drugs (Safe Custody) (Amendment) Regulations (2007) Available at: www.legislation.gov.uk/uksi/2007/2154/made

Misuse of Drugs Regulations (2001) Available at: www.legislation.gov.uk/uksi/2001/3998/contents/made

Misuse of Drugs (Safe Custody) Regulations (1973) Available at: www.legislation.gov.uk/uksi/1973/798/made

Moriarty, D. & Hudson, E. (2001) Hypodermoclysis for rehydration in the community. *British Journal of Community Nursing*, 6(9), 437–443.

Mouridsen, H.T., Langer, S.W., Buter, J., et al. (2007) Treatment of anthracycline extravasation with Savene (dexrazoxane): Results from two prospective clinical multicentre studies. *Annals of Oncology*, 18(3), 546–550.

Mraz, M., Thomas, C. & Rajcan, L. (2018) Intramuscular injection CLIMAT pathway: A clinical practice guidance. *British Journal of Nursing*, 27(13), 752–756.

Murray, W. & Glenister, H. (2001) How to use medical devices safely. *Nursing Times*, 97(43), 36–38.

Naylor, W. (2005) Extravasation of wounds: Aetiology and management. In: Brighton, D. & Wood, M. (eds) *The Royal Marsden Hospital Handbook of Cancer Chemotherapy: A Guide for the Multidisciplinary Team*. Edinburgh: Elsevier Churchill Livingstone, pp.109–112.

NES (NHS Education for Scotland) (2018) *Patient Group Directions*. Available at: https://www.hps.scot.nhs.uk/publications/patient-group-directions

NEWT (2018) *NEWT Guidelines*. Available at: www.newtguidelines.com

NHS Employers (2007) *The Management of Health, Safety and Welfare Issues for NHS Staff*. London: NHS Confederation (Employers).

NHS Employers (2015) *Managing the Risks of Sharps Injuries*. Available at: https://www.nhsemployers.org/-/media/Employers/Documents/Retain-and-improve/Health-and-wellbeing/Managing-the-risks-of-sharps-injuries-v7.pdf

NHS England (2014) *Patient Safety Alert NHS/PSA/2014/005: Improving Medication Error Incident Reporting and Learning*. London: NHS England.

NHS England (2015a) *Patient Safety Alert NHS/PSA/W/2015/004: Managing Risks during the Transition Period to New ISO Connectors for Medical Devices*. London: NHS England.

NHS England (2015b) *Patient Safety Alert NHS/PSA/RE/2015/009: Support to Minimize the Risk of Distress and Death from Inappropriate Doses of Naloxone*. London: NHS England.

NHS England (2016) *Patient Safety Alert NHS/PSA/W/2016/008: Restricted Use of Open Systems for Injectable Medication*. London: NHS England.

NHS England and NHSI (NHS Improvement) (2019) *Standard Infection Control Precautions: National Hand Hygiene and Personal Protective Equipment Policy*. Available at: https://improvement.nhs.uk/documents/4957/National_policy_on_hand_hygiene_and_PPE_2.pdf

NHS PQAC (NHS Pharmaceutical Quality Assurance Committee) (2015) *Guidance on the Safe Handling of Monoclonal Antibody (mAb) Products*, 5th edn. Available at: https://docplayer.net/19013058-Guidance-on-the-safe-handling-of-monoclonal-antibody-mab-products.html

NHSI (NHS Improvement) (2016) *Risk of Severe Harm and Death Due to Withdrawing Insulin from Pen Devices*. London: NHS Improvement.

NHSI (2017) *Patient Safety Alert NHS/PSA/RE/2017/004: Resources to Support Safe Transition from the Luer Connector to NRFit for Intrathecal and Epidural Procedures, and the Delivery of Regional Blocks*. London: NHS Improvement.

NHSI (2018a) *Patient Safety Alert NHS/PSA/W/2018/002: Risk of Death or Severe Harm from Inadvertent Intravenous Administration of Solid Organ Perfusion Fluids*. London: NHS Improvement.

NHSI (2018b) *Recommendations from National Patient Safety Alerts that Remain Relevant to Never Events List 2018*. Available at: https://improvement.nhs.uk/documents/2267/Recommendations_from_NPSA_alerts_that_remain_relevant_to_NEs_FINAL.pdf

NHSI (2018c) *Revised Never Events Policy and Framework*. Available at: https://improvement.nhs.uk/documents/2265/Revised_Never_Events_policy_and_framework_FINAL.pdf

NICE (National Institute for Health and Care Excellence) (2003) *Guidance on the Use of Continuous Subcutaneous Insulin Infusion for Diabetes* [TAG57]. London: National Institute for Health and Care Excellence.

NICE (2009) *Medicines Adherence: Involving Patients in Decisions about Prescribed Medicines and Supporting Adherence* [CG76]. Available at: www.nice.org.uk/guidance/CG76

NICE (2010) *Chronic Obstructive Pulmonary Disease: Management of Chronic Obstructive Pulmonary Disease in Adults in Primary and Secondary Care (Partial Update)* [CG101]. Available at: www.nice.org.uk/guidance/CG101

NICE (2012) *Palliative Care for Adults: Strong Opioids for Pain Relief* [CG140]. Available at: https://www.nice.org.uk/guidance/CG140

NICE (2014) *Drug Allergy: Diagnosis and Management of Drug Allergy in Adults, Children and Young People* [CG183]. London: National Institute for Health and Care Excellence.

NICE (2015a) *Medicines Management in Care Homes* [QS85]. London: National Institute for Health and Care Excellence.

NICE (2015b) *Medicines Optimisation Overview*. Available at: https://pathways.nice.org.uk/pathways/medicines-optimisation

NICE (2015c) *Medicines Optimisation: The Safe and Effective Use of Medicines to Enable the Best Possible Outcomes* [NG5]. London: National Institute for Health and Care Excellence.

NICE (2016a) *Controlled Drugs: Safe Use and Management* [NG46]. London: National Institute for Health and Care Excellence.

NICE (2016b) *Ensuring Appropriate Use of Monitored Dosage Systems: Reducing Unnecessary Pharmacy Workload QE Case Study*. London: National Institute for Health and Care Excellence.

NICE (2017a) *Managing Medicines for Adults Receiving Social Care in the Community* [NG67]. London: National Institute for Health and Care Excellence.

NICE (2017b) *Patient Group Directions* [MPG2]. Available at: https://www.nice.org.uk/guidance/mpg2/chapter/Recommendations

NICE (2017c) *Safer Insulin Prescribing*. London: National Institute for Health and Care Excellence.

NICE (2017d) *Safer Insulin Prescribing*. Available at: https://www.nice.org.uk/advice/ktt20/resources/safer-insulin-prescribing pdf 58758006482620

Nichols, C. & O'Brien, E. (2012) Ear irrigation. In: O'Brien, L. (ed) *District Nursing Manual of Clinical Procedures*. Oxford: John Wiley & Sons, pp.84–92.

Nisbet, A. (2006) Intramuscular gluteal injections in the increasingly obese population: Retrospective study. *BMJ*, 332, 637–638.

NIVAS (National Infusion and Vascular Access Society) (2019) *Intravenous Infusion Drug Administration: Flushing Guidance*. Marlow, UK: National Infusion and Vascular Access Society.

NMC (Nursing and Midwifery Council) (2018) *The Code: Professional Standards of Practice and Behaviour for Nurses, Midwives and Nursing Associates*. Available at: https://www.nmc.org.uk/standards/code

NPC (National Prescribing Centre) (2003) *Supplementary Prescribing: A Resource to Help Healthcare Professionals to Understand the Framework and Opportunities*. London: NHS.

NPSA (National Patient Safety Agency) (2002) *Patient Safety Alert: Potassium Chloride Concentrate Solutions*. Available at: https://www.sps.nhs.uk/wp-content/uploads/2018/02/2002-NRLS-1051A-Potassium-chloue-PSA-2002-10-31-v1.pdf

NPSA (2003) *Risk Analysis of Infusion Devices*. London: National Patient Safety Agency.

NPSA (2004) *Improving Infusion Device Safety*. Available at: https://www.sps.nhs.uk/articles/npsa-alert-improving-infusion-device-safety-2004

NPSA (2005) *Wristbands for Hospital Inpatients Improve Safety* [Safer Practice Notice 11]. London: National Patient Safety Agency.

NPSA (2006a) *Ensuring Safer Practice with High Dose Ampoules of Morphine and Diamorphine* [Alert No. 2006/12]. London: National Patient Safety Agency.

NPSA (2006b) *Patient Safety Alert: Improving Compliance with Oral Methotrexate Guidelines*. London: National Patient Safety Agency.

NPSA (2007a) *Rapid Response Report: Fire Hazard with Paraffin Based Skin Products on Dressings and Clothing*. London: National Patient Safety Agency.

NPSA (2007b) *Safer Practice Notice 0507: Standardising Wristbands Improves Patient Safety*. London: National Patient Safety Agency.

NPSA (2007c) *Patient Safety Alert 19: Promoting Safer Measurement and Administration of Liquid Medicines via Oral and Other Enteral Routes*. London: National Patient Safety Agency.

NPSA (2007d) *Promoting Safer Use of Injectable Medicines* [Alert No. 2007/20]. London: National Patient Safety Agency. Available at: https://www.sps.nhs.uk/wp-content/uploads/2016/12/2474_Inject_Multi-prof-1.pdf

NPSA (2007e) *Patient Safety Alert: Safer Practice with Epidural Injections and Infusions*. Available at: https://www.sps.nhs.uk/wp-content/uploads/2018/02/2007-NRLS-0396-Epidural-injectns-PSA-2007-03-28-v1.pdf

NPSA (2008a) *Rapid Response Report 05: Reducing Dosing Errors with Opioid Medicines*. London: National Patient Safety Agency.

NPSA (2008b) *Rapid Response Report 11: Reducing Risk of Overdose with Midazolam Injection in Adults*. London: National Patient Safety Agency.

NPSA (2008c) *Rapid Response Report: Using Vinca Alkaloid Minibags (Adult/Adolescent Units)* [NPSA/2008/RRR004]. London, National Patient Safety Agency

NPSA (2009) *Safety in Doses: Improving the Use of Medicines in the NHS*. London: National Patient Safety Agency.

NPSA (2010a) *Rapid Response Report: Reducing Treatment Dose Errors with Low Molecular Weight Heparins* [NPSA/2010/RRR014]. London: National Patient Safety Agency.

NPSA (2010b) *Rapid Response Report: Safer Administration of Insulin*. London: National Patient Safety Agency.

NPSA (2011) *Safer Spinal (Intrathecal), Epidural and Regional Devices* [NPSA/2011/PSA001]. Available at: https://www.sps.nhs.uk/wp-content/uploads/2018/02/NRLS-1310-Neuraxial-Alertupdate-2011.01.27-v1.pdf

Ostendorf, W. (2015) Administration of parenteral medication. In: Perry, A.G., Potter, P.A. & Ostendorf W. (eds) *Nursing Interventions & Clinical Skills*, 6th edn. St Louis, MO: Elsevier, pp.597–641.

Paparella, S.F. (2012) Accurate patient identification in the emergency department: Meeting the safety challenges. *Journal of Emergency Nursing*, 38(4), 364–367.

Peragallo-Dittko, V. (1997) Rethinking subcutaneous injection technique. *American Journal of Nursing*, 97(5), 71–72.

Pérez Fidalgo, J.A., García Fabregat, L., Cervantes, A., et al., on behalf of the ESMO Guidelines Working Group (2012) Management of chemotherapy extravasation: ESMO–EONS Clinical Practice Guidelines. *Annals of Oncology*, 23(Suppl. 7), vii167–vii173.

Perry A.G. (2015) Administration of nonparenteral medications. In: Perry, A.G., Potter, P.A. & Ostendorf, W. (eds) *Nursing Interventions & Clinical Skills*, 6th edn. St Louis, MO: Elsevier, pp.555–596.

Perry, A.G., Potter, P.A. & Ostendorf, W. (eds) (2015) *Nursing Interventions & Clinical Skills*, 6th edn. St Louis, MO: Elsevier.

Perucca, R. (2010) Peripheral venous access devices. In: Alexander, M., Corrigan, A., Gorski, L., et al. (eds) *Infusion Nursing: An Evidence-Based Approach*, 3rd edn. St Louis, MO: Saunders Elsevier, pp.456–479.

Pickstone, M. (1999) *A Pocketbook for Safer IV Therapy*. Broadstairs, UK: Scitech Educational.

Pickstone, M. (2000) Using the technology triangle to assess the safety of technology-controlled clinical procedures in critical care. *International Journal of Intensive Care*, 7(2), 90–96.

Police Reform and Social Responsibility Act (2011) Available at: www.legislation.gov.uk/ukpga/2011/13/notes

Polovich, M., Whitford, J.M. & Olsen, M. (eds) (2014) *Chemotherapy and Biotherapy Guidelines and Recommendations for Practice*, 4th edn. Pittsburgh: Oncology Nursing Society.

Pope, B.B. (2002) How to administer subcutaneous and intramuscular injections. *Nursing*, 32(1), 50–51.

Potter, P. & Perry, A. (2016) *Fundamentals of Nursing*, 9th edn. St Louis, MO: Elsevier.

Prescription Only Medicines (Human Use) Order (1997) Available at: https://www.legislation.gov.uk/uksi/1997/1830/contents/made

Public Health England (2006) Yellow fever. In: *Immunisation against Infectious Disease: The Green Book*. Available at: www.gov.uk/government/publications/yellow-fever-the-green-book-chapter-35

Quinn, C. (2000) Infusion devices: Risks, functions and management. *Nursing Standard*, 14(26), 35–41.

Quinn, C. (2008) Intravenous flow control and infusion devices. In: Dougherty, L. & Lamb, J. (eds) *Intravenous Therapy in Nursing Practice*, 2nd edn. Oxford: Blackwell, pp.197–224.

Rang, H.P., Ritter, J.M., Flower, R.J., et al. (2015) *Rang & Dale's Pharmacology*, 8th edn. Edinburgh: Elsevier Churchill Livingstone.

RCN (Royal College of Nursing) (2016) *Standards for Infusion Therapy*, 4th edn. London: Royal College of Nursing.

Regnard, C. & Hockley, J. (2004) *A Guide to Symptom Relief in Palliative Care*, 5th edn. Oxford: Radcliffe Medical Press.

Reid, A. (2012) Changing practice for safe insulin administration. *Nursing Times*, 108(10), 22–26.

Relihan, E., O'Brien, V., O'Hara, S. & Silke, B. (2010) The impact of a set of interventions to reduce interruptions and distractions to nurses during medication administration. *Quality & Safety in Health Care*, 19, e52.

Resuscitation Council (2015) *Resuscitation Guidelines*. Available at: https://www.resus.org.uk/resuscitation-guidelines

Reynolds, P., MacLaren, R., Mueller, S., et al. (2014) Management of extravasation injuries: A focused evaluation of noncytotoxic medications. *Pharmacotherapy*, 34(6), 617–632.

Riedl, M.A. & Casillas, A.M. (2003) Adverse drug reactions: Types and treatment options. *American Family Physician*, 68, 1781–1790.

Roberts, I.F. & Roberts, J.G. (1979) Relation between medicines sweetened with sucrose and dental disease. *BMJ*, 2(14), 14–16.

Rodger, M.A. & King, L. (2000) Drawing up and administering intra-muscular injection: A review of the literature. *Journal of Advanced Nursing*, 31(3), 574–582.

Rodrigues, C.C., Guilherme, C., Lobo da Costa, M., et al. (2012) Risk factors for vascular trauma during antineoplastic chemotherapy: Contributions of the use of relative risk. *Acta Paulista de Enfermagem*, 25(3), 448–452.

Rodriguez-Monguio, R., Otero, M.J. & Rovira, J. (2003) Assessing the economic impact of adverse drug effects. *Pharmacoeconomics*, 21(9), 623–650.

Roe, H. (2011) Anthracycline extravasations: Prevention and management. *British Journal of Nursing*, 20(17), S18–S22.

Roth, D. (2003) Extravasation injuries of peripheral veins: A basis for litigation. *Journal of Vascular Access Devices*, 8(1), 13–20.

Rotherham NHS Foundation Trust (2019) *Protocols*. Available at: http://www.earcarecentre.com/professionals/protocols

Rothschild, J.M., Keohane, C.A., Cook, E.F., et al. (2005) A controlled trial of smart infusion pumps to improve medication safety in critically ill patients. *Critical Care Medicine*, 33, 533–540.

RPS (Royal Pharmaceutical Society) (2005) *The Safe and Secure Handling of Medicines: A Team Approach*. Available at: https://www.rpharms.com/Portals/0/RPS%20document%20library/Open%20access/Publications/Safe%20and%20Secure%20Handling%20of%20Medicines%202005.pdf

RPS (2011) *Pharmaceutical Issues when Crushing, Opening or Splitting Oral Dosage Forms*. London: Royal Pharmaceutical Society.

RPS (2012) *Medicines, Ethics and Practice: The Professional Guide for Pharmacists*, 36th edn. London: Royal Pharmaceutical Society.

RPS (2013a) *Improving Patient Outcomes: The Better Use of Multi-compartment Compliance Aids*. London: Royal Pharmaceutical Society.

RPS (2013b) *Medicines Optimisation: Helping Patients Make the Most of Their Medicines*. London: Royal Pharmaceutical Society.

RPS (2016) *The Handling of Medicines in Social Care*. London: Royal Pharmaceutical Society.

RPS (2018) *Professional Guidance on the Safe and Secure Handling of Medicines*. Available at: https://www.rpharms.com/recognition/setting-professional-standards/safe-and-secure-handling-of-medicines/professional-guidance-on-the-safe-and-secure-handling-of-medicines

RPS (2019a) *Professional Guidance on the Administration of Medicines in Healthcare Settings*. Available at: https://www.rpharms.com/Portals/0/RPS%20document%20library/Open%20access/Professional%20standards/SSHM%20and%20Admin/Admin%20of%20Meds%20prof%20guidance.pdf?ver=2019-01-23-145026-567

RPS (2019b) *Prescribing Competency Framework*. Available at: www.rpharms.com/resources/frameworks/prescribers-competency-framework

Rudolph, R. & Larson, D.L. (1987) Etiology and treatment of chemotherapeutic agent extravasation injuries: A review. *Journal of Clinical Oncology*, 5(7), 1116–1126.

Sabin, M., Weeks, K., Rowe, D., et al. (2013) Safety in numbers 5: Evaluation of computer-based authentic assessment and high fidelity simulated OSCE environments as a framework for articulating a point of registration medication dosage calculation benchmark. *Nurse Education in Practice*, 13, e55–e65.

Sasson, M. & Shvartzman, P. (2001) Hypodermoclysis: An alternative infusion technique. *American Family Physician*, 64(9), 1575–1578.

Sauerland, C., Engelking, C., Wickham, R. & Corbi, D. (2006) Vesicant extravasation part I: Mechanisms, pathogenesis, and nursing care to reduce risk. *Oncology Nursing Forum*, 33(6), 1134–1142.

Savage, P. & Tripp, K. (2008) A study of independent double-checking processes for chemotherapy administration via an ambulatory infusion pump. 15th International Conference on Cancer Nursing abstract Q116, 17–21 August, Singapore.

Scales, K. (2011) Use of hypodermoclysis to manage dehydration. *Nursing Older People*, 23(5), 16–22.

Schrijvers, D.L. (2003) Extravasation: A dreaded complication of chemotherapy. *Annals of Oncology*, 14(Suppl. 3), 26iii–30iii.

Schug, S.A., Palmer, G.M., Scott, D.A., et al (2015) *Acute Pain Management: Scientific Evidence*, 4th edn. Melbourne: Working Group of the Australian and New Zealand College of Anaesthetists and Faculty of Pain Medicine.

Schulmeister, L. (1998) A complication of vascular access device insertion: A case study and review of subsequent legal action. *Journal of Intravenous Nursing*, 21(4), 197–202.

Schulmeister, L. (2008) Patient misidentification. *Clinical Journal of Oncology Nursing*, 12(3), 495–498.

Schulmeister, L. (2009) Antineoplastic therapy. In: Alexander, M., Corrigan, A., Gorski, M.S., et al. (eds) *Infusion Nursing: An Evidence-Based Approach*, 3rd edn. St Louis, MO: Saunders Elsevier, pp.351–371.

Sewell, G., Summerhayes, M. & Stanley, A. (2002) Administration of chemotherapy. In: Allwood, M., Stanley, A. & Wright, P. (eds) *The Cytotoxics Handbook*, 4th edn. Oxford: Radcliffe Medical Press, pp.85–115.

Shelton, B.K. & Shivnan, J. (2011) *Acute Hypersensitivity Reactions: What Nurses Need to Know*. Available at: http://magazine.nursing.jhu.edu/2011/04/acute-hypersensitivity-reactions-what-nurses-need-to-know

Shepherd, M. (2002) Medicines 2: Administration of medicines. *Nursing Times*, 98(16), 45–48.

Sherriff, K., Wallis, M. & Burston, S. (2011) Medication calculation competencies for registered nurses: A literature review. *Australian Journal of Advanced Nursing*, 28(4), 75–83.

Shipman Enquiry (2004) *The Fourth Report*. Available at: https://webarchive.nationalarchives.gov.uk/20090808163828/www.the-shipman-inquiry.org.uk/4r_page.asp

Skryabina, E.A. & Dunn, T.S. (2006) Disposable infusion pumps. *American Journal of Health-System Pharmacy*, 63(13), 1260–1268.

Small, S.P. (2004) Preventing sciatic nerve injury from intramuscular injections: Literature review. *Journal of Advanced Nursing*, 47(3), 287–296.

Smyth, J. (ed) (2006) *The NEWT Guidelines for Administration of Medication to Patients with Enteral Feeding Tubes and Swallowing Difficulties*. Wrexham, UK: North East Wales NHS Trust.

Springhouse (2009) *Intravenous Therapy Made Incredibly Easy*, 4th edn. Philadelphia: Lippincott Williams & Wilkins.

SPS (Specialist Pharmacy Service) (2016) Quality PGDs: 7 steps to success. *Specialist Pharmacy Service*, 9 July. Available at: https://www.sps.nhs.uk/articles/quality-pgds-7-steps-to-success

Stanley, A. (2002) Managing complications of chemotherapy administration. In: Allwood, M., Stanley, A. & Wright, P. (eds) *The Cytotoxics Handbook*, 4th edn. Oxford: Radcliffe Medical Press, pp.119–192.

Stolic, S. (2014) Educational strategies aimed at improving student nurse's medication calculation skills: A review of the research literature. *Nurse Education in Practice*, 14, 491–503.

Stollery, R., Shaw, M. & Lee, A. (2005) *Ophthalmic Nursing*, 3rd edn. Oxford: Blackwell.

Susser, W.S., Whitaker-Worth, D.L. & Grant-Kels, J.M. (1999) Mucocutaneous reactions to chemotherapy. *Journal of the American Academy of Dermatology*, 40(3), 367–398.

Suzuki, M., Cato, C. & Cato, A. (2015) Therapeutic antibodies: Their mechanisms of action and the pathological findings they induce in toxicity studies. *Journal of Toxicologic Pathology*, 28(3), 133–139.

Take 5 (2006) *Z-Track Injections*. Nursing2006. Available at: www.nursingcenter.com/upload/static/592775/Take5_Ztrack.pdf

Taxis, K., Dean, B. & Barber, N. (1999) Hospital drug distribution systems in the UK and Germany: A study of medication errors. *Pharmacy World & Science*, 21(1), 25–31.

Terry, A. (2017) Antineoplastic therapy. In: *Infusion Therapy Made Incredibly Easy*. Philadelphia: Wolters Kluwer Health, pp.269–304.

Thomas, C., Mraz, M. & Rajcan, L. (2016) Blood aspiration during IM injection. *Clinical Nursing Research*, 25(5), 549–559.

Thomas, J.R., Wallace, M., Yocum, R., et al. (2009) The INFUSE morphine study: Use of recombinant human hyaluronidase (rHuPH20) to enhance the absorption of subcutaneously administered morphine in patients with advanced illness. *Journal of Pain and Symptom Management*, 38, 663–672.

Toft, B. (2001) *External Inquiry into the Adverse Incident that Occurred at Queen's Medical Centre, Nottingham, 4th January 2001*. Available at: https://webarchive.nationalarchives.gov.uk/20120524040348/www.dh.gov.uk/prod_consum_dh/groups/dh_digitalassets/@dh/@en/documents/digitalasset/dh_4082098.pdf

Torrance, C. (1989) Intramuscular injection, parts 1 and 2. *Surgical Nurse*, 2(5), 6–10; 2(6), 24–27.

Torre, M. (2002) Subcutaneous infusion: Non-metal cannulae vs metal butterfly needles. *British Journal of Community Nursing*, 7(7), 365–369.

Tortora, G.J. & Derrickson, B. (2011) *Principles of Anatomy & Physiology*, 13th edn. Hoboken, NJ: John Wiley & Sons.

Trounce, J. & Gould, D. (2000) *Clinical Pharmacology for Nurses*, 16th edn. London: Churchill Livingstone.

Turner, M.S. & Hankins, J. (2010) Pharmacology. In: Alexander, M., Corrigan, A., Gorski, L., Hankins, J. & Perucca, R. (eds) *Infusion Nursing: An Evidence-Based Approach*, 3rd edn. St Louis, MO: Saunders Elsevier, pp.263–298.

Twycross, R., Wilcock, A., Dean, M. & Kennedy, B. (2007) *Palliative Care Formulary*, 3rd edn. Available at: https://about.medicinescomplete.com/#

Ulutin, H.C., Guden, M., Dede, M. & Pak, Y. (2000) Comparison of granulocyte-colony, stimulating factor and granulocyte macrophage-colony stimulating factor in the treatment of chemotherapy extravasation ulcers. *European Journal of Gynaecological Oncology*, 21(6), 613–615.

Verrue, C., Mehuys, E., Boussery, K., et al. (2010) Tablet splitting: a common but not so innocent practice. *Journal of Advanced Nursing*, 67, 26–32.

Vidall, C., Roe, H., Dougherty, L. & Harrold, K. (2013) Dexrazoxane: A management option for anthracycline extravasations. *British Journal of Nursing*, 22(17), S6–S12.

Vizcarra, C. & Clum, S. (2010) Intraosseous route as alternative access for infusion therapy. *Journal of Infusion Nursing*, 33(3), 163–171.

Walsh, G. (2005) Hypodermoclysis: An alternate method for rehydration in long-term care. *Journal of Infusion Nursing*, 28(2), 123–129.

Watt, S. (2003) Safe administration of medicines to children: Part 2. *Paediatric Nurse*, 15(5), 40–44.

Weinstein, S. & Hagle, M.E. (2014) *Plumer's Principles and Practices of Intravenous Therapy*, 9th edn. Philadelphia: Lippincott Williams & Wilkins.

Werawatganon, T. & Charuluxanun, S. (2005) Patient controlled intravenous opioid analgesia versus continuous epidural analgesia for pain after intra-abdominal surgery. *Cochrane Database of Systematic Reviews*, 1, CD004088.

Westbrook, J., Woods, A., Rob, M., et al. (2010) Association of interruptions with an increased risk of severity of medication administration errors. *Archives of Internal Medicine*, 170(8), 683–690.

Westbrook, J., Rob, M., Woods, A. & Parry, D. (2011) Errors in the administration of intravenous medications and the role of correct procedures and nurse experience. *BMJ Quality & Safety*, 20, 1027–1034.

Wheatley, R., Schug, S. & Watson, D. (2001) Safety and efficacy of postoperative epidural analgesia. *British Journal of Anaesthesia*, 87(1), 47–61.

Whittington, Z. (2008) Pharmacological aspects of intravenous therapy. In: Dougherty, L. & Lamb, J. (eds) *Intravenous Therapy in Nursing Practice*, 2nd edn. Oxford: Blackwell, pp.117–140.

Whittlesea, C. & Hodson, K. (eds) (2018) *Clinical Pharmacy and Therapeutics*, 6th edn. London: Elsevier.

WHO (World Health Organization) (2004) *Immunization in Practice: Module 6 – Holding an Immunization Session.* Geneva: World Health Organization.

WHO (2008) *Medicines: Safety of Medicines – Adverse Drug Reactions.* Available at: https://www.who.int/medicines/regulation/medicines-safety/M_SBN_Jun18.pdf?ua=1 or https://apps.who.int/medicinedocs/en/d/Jh2992e/2.html

Wilkes, G. (2018) Chemotherapy: Principles of administration. In: Yarbro, C.H., Wujcik, D. & Holmes Gobel, B. (eds) *Cancer Nursing: Principles and Practice*, 8th edn. Burlington, MA: Jones & Bartlett, pp.417–496.

Wilkes, G. & Barton-Burke, M. (2018) *2018 Oncology Nursing Drug Handbook.* Sudbury, MA: Jones & Bartlett.

Wilson, K. & Sullivan, M. (2004) Preventing medication errors with smart infusion technology. *American Journal of Health System Pharmacists*, 61(2), 177–183.

Wolf, R., Matz, H., Orion, E. & Marcos, B. (2005) Preparing the skin before injecting botulinum toxin: More myth than evidence-based good judgement. *SKINmed: Dermatology for the Clinician*, 4(6), 385–396.

Workman, B. (1999) Safe injection techniques. *Nursing Standard*, 13(39), 47–52.

Wright, D., Begent, D., Crawford, H., et al. (2017) *Medicines Management of Adults with Swallowing Difficulties.* Guidelines. Available at: https://www.guidelines.co.uk/dysphagia/swallowing-difficulties-medication-management-guideline/453844.article

Wright, K. (2010) Do calculation errors by nurses cause medication errors in clinical practice? A literature review. *Nurse Education Today*, 30(1), 85–97.

Zeind, C.S. & Carvalho, M.G. (eds) (2018) *Applied Therapeutics. The Clinical Use of Drugs*, 11th edn. Philadelphia: Wolter Kluwer.

Chapter 16

Perioperative care

Justine Hofland with Hayley Grafton, Pascale Gruber, Tina Kitcher and Lian Lee

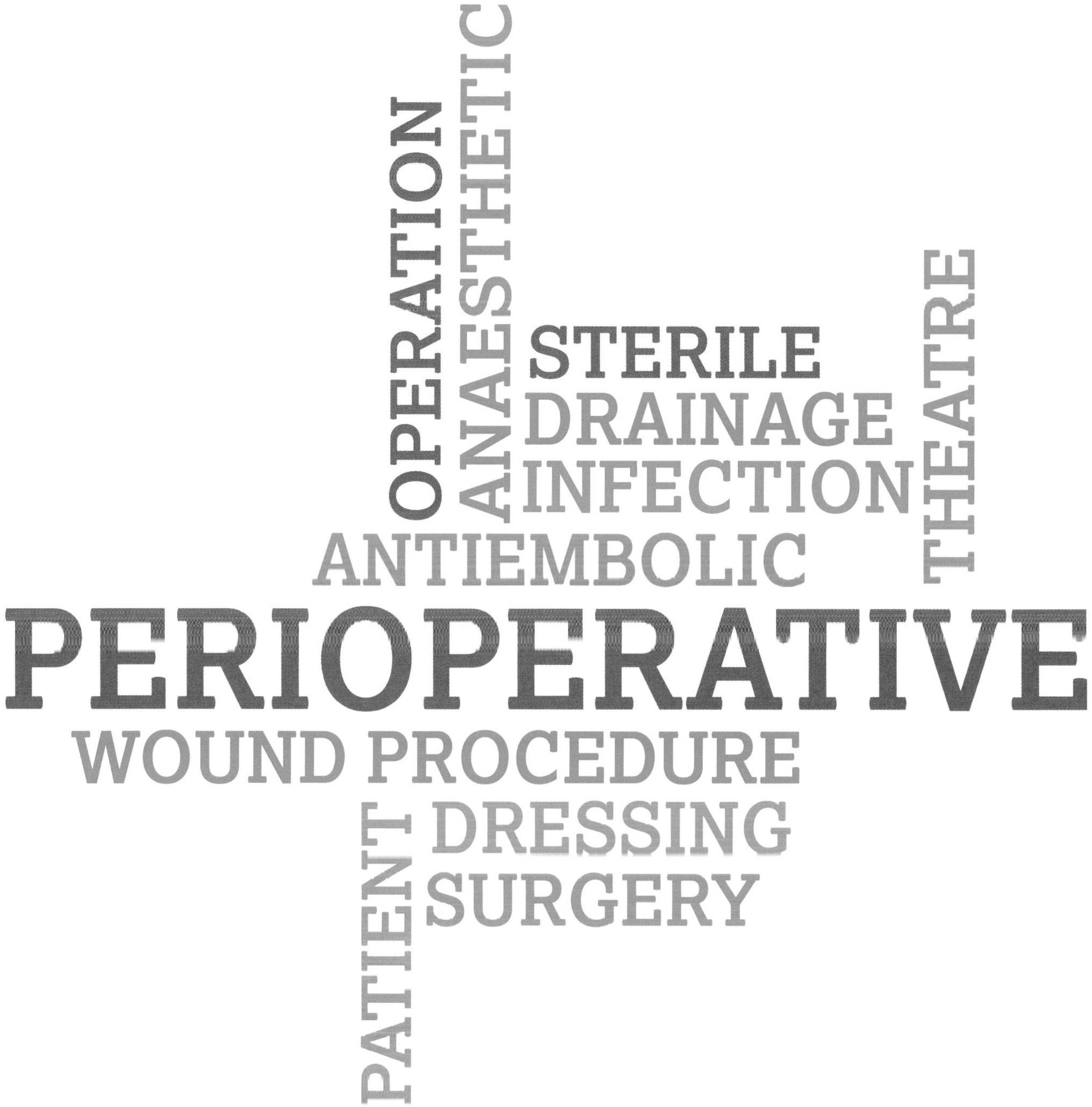

The Royal Marsden Manual of Clinical Nursing Procedures, Professional Edition, Tenth Edition. Edited by Sara Lister, Justine Hofland and Hayley Grafton.

Procedure guidelines

Overview

Care of patients undergoing any surgical procedure has three main phases: pre-operative (prior to the procedure), intraoperative (during the procedure) and post-operative (immediately following completion of the procedure).

Pre-operative care is delivered over two (or more) different episodes of contact with the patient. The first is pre-assessment, which usually takes place within days (in elective or semi-elective surgery), but sometimes minutes or hours (in emergency surgery), before the surgery. The aims of this phase are to assess the patient, carry out any necessary investigations to ensure they are physically and mentally able to have the procedure, and provide information about the anaesthetic and proposed surgery. The second is the immediate phase prior to the commencement of the procedure. The aims of this phase are to ensure the patient is prepared adequately for the surgical procedure and to mitigate any associated risks.

Intraoperative care usually consists of three phases: induction of anaesthesia, surgery and finally the recovery of the patient within the post-anaesthetic care unit (PACU). As care within surgery is delivered by a multidisciplinary team, a thorough handover of the patient is essential at every stage.

Finally, the care continues beyond the intraoperative phase when the patient receives *post-operative* care both before and after discharge from hospital. The amount and complexity of post-operative care required will vary significantly according to the nature of the surgery (e.g. minor, major, laparoscopic or robotic) and the physical, mental and social status of the patient.

Pre-operative care

Definition

Pre-operative care is the physical and psychosocial care provided to patients to help them prepare to safely undergo surgery. Psychosocial preparation includes assessing and managing patient stress, educating patients, and gaining informed consent for the procedure. Physical preparation is concerned with the prevention of peri- and post-operative complications (Liddle 2012, Turunen et al. 2017).

The pre-operative phase of care begins when the patient is informed of the need for surgery and subsequently makes the decision to undergo the procedure. This phase may be slightly longer than for a patient undergoing a minor day procedure.

Related theory

Optimal pre-operative care is underpinned by thorough assessment and planning. While physical preparation is concerned with the prevention of peri- and post-operative complications (Malley et al. 2015), attention should also be given to the patient's psychosocial needs and how the surgical procedure may affect their overall wellbeing.

The patient's pre-assessment includes a medical or adequately trained nurse review, which may prompt further diagnostic intervention or investigations (Boehm et al. 2016). Pre-assessment aims to assess the patient's fitness for surgery; provide information to the patient and their family about their upcoming anaesthetic and surgery; and provide advice about diet, exercise and lifestyle (e.g. smoking and alcohol cessation) to ensure the patient is fit and optimized for surgery. Pre-assessment is important in preparing patients physically and mentally for surgery, and it is key in improving post-operative outcomes and reducing cancellations on the day of surgery (Pritchard 2012).

Optimizing any co-morbidities pre-operatively that may affect the perioperative care of the patient is a key part of the review. The patient's current health status, performance and quality of life need to be considered, and the benefits of the surgery must outweigh the potential risks (Wood et al. 2016).

Traditionally, patients were admitted to hospital 1–2 days pre-operatively to allow for appropriate assessment, tests and investigations to be completed prior to their surgery; as such, they were not pre-assessed in dedicated clinics. However, once they were admitted it was frequently found that patients were presenting with complicated, newly identified or inappropriately managed co-morbidities, so surgeries were often delayed or cancelled. It was also found that a large number of cancelled operations occurred because patients did not arrive for their scheduled operation fasted. Some did not arrive because the date provided was inconvenient (due to childcare or work-related concerns) or the surgery was no longer wanted or needed.

In light of this, pre-operative assessment (POA) clinics were established to address these issues. The POA and planning carried out in these clinics aim to improve patient care and safety but also make the most efficient use of theatre resources and ward beds (K. Yu et al. 2017). POA is an essential part of the planned surgical care pathway. Subsequently, it has been found that providing patients with a time and place to explore their concerns and gain the information they need has increased the attendance of patients and therefore made more effective use of operating theatre time and other associated resources (NHS England 2017, NHS Modernization Agency 2003).

Any data obtained during the POA provides the foundation for producing an individualized patient care plan. This may consider the patient's frailty, risk of post-operative cognitive dysfunction, risk of infection, risk of pressure damage and risk of venous thromboembolism (VTE). A conversation with the patient during this POA is an effective way to increase the patient's awareness of certain risk factors (Almodaimegh et al. 2017, Haymes 2016).

The perioperative care documentation forms an important communication tool for the perioperative practitioners. It provides detailed records of the care delivered to the patient during their surgical journey. These records are maintained and handed over to various practitioners during each perioperative phase of care.

Depending on the complexity of the surgery, the POA can be undertaken either during a face-to-face conversation or via telephone clinics, which are increasingly nurse led.

Evidence-based approaches

Principles of care

POAs provide an effective screening process and help to identify the patient's overall risk of surgery-related complications. A POA should include three key stages:

1 comprehensive pre-operative history taking
2 physical examination
3 pre-operative investigations.

Pre-operative history taking

Medical history

A patient's medical history is an important component of any pre-operative evaluation. The history should start with current illness. This starts with the reason why the patient is having the planned procedure. It is important to include how the patient first presented with the symptoms of the condition, and any treatments that have been provided. It is important to obtain details of treatments such as previous chemotherapy or radiotherapy within the health history. A full history of current and previous medical problems should also be taken.

The history should also include a complete review of the patient's systems in order to look for undiagnosed disease or inadequately controlled chronic disease (see Chapter 2: Admissions and assessment). Diseases associated with an increased risk of surgical complications include respiratory and cardiac disease, malnutrition, and diabetes mellitus (Böhmer et al. 2014, Song et al. 2015). Diseases of the cardiovascular and respiratory systems are the most relevant in respect of a patient's fitness for anaesthesia and surgery (Kolh et al. 2016, [illegible] et al. 2015). It is valuable to obtain information such as dates of diagnosis, severity, ongoing treatment and any history of hospitalization for the disorders. A clear record of the patient's medical history produces the foundations for a substantial plan of care. 'This ensures the patient's surgical journey is effective, reducing the risk of suboptimal management and increasing safety with the least possible distress for the patient and their significant others' (Walsgrove 2011, p.33).

Family history

Asking the patient about illnesses that run in their family, such as hypertension, coronary artery disease, stroke, diabetes and hypercholesterolaemia, will alert the anaesthetist to any potential medical problems. A family history of adverse reactions associated with anaesthesia should also be obtained.

Surgical and anaesthetic history

A history of previous major surgeries and recent anaesthetics gives the assessor a comprehensive idea of the fitness of the patient. It is vital to find out about previous anaesthetic problems, such as post-operative nausea and vomiting. Patients with a history of bleeding complications should be carefully assessed for coagulation disorders (Gilbert-Kawai and Montgomery 2017), and a history of adverse anaesthetic reactions (in a patient or family members) should raise concerns about susceptibility to malignant hyperthermia (Chan et al. 2017). Patients susceptible to malignant hyperthermia (a rare, life-threatening progressive hyperthermic reaction during anaesthesia) require an anaesthesia consultation, appropriate preparation of the operating room, and adequate equipment and expertise in the event of a reaction during surgery. The Association of Anaesthetists of Great Britain and Ireland (AAGBI) (2011, 2013) offers guidance on the management of a malignant hyperthermia crisis (Figure 16.1).

The American Society of Anesthesiologists (ASA) (2014) has developed a scale with which to classify patients on the basis of their existing co-morbidities (Table 16.1). The scale is a well-established scoring tool that is useful for calculating patient risk of anaesthetic complications in relation to existing conditions (Doyle and Garmon 2019, Helkin et al. 2017).

Medications and allergies

A full list of the patient's current medications, including over-the-counter medications as well as vitamin and herbal supplements, is essential. Many medications interact with anaesthetic agents or negatively affect the patient in the intra- or post-operative period. These include anticoagulants, diabetic medications, calcium channel antagonists, beta blockers and some antidepressants. If a patient is taking steroids or opiates, these require careful titration intra- or post-operatively.

Generally, administration of most drugs should be continued up to and including on the morning of an operation, although some adjustments to dosage may be required (e.g. for anti-hypertensives and insulin). Some drugs should be discontinued pre-operatively, potentially days or weeks prior to surgery (Figure 16.2). Any monoamine oxidase inhibitors should be withdrawn 2–3 weeks before surgery because of the risk of interactions with drugs used during anaesthesia. The use of the oral contraceptive pill should be discontinued at least 4 weeks before elective surgery because of the increased risk of venous thrombosis. An assessment of any medications or herbal treatments that a patient consumes is included as part of the POA, and a decision is made on whether a further haematological work-up is required before surgery (Tassler and Kaye 2016). Some herbal supplements may have to be discontinued prior to surgery (Abe et al. 2014, Wang et al. 2015). Attributable side-effects of herbal medicines include cardiovascular instability, electrolyte disturbance, coagulation disturbance, coagulation disorder, endocrine effects, hepatotoxicity and renal failure (Batra and Rajeev 2007, Byard 2010).

The patient's allergy status should be obtained and specific details of reactions recorded in the care plan (particularly allergies to rubber products and to foods associated with latex reactions, such as bananas, avocados, kiwis, apricots and chestnuts). Medication 'intolerance' should also be documented to avoid severe side-effects such as nausea and vomiting. A history of previous anaphylactic reactions should be thoroughly documented to avoid potential incidents. Patients who are allergic to latex will need to be first on the theatre list, and theatre staff will need to be alerted to avoid complications (see 'Latex sensitivity and allergy' below).

Social history

A social history encompasses social situations such as home life and occupation. It provides a general picture of the social practices of the patient that may affect their fitness for surgery but also influence their recovery. A patient's past and current occupational background will provide an insight into their home and financial situation, as well as potential occupational disorders such as respiratory or musculoskeletal problems.

Understanding the patient's support systems (e.g. in their family or the wider community) is important. It will provide clues to potential 'road blocks' for a timely discharge. If the patient is found to have little or no available support in the community, the POA practitioner will have the opportunity to initiate any necessary discharge planning or social services referrals prior to admission. This will allow the patient to avoid any potential delays in their discharge.

The social history component of the POA includes a further assessment of smoking, drug and alcohol use. Long-term abuse of alcohol, tobacco products or drugs can result in organ damage, related medical complications, and therefore a higher incidence of perioperative morbidity and mortality. Intra- and post-operative events such as delirium tremens (an acute episode of delirium) are considered medical emergencies.

Alcohol

It is important to assess the amount of alcohol the patient consumes on a daily or weekly basis. Alcohol guidelines from the Department of Health (DH) (2016) recommend that both men and women should not drink more than 14 units of alcohol each week. Excessive alcohol consumption is a risk factor for post-operative delirium and withdrawal symptoms.

Smoking

It is important to assess smoking behaviour. There is strong evidence to suggest that higher risks and worse surgical outcomes occur when a patient continues to smoke (ASH 2016). Smoking causes increased cardiorespiratory complications, more intensive care admissions, higher rates of mortality, higher rates of wound infections and poorer wound healing after surgery (Thomsen et al. 2014). The POA practitioner should assess the length of time an individual has smoked, the number of tobacco products smoked per week, and the pattern of their smoking (i.e. times of day, and whether they smoke alongside specific activities, such as waking up, going to sleep or managing stress).

Pre-operative smoking cessation is important, and help with this should be offered during the assessment. Smoking cessation before elective surgery can significantly improve post-operative outcomes (Prestwich et al. 2017). The extent of smoking-related effects is dependent upon the amount and the length of time of smoking. Smokers have hyper-reactive airways that lead them to become more susceptible to incidents of laryngospasm and bronchospasm. They have an increased chance of developing post-operative lung infections due to a compromised ability to clear secretions. Post-operative healing is also affected by smoking as nicotine is a vasoconstrictor. Action on Smoking and Health (ASH) (2016) states that stopping smoking prior to surgery can reduce risks and improve outcomes. The National Institute for Health and Care Excellence (NICE) (2018b) offers guidance on stopping smoking interventions and services. The POA is an ideal opportunity to explore the smoking habits of the patient and provide advice on cessation.

Malignant Hyperthermia Crisis

AAGBI Safety Guideline

Successful management of malignant hyperthermia depends upon early diagnosis and treatment, onset can be within minutes of induction or may be insidious. The standard operating procedure below is intended to ease the burden of managing this rare but life threatening emergency.

1 Recognition

- Unexplained increase in $ETCO_2$ **AND**
- Unexplained tachycardia **AND**
- Unexplained increase in oxygen requirement
  (Previous uneventful anaesthesia does **not** rule out MH)
- Temperature changes are a late sign

2 Immediate management

- **STOP** all trigger agents
- **CALL FOR HELP.** Allocate specific tasks (action plan in MH kit)
- Install clean breathing system and **HYPERVENTILATE** with **100% O_2 high flow**
- Maintain anaesthesia with intravenous agent
- **ABANDON/FINISH** surgery as soon as possible
- Muscle relaxation with non-depolarising neuromuscular blocking drug

3 Monitoring & treatment

- Give **dantrolene**
- Initiate active **cooling** avoiding vasoconstriction
- **TREAT:**
  - **Hyperkalaemia:** calcium chloride, glucose/insulin, $NaHCO_3^-$
  - **Arrhythmias:** magnesium/amiodarone/metoprolol **AVOID** calcium channel blockers - interaction with dantrolene
  - **Metabolic acidosis:** hyperventilate, $NaHCO_3^-$
  - **Myoglobinaemia:** forced alkaline diuresis (mannitol/furosemide + $NaHCO_3^-$); may require renal replacement therapy later
  - **DIC:** FFP, cryoprecipitiate, platelets
- Check plasma CK as soon as able

DANTROLENE
2.5 mg/kg immediate iv bolus. Repeat 1 mg/kg boluses as required to max 10 mg/kg

For a 70 kg adult

- **Initial bolus: 9 vials dantrolene** 20 mg (each vial mixed with 60 ml sterile water)
- Further boluses of 4 vials dantrolene 20 mg repeated up to 7 times.

Continuous monitoring
Core & peripheral temperature
$ETCO_2$
SpO_2
ECG
Invasive blood pressure
CVP

Repeated bloods
ABG
U&Es (potassium)
FBC (haematocrit/platelets)
Coagulation

4 Follow-up

- Continue monitoring on ICU, repeat dantrolene as necessary
- Monitor for acute kidney injury and compartment syndrome
- Repeat CK
- Consider alternative diagnoses (sepsis, phaeochromocytoma, thyroid storm, myopathy)
- Counsel patient & family members
- Refer to MH unit (see contact details below)

The UK MH Investigation Unit, Academic Unit of Anaesthesia, Clinical Sciences Building, Leeds Teaching Hospitals NHS Trust, Leeds LS9 7TF. Direct line: 0113 206 5270. Fax: 0113 206 4140. Emergency Hotline: 07947 609601 (usually available outside office hours). Alternatively, contact Prof P Hopkins, Dr E Watkins or Dr P Gupta through hospital switchboard: 0113 243 3144

Your nearest MH kit is stored ....

This guideline is not a standard of medical care. The ultimate judgement with regard to a particular clinical procedure or treatment plan must be made by the clinician in the light of the clinical data presented and the diagnostic and treatment options available.

Figure 16.1 Malignant hyperthermia crisis. AAGBI safety guideline. Source: Adapted from AAGBI (2011) with permission of the Association of Anaesthetists.

Table 16.1 Modified American Society of Anesthesiologists physical status classification system

Class	Physical status	Example
I	A healthy patient	A fit patient with an inguinal hernia
II	A patient with mild systemic disease	A patient with essential hypertension and mild diabetes without end organ damage
III	A patient with severe systemic disease that is a constant threat to life	A patient with angina and moderate to severe chronic obstructive pulmonary disease (COPD)
IV	A patient with an incapacitating disease that is a constant threat to life	A patient with advanced COPD and cardiac failure
V	A moribund patient who is not expected to live 24 hours with or without surgery	A patient with a ruptured aortic aneurysm and a massive pulmonary embolism
VI	A declared brain-dead patient whose organs are being removed for donor purposes	(Brain dead is defined as irreversible brain damage causing the end of independent respiration, regarded as indicative of death.)
E	Emergency case	(An emergency exists when delay in treatment of the patient would lead to a significant increase in the threat to life or a body part.)

Source: Adapted from American Society of Anesthesiologists (2014).

Physical examination

Within the POA, the physical examination should build on the information gathered during the history taking. Baseline vital signs and physical assessment should be completed by a trained assessor. All patients should receive a thorough cardiovascular and pulmonary examination and should be asked about chronic or recent infections. The physical examination should pay specific attention to the respiratory and cardiovascular systems, as they are the systems that are most directly influenced by anaesthetics throughout the surgery and during the post-operative recovery period (Wijeysundera and Sweitzer 2015). Examination of further organ systems, such as abdominal or neurological systems, should also be completed if indicated by the patient's history. For example, patients with known alcohol or drug abuse should be further examined for hepatic and neurological impairments.

Patients with identified chronic organ diseases, such as congestive heart failure or chronic obstructive pulmonary disease, should be evaluated for any uncompensated disease. Patients with a history of heavy alcohol use should be assessed for signs of chronic liver disease with concomitant concern for post-operative alcohol withdrawal syndromes and delirium. Any abnormality detected in the review of all body systems (see Chapter 2: Admissions and assessment) should be characterized, investigated and addressed prior to surgery (particularly a new cough, fever or symptoms of an infection).

Finally, any airway problems must be recognized and addressed during the POA. The anaesthetic assessment also includes any cardiovascular, hepatic or pulmonary impairment; bleeding disorders; significant history of reflux or a hiatus hernia; and breathing difficulties such as sleep apnoea, paroxysmal nocturnal dyspnoea or orthopnoea. A failure to provide adequate ventilation can lead to hypoxia, a common anaesthetic problem that can result in morbidity and mortality during the perioperative phase. An airway assessment includes:

- range of motion of the neck and jaw
- mouth opening, including ability to protrude lower incisors in front of the upper incisors
- dentition (condition of teeth)
- history of temporomandibular joint dysfunction and other airway abnormalities.

If there are any problems with the airway, the anaesthetist needs to be informed so that appropriate equipment can be ordered for the day of surgery. Alert the anaesthetist if the patient has previously experienced a difficult intubation or if they currently have:

- disease
- surgical or radiotherapy scarring of the head, neck or mediastinum
- difficult or noisy breathing
- morbid obesity
- a poor mouth opening
- a rigid or deformed neck
- a receding chin or an overbite (Ong and Pearce 2011).

Further explanation of physical assessment can be found in Chapter 2: Admissions and assessment and Chapter 3: Discharge care and planning.

Pre-operative investigations

Laboratory investigations

Investigations are often ordered to establish baseline values, support or refute differential diagnoses, and support or monitor the management of existing disease processes. Laboratory tests should be ordered based on information obtained from both the patient history and the physical examination (Table 16.2). They should also take into account the patient's age and the complexity of the surgical procedure. NICE (2016b) offers an evidence-based guide for the ordering and use of routine pre-operative testing in elective surgeries. The investigations are based on ASA status (see Table 16.1), the age of the patient and their co-morbidities.

Non-laboratory investigations

Electrocardiograms

A standard 12-lead electrocardiogram (ECG) (Figure 16.3) is frequently performed if indicated by the age of the patient, risk factors, co-morbidities or findings of the physical examination. The patient's ASA grading (see Table 16.1) and the surgical grading of the planned surgery may also indicate an ECG. The proportion of patients with an abnormal ECG increases with age and the presence of co-morbidities. An ECG can also be completed to establish a baseline prior to surgery for post-operative comparison.

Imaging: chest X-ray

A chest X-ray can give the practitioner valuable information to support or refute potential diagnoses or further assess the severity of

The ROYAL MARSDEN
NHS Foundation Trust

Medication to Continue	Query	Medication to Omit

Pharmacological class of medication	Pre-operative management	Comments
Gastro-intestinal System	**H_2 antagonists** e.g. ranitidine Continue but for cimetidine see comments	Cimetidine: Caution: can lead to increased bupivacaine toxicity. Has been shown to raise plasma lidocaine levels, especially when used as an anti-arrhythmic
	Proton pump inhibitors e.g. lansoprazole, omeprazole	
	Aminosalicylates e.g. mesalazine, sulphasalazine	
Cardiovascular System	**Alpha antagonists** e.g. doxazosin Continue for anti-hypertensive indication but for urological indication see comments	Continue all, EXCEPT alfuzosin Stop alfuzosin 24 hours prior to operation
	Anti-arrythmics e.g. digoxin, amiodarone, flecainide	Refer to anaesthetist if hypokalaemic, hypomagnesaemic or hypercalcaemic
	Beta-blockers e.g. atenolol, bisoprolol, metoprolol, propranolol	Avoid stopping suddenly. Continue IV if prolonged NBM
	Calcium antagonists e.g. amlodipine, nifedipine, diltiazem	
	Centrally acting anti-hypertensives e.g. clonidine, moxonidine	
	Loop and Thiazide Diuretics e.g. furosemide, bendroflumethiazide, bumetamide, indapamide	Correct any electrolyte imbalances prior to surgery
	Nitrates e.g. isosorbide mononitrate, isosorbide dinitrate, glyceryl trinitrate (GTN)	

Figure 16.2 Guide to preoperative medication.

Pharmacological class of medication	Pre-operative management	Comments
	Potassium channel activator e.g. nicorandil	
	ACE inhibitors e.g. lisinopril, ramipril, enalapril: omit 24 hours prior to major surgery except for patients with exisiting heart failure – discuss with anaethetist	
	Angiostensin receptor II antagonists e.g. losartan, candesartan, irbesartan	
	Aspirin	Patients taking aspirin for primary prevention of heart disease can stop 7 days before surgery. All others please follow local **perioperative anti-platelet drug guidelines**
	Clopidogrel (Plavix) and prasugrel (Effient)	**See local perioperative anti-platelet drug guidelines** Discuss all patients taking these drugs with consultant anaesthetist. DO NOT STOP IN RECENT CORONARY STENTS (3 months for bare metal, and 12 months for drug eluting)
	Dipyridamole	Discuss with surgeons. If procedure high risk, omit on day of surgery
	Low-molecular-weight heparin e.g. tinzaparin, enoxaparin	**See local anticoagulant guidelines.** Therapeutic dose should not be given less than 24 hours before surgery
	Potassium sparing diuretics e.g. spironalactone, amiloride, co-amilofruse, co-amiloride	Omit on day of surgery. May contribute to hyperkalaemia post-op
	Oral anticoagulant e.g. warfarin, phenidione	**See local perioperative anticoagulation guidelines** Patients having minor procedures may be able to continue after discussion with surgical team
Respiratory System	**Aminophylline / Theophylline**	
	Inhalers e.g. salbutamol, beclometasone	Optimize treatment at pre-operative assessment

Figure 16.2 *Continued*

Pharmacological class of medication	Pre-operative management	Comments
Central Nervous System	**Anti-epileptics** e.g. phenytoin, sodium valproate, carbamazepine, lamotrigine, topiramate, tiagabine	For epilepsy MUST continue. Very important to maintain therapeutic concentrations to avoid seizures.
	Antipsychotics e.g. chlorpromazine, haloperidol, olanzapine, risperidone For clozapine see notes	Clozapine: stop on the day of operation Please note the last dose should be administered no later than 8 pm on the night before surgery; *can increase VTE risk and hypotension*
	Barbiturates e.g. phenobarbital	
	Benzodiazepines e.g. diazepam, temazepam, lorazepam	
	Opioid analgesics e.g. morphine, methadone, codeine, fentanyl	Consult anaesthetist to plan post-op analgesia. Must confirm dose of methadone with usual prescribing doctor/dispensing chemist.
	Paracetamol	
	Parkinson's treatment e.g. co-careldopa, co-beneldopa, cabergoline, selegiline, entacapone, procyclidine	Continue oral medications up to 2 hours before surgery. Must inform anaesthetist of patients on anti-Parkinsonian medicines. Selegiline interacts with pethidine to cause hyperpyrexia and CNS toxicity.
	Selective serotonin re-uptake Inhibitors (SSRIs) e.g. paroxetine, fluoxetine, citalopram, sertraline	
	Venlafaxine (Effexor), Mirtazapine (Zispin)	
	Lithium	Check levels pre-op. Continue for minor surgery. Discuss with anaesthetist plan for major surgery. Restart ASAP post-op
	Tricyclic antidepressants e.g. amitriptyline, lofepramine, dosulepin	Continue, but increased risk of arrhythmias
	Anti-dementia drugs e.g. donepezil, rivastigmine, galantamine (acetylcholinesterase inhibitors)	May prolong neuromuscular blockade and exaggerate muscle relaxation with succinylcholine-type muscle relaxants. Alert anaesthetist to the potential for prolonged neuromuscular blockade.

Figure 16.2 *Continued*

Pharmacological class of medication	Pre-operative management	Comments
		Omit rivastigmine and glantamine 24–48 hours prior to surgery. It is recommended to stop donepezil 2–3 weeks prior to surgery; however these patients may not return to their baseline mental function, so it may be unethical to stop
	Clozapine	Stop 12 hours pre-op. Restart ASAP; if discontinued for longer than 48 hours contact pharmacist for advice
	Monoamine-oxidase inhibitors (non-reversible) e.g. phenelzine, [illegible]	Stop 14 days pre-op (discuss with psychiatrist). If not withdrawn, inform [illegible]
	Reversible MAOIs e.g. moclobemide	Last dose 24 hours before surgery
Infections	**Antibiotics, antifungals, antivirals**	
	HIV antiretroviral drugs e.g. ritonavir	Wherever possible, treatment should not be interrupted due to concerns with developing resistance
Endocrine System	**Corticosteroids** e.g. prednisolone (Current or stopped within last 3 months) **See above for more details**	May need additional hydrocortisone bolus intra/post-operation: **Minor surgery**: 25 mg hydrocortisone at induction (or usual oral dose) **Moderate surgery**: 25 mg hydrocortisone at induction (or usual oral dose) then 25 mg hydrocortisone TDS for 24 hours and then restart usual steroid dose **Major surgery**: 50 mg hydrocortisone at induction (or usual oral dose) then 50 mg TDS hydrocortisone for 48–72 hours and then restart usual steroid dose
	Desmopressin (DDAVP) Continue but **see comments**	Continue and discuss with endocrinologist consultant for specialist advice in the peri-operative period
	Hormone antagonists e.g. tamoxifen, anastrazole	Specialist advice should be sought; VTE risk is increased

Figure 16.2 *Continued*

Pharmacological class of medication	Pre-operative management	Comments
	Hormone replacement therapy (HRT)	Specialist advice should be sought, VTE risk is increased
	Levothyroxine (thyroxine)	
	Progesterone-only oral contraceptives	Thromboprophylaxis and TEDS
	Combined oral contraceptives (i.e. containing oestrogen) **See above for more details**	Consult gynae team on individual patient basis Omit 4 weeks prior to major surgery; institute thromboprophylaxis and TEDS as per **local VTE guidelines**. Advise on alternative family planning
	Oral antidiabetics e.g. glibenclamide, glipizide, gliclazide, tolbutamide, pioglitazone	See local **diabetic guidelines**
	Insulin	See local **diabetic guidelines** Refer to anaesthetist. Continue until morning of surgery. Omit morning dose and breakfast **Minor surgery**: Restart s/c insulin post-op with first meal **Major surgery:** Omit breakfast and S/C insulin and start intravenous sliding-scale insulin
	Metformin	See **local diabetic guidelines**
	Bisphosphonates eg. alendronate, risedronate **For strontium see comments**	Restart when patient can sit upright and swallow the tablets whole with a glass of water For strontium: stop 14 days prior to operation
Malignant Disease and Immunosuppression	**Drugs to prevent adverse effects** e.g. allopurinol	Seek advice from oncologist/ haematologist
	Immunosuppressants e.g. azathioprine, ciclosporin, mycophenolate, tacrolimus	Seek advice from oncologist/ haematologist

Figure 16.2 *Continued*

Pharmacological class of medication	Pre-operative management	Comments
	Cytotoxics e.g. alkylating agents, antimetabolites	Seek advice from oncologist/ haematologist
Musculoskeletal and Joint Diseases	**Baclofen**	Continue if important for patients
	COX II inhibitors e.g. celecoxib	Continue if patient is taking
	DMARDS e.g. methotrexate for rheumatoid arthritis, penicillamine	Continue unless at risk of renal complications. Discuss with specialist
	Non-steroidal anti-inflammatory drugs (NSAIDs) e.g. diclofenac, ibuprofen	Increased risk of bleeding. Reduce intake if symptoms permit Minor surgery: continued if needed Major surgery: if increased risk of post-op bleeding or when a bleed could result in significant problems, stop pre-op • For drugs with a short half-life (e.g. diclofenac, ibuprofen, indomethacin) stop 1 day pre-op • For drugs with a longer half-life (e.g. naproxen) stop 3 days pre-op Restart when risk of bleeding no longer significant
Complimentary Alternative Medicines	Ideally these should be stopped at least 2 weeks prior to surgery. Refer to local guidance and consult local pharmacy services	
Homoeopathic Medicines	If the dilution of the remedy is not known or less than 12c or 24c then it may contain active ingredients and could potentially interact with conventional medicines. Therefore it should be stopped 2 weeks prior to surgery	
Nutrition and Blood	Drugs for nutrition (e.g. iron, folic acid, calcium, magnesium): continue unless specifically advised not to	

Figure 16.2 *Continued*

Table 16.2 Pre-operative laboratory tests

Pre-operative test	Rationale
Haematology	
Full blood count (FBC), including haemoglobin and haematocrit	Patients with a history of: • smoking • malignancy • respiratory disease • cardiac disease. *These patients may be at increased risk of anaemia and polycythaemia.*
White blood cell count	Patients with a history of: • recent chemotherapy and/or radiotherapy • malignancy • recent infection. *These patients may have either raised or lowered white blood cell count.*
Platelet count	Platelet count should be checked in patients with a history of: • bleeding tendencies • renal or hepatic disease • recent treatment with chemotherapy.
Coagulation screening, including prothrombin and activated partial thromboplastin time	This is not recommended unless the patient: • is taking anticoagulants • has a history of bleeding disorders • has a history of post-surgical bleeding • has a bleeding history (such as liver disease or malignancy) (Chee et al. 2008).
Group and save or cross-match	Having the blood tested prior to the date of surgery gives the blood bank more time to find the appropriate blood required for the specific patient. Patients with unusual blood typing or rare antibodies may need to have blood specially obtained from a national blood bank, and having the sample collected in advance will decrease the chance of errors and of the patient having their surgery postponed
Serum biochemistry	
Glycosylated haemoglobin (HbA1c) level	Patients presenting with a history of: • steroid use • obesity • cardiovascular disease • symptoms suggestive of diabetes. *The HbA1c provides a more accurate measurement of the patient's long-term glucose control and compliance compared with random glucose testing.*
Baseline serum creatinine and blood urea nitrogen level	Patients with a history of: • renal dysfunction • diabetes • cardiovascular disease • obesity • use of medications such as steroids or diuretics.
Liver function tests, such as albumin	Patients presenting with: • liver disease • malignancy • alcohol abuse • malnutrition • jaundice. *The liver and kidneys aid the metabolism and elimination of many anaesthetics and medications. Therefore, it is vital to ensure these are checked pre-operatively to ensure adequate organ function.*
Electrolyte levels	Electrolyte levels should be checked pre-operatively in patients with a history of: • renal dysfunction • diabetes • malignancy • malnutrition • vomiting or diarrhoea • use of medications such as diuretics or chemotherapy. *These patients may require pre-operative prescribing of supplements such as potassium to optimize their electrolyte levels prior to surgery. Electrolyte imbalances such as hypokalaemia or hyponatraemia can be life threatening.*

Pre-operative test	Rationale
Other tests	
Thyroid function testing	Patients with a history of: • hypothyroidism • hyperthyroidism. *Patients with untreated or severe thyroid disease are at increased risk of developing 'thyroid storm' (dangerously raised heart rate, blood pressure and temperature) relating to the stress of surgery or illness (Weinberg et al. 1983).*
Urinalysis	Patients presenting with symptoms of a urinary tract infection or those presenting for procedures of the urinary tract, e.g. cystoscopy.
Pregnancy testing	Pregnancy testing should be completed based on the findings of the medical history and the date of the last menstrual cycle. This should ideally be done on the day of admission unless the patient suspects she might be pregnant during pre-assessment.

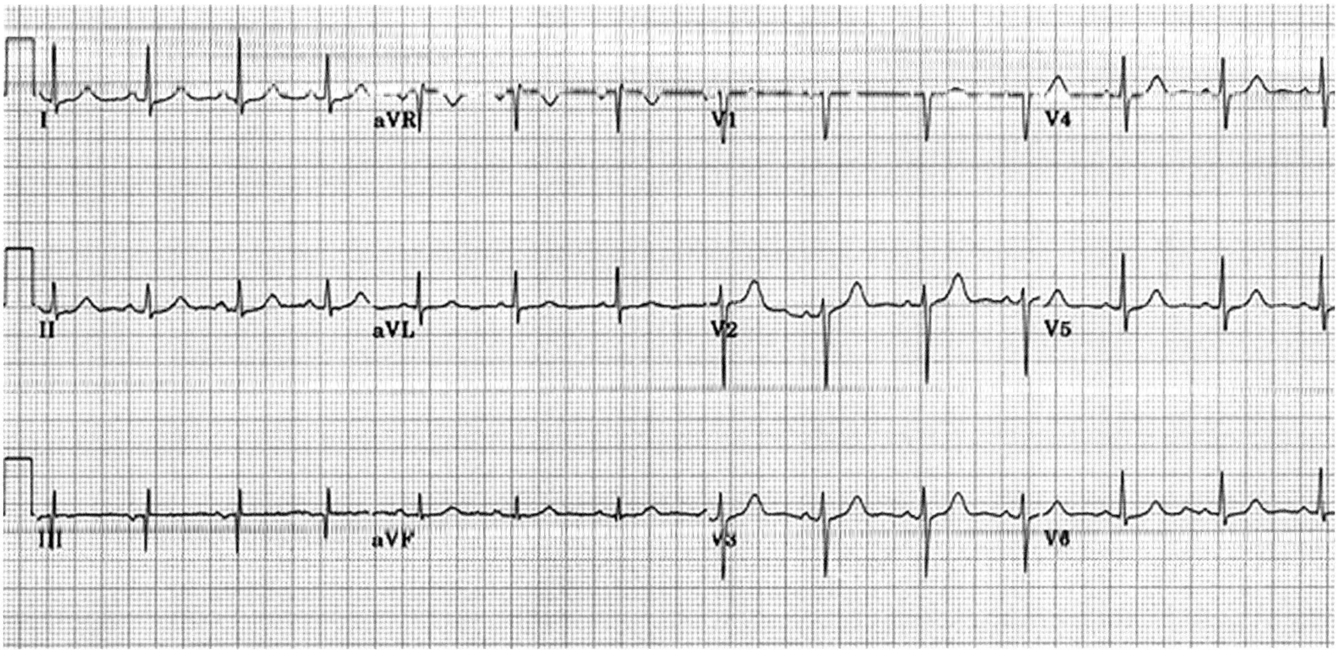

Figure 16.3 An example of a 12-lead electrocardiogram (ECG).

a specific disease. Patients presenting with history of cardiovascular or respiratory symptoms or with disease processes should have a chest X-ray completed pre-operatively. If the patient has had a chest X-ray within the past 6 months, it does not need to be repeated unless new problems have arisen or the existing problems have worsened.

Cardiopulmonary exercise testing

Older et al. (1993) introduced the concept of cardiopulmonary exercise testing (CPET) (Figure 16.4). CPET is a dynamic, non-invasive test involving the use of an exercise bicycle (cycle ergometer) where the work rate is gradually and imperceptibly increased in a stepped or ramped manner until the patient is unable to continue. This enables examination of the ability of the patient's cardiorespiratory system to adapt to a 'stress' situation of increased oxygen demand, in effect mimicking the conditions of surgery.

CPET relies upon accurate breath-by-breath measurements of pulmonary gas exchange through a mouthpiece that measures respiratory gas exchange. In addition, electrocardiography, blood pressure, pulse oximetry and heart rate are monitored during the exercise. From the CPET, two key indicators are derived: the body's maximum oxygen uptake (VO_2 max) and the point at which anaerobic metabolism exceeds aerobic metabolism (anaerobic threshold, or AT). Together these broadly indicate the ability of the cardiovascular system to deliver oxygen to the peripheral tissues and the ability of the tissues to use that oxygen. In addition, the AT has been shown to be a useful predictor of post-operative cardiac complications in abdominal surgery (Lanier et al. 2018).

CPET is often referred to as the gold standard for measuring exercise tolerance. It enables clinicians to triage patients to the appropriate level of care after surgery, allowing the efficient use of intensive care facilities (Mezanni 2017). It also assists surgeons in assessing treatment options more easily. The patient is then in a better position to evaluate their own risk–benefit ratio for surgery and thus make a more informed decision on consent for an operation (Guazzi et al. 2017).

Indications for CPET include:

- to estimate the likelihood of perioperative morbidity and mortality and contribute to pre-operative risk assessment
- to inform the processes of multidisciplinary shared decision making and consent
- to guide clinical decisions about the most appropriate level of perioperative care (ward versus critical care)
- to direct pre-operative referrals and interventions so as to optimize the detection and management of co-morbidities
- to identify previously unsuspected pathology
- to evaluate the effects of neoadjuvant cancer therapies, including chemotherapy and radiotherapy

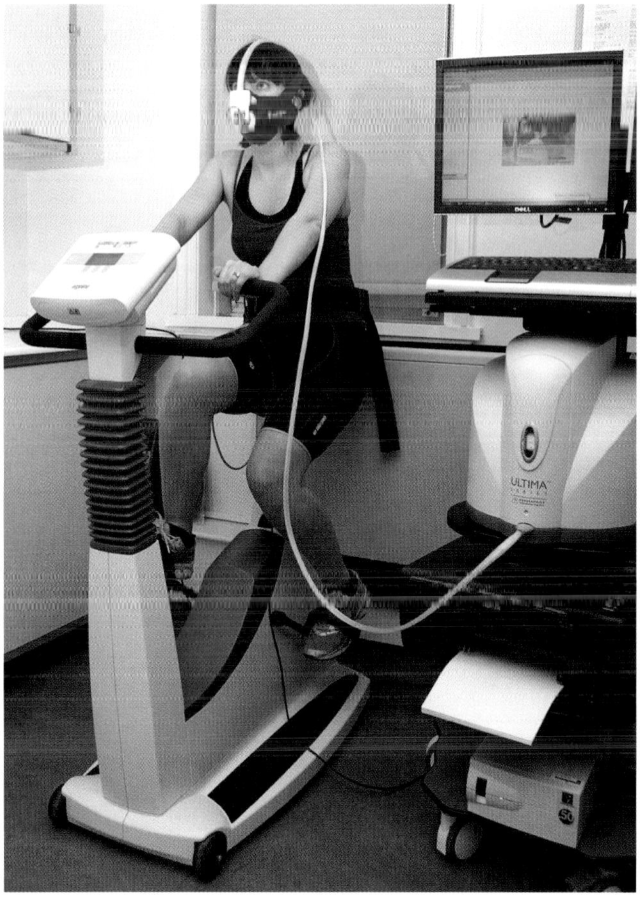

Figure 16.4 Cardiopulmonary exercise testing (CPET).

- to guide prehabilitation and rehabilitation training programmes
- to guide intraoperative anaesthetic practice (Levett et al. 2018, p.486).

Further referrals

During the POA, it is often deemed necessary to refer the patient for further expert assessment or advice. This is helpful in providing valuable information regarding the patient's condition and creating an appropriate plan of action for the patient in the perioperative or post-operative period. When referral is deemed necessary, patients are seen by a specialist to further assess whether they are in the optimum condition for the desired surgery and/or whether their health can be 'optimized' prior to surgery to improve their post-operative outcomes.

Anticipated patient outcomes

POA and planning is a holistic process, and the anticipated patient outcome is to ensure that the patient is safe to proceed with anaesthesia and surgery and/or optimize their health for surgery.

POA clinics and anaesthetists play an important role in ensuring the patient's surgical plan becomes a reality. This is a collaborative decision-making process in which clinicians and patients work together to select tests, treatments and management that are based on clinical evidence and the patient's informed preferences. POA clinics have several key objectives, referred to by the Royal College of Anaesthetists (RCoA) (2019):

- Provide the opportunity to further explain and discuss the upcoming surgery and recovery phase with the patient, with the aim of minimizing any fears, anxieties or stress and therefore aiding recovery.
- Assess the patient's fitness for the surgery, anaesthesia and post-operative recovery. This is achieved through a comprehensive medical history, physical examination and the ordering of appropriate investigations (NICE 2016b).
- Identify any co-morbidities that may require intervention prior to admission and surgery and that are likely to affect the intra- and post-operative care of the patient, such as discontinuation of anticoagulants or implementation of antihypertensive medications.
- Assist in ensuring that the patient is in optimum health prior to surgery, making further referrals to secondary care specialists as necessary, such as cardiologists.
- Identify the need for and arrange for the supply of any specialist equipment (e.g. bariatric equipment or critical care bed), and ensure that any other special requirements are planned for.
- Provide information to the patient about any specific pre-operative preparation that may be required (e.g. fasting or bowel preparation). This may require involving members of the multidisciplinary team, such as clinical nurse specialists, physiotherapists or dieticians.
- Give the patient a point of contact for further questions or concerns, or if they want to postpone or cancel the surgery.
- Provide the patient with information on what to expect in the post-operative period. This may include leaflets and videos to help the patient understand the planned procedure. They should also talk to the anaesthetist about pain control, intubation and potential critical care admission.
- Provide any assistance with health promotion activities such as smoking cessation, weight loss and alcohol awareness that will help to improve the patient's outcome in the perioperative and post-operative periods. This may include further referrals to primary care services, such as stop smoking services or dietetic advice.
- Identify any cultural, religious or communication needs of the patient.
- Assess older patients for risk of post-operative delirium (AAGBI 2014).
- Conduct individualized admission and discharge planning, ensuring that the patient and carer(s) know what to expect. This facilitates earlier discharge and enables follow-up care to be undertaken in the primary care setting.
- Identify patients who might benefit from a targeted exercise program prior to surgery (i.e. prehabilitation).
- Clearly define the risks of surgery and counsel patients on the risks of post-operative mortality and morbidity.
- Provide the appropriate pre-operative documentation to the multidisciplinary team (Liddle 2013, NICE 2016b, Oakley and Bratchell 2010).

A thorough POA results in good clinical outcomes and an enhanced patient experience, as evidenced by the success of the Enhanced Recovery Partnership Programme. This initiative has transformed elective surgical care pathways across the NHS since 2009 (DH 2011) (Box 16.1). It also minimizes length of hospital stay through:

- reduced cancellations due to patient ill health or DNAs (did not attend)
- increased number of same-day surgery admissions
- earlier discharge.

Clinical governance

The POA should generally only be performed by one of the following trained professional groups:

- a nurse or operating department practitioner
- an anaesthetist
- a doctor.

However, this list is not exhaustive due to the ever-expanding clinical complexity of surgical patients. The role of a POA practitioner

Box 16.1 The Enhanced Recovery Programme

The Enhanced Recovery Programme includes the following.

- *Pre-operative assessment, planning and preparation before admission*:
  - optimization of health (including encouraging patients to exercise and eat well) and pre-existing medical conditions (e.g. diabetes)
  - discharge planning
  - information giving.
- *Reduction of the physical stress of the operation*:
  - use of minimally invasive surgical techniques (e.g. laparoscopic)
  - individualized goal-directed fluid therapy
  - use of quick-offset anaesthetic agents, allowing quick recovery
  - prevention of hypothermia
  - use of effective, opiate-sparing analgesia to facilitate early mobilization (e.g. nerve blocks)
  - minimization of the risk of post-operative nausea and vomiting
  - minimization of the use of drains and nasogastric tubes.
- *Post-operative rehabilitation*:
  - early nutrition
  - early mobilization
  - early removal of catheters
  - post-operative education and support (e.g. with stoma care)
  - follow-up advice and support.

is broad (Box 16.2), and they should be competent in the following three principles of care (as previously outlined):

- conducting a comprehensive health history
- conducting a physical examination
- ordering appropriate laboratory and non-laboratory investigations.

Additionally, a POA practitioner should have knowledge of the Enhanced Recovery Programme (see Box 16.1) if it is required to support the patient along their perioperative care pathway.

The AAGBI (2018) states that trained POA staff 'play an essential role when, by working to agreed protocols, they screen and assess patients for fitness for anaesthesia and surgery' (p.6). Although they are not qualified to make the final decision about a patient's fitness for surgery, they play an important role in 'identifying potential problems' (p.6).

Non-complicated patients often do not require further assessment by an anaesthetist until the day of admission. Patients considered complicated by the trained assessor are further reviewed by an anaesthetist. This is supported by Kenny (2011), who found that approximately 20% of patients assessed by pre-assessment nurses were referred to the anaesthetic clinic. Of these referrals, half were due to the discovery of poorly controlled, undiagnosed or complex health problems and half were due to the nature of the surgery required.

While the POA can be performed by non-anaesthetic personnel such as nurses, it is vital that the anaesthetist in charge of the patient's case is aware of the patient's co-morbidities.

Competencies

Competency assessment is also carried out in pre-assessment in the form of a competency portfolio, as advocated by Walsgrove (2011). The competency portfolio was designed in correlation with the NHS Modernization Agency's (2003) guidance on POA. The portfolio covers administrative function, physical assessment (medical and nursing history), psychological and social assessment, decision making, and interventions (referral, pre-operative counselling, and ordering and performing tests and investigations). To ensure quality, regular audits of the pre-assessment documentation should be carried out.

Box 16.2 Role of the assessor in the pre-operative assessment (POA) clinic

- Work to guidelines and competencies agreed by anaesthetists, surgeons and other allied health professionals to ensure a consistent approach.
- Take a targeted history and conduct a relevant physical examination of the patient, including airway assessment.
- Refer patients who fall outside the agreed criteria to the anaesthetist, who may then make further referrals.
- Arrange and perform investigations in accordance with local and national guidance (NICE 2016b).
- Ensure that the results of tests are evaluated and address any abnormal investigation results with the available anaesthetist, surgeon and/or primary care professional, according to local guidelines.
- Refer patients back to primary care or another healthcare professional to optimize their medical condition, according to local guidelines.
- Take responsibility for following up referrals to ensure the patient remains in the pre-operative system.
- Liaise actively with the anaesthetic department.
- Arrange and co-ordinate any assessment and/or investigations needed nearer the time of surgery. Take responsibility for all communication with the patient throughout their pre-operative journey.
- Commence necessary planning for the perioperative stay and ensure a timely discharge.
- Identify factors that may influence the dates of surgery offered, for example school holidays.
- Collate all information prior to surgery and ensure that the multidisciplinary documentation is available for anaesthetists to see at least 48 hours prior to admission.
- Communicate the approximate length of an operation, any special requirements and essential resources to the waiting list office, bed management office, operating theatre department and/or theatre scheduler.
- Contact all patients who fail to attend POA to identify the reason. Act on the reason, following local protocols for the management of DNAs (did not attend) in POA.

Patient information and education

Related theory

Patients undergoing surgery have information and supportive care needs before and after their surgery. Providing information to patients is considered a crucial element of their surgical pathway. Patients require information that is meaningful for them as individuals. It is necessary to educate patients on the nature of the benefits and risks of procedures so they can be involved in the decision-making process and enabled to give fully informed consent. Accurate, reliable and complete information plays a pivotal role in helping patients to make informed decisions.

Evidence-based approaches

Principles of care

The way in which information is delivered and understood will help to determine whether a patient's actual post-operative experiences are congruent with the expected ones. Therefore, it is essential that information is provided at the right time and in a variety of formats. Information materials must contain scientifically reliable information and be presented in a form that is acceptable and useful to patients (i.e. suitable for the patient's educational level).

Providing patient education has been found to be extremely beneficial by reducing anxiety levels and promoting wellbeing (Guo 2015), which may ultimately result in patients requiring less analgesia. It is important that any form of education is tailored to

Table 16.3 Forms of patient education

Patient education	Definition	Advantages	Disadvantages
Face to face	Includes any education delivered verbally by a healthcare provider to a single patient or group of patients. This remains the most common form of patient education. See 'Verbal communication' below.	• Can be tailored to individual patient needs	• Time consuming • Consistency problems • Relies on the patient's ability to absorb, understand and retain the verbal information
Paper based	Includes any written information, such as patient information leaflets.	• Can develop comprehensive educational materials that are consistently presented • Patients can refer back to the materials	• Unable to tailor to individual patient needs
Web based	Includes any verbal or written patient information. Examples include web-based seminars, patient groups, programmes of care, interactive websites, podcasts, and videos (e.g. on YouTube).	• Wide-ranging and current information • Variety of teaching formats • Patient empowerment: patients can search for information themselves, look up research and help to generate questions for healthcare professionals. • Available 24 hours a day • Can develop comprehensive educational materials that are consistently presented • Patients can refer back to the materials • Can be accessed all over the world	• Potential for inaccurate information • Lack of access • Poor quality of online resources • Security and privacy issues

individual patients. There are currently three main forms of patient education: face to face, paper based and web based (Table 16.3).

Verbal communication

Any verbal information should be supported by paper-based or web-based written information from reliable, evidence-based sources and tailored to the patient's educational level. Written patient information in particular can:

- help patients to gain a greater understanding of surgery and what is expected of them
- ensure patients arrive on time and are properly prepared for surgery (e.g. pre-operative fasting)
- increase patient confidence, improving their overall experience
- refamiliarize patients with what they have already been told
- enhance patient and carer involvement in the patient's treatment and condition.

Consent

Definition

Consent can be defined as permission for something to happen or agreement to do something. NHS Choices (2016) states that 'consent to treatment means a person must give permission before they receive any type of medical treatment, test or examination'.

Evidence-based approaches

There are different types of consent in healthcare: written, verbal (explicit) and non-verbal (implied or implicit). The requirement to gain consent has two purposes, one legal and the other clinical (Richardson 2013). Sufficient evidence based information must be provided to the patient to allow them to make a balanced and informed decision about their care and treatment (GMC 2008, 2014, RCN 2017).

Principles of care

It is important to recognize that seeking consent for a surgical intervention is not merely the signing of a form. It is the process of providing the information that enables the patient to make a decision to undergo a specific treatment. Consent should be a considered and informed decision-making process. For major operations, it is good practice to gain a person's consent to the proposed procedure well in advance, ideally prior to pre-assessment. This allows time to respond to the person's questions and provide adequate information so that the person has time to develop an understanding and thereby make an informed decision (Hughes 2011). For patients with learning disabilities or mental health problems, it is advisable that a relative or carer is present so that consent, capacity and any reasonable adjustments (e.g. to equipment or psychological support) can be discussed depending on the needs of the patient (RCN 2017). For consent to be valid, it must be given voluntarily and freely, without pressure or undue influence, by an appropriately informed person who has the capacity to consent to the intervention in question (NMC 2018, RCN 2017). Informed consent is a legal requirement (*Montgomery v Lanarkshire Health Board* 2015).

While the validity of consent does not depend on the way in which it is given (RCN 2017), it is good practice to use forms for written consent where an intervention such as surgery is to be undertaken. Most hospitals' local consent policies will require written consent to be obtained in these circumstances.

However, the procedure and risks must be written down for the patient to read and understand, before signing the form; their signature alone does not make the consent valid. For example, if a person's signature to confirm their consent is gained immediately before the surgical procedure is due to start, at a time when they may be feeling particularly vulnerable, this would raise concerns about its validity (GMC 2014, RCN 2017). Furthermore, patients should not in any situation be given routine pre-operative medication before being asked for their consent to proceed with the treatment (RCN 2017).

Clinical governance

It is accepted that when a patient gives valid consent, this is valid indefinitely unless it is withdrawn by the patient; therefore, no specific time limit is designated from signature to procedure (Hughes 2011). However, it is good practice to confirm the patient's wishes if significant time has elapsed since the initial process. The patient is entitled to withdraw consent at any time (Hughes 2011).

For consent to be valid, it must encompass several factors:

- *Consent must be given willingly*: this means without pressure or undue influence to either undertake or not undertake treatment.
- *Consent must be informed*: the person must have an understanding of the procedure and the purpose behind it, and have been

given relevant information about the benefits and risks of the procedure as well as potential alternatives. This information needs to be explained or presented in a way that is meaningful and easy to understand by the person in a variety of formats (both verbal and written) to enable them to make an informed decision.
- *The person must have the capacity to consent to the procedure in question*: that is, they must have the ability to understand and retain the information provided, especially around the consequences of having or not having the procedure (NMC 2018, RCN 2017). An assessment of a person's capacity must be based on their ability to make a specific decision at the time it needs to be made, and not their ability to make a decision in general (DH 2009b). Under the Mental Capacity Act (2005), which became fully effective in England and Wales in 2007, a person must be presumed to have capacity unless it is established that they lack capacity. If there is any doubt, then the healthcare professional should assess the capacity of the patient to make a decision in general (see Chapter 5: Communication, psychological wellbeing and safeguarding).

During every discussion about consent, it is important to provide all relevant information about the procedure and its implications. In particular, discussions should include information on the following:

- the patient's diagnosis and prognosis
- options for treatment, including non-operative care and the option of no treatment
- the purpose and expected benefit of the treatment
- the likelihood of success
- the clinicians involved in the patient's treatment
- the risks inherent with the procedure, however small the possibility of their occurrence
- all potential side-effects and complications
- the consequences of non-operative alternatives
- potential follow-up treatment (RCS 2014).

The patient and their family should also be provided with information on post-operative care and expected recovery. This should include the following:

- Explain what patients can expect to have *in situ* after surgery, such as intravenous lines or drains, and pumps that may sound alarms.
- For patients who are expected to be transferred to the intensive care or high-dependency unit after surgery, offer for them to visit the unit beforehand.
- Explain that the patient's bed may be moved when they return to the ward so they can be observed more closely by nursing staff immediately after surgery.
- Discuss analgesia.
- Measure the patient for antiembolism stockings (see Procedure guideline 16.1: Measuring and applying antiembolic stockings), foot impulse devices and/or intermittent pneumatic compression devices (NICE 2018a).
- Explain the importance of deep breathing and coughing, regular gentle leg exercises and early mobilization to reduce the risk of complications such as chest infection, deep vein thrombosis and pulmonary embolism.
- Explain the need for post-operative physiotherapy.

Competencies

All healthcare professionals should be aware of the different types of consent and the importance of ensuring that patients understand what is going to happen to them and what is involved. Healthcare professionals should also be familiar with their local hospital consent policy and be aware of and understand what to do if people refuse care or treatment, or when consent is not valid or is no longer valid.

Current guidance states that the person obtaining consent must either be capable of performing the procedure themselves or have received specialist training in advising patients about the procedure (GMC 2014). The person who obtains the patient's consent for surgery should ideally be the surgeon performing the procedure. The anaesthetist should also discuss with the patient the risks related to the chosen method of anaesthesia and obtain consent from them (Hughes 2011).

Physical pre-operative preparation

Definition

Physical pre-operative preparation is concerned with reducing harm and complications in the peri- and post-operative period (NHSI 2018, Scott et al. 2007).

Related theory

For many patients, waiting for surgery can be a stressful time. Where possible, having someone to sit with patients before surgery (perhaps a relative) may help to reduce anxiety. Patients with learning disabilities or mental health problems can find new environments difficult, so it is preferable if the person with them is familiar.

Upon the patient's admission to the clinical area, a patient identity band (see below) should be placed on their dominant arm with printed information, in line with recommendations from NHS Improvement (NHSI) (2018). Any assessments not performed at the pre-assessment clinic should be completed and documented by the admitting practitioner.

The following risk assessments should be included as part of pre-operative patient checks and recorded in the perioperative care documentation (this is not an exhaustive list, as dependent on institutional protocol):

- pressure ulcer
- venous thromboembolism (VTE)
- falls
- nutrition screening
- baseline observations are required and should be recorded:
  - blood pressure
  - pulse
  - respirations
  - temperature
  - oxygen saturations
- blood glucose (if appropriate).

Box 16.3 outlines additional safety measures that may be necessary.

Identity bands

Identity bands (or name bands) are fundamental in the identification of patients. Patient misidentification contributes to errors and is a cause of patient safety incidents with potentially grave consequences. NHS Improvement (2018) highlights the importance of name bands. Since 1 July 2011, it has been mandatory for all hospitals to have electronically printed name bands. Key information should be clearly labelled on a patient's name band (NPSA 2007); see Box 16.4 for details.

Where possible, colour coding for individual risks should be avoided. If a healthcare organization believes colour coding is necessary to alert healthcare professionals to a known risk

Box 16.3 Pre-operative patient safety measures

- Identity bands
- Antiembolic stockings and prophylactic anticoagulation
- Pre-operative fasting
- Skin preparation
- Marking skin for surgery
- Pre-operative pregnancy testing
- Preventing toxic shock syndrome from tampons
- Assessment for latex allergy
- Comprehensive pre-operative checks

Box 16.4 Information to be included on an identity band

- Date of birth in the format dd-mmm-yyyy (e.g. 01-Mar-2013)
- Name (surname first in capitals followed by the first name with the first letter in capitals, e.g. MARSDEN, William)
- Patient's 10 digit NHS number

(e.g. patient allergy), then the National Patient Safety Agency (2007) recommends the use of only one colour: red.

Mechanical and pharmacological thromboembolism prophylaxis

Definition

Venous thromboembolism (VTE) is a condition where a thrombus (clot) forms within a vein (often the deep veins of the lower limbs). It can be very dangerous as the clot can dislodge and travel in the blood to the pulmonary circulation (NICE 2016c).

Related theory

VTE is normally caused by stasis of blood within a vessel, trauma to a vessel or an increase in the ability of the blood to clot (Figures 16.5 and 16.6). This most frequently happens in the deep veins of the leg, when it is termed a 'deep vein thrombosis' or DVT. If one of these clots dislodges from the leg and travels to the lungs via the bloodstream, it is called a 'pulmonary embolus' or PE (Figure 16.7); this can be a fatal event (NICE 2018a). Potential clinical signs of DVT and PE are outlined in Box 16.5.

Prevention of post-operative VTE is considered a quality and patient safety measure in most mandated quality-improvement initiatives. Various interventions have been used for prophylaxis of VTE (Roberts and Lawrence 2017). These include mechanical devices such as graduated antiembolic stockings (Figure 16.8), intermittent pneumatic compression (IPC) devices, and pharmacological agents such as unfractionated heparin, low-molecular-weight heparin and fondaparinux. Most of the strategies employ a combination of mechanical methods and pharmacological agents (Ma et al. 2017).

NICE (2018a) guidance on venous thrombosis recommends that all patients admitted to hospital must have a VTE risk assessment. They should then be reassessed within 24 hours of admission. A specific risk assessment tool (NICE 2018a) (Figure 16.9) forms the basis of hospitals' local patient perioperative documentation in the management of VTE.

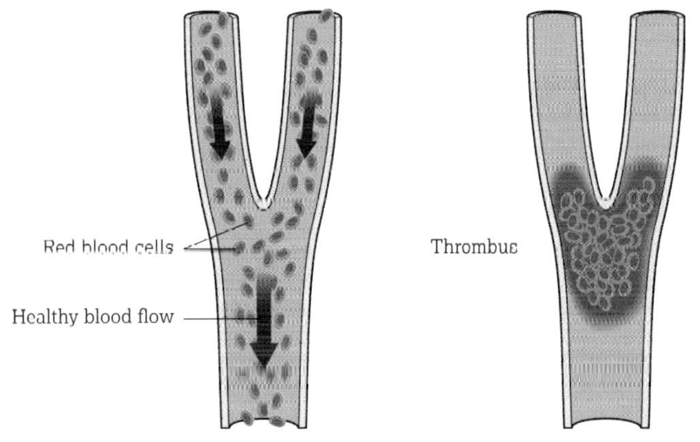

Figure 16.5 Pulmonary embolism.

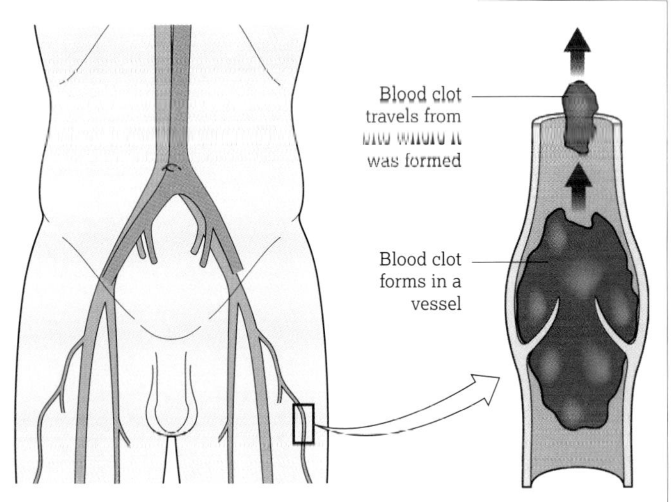

Figure 16.6 Deep vein thrombosis.

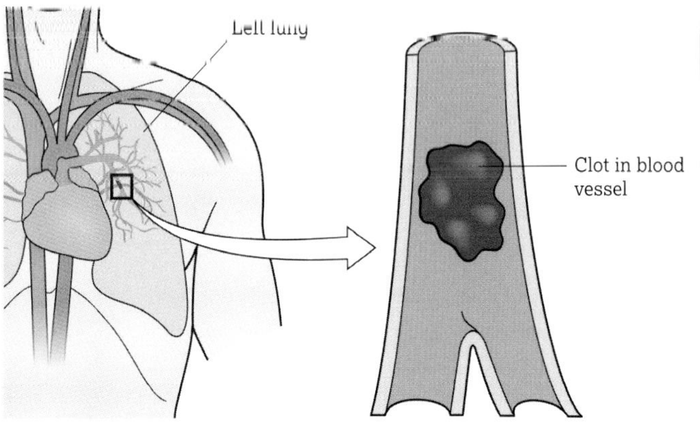

Figure 16.7 Thrombus.

Box 16.5 Signs of deep vein thrombosis or pulmonary embolism

- Complaints of calf or thigh pain
- Erythema, warmth, tenderness and abnormal swelling of the calf or thigh in the affected limb
- Numbness or tingling of the feet
- Dyspnoea, chest pain or signs of shock
- Pain in the chest, back or ribs that gets worse when the patient breathes in deeply
- Coughing up blood

Venous thrombosis risk factors include the following:

- surgery, including day surgery, where total anaesthetic and surgery time is over 90 minutes, or 60 minutes if the surgery involves the pelvis or lower limbs
- immobility, for example prolonged bedrest
- active cancer
- severe cardiac failure or recent myocardial infarction
- acute respiratory failure
- older age (i.e. elderly)
- previous history of DVT or PE
- acute infection or inflammation
- diabetes
- smoking

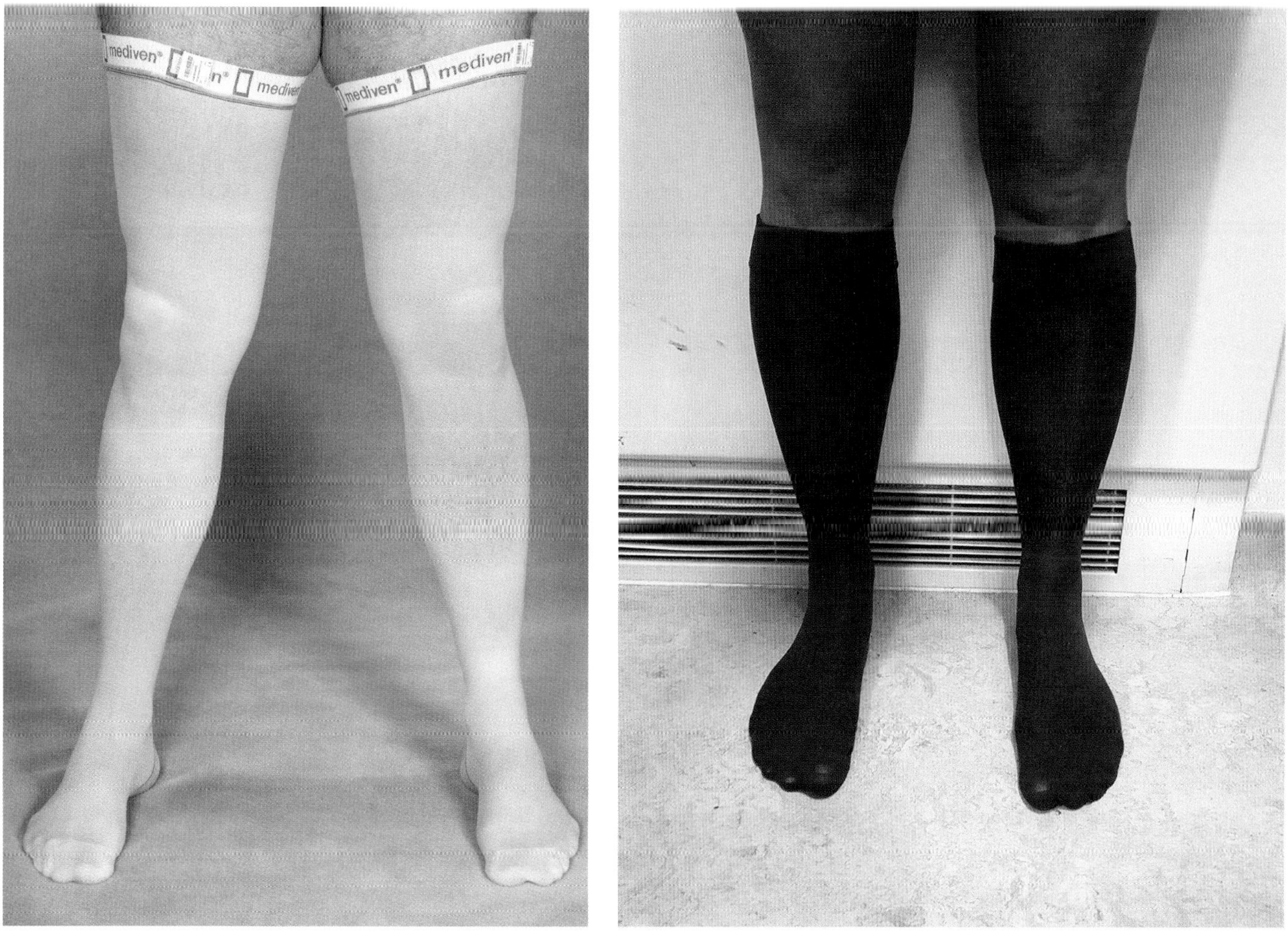

(a) (b)

Figure 16.8 Antiembolic stockings. (a) Thigh length. (b) Knee length.

- obesity
- gross varicose veins
- paralysis of lower limbs
- clotting disorders
- hormone replacement therapy
- oral contraceptives (Swanepoel et al. 2018).

All patients requiring an inpatient stay for surgery should have prophylactic treatment to reduce the risk of DVT, which may include prophylactic anticoagulation (e.g. low-molecular-weight heparin) and mechanical compression methods. Antiembolic stockings (see Figure 16.8) are the most common mechanical compression method, but extremely high-risk patients may also use intermittent pneumatic compression devices or venous foot pumps (NICE 2018a) in the intraoperative and post-operative periods (Figure 16.10). If antiembolic stockings are contraindicated (Box 16.6) then alternative forms of mechanical compression may need to be considered by the surgical team.

Patients should be given verbal and written information before surgery about the risks of VTE and the effectiveness of prophylaxis (NICE 2018a) (see Figure 16.11 for an example of a patient information leaflet). It is estimated that 10–40% of patients undergoing major surgery will develop a DVT, with the risk increasing to 40–60% of patients undergoing major orthopaedic surgery (Flevas et al. 2018).

Mechanical compression methods reduce the risk of DVT by about two-thirds when used as monotherapy and by about half when added to pharmacological methods (Bates et al. 2012, Roderick et al. 2005). Mechanical VTE prophylaxis will be continued until the patient no longer has significantly reduced mobility relative to their normal or anticipated mobility (NICE 2018a).

Graduated antiembolic stockings promote venous flow and reduce venous stasis not only in the legs but also in the pelvic veins and inferior vena cava (Pavon et al. 2016). There are two types of graduated antiembolic stocking: knee high and thigh high (see Figure 16.8). Thigh-length stockings appear to have superior efficacy; however, practical issues such as patient acceptability may prevent their wide use in clinical practice (Wade et al. 2016, 2017). Stockings should be applied according to the manufacturer's instructions and must be removed daily to assess the condition of the skin and tissues.

Alternatively, an intermittent pneumatic compression device provides sequential application of external compression on the lower extremities. It is believed to increase pulsatile venous flow (Pavon et al. 2016). This leads to improved emptying of the veins, decreasing venous pressure and increasing the arteriovenous pressure gradient, with subsequent increase in arterial flow.

RISK ASSESSMENT FOR VENOUS THROMBOEMBOLISM (VTE)

All patients should be risk assessed on admission to hospital. Patients should be reassessed within 24 hours of admission and whenever the clinical situation changes.

STEP ONE

Assess all patients admitted to hospital for level of mobility (tick one box). All surgical patients, and all medical patients with significantly reduced mobility, should be considered for further risk assessment.

STEP TWO

Review the patient-related factors shown on the assessment sheet against **thrombosis** risk, ticking each box that applies (more than one box can be ticked).

Any tick for thrombosis risk should prompt thromboprophylaxis according to NICE guidance.

The risk factors identified are not exhaustive. Clinicians may consider additional risks in individual patients and offer thromboprophylaxis as appropriate.

STEP THREE

Review the patient-related factors shown against **bleeding risk** and tick each box that applies (more than one box can be ticked).

Any tick should prompt clinical staff to consider if bleeding risk is sufficient to preclude pharmacological intervention.

Guidance on thromboprophylaxis is available at:

National Institute for Health and Clinical Excellence (2010) Venous thromboembolism: reducing the risk of venous thromboembolism (deep vein thrombosis and pulmonary embolism) in patients admitted to hospital. NICE clinical guideline 92. London: National Institute for Health and Clinical Excellence.

http://www.nice.org.uk/guidance/CG92

This document has been authorised by the Department of Health
Gateway reference no: 10278

Department of Health

Figure 16.9 Example of a venous thromboembolism (VTE) risk assessment form. *Source*: Reproduced from DH (2010) with permission of the National Institute for Health and Care Excellence.

Department of Health

RISK ASSESSMENT FOR VENOUS THROMBOEMBOLISM (VTE)

Mobility – all patients (tick one box)	Tick		Tick		Tick
Surgical patient		Medical patient expected to have ongoing reduced mobility relative to normal state		Medical patient NOT expected to have significantly reduced mobility relative to normal state	
Assess for thrombosis and bleeding risk below				**Risk assessment now complete**	

Thrombosis risk			
Patient related	**Tick**	**Admission related**	**Tick**
Active cancer or cancer treatment		Significantly reduced mobility for 3 days or more	
Age >60		Hip or knee replacement	
Dehydration		Hip fracture	
Known thrombophilias		Total anaesthetic + surgical time >90 minutes	
Obesity (BMI >30 kg/m^2)		Surgery involving pelvis or lower limb with a total anaesthetic + surgical time >60 minutes	
One or more significant medical comorbidities (e.g. heart disease; metabolic, endocrine or respiratory pathologies; acute infectious diseases; inflammatory conditions)		Acute surgical admission with inflammatory or intra-abdominal condition	
Personal history or first-degree relative with a history of VTE		Critical care admission	
Use of hormone replacement therapy		Surgery with significant reduction in mobility	
Use of oestrogen-containing contraceptive therapy			
Varicose veins with phlebitis			
Pregnancy or <6 weeks post-partum (see NICE guidance for specific risk factors)			

Bleeding risk			
Patient related	**Tick**	**Admission related**	**Tick**
Active bleeding		Neurosurgery, spinal surgery or eye surgery	
Acquired bleeding disorders (such as acute liver failure)		Other procedure with high bleeding risk	
Concurrent use of anticoagulants known to increase the risk of bleeding (such as warfarin with INR >2)		Lumbar puncture/epidural/spinal anaesthesia expected within the next 12 hours	
Acute stroke		Lumbar puncture/epidural/spinal anaesthesia within the previous 4 hours	
Thrombocytopaenia (platelets< 75×10^9/L)			
Uncontrolled systolic hypertension (230/120 mmHg or higher)			
Untreated inherited bleeding disorders (such as haemophilia and von Willebrand's disease)			

Figure 16.9 *Continued*

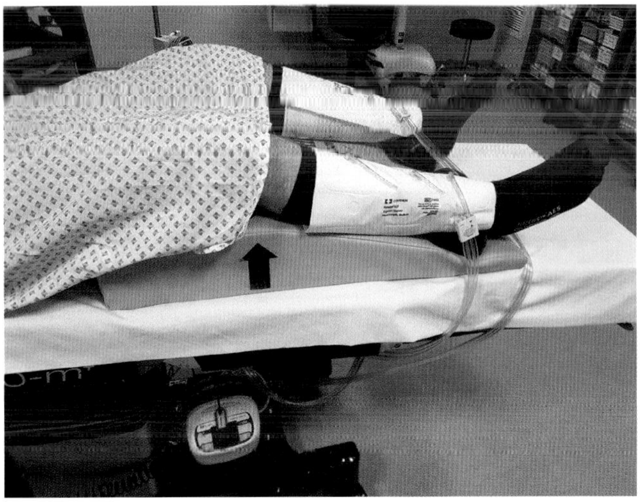

Figure 16.10 Intermittent compression device and boots.

Box 16.6 Contraindications for antiembolism stockings

- Suspected or proven peripheral arterial disease
- Peripheral arterial bypass grafting
- Peripheral neuropathy or other causes of sensory impairment
- Local condition in which stockings may cause damage, such as fragile tissue-paper skin
- Allergy to the material of manufacture
- Severe leg oedema
- Major limb deformity or unusual leg size or shape preventing correct fit
- Venous ulcers, wounds or pressure areas (not an absolute contraindication, but caution is required)

Source: Adapted from NICE (2018a).

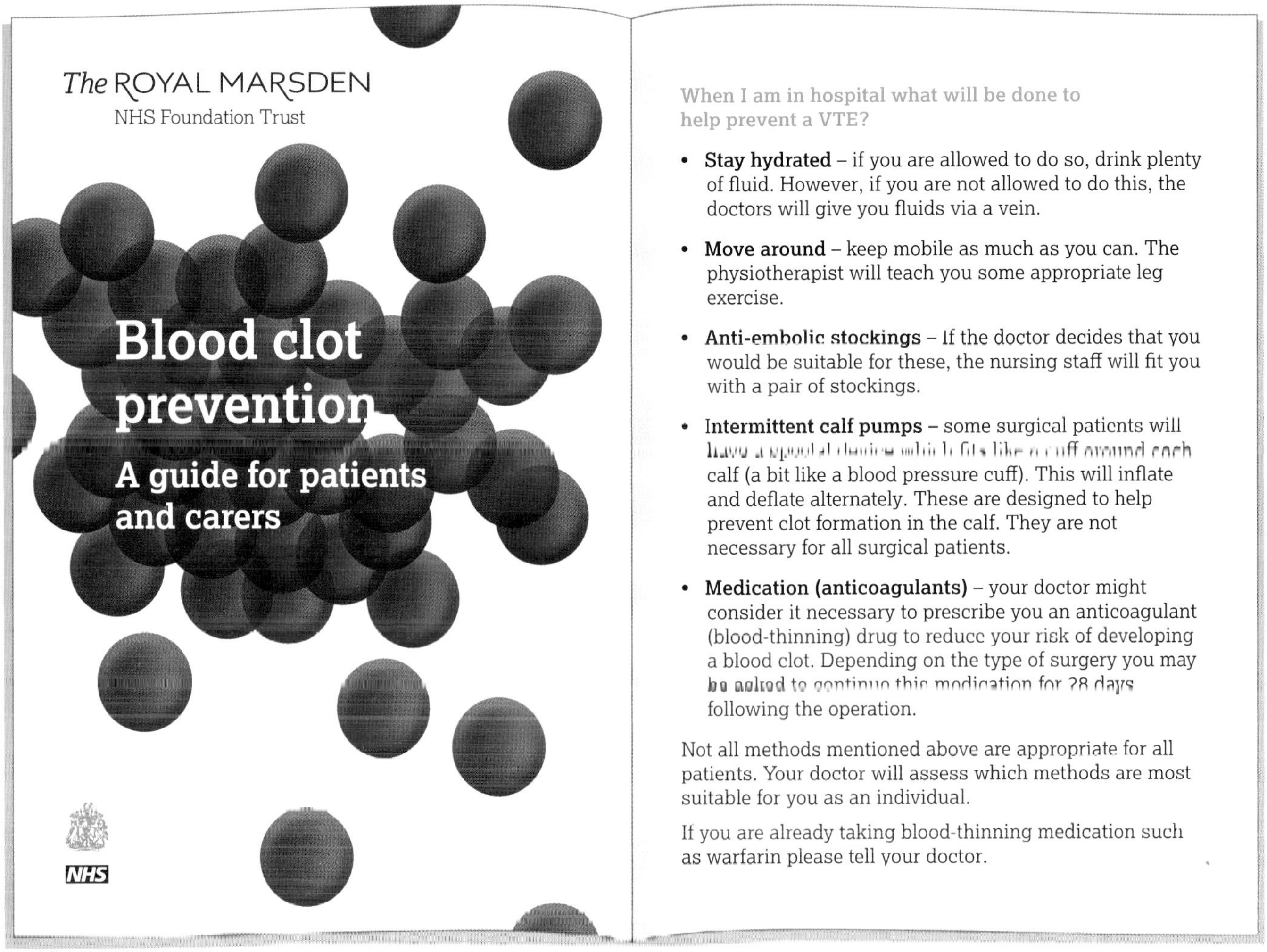

The ROYAL MARSDEN
NHS Foundation Trust

Blood clot prevention

A guide for patients and carers

NHS

When I am in hospital what will be done to help prevent a VTE?

- **Stay hydrated** – if you are allowed to do so, drink plenty of fluid. However, if you are not allowed to do this, the doctors will give you fluids via a vein.
- **Move around** – keep mobile as much as you can. The physiotherapist will teach you some appropriate leg exercise.
- **Anti-embolic stockings** – If the doctor decides that you would be suitable for these, the nursing staff will fit you with a pair of stockings.
- **Intermittent calf pumps** – some surgical patients will have a special device which fits like a cuff around each calf (a bit like a blood pressure cuff). This will inflate and deflate alternately. These are designed to help prevent clot formation in the calf. They are not necessary for all surgical patients.
- **Medication (anticoagulants)** – your doctor might consider it necessary to prescribe you an anticoagulant (blood-thinning) drug to reduce your risk of developing a blood clot. Depending on the type of surgery you may be asked to continue this medication for 28 days following the operation.

Not all methods mentioned above are appropriate for all patients. Your doctor will assess which methods are most suitable for you as an individual.

If you are already taking blood-thinning medication such as warfarin please tell your doctor.

Figure 16.11 Example of a patient information sheet for deep vein thrombosis (DVT). *Source*: Adapted from Royal Marsden NHS Foundation Trust (2010) with permission of The Royal Marsden NHS Foundation Trust.

Procedure guideline 16.1 Measuring and applying antiembolic stockings

Essential equipment

- Personal protective equipment
- Disposable tape measure (patient specific)
- Antiembolic stocking sizing chart
- Patient records/documentation

Action	Rationale
Pre-procedure	
1 Assess and record in the patient's documentation the patient's risk factors for VTE (DVT and PE).	All patients admitted to hospital should undergo a risk assessment for venous thrombosis to determine the most appropriate thromboprophylaxis (Farge et al. 2013, **R**; NICE 2018a, **C**; SIGN 2014, **C**). The higher the number of risk factors, the greater the risk of VTE (NICE 2018a, **C**; SIGN 2014, **C**).
2 Assess and record in the patient's documentation the patient's suitability for antiembolic stockings, identifying whether the patient has any contraindications to wearing antiembolic stockings (see Box 16.6).	To comply with national guidelines and hospital policy/guidelines. To ensure that antiembolic stockings are used appropriately (All Wales Tissue Viability Nurse Forum 2009, **E**; Farge et al. 2013, **R**; NICE 2018a, **C**; SIGN 2014, **C**).
3 Introduce yourself to the patient, explain and discuss the procedure with them, and gain their consent to proceed.	To ensure that the patient feels at ease, understands the procedure and gives their valid consent (NMC 2018, **C**).
Procedure	
4 Perform hand hygiene and put on an apron prior to the procedure.	To prevent cross-infection (NHS England and NHSI 2019, **C**).
5 *Measurement for thigh-length stockings:* a Measure upper thigh circumference at the widest part of the thigh (**Action figure 5a**). b Measure calf circumference at the widest part of the calf (**Action figure 5b**). *Note*: refer to individual manufacturers' instructions to ensure that no other measurements are necessary, e.g. length of leg. c Consult the product packaging to determine the appropriate size. • If right and left legs measure differently, order two different stocking sizes. • If thigh or calf circumference is greater than that stocked by the manufacturer, then refer to local trust guidelines to determine the appropriate course of action. In some cases, knee-length stockings may be more appropriate. *Measurement for knee-length stockings:* a Measure calf circumference at the widest part of the calf. *Note*: refer to individual manufacturers' instructions to ensure that no other measurements are necessary, e.g. length of leg. b Consult the product packaging to determine the appropriate size. c If the right and left legs measure differently, order two different stocking sizes. Order two pairs of stockings.	To comply with the manufacturer's instructions. **E** Incorrect sizing causes swelling and bruising to ankles and can constrict blood supply, leading to long-term complications. **E** It has also been suggested that 15–20% of patients cannot effectively wear thigh-length antiembolic stockings because of unusual limb size or shape (SIGN 2014, **C**).
6 Apply the stockings: a Insert hand into stocking as far as the heel pocket. b Grasp centre of heel pocket and turn stocking inside out to heel area. c Position stocking over foot and heel, ensuring the patient's heel is centred in the heel pocket (**Action figure 6a**). d Pull a few inches of the stocking up around the ankle and calf (**Action figure 6b**). e Continue pulling the stocking up the leg as described in the manufacturer's instructions. When using thigh-length stockings, the top band rests in the gluteal furrow. f Smooth out wrinkles. g Align the inspection window to fall under the toes (toes should not stick out).	To ensure the appropriate size of stocking is fitted correctly. **E** Thigh-length stockings are difficult to put on and can roll down, creating a tourniquet just above the knee that restricts blood supply, so patient monitoring and/or assistance should take place to ensure that stockings are fitted smoothly, are not rolled down or have the top band folded down (SIGN 2014, **R**; Todd 2015, **R**; Wounds UK 2015, **R**).

(continued)

Action	Rationale
Post-procedure	
7 Document the leg measurements and the size of stockings applied in the nursing records. Instruct the patient and provide written information about the following: a reasons for wearing antiembolic stockings b how to fit and wear stockings c what to report to the nurse, e.g. any feelings of pain or numbness and any skin problems d skin care: wash and dry legs daily, applying emollient if clinically indicated e reasons for early mobilization and adequate hydration f reasons for not crossing legs or ankles: to prevent constriction of blood supply g length of time that the stockings should be worn, e.g. stockings should be removed for a *maximum of 30 minutes daily* and worn until the patient returns to their usual level of mobility.	To ensure that the patient understands how to fit and wear stockings, including self care measures and what to report to the nurse so as to detect complications early (e.g. pressure sores or circulation difficulties of wearing antiembolic stockings) (NICE 2018a, **C**; Wade et al. 2017, **R**).

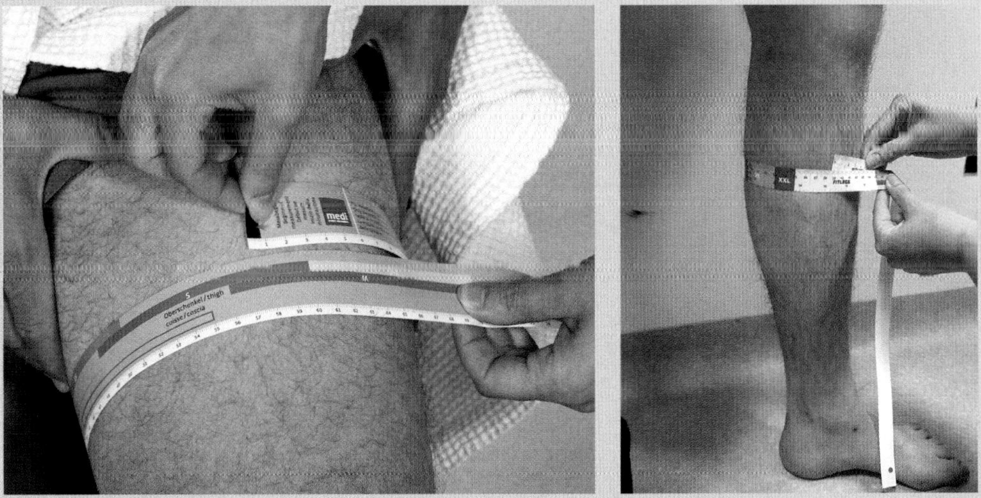

(a) (b)

Action Figure 5 Measure (a) thigh circumference and (b) mid-calf circumference.

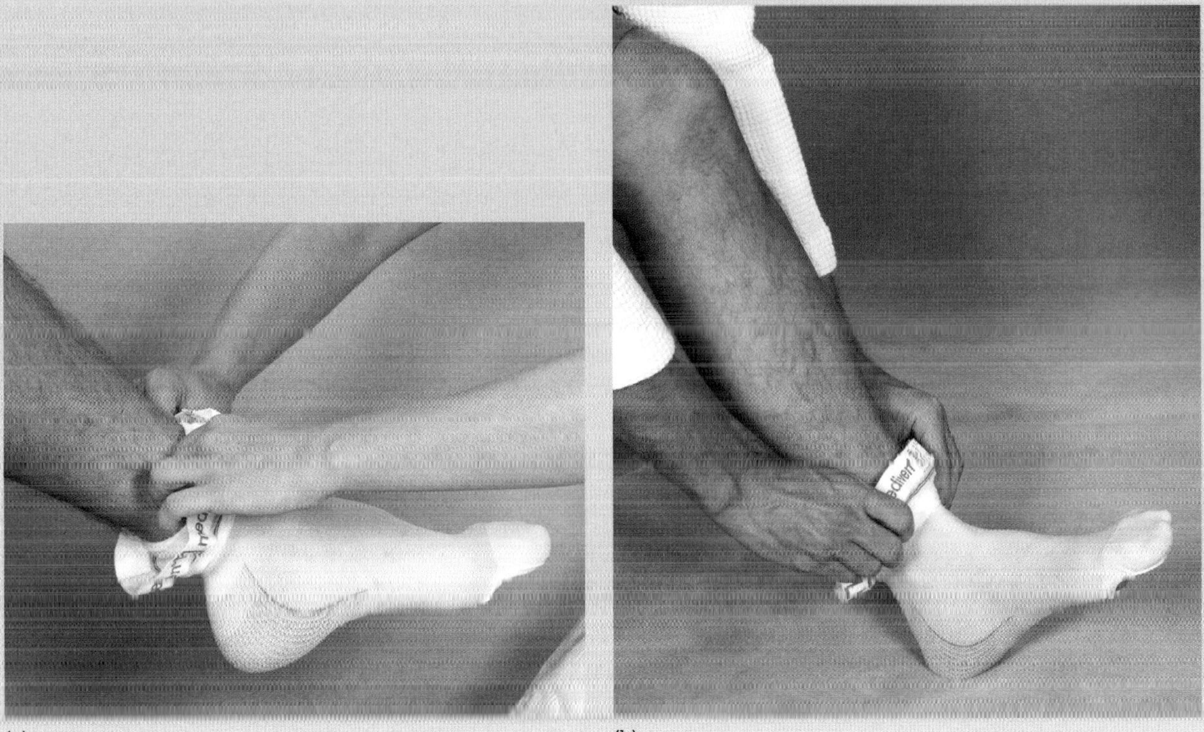
(a) (b)

Action Figure 6 (a) Ensure the heel is centred in the heel pocket. (b) Pull the stocking up over the ankle.

Pre-operative fasting

Definition

Pre-operative fasting is defined as a prescribed period of time before a procedure when patients are not allowed oral intake of liquids or solids.

Related theory

General anaesthesia carries the risk of the patient inhaling gastric contents during induction, due to airway reflexes (such as coughing or laryngospasm) or gastrointestinal motor responses (such as gagging or recurrent swallowing) (AAGBI 2010). Aspiration of gastric contents can result in respiratory problems (including aspiration pneumonitis and aspiration pneumonia) or at worst acute respiratory failure and death (Van de Putte et al. 2017). Risk factors for aspiration are outlined in Table 16.4, and Box 16.7 outlines current best practice pre-operative fasting guidelines for healthy adults undergoing elective surgery.

It is important to be aware that several factors can delay gastric emptying (Van de Putte et al. 2017). These include:

- reduced consciousness level
- systemic opiate therapy
- recent history of difficulty in eating, swallowing or digesting food
- recent history of dyspepsia (heartburn), particularly on lying down or bending over
- upper gastrointestinal surgery
- anxiety
- pregnancy or labour
- abdominal pain
- renal failure
- diabetes.

There are various techniques that can be used to prevent gastric aspiration during the induction period. These include a rapid-sequence induction/endotracheal intubation technique, or awake endotracheal intubation technique, which may be useful to prevent this problem during the induction of anaesthetic.

The American Society of Anesthesiologists (2011) has recognized that fasting times may be prolonged due to alterations in the operating list. Some alterations are unavoidable, but patients should be kept informed of changes to the theatre list and those without disorders of gastric emptying allowed to continue drinking clear fluids up to 2 hours prior to rescheduled surgery (Box 16.8) (Powell-Tuck et al. 2011). Where patients have disorders of gastric emptying or where the theatre time is difficult to ascertain, patients should be offered mouthwashes to keep their mouths moist and intravenous fluids considered if not contraindicated for the surgery being performed (e.g. liver surgery).

Table 16.4 Predisposing factors for aspiration under general anaesthesia

Patient factors	Increased gastric content	Intestinal obstruction Non fasted Drugs Delayed gastric emptying
	Lower oesophageal sphincter incompetence	Hiatus hernia Gastro-oesophageal reflux Pregnancy Morbid obesity Neuromuscular disease
	Decreased laryngeal reflexes	Head injury Bulbar palsy
	Sex	Male
	Age	Elderly
Operation factors	Procedure	Emergency Laparoscopic
	Position	Lithotomy
Anaesthetic factors	Airway	Difficult intubation Gas insufflation
	Maintenance	Inadequate depth

Source: Adapted from King (2010).

Box 16.7 Pre-operative fasting guidelines

- 6 hours fasting from solid food, provided the last meal is light (refer to local trust guidelines for examples of suitable light meal).
- Sweets, including lollipops, are solid food. A minimum pre-operative fasting time of 6 hours is recommended.
- Tea and coffee with milk are acceptable up to 6 hours before surgery.
- Clear fluids (those through which newsprint can be read) are acceptable up to 2 hours before (see Box 16.8).
- Patients being fed by nasogastric or gastrostomy tube should have their feed stopped 6 hours prior to surgery and water 2 hours prior to surgery.
- Chewing gum should be avoided on the day of surgery.
- Regular medication taken orally should be continued pre-operatively unless there is advice to the contrary. Patients can have up to 30 mL of water orally to help them take medication.

Box 16.8 Examples of clear fluids

- Water
- Tea or coffee *without* milk
- Fruit or herbal tea
- Fruit squash
- Polycal diluted half and half with water
- Fortijuice
- Enlive (clear liquids only)

Skin preparation

Definition

The purpose of pre-operative skin preparation is to remove visible contaminants and to reduce the levels of naturally occurring skin flora, particularly *Staphylococcus aureus*, so as to reduce the risk of surgical site infection (Wicker and O'Neill 2010). Surgical site preparation is the treatment of the intact skin of the intended surgical site and surrounding area, and this takes place once the patient is in the operating room, on the operating table (Allegranzi et al. 2016).

Related theory

Normal bacterial flora live in the nose, groin, armpit, gut, skin and hair of everybody. Organisms may become pathogenic when they move out of their normal area on the body to an open wound (Wicker and O'Neill 2010). NICE (2019) guidelines advise patients to shower or have a bath using soap either the day before or on the day of surgery. While there is no evidence concerning patient theatre attire, NICE (2019) advises that patients are given a clean theatre gown to wear and asked to remove their own clothing (depending on the operation). Theatre gowns should maintain the patient's comfort and dignity while allowing easy access to the operative site. Furthermore, theatre gowns avoid placing the patient's own clothes at risk of contamination from blood, body fluid and washout fluids (Pudner 2010).

The most widely used antiseptic skin preparation agents are 2% chlorhexidine gluconate and iodophors (e.g. povidone-iodine) in alcohol-based solutions. These are effective against a wide range of bacteria, fungi and viruses (NICE 2019). NICE (2019) has set out recommendations for surgical site preparation; these can be found in Table 16.5. Currently, some preparation solutions also

Table 16.5 Options for antiseptic skin preparation

Choice of antiseptic skin preparation	When
Alcohol-based solution of chlorhexidine	First choice unless contraindicated or the surgical site is next to a mucous membrane
Aqueous solution of chlorhexidine	If the surgical site is next to a mucous membrane
Alcohol-based solution of povidone-iodine	If chlorhexidine is contraindicated
Aqueous solution of povidone-iodine	If both an alcohol-based solution and chlorhexidine are unsuitable

Source: Adapted from NICE (2019).

contain colouring agents, which are helpful for indicating where the products have been applied (WHO 2018).

Surgical site hair removal

Pre-operative hair removal is used to prevent surgical site infection or to prevent interference with the incision site (Lefebvre et al. 2015). NICE (2019) guidance advises against routine hair removal in order to reduce the risk of surgical site infection. Hair removal should only be carried out if necessary (Loveday et al. 2014), which minimizes the potential risk of skin trauma. To further reduce the risk of skin trauma, the use of clippers instead of razors has been proposed (NICE 2019, Shi et al. 2017). Table 16.6 illustrates specific considerations to be made during skin preparation and explains the best practice of hair removal.

Marking skin for surgery

Definition

Skin marking is carried out to unambiguously identify the intended site of surgical incision. Any markings should be arrows; should be drawn with an indelible, latex-free marker pen; and should extend to, or near to, the exact incision site (Figure 16.12).

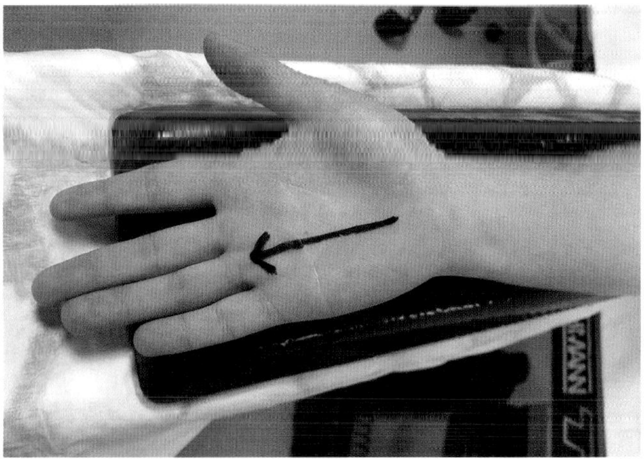

Figure 16.12 Example of skin marked for surgery.

Related theory

The surgeon may need to mark an area of the body for surgery (e.g. a limb to be operated on) or the position of an organ (e.g. a specific kidney in a patient undergoing a nephrectomy). Marking the surgical site is essential for the planning of any surgical procedure and for the prevention of wrong-site surgery (Table 16.7) (Bathla et al. 2017). The incidence of wrong-site surgery is low but any error can be devastating and in some cases fatal.

The marking should be undertaken by the surgeon performing the operation or a competent deputy (i.e. an individual capable of performing the procedure themselves) who will be present at the surgery, to ensure the correct site is marked; the site should be checked against the patient's consent form (Schäfli-Thurnherr et al. 2017). The mark should be an arrow, drawn with an indelible, latex-free marker pen, and should extend to, or near to, the exact incision site. The majority of surgical site marking pens contain gentian violet ink, which has antifungal properties (Maley and Arbiser 2013, Wise et al. 2016). Other types of marker pen include permanent ink markers, which despite their lack of antifungal properties have not been found to affect the sterility of the surgical field (Zhao et al. 2009). Marking must be undertaken before premedication or anaesthesia so that patients can be involved in ensuring the mark is in the correct place. It needs to remain visible after the application of antiseptic (aqueous or alcohol-based) skin preparation (e.g. povidone-iodine or chlorhexidine) and after the application of theatre drapes (Mears et al. 2009). The surgical site mark should not be easily removed with skin preparation but should not be so permanent as to last weeks or months after the surgical procedure.

Following surgery, once the wound has healed, residual traces of the marker pen can be gently removed using warm, soapy water. It

Table 16.6 Hair removal prior to surgery

Principle	Rationale
Electric clippers with a single-use disposable head should be used	Clippers do not come into contact with the skin and therefore reduce the risk of cuts and abrasions (NICE 2019, C; Pudner 2010, R). A single-use head prevents cross infection (AORN 2008, C). Electric clippers with single use disposable heads are the most cost-effective method of hair removal (NICE 2019, C).
If hair removal is required to facilitate access or view of the surgical site then, where possible, this should be undertaken on the day of surgery	Earlier removal would allow time for the hair to regrow (NICE 2019, C).
Only hair interfering with the surgical procedure should be removed	To prevent unnecessary trauma and shaving (NICE 2019, C; Shi et al. 2017, R).

Table 16.7 Pre-operative marking recommendation

How should marking be carried out?	• Use an indelible marker pen. • Mark an arrow that extends to, or near to, the incision site. • This mark must remain visible after the application of skin preparation and after the application of theatre drapes.
Where should be marked?	• Any surgical operations involving one side (laterality) of the body should be marked at, or near, the intended incision. • For digits on the hand or foot, the mark should extend to the specific digit.
Who should be involved in the pre-operative marking?	• Marking must be carried out by the operating surgeon or by a nominated deputy who will be present in the operating theatre at the time of the patient's procedure. • Pre-operative marking of the intended site should involve the patient and/or their family members or significant others wherever possible.
When should marking be carried out?	• The marking of the surgical site should be carried out on the ward or in the day care area prior to the patient's transfer to the operating theatre. • The marking should take place before pre-medication.
Verification of the mark	The surgical site mark should subsequently be checked against the patient's documentation, such as consent form or X-ray. This check should confirm the mark is (a) correctly located and (b) still legible. This check should occur at each transfer of the patient's care and end with a final verification prior to commencement of surgery. Confirmation of the site marking happens at the following pre-operative stages: • when ward staff are preparing the patient for the operating room • when ward staff hand over the patient to the anaesthetic practitioner • during the 'Sign In' stage of the WHO Surgical Safety Checklist (see 'Intraoperative care: anaesthesia' below) by the anaesthetist and anaesthetic practitioner (before any needle-to-skin in the anaesthetic room) • during the 'Time Out' stage of the WHO Surgical Safety Checklist, when the patient is on the operating table before the surgical procedure begins (carried out by the operating surgeon with the presence of all team members). All team members should be involved in checking the mark.

Source: Adapted from Bathla et al. (2017), NPSA (2005).

is important not to rub too hard to prevent irritating the skin or sinking the ink deeper into skin tissues, making it harder to extract. This process may need to be repeated over a series of days.

There are circumstances where marking may not be appropriate:

- emergency surgery
- surgery on teeth or mucous membranes
- bilateral procedures such as tonsillectomy or squint surgery
- situations where laterality of surgery will be confirmed during the procedure (NPSA 2005).

If a patient refuses pre-operative skin marking, local policy should be followed and documentation should clearly state that the patient refused marking, particularly on the WHO Surgical Safety Checklist (see 'Intraoperative care: anaesthesia' below).

There are some situations in which a specialist nurse may mark the skin. For example, stoma therapists mark the position on the patient's skin that is the optimum place for the stoma to be placed (see Chapter 6: Elimination).

Pre-operative pregnancy testing

Related theory

There is an increased risk of miscarriage, stillbirth or low birthweight when a patient undergoes surgery during pregnancy (Balinskaite et al. 2017). It is possible that this is caused by surgical manipulation and the patient's underlying medical condition rather than exposure to anaesthesia.

Prior to consenting to surgery, all female patients who have commenced menstruation (menarche) need to be informed of the risks surgery may pose to a pregnancy (NICE 2016b). The clinician performing the procedure or the appropriately delegated representative (i.e. an individual capable of performing the procedure themselves) is responsible for informing patients of the risks of surgery and is therefore responsible for ensuring that a female patient has had her pregnancy status assessed (NICE 2016b). Once she has been informed of the risks, the patient will need to take responsibility for her own contraception (NICE 2016b).

All female patients of child-bearing age should be considered for pregnancy testing if they express a concern that they may be pregnant or are undergoing gynaecology surgery (NICE 2016b). Any pregnancy testing requires informed consent and documentation in the patient's medical record, including test results or patient refusal, and the responsible surgical team must be informed prior to the initiation of the surgery (NICE 2016b). If a previously unknown pregnancy is detected, the risks and benefits of the surgery can be discussed with the patient. Surgery may be postponed or, if the decision is made to go ahead, the anaesthetic and surgical approaches can be modified if necessary (NPSA 2010). In emergency situations, confirmation of pregnancy should not delay treatment and should be taken into account within the clinical assessment of risk.

Clinical governance

The practice of checking and documenting current pregnancy status in the immediate pre-operative period has been shown to be inconsistent (NPSA 2010). Pre-operative assessment may take place weeks in advance of a planned operation but pregnancy status may change in the intervening time, so pregnancy status must be rechecked by asking the patient in the immediate pre-operative period on the ward and documented in the perioperative records used by staff performing the final clinical and identity checks (NICE 2016b, NPSA 2010). If there is a chance the patient could be pregnant, a test should be carried out again at this point.

Prevention of toxic shock syndrome from tampon use

Definition

Staphylococcal toxic shock syndrome (TSS) is a rare, life-threatening systemic bacterial infection, historically associated with the use of superabsorbent tampons. TSS is characterized by high fever, hypotension, rash and multiorgan dysfunction (NHS 2016).

Related theory

TSS occurs when the bacteria *Staphylococcus aureus* and *Streptococcus pyogenes*, which normally live harmlessly on the skin, enter the bloodstream and produce poisonous toxins. These toxins cause severe vasodilation, which in turn causes a large drop in blood pressure (shock), resulting in dizziness and confusion. They also begin to damage tissue, including skin and organs, and can disturb many vital organ functions. If TSS is left untreated, the combination of shock and organ damage can result in death. Symptoms usually occur together and get progressively worse over time. They include:

- high fever
- vomiting
- diarrhoea
- severe muscle aches
- feeling extremely weak or dizzy
- sunburn-like rash.

TSS can also affect men and children, and currently nonmenstrual TSS is more common (Sharma et al. 2018). However, the first reported cases of TSS involved women who were using tampons during menstruation (Eckert and Lentz 2012), and this risk must be taken into account in relation to surgery. Female patients of menstruating age therefore need to be made aware of the dangers of using tampons, which can cause infection leading to TSS. At the time of admission, it is important to ask female patients whether they are menstruating and to highlight the dangers of using tampons during surgery. If tampons are left *in situ* for longer than 6 hours, infection may develop. Nurses can offer a sanitary pad as an alternative.

Latex sensitivity and allergy

Related theory

Latex is a natural rubber composed of proteins and added chemicals. Its durable, flexible properties give it a high degree of protection from many micro-organisms, which makes it an ideal fibre to use for many healthcare products. It currently provides the best protection against infection in the healthcare field. It is found in the following products:

- gloves
- airways
- intravenous tubing
- stethoscopes
- catheters
- wound drains
- dressings and bandages (HSE 2018).

Some of the proteins in the natural rubber latex can cause sensitivity and allergic reactions, and the incidence of latex hypersensitivity seems to be increasing (Wu et al. 2016). Powdered gloves can create the greatest risk as proteins leak into the powder, which can become airborne when gloves are removed, and inhaling the powder may lead to respiratory sensitization. The amount of latex exposure needed to produce sensitization is unknown. Sensitivity can be described as the development of an immunological memory for specific latex proteins, which can be asymptomatic. A substance that causes sensitization is one that is capable of causing an allergic reaction in certain people. Allergy is the visible manifestation of the sensitivity (e.g. hives, rhinitis, conjunctivitis or anaphylaxis), which can be serious and potentially life threatening (Table 16.8) (Hauk 2018, HSE 2018).

Once sensitization has taken place, further exposure will cause symptoms to recur, and increasing exposure to latex proteins increases the risk of developing allergic symptoms (HSE 2018). Therefore, sensitivities and allergies should be treated in the same way (Hauk 2018). Routes of exposure include:

- direct external contact (i.e. with gloves or other latex products)
- airborne exposure

Table 16.8 Allergic reactions

Reaction*	Description	Symptoms
Irritation	Irritant contact dermatitis, a non-allergenic reaction caused by soaps, gloves, glove powder and hand creams	Dry, crusty and itchy skin Rashes and inflammation
Type I reaction: immediate hypersensitivity – occurs within minutes and can fade rapidly after removal of the latex	Immediate hypersensitivity, sometimes called immunoglobulin E response; caused by exposure to proteins in latex on glove surface and/or bound to powder	Most severe reaction Wheal and flare response Irritant and allergic contact Dermatitis Facial swelling Rhinitis Urticaria Respiratory distress and asthma Rarely, anaphylactic shock
Type IV reaction: delayed hypersensitivity – usually occurring within 6–48 hours of contact	Sometimes known as 'allergic contact dermatitis', caused by exposure to chemicals used in latex manufacturing	Red, raised, palpable area with bumps, sores and cracks

* Type II and type III reactions are not relevant to latex.
Source: Adapted from AORN (2018), HSE (2018).

- direct contact with the mucous membranes
- internal patient exposure from healthcare provider use of natural rubber latex gloves during surgical procedures
- internally placed devices (e.g. wound drains) (AORN 2018).

Latex allergies are classified as irritant contact dermatitis, type I and type IV reactions (see Table 16.8).

Clinical governance

Healthcare providers have an ethical responsibility to prevent latex sensitization; because there is no cure, protection must be paramount. Employers should have a latex allergy policy and procedure, which should provide information and instruction on measures to identify patients at risk, patient education, interventions to reduce undue latex exposure, recognizing symptoms of sensitization and the action to be taken if a sensitization is suspected (HSE 2018).

Assessment and monitoring for symptoms of latex allergy in both conscious and unconscious patients are required at all stages of perioperative care. The assessment should cover the following known risk factors for latex allergy:

- history of multiple surgeries beginning at an early age (e.g. spina bifida or urinary malformation)
- history of hayfever or asthma
- history of an allergic reaction to latex: for example, a history suggestive of reactivity to latex may be gained by anecdotal accounts of swelling or itching of the lips when blowing up balloons or following dental examinations, or swelling and itching of the hands when using household gloves
- history of an allergic reaction during an operation
- past experience of itchy skin, skin rash or redness when in contact with rubber products
- past skin irritation from an examination by a doctor or dentist wearing rubber gloves
- past sneezing, wheezing or chest tightness when exposed to rubber (AORN 2010).

Box 16.9 Pre-operative actions to be taken when patients have a potential or confirmed latex allergy

- Notify operating theatre of potential or confirmed latex allergy 24–48 hours (or as soon as possible) before the scheduled procedure.
- Identify the patient's risk factors for latex allergy and communicate them to the healthcare team.
- Schedule the procedure as the first case of the day if the facility is not latex safe.
- Plan for a latex-safe environment of care.
- The theatre must be cleaned with latex-free gloves and equipment.
- All latex products must be removed or covered with plastics so that the rubber elements are not exposed.
- All healthcare staff in direct contact with the patient must wear vinyl gloves during procedures and in the vicinity of the patient.
- Use latex-free replacements for all latex-containing items used by surgeons and anaesthetists.
- A latex-free contents box or trolley (containing stock of all latex-free products that will be required during surgery and anaesthetic) should be ready in every theatre department and recovery room. There should be a list of all latex-free equipment (including each item's manufacturer) available in the box or trolley.
- Notify the surgeon if no alternative product is available.
- Notify the anaesthetist if a latex-containing product must be used and develop a plan of emergency care if necessary.
- Where a type I (immediate hypersensitivity reaction; see Table 16.8) allergy is suspected, suitable clinical management procedures must be ready for use in the event of the patient having a hypersensitivity reaction.

Source: Adapted from AORN (2018).

If a suspected or confirmed latex sensitivity or allergy is found, this information must be documented in the patient's medical notes and communicated to all members of the healthcare team and departments that the patient may visit, including theatre, recovery, pathology and radiology (Liberatore 2019). Box 16.9 outlines the pre-operative actions to be taken when a patient has a potential or confirmed latex allergy. The anaesthetist will need to be informed so that decisions can be made regarding potential allergy prophylaxis pre-operatively. A latex-safe environment is recommended – one where every reasonable effort has been made to prevent high-allergen and airborne latex sources from coming into direct contact with affected individuals. Latex-free alternative items should be collected and stored in a quick-access location for ease of access and identification. At present, best practice dictates that patients with a suspected or confirmed latex allergy be scheduled first on the morning list because it is assumed that the inactivity in the room during the previous evening hours causes the content of latex-coated powder in the ambient air to be lowest in the morning (AORN 2018, Hauk 2018). Further guidance may be sought online from the Association of periOperative Registered Nurses (www.aorn.org).

There is a voluntary scheme in place for reporting cases of latex sensitization, both of staff and patients, to the Medical Devices Agency, which is an executive agency of the Department of Health (HSE 2018).

Pre-operative theatre checklist

Related theory

The pre-operative theatre checklist (Figure 16.13) is the final check after a patient has been moved from the ward to the operating theatre. It should be completed clearly and in full, in order to reduce the possibility of any complications during the period that the patient is put under anaesthetic or during the surgical procedure.

These checks include ensuring that blood results and X-rays or imaging accompany the patient. The blood results are important for assessing the patient's haemoglobin levels, which in turn help the body to transport oxygen and electrolytes to identify any imbalances, such as low sodium or potassium. Such deficiencies can interfere with anaesthetic agents and cause cardiovascular disturbances such as arrhythmias (Higgins and Higgins 2013) (Table 16.9).

Patients should not be given routine pre-operative medication before being asked for their consent to proceed with the treatment (NMC 2018) (see 'Consent' above).

The ROYAL MARSDEN
NHS Foundation Trust

Pre-operative care plan

Allergy status

Is the patient allergic or sensitive to: drugs and/or solutions (e.g. povidone-iodine) and/or dressings (e.g. elastoplast) and/or other products (e.g. latex)?

No known allergies or sensitivities OR specify allergies/sensitivities *(see medical notes/prescription chart and confirm on EPR)*

Baseline observations

Date		Time
Blood pressure (mmHg)	Pulse (rate/min)	Respirations (breaths/min)
Temperature (°C)	Peak flow (litres/min) **if required**	Oxygen (O_2) saturations (on air)
Urinalysis needed *(circle)* YES / NO Result:		Blood glucose level *(circle)* YES / NO Result:

Medications taken on the day of surgery:

Antiembolic prevention

☐ **Measure and fit thigh-length anti-embolism stockings on the morning of the operation**		
Two fingers width above the ankle bone (cm)	Left	Right
Stocking size *(circle)* EXTRA SMALL / SMALL / MEDIUM / LARGE / EXTRA LARGE / OTHER:		

Pressure area assessment

Skin intact *(circle)* YES / NO If NO, complete Waterlow Risk Assessment

Bowel preparation *(if applicable)*

YES / NO *(circle)*		
Preparation	Time	Result

Figure 16.13 Example of a pre-operative and theatre checklist.

The ROYAL MARSDEN

NHS Foundation Trust

Pre-operative checklist

Each entry below must be ticked to indicate Yes, No, or N/A (not applicable) with the relevant details

	1st Check by Ward/ Unit Nurse before pre-medication if prescribed or prior to leaving the ward			2nd Check by Operating Department Professional/ Theatre Nurse		
Section A - To be checked from nursing/medical notes/EPR	**Yes**	**No**	**N/A**	**Yes**	**No**	**N/A**
Consent to operation form signed/patient understands procedure						
Patient has undergone pre-anaesthetic consent						
Medical case notes/adult peri-operative care plan to accompany patient						
Blood results available on *(circle)*: EPR: YES / NO / N/A Date: Group & Save: YES / NO / N/A Date: Electrocardiogram (ECG): YES / NO / N/A Date:						
Confirm infection status and microbiology results *(circle)* Infection risk: YES / NO If YES, specify infection risk code: Active infection: YES / NO / N/A Precautions required: If positive, treatment given: YES / NO MRSA negative / positive *(circle)* MSSA negative / positive *(circle)* If positive, treatment given YES / NO Date commenced: If NO treatment commenced, surgical team informed						
Section B - To be checked by observing/asking patient	**Yes**	**No**	**N/A**	**Yes**	**No**	**N/A**
Attach identification bands to wrist/ankle						
Use red identification bands in case of allergy						
Operation site marked if appropriate						
Date/time of last food (24 hour clock):	Date/time of last drink (24 hour clock):					
Type of drink:						
Braces / Caps / Crowns / Bridge work / Loose teeth *(circle)*						
Dentures: YES / NO Dentures removed in DSU: YES / NO If NO, supply denture pot with patient's details						
Theatre gown and anti-embolic stockings						
Check and confirm status on all women of childbearing age: **Note:** pregnancy tests to be performed on all gynaecology surgical patients and patients undergoing laparotomy. Could you be pregnant? YES / NO / N/A Pregnancy test result: Date of last menstrual period:						
Cotton underwear worn or consent for removal of underwear						
Contact lenses removed / worn (circle)						
Glasses removed / worn *(circle)* Kept on ward / Kept in operating theatre *(circle)*						
Left / Right hearing aid removed / worn *(circle)* Kept on ward / Kept in operating theatre *(circle)*						
False nails / Nail varnish / Make-up removed *(circle)*						
Jewellery / Ring(s) / Metal hair accessories / Body piercing removed or taped *(circle)*						
Prosthesis e.g. knee replacements, implants, pacemaker *(specify)*:						

DSU/Unit Nurse *(circle)* (On handover to theatre staff)	Signature	Full Name *(PRINT)*	Date	Time
Theatre Practitioner/Nurse *(circle)*	Signature	Full Name *(PRINT)*	Date	Time

Figure 16.13 *Continued*

The ROYAL MARSDEN
NHS Foundation Trust

Anaesthetic room

Patient Care Need

Altered protection related to anaesthesia.

Anticipated outcome

- Patient safety will be maintained during anaesthesia .
- Patient will receive the anaesthesia in a safe and appropriate manner with the early detection of complications/side effects, which will be managed/treated effectively.

Patient Care Interventions

A - Consent and information giving

- Ensure valid consent has been given for the procedure and confirm patient identity in relation to the operating list.
- Provide the patient with accurate information about the anaesthesia.
- Part 1 of the Surgical Safety Checklist completed.

B - Venous access, patient monitoring and medical device management

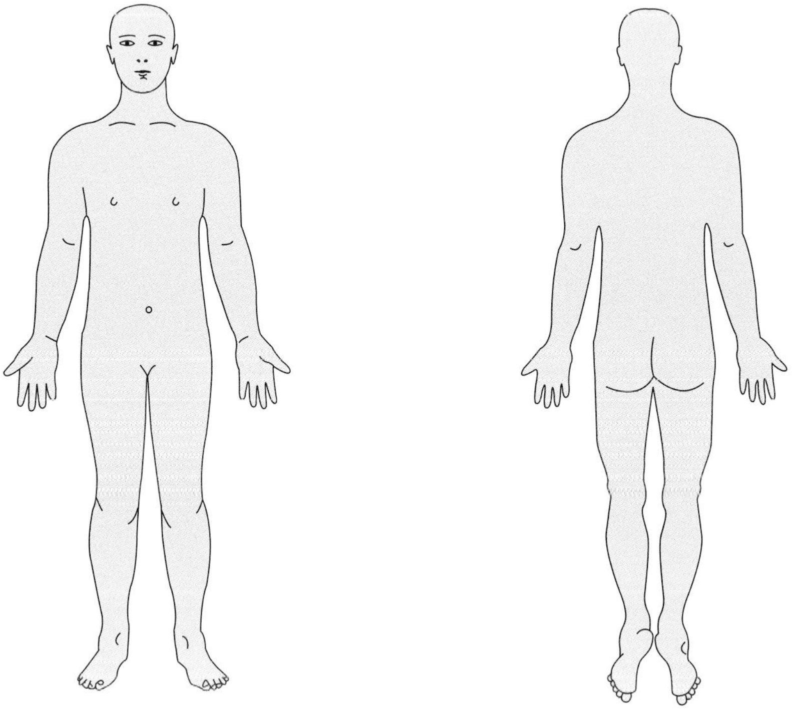

Indicate on the diagram the number of the corresponding item's and tick as appropriate:

1	Blood Pressure Cuff	**7**	Peripheral Cannula Size: ☐ Introcan ☐ Nexiva ☐ Other: Secured with:
2	Pulse Oximetry		
3	ECG Electrodes		
4	Diathermy Site *(operating staff to complete)* ☐ Site shaved ☐ Monopolar ☐ Bipolar ☐ Both	**8**	Central Venous Access Device *(circle)* LEFT / RIGHT NECK / FEMORAL Secured with:
5	Tourniquet *(operating staff to complete)*	**9**	Arterial Cannula *(circle)* LEFT / RIGHT RADIAL / FEMORAL / PEDAL Secured with: IV 3000 / STAT LOCK / ....
6	Nasogastric Tube Size:		

Figure 16.13 *Continued*

C - Type of anaesthesia

Induction time of anaesthetic:

☐ General	☐ Epidural	☐ Spinal	☐ Caudal
☐ Sedation	☐ Infiltration	☐ Local Block	☐ Throat Sprayed
☐ Rapid Sequence Induction			

D - Airway

☐ Laryngeal Mask Airway	☐ Oral Airway	☐ Nasopharyngeal Airway
☐ Oral Endotracheal Tube	☐ Tracheostomy Tube	☐ Naso-endotracheal Tube

State size:

☐ Throat pack inserted

E - Eyes taped / covered with pad *(circle as appropriate)*

F - Temperature management *(tick as appropriate)*

Temperature: °C **If less than 36°C commence warming prior to proceeding with surgery**

☐ Temperature probe — If **ticked**, state site: nasopharyngeal / axilla / rectal / skin probe

☐ Warming blanket — If **ticked**, specify: ☐ Bair Hugger ☐ Warming Mattress

☐ Hot line

Additional interventions

G/VTE: ☐ Stockings ☐ Sequential Compression Devices (SCD)

Document infection risk status:

Anaesthetic Practitioner	Signature	Full Name (PRINT)	Date	Time

Figure 16.13 *Continued*

Table 16.9 Haematology values

Test	Reference range	Functions and additional information
Red blood cells (RBC)	Men: 4.5–6.5 × 10^{12}/L Women: 3.9–5.6 × 10^{12}/L	The main function of the RBC is the transport of oxygen and carbon dioxide.
Haemoglobin (Hb)	Men: 130–170 g/dL Women: 120–150 g/dL	Hb is a protein pigment found within the RBC that carries oxygen. *Anaemia* (deficiency in the number of RBC or in the Hb content) may occur for many reasons. Changes to cell production, deficient dietary intake or blood loss may be relevant and need to be investigated further.
White blood cells (WBC)	Men: 3.7–9.5 × 10^{9}/L Women: 3.9–11.1 × 10^{9}/L	The function of the WBC is defence against infection. There are different kinds of WBC: neutrophils, lymphocytes, monocytes, eosinophils and basophils. *Leucopenia* is a WBC count lower than 3.7 and is usually associated with the use of cytotoxic drugs. *Leucocytosis* (high levels of neutrophils and lymphocytes) occurs as the body's normal response to infection and after surgery. *Leukaemia* involves an increased WBC count caused by changes in cell production in the bone marrow. The leukaemic cells enter the blood in increased numbers in an immature state.
Platelets	150–400 × 10^{9}/L	Clot formation occurs when platelets and the blood protein fibrin combine. A patient may be *thrombocytopenic* (low platelet count) due to drugs or poor production, or have a raised count (*thrombocytosis*) with infection or autoimmune disease.
Coagulation/ international normalized ratio (INR)	INR range 2–3 (in some cases a range of 3–4.5 is acceptable)	Coagulation occurs to prevent excessive blood loss by the formation of a clot (thrombus). However, a clot that forms in an artery may block the vessel and cause an infarction or ischaemia, which can be fatal. Aspirin, warfarin and heparin are three drugs used for the prevention and/or treatment of *thrombosis*. It is imperative that patients on warfarin therapy receive regular monitoring to ensure a balance of slowing the clot-forming process and maintaining the ability of the blood to clot.
Sodium	135–145 mmol/L	The main function of sodium is to maintain extracellular volume (water stored outside the cells), acid-base balance and the transmitting of nerve impulses. *Hypernatraemia* (serum sodium >145 mmol/L) may be an indication of dehydration due to fluid loss from diarrhoea, excessive sweating, increased urinary output or a poor oral intake of fluid. An increased salt intake may also cause an elevation. *Hyponatraemia* (serum sodium <135 mmol/L) may be indicated in fluid retention (oedema).
Potassium	3.5–5.2 mmol/L	Potassium plays a major role in nerve conduction, muscle function, acid-base balance and osmotic pressure. It has a direct effect on cardiac muscle, influencing cardiac output by helping to control the rate and force of each contraction. The most common cause of *hyperkalaemia* (serum potassium >5.2 mmol/L) is chronic renal failure, in which the kidneys are unable to excrete potassium. The level may be elevated due to an increased intake of potassium supplements during treatment. Tissue cell destruction caused by trauma or cytotoxic therapy may cause a release of potassium from the cells and an elevation in the potassium plasma level. It may also be observed in untreated diabetic ketoacidosis. Urgent treatment is required as hyperkalaemia may lead to changes in cardiac muscle contraction and cause subsequent cardiac arrest. The main cause of *hypokalaemia* (serum potassium <3.5 mmol/L) is the loss of potassium via the kidneys during treatment with thiazide diuretics. Excessive or chronic diarrhoea may also cause a decreased potassium level.
Urea	2.5–6.5 mmol/L	Urea is a waste product of metabolism that is transported to the kidneys and excreted as urine. Elevated levels of urea may indicate poor kidney function.
Creatinine	55–105 μmol/L	Creatinine is a waste product of metabolism that is transported to the kidneys and excreted as urine. Elevated levels of creatinine may indicate poor kidney function.
Calcium	2.20–2.60 mmol/L	Most of the calcium in the body is stored in the bone but ionized calcium, which circulates in the blood plasma, plays an important role in the transmission of nerve impulses and the functioning of cardiac and skeletal muscle. It is also vital for blood coagulation. High calcium levels, or *hypercalcaemia* (>2.6 mmol/L), can be caused by hyperthyroidism, hyperparathyroidism or malignancy. Elevation in calcium levels may cause cardiac arrhythmia, potentially leading to cardiac arrest. Tumour cells can cause excessive production of a protein called parathormone-related polypeptide (PTHrP), which causes loss of calcium from the bone and an increase in blood calcium levels. This is a major reason for hypercalcaemia in cancer patients (Higgins and Higgins 2013). *Hypocalcaemia* (<2.20 mmol/L) is often associated with vitamin D deficiency due to inadequate intake or increased loss due to gastrointestinal disease. Mild hypocalcaemia may be symptomless but severe disease may cause increased neuromuscular excitability and cardiac arrhythmias. It is also a common feature of chronic renal failure (Higgins and Higgins 2013).

Test	Reference range	Functions and additional information
C-reactive protein (CRP)	<10 mg/L	Elevation in the CRP level can be a useful indication of bacterial infection. CRP is monitored after surgery and for patients who have a high risk of infection. The CRP level can help to monitor the severity of inflammation and assist in the diagnosis of conditions such as systemic lupus erythematosus, ulcerative colitis and Crohn's disease (Higgins and Higgins 2013).
Albumin	35–50 g/L	Albumin is a protein found in blood plasma that assists in the transport of water-soluble substances and the maintenance of blood plasma volume.
Bilirubin	(total) <13 μmol/L	Bilirubin is produced from the breakdown of haemoglobin; it is transported to the liver for excretion in bile. Elevated levels of bilirubin may cause jaundice.

Procedure guideline 16.2 Pre-operative care: checking that the patient is fully prepared for surgery

Essential equipment

- Personal protective equipment
- Two name bands
- Theatre gown
- Cotton-based underwear or disposable pants (if these do not interfere with surgery)
- Antiembolic stockings
- Labelled containers for dentures, glasses and/or hearing aid (if necessary)
- Hypoallergenic tape
- Patient records/documentation including medical records, consent form, drug chart, X-ray films, blood test results, anaesthetic assessment and pre-operative checklist

Action	Rationale
Procedure	
1 Introduce yourself to the patient, explain and discuss the procedure with them, and gain their consent to proceed.	To ensure that the patient feels at ease, understands the procedure and gives their valid consent (NMC 2018, **C**).
2 Discuss with the patient: • if they know what surgery they are having and why • if they can tell you about the wound, any intravenous infusions or drains, etc. that they may expect after the surgery • if they have been told about levels of pain and how it will be controlled • how they can be involved in ensuring they recover as quickly as possible.	To ensure that the patient understands the nature and outcome of the surgery, to reduce anxiety and possible post-operative complications (Turunen et al. 2017, **E**).
3 Check that the patient has undergone relevant investigative procedures and that the results are included with the patient's notes. Examples include X-ray, ECG, MRI, CT, ECHO, blood test and urinalysis.	To ensure all relevant information is available to the nurses, anaesthetists and surgeons (AORN 2000, **C**).
4 Confirm and document when the patient last had food or drink, ensuring that this complies with pre-operative instructions. Record this in the pre-operative documentation.	To reduce the risk of regurgitation and inhalation of stomach contents on induction of anaesthesia. It can take 9 hours or more for a substantial meal to be emptied from the stomach (AAGBI 2015, **C**; King 2010, **C**; RCN 2017, **C**).
5 Confirm and document which medications the patient has taken and when. Ensure this complies with pre-operative instructions and record in the pre-operative documentation.	To ensure the patient does not take and/or omit any medication that could adversely affect surgery (e.g. continuation of high-dose warfarin). **E**
6 If the patient is female and of child-bearing age:	
a Check her pregnancy status and record the result in the pre-operative documentation. If a pregnancy test is required (e.g. if the patient expresses a concern that she may be pregnant or she is undergoing gynaecology surgery) (NICE 2016b), the test results should be given to the patient and record in the pre-operative documentation.	To eliminate the possibility of unknown pregnancy prior to the planned surgical procedure (NPSA 2010, **E**).
b If appropriate, ask the patient whether she is menstruating and ensure that she has a sanitary towel in place and not a tampon.	To prevent infection if the tampon is left in place for longer than 6 hours (www.tamponalert.org.uk, **C**).
7 In the presence of the patient, check the consent form is correctly completed, signed and dated.	To comply with legal requirements and hospital policy and to ensure that the patient has understood the surgical procedure (NMC 2018, **C**).
8 If applicable, check the operation site has been marked correctly with the patient and the consent form.	To ensure the patient undergoes the correct surgery for which they have consented (AORN 2000, **C**; Schäfli-Thurnherr et al. 2017, **R**).

(continued)

Procedure guideline 16.2 Pre-operative care: checking that the patient is fully prepared for surgery *(continued)*

Action	Rationale
9 Check that the patient has undergone pre-anaesthetic assessment by the anaesthetist.	To ensure that the patient can be given the most suitable anaesthetic and that any special requirements for anaesthetic have been highlighted (AORN 2000, **C**).
10 Measure and record the patient's pulse, blood pressure, respirations, oxygen saturations, temperature, weight and blood sugar (if required) in the pre-operative documentation.	To provide baseline data for comparison intra- and post-operatively. The weight is recorded so that the anaesthetist can calculate the correct dose of drugs to be administered (AORN 2000, **C**).
11 Ask the patient to remove all jewellery, cosmetics and nail varnish. Wedding rings may be left on fingers but must be covered and secured with hypoallergenic tape. Patients requesting to wear other forms of metal jewellery (e.g. chains) for personal or religious reasons will need to discuss this with the operating team.	Metal jewellery may be accidentally lost or may cause harm to the patient. Facial cosmetics make the patient's colour difficult to assess. Nail varnish makes the use of the pulse oximeter (which monitors the patient's pulse and oxygen saturation levels) impossible and masks peripheral cyanosis (Vedovato et al. 2004, **C**).
12 If the patient has valuables, these must be recorded and stored away securely according to hospital policy.	To prevent loss of valuables. **E**
13 Ensure the patient has showered or bathed as close to the planned time of the operation as possible and before a pre-medication is administered (if this has been prescribed). If the patient has long hair, this needs to be tied back with a non-metallic tie.	To minimize the risk of post-operative wound infection (Loveday et al. 2014, **C**). For safety, to prevent hair getting caught in equipment and to reduce the risk of infection. **E**
14 Apply antiembolic stockings according to local trust procedure (see Procedure guideline 16.1: Measuring and applying antiembolic stockings)	To reduce the risk of post-operative deep vein thrombosis or pulmonary emboli (NICE 2018a, **C**).
15 Ensure the patient is wearing two electronic/barcoded name bands containing their full name, date of birth and NHS number. One should be placed on the patient's wrist and the other on the ankle. Prior to placing the name bands on the patient, the details should be verbally checked and confirmed as accurate by the patient and against the patient's medical notes. The name bands should be white unless local trust policy stipulates that colour coding is necessary to alert healthcare professionals to a risk (e.g. allergy), in which case the wristbands should be red (NPSA 2007).	To ensure correct identification and prevent possible patient misidentification (AORN 2000, **C**). To reduce allergic reactions to known causative agents and to alert all involved in the care of the patient in the operating theatre (AORN 2010, **C**).
16 Record whether the patient has dental caps, crowns, bridge work or loose teeth in the pre-operative checklist.	The anaesthetist needs to be informed to prevent accidental damage. Loose teeth or a dental prosthesis could be inhaled by the patient when an endotracheal tube is inserted. **E**
17 Document any patient prostheses in the pre-operative checklist and whether they are removable (e.g. artificial limb, dentures or hearing aid) or irremovable (e.g. pacemaker or knee replacement). Removable prostheses may be retained until the patient is in the anaesthetic room. Spectacles and hearing aids may be retained until the patient has been anaesthetized (these may be left in position if a local anaesthetic is used). Any prosthesis that is removed should be labelled clearly (ideally with a patient identifier) and retained in the recovery room.	To promote patient safety during surgery. For example, dentures may obstruct the airway and contact lenses can cause corneal abrasions. Internal non-removable prostheses may be affected by the electric current used in diathermy. **C** To enable the patient to communicate fully, thus reducing anxiety and enabling the patient to understand any procedures carried out. **E** To enable patients with prosthetic limbs to mobilize independently to theatre. **C**
18 Check whether the patient passed urine before pre-medication or anaesthetic.	For patient comfort and because a full bladder may impede the surgeon's view during abdominal surgery. To prevent catheterization. To prevent urinary incontinence when sedated and/or unconscious and possible contamination of sterile area. **E**
19 Once the pre-operative checklist has been fully completed, administer any pre-medication, if prescribed, in accordance with the anaesthetist's instructions. Patients who receive a sedative pre-medication should be advised to remain in bed and to use the nurse call system if assistance is needed.	Specific drugs may be prescribed to complement the anaesthetic to be given (e.g. temazepam to reduce patient anxiety by inducing sleep and relaxation). **E** Questioning premedicated patients is not a reliable source of checking information as the patient may be drowsy and/or disorientated (AfPP 2017, **C**). To reduce the risk of accidental patient injury as the pre-medication may make the patient drowsy and disorientated. **E**

20	Accompany the patient to theatre, taking with you their notes, medication chart, X-rays/scans, blood results, completed consent form and pre-operative checklist. The patient should be accompanied to the theatre by a qualified nurse. Mobile patients who have not received a sedative pre-medication will be able to walk to theatre wearing appropriately fitting footwear. Immobile patients or patients who have received a sedative pre-medication will need to be taken to theatre on a theatre trolley.	To prevent delays, which can increase the patient's anxiety, and to ensure that the anaesthetist and surgeon have all the information they require for safe treatment of the patient. **E** To reduce patient anxiety and ensure a safe environment during anaesthetic induction. **E** To reduce the risk of accidental patient injury as pre-medication may make a patient drowsy and disorientated. **E**
21	Give a full handover to the anaesthetic nurse or operating department practitioner on arrival in the anaesthetic room, using the patient's records and the pre-operative checklist. Stay with the patient until they have been fully checked in by the anaesthetic assistant or nurse.	To ensure the patient has the correct operation. To ensure continuity of care and to maintain the safety of the patient by exchanging all relevant information (AfPP 2017, **C**).

Intraoperative care

Definition

Intraoperative care encompasses the following three phases: induction of anaesthesia, surgery and finally recovery. This phase of care begins when the patient arrives in the anaesthetic room or operating theatre and ends when the patient is transferred to the post-anaesthesia care area, where immediate post-surgical care is delivered to the patient.

Anaesthesia

Definition

Intraoperative care is the physical and psychological care given to the patient in the anaesthetic room and operating theatre, prior to their transfer to the post-anaesthetic care unit. General anaesthesia is usually described as a triad of components that include hypnosis (sleep), analgesia and muscle relaxation.

Evidence-based approaches

In the anaesthetic room, patients are admitted and checked into the operating suite. The patient is normally transferred (already anaesthetized) into the theatre on a trolley and moved across to the operating table. For some life-threatening emergency surgery (e.g. ruptured abdominal aortic aneurysm repair), it may be preferable to induce anaesthesia inside the operating theatre with the patient already positioned on the operating table (Leonard and Thompson 2008). A crucial role of the anaesthetic nurse is to support the patient, who is often frightened or anxious due to the unfamiliar, often intimidating environment and apprehensive about both the anaesthesia and the impending surgery (Turunen et al. 2017).

The patient should be carefully checked by the anaesthetist and an anaesthetic practitioner with reference to the 'Sign In' portion of the WHO Surgical Safety Checklist (WHO 2009). The patient should be comfortably positioned on a trolley or an operating table with the relevant monitoring devices attached (i.e. ECG leads, blood pressure cuff and pulse oximeter) (AAGBI 2015).

The patient may undergo surgery under general anaesthesia, regional anaesthesia or sedation; they may also have both general and regional anaesthesia. Depending on the nature of the surgery and the patient's co-morbidities, the anaesthetist may require additional invasive monitoring, such as large-bore intravenous cannula, arterial line or central venous catheter. After induction of general anaesthesia or performance of regional anaesthesia, and with the patient's cardiorespiratory stability ensured, the patient is carefully transferred to the operating table.

Depending on the nature of the surgery, the patient's position may need to be altered (e.g. moved into the prone or lateral position). Meticulous care of the patient's eyes, skin, joints and nerves must be taken during this positioning and throughout the surgery to avoid complications associated with prolonged immobility. The 'Time Out' portion of the WHO Surgical Safety Checklist (WHO 2009) is then completed before commencing the surgical procedure. Nursing activities during the intraoperative period are focused on patient safety, ensuring surgical swab counts are managed safely in accordance with the recommended safety practice, facilitating the procedure and adherence to infection control recommendations. It is then mandatory to complete the 'Sign Out' portion of the WHO Surgical Safety Checklist (WHO 2009) to confirm that all surgical counts are correct and to ensure any specific post-operative concerns from the surgical and anaesthetic team are relayed to the post-operative nursing care team.

General anaesthesia

The proportion of each of the three components of general anaesthesia (hypnosis/sleep, analgesia and muscle relaxation) may vary according to the surgery. For example, modern muscle relaxants, which emerged in the 1940s, enable adequate relaxation of the abdomen (for example) without relying on very deep anaesthesia (from a single agent) to achieve the same effect (Simpson et al. 2002). Today, anaesthesia is very safe, and there are very few deaths – less than 1 in 250,000 directly related to anaesthesia (RCoA 2013).

Anticipated patient outcomes

The anticipated patient outcomes of the anaesthesia phase of intraoperative care are:

- to ensure that the patient understands what will happen in the operating theatre in order to minimize anxiety
- to ensure that the patient has the correct surgery for which the consent form was signed
- to ensure patient safety at all times and minimize post-operative complications by:
  - giving the required care for the unconscious patient
  - ensuring injury is not sustained from hazards associated with the use of swabs, needles, instruments, diathermy and power tools
  - minimizing post-operative problems associated with patient positioning, such as nerve or tissue damage
  - maintaining asepsis during surgical procedures to reduce the risk of post-operative wound infection in accordance with hospital policies on infection control.

Clinical governance

The WHO Surgical Safety Checklist (WHO 2009) is a structured aid used to enhance communication and improve safety within surgery. It was first implemented in 2008 and is mandated in many countries, including the UK. The aim of the checklist is to decrease the numbers of errors and adverse events, and increase teamwork and communication in surgery. The checklist comprises three parts: before induction of anaesthesia ('Sign In'), before skin incision ('Time Out') and before the patient leaves the operating room ('Sign Out') (Figure 16.14).

World Health Organization

SURGICAL SAFETY CHECKLIST (FIRST EDITION)

Before induction of anaesthesia ▸▸▸▸▸▸▸▸▸▸ Before skin incision ▸▸▸▸▸▸▸▸▸▸▸▸▸▸ Before patient leaves operating room

SIGN IN

☐ PATIENT HAS CONFIRMED
- IDENTITY
- SITE
- PROCEDURE
- CONSENT

☐ SITE MARKED/NOT APPLICABLE

☐ ANAESTHESIA SAFETY CHECK COMPLETED

☐ PULSE OXIMETER ON PATIENT AND FUNCTIONING

DOES PATIENT HAVE A:

KNOWN ALLERGY?
☐ NO
☐ YES

DIFFICULT AIRWAY/ASPIRATION RISK?
☐ NO
☐ YES, AND EQUIPMENT/ASSISTANCE AVAILABLE

RISK OF >500 ML BLOOD LOSS (7 ML/KG IN CHILDREN)?
☐ NO
☐ YES, AND ADEQUATE INTRAVENOUS ACCESS AND FLUIDS PLANNED

TIME OUT

☐ CONFIRM ALL TEAM MEMBERS HAVE INTRODUCED THEMSELVES BY NAME AND ROLE

☐ SURGEON, ANAESTHESIA PROFESSIONAL AND NURSE VERBALLY CONFIRM
- PATIENT
- SITE
- PROCEDURE

ANTICIPATED CRITICAL EVENTS

☐ SURGEON REVIEWS: WHAT ARE THE CRITICAL OR UNEXPECTED STEPS, OPERATIVE DURATION, ANTICIPATED BLOOD LOSS?

☐ ANAESTHESIA TEAM REVIEWS: ARE THERE ANY PATIENT-SPECIFIC CONCERNS?

☐ NURSING TEAM REVIEWS: HAS STERILITY (INCLUDING INDICATOR RESULTS) BEEN CONFIRMED? ARE THERE EQUIPMENT ISSUES OR ANY CONCERNS?

HAS ANTIBIOTIC PROPHYLAXIS BEEN GIVEN WITHIN THE LAST 60 MINUTES?
☐ YES
☐ NOT APPLICABLE

IS ESSENTIAL IMAGING DISPLAYED?
☐ YES
☐ NOT APPLICABLE

SIGN OUT

NURSE VERBALLY CONFIRMS WITH THE TEAM:

☐ THE NAME OF THE PROCEDURE RECORDED

☐ THAT INSTRUMENT, SPONGE AND NEEDLE COUNTS ARE CORRECT (OR NOT APPLICABLE)

☐ HOW THE SPECIMEN IS LABELLED (INCLUDING PATIENT NAME)

☐ WHETHER THERE ARE ANY EQUIPMENT PROBLEMS TO BE ADDRESSED

☐ SURGEON, ANAESTHESIA PROFESSIONAL AND NURSE REVIEW THE KEY CONCERNS FOR RECOVERY AND MANAGEMENT OF THIS PATIENT

THIS CHECKLIST IS NOT INTENDED TO BE COMPREHENSIVE. ADDITIONS AND MODIFICATIONS TO FIT LOCAL PRACTICE ARE ENCOURAGED.

Figure 16.14 The World Health Organization's Surgical Safety Checklist. *Source*: Reproduced from WHO (2009) with permission of the World Health Organization.

Pre-procedural considerations

Pharmacological support

Prior to commencing anaesthesia, the patient is assessed by the anaesthetist. The type of anaesthetic administered will depend on multiple factors, including co-morbidities, the age and risks of the patient, the nature of the planned surgery, and the patient's and clinician's preferences. However, the following components are usually included.

Analgesia

This is an effective form of pain relief and is essential in the post-operative period. Analgesic drugs are given intravenously intraoperatively in anticipation of post-operative requirements. Commonly used drugs include paracetamol, non-steroidal anti-inflammatory drugs, opioids such as fentanyl and morphine, and ketamine. Peripheral nerve blockade using local anaesthetic agents (regional anaesthesia) is also widely used to render the operative site numb and pain free. Surgeons may also infiltrate local anaesthetic into wounds to help with post operative analgesia.

Antiemetics

Antiemetics are given with analgesia. Various factors influence the incidence of post-operative nausea and vomiting, and these may be pre-existing patient factors, surgical factors and anaesthetic-related factors. Antiemetic drugs have various mechanisms of action: commonly used agents include ondansetron, cyclizine, prochlorperazine and dexamethasone. The anaesthetic technique can also be adapted to reduce the risk of post-operative nausea and vomiting. The use of total intravenous anaesthesia using drugs such as propofol and remifentanil is associated with lower incidence of post-operative nausea and vomiting compared with volatile anaesthesia. Another anaesthetic alternative may be to perform the surgery under regional or local anaesthesia, thus avoiding the need for general anaesthesia completely.

Induction agents

Induction agents are drugs that induce unconsciousness. The most commonly used intravenous agent is propofol, a short acting drug that can also be used to maintain anaesthesia as an intravenous infusion in total intravenous anaesthesia. Other intravenous induction agents include the barbiturate thiopentone, etomidate and ketamine (each of which can also be administered intramuscularly). General anaesthesia may also be induced through inhalation of volatile anaesthetic agents, such as sevoflurane.

Inhalational agents

After induction, anaesthesia can be maintained by either inhalational anaesthetic agents or intravenous infusion (e.g. propofol).

Examples of modern inhalational agents are sevoflurane, desflurane and isoflurane. These volatile gases are administered through vaporizers, which are integrated into modern anaesthetic machines (Figure 16.15).

Muscle relaxants

Drugs that cause relaxation of the skeletal muscles (temporary paralysis) may be administered intravenously when the patient is unconscious in order to aid tracheal intubation and/or to improve conditions for the surgeon during the operation. Commonly used relaxants are suxamethonium, atracurium, vecuronium and rocuronium. The degree of muscle paralysis must be monitored with a peripheral nerve stimulator.

Specific patient preparation

When the patient arrives in the anaesthetic room, their identity is checked and the safety checklist is completed. At this point, consent is verified with the patient in order to confirm the planned operation. This should include the correct side of the body to be operated on, if relevant. A competent anaesthetic assistant must be present, and the surgeon must be ready. This completes the final phase of the pre-anaesthetic checklist.

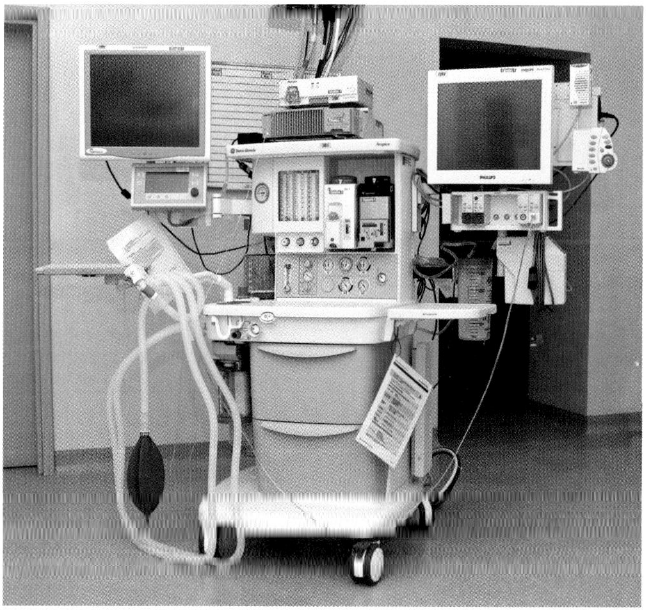

Figure 16.15 Anaesthetic machine.

Procedure guideline 16.3 Caring for the patient in the anaesthetic room

Essential equipment

- Personal protective equipment
- Suction
- Anaesthetic machine
- Airway equipment
- Medical gases (including back-up oxygen cylinders)
- Monitoring equipment
- Emergency drugs

Action	Rationale
Pre-procedure	
1 Introduce yourself to the patient, explain and discuss the procedure with them, and gain their consent to proceed. Confirm with the ward nurse that you have identified the correct patient for the scheduled operation.	To ensure that the patient feels at ease, understands the procedure and gives their valid consent (NMC 2018, **C**).
Procedure	
2 Identify the patient by checking the identification band (name and patient number) against the patient's notes and the operating list.	To safeguard against patient misidentification (AfPP 2017, **C**).
3 Check and confirm the correct completion of the pre-operative checklist.	To ensure that all the listed measures have been completed and that any additional information has been recorded. **E**
4 Check that the results of the investigative procedures (e.g. blood results and X-rays) are included with the patient's notes.	To ensure that all the required results are available for the theatre team's use. **E**
5 Maintain a calm, quiet environment and explain all the procedures to the patient, including the monitoring of blood pressure, pulse and oxygen saturation.	To reduce anxiety and enhance the smooth induction of anaesthesia (Turunen et al. 2017, **E**).
6 When the patient has been anaesthetized, ensure that the eyes are closed and secured with hypoallergenic tape or padding.	To prevent corneal damage due to eyes drying out or accidental abrasion. For longer surgical procedures a sterile lubricant may also be applied to the surface of the eye (Lillienthal et al. 2016, **E**; Malafa et al. 2016, **R**).
Post-procedure	
7 When the patient has been anaesthetized, they are transferred into the operating theatre.	To commence the surgical procedure. **C**

Airway management

Definition

Airway management is the planning and performance of manoeuvres and procedures that anticipate, prevent and relieve airway obstruction. It is one of the cornerstones of safe anaesthetic practice.

Related theory

When a supine patient is rendered unconscious with anaesthesia, the soft tissues of the tongue and neck relax, and occlude the laryngeal inlet. This can cause an obstruction of the airway.

The purpose of airway management during anaesthesia and surgery is to maintain patency of the airway, thereby facilitating effective ventilation of the patient's lungs. Assessment of the patient's airway prior to anaesthesia is vital in order for the anaesthetist to plan and prepare the most appropriate airway management strategy (Bradley et al. 2016). A complete airway assessment includes the patient's history (e.g. history of previous airway difficulties during anaesthesia or history of obstructive sleep apnoea) and a bedside examination (looking for congenital or acquired features that may make face-mask ventilation, airway adjunct placement or tracheal intubation difficult). The Mallampati test is a subjective evaluation of the ratio of oral cavity volume to tongue volume (Mahmoodpoor et al. 2017). The test is performed on a sitting patient with the head in a neutral position, mouth fully opened and tongue extended. It involves evaluating the visibility of the uvula, as shown in Figure 16.16. Any potential difficulties of laryngoscopy and tracheal intubation can then be assessed, with a class 1 airway being the easiest to manage and control by intubation, and a class 4 airway being potentially the most difficult.

There are several techniques for planning for airway management during the induction period. A combination of these techniques can be used if one is inadequate during a difficult intubation:

- face-mask ventilation
- supraglottic airway ventilation
- endotracheal intubation
- fibreoptic intubation.

Face-mask ventilation

This is a fundamental technique for safe anaesthesia and requires the practitioner to use simple airway manoeuvres (such as jaw thrust, chin lift) to open the airway. Simple adjuncts such as a Guedel airway may be useful at this stage. If the patient is apnoeic, the practitioner can deliver ventilation via an appropriate breathing circuit and a face-mask that is held to create a tight seal with the patient's face. Difficulties with face-mask ventilation may be encountered in a number of scenarios: inexperienced practitioner, high body mass index, the presence of a beard, facial deformities or an edentulous patient.

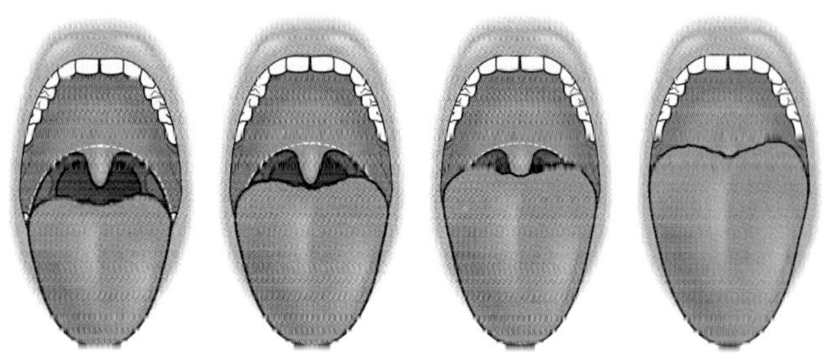

Figure 16.16 Mallampati classification of the airway.

Supraglottic airways

The laryngeal mask airway (LMA) was developed in 1988 by Dr Archie Brain and provides an effective alternative to face-mask ventilation in a starved patient. It is a type of supraglottic airway, which means that nothing passes through the vocal cords. Second- and third-generation LMAs have since been developed offering improved seals around the laryngeal inlet and increased flexibility in their applications. Different sizes are available depending on the patient's weight.

Endotracheal intubation

Endotracheal tubes have become fundamental to the practice of anaesthesia with the advent of neuromuscular blockade. Tubes are available in a number of sizes and styles depending on the weight of the patient and also features of the airway and surgical requirements. The trachea can be intubated with an endotracheal tube in a number of different ways: conventional direct laryngoscopy, video laryngoscopy, fibreoptic laryngoscopy or through a supraglottic airway, to name just a few.

Endotracheal intubation is a skill that requires specialist training. Techniques and devices to facilitate successful intubation of the trachea include optimal patient positioning, external laryngeal manipulation, stylets or bougies, and use of advanced airway equipment.

Theatre

Related theory

Before surgical intervention (skin incision)

The theatre team normally consists of:

- surgeon (at least one lead surgeon, often more including surgical trainees)
- surgical assistant
- anaesthetist
- scrub or anaesthetic practitioner: registered nurse (RN) or operating department practitioner (ODP)
- circulating practitioner(s): RN(s) and healthcare assistant.

The role of the scrub practitioner (RN or ODP) working in the sterile field is to manage the instrumentation, swabs and sutures and to assist as part of the surgical team without carrying out dual role responsibility (AfPP 2017). There will normally be at least one circulating person who remains outside the sterile field and provides items as required for the scrub practitioner. There will also be a designated anaesthetic practitioner (RN or ODP) who assists the anaesthetist (Figure 16.17).

Once the patient has been positioned on the operating table and before surgical intervention, the theatre team completes the 'Time Out' portion of the WHO Surgical Safety Checklist (WHO 2009);

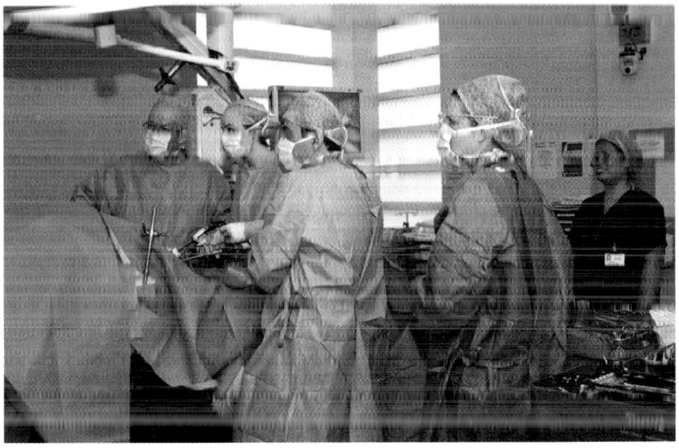

Figure 16.17 Surgical team.

the entire theatre team must pause to participate in this check in order to adhere to the recommendation of the National Safety Standards for Invasive Procedures (NatSSIPs) and Local Safety Standards for Invasive Procedures (LocSSIPs) (Lo 2016, Sevdalis and Arora 2016). This ensures that the team is fully aware and readily equipped for any problems that may arise during the procedure. Any discrepancies noted during this stage with regard to the consent, the patient's identification or any matters discussed in the checklist must be rectified before the procedure can begin.

It is imperative that pre-operative checks are completed thoroughly and in detail, in accordance with the NatSSIPs. The NatSSIPs (NHSI 2015) aim to reduce the number of patient safety incidents related to invasive procedures in which surgical 'Never Events' could occur (NHS England 2014). The NatSSIPs build on the existing WHO Surgical Safety Checklist (WHO 2009) and promote the effective performance of the Five Steps to Safer Surgery guidance (Vickers 2011).

Control of infection and asepsis in the operating theatre

As part of intraoperative care, the aim of operating theatres is to provide an environment that minimizes the presence of pathogens (both airborne and surface). The general principle is that the actual operating theatre is the cleanest area within the suite as this is the area where patients are at most risk of surgical site infection. Ventilation systems within theatres support this principle by using positive pressure ventilation to carry pathogens away from the surgical wound (Agodi et al. 2015, Bischoff et al. 2017, Parvizi et al. 2017).

Large quantities of bacteria are present in the nose and mouth, and on the skin, hair and the attire of personnel. The skin cells of staff become dispersed in the air and are a potential source of wound infection (Sivanandan et al. 2011). Therefore, staff working in operating theatres wear clean scrub suits and lint-free surgical hats to eliminate the possibility of bacteria, hair, dandruff or skin cells being shed into the environment (AfPP 2017). Well fitting shoes with impervious soles should be worn and regularly cleaned to remove splashes of blood and body fluids (AfPP 2017). Face-masks are worn to prevent droplets falling from the mouth into the operating field. The extent to which face-masks are capable of preventing droplet spread is disputed (Vincent and Edwards 2016). It is, however, accepted that masks offer protection to the wearer from blood splashes and for safety reasons should be worn by the scrub team. Instruments must be handled carefully, with needle holders and forceps used to manipulate sutures to minimize the risk of needle stick or sharps injury.

Laparoscopic surgery

Definition

Laparoscopic surgery, also called minimally invasive surgery or keyhole surgery, is a modern surgical technique in which operations are performed through small incisions (usually measuring 0.5–1.5 cm), which are made through the skin and tissues to allow access to the required internal site.

Related theory

Laparoscopy is a type of surgical procedure that allows a surgeon to access the inside of the abdomen and pelvis without having to make large incisions in the skin. It involves the introduction of a number of small ports through the skin to allow access into the abdominal cavity (Figure 16.18). Specialized cameras, lights and instruments are introduced through these ports in order to perform this minimally invasive surgery.

Laparoscopy involves the insufflation of the abdomen with carbon dioxide. This is necessary in order to expand the space in which the surgeon is operating to facilitate the surgery, and is known as 'pneumoperitoneum' (Figure 16.18). Carbon dioxide is used because unlike air or oxygen is does not support combustion in the presence of electricity and is readily excreted by the patient's respiratory system. However, it is not without risk as

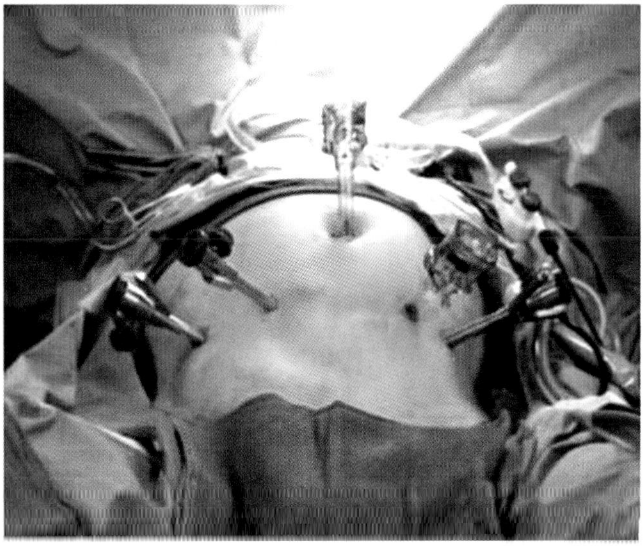

Figure 16.18 Port placement for pneumoperitoneum in laparoscopic or robotic surgery.

carbon dioxide absorption may be associated with adverse events such as hypercapnia and acidosis (T. Yu et al. 2017). Prolonged insufflation may also lead to hypothermia (Mason et al. 2017) as the gas flow causes the temperature in the abdomen to decrease. Surgical emphysema is also a risk when a large volume of carbon dioxide is used for a long procedure. Careful monitoring and recording of the patient's vital signs, including oxygen saturation and expiratory gas levels, are therefore essential during laparoscopic surgery.

It is important to carefully evaluate patients with known or suspected pulmonary disease prior to undertaking a laparoscopic procedure, as pneumoperitoneum and hypercarbia may be poorly tolerated. It is important to determine the baseline $PaCO_2$ (partial pressure of carbon dioxide) in patients with known pulmonary disease so that the extent of hyperventilation can be better evaluated intraoperatively (see Chapter 12: Respiratory care, CPR and blood transfusion and Chapter 14: Observations).

Pre-procedural considerations

Equipment

Insufflation system

An insufflation system is a device that allows the flow of gas into the required space. This system enables the adjustment of gas flow and displaces the intraperitoneal pressure. The intraperitoneal pressure should be maintained between 10 and 15 mmHg; pressures above 25 mmHg increase the risk of gas absorption, air embolism and venous return impedance (resulting from compression of the inferior vena cava filter) and impaired ventilation secondary to pressure on the diaphragm.

Imaging system

The imaging system functions as the eye of the operating team; components include the laparoscope, camera, monitor and light source. The laparoscope allows light transmission into the peritoneal cavity to the surgical field and the transmission of images out of the peritoneal cavity to the camera and monitor. Most laparoscopes consist of a rigid rod lens imaging system, an eyepiece and a flexible fibreoptic light-conducting cable. The camera magnifies the endoscopic view by a factor of 15, allowing high-resolution imaging of anatomical details. The camera attaches to the eyepiece of the laparoscope and transmits digitized optical information from the scope via a cable to the video box. The digital image data are then reconstructed and displayed on the monitor.

Irrigation/aspiration unit

The irrigation/aspiration unit is used to keep the field clean and clear. The irrigation fluid can flow by gravity, but the use of a pressurized bag provides more active flow. The most common irrigations are sterile normal saline and sterile water.

Electrocautery unit

An electrocautery unit (monopolar or bipolar; see 'Diathermy machine' below) is used for tissue cutting and coagulation. It is controlled by the surgeon using either a foot pedal or a hand switch. A variety of tips are available.

Basic laparoscopic instruments come in various handle types, the most common being the ring handle, which may or may not have a ratchet. The type of trocar used during a procedure depends upon surgical preference and technique. The type of trocar used will determine the diameter of the instruments required during the procedure.

The most common types of laparoscopic instrument used in a general procedure are as follows:

- electrocautery L hook (monopolar)
- electrocautery spatula (monopolar)
- monopolar graspers
- bipolar graspers
- monopolar scissors
- Johan bowel graspers
- vascular clamps
- needle holders
- suture knot pusher
- trocars and cannulas (3, 5, 10, 12 and 15 mm).

Figures 16.19, 16.20 and 16.21 show the variety of equipment required for laparoscopic surgery.

Haemorrhage can occur during any surgical procedure and may be difficult to detect and control in laparoscopic procedures. Therefore, theatre staff must always have the equipment necessary to convert to an open procedure. Theatre staff must also ensure that equipment is used safely and according to the manufacturer's instructions.

The principle of checking instruments applies to both open and laparoscopic instruments. However, extra care should be taken to inspect the insulation part of each laparoscopic instrument to ensure there are no cracks or breakage.

Complications

Electrosurgery is the application of a high-frequency (radio frequency) alternating-polarity electrical current to biological tissue as a means to cut, coagulate, desiccate or fulgurate tissue. Electrosurgery complications during laparoscopic surgery are primarily related to the number of instruments and cannulas within the operative field (AfPP 2017). The principal hazards associated with these procedures are:

- direct coupling, which occurs when an active instrument touches an inactive one
- capacitive coupling, which occurs when current is conducted from one instrument to another where there is no direct contact
- insulation failure, where breaks in insulation materials are not noticed prior to use.

Robotic surgery

Robotic surgery has now been established for some time (the Da Vinci system was licensed in 2000). Robotic surgery is another type of minimally invasive surgery; it uses miniaturized surgical instruments and a series of 5 or 8 mm incisions.

Related theory

Robotic arms have for some time been used to replace surgical assistants holding retractors, and more advanced devices are now in use. Telemanipulation systems exist, by which the surgeon's

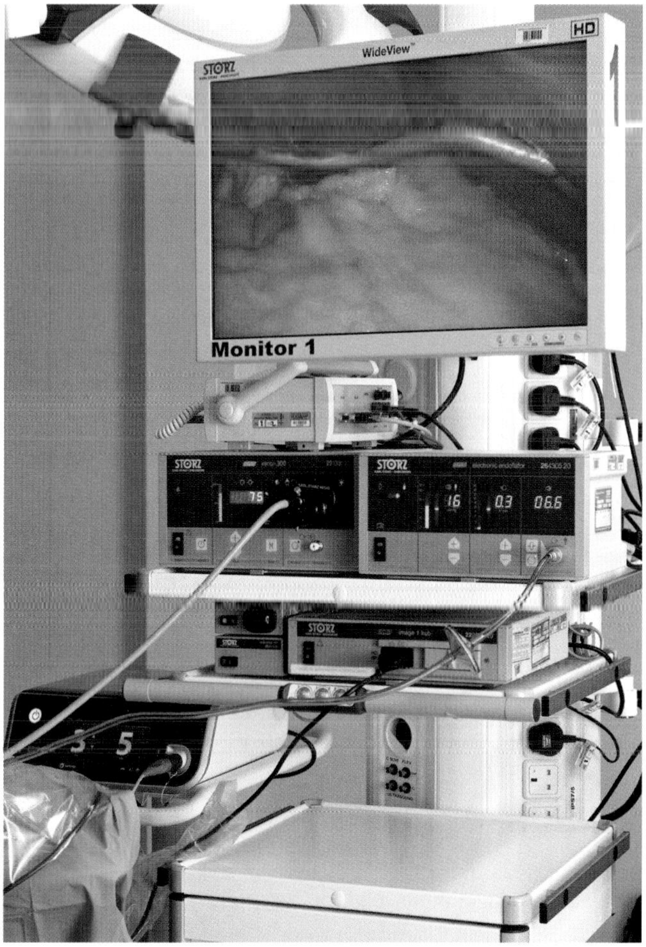

Figure 16.19 Laparoscopic stack system.

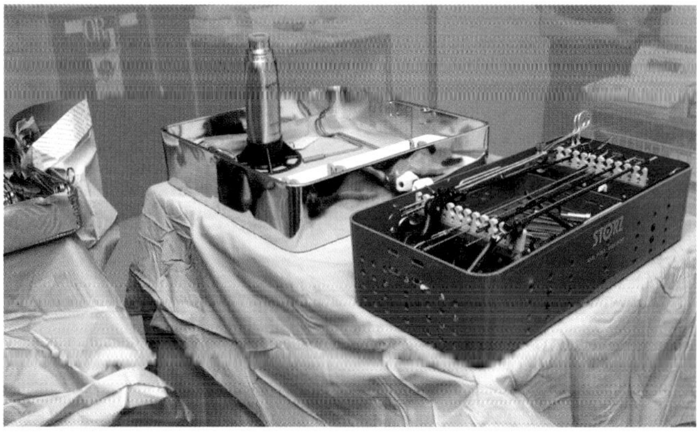

Figure 16.20 Laparoscopic telescope.

hand movements are accurately reproduced within the patient's body. The surgeon controls these instruments and the camera from a console located in the operating room. The surgeon controls all four arms of the robot simultaneously.

The Da Vinci Surgical System (Figure 16.22) is able to manipulate instruments through 360°, which is something that even the most talented and dextrous surgeon cannot do. Its endo-wrist allows better manipulation of the tissue retraction or dissection, in areas that are hard to reach compared to in laparoscopic or conventional open surgery. As with regular laparoscopic surgery, those patients having robotic surgery will have a shorter recovery

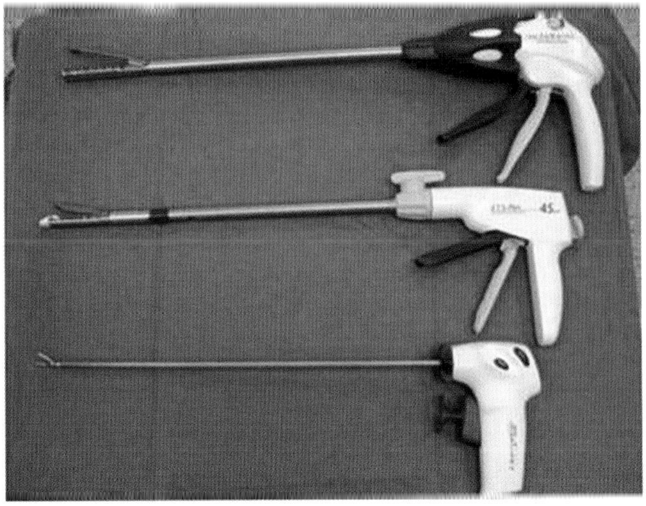

Figure 16.21 Laparoscopic stapling and energy instruments.

time in hospital compared to those having open surgery for the same procedure.

Clinical governance

Competencies

Staff involved with robotic surgery must have additional special training in order to set up and assist with robotic procedures (Figure 16.23). Robotic equipment requires a skilled practitioner who has the technical knowledge to operate the device competently. This is achieved through comprehensive technical training, which must be completed before a practitioner can assist in a robotic procedure (Figure 16.24)

Endoscopy

Definition

Endoscopy is the procedure of examining the interior of a hollow organ or body cavity using special equipment referred to as an 'endoscope'.

Related theory

An endoscope consists of a rigid or flexible tube that carries fibreoptic cables to transmit light. It relays images to a camera and provides channels for instruments to be inserted to carry out procedures. The images are usually displayed on a monitor (Figure 16.25) and there is provision to take still photographs as well as video so that the whole procedure can be recorded.

Endoscopy can be used both for diagnosis and for therapy, such as controlling bleeding in hollow organs. There are various types of endoscopy that can be performed in an operating room:

- *Flexible endoscopy* includes gastroscopy, colonoscopy, bronchoscopy and cystoscopy.
- *Rigid endoscopy* includes rigid cystoscopy, rigid hysteroscopy, colposcopy and rigid sigmoidoscopy.

The use of an endoscope is much less invasive than open or laparoscopic surgery because these instruments are inserted through the natural orifices leading to various organs. This also means that recovery is quicker and there are fewer complications (Kumar et al. 2016).

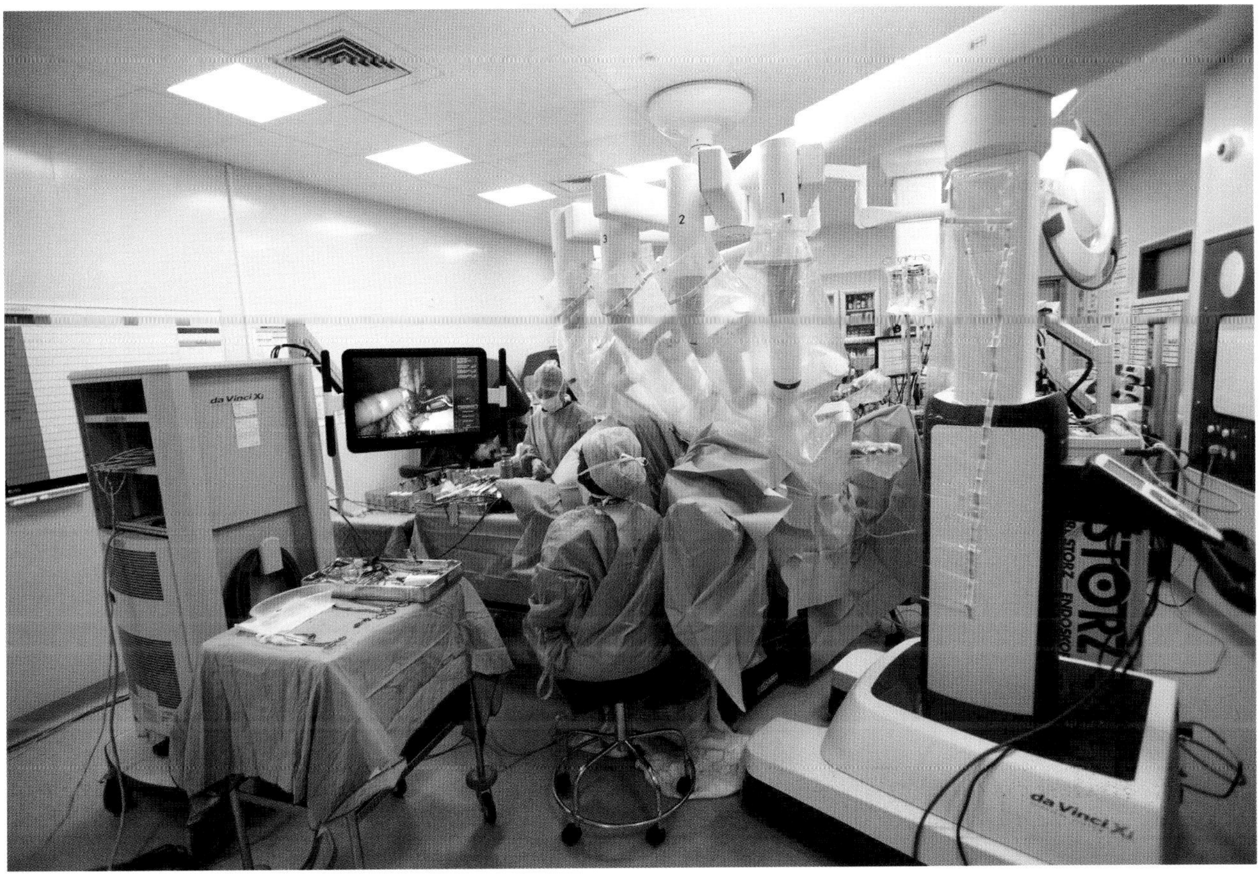

Figure 16.23 Da Vinci surgical robotic operating theatre.

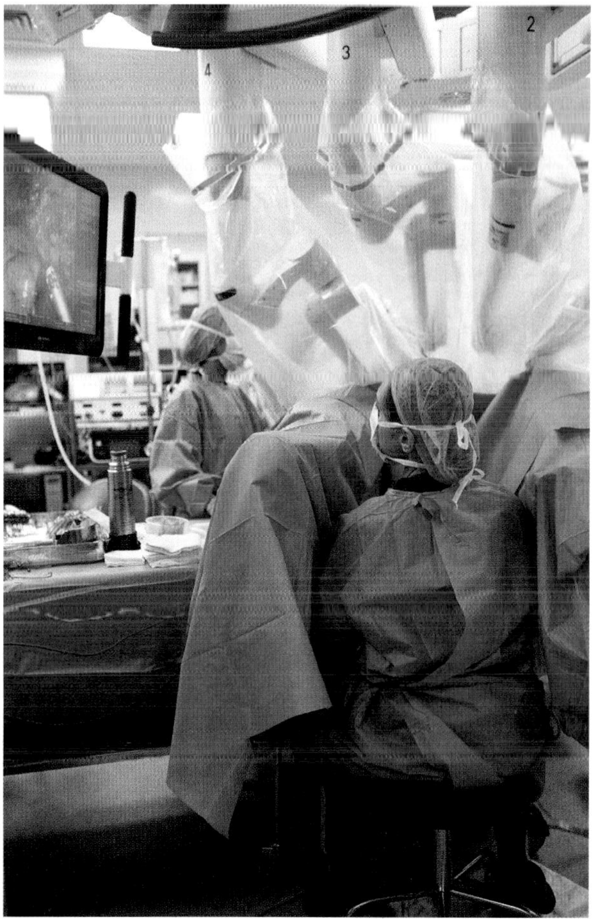

Figure 16.23 Specialist staff using Da Vinci robotic equipment.

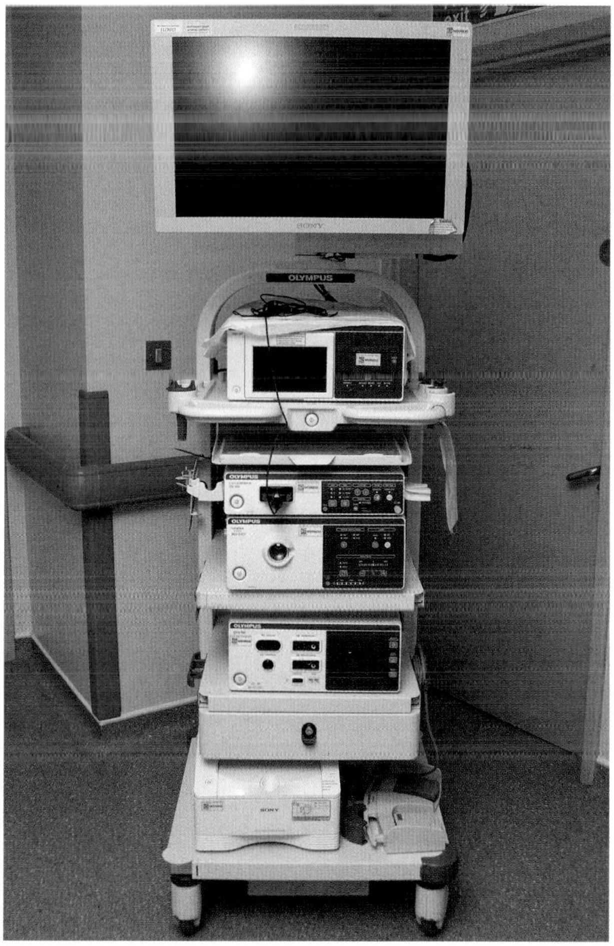

Figure 16.25 Example of a complete endoscopy stack system.

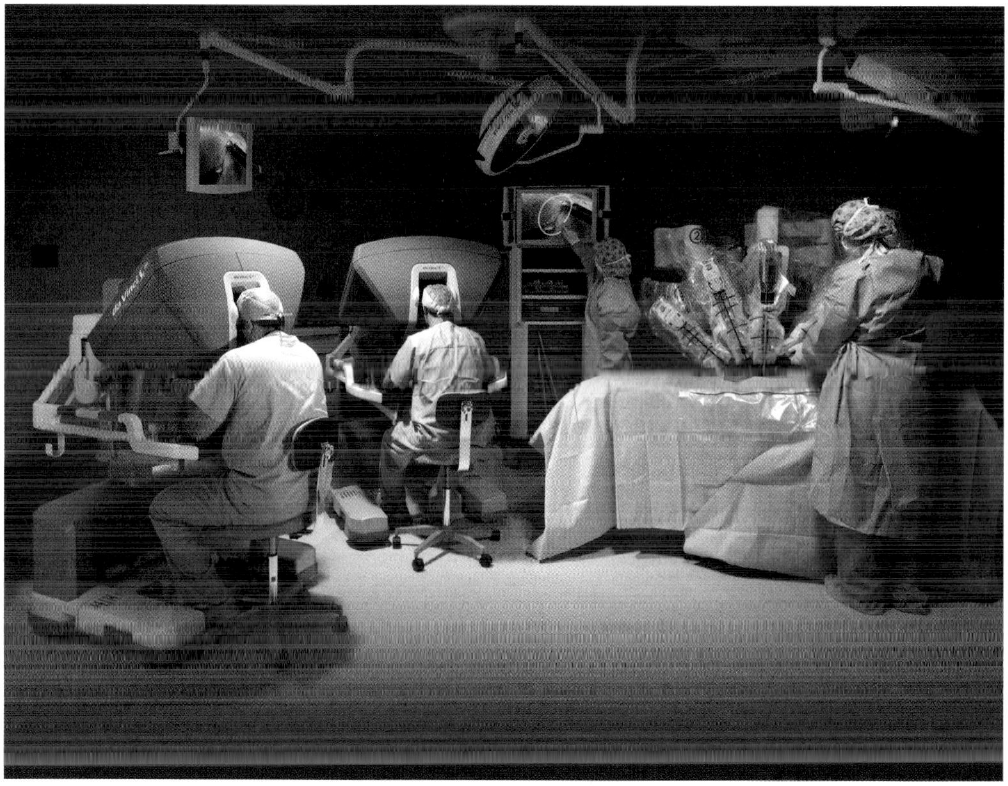

Figure 16.24 Robotic surgical team. *Source*: Reproduced with permission of Intuitive Medical, Inc. © 2014 Intuitive Surgical, Inc.

Endoscopy can be performed in a number of different areas of the body and also to examine the internal state of various organs, such as the oesophagus, stomach and large intestine. Advances in endoscopy have significantly altered the approach to the management of various surgical conditions (BSG 2018). The perioperative care of patients undergoing endoscopy follows the same principles of care as any other surgical intervention.

Head and neck

The nasal cavity, oral cavity, pharynx and larynx are all accessible to endoscope examination and procedures, and both rigid and flexible endoscopes can be used. The flexible scopes consist of two types. One is mainly used to provide vision. The other has working channels that allow specialized instruments to pass through to carry out treatment and also to allow irrigation and suction of any aspirates.

Oesophagus

The oesophagus can be examined using both rigid and flexible scopes, which are used to diagnose tumours, obtain biopsies, remove foreign bodies, and dilate or insert stents to overcome blockages.

Stomach

The stomach is usually examined using a flexible endoscope. The main aims are to provide diagnosis, obtain biopsies or aspiration of gastric fluids, remove foreign bodies and control bleeding from ulcers.

Large bowel

The large bowel consists of the rectum, colon and caecum. The rectum is usually examined using a rigid rectoscope or sigmoidoscope. The colon and caecum are examined using a flexible colonoscope.

Large bowel endoscopy is used for the diagnosis of inflammatory disease, polyps and tumours. Where necessary, endoscopic dilatation of the large bowel is carried out with the aid of a flexible endo-balloon (to dilate a narrowed channel, which could be due to obstruction from stricture) or the insertion of a stent (to open a passage that is blocked by a tumour).

Urinary system

Endoscopy of the urinary system usually involves examination and therapy relating to the urethra and bladder. Occasionally the ureter and kidney can also be examined using specialized flexible endoscopes. The urethra and bladder are generally examined using rigid endoscopes. However, a flexible endoscope (such as a cystoscope or ureteroscope) would be used for specific interventions. In patients with kidney stones, flexible endoscopes combined with rigid endoscopes are used to remove the stones using the percutaneous approach (percutaneous nephrolithotomy) (Ganpule et al. 2016).

Endoscopy plays a major role in the treatment of urinary tract problems such as enlarged prostate and bladder tumours. In patients with benign prostatic hyperplasia, transurethral resection has revolutionized the treatment, making possible removal of the obstruction without open surgery. It is one of the most commonly performed procedures in many surgical centres.

Gynaecology

In the field of gynaecology, rigid endoscopy is generally the preferred choice of procedure. It is used to carry out diagnosis or treatment of the female reproductive organs. Colposcopy in gynaecology refers to viewing the cervix, vagina and/or vulva with a specialized rigid instrument. The aim of colposcopy is to examine for any cancer in the organ (Khan et al. 2017).

Positioning the patient on the table

Evidence-based approaches

The position of the patient on the operating table must be such as to facilitate access to the operative site(s) by the surgeon and to the patient's airway for the anaesthetist. It will also be dependent upon the type of surgery being performed, the position of the monitoring equipment and any intravenous devices *in situ*. It should not compromise the patient's circulation or respiratory system or cause damage to the skin or nerves.

Pre-operative assessment will identify patients who may need extra precautions during positioning because of their weight, nutritional state, age, skin condition or pre-existing disease. The increased numbers of obese patients requiring surgery present specific challenges, and staff must be familiar with the weight limits of patient trolleys and operating tables. Many departments now have specialist bariatric equipment for the safe positioning of obese patients (Fencl et al. 2015).

Pre-existing conditions (such as backache or sciatica) can be exacerbated, particularly if the patient is in the lithotomy position (Figure 16.26), as the sciatic nerve can be compressed against the poles (AfPP 2017). Most post-operative palsies are caused by incorrect positioning of the patient on the operating table (Beckett 2010). Consideration by and co-operation of all theatre personnel can help to prevent many of the post-operative complications related to intraoperative positioning; this remains a team responsibility (AfPP 2017, Beckett 2010).

All movements of the limbs of the unconscious patient should take into account the anatomy and natural planes of movement of each limb to avoid stretching and pressure on the related nerve planes (AfPP 2017). Hyperabduction of the arm when placed on a board, for example, can stretch the brachial plexus, causing some post-operative loss of sensation and reduced movement of the forearm, wrist and fingers. To prevent this, the board should be angled at 45° and not 90°, with the patient's hands facing more towards the feet rather than the head (Figure 16.27). The ulnar and radial nerves may be affected by direct pressure as a result of insufficient padding on arm supports.

Compartment syndrome is a serious complication of the Lloyd-Davies position (Figure 16.28) and occurs when perfusion falls below tissue pressure in a closed anatomical space or compartment, such as a hand, forearm, buttock, leg, upper arm or foot. It develops through a combination of prolonged ischaemia and reperfusion of muscle within a tight osteofascial compartment (Schmidt 2016). Untreated, it can lead to necrosis, functional impairment, renal failure and death (Schinco and Hassid 2018).

If patients are placed in the Lloyd-Davies position and Trendelenburg tilt for longer than 4 hours, it is recommended that their legs should be removed from the support every 2 hours, or as close to 2 hours as possible, for a short period of time to prevent reperfusion injury (Raza et al. 2004). However, approaches vary according to local hospital policy, and clinical decisions are based on the patient's co-morbidity. Antiembolic stockings and intermittent compression devices used in the Lloyd-Davies position must be carefully inspected during patient positioning. Otherwise, if the

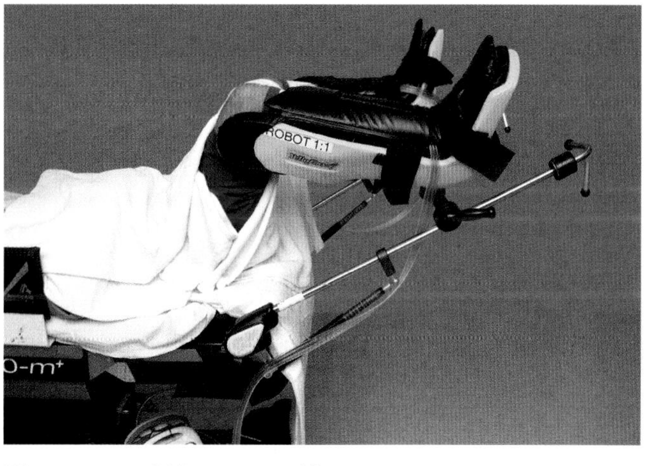

Figure 16.26 Lithotomy position.

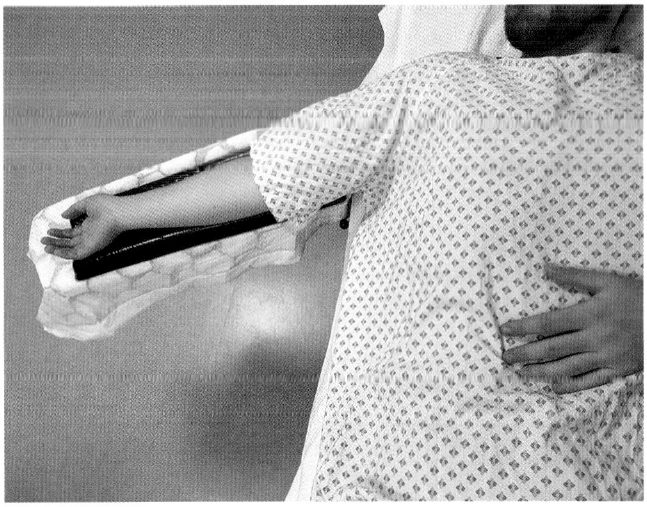

Figure 16.27 Armboard.

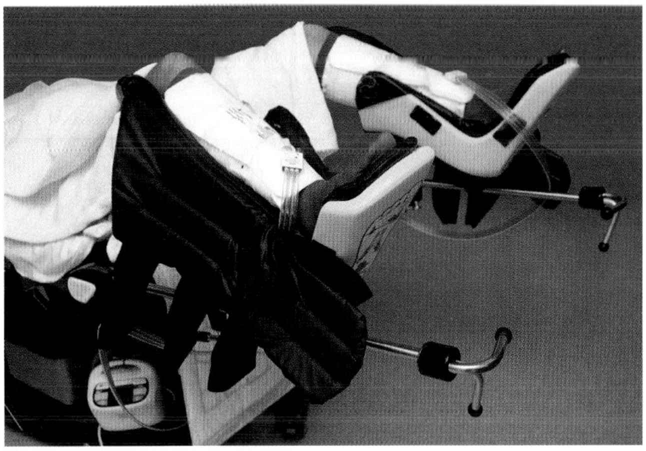

Figure 16.28 Lloyd-Davies position.

position is not implemented correctly, these devices may contribute to compartment syndrome (Malik et al. 2009). The use of these devices will depend on the clinical judgement of the surgeon and anaesthetist, the physical status of the patient, and the hospital protocol and recommendations.

Infection prevention

Evidence-based approaches

It is imperative that during surgical procedures, infection control and prevention are maintained at all times. The area immediately around the patient and the instrument trolley is known as the 'sterile field'. Only those staff who have put on sterile gloves and gowns after washing and decontaminating their hands and forearms ('scrubbing up') can enter the sterile field. Pre-surgical hand washing or scrubbing up (Figure 16.29) is an essential step in the prevention of infection during surgery (see Chapter 4: Infection prevention and control).

The aims of surgical hand antisepsis are to remove dirt and transient micro-organisms and to reduce (to a minimum) resident micro-organisms on the hands, nails and forearms (AORN 2013). For minor surgical procedures, current research supports 1 minute hand washing with a non-antiseptic soap followed by hand rubbing with liquid aqueous alcoholic solution prior to the first procedure of the day and before any subsequent procedures (Liu and Mehigan 2016, Santacatalina Mas et al. 2016, Tanner et al. 2016). This has been shown to be as effective as traditional hand scrubbing with an antiseptic soap containing 4% chlorhexidine gluconate or 7.5% povidone-iodine in preventing surgical site infection (Santacatalina Mas et al. 2016, Tanner et al. 2016). However, for more major cases it is usual to perform surgical hand antisepsis using a solution containing either chlorhexidine or iodine. The duration of the wash is usually 2–5 minutes (AfPP 2017). The steps of hand scrubbing and hand rubbing are demonstrated in Figure 16.30.

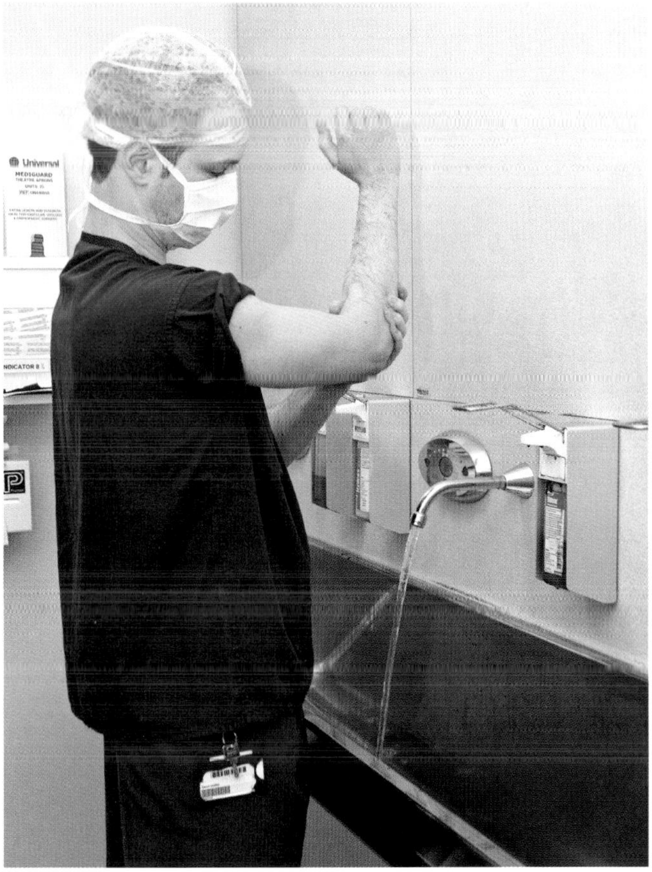

Figure 16.29 Surgical scrub.

Surgeons and staff who are working within the sterile field wear sterile surgical gowns. These gowns are designed to function as a sterile barrier between the wearer's body and the surgical field, and as protection for the wearer against exposure to blood, body fluids and tissue. The gown should be resistant to microbial and liquid penetration and minimize the release of particles (AfPP 2017).

Surgical gloves have a dual role, acting as a barrier to personal protection from the patient's blood and other exudates and preventing bacterial transfer from the surgeon's hands to the operating site. Surgical gloves must conform to international standards and different types are used for different procedures. It is essential that the glove is the correct size, not only for reasons of comfort but also for dexterity and sensitivity. It is common practice for surgeons and theatre staff to double glove. Evidence suggests that double gloving significantly reduces the number of perforations to the innermost glove, thus possibly reducing infection rates during surgical procedures (Tanner and Parkinson 2006).

Prior to skin incision, the skin of the patient is cleaned with an antiseptic solution. The purpose of this is to reduce the number of both transient and resident skin bacteria. Most surgical wound infections are caused by bacteria living on the patient's own skin. Several types of skin preparation are used; common choices include povidone-iodine and chlorhexidine gluconate. These agents are included in either aqueous or alcoholic solutions. Which is used depends on both the condition of the patient's skin and whether they are allergic to either of the agents (AfPP 2017).

1

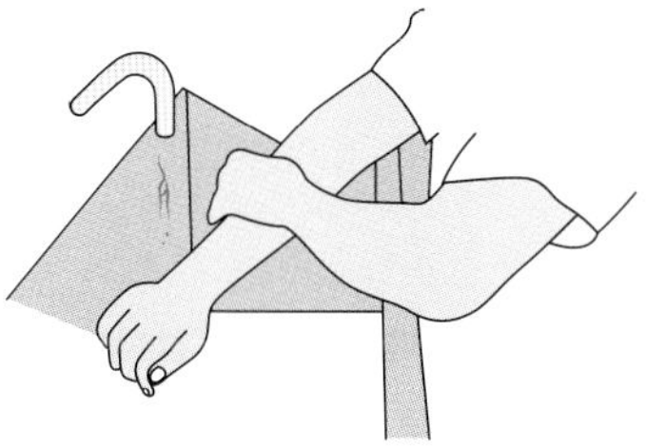

Wet hands and forearms.*

2

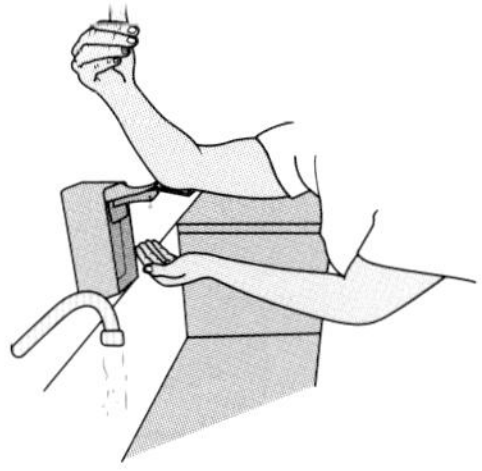

Put antimicrobial liquid soap onto the palm of each hand/arm using the elbow of your other arm to operate the dispenser.

3

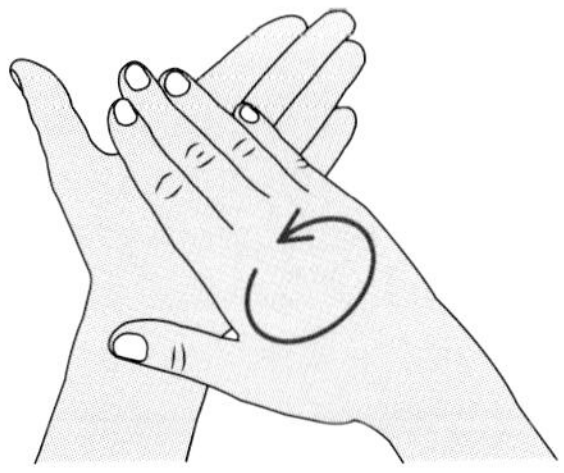

Rub hands palm to palm. Steps 3–8 should take a minimum of 2 minutes.

4

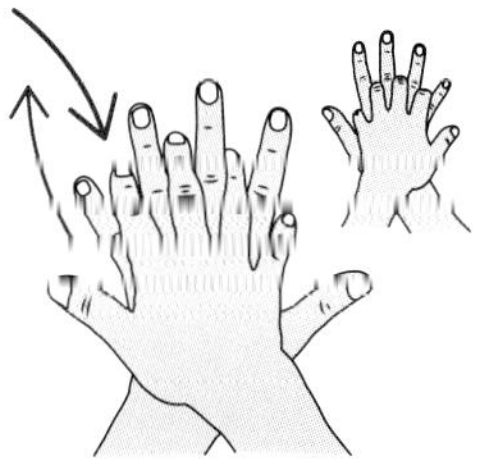

Right palm over the back of the other hand with interlaced fingers and vice versa.

5

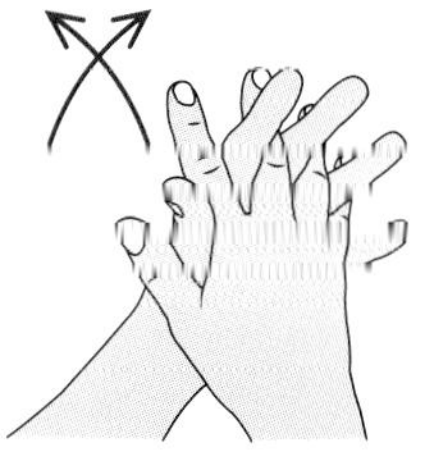

Palm to palm with fingers interlaced.

6

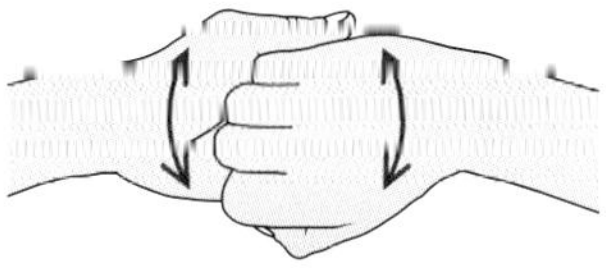

Backs of fingers to opposing palms with fingers interlocked.

7

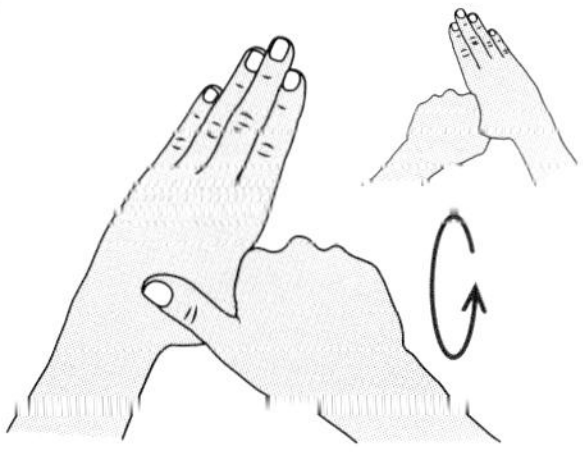

Rotational rubbing of left thumb clasped in right palm and vice versa.

8

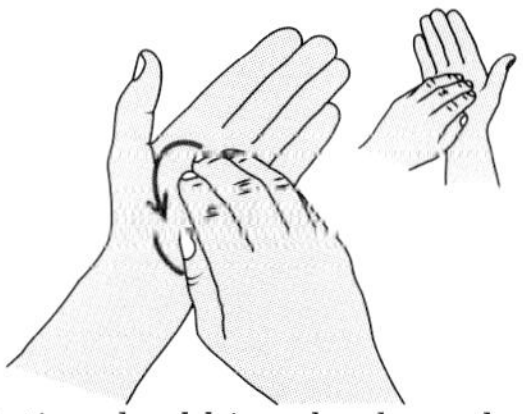

Rotational rubbing, backwards and forwards with clasped fingers of right hand in left palm and vice versa. Rinse hands between steps 8–9, passing them through the water in one direction only.

9

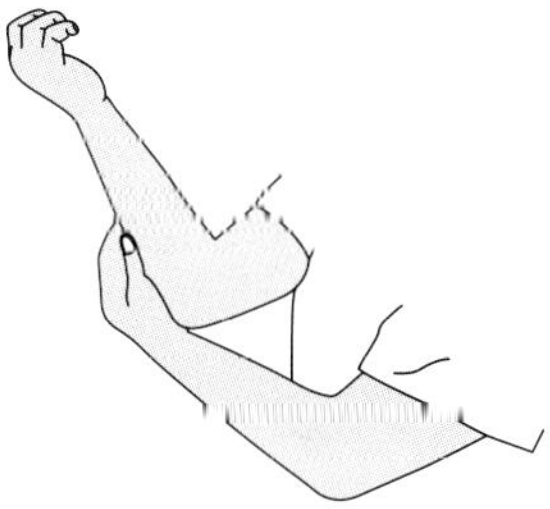

Put antimicrobial liquid soap onto the palm of your left hand using the elbow of your other arm to operate the dispenser. Use this to scrub the right arm for 1 minute using a rotational method keeping the hand higher than the arm at all times.

10

Repeat the process for the other hand and arm keeping hands above elbows at all times.

If the hand touches anything at any time, the scrub must be lengthened by 1 minute for the area that has been contaminated.

11

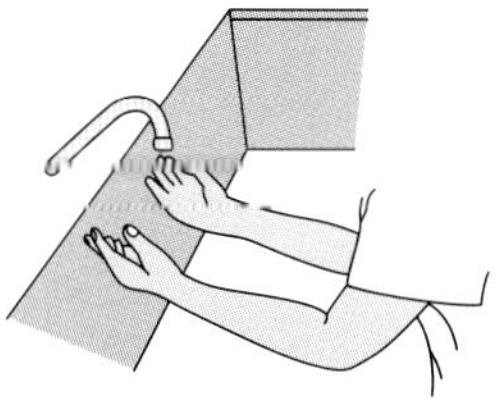

Rinse hands and arms by passing them through the water in one direction only, from fingertips to elbow. Do not move the arm back and forth through the water.

12

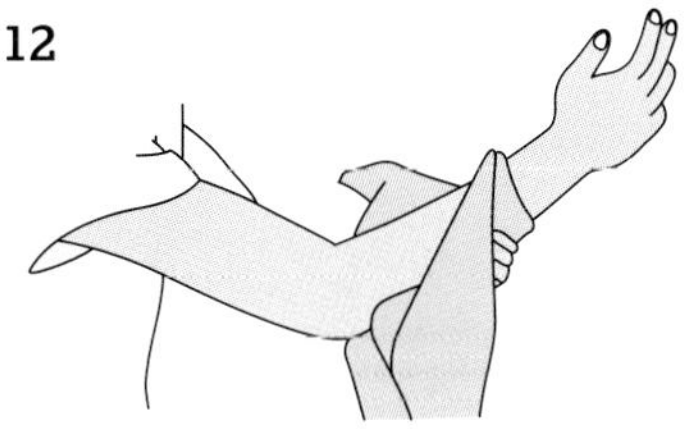

Hold hands above the elbow. Use one sterile, disposable tower per hand and arm. Blot the skin of the hand, then use a corkscrew movement to dry from the hand to the elbow.
The towel must not be returned to the hand once the arm has been dried and must be discarded immediately.

*Nails should be cleaned using a soft, single-use disposable nail brush or nail pick before the first scrub of the day or if visibly dirty. Any skin complaints should be referred to local occupational health or GP.

NHS SCOTLAND

Acknowledgement: With thanks to staff at the Golden Jubilee Foundation for their assistance producing this appendix.

Part of the National Infection Prevention and Control Manual (NIPCM), available at: http://www.nipcm.hps.scot.nhs.uk/. Produced by: Health Protection Scotland, July 2018.

(a)

Figure 16.30 (a) Surgical scrubbing technique. (b) Surgical rubbing technique. *Source*: Adapted from Health Protection Scotland (2018) with permission of the NHS.

Best Practice: Appendix 4 - Surgical rubbing: surgical hand preparation technique using alcohol based hand rub (ABHR) - step by step images

- The hand rubbing technique for surgical hand preparation must be performed on clean, dry hands.
- On arrival in the operating theatre and after having donned theatre clothing (cap/hat/bonnet and mask), hands must be washed with soap and water.
- After the operation when removing gloves, hands must be rubbed with an alcohol based formulation or washed with soap and water if any residual talc or biological fluids are present (e.g. the glove is punctured).
- Surgical procedures may be carried out one after the other without the need for hand washing, provided that the hand rubbing technique for surgical hand preparation is followed (images 1 to 15).

1
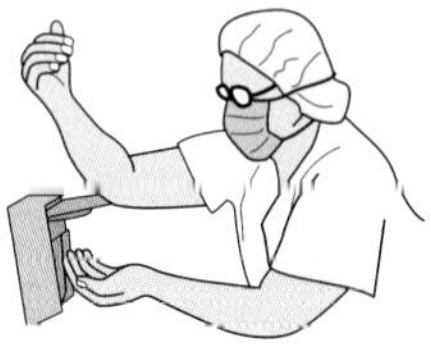
Put approximately 5 ml (3 doses) of alcohol-based handrub in the palm of your left hand, using the elbow of your other arm to operate the dispenser.

2
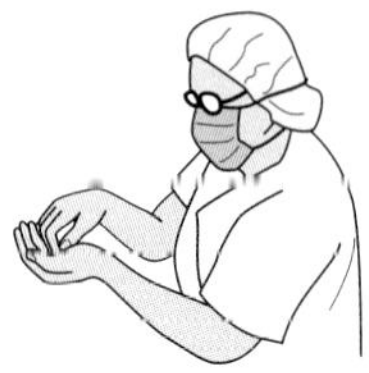
Dip the fingertips of your right hand in the handrub to decontaminate under the nails (5 seconds).

3
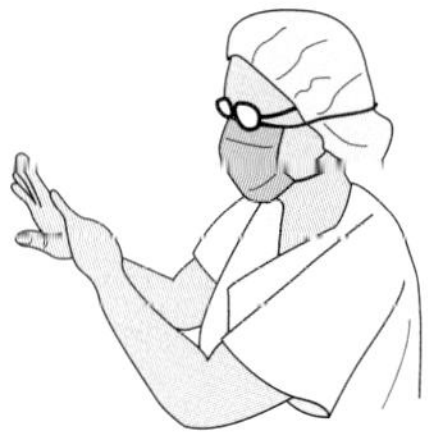 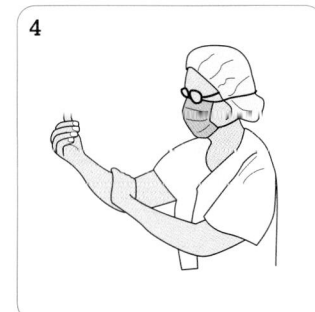
Steps 3–4. Smear the handrub on the right forearm up to the elbow.

4

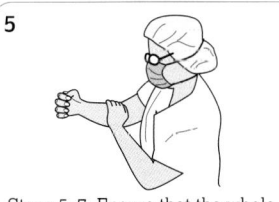

5

Steps 5–7. Ensure that the whole skin area is covered by using circular movements around the forearm until the handrub has fully evaporated (10–15 seconds).

6

7
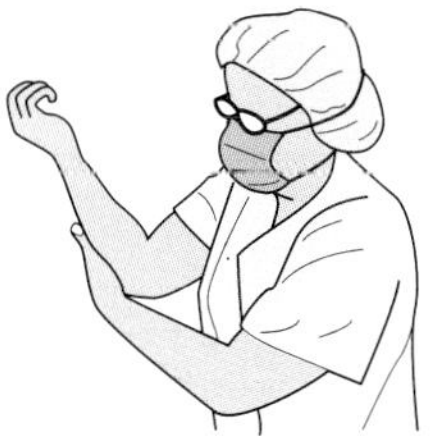

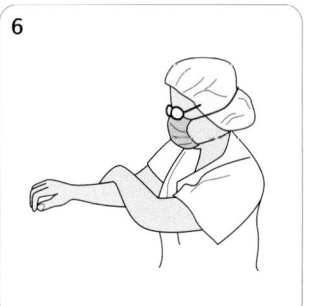

8
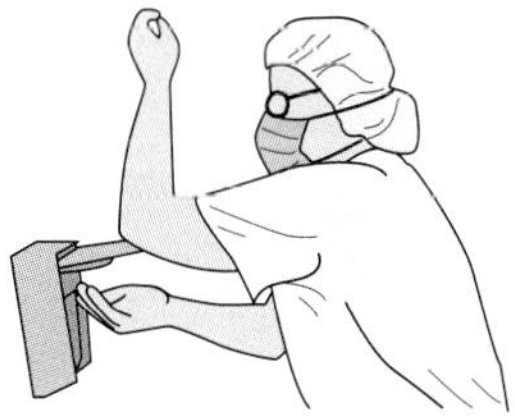
Repeat steps 1 to 7 for the left hand nails and arm.

9
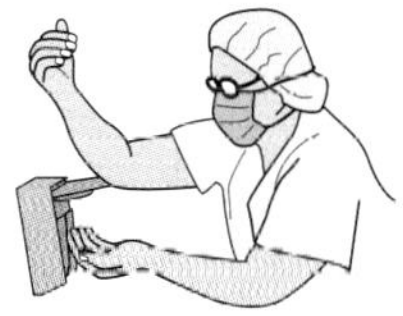
Put approximately 5 ml (3 doses) of alcohol-based handrub in the palm of your left hand, using the elbow of your other arm to operate the distributor. Rub both hands at the same time up to the wrists, and ensure that all the steps presented in steps 9–14 are followed.

10
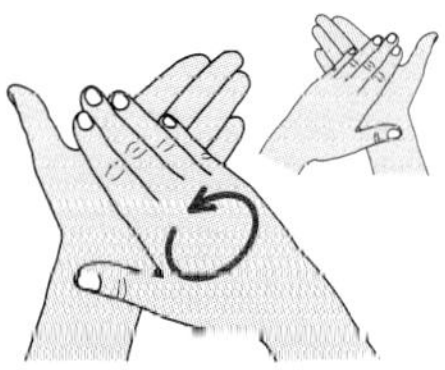
Cover the whole surface of the hands up to the wrist with alcohol-based handrub, rubbing palm against palm with a rotating movement.

11
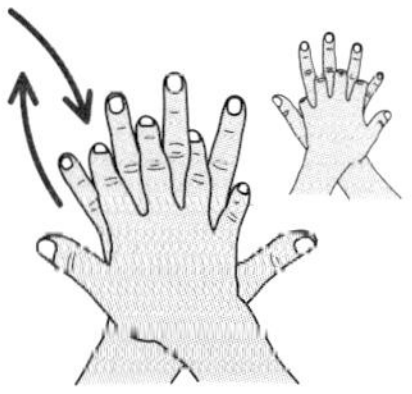
Rub the back of the hands up to the wrist with alcohol-based handrub, rubbing palm against palm with a rotating movement.

12
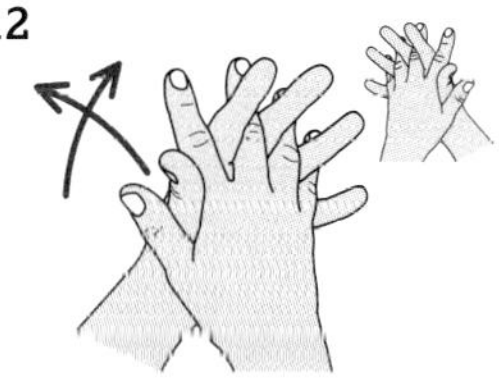
Rub the back of the left hand, including the wrist, moving the right palm back and forth and vice-versa.

13
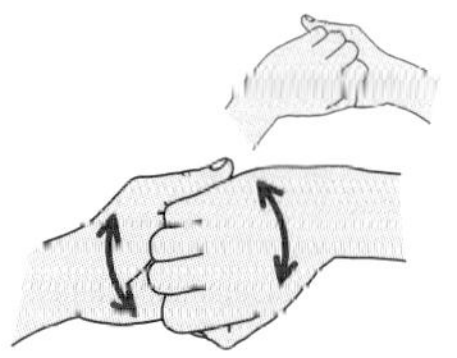
Rub palm against palm back and forth with fingers interlinked.

14
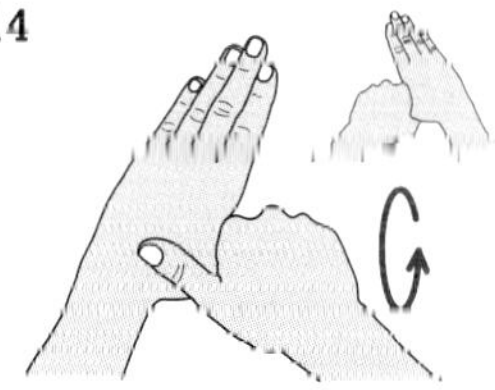
Rub the thumb of the left hand by rotating it in the clasped palm of the right hand and vice versa.

15
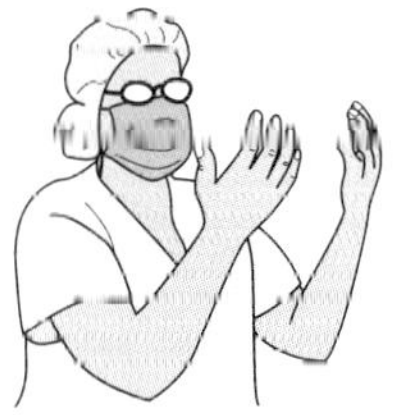
When the hands are dry, sterile surgical clothing and gloves can be donned.

Adapted from the World Health Organization

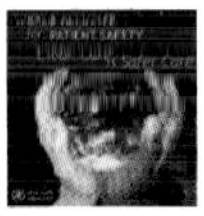

Germs. Wash your hands of them.

NHS SCOTLAND

Part of the National Infection Prevention and Control Manual (NIPCM), available at: http://www.nipcm.hps.scot.nhs.uk/.
Produced by Health Protection Scotland, July 2016.

(b)

Figure 16.30 *Continued*

Clinical governance

When a patient is transferred between the trolley or bed and the operating table, appropriate personnel should be present to ensure patient and staff safety (AfPP 2017). It is recommended that an approved sliding device is used to transfer patients from trolley to operating table, in compliance with national legislation on manual handling and local hospital policy and guidelines.

Safe manual handling and the safety of the patient depend on the participation of the correct number of staff in the specified handling manoeuvre. There should be a minimum of four staff: one at either end of the patient to support the head and the feet, and one on either side (Figure 16.31). Additional staff and/or specialist transfer devices may be required if the patient weighs over 90 kg.

Once the patient is in position, thromboprophylaxis devices can be applied (antiembolic stockings and/or pneumatic intermittent compression machine), as well as any pressure-relieving devices (Figure 16.32).

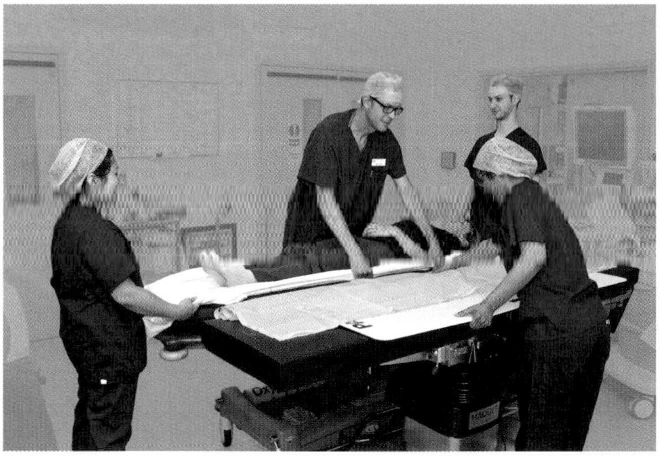
(a)

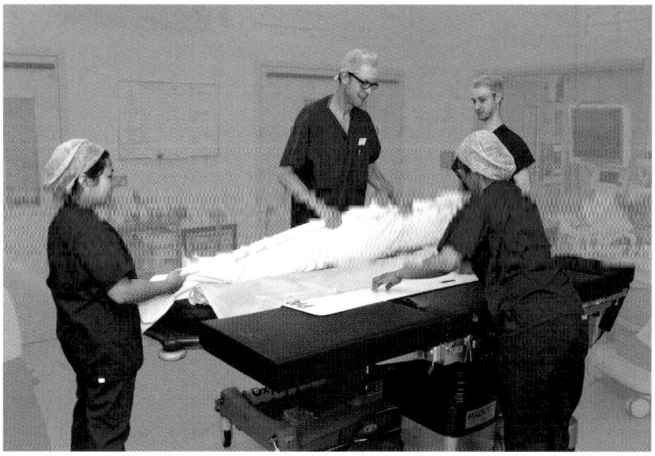
(b)

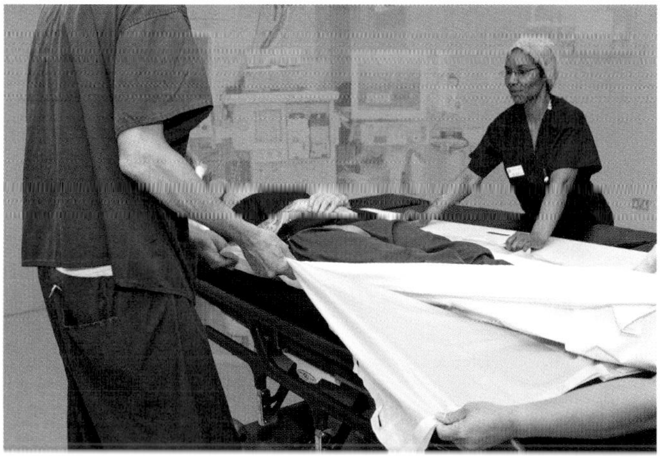
(c)

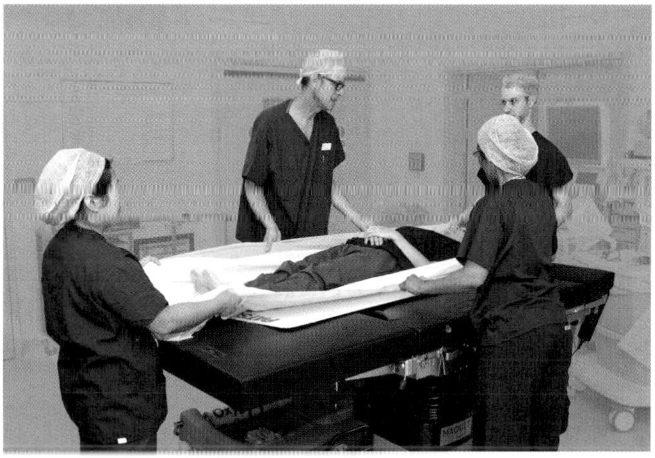
(d)

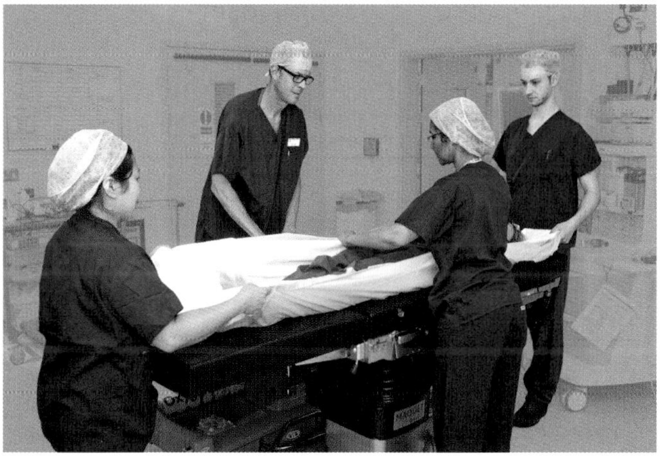
(e)

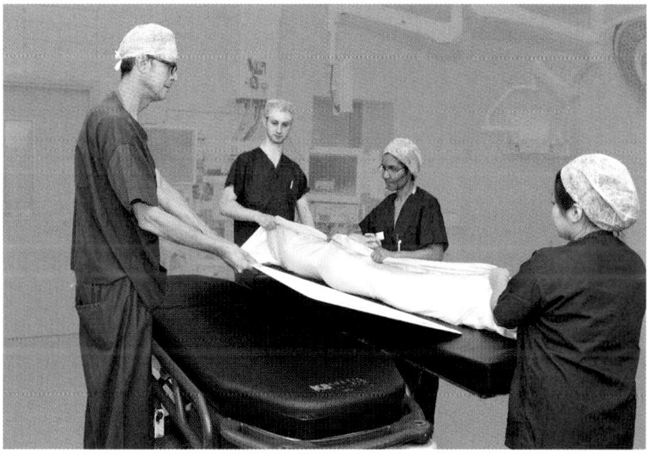
(f)

Figure 16.31 Lateral transfer, carried out in order from (a) to (f)

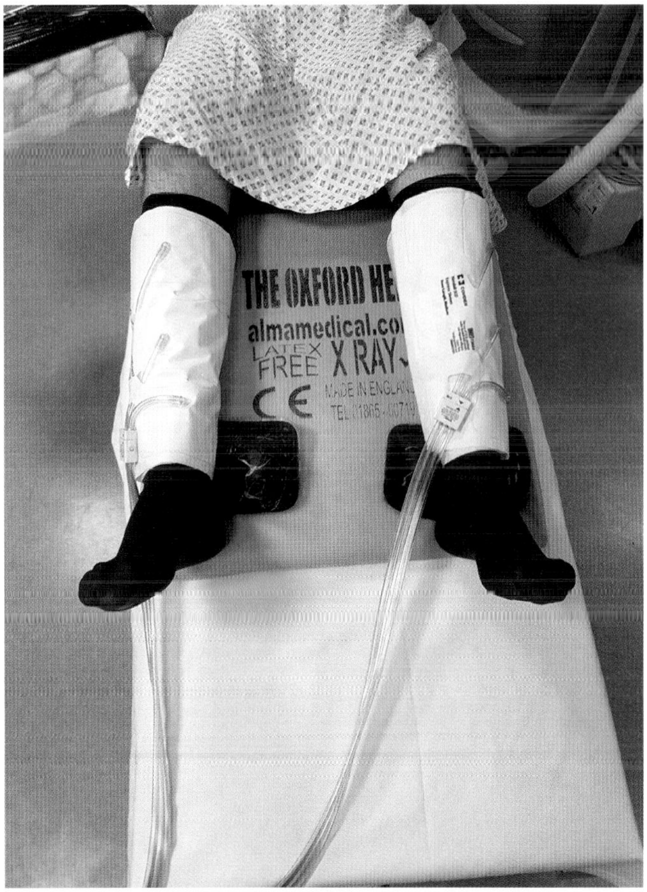

Figure 16.32 Thromboprophylaxis and pressure area prevention devices.

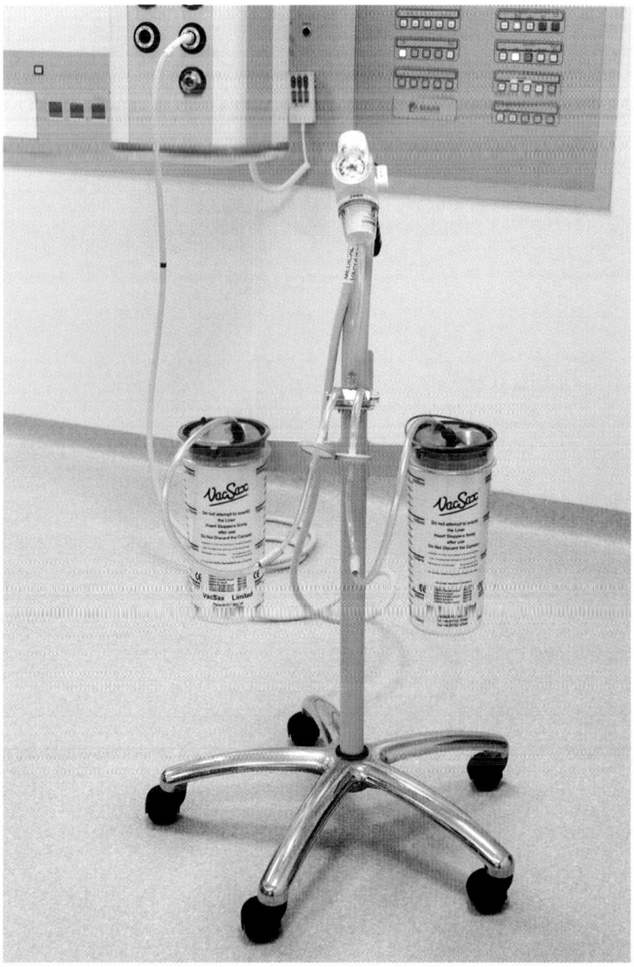

Figure 16.33 High vacuum suction unit.

Pre-procedural considerations

Equipment

In the operating room, the staff should ensure that all equipment is ready and checked before the first patient is sent for.

Anaesthetic machine and patient monitoring

The anaesthetic machine and monitoring equipment allow the anaesthetist to administer the correct proportions of oxygen, air and inhalational agents. Cardiovascular and respiratory monitoring is essential throughout the anaesthetic and surgery, and includes ECG, blood pressure, respiratory rate and volume, oxygen saturation and expired carbon dioxide monitoring. To ensure adequate depth of anaesthesia, either the expired anaesthetic agent or brain electrical activity are monitored by the anaesthetist (depending on the anaesthetic technique).

Suction unit

A suction unit (Figure 16.33) is attached to the anaesthetic machine and is used in the event of obstruction (to clear secretions) or to remove regurgitated stomach contents.

Vaporizer

A vaporizer is also attached to the anaesthetic machine and is used to administer inhalational anaesthetic agents.

Scavenging system

A scavenging system removes the inhalational agents that the patient exhales as contamination of the atmosphere with these agents can be harmful to staff (Braz et al. 2017).

Operating table

As part of the equipment check, the operating table (Figure 16.34) is assessed to ensure it is fully operational and performs all the required functions to enable correct positioning of the patient. The height of the operating table is adjusted in relation to the height of the surgeon and team to prevent any unnecessary strain on the back and neck. Modern operating tables are powered by a battery that needs to be charged when not in use. Therefore, it is essential that the table is plugged into the mains power supply at the end of the operating list.

Diathermy machine

Diathermy (or electrosurgery) is used routinely during surgery to cut tissue and control haemorrhage by sealing bleeding vessels (Figure 16.35). It uses heat from electricity, which is achieved by passing a normal electrical current through the diathermy machine, which converts the electricity into a high-frequency alternating current. There are two types of diathermy:

- *Monopolar*: this works by producing current from an active electrode (such as the diathermy forceps), which is then returned back to the machine through the patient's body via another electrode (such as a patient diathermy plate or pad), which creates a complete circuit. It is the most commonly used type of electrosurgery as a wide range of effects can be achieved (e.g. cutting, coagulating and fulgurating). The current is delivered by the surgeon operating a hand switch or foot pedal.
- *Bipolar*: this does not require a patient diathermy plate or pad to complete the circuit. The current produced by the machine passes down one side of the forceps prong, through the tissue and back to the machine via the other side of the forceps prong (rather than

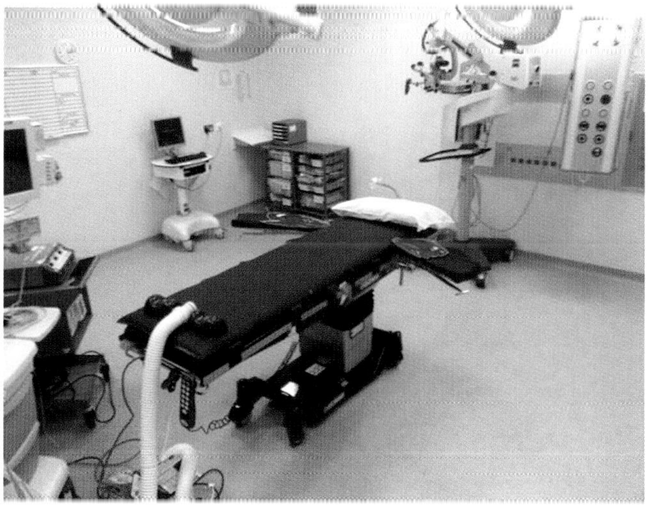

Figure 16.34 Operating table.

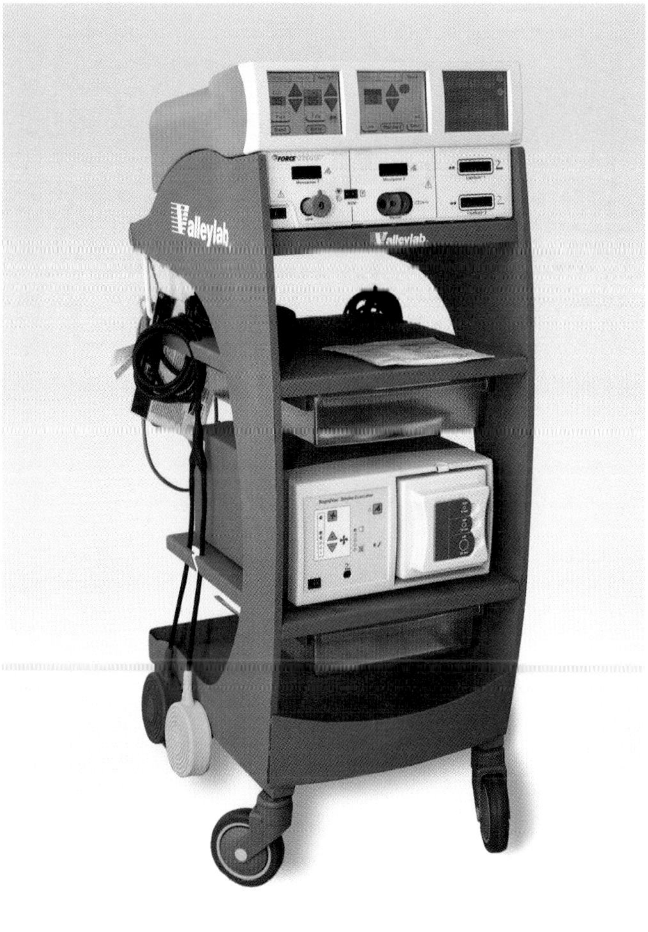

Figure 16.35 Diathermy equipment.

through the patient's body and returning to the machine via the plate or pad). Again, the surgeon operates the device using a hand switch or foot pedal. Bipolar diathermy is often used in laparoscopic surgery and in hand and foot surgery (AfPP 2017).

Diathermy is potentially hazardous to patients if used incorrectly. The main risk when using diathermy is of thermoelectrical burns. The most common causes are incorrect application of the patient plate or pad and a break in the connecting lead (Eder 2017); burns can also be caused if the patient comes into contact with metal, which allows the current to earth through the patient's skin. The machine automatically switches off or alarms if the neutral electrodes come loose from the patient. However, if the patient is in contact with metal, this is harder to identify. Care must therefore be taken during positioning that no part of the patient's body is in contact with metal and that the return electrode (plate or pad), if used, is placed close to the operative site (AfPP 2017).

It is important that theatre staff know how to test and use diathermy equipment to prevent patient injury (Eder 2017). This involves checking that the cables and plugs are not damaged and that the indicator lights are all in working order. It is also important that the theatre staff check the equipment before every operating list to ensure that the alarms are operational (these should alert the surgical team if the circuit is broken, e.g. if the plate or pad detaches from the patient) (AfPP 2017). If the patient's position is changed during the operation, the plate or pad should be rechecked to ensure that it is still in contact and that the connecting clamp or lead is not causing pressure on the skin. Use of diathermy and the position of the plate or pad should be documented on the nursing care plan, and the patient's skin condition (plate or pad site, pressure areas, and other areas where exposure to metal could have occurred) must be checked post operatively.

Other causes of burns include alcohol-based skin preparations and other liquids pooling around the plate or pad site. When using alcohol-based skin preparations, the skin should be dried or the alcohol allowed to evaporate before diathermy is used to avoid the risk of ignition (AfPP 2017, ECRI Institute 2012). The use of diathermy during surgical procedures results in a smoke by-product from the coagulation or cutting of the tissue. This smoke plume can be harmful to the perioperative team as it may contain:

- toxic gases and vapours such as benzene, hydrogen cyanide or formaldehyde
- bio-aerosols
- dead and live cellular material, including blood fragments
- viruses (Okoshi et al. 2015).

To reduce the risk to staff and patients, an efficient filtered evacuation system should be used, such as a smoke evacuation machine; piped hospital suction must not be used (Dalal and McLennan 2017). The patient suction unit must also be checked to ensure that it is patent and the suction power is adequate to withdraw large amounts of body fluids from the operating site.

Operating lights

The lights must be bright enough to ensure that the procedure is fully illuminated but not generate excess heat, which would dry the exposed tissue (Figure 16.36). The lights must be checked prior to every operation to ensure they are bright and in working order.

Equipment for laparoscopic procedures

The equipment used for laparoscopic surgery is very specialized and includes:

- camera system (consisting of light source, camera, insufflator, DVD recorder and two monitors)
- laparoscope
- other laparoscopy-specific instruments (scissors, biopsy forceps, grabbers, dissectors, ports, retrieval pouches, insufflating tube and light lead).

The Association of periOperative Registered Nurses recommends that all equipment is regularly and competently maintained and a maintenance record kept in a log (Cowperthwaite and Holm 2015). Policies should be developed for the checking procedure, and all staff must be thoroughly instructed in the operation of laparoscopic equipment. Staff must be able to properly check the equipment prior to use to ensure the clarity of colour and picture and in order to set the pressure and flow rate of the insufflator for inflating the abdomen with carbon dioxide. The surgeon will determine the level to achieve and this will be activated at the beginning of the procedure.

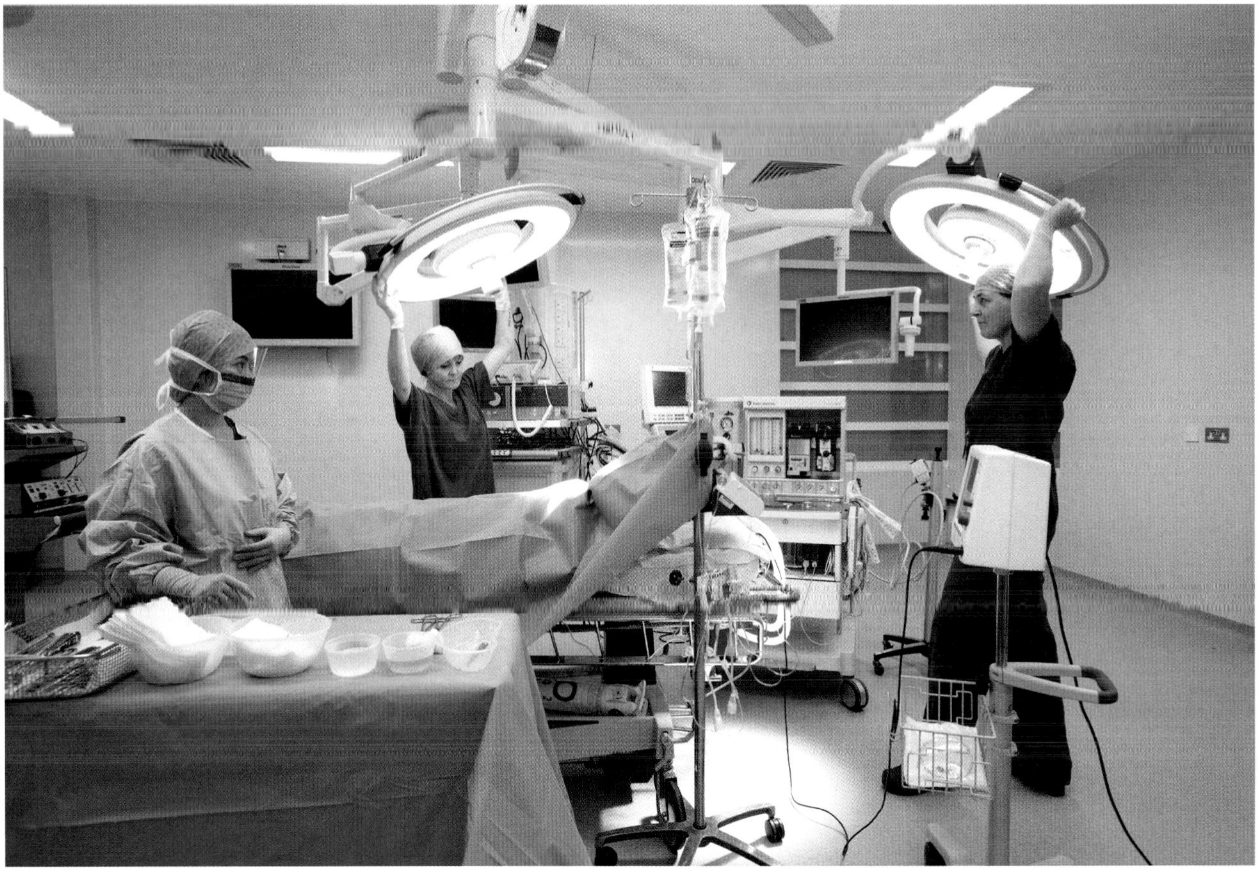

Figure 16.36 Operating lights.

Procedure guideline 16.4 Operating theatre procedure: maintaining the safety of a patient during surgery

- Personal protective equipment
- All equipment relevant to the patient's specific procedure

Action	Rationale
Pre-procedure	
1 Introduce yourself to the patient, explain and discuss the procedure with them, and gain their consent to proceed if possible.	To ensure that the patient feels at ease, understands the procedure and gives their valid consent as far as possible (NMC 2018, **C**).
2 Prior to transferring the patient from the trolley to the operating table, check with the anaesthetist that the patient's airway is protected, patent and safe.	To prevent complications with airway or breathing. **E**
3 There must be adequate staff (a minimum of four is recommended) to transfer the patient onto the operating table. The team must ensure that the brakes on the trolley and operating table have been applied. Ensure the patient's head and limbs are supported when transferring them to the operating table. When transferring anaesthetized patients, the anaesthetist takes charge of the patient's head and airway and co-ordinates the transfer.	To prevent patient injury during the transfer between trolley and operating table (AORN 2017, **C**).
4 When positioning the patient, the theatre staff must ensure that the limbs are supported and secure on the table and that bony prominences are padded or cushioned.	If the patient is unconscious and unable to maintain a safe environment, support is necessary to prevent injury. Nerve damage due to compression or stretching must be prevented (Welch 2019, **E**)
5 The patient's position will be dictated by the nature of the surgery and can include lateral (**Action figure 5a**) and prone (**Action figure 5b**) positions. The theatre staff must verify the position with the surgeon and anaesthetist, and prepare any required positioning equipment and devices.	The patient is at risk from skin and nerve damage during surgery, especially if it is prolonged. Measures must be taken to preserve the integrity of the skin (e.g. use of pressure-relieving mattress or pads). Positioning must take into account the natural movement of the back, neck and limbs to safeguard against injury (Rothrock 2018, **E**).

Procedure

6 Cover the patient with a gown or blanket. The patient must remain covered until immediately before surgery.	To maintain the patient's dignity. To help prevent a reduction in body temperature or inadvertent hypothermia. **E**
7 Use a warming mattress and/or blanket on the operating table (**Action figure 7**). Both intravenous and irrigation fluids should be warmed prior to administration. The theatre staff must ensure that patient- and fluid-warming devices are available for every operating list.	To help maintain the patient's body temperature, prevent inadvertent perioperative hypothermia and reduce post-operative complications due to hypothermia (NICE 2016a, **C**; Rothrock 2018, **E**).
8 Ensure the diathermy patient plate is attached securely in accordance with the manufacturer's instructions and sited correctly as close to the operative site as possible (**Action figure 8**).	To ensure that no injury is sustained from the use of diathermy during surgery. **E**
9 Before, during and at the end of surgery, theatre staff must perform thorough counts of surgical instruments, swabs, sutures, needles and blades (**Action figure 9**). If an item is not accounted for prior to closure of the surgical wound, the surgeon must be notified.	To ensure that all items used in surgery are accounted for at the end of the operation in order to guard against items being retained inside the patient's body following surgery (AfPP 2017, **C**).
10 The scrub nurse or operating department practitioner (ODP) is responsible for ensuring the wound(s) are covered with an appropriate surgical dressing (**Action figure 10**).	The dressing facilitates healing by preventing wounds from drying out and also acting as a barrier against external contaminants, which can cause wound infection (Wicker and O'Neill 2010, **E**). To reduce the risk of injury/infection to the patient and contamination of staff (Loveday et al. 2014, **C**).

Post-procedure

11 After the surgery has concluded, the theatre staff must follow hospital policy regarding the disposal of sharps and clinical waste that are no longer required.	To protect staff from injury and contamination as per all health and safety policies. **E**
12 Any swab that is intended to be packed inside the patient (e.g. vaginal pack or abdomen pack) must be recorded clearly in the patient's care plan. The swab used as packing must be X-ray detectable (e.g. Raytec) and clearly identified in the patient's notes, as per local policy. Orange 'Raytec stickers' are commonly applied to patients' notes.	X-ray detectable material allows easy location of the swab for retrieval. To alert all teams caring for a patient that they have packing or a foreign body *in situ*. **E**
13 The scrub nurse or ODP is responsible for ensuring that any tissue samples, organs or swabs taken from the patient during the surgery are correctly labelled with the patient's details and the exact nature of the specimen before being sent for histological or microbiological examination as specified by the operating surgeon.	Laboratory examination of specimens will determine any subsequent treatment for the patient. It is essential that labelling and documentation accompanying the specimen are accurate and that it arrives in the laboratory within the specified time frame (AfPP 2017, **C**).

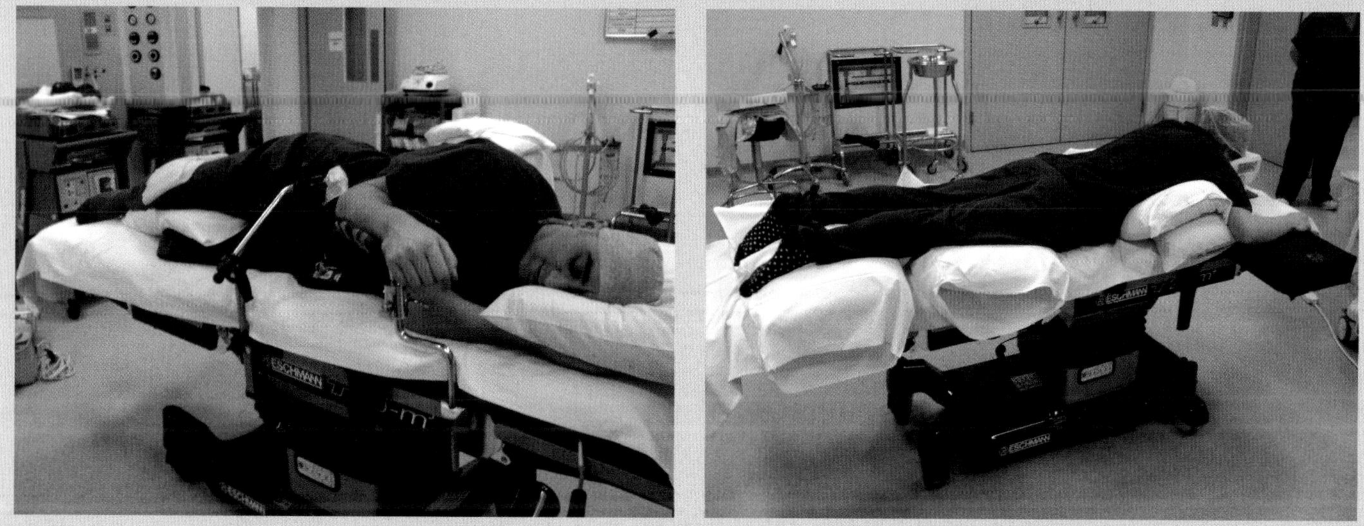

(a) (b)

Action Figure 5 (a) Lateral position. (b) Prone position.

(continued)

Procedure guideline 16.4 Operating theatre procedure: maintaining the safety of a patient during surgery *(continued)*

Action	Rationale
14 The scrub nurse or ODP together with the anaesthetist and the other theatre staff take responsibility for the safety, wellbeing and dignity of the patient during the phase between the surgery finishing and the transfer to the post-operative care team. During this period, when patients who have undergone general anaesthesia are usually emerging from the anaesthetic, the theatre staff prepare to hand over the patient and ensure that the relevant documentation has been completed. This is also when the 'Time Out' phase of the WHO Surgical Safety Checklist is completed by the whole theatre team (see Figure 16.14). The patient will require reassurance and safe transfer from the operating table to a trolley or bed.	To maintain the safety and dignity of the patient (NMC 2018, **C**).

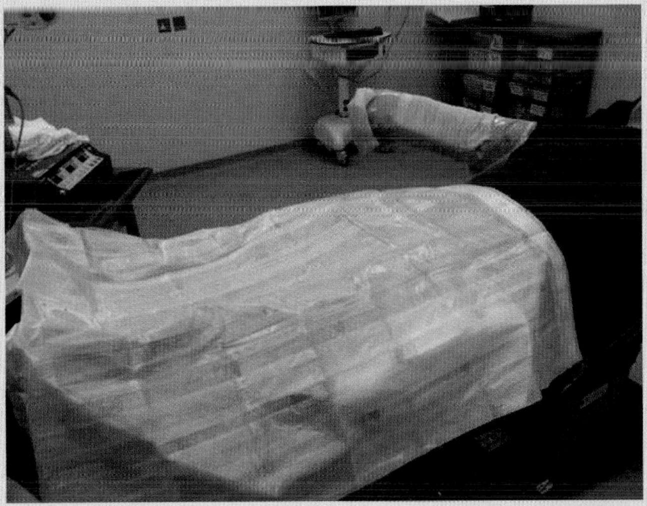

Action Figure 7 Warming blanket

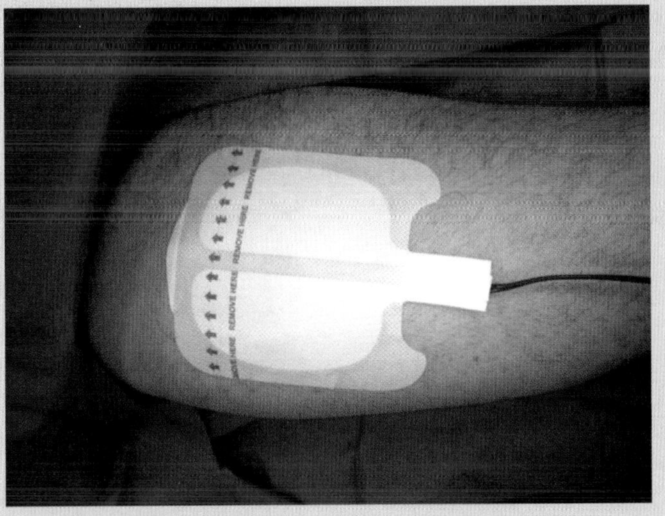

Action Figure 8 Diathermy plate in position.

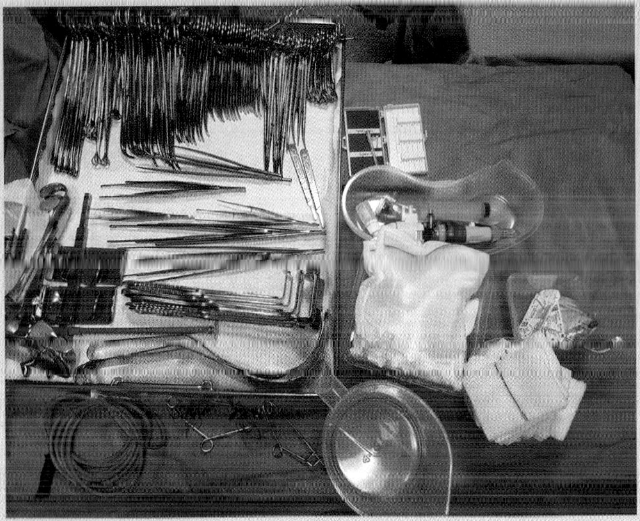

Action Figure 9 Surgical equipment in sterile field.

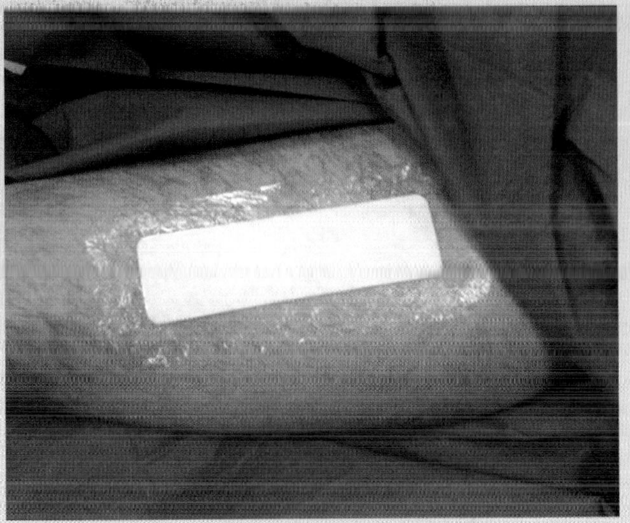

Action Figure 10 Surgical dressing *in situ*.

Post-anaesthetic care unit (PACU)

Definition

The post-operative phase of care begins with the transfer of the patient to the recovery unit and ends with the resolution of the surgical procedure.

Post-anaesthetic recovery involves the short- to medium-term care required by patients (following general, epidural or spinal anaesthesia) during the immediate post-operative period until they are stable, conscious, orientated and safe to transfer back to the ward, day unit or high-dependency area. The post-anaesthetic recovery room is an area within the operating department specifically designed, equipped and staffed for the support, monitoring and assessment of patients immediately following anaesthesia and surgery.

Evidence-based approaches

Transfer of the patient from the operating theatre to the PACU

The patient is transferred from the operating theatre to the PACU by one or more of the anaesthetist, anaesthetic nurse, scrub nurse or operating department practitioners. It is the anaesthetist's responsibility to ensure the safe transfer of the patient. The patient should be assessed as stable prior to leaving the operating theatre and the anaesthetist will decide on the level of monitoring required, which will depend on the distance of the transfer, the patient's level of consciousness, and the patient's cardiovascular and respiratory status.

Oxygen is usually administered to the patient during the transfer unless they did not receive supplemental oxygen during the procedure. It is vital that the anaesthetist flushes the patient's intravenous lines to ensure that there are no residual anaesthetic drugs remaining (AAGBI 2015).

Post-anaesthetic care

Post-anaesthetic care can best be described and understood as a series of nursing procedures performed sequentially and simultaneously on patients immediately after anaesthesia or surgery. Such patients will display varying degrees of responsiveness and physical and emotional states.

The recovery period is potentially hazardous. Therefore, when the patient arrives in the PACU, individual nursing care is required until the nurse is satisfied that the patient can maintain their own airway and is sufficiently oxygenated (AAGBI 2015, AfPP 2017).

Pre-procedural considerations

Equipment required in the PACU

Whereas in the past, post-anaesthetic care meant a relatively brief period of observation in an area close to theatres, it has now evolved into a distinct critical care area where patients of varying dependencies receive specialist clinical care from trained staff using a variety of drugs, monitoring and equipment (AAGBI 2015). The following items are the minimum required in each bed space or recovery bay (Figure 16.37):

- *Patient monitoring*: pulse oximetry, non-invasive blood pressure monitoring, ECG, invasive pressure monitoring, temperature monitoring and capnography.

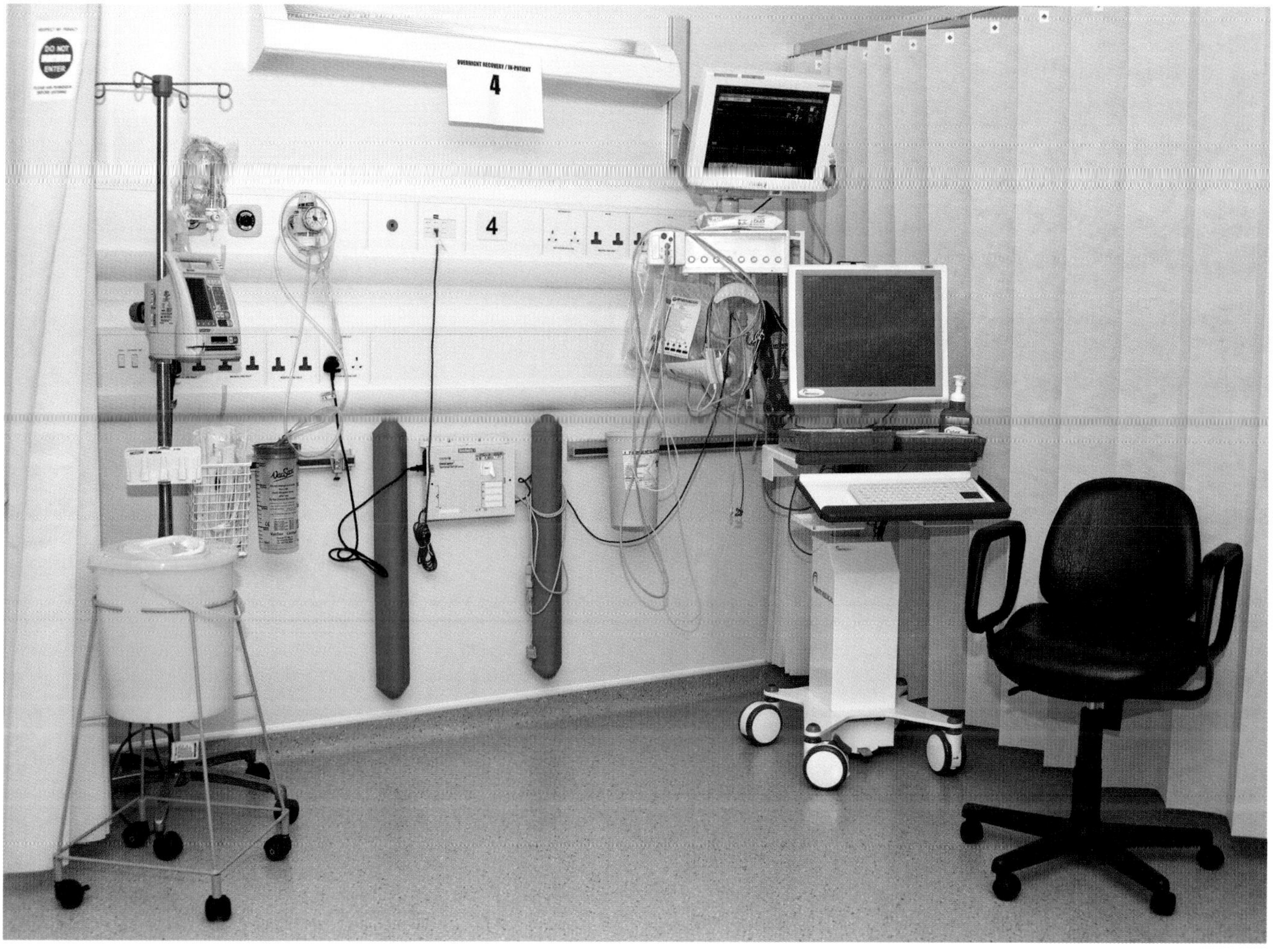

Figure 16.37 Recovery bay.

- *Basic equipment for airway maintenance*: wall-mounted piped oxygen with tubing and face-mask (with both fixed and variable settings), a Mapleson C breathing circuit and a self-inflating resuscitator bag (e.g. Ambu bag with face-mask, and a full range of oral and nasopharyngeal airways). These allow for maintenance of the airway, delivery of oxygen and artificial ventilation of the patient should it be necessary. Spare oxygen cylinders with flow meters should also be available in case of piped oxygen failure.
- *Suction*: a regulator with tubing and a range of oral and endotracheal suction catheters. An electricity-powered portable suction machine should also be available in case of pipeline vacuum failure.
- *Sphygmomanometer and stethoscope*: in case of failure of the electronic patient monitor, manual blood pressure monitoring equipment must always be available.
- *Electrical sockets and individual lights.*
- *Miscellaneous items*: receivers, tissues, disposable gloves, sharps container and waste receptacles (AAGBI 2015, AfPP 2017).

The equipment should be compatible between the operating theatres and the PACU. It must be arranged for ease of access and always be clean and in full working order.

Additionally, other equipment should be available centrally for respiratory and cardiovascular support:

- *Intubation and difficult airway equipment*: fibreoptic laryngoscopes with spare batteries and a range of blades (including McCoy tip), a range of endotracheal tubes, bougies, Magill forceps, syringe and catheter mount. This is to ensure that patients can be intubated quickly during an emergency.
- *Ventilator*: to ensure that patients can be mechanically ventilated if extubated too early or not fully reversed from the anaesthetic.
- *Range of tracheostomy tubes and tracheal dilator*: in case an emergency tracheostomy needs to be performed.
- *Intravenous infusion sets, cannula, central venous catheters and a range of intravenous fluids.*
- *Defibrillator*: required during a cardiac arrest to restart the heart.
- *Nerve stimulators*: to monitor level of neuromuscular blockade.
- *Patient- and fluid-warming devices*: to maintain normothermia and correct inadvertent perioperative hypothermia.

The relevant resuscitation equipment, drugs, fluids and algorithms should be immediately available for the management of both surgical and anaesthetic complications. Ideally these items should be contained in dedicated trolleys (AAGBI 2015, AfPP 2017).

Box 16.10 Minimum information to be recorded for patients in the post-anaesthesia care unit

- Level of consciousness
- Patency of the airway
- Respiratory rate and adequacy
- Oxygen saturation
- Oxygen administration
- Blood pressure
- Heart rate and rhythm
- Pain intensity on an agreed scale
- Post-operative nausea and vomiting (PONV)
- Intravenous infusions
- Drugs administered
- Core temperature
- Other parameters depending on circumstances, such as urinary output, central venous pressure, expired carbon dioxide and surgical drainage volume

Source: Reproduced from AAGBI (2015) with permission of John Wiley & Sons.

PACU staff

No fewer than two staff (at least one must be a registered practitioner) should be present when there is a patient in the PACU who does not fulfil the discharge criteria. The staffing level should allow one-to-one observation of every patient by an anaesthetist or registered PACU practitioner until patients have regained control of their airway, are haemodynamically and respiratorily stable, and are able to communicate. One member of staff present should be a certified acute life support (ALS) provider. Life-threatening complications can occur during the immediate post-operative and post-anaesthesia phase. Any failure to provide adequate care can have devastating consequences for patients, their families and staff. Patients must be kept under clinical observation at all times. The frequency of the observations is dependent on the procedure performed, the physical status of the patient and the stage of recovery. Box 16.10 outlines the minimum information that should be routinely monitored and recorded for patients in the PACU.

Procedure guideline 16.5 Handover in the post-anaesthetic care unit (PACU): scrub nurse or operating department practitioner to recovery practitioner

- Personal protective equipment
- All equipment relevant to the patient's specific procedure

Action	Rationale
Procedure	
1 Introduce yourself to the patient, explain and discuss the procedure with them, and gain their consent to proceed if possible.	To ensure that the patient feels at ease, understands the procedure and gives their valid consent as far as possible (NMC 2018, **C**).
2 Accompany the patient with the anaesthetist to the recovery area. Hand over information on the following:	To ensure continuity and effective communication of care for the patient. To ensure that the recovery practitioner has all the information required to assess the patient's recovery needs. **C**
• the surgical procedure performed	The actual procedure performed may be different from the proposed procedure. **E**
• allergies or pre-existing medical conditions, e.g. diabetes mellitus	To highlight specific potential post-operative complications to be assessed and monitored. **E**
• the patient's cardiovascular state and type of anaesthesia administered	To safely maintain the patient's cardiovascular system and airway immediately post-operatively. **E**
• the presence, position and nature of any drains, infusions, or intravenous or arterial devices	To ensure care and management of these drains are continued and that the positioning of the patient is assessed to prevent any occlusion of drains or infusions. **E**

• the presence of any surgical wound with a swab packed (this will need to be removed either on the ward post-operatively or during a second trip to the operating theatre on another day for pack removal)	To ensure care and management of the wound pack is continued as part of the safety process during the patient care pathway. This will avoid retention of foreign bodies. **E**
• confirmation of flushing of the intravenous line and cannula by the anaesthetist	To ensure that there is no residual anaesthetic drug in the intravenous system, thus avoiding a delayed recovery, and to avoid a potential anaesthetic complication in the recovery area (NHSI 2018, **R**).
• any anxieties the patient expressed before surgery, such as a fear of not waking after anaesthesia or fear of coping with pain	To ensure that the recovery practitioner can respond appropriately as the patient regains consciousness and to enable assessment of the efficacy of subsequent nursing interventions. **E**
• specific instructions from the surgeon or anaesthetist for post-operative care.	To facilitate effective communication of the patient's care and treatment and to ensure that the appropriate post-operative clinical care is delivered. **E**
Post-procedure	
3 Record all information in the perioperative nursing care plan.	To ensure accurate and up-to-date patient documentation (NMC 2018, **C**).

Procedure guideline 16.6 Safe management of patients in the post-operative care unit (PACU)

The following recommended actions are not necessarily listed in order of priority. Many will be carried out simultaneously and will depend on the patient's condition, type of surgery and level of consciousness.

- Personal protective equipment
- All equipment relevant to the patient's specific procedure

Action	Rationale
Pre-procedure	
1 Introduce yourself to the patient, explain and discuss the procedure with them, and gain their consent to proceed if possible.	To ensure that the patient feels at ease, understands the procedure and gives their valid consent as far as possible (NMC 2018, **C**).
2 Obtain a full handover from the surgical and anaesthetic team.	To ensure effective communication of the patient's care and treatment and to aid the planning of subsequent care. **E**
Procedure	
3 Assess the patency of the airway by feeling for movement of expired air.	To determine the presence of any respiratory depression or neuromuscular blockade. Observe chest and abdominal movement, respiratory rate, depth and pattern (Urbankowski and Przybyłowski 2016, **R**).
4 Listen for inspiration and expiration. Observe any use of accessory muscles of respiration and check for tracheal tug, which might indicate airway obstruction.	To ensure the airway is clear and laryngeal spasm is not present. **E**
5 If indicated, support the chin with the neck extended (head tilt, chin lift manoeuvre).	In unconscious patients, the tongue is liable to fall back and obstruct the airway, and protective reflexes are absent. **E**
6 Suctioning of the upper airway is indicated if: • gurgling sounds are present on respiration • blood secretions or vomitus are evident or suspected • the patient is unable to swallow • the patient is unable to cough adequately or at all. Suction must be applied with care to avoid damage to mucosal surfaces and further irritation or initiation of a gag reflex or laryngeal spasm.	Foreign matter can obstruct the airway or cause laryngeal spasm during induction of or emergence from anaesthesia. Foreign matter can also be inhaled when protective laryngeal reflexes are absent (Gavel and Walker 2014, **E**).
7 a Apply a face-mask and administer oxygen at the rate prescribed by the anaesthetist. b If an endotracheal tube or laryngeal mask is in position, check whether the cuff or mask is inflated and administer oxygen by means of a T-piece system.	To maintain adequate oxygenation. Oxygen should be administered to all patients in the recovery room (AAGBI 2013, **C**).
8 Check the colour of the lips and conjunctiva, then peripheral colour and perfusion (skin temperature and peripheral pulse).	Central cyanosis indicates impaired gaseous exchange between the alveoli and pulmonary capillaries. Peripheral cyanosis indicates low cardiac output (Adeyinka and Kondamundi 2019, **E**).

(continued)

Procedure guideline 16.6 Safe management of patients in the post-operative care unit (PACU) *(continued)*

Action	Rationale
9 Record blood pressure, pulse and respiratory rate measurements on admission to the PACU and at a minimum of 5 minute intervals unless the patient's condition dictates otherwise.	To enable any fluctuations or gross abnormalities in cardiovascular and respiratory functions to be detected immediately (AAGBI 2013, **C**).
10 Check the temperature of the patient.	Peri- and post-operative hypothermia is common and preventable (NICE 2016a, **C**).
11 Check and observe wound site(s), dressings and drains on admission to the PACU and at regular intervals. Note and record leakage/drainage on the post-operative chart and also on the drain bottle/bag.	To assess and monitor for signs of haemorrhage (RCoA 2019, **R**).
12 Check that intravenous infusions are running at the correct prescribed rate in accordance with local policy and that the site of the venous access device is assessed as patent in accordance with local protocol.	Care of venous devices and sites prevents complications and ensures that fluid replacement and balance are achieved safely. **E**
13 Check the prescription chart for medications to be administered during the immediate post-operative period, e.g. analgesia and antiemetics.	To treat and prevent symptoms such as pain and nausea swiftly and appropriately and further monitor their effectiveness. **E**
14 Orientate the patient to time and place as frequently as is necessary.	To alleviate anxiety, provide reassurance, and gain the patient's confidence and co-operation. Pre-medication and anaesthesia can induce a degree of amnesia and disorientation. **C**
15 Give mouth care including moistened mouth swabs, sips of water and petroleum jelly for the lips.	Pre-operative fasting, drying gases, manipulation of lips, etc. leave mucosa vulnerable, sore and foul tasting. **E**
16 After regional and/or spinal anaesthesia, assess the return of sensation and mobility of limbs. Check that the limbs are anatomically aligned.	To prevent inadvertent injury following sensory loss (AAGBI 2015, **C**).

Problem-solving table 16.1 Prevention and resolution (Procedure guideline 16.6)

Problem	Cause	Prevention	Action
Airway obstruction	Tongue occluding the airway	Do not remove the laryngeal mask or the Guedel airway until the patient starts responding to commands.	Support the chin forward from the angle of the jaw. If necessary, insert a Guedel airway. Use a nasopharyngeal airway if the teeth are clenched or crowned.
	Foreign material, blood, secretions or vomitus	Use suction to remove secretions when removing the airway.	Apply suction. Always check for the presence of a throat pack.
	Laryngeal spasm	Do not remove the airway until the patient responds to commands, and ensure oxygen flow is high (5–10 L per minute) on arrival in PACU.	Increase the rate of oxygen. Assist ventilation with an Ambu bag and face-mask. If there is no improvement, inform the anaesthetist and have intubation equipment ready. Offer the patient reassurance by talking to them and telling them what you are doing.
Hypoventilation	Respiratory depression from medications, for example opiates, inhalations or barbiturates	Monitor depth and rate of respiration before administering analgesia.	Inform the anaesthetist, keeping oxygen on, and administer antagonist on instruction, for example naloxone (opiate antagonist) or doxapram (respiratory stimulant). *Note*: if naloxone is given it can reverse the analgesic effects of opiates and has a duration of action of only 20–30 minutes. The patient must be observed for signs of returning hyperventilation (Nimmo et al. 1994).
	Decreased respiratory drive from a low partial pressure of carbon dioxide ($PaCO_2$), or loss of hypoxic drive in patients with chronic pulmonary disease	Ensure that Venturi masks are available and close to hand in the recovery bay.	Administer oxygen using a Venturi mask with graded low concentrations (as little as possible to achieve the desired peripheral oxygen saturations) (BNF 2019).

Problem	Cause	Prevention	Action
	Residual neuromuscular blockade from continued action of non-depolarizing muscle relaxants; signs include difficulty breathing and speaking, generalized weakness, visual disturbances and patient distress	Ensure an appropriate dose of neuromuscular blockade is given as part of anaesthesia.	Inform the anaesthetist, have available neostigmine and glycopyrrolate, or sugammadex. Often the blockade is mild and will wear off in minutes without treatment, but it is extremely frightening and patients will need continuous reassurance that their condition is not unnoticed and is resolving, and that they will not be left alone.
Hypotension	Hypovolaemia	Increase the rate of fluids (as prescribed) and ensure more fluids are prescribed.	Take manual reading of the blood pressure. Take central venous pressure (CVP) readings if a catheter is in place. Give oxygen. Lower the head of the trolley unless contraindicated, for example hiatus hernia or gross obesity. Check the record of anaesthetic agents used that might cause hypotension, for example beta blockers or sympathetic blockade following spinal anaesthesia. Check the peripheral perfusion. If the CVP is low, increase intravenous infusion unless contraindicated, for example in congestive cardiac failure. Check drains and dressings for visible bleeding and haematoma. Inform the anaesthetist or surgeon.
Hypertension	Pain	Ensure pain is assessed as soon as the patient is responding to commands. Record the scores.	Treat pain with prescribed analgesia and provide a quiet environment to enable the patient to rest or sleep. Pain from certain operation sites can be alleviated by changing the patient's position.
	Fluid overload	Slow the intravenous rate.	Check the fluid balance sheet and the rate of intravenous infusion.
	Distended bladder	Check whether the bladder is distended and the catheter is patent.	Offer a bedpan or urinal and if necessary catheterize the patient.
	Some anaesthetic drugs given during reversal of an anaesthetic	Ensure the anaesthetist monitors the patient when reversing the effects of anaesthetic drugs.	Check the prescription chart for those patients on regular antihypertensive therapy. If the situation is not resolved, inform the anaesthetist. Also check the patient's past medical history.
Bradycardia	Very fit patient, opiates, reversal agents, beta blockers, pain, vagal stimulation, or hypoxaemia from respiratory depression	Ensure that oxygen is administered and that the anaesthetist identifies any adverse episodes of bradycardia during surgery.	Connect the patient to an ECG monitor to exclude heart block and monitor cardiac activity. Ascertain pre-operative cardiac function. Check the prescription chart and anaesthetic sheet for medication administered that may cause bradycardia. Inform and liaise with the anaesthetist.
Tachycardia	Pain, hypovolaemia, some anaesthetic drugs (e.g. ephedrine), septicaemia, fear or fluid overload	Ensure pain is managed and intravenous fluids are administered.	Assess the patient's pain and provide analgesia. Check the anaesthetic chart to ascertain which anaesthetic drugs were used. Connect the patient to the ECG monitor to exclude ventricular tachycardia. Provide reassurance for the patient. Assess fluid balance.
Pain	Surgical trauma worsened by fear, anxiety and/or restlessness	Administer analgesia after assessing the patient's pain.	Provide prescribed analgesia and assess its efficacy. Reassure and orientate the patient. Try positional changes where feasible; for example, after breast surgery raise the back support by 20–40°; after abdominal or gynaecological surgery patients may be more comfortable lying on their side. Elevate limbs to reduce swelling where appropriate. If significant relief is not obtained, inform the anaesthetist and the pain control specialist nurse.
Nausea and vomiting	Anaesthetic agents, opiates, hypotension, abdominal surgery or pain; high-risk patients who have a history of post-operative nausea and vomiting	Administer antiemetics with the analgesia and ensure intravenous fluids are administered as prescribed.	Administer intravenous antiemetics and monitor their effectiveness. Encourage slow, regular breathing. If the patient is unconscious, turn them onto their side, tip their head down and suck out the pharynx; give oxygen.

(continued)

Problem-solving table 16.1 Prevention and resolution (Procedure guideline 16.6) *(continued)*

Problem	Cause	Prevention	Action
Hypothermia	Depression of the heat-regulating centre or vasodilation following abdominal surgery, large infusions of unwarmed blood and fluids	Measure and record the patient's temperature upon arrival in the PACU and maintain their temperature using a Bair Hugger.	Use extra blankets or a Bair Hugger (Madrid et al. 2016). Monitor the patient's temperature. Administer warm intravenous fluids. Bladder irrigation may also be warmed to normal body temperature.
Shivering	Some inhalational anaesthetics or hypothermia	Measure and record the patient's temperature on arrival in the PACU and maintain their temperature using a Bair Hugger. Measure temperature every 30–60 minutes.	Give oxygen, reassure the patient and take their temperature. Provide a Bair Hugger and warm blankets.
Hyperthermia	Infection or blood transfusion reaction	Measure and record the patient's temperature at least every 30–60 minutes.	Give oxygen; use a fan or tepid sponging if this is warranted. Obtain a medical assessment of antibiotic therapy and blood cultures. Administer intravenous paracetamol if prescribed.
	Malignant hyperpyrexia (above 40°C)	This may be identified during the anaesthetic. All anaesthetic and theatre personnel must know the location of the relevant emergency drug (dantrolene), which should be kept in every operating theatre suite.	Malignant hyperpyrexia is a medical emergency. Dantrolene is used to treat this life-threatening condition.
Oliguria	Mechanical obstruction of catheter, for example clots or kinking	Check patency and drainage upon arrival in the PACU and every 30–60 minutes.	Check the patency of the catheter. Consider bladder irrigation. If clots present, inform the surgeon.
	Inadequate renal perfusion, for example due to hypotension, systolic pressures under 60 mmHg, hypovolaemia or dehydration	Ensure adequate blood pressure and intravenous fluid input are maintained.	Take blood pressure and CVP if available. Increase intravenous fluids. Inform the anaesthetist.
	Renal damage, for example from blood transfusion, infection, drugs or surgical damage to the ureters	Check the drugs given do not adversely affect renal function, and that surgery does not damage the ureters.	Inform the anaesthetist or surgeon.

ECG, electrocardiogram; PACU, post-anaesthetic care unit.

Post procedural considerations

Discharge from the PACU

Discharge from the PACU is ultimately the responsibility of the anaesthetist but is usually delegated to PACU practitioners, who use discharge criteria to assess whether the patient has achieved the optimum recovery, enabling them to return to the ward safely. In the event of complications or deterioration, the anaesthetist must be informed and should assess the patient before their return to the ward (AAGBI 2015, AfPP 2017).

The PACU must adhere to minimum criteria that patients must meet prior to their discharge to the general ward or other clinical areas (Box 16.11).

Complications

Pain

Pain is the most common adverse effect of surgery for the majority of patients (Chou et al. 2016). Pain is a subjective experience and patients in the PACU should receive both effective and empathetic care to relieve their pain (AfPP 2017). A patient should not be discharged from the PACU until satisfactory pain control has been achieved. PACU staff must be trained and competent in the use of intravenous analgesia, patient-controlled analgesia, epidurals, spinals and peripheral nerve blocks (AAGBI 2015). It is important to recognize that pain may not only be caused by the surgery. Other reasons include pre-existing medical conditions, poor positioning during surgery, headache as a result of anaesthetic drugs, and muscle aches from the use of depolarizing muscle relaxants (e.g. suxamethonium) (Chou et al. 2016).

Nausea and vomiting

Post-operative nausea and vomiting may arise from many causes. These include hypotension, swallowing of blood (e.g. in oral surgery), abdominal surgery and anxiety, but most commonly as a side-effect of opioid administration. Nausea, vomiting and retching may exist independently and therefore require individual assessment (AfPP 2017). Patients should not be discharged from the PACU unless their post-operative nausea and/or vomiting are controlled and suitable medication has been prescribed (AAGBI 2013).

Box 16.11 Minimum criteria for discharge of patients from the post-anaesthesia care unit

- The patient is fully conscious, is able to maintain a clear airway and has protective airway reflexes.
- Breathing and oxygenation are satisfactory.
- The cardiovascular system is stable, with no unexplained cardiac irregularity or persistent bleeding. The specific values of pulse and blood pressure should approximate to normal pre-operative values or be at acceptable levels, ideally within parameters set by the anaesthetist, and peripheral perfusion should be adequate.
- Pain and post-operative nausea and vomiting should be adequately controlled, and suitable analgesic and antiemetic regimens prescribed.
- Temperature should be within acceptable limits. Patients should not be returned to the ward if significantly hypothermic.
- Oxygen therapy should be prescribed if appropriate.
- Intravenous cannulas should be patent and flushed if necessary to ensure removal of any residual anaesthetic drugs. Intravenous fluids should be prescribed if appropriate.
- All surgical drains and catheters should be checked.
- All health records should be complete and medical notes present.

Source: Reproduced from AAGBI (2015) with permission of John Wiley & Sons.

Hypothermia

Inadvertent perioperative hypothermia (below 36.0°C) is a common but preventable complication of surgery and is associated with poor outcomes for patients. Adult surgical patients may develop hypothermia at any stage of the perioperative journey, though the elderly, the malnourished and those who have undergone long surgery or where large amounts of blood or fluid replacement therapy have been used are especially at risk (Williams and El-Houdiri 2018).

During the first 30–40 minutes of anaesthesia, a patient's temperature can fall to below 35.0°C. Reasons for this include:

- loss of the behavioural response to cold
- impairment of thermoregulatory heat-preserving mechanisms (due to general or regional anaesthesia)
- anaesthesia-induced peripheral vasodilation (with associated heat loss)
- the patient becoming cold while waiting for surgery in the pre-operative area (NICE 2016a).

On admission to the PACU, the patient's temperature must be measured and documented. If it is below 36.0°C, active warming should be commenced until the patient is warm. They should not be discharged until their temperature is 36.0°C or above (NICE 2016a). Hypothermia produces symptoms that mimic those of other post-operative complications, which may result in inappropriate treatment. Hypothermia interferes with the effective reversal of muscle relaxants, so patients who are shivering, restless or confused, or who have respiratory depression, should be monitored. Shivering puts an increased demand on cardiopulmonary systems as oxygen consumption is increased (Feldmann 1988, Frank et al. 1993). Cardiac complications such as arrhythmias or myocardial infarction are some of the principal causes of post-operative morbidity (Warttig et al. 2014).

Other complications

When emerging from the final stage of anaesthesia, some patients can behave in an emotional and disinhibited fashion, at variance with their normal behaviour (Eckenhoff et al. 1961, Radtke et al. 2008). Therefore, it is important to establish a rapport with each individual to gain the patient's confidence and co-operation and to aid assessment. These displays are always transient and fortunately patients seldom have any recollection of them. All actions must be accompanied by commentary and explanation regardless of the patient's apparent responsiveness, as the sense of hearing returns before the patient's ability to respond (Levinson 1965, Starritt 1999).

Post-operative care

Definition

Post-operative care is the physical and psychological care given to a patient immediately after transfer from the recovery room to the ward. Post-operative care continues until the patient is discharged from hospital, and in some cases continues as ambulatory care provided to outpatients.

Evidence-based approaches

Principles of care

Although different surgical procedures require specific and specialist nursing care, the principles of post-operative care remain the same, underpinned by the application of evidence-based care. Optimal management of patients throughout the post-operative phase requires appropriate clinical assessment and monitoring, and timely and accurate documentation. The nursing care given during the post-operative period is directed towards the prevention of complications that may arise from surgery and anaesthesia. Potential complications are outlined in Figure 16.38.

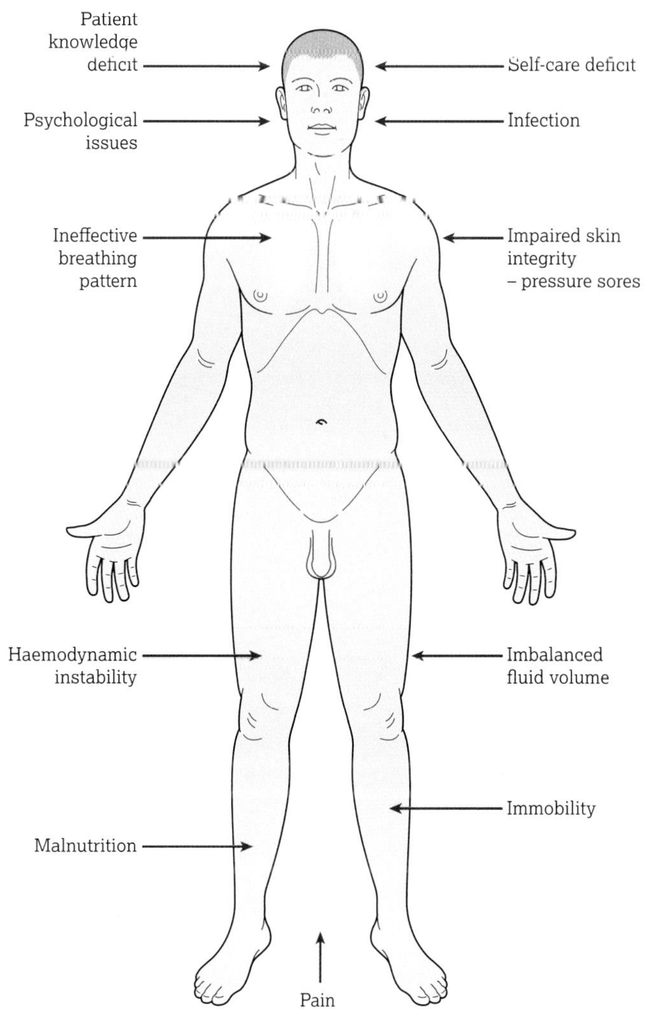

Figure 16.38 Potential post-operative complications.

Anticipated patient outcomes

The patient's safety will be maintained at all times and post-operative complications will be minimized by:

- *Following the required nursing care for post-operative patients*: this includes fully informing the patient of the post operative care requirements so that they can enhance their recovery, facilitating earlier discharge home.
- *Optimizing the patient's post-operative physical and psychological condition to minimize the risk of post-operative complications occurring*: this is achieved through comprehensive nursing assessment and planning to ensure early identification and management of any post-operative complications.

Post-operative observations

Evidence-based approaches

Principles of care

Regular monitoring and accurate reporting of patients' clinical observations in the post-operative period are essential parts of the planned surgical care pathway and can serve to identify potential complications. Post-operative observations are outlined in Table 16.10. A clear physiological monitoring plan should be made for each patient, detailing frequency of observations and parameters (NCEPOD 2011). All nurses should be aware of the parameters for these observations and what is normal for the patient under observation. Post-operative observations should be compared with baseline observations taken pre-operatively, during surgery and in the recovery area (Liddle 2013). The frequency of post-operative observations should be determined in accordance with local policies and guidelines and will be affected by the type of surgery performed, the method of pain control (e.g. epidural) and the patient's clinical condition. All vital signs and assessments should be documented in accordance with guidelines for record keeping (NMC 2018).

Table 16.10 Post-operative observations

Observations	Normal range
Routine post-operative observations	
Blood pressure	101–149 mmHg systolic
Pulse (rate, rhythm and amplitude)	51–100 beats per minute
Respiration rate (rate, depth, effort and pattern)	9–14 respirations per minute
Peripheral oxygen saturation	>95% on room air (less if patient has chronic obstructive pulmonary disease)
Temperature	36.1–37.9°C
Accurate fluid balance (input and output)	Desired balance guided by surgeons and surgery performed
Pain score	Verbal numeric pain scale: 0–1/10 at rest; 3/10 on movement/coughing
Sedation score	Sedation score: 0/4 (see Chapter 14: Observations)
Additional observations (if clinically indicated)	
Blood glucose	4–7 mmol/L
Central venous pressure	5–10 cmH_2O
Neurological response	Glasgow Coma Scale: 14–15/15

Source: Adapted from Bickley et al. (2009), DH (2000), Liddle (2013).

Critical care outreach and acute care teams have long encouraged the use of early warning scoring (EWS) systems to enable a more timely response to, and assessment of, acutely ill patients (RCP 2017). EWS is a simple physiological scoring system, based on the observations outlined in Table 16.10, that identifies patients at risk of deterioration who may require increased levels of care (NHS England 2019) (see Chapter 14: Observations).

Clinical governance

The National Confidential Enquiry into Patient Outcome and Death (NCEPOD 2011) report established that patients whose clinical condition was deteriorating post-operatively were not always identified and referred for a higher level of care. When assessing post-operative patients, it is vital to observe for signs of haemorrhage, shock, sepsis, and the effects of analgesia and anaesthetic (Liddle 2013). It is therefore imperative that nurses are able to interpret the results of post-operative observations and, if they are reliant on appropriately trained healthcare assistants to take the observations, that nurses themselves interpret the results, thereby ensuring that patients who require a higher level of care are given immediate priority. Refer to Chapter 14: Observations for further details on methods of obtaining observations and for troubleshooting.

Haemodynamic instability

Related theory

Haemodynamic instability is most commonly associated with an abnormal or unstable blood pressure, especially hypotension (Minokadeh and Pinsky 2016). A reduction in systolic blood pressure following surgery can indicate hypovolaemic shock, a condition in which the blood vessels do not contain sufficient blood (Hatfield and Tronson 2009). Bleeding is the most common cause but other causes can arise when tissue fluid is lost from the circulation, for example through bowel obstruction or nausea and vomiting. Ho et al. (2016) outline three stages of hypovolaemic shock:

- *Compensated shock*: blood flow to the brain and heart is preserved at the expense of the kidneys, gastrointestinal system, skin and muscles.
- *Decompensated shock*: the body's compensatory mechanisms begin to fail and organ perfusion is severely reduced.
- *Irreversible shock*: tissues become so deprived of oxygen that multiorgan failure occurs.

Evidence-based approaches

Principles of care

During compensated shock, some patients can lose up to 30% of their circulatory volume before the effects of hypovolaemia are reflected in their systolic blood pressure measurements or heart rate (Ho et al. 2016). Therefore, when assessing post-operative patients, it is also useful to consider the early signs of reduced tissue perfusion in detecting signs of hypovolaemic shock. These include:

- restlessness, anxiety or confusion (as a result of cerebral hypoperfusion or hypoxia)
- increased respiratory rate, becoming shallow (frequently occurring before signs of tachycardia and hypotension)
- rising pulse rate (tachycardia as the heart attempts to compensate for the low circulatory blood volume)
- low urine output of below 0.5 mL/kg/hour (as the kidneys experience a reduction in perfusion and pressure, which activates the renin–angiotensin system in an attempt to conserve fluid and increase circulatory blood volume)
- pallor (pale, cyanotic skin) and later sweating
- cool peripheries (pale, cyanotic lips and nailbed), resulting in a poor signal on the pulse oximeter
- visible bleeding and haematoma from drains and wounds (Anderson 2003, Hatfield and Tronson 2009, Jameson 2017, Jevon and Ewens 2012).

In most cases, if impending hypovolaemic shock is recognized and treated promptly, its progression through the aforementioned stages of shock can be circumvented (Kalkwarf and Cotton 2017). Irrespective of the cause of hypovolaemic shock, the aim of treatment is to restore adequate tissue perfusion (Ho et al. 2016). Excessive blood loss may require blood transfusion and occasionally surgical intervention. However, if signs indicate that the patient is in the compensated phase, fluid resuscitation with crystalloids or colloids and increased oxygenation to maintain saturation above 95% will often be sufficient to promote recovery.

Ineffective breathing pattern

Related theory

Post-operatively, respiratory function can be influenced by a number of factors:

- increased bronchial secretions from inhalation anaesthesia
- decreased respiratory effort from opiate medication
- pain or anticipated pain from surgical wounds
- surgical trauma to the phrenic nerve
- pneumothorax as a result of surgical or anaesthetic procedures
- co-morbidity, for example asthma or chronic obstructive pulmonary disease.

All factors affecting adequate expansion of the lungs and the ejection of bronchial secretions will encourage the development of atelectasis and consolidation of the affected lung tissue (AAGBI 2015). To prevent this, deep breathing exercises (DBEs), coughing exercises and early mobilization may be undertaken post-operatively. DBEs help to remove mucus, which can form and remain in the lungs due to the effects of general anaesthetic and analgesics (which depress the action of the cilia of the mucous membranes lining the respiratory tract and also depress the respiratory centre in the brain). DBEs prevent pneumonia by increasing lung expansion and preventing the accumulation of secretions. They also initiate the coughing reflex; voluntary coughing in conjunction with DBEs facilitates the expectoration of respiratory tract secretions. A physiotherapist will often provide pre-operative and/or post-operative advice and/or assessment for DBEs. Note that patients will require adequate analgesia and support for their wound to enable DBEs and mobilization.

Evidence-based approaches

Principles of care

Respiratory rate and function is often the first vital sign to be affected if there is a change in cardiac or neurological state. It is therefore imperative that this observation is performed accurately; however, studies show that it is often omitted or poorly assessed (NHS England and NHSI 2018). Routine post-operative respiratory observations will include:

- airway
- respiratory rate (regular and effortless), rhythm and depth (chest movements symmetrical)
- respiratory depression: indicated by hypoventilation or bradypnoea; may be opiate induced or due to anaesthetic gases
- listening for audible signs of stridor, wheeze or secretions
- observing any changes in the patient's colour for signs of peripheral or central cyanosis
- pulse oximetry: should be above 95% on air (unless the patient has lung disease) and maintained above 95% if oxygen therapy is prescribed to prevent hypoxia or hypoxaemia
- use of oxygen therapy: flow and method of delivery
- any chest drains (if applicable).

Oxygen is administered to enable the anaesthetic gases to be transported out of the body, and is prescribed when patients have an epidural, patient controlled analgesia or morphine infusion. Nurses should ensure and record the following.

- Oxygen therapy is prescribed.
- Oxygen is administered at the correct rate.
- Continuous oxygen therapy is humidified to prevent mucous membranes from drying out.
- The skin above the ears is protected from the elastic on the mask or nasal prongs.

Fluid balance

Definition

Fluid balance involves balancing the input and output of fluids in the body to allow metabolic processes to function correctly (Welch 2010).

Evidence-based approaches

Principles of care

Iatrogenic factors potentially contributing to fluid imbalance (circulating and tissue fluid volumes) in post-operative patients are outlined in Box 16.12. Some patients require fluid replacement in the post-operative period to ensure an adequate fluid balance, avoiding dehydration (NICE 2018a).

Post-operative fluid replacement should be based on the following considerations:

- maintenance requirements
- extra needs resulting from systemic factors (e.g. pyrexia or losses from surgical drains)
- requirements resulting from third-space losses (e.g. oedema and ileus) (Levinson 2006, NICE 2013, Powell-Tuck et al. 2011).

Daily maintenance fluids for sensible losses (i.e. measurable losses, e.g. urine output) and insensible losses (i.e. not measurable, e.g. sweating) will be dependent upon age, gender, weight and body surface area and will increase with pyrexia, hyperventilation and conditions that increase the catabolic rate.

Deciding on the optimal amount and composition of intravenous fluids to be administered and the best rate at which to give them can be a difficult and complex task, and decisions must be based on careful assessment of the patient's individual needs (NICE 2018a). Where possible and clinically indicated, euvolaemic and haemodynamically stable patients should return to oral fluids as soon as possible (Powell-Tuck et al. 2011). If intravenous fluids are required, the most commonly used replacement fluids are crystalloids and colloids, which have various effects on a range of important physiological parameters (Perel et al. 2013). All patients receiving intravenous fluids need regular monitoring. This should initially include at least daily reassessments of clinical fluid status, laboratory values (urea, creatinine and electrolytes) and fluid balance charts, along with weight measurement twice weekly (NICE 2016c).

In December 2013, NICE published guidance outlining recommendations and algorithms covering the general principles for

Box 16.12 Iatrogenic factors with the potential to contribute to fluid imbalance

- Pre-operative bowel preparation
- Pre-operative fasting times
- Potential fluid volume excess
- Fluid loss perioperatively
- Inappropriate fluid prescription
- Reduced fluid intake post-operatively
- Ongoing losses from bleeding
- Paralytic ileus and/or vomiting

Source: Adapted from Anderson (2003), Hatfield and Tronson (2009).

Table 16.11 Open and closed drains

Type of drain	Description	Examples
Open drains	Open drains are 'open' to the air with the exudate 'passively' collecting onto a sterile dressing, such as gauze (if only minimal) or a drainage bag (if copious), from the surgical wound bed. These drains are cheap, simple and versatile, and can be used in any part of the body in both clean and infected wounds. They can be brought out through the end of a wound or more commonly through a separate stab incision. It is important to suture open drains to the skin to prevent them from falling out. As these drains are 'open', there is an associated risk of infection; however, the development of deep infection from retrograde tracking of micro-organisms is rare owing to the continuous outward flow of exudate.	*Penrose drains*: thin walled soft rubber latex tubes that collapse to resemble a flat ribbon. Being very soft, they are considered safe to lay adjacent to bowel or other internal organs. *Yates drains*: quite flat but composed of multiple small tubules stuck side by side; much stiffer than Penrose drains. The tubules can be peeled off longitudinally to create any width of drain required. *Corrugated drain*: wavy strips of PVC (polyvinyl chloride), still relatively stiff. They usually have a radiopaque strip down the middle (see Figure 16.39a).
Closed drains	Closed drains are 'closed' to the air with the fluid collecting into a sealed collection system (bags or bottles); thus, the drain contents remain clean. Closed drains can be divided broadly into those that employ suction (active drains, e.g. Redivac, chest) and those that do not (passive drains).	Redivac, exudrain.
Closed non-suction drains (passive)	Closed non-suction drains (passive) are dependent on gravity and the pressure differential between the body cavity and the exterior in order for fluid to be drained (Brooks et al. 2008). They are commonly used after abdominal and pelvic surgery. They are characterized by a collapsible plastic bag on the end of the drainage tubing.	Examples include urinary catheter (Foley), nasogastric tube (Ryle), Robinson's drain and Bonanno catheter (see Figure 16.39b).
Closed suction drains (active)	Closed suction drains (active) combine gravity drainage with active suction created by the drainage system, which also acts as a reservoir for the drained fluid. They are commonly used in the subcutaneous tissues after abdominal, breast, plastic or orthopaedic surgery to obliterate dead spaces and prevent blood or serous fluid collections. They typically comprise a fine-bore tube with an end hole and multiple side perforations/drainage holes. For suction to be effective, all drainage holes must be located inside the drainage cavity (i.e. inside the skin).	Examples include drains connected to either a pre-vacuumed hard plastic bottle (e.g. Redivac; see Figure 16.39c) or to a soft concertina-style bottle (designed to be squeezed before connection to generate negative pressure; see Figure 16.39d).

managing intravenous fluids for adults in hospital (see NICE 2017a). See also Chapter 8: Nutrition and fluid balance.

Surgical drains

Definition

A surgical drain is a device, such as a tube, inserted intraoperatively into a body cavity (e.g. bladder or chest wall) or opening of a surgical wound to facilitate discharge of fluid or air.

Related theory

Surgical drains are used in many different types of surgery with the aim of decompressing, draining or diverting either fluid (blood, pus, gastric fluids, lymph or urine) or air from the site of the surgery (Mayerson 2016, Vecchio et al. 2016, Wong et al. 2016) to help prevent infection and facilitate healing (Knowlton 2015).

Drains can be open or closed and are made from latex, silicone or PVC (polyvinyl chloride) (Table 16.11, Figure 16.39). All drains induce some degree of tissue reaction (e.g. inflammation or fibrosis) as they are foreign bodies; however, the softer the drain, the less likely it is to cause tissue erosion. The type of drain used will be determined by the substance being drained (e.g. viscous versus thin fluid), the reason for the drain, the drain location and the volume of drainage (Mayerson 2016).

An open drain allows the drainage of fluids outside the body. For example, in a Penrose drain (a closed drain), an artificial conduit is left in the wound and connected to a container that is placed outside the body. A closed drain may be classified as passive, meaning it relies on gravity (e.g. a Robinson drain), or active, meaning it relies on negative pressure (e.g. a Redivac drain) (Khan et al. 2015) (Table 16.11).

Evidence-based approaches

Principles of care

Drains serve an important function as they allow the movement of fluid (e.g. blood, pus and serum) and air that has collected within a cavity in the body to pass outside the body. They reduce the risk of infection, promoting wound healing and making the cavity smaller (Wiker and Dalby 2016). However, they are also associated with complications such as haemorrhage, tissue inflammation, retrograde bacterial migration and drain entrapment (Walker 2007). It is essential that nurses are familiar with the monitoring and management of surgical drains and also the processes involved in their removal.

The management of a surgical drain is determined by its type, purpose and location; individual trusts' local procedural guidelines should be referred to. If a patient has more than one drain, each one should be numbered to prevent confusion. Drains should be firmly secured at the exit site (e.g. with a suture), and, if attached to a drainage bag or bottle, they should also be secured at one other point (e.g. with adhesive tape).

To minimize the risk of cross infection, the drainage bag or bottle should not be placed directly on the floor but should be placed below the level of the wound to facilitate drainage. Drainage output should be measured and recorded on the fluid balance chart or wound drainage chart, as accurate 24-hour totals are necessary for making decisions about drain management. Drains should be monitored regularly throughout a shift; this should be undertaken as clinically indicated (e.g. each time clinical observations are recorded). Nurses must monitor changes in the character (colour, viscosity and odour) and volume of drainage fluid. Unexpected

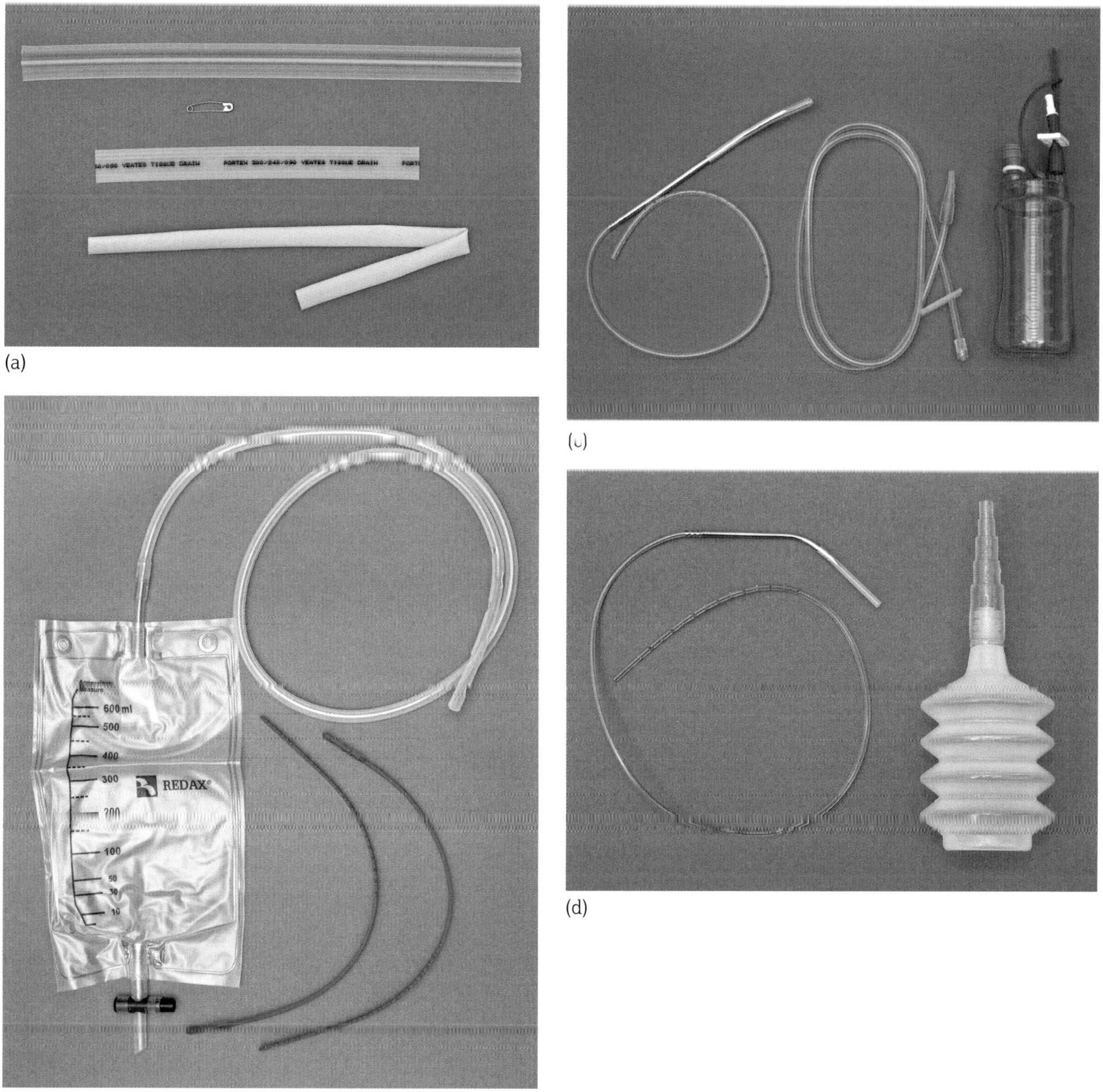

Figure 16.39 (a) Top to bottom: corrugated, Yates and Penrose drains. (b) Robinson's drain attached to a sterile closed drainage bag. (c) Redivac drain. (d) Concertina drain.

drainage volume (too high or too low) or type (unexpected fluids, e.g. blood in urinary catheter) should always prompt further investigation by the clinical team and could indicate that something is wrong (see Problem-solving table 16.2). The length of the drainage tubing (from drain exit point) should also be recorded on surgery documentation and regularly observed for signs of dislodgement (withdrawal or retraction). Furthermore, drain tubing and connections should regularly be inspected for signs of disconnection (e.g. suction pressure source), damage, blockages (viscous fluid, e.g. blood clots, pus or gastric contents) or kinks. For wound drains, it is also important that nurses observe the skin surrounding the drain site for signs of swelling, infection or haematoma. Swabs of wound and drain sites should only be taken if infection is suspected (e.g. due to inflammation of wound margins, pain, oedema, pyrexia and/or purulent exudates). Procedure guideline 16.7: Drainage systems: changing the dressing around the drain site for both open and closed drains offers guidance on dressing the drain site of both open and closed drains.

The Daily Drain Drill was created by Brooks et al. (2008) and outlines regularly and daily drain checks (Box 16.13).

Drains should be emptied frequently using clean technique or standard precautions to reduce the strain on the suture line and ensure maximum drainage (Lippincott Williams & Wilkins 2018). However, the dangers of introducing infection should be weighed against the need to empty the drain. Vacuum bottles (e.g. Redivac bottles) and underwater sealed drains (e.g. chest drains) are not emptied but renewed when full (see Procedure guideline 16.8: Closed drainage systems: changing a vacuum bottle).

Box 16.13 The DDD (Daily Drain Drill)

1 Volume of fluid (24-hour total)?
2 Type of fluid?
3 Blocked, kinked, leaking or displaced?
4 Adequately secured?
5 Adequate suction?
6 Ready for removal?

Source: Reproduced from Brooks et al. (2008) with permission of John Wiley & Sons.

With the exception of urinary catheters and Ryle's tubes, surgical drains are usually removed once the drainage has stopped or become less than approximately 25–50 mL/day. In some instances drains are 'shortened' by withdrawing them gradually (typically 2 cm/day) before they are completely removed or fall out, to promote gradual closure of the tract. The drain may also be 'cut and bagged' to facilitate easier mobilization. In each of these circumstances, the decision is taken by the surgical team. See Procedure guideline 16.10: Wound drain shortening for open drainage systems and Procedure guideline 16.11: Wound drain shortening for closed drainage systems for instructions concerning surgical wound drain shortening and removal.

Procedure guideline 16.7 Drainage systems: changing the dressing around the drain site for both open and closed drains

Essential equipment

- Personal protective equipment
- Dressing trolley or other suitable surface
- Detergent wipe
- Sterile fluids for cleaning and/or irrigation, e.g. 0.9% sodium chloride
- Appropriate absorbent dry dressing (required special features of a dressing should be referred to in the patient's nursing care plan)
- Dressing pack, including sterile towel, gauze, gallipot and disposable bag
- Gloves: one disposable pair, one sterile pair
- Hypoallergenic tape

Optional equipment

- Any extra equipment that may be needed during the procedure, e.g. sterile scissors, forceps and microbiological swab

Action	Rationale
Pre-procedure	
1 Check the medical notes to identify which drain is to be removed. Introduce yourself to the patient, explain and discuss the procedure with them, and gain their consent to proceed.	To ensure that the patient feels at ease, understands the procedure and gives their valid consent (NMC 2018, **C**; Walker 2007, **C**).
2 Check patient comfort, for example position and pain level. Offer the patient analgesia as described on their chart or encourage self-administration via a patient-controlled analgesia pump (if applicable) and allow appropriate time for the medication to take effect.	To promote patient comfort (NMC 2018, **C**).
3 Clean the trolley/tray per local trust guidelines and gather the equipment, checking the sterility and expiry date of equipment and solutions, and place everything on the bottom of the trolley.	To minimize the risk of infection (Loveday et al. 2014, **R**).
4 Take the trolley/tray to the bed and adjust the bed to the correct height to avoid stooping.	To promote good manual handling. **E**
5 Wash and dry hands thoroughly and put on an apron.	To minimize the risk of infection (NHS England and NHSI 2019, **C**).
Procedure	
6 Remove the dressing pack from the outer pack and place it on top of the clean dressing trolley/tray. Using aseptic technique, open the packaging of the other equipment required during the procedure (sterile gloves, dressing, etc.) and place the contents onto the sterile field of the opened dressing pack.	To minimize the risk of infection (Loveday et al. 2014, **R**).
7 Expose the drain site, adjusting the patient's clothes to expose the wound, taking care to maintain their dignity.	To minimize the amount of skin exposed; to maintain dignity. **E**
8 Wearing disposable gloves, remove the dressing covering the drain site and place it in a soiled dressing bag away from the sterile field. a Closed drains may have a small sterile gauze dressing surrounding the exit site. b Open drains will be covered with either a wound drainage bag (if copious exudate) or a small, absorbent, non-adhesive sterile gauze dressing (if only minimal exudate). Once the drainage bag/dressing has been removed from an open drain, the volume and character of exudate should be measured and recorded. If requested by the surgical team, gauze dressings can be weighed once saturated to ascertain the volume of drainage.	To minimize the risk of infection (Loveday et al. 2014, **R**).

9 Observe the drain to ensure the skin suture holding the drain in position is intact.	To ensure the drain is well secured and not withdrawn or retracted. Dislodgement can increase the risk of infection, erosion into adjacent structures (e.g. blood vessels or organs) and irritation to surrounding skin. **E**
10 Observe the skin surrounding the drain site for signs of excoriation, fluid collection or infection (inflammation of wound margins, pain, oedema, purulent exudate or pyrexia). *Note*: swabs of wound and drain sites should only be taken if infection is suspected.	To recognize and treat suspected complications (Fraise and Bradley 2009, **E**; Walker 2007, **E**).
11 Using aseptic technique, clean the surrounding skin with an appropriate sterile solution, such as 0.9% sodium chloride.	To minimize the risk of infection (Loveday et al. 2014, **R**; Wilkins and Unverdorben 2013, **E**).
12 If appropriate, cover the drain site as follows. a Closed drains should only be covered with a non-adherent, absorbent dressing if there is exudate or to promote patient comfort. b Open drains should be covered with a wound drainage bag (if exudate copious) or a small, absorbent, non-adhesive sterile gauze dressing (if only minimal exudate).	To allow effluent to drain, prevent excoriation of the skin, promote patient comfort and contain any odour. **E**
Post-procedure	
13 If applicable, tape the dressing securely. If the drain is attached to a drainage bag or bottle, it should also be secured at one other point (e.g. with adhesive tape).	To prevent the drain coming loose. **E**
14 If the drain is attached to a drainage bag or bottle, this should not be placed on the floor but placed below the level of the wound to allow drainage. If the drain is attached to a suction drain, ensure this is working correctly.	To ensure continuity of drainage. Ineffective drainage can result in oedema or haematoma. To minimize the risk of cross-infection (Hess 2012, **E**).
15 Check dressing/bag is secure and comfortable for the patient.	For patient comfort. **E**
16 Dispose of all clinical equipment in clinical waste bag or sharps bin according to local trust guidelines.	To ensure safe disposal. **E**
17 Document in the patient's notes that the dressing has been changed, and report any unusual signs or complications to surgical colleagues (NMC 2018). If the volume of exudate on the dressing has been measured, this should be documented on the fluid balance chart.	To ensure effective communication and instructions for ongoing care. For accurate documentation of drainage (NMC 2018, **C**).

Procedure guideline 16.8 Closed drainage systems: changing a vacuum bottle

This guideline is not to be used for underwater sealed drains (e.g. chest drains). See Chapter 12: Respiratory care, CPR and blood transfusion for such drains.

Essential equipment

- Personal protective equipment
- Dressing trolley or other suitable surface
- Alcohol/chlorhexidine wipe
- Sterile fluids for cleaning and/or irrigation, e.g. 0.9% sodium chloride
- Vacuum drainage bottle, e.g. Redivac
- Dressing pack, including sterile towel, gauze, gallipot and disposable bag
- Gloves: one disposable pair, one sterile pair

Optional equipment

- Any extra equipment that may be needed during the procedure, e.g. a clamp (although this is usually part of the drainage system in place) or hypoallergenic tape (to place on the side of the vacuum bottle to facilitate measurement of drain exudate)

Action	Rationale
Pre-procedure	
1 Introduce yourself to the patient, explain and discuss the procedure with them, and gain their consent to proceed.	To ensure that the patient feels at ease, understands the procedure and gives their valid consent (NMC 2018, **C**; Walker 2007, **C**).
2 Clean the trolley/tray and gather the equipment, checking the sterility and expiry date of the equipment and solutions, and place everything on the bottom of the trolley.	To minimize the risk of infection (Loveday et al. 2014, **R**).
3 Take the trolley/tray to the bed and adjust the bed to the correct height to avoid stooping.	To promote good manual handling. **E**

(continued)

Procedure guideline 16.8 Closed drainage systems: changing a vacuum bottle *(continued)*

Action	Rationale
4 Wash and dry hands thoroughly and put on apron and disposable gloves.	To minimize the risk of infection (NHS England and NHSI 2019, **C**).
Procedure	
5 Remove the dressing pack from the outer pack and place it on the top of the clean dressing trolley/tray. Using aseptic technique, open the packaging of the other equipment required during the procedure (sterile gloves, vacuum bottle, etc.) and place the contents onto the sterile field of the opened dressing pack.	To minimize the risk of infection (Fraise and Bradley 2009, **E**).
6 Clean hands with an alcohol-based handrub.	To prevent cross-contamination (NHS England and NHSI 2019, **C**).
7 Seal off the bottle by closing both sliding clamps on the drainage tubing leading from the patient and the bottle connector.	To prevent air and contamination entering the wound via the drain and to maintain the vacuum. **E**
8 Put on sterile gloves and, using a non-touch technique, place the sterile field/towel under the drain tubing at the connection point between the vacuum bottle and drain tubing.	To minimize the risk of infection (Loveday et al. 2014, **R**).
9 Disconnect the bottle by unscrewing the Luer-Lok, clean the end of the tube with an alcohol/chlorhexidine wipe and securely screw the new sterile bottle into the connecting tube at the Luer-Lok.	To maintain sterility. **E**
10 Unclamp both tubing clamps. Suction is established if the concertina bung remains compressed.	To re-establish the drainage system. **E**
11 The vacuum bottle should not be placed on the floor but placed below the level of the wound to allow drainage.	To ensure continuity of drainage. Ineffective drainage can result in oedema or haematoma. To minimize the risk of cross-infection (Hess 2012, **E**).
Post-procedure	
12 Measure the contents of the used drainage system and record any additional drainage in the appropriate documents.	To maintain an accurate record of drainage from the wound (NMC 2018, **C**).
13 Place the used vacuum drainage system into the clinical waste bag and dispose of it according to local trust policy.	To safely dispose of the used system. **E**
14 Document in patient's notes that the vacuum bottle has been changed.	To ensure effective communication and instructions for ongoing care and accurate documentation of drainage (NMC 2018, **C**).

Procedure guideline 16.9 Wound drain removal: closed drainage system

Essential equipment

- Personal protective equipment
- Dressing trolley or other suitable surface
- Detergent wipe
- Stitch cutter
- Sterile fluids for cleaning and/or irrigation, e.g. 0.9% sodium chloride
- Appropriate absorbent dry dressing (required special features of a dressing should be referred to in the patient's nursing care plan)
- Dressing pack, including sterile towel, gauze, gallipot and disposable bag
- Gloves: one disposable pair, one sterile pair
- Sterile dressing
- Hypoallergenic tape

Optional equipment

- Any extra equipment that may be needed during the procedure, e.g. microbiological swab or sterile specimen pot

Action	Rationale
Pre-procedure	
1 Introduce yourself to the patient, explain and discuss the procedure with them, and gain their consent to proceed.	To ensure that the patient feels at ease, understands the procedure and gives their valid consent (NMC 2018, **C**; Walker 2007, **C**).

2	Check patient comfort, for example position and pain level. Offer the patient analgesia as described on their chart or encourage self-administration via a patient-controlled analgesia pump (if applicable) and allow appropriate time for the medication to take effect. Another member of staff may be needed to reassure the patient during the procedure.	To promote patient comfort (NMC 2018, **C**).
3	If applicable, release the vacuum on the drainage bottle by clamping the tubing coming from the patient; keep the clamp on the bottle open. Loosen the Luer-Lok to allow air into the bottle. Reattach the Luer-Lok and release the clamp coming from the patient. Leave for 2–3 minutes. Note the amount of drainage in the bottle.	This releases the vacuum and prevents suction during the removal of the drain, which may cause tissue damage or pain (Walker 2007, **C**).
4	Clean the trolley/tray and gather the equipment, checking the sterility and expiry date of the equipment and solutions, and place everything on the bottom of the trolley.	To minimize the risk of infection (Loveday et al. 2014, **E**).
5	Take the trolley/tray to the bed and adjust the bed to the correct height to avoid stooping.	To promote good manual handling. **E**
6	Wash and dry hands thoroughly and put on an apron.	To minimize the risk of infection (NHS England and NHSI 2019, **C**).
Procedure		
7	Remove the dressing pack from the outer pack and place it on the top of the clean dressing trolley/tray. Using aseptic technique, open the packaging of the other equipment required during the procedure (sterile gloves, vacuum bottle, etc.) and place the contents onto the sterile field of the opened dressing pack.	To minimize the risk of infection (Loveday et al. 2014, **R**).
8	Expose the drain site, adjusting the patient's clothes to expose the wound, taking care to maintain their dignity.	To minimize the amount of skin exposed; to maintain dignity. **E**
9	Wearing disposable gloves, remove the dressing covering the drain site and place it in a soiled dressing bag away from the sterile field.	To minimize the risk of cross-infection (Loveday et al. 2014, **R**).
10	Wash and dry hands thoroughly and put on a fresh apron and sterile gloves using aseptic technique.	To minimize the risk of infection. Use of aseptic technique is essential when caring for and removing drains because micro-organisms may pass through the drain to tissue and body cavities, which may result in infection and surgical complications (Fraise and Bradley 2009, **E**; NHS England and NHSI 2019, **C**; Walker 2007, **C**).
11	Observe the skin surrounding the drain site for signs of excoriation, fluid collection or infection (inflammation of wound margins, pain, oedema, purulent exudate or pyrexia). If the drain site appears inflamed or purulent, a swab should be obtained and sent for microbiology and sensitivity analysis.	To assess the site for any signs and symptoms of infection and report findings to surgeons as needed (Knowlton 2015, **E**). To recognize and treat suspected complications (Fraise and Bradley 2009, **E**; Walker 2007, **C**).
12	The skin surrounding the drain site should only be cleansed (with 0.9% sodium chloride) if necessary – that is, if the drain site is purulent or to ensure the suture is visible and accessible.	To reduce the risk of infection (Fraise and Bradley 2009, **E**; Walker 2007, **C**).
13	Using a non-touch technique, place the sterile field under the drain tubing and gently lift up the knot of the suture with sterile forceps. Use the stitch cutter to cut the shortest end of the suture as close to the skin as possible and remove the suture with the forceps.	To allow space for the scissors or stitch cutter to be placed underneath. To minimize cross-infection by allowing the suture to be liberated from the drain without drawing the exposed part through tissue (Pudner 2010, **E**).
14	Warn the patient of the pulling sensation they will experience and reassure them throughout.	To promote comfort and co-operation (Walker 2007, **C**).
15	Fold up a sterile gauze swab several times to create an absorbent pad (Hess 2012). Loosening up of the drain should be done if possible, especially for a drain that has been in for some time. For round drains, this can be done by gently rotating the drain to 'break' it free. For flat ones, gentle movement from side to side can achieve this.	To minimize pain and reduce trauma. **E** Drains that have been left in for an extended period will sometimes be more difficult to remove due to tissue growing around the tubing (Walker 2007, **C**).
16	With gloved hand, place one finger on each side of the drain exit site, first stabilizing the skin around the drain with firm pressure. With the other hand, firmly grasp the drain as close to the skin as possible and gently remove it. Steady, gentle traction should be used to remove the drain rather than sudden, jerky movements. If there is resistance, place free gloved hand against the tissue to oppose the removal from the wound.	A firm grasp of the shortest length minimizes patient discomfort. This is especially important for supple drains such as those made from silicone or rubber, which can stretch for some distance and then suddenly break free (Walker 2007, **C**).

(continued)

Procedure guideline 16.9 Wound drain removal: closed drainage system *(continued)*

Action	Rationale
17 Maintain gentle pressure over the site for a few seconds until the drainage and/or bleeding has stopped or is minimal.	To prevent bleeding or leakage from the drain site. **E**
18 The edge of the drain should be clean cut and not jagged. The drain should be inspected to ensure that it is intact. If there is any doubt that the drain is intact, the surgeon should be contacted to inspect the drain before disposal.	This clean appearance ensures that the whole drain has been removed. **E**
19 Cover the drain site securely with a sterile dressing and tape. A wound management bag may be placed over a mature exit site if fluid discharge remains high after drain removal.	To prevent infection entering the drain site. **E** To prevent fluid collection or haematoma. A dressing may be necessary for 3–5 days to manage residual wound drainage (Knowlton 2015, **E**).
20 If the site is inflamed or there is a request for the tip of the drain to be sent to microbiology, cut the drain cleanly with sterile scissors and place the tip a sterile specimen container, maintaining asepsis.	To recognize and treat suspected infection (Fraise and Bradley 2009, **E**; Walker 2007, **C**).
21 Check the dressing/bag is secure and comfortable for the patient.	To promote patient comfort. **E**
Post-procedure	
22 Measure and record the contents of the drainage bottle in the appropriate documents.	To maintain an accurate record of drainage from the wound and enable evaluation of the state of the wound (NMC 2018, **C**).
23 Dispose of all clinical equipment in the clinical waste bag or sharps bin according to local trust guidelines.	To safely dispose of used equipment. **E**
24 Document in patient's notes that the drain has been removed, reporting complications to surgical colleagues.	To ensure effective communication and instructions for ongoing care. To ensure accurate documentation (NMC 2018, **C**).
25 Observe the drain site dressing for signs of excess fluid discharge (soaked dressing). On routine dressing change, observe the site for signs of infection (inflammation, oedema, purulent exudate or pyrexia) and obtain a wound swab if appropriate. Report any unusual signs or complications and record them in the appropriate documentation.	To recognize and treat potential complications (Fraise and Bradley 2009, **E**; Walker 2007, **C**). To ensure accurate documentation of any unusual signs or complications (NMC 2018, **C**).

Procedure guideline 16.10 Wound drain shortening for open drainage systems

Essential equipment

- Personal protective equipment
- Dressing trolley or other suitable surface
- Detergent wipe
- Stitch cutter
- Sterile fluids for cleaning and/or irrigation, e.g. 0.9% sodium chloride
- Appropriate absorbent dry dressing (required special features of a dressing should be referred to in the patient's nursing care plan)
- Sterile safety pin
- Dressing pack, including sterile towel, gauze, gallipot and disposable bag
- Gloves: one disposable pair, one sterile pair
- Sterile dressing
- Hypoallergenic tape

Optional equipment

- Any extra equipment that may be needed during the procedure, e.g. microbiological swab or sterile specimen pot

Action	Rationale
Pre-procedure	
1 Check the medical notes to identify which drain is to be shortened. Introduce yourself to the patient, explain and discuss the procedure with them, and gain their consent to proceed.	To ensure that the patient feels at ease, understands the procedure and gives their valid consent (NMC 2018, **C**).
2 Check patient comfort, for example position and pain level. Offer the patient analgesia as described on their chart or encourage self-administration via a patient-controlled analgesia pump (if applicable) and allow appropriate time for the medication to take effect. Another member of staff may be needed to reassure the patient during the procedure.	To promote patient comfort (NMC 2018, **C**).

3 Clean the trolley/tray and gather the equipment, checking the sterility and expiry date of the equipment and solutions, and place everything on the bottom of the trolley.	To minimize the risk of infection (Loveday et al. 2014, **R**).
4 Take the trolley/tray to the bed and adjust the bed to the correct height to avoid stooping.	To promote good manual handling. **E**
5 Wash and dry hands thoroughly and put on apron.	To minimize the risk of infection (NHS England and NHSI 2019, **C**).
Procedure	
6 Remove the dressing pack from the outer pack and place it on the top of the clean dressing trolley/tray. Using aseptic technique, open the packaging of the other equipment required during the procedure (sterile gloves, dressing, etc.) and place the contents onto the sterile field of the opened dressing pack.	To minimize the risk of infection (Loveday et al. 2014, **R**).
7 Expose the drain site, adjusting the patient's clothes to expose the wound, taking care to maintain their dignity.	To minimize the amount of skin exposed; to maintain dignity. **E**
8 Wearing disposable gloves, remove the dressing covering the drain site and place it in a soiled dressing bag away from the sterile field.	To minimize the risk of cross-infection (Loveday et al. 2014, **R**).
9 Wash and dry hands thoroughly and put on a fresh apron and sterile gloves using aseptic technique.	To minimize the risk of infection (NHS England and NHSI 2019, **C**). Use of an aseptic technique is essential when caring for and removing drains because micro-organisms may pass through the drain to tissue and body cavities, which may result in infection and surgical complications (Walker 2007, **E**).
10 Observe the skin surrounding the drain site for signs of excoriation, fluid collection or infection (inflammation of wound margins, pain, oedema, purulent exudate or pyrexia). If the drain site appears inflamed or purulent, a swab should be obtained and sent for microbiology and sensitivity analysis.	To recognize and treat suspected complications (NICE 2019, **E**).
11 The skin surrounding the drain site should only be cleansed (with 0.9% sodium chloride) if necessary – that is, if the drain site is purulent or to ensure the suture is visible and accessible.	To reduce the risk of infection (Loveday et al. 2014, **R**).
12 Using a non-touch technique, place the sterile field under the drain tubing. If the drain is sutured in place, gently lift up the knot of the suture with sterile forceps (**Action figure 12**). Use the stitch cutter to cut the shortest end of the suture as close to the skin as possible and remove the suture with the forceps.	To allow space for the scissors or stitch cutter to be placed underneath. To minimize cross-infection by allowing the suture to be liberated from the drain without drawing the exposed part through tissue (Pudner 2010, **E**).
13 Warn the patient of the pulling sensation they will experience and reassure them throughout.	To promote comfort and co-operation (Walker 2007, **E**).
14 With a gloved hand, place one finger on each side of the drain exit site, first stabilizing the skin around the drain with firm pressure. With the other hand, grasp the drain firmly as close to the skin as possible and gently ease the drain out of the wound to the length requested by the surgeon. Steady, gentle traction should be used to ease the drain out rather than sudden, jerky movements. If there is resistance, place free gloved hand against the tissue to oppose the removal from the wound.	A firm grasp of the shortest length minimizes patient discomfort. This is especially important for supple drains such as those made from silicone or rubber, which can stretch for some distance and then suddenly break free (Walker 2007, **E**). To allow healing to take place from the base of the wound. **E**
15 Using gloved hand, place a sterile safety pin through the drain as close to the skin as possible, taking great care not to stab either yourself or the patient (**Action figure 15**). Sterile tape should be used to secure the drain to the skin.	To prevent retraction of the drain into the wound and minimize the risk of cross-infection and sharps injury. **E** The tape is used as an additional measure to prevent the drain from falling out. **E**
16 Cover the drain site with a suitably sized sterile gauze dressing (taped securely) or a wound drainage bag (depending upon volume of exudate).	To prevent infection entering the drain site. **E** To prevent fluid collection or haematoma. **E**
17 Check dressing/bag is secure and comfortable for the patient.	To promote patient comfort. **E**

(continued)

Procedure guideline 16.10 Wound drain shortening for open drainage systems *(continued)*

Action	Rationale
Post-procedure	
18 Dispose of all clinical equipment in the clinical waste bag or sharps bin according to local trust guidelines.	To safely dispose of used equipment. **E**
19 Document in the patient's notes that the drain has been withdrawn, clearly stating: • length of drain withdrawn (in centimetres) • length of drain left visible from wound exit site to end of drain (in centimetres) • any complications during the procedure. Report complications to surgical colleagues.	To ensure effective communication and instructions for ongoing care (NMC 2018, **C**).
20 Observe the drain site dressing for signs of excess fluid discharge (soaked dressing). On routine dressing change, observe the site for signs of drain retraction, withdrawal or infection (inflammation, oedema, purulent exudate or pyrexia) and obtain a wound swab if appropriate. Report any unusual signs or complications and record in appropriate documentation.	To recognize and treat potential complications (Fraise and Bradley 2009; Walker 2007, **E**). To ensure accurate documentation of any unusual signs or complications (NMC 2018, **C**).

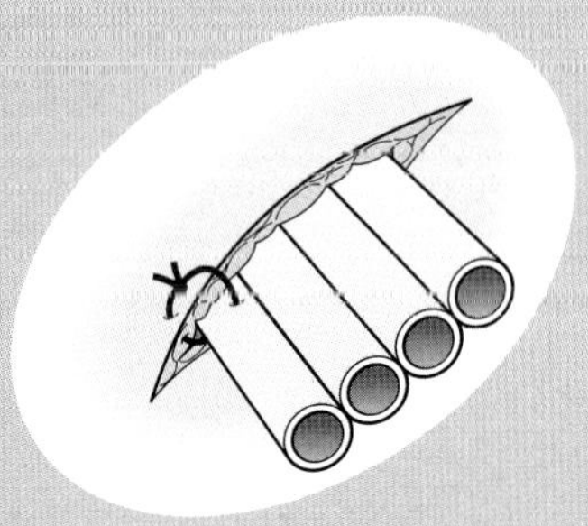

Action Figure 12 Use forceps to gently lift the knot of the suture.

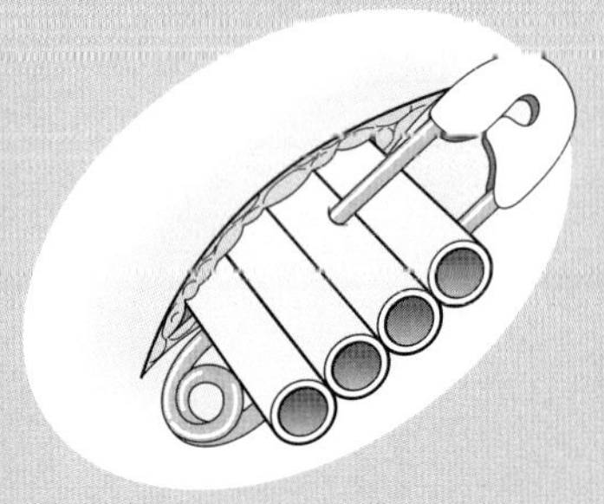

Action Figure 15 Position of safety pin through open drain to prevent retraction.

Procedure guideline 16.11 Wound drain shortening for closed drainage systems

This is also known as the 'cut and bag' procedure.

Essential equipment

- Personal protective equipment
- Dressing trolley or other suitable surface
- Detergent wipe
- Stitch cutter
- Sterile fluids for cleaning and/or irrigation, e.g. 0.9% sodium chloride
- Appropriate absorbent dry dressing (required special features of a dressing should be referred to in the patient's nursing care plan)
- Sterile safety pin
- Dressing pack, including sterile towel, gauze, gallipot and disposable bag
- Gloves: one disposable pair, one sterile pair
- Two-piece wound drainage bag
- Hypoallergenic tape

Optional equipment

- Any extra equipment that may be needed during the procedure, e.g. microbiological swab or sterile specimen pot

Action	Rationale
Pre-procedure	
1 Check the medical notes to identify which drain is to be shortened (cut and bagged). Introduce yourself to the patient, explain and discuss the procedure with them, and gain their consent to proceed.	To ensure that the patient feels at ease, understands the procedure and gives their valid consent (NMC 2018, **C**).
2 Check patient comfort, for example position and pain level. Offer the patient analgesia as described on their chart or encourage self-administration via a patient-controlled analgesia pump (if applicable) and allow appropriate time for the medication to take effect. Another member of staff may be needed to reassure the patient during the procedure.	To promote patient comfort (NMC 2018, **C**).

3 Clean the trolley/tray and gather the equipment, checking the sterility and expiry date of the equipment and solutions, and place everything on the bottom of the trolley.	To minimize the risk of infection (Loveday et al. 2014, **E**).
4 Take the trolley/tray to the bed and adjust the bed to the correct height to avoid stooping.	To promote good manual handling. **E**
5 Wash and dry hands thoroughly and put on apron.	To minimize the risk of infection (NHS England and NHSI 2019, **C**).

Procedure

6 Remove the dressing pack from the outer pack and place it on the top of the clean dressing trolley/tray. Using aseptic technique, open the packaging of the other equipment required during the procedure (sterile gloves, dressing, etc.) and place the contents onto the sterile field of the opened dressing pack.	To minimize the risk of infection (Loveday et al. 2014, **R**).
7 Expose the drain site, adjusting the patient's clothes to expose the wound, taking care to maintain their dignity.	To minimize the amount of skin exposed; to maintain dignity. **E**
8 Wearing disposable gloves, remove the dressing covering the drain site and place it in a soiled dressing bag away from the sterile field.	To minimize the risk of cross-infection (Loveday et al. 2014, **C**).
9 Wash and dry hands thoroughly and put on a fresh apron and sterile gloves using aseptic technique.	To minimize the risk of infection (Loveday et al. 2014, **R**; NHS England and NHSI 2019, **C**). Use of an aseptic technique is essential when caring for and removing drains because micro-organisms may pass through the drain to tissue and body cavities, which may result in infection and surgical complications (Walker 2007, **E**).
10 Observe the skin surrounding the drain site for signs of excoriation, fluid collection or infection (inflammation of wound margins, pain, oedema, purulent exudate or pyrexia). If the drain site appears inflamed or purulent, a swab should be obtained and sent for microbiology and sensitivity analysis.	To recognize and treat suspected complications (Fraise and Bradley 2009, **E**; Walker 2007, **E**).
11 The skin surrounding the drain site should only be cleansed (with 0.9% sodium chloride) if necessary – that is, if the drain site is purulent or to ensure the suture is visible and accessible.	To reduce the risk of infection (Loveday et al. 2014, **R**).
12 Using a non-touch technique, place the sterile field under the drain tubing. Using sterile scissors, cut the drain approximately 7–10 cm from the patient's skin, taking care to securely hold the drain in place at the patient's side with a gloved hand.	To prevent retraction of the drain back into the body (retained drain) if the drain is cut too short. **E**
13 Measure the contents of the drainage bag and place it in a soiled dressing bag away from the sterile field.	To maintain an accurate record of drainage from the wound (NMC 2018, **C**).
14 Remove the sticky backing from the flange of the two-piece drainage bag and carefully place the flange over the drainage tube and onto the skin. Check the aperture on the flange fits snugly around the drain tube. Hold the flange in place for a few minutes to ensure a good seal.	To prevent excoriation of the surrounding skin. **E**
15 Using gloved hand, place a sterile safety pin through the drain as close to the skin as possible, taking great care not to stab either yourself or the patient.	To prevent retraction of the drain into the wound and minimize the risk of cross-infection and sharps injury. **E**
16 Carefully place the drainage bag over the drain and click it into place.	To prevent infection entering the drain site. **E** To prevent fluid collection or haematoma. **E**
17 Check the dressing/bag is secure and comfortable for the patient.	To promote patient comfort. **E**

Post-procedure

18 Measure and record the contents of the drainage bag in the appropriate documentation.	To maintain an accurate record of drainage from the wound and enable evaluation of the state of the wound (NMC 2018, **C**).
19 Dispose of all clinical equipment in the clinical waste bag or sharps bin according to local trust guidelines.	To safely dispose of used equipment. **E**

(continued)

Procedure guideline 16.11 Wound drain shortening for closed drainage systems *(continued)*

Action	Rationale
20 Document in the patient's notes that the drain has been cut and bagged, clearly stating: • length of drain left visible from wound exit site to end of drain (in centimetres) • any complications during the procedure. Report complications to surgical colleagues.	To ensure effective communication and instructions for ongoing care (NMC 2018, **C**).
21 Observe the drain site dressing for signs of excess fluid discharge (soaked dressing). On routine dressing change, observe the site for signs of drain retraction, withdrawal or infection (inflammation, oedema, purulent exudate or pyrexia) and obtain a wound swab if appropriate. Report any unusual signs or complications and record in appropriate documentation.	To recognize and treat potential complications (Fraise and Bradley 2009, **E**; Walker 2007, **E**). To ensure accurate documentation of any usual signs or complications (NMC 2018, **C**).

Problem-solving table 16.2 Prevention and resolution (Procedure guidelines 16.7, 16.8, 16.9, 16.10 and 16.11)

This refers to open and closed drainage systems only (not chest drains). The surgical team must be contacted in the event of any of the following problems occurring.

Problem	Cause	Prevention	Action
Blocked drain Blockage should be suspected when there is a sudden drop in drainage output, lower output than expected, or no output at all.	Overly tight sutures, kinking. Ingrowth or collapse of surrounding tissues. Debris accumulation and blood clots in the lumen. Commonly a drain is blocked due to lumenal debris, which may not be visible from external inspection.	Drain tubing and connections should be regularly inspected for blockages or kinks.	**The surgical team should be informed prior to any action being taken.** *'Milk'* Manual 'milking' of debris out through the drain can help to dislodge the obstruction or break it up into smaller debris. This can be done by gently squeezing the tube between your thumb and index finger while moving your fingers along the tubing towards the suction bottle.
Unexpected fall in drain output may result from drain dislodgement rather than blockage. Advice should be obtained from the surgical team prior to any intervention.			*Aspirate* After ruling out external compression, a drain can usually be unblocked by aspirating the drain according to local trust guidelines. **This should not be undertaken without instruction from the surgical team.** *Flush* Failing aspiration and milking, an attempt can be made to flush the drain with sterile saline using aseptic technique according to local trust guidelines. This can push back in any debris too large to be aspirated through the drain. Flushing also helps to re-establish drainage where tissue collapse or adhesion around the drain interferes with its function. **No attempt should be made to flush a drain without instruction and guidance from the surgical team that inserted the drain.**
Leaking drain	Determined by site of leakage. Leakage occurring around the exit site of a suction drain is usually due to a blocked drain rather than a perforation in the drain. The drainage fluid may find its way out along the external surface of the drain when the lumen is blocked. Leakage around the tubing or connections is due to damaged tubing or connections. Skin incision too big for the drain.	Drain tubing and connections should be regularly inspected for blockages, kinks or damaged tubing/connectors. Ensure the drainage bag is lower than the drain site.	**The surgical team should be informed prior to any action being taken.** *Blocked drain* Unblock the drain using the methods outlined above for blocked drains. *Connections* Using aseptic technique, replace the tubing according to the manufacturer's instructions and tighten the connections as appropriate. *Reduce the size of the skin incision* If the skin incision is too big, report this to the surgical team for guidance. They may consider an additional suture or may cut and bag the drain to collect the leaking exudate. See Procedure guideline 16.11: Wound drain shortening for closed drainage systems for information on the 'cut and bag' procedure.

Problem	Cause	Prevention	Action
Loose drain	Causes may include the drain-securing suture cutting through the skin, loose knot tying or traction on the drain.	The majority of drains need to be well secured, preferably at two points. Ensure regular observation of the drain to check it is firmly secured at its exit site (e.g. with a suture) and one other point (e.g. with adhesive tape). Be aware of the length of the drain from exit site at the skin to the drainage bag (if applicable); this should be documented in nursing/medical notes.	**The surgical team should be informed prior to any action being taken.** Loose drains must be re-secured appropriately and promptly. If the suture around the drain appears loose, the surgical team should be contacted immediately, and they may consider placing a stitch through the skin next to the drain exit site under local anaesthetic, then tying the suture securely around the drain. Extra security can be provided by taping the drain/ tubing to the skin. Open drains should be prevented from falling into the drainage cavity, e.g. by passing a large sterile safety pin through the drain. See step 15 in Procedure guideline 16.10: Wound drain shortening for open drainage systems for guidance on how to perform this procedure.
Drain retraction	Drain retraction is caused by a loose drain being pushed inwards, e.g. during dressing change or from patient movement.	The majority of drains need to be well secured, preferably at two points. Ensure regular observation of the drain to check it is firmly secured at its exit site (e.g. with a suture) and one other point (e.g. with adhesive tape). Be aware of the length of the drain from exit site at the skin to the drainage bag (if applicable); this should be documented in nursing/medical notes.	**The surgical team should be informed prior to any action being taken**. *Re-secure* This should be dealt with as a loose drain (see 'Loose drain' above). **Alert:** Drains suspected to have partially retracted inside a wound should be left in place and properly re-secured by a member of the surgical team and a safety pin placed through the tubing to prevent further retraction (see Procedure guidelines 16.10 and 16.11). **Alert:** Attempts to pull the drain back out **should be avoided** unless the distance of retraction is known (e.g. drain retraction witnessed or length at skin surface marked). Otherwise any attempt to pull the drain back out may lead to it being dislodged altogether. *Reposition* Drains that have clearly retracted inwards should be pulled out by a member of the surgical team to a length that allows removal at a later date before being re-secured. **Alert:** A drain that is 'cut and bagged' must always be secured with a large, sterile safety pin placed through the external tubing close to the skin to prevent retraction (see Procedure guideline 16.10).
Drain appears to be falling out or has fallen out	This may be due to: • failure of the sutures to secure the drain • tethering of the drain or drainage bottle/bag • breakage of the drain • tugging of the drain by the patient or staff • retraction of the drain.	The majority of drains need to be well secured, preferably at two points. Ensure regular observation of the drain to check it is firmly secured at its exit site (e.g. with a suture) and one other point (e.g. with adhesive tape). Be aware of the length of drain the from exit site at the skin to the drainage bag (if applicable); this should be documented in nursing/medical notes.	**In this event a member of the surgical team should be contacted immediately for guidance.** *Re-secure* A drain that has only partially migrated out should be re-secured and the surgical team informed. **It should not be pushed back in** as the externalized part is now contaminated. *Examine* If a drain has fallen out completely, the tube must be inspected to ensure that the drain is intact and saved for inspection by the surgeon. Also ensure that no part of the drain is left inside. If there is any doubt, an X-ray should be performed to ensure no part of the drain remains inside the body. The surgeon will decide if the drain requires replacement and make the necessary arrangements. A wound management bag may be placed over the exit site to catch any ongoing drainage from a mature tract.

(continued)

Problem-solving table 16.2 Prevention and resolution (Procedure guidelines 16.7, 16.8, 16.9, 16.10 and 16.11) *(continued)*

Problem	Cause	Prevention	Action
Broken drain or tubing, or retained drain	This is usually caused by repetitive physical trauma with potential contributing factors including: • manufacturing defects • drain weakness as a result of prolonged use • contact with digestive enzymes in body fluids • accidental tethering of the tube/bag. A high-risk factor is a drain that is 'cut and bagged' without use of a safety pin.	The majority of drains need to be well secured, preferably at two points. Ensure regular observation of the drain to check it is firmly secured at its exit site (e.g. with a suture) and one other point (e.g. with adhesive tape).	**In this event a member of the surgical team should be contacted immediately for guidance.** *Replacement* If breakage occurs to the external part of the drain or tubing, then the drain might still be able to function. It may be reconnected to a new reservoir or have tubing replaced as appropriate. A safety pin should be placed through the tubing to prevent retraction. *Removal* If the break is flush with the skin exit site, the surgeon should be contacted immediately and then it should be removed by the surgeon so as not to push it further inside the wound. The surgeon will do this using aseptic technique, taking care to avoid pushing the broken part further inside or creating tissue bleeding, which may further obscure vision. If the surgeon is unable to remove the drain, intraoperative removal under X-ray guidance or an open procedure may be necessary.
Inflamed drain exit site	Minimal redness can often be seen around drain exit sites due to local irritation. Cellulitis at the drain exit site may appear as a more pronounced zone of redness, warmth and tenderness. Fever and/or tachycardia may also be present as part of the systemic inflammatory response. Purulent discharge at the drain exit site may persist around drains that have been in place beyond the acute post-operative phase. However, the discharge must be examined by the surgical team to distinguish between purulent drainage fluid coming up around the outside of the drain and local abscess collection (unusual).	The majority of drains need to be well secured, preferably at two points. Ensure regular observation of the drain to check it is firmly secured at its exit site (e.g. with a suture) and one other point (e.g. with adhesive tape). Cleanliness of site.	*Irritation* If local irritation is suspected, no treatment is required other than good wound care according to local trust guidelines to keep the drain exit site clean and dry, and regular monitoring of the drain to ensure it is firmly secured at the exit site (e.g. with a suture) and one other point (e.g. with adhesive tape). *Cellulitis* The surgical team should be informed if cellulitis is suspected as this can indicate inadequate drainage. Antibiotics are **not** indicated unless there is significant associated cellulitis or systemic immunosuppression. *Purulent discharge* If an abscess has been excluded, then local care for a small wound should be given according to local trust guidelines. Where there is an abscess collection, the treatment in some cases is drainage by a member of the surgical team using appropriate aseptic technique. This can usually be done via a simple incision after infiltration with local anaesthetic. Antibiotics are **not** indicated unless there is significant associated cellulitis or systemic immunosuppression.
Atypical drainage fluids	Unexpected fluids coming up from around a drain or in the drain lumen may be due to: • anastomotic leaks • drain erosion into adjacent structures, e.g. bowel, bladder or blood vessels; the likelihood of tissue erosion is increased by the fragility of the local tissues (e.g. in the presence of local inflammation, infection or necrosis), the use of large or rigid drains, and the use of continuous high pressure suction, which sucks surrounding tissues into the drain holes.	Ensure the drain is well secured to minimize the risk of tissue erosion into adjacent structures.	**In this event a member of the surgical team should be contacted immediately for guidance.** *Bleeding or early bleeding* The team registrar or consultant must be notified of any significant bleeding. Superficial bleeding will usually settle with local pressure but on occasion may require additional suturing by a member of the surgical team. Deep bleeding may need angiography or surgery.

Problem	Cause	Prevention	Action
	Blood Bleeding can be deep or superficial, early or delayed. *Early bleeding* This usually results from a vessel being accidentally pierced by the trocar during insertion or by the drain stitch.		
	Delayed bleeding May indicate erosion of a vessel by the drain anywhere along the drain tract. Erosion into blood vessels may appear as an initial 'herald bleed' consisting of a brief and bright fresh bleed, which may be followed by a more catastrophic haemorrhage at a later stage.	Ensure the drain is well secured to minimize the risk of tissue erosion into adjacent structures.	*Anastomotic leak or tissue erosion* There are several possible approaches, including observation only, reducing or stopping suction (if applicable), partial withdrawal of the drain, removal of the drain or intraoperative repair. The approach taken will be determined by the surgical team. Anastomotic leaks may be verified by testing for appropriate biochemical markers (e.g. amylase for suspect pancreatic anastomotic leak or creatinine for urinary tract anastomotic leak). If the concentration of the particular biochemical marker in the drainage fluid is significantly higher than the serum concentration, then leakage should be suspected.
High drainage output	Unless it is suspected that the drain is blocked, a sudden increase in drain output usually signifies a complication, such as an anastomotic leak or erosion into adjacent organs (see 'Atypical drainage fluids' above).	n/a	**In this event a member of the surgical team should be contacted immediately for guidance.** Management steps appropriate to the cause should be undertaken.
Vacuum failure for suction drains When the vacuum suction reservoir fills with air, loss of vacuum has occurred.	This may be the result of: • an air leak in the actual drain or the connecting tubing • a problem with the actual reservoir, e.g. failure to close a cap or presence of a puncture in the reservoir • less commonly, this may be due to the development of a communication between the drainage cavity and the external environment (e.g. wound dehiscence) or an adjacent hollow viscus (e.g. fistula development).	The drain's tubing and connections should be regularly inspected to ensure the maintenance of the vacuum within the bottle (according to the manufacturer's instructions).	If the vacuum of the drainage system is continually being lost, check all connections for evidence of an air leak and for any wound drain perforations exposed above skin level. Any drain hole outside the skin should be covered with an occlusive dressing or bandaging using aseptic technique to stop the air leak. Air leaks elsewhere in the system should be stopped, preferably by tightening of connections and/or replacement of any defective component. Otherwise occlusive tape may also be used to seal such defects. If no air leak or suction reservoir defect is found, an opened wound edge or some abnormal communication from the drainage cavity ought to be suspected. The surgical team must be notified.
Drain appears stuck and will not come out on attempted removal.	Potential causes include: • stitches remain *in situ* • the drain may just have been in for so long that tissue has grown into it, or perhaps tissue has been sucked into the side holes.	Check operation notes to determine number and types of sutures *in situ* prior to attempting drain removal.	Recheck operation notes to ensure all non-absorbable stitches have been removed. Loosening up of the drain should be done if possible, especially for a drain that has been in for some time. For round drains, this can be done by gently rotating the drain to release it. For flat drains, gentle movement from side to side can achieve this. *Note*: removal using excess force should not be attempted. Assistance from the surgical team should be sought if the drain does not loosen easily.

Source: Adapted from Ngo et al. (2004) and Nottingham University Hospital and Rushcliffe PCT (2006).

Surgical wounds

Definition

Surgical wounds are incisions through the skin that are made by a cutting instrument (e.g. scalpel). This allows a surgeon to gain access to the deeper tissues or organs. Surgical incisions are usually clean and cause minimal tissue loss and disruption. They are made in a sterile environment, where many variables can be controlled, such as bacteria, size, location and the nature of the wound itself (Toon et al. 2015).

A wound results in tissue damage, which stimulates a co-ordinated physiological response to provide haemostasis and initiate the processes of inflammation. A surgical wound is classified as an 'acute wound', which is a controlled form of trauma (Singh et al. 2017).

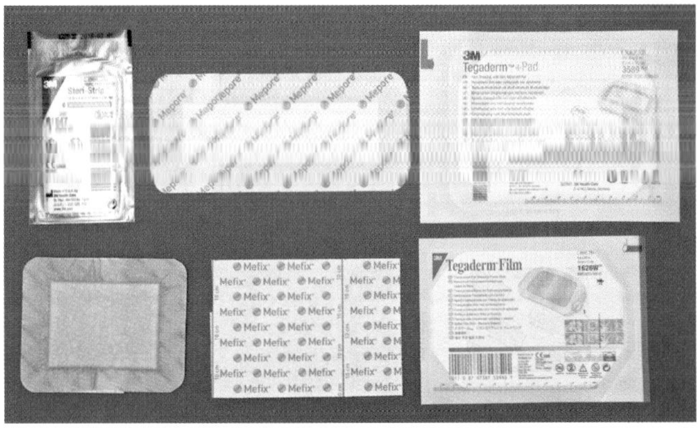

Figure 16.40 Surgical wound dressings.

Related theory

Surgical wounds are usually closed fully at the end of the procedure. This is known as 'primary closure' and is done using one of four devices, depending on the type of surgery and the surgeon's preference. They are:

- sutures (absorbable and non-absorbable)
- adhesive skin closure strips (e.g. Steri-Strips)
- tissue adhesive
- staples.

Non-absorbable sutures, Steri-Strips and staples need to be removed but only on the advice of the surgical team, usually 7–10 days post-operatively.

Dressings for surgical wounds

The location of the wound and the method of wound closure usually determine whether the wound is dressed or not. In a closed surgical wound (i.e. one closed by sutures or clips), the main functions of a wound dressing are to:

- promote healing by providing a moist environment without causing maceration (softening and deterioration) of the surrounding skin
- protect the wound from potentially harmful agents (e.g. bacterial contamination) or injury
- allow appropriate assessment of the wound post-operatively
- absorb exudates (e.g. blood or haemoserous fluids)
- ease discomfort (preventing the wound rubbing on clothing) (NICE 2019).

NICE (2015) describes three categories of wound dressing (Figure 16.40) that are used post-operatively:

- *passive*: designed solely to cover the wound, neither promoting nor intentionally hindering the wound-healing process (e.g. 'gauze-like' materials)
- *interactive*: designed to promote the wound-healing process through the creation and maintenance of a warm, moist environment underneath the chosen dressing (e.g. alginates, foams, hydrocolloids and semi-permeable film)
- *active*: designed to manipulate or alter the wound-healing environment to either re-stimulate or further promote the healing process (e.g. collagen and negative pressure therapy) (see Chapter 18: Wound management).

Current guidance states that surgical incisions should be covered with an appropriate interactive dressing at the end of an operation (NICE 2015). However, a systematic review published in 2011 that evaluated the clinical effectiveness of wound dressings for preventing surgical site infection concluded that there is no evidence to suggest that applying a wound dressing to a surgical wound healing by primary intention reduces the risk of surgical site infection (Dumville et al. 2011).

When dressings are applied in theatre, it is recommended that they are not removed unless exudate, commonly termed 'strike-through', is evident or clinical signs of local or systemic infection (e.g. malodour or fever) occur. Unless contraindicated, dressings changes required within 48 hours of surgery should be undertaken using aseptic non-touch technique and sterile normal saline (see Chapter 4: Infection prevention and control). While some dressings allow early bathing or showering of the rest of the patient after 48 hours, this should be confirmed with the surgeon performing the procedure (NICE 2015).

Studies have demonstrated that it is unnecessary to dress surgical wounds after 72 hours as a surgical wound that has good apposition is sealed against pathogenic invasion by epithelialization in approximately 48–72 hours (Dumville et al. 2011, Toon et al. 2015); however, the application of wound dressings and their removal and subsequent renewal will depend upon local trust protocols. Careful assessment of the wound and the peri-wound tissues is vital to monitor wound healing and to aid dressing selection; this should be evaluated at each dressing change (Vowden and Vowden 2017). If a dressing is required, it should be changed using aseptic non-touch technique, to prevent micro-organisms being introduced into the wound (NICE 2019).

The choice of dressing will depend on which qualities are required (i.e. absorptive or supportive) and should be made according to surgical recommendation (Dumville et al. 2011). Gauze-based dressings should not be used to dress surgical wounds as these can completely adhere to the wound and become part of the healing tissue, causing excessive pain and wound damage (Vermeulen et al. 2005).

Patient education and psychological support will be required prior to exposing a wound as it may cause patient distress. On discharge, the patient should be referred to a community nurse and/or be educated about how to care for the surgical wound. Verbal and written information should be given to the patient; it should include the need to observe for signs of infection and swelling or seroma formation, and information on how to seek support and advice if such an event arises.

Complications

Surgical wound complications are important causes of early and late post-operative morbidity (Mizell 2012). Surgical wounds in normal, healthy individuals heal through an orderly sequence of physiological events that include inflammation, epithelialization, fibroplasia and maturation. Failure of wound healing following surgery can lead to various complications, including dehiscence, surgical site infection, seroma and haematoma.

Problem solving table 16.3 Surgical wound complications: prevention and resolution

The surgical team must be contacted in the event of any of the following problems occurring.

Problem	Cause	Prevention	Action
Dehiscence: partial or total disruption of any or all layers of the surgical wound.	Systemic factors such as diabetes mellitus, cancer, immunosuppression. Local factors: • inadequate closure of surgical wound site • tight suturing, which can tear the skin and affect the vascularity of the wound edges, and may result in necrosis and wound breakdown • increased intra-abdominal pressure (ileus) • suboptimal wound care • impaired wound healing caused by infection, seroma, haematoma or drains • impaired wound healing caused by poor perfusion of the wound bed due to risk factors including smoking, male sex, obesity, rheumatoid arthritis or malnutrition.	Reduce risk factors (see the 'Cause' column) via comprehensive pre-assessment. Ensure adequate closure of the surgical wound intraoperatively.	Action is dependent upon level of dehiscence, which may consist of any of the following: • a sudden discharge of fluid or cellulitis along the suture line • the splitting open of the skin layers • complete dehiscence of the muscle and fascia, exposing internal organs, and occasionally incisional hernia with outer layers intact. *Note*: if dehiscence is suspected then a member of the surgical team should be contacted immediately for guidance. *Minor dehiscence* Local care for a small wound should be given according to local trust guidelines. Wound manager bags are occasionally indicated to drain the excessive exudate from a partially dehisced wound, particularly if skin integrity is compromised. *Partial (deep) or full dehiscence* In this event, a member of the surgical team should be contacted **immediately** for guidance. Management steps appropriate to the cause should be undertaken.
Surgical site infection (SSI): when pathogenic organisms multiply in a wound, giving rise to local and systemic signs and symptoms. SSI can occur at the incision site or in subcutaneous dead space. Symptoms include localized erythema, purulent exudates, tenderness and wound odour at the incision site. In more serious cases, systemic signs of infection (including raised temperature and raised white cell count) may be present. Infection in the surgical wound may prevent healing taking place so that the wound edges separate or it may cause an abscess to form in the deeper tissues.	Systemic factors such as diabetes mellitus, cancer or immunosuppression. Local factors: • inadequate closure of surgical wound site • suboptimal wound care • impaired wound healing caused by poor perfusion of the wound bed due to risk factors including smoking, male gender, rheumatoid arthritis or malnutrition. Obesity, which causes increased subcutaneous dead space, rendering the patient more susceptible to infection. Drains and sutures. Poor hand hygiene contaminating the surgical site.	Reduce risk factors (see the 'Cause' column) via comprehensive pre-assessment. Ensure adequate closure of the surgical wound intraoperatively. Ensure optimal wound care is provided.	Some signs of SSI (including erythema and tenderness) are also seen in the normal post-operative inflammatory response, lasting up to 48 hours. Persistent inflammation beyond this period, the presence of pus or purulent discharge, or pyrexia may indicate infection. *Note*: if infection is suspected then a member of the surgical team should be contacted **immediately** for guidance. A swab, pus sample and blood cultures (if systemic signs of infection, e.g. pyrexia, are present) should be taken to identify the causative micro-organism and appropriate treatment commenced to eradicate it. Antibiotics will usually only be given if adjacent tissue is inflamed or there are systemic signs of infection. In more serious cases, infected wounds may need to be opened and explored or debrided.

(continued)

Problem-solving table 16.3 Surgical wound complications: prevention and resolution *(continued)*

Problem	Cause	Prevention	Action
Haematoma: collection of blood. The blood seeps from blood vessels that are cut during the operation to remove tissue.	Inadequate haemostasis. Use of coagulants. Obesity, which causes increased subcutaneous dead space, rendering the patient more susceptible to haematoma formation.	Ensure adequate haemostasis. Reduce risk factors (see the 'Cause' column) via comprehensive pre-assessment.	Action is dependent upon manifestation. Haematomas can be asymptomatic or manifest as swelling with pain. They can cause the incision to separate and become predisposed to wound infection, since bacteria can gain access to deeper layers and multiply uninhibited in the stagnant blood. *Small haematomas* These can be managed expectantly and may resolve with no intervention as, once the small vessels heal, no further blood collects and the haematoma will gradually be absorbed by the body. *Large haematomas* These may require drainage under sterile conditions by needle aspiration. This will be undertaken by a member of the surgical team.
Seroma: collection of serous fluid. The fluid seeps from small blood and lymph vessels that are cut during the operation to remove the tissue or lymph nodes. Most frequently seen under split-thickness skin grafts and in areas with large dead spaces (e.g. axilla, groin, neck or pelvis).	Difficult surgery. Obesity, which causes increased subcutaneous dead space, rendering the patient more susceptible to seroma formation.	Reduce risk factors (see the 'Cause' column) via comprehensive pre-assessment.	Action is dependent upon manifestation. Seromas can be asymptomatic or manifest as swelling with pain. Seromas can cause the incision to separate and become predisposed to wound infection since bacteria can gain access to deeper layers and multiply uninhibited in the stagnant fluid. *Small seromas* These can be managed expectantly and may resolve with no intervention as, once the small vessels heal, no further fluid collects and the seroma will gradually be absorbed by the body, usually over 1 month. *Large seromas* These may require drainage under sterile conditions by needle aspiration. This will be undertaken by a member of the surgical team.
Allergic reaction: local rash, redness and/or itching at the site of the surgical wound.	Allergic reaction to surgical dressing or topical ointment applied intraoperatively.	Ensure identification of allergies via comprehensive pre-assessment.	Remove the allergen (dressing or ointment). If the allergic reaction is severe, give antihistamine. Document the allergy according to local policy, e.g. update the patient's records to alert other healthcare professionals. Inform the patient.

Source: Adapted from Escobar and Knight (2012), Mizell (2012), NICE (2015), Sørensen et al. (2005).

Urinary output and catheters

Related theory

It is important that patients pass urine within 6–8 hours of surgery or pass more than 0.5 mL/kg/hour (i.e. half the patient's bodyweight in kilograms converted to millilitres, for example 60 kg = 30 mL, per hour) if a urinary catheter is *in situ* (Liddle 2013). Urinary catheters are used to relieve or prevent urinary retention and bladder distension, or to monitor urine output. Most urinary catheters are inserted urethrally but, where this is contraindicated, suprapubic catheters can be used (see Chapter 6: Elimination).

Evidence-based approaches

Principles of care

Urine output should be measured and accurately recorded on the fluid balance chart. This should be undertaken as clinically indicated (e.g. hourly in the immediate post-operative period). Nurses should also monitor and report changes in the character (colour, viscosity or odour) or volume of urine output; for example, oliguria (urine output of less than 0.5 mL/kg/hour for 2 consecutive hours in a catheterized patient) could indicate the patient is hypovolaemic and should be reported to surgical staff immediately (once catheter tubing has been checked to confirm it is not kinked or blocked). If a patient does not have a catheter *in situ*, it is important that the patient is asked to pass urine into a jug or commode so that the volume of urine can be measured and recorded.

The inability to pass urine post-operatively is usually caused by a condition called 'neurogenic bladder', a type of bladder dysfunction that interferes with the nerve impulses from the brain to the bladder, preventing it from emptying. For patients with no history of difficulty urinating prior to surgery, the problem is often attributed to a combination of risk factors that include abdominal surgery, general anaesthesia, and pain medications and fluids given perioperatively. Signs that a patient is in urinary retention include the patient reporting discomfort, pain, a full bladder and/or inability to urinate despite feeling the urge. A bladder scan can be used to determine the residual volume of urine in the bladder. If encouraging the patient to urinate on several occasions is unsuccessful, then an in/out urinary catheter can be inserted to drain the bladder. No attempts should be made to catheterize the patient without seeking confirmation from the surgical team that this is the appropriate course of action to take.

Bowel function

Related theory

Patients undergoing abdominal surgery experience reduced gastrointestinal (GI) peristalsis due to surgical manipulation of the bowel and post-operative opioid medication (Litkouhi 2013). The motility of the small intestine is affected to a lesser degree, except in patients who have had small bowel resection or who were operated on to relieve small bowel obstruction (Crainic et al. 2009). GI peristalsis usually returns within 24 hours after most operations that do not involve the abdominal cavity and within 48 hours after laparotomy (Crainic et al. 2009). Prolonged inhibition of GI peristalsis (more than 3 days post-surgery) is referred to as 'paralytic ileus' (Litkouhi 2013). Post-operative ileus is an abnormal pattern of GI motility whose principal features include a combination of nausea and vomiting, inability to tolerate oral diet, abdominal distention, and delayed passing of flatus or stool (Vather et al. 2013). The duration of post-operative ileus correlates with the degree of surgical trauma, occurring less frequently following laparoscopic than open surgery (Baig and Wexner 2004). Traditional interventions to prevent post-operative ileus or stimulate bowel function after surgery include:

- decompression of the stomach until return of bowel function with a nasogastric tube
- reduction in opioid use
- early mobilization of the patient to stimulate bowel function
- early post-operative feeding (Crainic et al. 2009, Nelson et al. 2005)
- chewing gum post-operatively, as this may help the digestive system to start to work (Short et al. 2015).

Return of peristalsis is often noted by patients as mild cramps, passage of flatus and return of appetite. Unless clinically indicated, both food and enteral feeds should be withheld until there is evidence of the return of normal GI motility.

Evidence-based approaches

Principles of care

Post-operatively, nurses should monitor and document when patients pass flatus, when the patient's bowels first open and ongoing bowel movements to facilitate early identification of a return to GI motility or if complications are arising (e.g. prolonged ileus or infection). Bowel motions should be documented according to the Bristol Stool Chart and any abnormalities (e.g. blood or pale stools) should be escalated to the surgical team. If the patient has undergone abdominal surgery or if clinically appropriate, the surgical team should also be made aware of any evidence of the return of GI motility so that food or enteral feeds can be recommenced if clinically indicated (see Chapter 6: Elimination).

Nutrition

Related theory

For normally nourished patients, the primary objective of post-operative care is restoration of normal GI function to allow adequate food and fluid intake and rapid recovery. Prolonged delays in oral feeding may compromise post-operative nutrition, which can lead to poor wound healing, susceptibility to infection and the need for nutritional support (Litkouhi 2013, NICE 2015). Post-operatively, energy and protein requirements depend on body composition, clinical status and mobility. Surgery places the body under extraordinary stressors (e.g. hypovolaemia or hypervolaemia, bacteraemia, and medications) and wound healing requires the intake of appropriate vitamins and minerals (e.g. vitamin A, vitamin C and zinc) and adequate calories from protein (see Chapter 8: Nutrition and fluid balance).

Evidence-based approaches

Principles of care

Surgery may exert a detrimental effect on appetite and the ability to maintain adequate nutritional intake post-operatively. Causative factors include:

- the surgery itself
- post-operative nausea and vomiting
- anorexia
- altered bowel movements (e.g. constipation, ileus or diarrhoea)
- medication
- oral candida
- sore mouth
- dysphagia
- early satiety.

Unless contraindicated by the surgery performed (e.g. major abdominal or head and neck surgery) or the patient's current clinical status (e.g. risk of pulmonary aspiration, vomiting and/or ileus), the majority of patients will be able to meet their nutritional requirements orally in the post-operative period. If clinically indicated, any food or drink taken by the patient should be accurately recorded (volume and type of food) on a food chart and fluid balance chart. It is essential that appropriately trained healthcare professionals do the following:

- undertake ongoing oral and nutritional screening assessments in accordance with local trust policy
- put preventive measures in place (e.g. providing good oral hygiene, offering appetizing food and drink, and providing assistance with eating and drinking)
- alert the dietician and/or surgeon when there is cause for concern.

Any patient unable to meet their nutritional requirements orally will require referral to a dietician, who will assess the patient's nutritional requirements and tailor any nutritional replacement – whether oral (e.g. nutritional supplements), enteral or parenteral – to their needs.

Post-operative nutritional support has potentially serious complications (NICE 2017b). Enteral nutrition uses the physiological route of nutrient intake, is cheaper and is generally safer, and should be the preferred method of nutritional support, in the presence of a functioning GI tract (Weimann et al. 2017). Types of enteral feed tubes include nasogastric, nasoduodenal, nasojejunal, gastrostomy and jejunostomy. While enteral feeding is the preferred route of nutritional support (NICE 2017b), parenteral nutrition may be indicated for some post-operative patients who have undergone major abdominal surgery or those with prolonged ileus, uncontrolled vomiting or diarrhoea, short bowel syndrome or GI obstruction.

More detailed information can be found in the Chapter 8: Nutrition and fluid balance.

Post-operative pain

Evidence-based approaches

Acute post-operative pain is a normal response to surgical intervention and must be managed effectively (Lovich-Sapola et al. 2015). Effective management of pain following surgery requires that information about the patient's goals for pain relief, previous history with analgesics and type of surgical procedure is used to guide decisions about analgesic regimens (Bell and Duffy 2009, Layzell 2008). It is imperative that the patient's pain is managed well, initially by the anaesthetist and then the ward staff and pain team to ensure that the patient has adequate analgesia but is alert enough to be able to communicate and co-operate with staff (Liddle 2013). Analgesics are selected based on the location of the surgery, the degree of anticipated pain and patient characteristics (e.g. co-morbidities); routes of administration and dosing schedules aim to maximize the effectiveness and safety of analgesia while minimizing the potential for adverse events (Layzell 2008).

Pain management can be delivered using the following routes: oral, rectal, epidural and intravenous (including patient-controlled analgesia and opioid continuous infusion) (Liddle 2013). A pain tool (e.g. verbal numeric rating score) should be used to assess the effectiveness of prescribed analgesia and action should be taken if the patient's pain is not controlled. See Chapter 10: Pain assessment and management for further information concerning effective management of pain following surgery, including assessment tools.

Immobility

Related theory

Post-operatively, patients are at increased risk of developing deep vein thrombosis (DVT); risk factors include muscular inactivity, post-operative respiratory and circulatory depression, abdominal and pelvic surgery, prolonged pressure on calves (e.g. from lithotomy poles), increased production of thromboplastin as a result of surgical trauma, and pre-existing coronary artery disease (Rashid et al. 2005). To prevent this complication, many patients undergoing surgery will be treated with anticoagulants, for example low-molecular weight heparin subcutaneous injections or a continuous heparin infusion if the patient was previously anticoagulated (NICE 2018a).

Unless contraindicated, patients will also wear antiembolic stockings. Stockings should usually only be removed for up to 30 minutes daily; however, they can be removed more frequently if clinically indicated (e.g. if the patient complains of pain or discomfort). Patients should be supported to provide daily skin hygiene by careful washing and application of an emollient cream if the skin is dry. See 'Mechanical and pharmacological thromboembolism prophylaxis' above for further information relating to DVTs and their prevention.

The surgeon's post-operative instructions should describe any required special positioning of the patient. Where a patient's condition allows, early mobilization (wearing non-slip slippers or shoes to reduce the risk of falls) is encouraged to reduce venous stasis. For patients on bedrest, a physiotherapist should provide the patient with verbal and written information about deep breathing and leg exercises (i.e. flexion, extension and rotation of the ankles). Furthermore, patients on bedrest should be encouraged to change position hourly to minimize the risk of atelectasis and circumvent the development of pressure sores (Jocelyn Chew et al. 2018). Patients on bedrest may also have intermittent pneumatic compression or foot impulse devices in addition to graduated antiembolic stockings while in hospital (NICE 2018a).

Ongoing care on discharge

Related theory

All patients – whether a day case or needing a short or long stay, and whether they have few needs or complex needs – should receive comprehensive discharge planning. Post-operatively, discharge planning must be tailored to the individual needs of the patient, particularly in relation to advice and information on recovery and self-management (DH 2004).

The increase in same-day surgical admissions combined with shorter hospital stays means that more post-operative recovery, including wound healing, now takes place at home. This means that where appropriate, patients need to have assimilated the knowledge of usual post-operative outcomes and management with the ability to recognize when professional intervention and/or advice are required.

Surgery can be physically and psychologically stressful, resulting in patients forgetting information and teaching provided pre-operatively (Mitchell 2005, Pereira et al. 2016). Nurses therefore need to reinforce pre-operative education post-operatively, ensuring that information and discussions are tailored to the patient's individual needs, taking into account their level of anxiety and distress (Mitchell 2005). Ongoing assessment of the patient's understanding of the information given should be carried out and documented. Nurses should teach patients and carers any necessary skills (including how to use equipment), allowing sufficient time for them to practise before discharge. This will enable patients to be as independent as possible post-operatively and promote an understanding of any self-care initiatives required on discharge. This should be supported with centralized evidence-based written information concerning post-discharge care at home (see Chapter 3: Discharge care and planning).

Websites

Association of periOperative Registered Nurses
www.aorn.org

Tampon Alert
www.tamponalert.org.uk

References

AAGBI (Association of Anaesthetists of Great Britain and Ireland) (2010) *Pre-operative Assessment and Patient Preparation: The Role of the Anaesthetist* [AAGBI Guideline 2]. London: Association of Anaesthetists of Great Britain and Ireland.

AAGBI (2011) *Malignant Hyperthermia Crisis AAGBI Safety Guideline.* Available at: https://anaesthetists.org/Home/Resources-publications/Guidelines/Malignant-hyperthermia-crisis

AAGBI (2013) AAGBI safety guideline: Immediate post-anaesthesia recovery. *Anaesthesia*, 68, 288–297.

AAGBI (2014) Peri-operative care of the elderly 2014. *Anaesthesia*, 69(Suppl. 1), 81–98.

AAGBI (2015) Recommendations for standards of monitoring during anaesthesia and recovery. *Anaesthesia*, 71, 85–93.

AAGBI (2018) *Guidelines: The Anaesthetic Team.* Available at: https://anaesthetists.org/Portals/0/PDFs/Guidelines%20PDFs/Guideline_The%20Anaesthesia%20Team_2018.pdf?ver=2019-01-08-163915-087&timestamp=1546967138246&ver=2019-01-08-163915-087&timestamp=1546967138246

Abe, A., Kaye, A.D., Gritsenko, K., et al. (2014) Perioperative analgesia and the effects of dietary supplements. *Best Practice & Research: Clinical Anaesthesiology*, 28(2), 183–189.

Adeyinka, A. & Kondamundi, N.P. (2019) *Cyanosis.* StatPearls. Available at: https://www.ncbi.nlm.nih.gov/books/NBK482247

AfPP (Association for Perioperative Practice) (2017) *Standards and Recommendations for Safe Perioperative Practice.* Harrogate: Association for Perioperative Practice.

Agodi, A., Auxilia, F., Barchitta, M., et al. (2015) Operating theatre ventilation systems and microbial air contamination in total joint replacement surgery: Results of the GISIO-ISChIA study. *Journal of Hospital Infection*, 90(3), 213–219.

All Wales Tissue Viability Nurse Forum (2009) Guidelines for best nursing: The nursing care of patients wearing anti-embolic stockings. *British*

Journal of Nursing. Available at: https://hrhealthcare.co.uk/downloads/carolon/All-Wales-Guidlines-for-Best-Practice.pdf

Allegranzi, B., Bischoff, P., de Jonge, S., et al. (2016) New WHO recommendations on preoperative measures for surgical site infection prevention: An evidence-based global perspective. *Lancet Infectious Diseases*, 6(12), e276–e287.

Almodaimegh, H., Alfehaid, L., Alsuhebany, N., et al. (2017) Awareness of venous thromboembolism and thromboprophylaxis among hospitalized patients: A cross-sectional study. *Thrombosis Journal*, 15, 19.

American Society of Anesthesiologists (2011) Practice guidelines for preoperative fasting and the use of pharmacologic agents to reduce the risk of pulmonary aspiration: Application to healthy patients undergoing elective procedures – An updated report by the American Society of Anesthesiologists Committee on Standards and Practice Parameters. *Anesthesiology*, 114(3), 495–511.

American Society of Anesthesiologists (2014) *ASA Physical Status Classification System*. Available at: https://www.asahq.org/standards-and-guidelines/asa-physical-status-classification-system

Anderson, I.D. (2003) *Care of the Critically Ill Surgical Patient*, 2nd edn. London: Arnold.

AORN (Association of periOperative Registered Nurses) (2000) Recommended practices for safety through identification of potential hazards in the perioperative environment. *AORN Journal*, 72(4), 690–692, 695–698.

AORN (2008) *Perioperative Standards and Recommended Practices*. Denver, CO: Association of periOperative Registered Nurses.

AORN (2010) *AORN Latex Guideline*. Denver, CO: Association of periOperative Registered Nurses.

AORN (2013) *Hand Antisepsis*. Denver, CO: Association of periOperative Registered Nurses.

AORN (2017) Recommended practices for positioning the patient in the perioperative practice setting. *AORN Journal*, 73(1), 231–235, 237–238.

AORN (2018) *Guidelines for Perioperative Practice*. Denver, CO: Association of periOperative Registered Nurses.

ASH (Action on Smoking and Health) (2016) *Joint Briefing: Smoking and Surgery*. Available at: https://www.rcoa.ac.uk/sites/default/files/Joint-briefing-Smoking-Surgery.pdf

Baig, M.K. & Wexner, S.D. (2004) Postoperative ileus: A review. *Diseases of the Colon & Rectum*, 47(4), 516–526.

Balinskaite, V., Bottle, A., Sodhi, V., et al. (2017) The risk of adverse pregnancy outcomes following nonobstetric surgery during pregnancy: Estimates from a retrospective cohort study of 6.5 million pregnancies. *Annals of Surgery*, 266(2), 260–266.

Bates, S.M., Greer, I.A., Middeldorp, S., et al. (2012) VTE, thrombophilia, antithrombotic therapy, and pregnancy: *Antithrombotic Therapy and Prevention of Thrombosis*, 9th ed: American College of Chest Physicians evidence-based clinical practice guidelines. *Chest*, 141(2 Suppl.), e691S–e736S.

Bathla, S., Chadwick, M., Nevins, E.J. & Seward, J. (2017) Preoperative site marking: Are we adhering to good surgical practice? *Journal of Patient Safety*. DOI: 10.1097/PTS.0000000000000398.

Batra, Y.K. & Rajeev, S. (2007) Effect of common herbal medicines on patients undergoing anaesthesia. *Indian Journal of Anaesthesia*, 51, 184–191.

Beckett, A.E. (2010) Are we doing enough to prevent patient injury caused by positioning for surgery? *Journal of Perioperative Practice*, 20(1), 26–29.

Bell, L. & Duffy, A. (2009) Pain assessment and management in surgical nursing: A literature review. *British Journal of Nursing*, 18(3), 153–156.

Bickley, L.S., Bates, B. & Szilagyi, P.G. (2009) *Bates' Pocket Guide to Physical Examination and History Taking*, 6th edn. Philadelphia: Lippincott Williams & Wilkins.

Bischoff, P., Kubilay, N.Z., Allegranzi, B., et al. (2017) Effect of laminar airflow ventilation on surgical site infections: A systematic review and meta-analysis. *Lancet Infectious Diseases*, 17(5), 553–561.

BNF (British National Formulary) (2019) *Oxygen*. Available at: https://bnf.nice.org.uk/treatment-summary/oxygen.html

Boehm, O., Baumgarten, G., & Hoeft, A. (2016) Preoperative patient assessment: Identifying patients at high risk. *Best Practice & Research: Clinical Anaesthesiology*, 30(2), 131–143.

Böhmer, A.B., Wappler, F. & Zwissler, B. (2014) Preoperative risk assessment: From routine tests to individualised investigation. *Deutsches Ärzteblatt International*, 111, 437–446.

Bradley, P., Chapman, G., Crooke, B. & Greenland, K. (2016) *Airway Assessment*. Australia and New Zealand College of Anaesthesiology. Available at: www.anzca.edu.au/documents/pu-airway-assessment-20160916v1.pdf

Braz, L.G., Braz, J.R.C., Cavalcante, G.A.S., et al. (2017) Comparison of waste anesthetic gases in operating rooms with or without a scavenging system in a Brazilian University Hospital. *Brazilian Journal of Anesthesiology*, 67(5), 516–520.

Brooks, A., Mahoney, P.F. & Rowlands, B. (2008) *The ABC of Tubes, Drains, Lines and Frames*. Oxford: Wiley Blackwell.

BSG (British Society of Gastroenterology) (2018) *BSG Guidelines*. Available at: https://www.bsg.org.uk/clinical/bsg-guidelines.html

Byard, R.W. (2010) A review of the potential forensic significance of traditional herbal medicines. *Journal of Forensic Sciences*, 55, 89–92.

Chan, T.Y., Bulger, T.F., Stowell, K.M., et al. (2017) Evidence of malignant hyperthermia in patients administered triggering agents before malignant hyperthermia susceptibility identified: Missed opportunities prior to diagnosis. *Anaesthesia and Intensive Care*, 45(6), 707–713.

Chee, Y., Crawford, J., Watson, H. & Greaves, M. (2008) Guidelines on the assessment of bleeding risk prior to surgery or invasive procedures: British Committee for Standards in Haematology. *British Journal of Haematology*, 140, 496–504.

Chou, R., Gordon, D.B., de Leon-Casasola, O.A., et al. (2016) Management of postoperative pain: A clinical practice guideline from the American Pain Society, the American Society of Regional Anesthesia and Pain Medicine, and the American Society of Anesthesiologists' Committee on Regional Anesthesia, Executive Committee, and Administrative Council. *Journal of Pain*, 17(2), 131–157.

Cowperthwaite, L. & Holm, R.L. (2015) Guideline implementation: Surgical instrument cleaning. *AORN Journal*, 101(5), 542–549.

Crainic, C., Erickson, K., Gardner, J., et al. (2009) Comparison of methods to facilitate postoperative bowel function. *MEDSURG Nursing*, 18(4), 235–238.

Dalal, A.J. & McLennan, A.S. (2017) Surgical smoke evacuation: A modification to improve efficiency and minimise potential health risk. *British Journal of Oral Maxillofacial Surgery*, 55(1), 90–91.

DH (Department of Health) (2000) *Comprehensive Critical Care: A Review of Adult Critical Care Services*. Available at: http://webarchive.nationalarchives.gov.uk/20130107105354/www.dh.gov.uk/prod_consum_dh/groups/dh_digitalassets/@dh/@en/documents/digitalasset/dh_4082872.pdf

DH (2004) *Achieving Timely Simple Discharge from Hospital: A Toolkit for the Multi-disciplinary Team*. Available at: http://webarchive.nationalarchives.gov.uk/+/www.dh.gov.uk/en/Publicationsandstatistics/Publications/PublicationsPolicyAndGuidance/DH_4088366

DH (2009) *Reference Guide to Consent for Examination or Treatment*, 2nd edn. Available at: http://webarchive.nationalarchives.gov.uk/20130107105354/www.dh.gov.uk/prod_consum_dh/groups/dh_digitalassets/documents/digitalasset/dh_103653.pdf

DH (2010) *Risk Assessment for Venous Thromboembolism (VTE)*. London: Department of Health.

DH (2011) *Enhanced Recovery Partnership Project Report*. Available at: www.gov.uk/government/uploads/system/uploads/attachment_data/file/215511/dh_128707.pdf

DH (2016) *Health Risks from Alcohol: New Guidelines*. Available at: https://www.gov.uk/government/consultations/health-risks-from-alcohol-new-guidelines

Doyle D.J. & Garmon E.H. (2019) *American Society of Anesthesiologists Classification (ASA Class)*. Treasure Island, FL: *Stat*Pearls.

Dumville, J.C., Walter, J., Sharp, A. & Page, T. (2011) Dressings for the prevention of surgical site infection. *Cochrane Database of Systematic Reviews*, 7, CD004423.

Eckenhoff, J.E., Kneale, D.H. & Dripps, R.D. (1961) The incidence and etiology of postanesthetic excitement: A clinical survey. *Anesthesiology*, 22, 667–673.

Eckert, L.O. & Lentz, G.M. (2012) Infections of the lower genital tract: Vulva, cervix, toxic shock syndrome, endometritis, and salpingitis. In: Lentz, G.M., Lobo, R.A., Gershenson, D.M. & Katz, V.L. (eds) *Comprehensive Gynecology*, 6th edn. Philadelphia: Elsevier Mosby, pp.519–560.

ECRI Institute (2012) *Health Devices: Top 10 Health Technology Hazards for 2013*. Available at: https://www.ecri.org/Resources/Whitepapers_and_reports/2013_Health_Devices_Top_10_Hazards.pdf

Eder, S.P. (2017) Guideline implementation: Energy-generating devices, Part 1: Electrosurgery. *AORN Journal*, 105(3), 300–310.

Escobar, P. & Knight, J. (2012) *Surgical Wounds. Strategies for Minimizing Complications.* Available at: https://www.contemporaryobgyn.net/modern-medicine-now/surgical-wounds-strategies-minimizing-complications

Farge, D., Debourdeau, P., Beckers, M., et al. (2013) International clinical practice guidelines for the treatment and prophylaxis of venous thromboembolism in patients with cancer. *Journal of Thrombosis and Haemostasis*, 11(1), 56–70.

Feldmann, M.E. (1988) Inadvertent hypothermia: A threat to homeostasis in the postanesthetic patient. *Journal of Post Anesthesia Nursing*, 3(2), 82–87.

Fencl, J.L., Walsh, A. & Vocke, D. (2015) The bariatric patient: An overview of perioperative care. *AORN Journal*, 102(2), 116–131.

Flevas, D.A., Megaloikonomoa, P.D., Dimopoulos, L., et al. (2018) Thromoboembolism prophylaxis in orthopaedics: An update. *Effort Open Reviews*, 3, 136–148.

Fraise, A.P. & Bradley, C. (2009) *Ayliffe's Control of Healthcare-Associated Infection: A Practical Handbook*, 5th edn. London: Hodder Arnold.

Frank, S.M., Beattie, C., Christopherson, R., et al. (1993) Unintentional hypothermia is associated with postoperative myocardial ischemia: The Perioperative Ischemia Randomized Anesthesia Trial Study Group. *Anesthesiology*, 78(3), 468–476.

Ganpule, A.P., Vijayakumar, M., Malpani, A. & Desai, M.R. (2016) Percutaneous nephrolithotomy (PCNL) a critical review. *International Journal of Surgery*, 36, 660–664.

Gavel, G. & Walker, R.W.M. (2014) Laryngospasm in anaesthesia. *Continuing Education in Anaesthesia, Critical Care & Pain*, 14(2), 47–51.

Gilbert-Kawai, E. & Montgomery, H. (2017) Cardiovascular assessment for non-cardiac surgery: European guidelines. *British Journal of Hospital Medicine*, 78(6), 327–332.

GMC (General Medical Council) (2008) *Consent: Patients and Doctors Making Decisions Together.* Available at: https://www.gmc-uk.org/-/media/documents/Consent___English_0617.pdf_48903482.pdf

GMC (2014). *Good Medical Practice.* Available at: https://www.gmc-uk.org/ethical-guidance/ethical-guidance-for-doctors/good-medical-practice

Guazzi, M., Bandera, F., Ozemek, C., et al. (2017) Cardiopulmonary exercise testing: What is its value? *Journal of the American College of Cardiology*, 70(13), 1618–1636.

Guo, P. (2015) Preoperative education interventions to reduce anxiety and improve recovery among cardiac surgery patients: A review of randomised controlled trials. *Journal of Clinical Nursing*, 24(1/2), 34–46.

Hatfield, A. & Tronson, M. (2009) *The Complete Recovery Room Book*, 4th edn. Oxford: Oxford University Press.

Hauk, L. (2018) Guidance for perioperative practice: Safe environment of care. *AORN Journal*, 108(3), P10–P12.

Haymes, J. (2016) Venous thromboembolism: Patient awareness and education in the pre-operative assessment clinic. *Journal of Thromboembolism and Thrombolysis*, 41(3), 459–463.

Health Protection Scotland (2018) *Appendix 3: Best Practice – Surgical Scrubbing / Appendix 4: Best Practice – Surgical Rubbing.* Available at: www.nipcm.hps.scot.nhs.uk/appendices/

Helkin, A., Jain, S.V., Gruessner, A., et al. (2017) Impact of ASA score misclassification on NSQIP predicted mortality: A retrospective analysis. *Perioperative Medicine*, 6, 23.

Hess, C.T. (2012) *Wound Care*, 7th edn. Philadelphia: Lippincott Williams & Wilkins.

Higgins, C. & Higgins, C. (2013) *Understanding Laboratory Investigations: A Guide for Nurses, Midwives and Healthcare Professionals*, 3rd edn. Oxford: John Wiley & Sons.

Ho, L., Lau, L., Churilov, L., et al. (2016) Comparative evaluation of crystalloid resuscitation rate in a human model of compensated haemorrhagic shock. *SHOCK*, 46(2), 149–157.

HSE (Health and Safety Executive) (2018) *Latex Allergy in Health and Social Care.* Available at: www.hse.gov.uk/healthservices/latex

Hughes, C. (2011) Consent and the perioperative patient. In: Radford, M., Williamson, A. & Evans, C. (eds) *Preoperative Assessment and Perioperative Management.* Keswick, UK: M&K Update, pp.303–318.

Jameson, J. (2017) *Care of the Critically Ill Surgical Patient: Participant Handbook*, 4th edn. London: Royal College of Surgeons of England.

Jevon, P. & Ewens, B. (2012) *Monitoring the Critically Ill Patient*, 3rd edn. Oxford: John Wiley & Sons.

Jocelyn Chew, H.S., Thiara, E., Lopez, V. & Shorey, S. (2018) Turning frequency in adult bedridden patients to prevent hospital-acquired pressure ulcer: A scoping review. *International Wound Journal*, 15(2), 225–236.

Kalkwarf, K.J. & Cotton, B.A. (2017) Resuscitation for hypovolemic shock. *Surgical Clinics of North America*, 97(6), 1307–1321.

Kenny, L. (2011) The evolving role of the preoperative assessment team. In: Radford, M., Williamson, A. & Evans, C. (eds) *Preoperative Assessment and Perioperative Management.* Keswick, UK: M&K Update, pp.1–13.

Khan, M.J., Werner, C.L., Darragh, T.M., et al. (2017) ASCCP colposcopy standards: Role of colposcopy, benefits, potential harms, and terminology for colposcopic practice. *Journal of Lower Genital Tract Disease*, 21(4), 223–229.

Khan, S.M., Smeulders, M.J.C. & Van der Horst, C.M. (2015) Wound drainage after plastic and reconstructive surgery of the breast. *Cochrane Database of Systematic Reviews*, 10, CD007258.

King, W. (2010) *Pulmonary Aspiration of Gastric Contents.* Available at: https://www.frca.co.uk/Documents/192%20Pulmonary%20aspiration%20of%20gastric%20contents.pdf

Knowlton, M.C. (2015) Nurse's guide to surgical drain removal. *Nursing*, 45(9), 59–61.

Kolh, P., De Hert, S. & De Rango, P. (2016) The concept of risk assessment and being unfit for surgery. *European Journal of Vascular & Endovascular Surgery*, 51(6), 857–866.

Kraiss, L.W., Beckstrom, J.L. & Brooke, B.S. (2015) Frailty assessment in vascular surgery and its utility in preoperative decision making. *Seminars in Vascular Surgery*, 28(2), 141–147.

Kumar, A., Yadav, N., Singh, S. & Chauchan, N. (2016) Minimally invasive (endoscopic-computer assisted) surgery: Technique and review. *Annals of Maxillofacial Surgery*, 6(2), 159–164.

Lanier, G.M., Fallon, J.T. & Naidu, S.S. (2018) Role of advanced testing: Invasive hemodynamics, endomyocardial biopsy, and cardiopulmonary exercise testing. *Cardiology Clinics*, 37(1), 73–82.

Layzell, M. (2008) Current interventions and approaches to postoperative pain management. *British Journal of Nursing*, 17(7), 414–419.

Lefebvre, A., Saliou, P., Lucet, J.C., et al. (2015) Preoperative hair removal and surgical site infections: Network meta-analysis of randomized controlled trials. *Journal of Hospital Infections*, 91(2), 100–108.

Leonard, A. & Thompson, J. (2008) Anaesthesia for ruptured abdominal aortic aneurysm. *Continuing Education in Anaesthesia, Critical Care & Pain*, 8(1), 11–15.

Levett, D.Z.H., Jack, S., Swart, M., et al. (2018) Perioperative cardiopulmonary exercise testing (CPET): Consensus clinical guidelines on indications, organization, conduct, and physiological interpretation. *British Journal of Anaesthesia*, 120(3), 484–500.

Levinson, B.W. (1965) States of awareness during general anaesthesia. Preliminary communication. *British Journal of Anaesthesia*, 37(7), 544–546.

Levinson, W.E. (ed) (2006) *Current Surgical Diagnosis and Treatment*, 12th edn. London: Lange Medical Books / McGraw-Hill.

Liberatore, K. (2019) Protecting patients with latex allergies. *AJN*, 119(1), 60–63.

Liddle, C. (2012) Preparing patients to undergo surgery. *Nursing Times*, 108(48), 12–13.

Liddle, C. (2013) Principles of monitoring postoperative patients. *Nursing Times*, 109(22), 24–26.

Lillienthal, K., Josue, A.M., Templonevo, M., et al. (2016) Scratching the surface: Prevention of corneal abrasion in the PACU. *Journal of PeriAnesthesia Nursing*, 31(4), e53.

Lippincott Williams & Wilkins (2018) *Lippincott Nursing Procedures*, 8th edn. Philadelphia: Lippincott Williams & Wilkins.

Litkouhi, B. (2013) Postoperative ileus. *UpToDate.* Available at: www.uptodate.com/contents/postoperative-ileus?source=search_result&search=postoperative&selectedTitle=3 %7E150

Liu, L.Q. & Mehigan, S. (2016) The effects of surgical hand scrubbing protocols on skin integrity and surgical site infection rates: A systematic review. *AORN Journal*, 103(5), 468–482.

Lo, Q. (2016) One step closer to safer surgery: The National Safety Standards for Invasive Procedures (NatSIPPs). *Journal of Perioperative Practice*, 26(6 Suppl, 8).

Loveday, H., Wilson, J., Pratt, R., et al. (2014) epic3: National evidence-based guidelines for preventing healthcare-associated infections in NHS hospitals in England. *Journal of Hospital Infection*, 86(Suppl. 1), S1–S70.

Lovich-Sapola, J., Smith, C.E. & Brandt, C.P. (2015) Postoperative pain control. *Surgical Clinics*, 95(2), 301–318.

Ma, K., Alhassan, S., Sharara, R., et al. (2017) Prophylaxis for venous thromboembolism. *Critical Care Nursing Quarterly*, 40(3), 219–229.

Madrid, E., Urrútia, G., Roqué i Figuls, M., et al. (2016) Active body surface warming systems for preventing complications caused by inadvertent perioperative hypothermia in adults. *Cochrane Database of Systematic Reviews*, 4, CD009016.

Mahmoodpoor, A., Soleimanpour, H., Golzari, S.E.J., et al. (2017) Determination of the diagnostic value of the modified Mallampati score, upper lip bite test and facial angle in predicting difficult intubation: A prospective descriptive study. *Journal of Clinical Anesthesia*, 37, 99–102.

Malafa, M.M., Coleman, J.E., Bowman, R.W. & Rohrich, R.J. (2016) Perioperative corneal abrasion: Updated guidelines for prevention and management. *Plastic and Reconstructive Surgery*, 137(5), 790e–798e.

Maley, A.M. & Arbiser, J.L. (2013) Gentian violet: A 19th century drug re-emerges in the 21st century. *Experimental Dermatology*, 22(12), 775–780.

Malik, A.A., Khan, W.S., Chaudhry, A., et al. (2009) Acute compartment syndrome: A life and limb threatening surgical emergency. *Journal of Perioperative Practice*, 19(5), 137–142.

Malley, A., Kenner, C., Kim, T. & Blakeney, B. (2015) The role of the nurse and the preoperative assessment in patient transitions. *AORN Journal*, 102(2), 181.e1–181.e9.

Mason, S.E., Kinross, J.M., Hendricks, J. & Arulampalam, T.H. (2017) Postoperative hypothermia and surgical site infection following peritoneal insufflation with warm, humidified carbon dioxide during laparoscopic colorectal surgery: A cohort study with cost-effectiveness analysis. *Surgical Endoscopy*, 31(4), 1923–1929.

Mayerson, J.M. (2016) A brief history of two common surgical drains. *Annals of Plastic Surgery*, 77(1), 4–5.

Mears, S.C., Davani, A.B. & Belkoff, S.M. (2009) Does the type of skin marker prevent marking erasure of surgical-site markings? *ePlasty*, 9, 342–346.

Mental Capacity Act (2005) Available at: www.legislation.gov.uk/ukpga/2005/9/contents

Mezanni, A. (2017) Cardiopulmonary exercise testing: Basics of methodology and measurements. *Annals of the American Thoracic Society*, 14(Suppl. 1), S3–S11.

Minokadeh, A. & Pinsky, M.R. (2016) Postoperative hemodynamic instability and monitoring. *Current Opinion in Critical Care*, 22(4), 393–400.

Mitchell, M.D. (2005) *Anxiety Management in Adult Day Surgery: A Nursing Perspective*. London: Whurr.

Mizell, J.S. (2012) Complications of abdominal surgical incisions. *UpToDate*. Available at: www.uptodate.com/contents/complications-of-abdominal-surgical-incisions

Montgomery v Lanarkshire Health Board [2015] *UKSC 11*.

NCEPOD (National Confidential Enquiry into Patient Outcome and Death) (2011) *Knowing the Risk: A Review of the Peri-operative Care of Surgical Patients*. Available at: www.ncepod.org.uk/2011report2/downloads/POC_fullreport.pdf

Nelson, R., Tse, B. & Edwards, S. (2005) Systematic review of prophylactic nasogastric decompression after abdominal operations. *British Journal of Surgery*, 92(6), 673–680.

Ngo, Q., Lam, V. & Deane, S. (2004) *Drowning in Drainage*. Liverpool Hospital. Available at: www.surgicaldrains.com/includes/DID.pdf

NHS (2016) *Toxic Shock Syndrome*. Available at: https://www.nhs.uk/conditions/toxic-shock-syndrome

NHS Choices (2016) *Consent to Treatment*. Available at: www.nhs.uk/conditions/consent-to-treatment/pages/introduction.aspx

NHS England (2014) *Summary of the Report of the NHS England Never Events Taskforce*. Available at: https://improvement.nhs.uk/documents/921/sur-nev-ev-tf-sum.pdf

NHS England (2017) *Theatres Benchmarking 2016: Findings Published*. Available at: https://www.nhsbenchmarking.nhs.uk/news/theatres-benchmarking-2016-findings-published

NHS England (2019) *National Early Warning Scores*. Available at: https://www.england.nhs.uk/ourwork/clinical-policy/sepsis/nationalearlywarningscore

NHS England and NHSI (NHS Improvement) (2018) *Resources to Support the Safe Adoption of the Revised National Early Warning Score (NEWS2)*. Available at: https://improvement.nhs.uk/documents/2508/Patient_Safety_Alert_-_adoption_of_NEWS2.pdf

NHS England and NHSI (NHS Improvement) (2019) *Standard Infection Control Precautions: National Hand Hygiene and Personal Protective Equipment Policy*. Available at: https://improvement.nhs.uk/documents/4957/National_policy_on_hand_hygiene_and_PPE_2.pdf

NHS Modernization Agency (2003) Definition of preoperative assessment. In: *National Good Practice Guideline on Preoperative Assessment for Inpatient Surgery*. London: NHS Modernization Agency, pp.2–3.

NHSI (NHS Improvement) (2015) *National Safety Standards for Invasive Procedures (NatSSIPs)*. Available at: https://improvement.nhs.uk/documents/923/natssips-safety-standards.pdf

NHSI (2018) *Enhanced Recovery*. Available at: https://improvement.nhs.uk/documents/2111/enhanced-recovery.pdf

NICE (National Institute for Health and Care Excellence) (2013) *Intravenous Fluid Therapy in Adults in Hospital*. Available at: www.nice.org.uk/nicemedia/live/14330/66015/66015.pdf

NICE (2015) *Wound Care Products*. Available at: https://www.nice.org.uk/advice/ktt14/resources/wound-care-products-pdf-58757952734917

NICE (2016a) *Hypothermia: Prevention and Management in Adults Having Surgery*. Available at: https://www.nice.org.uk/guidance/cg65/resources/hypothermia-prevention-and-management-in-adults-having-surgery-pdf-975569636293

NICE (2016b) *Routine Preoperative Tests for Elective Surgery* [NG45]. Available at: https://www.nice.org.uk/guidance/ng45

NICE (2016c) *Venous Thromboembolism in Adults: Diagnosis and Management* [QS29]. Available at: https://www.nice.org.uk/guidance/qs29/chapter/introduction-and-overview

NICE (2017a) *Intravenous Fluid Therapy in Adults in Hospital* [CG174]. Available at: https://www.nice.org.uk/guidance/cg174

NICE (2017b) *Nutrition Support in Adults: Oral Nutrition Support, Enteral Tube Feeding and Parenteral Nutrition* [CG32]. Available at: https://www.nice.org.uk/guidance/cg32

NICE (2018a) *Venous Thromboembolism in Over 16s: Reducing the Risk of Hospital-Acquired Deep Vein Thrombosis or Pulmonary Embolism* [NG89]. Available at: https://www.nice.org.uk/guidance/ng89

NICE (2018b) *Stop Smoking Interventions and Services* [NG92]. Available at: https://www.nice.org.uk/guidance/ng92

NICE (2019) *Surgical Site Infections: Prevention and Treatment* [NG125]. Available at: https://www.nice.org.uk/guidance/NG125

Nimmo, W.S., Rowbotham, D.J. & Smith, G. (1994) *Anaesthesia*, 2nd edn. Oxford: Blackwell Scientific.

NMC (Nursing and Midwifery Council) (2018) *The Code: Professional Standards of Practice and Behaviour for Nurses, Midwives and Nursing Associates*. Available at: https://www.nmc.org.uk/standards/code

Nottingham University Hospital and Rushcliffe PCT (2006) *Nursing Practice Guidelines: General Principles for all Guidelines*. Available at: https://www.nottingham.ac.uk/mhs/documents/clinical-skills/general-principles-guidelines.pdf

NPSA (National Patient Safety Agency) (2005) *Patient Safety Alert 06: Correct Site Surgery* [0169DEC04]. London: NPSA / Royal College of Surgeons.

NPSA (2007) *Fifth Report from the Patient Safety Observatory: Safer Care for the Acutely Ill Patient – Learning from Serious Incidents*. London: National Patient Safety Agency.

NPSA (2010) *Checking Pregnancy before Surgery: Rapid Response Report* [NSPA/2010RRR011]. London: National Patient Safety Agency.

Oakley, M. & Bratchell, J. (2010) Preoperative assessment. In: Pudner, R. (ed) *Nursing the Surgical Patient*, 3rd edn. Edinburgh: Baillière Tindall / Elsevier, pp.3–16.

Okoshi, K., Kobayashi, K., Kinoshita, K., et al. (2015) Health risks associated with exposure to surgical smoke for surgeons and operation room personnel. *Surgery Today*, 45(8), 957–965.

Older, P., Smith, R., Courtney, P. & Hone, R. (1993) Preoperative evaluation of cardiac failure and ischemia in elderly patients by cardiopulmonary exercise testing. *Chest*, 104(3), 701–704.

Ong, C. & Pearce, A. (2011) Assessment of the airway. In: Radford, M., Williamson, A. & Evans, C. (eds) *Preoperative Assessment and Perioperative Management*. Keswick, UK: M&K Update.

Parvizi, J., Barnes, S., Shohat, N. & Edmiston, C.E. Jr. (2017) Environment of care: Is it time to reassess microbial contamination of the operating room air as a risk factor for surgical site infection in total joint arthroplasty? *American Journal of Infection Control*, 45(11), 1267–1272.

Pavon, J.M., Adam, S.S., Razouki, Z.A., et al. (2016) Effectiveness of intermittent pneumatic compression devices for venous thromboembolism prophylaxis in high-risk surgical patients: A systematic review. *Journal of Arthroplasty*, 31(2), 524–532.

Pereira, L., Figueiredo Braga, M. & Carvalho, I.P. (2016) Preoperative anxiety in ambulatory surgery: The impact of an empathic patient-centered approach on psychological and clinical outcomes. *Patient Education and Counseling*, 99(5), 733–738.

Perel, P., Roberts, I. & Ker, K. (2013) Colloids versus crystalloids for fluid resuscitation in critically ill patients. *Cochrane Database of Systematic Reviews*, 2, CD000567.

Powell-Tuck, J., Gosling, P., Lobol, D., et al. (2011) *British Consensus Guidelines on Intravenous Fluid Therapy for Adult Surgical Patients*. British Association for Parenteral and Enteral Nutrition. Available at: www.bapen.org.uk/pdfs/bapen_pubs/giftasup.pdf

Prestwich, A., Moore, S., Kotze, A., et al. (2017) How can smoking cessation be induced before surgery? A systematic review and meta-analysis of behavior change techniques and other intervention characteristics. *Frontiers in Psychology*, 8, 915.

Pritchard, M.J. (2012) Pre-operative assessment of elective surgical patients. *Nursing Standard*, 26(30), 51–56, quiz 58.

Pudner, R. (2010) *Nursing the Surgical Patient*, 3rd edn. Edinburgh: Baillière Tindall.

Radtke, F.M., Franck, M., Schneider, M., et al. (2008) Comparison of three scores to screen for delirium in the recovery room. *British Journal of Anaesthesia*, 101(3), 338–343.

Rashid, S.T., Thursz, M.R., Razvi, N.A., et al. (2005) Venous thromboprophylaxis in UK medical inpatients. *Journal of the Royal Society of Medicine*, 98(11), 507–512.

Raza, A., Byrne, D. & Townell, N. (2004) Lower limb (well leg) compartment syndrome after urological pelvic surgery. *Journal of Urology*, 171(1), 5–11.

RCN (Royal College of Nursing) (2017) *Principles of Consent Guidance for Nursing Staff*. London: Royal College of Nursing.

RCoA (Royal College of Anaesthetists) (2013) *Risks Associated with Your Anaesthetic: Section 14 – Death or Brain Damage*. London: Royal College of Anaesthetists.

RCoA (2019) *Guidelines for the Provision of Anaesthesia Services (GPAS): Guidelines for the Provision of Postoperative Care 2019*. Available at: https://www.rcoa.ac.uk/system/files/GPAS-2019-04-POSTOP.pdf

RCP (Royal College of Physicians) (2017) *National Early Warning Scores (NEWS): Standardising the Assessment of Acute-Illness Severity in the NHS*. Available at: www.rcplondon.ac.uk/sites/default/files/documents/national-early-warning-score-standardising-assessment-acute-illness-severity-nhs.pdf

RCS (Royal College of Surgeons) (2014) *Good Surgical Practice England*. Available at: https://www.rcseng.ac.uk/-/media/files/rcs/standards-and-research/gsp/gsp-2014-web.pdf

Richardson, V. (2013) Patient comprehension of informed consent. *Journal of Perioperative Practice*, 23(1/2), 26–30.

Roberts, H.S. & Lawrence, S.M. (2017) CE: Venous thromboembolism. *AJN*, 117(5), 38–47.

Roderick, P., Ferris, G., Wilson, K., et al. (2005) Towards evidence-based guidelines for the prevention of venous thromboembolism: Systematic reviews of mechanical methods, oral anticoagulation, dextran and regional anaesthesia as thromboprophylaxis. *Health Technology Assessment*, 9(49), 1–78.

Rothrock, J.C., (2018) *Alexander's Care of the Patient in Surgery*, 16th edn. St Louis, MO: Elsevier.

Royal Marsden NHS Foundation Trust (2010) *Blood Clot Prevention: A Guide for Patients and Carers*. London: Royal Marsden NHS Foundation Trust.

Santacatalina Mas, R., Peix Sagues, M.T., Miranda Salmerón, J., et al. (2016) Surgical hand washing: Handscrubbing or handrubbing [in Spanish]. *Revista de Enfermeria*, 39(2), 8–16.

Schäfli-Thurnherr, J., Biegger, A., Soll, C. & Melcher, G.A. (2017) Should nurses be allowed to perform the pre operative surgical site marking instead of surgeons? A prospective feasibility study at a Swiss primary care teaching hospital. *Patient Safety in Surgery*, 11, 9.

Schinco, M.A. & Hassid, V.J. (2018) Compartment syndrome of extremities. *BMJ Best Practice*. Available at: https://bestpractice.bmj.com/topics/en-gb/500

Schmidt, A.H. (2016) Acute compartment syndrome. *Orthopedic Clinics of North America*, 47(3), 517–525.

Scott, C., McArthur-Rouse, F. & Prosser, S. (2007) Pre-operative assessment and preparation. In: McArthur-Rouse, F.J. & Prosser, S. (eds) *Assessing and Managing the Acutely Ill Adult Surgical Patient*. Oxford: Blackwell, pp.3–16.

Sevdalis, N. & Arora, S. (2016) Safety standards for invasive procedures. *BMJ*, 29, 352.

Sharma, H., Smith, D., Turner, C.E., et al. (2018) Clinical and molecular epidemiology of staphylococcal toxic shock syndrome in the United Kingdom. *Emerging Infectious Diseases*, 24(2), 258.

Shi, D., Yao, Y. & Yu, W. (2017) Comparison of preoperative hair removal methods for the reduction of surgical site infections: A meta-analysis. *Journal of Clinical Nursing*, 26(19/20), 2907–2914.

Short, V., Herbert, G., Perry, R., et al. (2015) Chewing gum for postoperative recovery of gastrointestinal function. *Cochrane Database of Systematic Reviews*, 2, CD006506.

SIGN (Scottish Intercollegiate Guidelines Network) (2014) *Prevention and Management of Thromboembolism: A National Guideline*. Edinburgh: Healthcare Improvement Scotland.

Simpson, P.J., Popat, M.T. & Carrie, L.E. (2002) *Understanding Anaesthesia*, 4th edn. Oxford: Butterworth-Heinemann.

Singh, S., Young, A. & McNaught, C.E. (2017) The physiology of wound healing. *Surgery (Oxford)*, 35(9), 473–477.

Sivanandan, I., Bowker, K.E., Bannister, G.C. & Soar, J. (2011) Reducing the risk of surgical site infection: A case controlled study of contamination of theatre clothing. *Journal of Perioperative Practice*, 21(2), 69–72.

Song, F., Brown, T.J., Blyth, A., et al. (2015) Identifying and recruiting smokers for preoperative smoking cessation: A systematic review of methods reported in published studies. *Systematic Reviews*, 4, 157.

Sørensen, L.T., Hemmingsen, U., Kallehave, F., et al. (2005) Risk factors for tissue and wound complications in gastrointestinal surgery. *Annals of Surgery*, 241(4), 654–658.

Starritt, T. (1999) Patient assessment in recovery. *British Journal of Theatre Nursing*, 9(12), 593–595.

Swanepoel, A.C., Roberts, H.C., Soma, P., et al. (2018) Hemorheological mechanisms for increased thrombosis in subjects using gestodene. *Microscopy Research and Technique*, 8(12), 1489–1500.

Tanner, J., Dumville, J.C., Norman, G. & Fortnam, M. (2016) Surgical hand antisepsis to reduce surgical site infection. *Cochrane Database of Systematic Reviews*, 1, CD004288.

Tanner, J. & Parkinson, H. (2006) Double gloving to reduce surgical cross-infection. *Cochrane Database of Systematic Reviews*, 3, CD003087.

Tassler, A. & Kaye, R. (2016) Preoperative assessment of risk factors. *Otolaryngologic Clinics of North America*, 49(3), 517–529.

Thomsen, T., Villebro, N. & Møller, A.M. (2014) Interventions for preoperative smoking cessation. *Cochrane Database of Systematic Reviews*, 27(3), CD002294.

Todd, M. (2015) Selecting compression hosiery. *British Journal of Nursing*, 24(4), 210–212.

Toon, C.D., Ramamoorthy, R., Davidson, B.R. & Gurusamy, K.S. (2015) Early versus delayed dressing removal after primary closure of clean and clean-contaminated surgical wounds. *Cochrane Database of Systematic Reviews*, 9, CD010259.

Turunen, E., Miettinen, M., Setälä, L., & Vehviläinen-Julkunen, K. (2017) An integrative review of a preoperative nursing care structure. *Journal of Clinical Nursing*, 26(7/8), 915–930.

Urbankowski, T. & Przybyłowski, T. (2016) Methods of airway resistance assessment [in Polish]. *Pneumonologia Alergologia Polska*, 84(2), 134–141.

Van de Putte, P., Vernieuwe, L., Jerjir, A., et al. (2017) When fasted is not empty: A retrospective cohort study of gastric content in fasted surgical patients. *British Journal of Anaesthesiology*, 118(3), 363–371.

Vather, R., Trivedi, S. & Bissett, I. (2013) Defining postoperative ileus: Results of a systematic review and global survey. *Journal of Gastrointestinal Surgery*, 17(5), 962–972.

Vecchio, R., Intagliata, E., Marchese, S. & Cacciola, E. (2016) The use of surgical drains in laparoscopic splenectomise: Consideration on a large series of 117 consecutive cases. *Annali Italiani di Chirurgia*, 87, 442–445.

Vedovato, J.W., Polvora, V.P. & Leonardi, D.F. (2004) Burns as a complication of the use of diathermy. *Journal of Burn Care & Rehabilitation*, 25(1), 120–123, discussion 119.

Vermeulen, H., Ubbink, D.T., Goossens, A., et al. (2005) Systematic review of dressings and topical agents for surgical wounds healing by secondary intention. *British Journal of Surgery*, 92(6), 665–672.

Vickers, R. (2011) Five steps to safer surgery. *Annals of The Royal College of Surgeons of England*, 93(7), 501–503.

Vincent, N. & Edwards, P. (2016) Disposable surgical face masks for preventing surgical wound infection in clean surgery. *Cochrane Database of Systematic Reviews*, 4, CD002929.

Vowden, K. & Vowden, P. (2017) Wound dressings: Principles and practice. *Surgery (Oxford)*, 35(9), 489–494.

Wade, R., Paton, F., Rice, S., et al. (2016) Thigh length versus knee length antiembolism stockings for the prevention of deep vein thrombosis in postoperative surgical patients: A systematic review and network meta-analysis. *BMJ Open*, 6(2), e009456.

Wade, R., Paton, F. & Woolacott, N. (2017) Systematic review of patient preference and adherence to the correct use of graduated compression stockings to prevent deep vein thrombosis in surgical patients. *Journal of Advanced Nursing*, 73(2), 336–348.

Walker, J. (2007) Patient preparation for safe removal of surgical drains. *Nursing Standard*, [illegible].

Walsgrove, H. (2011) History taking. In: Radford, M., Williamson, A. & [illegible] (eds) *Preoperative Assessment and Perioperative Management*. Keswick, UK: M&K Update, pp.[illegible].

Wang, C.Z., Moss, J. & Yuan, C.S. (2015) Commonly used dietary supplements on coagulation function during surgery. *Medicines*, 2(3), 157–185.

Warttig, S., Alderson, P., Campbell, G. & Smith, A.F. (2014) Interventions for treating inadvertent postoperative hypothermia. *Cochrane Database of Systematic Reviews*, 11, CD009892.

Weimann, A., Braga, M., Carli, F., et al. (2017) ESPEN guideline: Clinical nutrition in surgery. *Clinical Nutrition*, 36(3), 623–650.

Weinberg, A.D., Brennan, M.D., Gorman, C.A., et al. (1983) Outcome of anesthesia and surgery in hypothyroid patients. *Archives of Internal Medicine*, 143(5), 893–897.

Welch, K. (2010) Fluid balance. *Learning Disability Practice*, 13(6), 33–38.

Welch, M.B. (2019) Patient positioning for surgery and anesthesia in adults. *UpToDate*. Available at: https://www.uptodate.com/contents/patient-positioning-for-surgery-and-anesthesia-in-adults

WHO (World Health Organization) (2009) *WHO Surgical Safety Checklist*. Available at: [illegible]_Checklist_finalJun08.pdf?ua=1

WHO (2018) *Global Guidelines for the Prevention of Surgical Site Infection*. Available at: https://apps.who.int/iris/bitstream/handle/10665/277399/9789241550475-eng.pdf?ua=1

Wicker, P. & Dalby, S. (2016) *Rapid Perioperative Care*. Chichester: John Wiley & Sons.

Wicker, P. & O'Neill, J. (2010) *Caring for the Perioperative Patient*, 2nd edn. Oxford: John Wiley & Sons.

Wijeysundera, D.N. & Sweitzer, B.J. (2015) Preoperative evaluation. In: Miller, R.D. (ed) *Miller's Anesthesia*. Philadelphia: Elsevier Saunders, pp.1085–1155.

Wilkins, R.G. & Unverdorben, M. (2013) Wound cleaning and wound healing: A concise review. *Advances in Skin Wound Care*, 26(4), 160–163.

Williams, M. & El-Houdiri, Y. (2018) Inadvertent hypothermia in hip and knee total joint arthroplasty. *Journal of Orthopaedics*, 15(1), 151–158.

Wise, E.S., Cheung-Flynn, J. & Brophy, C.M. (2016) Standard surgical skin markers should be avoided for intraoperative vein graft marking during cardiac and peripheral bypass operations. *Frontiers in Surgery*, 3, 36.

[illegible] antibiotic use following ventral hernia repair with placement of surgical [illegible] *Reconstructive Surgery*, [illegible].

Wood, F., Martin, S.M., Carson-Stevens, A., et al. (2016) Doctors' perspectives of informed consent for non-emergency surgical procedures: A qualitative interview study. *Health Expectations*, 19(3), 751–761.

Wounds UK (2015) *Best Practice Statement: Compression Hosiery*. Available at: https://www.wounds-uk.com

Wu, M., McIntosh, J. & Liu, J. (2016) Current prevalence rate of latex allergy: Why it remains a problem? *Journal of Occupational Health*, 58(2), 138–144.

Yu, K., Xie X., Luo L., & Gong, R. (2017) Contributing factors of elective surgical case cancellation: A retrospective cross sectional study at a single site hospital. *BMC Surgery*, 17(1). DOI: 10.1186/s12893-017-0296-9.

Yu, T., Cheng, Y., Wang, X., et al. (2017) Gases for establishing pneumoperitoneum during laparoscopic abdominal surgery. *Cochrane Database of Systematic Reviews*, 6, CD009569.

Zhao, X., Chen, J., Fang, X.Q. & Fan, S.W. (2009) Surgical site marking [illegible], 319–320.

Chapter 17

Vascular access devices: insertion and management

Gema Munoz-Mozas with Lorraine Hyde and Hannah Overland

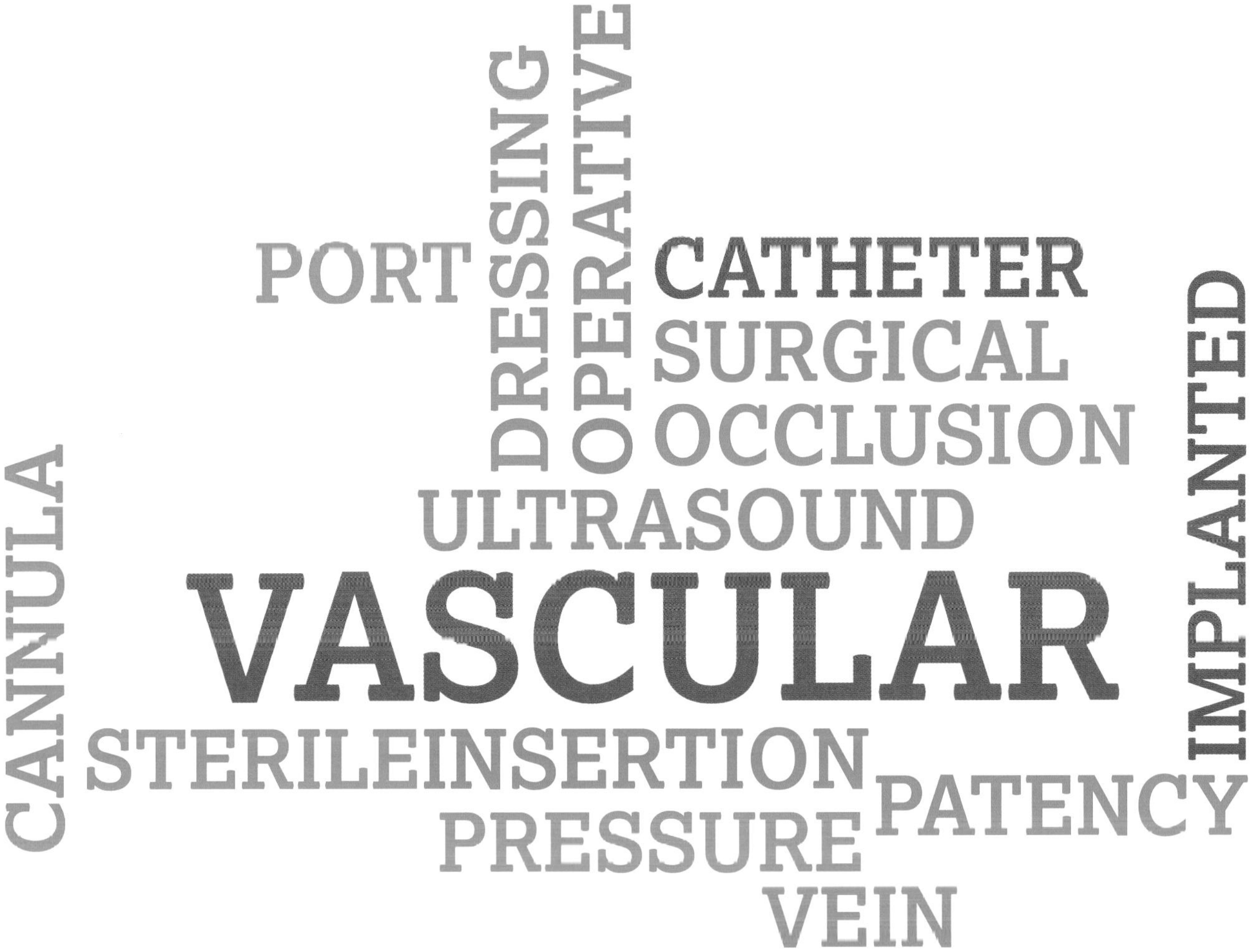

The Royal Marsden Manual of Clinical Nursing Procedures: Professional Edition, Tenth Edition. Edited by Sara Lister, Justine Hofland and Hayley Grafton.

Procedure guidelines

Being an accountable professional

At the point of registration, the nurse will:

2. Use evidence-based, best practice approaches to undertake the following procedures:

2.2 undertake venepuncture and cannulation and blood sampling, interpreting normal and common abnormal blood profiles and venous blood gases

11. Have procedural competencies required for best practice, evidence-based medicines administration and optimisation

Future Nurse: Standards of Proficiency for Registered Nurses (NMC 2018)

Overview

This chapter provides an overview of vascular access devices inserted in a vein or an artery. It describes the variety of common devices used for both peripheral and central access along with their insertion, care and removal. Taking blood samples is covered in Chapter 13: Diagnostic tests.

Vascular access devices

Definition

A vascular access device (VAD) is a device that is inserted into either a vein or an artery, via the peripheral or central vessels, to provide for either diagnostic (blood sampling or central venous pressure reading) or therapeutic (administration of medications, fluids and/or blood products) purposes (pressure is measured in mmHg or pounds per square inch (psi)). There is now a comprehensive range of VADs available, which allows selection to be made based on the device, the required therapy and the quality-of-life needs of the patient (RCN 2016a). Table 17.1 lists the main types of VAD.

Anatomy and physiology

Anatomy of veins

Veins consist of three layers.

Tunica intima

The tunica intima is a smooth endothelial lining that allows the passage of blood cells (Jenkins and Tortora 2014). If it becomes damaged, the lining may become roughened and there is an increased risk of thrombus formation (Hadaway 2010, Scales 2008). Within this layer are thin folds of endothelium called valves (flap-like cusps), which keep blood moving towards the heart by preventing backflow (Jenkins and Tortora 2014). Valves are present in larger vessels and at points of branching, and can be seen as noticeable bulges in the veins (Weinstein and Hagle 2014).

Tunica media

The middle layer of the vein wall is composed of muscular tissue and nerve fibres, both vasoconstrictors and vasodilators, which can stimulate the vein to contract or relax. This layer is not as strong or stiff as in an artery and therefore veins can distend or collapse as the pressure rises or falls (Jenkins and Tortora 2014). Stimulation of this layer by a change in temperature (cold) or by a mechanical or chemical stimulus can produce venous spasm, which can make insertion of a needle more difficult.

Tunica adventitia or externa

The tunica adventitia (also known as the tunica externa) is the tough outer layer and consists of connective tissue, which surrounds and supports the vessel (Tortora and Derrickson 2017).

Anatomy of arteries

Arteries tend to be placed more deeply than veins and can be distinguished by their thicker walls (which do not collapse), the presence of a pulse and bright red blood. It should be noted that aberrant arteries may be present. These are arteries that are located superficially in an unusual place (Jenkins and Tortora 2014).

There are two main types of arteries – muscular and elastic – and they are composed of three layers:

- the tunica intima, which has elongated endothelial cells
- the tunica media, which in elastic arteries is thicker, with more elastic and fibrous tissue arranged in circular bands, while in

Table 17.1 Vascular access devices

Type of device	Possible materials	Features	Common insertion site (veins)	Recommended indwelling life and common uses
Peripheral intravenous cannula (PIVC)	Teflon (PTFE) Polyurethane Vialon	Winged or non-winged Ported or non-ported Closed system, single ported or dual ported	Cephalic or basilic Dorsal venous network	Removed when clinically indicated for short-term access
Midline catheter	Silicone Polyurethane	Single lumen Dual lumen	Basilic Median cubital Cephalic	Used for 1–6 weeks for short- to intermediate-term access
Peripherally inserted central catheter (PICC)	Polyurethane Silicone	Triple lumen Dual lumen Single lumen Valved or non-valved	Basilic Cephalic Brachial	Used primarily for patients requiring several weeks or months of intravenous access
Short-term percutaneous central venous catheter (non-tunnelled)	Polyurethane Silicone	Heparin, antibiotic and antiseptic coatings; multiple lumen	Jugular Subclavian Femoral	Intended for days to weeks of intravenous access
Skin-tunnelled catheter (STC)	Polyurethane Silicone	Valved or non-valved Antimicrobial/silver cuff Multiple lumen Computed tomography compatible	Jugular Axillary Subclavian Femoral	Indefinite: used for long-term intermittent, continuous or daily intravenous access; may be appropriate for short-term use if reliable access needed
Implanted ports	*Catheter*: silicone or polyurethane *Port*: titanium or plastic	Single or dual ports Peripheral or chest ports Valved or non-valved Low profile Computed tomography compatible	Veins of the upper arm (basilic, brachial) Jugular Axillary Subclavian Femoral	Indefinite: used for long-term access Intermittent, continuous or daily intravenous access

muscular arteries it is a large mass of smooth muscle fibres that control constriction and relaxation
- the tunica adventitia, which contains both collagen and elastic fibres, nerve bundles and lymphatic vessels (Tortora and Derrickson 2017).

Veins of the peripheral circulation

The superficial veins of the upper limbs are most commonly chosen for cannulation and insertion of midlines and peripherally inserted central catheters (PICCs). These veins are numerous and accessible, which ensures that the procedure can be performed safely and with minimum discomfort (Garza and Becan-McBride 2019, Hoeltke 2017). They are:

- the cephalic vein
- the basilic vein
- the metacarpal veins (used only when the others are not accessible) (Figure 17.1).

On the lateral aspect of the wrist, the cephalic vein rises from the lateral aspect of the dorsal venous network of the hand and flows upwards along the radial border of the forearm as the median cephalic, crossing the antecubital fossa as the median cubital vein (Jenkins and Tortora 2014). Care must be taken to avoid accidental arterial puncture, as this vein crosses the brachial artery (Jenkins and Tortora 2014). It is also in close proximity to the radial nerve (Dougherty 2008, Jenkins and Tortora 2014, Masoorli 2007).

The basilic vein begins on the medial aspect of the dorsal venous network of the hand and ascends the forearm and antemedial surface of the arm (Jenkins and Tortora 2014). It may be prominent but is not well supported by subcutaneous tissue, which makes it roll easily. Owing to its position, a haematoma may occur if the patient flexes the arm on removal of the needle, as this squeezes blood from the vein into the surrounding tissues (McCall and Tankersley 2019, Weinstein and Hagle 2014). Care must also be taken to avoid accidental puncture of the median nerve and brachial artery (Garza and Becan-McBride 2019).

The metacarpal veins are easily visualized and palpated. However, the use of these veins is contraindicated in the elderly, where skin turgor and subcutaneous tissue are diminished (Weinstein and Hagle 2014).

Veins of the central venous circulation

A central vein is one near the centre of the circulation: the heart (Chantler 2009). Those more commonly used for central venous catheterization are the internal jugular, subclavian and femoral veins (Figure 17.2). The internal jugular vein emerges from the skull through the jugular foramen and runs down the neck into the carotid sheath (Farrow et al. 2009, Tortora and Derrickson 2017). The axillary vein is a continuation of the basilic vein. From the lateral edge of the ribs to the sternal edge of the clavicle, the continuation of the axillary becomes the subclavian. It angles upwards as it arches over the first rib and passes under the clavicle, forming a narrow passage for the vein (Galloway and Bodenham 2004, 2009, Hadaway 2010). Here it joins the internal jugular vein to form the brachiocephalic vein behind the sternoclavicular joint. The left brachiocephalic vein is 6 cm in length, twice as long as the right (Hadaway 2010, Jenkins and Tortora 2014).

The superior vena cava (SVC) drains venous blood from the upper half of the body and is formed from the confluence of the two brachiocephalic (innominate) veins (2 cm wide) (Farrow et al. 2009). The SVC is 7 cm long in normal adults and descends vertically to the upper part of the right atrium of the heart (Farrow et al. 2009).

The femoral vein drains the majority of blood from the lower limb and enters the thigh as a continuation of the popliteal vein. It ascends through the thigh and becomes the external iliac vein and drains into the inferior vena cava. The inferior vena cava drains the lower half of the body and is formed by the two common iliac veins (Jenkins and Tortora 2014).

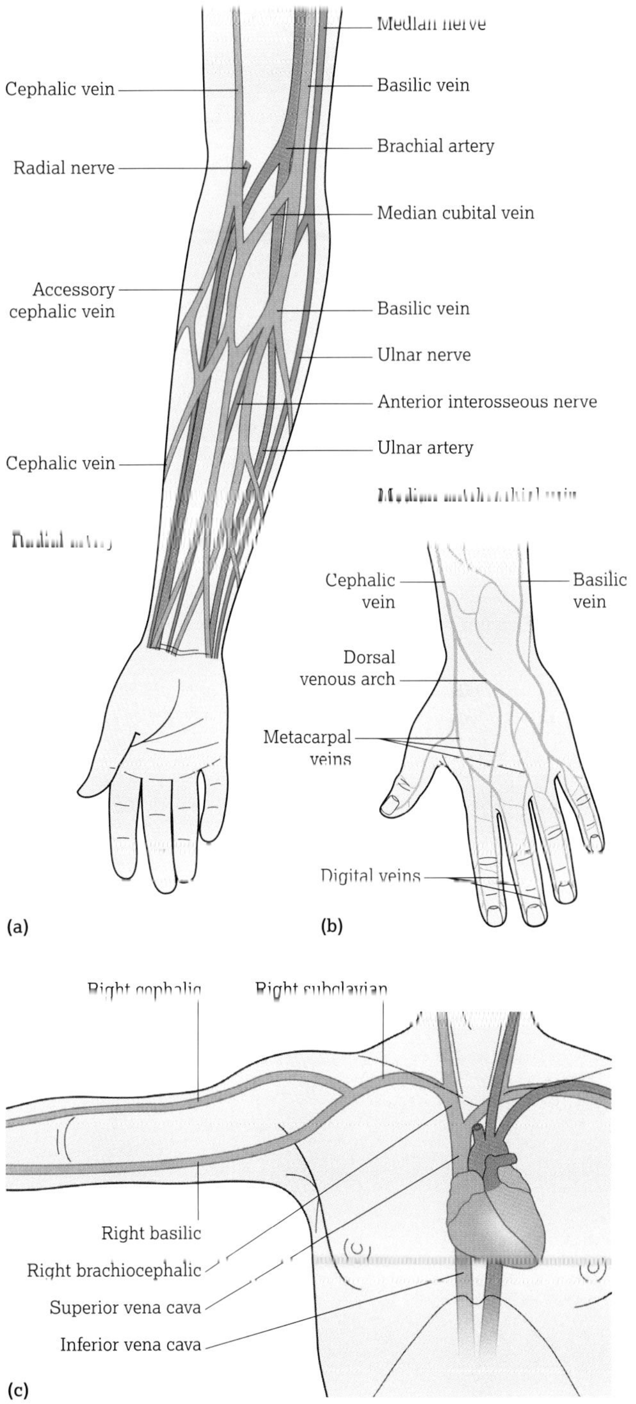

Figure 17.1 (a) Superficial veins of the forearm. (b) Superficial veins of the dorsal aspect of the hand. (c) Central veins and veins of the upper arm.

Evidence-based approaches

Rationale

Indications

VADs are used:

- to obtain venous and arterial blood samples
- to administer fluids, nutrition, medication or blood products
- to monitor central venous pressure and arterial pressure.

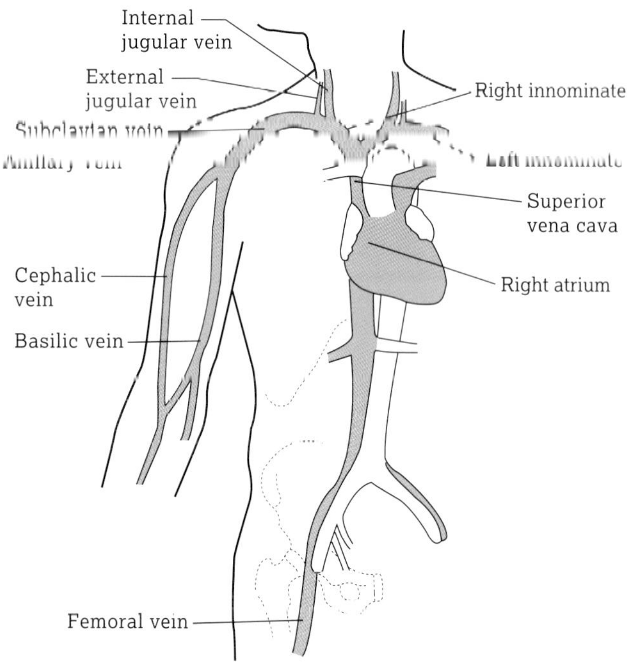

Figure 17.2 The main veins used for central venous access device placement. *Source*: Reproduced from Dougherty (2006) with permission of John Wiley & Sons.

Contraindications

There are no specific contraindications for inserting a VAD but there may be contraindications for location of the device and the type of medication that can be administered (very few can be administered via an artery).

Principles of care

Regardless of the type of VAD used, the principles of care for the device remain the same:

- to prevent infection
- to maintain a 'closed' intravenous system with minimal connections to reduce the risk of contamination
- to prevent damage to the device and associated intravenous equipment
- to maintain a patent and correctly positioned device.

Each of these principles will be discussed generally and then in more detail under each type of access device.

Methods of preventing infection at the insertion site

Aseptic technique and compliance with recommendations for equipment and dressing changes are essential if microbial contamination is to be prevented (Gorski et al. 2016, Loveday et al. 2014, O'Grady et al. 2011, RCN 2016a). Whenever the insertion site is exposed or the intravenous system is broken, standard aseptic non-touch technique (ANTT) should be practised. ANTT is basic in nature and clearly defined, focusing on the essentials of all intravenous therapy regardless of the intravenous device (Rowley et al. 2010) and it is now the de facto standard aseptic technique in the UK (Rowley and Clare 2011), used for all techniques relating to VADs regardless of whether they are peripherally or centrally inserted (Loveday et al. 2014, Rowley et al. 2010). Where blood or body fluids may be present, gloves should be worn to comply with safe practice guidelines (Rowley 2001). It is not necessary to wear sterile gloves when accessing a central venous access device (CVAD); clean gloves are adequate (Hemsworth et al. 2007). The use of well-fitting gloves is key in ANTT: they should be neither too small nor too large as they may otherwise impede manual dexterity (RCN 2016a) (see also Chapter 4: Infection prevention and control).

Cleaning solutions

Most transient flora can be removed from the skin with soap and water using mechanical friction. It is also important to remove dirt, which renders antiseptic solutions less effective as they cannot penetrate surface dirt (McGoldrick 2010). Use of a chlorhexidine bath or shower prior to insertion of a central venous catheter has been shown to reduce infection (Lopez 2011, Montecalvo et al. 2012). 2% chlorhexidine in 70% alcohol has been shown to be the most effective agent for skin cleaning around the VAD insertion site prior to insertion and between dressing changes (Cobbett and LeBlanc 2000, DH 2010, Kim and Lam 2008, Maki et al. 1991, Nishihara et al. 2012, O'Grady et al. 2011, Soothill et al. 2009, Timsit et al. 2012). The 70% alcohol acts by denaturing protein and so has excellent properties for destruction of gram-positive and gram-negative bacteria, as well as being active against fungi and viral organisms. Alcohol concentrations between 70% and 92% provide the most rapid and greatest reduction in microbial counts on skin but do not have any residual activity (Larson 1988). This is where chlorhexidine in alcohol has an advantage over alcohol used alone (Loveday et al. 2014, Nishihara et al. 2012). Therefore, chlorhexidine (>0.5% concentration) in 70% alcohol is recommended (Moureau 2013) as alcohol has an immediate effect and dries quickly, but chlorhexidine has ongoing antimicrobial action for 7–10 days; when used together, they also kill a wide variety of micro-organisms (Rickard et al. 2017). It is important to be aware of patient sensitivity to chlorhexidine gluconate (Loveday et al. 2014, MHRA 2012), both in cleaning solutions and within coatings of CVADs. For patients with sensitivities to chlorhexidine, consider tincture of iodine, povidone-iodine or 70% alcohol (Gorski et al. 2016). In patients with very delicate skin, cleaning with 70% alcohol followed by sterile saline and 0.5% chlorhexidine in aqueous solution is recommended in practice (Rickard et al. 2017).

Solutions should be applied with friction in back-and-forth strokes for at least 30 seconds and allowed to air dry for 30–60 seconds (DH 2010, Gorski et al. 2016, McGoldrick 2010, O'Grady et al. 2011, Scales 2009). It has been found that 1 minute of application with alcohol is as effective as 12 minutes of scrubbing and reduces bacterial counts by 75%. However, a quick wipe fails to reduce bacterial counts prior to peripheral cannulation (Gorski et al. 2016, Weinstein and Hagle 2014). Allowing any cleaning solution to dry is vital in order for disinfection to be completed and, in the case of alcohol, which is a plasticizer, it ensures that plastic equipment will not 'glue together' (Dougherty 2006). Dressings placed on moist skin are the true cause of many so-called 'dressing allergies', where skin becomes red, painful and/or itchy (Rickard et al. 2017).

Inspection of insertion site and cleaning of equipment

Cleaning solutions should be used not only on insertion sites but also to clean junctions, connections and so on. It is recommended that injection caps should be cleaned vigorously with appropriate cleaning agents such as 2% chlorhexidine in alcohol (Brown et al. 1997, DH 2010, Loveday et al. 2014, NICE 2012, Wright et al. 2013). The optimal frequency for cleaning the insertion site is debatable; peripheral sites are rarely cleaned once the device is sited because the device is *in situ* for such a short period of time. However, central venous access sites (e.g. PICCs) may be cleaned weekly (at dressing change), and short-term central venous catheters (CVCs) may be cleaned weekly, daily or more frequently (as these are associated with the highest infection risk). The insertion site should be checked regularly for signs of phlebitis (erythema, pain and/or swelling) or infection using the Visual Infusion Phlebitis (VIP) scoring system or similar (DH 2003, Gorski et al. 2016, Jackson 1998, RCN 2016a). Complaints of soreness, unexpected pyrexia, and damaged, wet or soiled dressings are reasons for immediate inspection and renewal of the dressing.

Securement and dressings

There are a number of securement devices and dressings available. The aim of a securement device is to secure the device to the skin and prevent movement of the device, which in turn will reduce the risk of mechanical phlebitis and infection. Decurement devices also prevent dislodgement. Types of securement include tape, sutures and self-adhesive anchoring devices applied to the skin (e.g. StatLock) (Luo et al. 2017, Moureau and Iannucci 2003) and anchor devices that are placed just beneath the skin at the insertion site (e.g. SecurAcath) (Egan et al. 2013). Suturing can result in inflammation and bacterial colonization of the exit site (Schears 2005) and is no longer recommended (Maki 2002), particularly with PICCs (Nakazawa 2010b). StatLocks have been shown to result in significantly longer duration *in situ* and fewer total complications (Luo et al. 2017, Schears 2005, Yamamoto et al. 2002) but adhesive devices can cause skin surface irritation. To avoid this, anchoring devices such as SecurAcath are now recommended for the securement of percutaneous catheters (NICE 2017) and they have been shown to save time and prevent catheter dislodgement during dressing change (Goossens et al. 2010). Alternatively, the use of tissue adhesives, traditionally used for wound closure (Singer and Thode 2004), has become a novel method of securing VADs and its clinical use continues to increase due to the ability to 'seal' the insertion site. This prevents ooze and entry of micro-organisms, has bacteriostatic properties and provides high tensile strength (Corley et al. 2017, Jeanes and Martinez-Garcia 2016, Scoppettuolo et al. 2015, Simonova et al. 2012). Cyanoacrylate (medical-grade superglue) applied directly to the exit site, and under the hub on insertion, is an effective way to reduce micro-movements, achieve haemostasis when there is oozing from the exit site and provide further infection prevention (Rickard et al. 2017).

Types of dressings include sterile gauze and transparent dressings. The recommendation for a CVAD site is an intact, dry, adherent semi-occlusive transparent dressing (DH 2010, Loveday et al. 2014). The RCN (2016a) recommends the use of transparent IV film dressings. These dressings allow observation of the exit site without the need to remove the dressing. They are also moisture permeable, thereby reducing the collection of moisture under the dressing (Casey and Elliott 2010). The key benefits of transparent IV film dressings (i.e. intravenous vapour-permeable film dressings) are their waterproof nature, conformability and moisture vapour transmission rate (CET 2018). The moisture vapour transmission rate (MVTR) is the measurement of water vapour diffusion through a material and it defines the breathability of IV film dressings. It is important that the skin under the dressing maintains its normal function to avoid skin irritation or maceration without excessive proliferation of skin flora (Rickard et al. 2017).

Newer chlorhexidine-impregnated dressings can be beneficial in preventing catheter colonization (Safdar et al. 2014). These products include a chlorhexidine gluconate antimicrobial transparent dressing, which contains a chlorhexidine gel pad, which is integral to the dressing and has been shown to allow visualization of the site, facilitating absorption of fluid under the dressing (Moureau et al. 2009, Pfaff et al. 2012). It has been shown to prevent the regrowth of microbial skin flora (Maki 2008) and reduce the incidence of bloodstream infection (Jeanes and Bitmead 2015). This can also be achieved by attaching a hydrophilic polyurethane absorptive foam patch impregnated with chlorhexidine gluconate under the transparent dressing, which has been shown to reduce the rate of catheter colonization and demonstrated significant reductions in the associated rate of catheter-related bloodstream infection (Ho and Litton 2006, Ruschulte et al. 2009, Timsit et al. 2009). However, the foam patch does not enable insertion site visualization.

Methods of maintaining a closed intravenous system

If equipment becomes accidentally disconnected, air embolism or profuse blood loss may occur, depending on the condition and position of the patient (Perucca 2010). Accidental disconnection poses a greater risk in patients with central venous or arterial access devices than in those with peripheral venous devices. This is because of the amount of air that may be introduced via a CVAD and the speed with which it may enter the pulmonary vessels or the speed of haemorrhage. Luer-Lok provides the most secure connection and all equipment should have these fittings: that is, administration sets, extension sets and injection caps (Dougherty 2006). Needle-free systems provide a closed environment, which further reduces the risk of air entry (Dougherty 2006, 2008, Kelly et al. 2017). Care should be taken to clamp the catheter firmly when changing equipment. Connections must be double checked and precautions taken to prevent the introduction of air into the system when making additions to, or taking blood from, a CVC (Dougherty 2006). Another way of maintaining a closed intravenous system is the use of newer peripheral intravenous cannulas with integrated extension tubing (closed system) (Shaw 2017) (see Figure 17.15).

Methods of preventing damage of the vascular access device and performing a repair

Catheters are made of non-resealable material, so penetration by a needle creates holes and a catheter can rupture if excessive force is exerted (Gorski et al. 2010). Pinch-off syndrome can also result in a transected and potentially embolized catheter segment (Gorski et al. 2010). Temporary and permanent repairs can be performed depending on where the catheter is damaged and the type of catheter (Dougherty 2006, 2014). Damaged catheters must be repaired or removed, as any opening in the catheter can act as a point of entry for bacteria or air (Dougherty 2014). The repair of a ruptured tunnelled CVAD is often the least invasive and most viable intervention for certain patient populations (Gordon and Gardiner 2013). Catheter repairs do not increase the rate of infection despite longer dwell times (Gordon and Gardiner 2013, Koh et al. 2012).

Artery forceps or sharp-edged clamps should not be used to clamp the catheter. A smooth clamp should be placed on the reinforced section of the catheter provided for clamping (Dougherty 2006). If a reinforced section is not present, placing a tape tab over part of the catheter can create one. A second alternative is to move the clamp up or down the catheter at regular intervals to reduce the risk of wear and tear in one place (Dougherty 2006).

Use of the correct syringe size in accordance with the manufacturer's guidelines will reduce the risk of catheter rupture (Gorski et al. 2016). However, appropriate syringe size alone will not be sufficient to prevent catheter rupture. If resistance is felt and more pressure is applied to overcome it, catheter fracture can result regardless of the syringe size (Hadaway 1998a, Macklin 1999). Nurses must be familiar with the action to be taken to minimize any risk to patient safety in this event. Immediate clamping of the catheter proximal to the fracture or split is essential to prevent blood loss or air embolism (Gorski et al. 2010). The split area should be cleaned vigorously using a chlorhexidine swab and friction for at least 30 seconds, left to air dry and then covered with an occlusive transparent dressing until emergency repair equipment has been collected (Gordon and Gardiner 2013). The procedure must be done using an aseptic technique. The repair should only be undertaken by a healthcare professional who has the necessary knowledge and skills, and according to the manufacturer's instructions (Dougherty 2014).

Methods of maintaining patency

Patency is defined as the ability to infuse through and aspirate blood from a VAD (Dougherty 2006). It is important for the patency of the device to be maintained at all times. Blockage can lead to device damage, infection, inconvenience to patients and disruption to drug delivery. Maintaining patency and avoidance of infections are key objectives in long-term CVAD usage (Kumwenda et al. 2018). Occlusion of a device is usually the result of one or more of the following:

- clot formation (Figure 17.3) due to (a) an administration set or electronic infusion device being turned off accidentally and left for a prolonged period or (b) insufficient or incorrect flushing of

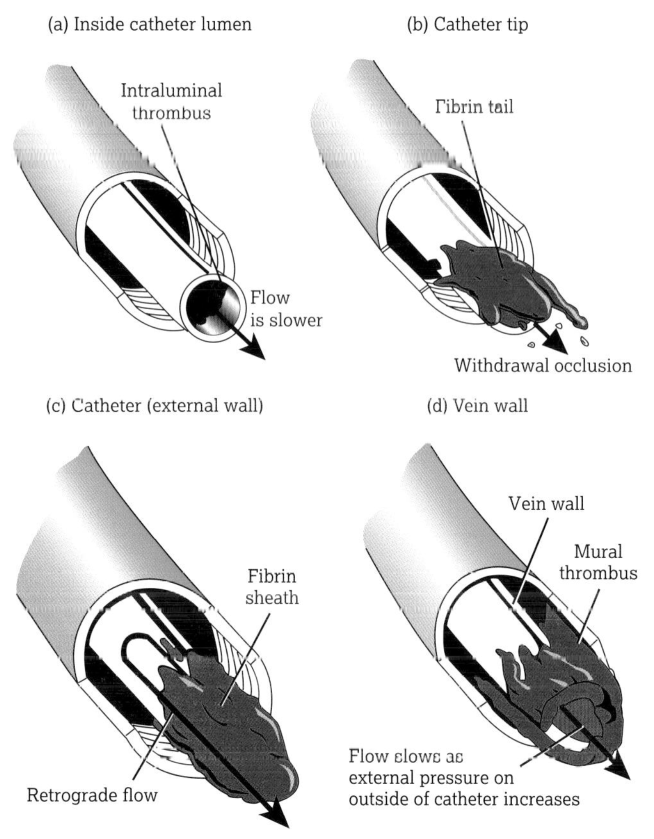

Figure 17.3 Clot formations. *Source*: Reproduced from Macklin and Chernecky (2004) with permission of Elsevier.

the device when not in use; thrombotic occlusions are responsible for up to 58% of all occlusions (Hadaway 2010)
- precipitate formation due to inadequate flushing between incompatible medications (Dougherty 2006).

Kinking or pinch-off syndrome may also impair the patency of the device. Meticulous intravenous technique will prevent the majority of these problems.

Two main types of solution are used to maintain patency in VADs: heparin and 0.9% sodium chloride. All devices should be flushed with 10–20 mL 0.9% sodium chloride after blood withdrawal and then flushed again with the appropriate flushing solution (Dougherty 2006, 2008, Gorski et al. 2016, RCN 2016a).

Maintaining patency can be achieved by one of the following:

- a continuous infusion to keep the vein open, either by the patient being attached to an infusion of 0.9% sodium chloride via a volumetric pump, which reduces comfort and mobility, or by use of an elastomeric device, which is less restrictive and has been able to reduce loss of patency by 50% (Heath and Jones 2001)
- intermittent flushing (previously known as a 'heparin lock') (Box 17.1).

When used for intermittent therapy, the device should be flushed after each use with the appropriate flushing solution (guidelines for volumes, concentrations and frequency of flushing are commonly established within individual institutions). It is now well established that flushing with 0.9% sodium chloride can also adequately maintain the patency of a cannula (Goode et al. 1991, White et al. 2011). This avoids side-effects such as local tissue damage, drug incompatibilities and iatrogenic haemorrhage, which can occur with heparin (Goode et al. 1991, NPSA 2008a). As well as being cost-effective, it appears that daily or twice-daily

Box 17.1 Advantages and disadvantages of intermittent flushing

The advantages of intermittent flushing compared with a continuous infusion are:
- it reduces the risk of circulatory overload
- it reduces the risk of vascular irritation
- it decreases the risk of bacterial contamination as it eliminates a continuous intravenous pathway
- it increases patient comfort and mobility
- it may reduce the cost of intravenous equipment (Phillips 2005).

The major disadvantage is the necessity for constant vigilance and regular flushing (Weinstein and Hagle 2014).

flushing with a volume of 2–5 mL 0.9% sodium chloride is appropriate (Goode et al. 1991, LeDuc 1997).

The consensus about the solution to use for maintaining patency of CVADs has changed in the past few years from heparinized saline to 0.9% sodium chloride (Dal Molin et al. 2014, 2015, Lopez-Briz et al. 2014, 2018, Pittiruti et al. 2016, Solinas et al. 2017, Zhong et al. 2017) and most guidelines favour the use of 0.9% sodium chloride for flush and lock purposes for any type of non-dialysis CVAD (Gorski et al. 2016, Loveday et al. 2014, RCN 2016a, Sousa et al. 2015). However, some local policies continue to recommend heparinized saline to maintain the patency of CVCs; in particular, for intermittent or infrequent use of implanted ports (Kefeli et al. 2009, Palese et al. 2014), it is recommended to use a stronger solution of heparin, usually 500 international units of heparin in 5 mL 0.9% sodium chloride (Berreth 2013a, Perucca 2010). There is a lack of consensus on the optimal frequency of flushing of CVADs (Conway et al. 2014, Goossens 2015, Green et al. 2008, Mitchell et al. 2009, Sona et al. 2011) and practice varies between organizations. Flushing regimens ranging from once daily to once weekly have been found to be effective. PICCs and skin-tunnelled catheters (STCs) normally require flushing once a week, while recommendations for implanted ports range from monthly (Vescia et al. 2008) to every 6 weeks (Kefeli et al. 2009) to every 8 weeks (Hoffman 2001, Palese et al. 2014) to every 3–4 months when not in use (Kuo et al. 2005, Solinas et al. 2017). The decision regarding which solution and frequency to use to maintain patency is often based on local data (Bolton 2013, Hadaway 2006).

Using the correct techniques to flush the VAD has been highlighted as one of the key issues in maintaining patency (Baranowski 1993, Goodwin and Carlson 1993). Flush efficiency is more about flushing technique than solution used (Ferroni et al. 2014, Goossens 2015). There are two stages in flushing:

1. A push–pause, pulsatile or turbulent technique is more effective when rinsing the internal diameter of a catheter than laminar or continuous low flow infusion (Goossens 2015, Guiffant et al. 2012). These techniques create turbulent flow when the solution is administered, regardless of type and volume. This removes debris from the internal catheter wall (Cummings Winfield and Mushani Kanji 2008, Goodwin and Carlson 1993, Guiffant et al. 2012).
2. The procedure is completed using the positive pressure technique. This is accomplished by maintaining pressure on the plunger of the syringe while disconnecting the syringe from the needle-free connector, which prevents reflux of blood into the tip, reducing the risk of occlusion (Berreth 2013a, Gorski et al. 2016, Hadaway 2010).

Manufacturers have now produced needle-free connectors, which are intended to reduce incidence of occlusion and infection (Blaiche et al. 2011, Chernecky and Walker 2011, Hadaway 2012, Macklin 2010a). Blood reflux is caused by changes in pressure within intravascular catheters upon connection or disconnection of a syringe or intravenous tubing from a needle-free connector (Hull et al. 2018). Some needle-free connectors enable a positive 'displacement' flush and achieve positive pressure without practitioners being required to actively achieve the positive pressure (Weinstein and Hagle 2014). They have been shown to reduce significantly the incidence of catheter occlusion (Berger 2000, Lenhart 2000, Mayo 2001, Rummel et al. 2001). However, changes in pressure, differing with type of needle-free connector, may result in fluid movement and blood reflux, which can contribute to intraluminal catheter occlusions and increase the potential for CVAD-associated bloodstream infections (Hull et al. 2018). Therefore, it is recommended to carry out a risk assessment prior to routine use and to change the needle-free connector regularly (e.g. once per week) (Casey et al. 2018, Hadaway 2010). Negative pressure devices require positive pressure on the syringe. Neutral displacement connectors allow no blood reflux to occur on disconnection and they are not dependent upon flushing technique so can be clamped before or after syringe disconnection (Casey et al. 2018, Chernecky et al. 2009).

Excessive force should never be used when flushing devices. When a catheter lumen is totally patent, internal pressure will not increase during flushing (Dougherty 2014, Hadaway 1998b). However, if resistance is felt (due to partial occlusion) and a force is applied to the plunger, particularly with a small-volume syringe, high pressure can result within the catheter, which may then rupture (Conn 1993, Dougherty 2014, Gorski et al. 2010, Hadaway 1998b, Macklin 1999). It is therefore recommended that the device is checked first with a 10 mL or larger syringe containing 0.9% sodium chloride (Hadaway 1998b, Macklin 2010b, RCN 2016a). However, smaller syringes should only be used to administer drugs where there is no pressure or occlusion and where it is not possible to further dilute drugs and administer them in a large syringe (Hadaway 1998a, Macklin 1999). The composition of the individual device determines the maximum pressure that can be exerted. There are now CVADs available (PICCs, STCs and implanted ports) and midlines that allow computed tomography (CT) contrast to be administered via a pressure injection pump at 3–5 mL per second without damaging the device.

If a catheter becomes occluded, the nurse should establish the cause of the clot, occlusion or precipitation (Bolton 2013, Gorski et al. 2016). If precipitation occurs, instillation of hydrochloric acid or ethyl chloride may be required (Doellman 2011, Hadaway 2010). Thrombus formation (both intraluminal and external) and formation of a fibrous connective tissue sheath (traditionally described as 'fibrin sheath') plays a central role in CVAD dysfunction and can limit the efficacy of treatment and the longevity of the CVAD, and create life-threatening situations where the relevant therapy cannot be provided (Gallieni et al. 2016, Kumwenda et al. 2018). There are two types of thrombotic occlusion:

- *Partial withdrawal occlusion* (Figure 17.4): this is usually caused by fibrin sheath formation and identified by absent or sluggish blood return while fluids can be infused (Nakazawa 2010b). Fibrin sheaths can result in seeding of bacteria and drug extravasation (Mayo 2000, 2001) and can be resolved by the instillation of a thrombolytic agent, such as urokinase or alteplase (Dougherty 2006, Fanikos et al. 2009, Haire and Herbst 2000, Kumwenda et al. 2018, Weinstein and Hagle 2014).
- *Total occlusion*: this is when there is an inability to withdraw blood or infuse fluids or medications. This can be resolved by instillation of a thrombolytic agent (Baskin et al. 2009, 2012, Deitcher et al. 2002, Kumwenda et al. 2018, Ponec et al. 2001, Syner-Kinase 2011, Timoney et al. 2002).

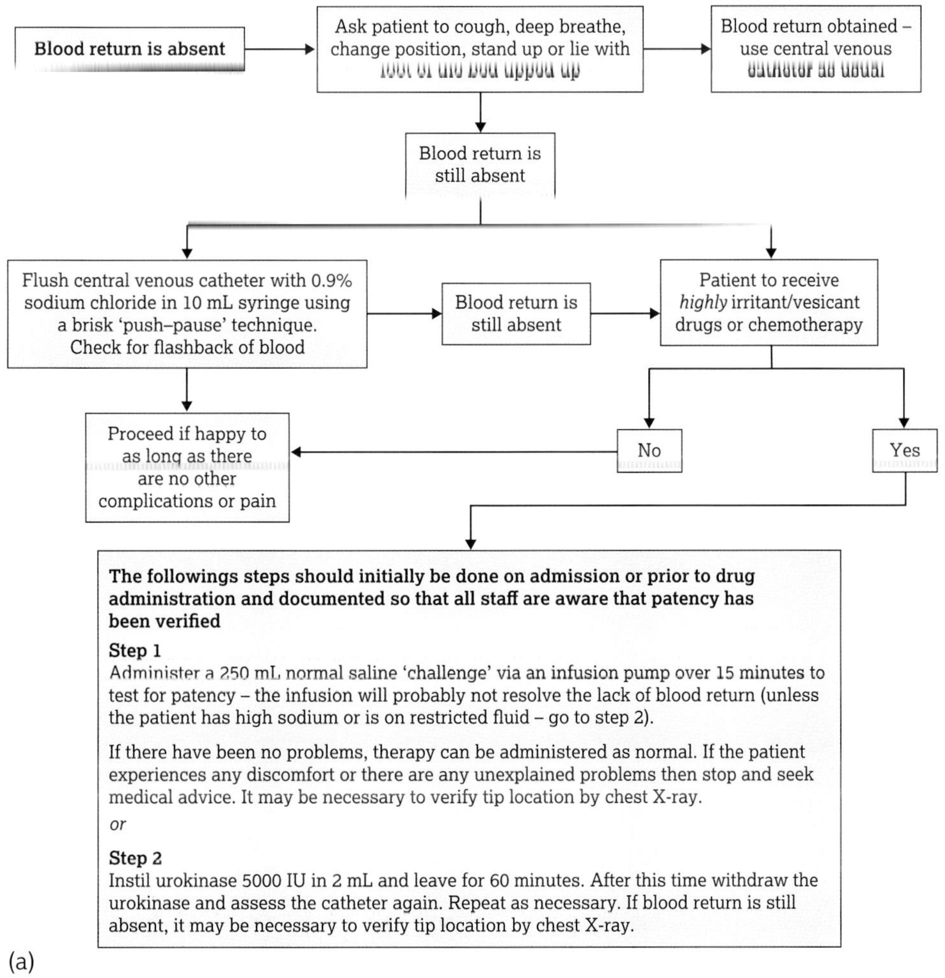

(a)

Figure 17.4 (a) Algorithm for partial withdrawal occlusion – that is, fluids can be infused freely by gravity but blood cannot be withdrawn from the catheter. (b) Evidence based protocol for management of occluded CVADs in non-renal settings. *Source*: (a) Adapted from UCL Hospital Central Venous Catheter Policy.

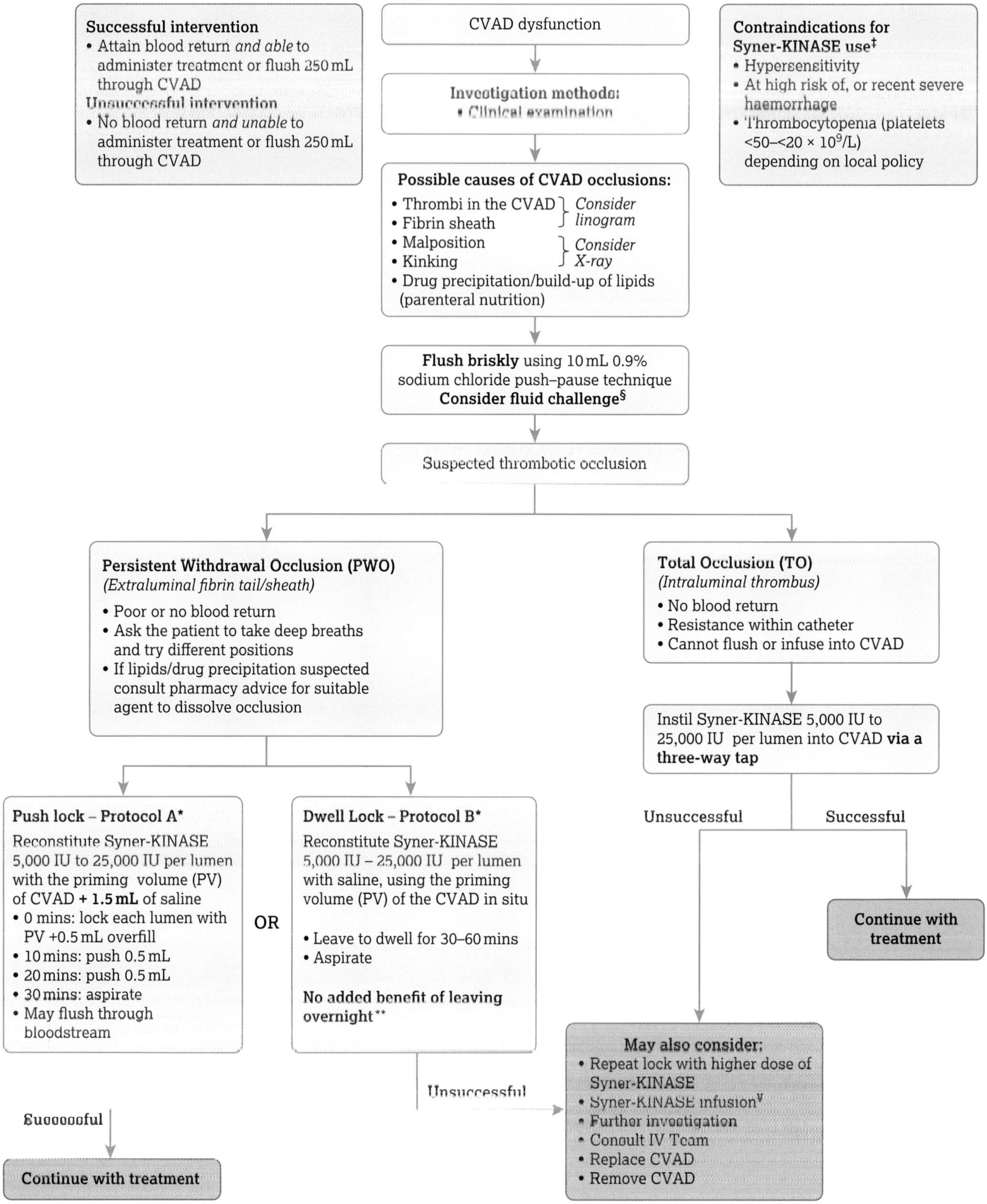
Successful intervention
• Attain blood return and able to administer treatment or flush 250 mL through CVAD
Unsuccessful intervention
• No blood return and unable to administer treatment or flush 250 mL through CVAD
CVAD dysfunction
Investigation methods:
• Clinical examination
Contraindications for Syner-KINASE use‡
• Hypersensitivity
• At high risk of, or recent severe haemorrhage
• Thrombocytopenia (platelets <50–<20 × 10⁹/L) depending on local policy
Possible causes of CVAD occlusions:
• Thrombi in the CVAD
• Fibrin sheath
Consider linogram
• Malposition
• Kinking
Consider X-ray
• Drug precipitation/build-up of lipids (parenteral nutrition)
Flush briskly using 10 mL 0.9% sodium chloride push–pause technique
Consider fluid challenge§
Suspected thrombotic occlusion
Persistent Withdrawal Occlusion (PWO)
(Extraluminal fibrin tail/sheath)
• Poor or no blood return
• Ask the patient to take deep breaths and try different positions
• If lipids/drug precipitation suspected consult pharmacy advice for suitable agent to dissolve occlusion
Total Occlusion (TO)
(Intraluminal thrombus)
• No blood return
• Resistance within catheter
• Cannot flush or infuse into CVAD
Instil Syner-KINASE 5,000 IU to 25,000 IU per lumen into CVAD via a three-way tap
Push lock – Protocol A*
Reconstitute Syner-KINASE 5,000 IU to 25,000 IU per lumen with the priming volume (PV) of CVAD + 1.5 mL of saline
• 0 mins: lock each lumen with PV +0.5 mL overfill
• 10 mins: push 0.5 mL
• 20 mins: push 0.5 mL
• 30 mins: aspirate
• May flush through bloodstream
OR
Dwell Lock – Protocol B*
Reconstitute Syner-KINASE 5,000 IU – 25,000 IU per lumen with saline, using the priming volume (PV) of the CVAD in situ
• Leave to dwell for 30–60 mins
• Aspirate
No added benefit of leaving overnight**
Unsuccessful
Successful
Continue with treatment
Successful
Continue with treatment
Unsuccessful
May also consider:
• Repeat lock with higher dose of Syner-KINASE
• Syner-KINASE infusion¥
• Further investigation
• Consult IV Team
• Replace CVAD
• Remove CVAD

‡For a full list of contraindications consult Syner-Kinase summary of product characteristics (Syner Med, 2018).
§Dougherty and Lister (2015, chapter 14).
*It is the discretion of the healthcare professional to use either protocol A or B, in discussion with the patient.
**Leaving lock on overnight has no added benefit, but it may be considered if more practical for the patient and centre.
¥Refer to descriptive protocol for information on Syner-KINASE infusion.

(b)

Figure 17.4 *Continued*

If the occlusion is caused by a clot, gentle pressure and aspiration may be sufficient to dislodge it. Silicone catheters expand on pressure and allow fluid to flow around the clot, facilitating its dislodgement. This should only be attempted using a 10 mL or larger syringe. Smaller syringes should never be used as they create a greater pressure (Camp-Sorrell et al. 2004, Gorski et al. 2010). This can result in rupture of the catheter, leading to loss of catheter integrity (Gorski et al. 2010). Clearance of a catheter occlusion and instillation of thrombolytic agents should be performed using a three-way tap and negative pressure (Gabriel 2008, Gallieni et al. 2008, McKnight 2004). The establishment of negative pressure involves creating a vacuum by aspiration of the air or dead space within a catheter (Gabriel 2008, Dougherty 2006, Moureau et al. 1999). Another method is use of the percussion technique (Johnston 2007, Stewart 2001). Unblocking a catheter is not a quick procedure and it can take some time to achieve success.

Methods of maintaining a correctly positioned catheter tip

A CVAD is defined as a catheter whose tip terminates in the lower third of the superior vena cava (SVC) (Gorski et al. 2016, RCN 2016a, Wilkes 2011). Optimal tip location is a subject of debate, although there are some common recommendations (Chantler 2009):

- The vein should be large with a high blood flow (this dilutes drugs and reduces the risk of damage to the vein intima).
- The end of the catheter should be in the long axis of the vein and not abutting the vessel wall (to reduce damage to the intima and avoid inaccurate pressure readings).
- The tip should be beyond the last venous valve.

Ideally, the tip of a CVAD should be positioned in the proximity of the cavo-atrial junction (CAJ), in a 'safe' area, such as the lower third of the SVC and the upper portion of the right atrium (Bodenham et al. 2016, Fletcher and Bodenham 2000, Lamperti and Pittiruti 2015).

The tip location of a CVAD will affect the catheter's performance; if the tip is too high or too far within the right atrium, it may be sucked against the adjacent wall when aspiration is applied (Vesely 2002, 2003), and this increases the risk of thrombosis (Gallieni et al. 2008). A catheter tip positioned against a vascular wall may also become a source of persistent irritation, potentially leading to the creation of a nidus for thrombus formation (Bodenham et al. 2016, Galloway and Bodenham 2004, Mayo 2001). This is reported more frequently in patients who have left-sided placements (Chantler 2009). The arguments for right atrial tip placement are that the tip is in a large chamber, thus preventing contact with the vein wall, and the rapid blood flow also prevents accumulation of thrombin and minimizes irritation of substances. The disadvantages of this tip position are an increase in cardiac arrhythmias (although this may be associated with the insertion of the guidewire as its incidence is reduced by image guidance) and catheter-induced perforation and cardiac tamponade (although this has been reduced by using softer materials and imaging guidance) (Chantler 2009, Lamperti and Pittiruti 2015, Vesely 2002).

The tip position can also change during its time *in situ*. The position of a CVAD tip moves with respiration and patient position (Bodenham et al. 2016). For example, the final position of a PICC is dependent on the insertion site and the position of the patient's arm, and the catheter can move at least 2 cm further into the right atrium on movement (Forauer and Alonzo 2000, Spencer 2017). PICCs placed in the left arm tend to move more than those placed in the right arm, and those placed in the basilic vein are more likely to move than those placed in the cephalic vein (Vesely 2003). Anatomical changes occur with subclavian and internal jugular insertion when patients sit upright following insertion and the catheter tip can move upward. In an STC this can be 2–3 cm, particularly in overweight patients of either sex or female patients with substantial breast tissue. Large-diameter catheters can move more than smaller ones and subclavian more than internal jugular placements.

The tip of the catheter can also move during high-flow flushing and power injection of contrast material (Morden et al. 2014, Spencer 2017). There have been reports of CT-PICC displacement events during power injection of contrast for CT scanning (Morden et al. 2014). This is less likely to happen if the tip of the catheter is placed in the distal SVC or within the CAJ (Spencer 2017).

A correctly placed catheter tip will probably be one that undergoes a range of movement between the SVC and upper right atrium (Dougherty 2006, Nakazawa 2010a, Spencer 2017). The direction of the catheter can be tracked with electromagnetic navigation devices and this prevents malposition (La Greca 2014). Tip position is determined by:

- taking a chest X-ray using the posterior anterior view (Wise et al. 2001) (Figure 17.5)
- using electrocardiogram (ECG) technology (intracavitary ECG), which has been shown to provide accurate and consistent guidance of the tip to the lower third of the SVC or CAJ; it also removes the time needed to interpret an X-ray and the cost of the X-ray, reduces patient exposure to radiation and saves time repositioning the tip or catheter (Moureau et al. 2010, Oliver and Jones 2014, Pittiruti et al. 2012) (Figure 17.6).

Catheter tip position can also be detected by transoesophageal echocardiogram (TOE) but this is expensive, invasive and impractical in most patients (Lamperti and Pittiruti 2015).

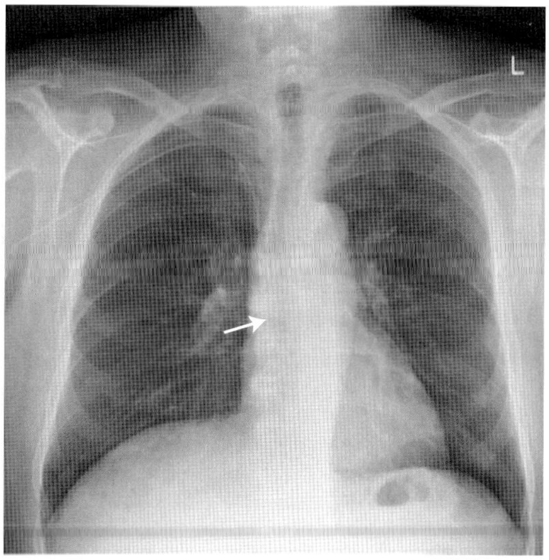

Figure 17.5 Chest X-ray showing catheter tip correctly positioned (arrow).

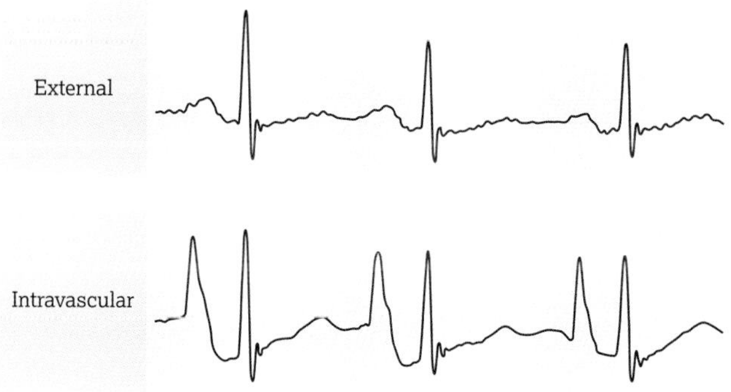

Figure 17.6 Electrocardiogram (ECG) pattern indicating raised P waves.

Anticipated patient outcomes

The patient will have a functioning VAD.

Clinical governance

Competencies

Nurses who insert devices and/or provide infusion therapy should be competent in all clinical aspects of infusion therapy and have validated competencies in clinical judgement and practice; they should also maintain their knowledge and skills in accordance with the Nursing and Midwifery Council's *Code* (Collins et al. 2006, Hyde 2008, NMC 2018, RCN 2016a).

The RCN (2016a) recommends that any registered nurses who undertake the insertion of VADs or those who manage VADs or administer infusion therapy should have undergone theoretical and practical training in a number of areas (Box 17.2) (Corrigan 2010, DH 2004, Hyde 2010, Loveday et al. 2014, MHRA 2015, Moureau et al. 2013, NICE 2003, NMC 2018, NPSA 2003, 2007, RCN 2016a). All staff have a professional obligation to maintain their knowledge and skills (HCPC 2016, NMC 2018). It is also the responsibility of the organization to support staff and provide them with training and education. This may be in the form of study days, practical sessions using a mannequin and a role development workbook, or simulation (Andreatta et al. 2011, Collins et al. 2006, Kokotis 2014, Phillips et al. 2011).

Consent

Prior to insertion of a peripheral cannula, it is usual to obtain verbal consent from the patient (Hyde 2010). However, prior to insertion of a CVAD, written consent should be obtained (unless required in an emergency) following an explanation of the procedure, the benefits, the alternatives, and the possible complications and the percentage risk of each (these would include pneumothorax, malposition, haemorrhage, thrombosis and infection). This information should be provided verbally and in written form (Hamilton 2009, HCPC 2016, NMC 2018) and it should follow local and national guidelines (Bodenham et al. 2016).

Pre-procedural considerations

Equipment

There are many different types of device available, made of a variety of materials and tip endings (see Table 17.1). There is also specific equipment associated with VADs, including securement devices and dressings. These will be discussed in more detail in each individual section.

Securement (stabilization) of device and dressings

Devices are secured to prevent movement, which reduces the risk of phlebitis, infiltration, infection and migration (Gorski et al. 2016, McGoldrick 2010, Moureau and Iannucci 2003, Schears 2005, Yamamoto et al. 2002). This can be achieved by suturing, taping or use of securing devices (Figure 17.7). These all require a dressing over them. The stabilization device should be used in a manner that does not interfere with the assessment and monitoring of the access site (McGoldrick 2010).

The choice of dressing is usually based upon what is most suitable for a particular VAD site or type of skin. An intravenous dressing is applied to minimize contamination of the insertion site and

Box 17.2 Knowledge and skills required of a nurse who inserts vascular access devices and/or provides infusion therapy

Vascular access device insertion

- Anatomy and physiology of the circulatory system, in particular the anatomy of the location in which the device is placed, including veins, arteries and nerves and the underlying tissue structures.
- Assessment of patients' vascular access needs, nature and duration of therapy, and quality of life.
- Improving venous access, for example the use of pharmacological and non-pharmacological methods.
- Selection of veins and problems associated with venous access due to thrombosed, inflamed or fragile veins; the effects of ageing on veins; disease processes; previous treatment; lymphoedema or presence of infection.
- Selection of device and other equipment.
- Infection control issues (e.g. hand washing and skin preparation).
- Pharmacological issues (e.g. use of local anaesthetics, management of anxious patients, management of haematoma and management of phlebitis).
- The patient's perspective on living with a vascular access device.
- Risk management in order to reduce the risk of blood spills and needle stick injury.
- Professional and legal aspects (e.g. consent, professional guidance, knowledge and skill maintenance, and documentation).
- Performing the procedure.
- Prevention and management of complications during insertion (e.g. nerve injury and haematoma).
- Monitoring and care of the site (e.g. flushing, dressing and removal).
- Product evaluation.
- Patient information and education.
- Documentation.
- Specific training for insertion of vascular access devices in certain groups (e.g. neonates, children and oncology patients).

Administration of intravenous medication and care of vascular access devices *in situ*

- Legal, professional and ethical issues.
- Anatomy and physiology.
- Fluid balance and blood administration.
- Mathematical calculations relating to medications.
- Pharmacology and pharmaceutics relating to reconstitution administration.
- Local and systemic complications.
- Infection control issues.
- Use of equipment, including infusion equipment.
- Drug administration.
- Risk management, and health and safety.
- Care and management of vascular access devices.
- Infusion therapy in specialist areas (e.g. paediatrics, oncology, parenteral nutrition or transfusion therapy).

Source: Adapted from [illegible] (2010) with permission of [illegible]

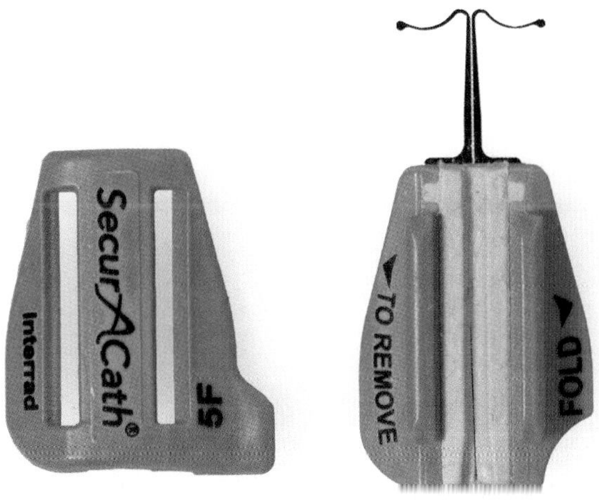

Figure 17.7 SecurAcath securing device. *Source:* Reproduced with permission of Interrad Medical, Inc.

provide stability of the device (Dougherty 2006, Jeanes and Martinez-Garcia 2016). Therefore, the ideal intravenous dressing should:

- provide an effective barrier to bacteria
- allow the catheter to be securely fixed
- be sterile
- be easy to apply and remove
- be waterproof
- adhere well
- be comfortable for the patient (Hitchcock and Savine 2017, Rickard et al. 2017, Ullman et al. 2015).

There are two main types of dressing: dry, sterile, low-linting gauze dressings and transparent dressings. A dry, sterile, low linting gauze dressing secured with the minimum of hypoallergenic tape is most suitable for patients with skin that is prone to allergy or is thin and tears easily, as transparent dressings can damage the skin if not removed correctly. Always follow the manufacturer's instructions when removing transparent IV film dressings. International and local clinical practice guidelines rarely acknowledge or provide recommendations for how to effectively dress and secure VADs within complex situations (Broadhurst et al. 2017). Medical adhesive-related skin injury (MARSI) is a term used for skin reactions or manifestations of cutaneous abnormality related to medical adhesive that persist for 30 minutes or more after removal of the adhesive (Hitchcock and Savine 2017, McNichol et al. 2013). The following can predispose patients to a high risk of skin injury:

- not allowing the skin decontamination product to dry completely prior to the application of an IV film dressing
- inappropriate removal of the dressing, causing some degree of skin damage
- inconsistent assessment and documentation of skin condition (Hitchcock and Savine 2017, Rickard et al. 2017).

Early recognition of MARSI enables early intervention and specialist advice and thus is key in order to prevent the loss of skin integrity. The use of algorithms that consider all elements of IV dressing (i.e. skin decontamination, skin protection, what to do in the event of a known sensitivity or allergy to specific decontamination or dressing products, and the appropriate referral for specialist input) has been found to be effective in preventing MARSI in clinical practice (Hitchcock and Savine 2017).

The benefits of transparent dressings are that:

- they allow inspection of the insertion site while the dressing is *in situ* and therefore do not require removal each time
- they are waterproof
- many are also moisture permeable (CET 2018, McGoldrick 2010).

This means that the dressing allows moisture vapour transmission, which is an important factor related to the risk of infection, as collection of moisture enhances the proliferation of micro-organisms and the risk of skin damage due to skin maceration (CET 2018, Loveday et al. 2014, O'Grady et al. 2011).

Comparisons of infection rates when transparent dressings and sterile gauze are used have shown that there is no significant difference in peripheral devices, and that infection rates may be reduced in CVADs (DH 2010, Maki and Ringer 1987, RCN 2016a). CVAD dressings must be removed and replaced within 24 hours following insertion of the catheter (Dougherty 2006, Ryder 2001, RCN 2016a). This is due to the bacterial colonization or 'biofilm', which occurs 6–18 hours following insertion (Ryder 2002). Transparent dressings should be changed every 7 days unless the manufacturer recommends otherwise or the integrity is compromised – that is, when the dressing is damp, loose or soiled (Gorski et al. 2016, Loveday et al. 2014, RCN 2016a). If gauze is used, it must be replaced when the dressing becomes damp, loose or soiled or when inspection of the site is necessary (Loveday et al. 2014, RCN 2016a). When the dressing is changed, the insertion site should be inspected for inflammation and/or discharge and the condition of the skin documented (DH 2010).

There are also dressings impregnated with chlorhexidine gluconate (CHG) (e.g. protective disc impregnated with CHG or CHG gel integrated into the dressing) and ionic silver alginate pads, both of which may also be considered for placement at the catheter skin junction. This is done to protect the extraluminal pathway and eliminate or reduce the incidence of infection (Hill et al. 2010, McGoldrick 2010). Tissue adhesives (surgical glue (cyanoacrylate) or metallic powder) can be applied to the site to reduce bleeding at the insertion site, which may enable the dressing to be left in place for at least 7 days following insertion and reduce extraluminal contamination (Corley et al. 2017, Jeanes and Martinez-Garcia 2016, Scoppettuolo et al. 2013, Simonova et al. 2012). There is no need to change a CVAD dressing 24 hours post-insertion if tissue adhesive was applied or impregnated discs were used post-CVAD insertion as they prevent bacterial contamination while facilitating haemostasis (Corley et al. 2017).

Assessment and recording tools

Tools have been developed to facilitate venous assessment and venous access device assessment. For example, the Venous Assessment Tool (VAT) consists of a series of risk factors and characteristics that can be assessed to determine whether cannulation will be easy, moderately difficult or hard (Figure 17.8). The VAT score can then be used in the algorithms 'Deciding On Intravenous Access' or 'DIVA (Difficult Intravenous Access)'. This helps practitioners to bring together the proposed therapy and the type of venous access in order to identify the most suitable VAD (Wells 2008). The Vessel Health Preservation (VHP) system involves carrying out an assessment to ensure that the right device is used in the right patient at the right time (Hallam et al. 2016, Moureau et al. 2012, Trick 2011) (Figure 17.9). The Michigan Appropriateness Guide for Intravenous Catheters (MAGIC) is another tool designed to inform and improve clinical decision making with respect to VADs, in particular the use of PICCs (Chopra et al. 2015). These tools and their implementation aim to improve patient outcomes by defining best practices for device insertion, care and management through a systematic process involving the patient and the multidisciplinary team (Chopra et al. 2015, Gorski et al. 2016, RCN 2016a, Swaminathan et al. 2016).

1. Patient characteristics		5. Evidence of previous use	
Needle phobia		Evidence of phlebitis	
Confusion		Evidence of infiltration or extravasation	
2. Limiting the number of available veins		Visible phlebitis or needle marks	
Hemiplegia, spasticity of upper limb(s), for example post-cerebrovascular accident		Bruising from vasculature use	
Radical mastectomy		Dark, stained veins	
Arteriovenous fistula		Cord-like, hard veins	
3. Changes in skin integrity		**6. Suitability of veins**	
Skin graft versus host disease		Flow visible veins	
Tattoos, burns, scars, eczema, over veins		Flow palpable veins	
		Few straight veins	
4. Changes in tissue		Veins are mobile	
Oedema		Only short veins identifiable or multiple valves are palpable	
Obesity		**7. History**	
Cachexia		Previous peripheral chemotherapy	
Radiotherapy to the upper limb(s)		Previous multiple courses of intravenous (IV) antibiotics	
Dark skin		Previous peripheral vesicant chemotherapy	

- For each risk factor score either 0, 1 or 2.
- 0 = risk factor not present.
- 1 = risk factor present
- 2 = risk factor present and will complicate a cannulation attempt now.
- Total points to give VAT score.
- Follow action specified below.
- Re-evaluate patient score at least every three days.

VAT score	Action
< 3 (easy)	Routine cannulation
4–8 (moderate)	Difficult cannulation Consider alternative IV access device for future therapy
> 9 (difficult)	Expert cannulation. Will require alternative IV access device for therapy to continue

Figure 17.8 Venous Assessment Tool (VAT) score. *Source*: Reproduced from Wells (2008) with permission of *Nursing Standard*.

Pharmacological support

Solutions to maintain patency

Heparin inhibits the conversion of prothrombin to thrombin and fibrinogen to fibrin, thus inhibiting coagulation, and is therefore used to prevent the build up of fibrin. The standard strength is 10 international units (IU) per mL up to a total of 5 mL (50 IU) for all CVADs with the exception of implanted ports, where it is usual for the dose to be 100 IU/mL (500 IU total). A higher dose (1000 IU/mL) is used to maintain patency in dialysis-type catheters. 0.9% sodium chloride is used to clean the internal diameter of the device of blood and drugs (Camp-Sorrell et al. 2004). Recent guidance favours the use 0.9% sodium chloride over heparinized saline for flush and lock purposes for any type of non-dialysis CVAD (Gorski et al. 2016, Loveday et al. 2014, RCN 2016a, Sousa et al. 2015). Urokinase is a fibrinolytic agent indicated for the lysis of blood clots in venous catheters that are occluded by fibrin clots. Usually, 10,000 IU is dissolved in sterile saline and instilled into the catheter every 10 minutes over 30 minutes. The drug and any clots are then aspirated and the process can be repeated if necessary (Syner-Med 2016) (see Figure 17.4b).

Specific patient preparation

Education

Involving the patient in the decision-making process is vital (Chittle et al. 2016, Dougherty 2006, Kelly 2017). Patients should be provided with individualized information and support in order to be involved in the clinical decision-making process (Sharp et al. 2014). Patient choice about the device or even the site of insertion, for example use of the non-dominant arm, results in better compliance with care of the device and monitoring of problems (Gabriel 2008). It also enables patients to cope better with the changes to their normal activities (Cooper et al. 2017, Daniels 1995) and the impact on body image can be reduced by involving the individual in the choice and management of the device (Cooper et al. 2017, Daniels 1995, Dougherty 2006, Kelly 2017).

Body image and a patient's lifestyle can be issues when a patient is living with a CVAD (Dougherty 2006). This is particularly true with an external catheter, which can be distressing and embarrassing for some patients (Hayden and Goodman 2005, Kelly 2017). It can result in restrictions to normal daily activities (e.g. bathing) or involvement in sporting activities (e.g. swimming) (Cooper et al. 2017, Gabriel 2000, Molloy et al. 2008, Robbins et al. 2000); some of these can be resolved by the use of an implanted device (Chernecky 2001, Johansson et al. 2009, Kelly 2017).

The following are ways in which a CVAD can affect body image:

- physical presence and alteration of body appearance and invasion of body integrity
- influence on the types of clothes that can be worn
- interference with physical expressions of closeness and sexuality (Daniels 1995).

The presence of a CVAD can also affect how others view the individual's roles and ability to function, particularly if the individual is attached to an infusion pump (Thompson et al. 1989). The psychological impact of an indwelling catheter on body image should not be overlooked, especially when patients are sexually active (Gabriel 2000, Kelly 2017, Oakley et al. 2000).

Post-procedural considerations

Immediate care

This will depend on the type of VAD that has been inserted (see sections on each individual VAD below in this chapter).

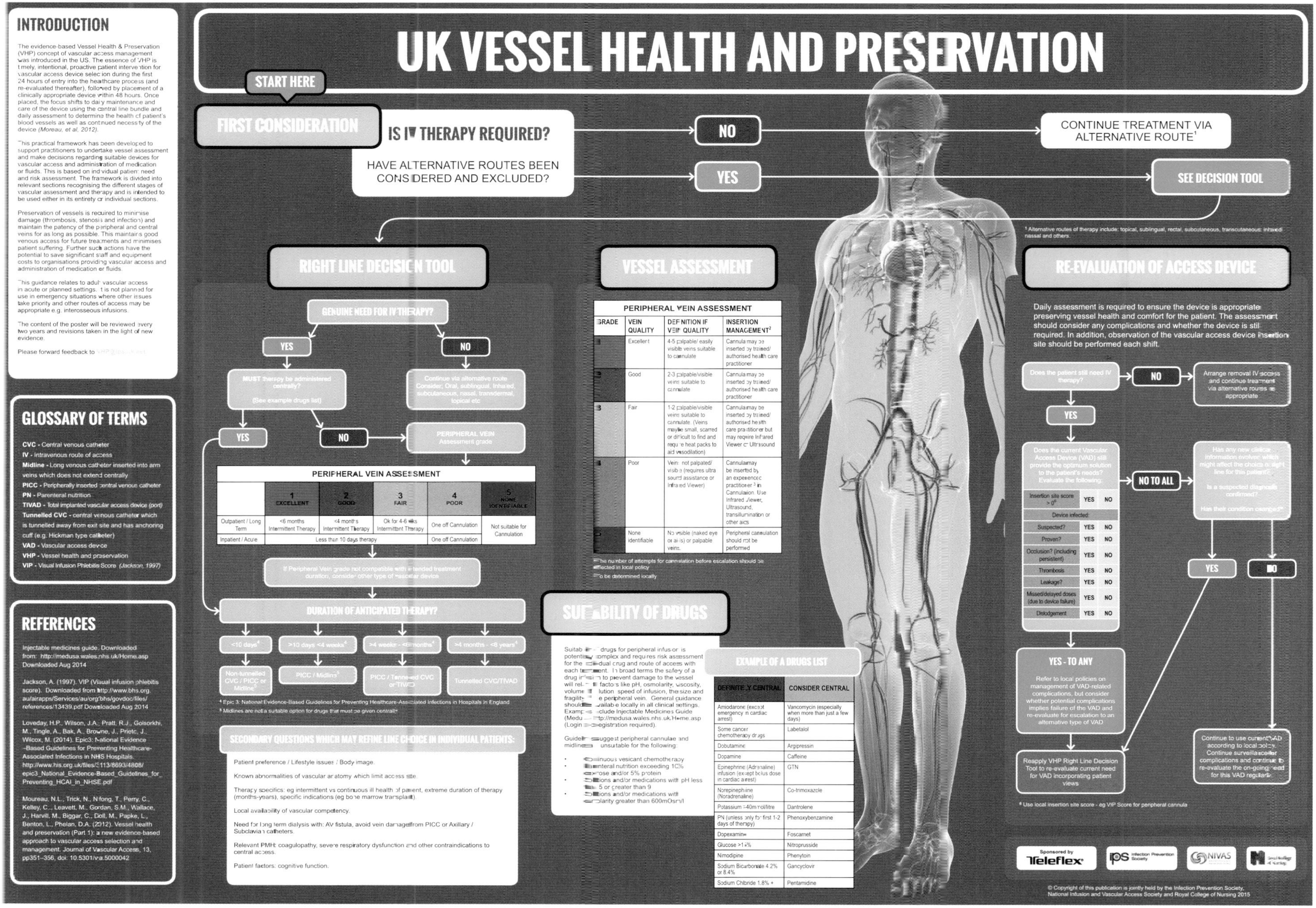

Figure 17.9 Vessel Health Preservation (VHP) framework. *Source*: Reproduced from Hallam et al. (2016) with permission of Sage Publications.

Procedure guideline 17.1 Central venous catheter: insertion site dressing change

This procedure can be adapted for changing a peripheral cannula dressing, although such dressings are rarely changed and are usually removed along with the cannula.

Essential equipment

- Personal protective equipment
- Sterile dressing pack (containing sterile towel, low-linting gauze and gloves)
- Alcohol-based skin-cleaning preparation, 2% chlorhexidine in 70% alcohol
- Semi-permeable transparent dressing (IV film dressing), sterile low-linting gauze or another appropriate dressing
- Hypoallergenic tape

Optional equipment

- Securing device
- Bacteriological swab

Action	Rationale
Pre-procedure	
1 Introduce yourself to the patient, explain and discuss the procedure with them, and gain their consent to proceed.	To ensure that the patient feels at ease, understands the procedure and gives their valid consent (NMC 2018, **C**).
Procedure	
2 This procedure should be performed using an aseptic non-touch technique.	To prevent infection (DH 2010, **C**). (For further information on asepsis, see Chapter 4: Infection prevention and control.)
3 Screen the bed. Assist the patient into a supine position, if possible.	To allow dust and airborne organisms to settle before the insertion site and the sterile field are exposed. **E**
4 Wash hands with soap and water, or an alcohol-based handrub, and dry.	To reduce the risk of cross-infection (DH 2010, **C**; Fraise and Bradley 2009, **E**).
5 Place all equipment required for the dressing on the bottom shelf of a clean dressing trolley.	To reduce the risk of cross-infection (DH 2010, **C**).
6 Take the trolley to the patient's bedside, disturbing the screens as little as possible.	To minimize airborne contamination (DH 2010, **C**).
7 Open the sterile dressing pack onto the top of the trolley.	To gain access to the equipment. **E**
8 Attach an orange clinical waste bag to the side of the trolley below the level of the top shelf.	So that contaminated material is below the level of the sterile field (DH 2010, **C**).
9 Open the other sterile packs, tipping their contents gently onto the centre of the sterile field. Pour lotions into gallipots or into an indented plastic tray where required.	To reduce the risk of contamination of contents. **E**
10 Wash hands with soap and water, or an alcohol-based handrub, and dry.	Hands may have become contaminated by handling the outer packs (DH 2010, **C**).
11 Place the sterile field under the patient's arm or on their chest.	To create a clean working area. **E**
12 Loosen the old dressing gently.	So that the dressing can be lifted off easily. **E**
13 Put on clean gloves.	For protection from any contact with the patient's blood. **E**
14 Using gloved hands, remove the old dressing and discard it. Remove tapes or the securing device if loose, contaminated or due to be changed.	To remove the old dressing without contaminating hands (DH 2010, **C**).
15 If the site is red or discharging, take a swab for bacteriological investigation.	For identification of pathogens. To select appropriate treatment (DH 2010, **C**).
16 Remove and dispose of gloves, clean hands with an alcohol-based handrub and put on sterile gloves from pack.	To minimize the risk of introducing infection (DH 2010, **C**).
17 Clean the wound with 2% chlorhexidine in 70% alcohol, using back-and-forth strokes with friction. Allow the area to dry prior to applying the dressing.	To enable the disinfection process to be completed. To prevent skin reaction in response to the application of a transparent dressing to moist skin (Loveday et al. 2014, **C**; NICE 2012, **C**).
18 Reapply tapes or the securing device if necessary. This may require skin preparation prior to application of the securing device.	To secure the device and prevent dislodgement and phlebitis (Rickard et al. 2017, **E**; Schears 2005, **R**).
19 Apply the appropriate dressing, moulding it into place so that there are no folds or creases.	To minimize skin irritation and reduce the risk of the dressing peeling or becoming damaged. **E** To ensure security of the device and prevent dislodgement. **E**
20 Document the date and time on the dressing.	To ensure the dressing is changed as required (DH 2010, **C**; Gorski et al. 2016 **C**; NICE 2012, **C**; RCN 2016a, **C**).

Action	Rationale
Post-procedure	
21 Remove gloves and dispose of in waste bag.	To dispose of waste. **E**
22 Fold up the sterile field, place it in the orange clinical waste bag and seal the bag before moving the trolley. Draw back the curtains. Dispose of waste in the appropriate containers.	To prevent environmental contamination (DH 2010, **C**).
23 Document the date and time of the dressing change, site observations and any relevant changes at the insertion site in the patient's records.	To ensure adequate records are maintained and to enable continued care of the patient and device (NMC 2018, **C**).

Procedure guideline 17.2 Vascular access devices: maintaining patency

Essential equipment

- Personal protective equipment
- Sterile pack (containing sterile towel and low-linting gauze)
- 2% chlorhexidine in 70% alcohol

Medicinal products

- Flushing solution ready prepared in a 10 mL syringe in a clinically clean container

Action	Rationale
Pre-procedure	
1 Introduce yourself to the patient, explain and discuss the procedure with them, and gain their consent to proceed.	To ensure that the patient feels at ease, understands the procedure and gives their valid consent (NMC 2018, **C**).
2 Wash hands with soap and water, or an alcohol-based handrub, and dry.	To reduce the risk of contamination (DH 2010, **C**; Fraise and Bradley 2009, **E**).
Procedure	
3 Open sterile pack and arrange equipment.	To gain access to equipment. **E**
4 Clean the needle-free connector using 2% chlorhexidine in 70% alcohol. Apply with friction, rubbing the cap in a clockwise and anticlockwise manner at least five times. Allow to air dry.	To minimize the risk of contamination at the connections (DH 2010, **C**; Loveday et al. 2014, **C**; NICE 2012, **C**).
5 Attach the syringe to the needle-free connector.	To establish a connection between the cap and syringe. **E**
6 Using a push–pause method, inject the contents of the syringe (inject 1 mL at a time).	To create turbulence in order to flush the catheter thoroughly (Goodwin and Carlson 1993, **E**; Guiffant et al. 2012, **E**).
7 Maintain pressure on the plunger as the syringe is disconnected from the connector, then clamp the device tubing if necessary.	To maintain positive pressure, thus preventing backflow of blood into the catheter and possible clot formation (Berreth 2013a, **E**; Dougherty 2006, **E**; Gorski et al. 2016, **C**).
Post-procedure	
8 Dispose of equipment safely.	To prevent contamination of others (DH 2010, **C**).
9 Record the procedure in the relevant care plan within the patient's records.	To maintain accurate records (NMC 2018, **C**).

Procedure guideline 17.3 Central venous access devices: unblocking an occlusion

Essential equipment

- Personal protective equipment
- Sterile pack (containing sterile towel and low-linting gauze)
- Alcohol-based skin-cleaning preparation, e.g. 2% chlorhexidine in 70% alcohol
- 10 mL syringes × 3
- 0.9% sodium chloride
- Fibrinolytic solution if required, e.g. urokinase
- Needles
- Three-way tap
- Extension set or needle-free connector

Action	Rationale
Pre-procedure	
1 Introduce yourself to the patient, explain and discuss the procedure with them, and gain their consent to proceed.	To ensure that the patient feels at ease, understands the procedure and gives their valid consent (NMC 2018, **C**).

(continued)

Action	Rationale
2 This procedure should be performed using an aseptic non-touch technique.	To minimize the risk of infection (DH 2010, **C**; Fraise and Bradley 2009, **E**; Rowley and Clare 2011, **E**). (For further information on asepsis see Chapter 4: Infection prevention and control.)
3 Wash hands with soap and water, or an alcohol-based handrub, and dry. Place all equipment required on the bottom shelf.	To minimize the risk of cross infection (DH 2010, **C**).
4 Open a sterile pack and empty the other equipment onto it.	To create a clean working area (DH 2010, **C**).
5 Wash hands with soap and water, or an alcohol-based handrub, and dry.	Hands may have become contaminated by handling the outer packs (DH 2010, **C**).
Procedure	
6 Clean the connections thoroughly with 2% chlorhexidine in 70% alcohol before disconnection.	To minimize infection risk at the connection site (DH 2010, **C**).
7 Remove any extension sets or needle-free connectors.	The occlusion may be in the extension set/cap and not in the catheter. **E**
8 Draw up 0.9% sodium chloride and attempt to flush the catheter using a 10 mL syringe.	Smaller syringes create excessive pressure, which can result in catheter rupture (Conn 1993, **E**).
9 If there is pressure within the device lumen, attempt to gently instil the 0.9% sodium chloride using a 'to and fro' motion (push–pull) over a few minutes.	To attempt to clear the catheter (Gabriel 2008, **E**).
10 If nothing can be aspirated: • If a peripheral device: remove the device and resite as necessary: • If a central venous access device: determine the cause of the occlusion: – If blood: discuss with doctors, who may prescribe a fibrinolytic agent, e.g. urokinase or alteplase (Box 17.3). – If precipitation: discuss with pharmacy to determine best antidote, e.g. ethyl alcohol or hydrochloric acid.	 To break down fibrin (BNF 2019, **C**; RCN 2016a, **C**). To break down drug precipitate or fat emulsion (BNF 2019, **C**).
11 Draw up the prescribed solution in a 10 mL syringe.	To prepare the appropriate treatment. **E**
12 Attach a three-way tap and attach an empty 10 mL syringe and the syringe containing the prescribed solution (**Action figure 12**).	To commence the negative pressure technique (Gabriel 2008, **E**; McKnight 2004, **E**).
13 Put on clean gloves.	To minimize the risk of introducing infection (DH 2010, **C**).
14 Instil the solution via a three-way tap using negative pressure technique (**Action figure 14**).	To prevent catheter rupture (Conn 1993, **E**).
15 Attach the syringe and inject the priming volume plus 0.5 mL extra into the catheter lumen (Box 17.3).	To allow the drug to come into contact with the fibrin (SynerMed 2016, **E**).
16 Wait 10 minutes.	To allow the drug to come into contact with the fibrin (SynerMed 2016, **E**).
17 Inject another 0.5 mL.	To allow the drug to come into contact with the fibrin (SynerMed 2016, **E**).
18 Wait 10 minutes.	To allow the drug to come into contact with the fibrin (SynerMed 2016, **E**).
19 Inject last 0.5 mL.	To allow the drug to come into contact with the fibrin (SynerMed 2016, **E**).
20 Attach an empty syringe to the catheter and attempt to aspirate any clots and solution.	To unblock the catheter and ensure no clots are administered into the patient (Gabriel 2008, **E**).

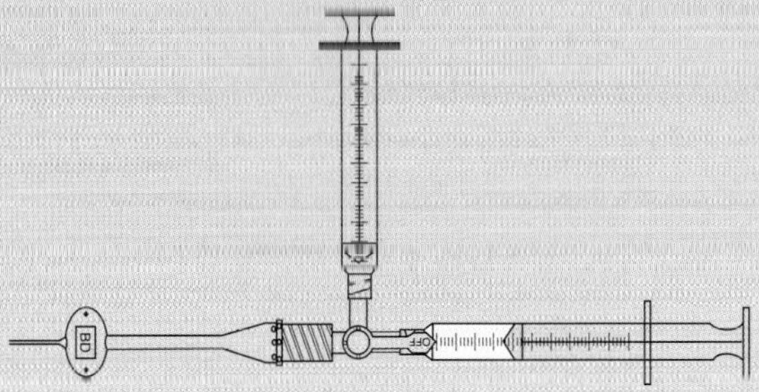

Action Figure 12 Turn the tap to close off the pre-filled syringe and open it to the empty syringe.

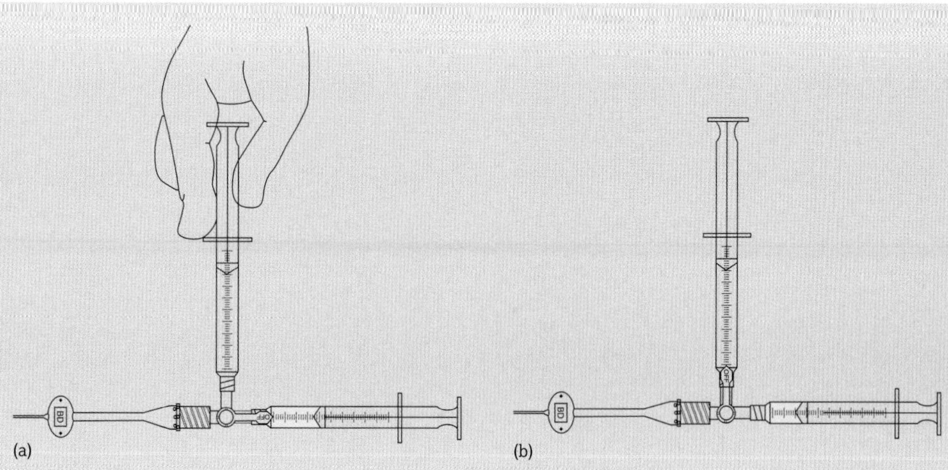

Action Figure 14 Unblocking an occluded catheter. (a) Aspirate on an empty syringe, which creates negative pressure. (b) Turn the tap to close off the empty syringe and open it to the pre-filled syringe. The medication will automatically be aspirated into the catheter. Repeat as necessary. *Source*: Adapted from Becton Dickinson First PICC Clinical Education Manual D11 952B 5/98.

21 If blood returns, withdraw at least 10 mL and discard.	To ensure no clots are flushed into the patient (Gabriel 2008, **E**).
22 Flush the catheter with 10 mL 0.9% sodium chloride using a pulsatile flush.	To ensure the catheter is flushed and patent (RCN 2016a, **C**).
Post-procedure	
23 Remove gloves and dispose of waste.	To prevent contamination of others (DH 2010, **C**).
24 If still unable to aspirate, consider the use of a second instillation of fibrinolytic agent at a higher dose or use an infusion. It may be necessary to remove the catheter (if a single lumen) or to refrain from using the occluded lumen and label 'not for use' (if multilumen).	To allow a higher dose of drug to be in contact with the clot (Syner-Med 2016, **E**). To maintain some venous access for the patient. If the occlusion cannot be resolved, the catheter is no longer patent. In multilumen catheters, there may be another patent lumen for use (Gabriel 2008, **E**). To follow the best evidence-based practice (i.e. an algorithm for the management of occluded CVADs) (Kumwenda et al. 2018, **E**).
25 Document the procedure in the patient's records.	To ensure adequate records are maintained and to enable continued care of device and patient (NMC 2018, **C**).

Box 17.3 Volumes for instillation of urokinase

Priming volumes

- PICC = 0.5 mL
- Skin-tunnelled catheter = 1 mL
- Port = 3 mL

Reconstitute

- Reconstitute Syner-Kinase: 10,000 units with the priming volume of the CVAD plus an additional 1.5 mL of 0.9% sodium chloride

Ongoing care

Discharging patients home with a VAD *in situ*

Patients may be discharged home with a VAD *in situ*, which will allow them to receive treatment at home (e.g. continuous chemotherapy or intermittent antibiotics) or allow for easier access on each admission (e.g. via a long-term CVAD). An early referral to the community nurses is crucial to ensure adequate support for the patient once they are at home (Kayley 2012).

Patients may now receive daily treatment over a 3–5-day period with an indwelling peripheral cannula (Shotkin and Lombardo 1996). The degree of care is minimal compared with a CVAD, but patients should receive adequate information about the early signs of phlebitis (such as pain, redness and swelling) and what to do in the case of accidental dislodgement or removal of the cannula.

The dressing of choice for PICC and skin-tunnelled catheter (when required) insertion sites is one that is moisture permeable and transparent (Loveday et al. 2014, NICE 2003) and that usually only requires changing once a week (following the initial change within the first 24 hours, if required) (RCN 2016a, Ryder 2001). This type of dressing may make it difficult for patients to change the dressing themselves and so a carer or community nurse will need to be involved. At the dressing change, the site should be inspected and any signs of erythema or inflammation should be reported to the hospital at once in order for appropriate treatment to be prescribed (DH 2010). The area should be cleaned using an aseptic technique with a 2% chlorhexidine-based solution (DH 2010, Loveday et al. 2014, NICE 2003).

If a patient wishes to be self-caring, the nurse should observe them carrying out the flushing procedure, either in hospital or in the home setting, until they are competent to do so without the supervision of a nurse (Dougherty 2006, Gorski et al. 2016). However, some patients prefer the community nurse to take responsibility for maintaining patency. Sufficient equipment (Boxes 17.4 and 17.5) must be supplied to enable the patient or nurse to care for the CVAD from the time of discharge until the patient's next admission (Kayley 2012).

Box 17.4 Example of a CVAD flushing kit

A CVAD flushing kit should contain the following when a patient has a skin-tunnelled catheter or PICC *in situ*:

- Needle-free connectors
- Ampoules of heparinized saline (50 international units heparin in 5 mL 0.9% sodium chloride) or pre-filled syringes (depending on local practice)
- 2% chlorhexidine in 70% alcohol wipes
- Sterile 10 mL Luer-Lok syringes
- Blunt drawing-up needles
- Instruction leaflet to provide both the community nurse and the patient with a point of reference, for example a patient information leaflet on central venous access devices
- Sharps container

Box 17.5 Contents of pack to take home for patients with a PICC

For PICC dressings, a pack containing the following should be sent home with the patient:

- Dressing packs (including gloves)
- Securing device (where required)
- Gauze
- Transparent dressings
- 2% chlorhexidine in 70% alcohol sponges
- Bandages or spare protective sleeves (e.g. tubular bandages)

Education of the patient and relevant others

Patients with long-term CVADs *in situ*, such as PICCs or skin-tunnelled catheters, will require instruction and supervision to ensure adequate understanding of the care and maintenance of their devices (Dougherty 2006, Kayley 2012). This must start early within the discharge planning process along with an assessment of the home environment, the patient's manual dexterity, and their physical and medical condition (Kayley 2012). Patient education is one of the most important aspects of care but, to make teaching effective, it is essential to recognize each patient's needs and limitations. It is also vital to acknowledge each patient's past experiences and readiness to learn (Czaplewski 2010, Kayley 2012). Education of the patient should encompass care and maintenance of the device as well as signs and symptoms of complications (Kayley 2012, RCN 2016a). Educational packages should be prepared in the form of practical demonstrations and clear, succinct handouts (Gorski et al. 2016, Kayley 2012, NICE 2012) (Figure 17.10). It is also important to recognize the need to prepare patients carefully to participate in their own self-care and therapy (Czaplewski 2010). The patient, their relatives and/or their carers should understand the following:

- how frequently to change the dressing and how to care for the site
- how to maintain patency
- how to inspect for signs of infection or other complications
- how to solve problems and where to seek help (RCN 2016a).

Patients should be taught what early signs and symptoms to look out for, what to do if the catheter becomes occluded or damaged, and when and who to contact (along with a contact name and number) if they need professional advice. This will help to alleviate any anxiety (Dougherty et al. 1998). Most problems can be managed at home with the involvement of community nurses and the patient's GP (Kayley 2012).

The most common complications associated with CVADs are infection and thrombosis (Dougherty 2006, Kayley 2008, RCN 2016a). The patient should be told to report:

- signs of redness and tracking at the exit site, along the skin tunnel or up the arm
- any oozing at the exit site
- fevers or rigors.

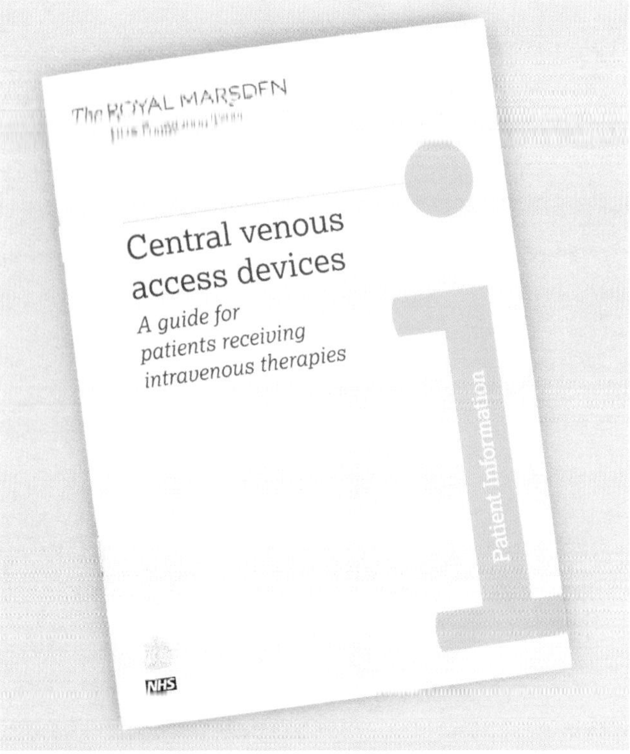

Figure 17.10 Patient information booklet on central venous access devices.

Patients are no longer routinely prescribed prophylactic warfarin as this has been shown to have no apparent benefit in the prevention of thrombosis (Couban et al. 2005, Young et al. 2005). Therefore, it should be stressed to the patient that any of the following signs or symptoms should be reported immediately: breathlessness, pain and/or swelling over the shoulder, across the chest, and/or into the neck and arm. Early reporting will enhance the effectiveness of treatment and may avoid the removal of the device (Bishop 2009).

Complications

The complications associated with VADs can be found in Box 17.6. Each complication will be discussed in more detail under each specific device later in this chapter.

Peripheral cannulas

Definition

A cannula is a flexible tube containing a needle (stylet) that may be inserted into a blood vessel (Dougherty 2008, RCN 2016a). Cannulas are usually placed in the peripheral veins in the lower arm but may also be placed in the veins of the foot (an area used particularly in paediatric care) (Weinstein and Hagle 2014). However, veins of the lower extremities should not be routinely used in adults due to the risk of embolism and thrombophlebitis (Gorski et al. 2016, RCN 2016a).

Anatomy and physiology

Choice of vein

The main factors to consider prior to inserting a peripheral cannula are the location for siting, the condition of the vein, the purpose of the infusion (i.e. the rate of flow required and the solution to be infused) and the duration of therapy (Dougherty 2008, Phillips 2005, RCN 2016a).

Box 17.6 Complications associated with vascular access devices

- Haematoma
- Arterial puncture
- Nerve injury
- Phlebitis
- Infiltration
- Extravasation
- Occlusion
- Infection
- Hydrothorax
- Brachial plexus injury
- Catheter embolism
- Arterial puncture and malposition
- Air embolism
- Haemorrhage
- Thoracic duct trauma
- Thrombosis
- Pneumothorax
- Haemothorax
- Misdirection or kinking
- Cardiac tamponade
- Cardiac arrhythmias

Source: Adapted from Dougherty (2006, 2008), Weinstein and Hagle (2014).

A suitable vein should always be determined prior to selection of the device. The vein should feel bouncy, refill when depressed, and be straight and free of valves to ensure easy advancement of the cannula. Valves can be felt as small lumps in the vein; some may be visualized at bifurcations, whereas some may be visible to the naked eye in certain vessels. It is best to avoid siting a cannula over a joint as this increases the risk of mechanical phlebitis and an infusion that will infuse intermittently due to the patient's movement (Dougherty 2008, Gorski et al. 2016, RCN 2016a, Witt 2010). It can also be very awkward for the patient and may restrict their ability to carry out activities (Macklin and Chernecky 2004, Marsigliese 2000).

The veins of choice are either the cephalic or the basilic veins, followed by the dorsal venous network (see Figure 17.1). The practitioner should choose distal veins and then cannulate at proximal points (Gorski et al. 2016, Perucca 2010). The best vein should always be used (Weinstein and Hagle 2014).

The cephalic vein

The size and position of the cephalic vein make it an excellent vessel for administration of transfusions. It readily accommodates a large-gauge cannula and, by virtue of its position on the forearm, provides a natural splint (Weinstein and Hagle 2014). However, its position at a joint may increase complications, such as mechanical phlebitis and even general discomfort. The tendons controlling the thumb obscure the vein during insertion (Hadaway 2010), and care must be taken not to touch the radial nerve (Dougherty 2008).

The basilic vein

The basilic vein is a large vessel that is often overlooked due to its inconspicuous position on the ulnar border of the hand and forearm. It is found on palpation when the patient's arm is placed across the chest, with the practitioner opposite the patient (Hadaway 2010). Cannulation can be awkward because of its position, mobility and tendency to have many valves (Dougherty 2008, Hadaway 2010).

The dorsal venous network

Using the veins of the dorsal venous network of the hand allows for cannulation proximally along the veins when re-siting a device (Weinstein and Hagle 2014). These veins can usually be visualized and palpated easily (Hadaway 2010):

- The *digital veins* are small and may be prominent enough to accommodate a small-gauge needle as a last resort for fluid administration. With adequate taping, the fingers can be immobilized, making them more comfortable as well as preventing the cannula from piercing the posterior wall of the vein (leading to bruising or infiltration) (Springhouse 2009).
- The *metacarpal veins* are accessible, and easily visualized and palpated. They are well suited for cannulation as the cannula lies flat and the metacarpal veins provide a natural splint (Weinstein and Hagle 2014). The veins tend to be smaller than those in the forearm and therefore may prove difficult to access in infants because they have higher amounts of subcutaneous fat than older children and adults. The use of these veins is contraindicated in the elderly as there is diminished skin turgor and loss of subcutaneous tissue, making the veins difficult to stabilize. They are also more fragile and venous distension is slower (Fabian 2010, Hadaway 2010, Springhouse 2009). Metacarpal veins are a better option for short-term or outpatient intravenous therapy.

Evidence-based approaches

Rationale

The advantages of using a peripheral cannula are that they are usually easy to insert and have few associated complications; however, they are associated with phlebitis (either mechanical or chemical) and require constant re-siting (Dougherty 2008, Gorski et al. 2016, RCN 2016a).

The insertion of a peripheral intravenous cannula (PIVC) is the most common invasive clinical procedure performed in hospitals worldwide (Ahlqvist et al. 2010, Alexandrou et al. 2018, Webster et al. 2008). Despite their prevalence, PIVCs are associated with high rates of complication, including insertion difficulty, phlebitis, infiltration, occlusion, dislodgement and catheter-related bloodstream infection (CRBSI), all of which are known to increase morbidity and mortality rates (Alexandrou et al. 2015, 2018). Recent VAD prevalence audits demonstrate substantial concerns with everyday practice, particularly relating to redundant devices, insertion site complications, substandard dressings, and documentation of site assessment and flushing practices (Ray-Barruel et al. 2018). The One Million Global Catheters study (Alexandrou 2014) assessed the prevalence of PIVCs and their management practices worldwide and reported that 59% of patients in hospital had at least one PIVC in place and 16% had other types of VAD. The prevalence of idle PIVCs was 16%, and 12% of those had at least one symptom of phlebitis (Alexandrou et al. 2015). Failure and complications of PIVCs commonly result in premature removal and replacement as well as increased patient pain and anxiety, particularly in patients with difficult venous access (Carr et al. 2017). Up to 90% of PIVCs are prematurely removed owing to failure before planned replacement of the device or before intravenous therapy has been completed (Alexandrou et al. 2018), resulting in increased healthcare costs associated with increased length of hospital stay (Alexandrou et al. 2015, 2018, Wallis et al. 2014). There are evidence-based guidelines and standards of practice (Gorski et al. 2016, RCN 2016a) to assist clinicians in managing these devices while reducing PIVC failure rate (Alexandrou et al. 2015, 2018). Reports suggest that a team approach to the assessment, insertion and maintenance of VADs improves clinical outcomes, patient experience and healthcare processes (Carr et al. 2018, Johnson et al. 2017).

Indications

Indications for the insertion of a PIVC include:

- short-term therapy lasting less than a week
- bolus injections or short infusions in the outpatient or day unit setting (Hadaway 2010, RCN 2016a).

Contraindications

Contraindications for the insertion of a PIVC include:

- long-term intravenous therapy
- longer-term or continous infusions of medications that are vesicant or those that have a pH below 5 or over 9 (Hadaway 2010).

Methods of improving venous access

Difficult peripheral access is traumatic for patients. Application of a tourniquet, tapping and stroking of veins, vigorous swabbing, clenching the hand to pump up veins, hanging the forearm downwards and application of local warmth are all commonly used aids for cannulation (Berreth 2013b, Dougherty 2008).

The application of a tourniquet promotes venous distension. The tourniquet should be tight enough to impede venous return while not affecting arterial flow (Garza and Becan-McBride 2018, Perucca 2010, RCN 2016a). There is strong evidence that reusable tourniquets are associated with the increased risk of infections such as MRSA (meticillin-resistant *Staphylococcus aureus*) (Elhassan and Dixon 2012), and, as such, the use of disposable tourniquets is recommended. The tourniquet should be applied around the upper forearm about 15–20 cm above the venepuncture site (McCall and Tankersley 2019) to promote dilation of the veins, and time should be allowed for the veins to fill. However, too tight application (particularly in older patients) can result in petechiae at the site of the tourniquet, haematoma, general bruising or venous high-pressure backflow of blood, resulting in vein 'blows' (Moureau 2008). To help reduce this, the tourniquet should be applied over clothing wherever possible (Hoeltke 2017, Toth 2002, Weinstein and Hagle 2014) or using a blood pressure cuff placed upside down and inflated just below diastolic pressure for effective compression. It may also be possible in some patients to avoid a tourniquet altogether by compressing a superficial vein with a finger above the insertion site (Dougherty 2013). Light tapping of the vein may be useful as this releases histamines beneath the skin and causes dilation (Frank 2018, Phillips 2005), but it can be painful and may result in the formation of a haematoma; again, older patients and those with fragile veins are most at risk (Garza and Becan-McBride 2018, Witt 2010). Other methods used to improve venous distension include lowering the extremity below the level of the heart and opening and closing the fist (the action of the muscles forces blood into the veins, causing them to distend) (Frank 2018, Phillips 2005).

When these methods fail, applying a warm compress in the form of a heat pack, warmed towels or electric heating blanket, or immersing the limb in a bowl of warm water for 10–15 minutes, helps to increase vasodilation and promote venous filling (Chen 2002, Fink et al. 2009, Weinstein and Hagle 2014). Ointments or patches containing small amounts of glycerol trinitrate have been used to improve vasodilation (Frank 2018, Gunwardene and Davenport 1990) as well as to reduce the incidence of chemical phlebitis and increase site survival time (Hecker 1988).

Vein locating devices

These are optional but useful portable devices that make it easier to locate veins that are difficult to visualize or palpate (Berreth 2013b). Transillumination devices enable visualization of veins by passing light (e.g. LED or infra-red light) through the walls and subcutaneous tissues to highlight the vessels. The haemoglobin in the blood absorbs the light, causing the vein to stand out as a dark line (Berreth 2013b, McCall and Tankersley 2019) (Figure 17.11). Ultrasound-guided peripheral cannulation is becoming the gold standard for complex and/or difficult-to-palpate peripheral veins (Bodenham et al. 2016, Gorski et al. 2016, Lamperti et al. 2012, Liu et al. 2014, Moureau and Chopra 2016, Walker 2009). Real-time ultrasound guidance techniques optimize the probability of inserting the needle into the vein upon the first attempt while minimizing the risk of complications (Bodenham et al. 2016, Lamperti et al. 2012, Liu et al. 2014, Moureau and Chopra 2016). They also allow the identification and demonstration of a patent and healthy vessel prior to cannulation (Blackburn 2014, Kumar and Chuan 2009, Lamperti et al. 2012).

Methods of insertion

Skin stabilization is one of the most important elements of successful cannulation (Dougherty 2008, Frank 2018, Perucca 2010) (Figure 17.12). Superficial veins tend to roll; to prevent this, the

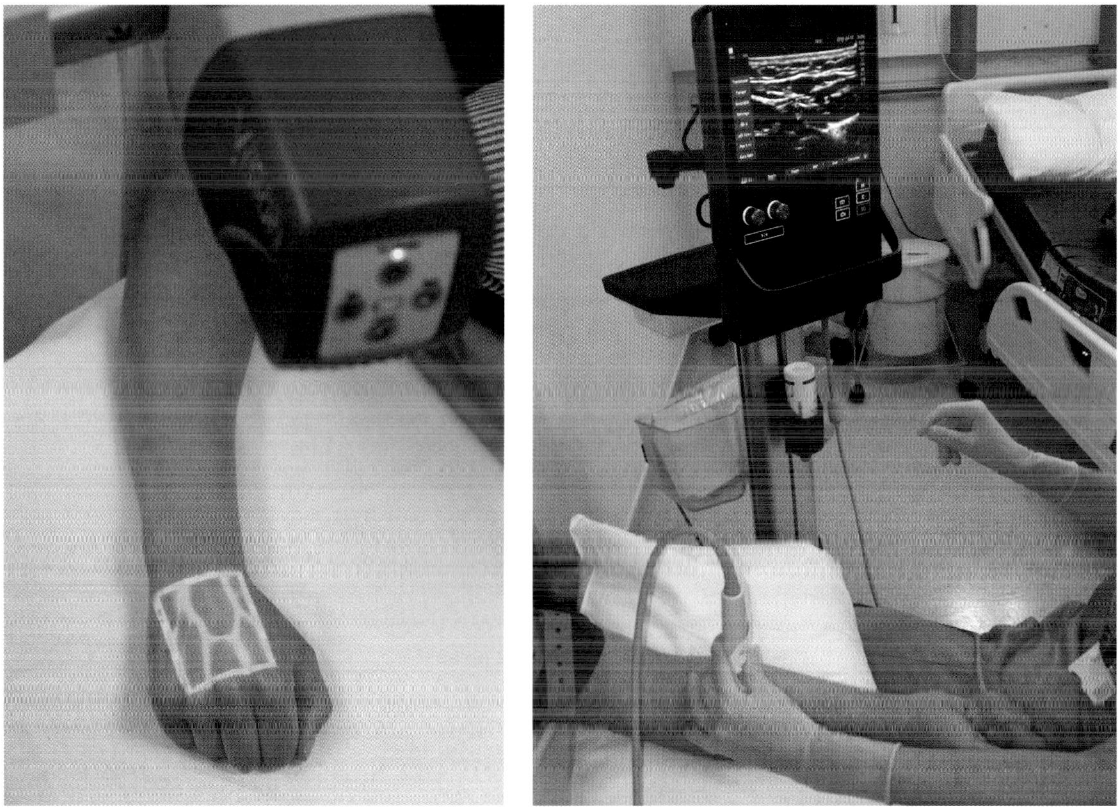

(a) (b)

Figure 17.11 (a) Vein visualization device. (b) Vascular access ultrasound scanner.

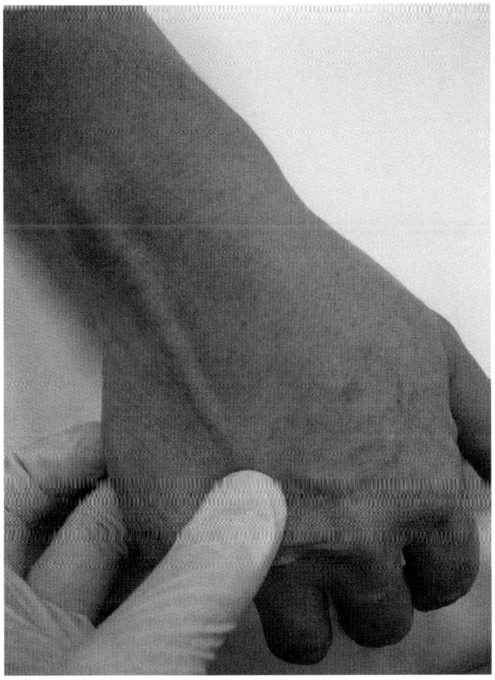

Figure 17.12 Anchoring the vein with the thumb. *Source*: Reproduced from Dougherty (2008) with permission of John Wiley & Sons.

vein must be stabilized by applying traction to the side of the insertion site or below it, using the practitioner's non-dominant hand. This also facilitates a smoother needle entry. Various methods are used (Dougherty 2008):

- The practitioner's thumb can be used to stretch the skin downwards.
- The practitioner's hand can be placed under the patient's arm and traction applied with the thumb and forefinger on either side, creating even traction.
- The vein can be stretched between the practitioner's forefinger and thumb.

Stabilization of the vein must be maintained throughout the procedure until the needle or cannula is successfully sited. If the tension is released halfway through the procedure, the needle may penetrate the opposite wall of the vein, resulting in the formation of a haematoma (De Verteuil 2010, Dougherty 2008).

It is important that the needle enters the skin with the bevel up, as this results in a smooth venepuncture as the sharpest part of the needle will penetrate the skin first, and it also reduces the risk of piercing the posterior wall of the vein (Weinstein and Hagle 2014). The angle at which the needle enters the skin varies with the type of device used and the depth of the vein in the subcutaneous tissue, from 10° to 45° (Dougherty 2008, Perucca 2010, Weinstein and Hagle 2014). Once the device is in the vein, the angle should always be reduced in order to prevent puncture of the posterior wall of the vein (Perucca 2010).

There are two main methods of approaching the vein:

- In the *direct method*, the device enters through the skin and immediately enters the vein. However, with smaller veins this method may result in puncture of the posterior wall (Dougherty 2008).
- In the *indirect method*, the device is inserted through the skin and then the vein is relocated and the device advanced into the vessel. This method enables a more gentle entry and may be useful in veins that are palpable and visible for only a short section (Dougherty 2008, Perucca 2010, Weinstein and Hagle 2014).

When blood appears in the chamber of a cannula, this is known as 'flashback' and it indicates that the initial entry into the vein has been successful. This may be accompanied by a 'giving way' sensation felt by the practitioner, which occurs because resistance from the vein wall decreases as the device enters the lumen of the vein. This usually occurs with thicker-walled cannulas (De Verteuil 2010, Weinstein and Hagle 2014). If the device punctures the posterior wall, the flashback will stop. However, the flashback may be slow with small-gauge cannulas or hypotensive patients.

The cannula should be advanced gently and smoothly into the vein, and practitioners use a number of techniques to achieve this. One method, which provides the least risk of through-puncture but can be difficult to learn initially, is the *one-handed technique* (De Verteuil 2010, Frank 2018, Perucca 2010). The same hand that performs the cannulation also withdraws the stylet and advances the cannula into the vein. This allows skin traction to be maintained while the device is advanced, and in older patients it also allows the practitioner to draw loose thick skin downward from underneath by using the hand in a 'C clamp' position (Rosenthal 2005). If one hand is not used to apply traction, then on cannula advancement there may be unnecessary damage to the endothelium, resulting in phlebitis (Hadaway 2010). This technique is also more suited to older patients (Hadaway 2000, Perucca 2010, Weinstein and Hagle 2014) because the connective tissue that anchors superficial veins is reduced with ageing and this makes veins more likely to roll, so it is important to firmly anchor older adult veins (Rosenthal 2005).

In the *one-step technique*, after the cannula has entered the vein, the practitioner slides the cannula off the stylet in one movement. The disadvantage of this method is that the stylet must remain completely still in order to prevent damage to the vein. It is best accomplished on a straight vein and when the cannula has a small fingerguard, which can be used to 'push' the cannula off (Dougherty 2008).

In the *two handed technique*, the practitioner performs the cannulation with one hand but releases the skin traction in order to advance the cannula off the stylet. This method prevents blood spill; however, as it necessitates the release of skin traction, it can often lead to puncturing of the vein wall (Dougherty 2008).

If the cannulation is unsuccessful, the stylet should not be reintroduced as this could result in catheter fragmentation and embolism (Perucca 2010). A practitioner should not make more than two attempts at cannulation before passing the patient on to a more experienced colleague (Dougherty 2008, Gorski et al. 2016, Perucca 2010).

Anticipated patient outcomes

The patient will receive their intravenous therapy and have a cannula placed that is comfortable and in a convenient position, enabling them to continue their daily activities. It will be secured and dressed to prevent any complications.

Clinical governance

Consent

Implied (presumed) consent is felt adequate for a procedure such as placement of a peripheral venous cannula; therefore, patients usually give verbal consent for cannulation (Frank 2018, Hyde 2010). Consent can also sometimes be assumed if the patient extends their arm for the procedure to be performed (Frank 2018).

Competencies

Nurses and other healthcare professionals who practise intravenous cannulation must ensure that they are operating within their scope of practice (HCPC 2016, NMC 2018). Pre-registration nurse education does not normally cover cannulation, necessitating post-registration training (Phillips et al. 2011). Post-registration nurses must follow professional guidelines and local policy prior to taking up these skills as they are classified as expanded practice. Nurses must be taught both theory and practical skills in cannulation (RCN 2016a). Competencies include:

- knowledge and skills in anatomy and physiology of the veins
- selection of the vein and equipment
- ability to improve venous access
- prevention and management of complications.

One way of gaining these skills is to use a structured learning programme (Collins et al. 2006) that provides supervised self-assessment using objective structured clinical examinations (Phillips et al. 2011). Additionally, less skilled practitioners can refer patients to more skilled practitioners who undertake cannulation on a regular basis, for example those in intravenous therapy teams; this can reduce pain and discomfort for patients and reduce local complications such as phlebitis (Dougherty 1994, McGowan 2014).

Pre-procedural considerations

Equipment

Sizing

A number of different types of peripheral cannula are available. It has been shown that the incidence of vascular complications increases as the ratio of the external diameter of the cannula to vessel lumen increases. The placement of large PIVCs is known to increase the incidence of malfunction that leads to failure (Alexandrou et al. 2018). Therefore, most of the literature recommends using the smallest, shortest gauge cannula possible in any given situation (Bitmead and Oliver 2018, Frank 2018, Gorski et al. 2016, Macklin and Chernecky 2004, RCN 2016a). The measurement used for needles and cannulas is standard wire gauge (swg), which measures the internal diameter; the smaller the gauge size, the larger the diameter. Standard wire gauge measurement is determined by how many cannulas fit into a tube with an inner diameter of 1 inch (25.4 mm) and uses consecutive numbers from 13 to 24. The diameter, for example 1.2 mm, may be expressed as a gauge, for example 18 G (Nauth-Misir 1998). Needles use odd numbers, for example 19 G or 21 G, while cannulas use even numbers, for example 18 G or 20 G (Weinstein and Hagle 2014). Therefore, a smaller gauge cannula will minimize trauma to the vein and increase blood flow around the device, promoting dilution and minimizing the risk of mechanical phlebitis (Bitmead and Oliver 2018, McGowan 2014) (Figures 17.13, 17.14 and 17.15).

The walls of the device should therefore be thin to provide the largest possible internal diameter without increasing the external diameter. This is to ensure that maximum flow rates may be achieved while reducing complications such as mechanical irritation. Flow rates vary with equipment from different manufacturers. Flow rate through a cannula is related to its internal diameter and is inversely proportional to its length (Table 17.2). However, as the length of the cannula increases, so does the likelihood of vascular complications. For example, a large-gauge device of longer length (1.6–2.0 cm) will fill the vessel, preventing blood flow around it, which could result in mechanical trauma to the vessel and encourage the development of phlebitis (Dougherty 2008, Tagalakis et al. 2002).

Materials

The most suitable material is one that is non-irritant and does not increase the risk of thrombus formation (Dougherty 2008). The material should also be radio-opaque or contain a stripe of radio-opaque material for radiographic visualization in the event of catheter embolus (Dougherty 2008, Perucca 2010). Types of material can vary and include PVC (polyvinyl chloride), Teflon, Vialon, and various polyurethane and elastomeric hydrogel materials (Bitmead and Oliver 2018, Dojcinovska 2010). Studies have compared the different types of material available to ascertain which is associated with the lowest potential risk of phlebitis (Karadag and Gorgulu 2000). When considering the results of these studies, however, it must be noted that investigators often use different phlebitis scales and calculations to create a total score for each device. Other inconsistencies relate to differences in catheter size, skin preparation, the use of dressings and the type of solution being infused. This makes it difficult to interpret research comparing catheter materials.

Table 17.2 Example of gauge sizes and average flow rates, using water (note that these may differ between manufacturers and cannula types)

Gauge (G)	Flow rate (mL/min)	General uses
14	350	In theatres and emergencies for rapid transfusion of blood or viscous fluids
16	215	As 14 G
18	104	Blood transfusions, parenteral nutrition, stem cell harvesting and cell separation, and large volumes of fluids
20	62	Blood transfusions and large volumes of fluids
22	35	Blood transfusions, and most medications and fluids
24	24	Medications, short-term infusions, fragile veins and children

Types of cannula

The 'over the needle' type of cannula is the most commonly used device for peripheral venous access and is available with various gauge sizes, lengths, compositions and design features (Dougherty 2008). The cannula is mounted on the needle (known as the stylet) and once the device has been pushed off the needle into the vein, the stylet is removed. A sharp-tipped stylet facilitates penetration into the vein and the type of graduation from the cannula to the needle can affect the degree of trauma to the vessel and the cannula tip (Dougherty 2008). A thin, smooth-walled cannula tapering to a scalloped end causes less damage than one that is abruptly cut off (Dougherty 2008, Macklin and Chernecky 2004).

Some peripheral cannulas have wings, which help with securing the device to the skin in order to prevent a piston-like movement within the vein and accidental removal (Dougherty 2008). Some devices have small ports on the top (these are favoured more in Europe than in the US) (Figure 17.13). The advantage of a ported device is the ability to administer drugs without interfering with a continuous infusion. However, the caps are often not replaced correctly, which leaves the system exposed to contamination and the risk of air entering, so where ported devices are used they should be capped off using a needle-free injection connector (Easterlow et al. 2010). It has also been found that the ports cannot be adequately sterilized with a swab, as there is no flat surface, so these devices are associated with an increased risk of infection (Easterlow et al. 2010).

Safety cannulas are now available and have either active or passive mechanisms. In the active devices the practitioner has to push a button in order to activate the safety feature, while in the passive devices the stylet has a blunting or shielding facility, which is automatically activated on removal from the cannula (Dojcinovska 2010, Dougherty 2008, Gorski et al. 2016, HSE 2013, RCN 2016a) (Figure 17.14). New closed system safety cannulas (Figure 17.15) can also reduce the healthcare professional's exposure to blood by introducing an integrated catheter tubing that prevents blood spillage (Bitmead and Oliver 2018). There is evidence that these integrated closed-cannula systems can reduce the risks of needle stick injury, blood leakage and exposure, as well as increase dwell time and patient comfort (Shaw 2017), making them safer, more convenient and more economical (Burton 2010, Bitmead and Oliver 2018).

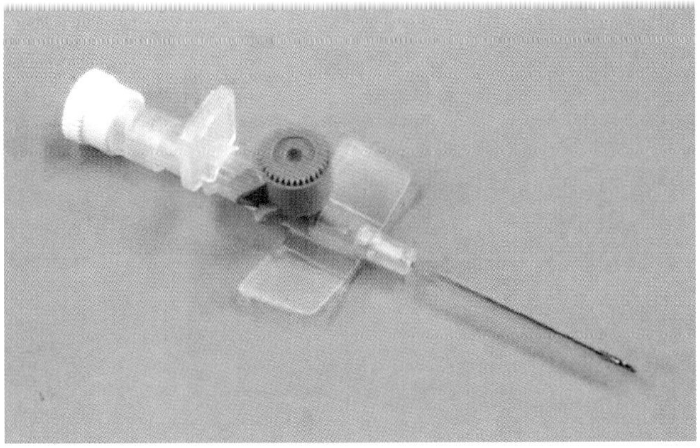

Figure 17.13 Ported cannula.

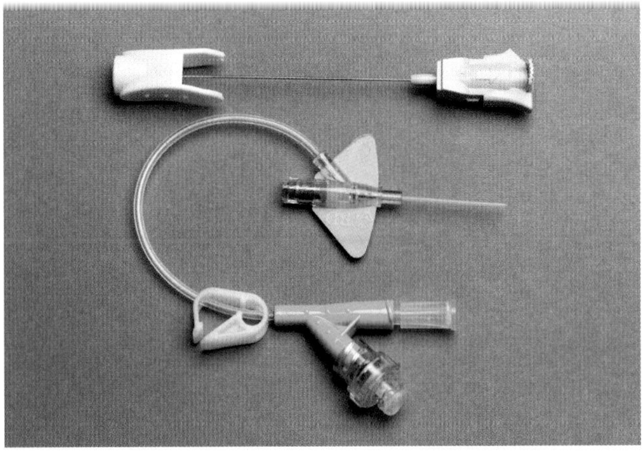

Figure 17.15 Safety integrated closed system.

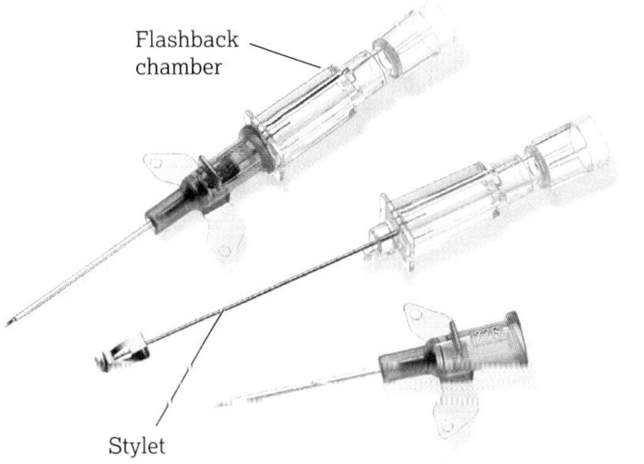

Figure 17.14 Safety non-ported cannula.

Assessment and recording tools

Proactive patient assessment and intentional device selection are fundamental to the successful placement and preservation of the PIVC (Bitmead and Oliver 2018). There are various models, for example:

- I-DECIDED: IV Assessment and Decision Tool (Ray-Barruel et al. 2018) (Figure 17.16)
- Vessel Health Preservation (VHP) framework (Hallam et al. 2016)
- Michigan Appropriateness Guide for Intravenous Catheters (MAGIC) (Chopra et al. 2015)
- UK Oncology Nursing Society's Cancer Therapy Venous Access Device Decision Guide (Flynn et al. 2014)

These all provide guidance on the selection and insertion of intravenous devices by offering a standardized pathway approach (Bitmead and Oliver 2018) and give guidance on how to select an

I-DECIDED™
IV ASSESSMENT & DECISION TOOL

IDENTIFY if an IV is *in situ*
If an IV has been removed in past 48 hours, observe site for post-infusion phlebitis.

DOES patient need the IV?
If not used in past 24 hours, or unlikely to be used in next 24 hours, consider removal. Consider change to oral medications.

EFFECTIVE function?
Does the IV infuse and/or flush well? Follow local policy for flushing and locking.

COMPLICATIONS at IV site?
Pain ≥ 2/10, redness > 1 cm, swelling > 1 cm, discharge, infiltration, extravasation, hardness, palpable cord or purulence.

INFECTION prevention
Hand hygiene, scrub the hub and allow to dry before each IV access. Careful use of administration sets.

DRESSING & securement
Clean, dry and intact. IV and lines secure.

EVALUATE & EDUCATE
Evaluate concerns. Educate as needed. Discuss IV plan with patient and family.

DOCUMENT your decision
Continue to monitor, change dressing/securement or remove IV.

Always consider local policy, and consult with team and patient as required.

Figure 17.16 I-DECIDED: IV Assessment and Decision Tool. *Source*: Reproduced from Ray-Barruel et al. (2018) with permission of *BMJ*.

intravenous device, based on the type and duration of therapy, vein health and the patient's medical condition. Using a care bundle for insertion helps to promote best practice and includes hand hygiene and ensuring the practitioner has the appropriate equipment (e.g. gloves, tourniquet, skin preparation, cannulas, dressings and sharps bins) (Burnett et al. 2010). Many PIVC infusion phlebitis scales and definitions are used internationally, for example the Visual Infusion Phlebitis (VIP) scale (Figure 17.17). The scale was developed by Jackson (1998) and measures the signs and symptoms of phlebitis, matching them to the appropriate management. Each stage has a numbered score; this is recorded by nursing staff at regular intervals and, where necessary, the corresponding action is taken (Groll et al. 2010, Morris 2011). However, there is now debate as to the lack of inter-rater agreement between these phlebitis assessment scales and the need for new approaches to evaluate vein irritation that demonstrate comprehensive reliability and validity (Marsh et al. 2015, Ray-Barruel et al. 2014, 2018).

Pharmacological support

The use of local anaesthetic prior to insertion of peripheral cannulas has been advocated to reduce pain and anxiety in children and specific adults (Scales 2005). It is recommended:

- if the cannula is larger than 18 G
- for use at a sensitive site, for example inner aspect of the wrist
- at the patient's request (Dougherty 2008, Moureau and Zonderman 2000).

When required, the agent that is the least invasive and/or carries the least risk for allergic reaction should be considered first (RCN 2016a). Local anaesthetic may be applied as follows:

- in a cream or gel
- as an intradermal injection (Anderson et al. 2010, Ganter-Ritz et al. 2012)
- by iontophoresis, which is a painless method in which a dry electrode pushes the local anaesthetic into the skin within 7–10 minutes to a depth of 10 mm (Dougherty 2011).

The most commonly used local anaesthetic creams are EMLA (eutectic mixture of local anaesthetics: lidocaine and prilocaine) and Ametop (topical amethocaine). These are applied to the skin 30–60 minutes prior to cannulation and covered with an occlusive dressing. A meta-analysis showed that EMLA cream significantly decreased the pain of intravenous cannulation in 85% of adults and children (Fetzer 2002). However, it causes vasoconstriction, making cannulation more difficult. Ametop has been shown to be more effective than EMLA and to cause significantly less vasoconstriction (Browne et al. 1999). However, it can result in an erythematous rash if left *in situ* for longer than the recommended time (BNF 2019).

Ethyl chloride is a fast-acting vapo-coolant spray that provides rapid, transient, topical local analgesia for minor invasive procedures such as cannulation. It has no anaesthetic properties but the sprayed liquid makes the skin cold and less sensitive as it evaporates, causing instant numbing. The effect lasts for about 30–45 seconds (Fossum et al. 2016).

Intradermal lidocaine 1% can be slowly injected around the vein to be cannulated after skin sterilization to minimize the discomfort of the procedure. Intradermal injection of lidocaine has been shown to reduce the pain of intravenous cannulation and be less painful than placement of the cannula itself (Brown and Larson 1999, Ganter-Ritz et al. 2012). However, it should be used with caution because of the potential to cause an allergic reaction, tissue damage and inadvertent injection of the drug into the vascular system, and it can even obliterate the vein (Dougherty 2011, Gorski et al. 2016). It is not recommended for routine use (Gorski et al. 2016, RCN 2016a).

Iontophoresis uses a painless electrical current to facilitate the movement of solute ions across the skin. It has been used to administer lidocaine prior to intravenous cannulation without the

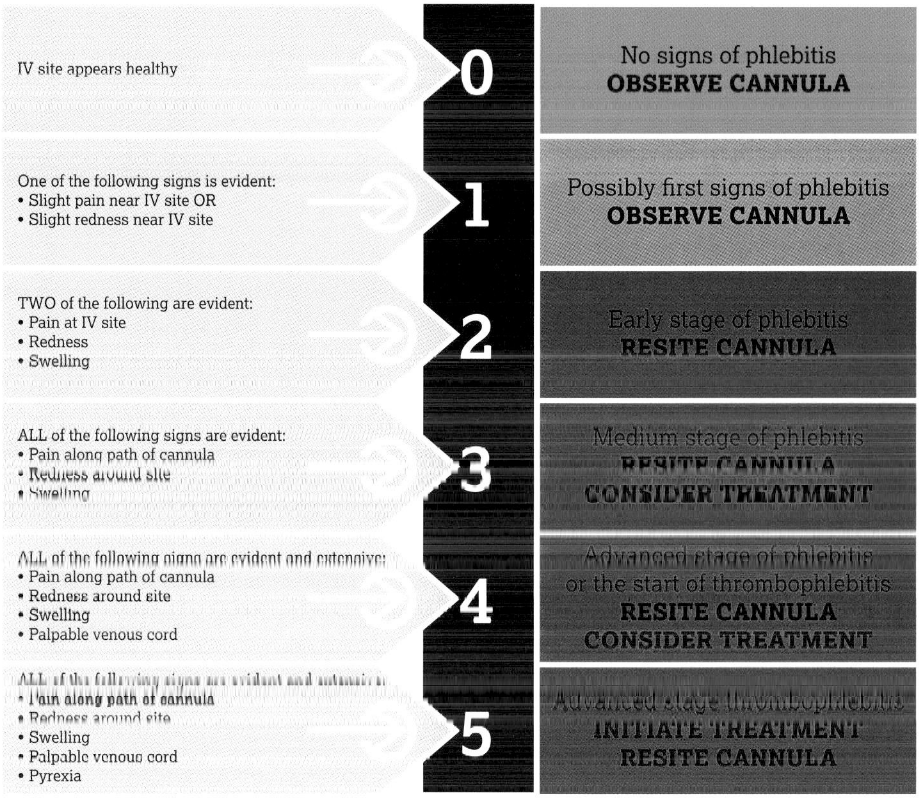

Figure 17.17 Visual Infusion Phlebitis (VIP) scale. *Source*: Reproduced from Jackson (1998) with permission of *Nursing Times*.

need for intradermal injection and has been shown to be as effective as EMLA (Dougherty 2011, Gallinkin et al. 2002).

Although local anaesthetic reduces the pain of intravenous cannulation, it is not without complications. Irrespective of the method of anaesthesia, there is a risk that the symptoms of extravasation may be obscured and it may even influence the risk of injury occurring (Stanley 2002).

Non-pharmacological support

There are a number of methods for relieving pain using a non-pharmacological approach (MacKereth et al. 2012). The provision of clear and comprehensive information about the procedure can help to alleviate any associated fear and anxiety the patient may have, and it also enables early consideration of interventions such as relaxation techniques, massage or distraction therapy (McGowan 2014). Distraction therapy includes techniques such as the cough trick (Usichenko et al. 2004), massage (Wendler 2003), transcutaneous electrical nerve stimulation (TENS) (Coyne et al. 1995) and visualization (Andrews and Shaw 2010).

Specific patient preparation

Skin preparation

As the most common cause of VAD infection is the patient's own skin flora, it is important to clean the skin adequately prior to cannulation (Figure 17.18). The patient's skin should be washed with soap and water if visibly dirty, which will remove most transient flora (Perucca 2010). Then an antiseptic solution, such as 2% chlorhexidine solution in 70% alcohol, should be applied with repeated up-and-down, back-and-forth strokes with friction for 30–60 seconds over an area of 4–5 cm diameter (Bitmead and Oliver 2018, Bodenham et al. 2016, DH 2010, Perucca 2010). A quick wipe fails to reduce bacteria count (Weinstein and Hagle 2014). The skin should then be allowed to air dry for up to 1 minute to ensure coagulation of the organism and to prevent stinging as the needle pierces the skin (Gorski et al. 2016, RCN 2016a, Weinstein and Hagle 2014). Fanning, blowing on and blotting the prepared area are contraindicated (Perucca 2010). Once the skin has been cleaned, it must not be touched or repalpated (Dougherty 2008). If it is necessary to repalpate, then the cleaning regimen should be repeated. The principles of aseptic non-touch technique must be adhered to at all times (Bitmead and Oliver 2018).

Shaving the skin prior to cannulation is not recommended (Gorski et al. 2016, RCN 2016a, Weinstein and Hagle 2014) as the supposed need to remove hair has not been substantiated by scientific evidence (Weinstein and Hagle 2014). Shaving with a razor should not be performed because of the potential to cause micro-abrasions, which increase the risk of infection (Gorski et al. 2016, Perucca 2010, RCN 2016a). Depilatories should not be used because of the potential for allergic reaction or irritation (Perucca 2010, RCN 2016a). If hair removal is felt to be necessary then this can be accomplished by clipping with scissors or clippers (Perucca 2010, RCN 2016a). These should be cleaned between patient use or only used once to prevent cross-infection (RCN 2016a).

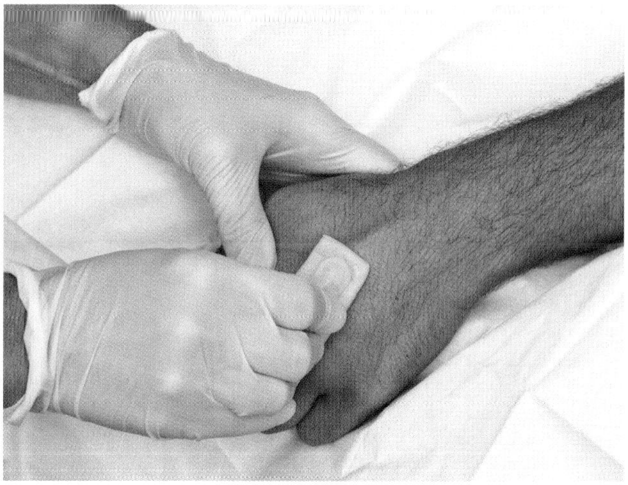

Figure 17.18 Cleaning the skin.

Psychological preparation

The influence of a bad experience can be overwhelming for a patient, and any practitioner performing venepuncture or cannulation must never underestimate either the impact for the patient of undergoing the procedure or how they may view these procedures in the future (Dougherty 2011). It has been found that 20% of adults experience mild to intense fear of injections and blood, with 10% having a profound fear of needles; this may be expressed as feelings of anxiety and/or a vasovagal episode with symptoms of bradycardia and hypotension (Dougherty 2008, Jenkins 2014). Anxiety can be caused by previous bad experiences, a degree of needle phobia or dislike of needle procedures (Andrews 2011, Andrews and Shaw 2010, Jenkins 2014, Lavery and Ingram 2005). Many patients will be apprehensive and this anxiety may cause vasoconstriction, making cannulation more difficult as well as more painful for the patient. How nurses approach the patient, and their manner and attitude, may have a direct bearing on the patient's response to the procedure (Dougherty 2011, McGowan 2014).

If the patient's history includes complications associated with any procedure, venepuncture or cannulation may be very difficult (Jenkins 2014, Weinstein and Hagle 2014). However, when a procedure is performed by an experienced practitioner and it is a positive experience for the patient, they may feel comfortable and relaxed. The nurse should ask patients about their past experiences and acknowledge their feelings and fears (Dougherty 2011, McGowan 2014). Provision of clear and comprehensive information on the procedure should reduce the patient's anxiety and pain (Dougherty 2011, Lüker and Stahlheber-Dilg 2003, Weinstein and Hagle 2014).

Procedure guideline 17.4 Peripheral cannula insertion

Essential equipment

- Personal protective equipment
- Sterile pack
- Various gauges of cannula
- Alcohol-based skin preparation, e.g. 2% chlorhexidine in 70% alcohol
- Extension set (if needed)
- Needle-free connector
- Semi-permeable transparent IV film dressing
- Bandage or tubular bandage (if needed)
- 5 mL syringe
- Blunt drawing-up needle
- Tourniquet (disposable)

(continued)

Procedure guideline 17.4 Peripheral cannula insertion *(continued)*

- Sharps container
- Labels

Optional equipment

- Securing device, e.g. StatLock
- Topical local anaesthetic

Medicinal products

- 0.9% sodium chloride: 5 mL

Action	Rationale
Pre-procedure	
1 Introduce yourself to the patient, explain and discuss the procedure with them, and gain their consent to proceed.	To ensure that the patient feels at ease, understands the procedure and gives their valid consent (NMC 2018, **C**).
2 If the patient requires topical local anaesthetic, apply it to the chosen venepuncture site and leave in place for 30–60 minutes prior to cannulation.	In order to give adequate time for the local anaesthetic to be effective (BNF 2019, **C**).
3 Assemble all the equipment necessary for cannulation.	To ensure that time is not wasted and that the procedure goes smoothly without unnecessary interruptions. **E**
4 Check all packaging before opening and preparing the equipment to be used.	To ensure all equipment is in date and not contaminated. **E**
Procedure	
5 Wash your hands using bactericidal soap and water or an alcohol-based handrub and dry.	To minimize the risk of infection (DH 2010, **C**; Fraise and Bradley 2009, **E**).
6 Check your hands for any visibly broken skin, and cover any breaks with a waterproof dressing.	To minimize the risk of contamination of the nurse by the patient's blood (Loveday et al. 2014, **C**).
7 Ensure adequate lighting and privacy, and assist the patient into a comfortable position.	To ensure that the nurse and patient are comfortable and that adequate light is available to illuminate the procedure. **E**
8 Support the chosen limb on a pillow.	To ensure the patient's comfort and give the nurse ease of access. **E**
9 Apply a tourniquet to the chosen limb, or use other methods if appropriate.	To dilate the veins by obstructing venous return (Dougherty 2008, **E**).
10 Assess the veins and select one for use (**Action figure 10**).	To select a vein (Dougherty 2008, **E**).
11 Release the tourniquet.	To ensure that the patient does not feel discomfort while the device is selected and equipment is prepared (Dougherty 2008, **E**).
12 Select a device based on the vein size.	To reduce damage or trauma to the vein. To reduce the risk of phlebitis (Dougherty 2008, **E**; RCN 2016a, **C**).
13 Wash hands with soap and water, or an alcohol-based handrub, and dry.	To minimize the risk of infection (DH 2010, **C**; Fraise and Bradley 2009, **E**).
14 Open a pack, empty all equipment onto the pack and place a sterile dressing towel under the patient's arm (**Action figure 14**).	To create a clean working area. **E**
15 Prime the extension set with a syringe containing 0.9% sodium chloride (unless taking blood samples immediately after cannulation). *Note*: when using a closed system integrated peripheral intravenous cannula, there is no need to prime the system.	To remove air from the set prior to connection. If taking blood then the sodium chloride will contaminate the sample (Dougherty 2008, **E**). To reduce the manipulation of components and minimize the risk of contamination. **E**
16 Reapply the tourniquet.	To promote venous filling (Dougherty 2008, **E**).
17 Clean the patient's skin over the selected vein for at least 30 seconds using 2% chlorhexidine using back and forth strokes with friction and allow to dry (see Figure 17.18). Do not repalpate the vein or touch the skin.	To maintain asepsis and remove skin flora (DH 2010, **C**; Dougherty 2008, **E**; RCN 2016a, **C**).
18 Put on gloves.	To prevent contamination of the nurse from any blood spill (DH 2010, **C**).
19 Remove the needle guard and inspect the device for faults (**Action figure 19**).	To detect faulty equipment, for example bent or barbed needles. If these are present, do not use and report to the manufacturer as faulty equipment (MHRA 2005, **C**; RCN 2016a, **C**).
20 Anchor the vein with the non-dominant hand by applying manual traction on the skin a few centimetres below the proposed site of insertion.	To immobilize the vein. To provide counter-tension, which will facilitate a smooth needle entry (Dougherty 2008, **E**).

21 Holding the cannula in the dominant hand, ensure that it is in the bevel-up position and place the device directly over the vein; insert the cannula through the skin at the selected angle according to the depth of the vein (**Action figure 21**).	To ensure a successful, pain-free cannulation (Dougherty 2008, **E**).
22 Wait for the first flashback of blood in the flashback chamber of the stylet (see **Action figure 21**).	To indicate that the needle has entered the vein (Dougherty 2008, **E**).
23 Level the device by decreasing the angle between the cannula and the skin. Advance the cannula slightly to ensure entry into the lumen of the vein.	To avoid advancing too far and causing damage to the vein wall. To stabilize the device (Dougherty 2008, **E**).
24 Withdraw the stylet slightly with the dominant hand and a second flashback of blood will be seen along the shaft of the cannula (**Action figure 24**).	To ensure that the cannula is still in a patent vein. This is called the 'hooded technique' (Dougherty 2008, **E**).
25 Maintaining skin traction with the non-dominant hand, slowly advance the cannula off the stylet and into the vein using the dominant hand.	To ensure that the vein remains immobilized, thus reducing the risk of a through-puncture (Dougherty 2008, **E**).
26 Release the tourniquet.	To decrease the pressure within the vein. **E**
27 Apply digital pressure to the vein above the cannula tip and remove the stylet (**Action figure 27**). *Note:* when using an integrated closed system peripheral intravenous cannula there is no need for digital pressure as blood is contained within the system by a vent plug.	To prevent blood spillage. **E** To minimize exposure to blood. **E**
28 Immediately dispose of the stylet in an appropriate sharps container (**Action figure 28**).	To reduce the risk of accidental needle stick injury (HSE 2013, **C**; NHS Employers 2010, 2015, **C**).

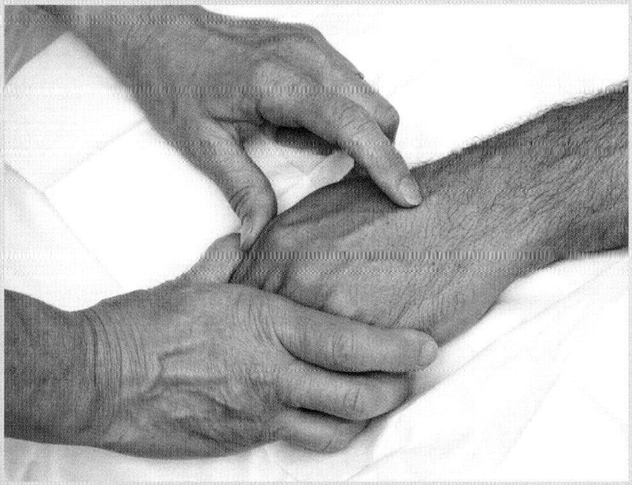

Action Figure 10 Palpating the vein.

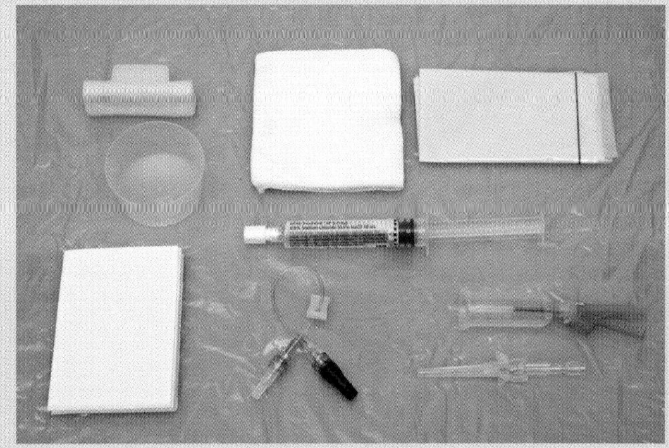

Action Figure 14 Opening the equipment.

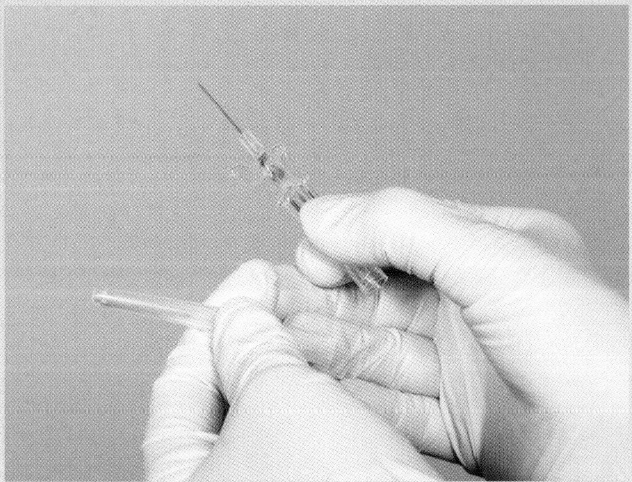

Action Figure 19 Checking the needle tip.

(continued)

Procedure guideline 17.4 Peripheral cannula insertion *(continued)*

Action	Rationale
29 Attach a primed extension set, needleless injection cap or administration set (**Action figure 29**). *Note*: when using an integrated closed system peripheral intravenous cannula, there is no need to attach an extension set as it is integrated.	To enable flushing of the cannula (Dougherty 2008, **E**). To minimize the risk of infection through manipulating the system (Bitmead and Oliver 2010, **E**).
30 Using the sterile tape provided in the dressing package, secure the cannula using, for example, the method illustrated in **Action figure 30**, always allowing visualization of the insertion site.	To ensure the device will remain stable and secure (Dougherty 2008, **E**). To visualize and monitor phlebitis score (RCN 2016a, **C**).
31 Aspirate to check for blood flashback then flush the cannula with 0.9% sodium chloride using a pulsatile flush ending with positive pressure.	To ascertain and maintain patency (Goode et al. 1991, **R**; RCN 2016a, **C**).
32 Observe the site for signs of swelling or leakage and ask the patient whether they are experiencing any discomfort or pain.	To check that the device is positioned correctly and is stable and secure (Dougherty 2008, **E**).
33 Cover the entry site with a semi-permeable transparent IV film dressing (unless contraindicated) and apply a date and time label (**Action figure 33**).	To ensure patient comfort and security of the device. To enable all staff to know when the dressing was applied (Loveday et al. 2014, **C**; RCN 2016a, **C**).

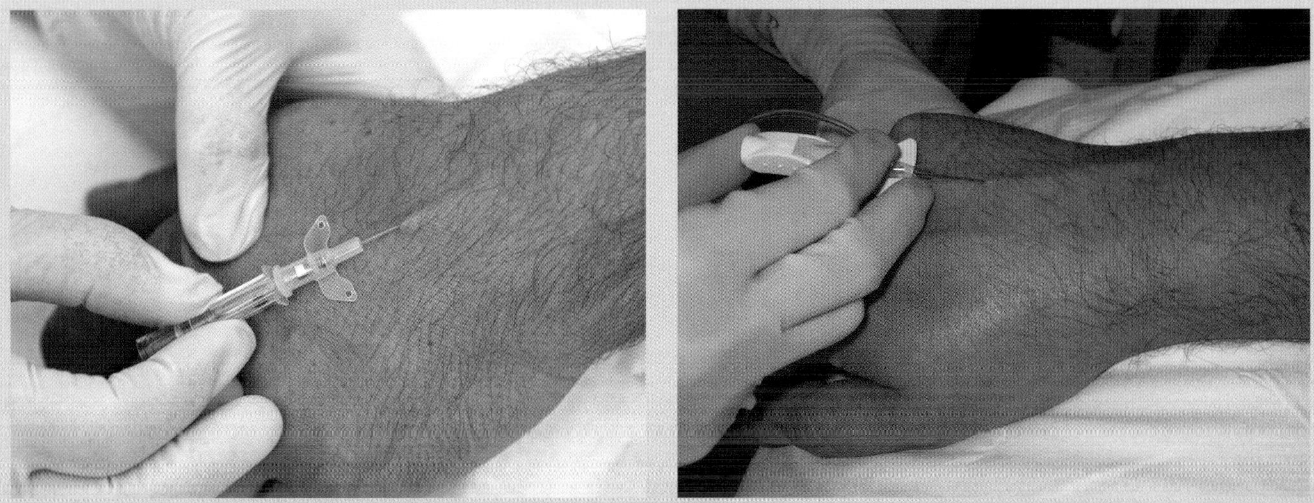

(a) (b)

Action Figure 21 Inserting the cannula and waiting for first flashback. (a) Open cannula. (b) Integrated closed system cannula.

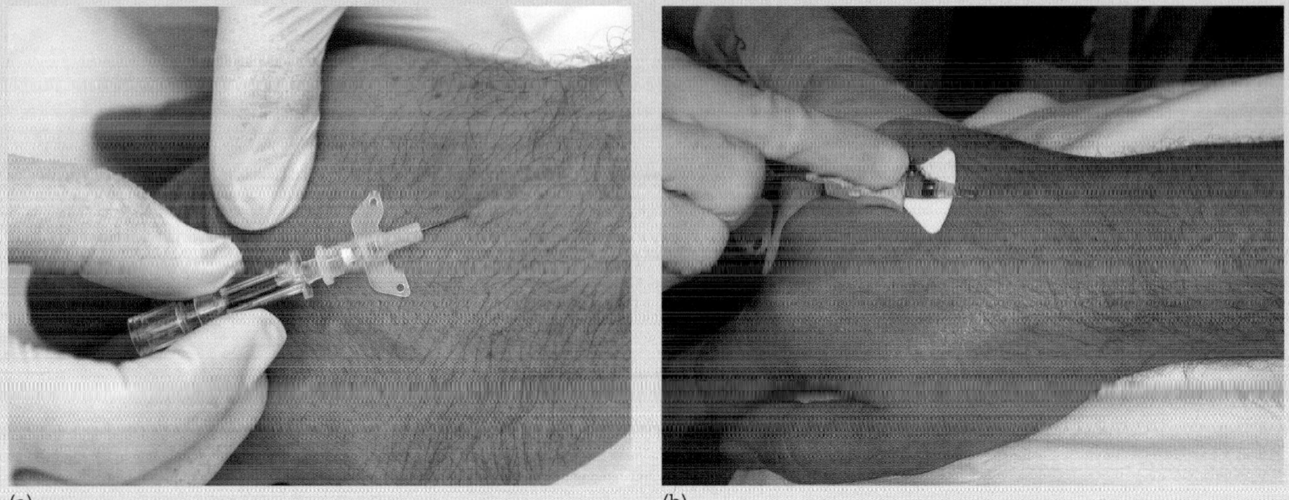

(a) (b)

Action Figure 24 Second flashback. (a) Open cannula. (b) Integrated closed system cannula.

Post procedure

34 Remove gloves and discard waste, making sure it is placed in the appropriate containers.	To ensure safe disposal in the correct containers and avoid laceration or injury of other staff. To prevent reuse of equipment (NHS Employers 2010, 2015, **C**). To prevent sharps injury (HSE 2013, **C**).
35 Document date and time of insertion, site, size of cannula, number of attempts, and volume and type of flushing solution, and sign in the patient's notes or care plan.	To ensure adequate records are maintained and to enable continued care of the patient and device (DH 2011, **C**; NMC 2018, **C**).

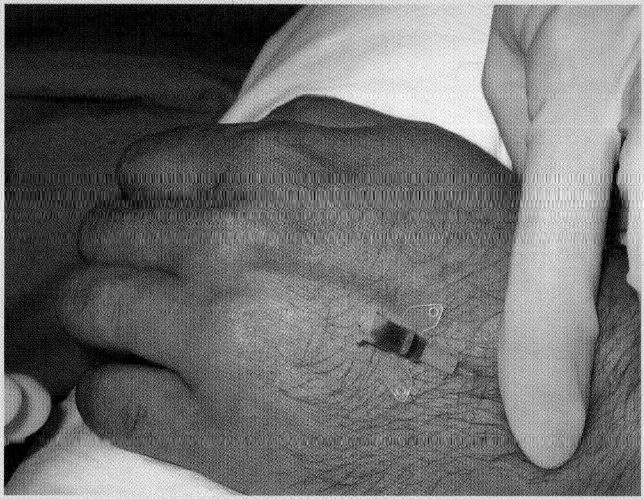

Action Figure 27 Applying digital pressure and removing the stylet.

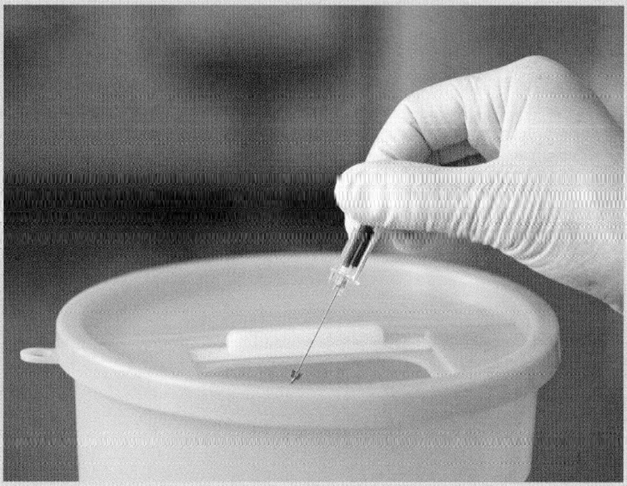

Action Figure 28 Disposing of the stylet into a sharps bin.

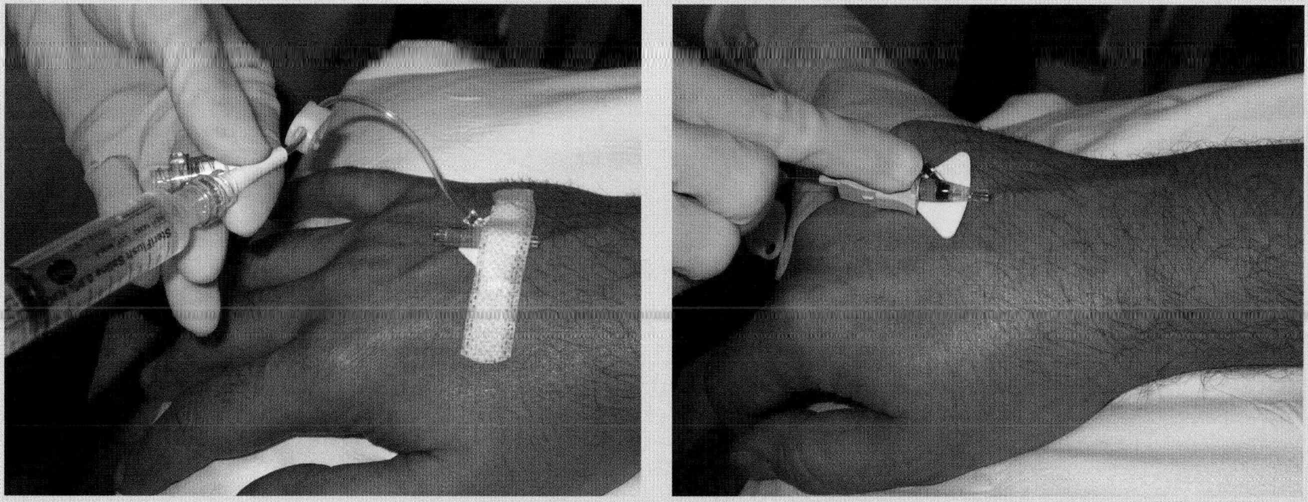

(a) (b)

Action Figure 29 Flushing the cannula. (a) Open cannula. (b) Integrated closed system cannula.

(continued)

Procedure guideline 17.4 Peripheral cannula insertion *(continued)*

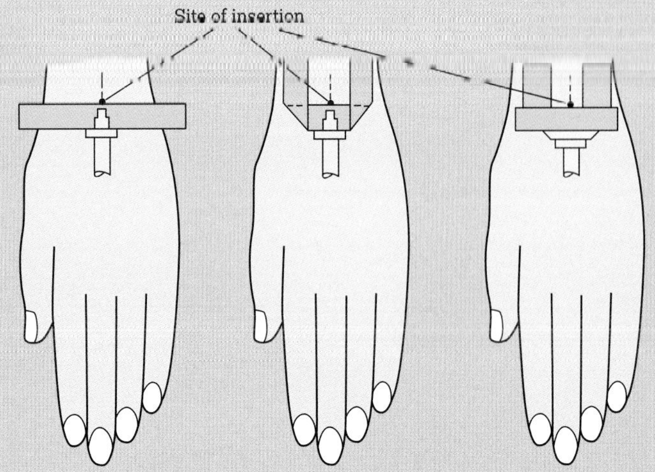

Action Figure 30 Method of taping a peripheral cannula.

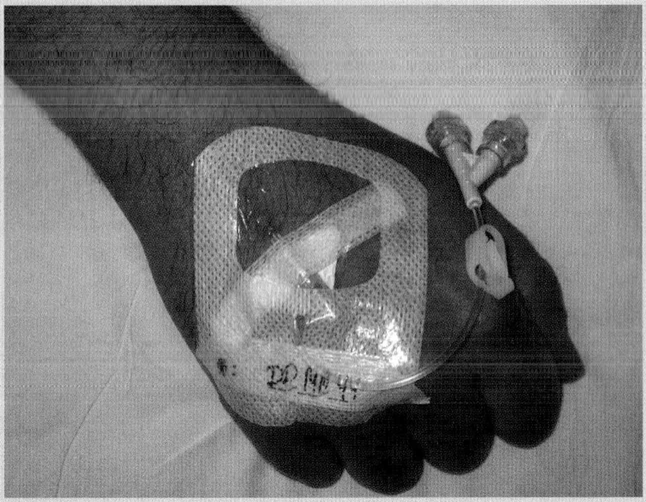

Action Figure 33 Semi-permeable transparent IV film dressing.

Problem-solving table 17.1 Prevention and resolution (Procedure guideline 17.4)

Problem	Cause	Prevention	Action
Anxious patient	Previous traumatic experiences Fear of needles or blood Ignorance about what the procedure involves	Approach the patient in a calm and confident manner. Listen to the patient's previous experiences and involve them in site selection. Offer a local anaesthetic (by gel or injection). Explain what the procedure involves and show them the equipment if appropriate. Offer the patient the opportunity to lie down or recline during the procedure. Use all methods of improving venous dilation to ensure success on the first attempt.	Refer the patient for psychological support if the anxiety and fear are of phobic proportions. It usually takes a few weeks to help a patient manage needle phobia.
Difficulty in locating a suitable vein	Excessive previous use Shock or dehydration. Anxiety Fragile, thready veins, for example in the elderly or in patients on anticoagulant therapy Thrombosed veins as a result of treatment, for example cytotoxic therapy	Alternate sites wherever possible to avoid overuse of certain veins. Use the methods described above to reduce anxiety.	Reassure the patient. Use all methods of improving venous access before attempting the procedure, for example use warm water or glyceryl trinitrate patches to encourage venous dilation, or use vein illumination or ultrasound devices. Assess the patient using an assessment tool to ascertain the likely degree of difficulty and refer for a central venous access device if necessary. Do not attempt the procedure unless experienced.
Missing the vein on insertion of the cannula	Inadequate anchoring Collapse of the vein Incorrect position of practitioner or patient Inadequate palpation Poor vein choice Lack of concentration Failure to penetrate the vein properly due to incorrect insertion angle	Ensure good position and lighting. Ensure optimal preparation and concentration. Use correct technique and accurate vein selection.	Withdraw the needle and manoeuvre it gently to realign it and correct the angle of insertion. Check during manoeuvring that the patient is not feeling any pain. If the patient complains of excessive pain, remove the needle. If unsuccessful then remove the needle. Where necessary, refer the patient to a colleague with more experience.

Problem	Cause	Prevention	Action
Blood flashback seen and then stops	Venospasm Bevel of needle up against a valve Penetration of the posterior vein wall by the device Possible vein collapse	Try to locate valves prior to insertion and insert the device just above the valve. Carefully level off once in the vein to prevent penetration of the posterior wall. Use a good angle of approach to the vein to prevent through-puncture.	Release and tighten the tourniquet (if possible). Gently stroke the vein above the needle to relieve venous spasm. Withdraw the needle slightly to move the bevel away from the valve. If the vein wall has been penetrated, remove the device.
Difficulty in advancing the cannula	Releasing the tourniquet too soon, causing the vein to collapse Removing the stylet too far and being unable to advance the cannula, which is now no longer rigid enough to be advanced Encountering a valve Not releasing the cannula from the needle prior to insertion according to the manufacturer's instructions Poor anchoring or stretching of the skin	Ensure the tourniquet remains sufficiently tight until insertion is completed. Ensure the cannula is released from the stylet prior to insertion, to allow for smooth advancement. Ensure that a sufficient length of the cannula is inserted into the vein before stylet withdrawal. Use good technique. Assess the vein accurately, observing for valves, and avoid them where possible.	In the event of early stylet removal or encountering a valve, connect a syringe of 0.9% sodium chloride, flush the cannula and advance at the same time in an effort to 'float' the device into the vein. Tighten the tourniquet and wait for the vein to refill.
Difficulty in flushing once the cannula is *in situ*	Sometimes, the cannula is successfully inserted but, on checking patency by flushing, the practitioner has difficulty due to one or more of the following: • the cannula tip is up against the valve • the cannula has pierced the posterior wall of the vein • the cannula tip is resting on the wall of the vein • there is an occlusion	Avoid areas along the vein where there may be valves. Ensure careful insertion to prevent puncturing the posterior wall of the vein.	Withdraw the cannula slightly to move it away from the vein wall or valve and attempt to flush. If the vein wall is pierced and any swelling is observed, remove the cannula. Attempt to withdraw the clot and clear the occlusion.

Procedure guideline 17.5 Ultrasound-guided peripheral cannula insertion

Essential equipment

- Personal protective equipment
- Sterile pack
- Various gauges of cannula
- Alcohol-based skin preparation, e.g. 2% chlorhexidine in 70% alcohol
- Extension set (if needed)
- Needle-free connector
- Semi-permeable transparent IV film dressing × 2
- Ultrasound machine
- Bandage or tubular bandage (if needed)
- 5 mL syringe
- Blunt drawing-up needle
- Tourniquet (disposable)
- Sharps container
- Labels

Optional equipment

- Securing device, e.g. StatLock
- Topical local anaesthetic

Medicinal products

- 0.9% sodium chloride: 5–10 mL

(continued)

Procedure guideline 17.5 Ultrasound-guided peripheral cannula insertion *(continued)*

Action	Rationale
Pre-procedure	
1 Introduce yourself to the patient, explain and discuss the procedure with them, and gain their consent to proceed.	To ensure that the patient feels at ease, understands the procedure and gives their valid consent (NMC 2018, **C**).
2 If the patient requires topical local anaesthetic, apply it to the chosen venepuncture site and leave in place for 30–60 minutes prior to cannulation.	In order to give adequate time for the local anaesthetic to be effective (BNF 2019, **C**).
3 Assemble all the equipment necessary for cannulation.	To ensure that time is not wasted and that the procedure goes smoothly without unnecessary interruptions. **E**
4 Check all packaging before opening and preparing the equipment to be used.	To ensure all equipment is in date and not contaminated. **E**
Procedure	
5 Wash your hands using bactericidal soap and water or an alcohol-based handrub and dry.	To minimize the risk of infection (DH 2010, **C**; Fraise and Bradley 2009, **E**).
6 Check your hands for any visibly broken skin, and cover any breaks with a waterproof dressing.	To minimize the risk of contamination of the nurse by the patient's blood (Loveday et al. 2014, **C**).
7 Ensure adequate lighting and privacy, and assist the patient into a comfortable position.	To ensure that the operator and patient are comfortable and that adequate light is available to illuminate the procedure. **E**
8 Support the chosen limb on a pillow.	To ensure the patient's comfort and give the nurse ease of access. **E**
9 Apply a tourniquet to the chosen limb, or use other methods if appropriate.	To dilate the veins by obstructing the venous return (Dougherty 2008, **E**).
10 Apply gel to the area and using the ultrasound probe assess and select the vein (**Action figure 10**).	To select a vein (Alexandrou et al. 2011, **E**; Gorski et al. 2016, **C**; Moureau 2014, **E**).
11 Release the tourniquet and wipe off the gel.	To ensure that the patient does not feel discomfort while the device is selected and equipment is prepared (Dougherty 2008, **E**).
12 Select a device based on the vein size and depth.	To reduce damage or trauma to the vein. To reduce the risk of phlebitis (Dougherty 2008, **E**; Moureau 2014, **E**; RCN 2016a, **C**).
13 Wash hands with soap and water, or an alcohol-based handrub, and dry.	To minimize risk of infection (DH 2010, **C**; Fraise and Bradley 2009, **E**).
14 Open a pack, empty all equipment onto the pack and place a sterile dressing towel under the patient's arm	To create a clean working area. **E**
15 Prime the extension set with a syringe of 0.9% sodium chloride (unless taking blood samples immediately after cannulation). *Note*: when using a closed system integrated peripheral intravenous cannula, there is no need to prime the system.	To remove air from the set prior to connection. If taking blood then the sodium chloride will contaminate the sample (Dougherty 2008, **E**). To reduce the manipulation of components and minimize the risk of contamination. **E**
16 Reapply the tourniquet.	To promote venous filling (Dougherty 2008, **E**).
17 Clean the patient's skin over the selected vein for at least 30 seconds using 2% chlorhexidine using back-and-forth strokes with friction and allow to dry (see Figure 17.18). Do not re-touch the skin.	To maintain asepsis and remove skin flora (DH 2010, **C**; Dougherty 2008, **E**; Loveday et al. 2014, **C**; RCN 2016a, **C**).
18 Put on gloves.	To prevent contamination of the nurse from any blood spill (DH 2010, **C**)
19 Using an aseptic non-touch technique, apply sterile gel to the transducer on the ultrasound probe and cover it with a sterile semi-permeable transparent IV film dressing (**Action figure 19**)	To maintain asepsis and minimize the risk of infection (DH 2010, **C**; Loveday et al. 2014, **C**).
20 Remove the needle guard and inspect the device for any faults.	To detect faulty equipment, for example bent or barbed needles. If these are present, do not use and report to the manufacturer as faulty equipment (MHRA 2005, **C**; RCN 2016a, **C**).
21 Apply sterile gel and, using the non-dominant hand, position the ultrasound probe 0.5–1.0 cm above the proposed site of insertion (**Action figure 21**).	To visualize the vein and facilitate a smooth needle entry (Moureau 2014, **E**)
22 Holding the cannula in the dominant hand, ensure that it is in the bevel-up position, and puncture through the skin, 0.5–1.0 cm below the probe, at the selected angle (normally 45°). Adapt the puncture angle according to the depth of the vein (**Action figure 22**).	To ensure optimum visualization of the echogenic needle tip during cannulation. **E**

23	Visualizing the vein under ultrasound, slowly slide the probe upwards using the non-dominant hand, while the dominant hand slowly advances the cannula tip towards the top of the vein wall.	To allow clear visualization of the echogenic needle tip. **E**
24	While continuing to visualize with ultrasound, advance the cannula tip and puncture the vein wall. At this point there will be a first blood flashback into the stylet chamber of the cannula (**Action figure 24**).	To continue to clearly visualize the echogenic needle tip. **E** To ensure that the needle has entered the vein. **E**
25	Level the cannula by decreasing the angle between the cannula and the skin. While continuing to visualize with ultrasound, advance the cannula slightly to ensure entry into the lumen of the vein (**Action figure 25**).	To avoid advancing too far and causing damage to the vein wall. To stabilize the device (Alexandrou et al. 2011, **E**; Dougherty 2008, **E**; Moureau 2014, **E**).
26	Withdraw the stylet slightly with the dominant hand and a second flashback of blood will be seen along the shaft of the cannula (**Action figure 26**).	To ensure that the cannula is still in a patent vein. This is called the 'hooded technique' (Dougherty 2008, **E**).
27	Using the dominant hand, continue to slowly advance the cannula off the stylet and into the vein (**Action figure 26**).	To ensure the vein remains immobilized, thus reducing the risk of a through-puncture (Dougherty 2008, **E**).
28	Release the tourniquet and remove the ultrasound probe from the skin.	To decrease the pressure within the vein. **E**

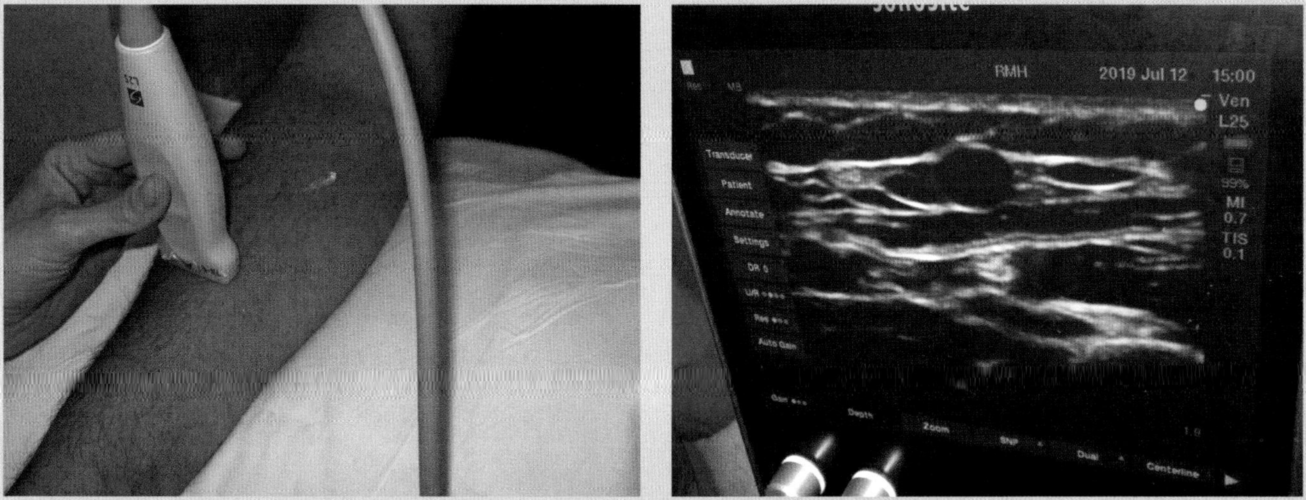

Action Figure 10 Apply gel to the area and, using the ultrasound probe, assess and select the vein.

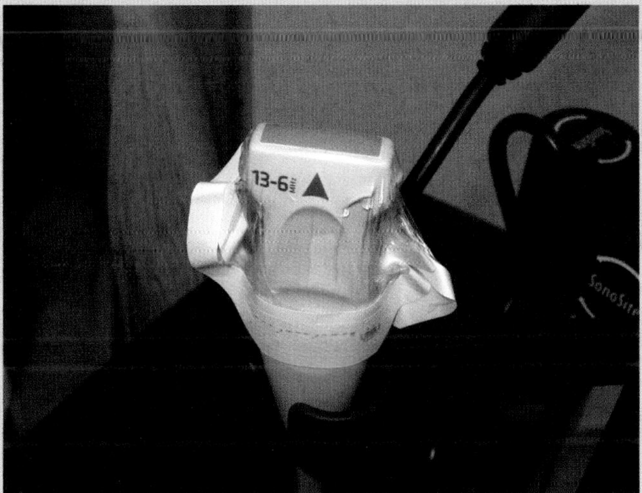

Action Figure 19 Using aseptic non-touch technique, apply sterile gel to the transducer on the ultrasound probe and cover it with a sterile semi-permeable transparent IV film dressing.

(continued)

Procedure guideline 17.5 Ultrasound-guided peripheral cannula insertion *(continued)*

Action	Rationale
29 Apply digital pressure to the vein above the cannula tip and completely remove the stylet. *Note*: when using an integrated closed system peripheral intravenous cannula, there is no need for digital pressure as blood is contained within the system by a vent plug (**Action figure 26**).	To prevent blood spillage. **E** To minimize exposure to blood. **E**
30 Immediately dispose of the stylet into an appropriate sharps container.	To reduce the risk of accidental needle stick injury (NHS Employers 2010, 2015, **C**).
31 Attach a primed extension set, needleless injection cap or administration set. *Note*: if using an integrated closed system peripheral intravenous cannula, there is no need to attach an extension set as it is integrated.	To enable flushing of the cannula (Dougherty 2008, **E**). To minimize the risk of infection through manipulating the system (Bitmead and Oliver 2018, **E**).
32 Using the sterile tape provided in the dressing package, secure the cannula using, for example, the method illustrated in **Action figure 32**, always allowing visualization of the insertion site.	To ensure the device will remain stable and secure (Dougherty 2008, **E**). To visualize and monitor phlebitis score (RCN 2016a, **C**).
33 Aspirate to check for blood flashback then flush the cannula with 0.9% sodium chloride using a pulsatile flush ending with positive pressure.	To ascertain and maintain patency (Goode et al. 1991, **R**; RCN 2016a, **C**).
34 Observe the site for signs of swelling or leakage and ask the patient whether they are experiencing any discomfort or pain.	To check that the device is positioned correctly and is stable and secure (Dougherty 2008, **E**).
35 Cover with semi-permeable transparent IV film dressing (unless contraindicated) and apply a date and time label (**Action figure 35**).	To ensure patient comfort and security of the device. To enable all staff to know when the dressing was applied (Loveday et al. 2014; **C**; RCN 2016a, **C**).

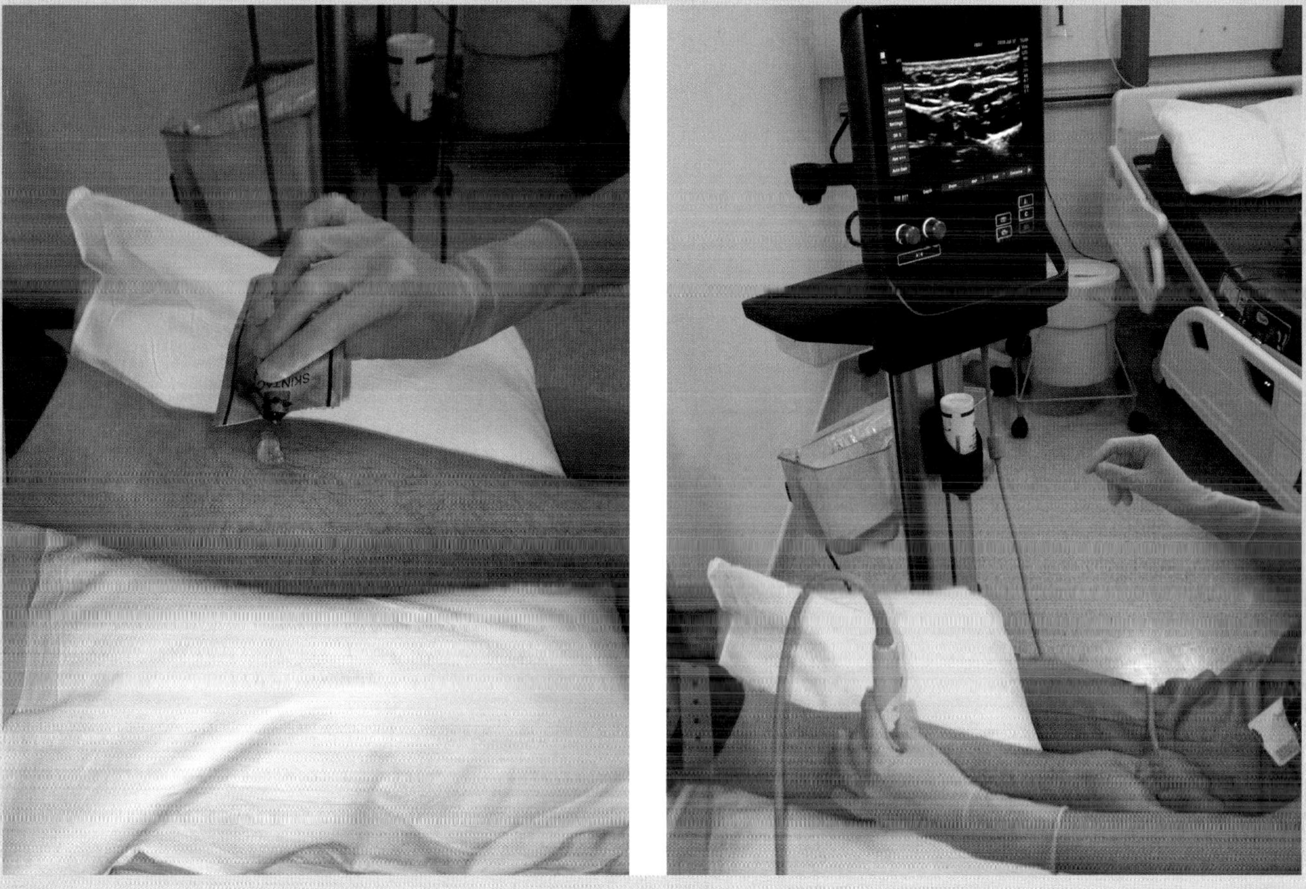

Action Figure 21 Apply sterile gel and using the non-dominant hand position the ultrasound probe 0.5–1.0 cm above the proposed site of insertion.

Post-procedure

36 Remove gloves and discard waste, making sure it is placed in the appropriate containers.	To ensure safe disposal in the correct containers and avoid laceration or injury of other staff. To prevent reuse of equipment (NHS Employers 2010, 2015, **C**). To prevent sharps injury (HSE 2013, **C**).
37 Clean and decontaminate the ultrasound equipment as per infection control guidelines. Label as cleaned.	To minimize the risk of cross-infection (Loveday et al. 2014, **C**).
38 Document date and time of insertion, site, size of cannula, number of attempts, and volume and type of flushing solution, and sign in the patient's notes or care plan.	To ensure adequate records are maintained and to enable continued care of the patient and device (DH 2011, **C**; NMC 2018, **C**).

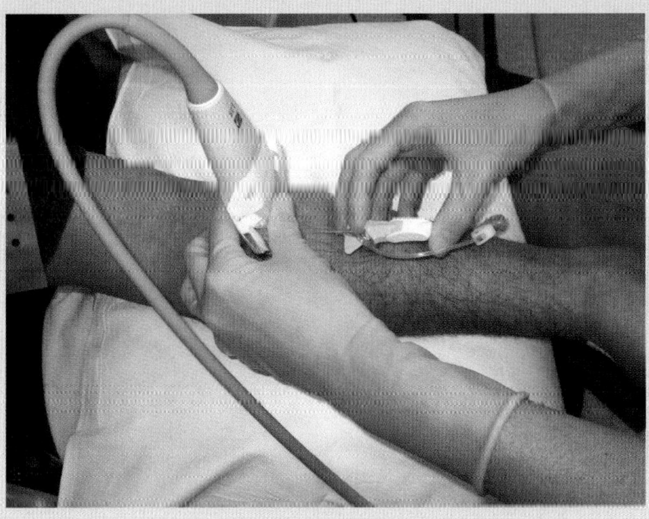

Action Figure 22 Puncture through the skin, 0.5–1.0 cm below the probe, at the selected angle.

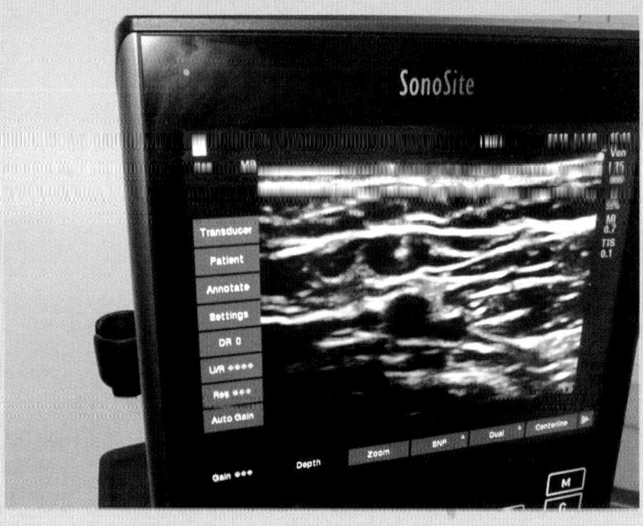

Action Figure 25 Ultrasound image of the cannula inside the vein.

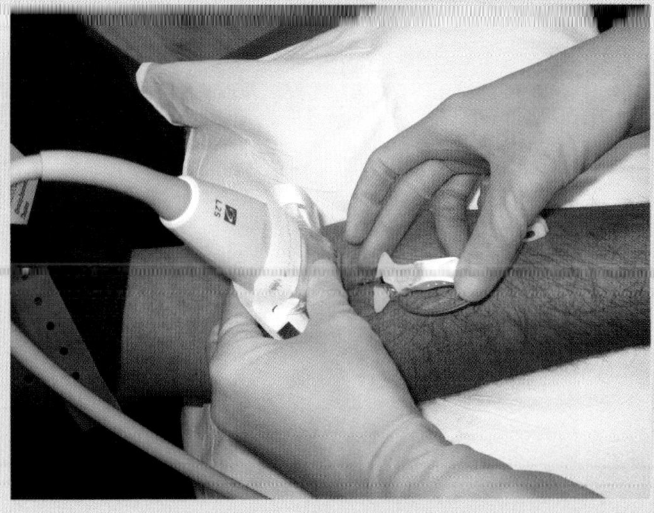

Action Figure 24 Flashback into the cannula chamber when the vein is punctured.

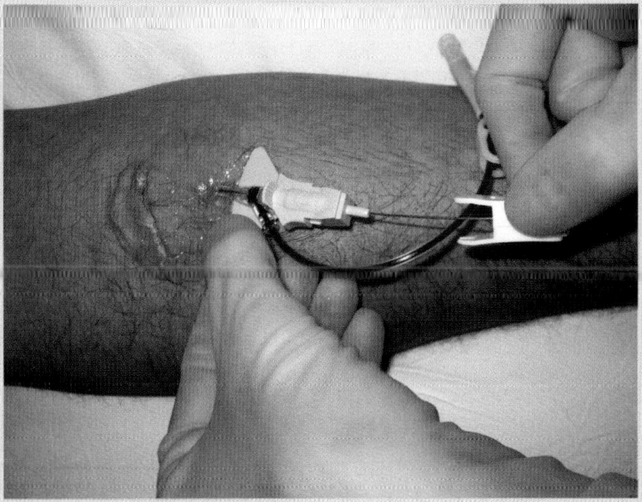

Action Figure 26 Withdraw the stylet while advancing the rest of the cannula.

(continued)

Procedure guideline 17.5 Ultrasound-guided peripheral cannula insertion *(continued)*

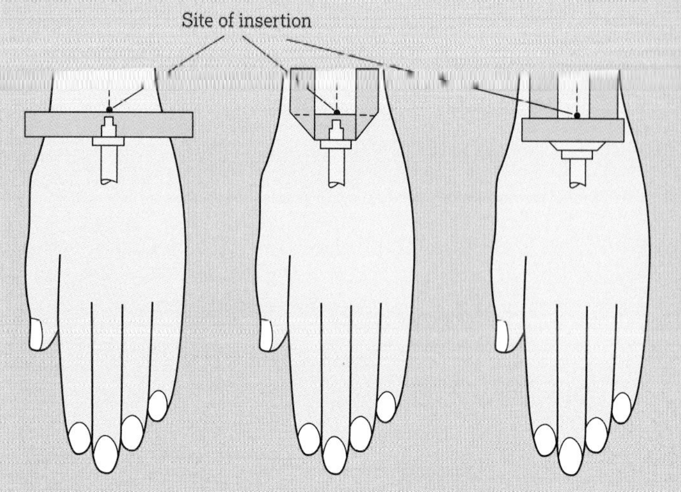

Action Figure 32 Method for taping a peripheral cannula.

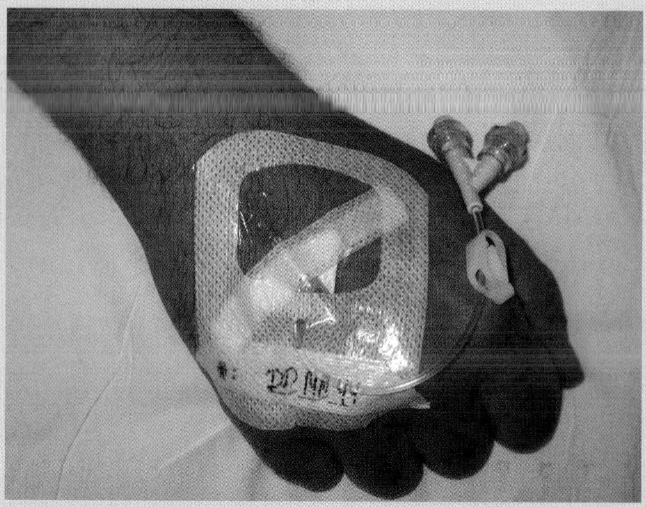

Action Figure 35 Semi-permeable transparent IV film dressing.

Post-procedural considerations

1066

Immediate care

Once sited, the peripheral cannula should be flushed using a pulsatile flush ending with positive pressure (Dougherty 2008, RCN 2016a, Weinstein and Hagle 2014). The cannula should be secured using an IV film dressing, clean tape or a securing device (Figure 17.19). Tape should not cover the insertion site, and taping with the sterile tape provided with the IV film dressing should enable the site to remain visible and the cannula stable (Figure 17.20). The approach shown in Procedure guideline 17.4: Peripheral cannula insertion, Action figure 30, is recommended (Dougherty 2008, Hadaway 2000). Securement devices are now available and reduce the risk of dislodgement and other complications (Bausone-Gazda et al. 2010, Higginson 2015, Moureau and Iannucci 2003, Ullman et al. 2017). Low-linting gauze should only be used if IV film dressing is contraindicated (Gorski et al. 2016, Loveday et al. 2014, RCN 2016a).

Ongoing care

A peripheral cannula should be flushed before and after each use to check for patency prior to administration of a medication, and at least daily if not in use, using 0.9% sodium chloride. The dressing should be changed as required (if transparent) or each time the device is manipulated (gauze). In order to determine skin health at the PIVC site, the clinician should inspect the skin for colour, texture, uniformity of appearance and integrity (Broadhurst et al. 2017). The site should be monitored daily or when the device is used. The site should be inspected for signs of infiltration, extravasation and leakage, using a recognized scale such as the VIP scale for signs of phlebitis or infection (Bitmead and Oliver 2018, DH 2010, Gorski et al. 2016, RCN 2016a, Ullman et al. 2017). To avoid contamination when accessing the cannula, good hand hygiene and aseptic non touch technique are required, and the needle-free connector should be disinfected with a wipe saturated with 2% chlorhexidine in 70% alcohol for 15 seconds and left to air dry (Bitmead and Oliver 2018). All ongoing care must be documented (DH 2010, Gorski et al. 2016, RCN 2016a).

Removal

Van Donk et al. (2009) and Webster et al. (2008) recommended the re-siting of cannulas based on clinical indication instead of time *in situ*. Lee et al. (2009) further state that this approach does not increase infection rates but they do recommend that insertion is done by highly skilled intravenous teams or rates could increase. Rickard et al. (2012), who conducted a study of over 1,000 peripheral cannulas, found no difference in phlebitis, infection or failure rates between replacing cannulas every 3 days compared with leaving them *in situ* and replacing them when clinically indicated. They concluded that peripheral devices need only be removed as clinically indicated and that this would save millions of unnecessary re-sites, reduce associated discomfort, and reduce costs of both equipment and staff time. This is supported by recent changes in guidelines that suggest that PIVCs should be re-sited only when clinically indicated and not routinely, unless device-specific recommendations from the manufacturer indicate otherwise (Gorski et al. 2016, Loveday et al. 2014, RCN 2016a).

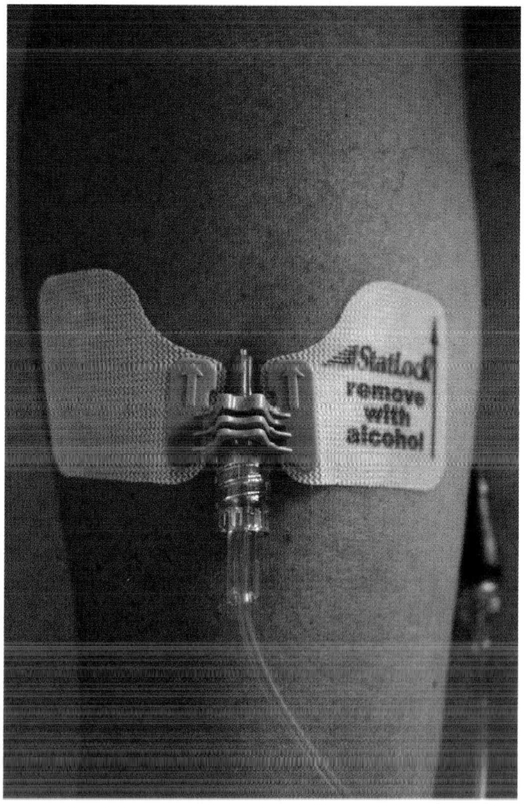

Figure 17.19 Peripheral cannula secured with StatLock.

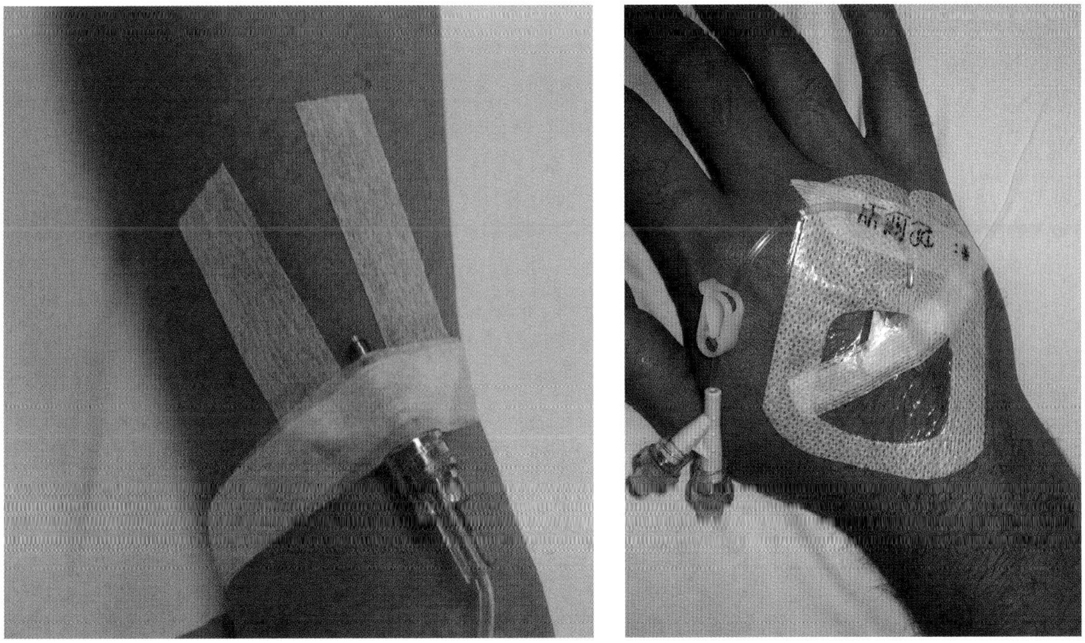

(a) (b)

Figure 17.20 (a) Cannula *in situ*. (b) Cannula secured with a semi-permeable transparent IV film dressing.

Removal of the peripheral intravenous device or cannula should be an aseptic procedure. The device should be removed carefully using a slow, steady movement keeping the hub parallel with the skin, and pressure should be applied until haemostasis is achieved. This pressure should be firm and not involve any rubbing movement. A haematoma will occur if the device is carelessly removed, causing discomfort and a focus for infection (Perucca 2010). The site should be inspected to ensure bleeding has stopped and should then be covered with a sterile dressing (Bitmead and Oliver 2018, Gorski et al. 2016). The cannula's integrity should be checked to ensure that a complete device has been removed (Dougherty 2008, Gorski et al. 2016, RCN 2016a).

Documentation

On insertion, the practitioner should document the date and time, the site and size of the cannula, the number of attempts and the flushing solution used. They should also date and time the dressing and sign their name. This can be done as part of a specific cannula care plan or by use of a sticker in the patient's notes (Figure 17.21) (DH 2010). If a tool is used to monitor the site, for example VIP score, then this should be recorded on a regular basis (e.g. every shift change or at least once a day) (Gorski et al. 2016, Loveday et al. 2014, RCN 2016a). The date, time and reason for removal of the cannula must also be documented in the patient's notes (DH 2011, Dougherty 2008, RCN 2016a). This documentation ensures adequate records for the continued care of the patient and device and also enables audit and gathering of statistics on rates of phlebitis, infiltration and so on.

Education of the patient and relevant others

See 'Discharging patients home with a VAD *in situ*' above.

Complications

On insertion

Pain

Pain can be caused by the following:

- tentative stop–start insertion (often associated with hesitant or new practitioners)
- hitting an artery, nerve or valve
- poor technique: inadequate anchoring causes skin to gather as the needle is inserted
- alcohol not allowed to dry adequately before insertion, resulting in stinging pain
- using a frequently punctured, recently used or bruised vein
- anxious patient, who may have a low pain threshold
- use of large-gauge device
- use of veins in sensitive areas (Dougherty 2008).

Pain can be prevented by using methods to relax and relieve anxiety, for example massage, distraction or the use of local anaesthetic creams or injections. The practitioner should avoid the use of bruised, recently used or sensitive areas. If the patient complains of pain, depending on the site (e.g. nerve or artery), it may be necessary to remove the device immediately. Reassure the patient and explain, especially in the case of nerve pain, that it may last for a few hours; provide the patient with an information leaflet (containing instructions on what to do if the pain gets worse or there is no improvement) and document the incident (Dougherty 2008).

Haematoma

Haematoma is leakage of blood into the tissues and is indicated by rapid swelling during the insertion procedure or after removal (McCall and Tankersley 2019, Perucca 2010). It can be caused by:

- penetration of the posterior vein wall
- incorrect choice of needle for the vein size
- fragile veins
- patients receiving anticoagulant therapy
- excessive or blind probing to locate the vein
- spontaneous rupture of the vessel on application of the tourniquet or cleaning of the skin
- inadequate pressure on the venepuncture site following removal of the cannula (Dougherty 2008, McCall and Tankersley 2019, Moini 2013).

Prevention includes good vein and device selection and using a careful technique. Practitioners should always be aware of when patients have fragile veins or are on anticoagulant therapy, and

The ROYAL MARSDEN

NHS Foundation Trust

Venous Access Devices

Name:	Hospital Number:	Date of birth:

Peripheral Cannula (PIVC – Peripheral Intra Venous Catheter)

Date & time:		**Reason for cannula:**	☐ Transfusion ☐ Antibiotics ☐ Fluids ☐ SACT ☐ Other:

Insertion:

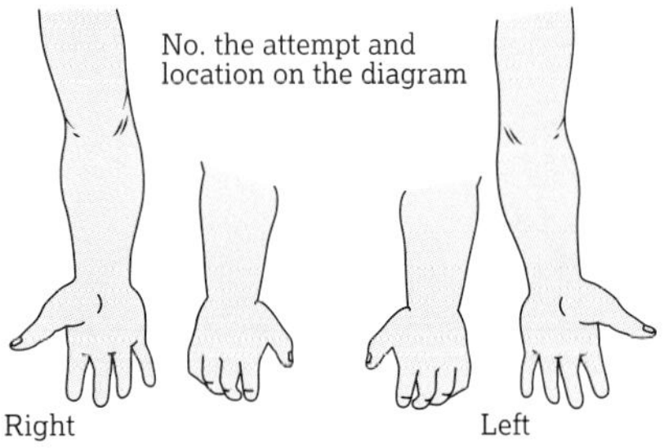

Attempt	**Site**	**Cannula gauge**	**Sign/print/designation**
1st			
2nd			
3rd			
4th			

Ongoing assessment	Day 1	Day 2	Day 3	Day 4	Day 5	Day 6	Day 7
(at least twice a day) **DATE**							
VIP score (0–5) (Day)							
Sign/print/designation							
VIP score (0–5) (Night)							
Sign/print/designation							
Removal reason							

Date & time:		**Reason for cannula:**	☐ Transfusion ☐ Antibiotics ☐ Fluids ☐ SACT ☐ Other:

Insertion:

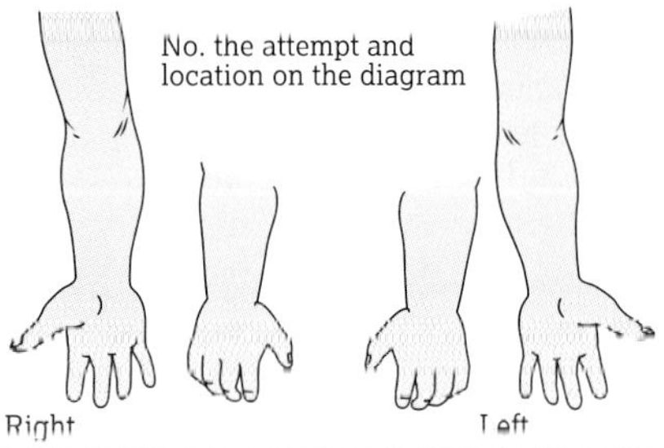

Attempt	**Site**	**Cannula gauge**	**Sign/print/designation**
1st			
2nd			
3rd			
4th			

Ongoing assessment	Day 1	Day 2	Day 3	Day 4	Day 5	Day 6	Day 7
(at least twice a day) **DATE**							
VIP score (0–5) (Day)							
Sign/print/designation							
VIP score (0–5) (Night)							
Sign/print/designation							
Removal reason							

Figure 17.21 Documentation example from The Royal Marsden NHS Foundation Trust's vascular access device documentation booklet. *Source:* Reproduced with permission of The Royal Marsden NHS Foundation Trust.

Central Venous Access Devices (CVADs)

Insertion details – *if not completed by the practitioner inserting the device refer to EPR for details*

Reason for insertion	
Insertion site (position)	

NON-Tunnelled Catheters	PICC ☐ Acute CVC ☐ Vascath ☐ Number of Lumens 1. ☐ 2. ☐ 3. ☐ 4. ☐	**Location where inserted** Theatres ☐	CCU ☐
Tunnelled Catheters	Skin Tunnelled Catheter e.g. Hickman ☐ LTS – Permcath Type ☐ Implanted PORT ☐ Number of Lumens 1. ☐ 2. ☐ 3. ☐	Procedure room ☐	Other ☐ (Specify)

MRSA/MSSA screen pre-insertion Yes ☐ No ☐ Result & action taken:...

Octenisan wash pre-insertion Yes ☐ No ☐ ....

CVAD secured by: Sutures ☐ Securement device ☐ Transparent dressing ☐

CXR / ECG tip location checked by competent practitioner prior to use ☐

Date inserted / /	Time *(24hr clock)*		Sign/print/designation

CVAD – already in situ ☐ *specify position, type and date inserted in section above*

Daily surveillance of Central Venous Access Device (CVADs) *(please tick)*

DATE (day/month/year)														
	Day	Night	Day	Night	Day	Night	Day	Night	Day	Night	Day	Night	Day	Night
CVC only: number of days in situ:_______														
Device Functioning														
Hand hygiene used when accessing the line device?														
ANTT: 2% chlorhexidine in 70% alcohol														
Flushed with 10 mL 0.9% sodium chloride before and after use														
Is the device **patent** (flushing & aspirating)?														
If flushing well but not aspirating, **fluid challenge** (*250 mL 0.9% sodium chloride)* given														
If **sluggish** or **not flushing**, *urokinase* used														
Exit site & exit dressing														
PORT ACESSS only: Needle size (specify)														
PORT ACESSS only: Accessed by														
PORT ACESSS only: Needle removed/reason														
Exit site **visible? Transparent dressing** in place? *If NO, change*														
Dressing intact, clean and dated?														
Exit site: inflammation/redness/ discharge? **VIP score (0–5)**														
Device Required														
Is the device needed? **Y/N** **If not, remove**														
Removal date *(day/month/year)*														
Removal reason														
Sign/print/ Designation														

Figure 17.21 *Continued*

inexperienced individuals should not attempt cannulation in these individuals (Perucca 2010). A tourniquet should not be applied to a limb where recent venepuncture has occurred and the tourniquet should not be left in place for any longer than necessary.

On removal of the cannula, adequate pressure should be applied to the site. Alcohol pads inhibit clotting and should not be used (Perucca 2010). In the event of a haematoma occurring, the needle should be removed immediately and pressure applied to the site for a few minutes (Garza and Becan-McBride 2018, McCall and Tankersley 2019). Elevate the extremity if appropriate, reassure the patient and explain the reason for the bruise. Apply a pressure dressing if required and an ice pack if the bruising is extensive (Moini 2013). Hirudoid or arnica ointment can help to reduce bruising and discomfort. Arnica is made of dried roots or flower of the arnica plant, which stimulates activity of the white blood cells, which in turn process congested blood and reduce the bruise (Goedemans et al. 2014). Hirudoid is a substance similar to heparin and acts by dissolving blood clots and improving blood supply to the skin (EMC 2015). They are both applied directly to the affected arm (BNF 2019). The incident should be documented and the patient given an information sheet with advice about when and whom to contact if the haematoma gets worse or they develop any numbness in the limb (Dougherty 2008, Moini 2013, Morris 2011, Perucca 2010).

Inadvertent arterial puncture

Inadvertent arterial puncture is characterized by pain and bright red blood caused by accidental puncture of an artery (Dougherty 2008, McCall and Tankersley 2019, Moini 2013). It can be prevented by adequate assessment and recognition of arteries prior to performing the procedure. It is rare when proper procedures are followed and can be associated with deep or blind probing (McCall and Tankersley 2019). However, should it occur, the device should be removed immediately and pressure applied to the puncture site for up to 5 minutes or until the bleeding has stopped (McCall and Tankersley 2019, Moini 2013). Reassure the patient but do not reapply the tourniquet to the affected limb. If an inadvertent arterial puncture goes undetected, accumulation of blood can result in compression injury and damage nearby nerves. The incident must be documented and the patient given an information sheet with advice about when and whom to contact if they develop numbness or tingling in the limb (Dougherty 2008).

Nerve injury

If a nerve is accidentally hit on insertion of the needle into the vein, this will result in pain, described as severe shooting pain (Masoorli 2003, Yuan and Cohen 1985), painful burning sensation (Moini 2013) or a sharp electric tingling sensation that radiates down the nerve (McCall and Tankersley 2019). It can occur due to poor vein selection, inserting the needle too deeply or quickly, or blind probing, and can lead to injury and possibly permanent damage (McCall and Tankersley 2019). Prevention may be achieved by ensuring that the location of superficial nerves is known; for example, a common place to hit a nerve is the cephalic vein but this can be avoided by placing three fingers at the wrist and inserting the needle above them (the nerve runs deeper at that point and therefore the practitioner will be less likely to touch it) (Boeson et al. 2000, Masoorli 2007). In the event of touching a nerve, release the tourniquet and remove the needle immediately (Garza and Becan-McBride 2018). Reassure the patient and explain that the pain may last for a few hours or days and that the area may feel numb. Explain that if the pain continues beyond a few days or gets worse, medical advice should be sought. Give the patient an information sheet with advice about when and whom to contact and document the incident (Dougherty 2008, Garza and Becan-McBride 2018).

Once *in situ*

Phlebitis

Phlebitis is inflammation of the intima of a vein (Perucca 2010, Washington and Barrett 2012). It is characterized by pain and tenderness along the cannulated vein, erythema, warmth, and streak formation with or without a palpable cord (a palpable thickening of the vein that occurs in relation to phlebitis) (Mermel et al. 2001).

There are three main types of phlebitis:

- *Mechanical* phlebitis is related to irritation and damage to a vein by a large gauge cannula, siting a cannula where there is movement (e.g. antecubital fossa), and securing the cannula inadequately, or increased dwell time.
- *Chemical* phlebitis is related to chemical irritation from drugs (extreme pHs) such as antibiotics and chemotherapy.
- *Bacterial* phlebitis occurs when the site becomes infected due to poor hand washing or aseptic technique (Lamb and Dougherty 2008, Morris 2011).

Phlebitis causes significant pain, PIVC failure and therapy interruption, and it requires the insertion of a new PIVC with associated increased equipment costs and staff time (Ray-Barruel et al. 2014, 2018). It compromises future venous access, and untreated bacterial phlebitis may lead to bloodstream infection; therefore, early detection of complications and removal of the PIVC is crucial (Alexandrou et al. 2018, Ray-Barruel et al. 2014). Influencing factors that increase the risk of phlebitis include being female, dwell time, large-gauge cannulas, higher number of doses of irritating medications such as antibiotics; factors that reduce risk include choice of vein (forearm), smaller-gauge cannulas and use of specialized vascular access teams (Alexandrou et al. 2018, Carr et al. 2018, Da Silva et al. 2010, Johnson et al. 2017, Mestre et al. 2013, Wallis et al. 2014, Washington and Barrett 2012). Prevention is key and includes appropriate device and vein selection, dilution of drugs, and pharmacological methods, for example application of glyceryl trinitrate patches (Alexandrou et al. 2018, Dougherty 2008). Treatment includes discontinuing the infusion at the first signs of phlebitis (grade 1) (see Figure 17.8). Warm or cold compresses can be applied to the affected site. The patient should be referred to a doctor if the phlebitis rating is over 3. If bacterial phlebitis is suspected then the insertion site should be cultured and the cannula tip sent to microbiology (Dougherty 2008, Morris 2011).

Infiltration and extravasation

See Chapter 15: Medicines optimization: ensuring quality and safety.

Midline catheters

Definition

A midline catheter can be defined as one that is between 7.5 and 20 cm in length (Bodenham et al. 2016, Cummings et al. 2011, Dougherty 2008, RCN 2016a). It provides vascular access in a larger peripheral vein without entering the central venous circulation. It is inserted into a vein in the upper arm, above the antecubital fossa, and the tip is extended into the vein for up to 20 cm, but it is not extended past the axilla (Bodenham et al. 2016, Hadaway 2010, RCN 2016a).

Anatomy and physiology

Choice of vein

The basilic vein is the vein of choice due to its larger size, straighter course for catheter advancement and higher haemodilution capability (Moureau and Chopra 2016, Perucca 2010, Weinstein and Hagle 2014). The cephalic and median cubital veins are the second and third choices, respectively (Gorski et al. 2016).

Evidence-based approaches

Rationale

A midline catheter offers an alternative to peripheral and central venous access. Where patients present with poor peripheral venous access and when the use of a central venous catheter (CVC) is contraindicated, a midline catheter provides venous accessibility along with easy, less hazardous insertion in veins of the upper arm, above the antecubital fossa (Dawson and Moureau 2013, Mushtaq et al. 2018, Weinstein and Hagle 2014). Because the tip of the catheter does not extend beyond the extremities in which it is placed, radiographic confirmation of tip placement is optional and recommended only when there is difficulty in insertion or flushing (Gorski and Czaplewski 2004, Weinstein and Hagle 2014).

Midlines are experiencing a resurgence of attention and usage due to improvements in catheter materials and product development. Newer midline catheters are 8–10 cm in length and can be placed using a modified Seldinger technique (MST). Some models are all-in-one devices with the needle, wire and introducer in a combined unit for ease and speed of access; for these, the insertion technique referred to as accelerated Seldinger (AST) should be used (Moureau and Chopra 2016). The growing evidence to support the use of midlines demonstrates lower phlebitis rates than those for peripheral intravenous cannulas and lower rates of infection than those for CVCs (Caparas and Hu 2014, Dawson and Moureau 2013, Moureau and Chopra 2016, Mushtaq et al. 2018, Warrington et al. 2012). Other benefits to patients include less frequent re-siting of peripheral intravenous cannulas and a subsequent reduction in associated venous trauma (Gorski and Czaplewski 2004, Moureau and Chopra 2016, Weinstein and Hagle 2014).

Indications

Midline catheters are indicated in the following circumstances:

- When patients do not have accessible peripheral veins in the lower arm.
- When patients will be undergoing therapy for 1–4 weeks (Carlson 1999, Chopra et al. 2015, Moureau and Chopra 2016), in order to preserve the integrity of the veins and increase patient comfort by removing the need for peripheral intravenous cannula re-sites, for example antibiotics. Michigan Appropriateness Guide for Intravenous Catheters (MAGIC) guidelines (Chopra et al. 2015) suggest the use of midlines for patients with peripherally compatible solution or medications where treatment will likely exceed 6 days (Chopra et al. 2015, Moureau and Chopra 2016).
- When patients are considered DIVAs (Difficult Intravenous Access) and ultrasound guided peripheral access has failed (Moureau and Chopra 2016).
- Patient preference (Cummings et al. 2011, Dougherty 2008, Hadaway 2010, Perucca 2010).

Contraindications

The following should not be used for administration via a midline catheter:

- vesicant medications, especially by continuous infusion
- parenteral nutrition
- solutions and/or medications with a pH of less than 5 or greater than 9
- solutions and/or medications with an osmolarity greater than 600 mOsmol/L (Chopra et al. 2015, Gorski and Czaplewski 2004, Gorski et al. 2016, Hadaway 2010, Moureau and Chopra 2016, RCN 2016a).

Methods of insertion

The insertion is performed via an introducer or using an MST (i.e. when venous access is established with a needle, a guidewire is threaded through the needle, the needle is removed, an introducer/peel-away sheath is threaded over the guidewire, the guidewire and dilator are then removed, and the catheter is advanced into the venous system through the introducer/peel-away sheath) (Hadaway 2010, Weinstein and Hagle 2014). Newer all-in-one midlines follow an AST as the needle, guidewire and introducer are combined (Moureau and Chopra 2016). Adequate ultrasound assessment of the patient's veins is vital to ensure vessel patency, identify any thrombosis and assess the diameter of the vein to be cannulated (Alexandrou et al. 2011, Gorski et al. 2016). Given the choice, the non-dominant arm should be used (Alexandrou et al. 2011).

Clinical governance

The procedure should only be performed by trained and competent healthcare professionals who have achieved a high standard in cannulation (NMC 2018, RCN 2016a, Weinstein and Hagle 2014) and have completed a formal educational program including theoretical and practical components (Moureau et al. 2013). Competencies include knowledge of the anatomy and physiology of the veins of the upper arm, ability to select veins and equipment, and ability to prevent and manage complications.

Pre-procedural considerations

Equipment

Silicone and polyurethane are the materials most frequently used in the manufacturing of midline catheters (de Lutio 2014, Hadaway 2010, Kupensky 1998). Catheters are available as single and dual lumen in lengths of up to 20 cm, which can be cut to the desired length following measurement of the arm from the selected vein towards the axilla. They are available in various sizes from 2 to 5 Fr (French; a larger Fr indicates a larger internal catheter diameter) (Dougherty 2008, Hadaway 2010). Newer all-in-one midline catheters come in a set measure of either 8 or 10 cm and they are available in 4 or 5 Fr (Moureau and Chopra 2016).

Procedure guideline 17.6 Midline catheter insertion

It is helpful to have an assistant when performing this procedure, if possible.

Essential equipment

- Personal protective equipment
- Sterile gloves
- Sterile minor operation pack (containing sterile drapes and scissors)
- Alcohol-based skin-cleaning preparation, e.g. 2% chlorhexidine in 70% alcohol
- Extension set (if needed) and needle-free connector
- Midline catheter
- Introducer, or needle, guidewire and peel-away introducer if using modified Seldinger technique (MST)
- Semi-permeable transparent IV film dressing
- Securing device and sterile tapes
- 10 mL syringes × 2–3
- 25 G safety needle
- Drawing-up needle
- Tape measure
- Sterile gown, theatre cap and mask
- Disposable tourniquet

(continued)

Procedure guideline 17.6 Midline catheter insertion *(continued)*

Optional equipment

- Ultrasound equipment (if using MST)

Medicinal products

- 0.9% sodium chloride
- Topical local anaesthetic and/or 1% lidocaine injection

Action	Rationale
Pre-procedure	
1 Introduce yourself to the patient, explain and discuss the procedure with them, and gain their consent to proceed.	To ensure that the patient feels at ease, understands the procedure and gives their valid consent (NMC 2018, **C**).
2 Apply a tourniquet to the arm. Assess venous access and locate veins using ultrasound guidance (if using MST), then release the tourniquet. Repeat for the other arm if needed.	To ensure the patient has adequate venous access and to select the vein for catheterization (Gorski et al. 2016, **C**; RCN 2016a, **C**).
3 If necessary (e.g. in very anxious or needle-phobic patients, or children), apply local anaesthetic cream or gel to the chosen venepuncture site and leave for the allotted time.	To minimize the pain of insertion (BNF 2019, **C**).
4 Apply apron, draw screens and assist the patient into a comfortable position.	To ensure privacy. To aid insertion and correct placement. **E**
5 Using the tape measure, measure from the selected venepuncture site up the arm to just below the axilla.	To enable selection of the most suitable catheter length and to know how far to advance the catheter in order for its tip to be located in the correct position. **E**
6 Take the equipment required to the patient's bedside. Open the outer pack.	To gain access to the equipment. **E**
Procedure	
7 Wash hands with soap and water, or an alcohol-based handrub, and dry.	To minimize the risk of infection (Fraise and Bradley 2009, **E**; NHS England and NHSI 2019, **C**).
8 Put on sterile gown and gloves; open sterile pack, arranging the contents as required. Draw up the syringe with 0.9% sodium chloride (provided by assistant if possible) or use sterile 0.9% sodium chloride pre-filled syringes.	To prevent contamination. **E**
9 Remove the cap from the extension set and attach the syringe of 0.9% sodium chloride; gently flush with 2 mL and leave the syringe attached.	To check that the catheter is patent and to enable easy removal of the guidewire. **E**
10 Using the graduated markings along the catheter, select the marking required and pull back the stylet (if present) 1 cm from the desired new tip, and using sterile scissors trim the catheter. *Never trim the stylet.*	To ensure the catheter will be the correct length for placement and to prevent damage to the vein if the stylet is damaged. **E**
11 Place a sterile towel under the patient's arm.	To provide a sterile field to work on. **E**
12 Clean the skin at the selected site with an appropriate disinfectant, for example 2% chlorhexidine in 70% alcohol, using back-and-forth strokes with friction. In this way, prepare an area of 15–25 cm².	To ensure skin flora is destroyed and to minimize the risk of infection (Fraise and Bradley 2009, **E**; Gorski et al. 2016, **C**; Loveday et al. 2014, C; RCN 2016a, **C**).
13 Allow the solution to dry thoroughly.	To ensure coagulation of bacteria and completion of disinfection process (Loveday et al. 2014, **C**).
14 Drape the patient with a fenestrated towel.	To provide a sterile field (Loveday et al. 2014, **C**).
15 Draw up and inject local anaesthetic intradermally, if required, using a 25 G safety needle and wait for a few minutes for it to take effect.	To provide adequate anaesthesia (BNF 2019, **C**).
16 Reapply the tourniquet.	To aid venous distension (Dougherty 2008, **E**).
17 *Either:*	
If not using MST (modified Seldinger technique), perform the venepuncture with the introducer by entering the skin 1 cm from the desired point of entry, at a 15–30° angle. Advance 0.5–1.0 cm once flashback is seen. Continue to step 24.	To gain venous access (Dougherty 2008, **E**).
Or:	
If using MST, while visualizing the vein under ultrasound, perform the venepuncture with a needle or cannula. (If using a cannula, when flashback is seen, advance the cannula into the vein.) Continue to step 18.	To gain venous access (Gabriel 2008, **E**; Moureau 2014, **E**). To prevent blood loss and through-puncture and enable advancement of the catheter (Gabriel 2008, **E**).

18 Remove the stylet and advance the guidewire through the needle (or cannula) until there is 10–15 cm of wire in the vein (**Action figure 18**).	To maintain venous access. **E**
19 Release the tourniquet.	To prevent blood loss and through-puncture, and enable advancement of catheter (Dougherty 2008, **E**).
20 Advance the introducer over the wire up to the puncture site. (If using a cannula, first remove it, applying digital pressure.)	To prepare for insertion. **E**
21 Reinfiltrate over the puncture site with 1% lidocaine (intrademally) if necessary, until a small bleb is observed (**Action figure 21**).	To achieve anaesthesia and minimize patient discomfort. **E**
22 Check the patient has no sharp sensations at the puncture site and then make a small incision by sliding the tip of the scalpel blade along the top of the wire (**Action figure 22**).	To ensure the area is anaesthetized before proceeding. **E**
23 Activate the safety function on the scalpel and place it back onto the sterile field.	To minimize the risk of sharp stick injury. **E**
24 Grip the introducer firmly and advance through the puncture site (**Action figure 24**).	To enable advancement of the dilator. **E**
25 Remove the guidewire and the dilator from the introducer/peel-away sheath. Grip the catheter a few centimetres from the tip and thread through the introducer/peel-away sheath.	To enable catheter insertion. **E**
26 Continue slow advancement of the catheter and aspirate (if possible) and flush to check for blood return or resistance.	To minimize damage to the tunica intima of the vein (Gabriel 2008, **E**). To check there is no obstruction and that the catheter advances into the correct location. **E**
27 Position fingers in a V, with index finger on wings and middle finger above sheath tip, and gently remove stylet. Apply pressure.	To contain flashback, prevent contamination of the area with blood and minimize the amount of blood loss from the patient (Dougherty 2008, **E**).
28 Grip the catheter at least 1 cm from the tip and thread through the introducer sheath.	To ensure the tip is not contaminated (Dougherty 2008, **E**).
29 Continue slow advancement of the catheter to the desired length.	To minimize damage to the intima of the vein (Dougherty 2008, **E**).
30 Apply pressure above the introducer and carefully withdraw the introducer and peel apart.	To ensure there is no movement of the catheter. To remove the peel-away introducer (Dougherty 2008, **E**).
31 Aspirate for blood return and flush the catheter with 0.9% sodium chloride.	To check the patency of the device and ensure continued patency (Dougherty 2008, **E**).
32 Apply gentle pressure on the catheter and slowly withdraw the stylet.	To ensure there is no withdrawal of the catheter (Dougherty 2008, **E**).
33 Attach a needle-free connector and flush as per local policy.	To ensure the patency of the device (Dougherty 2008, **E**).
34 Secure the catheter with sterile tape or another securing device and a small pressure dressing over the insertion site. Apply a semi-permeable transparent IV film dressing. Add the insertion date to the dressing. Apply gauze and a bandage or a tubular bandage.	To ensure stability of the device and protection of the site (Dougherty 2008, **E**). To know when the dressing needs to be changed (RCN 2016a, **C**).
Post-procedure	
35 Remove gloves and gown, and dispose of equipment appropriately. Dispose of sharps and clinical waste.	To ensure safe disposal in the correct containers and avoid laceration or injury of other staff. To prevent reuse of equipment (NHS Employers 2010, 2015, **C**). To reduce the risk of sharps injury (HSE 2013, **C**).
36 Document the procedure in the patient's notes: • type, length and gauge of catheter • where it was inserted • any problems • how it was secured.	To ensure adequate records are maintained and enable continued care of the patient and device (NMC 2018, **C**).

(continued)

Procedure guideline 17.6 Midline catheter insertion *(continued)*

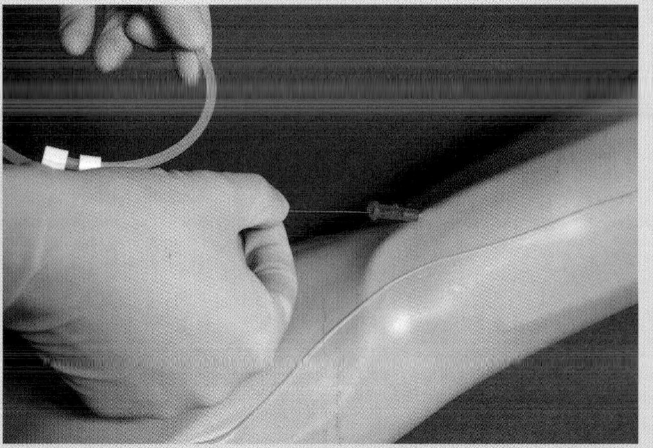

Action Figure 18 Wire being threaded in the cannula.

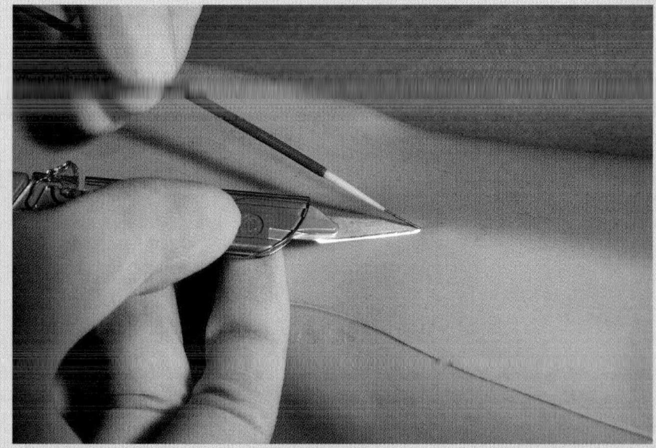

Action Figure 22 Making an incision with a scalpel.

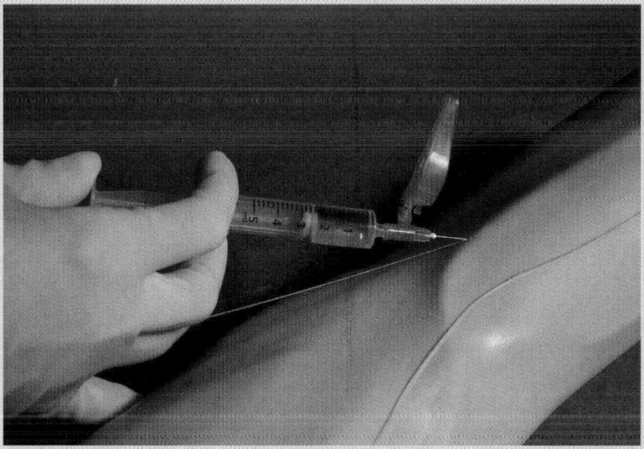

Action Figure 21 Local anaesthetic injection.

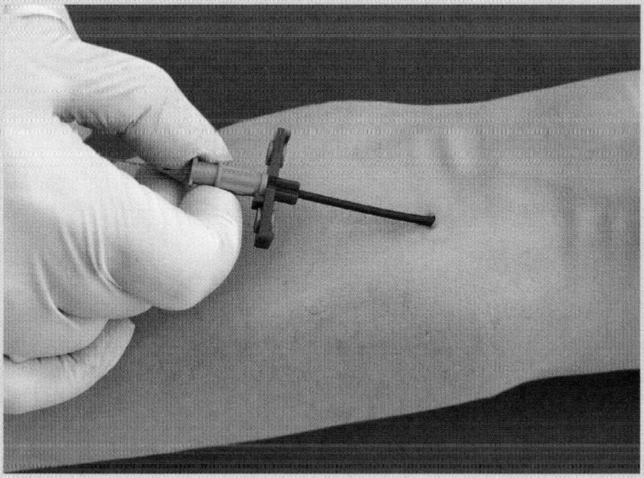

Action Figure 24 Advancing the introducer.

Problem-solving table 17.2 Prevention and resolution (Procedure guideline 17.6)

Problem	Cause	Prevention	Action
Missed vein: see 'Missing the vein on insertion of the cannula' in Problem-solving table 17.1			
Unable to advance catheter	Valves Choice of vein, for example the cephalic narrows above the antecubital fossa	Select a vein with fewer valves or one with a large lumen.	Flush and attempt to advance the catheter. Depending on the length advanced, it may be acceptable to leave it and use it for a short period of time.

Post-procedural considerations

Immediate care

It is not usually appropriate to suture these devices *in situ*, as they can be adequately secured with Steri Strips or catheter securement devices such as a StatLock or Grip-Lok (Luo et al. 2017, Perucca 2010, Ullman et al. 2017). The insertion site can then be covered with a semi-permeable transparent IV film dressing and changed according to the manufacturer's recommendations, for example once a week. The device should be flushed with 0.9% sodium chloride after each use and according to the manufacturer's recommendations, for example weekly.

Ongoing care

Midline catheters can be left *in situ* for extended periods of time; the optimal time interval for removal of a midline catheter is unknown (Hadaway 2010), although most manufacturers advise an indwelling time of 30 days. Therefore, it is recommended that maximum dwell times should be limited to 2–4 weeks (Chopra et al. 2015, Gorski et al. 2016, RCN 2016a). Longer dwell times should be decided on the basis of a site assessment, the anticipated duration of the therapy and the patient's condition (Gorski et al. 2016, Kupensky 1998). Once *in situ*, the catheter should be managed exactly like a CVC. If a patient goes home with a midline then they should receive information about all aspects of the care of the catheter, including equipment and support (see 'Discharging patients home with a VAD *in situ*' above).

Removal

With gentle, firm traction, the catheter will slide out from the insertion site. After removal, pressure should be applied for at least 3–4 minutes and the site inspected prior to applying a dressing to ensure bleeding has stopped. The catheter's integrity should be checked and its length measured to ensure that a complete device has been removed (RCN 2016a).

Complications

Mechanical phlebitis is a common side-effect. Close observation and appropriate management, such as the application of heat, are indicated (see the section on complications in 'Peripheral cannulas' above for more details on management).

Peripherally inserted central catheters

Definition

A peripherally inserted central catheter (PICC) is a catheter that is inserted percutaneously via the veins in the arm and advanced into the central veins, with the tip located in the superior vena cava (SVC) (usually the lower third) or cavo-atrial junction (Gorski et al. 2016, Hadaway 2010, Nakazawa 2010a, RCN 2016a). It is not to be confused with a mid-clavicular catheter (often referred to as a 'long line'), where the tip is located in a central vein leading to the SVC, such as the subclavian or proximal axillary vein (Carlson 1999, Dougherty 2006). Because of the increasing evidence that mid-clavicular catheters are associated with a high incidence of thrombotic complications (up to 60%), mid-clavicular placement should only be considered if there are anatomical or pathophysiological reasons, for example SVC syndrome (Carlson 1999, Gallieni et al. 2008).

PICCs have been a popular vascular access device (VAD) since the early 1990s in both, adults and children. They can deliver drugs, liquids or parenteral nutrition via a central vein with the safety of conventional peripheral venous access. Therefore, PICCs can be considered as a hybrid of conventional peripheral venous access devices and central venous catheters (Mussa 2014).

Anatomy and physiology

Choice of vein

Careful evaluation and adequate assessment of the patient prior to attempting catheter placement go a long way to ensuring success. Both arms should be examined using ultrasound with a tourniquet in place (Figure 17.22). The PICC should preferably be inserted in the non-dominant arm, although the use of the non-dominant arm for PICC insertion has only a marginal impact on activities of daily living for patients (Sharp et al. 2014). It has been shown that ultrasonography can increase the chance of successful cannulation of the vein on the first attempt (Bodenham et al. 2016, Lamperti et al. 2012, LaRue 2000, Moureau 2014) compared with using the traditional landmark method (using surface anatomical landmarks and knowing the expected anatomical relationship between the vein and its palpable companion artery) (Dougherty 2006, NICE 2002). By using ultrasound, the nurse can position the transducer to obtain a transverse (cross-sectional) or horizontal view of the vein, which may aid in the identification of arterial vessels as well as facilitating visualization of solid material, such as a thrombus, in the lumen of the vessel (Hadaway 2010, Moureau 2014, Weinstein and Hagle 2014) (Figures 17.23 and 17.24). Ultrasound can be used to assess vein health and lack of scar tissue or thrombosis by compressing veins with light to moderate pressure (healthy veins should easily compress); if the vein does not compress or collapse to light to moderate pressure or compresses in a lopsided way, thrombosis may be present in the vein (Dawson 2014).

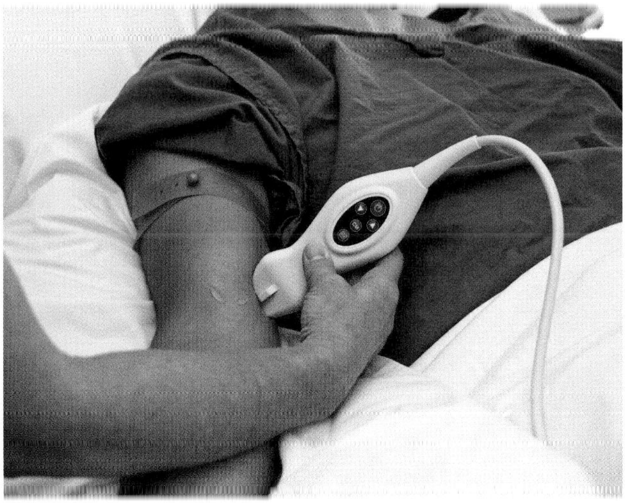

Figure 17.22 Applying an ultrasound probe to the arm to locate veins

The size of the vessels can be improved by use of a blood pressure cuff (Mahler et al. 2011). Choice of vein and vein diameter are vital to avoid thrombosis (Meyer 2011). Dawson (2011) found that thrombosis rates were 57% in cephalic veins, 14% in basilic veins and 10% in brachial veins. Veins more suitable for venous access are ideally three times the diameter of the selected catheter (e.g., a 4 Fr catheter has a diameter of 1.33 mm and so requires a 4 mm or larger vein), which allows for adequate blood flow around the catheter, enables abundant dilution of infused drugs with the blood as they enter the circulation, and protects the vein walls from the catheter (Moureau 2014). Spencer and Mahoney (2017) defined the catheter-to-vessel ratio as 'the indwelling space or area occupied by an intravascular device inserted and positioned within a venous or arterial blood vessel' (p.428). Measuring the vein diameter and choosing a catheter to vein (vessel) ratio of 45% or less may reduce thrombosis risk in PICCs and midlines (Gorski et al. 2016, Moureau and Chopra 2016, Nifong and McDevit 2011, Sharp et al. 2015).

Movement of the catheter in and out of the insertion site contributes to the development of phlebitis and other complications. It is important to find a stable location at least 4 cm above the antecubital fossa to reduce the amount of catheter movement associated with this location (Dawson 2011, Moureau 2014). Veins in the upper arm and specifically on the middle section of the upper arm offer stability and give the best results. Dawson (2011) proposed the PICC Zone Insertion Method (ZIM) as a traffic-light (red, green and yellow) system to enable a systematic approach to determining the ideal insertion site for PICCs in the upper arm. The green area is the ideal target zone and is located in the mid-upper arm, above the antecubital fossa (red zone) and below the axilla (yellow zone). The final determination for the PICC insertion site should include ultrasound visualization of the best vein within the green zone (Dawson 2011) (Figure 17.25).

The basilic and brachial veins

The upper basilic vein is the vein of choice for PICC insertions owing to its larger size, straighter course for catheter advancement and higher haemodilution capability (Bullock-Corkhill 2010, Gorski et al. 2016, RCN 2016a) (Figure 17.26). The basilic vein begins in the ulnar (inner aspect) part of the forearm, runs along the posterior, medial surface (back of the arm) and then curves towards the antecubital region, where it is joined by the median cubital vein. It then progresses straight up the upper arm for approximately 5–8 cm and enters the deep tissues. It ascends medially to form the axillary vein (Dougherty 2006, Hadaway 2010, Tortora and Derrickson 2017). This vein is the largest and

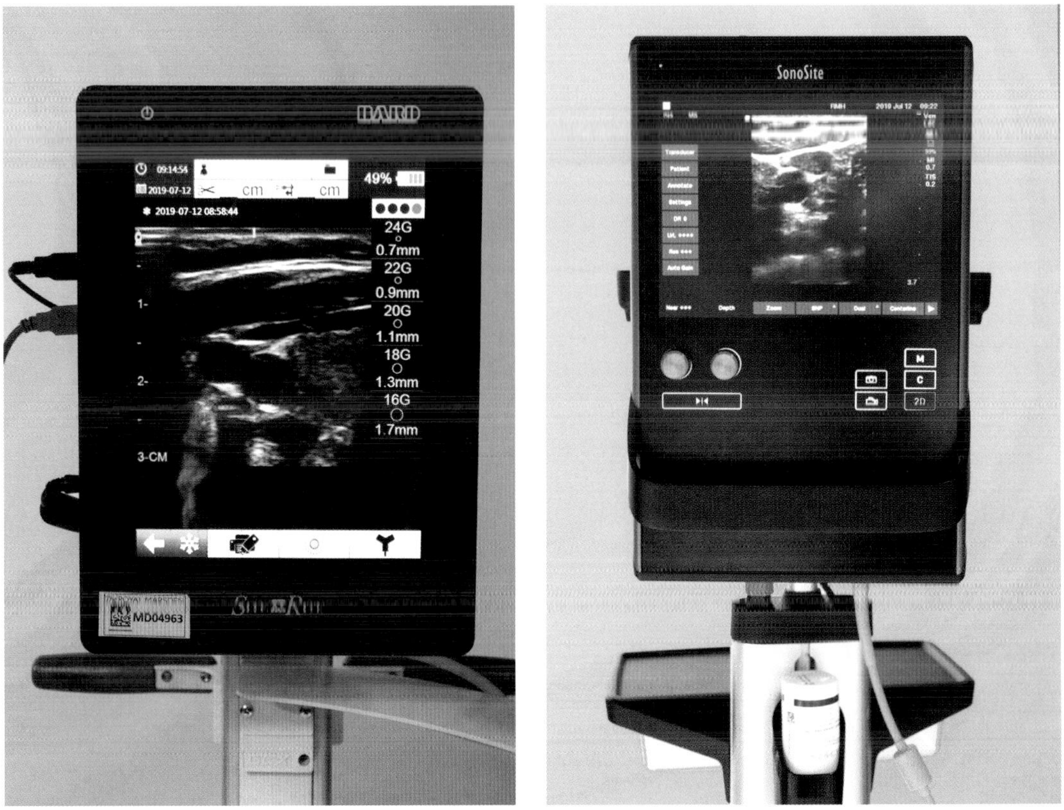

Figure 17.23 Ultrasound images of veins on screen.

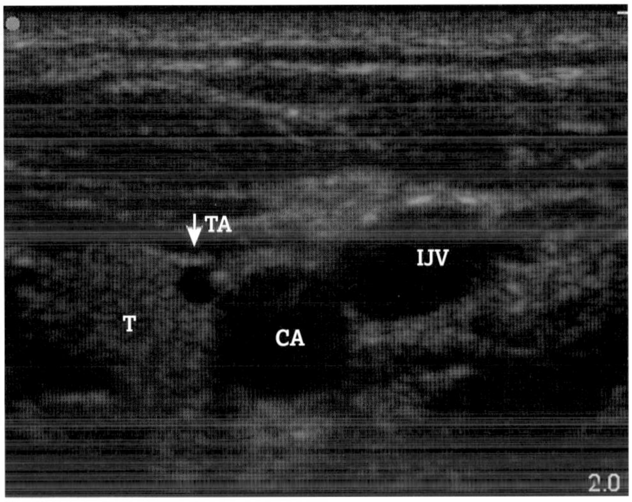

Figure 17.24 Ultrasound cross-sectional image of the right internal jugular vein (IJV) without compression through the probe. Image orientation as seen from the head of the patient. The depth of field of the image is only 2.8 cm, so all structures are very superficial. CA, carotid artery; T, thyroid; TA, thyroid artery. *Source*: Reproduced from Hamilton (2009) with permission of John Wiley & Sons.

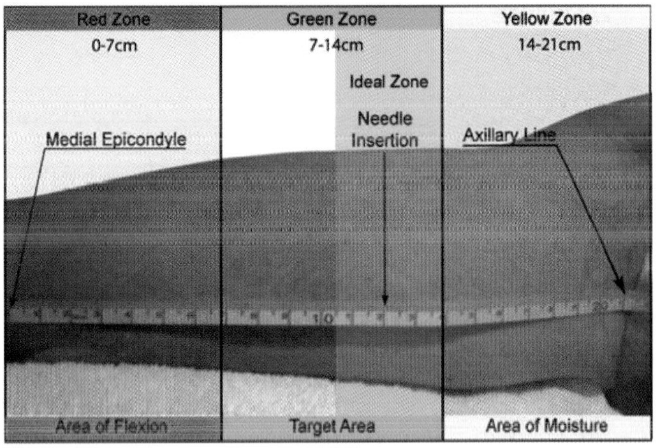

Figure 17.25 PICC Zone Insertion Method (ZIM). *Source*: Reproduced from Dawson (2011) with permission of Elsevier.

straightest vein in the arm and presents lower risk of complication relating to access as it is not generally accompanied by an artery or a nerve.

The brachial veins (Figure 17.27) are located deep in the arm alongside the brachial artery and the median nerve (together, they form the brachial bundle) and are slightly smaller than the basilic vein (Hadaway 2010, Tortora and Derrickson 2017). The brachial bundle is easy to locate with ultrasound as it has a configuration that resembles Mickey Mouse's head (i.e. one larger 'head' circle below and adjoining two larger 'ear' circles). The brachial veins advance up the arm deep within the muscle and join with the basilic vein or directly into the axillary vein (Moureau 2014, Tortora and Derrickson 2017). Their proximity to the brachial artery means that there is a greater chance of arterial puncture and touching the median nerve.

The median cubital vein

The median cubital vein (see Figure 17.27) ascends from just below the middle of the antecubital region and commonly divides into two vessels, one of which joins the basilic and the

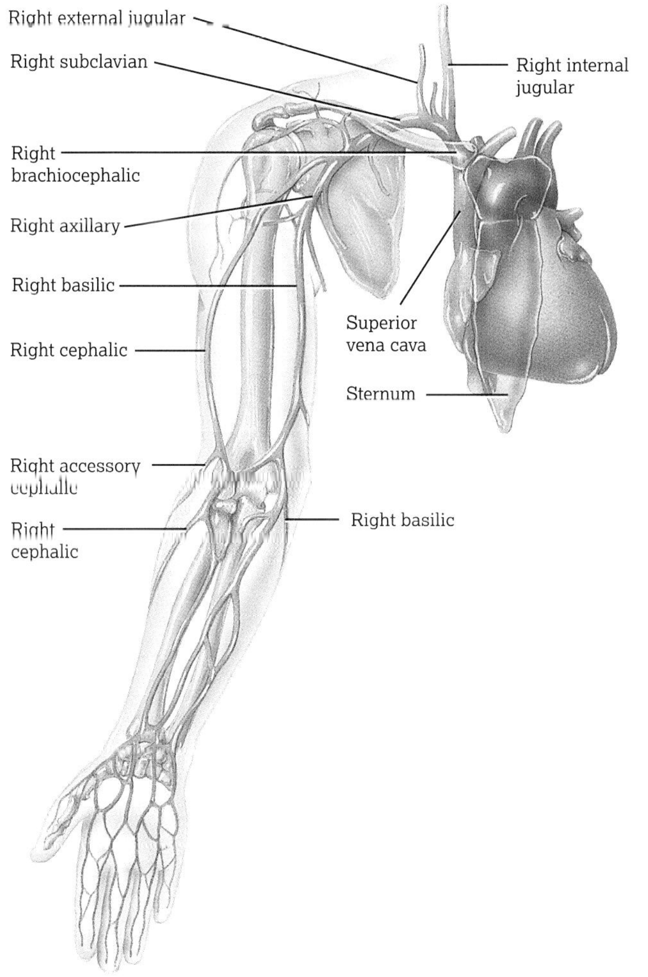

Figure 17.26 Anterior view of the superficial veins.

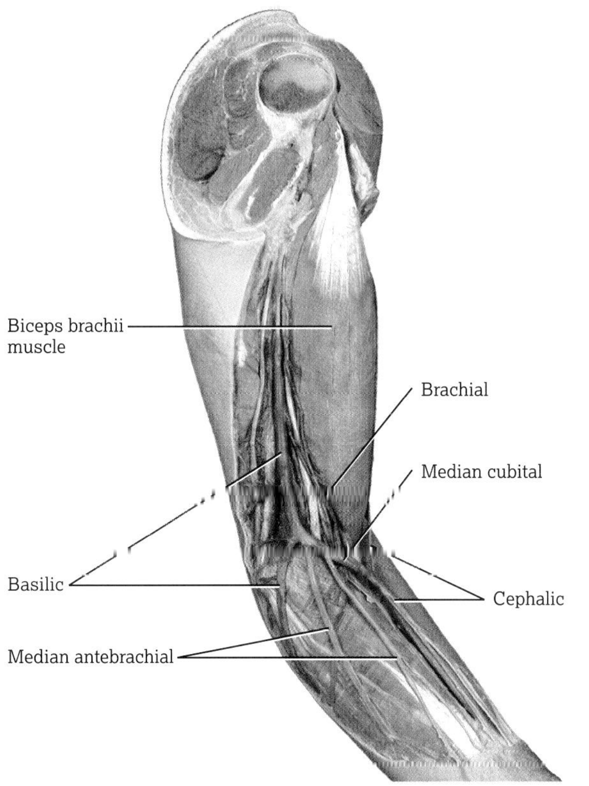

Figure 17.27 Anteromedial view of the superficial veins of the arm and forearm. *Source*: Reproduced from Tortora and Derrickson (2017) with permission of John Wiley & Sons.

other the cephalic vein (Tortora and Derrickson 2017). The median cubital vein is commonly used for blood sampling owing to its size and ease of needle entry. If a practitioner is having difficulty locating and/or cannulating the basilic vein, then the median cubital vein may be used as an alternative insertion route (Sansivero 1998). The catheter will then advance into the basilic (or cephalic) vein.

The cephalic vein

The cephalic vein begins in the radial side (thumb side) of the hand and ascends laterally (along the outer region of the forearm) into the antecubital region, where it forms a junction with the axillary vein. This vein is usually more accessible than the basilic but its size, its tortuous path and the sharp angle where it anastomoses with the subclavian make it more difficult to advance the catheter (Dougherty 2006, Moureau 2014). Therefore, it presents a greater potential for catheter tip malposition (Dougherty 2006, Weinstein and Hagle 2014).

Evidence-based approaches

Rationale

PICCs have many advantages over the other CVADs. Firstly, they eliminate the mechanical complications associated with CVC placement, particularly pneumothorax (Bodenham et al. 2016, Dougherty 2006, Gallieni et al. 2008). Secondly, PICCs have been shown to be associated with a reduction in catheter sepsis. This may be related to the temperature of the skin; it has been reported that peripheral sites rarely have more than 50–100 colony-forming units (cfu) of bacteria per 10 cm^2 of skin compared with 1000–10,000 cfu/cm^2 on the neck and chest (Carlson 1999, Moureau and Gabriel 2009, Mussa 2014). Thirdly, PICCs are easy to use for both staff and patients (Dougherty 2006, Mussa 2014) and they also help to preserve peripheral veins (Gabriel 2000, Mussa 2014, Oakley et al. 2000). They have been shown to cause less discomfort than other central venous access devices and provide a reliable form of access (Costa and Ferguson 2002, Oakley et al. 2000, Mussa 2014). They are also cost-effective when compared with other long-term and short-term catheters and can be inserted at the bedside (Mussa 2014, Snelling et al. 2001, Wilkes 2011). With proper care and maintenance, PICCs may last for up to a year, without changing the entry site and with minimal risk of complications (Mussa 2014).

Disadvantages of PICCs include an increased need for self-care, potentially increased difficulty of blood withdrawal with catheters smaller than 4 Fr, and increased chance of occlusion (Dougherty 2006, Molloy et al. 2008). Another issue can be flow rate: the diameter of PICCs ordinarily ranges from 3 to 6 Fr, whereas the diameter of other CVCs ranges from 5 to 12 Fr, which explains PICCs' lower flow rate. However, new CT-rated technology and newer PICC materials allow higher flow rates, and high-density solutions (blood, nutritional solutions and/or contrast media) can safely be delivered via PICCs using an infusion pump (Mussa 2014). A further problem is that over time, multiple insertions can cause venous scarring and decrease the ability to reuse the site (Wilkes 2011). It has also been found that compared with skin-tunnelled catheters in patients with gastrointestinal cancers, the advantages of a PICC decrease significantly if treatment lasts longer than 120 days (Snelling et al. 2001). PICCs should not be considered as a last resort but introduced early in treatment (Blackburn 2014, Chopra et al. 2015, Moureau and Chopra 2016, Springhouse 2009).

Indications

Indications for the use of a PICC include the following:

- lack of peripheral access
- infusions of vesicant, irritant, parenteral nutrition or hyperosmolar solutions
- intermediate to long-term venous access
- patient preference
- patients with needle phobia, to prevent repeated cannulation
- clinician preference if patients are at risk of complications associated with CVAD insertion, for example haemorrhage or pneumothorax
- if other types of device are contraindicated (Chopra et al. 2015, Dougherty 2006, Lin et al. 2010, Moureau and Chopra 2016, Moureau and Gabriel 2009, Yamada et al. 2010).

Contraindications

Contraindications and issues for the use of a PICC include the following:

- anatomical distortions from surgery, injury or trauma, for example scarring from a previous CVAD insertion or removal, mastectomy, lymphoedema or burns, which may prevent advancement of the catheter to the desired tip location (Chopra et al. 2015, Dougherty 2006)
- cardiac pacemaker *in situ*
- enlarged axillary or supraclavicular lymph nodes
- tumour mass
- previous history of thrombosis
- history of fractured clavicle (may be necessary to avoid that side of the patient's body).

Methods of insertion

Ultrasound guidance aids the clinician in vein identification, assessment and insertion while reducing the risk of complications and stress to patients (Moureau 2014). Venous assessment and selection play key roles in the successful insertion of a PICC, along with correct positioning of the patient and careful measurement of the patient and the device. To obtain the correct measurement of the length of catheter to be inserted based on anatomical landmarks, one option is to use a tape measure and with the patient's arm at a 90° angle to their torso, measure from the selected point for venepuncture to the axilla, and then measure the total distance across the clavicle and down to the intercostal space. Alternatively, Lum (2004) has developed a formula-based measurement guide based on the patient's height, which provides a more accurate way to achieve optimal tip placement (Dougherty 2006) (Box 17.7). Arm adduction and bending can influence PICC depth and movement (Connolly et al. 2006). Another simple option is measuring the distance from the selected venepuncture site to the sternoclavicular notch, and then adding the result to a standard value of 10 cm (in right arm insertions) or 15 cm (in left arm insertions). However, these methods, although useful and included in the insertion protocols of most working groups, remain merely predictive and do not give any information about the actual tip location (La Greca 2014).

Box 17.7 Formula for calculating length of PICC

This formula assumes the PICC is to be located 2.5 cm below the antecubital fossa. It can be used as an orientation guide when placing a PICC in the upper arm with ultrasound guidance. *Note*: the distance to the venepuncture site should be subtracted from the result.

- Right PICC: height (cm) × 3 ÷ 10
- Left PICC: height (cm) × 3 ÷ 10 + 4 cm

Source: Adapted from Lum (2004).

The catheter tip position may be checked during the procedure, after the procedure or both. Anteroposterior chest X-ray film continues to be the gold standard method for checking tip position after insertion. However, checking the tip position during catheter insertion is preferable as it avoids repositioning the device and also provides accuracy regarding the exact tip position (La Greca 2014, Pittiruti et al. 2012).

Catheter tip position can be checked during insertion using various methods:

- navigating or tracking devices with electromagnetic technology
- intraoperative fluoroscopy
- transthoracic echocardiography
- transoesophageal echocardiography
- electrocardiographic/intracavitary ECG method
- a combination of the above (La Greca 2014).

Among these intraprocedural methods, fluoroscopy remains the gold standard but it has cost implications and its use may be limited due to logistical issues. ECG-based tip verification systems offer a safe, accurate, cheap and universally applicable alternative (La Greca 2014, Oliver and Jones 2014, 2016, Pittiruti et al. 2012). The ECG method uses the catheter itself as an intravascular (intracavitary) electrode, which replaces the 'red' or 'right shoulder' electrode (lead II in a bipolar three-lead ECG according to the classical Einthoven triangle) of a standard surface ECG (see Chapter 14: Observations for further information on ECG types and lead placement). When the ECG is connected to the intravascular electrode (using either a guidewire/stylet or a saline adapter), the reading of electrode II will show a P wave whose shape and height will change while the catheter is advanced from the peripheral venous system towards the heart. As the catheter tip approaches the sinoatrial node at the cavo-atrial junction, the P wave starts to elevate, reaching its maximum height at the cavo-atrial junction. When the tip passes through into the right atrium, the P wave starts to invert, indicating that the catheter tip is in too far. The ideal position for the catheter tip is where the ECG reading shows 'maximal P' or where the P wave is at its maximum height without any inversion or negative deflection (La Greca 2014, Pittiruti et al. 2012). Changes in the P wave as the catheter tip advances are shown in Figure 17.28.

The accuracy of this method has been proven in numerous international studies (Barton 2016, Feng et al. 2010, La Greca 2013, Moureau et al. 2010, Oliver and Jones 2014, 2016, Pittiruti et al. 2012) and new dedicated ECG tip position devices have been introduced to clinical practice. The combination of the ECG method with a navigation system is now recommended (NICE 2015). Navigation systems are mainly based on electromagnetic tracking of the catheter tip. The catheter tip is assembled with a magnetic-tip stylet, which can be located with a magnetic sensor placed on the patient's chest surface, either fixed on the chest area or hand-held by the operator. This allows the catheter tip to be followed as it is progressing through the venous system by a virtual image on a specific screen, using a visual or acoustic alert on the sensor surface, or both (La Greca 2014).

Clinical governance

Nurses who wish to undertake this role must be competent in cannulation, and they must receive additional training in theory and practical hands-on instruction at the bedside (Bullock-Corkhill 2010, NMC 2018, RCN 2016a). Moureau et al. (2013) developed evidence-based guidelines for training in CVAD insertion and insertion itself, and highlighted the need for standardized

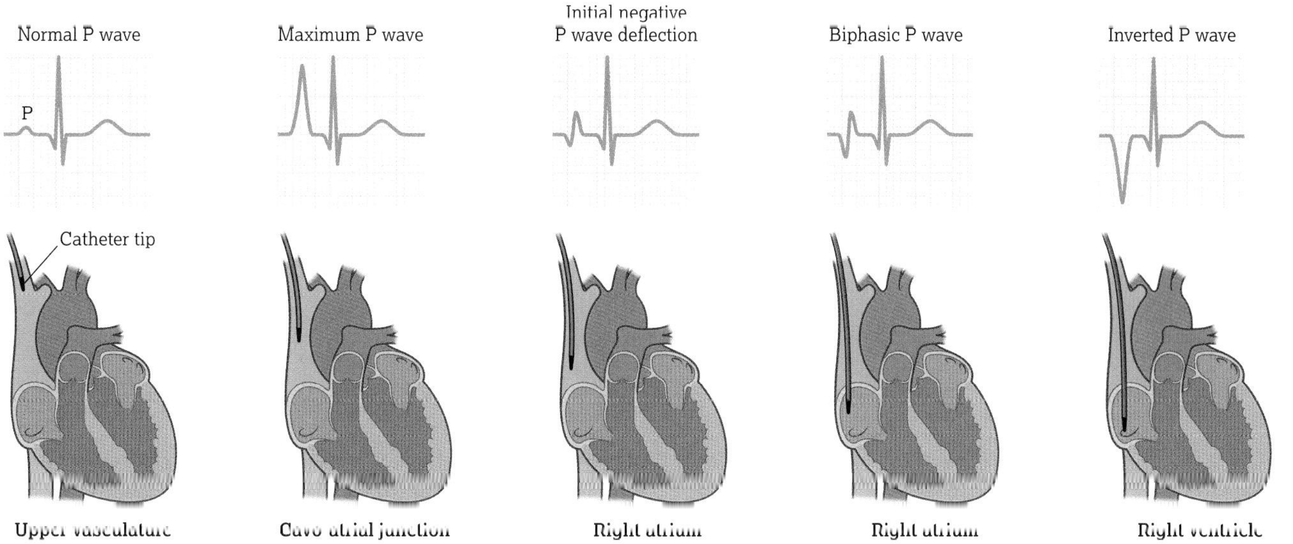

Figure 17.28 Electrocardiogram (ECG) tracing showing P wave changes depending on catheter tip position.

education, simulation practice and supervised insertions in order for nurses to achieve clinical competency.

Competencies include:

- knowledge and skills in anatomy and physiology of the veins of the upper arm and central veins
- selection of the vein and equipment
- use of ultrasound and local anaesthetic
- prevention and management of complications.

A number of hospitals and organizations now provide PICC training days and programmes that combine theory and practice and that may also include the use of ultrasound and ECG technology. Dedicated PICC or vascular access teams are developing globally in most healthcare settings as they successfully contribute to the implementation of best practices and the achievement of improved outcomes for patients while reducing cost and complications (Alexandrou et al. 2010a, Johnson et al. 2017, Kokotis 2014).

Consent

The benefits (the ability to withdraw blood and infuse medications over the long term), risks (bleeding, thrombosis, infection and malposition) and possible alternatives must be explained to patients prior to insertion. Patients must be given sufficient information, in a way that they can understand, in order to enable them to make an informed decision (Celli 2014). Written consent must be obtained. An example of a PICC consent form is shown in Figure 17.29.

Pre-procedural considerations

Equipment

PICCs are available as single, double and triple lumen; may be non-valved or valved (the latter may reduce occlusions) (Bartock 2010, Johnston et al. 2012); and may be made of silicine, polyurethane or newer polymers of polyurethane (de Lutio 2014, Dougherty 2006). A stylet within a silicone catheter adds firmness, which makes advancement easier. Stylets are not usually required with a polyurethane catheter because of catheter stiffness (Perucca 2010). Newer polyurethane polymers have improved material stiffness and biocompatibility while mechanical strength is preserved (de Lutio 2014). These newer catheters are available as power-injectable devices that can tolerate up to 300 psi (de Lutio 2014, Wilkes 2011). Catheters usually measure 55 cm long, with a diameter of 2–7 Fr (Figure 17.30). PICCs can be cut to the required length, if required, unless valved at the tip (Dougherty 2006). Valved catheters may have valves either proximally or distally; these open and close depending on the pressure. If a PICC is damaged or disconnected, or at the end of an infusion, the low pressure closes the valve, thereby preventing backflow and occlusion. This safety feature and ease of use make valved PICCs preferred for home-care and outpatient settings (Mussa 2014).

The catheter is inserted using a modified Seldinger technique, in which venous access is established via a needle or cannula; a guidewire is threaded through the needle, which is then removed; a dilator, introducer or peel-away sheath is threaded over the guidewire (frequently a scalpel is used to enlarge the skin puncture site and facilitate the advancement of the introducer); the guidewire and dilator are then removed; and the catheter is advanced into the venous system through the introducer or peel-away sheath (Dougherty 2006, Gabriel 2008, Hadaway 2010, Sansivero 1998, Weinstein and Hagle 2014). The benefit of this technique is that it reduces the trauma to the vein and lowers the risk of arterial or nerve damage (Bullock-Corkhill 2010). It can also be used to facilitate placement in smaller difficult veins, as well as ultrasound-guided upper arm placement (Bullock-Corkhill 2010, Moureau 2014, Sansivero 1998). The use of an ECG navigating system is recommended to ascertain tip position at the time of insertion and minimize the need to reposition catheters (NICE 2015).

Pharmacological support

The use of local anaesthetic by injection reduces the pain associated with the initial venepuncture and ensures that the area where the incision is made (or deeper tissues) are anaesthetized to reduce pain and discomfort (Dwyer and Rutkowski 2013, Hartley-Jones 2009). Injectable local anaesthetic, such as 1% lidocaine, is commonly used, and it has been found that intradermal lidocaine is superior to EMLA (eutectic mixture of local anaesthetics: lidocaine and prilocaine) prior to insertion of PICCs (Fry and Aholt 2001).

Patient identifier/label:

Consent Form 1

THE ROYAL MARSDEN
NHS FOUNDATION TRUST

Insertion of a peripherally inserted central catheter (PICC)

Patient Agreement to Investigation or Treatment

Patient's surname/family name

Patient's first names

Date of birth

Health professional seeking consent

Job title

NHS number (or other identifier)

☐ Male ☐ Female

Special requirements
(e.g. other language/other communication method)

Name of proposed procedure (include brief explanation if medical term not clear)

Insertion of a peripherally inserted central catheter (PICC)

The PICC is a long thin tube (catheter) that is inserted into a vein in your upper arm and threaded up into the main vein to your heart called the superior vena cava. Before insertion, local anaesthetic will be administered (usually as an injection) around the vein to minimise pain during the procedure. The procedure takes about 30 minutes, and we will use a tracking device to ensure correct placement; however, you may still need to have a chest X-ray to confirm the final position of the PICC tip. The PICC is secured using a small anchoring device that clips under the skin.

Statement of health professional seeking consent (to be filled in by health professional with appropriate knowledge of proposed procedure, as specified in consent policy)

I have explained the procedure to the patient. In particular, I have explained:

The intended benefits:

This catheter:

☐ provides a reliable way to administer your therapy or diagnostic tests into your vein

☐ can be used to take blood samples

☐ ....
....
....

To be retained in patient's notes

Figure 17.23 Example peripherally inserted central catheter (PICC) consent form.

Patient identifier/label:

Minor side effects or complications:

☐ The needle could cause a bruise or swelling (haematoma). This is more likely if you are on blood thinning medicines or you have low levels of the blood cells that help with clotting (platelets).

Significant, unavoidable or frequently occurring risks based on experience at The Royal Marsden

On insertion:

☐ In less than 1 in 1,000 patients, the PICC may not thread into the correct position and the tip may not be in the correct vein. This is, however, unlikely with use of tracking technology. You will have a Y shaped device placed on your chest which tracks the location of the catheter using a small magnet in the tip, until it reaches its ideal position.

☐ Damage to an artery (arterial puncture); occurs in less than 1 in 1,000 patients.

☐ Damage to a nerve; occurs in less than 1 in 1,000 patients.

Other problems that may arise when the PICC is IN USE include:

☐ Once the PICC is in place there is a risk of infection. The risk is usually less than 4 in 100 but can be higher depending on many other factors, such as your diagnosis or treatment. Your doctor or nurse will be able to explain the risk to you. You may be able to have antibiotics to treat the infection if it is local around the PICC site. If not, the PICC may need to be removed.

☐ Once the PICC is in place there is a risk of a clot (thrombosis) forming around the PICC. This occurs in less than 3 of every 100 patients depending on your diagnosis, treatment or if you have had a clot before. Your doctor or nurse will be able to explain the risk to you. You may need to take blood thinning medication (anticoagulants) but the PICC may only need to be removed if the blood clot does not respond to the medication.

☐ There is a possibility that the catheter may irritate the heart causing palpitations (arrhythmias). This may require minor adjustments to be made to the position of the catheter. This occurs uncommonly (in approximately 2 in every 1,000 patients).

Other problems that may arise when the PICC is in place include:

☐ Sometimes the PICC does not provide blood samples easily or can become blocked. This can usually be unblocked by instilling a medication by the nursing staff but if it cannot be unblocked it may necessitate removing the PICC. This occurs in less than 2 of every 100 patients.

☐ The PICC may split or become damaged. This occurs in less than 1 of every 100 patients. We cannot repair PICCs and it will have to be removed and replaced.

☐ The PICC may become dislodged. This occurs in less than 1 of every 100 patients and, if no longer in the correct position, it will need to be removed and replaced.

To be retained in patient's notes

Figure 17.29 *Continued*

Patient identifier/label:

When the PICC needs removing

The catheter is usually removed with ease but on rare occasions (less than 1 in 1,000) there may be difficulty removing it (especially if it has been in place for over a year). This can be resolved by using heat. The anchoring device that holds the PICC in place can also be difficult to remove (occurs about 1 in a 100). If it is painful, we will inject some local anaesthetic at the site before removal.

Any other risks: ....
....
....

Any extra procedures which may become necessary during the procedure

☐ other procedure (please specify) ....
....

I have also discussed what the procedure is likely to involve, the benefits and risks of any available alternative treatments (including no treatment) and any particular concerns of this patient.

The following leaflet has been provided as part of the patient's information prescription:

☐ Central venous access devices - a guide for patients PI-0084 (version no________)

☐ .... (version no________)

This procedure will involve:

☐ local anaesthesia ☐ sedation

Signed: .... Date ....

Name (PRINT) .... Job title ....

☐ I am capable of performing this procedure or prescribing this treatment.

☐ I am trained and authorised to obtain consent for this procedure or treatment which I cannot perform or prescribe by myself. I have been delegated to take your consent by .... (name of supervising consultant).

While under the care of The Royal Marsden you will be treated by a team of healthcare professionals (clinicians), working with the consultant(s) responsible for your care. Team members may include registered nurses, allied health professionals and qualified doctors in training.

All clinical procedures or treatments will be performed by clinicians who are fully competent to do so, but they may also be supervising team members who are in training. The presence of any particular clinician at any given time cannot be guaranteed.

To be retained in patient's notes

Figure 17.00 Continued

Patient identifier/label:

Contact details (if patient wishes to discuss options later) ....
....
....

Statement of interpreter (where appropriate)

I have interpreted the information above to the patient to the best of my ability and in a way in which I believe s/he can understand.

Signed .... Date ....

Name (PRINT) ....

Figure 17.29 *Continued*

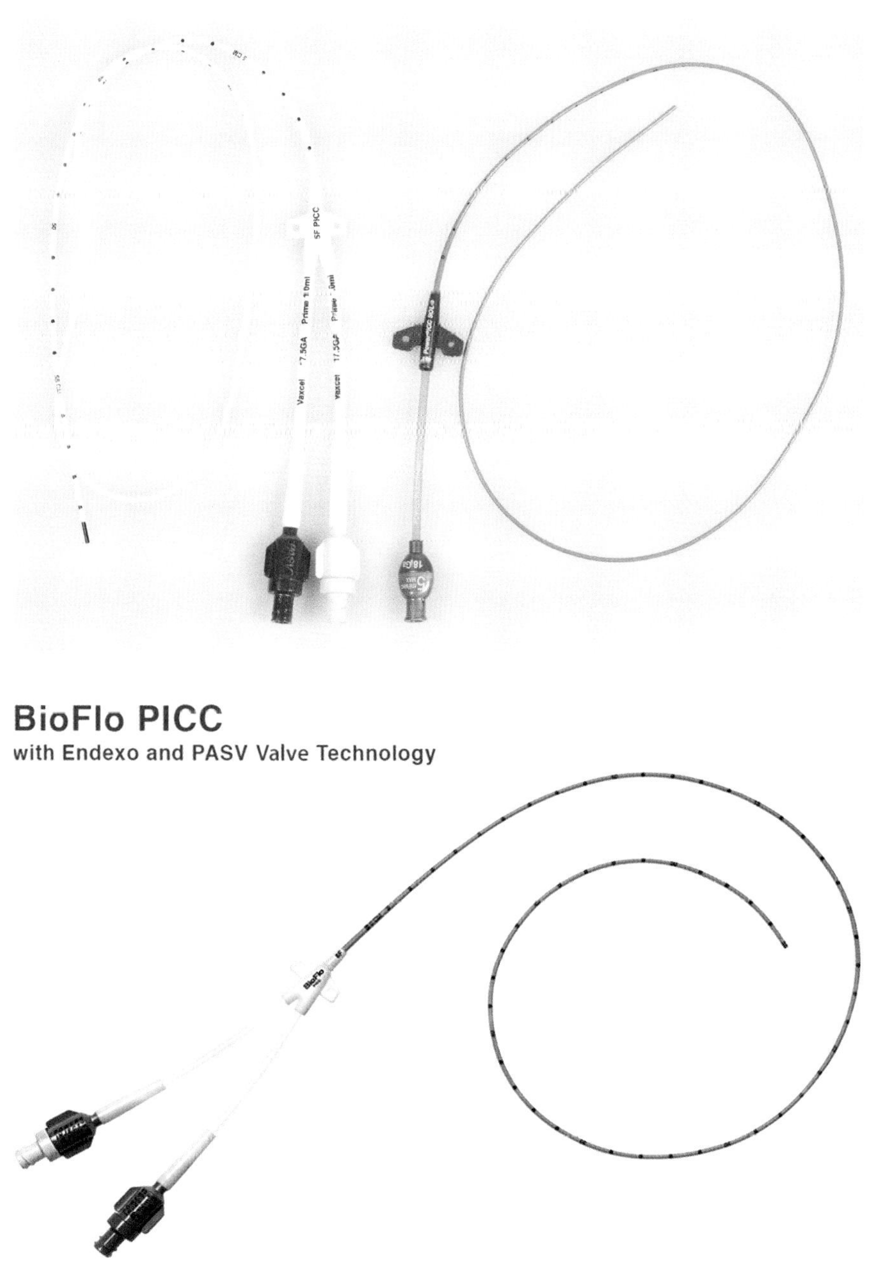

Figure 17.30 Peripherally inserted central catheter (PICC) types.

Procedure guideline 17.7 PICC insertion using modified Seldinger technique (MST) with ultrasound

It is helpful to have an assistant when performing this procedure, if possible.

Essential equipment

- Personal protective equipment
- One or two pairs of sterile gloves (according to practitioner preference)
- Sterile pack containing sterile gown, mask with visor, theatre cap, sterile drapes and scissors
- Alcohol-based skin-cleaning preparation, e.g. 2% chlorhexidine in 70% alcohol
- 10 mL syringes × 2–3
- Needle-free connector
- MST kit (containing needle, guidewire, 5 mL syringe, dilator/introducer/peel-away sheath, safety scalpel, and a 22 or 20 G cannula)
- PICC
- Transparent semi-permeable IV film dressing
- Securing device and sterile tapes
- 25 G safety needle
- Blunt drawing-up needles
- Tape measure
- Disposable tourniquet
- Sharps container
- Ultrasound machine, sterile gel and sterile probe cover
- ECG leads, electrodes and monitor
- Labels

Medicinal products

- Sterile pre-filled 10 mL syringes of 0.9% sodium chloride × 2–3
- 1% lidocaine

Action	Rationale
Pre-procedure	
1 Introduce yourself to the patient, explain and discuss the procedure with them, and gain their consent to proceed.	To ensure that the patient feels at ease, understands the procedure and gives their valid consent (NMC 2018, **C**).
2 Assess the patient's medical and intravenous device history.	To ensure the patient has no underlying medical problems (e.g. taking anticoagulants or previous surgery to arm or chest) and so is suitable to undergo the procedure (Hamilton 2009, **E**; Moureau 2014, **E**).
3 Draw screens and assist the patient into a (semi)supine position, with the patient's arm at a 90° angle to their torso.	To ensure privacy. To aid insertion of the introducer and then advancement of the catheter (Gabriel 2008, **E**; Moureau 2014, **E**).
4 Take the ultrasound equipment to the patient. Apply a tourniquet and gel to one of the patient's upper arms and use the ultrasound probe to assess venous access. Repeat for the other arm. Locate the most suitable vein, potentially using the Zone Insertion Method (Dawson 2011) (see Figure 17.25).	To ensure the patient has adequate venous access and to select the vein for catheterization (Gabriel 2008, **E**; Moureau 2014, **E**). To select the best area for PICC insertion (Dawson 2011, **E**).
5 If necessary (e.g. in very anxious or needle-phobic patients, or children), apply local anaesthetic cream or gel to the chosen venepuncture site and leave for the allotted time.	To minimize the pain of insertion (BNF 2019, **C**).
6 Ascertain the length of the catheter by using Lum's (2004) formula (which is based on the height of the patient; see Box 17.7) or by measurement. Measure from the selected venepuncture site to the sternoclavicular notch, adding 10 cm for right arm insertions or 15 cm for left arm insertions. If using an anchoring stabilization device then additional centimetres will need to be added depending on whether the right or left arm is used.	To enable selection of the most suitable catheter length and to establish how far to advance the catheter in order for its tip to be located in the correct position – that is, the superior veva cava (SVC) (La Greca 2014, **E**; Lum 1999, **E**; Lum 2004, **E**).
7 Take the equipment required to the patient's bedside. Open the outer pack.	To ensure the appropriate equipment is available for the procedure. **E**
8 Attach ECG leads to electrodes and monitor, and apply to the patient: black lead to right shoulder and red lead to left thigh.	To ensure an ECG tracing can be obtained and used as a comparison once PICC inserted (La Greca 2014, **E**; manufacturer's instructions, **C**; Oliver and Jones 2014, **E**; Oliver and Jones 2016, **E**).
9 If using a tracking device, attach it to the patient's chest area.	To track the tip of the catheter as it advances into the venous system (La Greca 2014, **E**; manufacturer's instructions, **C**; Oliver and Jones 2014, **E**; Oliver and Jones 2016, **E**).
10 Apply a theatre cap and face-mask with visor.	To minimize the risk of infection during the procedure and to protect the practitioner from blood splash contamination (Loveday et al. 2014, **E**).

Procedure

11	Wash hands with soap and water, or an alcohol-based handrub. Dry using sterile paper towels from the sterile pack.	To minimize the risk of infection (Fraise and Bradley 2009, **E**; NHS England and NHSI 2019, **C**).
12	Put on sterile gown and sterile gloves. Open the inner pack, arranging the contents as required.	To prevent contamination (Elliott 1993, **E**; Loveday et al. 2014, **C**). To have medications prepared for use. **E**
13	If not using pre-filled syringes then draw up 0.9% sodium chloride into a 10 mL syringe (provided by assistant if possible). Label the syringe.	To prevent contamination (Elliott 1993, **E**; Loveday et al. 2014, **C**). To have medications prepared for use. **E**
14	Draw up 1% lidocaine into a 5 mL syringe and attach a 25 G safety needle. Label the syringe.	To have medications prepared for use and avoid confusion or medication errors. **E**
15	Remove the cap from the extension set and attach a syringe of 0.9% sodium chloride; gently flush to the end of each lumen and leave the syringe attached.	To check that the catheter is patent and to enable easy removal of the guidewire (manufacturer's guidelines, **C**).
16	Place a sterile towel under the patient's arm.	To provide a sterile field to work on. **E**
17	Clean the skin at the selected site with 2% chlorhexidine in 70% alcohol, with friction, for 30 seconds, and prepare an area of 15–25 cm².	To ensure the removal of skin flora and to minimize the risk of infection (Fraise and Bradley 2009, **E**; Loveday et al. 2014, **C**).
18	Allow the solution to dry thoroughly.	To ensure coagulation of bacteria and disinfection (Loveday et al. 2014, **C**).
19	Drape the patient with a full-body sterile fenestrated drape.	To provide a sterile field (Loveday et al. 2014, **C**).
20	Add sterile gel to the ultrasound probe cover. Then apply the sterile ultrasound probe cover over the probe head and pull down along the cable.	To ensure all equipment that is in contact with the patient is sterile (Loveday et al. 2014, **C**).
21	Re-tighten the disposable tourniquet through the sterile drapes or ask an assistant to do this.	To aid venous distension (Dougherty 2008, **E**).
22	Apply gel to the skin and scan for the chosen vein.	To visualise the chosen vein. **E**
23	*Keeping the probe in position*, inject local anaesthetic intradermally using a 25 G needle and wait for it to take effect.	To provide adequate anaesthesia (BNF 2019, **C**).
24	*While visualizing the vein under ultrasound*, perform venepuncture with a needle or cannula. (If using a cannula, when flashback is seen, advance the cannula into the vein.)	To gain venous access (Gabriel 2008, **E**; Moureau 2014, **E**). To prevent blood loss and through-puncture and enable advancement of the catheter (Gabriel 2008, **E**).
25	Remove the stylet and advance the guidewire through the needle (or cannula) until there is 10–15 cm of wire in the vein (**Action figure 25**).	To maintain venous access. **E**
26	Release the tourniquet and remove the probe.	To contain flashback, prevent contamination of the area with blood and minimize the amount of blood loss from the patient (Gabriel 2008, **E**).
27	Advance the introducer over the wire up to the puncture site. (If using a cannula, remove it first applying digital pressure.)	To prepare for insertion. **E**
28	Reinfiltrate over the puncture site with 1% lidocaine (intrademally) if necessary, until a small bleb is observed (**Action figure 28**).	To achieve anaesthesia and minimize patient discomfort. **E**
29	Check the patient has no sharp sensations at the puncture site and then make a small incision by sliding the tip of the scalpel blade along the top of the wire (**Action figure 29**).	To ensure the area is anaesthetized before proceeding. **E**
30	Activate the safety function on the scalpel and place it back onto the sterile field.	To minimize the risk of sharp stick injury. **E**
31	Grip the introducer firmly and advance through the puncture site (**Action figure 31**).	To enable advancement of the dilator. **E**
32	Measure using the desired method to ascertain the final length of the catheter.	To ensure the correct length of catheter is used. **E**
33	If the catheter tip can be trimmed, using the graduated markings along the catheter, select the marking required and pull back the stylet (if required) 1 cm from the desired new tip. Using sterile scissors, trim the catheter. *Be careful not to trim the stylet.*	To ensure the catheter will be the correct length for SVC tip placement and to prevent damage to the vein if the guidewire is damaged (manufacturer's guidelines, **C**).

(continued)

Procedure guideline 17.7 PICC insertion using modified Seldinger technique (MST) with ultrasound *(continued)*

Action	Rationale
34 Remove the guidewire and the dilator from the introducer/peel-away sheath. Grip the catheter a few centimetres from the tip and thread through the introducer/peel-away sheath.	To enable catheter insertion. **E**
35 Continue slow advancement of the catheter and aspirate (if possible) and flush to check for blood return or resistance.	To minimize damage to the tunica intima of the vein (Gabriel 2008, **E**). To check there is no obstruction and that the catheter advances into the correct location. **E**
36 Ask the patient to turn their head towards the arm of insertion and place their chin on their shoulder if possible.	To prevent the catheter entering the jugular vein and to ensure correct advancement of the catheter downwards to the SVC (Gabriel 2008, **E**).
37 Ask the patient if they have any aural (behind the ear) sensations on the side of the catheter insertion. If using a tracking device, observe the direction of the catheter on the screen.	Aural sensations could indicate that the catheter has advanced along the internal jugular vein and needs to be withdrawn and readvanced (Dougherty 2006, **E**; manufacturer's instructions, **C**).
38 Continue slow advancement of the catheter until unable to advance any further. If using a tracking device, check the catheter is in the expected position.	To minimize damage to the intima of the vein (Gabriel 2008, **E**). To make sure the catheter has entered the SVC (manufacturer's instructions, **C**; Mussa 2014, **E**).
39 Apply pressure above the introducer. Carefully withdraw the introducer and peel apart.	To ensure there is no movement of the catheter. To remove the peel-away introducer (Gabriel 2008, **E**).
40 Advance the catheter to the hub and do a final check for any aural sensations. If using ECG technology, gently manipulate the catheter, observing the ECG trace for changes in the P wave. When the highest P wave without deflection is observed, the catheter tip is in the correct position (cavo-atrial junction).	To check for malposition. **E** To ascertain tip position (La Greca 2014, **E**; manufacturer's instructions, **C**; Moureau et al. 2010, **E**; Oliver and Jones 2014, **E**; Pittiruti et al. 2012, **E**).
41 Apply gentle pressure on the catheter and slowly withdraw the stylet.	To ensure there is no withdrawal of the catheter (Gabriel 2008, **E**).
42 Aspirate for blood return and flush the catheter with 0.9% sodium chloride.	To check the patency of the device and ensure continued patency (Gabriel 2008, **E**; Loveday et al. 2014, **C**).
43 Attach a needle-free connector and flush as per local policy.	To ensure the patency of the device (Gabriel 2008, **E**; Loveday et al. 2014, **C**).
44 Secure the catheter with a securing adhesive device (e.g. StatLock) or anchoring device (e.g. SecurAcath). Fold the device and then slide the prongs down the side of the venotomy and release (**Action figure 44**).	To ensure stability of the device (Gabriel 2008, **E**; Hughes 2014, **E**; Moureau and Iannucci 2003, **E**; NICE 2017, **C**; RCN 2016a, **C**).
45 Apply a small pad of sterile low-linting gauze or an absorbent pad (impregnated with chlorhexidine gluconate or ionic silver alginate) directly over the insertion site and secure with sterile tape if required. If an absorbent pad is used, there is no need to change the dressing after 24 hours.	To minimize blood leakage at the site, which occurs following insertion (Gabriel 2008, **E**; Loveday et al. 2014, **C**; RCN 2016a, **C**).
46 Apply a semi-permeable transparent IV film dressing. Date the dressing.	To ensure protection of the site while enabling observation of the exit site at all times (Loveday et al. 2014, **C**; RCN 2016a, **C**). To know when the dressing is due to be changed. **E**
47 Apply low-linting gauze over the lumens (optional), then bandage or apply a tubular bandage.	To prevent the tubing pressing into the patient's skin (Gabriel 2008, **E**; RCN 2016a, **C**).

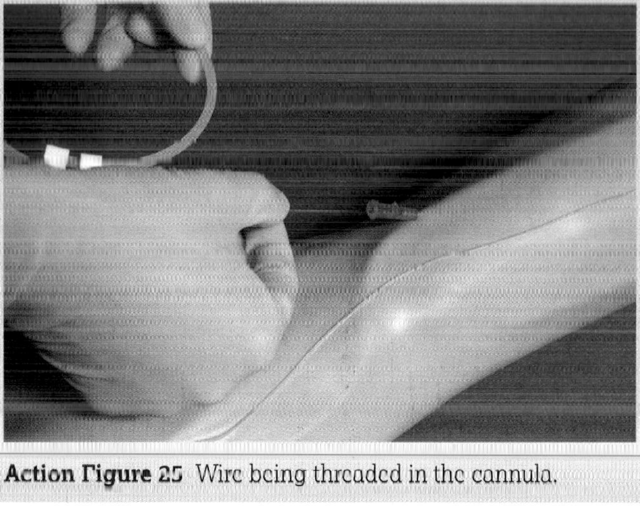

Action Figure 25 Wire being threaded in the cannula.

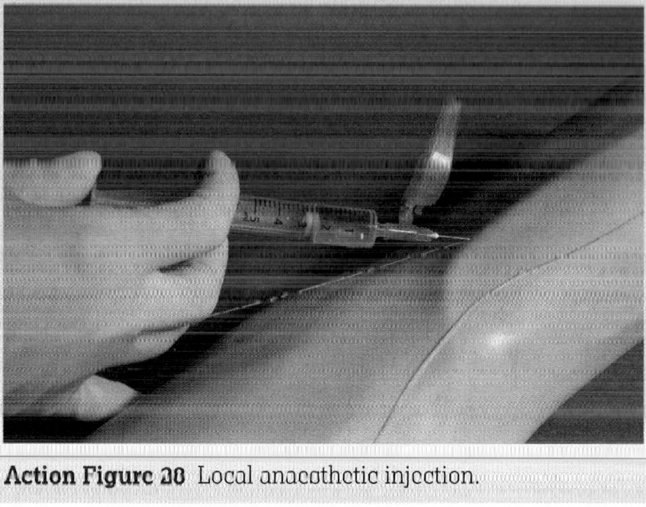

Action Figure 20 Local anaesthetic injection.

Post-procedure

48 Dispose of sharps and clinical waste. Remove gloves, gown, mask and theatre cap and dispose of equipment appropriately.	To prevent sharps injury. To ensure safe disposal in the correct containers and avoid laceration or injury to other staff. To prevent reuse of equipment (HSE 2013, **C**; NHS Employers 2010, 2015, **C**).
49 Send the patient for a chest X-ray if necessary. Ensure the position of the catheter is assessed and documented by the appropriate healthcare professional (see Figure 17.5).	To ensure that the catheter tip is in the correct position (Wise et al. 2001, **E**).
50 If ECG tip positioning technology was used during catheter insertion (*recommended*), a chest X-ray is not required provided that a good ECG tracing is obtained showing maximal P wave elevation. This must be verified by the operator, who should be proficient in the use of this type of technology.	To ensure correct tip position and minimize unnecessary patient exposure to radiation (La Greca 2014, **E**; NICE 2017, **C**; Oliver and Jones 2016, **E**; Pittiruti et al. 2012, **E**; RCN 2016a, **C**).
51 Document the procedure in the patient's notes: • type, length and gauge (Fr) of catheter • where it was inserted • tip confirmation by ECG and/or chest X-ray • batch number of catheter and lot number of sterile packs • ECG trace • any problems • how it was secured • patient education given.	To ensure adequate records are maintained and enable continued care of the patient and device (NMC 2018, **C**; RCN 2016a, **C**). To enable any faulty equipment to be traced back to the manufacturer (MHRA 2004, **C**).

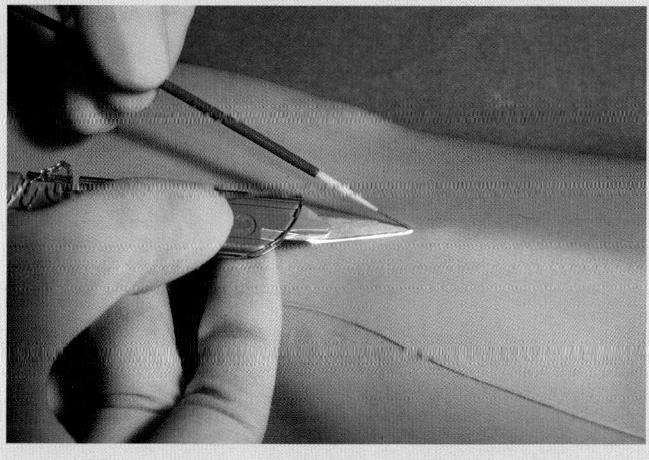

Action Figure 29 Making an incision with a scalpel.

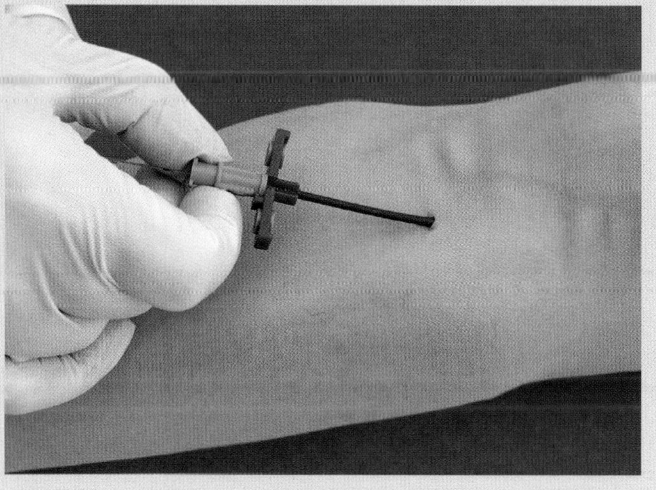

Action Figure 31 Advancing the introducer.

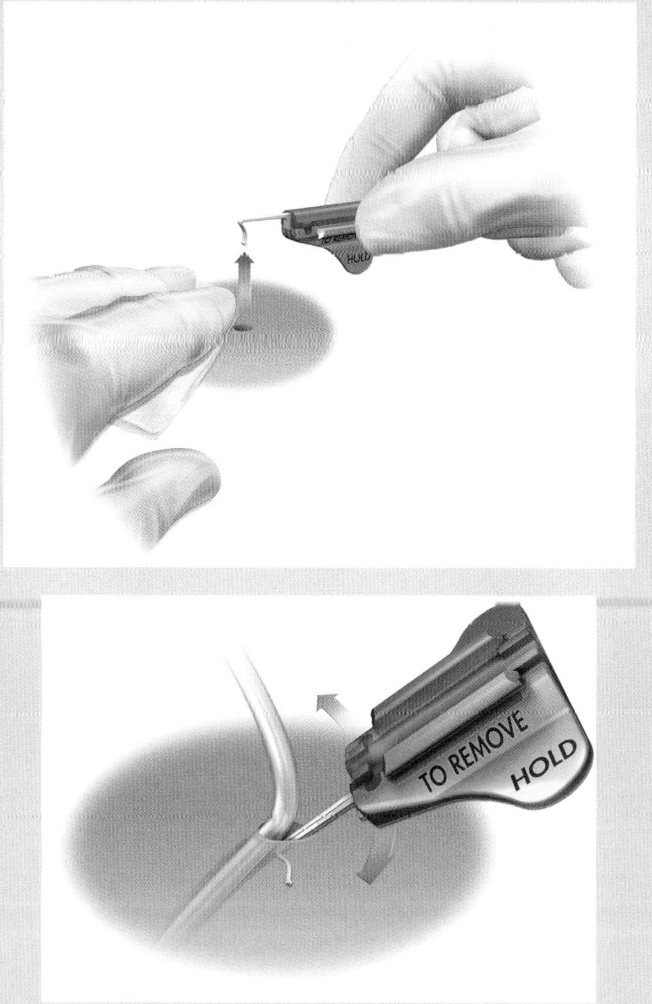

Action Figure 44 Attaching the securing device to the skin. *Source*: Reproduced with permission of Interrad Medical, Inc.

Problem-solving table 17.3 Prevention and resolution (Procedure guidelines 17.6 and 17.7)

Problem	Cause	Prevention	Action
Difficulty when advancing the catheter (this may be indicated by resistance when advancing the catheter with or without blood return)	Valves Chosen vein, for example cephalic (size or problems when at junction of axillary vein into subclavian) Muscle spasm in neck	Select a vein with fewer valves or one with a large lumen.	Flush and attempt to advance the catheter. Ask the patient to turn their head to the normal position and allow their neck muscles to relax.
Aural sensations when flushing	Catheter has advanced into the jugular vein	Ask the patient to turn their head to the side of the insertion and tuck their chin down on the clavicle to help prevent tip malposition.	Withdraw the catheter until the sensations have disappeared, ask the patient to turn their head to the side of the insertion and tuck their chin down on the clavicle. Attempt to readvance, checking for sensations. If the sensations continue, it may be necessary to abandon placement in that vein.
Malposition (coiled in vessels, or advanced into jugular or accessory veins)	Patient has deviant anatomy Patient not correctly positioned Catheter deflected by valves	Check the patient's previous history in case they have had previous problems in that vein. Position the patient correctly. Advance the catheter slowly.	Sit the patient upright. Withdraw the wire a few centimetres to allow the tip to be more flexible and flush vigorously.

Post-procedural considerations

Immediate care

Most PICCs are designed with suture wings, so the PICC can be sutured to the patient's skin. However, patients have reported long-term suturing to be uncomfortable; there may also be scarring when the device is removed (Gabriel 2000, 2001) and inflammation and bacterial colonization of the exit site (Schears 2005). Therefore, suturing is no longer recommended (Maki 2002). PICCs can be adequately secured using Steri-Strips, securement devices (such as self-adhesive stabilization devices applied to the skin, e.g. StatLock) or anchoring devices (such as SecurAcath) (Figure 17.31). These have been shown to result in significantly longer catheter dwell times and fewer total complications (Gabriel 2001, Hughes 2014, Maki 2002, Schears 2005, Yamamoto et al. 2002). NICE (2017) recommends the use of SecurAcath. Bleeding occurs in the first 24 hours so a fold of sterile gauze should be placed over the site under the dressing (Philpot and Griffiths 2003). Alternatively, an absorbent pad (impregnated with CHG or silver alginate) can be used (Hill et al. 2010, McGoldrick 2010). The insertion site is then covered with a semi-permeable transparent IV film dressing (Gorski et al. 2016, Loveday et al. 2014, RCN 2016a).

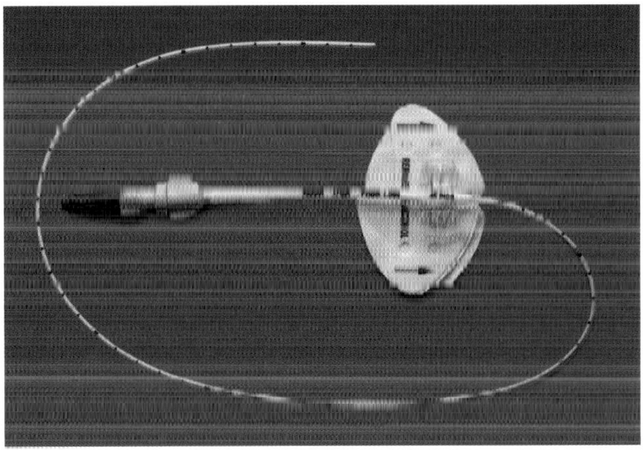

Figure 17.31 Peripherally inserted central catheter (PICC) with adhesive securing device.

The position of the tip of the PICC should be verified immediately after insertion before any infusion. This can be done during insertion using ECG tip position technology (La Greca 2014, NICE 2017, Oliver and Jones 2016, Pittiruti et al. 2012) or by a chest X-ray post-procedure. Ascertaining correct placement is the major reason for ordering a chest X-ray, but a chest X-ray also rules out malposition and confirms acceptable tip location for the type of medication being administered (Dougherty 2006, Gorski et al. 2016, RCN 2016a, Royer 2001, Wise et al. 2001). Tip malposition can be avoided by using navigating methods or tip location technology (e.g. Sherlock or Navigator), which enables tracking of the PICC during insertion to identify malposition (La Greca 2014, Naylor 2007). If using the ECG method to ascertain tip location, the print-out and relevant information must be documented.

Ongoing care

If the initial dressing consists of sterile gauze, it should be changed after 24 hours and then according to the dressing manufacturer's recommendations, for example once a week, to minimise the potential for infection and catheter migration (Loveday et al. 2014, NICE 2003, RCN 2016a). If a CHG-impregnated patch or ionic silver alginate pad is *in situ* following insertion, there is no need to change the initial dressing after 24 hours (Corley et al. 2017, RCN 2016a).

Flushing solution and frequency are usually dependent on the type of catheter and so the manufacturer's recommendations should be followed. For example, PICCs are usually flushed once a week with 0.9% sodium chloride (Gorski et al. 2016, Loveday et al. 2014, RCN 2016a). Care should be taken when using devices such as power injectors to administer intravenous contrast agents via a PICC as the pressure created may lead to catheter rupture. The likelihood of rupture will depend on the Fr and material of the catheter (de Lutio 2014, Williamson and McKinney 2001) but most manufacturers now provide CT-compatible PICCs, made specifically to withstand the pressure created during CT scanning. The Medicines and Healthcare products Regulatory Agency recommends that CT contrast using a pressure injector should not be performed via any CVAD that is not CT rated (MHRA 2004).

Documentation

The following should be documented on insertion (Chopra et al. 2015, Gorski et al. 2016, Moureau and Gabriel 2009, RCN 2016a):

- vein used
- insertion date and time
- length of catheter inserted and external length
- size of catheter, manufacturer and batch number
- number of cannulation attempts, vein(s) used and problems encountered
- flushing solution used
- securement method and dressing type
- ECG or X-ray confirmation and tip location
- type of local anaesthetic used
- type of cleaning solution used
- signature of practitioner who inserted the PICC.

Education of the patient and relevant others

See 'Discharging patients home with a VAD *in situ*' above.

Complications

On insertion

Haematoma, arterial puncture or hitting a nerve

See the relevant sections in the 'Complications' section under 'Peripheral cannulation' above.

Once *in situ*

Mechanical phlebitis

See 'Phlebitis' in the 'Complications' section under 'Peripheral cannulation' above.

Thrombosis

A venous thrombosis is a clot of blood that can be present at the tip of a catheter or can surround the catheter, for example a thrombosis in the upper arm caused by the presence of a PICC (Dougherty 2014). A SVC thrombus occurs when a catheter chronically rubs against the wall of the SVC, provoking a thrombosis at the site, and is often associated with a fibrin sheath. In order for a thrombosis to develop, three factors are required, known as Virchow's triad:

- stasis
- endothelial damage
- hypercoagulable state, caused by one or more of the following conditions: diabetes, malnutrition, dehydration, pregnancy, osteomyelitis, smoking, chronic renal failure, cirrhosis, cancer, obesity, sickle cell, surgery, congestive heart failure or oestrogen therapies (Gorski et al. 2010, Qinming 2012, Wall et al. 2016, Wilkes 2011).

The incidence of thrombotic catheter disfunction can be 3–7% (Dougherty 2014), with rates in PICCs normally ranging from 4% to 5% (Aw et al. 2012, Chopra et al. 2015, 2016, Lobo et al. 2009). A review of the literature by Fallouh et al. (2015) showed that the incidence could be as high as 75%. The risk is highest with suboptimal tip position in the high SVC and the brachiocephalic vein, and there are lower risks with small-bore catheters, basilic rather than cephalic vein and a secure fixation (Bodenham and Simcock 2009, Chopra et al. 2015, Garrino 2014). Thrombosis may initially present as partial withdrawal occlusion, inability to aspirate blood or resistance to flushing (Bodenham and Simcock 2009). Symptoms can be very acute or vague. The majority of cases of catheter-related thrombosis (two-thirds) are asymptomatic, which can make diagnosis difficult (Wall et al. 2016). When symptoms are present, the patient will usually complain of pain in the area (such as the arm or neck); oedema of the neck, chest and upper extremity; periorbital oedema; facial tenderness; tachycardia; shortness of breath and sometimes a cough; signs of a collateral circulation over the chest area; jugular venous distension; and/or discoloration of the limb (Bodenham and Simcock 2009, Qinming 2012, Wall et al. 2016).

Thrombosis can be prevented by correct placement of the tip in the lower third of the superior vena cava, cavo-atrial junction, inferior vena cava or right atrium (Bodenham and Simcock 2009), monitoring the catheter's function and flushing with pulsatile positive pressure flush (Dougherty 2014, Mayo 2000). The use of prophylactic anticoagulants, such as low-dose warfarin, has been shown to be of no apparent benefit (Couban et al. 2005, Wall et al. 2016, Young et al. 2005). Full anticoagulation may be necessary if the patient has had previous thromboembolic events (Bishop 2009, Dougherty 2014, Wall et al. 2016).

If a thrombosis is suspected, the patient should have a Doppler ultrasound. A venogram should be performed if suspicion of thrombosis is high despite a negative Doppler ultrasound (Dougherty 2006, Wall et al. 2016). Treatment can be either catheter removal or leaving the CVAD *in situ* and commencing anticoagulation, as thrombolytic therapy has proved successful in extreme cases and is often dependent on the size of the clot and the area of impaired circulation (Bodenham and Simcock 2009, Gorski et al. 2010, Wall et al. 2016). The current recommendations state that if the catheter is still required and functioning well, it does not need to be removed provided that it is well positioned, is infection free and demonstrates good resolution of symptoms on surveillance (Debourdeau et al. 2013, Wall et al. 2016). If the catheter is to be removed, patients will be prescribed injectable low-molecular-weight heparin for 6 weeks to 6 months and up to 3 months following removal (Gorski et al. 2010, Wall et al. 2016) (see Figure 17.32).

Sepsis

Infection is one of the most common and most serious complications associated with a central venous catheter (Dougherty 2006). Colonization by micro-organisms primarily occurs via two mechanisms: extraluminal and intraluminal (Scoppettuolo 2014). The catheter provides the ideal opportunity for micro-organisms to either track along the outside of the catheter (extraluminal) or be administered via the hub (intraluminal) internally into the central venous system. Infections can occur locally on the skin at the insertion site, in the skin tunnel or port pocket, or systemically (Wilkes 2011). Signs of infection at the insertion site include erythema, oedema, tracking along the length of the catheter, tenderness at the site, exudate (such as pus) and offensive smell (Wilkes 2011).

Septicaemia is a systemic infection that is usually characterized by pyrexia, flushing, sweating and rigors (rigors occur particularly when the catheter is flushed) (Wilkes 2011). The aim of extraluminal prevention is to lower the microbial load present on the patient's skin and on the hands of people who manipulate the catheter insertion site (i.e. via effective hand washing, skin antisepsis at insertion and after insertion, good aseptic non-touch technique (ANTT) for dressing changes and catheter maintenance). Intraluminal prevention focuses on good ANTT, and proper disinfection of the hub or needle-free connectors (Scoppettuolo 2014). Further means of preventing catheter-related bloodstream infections (Scoppettuolo 2014) include:

- the use of evidence-based guidelines, for example CVC care bundles with an emphasis on education (DH 2010, Loveday et al. 2014, Wilkes 2011)

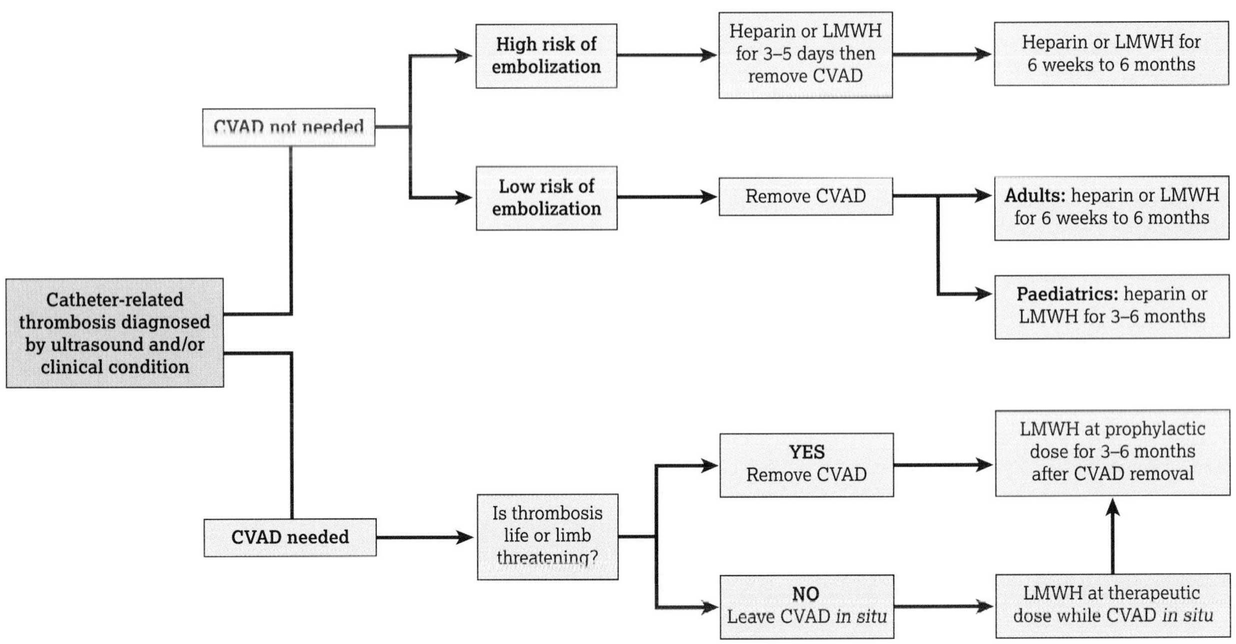

Figure 17.32 Royal Marsden NHS Foundation Trust algorithm for the management and treatment of CVAD-related thrombosis. CVAD, central venous access device; LMWH, low-molecular-weight heparin. *Source*: Reproduced with permission of The Royal Marsden NHS Foundation Trust.

- the use of catheters with antiseptic properties (e.g. impregnated, bonded or coated with antibiotics or chlorhexidine, or the addition of chlorhexidine or ionic silver to an impregnated patch or integrated in a gel dressing) (DH 2007, Wilkes 2011).

If a patient develops symptoms of an infection, then site swabs should be taken along with blood cultures (from the device and peripheral veins). The needle should be removed from the port if there is a skin infection and the port should not be reaccessed until the skin infection has cleared (Wilkes 2011). Depending on the clinical condition of the patient, the CVAD may be removed and/or intravenous antibiotics may be commenced (Gorski et al. 2010).

Removal of peripherally inserted central catheters

Pre-procedural considerations

With gentle, firm traction, the catheter will slide out from the insertion site. A PICC may resist removal because of venous spasm, vasoconstriction, phlebitis, valve inflammation, thrombophlebitis or the presence of a fibrin sheath (Gorski et al. 2010). Difficulty may occur in 1% of removals (Drewett 2000). Gentle traction and a warm, moist compress can be applied to alleviate venous spasm, resulting in easier removal of the catheter (Gorski et al. 2010, Marx 1995). If there is difficulty with removal, the practitioner should wait for 20–30 minutes and try again, or wait for 12–24 hours (Dougherty 2006). Other interventions that can be used to aid removal include smooth muscle relaxants, hand and arm exercises, and relaxation techniques (Gorski et al. 2010, Marx 1995).

If SecurAcath was used to secure the PICC, there may be difficulty at removal. Granulation at the anchor site can result in resistance as the device becomes embedded in the tissue. Cutting through the middle of the SecurAcath and pulling each prong out separately can help removal and avoid discomfort (see Action figure 8 in Procedure guideline 17.8: PICC removal; see also Figure 17.33).

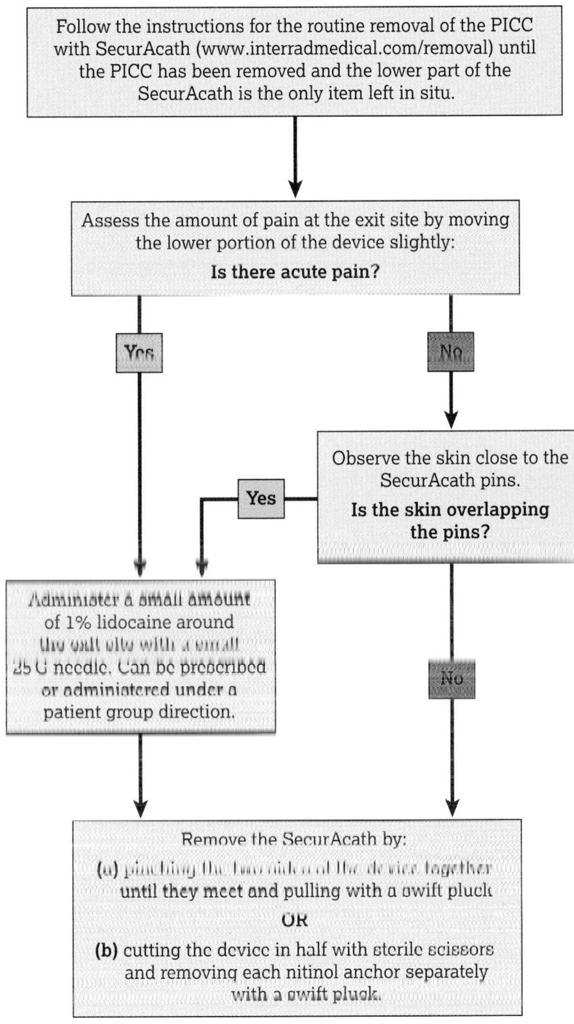

Figure 17.33 Algorithm for the removal of a peripherally inserted central catheter (PICC). *Source*: Adapted from Hughes (2014).

Procedure guideline 17.8 PICC removal

Essential equipment

- Personal protective equipment
- Dressing pack containing gauze and sterile gloves
- Cleaning solution
- Occlusive dressing
- Sterile scissors

Optional equipment

- Specimen container

Action	Rationale
Pre-procedure	
1 Introduce yourself to the patient, explain and discuss the procedure with them, and gain their consent to proceed.	To ensure that the patient feels at ease, understands the procedure and gives their valid consent (NMC 2018, **C**).
2 Ask the patient to lay supine if possible.	To reduce the risk of air embolism (Scales 2008, **E**).
Procedure	
3 Wash hands with soap and water, or an alcohol-based handrub, and dry. Gather the equipment required. Apply apron and clean gloves.	To minimize the risk of infection (DH 2010, **C**; Fraise and Bradley 2009, **E**).
4 Remove the transparent dressing and gently remove adhesive securing devices and/or sterile tapes as necessary.	To prepare for catheter removal. **E**
5 Apply sterile gloves and clean the insertion site. If there is a SecurAcath *in situ*, remove the top of the device.	To prevent contamination of the site. **E** To facilitate the removal of the catheter. **E**
6 Using a steady and constant motion, gently pull the catheter until it has been completely removed from the exit site.	To remove the catheter and prevent vein damage. **E**
7 Apply pressure with a finger (digital pressure) on a gauze square over the exit site for about 2–3 minutes or until the bleeding stops.	To minimize blood loss and bruising. **E**
8 Cut down the centre of the SecurAcath and remove the device (**Action figure 8**).	To facilitate the removal of the device. **E**
9 Apply an occlusive dressing.	To provide protection of the entry site. **E**
Post-procedure	
10 Check the markings on the length removed and ensure they show that the same length has been removed as the length that was inserted.	To ensure that the whole catheter has been removed (RCN 2016a, **C**).
11 If the catheter has been removed because of infection, carefully cut off the tip (approximately 5 cm) of the catheter using sterile scissors and place it in a sterile container for microbiological investigation.	To detect any infection related to the catheter and thus provide necessary treatment (DH 2010, **C**).
12 Remove gloves and dispose of waste.	To ensure safe disposal in the correct containers and avoid laceration or injury of other staff. To prevent reuse of equipment (NHS Employers 2010, 2015, **C**).
13 Document the length of the catheter removed and the reason for removal in the patient's care plan, as well as any problems or complications.	To ensure adequate records are maintained and to enable continued care of the patient and device (DH 2011, **C**; NMC 2018, **C**).

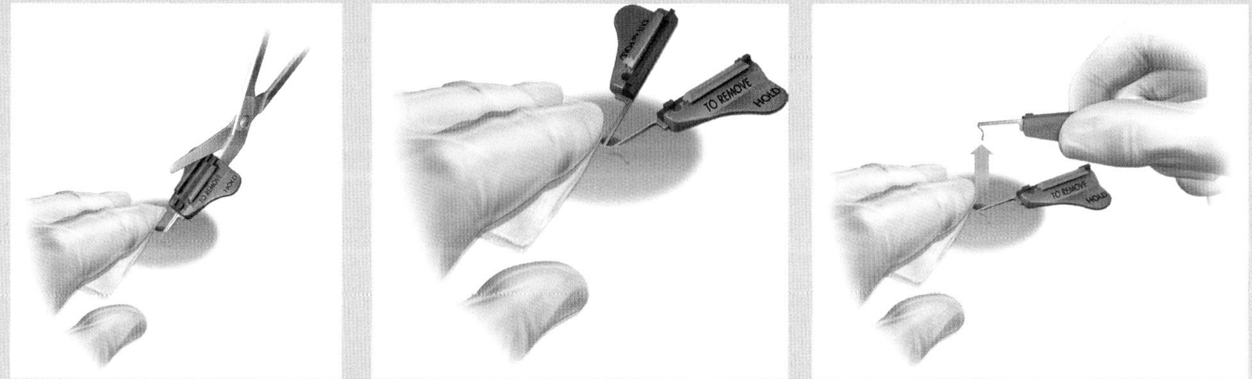

Action Figure 8 Removing the SecurAcath device. *Source*: Reproduced with permission of Interrad Medical, Inc.

Post-procedural considerations

Following removal of the PICC, pressure should be applied for at least 2–3 minutes. The site should then be inspected and a sterile occlusive dressing should be applied to ensure the bleeding has stopped. The catheter's integrity should be checked and its length measured to ensure an intact device has been removed (Dougherty 2006).

Documentation

On removal, the following should be documented:

- catheter length and integrity
- site appearance
- dressing applied
- reason for removal (Gorski et al. 2010, 2016, RCN 2016a).

Short-term percutaneous central venous catheters (non-tunnelled)

Definition

A short-term non-tunnelled percutaneous central venous catheter (CVC) is a device that enters through the skin directly into a central vein (Dougherty 2006, Hamilton 2009).

Evidence-based approaches

Rationale

Percutaneous non-tunnelled CVCs are commonly used for patients in acute settings and insertion may be in response to an emergency or planned event (Hamilton 2009, Wilkes 2011). Their multilumen configuration allows administration of several solutions at once and they are easy to remove (Dougherty 2006, Ives 2009). However, these catheters are associated with an increased risk (e.g. compared to PICCs) of complications such as pneumothorax and infection (Chantler 2009). Additionally, the catheter material results in irritation of the inner lumen of the vessel and is more thrombogenic than softer silicone catheters (Dougherty 2006, Springhouse 2009).

Indications

Percutaneous non-tunnelled CVCs are indicated for:

- short-term therapy (a few days up to several weeks)
- haemodynamic monitoring
- emergency use, for example fluid replacement
- absence of peripheral veins (Brockmeyer et al. 2009, Dougherty 2006).

Contraindications

There are few absolute contraindications to the use of percutaneous non-tunnelled CVCs, but where possible they should be avoided in the following patients:

- patients who have an existing infection
- patients with an existing pneumothorax or poor respiratory function
- patients with radiation burns to the insertion site, a fractured clavicle, or a malignant lesion at the base of the neck or apex of the lungs (Dougherty 2006, Scales 2008)
- patients with SVC syndrome or a history of central placement problems (Hamilton 2009, Smith and Nolan 2013).

Vein selection

These catheters are usually placed in the jugular, subclavian or femoral veins. The shortest catheter and the most direct route are required to create rapid blood flow around the catheter, which reduces irritation and obstructions and the risk of complications, and increases the dwell time of the catheter (Loveday et al. 2014, O'Grady et al. 2011, Weinstein and Hagle 2014). The preferred veins for most short-term CVCs are the subclavian and internal jugular (Smith and Nolan 2013, Weinstein and Hagle 2014). The subclavian route has a lower risk of infection (Chantler 2009, Parienti et al. 2015), allows greatest patient mobility after insertion and provides a flatter surface on which to maintain a dressing (Hadaway 2010). Its disadvantages are an increased risk of pneumothorax and difficulty controlling bleeding (Bodenham et al. 2016, Chantler 2009).

The jugular vein approach can be via the internal or external jugular vein. The anatomical location of the internal jugular vein makes it easier to catheterize than the subclavian vein and there is less risk of pneumothorax (Bodenham et al. 2016, Chantler 2009, Hadaway 2010, Smith and Nolan 2013). The external jugular vein is observable and easily entered, with rare insertion complications (Weinstein and Hagle 2014), but central catheter positioning can be difficult when using this route (Bodenham et al. 2016). Disadvantages include catheter occlusion and venous irritation as a result of head movement, difficulty in maintaining an intact dressing, and the position of the catheter being disturbing for the patient and their family (Chantler 2009, Dougherty 2006, Weinstein and Hagle 2014).

The femoral veins are primarily only used for short-term access when other sites are not suitable (O'Grady et al. 2011) but they are preferred to the subclavian route for short-term dialysis catheters (Smith and Nolan 2013). This route is associated with an increased risk of infection and thrombosis, difficulty in maintaining an intact dressing and inhibiting the patient's mobility (Chantler 2009, Dougherty 2006, Hadaway 2010). Although the groin may have a higher microbial colonization rate, tunnelling devices away from the groin may reduce such risks (Bodenham et al. 2016).

Central venous catheter insertion is a sterile procedure and the insertion should be performed following a central venous catheter care bundle, which should include the use of a theatre cap, mask, sterile gloves, a gown and sterile full-body drapes (DH 2011, Gorski et al. 2016, Loveday et al. 2014, O'Grady et al. 2011, RCN 2016a). These catheters should be inserted in a controlled environment to reduce the risk of contamination (Dougherty 2006). This procedure is performed by doctors, nurses and allied health professionals who have been taught all aspects of catheter insertion principles and practice (Alexandrou et al. 2010b, Smith and Nolan 2013).

Ultrasound guidance should be used routinely when a CVC is being inserted via the jugular or femoral vein, whether in an elective or emergency situation (NICE 2002, Smith and Nolan 2013, Wigmore et al. 2007). Ultrasound-guided catheterization of the subclavian vein is possible with the use of a slightly more lateral approach (Smith and Nolan 2013). In fact, entry is more into the axillary vein (Schmidt et al. 2015). Ultrasound provides the operator with visualization of the target veins as well as other surrounding anatomical structures, including any variations that the patient may have in their anatomy. It increases first-time puncture success rates while decreasing complication rates (Kelly 2014, NICE 2002).

The Trendelenburg position and Valsalva manoeuvre

Placing the patient in the Trendelenburg position facilitates entry to the vein by distending the vein, increasing central venous pressure and venous blood supply, and making veins more visible and accessible (Farrow et al. 2009). It also reduces the chance of air embolism because the venous pressure is higher than the atmospheric pressure. This is especially important when the catheter is placed using the subclavian approach (Dougherty 2006). A rolled towel may be placed under the patient's back along the spinal cord and between the shoulders to hyperextend the neck and clavicle (Weinstein and Hagle 2014).

The Valsalva manoeuvre can be performed by conscious patients to aid insertion of the catheter and to prevent air embolism (Cowlishaw and Ballard 2007, Dougherty 2006, Verghese et al. 2002, Weinstein and Hagle 2014). The patient is asked to breathe in and then try to force the air out with the mouth and nose closed (i.e. against a closed glottis). This increases the intrathoracic pressure so that the return of blood to the heart is reduced momentarily and the veins in the neck region become engorged (Dougherty 2006).

Clinical governance

Nurses and other healthcare professionals who wish to undertake this role must receive additional training in theory and practical hands-on instruction in insertion techniques and ultrasound (Alexandrou et al. 2010a, Bullock-Corkhill 2010). They must also ensure that they are operating within their scope of practice (HCPC 2016, NMC 2018). Competencies include:

- knowledge of the anatomy and physiology of the vasculature of the neck and chest
- selection of the vein and equipment
- use of ultrasound and local anaesthetic
- prevention, recognition and management of complications (Leung 2011, Paolucci et al. 2011, RCN 2016a, Wilbeck 2011).

Periodic assessments of continued competency and proficiency in CVC insertion should take place to ensure safe practice (Alexandrou et al. 2010a, 2010b, Moureau et al. 2013). Previous training in critical care, theatre or advanced life support skills is recommended in order to assist clinicians to respond appropriately in the event of an emergency during insertion (Hamilton 2009).

Pre-procedural considerations

Equipment

Catheters

Most catheters are made of polyurethane and may be single or multi-lumen (up to five) devices (Figure 17.34). There is a variety of lumen gauges and the catheters vary in length. They are usually open-ended but lumens can exit at staggered points along the catheter (Figure 17.35) (Dougherty 2006, Ives 2009). Multilumen catheters may carry a higher risk of infection than single-lumen ones (Smith and Nolan 2013), which has resulted in the manufacture of coated and impregnated catheters, which may have antimicrobial agents such as chlorhexidine, silver sulphadiazine or antibiotics bonded onto the surface (Hill et al. 2010, Monzillo et al. 2012). It has been shown that this can reduce the incidence of catheter-related bloodstream infections, and the use of such devices is strongly recommended by the Department of Health (Bassetti et al. 2001, Loveday et al. 2014, RCN 2016a, Sampath et al. 2001). Care must be taken as patients have been known to develop sensitivity to chlorhexidine (MHRA 2012) or the medications impregnated in the catheter (Lai et al. 2013).

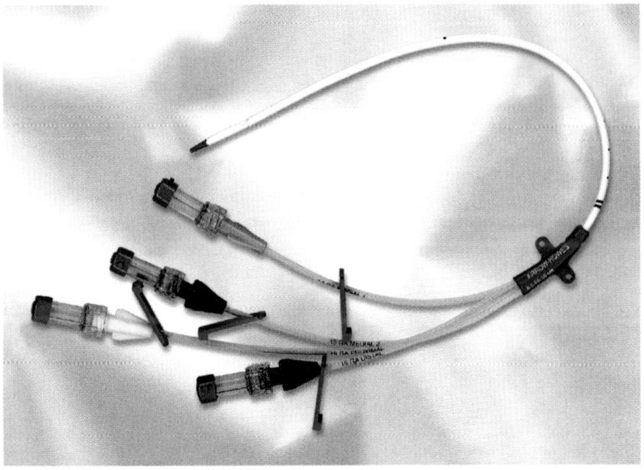

Figure 17.34 Non-tunnelled multilumen central venous catheter.

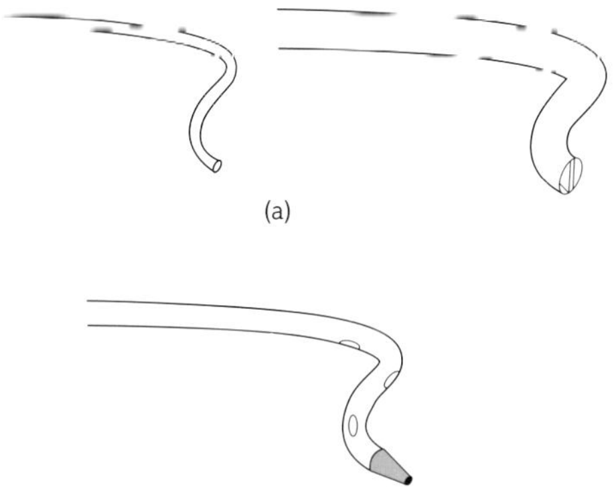

Figure 17.35 Types of catheter tip. (a) Open-ended catheter (single and double lumen). (b) Staggered-exit open-ended catheter.

Pharmacological support

Since these devices are usually in constant use, 0.9% sodium chloride is the flushing solution of choice to reduce the risk of occlusion (Loveday et al. 2014, RCN 2016a). It may be appropriate to use continuous infusions to keep the vein open. 1% lidocaine is often used to provide anaesthesia prior to cannulation and advancement of the introducer.

Specific patient preparation

Prior to inserting the catheter, the following should be carried out (Hamilton 2009):

- assessment of allergies
- physical examination, for example of physique, weight (e.g. obesity or cachexia) and relevant physical features (e.g. bull neck, lymphoedema or tracheostomy)
- vascular assessment
- assessment of respiratory, cardiovascular and neurological function
- assessment for fractures, arthritis and shape of sternum
- assessment for infection issues
- radiological assessment (e.g. to check for thrombosis)
- laboratory assessment (e.g. biochemistry, coagulation and platelets).

In general, the nurse's responsibilities when assisting another practitioner include the following:

- ensuring, where possible, that the patient understands and has been given a full explanation of the procedure and had the opportunity to discuss any aspects of it that they wish (DH 2009, NMC 2018, RCN 2016b)
- explaining any specific pre- and post-procedure instructions and the appearance and function of the catheter
- teaching the patient techniques that may be required during insertion (e.g. the Valsalva manoeuvre) and explaining that they may be placed in the Trendelenburg position (where the patient lies flat with the head lower than the feet, potentially with their knees bent) (Dougherty 2006, Weinstein and Hagle 2014) (Figure 17.36)
- assembling the equipment requested
- preparing local anaesthesia and dressing materials
- ensuring the correct positioning of the patient during insertion (i.e. in the supine or Trendelenburg position)
- attending to the physical and psychological comfort of the patient during and immediately following the procedure
- ensuring that no fluid or medication is infused before the correct position of the catheter has been confirmed on X-ray by an appropriate clinician and the tip location has been documented in the patient's notes.

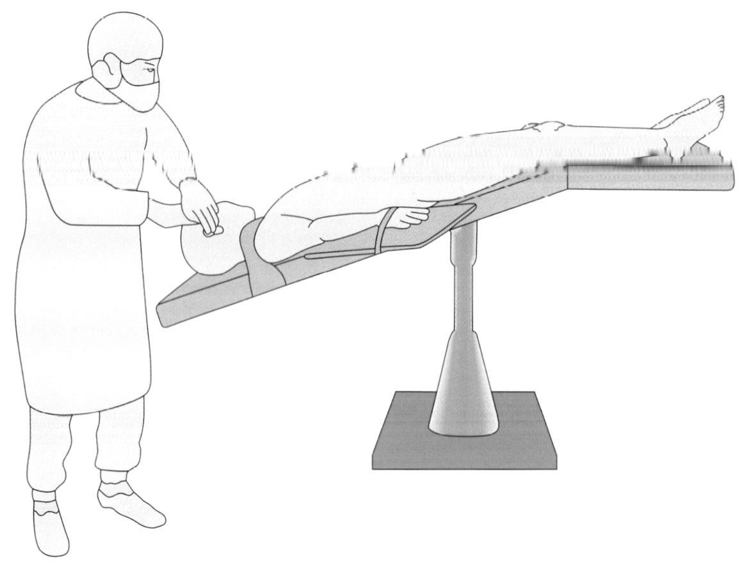

Figure 17.36 One way to achieve the Trendelenburg position.

Procedure guideline 17.9 Short-term central venous catheter (non-cuffed and non-tunnelled) insertion into the internal jugular vein

It is helpful to have an assistant when performing this procedure, if possible.

Essential equipment

- Personal protective equipment
- One or two pairs of sterile gloves (powder free) (quantity according to practitioner preference)
- Sterile pack containing sterile gown and drapes
- Alcohol-based skin-cleaning preparation, e.g. 2% chlorhexidine in 70% alcohol
- 10 mL syringes × 2–3
- 5 mL syringe
- Needle-free connectors (quantity to match the number of lumens)
- Introducer
- Central venous catheter and kit
- Semi-permeable transparent IV film dressing
- Sutures or securing device
- Blunt drawing-up needle
- 23 G safety needle
- 25 G safety needle
- Ultrasound machine
- Sterile ultrasound gel
- Sterile ultrasound probe cover
- Labels

Medicinal products

- 0.9% sodium chloride
- 1% lidocaine: 10 mL

Action	Rationale
Pre-procedure	
1 Gain consent from medical team to carry out the procedure and assess the patient's medical and intravenous device history.	To ensure the patient has no underlying medical problems and is suitable to undergo the procedure. **E**
2 Introduce yourself to the patient, explain and discuss the procedure with them, and gain their consent to proceed.	To ensure that the patient feels at ease, understands the procedure and gives their valid consent (NMC 2018, **C**).
3 Draw screens and assist the patient into a supine position.	To ensure privacy. To aid insertion of the introducer and then advancement of the catheter (Gabriel 2008, **E**).
4 Wash hands with soap and water, or an alcohol-based handrub, and dry.	To minimize the risk of infection (Fraise and Bradley 2009, **E**; NHS England and NHSI 2019, **C**; RCN 2016a, **C**).

5 Take the equipment required to the patient's bedside. Open the outer pack. Put on theatre cap and mask with visor.	To ensure appropriate equipment is available for the procedure. **E** To prevent contamination (Loveday et al. 2014, **C**).
Procedure	
6 Wash hands with soap and water, or an alcohol-based handrub, and dry.	To minimize the risk of infection (Fraise and Bradley 2009, **E**; NHS England and NHSI 2019, **C**; RCN 2016a, **C**).
7 Put on sterile gown and powder-free sterile gloves; open sterile tray, arranging and preparing the contents as required.	To prevent contamination. Powder on gloves can increase the risk of mechanical phlebitis (Elliott 1993, **E**; Loveday et al. 2014, **C**).
8 Pre-fill a 10 mL syringe with 0.9% sodium chloride and flush each lumen of the catheter. Then slide the clamp across the lumens.	To prevent blood loss and reduce risk of air entry. To ascertain that all lumens are patent. **E**
9 Draw up lidocaine into a 5 mL syringe and apply identifying label to it.	To ascertain which syringe contains the local anaesthetic. **E**
10 Place a sterile towel under the intended site for insertion.	To provide a sterile field to work on. **E**
11 Clean the skin at the selected site with 2% chlorhexidine in 70% alcohol, with friction, and prepare an area of 15–25 cm^2.	To ensure the removal of skin flora and to minimize the risk of infection (Loveday et al. 2014, **C**).
12 Allow the solution to dry thoroughly.	To ensure coagulation of bacteria and disinfection (Loveday et al. 2014, **C**).
13 Drape the patient with a sterile full-body fenestrated towel.	To provide a sterile field (Loveday et al. 2014, **C**).
14 Ask assistant to tip the patient's head down into the Trendelenburg position.	To encourage venous filling and reduce the risk of air embolism (Farrow et al. 2009, **E**).
15 Apply sterile ultrasound gel inside the ultrasound probe cover. Then cover the probe with the sterile ultrasound probe cover.	To improve conductivity. **E** To maintain sterility during the procedure. **E**
16 Apply ultrasound gel to the patient's neck and scan the side of the neck from below the ear lobe to the clavicle to locate the internal jugular vein and other vessels.	To identify and select a suitable vein and vessels to avoid, for example thrombosed vessels or arteries (Kelly 2014, **E**; Moureau 2014, **E**; NICE 2002, **C**).
17 Inject local anaesthetic intradermally using a 25 G safety needle to the area over the selected vessel and wait for it to take effect.	To ensure that the area is anaesthetized and reduce patient discomfort. **E**
18 Attach an empty 5 mL syringe to the seeker needle.	To prepare equipment. **E**
19 While visualizing the vein on the ultrasound machine, insert the needle directly into the vein at a downward angle of 30–50° (or steeper, up to 60–70°, to get clear visualization on the screen), maintaining gentle suction with the syringe plunger.	To gain venous access (Gabriel 2008, **E**), reduce the risk of arterial puncture and to know when the needle is in the vein. Apposition of the anterior and posterior walls of the vein can occur so blood is often only aspirated on withdrawal rather than insertion (Farrow et al. 2009, **E**).
20 When blood is observed in the syringe, check that the blood is dark and non-pulsatile.	To ensure the needle is in the vein and not the artery as it would then be bright red and pulsatile, although the most reliable method of checking is to perform a blood gas analysis (Farrow et al. 2009, **E**).
21 Remove the syringe from the needle, apply a digit over the entry and thread the guidewire through the needle until the selected depth is reached (this will depend on the side used and the anatomy of the patient). Keep hold of the guidewire at all times.	To prevent air entry and contamination of the area with blood, and to minimize the amount of blood loss from the patient (Gabriel 2008, **E**). If the guidewire is placed too deeply, the patient will have arrhythmias (Farrow et al. 2009, **E**).
22 Advance the dilator over the wire up to the puncture site.	To prepare for advancement of the dilator. **E**
23 Make a small incision in the skin at the puncture site.	To aid the advancement of the dilator through the skin. **E**
24 Advance the dilator using a gentle corkscrew motion to dilate the soft tissues. Advance to about the same depth as the venepuncture and then remove.	To facilitate the passage of the catheter (Farrow et al. 2009, **E**).
25 Remove the catheter from the plastic cover and advance it over the wire and into the vein via the puncture site.	To maintain sterility until required. To commence insertion of the catheter. **E**
26 As the catheter is advanced along the wire, keep hold of the guidewire from the end of the lumen and ensure it moves freely.	To ensure that the wire is not kinked or stuck within the vessels (Farrow et al. 2009, **E**).

(continued)

Procedure guideline 17.9 Short-term central venous catheter (non-cuffed and non-tunnelled) insertion into the internal jugular vein *(continued)*

Action	Rationale
27 Continue slow advancement of the catheter to the desired length (15 cm on right or 17 cm on left) then remove the guidewire.	To minimize damage to the intima of the vein (Gabriel 2008, **E**). To check there is no obstruction and that the catheter advances into the correct location (Farrow et al. 2009, **E**).
28 Aspirate and flush all lumens with 0.9% sodium chloride. Clamp each lumen after flushing.	To check for blood return or resistance. To check the patency of the device and ensure continued patency. To prevent air embolism (Gabriel 2008, **E**; Loveday et al. 2014, **C**).
29 Return the patient to a supine position.	To aid patient comfort. **E**
30 Attach needle-free connectors.	To ensure a closed system. **E**
31 Clean the insertion site and attach the wings of the catheter to the securing device.	To ensure protection of the site. To prevent the tubing pressing into the patient's skin (Gabriel 2008, **E**; RCN 2016a, **C**).
32 Attach the wings to a securing device (preferably), or alternatively stitch them to the skin with polypropylene sutures. Cover with a semi-permeable transparent IV film dressing.	To ensure the stability of the device (Gabriel 2008, **E**; RCN 2016a, **C**).
Post-procedure	
33 Remove gloves, hat, mask and gown and dispose of equipment appropriately. Dispose of sharps and clinical waste.	To prevent sharps injury. To ensure safe disposal in the correct containers and avoid laceration or injury of other staff. To prevent reuse of equipment (HSE 2013, **C**; NHS Employers 2010, 2015, **C**).
34 Send the patient for a chest X-ray. Ensure the position of the catheter is assessed and documented by a doctor or qualified practitioner. The X-ray should also be checked to ensure there is no pneumothorax.	To ensure that the catheter tip is in the correct position and that there is no pneumothorax (Wise et al. 2001, **E**).
35 Document the procedure in the patient's notes: • type of catheter (number of lumens) • number of passes (times needle inserted) • vein used • any problems • ability to aspirate blood • how it was secured • confirmation tip • patient education • serial number of catheter and ultrasound machine used.	To ensure adequate records are maintained and enable continued care of the patient and device (NMC 2018, **C**).

Problem-solving table 17.4 Prevention and resolution (Procedure guideline 17.9)

Problem	Cause	Prevention	Action
Unable to advance wire, dilator or catheter	Anatomical deviation Valves	Use ultrasound prior to insertion. Ensure good history taking and physical examination prior to commencing the procedure.	Do not force the wire, dilator or catheter as this may rupture a vessel. Remove the wire/catheter and reposition the patient. If problems persist, remove the wire/catheter and change site or contact a more experienced colleague.
Unable to achieve blood flashback	Vein may be transfixed Vein missed	Use ultrasound to visualize the vein.	Only aspirate blood on withdrawal, not on insertion. Withdraw the needle slowly, aspirating gently until flashback is seen.
Arterial blood aspirated	Arterial puncture	Ensure accurate use of ultrasound and steep needle insertion to avoid past pointing.	Withdraw the needle and press on the site firmly for at least 5 minutes to prevent major haematoma formation.
Occurrence of arrhythmias on inserting the wire	Wire inserted too far	Assess likely distance to the heart prior to insertion.	Withdraw the wire 2–3 cm.
Air aspirated from needle	Pleural space entered during insertion	Ensure accurate use of ultrasound.	Abandon the procedure. Contact the medical team urgently to request insertion of a chest drain.
Pneumothorax on post procedure chest X-ray	Pleural space entered during insertion	Ensure accurate use of ultrasound.	Contact the medical team urgently to request insertion of a chest drain.

Post-procedural considerations

Immediate care

The catheter may be sutured in place but this is no longer recommended due to the risk of infection and the need to reduce the use of sharps (Crnich and Maki 2002, HSE 2013, Maki 2005). The use of other securement devices is recommended, such as a StatLock (Figure 17.37) or SecurAcath (Ullman et al. 2017).

Ongoing care

Flushing is recommended after each use of the catheter. The types of dressing used at the insertion site may vary according to the type of patient and unit. A transparent dressing should be used and changed every 7 days or according to the manufacturer's instructions or local policy (NICE 2012, RCN 2016a). This enables staff to observe the site regularly for any signs of infection.

These types of catheter can remain *in situ* for up to 3–4 weeks (follow the manufacturer's instructions). However, actual practice will depend on local policy: some units will remove and reinsert if necessary every 10–14 days.

Complications

Air embolism

Air embolism may be fatal and can occur in conjunction with any entry into the vascular system at any time, but it commonly occurs at insertion and removal of central venous catheters (Bodenham et al. 2016, Cook 2013). For air to enter the vascular system, a pressure gradient between the vascular space and atmospheric air must exist, giving a direct line of access to the blood vessel (Cook 2013). The severity of the embolism depends on:

- *The volume of air that enters the vessel*: there is not an exact volume of air that is significant but usually any volume of air greater than 50 mL is considered potentially lethal, although patients are likely to experience symptoms at 20 mL of air per second (Bodenham et al. 2016).
- *The rate of entry*: rapid bolus injection may cause cardiovascular collapse whereas gradual accumulations (of microbubbles) may go unnoticed.

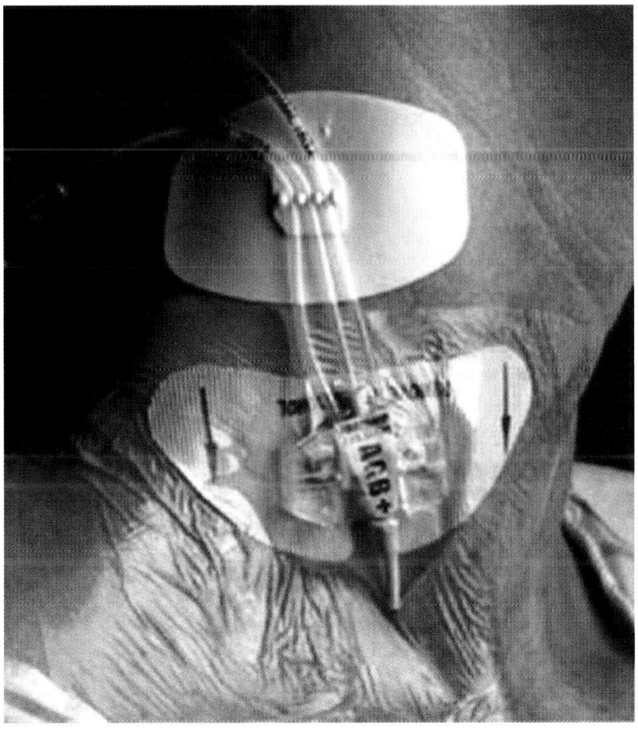

Figure 17.37 StatLock securement device.

- *The patient's position at the time of entry*: patients sitting upright during removal are at greater risk (due to passive air entry). Active air entry may occur when using pressure bags or if tubing has not been primed correctly or syringes are not purged of air (Cook 2013).

Incidence is considered low and while the true frequency is unknown, it is estimated to fall between 1:47 and 1:3000 (Cook 2013). Prevention of air embolism requires careful insertion and removal techniques, adequate fixation, and safe handling when accessing the catheter (Bodenham et al. 2016). For prevention see Box 17.8. Presentations range from subtle neurological, respiratory or cardiovascular signs to shock, loss of consciousness and cardiac arrest (Bodenham et al. 2016). The most common signs and symptoms include sudden dyspnoea, light-headedness, shoulder and chest pain, tachypnoea, tachycardia and hypotension (Cook 2013). Management includes turning the patient onto the left side and moving them into the Trendelenburg position. This is the optimal position as it decreases the gradient between the atmospheric air and the vessels and holds the entrapped air in the apex of the right atrium to prevent occlusion of the pulmonary artery (Cook 2013). The patient's vital signs should be monitored, and they should have 100% oxygen administered via a mask.

Pneumothorax

Pneumothorax is the presence of air in the pleural space between the lungs and the chest wall (Bodenham and Simcock 2009, Scales 2008). It can occur for a number of reasons but is the most common complication with central venous catheterization. It results when a needle, guidewire, dilator or catheter inadvertently punctures the lungs during insertion of a central venous catheter. Incidence is 0.3–2.3%, and is highest using the subclavian route (Bodenham et al. 2016). It also depends on the experience of the operator, the site and the technique used (Biffi 2012a). It is more common with the subclavian approach due to this vein's anatomical proximity to the lung. It is characterized by shortness of breath and sudden onset of chest pain but it may be clinically silent (Bodenham and Simcock 2009, Bodenham et al. 2016) and only be discovered on the chest X-ray performed following the procedure. It may be invisible on initial post-procedure image and therefore staff and patients should be warned to report late signs and symptoms. Pneumothorax may also be diagnosed by ultrasound (Lichenstein et al. 2005, Volpicelli 2011). Other symptoms include tachycardia, persistent cough and diaphoresis (Dougherty 2006).

Prevention is based on the skill level of the inserting practitioner (Biffi 2012a, Wigmore et al. 2007) as well as the use of ultrasound (Bodenham et al. 2016, NICE 2002). If symptoms are noted during insertion, the practitioner should stop the procedure. The patient's colour, respirations and pulse should be monitored and oxygen

Box 17.8 Prevention of air embolism

During insertion and removal	Position the patient supine or in the Trendelenburg position
	Ask the patient to perform the Valsalva manoeuvre
	Use an air-occlusive dressing for 24 hours
During use and maintenance	Expel air from all intravenous systems before attaching to the patient
	Use Luer-Lok connections to prevent accidental disconnection of tubing
	Examine equipment for cracks or leaks, which may allow ingress of air
	Use infusion devices that have air-in-line alarms
	Do not allow collapsible intravenous fluid bags to run dry

should be administered. In the case of a small pneumothorax (up to 30% of the pleural cavity), the patient may be asymptomatic or feel slightly breathless but no intervention is required and the pneumothorax will heal spontaneously (Bodenham and Simcock 2009, Bodenham et al. 2016). However, a large pneumothorax will necessitate the insertion of a chest drain (Biffi 2012a, Bodenham et al. 2016, Scales 2008).

Haemorrhage

Haemorrhage results from damage to a vein and/or artery during or following insertion of a CVAD. It is not usually a serious problem unless the carotid artery is punctured (Bodenham and Simcock 2009, Scales 2008). The incidence of arterial puncture is 0–15% (Qinming 2012). The use of ultrasound can help to reduce the risk of arterial puncture as the artery can be visualized during insertion (Bodenham and Simcock 2009, Lamperti et al. 2012, Qinming 2012).

The incidence of accidental arterial cannulation is estimated as 0.1–1% (Bodenham et al. 2016) and it can be recognized by excessive bleeding along the guidewire or on passing dilators and introducers. It is important to ensure that the patient is not compromised by having a high international normalized ratio (INR) or a low platelet count, or receiving anticoagulant therapy (Bodenham and Simcock 2009). These should all be corrected prior to CVAD insertion by administration of platelets and vitamin K, stopping medication a few days prior to insertion, or changing the patient from warfarin to subcutaneous injectable low-molecular-weight heparin, for example tinzaparin (Bodenham and Simcock 2009, Dougherty 2006). If symptoms are noted at the time of insertion and the artery can be located, then digital pressure should be applied for at least 5 minutes (10 minutes if the patient has a bleeding disorder), or until haemostasis is achieved; the patient should then have 6 hours of bedrest if the procedure was an arterial cannulation (Bodenham et al. 2016). Pressure is not always possible as the ability to apply pressure depends on the location of the artery (Bodenham and Simcock 2009, Qinming 2012). If symptoms are not recognized immediately then the patient may develop a mediastinal haematoma, which can then lead to tracheal compression and respiratory distress and require surgical intervention (Bodenham and Simcock 2009, Bodenham et al. 2016).

Removal of short-term percutaneous central venous catheters (non-tunnelled)

Pre-procedural considerations

Central venous catheters should not be removed and replaced routinely as there is no evidence that this prevents catheter-related infection (Loveday et al. 2014). Devices should be removed when they are no longer required or are causing problems (Bodenham et al. 2016).

Procedure guideline 17.10 Short-term central venous catheter (non-cuffed and non-tunnelled): removal

Essential equipment

- Personal protective equipment
- Sterile dressing pack (containing sterile gloves)
- Occlusive dressing or another appropriate dressing
- Hypoallergenic tape
- Sterile scissors
- Small sterile specimen container
- Stitch cutter
- Sterile low-linting gauze swab
- Dressing trolley

Medicinal products

- Alcohol-based skin-cleaning preparation, e.g. 2% chlorhexidine in 70% alcohol

Action	Rationale
Pre-procedure	
1 Introduce yourself to the patient, explain and discuss the procedure with them, and gain their consent to proceed.	To ensure that the patient feels at ease, understands the procedure and gives their valid consent (NMC 2018, **C**).
2 Screen the bed.	To allow dust and airborne organisms to settle before the insertion site and the sterile field are exposed. **E**
3 Wash hands with soap and water, or an alcohol-based handrub, and dry. Place all equipment required for the dressing on the bottom shelf of a clean dressing trolley.	To reduce the risk of cross-infection (DH 2010, **C**; Fraise and Bradley 2009, **E**).
Procedure	
4 Take the trolley to the patient's bedside, disturbing the screens as little as possible.	To minimize airborne contamination (DH 2010, **C**).
5 Open the sterile dressing pack.	To gain access to the sterile field. **E**
6 Attach an orange clinical waste bag to the side of the trolley below the level of the top shelf.	So that contaminated material is below the level of the sterile field (DH 2010, **C**).
7 Open the other sterile packs, tipping their contents gently onto the centre of the sterile field. Pour lotions into gallipots or an indented plastic tray where required.	To reduce the risk of contamination of contents. **E**
8 Discontinue the infusion, if in progress, and disconnect the infusion system from the catheter. Clamp the catheter.	To prevent entry of air or leakage of blood when the catheter is disconnected. **E**

9	Assist the patient into the Trendelenburg position – that is, head slightly lower than feet.	To prevent air entering the vein on catheter removal (Drewett 2009, **E**).
10	Wash hands with soap and water, or an alcohol-based handrub, and dry.	To reduce the risk of cross-contamination (Fraise and Bradley 2009, **E**).
11	Loosen the old dressing gently.	So that the dressing can be lifted off easily. **E**
12	Put on clean gloves.	To protect the nurse from any contact with the patient's blood. **E**
13	Using gloved hands, remove the old dressing and discard it. Remove tapes or securing device.	To remove the old dressing without contaminating hands (DH 2010, **C**).
14	Remove gloves, clean hands with an alcohol-based handrub and put on sterile gloves from pack.	To minimize the risk of introducing infection (DH 2010, **C**; Fraise and Bradley 2009, **E**).
15	Clean the wound with 2% chlorhexidine in 70% alcohol using back-and-forth strokes, with friction.	To prevent contamination of the catheter on removal and a false-positive culture result (DH 2010, **C**; Loveday et al. 2014, **C**).
16	Cut and remove any skin suture securing the catheter.	To facilitate removal. **E**
17	Cover the insertion site with low-linting gauze.	Swabs are used to discourage the entry of organisms into the insertion site and to absorb any leakage of blood. **E**
18	Ask the patient to perform the Valsalva manoeuvre.	To reduce the risk of air embolism (Drewett 2009, **E**).
19	Hold the catheter with one hand near the point of insertion and pull firmly and gently. As the catheter begins to move, press firmly down on the site with the swabs. Maintain pressure on the swabs for about 5 minutes after the catheter has been removed.	Pressure is applied to prevent haemorrhage and to encourage resealing of the vein wall. It also prevents the entry of air into the vein. **E** Continued pressure is necessary to allow time for the puncture in the vein to close. **E**
20	Remove the catheter and check the tip is intact.	To ensure that all of the catheter has been removed. **E**
21	If the catheter has been removed because of infection, carefully cut off the tip (approximately 5 cm) of the catheter using sterile scissors and place it in a sterile container for microbiological investigation.	To detect any infection related to the catheter and thus provide necessary treatment (DH 2010, **C**; Loveday et al. 2014, **C**).
Post-procedure		
22	When bleeding has stopped (approximately 5 minutes), cover the site with a small gauze pad and a transparent dressing.	To detect any infection at the exit site. To prevent air entering the vein via the site (Scales 2008, **E**).
23	Fold up the sterile field, place it in the orange clinical waste bag and seal the bag before moving the trolley. Dispose of the equipment in the appropriate containers.	To reduce the risk of environmental contamination (DH 2010, **C**).
24	Make the patient comfortable.	To ensure patient comfort. **E**
25	Document the date and time and reason for removal in the patient's notes or care plan.	To ensure adequate records are maintained and to enable continued care of the patient and device (NMC 2018, **C**).

Post-procedural considerations

Immediate care

The patient should lie flat with the exit site below the heart to reduce the risk of air embolism. Major vessels usually heal quickly, but firm and direct digital pressure must be applied to the site to help this process for at least 5 minutes or until cessation of bleeding (Bodenham et al. 2016, Dougherty 2015, Gorski et al. 2016). A sterile transparent occlusive dressing should be applied (Bodenham et al. 2016, Dougherty 2015, RCN 2016a, Scales 2008). Patients should remain flat for a short time after catheter removal, usually 30 minutes (Dougherty 2015), to maintain positive intrathoracic pressure and allow the tissue tract time to seal (Bodenham et al. 2016, Drewett 2009).

Ongoing care

The dressing should remain intact for 72 hours, until the tract is epithelialized, to minimize the risk of air embolism following CVC removal (Dougherty 2015, Gorski et al. 2016, RCN 2016a). The integrity of the catheter should be ascertained, and the date, time and reason for removal must be documented (NMC 2018, RCN 2016a).

Skin-tunnelled catheters

Definition

A skin-tunnelled catheter is a long-term catheter that lies in a subcutaneous tunnel before entering a central vein (usually subclavian) (Hadaway 2010). The tunnel commonly exits between the sternum and the nipple. The tip lies at the junction of the superior vena cava (SVC) and the right atrium or within the lower portion of the SVC or the upper right atrium (Dougherty 2006, Galloway and Bodenham 2004) (Figure 17.38).

Evidence-based approaches

Rationale

Tunnelled silicone catheters were first described by Broviac in Seattle in 1973 and were subsequently modified by Hickman and colleagues, who created a larger lumen of 1.6 mm internal diameter (Bjeletich and Hickman 1980). The special features added included an inert antithrombogenic flexible material and a subcutaneous Dacron cuff attached to the catheter (Ives 2009). The cuff has two functions: to secure the catheter and prevent

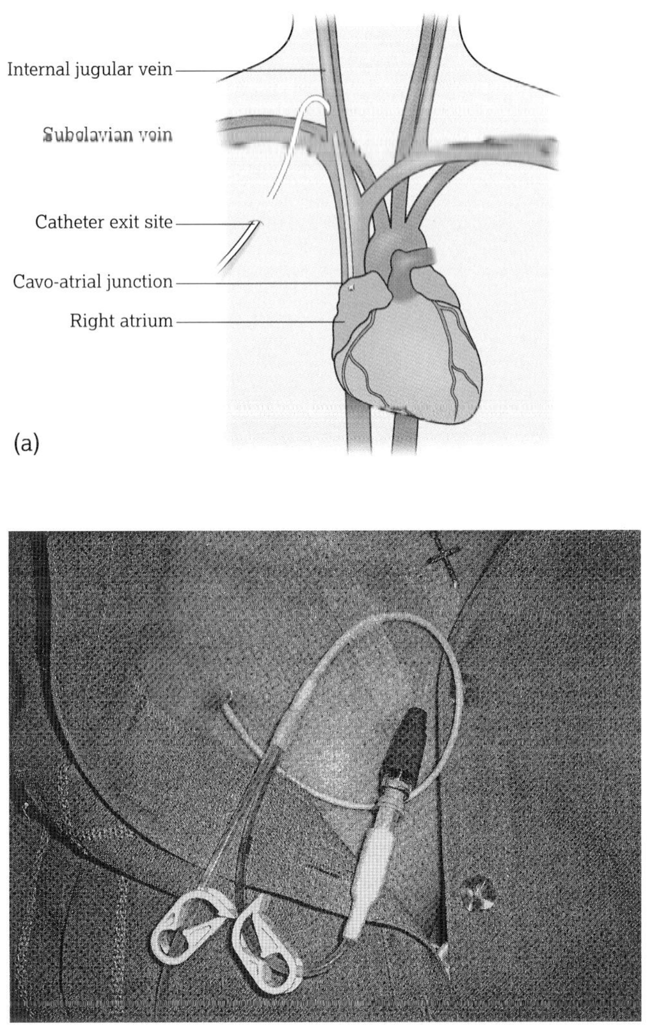

Figure 17.38 Tunnelled catheter. (a) Anatomical positioning of tunnelled catheter. (b) Patient with tunnelled catheter *in situ*.

infection; it achieves these by increasing the length of the subcutaneous tunnel – that is, the distance between the point of insertion of the catheter into the vessel and the exit site from the skin (Singh Vats 2012).

Indications

A skin-tunnelled catheter is used when safe and reliable long-term venous access is required (e.g. for total parenteral nutrition, chemotherapy, haemodialysis or antimicrobial treatment) or if peripheral vascular access is problematic (Dougherty 2006, Light et al. 2014, Wilkes 2011).

Contraindications

These are the same as for other CVADs.

Methods of insertion

The insertion of a skin-tunnelled catheter is a surgical procedure usually carried out in an operating theatre or designated area, under aseptic conditions, using fluoroscopy and monitoring of the patient by pulse oximetry and ECG to detect arrhythmias (Benton and Marsden 2002, Dougherty 2006, Galloway and Bodenham 2004, Weinstein and Hagle 2014). The procedure is now also performed by nurse specialists at the bedside and within radiology departments (Benton and Marsden 2002, Boland et al. 2003, Fitzsimmons et al. 1997, Hamilton et al. 1995, Light et al. 2014). The procedure is usually performed under sedation along with the use of local anaesthesia (Dougherty 2006). In some patients, for example children, the procedure is carried out under general anaesthesia.

The aim of the insertion is to place the catheter tip in the cavo-atrial junction or right atrium via the internal jugular vein or the subclavian vein (Bodenham et al. 2016, Galloway and Bodenham 2004). The internal jugular vein route presents the lowest incidence of mechanical and thrombotic complications (Biffi et al. 2014, Bodenham et al. 2016, Granziera et al. 2014). When there is an SVC obstruction from thrombosis or compression, the femoral vein can be used to access the inferior vena cava. Selection of vessels is as for non-tunnelled CVCs (refer to 'Vein selection' within 'Short-term percutaneous central venous catheters (non-tunnelled)' above). Access may be gained percutaneously using a needle and guidewire or via an open surgical cutdown procedure.

The catheter can be inserted percutaneously when the venepuncture site is near the subclavian or internal jugular. The tunnelling rod is then passed under the skin and exits at a predetermined point on the chest. The catheter is then attached to the tunnelling rod and drawn through the subcutaneous tunnel. The catheter is then passed into the vein via a peel-away sheath introducer (Davidson and Al Mufti 1997, Galloway and Bodenham 2004, Hadaway 2010). Position is confirmed by the easy aspiration of blood from each lumen and these are then flushed with heparin until correct tip placement has been confirmed. A chest X-ray should be performed after insertion to check for correct placement and rule out pneumothorax (Bodenham et al. 2016, Davidson and Al Mufti 1997, Stacey et al. 1991).

Methods of removal

Removal techniques for skin-tunnelled catheters vary. Removal should only be performed by specially trained nurses or doctors. It is recommended that the patient is placed supine and that aseptic technique is used throughout. There are two methods of removal: surgical excision and the traction method.

Surgical excision

This method involves locating the cuff and performing a minor surgical excision under local anaesthetic. Most cuffed devices need surgical cut-downs as they develop complex adherent fibrin sleeves and scar tissue (Bodenham et al. 2016). A small incision is made over the site of the cuff and blunt dissection (i.e. using forceps) is carried out to prise the tissues apart (Galloway and Bodenham 2004, Hudman and Bodenham 2013); this causes less damage to the tissues than using a scalpel. The cuff and the catheter are freed from the surrounding fibrous tissue (Dougherty 2006). The proximal section of the catheter is then removed and cut, and the distal end is removed via the exit site. Once the catheter has been removed, the wound is sutured using interrupted sutures, which can be removed after 7 days (Drewett 2009, Galloway and Bodenham 2004).

Traction method

With the traction method, there is a greater risk of the catheter breaking, which can result in a catheter embolism. This method should only be used if the catheter has been *in situ* for less than 3–4 weeks, if healing is delayed or if the site is heavily infected, as in all of these situations the cuff may not be fixed and is easier to pull out (Light et al. 2014). If movable, the cuff will pull out with a series of tugs, as it passes through the tissues. If immovable, proceed to surgical removal to avoid breaking the catheter (Drewett 2009). Very long-term catheters may become attached to the wall of the SVC or right atrium and cannot be removed by traction alone; cutting off and leaving *in situ* or surgical removal may be required (Bodenham et al. 2016).

Clinical governance

Nurses and other healthcare professionals who wish to undertake this role must receive additional training in theory and practical hands-on instruction at the bedside in the removal technique and training ([illegible] 2018). The [illegible] that they are operating within their scope of practice (HCPC 2016, NMC 2018). Competencies include:

- using local anaesthetic
- making an incision and using a scalpel
- suturing
- preventing and managing complications.

Periodic assessments of continued competency and proficiency should take place to ensure safe practice (Moureau et al. 2013).

Pre-procedural considerations

Equipment

Polyurethane or silicone skin-tunnelled catheters are available in single-, double- and triple-lumen versions with a Dacron cuff (Wilkes 2011). The cuff is used to secure the catheter as fibrous tissue grows around it and obliterates part of the subcutaneous tunnel within 1–2 weeks of insertion. As it becomes overgrown with epithelial cells, this also serves to prevent easy passage of micro-organisms from the skin along the catheter into the vein (Light et al. 2014, Wilkes 2011). The cuff is about 1 cm wide (Hadaway 2010) and is usually located about 3–5 cm from the exit site (Stacey et al. 1991, Weinstein and Hagle 2014). Knowledge of the distance from the cuff to the bifurcation may assist the practitioner in locating the cuff during removal of the catheter, although the distance will vary according to the brand of catheter.

The tip of the catheter may be valved or non-valved (Dougherty 2006, Ives 2009). The disadvantage of a non-valved catheter is the problem of blood reflux, which can result in occlusion. Valved catheters can have the valves in a round closed tip (such as in the Groshong catheter) or in the hub. Valves (proximal or distal) close and open the catheter depending on the pressure, so if a catheter is damaged or disconnected, or at the end of an infusion, the low pressure closes the valve, thereby preventing backflow and occlusion. The valve opens with minimal positive pressure for infusion but requires [illegible] pressure for aspiration (Weinstein and Hagle 2014). This feature reduces the risk of air embolism or bleeding resulting from accidental disconnection; it also eliminates the need for catheter clamping and the need for heparin, and reduces the frequency of flushing (Ives 2009, Mussa 2014). The valve is usually a two-way valve that remains closed at normal vena caval pressure. Application of a vacuum in order to withdraw blood enables the valve to open inwards, whereas positive pressure into the catheter forces the valve to open outwards (Figure 17.39) (Dougherty 2006). When a valve is incorporated within the hub and not the tip, it may reduce the risk of reflux even during periods of raised central venous pressure (Weinstein and Hagle 2014). However, if a thrombus forms around the tip, it can result in malfunction and loss of valve competence (Dougherty 2006).

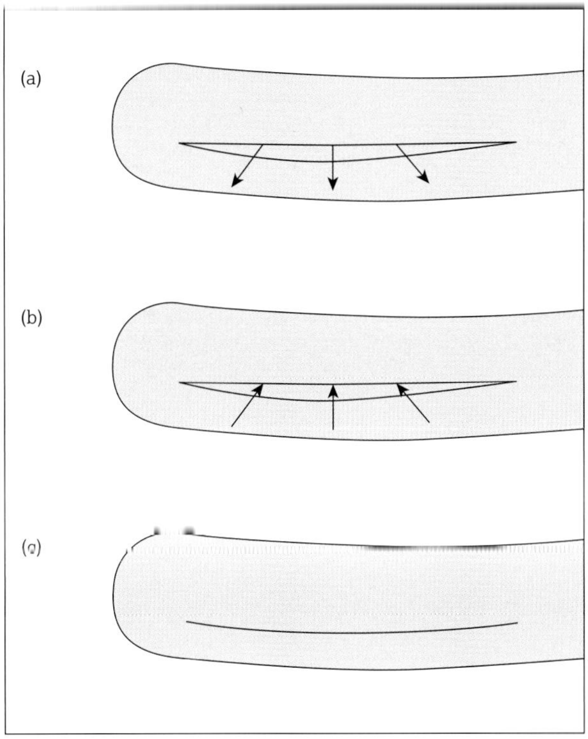

Figure 17.39 Groshong two-way valve catheter. (a) Infusion (positive pressure). (b) Aspiration (negative pressure). (c) Closed (neutral pressure).

Procedure guideline 17.11 Central venous catheter (skin tunnelled): surgical removal

Essential equipment

- Personal protective equipment
- Minor operations set
- 10 mL Luer-Lok syringe
- 25 G safety needle
- 23 G safety needle
- Blunt drawing-up needle
- 10×10 cm low-linting gauze swabs × 5
- 3-0 prolene suture on a curved needle
- Transparent dressing

Optional equipment

- Steri-Strips (if necessary)
- Specimen container

Medicinal products

- 1% lidocaine: 10 mL
- 2% chlorhexidine in 70% alcohol

(continued)

Procedure guideline 17.11 Central venous catheter (skin tunnelled): surgical removal *(continued)*

Action	Rationale
Pre-procedure	
1 Check the patient's full blood count and clotting profile for that day.	To ensure that the patient is not at risk of bleeding or infection from this invasive procedure. The patient's platelets should be above 100 × 10^9/L, their white blood count should be above 2 and their international normalized ratio (INR) should be less than 1.3. In haematology patients, the platelets should be above 50 and the INR less than 1.5 (Dougherty 2006, **E**). *Note platelet transfusion guidelines and always follow local policy.*
2 Introduce yourself to the patient, explain and discuss the procedure with them, and gain their consent to proceed.	To ensure that the patient feels at ease, understands the procedure and gives their valid consent (NMC 2018, **C**).
3 Screen the bed and ask the patient to remove their clothing down to the waist.	To ensure ease of access to the patient's chest. **E**
4 Ask the patient to lie as flat as possible with their arms by their sides.	To minimize the risk of bleeding from gravitational pressure and to dissuade the patient from touching the sterile field (Dougherty 2015, **E**; Drewett 2009, **E**).
Procedure	
5 Wash or decontaminate hands as per World Health Organization guidelines.	To reduce the risk of infection (DH 2010, **C**; Fraise and Bradley 2009, **E**; WHO 2009, **E**).
6 Palpate and identify the position of the cuff in the patient. This can be done by gently pulling on the catheter and observing for skin pucker.	To locate the area for the incision (Drewett 2009, **E**; Galloway and Bodenham 2004, **E**).
7 If the cuff cannot easily be felt, measure up from the bifurcation or hub at the end of the catheter distal to the patient, dependent on the type of catheter *in situ*, then palpate again. If it still cannot be felt, ask for assistance from a more experienced colleague.	The cuff will be positioned differently depending on the type of catheter. To locate the probable site of the cuff. To guard against malplaced incisions (Dougherty 2006, **E**).
8 Open the outer bag of the minor operation pack.	To gain access to the contents. **E**
9 Put on a plastic apron and wash hands with soap and water, or an alcohol-based handrub. Dry hands on the sterile towel provided in the pack.	To reduce the risk of infection (DH 2010, **C**; Fraise and Bradley 2009, **E**).
10 Put on sterile gloves and assemble all necessary equipment on the sterile pack.	To maintain asepsis, prepare for the procedure and maximize efficiency (DH 2010, **C**).
11 Advise the patient that you will explain each step of the procedure as you go along if the patient wishes.	This should take into account the patient's individual wish for information. **E**
12 Clean the area directly over the cuff with 2% chlorhexidine in 70% alcohol, using back-and-forth strokes, working out from the centre directly over the cuff. Allow the area to dry.	To reduce the risk of infection. To enable the disinfection process to be completed. To prevent stinging on insertion of the needle (Dougherty 2006, **E**).
13 Apply a fenestrated drape.	To create a sterile field to operate within and thereby reduce the risk of infection (Dougherty 2006, **E**).
14 Inform the patient that you are about to administer the local anaesthetic and that this will cause a stinging sensation.	To prepare the patient. The first injection can be painful and causes a stinging sensation (BNF 2019, **C**, **P**).
15 With a 25 G needle, administer the first millilitre of local anaesthetic intradermally directly over the cuff site, causing a raised bleb.	To commence the numbing of the area to be incised. To provide a raised area for the next injection and identification of the site (Macklin and Chernecky 2004, **E**).
16 Give a further 1–2 mL of local anaesthetic subcutaneously, using the bleb as the area for insertion of the needle but directing the needle out and around the area of the cuff site.	To reduce pain for the patient with repeated injections. To ensure the whole incision area is numb (Dougherty 2011, **E**).
17 Attach the 23 G needle and with the remaining 4 mL of local anaesthetic give two deeper injections to either side of the cuff area.	To ensure anaesthesia at a deeper level during the blunt dissection around the cuff (Macklin and Chernecky 2004, **E**).
18 Test the area above the cuff for numbness and then make the incision over the cuff site (but slightly to the side of the cuff site in very thin patients). The incision should be longitudinal and about 2 cm in length. Ensure that the incision is through the epidermis and dermis.	To ensure that the patient will not experience any pain. To facilitate identification and removal of the cuff. To allow access to the cuff, which is situated below the dermis. To reduce the risk of cutting through the cuff before the cuff has been identified (Dougherty 2006, **E**; Drewett 2009, **E**).
19 With one pair of small artery forceps, commence blunt dissection of tissue from around the cuff. At intervals, place your finger (if possible) into the site and feel the cuff.	To free the cuff from the surrounding fibrous tissue. To assess the mobility of the cuff. To reduce the risks of bleeding and damaging the catheter (Dougherty 2006, **E**; Drewett 2009, **E**).

20	Continue with blunt dissection around and under the cuff until it feels mobile.	To facilitate the loosening of the cuff (Dougherty 2006, **E**).
21	With one pair of artery forceps or the dissecting hook, loop under the cuff and lift it up out of the incision.	To identify the catheter so as to allow removal (Dougherty 2006, **E**).
22	Once the cuff is free, still maintaining a grip on the cuff, gently and carefully peel away the thin straw-coloured tissue from the catheter with the blade, ensuring the blade is pulled away from the catheter.	To free the catheter from the anchoring fibrous bands and enable removal. To reduce the risk of accidental incision of the catheter (Dougherty 2006, **E**).
23	As the last strands of fibre are separated, the catheter should become free and the white material of the catheter should become visible.	To ensure that the catheter is completely freed for removal (Dougherty 2006, **E**).
24	Ask the patient to perform the Valsalva manoeuvre as the proximal portion of the catheter is withdrawn from the vein. Apply gentle pressure at the vein exit site.	To remove the catheter and prevent bleeding or air entry (Drewett 2009, **E**).
25	Cut through the catheter using a blade or scissors and remove the distal portion via the skin exit site.	To remove the distal half of the catheter below the cuff (Dougherty 2006, **E**).
26	If the catheter has been removed because of infection, carefully cut off the tip (approximately 5 cm) of the catheter using sterile scissors and place it in a sterile container for microbiological investigation.	To detect any infection related to the catheter and thus provide necessary treatment (DH 2010, **C**).
27	Close the incision with three sutures (3-0 prolene). Commence the first suture in the middle of the incision, with the remaining sutures evenly on either side.	To close the incision efficiently. To ensure that the skin edges and insert are brought together in alignment (Dougherty 2006, **E**).
28	If there continues to be any bleeding, Steri-Strips can be applied across the incision over the sutures.	To minimize blood loss (Dougherty 2006, **E**).
29	It is not usually necessary to suture the exit site.	To leave the exit site to granulate without a suture (Drewett 2009, **E**).
Post-procedure		
30	Apply a small pressure dressing and cover with an airtight dressing.	To absorb any slight bleeding and to maintain a clean site (Dougherty 2015, **E**; Scales 2008, **E**).
31	Advise the patient that there might be some oozing and to reapply a dry dressing after 24 hours and thereafter once a day until the sutures are removed. Advise the patient that the sutures should be removed in 7–10 days.	To ensure that the incision has fully closed and healed (Dougherty 2006, **E**; Drewett 2009, **E**).
32	Dispose of the equipment in the appropriate containers.	To reduce the risk of environmental contamination (DH 2010, **C**). To ensure safe disposal in the correct containers and avoid laceration or injury of other staff. To prevent reuse of equipment (NHS Employers 2010, 2015, **C**).
33	Ask the patient to rest on the bed for the next 30–60 minutes, or longer if required, especially patients who are prone to bleeding.	To reduce the risk of bleeding and air embolism as the patient sits or gets up (Dougherty 2006, **E**; Dougherty 2015, **E**).
34	Liaise with the nursing team and document the date, time and reason for removal; type of local anaesthetic used (volume and percentage); and any problems in the nursing and medical notes.	To ensure there is good communication between all teams and a written record of the procedure (NMC 2018, **C**).

Problem-solving table 17.5 Prevention and resolution (Procedure guideline 17.11)

Problem	Cause	Prevention	Action
Unable to locate cuff	Cuff too deep Lack of knowledge of cuff location	Ensure knowledge of all types of catheter and where the cuff is located on each, as measurements differ between manufacturers.	Contact the catheter manufacturer for cuff details.
Bleeding at site	Low platelets or raised international normalized ratio Small vessels cut	Never undertake this procedure unless the patient's levels have been corrected.	Apply pressure to site until bleeding stops. May need vessel to be tied off.
Cut through catheter or catheter breaks	Removing catheter by traction	Only remove the catheter using a surgical technique.	Attempt to clamp any remaining part of the catheter with artery forceps.
	Incision made too deeply directly over cuff	Make the incision to the side of the cuff.	Contact surgical team for assistance.

Post-procedural considerations

Immediate care

Following insertion

The dressing should be left intact and changed 24 hours after insertion.

Following removal

Since the vein closes following removal of the catheter, there is usually no bleeding. However, there may be slight bleeding at the exit site immediately after removal because of the passage of the cuff.

Following either removal method, pressure should be applied to the site until the bleeding stops, and a dressing may be required for 24–48 hours. The patient should be encouraged to rest flat for 30–60 minutes to allow the tissue tract time to seal and prevent possible air embolism (Dougherty 2015, Galloway and Bodenham 2004, McCarthy et al. 2016).

Ongoing care

Following insertion

Healing of the skin tunnel takes approximately 7 days, so at this time the sutures at the entry site may be removed (Dougherty 2006). The exit site sutures should be retained until the fibroblastic response to the Dacron cuff is adequate to secure the catheter, usually within 2–3 weeks (Perucca 2010, Stacey et al. 1991, Weinstein and Hagle 2014). A transparent dressing should cover the site and be changed weekly until removal of the sutures.

Following removal

Sutures at the incision site should be removed after 7 days (Dougherty 2006).

Education of the patient and relevant others

See 'Discharging patients home with a VAD *in situ*' above.

Complications

Infection and thrombosis are the main complications; see the 'Complications' section under 'Peripherally inserted central catheters' above.

Implanted ports

Definition

An implanted port is a totally implanted vascular access device (TIVAD) made of two components: a reservoir with a self-sealing septum, which is attached to a silicone catheter (Figure 17.40). The port is usually placed subcutaneously on either the chest or the arm but it can be placed on the lower chest wall, abdomen or thigh, depending on the patient's needs (Busch et al. 2012, Wilkes 2011). It is accessed percutaneously using a special non-coring (Huber) needle (Dougherty 2006, Weinstein and Hagle 2014, Wilkes 2011).

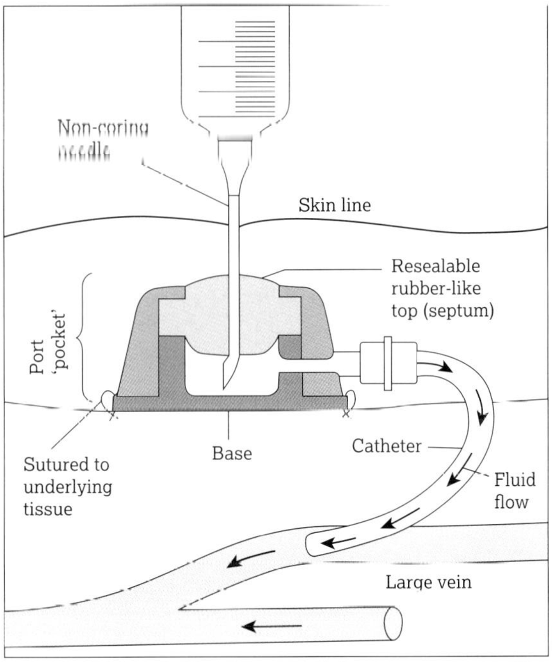

Figure 17.40 Implantable port cross-section, accessed with non-coring needle.

Evidence-based approaches

Rationale

Ports are implanted subcutaneously to provide repeated long-term access (Weinstein and Hagle 2014) to the vascular system (other ports include arterial, epidural and peritoneal). Implanted ports require little care of the site because of the intact skin layer over the port, except when accessed. When not in use, the only care required is a regular flush to maintain patency (Weinstein and Hagle 2014). Other benefits include a reduced risk of infection (Bow et al. 1999, Mirro et al. 1989, Moureau et al. 1999), less interference with daily activities such as bathing or swimming (Wilkes 2011), and less of a threat to body image than with the presence of an external catheter (Biffi et al. 2011, Bow et al. 1999, Mirro et al. 1989). Patients with ports are often very satisfied with their access devices (Chernecky 2001, Johansson et al. 2009).

Disadvantages of ports include discomfort when accessing is performed (particularly if placed deeply or in a difficult-to-access area). This can be overcome with the use of topical local anaesthetic. However, the tissue over the septum becomes callused or scarred and over time there is loss of sensitivity (Fougo 2012a, Hadaway 2010). Needle dislodgement with resulting extravasation and needle stick injury are well-documented problems associated with ports (Dougherty 2012, Schulmeister and Camp-Sorrell 2000, Viale 2003). There are also issues related to occlusion and 'sludge' build-up, although newer designs are attempting to reduce these issues (Stevens et al. 2000). Finally, there can be problems with obtaining blood return (Moureau et al. 1999).

Indications

An implanted port can be used for long-term venous access for all types of therapy, both continuous and intermittent, and if patients have problematic venous access (Dassi et al. 2012, Dougherty 2006, Heibl et al. 2010).

Contraindications

Contraindications are primarily related to the location of the port. For example, ports should not be located on the chest if there has been bilateral mastectomy or radiation burns. A further contraindication is a patient's inability to undergo a general anaesthetic for insertion if required (Di Carlo 2012).

Methods of insertion

Implantation is a surgical procedure carried out under general anaesthetic, or sedation and local anaesthetic (Goossens et al. 2011). Some catheters are pre-attached to the reservoir while others require attachment on insertion (Dougherty 2006, Wilkes 2011).

The most common veins used are the subclavian, the internal jugular, the femoral and the veins of the upper arm (Bodenham et al. 2016, Hadaway 2010, Pittiruti et al. 2012, Weinstein and Hagle 2014). Samman et al. (2015) recommend the jugular vein as the first site for access unless the patient's circumstances do not permit this approach. Ports must be implanted over a bony prominence and most commonly over the bony area below the clavicle; less commonly, they are implanted on the ribs or the forearm (Biffi 2012b, Wilkes 2011). Arm ports are becoming a viable alternative as they are easy to implant and have very low complication rates (Burbridge and Goyal 2016, Goltz et al. 2012, Krieger and Burbridge 2000, Shiono et al. 2014).

The catheter is introduced into the superior vena cava via the subclavian or jugular vein (chest ports) or the basilic or brachial vein (upper arm ports), and fluoroscopy or ECG technology (for arm ports) is used to verify the placement of the tip. The catheter is then tunnelled to the pocket (Dougherty 2006). The pocket is made just under the skin, usually on a bony prominence for stabilization (Wilkes 2011). The port is then sutured into place to the underlying fascia. The suture line can be lateral, medial, superior or inferior to the port septum to remove it from the area where the port will be accessed because repeated access could cause stress to the suture line (Dougherty 2006, Weinstein and Hagle 2014). The area is tender and oedematous for up to a week following implantation, and any manipulation or accessing may be painful. When immediate use is indicated, the port should be accessed and dressed immediately following insertion (Wilkes 2011).

Ports are associated with a low rate of complication, particularly infection (Barbetakis et al. 2011, Beckers et al. 2010, Biffi et al. 2014, Dal Molin et al. 2011).

Clinical governance

Some nurses insert ports (Hadaway 2010, Pittiruti et al. 2012), and many are responsible for accessing and deaccessing ports. It is vital that the needle is placed in the port because if it is not, there is a risk of the medications extravasating or infiltrating. Therefore, any nurse who wishes to access ports must undergo specific training to gain the necessary knowledge and skills to select the correct type and length of needle and access the port successfully with little patient discomfort (NMC 2018).

Pre-procedural considerations

Equipment

A variety of ports are available, and the choice is dependent on a number of factors, for example whether the patient is a child or an adult, the amount of access required and where the port will be located (Fougo 2012a). Ports are usually single lumen, although dual lumen ports are available (Dougherty 2006). However, dual-lumen ports have two septums and therefore require needle access into each septum (Wilkes 2011). Port reservoirs (Figure 17.41) are about 2.5 cm in height and 0.625 cm in diameter and can weigh from 21 to 28 g; low-profile ports are smaller and often placed in the arm (Ives 2009). Entry can be gained via the side or top but most are accessed via the top (Weinstein and Hagle 2014). There are now also CT-rated ports that allow CT contrast to be administered through the port without causing damage.

Port catheters are made of silicone or polyurethane and may be valved or non-valved (Biffi et al. 2011, 2014). The port body may be made of stainless steel, plastic or titanium, although stainless steel is rarely used now as it interferes with electromagnetic imaging procedures and is quite heavy in comparison with other materials (Dougherty 2006). The self-sealing silicone septum can be accessed approximately 2000 times (regular size; small ports may take only 750), often dependent on the size of the needle used (Hadaway 2010, Wilkes 2011).

Non-coring needles have the penetration style of a knife so when the needle is removed, the septum closes behind it (Fougo 2012b, Hadaway 2010) (Figure 17.42). The bevel opens on the side of the needle instead of the end (Gabriel 2008, Weinstein and Hagle 2014). Needles are available in straight or 90° angle configurations with or without extension sets (Wilkes 2011) and with a metal or plastic hub in gauges 19–24 and lengths from 0.65 to 2.5 cm. Needle gauge is selected dependent on the type and rate of infusate as well as the location of the port (Dougherty 2006, Fougo 2012b). Safety needles are also now available and activate on withdrawal from the port; they are recommended for use (HSE 2013).

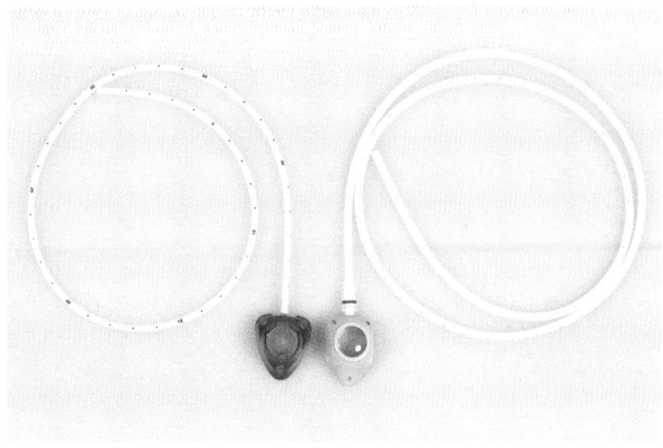

Figure 17.41 Implanted ports.

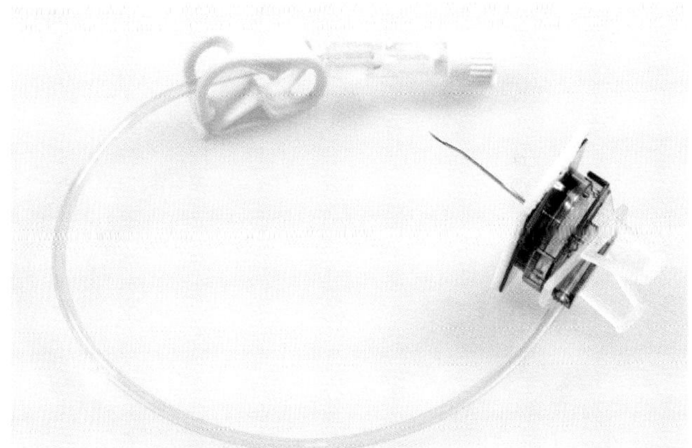

Figure 17.42 Non-coring needles have the penetration style of a knife so when the needle is removed, the septum closes behind it.

Pharmacological support

Prior to accessing a port, topical local anaesthetic may be used over the site (Gorski et al. 2010). While the port is accessed, it is usual to flush it with 0.9% sodium chloride and heparinized saline (50 international units in 5 mL); however, when the needle is due to be removed, a higher strength of heparin is recommended – 100 international units of heparin per millilitre to a total of 5 mL (500 international units) (Blackburn and van Boxtel 2012, Wilkes 2011). There is now evidence to suggest that ports can be flushed with 0.9% sodium chloride (Bertoglio et al. 2012) and that flushing less frequently than monthly is both safe and beneficial (Goossens 2015, Ignatov et al. 2010, Kefeli et al. 2009, Kuo et al. 2005).

Procedure guideline 17.12 Implanted arm PORT insertion using modified Seldinger technique (MST) with ultrasound guidance and ECG technology

It is helpful to have an assistant when performing this procedure, if possible.

Essential equipment

- Personal protective equipment
- One or two pairs of sterile gloves (according to practitioner preference)
- Sterile pack containing sterile gown, mask with visor, theatre cap, sterile drapes and scissors
- Sterile minor operation pack containing a variety of forceps and a needle holder
- Alcohol-based skin-cleaning preparation, e.g. 2% chlorhexidine gluconate in 70% alcohol
- 10 mL syringes × 2–3
- 5 mL syringes × 2
- MST kit (containing needle, guidewire, 5 mL syringe, dilator/introducer/peel-away sheath, safety scalpel, and 22 or 20 G cannula)
- Arm PORT kit (containing catheter, PORT and tunneller)
- Sutures
- Surgical glue
- Padded semi-permeable IV film dressing
- Small transparent semi-permeable IV film dressing
- 25 G safety needle
- 23 G safety needle
- Blunt drawing-up needles
- Tape measure
- Disposable tourniquet
- Sharps container
- Ultrasound machine, sterile gel and sterile probe cover
- ECG leads, electrodes and monitor
- Labels

Medicinal products

- Sterile pre-filled 10 mL syringes of 0.9% sodium chloride × 2–3
- 1% lidocaine with adrenaline

Action	Rationale
Pre-procedure	
1 Introduce yourself to the patient, explain and discuss the procedure with them, and gain their consent to proceed.	To ensure that the patient feels at ease, understands the procedure and gives their valid consent (NMC 2018, **C**).
2 Assess the patient's medical and intravenous device history. Assess the patient's arms for suitability of port implantation.	To ensure the patient has no underlying medical problems such as taking anticoagulants or previous surgery to the arm or chest and so is suitable to undergo the procedure (Hamilton 2009, **E**; Moureau 2014, **E**). To ensure suitability for an implanted arm port (Goltz et al. 2012, **E**; Shiono et al. 2014, **E**).
3 Draw screens and assist the patient into a (semi)supine position, with their arm at a 90° angle to their torso.	To ensure privacy. To aid insertion of the introducer and then advancement of the catheter (Gabriel 2008, **E**; Moureau 2014, **E**). To help in creating a subcutaneous pocket and insertion of the port (Shiono et al. 2014, **E**).
4 Take the ultrasound equipment to the patient. Apply a tourniquet and gel and assess venous access using ultrasound, assessing both extremities. Locate and select the most suitable vein.	To ensure the patient has adequate venous access and to select the vein for catheterization (Gabriel 2008, **E**; Goltz et al. 2012, **E**; Krieger and Burbridge 2000, **E**; Moureau 2014, **E**; Shiono et al. 2014, **E**).
5 Where required, apply local anaesthetic cream or gel to the chosen venepuncture site and leave for the allotted time.	To minimize the pain of insertion (BNF 2019, **C**).
6 Take the equipment required to the patient's bedside. Open the outer pack.	To ensure the appropriate equipment is available for the procedure. **E**
7 Attach ECG leads to electrodes and monitor, and apply to the patient as per the manufacturer's instructions.	To ensure an ECG tracing can be obtained and used as a comparison once the catheter has been inserted (La Greca 2014, **E**; manufacturer's instructions, **C**; Oliver and Jones 2014, **E**; Oliver and Jones 2016, **E**).
8 If using a tracking device, attach it to the patient's chest area.	To track the tip of the catheter as it advances into the venous system (La Greca 2014, **E**; manufacturer's instructions, **C**; Oliver and Jones 2014, **E**; Oliver and Jones 2016, **E**).
9 Apply a theatre cap and face-mask with visor.	To minimize the risk of infection during the procedure and to protect the practitioner from blood splash contamination (Loveday et al. 2014, **C**, **E**).

Procedure

10	Wash hands with soap and water, or an alcohol-based handrub. Dry hands using sterile paper towels from the pack.	To minimize the risk of infection (Fraise and Bradley 2009, **E**; Loveday et al. 2014, **C**).
11	Put on sterile gown and sterile gloves; open the inner pack, arranging the contents as required.	To prevent contamination (Elliott 1993, **E**; Loveday et al. 2014, **C**). To have medications prepared for use. **E**
12	If not using pre-filled syringes then draw up 0.9% sodium chloride into a 10 mL syringe (provided by assistant if possible). Label the syringe.	To prevent contamination (Elliott 1993, **E**; Loveday et al. 2014, **C**). To have medications prepared for use. **E**
13	Draw up 1% lidocaine with adrenaline into two 5 mL syringes (provided by assistant if possible) and attach 25 G safety needles. Label the syringes.	To have medications prepared for use and avoid confusion and medication errors. **E**
14	Remove the cap from the extension set and attach the syringe containing 0.9% sodium chloride; gently flush to the end of the catheter lumen and leave the syringe attached. Prepare the port as per the manufacturer's guidelines.	To check that the catheter is patent and to enable easy removal of the guidewire (Krieger and Burbridge 2000, **E**; manufacturer's instructions, **C**; Shiono et al. 2014, **E**).
15	Place a sterile towel under the patient's arm.	To provide a sterile field to work on. **E**
16	Clean the skin at the selected site with 2% chlorhexidine gluconate in 70% alcohol, with backwards and forwards movements and friction, for 30 seconds, and prepare an area of 15–25 cm^2.	To ensure the removal of skin flora and to minimize the risk of infection (Fraise and Bradley 2009, **E**; Loveday et al. 2014, **C**).
17	Allow the solution to dry thoroughly.	To ensure coagulation of bacteria and disinfection (Loveday et al. 2014, **C**).
18	Drape the patient with a full-body sterile fenestrated drape.	To provide a sterile field (Loveday et al. 2014, **C**).
19	Apply sterile gel to the ultrasound probe cover. Then apply the sterile ultrasound probe cover over the probe head and pull down along the cable.	To ensure all equipment that is in contact with the patient is sterile (Loveday et al. 2014, **C**).
20	Retighten the disposable tourniquet through the sterile drapes or ask assistant to do this.	To aid venous distension (Dougherty 2008, **E**).
21	Apply sterile gel to the skin and scan to find the chosen vein.	To identify the most suitable vein. **E**
22	Keeping the probe in position, inject local anaesthetic intradermally using a 25 G needle and wait for it to take effect.	To provide adequate anaesthesia (BNF 2019, **C**).
23	While visualizing the vein under ultrasound, perform venepuncture with a needle or cannula. (If using a cannula, when flashback is seen, advance the cannula into the vein.)	To gain venous access (Gabriel 2008, **E**; Goltz et al. 2012, **E**; Moureau 2014, **E**; Shiono et al. 2014, **E**). To prevent blood loss and through-puncture, and enable advancement of the catheter (Gabriel 2008, **E**).
24	Remove the stylet and advance the guidewire through the needle (or cannula) until there is 10–15 cm of wire in the vein.	To maintain venous access (Goltz et al. 2012, **E**; Krieger and Burbridge 2000, **E**; Shiono et al. 2014, **E**)
25	Release the tourniquet and remove the probe.	To contain flashback, prevent contamination of the area with blood and minimize the amount of blood loss from the patient (Gabriel 2008, **E**).
26	Reinfiltrate over the puncture site with 1% lidocaine with adrenaline (intrademally) if necessary.	To achieve anaesthesia and minimize patient discomfort. **E**
27	Inject 1% lidocaine with adrenaline intradermally using a 23 G needle and making an L-shape in a fanning motion to a lateral and distal area approximately 4 cm away from the cannulation site until a bleb is observed.	To allow for subcutaneous pocket formation (Goltz et al. 2012, **E**; Krieger and Burbridge 2000, **E**; Shiono et al. 2014, **E**).
28	Further inject 1% lidocaine with adrenaline intradermally between the cannulation site and the subcutaneous pocket area.	To create a subcutaneous tunnel between the puncture site and subcutaneous pocket (Krieger and Burbridge 2000, **E**; Shiono et al. 2014, **E**).
29	Check the patient has no sharp sensations at the anaesthetized areas	To ensure area is anaesthetized before proceeding. **E**
30	Make a small incision by sliding the tip of the scalpel blade along the top of the wire.	To ensure that connective tissues between the skin and guidewire are free with the purpose of facilitating the introduction of the dilator/peel-away sheath and to place the catheter route deeper to reduce the risk of catheter erosion (Shiono et al. 2014, **E**).
31	With the scalpel at 60–90° to the skin, make a 2–3 cm incision perpendicular to the long axis of the arm to the previously anaesthetized L-shaped area.	To facilitate entrance and to allow for subcutaneous pocket formation (Goltz et al. 2012, **E**; Krieger and Burbridge 2000, **E**; Shiono et al. 2014, **E**).

(continued)

Procedure guideline 17.12 Implanted arm PORT insertion using modified Seldinger technique (MST) with ultrasound guidance and ECG technology *(continued)*

Action	Rationale
32 Activate the safety function on the scalpel and replace it onto the sterile field.	To minimize the risk of sharp stick injury (HSE 2013, **C**; NHS Employers 2015, **C**).
33 Grip the dilator/peel-away introducer firmly and advance it over and along the guidewire.	To enable advancement of the introducer/peel-away sheath (Goltz et al. 2012, **E**; Shiono et al. 2014, **E**).
34 Withdraw the guidewire and dilator and leave the peel-away introducer *in situ*.	To enable catheter insertion (Goltz et al. 2012, **E**; Krieger and Burbridge 2000, **E**; Shiono et al. 2014, **E**).
35 Grip the catheter a few centimetres from the tip and thread through the peel-away introducer sheath.	To facilitate catheter insertion. **E**
36 Continue slow advancement of the catheter and aspirate (if possible) and flush to check for blood return or resistance.	To minimize damage to the tunica intima of the vein (Gabriel 2008, **E**). To check there is no obstruction and that the catheter advances into the correct location. **E**
37 Ask the patient to turn their head towards the arm of insertion and place their chin on their shoulder if possible.	To prevent the catheter entering the jugular vein and to ensure correct advancement of the catheter downwards to the superior vena cava (Gabriel 2008, **E**).
38 Ask the patient whether they have any aural (behind the ear) sensations on the side of catheter insertion. If using a tracking device, observe the direction of the catheter on the screen.	This could indicate that the catheter has advanced along the internal jugular vein and needs to be withdrawn and readvanced (Dougherty 2006, **E**; manufacturer's instructions, **C**).
39 Using the ECG technology, gently manipulate the catheter, observing the ECG trace for changes in the P wave. When the highest P wave without deflection is observed, the catheter tip is in the correct position (cavo-atrial junction). If using a tracking device, track to see the catheter heading down and then verify the exact position using ECG technology.	To ascertain tip position (La Greca 2014, **E**; manufacturer's instructions, **C**; Moureau et al. 2010, **E**; Oliver and Jones 2014, **E**; Pittiruti et al. 2012, **E**). To track the tip of the catheter as it advances into the venous system (La Greca 2014, **E**; manufacturer's instructions, **C**; Oliver and Jones 2014, **E**; Oliver and Jones 2016, **E**).
40 Carefully withdraw the peel-away/ introducer sheath and peel apart.	To ensure there is minimal movement of the catheter. To remove the peel-away introducer (Gabriel 2008, **E**; Goltz et al. 2012, **E**; Moureau 2014, **E**; Shiono et al. 2014, **E**).
41 Aspirate for blood return and flush the catheter with 0.9% sodium chloride.	To check the patency of the device and ensure continued patency (Gabriel 2008, **E**; Loveday et al. 2014, **C**).
42 Using the ECG technology, gently manipulate the catheter, observing the ECG trace for changes in the P wave. Ensure the highest P wave without deflection is observed.	To ensure that the catheter tip remains in the correct position (cavo atrial junction) (La Greca 2014, **E**; manufacturer's instructions, **C**; Moureau et al. 2010, **E**; Oliver and Jones 2014, **E**; Pittiruti et al. 2012, **E**).
43 Acknowledge the catheter's length (from the cannulation site to the cavo-atrial junction) by looking at the catheter markings.	To determine catheter length when the tip is positioned at the cavo-atrial junction. **E**
44 Make a subcutaneous pocket through the incision made to the anaesthetized L-shaped area by blunt dissecting using forceps. The pocket needs to accommodate a snug implantation of the port.	To facilitate the port implantation (Goltz et al. 2012, **E**; Krieger and Burbridge 2000, **E**; Shiono et al. 2014, **E**).
45 Apply gentle pressure on the catheter and slowly withdraw the stylet.	To ensure there is no withdrawal of the catheter (Gabriel 2008, **E**).
46 Attach the distal end of the catheter to the tunneller and tunnel under the subcutaneous tissue from the venotomy (cannulation) site to the already formed subcutaneous pocket. The tunneller will come out at the pocket incision.	To make a subcutaneous tunnel between the venotomy site and the subcutaneous port pocket (Goltz et al. 2012, **E**; Krieger and Burbridge 2000, **E**). To minimize infection risk as the tunnel increases the distance from the venotomy site to the implantation site (Singh Vats 2012, **E**).
47 Remove the tunneller and trim the distal catheter end accordingly.	To ensure correct catheter length and appropriate assembly of parts (Goltz et al. 2012, **E**; Krieger and Burbridge 2000, **E**; manufacturer's instructions, **C**; Shiono et al. 2014, **E**).
48 Connect the catheter to the port as per the manufacturer's instructions.	To ensure correct assembly of the catheter and reservoir (manufacturer's instructions, **C**).
49 Place the port into the subcutaneous pocket (suturing of the port to the connective tissue through the suture hole is optional).	To implant the port into the subcutaneous pocket and ensure the stability of the device (Goltz et al. 2012, **E**; Krieger and Burbridge 2000, **E**; manufacturer's instructions, **C**; Shiono et al. 2014, **E**)
50 After percutaneously accessing the port with a non-coring needle, aspirate and flush with at least 10 mL of 0.9% sodium chloride.	To ascertain device function and to ensure continued patency (Gabriel 2008, **E**; Loveday et al. 2014, **C**).

51 Remove the non-coring needle and activate its safety mechanism.	To minimize the risk of sharp stick injury (HSE 2013, **C**; NHS Employers 2015, **C**).
52 Suture the port insertion site with a curved needle. Use 2-0 vicryl to close the subcutaneous pocket and 4-0 monocryl to close the skin subcuticularly. (Refer to the section on suturing in Chapter 18: Wound management.)	To ensure the stability of the device (Gabriel 2008, **E**; Hughes 2014, **E**; Moureau and Iannucci 2003, **E**; NICE 2017, **C**; RCN 2016a, **C**).
53 Clean the area with 2% chlorhexidine gluconate in 70% alcohol and leave to air dry.	To minimize the risk of infection (Fraise and Bradley 2009, **E**; Loveday et al. 2014, **C**).
54 Apply a small amount of surgical glue to both the small venotomy incision and the subcutaneous pocket exit site, and leave to air dry.	To minimize bleeding at the implantation site and reduce extraluminal contamination (Corley et al. 2017, **E**; Jeanes and Martinez-Garcia 2016, **E**; Scoppettuolo et al. 2013, **E**; Simonova et al. 2012, **E**).
55 If the patient needed the device for immediate use, insert a safety non-coring needle and fix it to the patient using an appropriate dressing.	To minimize pain and discomfort and to decrease the risk of infection from early manipulation of the implantation site (Krieger and Burbridge 2000, **E**; Wilkes 2011, **E**).
56 Apply a semi-permeable transparent IV film dressing (using a padded semi-permeable IV film dressing is optional). Date the dressing.	To ensure protection of the site (Loveday et al. 2014, **C**; RCN 2016a, **C**). To see when the dressing is due for changing if appropriate. **E**
Post-procedure	
57 Dispose of sharps and clinical waste. Remove gloves, gown, mask and theatre cap and dispose of equipment appropriately.	To prevent sharps injury (HSE 2013, **C**; NHS Employers 2015, **C**).
58 If necessary, send the patient for a chest X-ray. The position of the catheter should be assessed and documented by an appropriate healthcare professional (see Figure 17.5).	To ensure that the catheter tip is in the correct position (Wise et al. 2001, **E**).
59 If ECG tip positioning technology was used during catheter insertion (recommended), a chest X-ray is not required provided that a good ECG tracing is obtained showing maximal P wave elevation. This must be verified by the operator, who should be proficient in the use of this type of technology.	To ensure correct tip position and minimize unnecessary patient exposure to radiation (La Greca 2014, **E**; NICE 2017, **C**; Oliver and Jones 2016, **E**; Pittiruti et al. 2012, **E**; RCN 2016a, **C**).
60 Document the procedure in the patient's notes: • size and type of port • depth and size of needle used to access or left *in situ* (as appropriate) • where the port was inserted • tip confirmation by ECG and/or chest X-ray • batch number of catheter and lot number of sterile packs • ECG trace • any problems • how the port was secured • patient education/booklets given.	To ensure adequate records are maintained and enable continued care of the patient and device (NMC 2018, **C**; RCN 2016a, **C**). To enable any faulty equipment to be traced back to the manufacturer (MHRA 2004, **C**).

Procedure guideline 17.13 Implanted ports: insertion and removal of non-coring needles

Essential equipment

- Personal protective equipment
- Sterile dressing pack (containing sterile gloves)
- 10 mL syringes containing 0.9% sodium chloride × 2
- Non-coring (Huber point) needle with extension set
- Needle-free connector
- Plaster

Optional equipment

- Semi-permeable transparent IV film dressing (if needle remaining *in situ*)

Medicinal products

- Heparinized saline in 10 mL syringe (if needed as part of local policy)
- 2% chlorhexidine in 70% alcohol

(continued)

Procedure guideline 17.13 Implanted ports: insertion and removal of non-coring needles *(continued)*

Action	Rationale
Pre-procedure	
1 Introduce yourself to the patient, explain and discuss the procedure with them, and gain their consent to proceed.	To ensure that the patient feels at ease, understands the procedure and gives their valid consent (NMC 2018, **C**).
2 If required, apply topical local anaesthetic cream to the area and leave for 30–60 minutes.	To reduce the feeling of pain on insertion of the needle. **E**
3 Assist the patient into a comfortable position.	To aid patient comfort and gain access to the port. **E**
4 Wash hands with soap and water, or an alcohol-based handrub, and dry.	To minimize the risk of contamination (DH 2010, **C**).
5 Locate the port and identify the septum; assess the depth of the port and thickness of the skin.	In order to select the correct length of needle (Dougherty 2006, **E**).
6 Check the duration and type of therapy required.	In order to select the correct gauge and configuration of the needle (Camp-Sorrell et al. 2004, **C**; Dougherty 2006, **E**).
Procedure	
7 Wash hands with soap and water, or an alcohol-based handrub, and dry. Open the pack and empty the equipment out onto the sterile field. Keep in mind the principles of aseptic non-touch technique and protect key parts at all times.	To minimize the risk of contamination (DH 2010, **C**; Fraise and Bradley 2009, **E**; Rowley and Clare 2011, **E**).
8 Put on apron and sterile gloves.	To minimize the risk of contamination (DH 2010, **C**).
9 Flush the port needle and extension set with 0.9% sodium chloride.	To check the patency of the needle and set (Dougherty 2006, **E**).
10 Clean the skin over the port with 2% chlorhexidine in 70% alcohol using back-and-forth strokes. Allow to dry.	To minimize the risk of contamination and destroy skin flora (DH 2010, **C**; Loveday et al. 2014, **C**). To ensure disinfection (DH 2010, **C**; Loveday et al. 2014, **C**).
11 Holding the needle in the dominant hand, stabilize the port between the thumb and index finger of the non-dominant hand (**Action figure 10**).	To ensure the port is stabilized and will not move on insertion of the needle (Dougherty 2006, **E**).
12 Inform the patient that you are about to insert the needle.	To prepare the patient for a pushing sensation. **P**, **E**
13 Push the needle through the skin at a perpendicular angle until it hits the back plate.	To ensure the needle is well inserted into the portal septum. **E**
14 Draw back on the syringe and check for blood return.	To check the needle is correctly placed and the port is patent (Camp-Sorrell et al. 2004, **C**; Dougherty 2006, **E**).
15 Flush with 0.9% sodium chloride and observe the site for any swelling or pain.	To check for patency and correct positioning (Camp-Sorrell et al. 2004, **C**; Dougherty 2006, **E**).
16 Administer the drug as required.	To carry out instructions as per the prescription. **E**
17 Flush with 10 mL 0.9% sodium chloride.	To ensure all of the drug is administered (RCN 2016a, **C**).
18 If the needle is to remain *in situ*, attach a needle-free connector and flush with an appropriate flushing solution (e.g. 0.9% sodium chloride or heparinized saline as per local policy) using a pulsatile flush and ending with positive pressure.	To maintain patency (Camp-Sorrell et al. 2004, **C**; Dougherty 2006, **E**; Goossens 2015, **E**).
19 Secure the needle by placing gauze under the needle (if necessary) and cover with a semi-permeable transparent IV film dressing.	To ensure the needle is well supported and will not become dislodged (Camp-Sorrell et al. 2004, **C**; Dougherty 2006, **E**).
20 If the needle is to be removed, lock with appropriate solution (5 mL 0.9% sodium chloride or 500 IU heparin in 5 mL 0.9% sodium chloride as per local policy).	To maintain patency over a longer period of time (Camp-Sorrell et al. 2004, **C**; Dougherty 2006, **E**; Goossens 2015, **E**).
21 Maintain pressure on the plunger as the syringe is disconnected from the injection cap.	To prevent backflow of blood and possible clot formation (Camp-Sorrell et al. 2004, **C**; Dougherty 2006, **E**).
22 Press down on either side of the portal of the implanted port with two fingers.	To support the port while removing the needle (Camp-Sorrell et al. 2004, **C**; Dougherty 2006, **E**).
23 Withdraw the needle using steady traction and activate the safety device where appropriate. Discard the needle in an appropriate sharps container.	To prevent trauma to the skin and reduce the risk of needle stick injury (HSE 2013, **C**).

Post-procedure

	Action	Rationale
24	No dressing is usually required, but a small plaster may be applied.	To prevent oozing at the site. **E**
25	Remove gloves and dispose of waste in the appropriate containers.	To reduce the risk of environmental contamination (DH 2010, **C**).
26	Document the date of access, size and length of needle, number of attempts and any problems encountered in the patient's notes or care plan.	To ensure adequate records are maintained and to enable continued care of the patient and device (NMC 2018, **C**).

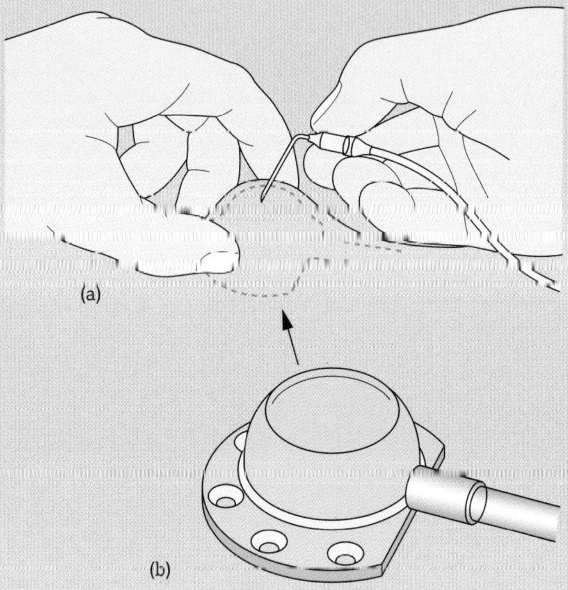

Action Figure 10 Flushing a port.

Problem-solving table 17.6 Prevention and resolution (Procedure guideline 17.13)

Problem	Cause	Prevention	Action
Unable to access port	Incorrect length of needle selected Port too deep or mobile Unable to locate port	Choose the correct length of needle. Skilled practitioners should access difficult ports	Ask for assistance from a colleague to locate the port and help to stabilize it.
Unable to withdraw blood	Needle not in port Fibrin sheath		Realign the needle, or remove it and ask a colleague to access the port. Instil urokinase to remove fibrin.

Post-procedural considerations

Immediate care

Once accessed

The needle should be supported with gauze (if necessary) and covered with a semi-permeable transparent IV film dressing to minimize the risk of needle dislodgement (Camp-Sorrell et al. 2004, Dougherty 2006).

Ongoing care

Regular assessment of the port when it is accessed is essential to check for signs of erythema, swelling or discomfort, which could indicate infection, infiltration or extravasation (Gorski et al. 2016). Most manufacturers recommend that only syringes of 10 mL or larger should be used for drug administration or when flushing; this prevents excessive pressure, which can result in separation of the catheter from the reservoir or rupture if the catheter is occluded (Conn 1993). When the port is accessed, the needle can remain *in situ* for 7 days (Dougherty 2006, Gorski et al. 2010), although Karamanoglu et al. (2003) found that leaving the needle in place for up to 28 days led to no increase in rates of infection or irritation. When not in use, the port only requires flushing once a month (Blackburn and van Boxtel 2012, Gorski et al. 2010, Vescia et al. 2008, Weinstein and Hagle 2014). Some local policies continue to recommend heparinized saline, usually 500 international units heparin in 5 mL 0.9% sodium chloride (Berreth 2013a, Perucca 2010) for intermittent or infrequent use of implanted ports (Kefeli et al. 2009, Palese et al. 2014). However, most guidelines favour the use of 0.9% sodium chloride for flush and lock purposes (Gorski et al. 2016, Loveday et al. 2014, RCN 2016a, Sousa et al. 2015).

Removal

Implanted ports must be removed using surgical technique. After removal, the site must be assessed for any signs of inflammation (Galloway and Bodenham 2004, LaBella and Tang 2012).

Education of the patient and relevant others

Patients can be taught to access their own ports. See 'Discharging patients home with a VAD *in situ*' above.

Complications

These are the same as for other CVADs.

'Twiddler's syndrome'

'Twiddler's syndrome' is a term used to describe patients who nervously touch and potentially dislodge their ports by turning them over so the septum cannot be accessed (Gorski et al. 2010). If this occurs then the port may need to be turned back surgically. Explain to patients who 'twiddle' their ports why it can result in problems.

Arterial cannulas

Definition

An arterial cannula is a plastic tube inserted and secured in a peripheral or central artery. They are most commonly used in intensive care units and during surgery to provide the means for continuous intra-arterial pressure monitoring and facilitate frequent blood sampling for blood gas and laboratory analysis (Koh et al. 2008).

Anatomy and physiology

Arteries are elastic, muscular blood vessels that carry oxygenated blood from the left side of the heart (Jarvis 2018). The large pressure generated by the heart and resistance in the arteries ensure that organs and tissues receive highly oxygenated blood (Scales 2008). The safest and most common peripheral sites for arterial cannulation are the radial artery or dorsalis pedis. If peripheral arterial cannulation is not possible, femoral cannulation is the central site of choice.

Arterial pressure waveforms

The arterial waveform has three separate components that reflect the cardiac cycle (Figure 17.43):

- *upstroke*: the positive deflection occurs at the peak of systole
- *dicrotic notch*: occurs with aortic valve closure and reflects the beginning of diastole
- *end-diastole*: the lowest point of the waveform.

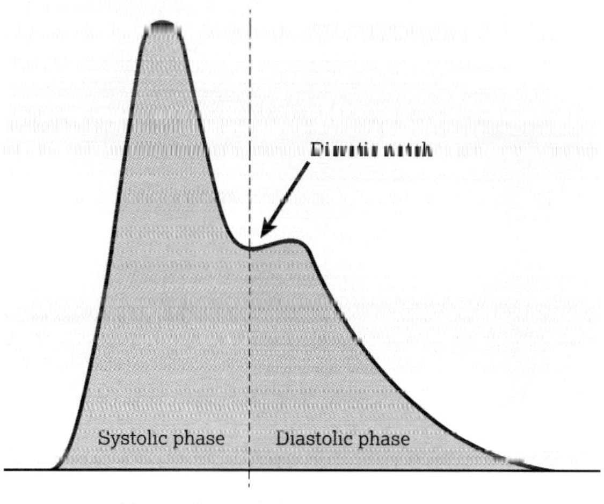

Figure 17.43 Normal arterial trace.

Peripheral artery waveforms differ from central arterial waveforms; their traces have a higher peak systolic pressure, a wider pulse pressure and a more prominent dicrotic notch, described as 'distal pulse amplification' (Azim and Saigal 2016). This is because peripheral arteries are smaller and less compliant than central arteries. Despite ongoing debate about whether central arterial cannulation (e.g. femoral) is superior to peripheral arterial cannulation when monitoring mean arterial blood pressure (MAP), it appears that there is no statistically significant evidence to corroborate this (Mignini et al. 2006).

In addition to the continuous arterial pressure readings, the shape of the arterial waveform can be very informative when assessing the haemodynamic status of a patient. The slope of the arterial upstroke gives an indication of myocardial contractility. Additionally, an exaggerated swing in systolic pressure is seen on the monitor in pulsus paradoxus, a term used when the difference in peak systolic pressure between inspiration and expiration is greater than 10 mmHg. This is caused by:

- pericardial disease, for example cardiac tamponade causing impeded ventricular filling
- exaggerated inspiration by the patient
- changes in intrathoracic pressure caused by lung pathology, such as asthma
- hypovolaemia, particularly when the patient has concurrent high airway pressures.

Evidence-based approaches

Rationale

It is worth noting that morbidity associated with arterial cannulation is less than that associated with five or more arterial punctures (Bersten et al. 2009, Cole and Johnson 2014). An arterial puncture is a one-off insertion of a needle attached to an appropriately heparinized syringe enabling the aspiration of blood from the artery for analysis. Arterial punctures are important and useful in the initial and short-term assessment of acid-base balance and respiratory function. However, multiple puncture attempts will increase the risk of injury, not only due to the direct trauma but also due to vasospasm (Lipsitz 2004). If repetitive blood sampling is necessary, it may be more appropriate to admit the patient into a more clinically suitable area where arterial cannulation is possible. This minimizes both the distress to the patient and the time taken by skilled personnel in obtaining each sample, and it also reduces the risks associated with multiple punctures.

An arterial cannula provides an invaluable tool in providing continuous monitoring of systemic blood pressure and facilitates frequent arterial blood gas (ABG) and laboratory sampling. Arterial cannulation is most commonly achieved and maintained in the critical care and theatre settings (Daud et al. 2013, Mignini et al. 2006). Ideally, prior to obtaining any ABG sample, patients should be in a respiratory steady state for 15 20 minutes. The oxygen should not be titrated, and, if ventilated, suction should not be attempted and ventilation parameters should not be adjusted (Weinstein and Hagle 2014).

The arterial device is attached to a transducer, which enables the mechanical energy of the arterial pressure to be transformed into an electrical signal. This is displayed as a waveform by a haemodynamic monitoring system. An amplifier enhances the signal, which is converted into a digital display and oscilloscope trace (Hazinski 2013). Arterial device tubing should be stiff with low compliance as this prevents the loss of pressure signals through tube expansion.

Indications

Use of an arterial cannula is indicated:

- during and following major anaesthesia
- for monitoring acid/base balance and respiratory status in:
  - acute respiratory failure
  - mechanical ventilation, especially in response to alteration of support and oxygenation

the period during and after cardiorespiratory arrest
- severe sepsis
- shock conditions
- major trauma
- acute poisoning
- acute renal failure
- severe diabetic ketoacidosis
- critically ill patients (Adam et al. 2017).

Contraindications

Use of an arterial cannula is contraindicated in patients with:

- previous upper extremity surgery (harvested for pedicled or free flaps)
- previous axillary clearance
- peripheral vascular disease
- Raynaud's syndrome
- diabetes
- collagen vascular disease
- active upper or lower limb infection (Dodenham et al. 2016).

Principles of care

In critical care, continuous arterial monitoring is invaluable in optimizing and evaluating treatments, particularly in patients receiving intravenous nitrates and inotropes, whose effects on mean blood pressure can be instantaneous, necessitating appropriate titration (Mignini et al. 2006). Arterial devices must be cared for, managed and interpreted by skilled personnel who are able to regularly access areas distal to the cannula, identify accurate waveforms, distinguish artefacts, troubleshoot complications and maintain safe practice (DH 2011, Loveday et al. 2014). The use of arterial devices is limited outside specialized areas due to the hazard of disconnection, the necessary monitoring systems, the potential consequences of severe haemorrhage and the risks associated with accidental intra-arterial drug administration.

Routes of cannulation

Radial arterial cannulation

The radial artery originates from the brachial artery at the neck of the radius and passes along the lateral aspect of the forearm (Jenkins and Tortora 2014). The radial artery gives off multiple fasciocutaneous perforators until it reaches the wrist, where it forms the deep palmar arch. It contributes to the main artery of the thumb and index finger (Wallach 2004). The radial pulse can be felt by gently palpating the radial artery against the underlying muscle and bone (Drake et al. 2005). Cannulation of the radial artery is the most common placement of arterial cannulas (Brezezinski et al. 2009, Mignini et al. 2006) and is performed in most acute care settings. The hand has a good collateral blood supply as the radial artery is near the skin surface; this artery is also readily accessible and easily secured, and the patient is disturbed less than when other sites are used (Adam et al. 2017, Brezezinski et al. 2009, Wallach 2004). Ideally, the cannula should not be positioned close to any intravenous cannulas as this may compromise blood flow around the adjoining structures.

Dorsalis pedis cannulation

The dorsalis pedis originates from the anterior tibial artery and arises at the anterior aspect of the ankle joint (Irwin and Rippe 2013). The dorsalis pedis route for arterial cannulation is no more or less risky than radial cannulation; it is more technically difficult, but it provides a safe and easily available alternative when radial arteries are not accessible (Chen et al. 2016).

Blood pressure measured from the dorsalis pedis and radial artery typically has higher systolic and lower diastolic pressures than centrally measured blood pressure (due to distal amplification), although the mean blood pressure is identical and clinically interchangeable (Mignini et al. 2006). Antiembolic stockings must be adapted to avoid any pressure on the device itself (which may dampen the waveform trace or cause a pressure sore) and also to leave the insertion site visible (Koyfman et al. 2018).

Femoral artery cannulation

The femoral artery may be cannulated if it is not possible to cannulate a peripheral artery. This is particularly useful if the patient is haemodynamically compromised as it can be palpated with relative ease even when there is only a weak pulse (Adam et al. 2017). Lower extremity insertion sites, such as the femoral artery, will increase the risk of infection and should be avoided if possible in favour of the radial artery (O'Horo et al. 2014). Femoral catheters should be positioned at a 45° angle, as there is an increased risk of catheter fracture (Ho et al. 2003). This is a particularly serious risk as there is no collateral blood supply to the leg and lower limb, and as such arterial fracture may have major long-term consequences for the patient (Chim et al. 2015).

Brachial artery cannulation

The brachial artery is the major artery of the arm and divides into the radial and ulnar branches (Irwin and Rippe 2013). A cannula inserted at the antecubital fossa into the brachial artery may risk cannula fracture in conscious patients due to arm flexion. Its placement may also be uncomfortable and cause inconvenience as the patient will be asked to reduce their arm flexion.

Ulnar artery cannulation

The ulnar artery, along with the radial artery, forms the blood supply to the forearm and hand (Irwin and Rippe 2013). It is often avoided as it is usually the dominant artery of the hand, providing the most collateral circulation. Cannulation of the ulnar artery is also technically challenging because of its deeper and more painful course, and its size associates it with more risk of bleeding on removal than the radial artery (Brezezinski et al. 2009). For these reasons the ulnar artery is an unfavourable peripheral site and generally avoided.

Clinical governance

In 2008 the National Patient Safety Agency (NPSA) published a rapid response report that highlighted the many potential errors associated with the use of arterial cannulas. Various recommendations were given and immediate actions mandated to be put in place by January 2009 (Thillainathan and Mariyaselvam 2017) (Box 17.9).

Box 17.9 Actions required by the National Patient Safety Agency when using arterial catheters

- Sampling from arterial devices is risky and should only be undertaken by competent trained staff. Trusts should raise awareness of the risks and review local guidelines. These should include criteria for requests for blood gas analysis, sampling technique, monitoring and interpretation of results (including unexpected findings).
- Arterial infusion sets must be identified clearly. This means labelling or use of safety solutions, such as marked sets, which have been adopted by some trusts.
- Any infusion (or additive) attached to the arterial catheter must be prescribed before administration. Further checks should be made at regular intervals and key points (such as shift handover).
- Staff should only use 0.9% sodium chloride to keep catheters open.
- Labels should clearly identify the contents of the infusion bags, even when pressure bags are used. Over time, the manufacturers should develop a universal system to address this problem.

Source: Adapted from National Patient Safety Agency (www.npsa.nhs.uk). For updates see www.england.nhs.uk.

In order to minimize the risks associated with arterial cannulation, sampling should only be done by competent trained staff (Cole and Johnson 2014, NPSA 2008b).

Pre-procedural considerations

Assessment

It is important prior to any cannulation that the circulation of the hand is assessed: temperature, capillary refill and the colour of the hand (RCN 2016a). The radial artery is the preferred access site because of adequate flow through collateral supply, which prevents ischaemia should either the radial or ulnar artery be interrupted (Handlogten et al. 2014). Although not fully reliable, the Allen test should be completed prior to radial arterial cannulation in order to establish whether there is adequate blood supply to the hand (Figure 17.44). The Allen test consists of simultaneously compressing both the radial and the ulnar arteries for approximately 1 minute (Tegtmeyer et al. 2006, Tiru et al. 2012). During this time, conscious patients rapidly open and close their hand to promote local exsanguination. Approximately 5 seconds after release of one of the arteries (usually the ulnar), the extended hand should blush owing to capillary refilling. If blanching occurs, palmar arch circulation is inadequate and a radial cannula could lead to ischaemia of the hand (Pierce 2006).

Due to the unreliability of the Allen test, ultrasound can be used to assess vessel patency and size (Bodenham et al. 2016, Moussa Pacha et al. 2018). Furthermore, Adam et al. (2017) recommend evaluation by a Doppler probe as the most reliable alternative. Shiloh et al. (2010) suggest that using ultrasound guidance may improve arterial cannulation. Indeed, Gu et al. (2016) advocate that the use of ultrasound reduces the incidence of first-attempt failure of arterial cannulation when compared to palpation alone. However, ultrasound is still not commonly used during arterial cannulation.

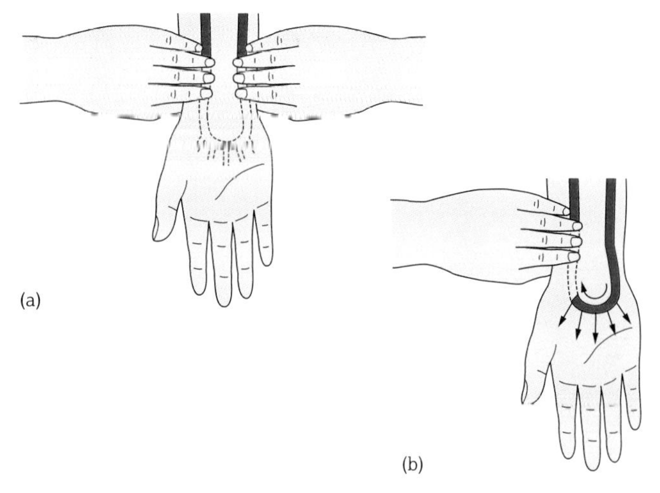

Figure 17.44 The Allen test.

Procedure guideline 17.14 Arterial cannula insertion: preparation and setting up of monitoring set

It is helpful to have an assistant when performing this procedure, if possible.

Essential equipment

- Personal protective equipment
- 500 mL pressure infuser cuff
- Pressure monitoring system equipment
- Designated arterial cannula
- Sterile intravenous pack
- Transparent dressing
- 10 mL syringe
- 5 mL syringe
- 2% chlorhexidine in alcohol swab
- Transpore tape
- Labels
- Trolley

Medicinal products

- 500 mL bag of 0.9% sodium chloride
- 1% lidocaine injection

Action	Rationale
Pre-procedure	
1 Introduce yourself to the patient, explain and discuss the procedure with them, and gain their consent to proceed.	To ensure that the patient feels at ease, understands the procedure and gives their valid consent (NMC 2018, **C**). *Note:* many patients are anaesthetized when arterial devices are inserted.
2 Wash hands with soap and water, or an alcohol-based handrub, and dry.	To minimize the risk of infection (DH 2010, **E**; NHS England and NHSI 2019, **C**).
3 Prepare the infusion and transducer sets using aseptic technique.	To minimize the risk of infection (DH 2010, **E**; Loveday et al. 2014, **C**).
4 Check that all Luer-Lok connections are secure.	To prevent disconnection, as equipment is often loose when taken straight from the packaging. **E**

Procedure

Action	Rationale
5 Connect the transducer to a 500 mL bag of 0.9% sodium chloride, which must be prescribed.	To prepare the infusion; saline is more effective than heparinized flush (Gamby and Bennett 1995, **R**; Kulkarni et al. 1994, **R**; O'Grady et al. 2011, **C**). Only 0.9% sodium chloride must be used as flush (NPSA 2008b, **C**). To prime the administration set and three-way tap ports. **E**
6 Open the roller clamp fully and squeeze the flush device actuator (see instructions with set).	To reduce the risk of air embolism, although retrograde air embolism is a rare event after routine radial artery cannula flushing. **E**
7 Check thoroughly for air bubbles in the circuit.	To reduce the risk of inaccurate pressure readings caused by bubbles in the set (Daily and Schroeder 1994, **R**).
8 Insert the bag into the pressure infuser, and inflate the pressure bag to 300 mmHg. An automatic flush mode is activated within the system, which delivers 3 mL per hour, which maintains the patency of the cannula.	To prevent backpressure of blood into the transducer set by ensuring the pressure is higher than the arterial blood pressure (Morton and Fontaine 2009, **R**).
9 Wash hands with soap and water, or an alcohol-based handrub, and dry.	To reduce the risk of cross-infection (DH 2010, **C**; NHS England and NHSI 2019, **C**).
10 Prepare a trolley near the patient.	To reduce the risk of cross-infection (DH 2010, **C**; Loveday et al. 2014, **E**).
11 Complete the Allen test (see Figure 17.44) if the radial artery is to be used.	To assess whether palmar arch circulation is adequate, although this assessment is not entirely reliable (Valgimigli et al. 2014, Wallach 2004, **R**).
12 Prepare the insertion site with a 2% chlorhexidine in 70% alcohol swab and place a sterile towel under the appropriate area.	To maintain asepsis. To provide a clean working area (DH 2010, **C**). To minimize the risk of infection (Loveday et al. 2014, **E**).
13 Administer adequate local anaesthetic.	To minimize pain during the procedure; this may reduce sudden movements by the patient, which could result in through-puncture (Lipsitz 2004, **R**; Zinchenko et al. 2016, **R**). Local vasodilation effects of the local anaesthetic may reduce vasospasm, making a successful cannulation more likely (Lipsitz 2004, **R**).
14 Put on gloves.	To prevent contamination of hands if blood spillage occurs (Loveday et al. 2014, **C**).
15 Another nurse may act as an assistant and hold the patient's foot or arm. If the radial artery is cannulated, the wrist must be hyperextended. Promptly return the wrist to the neutral position following cannulation.	To prevent movement and to flex the hand or foot slightly to facilitate insertion. **E** Prolonged hyperextension may be associated with changes in median nerve conduction (Chowet et al. 2004, **R**).
16 Insert the cannula and observe for blood flashback.	To ascertain that the cannula is in the artery. **E**
17 Attach the transducer set and fully open the roller clamp.	To commence the flush infusion system and prevent backflow of blood. **E**
18 Apply a transparent dressing over the cannula and tape the tubing securely.	To leave the site visible and secure, and to allow observers to immediately recognize any dislodgement, inflammation or disconnection (Healy et al. 2018, **E**).
19 Clearly label the device as arterial, on the dressing as well as on the tubing.	To ensure the device is not mistaken for a venous cannula, preventing accidental intra-arterial injection of drugs (**E**), particularly if the tubing is disconnected and the cannula capped off in the event of a transfer (NPSA 2008b, **C**), although this practice should be discouraged.
20 Loop the tubing around the thumb, ensuring this is not too tight (**Action figure 20**).	To minimize movement of the cannula and damage to the vessel, and to prevent ulcer formation. **E**
21 Connect the transducer to the monitoring equipment.	To allow the arterial waveform to be checked and to obtain continuous blood pressure measurements. **E**
22 Calibrate the arterial device (the transducer will read an arterial pressure calibrated to atmospheric air, which offsets the extraneous atmospheric and hydrostatic pressures).	To make sure that readings are accurate. **E**

Post-procedure

Action	Rationale
23 Remove gloves and dispose of equipment and clinical waste appropriately.	To prevent sharps injury (NHS Employers 2015, **C**).
24 Clearly document the date of insertion and the placement of the arterial cannula in the patient's records.	To maintain accurate records and provide appropriate reference (NMC 2018, **C**).

(continued)

Procedure guideline 17.14 Arterial cannula insertion: preparation and setting up of monitoring set *(continued)*

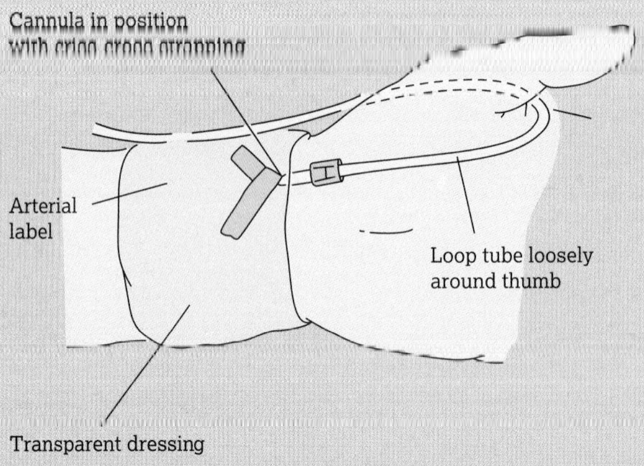

Action Figure 20 Positioning, securing and labelling the cannula.

Post-procedural considerations

Ongoing care

Arterial cannulas are not replaced routinely so frequent and accurate assessment is essential in order to minimize complications. In the event of a spike in temperature and raised inflammatory markers, removal may be considered.

The arterial cannula site must be assessed at regular intervals to check for appropriate labelling of the device, use of the correct flush fluid, and any pain or erythema at the site. The arterial site should (where appropriate) be left exposed to minimize any delay in detecting dislodgement of the device or exsanguination from the artery. There should always be vigilance if the sample taken from the arterial cannula is not within the expected range, and staff must be trained in considering and eliminating any risk of contamination as this may affect blood results, which could in turn determine changes in consequent therapies. The NPSA (2008b) described a number of serious incidents associated with changes in treatment directly related to arterial blood sampling results. These incidents occurred because of the use of inappropriate flush agents, predominantly dextrose; for example, patients had insulin sliding-scale infusions titrated in response to contaminated samples where blood glucose was abnormally high and not reflective of the patient's actual serum glucose.

The following volumes of blood should be withdrawn and discarded in order to clear 0.9% sodium chloride, old blood and small emboli from the dead space, the cannula and the three-way tap:

- *Peripheral artery cannula*: generally, 3–5 mL must be taken and discarded.
- *Femoral artery cannula*: these devices are longer and commonly 5 mL should be taken and discarded, but always check the manufacturer's instructions.

On each shift it is advisable that the following are checked and documented:

- site of the cannulated artery
- appropriate flush agent prescribed
- labelling is appropriate
- any pain or colour changes distal to the cannula.

Arterial administration sets should be replaced every 24–72 hours, depending on local policy (Daud et al. 2013, Loveday et al. 2014).

Procedure guideline 17.15 Arterial cannula: removal

Essential equipment

- Personal protective equipment
- Sterile dressing pack
- Hypoallergenic tape
- 2% chlorhexidine in 70% alcohol swab
- Trolley

Action	Rationale
Pre-procedure	
1 Introduce yourself to the patient, explain and discuss the procedure with them, and gain their consent to proceed.	To ensure that the patient feels at ease, understands the procedure and gives their valid consent (NMC 2018, **C**).
2 Check the patient's platelet and coagulation screen.	To prevent delay in removal while coagulation is corrected. **E**
3 Prepare a trolley.	To reduce the risk of cross-infection (DH 2010, **C**; Fraise and Bradley 2009, **E**).

4 Wash hands with soap and water, or an alcohol-based handrub, and dry before leaving the clinical room.	To reduce the risk of cross-infection (DH 2010, **C**; Fraise and Bradley 2009, **E**).
Procedure	
5 Turn the three-way tap diagonally or turn off the flow switch, depending on the arterial product.	To prevent backflow of blood into the cannula. **E**
6 Turn off the flush set.	To prevent spillage when removing the cannula. **E**
7 Deflate the pressure cuff.	Pressure is no longer required. **E**
8 Loosen the transparent dressing and tape from the cannula site.	To facilitate removal of the cannula. **E**
9 Clean hands with an alcohol-based handrub.	To minimize the risk of infection (DH 2010, **C**; Fraise and Bradley 2009, **E**).
10 Apply gloves.	To prevent contamination of hands with blood (Loveday et al. 2014, **C**).
11 Remove dressing and tape. Clean the cannula site area with a 2% chlorhexidine in 70% alcohol swab.	To reduce the risk of infection (DH 2010, **C**; Fraise and Bradley 2009, **E**).
12 Place sterile gauze over the area and gently remove the cannula.	To minimize bleeding and blood spillage (Loveday et al. 2014, **C**).
13 Apply pressure for a minimum of 5 minutes.	To prevent haematoma and blood loss (RCN 2016a, **C**).
14 Apply a clean, sterile, low-linting gauze dressing.	To maintain asepsis and minimize blood loss. **E**
15 Secure with tape. Do not create a tourniquet-type dressing.	To ensure pressure and to prevent haematoma and blood loss. **E**
Post-procedure	
16 Remove gloves and dispose of equipment appropriately.	To prevent sharps injury (NHS Employers 2015, **C**).
17 Document the date and time of removal in the patient's notes.	To ensure adequate records are maintained and enable continued care of the patient (NMC 2018, **C**).

Problem-solving table 17.7 Prevention and resolution (Procedure guideline 17.15)

Problem	Cause	Prevention	Action
Backflow of blood into the cannula	The pressure infusor cuff may not be inflated to the optimum level	Ensure that the pressure infusor cuff is inflated to 300 mmHg.	Check that the pressure infusor cuff is inflated to 300 mmHg and, if not, inflate it to the correct level.
Arterial spasm	Forceful flushing or forceful aspiration when withdrawing blood	When the flushing pressure is higher than arterial blood pressure, an automatic flush mode is activated in the system that delivers 3 mL per hour. This maintains the patency of the circuit, cannula and artery (Allan 1984).	Check that the pressure infusor cuff is inflated to 300 mmHg and, if not, inflate it to the correct level.
Cerebral embolism	Prolonged, high-pressure flushing can drive a clot or gas bubbles retrograde to produce cerebral embolism	Avoid forceful flushing or aspiration and maintain slow, even pressure when withdrawing blood.	Check that the pressure infusor cuff is inflated to 300 mmHg and, if not, inflate it to the correct level.

Removal of an arterial cannula

Post-procedural considerations

Immediate care

Following the procedure, check the patient's hand, and assess and document the temperature, colour, swelling and any signs of bleeding. Avoid taking blood pressure measurement manually on the arm where the arterial cannula was removed for 12–24 hours to minimize bleeding or haematoma formation. Medical staff must be informed immediately if the hand or forearm becomes discoloured or swollen, or if the patient complains of pain in the limb. In the event of any complication, careful documentation is essential; consider a request for medical photography of the affected area.

Specific patient preparation

Education

Ask the patient to apply pressure if they notice any oozing from the dressing and immediately inform a member of staff.

Complications

There are a number of complications that can occur as a result of arterial cannulation: see Box 17.10.

Infections

If the arterial device is inserted under emergency conditions and asepsis has been compromised, O'Grady et al. (2011) recommend that the cannula should be replaced within 24 hours. Colonization

Box 17.10 Complications of arterial cannulation

- Vascular thrombosis
- Distal embolization (see Box 17.11)
- Proximal embolization: digital ischaemia
- Local or systemic infection
- Vascular spasm
- Skin necrosis of the catheter site due to accidental intra-arterial injection
- Hypovolaemia secondary to accidental disconnection
- Cannula fracture or breakage
- Pseudo-aneurysm formation
- Median nerve palsy (Bersten et al. 2009)
- Damage to nearby structures

Box 17.11 Treatment of distal embolism

- Remove the cannula
- Arrange for Doppler imaging
- After consultation with a consultant, heparinize (if no contraindications)
- Consider a peripheral vasodilator

and infection of arterial devices are rare (Minnaganti and Cunha 2000) and are usually related to duration of cannulation. However, arterial cannulas do represent a potential source of bloodstream infection that is often underappreciated (O'Horo et al. 2014).

Historically, arterial cannulas were associated with a significantly lower risk of local cannula-related infection when compared to short-term peripheral venous cannulas that had been left *in situ* for the equivalent length of time. Despite a common risk of catheter colonization, serious soft tissue infections are very rare, which may be related to exposure to high vascular pressures and subsequent local turbulence experienced in arterial cannulas (Koh et al. 2008, O'Grady et al. 2011, RCN 2016a). Additionally, if the puncture site is well stabilized and treated with asepsis and all samples are obtained using aseptic technique, this will further minimize the risk of soft tissue infection (Marini and Wheeler 2010). However, more recent studies have begun to challenge this assertion and suggest that the infection risks of arterial cannulas are actually comparable to those of central venous catheters (Gowardman et al. 2010, O'Horo et al. 2014). The site of arterial cannulation has relevance in preventing possible infection, and it is advisable to avoid the femoral site, when feasible (O'Horo et al. 2014). Regular observation of the arterial cannula insertion site is imperative to identify signs of inflammation, which may predispose patients to cannula-related infection. Leaving cannulas *in situ* for more than 4 days increases the risk of infection (O'Grady et al. 2011, O'Horo et al. 2014).

There is the potential for administration sets attached to the arterial device to provide pathways for micro-organisms into the bloodstream, exposing the patient to catheter-related bloodstream infections (CRBSIs). Current practices related to changing the administration sets of arterial devices are based on the Saving Lives guidelines for infections in central venous devices (DH 2010); they advocate changing sets every 72 hours (Loveday et al. 2014). There are no specific recommendations set out by any British governing body for when to change administration sets in peripheral artery devices. In a systematic review (mainly of Canadian and American studies), it was clearly found that practices around routinely changing arterial administration sets ranged from 24 to 96 hours (Daud et al. 2013). There is some evidence to suggest that changing the administration set between 24 and 72 hours is associated with less risk of infection among critically ill patients but there is not enough evidence to suggest a definitive lifetime of the sets (Daud et al. 2013).

Hypovolaemia

Hypovolaemia can occur as a result of severe haemorrhage, which can be caused by (a) accidental disconnection of tubing from the cannula or from one of the connections within the system or (b) dislodgement of the cannula.

The flow from an 18 G cannula can result in blood loss of 350 mL per minute (Bersten et al. 2009). Unconscious or delirious patients and children are at particular risk. The risk can be minimized by clearly labelling the arterial cannula (Zideman and Morgan 1981), ensuring that arterial tubing and sets are predominantly red in colour, and ensuring that alarm settings on the monitor are turned on and audible (Adam et al. 2017). Further ways of reducing the risk of this complication occurring include the use of Luer-Lok connections, ensuring visibility of the cannula, appropriate nurse–patient ratios, and adequate training and competency of nurses caring for patients with arterial cannulas.

The cannula may become dislodged, particularly if the patient is diaphoretic, in which case dressings tend to lift. Securing the cannula using an appropriate cannula-securing device may be useful. Inform the patient about the danger of dislodging the cannula and the amount of movement that is preferred. Staff must also take care when moving the patient, and avoid putting stress on the arm and connections. Ideally, non-invasive blood pressure readings should not be taken on the same arm as the arterial cannula. Marini and Wheeler (2010) recommend attempting a minimum of once-daily sphygmomanometry in order to confirm cannula pressure, especially in patients whose vasopressors are titrated to these pressures, and particularly in those patients who are elderly, are hypertensive or have underlying vascular disease.

Accidental intra-arterial injection of drugs

Accidental intra-arterial injection of drugs intended for administration through a central or peripheral venous device may cause distal ischaemia and necrosis, sometimes resulting in permanent functional damage (Marieb and Hoehn 2018, Teplitz 1990, Tinker and Zapol 1992). Drugs such as calcium channel blockers and vasopressors are particularly harmful if injected intra-arterially (Marini and Wheeler 2010). Careful and appropriate labelling and appropriate staff training can minimize this risk. In the event of accidental injection of any drug, stop administering the drug and immediately report the incident to medical staff and the senior nurse. The nurse should then attempt to withdraw blood from the three-way tap in order to aspirate any of the drug. Then assess the limb pulse, colour and temperature hourly, or more frequently if required, and complete an accident form and/or other relevant documentation.

Ischaemia

Radial artery catheterization is considered a relatively safe procedure with an incidence of permanent ischaemic complications of only 0.09% (Chim et al. 2015, Scheer et al. 2002). However, it is believed that many cases of hand ischaemia go unreported and hence it remains difficult to estimate its true incidence (Brezezinski et al. 2009). Local damage to the artery is the most common complication of arterial cannulation (Marieb and Hoehn 2018). Cannulation for as little as 6 hours has been associated with arterial wall scarring (Brezezinski et al. 2009). Regular close inspection and assessment of the limb and areas distal to the cannula must be carried out as there is a risk of thrombosis and embolism. Arterial catheter-related ischaemia can present as:

- absent pulse
- dampened waveform
- mottled or blanched skin
- delayed capillary refill
- painful or cold hand
- motor weakness.

To minimize such risks, cannulation of the non-dominant hand should be attempted whenever possible (Wallach 2004).

The medical team should be informed if any of the above are discovered (Adam et al. 2017). If a distal embolism is suspected, the cannula may have to be removed and limb warming attempted in order to avoid permanent damage (see Box 17.11). The risk of ischaemia distal to the cannula is increased when it is associated with low cardiac output, shock, sepsis or prolonged cannulation (Bersten et al. 2009, Gamby and Bennett 1995).

References

Adam, S.K., Osborne, S. & Welch, J. (2017) *Critical Care Nursing: Science and Practice*, 3rd edn. Oxford: Oxford University Press.

Ahlqvist, M., Berglund, B., Norsdtrom, G., et al. (2010) A new reliable tool (PVC access) for assessment of peripheral venous catheters. *Journal of Evaluation in Clinical Practice*, 16(6), 1108–1115.

Alexandrou, E. (2014) The One Million Global Catheters PIVC worldwide prevalence study. *British Journal of Nursing*, 23(8), S16–S17.

Alexandrou, E., Ramjan, L.M., Spencer, T., et al. (2011) The use of midline catheters in the adult acute care setting: Clinical implications and recommendations for practice. *Journal of the Association for Vascular Access*, 16(1), 35–41.

Alexandrou, E., Ray-Barruel, G., Carr, P.J., et al. (2015) International prevalence of the use of peripheral intravenous catheters. *Journal of Hospital Medicine*, 10(18), 530–533.

Alexandrou, E., Ray-Barruel, G., Carr, P.J., et al. (2018) Use of short peripheral intravenous catheters: Characteristics, management and outcomes worldwide. *Journal of Hospital Medicine*, 13(5). DOI: 10.12788/jhm.3039.

Alexandrou, E., Spencer, T., Frost, S.A., et al. (2010a) Establishing a nurse-led central venous catheter insertion service. *Journal of the Association for Vascular Access*, 15(1), 21–27.

Alexandrou, E., Spencer, T., Frost, S.A., et al. (2010b) A review of the nursing role in central venous cannulation: Implications for practice policy and research. *Journal of Clinical Nursing*, 19(11/12), 1485–1495.

Allan, D. (1984) Care of the patient with an arterial catheter. *Nursing Times*, 80(46), 40–44.

Anderson, S., Cockrell, J., Beller, P., et al. (2010) Administration of local anesthetic agents to decrease pain associated with peripheral vascular access. *Journal of Infusion Nursing*, 33(6), 353–361.

Andreatta, P., Chen, Y., Marsh, M. & Cho, K. (2011) Simulation-based training improves applied clinical placement of ultrasound-guided PICCs. *Supportive Care in Cancer*, 19(4), 539–543.

Andrews, G.J. (2011) 'I had to go to the hospital and it was freaking me out': Needle phobic encounter space. *Health Place*, 17(4), 875–884.

Andrews, G.J. & Shaw, D. (2010) 'So we started talking about a beach in Barbados': Visualization practices and needle phobia. *Social Science & Medicine*, 71(10), 1804–1810.

Aw, A., Carrier, M., Koczerginski, J., et al. (2012) Incidence and predictive factors of symptomatic thrombosis related to peripherally inserted central catheters in chemotherapy patients. *Thrombosis Research*, 130(3), 323–326.

Azim, A. & Saigal, S. (2016) Arterial blood sampling and cannulation. In: Gurjor, M. (ed) *Manual of ICU Procedures*. Philadelphia: Jaypee Brothers Medical Publishers, pp.298–308.

Baranowski, L. (1993) Central venous access devices: Current technologies, uses, and management strategies. *Journal of Intravenous Nursing*, 16(3), 167–194.

Barbetakis, N., Asteriou, C., Kleontas, A. & Tsilikas, C. (2011) Totally implantable central venous access ports: Analysis of 700 cases. *Journal of Surgical Oncology*, 104(6), 654–656.

Bartock, L. (2010) An evidence-based systematic review of literature for the reduction of PICC line occlusions. *Journal of the Association for Vascular Access*, 15(2), 58–63.

Barton, A. (2016) Confirming PICC tip position during insertion with real-time information. *British Journal of Nursing*, 25(2), S17–S21.

Barton, A. (2018) Clinical use of closed-system safety peripheral intravenous cannulas. *British Journal of Nursing*, 27(8), S22–S27.

Baskin, J.L., Pui, C.H., Reiss, U., et al. (2009) Management of occlusion and thrombosis associated with long-term indwelling central venous catheters. *Lancet*, 374(9684), 159–169.

Baskin, J.L., Reiss, U., Wilimas, J.A., et al. (2012) Thrombolytic therapy for central venous catheter occlusion. *Haematologica*, 97(5), 641–650.

Bassetti, S., Hu, J., D'Agostino, R.B. Jr., et al. (2001) Prolonged antimicrobial activity of a catheter containing chlorhexidine-silver sulfadiazine extends protection against catheter infections in vivo. *Antimicrobial Agents and Chemotherapy*, 45(5), 1535–1538.

Bassi, K.K., Giri, A., Pattanayak, M., et al. (2012) Totally implantable venous access ports: Retrospective review of long term complications of 81 patients. *Indian Journal of Cancer*, 49(1), 114–118.

Bausone-Gazda, D., Lefaiver, C.A. & Walters, S.A. (2010) A randomized controlled trial to compare the complications of 2 peripheral intravenous catheter-stabilization systems. *Journal of Infusion Nursing*, 33(6), 371–384.

Beckers, M.M., Ruven, H., Seldenrijk, C., et al. (2010) Risk of thrombosis and infections of central venous catheters and totally implanted access ports in patients treated for cancer. *Thrombosis Research*, 125(4), 318–321.

Benton, S. & Marsden, C. (2002) Training nurses to place tunnelled central venous catheters. *Professional Nurse*, 17(9), 531–533.

Berger, L. (2000) The effects of positive pressure devices on catheter occlusions. *Journal of Vascular Access Devices*, 5(4), 31–34.

Berreth, M. (2013a) Clinical concepts of infusion therapy: Flushing and locking – Part 2. *INS Newsline*, 35(1), 6–7.

Berreth, M. (2013b) Clinical concepts of infusion therapy: Vein visualisation technology. *INS-Newsline*, 35(2), 6–7.

Bersten, A.D., Soni, N. & Oh, T.E. (2009) *Oh's Intensive Care Manual*, 6th edn. Oxford: Butterworth Heinemann.

Bertoglio, S., Solari, N., Meszaros, P., et al. (2012) Efficacy of normal saline versus heparinized saline solution for locking catheters of totally implantable long-term central vascular access devices in adult cancer patients. *Cancer Nursing*, 35(4), E35–E42.

Biffi, R. (2012a) Pneumothorax. In: Di Carlo, I. & Biffi, R. (eds) *Totally Implantable Venous Access Devices*. Milan: Springer, pp.107–114.

Biffi, R. (2012b) Power technology: How to use ports and central catheters to deliver contrast medium in radiology procedures. In: Di Carlo, I. & Biffi, R. (eds) *Totally Implantable Venous Access Devices*. Milan: Springer, pp.239–246.

Biffi, R., Orsi, F., Pozzi, S., et al. (2011) No impact of central venous insertion site on oncology patients' quality of life and psychological distress: A randomized three-arm trial. *Supportive Care in Cancer*, 19(10), 1573–1580.

Biffi, R., Toro, A., Pozzi, S., et al. (2014) Totally implantable vascular access devices 30 years after the first procedure. What has changed and what is still unsolved? *Supportive Care Cancer*, 22, 1705–1714.

Bishop, L. (2009) Aftercare and management of central access devices. In: Hamilton, H. & Bodenham, A. (eds) *Central Venous Catheters*. Oxford: John Wiley & Sons, pp.221–237.

Bjeletich, J. & Hickman, R.O. (1980) The Hickman indwelling catheter. *American Journal of Nursing*, 80(1), 62–65.

Bitmead, J. & Oliver, G. (2018) A safe procedure: Best practice for intravenous peripheral cannulation. *British Journal of Nursing*, 27(2), S1–S8.

Blackburn, P.L. (2014) Vessel health and preservation. In: Sandrucci, S. & Mussa, B. (eds) *Peripherally Inserted Central Venous Catheters*. Milan: Springer, pp.21–29.

Blackburn, P.L. & van Boxtel, T. (2012) Nursing of vascular access: Highlights of hot issues. In: Di Carlo, I. & Biffi, R. (eds) *Totally Implantable Venous Access Devices*. Milan: Springer, pp.227–230.

BNF (British National Formulary) (2019) *British National Formulary*. National Institute for Health and Care Excellence. Available at: https://bnf.nice.org.uk

Bodenham, A., Babu, S., Bennett, J., et al. (2016) Association of Anaethetists of Great Britain and Ireland: Safe vascular access 2016. *Anaesthesia*, 71(5), 573–585.

Bodenham, A.R. & Simcock, L. (2009) Complications of central venous access. In: Hamilton, H. & Bodenham, A. (eds) *Central Venous Catheters*. Oxford: John Wiley & Sons, pp.175–205.

Boeson, M.B., Hranchook, A. & Stoller, J. (2000) Peripheral nerve injury from intravenous cannulation: A case report. *AANA Journal*, 68(1), 53–57.

Boland, A., Haycox, A., Bagust, A. & Fitzsimmons, L. (2003) A randomised controlled trial to evaluate the clinical and cost-effectiveness of Hickman line insertions in adult cancer patients by nurses. *Health Technology Assessment*, 7(36), iii, ix–x, 1–99.

Bolton, D. (2013) Preventing occlusion and restoring patency to central venous catheters. *British Journal of Community Nursing*, 18(11), 539–544.

Bow, E.J., Kilpatrick, M.G. & Clinch, J.J. (1999) Totally implantable venous access ports systems for patients receiving chemotherapy for solid tissue malignancies: A randomized controlled clinical trial examining the safety, efficacy, costs, and impact on quality of life. *Journal of Clinical Oncology*, 17(4), 1267.

Brezezinski, M., Thomas, L. & Martin, J. (2009) Radial artery cannulation: a comprehensive review of recent anatomic and physiological interventions. *Anesthesia & Analgesia*, 109(6), 1763–1781.

Broadhurst, D., Moureau, N. & Ullman, A.J. (2017) Management of central venous access devices-associated skin impairment: An evidence based algorithm. *Journal of Wound, Ostomy and Continence Nursing*, 44(3), 211–220.

Brockmeyer, J., Simon, T., Seery, J., et al. (2009) Cerebral air embolism following removal of central venous catheters. *Military Medicine*, 174(8), 878–881.

Brown, J. & Larson, M. (1999) Pain during insertion of peripheral intravenous catheters with and without intradermal lidocaine. *Clinical Nurse Specialist*, 13(6), 283–285.

Brown, J.D., Moss, H.A. & Elliott, T.S. (1997) The potential for catheter microbial contamination from a needleless connector. *Journal of Hospital Infection*, 36(3), 181–189.

Browne, J., Awad, I., Plant, R., et al. (1999) Topical ametocaine (Ametop) is superior to EMLA for intravenous cannulation. *Canadian Journal of Anesthesia*, 46(11), 1014–1018.

Btaiche, I.F., Kovacevich, D.S., Khalidi, N. & Papke, L.F. (2011) The effects of needleless connectors on catheter-related bloodstream infection. *American Journal of Infection Control*, 39(4), 277–283.

Bullock-Corkhill, M. (2010) Central venous access devices: Access and insertion. In: Alexander, M., Corrigan, A., Gorski, L., et al. (eds) *Infusion Nursing: An Evidence-Based Approach*, 3rd edn. St Louis, MO: Saunders Elsevier, pp.480–494.

Burbridge, B. & Goyal, K. (2016) Quality of life assessment: Arm TIVAD versus chest TIVAD. *Journal of Vascular Access*, 17(6), 527–534.

Burnett, S., Cooke, M., Deelchand, V., et al. (2010) *Evidence in Brief: How Safe Are Clinical Systems? Primary Research into the Reliability of Systems within Seven NHS Organisations and Ideas for Improvement.* London: Health Foundation.

Busch, J., Hermann, J., Heller, F., et al. (2012) Follow-up of radiologically totally implanted central venous access ports of the upper arm: Long term complications in 127750 catheter days. *American Journal of Roentgenology*, 199(2), 447–452.

Camp-Sorrell, D., Cope, D.G. & Oncology Nursing Society (2004) *Access Device Guidelines: Recommendations for Nursing Practice and Education*, 2nd edn. Pittsburgh: Oncology Nursing Society.

Caparas, J.V. & Hu, J.-P. (2014) Safe administration of vancomycin through a novel midline catheter: A randomized, prospective clinical trial. *Journal of Vascular Access*, 15(4), 251–256.

Carlson, K.R. (1999) Correct utilization and management of peripherally inserted central catheters and midline catheters in the alternate care setting. *Journal of Intravenous Nursing*, 22(6 Suppl.), S46–S50.

Carr, P.J., Higgins, N.S., Cooke, M.L., et al. (2017) Tools, clinical prediction rules, and algorithms for the insertion of peripheral intravenous catheters in adult hospitalised patients: A systematic scoping review of literature. *Journal of Hospital Medicine*, 12(10), 851–858.

Carr, P.J., Higgins, N.S., Cooke, M.L., et al. (2018) Vascular access specialist teams for device insertion and prevention of failure. *Cochrane Database of Systematic Reviews*, 3, CD011429.

Casey, A.L. & Elliott, T.S. (2010) Prevention of central venous catheter-related infection. Update. *British Journal of Nursing*, 19(2), 78–87.

Casey, A.L., Karpanen, T.J., Nightingale, P., et al. (2018) The risk of microbial contamination associated with six different needle free connectors. *British Journal of Nursing*, 27(2), S18–S26.

Cerri, R. (2014) Peripheral inserted central catheters: Medico-legal aspects. In: Sandrucci, S. & Mussa, B. (eds) *Peripherally Inserted Central Catheters*. Milan: Springer, pp.155–164.

CET (NHS Clinical Evaluation Team) (2018) *Clinical Review: Intravenous Vapour Permeable Film Dressings (IV Films) – Part One: Securing Peripheral Cannulae in Adults.* NHS Clinical Evaluation Team. Available at: https://wwwmedia.supplychain.nhs.uk/media/Clinical-Review-for-IV-Film-Dressings-March-2018.pdf

Chantler, J. (2009) Applied anatomy of the central veins. In: Hamilton, H. & Bodenham, A. (eds) *Central Venous Catheters*. Oxford: John Wiley & Sons, pp.14–33.

Chen, B.H. (2002) Active hand warming eases peripheral intravenous catheter insertion. *BMJ*, 325, 409–410.

Chen, Y., Cui, J., Sun, J.J., et al. (2016) Gradient between dorsalis pedis and radial arterial blood pressures during sevoflurane anaesthesia: A self-control study in patients undergoing neurosurgery. *European Journal of Anaesthesiology*, 33(2), 110–117.

Chernecky, C. (2001) Satisfaction versus dissatisfaction with venous access devices in outpatient oncology: A pilot study. *Oncology Nursing Forum*, 28(10), 1613–1616.

Chernecky, C., Macklin, D., Casella, L., et al. (2009) Caring for patients with cancer through nursing knowledge of IV connectors. *Clinical Journal of Oncology Nursing*, 13(6), 630–633.

Chernecky, C. & Walker, J. (2011) Comparative evaluation of five needleless intravenous connectors. *Journal of Advanced Nursing*, 67(7), 1601–1613.

Chim, H., Bahkri, K. & Moran, S.L. (2015) Complications related to radial artery occlusion, radial artery harvest, and arterial lines. *Hand Clinics*, 31(1), 93–100.

Chittle, M.D., Oklu, R., Pino, R.M., et al. (2016) Sedation shared decision-making in ambulatory venous access device placement: Effects on patient choice, satisfaction and recovery time. *Vascular Medicine*, 21(4), 355–360.

Chopra, V., Flanders, S.A., Saint, S., et al. (2015) The Michigan Appropriateness Guide for Intravenous Catheters (MAGIC): Results from a multispeciality panel using RAND/UCLA appropriateness method. *Annals of Internal Medicine*, 163(6), S1–S40.

Chopra, V., Smith, S., Swaminathan, L., et al. (2016) Variations in peripherally inserted central catheter use and outcomes in Michigan hospitals. *Journal of the American Medical Association*, 176(4), 548–551.

Chowet, A.L., Lopez, J.R., Brock-Utne, J.G., et al. (2004) Wrist hyperextension leads to median nerve conduction block: Implications for intra-arterial catheter placement. *Anesthesiology*, 100(2), 287–291.

Cobbett, S. & LeBlanc, A. (2000) Minimising IV site infection while saving time and money. *Australian Infection Control*, 5, 8–14.

Cole, K.E. & Johnson, L.M. (2014) Impact of improving patient access time: Arterial cannulation. *Intensive Critical Care Nursing*, 30(3), 167–174.

Collins, M., Phillips, S., Dougherty, L., et al. (2006) A structured learning programme for venepuncture and cannulation. *Nursing Standard*, 20(26), 34–40.

Conn, C. (1993) The importance of syringe size when using an implanted vascular access device. *Journal of Vascular Access Networks*, 3(1), 11–18.

Connolly, B., Amaral, J., Walsh, S., et al. (2006) Influence of arm movement on central tip location of peripherally inserted central catheters (PICCs). *Pediatric Radiology*, 36(8), 845–850.

Conway, M.A., McCollom, C. & Bannon, C. (2014) Central venous catheter flushing recommendations: A systematic evidenced-based practice review. *Journal of Pediatric Oncology Nursing*, 31(4), 185–190.

Cook, L.S. (2013) Infusion-related air embolism. *Journal of Infusion Nursing*, 36(1), 26–36.

Cooper, A.L., Kelly, C.M. & Brown, J.A. (2017) Exploring the patient experience of living with a peripherally inserted central catheter (PICC): A pilot study. *Australian Journal of Cancer Nursing*, 10(1), 10–14.

Corley, A., Marsh, N., Ullman, A.J., et al. (2017) Tissue adhesive for vascular access devices: Who, what, where and when? *British Journal of Nursing*, 26(19), S4–S17.

Corrigan, A. (2010) Infusion therapy in children. In: Alexander, M. & Corrigan, A. (eds) *Infusion Nursing as a Specialty*, 3rd edn. St Louis, MO: Saunders Elsevier, pp.1–9.

Costa, N. & Ferguson, E. (2002) Placement of triple lumen peripherally inserted central catheters in critical patients. *Journal of Vascular Access Devices*, 7(4), 27–30.

Couban, S., Goodyear, M., Burnell, M., et al. (2005) Randomized placebo-controlled study of low-dose warfarin for the prevention of central venous catheter-associated thrombosis in patients with cancer. *Journal of Clinical Oncology*, 23(18), 4063–4069.

Cowlishaw, P. & Ballard, P. (2007) Valsalva manoeuvre for central venous cannulation. *Anaesthesia*, 62(6), 640.

Coyne, P.J., MacMurren, M., Izzo, T., et al. (1995) Transcutaneous electrical nerve stimulator for procedural pain associated with intravenous needlesticks. *Journal of Intravenous Nursing*, 18(5), 263–267.

Crnich, C.J. & Maki, D.G. (2002) The promise of novel technology for the prevention of intravascular device-related bloodstream infection. II. Long-term devices. *Clinical Infectious Diseases*, 34(10), 1362–1368.

Cummings, M., Hearse, N., McCutcheon, H., et al. (2011) Improving antibiotic treatment outcomes through the implementation of a midline: Piloting a change in practice for cystic fibrosis patients. *Journal of Vascular Nursing*, 29(1), 11–15.

Cummings-Winfield, C. & Mushani-Kanji, T. (2008) Restoring patency to central venous access devices. *Clinical Journal of Oncology Nursing*, 12(6), 925–934.

Czaplewski, L. (2010) Clinician and patient education. In: Alexander, M., Corrigan, A., Gorski, L., et al. (eds) *Infusion Nursing: An Evidence-Based Approach*, 3rd edn. St Louis, MO: Saunders Elsevier, pp.71–94.

Da Silva, G.A., Priebe, S. & Dias, F.N. (2010) Benefits of establishing an intravenous team and the standardisation of peripheral intravenous catheters. *Journal of Infusion Nursing*, 33(3), 156–160.

Daily, E.K. & Schroeder, J.S. (1994) *Techniques in Bedside Hemodynamic Monitoring*, 5th edn. St Louis, MO: Mosby.

Dal Molin, A., Allara, E., Montani, D., et al. (2014) Flushing the central venous catheter: Is heparin necessary? *Journal of Vascular Access*, 15(4), 241–248.

Dal Molin, A., Clericco, M., Baccini, M., et al. (2015) Normal saline versus heparin solution to lock totally implanted venous access devices: Results from a multicenter randomized trial. *European Journal of Oncology Nursing*, 19(6), 638–643.

Dal Molin, A., Rasero, L., Guerretta, L., et al. (2011) The late complications of totally implantable central venous access ports: The results from an Italian multicenter prospective observation study. *European Journal of Oncology Nursing*, 15(5), 377–381.

Daniels, L.E. (1995) The physical and psychosocial implications of central venous access devices in cancer patients: A review of the literature. *Journal of Cancer Care*, 4(4), 141–146.

Daud, A., Rickard, C., Cooke, M. & Reynolds, H. (2013) Replacement of administration sets (including transducers) for peripheral artery catheters: A systematic review. *Journal of Clinical Nursing*, 22, 303–317.

Davidson, T. & Al Mufti, R. (1997) Hickman central venous catheters in cancer patients. *Cancer Topics*, 10(8), 10–14.

Dawson, R.B. (2011) PICC Zone Insertion Method™ (ZIM™): A systematic approach to determine the ideal insertion site for PICCs in the upper arm. *Journal of the Association for Vascular Access*, 16(3), 156–165.

Dawson, R.B. (2014) Driving performance improvement in ultrasound guided peripheral access: Navigating the procedure and process. World Congress Vascular Access presentation. Available at: https://www.bbraun.ca/content/dam/b-braun/us/website/products-and-therapies/infusiontherapy/Rob_Dawson_Final_Presentation.pdf.bb-.07738563/Rob_Dawson_Final_Presentation.pdf

Dawson, R.B. & Moureau, N.L. (2013) Midline catheters: An essential tool in CLASBI reduction. *Infection Control Today*, 15 March. Available at: https://www.infectioncontroltoday.com/clabsi/midline-catheters-essential-tool-clabsi-reduction

de Lutio, E. (2014) Which material and device? The choice of PICC. In: Sandrucci, S. & Mussa, B. (eds) *Peripherally Inserted Central Catheters*. Milan: Springer, pp.7–20.

De Verteuil, A. (2010) Procedures for venepuncture and cannulation. In: Phillips, S., Collins, M. & Dougherty, L. (eds) *Venepuncture and Cannulation*. Oxford: John Wiley & Sons, pp.131–174.

Debourdeau, P., Farge, D., Beckers, M., et al. (2013) International clinical practice guidelines for the treatment and prophylaxis of thrombosis associated with central venous catheters in patients with cancer. *Journal of Thrombosis and Haemostasis*, 11, 71–80.

Deitcher, S.R., Fesen, M.R., Kiproff, P.M., et al. (2002) Safety and efficacy of alteplase for restoring function in occluded central venous catheters: Results of the cardiovascular thrombolytic to open occluded lines trial. *Journal of Clinical Oncology*, 20(1), 317–324.

DH (Department of Health) (2003) *Winning Ways: Working Together to Reduce Healthcare Associated Infection in England – Report of the Chief Medical Officer*. London: Department of Health.

DH (2004) *Building a Safer NHS for Patients: Improving Medication Safety*. London: Department of Health.

DH (2007) *Saving Lives: Reducing Infection, Delivering Clean and Safe Care – High Impact Intervention No. 1 (Central Venous Bundle) and No. 2 (Peripheral IV Cannula Care Bundle)*. London: Department of Health.

DH (2009) *Reference Guide to Consent for Examination or Treatment*, 2nd edn. London: Department of Health.

DH (2010) *Clean Safe Care: High Impact Intervention – Central Venous Catheter Care Bundle and Peripheral IV Cannula Care Bundle*. London: Department of Health.

DH (2011) *High Impact Intervention: Central Venous Catheter Care Bundle*. Available at: http://webarchive.nationalarchives.gov.uk/20120118164404/hcai.dh.gov.uk/files/2011/03/2011-03-14-HII-Central-Venous-Catheter-Care-Bundle-FINAL.pdf

Di Carlo, I. (2012) Skin incision to implant the port: Could this be the real reason to prefer the surgical cut down to implant a totally implantable venous access device? *Annals of Surgery*, 255(5), e9.

Doellman, D. (2011) Prevention, assessment and treatment of central venous occlusions in neonatal and young pediatric patients. *Journal of Infusion Nursing*, 34(4), 251–259.

Dojcinovska, M. (2010) Selection of equipment. In: Phillips, S., Collins, M. & Dougherty, L. (eds) *Venepuncture and Cannulation*. Oxford: John Wiley & Sons, pp.68–90.

Dougherty, L. (1994) *A Study to Discover How Cancer Patients Perceive the Intravenous Cannulation Experience* [MSc thesis]. University of Guildford.

Dougherty, L. (2006) *Central Venous Access Devices: Care and Management*. Oxford: Blackwell.

Dougherty, L. (2008) Obtaining peripheral vascular access. In: Dougherty, L. & Lamb, J. (eds) *Intravenous Therapy in Nursing Practice*, 2nd edn. Oxford: Blackwell, pp.225–270.

Dougherty, L. (2011) Patients' perspective. In: Phillips, S., Collins, M. & Dougherty, L. (eds) *Venepuncture and Cannulation*. Oxford: John Wiley & Sons, pp.281–296.

Dougherty, L. (2012) Extravasation. In: Di Carlo, I. & Biffi, R. (eds) *Totally Implantable Venous Access Devices*. Milan: Springer, pp.221–226.

Dougherty, L. (2013) Intravenous therapy in older patients. *Nursing Standard*, 28(6), 50–58.

Dougherty, L. (2014) Frequency, diagnosis, and management of occlusive and mechanical PICC complications. In: Sandrucci, S. & Mussa, B. (eds) *Peripherally Inserted Central Venous Catheters*. Milan: Springer, pp.90–92.

Dougherty, L. (2015) How to remove a non-tunnelled central venous catheter. *Nursing Standard*, 30(16/18), 36–38.

Dougherty, L. & Lister, S. (2015) *The Royal Marsden Manual of Clinical Nursing Procedures*, 9th edn. Chichester: John Wiley & Sons.

Dougherty, L., Viner, C. & Young, J. (1998) Establishing ambulatory chemotherapy at home. *Professional Nurse*, 13(6), 356–358.

Drake, R.L., Vogl, W. & Mitchell, A.W.M. (2005) *Gray's Anatomy for Students*. Philadelphia: Elsevier.

Drewett, S.R. (2000) Central venous catheter removal: Procedures and rationale. *British Journal of Nursing*, 9(22), 2304–2315.

Drewett, S.R. (2009) Removal of central venous access devices. In: Hamilton, H. & Bodenham, A. (eds) *Central Venous Catheters*. Oxford: John Wiley & Sons, pp.238–248.

Dwyer, V. & Rutkowski, B. (2013) Intradermal lidocaine for peripheral IV insertion: A change in practice. *Journal of PeriAnesthesia Nursing*, 28(3), e49–e50.

Easterlow, D., Hoddinott, P. & Harrison, S. (2010) Implementing and standardising the use of peripheral vascular access devices. *Journal of Clinical Nursing*, 19, 721–727.

Egan, G.M., Siskin, G.P., Weinmann, R.T., et al. (2013) A prospective postmarket study to evaluate the safety and efficacy of a new peripherally inserted central catheter stabilization system. *Journal of Infusion Nursing*, 36(3), 181–188.

Elhassan, H.A. & Dixon, T. (2012) MRSA contaminated venepuncture tourniquets in clinical practice. *Postgraduate Medical Journal*, 88(1038), 194–197.

Elliott, T.S. (1993) Line-associated bacteraemias: Communicable disease report. *CDR Review*, 3(7), R91–R96.

EMC (Electronic Medicines Compendium) (2015) *Hirudoid Cream*. Available at: https://www.medicines.org.uk/emc/product/1341/smpc

Fabian, B. (2010) Infusion therapy in the older adult. In: Alexander, M., Corrigan, A., Gorski, L., et al. (eds) *Infusion Nursing: An Evidence Based Approach*, 3rd edn. St Louis, MO: Saunders Elsevier, pp.571–582.

Fallouh, N., McGuirk, H.M., Flanders, S.A. & Chopra, V. (2015) Peripherally inserted central catheter-associated deep vein thrombosis: A narrative review. *American Journal of Medicine*, 128, 722–738.

Fahlkos, J., Fudyma, C. & Herbst, S.F. (2009) To aliquot or not? Optimising use of fibrinolytic agents in the management of catheter occlusions. *Clinical Courier*, 26(18), 1–4.

Farrow, C., Bodenham, A. & Millo, J. (2009) Cannulation of the jugular veins. In: Hamilton, H. & Bodenham, A. (eds) *Central Venous Catheters*. Oxford: John Wiley & Sons, pp.78–91.

Feng, B., Yao, S., Zhou, S., et al. (2010) The changes and role of intracavitary electrocardiogram in the placement of peripherally inserted central catheters. *Chinese Journal of Nursing*, 45(1), 26–28.

Ferroni, A., Gaudin, F., Guiffant, G., et al. (2014) Pulsative flushing as a strategy to prevent bacterial colonization of vascular access devices. *Medical Devices: Evidence and Research*, 7, 379–383.

Fetzer, S.J. (2002) Reducing venipuncture and intravenous insertion pain with eutectic mixture of local anesthetic: A meta-analysis. *Nursing Research*, 51(2), 119–124.

Fink, R.M., Hjort, E., Wenger, B., et al. (2009) The impact of dry versus moist heat on peripheral IV catheter insertion in a hematology-oncology outpatient population. *Oncology Nursing Forum*, 36(4), E198–E204.

Fitzsimmons, C.L., Gilleece, M.H., Ranson, M.R., et al. (1997) Central venous catheter placement: Extending the role of the nurse. *Journal of the Royal College of Physicians of London*, 31(5), 533–535.

Fletcher, S. & Bodenham, A. (2000) Safe placement of central venous catheters: Where should the tip of the catheter lie? *British Journal of Anaesthesiology*, 110, 188–191.

Flynn, M., Dougherty, L., Freires, M., et al. (2014) *Cancer Therapy Venous Access Devices Decision Guide*. Marlow, UK: UK Oncology Nursing Society.

Forauer, A.R. & Alonzo, M. (2000) Change in peripherally inserted central catheter tip position with abduction and adduction of the upper extremity. *Journal of Vascular and Interventional Radiology*, 11(10), 1315–1318.

Fossum, K., Love, S.L. & April, M.D. (2016) Topical ethyl chloride to reduce pain associated with venous catheterization: A randomized crossover trial. *American Journal of Emergency Medicine*, 34, 845–850.

Fougo, J.L. (2012a) Quality of life and patients' satisfaction. In: Di Carlo, I. & Biffi, R. (eds) *Totally Implantable Venous Access Devices*. Milan: Springer, pp.265–268.

Fougo, J.L. (2012b) Huber needle: Different types, uses, prevention of accidents. In: Di Carlo, I. & Biffi, R. (eds) *Totally Implantable Venous Access Devices*. Milan: Springer, pp.29–33.

Fraise, A.P. & Bradley, C. (2009) *Ayliffe's Control of Healthcare-Associated Infection: A Practical Handbook*, 5th edn. London: Hodder Arnold.

Frank, R.L. (2018) Peripheral venous access in adults. *UpToDate*. Available at: https://www.uptodate.com/contents/peripheral-venous-access-in-adults

Fry, C. & Aholt, D. (2001) Local anesthesia prior to the insertion of peripherally inserted central catheters. *Journal of Infusion Nursing*, 24(6), 404–408.

Gabriel, J. (2000) What patients think of a PICC. *Journal of Vascular Access Devices*, 5(4), 26–30.

Gabriel, J. (2001) PICC securement: Minimising potential complications. *Nursing Standard*, 15(43), 42–44.

Gabriel, J. (2008) Long-term central venous access. In: Dougherty, L. & Lamb, J. (eds) *Intravenous Therapy in Nursing Practice*, 2nd edn. Oxford: Blackwell, pp.321–351.

Galinkin, J.L., Rose, J.B., Harris, K., et al. (2002) Lidocaine iontophoresis versus eutectic mixture of local anesthetics (EMLA) for IV placement in children. *Anesthesia & Analgesia*, 94(6), 1484–1488.

Gallieni, M., Giordano, A., Rossi, U., et al. (2016) Optimisation of dialysis catheter function. *Journal of Vascular Access*, [illegible]

Gallieni, M., Pittiruti, M. & Biffi, R. (2008) Vascular access in oncology patients. *CA: A Cancer Journal for Clinicians*, 58(6), 323–346.

Galloway, S. & Bodenham, A. (2004) Long-term central venous access. *British Journal of Anaesthesia*, 92(5), 722–734.

Galloway, S. & Bodenham, A.R. (2009) Central venous access via subclavian and axillary veins. In: Hamilton, H. & Bodenham, A. (eds) *Central Venous Catheters*. Oxford: John Wiley & Sons, pp.101–113.

Gamby, A. & Bennett, J. (1995) A feasibility study of the use of non-heparinised 0.9% sodium chloride for transduced arterial and venous lines. *Intensive and Critical Care Nursing*, 11(3), 148–150.

Ganter-Ritz, V., Speroni, K.G. & Atherton, M. (2012) A randomized double-blind study comparing intradermal anesthetic tolerability, efficacy, and cost effectiveness of lidocaine, buffered lidocaine, and bacteriostatic normal saline for peripheral intravenous insertion. *Journal of Infusion Nursing*, 35(2), 93–99.

Garrino, C. (2014) Clinical problems associated with the use of peripheral venous approaches in clinical practice: Thrombosis. In: Sandrucci, S. & Mussa, B. (eds) *Peripherally Inserted Central Venous Catheters*. Milan: Springer, pp.111–120.

Garza, D. & Becan-McBride, K. (2018) *Phlebotomy Handbook: Blood Specimen Collection from Basic to Advanced*. New York: Pearson.

Garza, D. & Becan-McBride, K. (2019) *Phlebotomy Simplified*, 3rd edn. Upper Saddle River, NJ: Pearson Education.

Goedemans, A., Liang, K., Cottell, B., et al. (2014) Topical arnica and mucopolysaccharide polysulphate (Hirudoid) to decrease bruising and pain associated with haemodialysis cannulation-related infiltration: A pilot study. *Renal Society of Australasia Journal*, 10(2), 62–65.

Goltz, J.P., Noack, C., Petritsch, B., et al. (2012) Totally implantable venous power ports of the forearm and the chest: Initial clinical experience with port devices approved for high pressure injections. *British Journal of Radiology*, 85, e966–e972.

Goode, C.J., Titler, M., Rakel, B., et al. (1991) A meta-analysis of effects of heparin flush and saline flush: Quality and cost implications. *Nursing Research*, 40(6), 324–330.

Goodwin, M.L. & Carlson, I. (1993) The peripherally inserted central catheter: A retrospective look at three years of insertions. *Journal of Intravenous Nursing*, 16(2), 92–103.

Goossens, E., Goossens, G.A., Stas, M., et al. (2011) Sensory perceptions of patients with cancer undergoing surgical insertion of a totally implantable venous access device: A qualitative, exploratory study. *Oncology Nursing Forum*, 38(1), E20–E26.

Goossens, G.A. (2015) Flushing and locking of venous catheters: Available evidence and evidence deficit. *Nursing Research in Practice*, 1(2), 985686.

Goossens, G.A., Grumiax, N., Janssens, C., et al. (2018) SecurAstaP trial: Securement with SecurAcath versus StatLock for peripherally inserted central catheters – A randomised open trial. *BMJ Open*, 8(2), e016058.

Gordon, S. & Gardiner, S. (2013) Central line infections in repaired catheters: A retrospective review. *Journal of Advanced Vascular Access*, 18(3), 164–166.

Gorski, L. & Czaplewski, L.M. (2004) Peripherally inserted central catheters and midline catheters for the homecare nurse. *Journal of Infusion Nursing*, 27(6), 399–409.

Gorski, L., Hadaway L., Hagle M., et al. (2016) Infusion therapy standards of practice. *Journal of Infusion Nursing*, 39(1 Suppl.), S1–S159.

Gorski, L., Perucca, R. & Hunter, M. (2010) Central venous access devices: Care, maintenance, and potential problems. In: Alexander, M., Corrigan, A., Gorski, L., et al. (eds) *Infusion Nursing: An Evidence-Based Approach*, 3rd edn. St Louis, MO: Saunders Elsevier, pp.495–515.

Gowardman, J.R., Lipman, J. & Rickard, C.M. (2010) Assessment of peripheral arterial catheters as a source of sepsis in the critically ill: A narrative review. *Journal of Hospital Infection*, 75, 12–18.

Granziera, E., Scarpa, M., Ciccarese, A., et al. (2014) Totally implantable venous access devices. Retrospective analysis of different insertion techniques and predictors of complications in [illegible] devices implanted in a single institution. *BMC Surgery*, 14(1). DOI: 10.1186/1471-2482-14-27.

Green, E., Macartney, G., Zwaal, C., et al. (2008) Managing central access devices in cancer patients. A clinical practice guideline. *Canadian Oncology Nursing Journal*, 18(2). DOI: 10.5737/1181912x18219.

Groll, D., Davies, B., MacDonald, J., et al. (2010) Evaluation of the psychometric properties of the phlebitis and infiltration scales for the assessment [illegible] *Journal of Infusion Nursing*, 33(6), 385–390.

Gu, W.J., Wu, X.D., Wang, F., et al. (2016) Ultrasound guidance facilitates radial artery catheterization: A meta-analysis with trial sequential analysis of randomized controlled trials. *Chest*, 149(1), 166–179.

Guiffant, G., Durussel, J.J., Merckx, J., et al. (2012) Flushing of intravascular access devices (IVADs): Efficacy of pulsed and continuous infusions. *Journal of Vascular Access*, 13(1), 75–78.

Gunwardene, R. & Davenport, H. (1990) Local application of EMLA and glyceryl trinitrate ointment before venepuncture. *Anaesthesia*, 45(1), 52–54.

Hadaway, L.C. (1998a) Catheter connection: Are large syringes necessary? *Journal of Vascular Access Devices*, 3(3), 40–41.

Hadaway, L.C. (1998b) Major thrombotic and nonthrombotic complications: Loss of patency. *Journal of Intravenous Nursing*, 21(5 Suppl.), S143–S160.

Hadaway, L.C. (2000) Peripheral IV therapy in adults. In: *Self-Study Workbook*. Milner, GA: Hadaway Associates.

Hadaway, L.C. (2006) Heparin locking for central venous catheters. *Journal of Vascular Access*, 11(4), 225–231.

Hadaway, L.C. (2010) Anatomy and physiology related to infusion therapy. In: Alexander, M., Corrigan, A., Gorski, L., et al. (eds) *Infusion Nursing: An Evidence-Based Approach*, 3rd edn. St Louis, MO: Saunders Elsevier, pp.139–177.

Hadaway, L.C. (2012) Short peripheral intravenous catheters and infections. *Journal of Infusion Nursing*, 35(4), 230–240.

Haire, W.D. & Herbst, S.F. (2000) Consensus conference on the use of alteplase (t-PA) for the management of thrombotic catheter dysfunction. *Journal of Vascular Access Devices*, 5(2), 28–36.

Hallam, C., Weston, V., Denton, A., et al. (2016) Development of the UK vessel health and preservation (VHP) framework: A multi organisational collaborative. *Journal of Infection Prevention*, 17(2), 65–72.

Hamilton, H. (2009) Patient examination and assessment: Choice of devices. In: Hamilton, H. & Bodenham, A. (eds) *Central Venous Catheters*. Oxford: John Wiley & Sons, pp.34–56.

Hamilton, H., O'Byrne, M. & Nicholai, L. (1995) Central lines inserted by clinical nurse specialists. *Nursing Times*, 91(17), 38–39.

Handlogten, K.S., Wilson, G.A., Clifford, L., et al. (2014) Brachial artery catheterization: An assessment of use patterns and associated complications. *Anesthesia & Analgesia*, 118(2), 288–295.

Hartley-Jones, C. (2009) Problems and practical solutions during insertion of catheters. In: Hamilton, H. & Bodenham, A. (eds) *Central Venous Catheters*. Oxford: John Wiley & Sons, pp.157–174.

Hayden, M.K. & Goodman, M. (2005) Chemotherapy: Principles of administration. In: Yarbro, C.H., Goodman, M. & Frogge, M.H. (eds) *Cancer Nursing: Principles and Practice*, 6th edn. Sudbury, MA: Jones & Bartlett, pp.351–411.

Hazinski, M.F. (2013) *Nursing Care of the Critically Ill Child*, 3rd edn. St Louis, MO: Mosby.

HCPC (Health and Care Professions Council) (2016) *Standards of Conduct, Performance and Ethics*. Available at: https://www.hcpc-uk.org/standards/standards-of-conduct-performance-and-ethics

Healy, C., Baldwin, J., & Driscoll, A. (2018) A randomized controlled trial to determine the effectiveness of a radial arterial catheter dressing. *Critical Care and Resuscitation*, 20(1), 61–67.

Heath, J. & Jones, S. (2001) Utilization of an elastomeric continuous infusion device to maintain catheter patency. *Journal of Intravenous Nursing*, 24(2), 102–106.

Hecker, J. (1988) Improved technique in I.V. therapy. *Nursing Times*, 84(34), 28–33.

Heibl, C., Trommet, V., Burgstaller, S., et al. (2010) Complications associated with the use of Port-a-Caths in patients with malignant or haematological disease: A single-centre prospective analysis. *European Journal of Cancer Care*, 19(5), 676–681.

Hemsworth, S., Selwood, K., van Saene, R., et al. (2007) Does the number of exogenous infections increase in paediatric oncology patients when sterile surgical gloves are not worn for accessing central venous access devices? *European Journal of Oncology Nursing*, 11(5), 442–447.

Higgingson, R. (2015) IV cannula securement: Protecting the patient from infection. *British Journal of Nursing*, 24(8), S23–S28.

Hill, M.L., Baldwin, L., Slaughter, J.C., et al. (2010) A silver-alginate-coated dressing to reduce peripherally inserted central catheter (PICC) infections in NICU patients: A pilot randomized controlled trial. *Journal of Perinatology*, 30(7), 469–473.

Hitchcock, J. & Savine, L. (2017) Medical adhesive-related skin injuries associated with vascular access. *British Journal of Nursing*, 26(8), S4–S12.

Ho, K.M. & Litton, E. (2006) Use of chlorhexidine-impregnated dressing to prevent vascular and epidural catheter colonization and infection: A meta-analysis. *Journal of Antimicrobial Chemotherapy*, 58(2), 281–287.

Ho, K.S., Chia, K.H. & Teh, L.Y. (2003) An unusual complication of radial artery cannulation and its management: A case report. *Journal of Oral and Maxillofacial Surgery*, 61(8), 955–957.

Hoeltke, L.B. (2017) *The Complete Textbook of Phlebotomy*, 5th edn. Clifton Park, NY: Delmar Cengage Learning.

Hoffman, K.R. (2001) Subcutaneous ports used for vascular access need only be flushed every eight weeks to maintain patency. *Proceedings of the American Society of Clinical Oncology*, 20, 1634.

HSE (Health and Safety Executive) (2013) *Health and Safety (Sharp Instruments in Healthcare) Regulations 2013: Guidance for Employers and Employees*. London: Health and Safety Executive.

Hudman, L. & Bodenham, A. (2013) Practical aspects of long-term venous access. *Continuing Education in Anaesthesia, Critical Care & Pain*, 13, 6–11.

Hughes, M. (2014) Reducing PICC migration and improving patient outcomes. *British Journal of Nursing*, 23(2), S12–S18.

Hull, G.J., Moureau, N.L. & Sengupta, S. (2018) Quantitative assessment of reflux in commercially available needle-free IV connectors. *Journal of Vascular Access*, 19(1), 12–22.

Hyde, L. (2008) Legal and professional aspects of intravenous therapy. In: Dougherty, L. & Lamb, J. (eds) *Intravenous Therapy in Nursing Practice*, 2nd edn. Oxford: Blackwell, pp.3–21.

Hyde, L. (2010) Legal and professional aspects. In: Phillips, S., Collins, M. & Dougherty, L. (eds) *Venepuncture and Cannulation*. Oxford: John Wiley & Sons, pp.5–15.

Ignatov, A., Hoffman, O., Smith, B., et al. (2010) An 11 year retrospective study of totally implanted central venous access ports: Complications and patient satisfaction. *European Journal of Surgical Oncology*, 35(3), 241–246.

Irwin, R.S. & Rippe, J.M. (2013) *Intensive Care Medicine*, 7th edn. Philadelphia: Lippincott Williams & Wilkins.

Ives, F. (2009) Catheter design and materials. In: Hamilton, H. & Bodenham, A. (eds) *Central Venous Catheters*. Oxford: John Wiley & Sons, pp.57–77.

Jackson, A. (1998) Infection control: A battle in vein – Infusion phlebitis. *Nursing Times*, 94(4), 68, 71.

Jarvis, S. (2018) Vascular system 2: Diseases affecting the arterial system. *Nursing Times*, 114(5), 58–62.

Jeanes, A. & Bitmead, J. (2015) Reducing bloodstream infection with a chlorhexidine gel IV dressing. *British Journal of Nursing*, 24(19), S14–S19.

Jeanes, A. & Martinez-Garcia, G. (2016) Intravenous securement devices: An overview. *British Journal of Healthcare Management*, 22(10), 488–492.

Jenkins, G.W. & Tortora, G.J. (2014) *Anatomy and Physiology: From Science to Life*, 3rd edn. Hoboken, NJ: John Wiley & Sons.

Jenkins, K. (2014) Needle phobia: A psychological perspective. *British Journal of Anaesthesia*, 113(1), 6–9.

Johansson, E., Engervall, P., Björvell, H., et al. (2009) Patients' perceptions of having a central venous catheter or a totally implantable subcutaneous port system: Results from a randomised study in acute leukaemia. *Supportive Care in Cancer*, 17(2), 137–143.

Johnson, D., Snyder, T., Strader, D., et al. (2017) Positive influence of a dedicated vascular access team in an acute care hospital. *Journal of the Association for Vascular Access*, 22(1), 35–37.

Johnston, A.J., Streater, C.T., Noorani, R., et al. (2012) The effect of peripherally inserted central catheter (PICC) valve technology on catheter occlusion rates: The 'ELeCTRiC' study. *Journal of Vascular Access*, 13(4), 421–425.

Johnston, C. (2007) *Restoring Patency Using POP Technique*. Intravenous Nursing New Zealand. Available at: https://ivnnz.co.nz/cvc-complications/restoring-patency-using-pop-technique

Karadag, A. & Gorgulu, S. (2000) Effect of two different short peripheral catheter materials on phlebitis development. *Journal of Intravenous Nursing*, 23(3), 158–166.

Karamanoglu, A., Yumuk, P.F., Gumus, M., et al. (2003) Port needles: Do they need to be removed as frequently in infusional chemotherapy? *Journal of Infusion Nursing*, 26(4), 239–242.

Kayley, J. (2008) Intravenous therapy in the community. In: Dougherty, L. & Lamb, J. (eds) *Intravenous Therapy in Nursing Practice*, 2nd edn. Oxford: Blackwell, pp.352–374.

Kayley, J. (2012) Intravenous therapy and central venous access devices. In: O'Brien, L. (ed) *District Nursing Manual of Clinical Procedures*. Oxford: John Wiley & Sons, pp.131–176.

Kefeli, U., Dane, F., Yumuk, P., et al. (2009) Prolonged interval in prophylactic heparin flushing for maintenance of subcutaneous implanted port care in patients with cancer. *European Journal of Cancer Care*, 18(2), 191–194.

Kelly, L.J. (2014) Getting the most from ultrasound guidance for CVC insertion. *British Journal of Nursing*, 23(1), S24–S28.

Kelly, L.J. (2017) The experience of patients living with a vascular access device. *British Journal of Nursing*, 26(19), S36.

Kelly, L.J., Jones, T. & Kirkham, S. (2017) Needle-free devices: Keeping the system closed. *British Journal of Nursing*, 26(2), S14–S19.

Kim, K.S. & Lam, L. (2008) Chlorhexidine: Pharmacology and clinical applications. *Anaesthesia and Intensive Care*, 36(4), 502–512.

Kokotis, K. (2014) The PICC team. In: Sandrucci, S. & Mussa, B. (eds) *Peripherally Inserted Central Catheters*. Milan: Springer, pp.165–187.

Koh, D., Robertson, I., Watts, M., et al. (2012) Density of microbial colonization on external and internal surfaces of concurrently placed intravascular devices. *American Journal of Critical Care*, 21(3), 162–171.

Koh, D.B.C., Gowardman, J.R. & Brown, A. (2008) Prospective study of peripheral arterial catheter infection and comparison with concurrently sited central venous catheters. *Critical Care Medicine*, 36, 397–402.

Koyfman, A., Radwine, Z., Sawyer, T.L., et al. (2018) Arterial line placement. In: Lopez-Rowe, V. (ed) *Clinical Procedures*. Available at: https://emedicine.medscape.com/article/1999586-overview#a1

Krieger, E. & Burbridge, B. (2000) Arm placement of vein ports: A viable alternative. *Canadian Journal of Medical Radiation Technology*, 31(1), 12–16.

Kulkarni, M., Elsner, C., Ouellet, D., et al. (1994) Heparinized saline versus normal saline in maintaining patency of the radial artery catheter. *Canadian Journal of Surgery*, 37(1), 37–42.

Kumar, A. & Chuan, A. (2009) Ultrasound guided vascular access: Efficacy and safety. *Best Practice & Research: Clinical Anaesthesiology*, 23, 299–311.

Kumwenda, M., Dougherty, L., Spooner, H., et al. (2018) Managing dysfunctional central venous access devices: A practical approach to urokinase thrombolysis. *British Journal of Nursing*, 27(2), S4–S10.

Kuo, Y.S., Schwartz, B., Santiago, J., et al. (2005) How often should a Port-a-Cath be flushed? *Cancer Investigations*, 23(7), 582–585.

Kupensky, D.T. (1998) Applying current research to influence clinical practice. *Journal of Intravenous Nursing*, 21(5), 271–274.

La Greca, A. (2013) Current recommendations for placement of long term VADs: Role of ultrasound, role of intracavitary EKG and the SIPTA-2 bundle in 2013. Presentation at the 8th GAVeCeLT Congress, 6–7 December, Turin, Italy.

La Greca, A. (2014) Evaluation techniques of the PICC tip placement. In: Sandrucci, S. & Mussa, B. (eds) *Peripherally Inserted Central Catheters*. Milan: Springer, pp.63–84.

LaBella, G.D. & Tang, J. (2012) Removal of totally implantable venous access devices. In: Di Carlo, I. & Biffi, R. (eds) *Totally Implantable Venous Access Devices*. Milan: Springer, pp.247–255.

Lai, N.M., Chaiyakunapruk, N., Lai, N.A., et al. (2013) Catheter impregnation, coating or bonding for reducing central venous catheter-related infections in adults (review). *Cochrane Database of Systematic Reviews*, 6, CD007878.

Lamb, J. & Dougherty, L. (2008) Local and systemic complications of intravenous therapy. In: Dougherty, L. & Lamb, J. (eds) *Intravenous Therapy in Nursing Practice*, 2nd edn. Oxford: Blackwell, pp.167–196.

Lamperti, M., Bodenham, A.R., Pittiruti, M., et al. (2012) International evidence-based recommendations on ultrasound-guided vascular access. *Intensive Care Medicine*, 38(7), 1105–1117.

Lamperti, M. & Pittiruti, M. (2015) Central venous catheter tip position: Another point of view. *European Journal of Anaesthesiology*, 32, 3–4.

Larson, E. (1988) Guideline for use of topical antimicrobial agents. *American Journal of Infection Control*, 16(6), 253–266.

LaRue, G.D. (2000) Efficacy of ultrasonography in peripheral venous cannulation. *Journal of Intravenous Nursing*, 23(1), 29–34.

Lavery, I. & Ingram, P. (2005) Venepuncture: Best practice. *Nursing Standard*, 19(49), 55–65.

LeDuc, K. (1997) Efficacy of normal saline solution versus heparin solution for maintaining patency of peripheral intravenous catheters in children. *Journal of Emergency Nursing*, 23, 306–309.

Lee, W., Chen, H., Tsai, T., et al. (2009) Risk factors for peripheral intravenous catheter infection in hospitalized patients: A prospective study of 3165 patients. *American Journal of Infection Control*, 37(8), 683–686.

Lenhart, C. (2000) Prevention versus treatment of venous access device occlusions. *Journal of Vascular Access Devices*, 5(4), 34–35.

Leung, T.K. (2011) A retrospective study on the long term placement of peripherally inserted central catheters and the importance of nursing care and education. *Cancer Nursing*, 34(1), e25–e30.

Lichenstein, D.A., Meziere, G., Lascols, N., et al. (2005) Ultrasound diagnosis of occult pneumothorax. *Critical Care Medicine*, 33(6), 1231–1238.

Light, D., Subramonia, S. & Krishna, A. (2014) Safe removal of long term venous catheters in the neck. *Scottish Medical Journal*, 59(3), e13–e15.

Lin, S.C., Wen, K.Y., Liu, C.Y., et al. (2010) The use of peripherally inserted central catheters in cancer patients. *Journal of the Association for Vascular Access*, 15(1), 16–19.

Lipsitz, E.C. (2004) Cannulation injuries of the radial artery. *American Journal of Critical Care*, 13(4), 314–319.

Liu, Y.T., Alsaawi, A. & Bjornsson, H.M. (2014) Ultrasound guided peripheral venous access: A systematic review of randomized-controlled trials. *European Journal of Emergency Medicine*, 21(1), 18–23.

Lobo, B., Vaidean, G., Broyles, J., et al. (2009) Risk of venous thromboembolism in hospitalised patients with peripherally inserted central catheters. *Journal of Hospital Medicine*, 4(7), 417–422.

Lopez, A.C. (2011) A quality improvement program combining maximal barrier precaution compliance monitoring and daily chlorhexidine gluconate baths resulting in decreased central line bloodstream infection. *Dimensions of Critical Care Nursing*, 30(5), 293–298.

Lopez-Briz, E., Ruiz-Garcia, V, Cabello, J.B., et al. (2014) Heparin versus 0.9% sodium chloride intermittent flushing for prevention of occlusion in central venous catheters in adults. *Cochrane Database of Systematic Reviews*, 10, CD008462.

López-Briz, E., Ruiz-Garcia, V., Cabello, J.B., et al. (2018) Heparin versus 0.9% sodium chloride locking for prevention of occlusion in central venous catheters in adults. *Cochrane Database of Systematic Reviews*, 7, CD008462.

Loveday, H.P., Wilson, J.A., Pratt, R.J., et al. (2014) epic3: National evidence-based guidelines for preventing healthcare-associated infections in NHS hospitals in England. *Journal of Hospital Infection*, 86(Suppl. 1), S1–S70.

Lüker, P. & Stahlheber-Dilg, B.A. (2003) Pain related to Optiva 2, Biovalve, and Venflon 2 intravenous catheters. *British Journal of Nursing*, 12, 1345–1354.

Lum, P. (1999) Techniques for optimizing catheter tip position. Presentation at the NAVAN 13th Conference, Orlando, FL.

Lum, P. (2004) A new formula-based measurement guide for optimal positioning of central venous catheters. *Journal of the Association for Vascular Access*, 9(2), 80–86.

Luo, X., Guo, Y., Yu, H., et al. (2017) Effectiveness, safety and comfort of StatLock securement for peripherally inserted central catheters: A systematic review and meta-analysis. *Nursing & Health Sciences*, 19, 403–413.

MacKereth, P., Hackman, E., Tomlinson, L., et al. (2012) Needle with ease: Rapid stress management techniques. *British Journal of Nursing*, 21(14), S18–S22.

Macklin, D. (1999) What's physics got to do with it? A review of the physical principles of fluid administration. *Journal of Vascular Access Devices*, 4(2), 7–11.

Macklin, D. (2010a) The impact of IV connectors on clinical practice and patient outcomes. *Journal of the Association for Vascular Access*, 15(3), 126.

Macklin, D. (2010b) Catheter management. *Seminars in Oncology Nursing*, 26(2), 113–120.

Macklin, D. & Chernecky, C.C. (2004) *IV Therapy*. St Louis, MO. Saunders.

Mahler, S.A., Massey, G., Meskill, L., et al. (2011) Can we make the basilic vein larger? Maneuvers to facilitate ultrasound guided peripheral intravenous access: A prospective cross sectional study. *International Journal of Emergency Medicine*, 4, 53.

Maki, D.G. (2002) The promise of novel technology for the prevention of intravascular device related blood stream infections. Presentation at the NAVAN Conference, San Diego, CA.

Maki, D.G. (2005) Renowned expert Dennis Maki addresses catheter related infections. *Infection Control Today*, 1 January. Available at: https://www.infectioncontroltoday.com/infections/renowned-expert-dennis-maki-md-addresses-catheter-relatedinfections

Maki, D.G. (2008) A novel integrated chlorhexidine impregnated transparent dressing for prevention of catheter related blood stream infection: A prospective comparative study in health volunteers. Presentation at the 18th Annual Scientific Meeting of the Society of Healthcare Epidemiology of America, Orlando, FL.

Maki, D.G. & Ringer, M. (1987) Evaluation of dressing regimens for prevention of infection with peripheral intravenous catheters: Gauze, a transparent polyurethane dressing, and an iodophor-transparent dressing. *JAMA*, 258(17), 2396–2403.

Maki, D.G., Ringer, M. & Alvarado, C.J. (1991) Prospective randomised trial of povidone-iodine, alcohol, and chlorhexidine for prevention of infection associated with central venous and arterial catheters. *Lancet*, 338(8763), 339–343.

Marieb, E.N. & Hoehn, K. (2018) *Human Anatomy & Physiology*, 11th edn. Harlow: Pearson.

Marini, J.L. & Wheeler, N.P. (2010) *Critical Care: The Essentials*, 3rd edn. Philadelphia: Lippincott Williams & Wilkins.

Marsh, N., Mihala, G., Ray-Barruel, G., et al. (2015) Inter-rater agreement on PIVC: Associated phlebitis signs, symptoms and scales. *Journal of Evaluation in Clinical Practice*, 21, [illegible].

Margiglicar, A.M. (2000) Evaluation of comfort levels and complication rates as determined by peripheral intravenous catheter sites. *Canadian Intravenous Nurses Association*, 17, 26–39.

Marx, M. (1995) The management of the difficult peripherally inserted central venous catheter line removal. *Journal of Intravenous Nursing*, 18(5), 246–249.

Masoorli, S. (2003) Extravasation injuries associated with the use of central vascular access devices. *Journal of Vascular Access Devices*, 8(1), 21–23.

Masoorli, S. (2007) Nerve injuries related to vascular access insertion and assessment. *Journal of Infusion Nursing*, 30(6), 346–350.

Mayo, D.J. (2000) Catheter-related thrombosis. *Journal of Vascular Access Devices*, 5(2), 10–20.

Mayo, D.J. (2001) Catheter-related thrombosis. *Journal of Intravenous Nursing*, 24(3 Suppl.), S13–S22.

McCall, R.E. & Tankersley, C.M. (2019) *Phlebotomy Essentials*, 6th edn. Philadelphia: Lippincott Williams & Wilkins.

McCarthy, C.J., Behravesh, S., Naidu, S.G. & Oklu, R. (2016) Air embolism: Practical tips for prevention and treatment. *Journal of Clinical Medicine*, 5(11), pii: e93.

McGoldrick, M. (2010) Infection prevention and control. In: Alexander, M., Corrigan, A., Gorski, L., et al. (eds) *Infusion Nursing: An Evidence-Based Approach*, 3rd edn. St Louis, MO: Saunders Elsevier, pp.204–228.

McGowan, D. (2014) Peripheral intravenous cannulation: Managing stress and anxiety. *British Journal of Nursing*, 23(19), S4–S9.

McKnight, S. (2004) Nurse's guide to understanding and treating thrombotic occlusion of central venous access devices. *MEDSURG Nursing*, 13(6), 377–382.

McNichol, L., Lund, C., Rosen, T. & Gray, M. (2013) Medical adhesives and patient safety: State of the science consensus statements for the assessment, prevention, and treatment of adhesive-related skin injuries. *Journal of the Dermatology Nurses' Association*, 5(6), 323–338.

Mermel, L.A., Farr, B.M., Sherertz, R.J., et al. (2001) Guidelines for the management of intravascular catheter-related infections. *Journal of Intravenous Nursing*, 24(3), 180–205.

Mestre G., Berbel, C., Tortajada, P., et al. (2013) Successful multifaceted intervention aimed to reduce short peripheral venous catheter related adverse events. *American Journal of Infection Control*, 41(6), 520–526.

Meyer, B.M. (2011) Managing peripherally inserted central catheter thrombosis risk: A guide for clinical best practice. *Journal of the Association for Vascular Access*, 16(3), 144–147.

MHRA (Medicines and Healthcare products Regulatory Agency) (2004) *Medical Device Alert MDA/2004/010: Central Venous Catheters (All Manufacturers) (25/2/04), 1–3.* London: Medicines and Healthcare products Regulatory Agency.

MHRA (2005) *Alert MDA 2005/01 and Device Bulletin DB 2005 (01): Reporting Adverse Incidents and Disseminating Medical Device Alerts.* London: Medicines and Healthcare products Regulatory Agency.

MHRA (2012) *Medical Device Alert MDA/2012/075 25: All Medical Devices and Medicinal Products Containing Chlorhexidine.* London: Medicines and Healthcare products Regulatory Agency.

MHRA (2015) *Managing Medical Devices: Guidance for Healthcare and Social Services Organisations.* Available at: https://assets.publishing.service.gov.uk/government/uploads/system/uploads/attachment_data/file/421028/Managing_medical_devices_-_Apr_2015.pdf

Mignini, M.A., Piacentini, E. & Dubin, A. (2006) Peripheral arterial blood pressure monitoring adequately tracks central arterial blood pressure in critically ill patients: An observational study. *Critical Care*, 10(2), R43.

Minnaganti, V.R. & Cunha, B.A. (2000) *Acinetobacter baumannii*-associated arterial line infection. *American Journal of Infection Control*, 28(5), 376–377.

Mirro, J. Jr., Rao, B.N., Stokes, D.C., et al. (1989) A prospective study of Hickman/Broviac catheters and implantable ports in pediatric oncology patients. *Journal of Clinical Oncology*, 7(2), 214–222.

Mitchell, M., Anderson, B., Williams, K. & Umscheid, A. (2009) Heparin flushing and other interventions to maintain patency of central venous catheters: A systematic review. *Journal of Advanced Nursing*, 65(10), 2007–2021.

Moini, J. (2013) *Phlebotomy: Principles and Practice.* Burlington, MA: Jones & Bartlett Learning.

Molloy, D., Smith, L.N. & Aitchison, T. (2008) Cytotoxic chemotherapy for incurable colorectal cancer: Living with a PICC line. *Journal of Clinical Nursing*, 17(18), 2398–2407.

Montecalvo, M.A., McKenna, D., Yarrish, R., et al. (2012) Chlorhexidine bathing to reduce central venous catheter associated bloodstream infection: Impact and sustainability. *American Journal of Medicine*, 125, 505–511.

Monzillo, V., Corona, S., Lanzarini, P., et al. (2012) Chlorhexidine-silver sulfadiazine-impregnated central venous catheters: In vitro antibacterial activity and impact on bacterial adhesion. *New Microbiology*, 35(2), 175–182.

Morden, P., Sokhandon, F., Miller, L., et al. (2014) The role of saline flush injection rate in displacement of CT-injectable peripherally inserted central catheter tip during power injection of contrast material. *American Journal of Roentgenology*, 202(1), W13–W18.

Morris, W. (2011) Complications. In: Phillips, S., Collins, M. & Dougherty, L. (eds) *Venepuncture and Cannulation.* Oxford: John Wiley & Sons, pp.175–222.

Morton, P.G. & Fontaine, D.K. (eds) (2009) *Critical Care Nursing: A Holistic Approach*, 11th edn. Philadelphia: Lippincott Williams & Wilkins.

Moureau, N.L. (2008) Tips for inserting an I.V. device in an older adult. *Nursing*, 38(12), 12.

Moureau, N.L. (2013) Safe patient care when using vascular access devices. *British Journal of Nursing*, 22(2), S14, S16, S18, passim.

Moureau, N.L. (2014) Ultrasound anatomy of peripheral veins and ultrasound-guided venipuncture. In: Sandrucci, S. & Mussa, B. (eds) *Peripherally Inserted Central Catheters.* Milan: Springer, pp.53–62.

Moureau, N.L. & Chopra, V. (2016) Indications for peripheral, midline and central catheters: Summary of the MAGIC recommendations. *British Journal of Nursing*, 25(8), S15–S24.

Moureau, N.L., Dennis, G.L., Ames, E., et al. (2010) Electrocardiogram (EKG) guided peripherally inserted central catheter placement and tip position: Results of a trial to replace radiological confirmation. *Journal of the Association for Vascular Access*, 15(1), 8–14.

Moureau, N.L., Deschneau, M. & Pyrek, J. (2009) Evaluation of the clinical performance of a chlorhexidine gluconate antimicrobial transparent dressing. *Journal of Infection Prevention*, 10(Suppl.), S13–S17.

Moureau, N.L. & Gabriel, J. (2009) Peripherally inserted central catheters. In: Hamilton, H. & Bodenham, A. (eds) *Central Venous Catheters.* Oxford: John Wiley & Sons, pp.114–126.

Moureau, N.L. & Iannucci, A.L. (2003) Catheter securement: Trends in performance and complications associated with the use of either traditional methods or adhesive anchor devices. *Journal of Vascular Access Devices*, 8(1), 29–33.

Moureau, N.L., Lamperti, M., Kelly, L.J., et al. (2013) Evidence-based consensus on the insertion of central venous access devices: Definition of minimal requirement for training. *British Journal of Anaesthesia*, 110, 347–356.

Moureau, N.L., McKinnon, B.T. & Douglas, C.M. (1999) Multidisciplinary management of thrombotic catheter occlusions in vascular access devices. *Journal of Vascular Access Devices*, 4(2), 22–29.

Moureau, N.L., Trick, N., Nifong, T., et al. (2012) Vessel health and preservation (Part 1): A new evidence-based approach to vascular access selection and management. *Journal of Vascular Access*, 3(3), 351–356.

Moureau, N.L. & Zonderman, A. (2000) Does it always have to hurt? Premedications for adults and children for use with intravenous therapy. *Journal of Intravenous Nursing*, 23(4), 213–219.

Moussa Pacha, H., Alahdab, F., Al-Khadra, Y., et al. (2018) Ultrasound-guided versus palpation: Guided radial artery catheterization in adult population – A systematic review and meta-analysis of randomized controlled trials. *American Heart Journal*, 204, 1–8.

Mushtaq, A., Navalkele, B., Kaur, M., et al. (2018) Comparison of complications in midlines versus central venous catheters: Are midlines safer than central venous lines? *American Journal of Infection Control*, 46, 788–792.

Mussa, B. (2014) Advantages, disadvantages, and indications of PICCs in inpatients and outpatients. In: Sandrucci, S. & Mussa, B. (eds) *Peripherally Inserted Central Catheters*. Milan: Springer, pp.43–53.

Nakazawa, N. (2010a) Challenges in the accurate identification of the ideal catheter tip location. *Journal of the Association for Vascular Access*, 15(4), 196–201.

Nakazawa, N. (2010b) Infectious and thrombotic complications of central venous catheters. *Seminars in Oncology Nursing*, 26(2), 121–131.

Nauth-Misir, N. (1998) Intravascular catheters. *Professional Nurse*, 13(7), 463–471.

Naylor, C.L. (2007) Reduction of malposition in peripherally inserted central catheters with tip location system. *Journal of the Association for Vascular Access*, 12(1), 29–31.

NHS Employers (2010) *Needlestick Injury*. London: NHS Employers.

NHS Employers (2015) *Managing the Risks of Sharps Injuries*. Available at: https://www.nhsemployers.org/-/media/Employers/Documents/Retain-and-improve/Health-and-wellbeing/Managing-the-risks-of-sharps-injuries-v7.pdf

NHS England and NHSI (NHS Improvement) (2019) *Standard Infection Control Precautions: National Hand Hygiene and Personal Protective Equipment Policy*. Available at: https://improvement.nhs.uk/documents/4957/National_policy_on_hand_hygiene_and_PPE_2.pdf

NICE (National Institute for Health and Care Excellence) (2002) *Guidance on the Use of Ultrasound Locating Devices for Placing Central Venous Catheters* [TA49]. Available at: https://www.nice.org.uk/guidance/ta49

NICE (2003) *Infection Control: Prevention of Healthcare-Associated Infection in Primary and Community Care* [CG2]. Available at: www.nice.org.uk/guidance/CG2

NICE (2012) *Infection: Prevention and Control of Healthcare-Associated Infections in Primary and Community Care* [CG139]. Available at: www.nice.org.uk/Guidance/CG139

NICE (2015) *The Sherlock 3CG Tip Confirmation System for Placement of Peripherally Inserted Central Catheters* [MTG24]. Available at: www.nice.org.uk/Guidance/mtg24

NICE (2017) *SecurAcath for Securing Percutaneous Catheters* [MTG34]. Available at: www.nice.org.uk/Guidance/MTG34

Nifong, T.P. & McDevit, T.J. (2011) The effect of catheter to vein ratio on blood flow rates in a simulated model of peripherally inserted central venous catheters. *Chest*, 140(1), 48–53.

Nishihara, Y., Kajiura, T., Yokota, K., et al. (2012) A comparative clinical study focusing on the antimicrobial efficacies of chlorhexidine gluconate alcohol for patient skin preparations. *Journal of Infusion Nursing*, 35(1), 44–50.

NMC (Nursing and Midwifery Council) (2018) *The Code: Professional Standards of Practice and Behaviour for Nurses, Midwives and Nursing Associates*. Available at: https://www.nmc.org.uk/standards/code

NPSA (National Patient Safety Agency) (2003) *Risk Analysis of Infusion Devices*. London: National Patient Safety Agency.

NPSA (2007) *Alert 20: Promoting the Safer Use of Injectable Medicines*. London: National Patient Safety Agency.

NPSA (2008a) *Risks with Intravenous Heparin Flush Solutions*. London: National Patient Safety Agency.

NPSA (2008b) *Infusions and Sampling from Arterial Lines*. London: National Patient Safety Agency.

Oakley, C., Wright, E. & Ream, E. (2000) The experiences of patients and nurses with a nurse-led peripherally inserted central venous catheter line service. *European Journal of Oncology Nursing*, 4(4), 207–218.

O'Grady, N.P., Alexander, M., Burns, L.A., et al. (2011) Guidelines for the prevention of intravascular catheter-related infections. *Clinical Infectious Diseases*, 52(9), e162–e193.

O'Horo, J.C., Maki, D.G., Krupp, A.E. & Safdor, N. (2014) Arterial catheters as a source of BSI: A systematic review and meta-analysis. *Critical Care Medicine*, 42(6), 1334–1339.

Oliver, G. & Jones, M. (2014) ECG or X-ray as the 'gold-standard' for establishing PICC-tip location? *British Journal of Nursing*, 23(19), S10–S16.

Oliver, G. & Jones, M. (2016) ECG-based PICC tip verification system: An evaluation 5 years on. *British Journal of Nursing*, 25(19), S4–S10.

Palese, A., Baldassar, D., Rupil, A., et al. (2014) Maintaining patency in totally implanted venous access devices (TIVAD): A time-to-event analysis of different lock irrigation intervals. *European Journal of Oncology Nursing*, 18(1), 66–71.

Paolucci, H., Nutter, B. & Albert, N.M. (2011) RN knowledge of vascular access devices management. *Journal of the Association for Vascular Access*, 16(4), 221–225.

Parienti, J.J., Mongardon, N., Mégarbane, B., et al. (2015) Intravascular complications of central venous catheterization by insertion site. *New England Journal of Medicine*, 373, 1220–1229.

Perucca, R. (2010) Peripheral venous access devices. In: Alexander, M., Corrigan, A., Gorski, L., et al. (eds) *Infusion Nursing: An Evidence-Based Approach*, 3rd edn. St Louis, MO: Saunders Elsevier, pp.456–479.

Pfaff, B., Heithouse, T. & Emanuelsen, M. (2012) Use of a 1-piece chlorhexidine gluconate transparent dressing on critically ill patients. *Critical Care Nurse*, 32(4), 35–40.

Phillips, L.D. (2005) *Manual of I.V. Therapeutics*, 4th edn. Philadelphia: F.A. Davis.

Phillips, S., Collins, M. & Dougherty, L. (eds) (2011) *Venepuncture and Cannulation*. Oxford: John Wiley & Sons.

Philpot, P. & Griffiths, V. (2003) The peripherally inserted central catheter. *Nursing Standard*, 17(44), 39–46.

Pierce, L.N.B. (2006) Non-invasive respiratory monitoring and invasive monitoring of direct and derived tissue oxygenation variables. In: *Management of the Mechanically Ventilated Patient*, 2nd edn. Philadelphia: Saunders Elsevier, pp.331–377.

Pittiruti, M., Bertello, D., Briglia, E., et al. (2012) The intracavitary ECG method for positioning the tip of central venous catheters: Results of an Italian multicenter study. *Journal of Vascular Access*, 13(3), 357–365.

Pittiruti, M., Bertoglio, S., Scoppettuolo, G., et al. (2016) Evidence-based criteria for the choice and the clinical use of the most appropriate lock solutions for central venous catheters (excluding dialysis catheters): A GAVeCeLT consensus. *Journal of Vascular Access*, 17(6), 453–464.

Ponec, D., Irwin, D., Haire, W.D., et al. (2001) Recombinant tissue plasminogen activator (alteplase) for restoration of flow in occluded central venous access devices: A double-blind placebo-controlled trial – The Cardiovascular thrombolytic to Open Occluded Lines (COOL) efficacy trial. *Journal of Vascular and Interventional Radiology*, 12(8), 951–955.

Qinming, Z. (2012) Thrombosis. In: Di Carlo, I. & Biffi, R. (eds) *Totally Implantable Venous Access Devices*. Milan: Springer, pp.173–182.

Ray-Barruel, G., Cooke, M., Mitchell, M., et al. (2018) Implementing the I-DECIDED clinical decision-making tool for peripheral intravenous catheter assessment and safe removal: Protocol for an interrupted time-series study. *BMJ Open*, 8, e021290.

Ray-Barruel, G., Polit, D.F., Murfield, J.E., et al. (2014) Infusion phlebitis assessment measures: A systematic review. *Journal of Evaluation in Clinical Practice*, 20, 191–202.

RCN (Royal College of Nursing) (2016a) *Standards for Infusion Therapy*, 4th edn. London: Royal College of Nursing.

RCN (2016b) *Principles of Consent*. Available at: https://www.rcn.org.uk/professional-development/publications/pub-006047

Rickard, C., Ullman, A., Kleidon, T., et al. (2017) Ten tips for dressing and securement of IV device wounds. *Australian Nursing & Midwifery Journal*, 24(10), 32–34.

Rickard, C.M., Webster, J., Wallis, M.C., et al. (2012) Routine versus clinically indicated replacement of peripheral intravenous catheters: A randomised controlled equivalence trial. *Lancet*, 380(9847), 1066–1074.

Robbins, T.L., Cromwell, P. & Korones, D.N. (2000) Swimming and central venous catheter-related infections in children with cancer. In: Nolan, M.T. & Mock, V. (eds) *Measuring Patient Outcomes*. Thousand Oaks, CA: Sage, pp.169–184.

Rosenthal, K. (2005) Tailor your I.V. insertion techniques: Special populations. *Nursing*, 35(5), 36–41.

Rowley, S. (2001) Theory to practice: Aseptic non-touch technique. *Nursing Times*, 97(7), VI–VIII.

Rowley, S. & Clare, S. (2011) ANTT: A standard approach to aseptic technique. *Nursing Times*, 107(36), 12–14.

Rowley, S., Clare, S., Macqueen, S. & Molyneux, R. (2010) ANTT v2: An updated practice framework for aseptic technique. *British Journal of Nursing*, 19(5), S5–S11.

Royer, T. (2001) A case for posterior, anterior, and lateral chest X-rays being performed following each PICC placement. *Journal of Vascular Access Devices*, 6(4), 9–12.

Rummel, M.A., Donnelly, P.J. & Fortenbaugh, C.C. (2001) Clinical evaluation of a positive pressure device to prevent central venous catheter occlusion: Results of a pilot study. *Clinical Journal of Oncology Nursing*, 5(6), 261–265.

Ruschulte, H., Franke, M., Gastmeier, P., et al. (2009) Prevention of central venous catheter related infections with chlorhexidine gluconate impregnated wound dressings: A randomized controlled trial. *Annals of Hematology*, 88(3), 267–272.

Ryder, M. (2001) The role of biofilm in vascular catheter related infections. *New Developments in Vascular Disease*, 2(2), 15–25.

Ryder, M. (2002) *Biofilm: Unlocking the mystery of catheter related infections*. Presentation at the NAVAN 15th Annual Conference, 19–22 January, Alexandria, VA.

Safdar, N., O'Horo, J.C., Ghufran, A., et al. (2014) Chlorhexidine-impregnated dressing for prevention of catheter-related bloodstream infection: A meta-analysis. *Critical Care Medicine*, 42(7), 1703–1713.

Samman, M., Mujo, T., Harris, J.J., et al. (2015) Subcutaneous port malfunction: A retrospective comparison between internal jugular and subclavian vein access. *Journal of the Association for Vascular Access*, 20(4), 229–234.

Sampath, L.A., Saborio, D.V., Yaron, I., et al. (2001) Safety and efficacy of an improved antiseptic catheter impregnated intraluminally with chlorhexidine. *Journal of Infusion Nursing*, 24(6), 395–403.

Sansivero, G.E. (1998) Venous anatomy and physiology: Considerations for vascular access device placement and function. *Journal of Intravenous Nursing*, 21(5 Suppl.), S107–S114.

Scales, K. (2005) Vascular access: A guide to peripheral venous cannulation. *Nursing Standard*, 19(49), 48–52.

Scales, K. (2008) Anatomy and physiology related to intravenous therapy. In: Dougherty, L. & Lamb, J. (eds) *Intravenous Therapy in Nursing Practice*, 2nd edn. Oxford: Blackwell, pp.23–48.

Scales, K. (2009) Correct use of chlorhexidine in IV practice. *Nursing Standard*, 24(8), 41–46.

Schears, G.J. (2005) The benefits of a catheter securement device on reducing patient complications. *Managing Infection Control*, 5(2), 14–25.

Scheer, B.V., Perel, A. & Pfeiffer, U.J. (2002) Clinical review: Complications and risk factors of peripheral arterial catheters used for haemodynamic monitoring in anaesthesia and intensive care medicine. *Critical Care*, 6, 198–204.

Schmidt, G.A., Maizel, J. & Slama, M. (2015) Ultrasound-guided central venous access: What's new? *Intensive Care Medicine*, 41, 705–707.

Schulmeister, L. & Camp-Sorrell, D. (2000) Chemotherapy extravasation from implanted ports. *Oncology Nursing Forum*, 27(3), 531–538.

Scoppettuolo, G. (2014) Clinical problems associated with the use of peripheral venous approaches: Infections. In: Sandrucci, S. & Mussa, B. (eds) *Peripherally Inserted Central Catheters*. Milan: Springer, pp.95–109.

Scoppettuolo, G., Annetta, M.G., Marano, C., et al. (2013) Cyanoacrylate glue prevents early bleeding of the exit site after CVC or PICC placement. *Critical Care*, 17(2), 1–6.

Scoppettuolo, G., Dolcetti, L., Emoli, A., et al. (2015) Further benefits of cyanoacrylate glue for central venous catheterisation. *Anaesthesia*, 70(6), 750–763.

Sharp, R., Cummings, M., Fielder, A., et al. (2015) The catheter to vein ratio and rates of symptomatic venous thromboembolism in patients with peripherally inserted central catheter (PICC): A prospective cohort study. *International Journal of Nursing Studies*, 52(3), 677–685.

Sharp, R., Grech, C., Fielder, A., et al. (2014) The patient experience of a peripherally inserted central catheter (PICC): A qualitative descriptive study. *Contemporary Nurse*, 48(1), 26–35.

Shaw, S.J. (2017) Use of closed cannula in peripheral intravenous cannulation. *Nursing Standard*, 31(36), 54–63.

Shiloh, A.L., Savel, R.H., Paulin, L.M. & Eisen, L.A. (2010) Ultrasound-guided catheterization of the radial artery: A systematic review and meta analysis of randomized controlled trials. *Chest*, 10, 919.

Shiono, M., Takahashi, S., Kakudo, Y., et al. (2014) Upper arm central venous port implantation: A 6 year single institutional retrospective analysis and pictorial essay of procedures for insertion. *PLOS ONE*, 9(3), e91335.

Shotkin, J.D. & Lombardo, F. (1996) Use of an indwelling peripheral catheter for 3–5 day chemotherapy administration in the outpatient setting. *Journal of Intravenous Nursing*, 19(6), 315–320.

Simonova, G., Rickard, C., Dunster, K., et al. (2012) Cyanoacrylate tissue adhesives: Effective securement technique for intravascular catheters – In vitro testing of safety and feasibility. *Anaesthesia and Intensive Care*, 40(3), 460–466.

Singer, A.J. & Thode, H.C.J. (2004) A review of the literature on octycyanoacrylate tissue adhesive. *American Journal of Surgery*, 187(2), 238–248.

Singh Vats, H. (2012) Complications of catheters: Tunnelled and non-tunnelled. *Advances in Chronic Kidney Disease*, 19(3), 188–194.

Smith, R.N. & Nolan, J.P. (2013) Clinical review: Central venous catheters. *BMJ*, 347, f6570.

Snelling, R., Jones, G., Figueredo, A., et al. (2001) Central venous catheters for infusion therapy in gastrointestinal cancer: A comparative study of tunnelled centrally placed catheters and peripherally inserted central catheters. *Journal of Intravenous Nursing*, 24(1), 38–47.

Solinas, G., Platini, F., Trivellato, M., et al. (2017) Port in oncology practice: 3-monthly locking with normal saline for catheter maintenance – A preliminary report. *Journal of Vascular Access*, 18(4), 325–327.

Sona, C., Prentice, D. & Schallom, L. (2011) National survey of CVC flushing in the intensive care unit. *Critical Care Nurse*, 32(1), 12–19.

Soothill, J.S., Bravery, K., Ho, A., et al. (2009) A fall in bloodstream infections followed a change to 2% chlorhexidine in 70% isopropanol for catheter connection antisepsis: A pediatric single center before/after study on a hemopoietic stem cell transplant ward. *American Journal of Infection Control*, 37(8), 626–630.

Sousa, B., Furlanetto, J., Hutka, M., et al. (2015) Central venous access in oncology: ESMO Clinical Practice Guidelines. *Annals of Oncology*, 26(5), v152–v168.

Spencer, T.R. (2017) Repositioning of central venous access devices using a high-flow flush technique: A clinical practice and cost review. *Journal of Vascular Access*, 18(5), 419–425.

Spencer, T.R. & Mahoney, K.J. (2017) Reducing catheter-related thrombosis using a risk reduction tool centred on catheter to vessel ratio. *Journal of Thrombosis and Thrombolysis*, 44(4), 427–434.

Springhouse (2009) *Intravenous Therapy Made Incredibly Easy*, 4th edn. Philadelphia: Lippincott Williams & Wilkins.

Stacey, R.G., Filshie, J. & Skewes, D. (1991) Percutaneous insertion of Hickman-type catheters. *British Journal of Hospital Medicine*, 46(6), 396–398.

Stanley, A. (2002) Managing complications of chemotherapy administration. In: Allwood, M., Stanley, A. & Wright, P. (eds) *The Cytotoxics Handbook*, 4th edn. Oxford: Radcliffe Medical Press, pp.119–192.

Stevens, B., Barton, S.E., Brechbill, M., et al. (2000) A randomized, prospective trial of conventional vascular ports vs the Vortex 'Clear-Flow' reservoir port in adult oncology patients. *Journal of Vascular Access Devices*, 5(2), 37–40.

Stewart, D. (2001) The percussion technique for restoring patency to central venous catheters. *Care of the Critically Ill*, 17(3), 106–107.

Swaminathan, L., Flanders, S., Rogers, M., et al. (2016) Improving PICC use and outcomes in hospitalised patients: An interrupted time series study using MAGIC criteria. *BMJ*, 27, 271–278.

Syner-Kinase (2011) Syner-Med (Pharmaceutical Products) Ltd. Available at: www.medicines.org.uk

Syner-Med (2016) *Summary of Product Characteristics*. Available at: https://www.syner-med.com

Tagalakis, V., Kahn, S.R., Libman, M., et al. (2002) The epidemiology of peripheral vein infusion thrombophlebitis: A critical review. *American Journal of Medicine*, 113(2), 146–151.

Tegtmeyer, K., Brady, G., Lai, S., et al. (2006) Videos in clinical medicine: Placement of an arterial line. *New England Journal of Medicine*, 354(15), e13.

Teplitz, L. (1990) Arterial line disconnection. *Nursing*, 20(5), 33.

Thillainathan, S. & Mariyaselvam, M.Z. (2017) Why has NHS England introduced an innovation and technology tariff to improve safer arterial systems in England? *British Journal of Anaesthesia*, 119(6), 1231–1244.

Thompson, A.M., Kidd, E., McKenzie, M., et al. (1989) Long term central venous access: The patient's view. *Intensive Therapy and Clinical Monitoring*, 10(5), 142–145.

Timoney, J.P., Malkin, M.G., Leone, D.M., et al. (2002) Safe and cost effective use of alteplase for the clearance of occluded central venous access devices. *Journal of Clinical Oncology*, 20(7), 1918–1922.

Timsit, J.F., Bouadma, L., Ruckly, S., et al. (2012) Dressing disruption is a major risk factor for catheter-related infection. *Critical Care Medicine*, 40, 1707–1714.

Timsit, J.F., Schwebel, C., Bouadma, L., et al. (2009) Chlorhexidine-impregnated sponges and less frequent dressing changes for prevention of catheter-related infections in critically ill adults: A randomized controlled trial. *JAMA*, 301(12), 1231–1241.

Tinker, J. & Zapol, W.M. (1992) *Care of the Critically Ill Patient*, 2nd edn. New York: Springer.

Tiru, B., Bloomstone, J.A. & McGee, W.T. (2012) Radial artery cannulation: A review article. *Journal of Anesthesia and Clinical Research*, 3(5).

Tortora, G.J. & Derrickson, B.H. (2017) *Principles of Anatomy & Physiology*, 15th edn. Hoboken, NJ: John Wiley & Sons.

Toth, L. (2002) Monitoring infusion therapy in patients residing in long-term care facilities. *Journal of Vascular Access Devices*, 7(1), 34–38.

Trick, N. (2011) *Overview: Vessel Health and Preservation*. Edinburgh: Infection Prevention Society.

Ullman, A.J., Cooke, M.L., Mitchell, M., et al. (2015) Dressings and securement devices for central venous catheters (CVC). *Cochrane Database of Systematic Reviews*, 9, CD010367. DOI: 10.1002/14651858.CD010367.pub2.

Ullman, A., Marsh, N. & Rickard, C. (2017) Securement for vascular access devices: Looking into the future. *British Journal of Nursing*, 26(8), S24–S26.

Usichenko, T.I., Pavlovic, D., Foellner, S., et al. (2004) Reducing venipuncture pain by a cough trick: A randomized crossover volunteer study. *Anesthesia & Analgesia*, 98(2), 343–345.

Valgimigli, M., Campo, C., Penzo, C., et al. (2014) Transradial coronary catheterization and intervention across the whole spectrum of Allen test results. *Journal of American College of Cardiology*, 63(18), 1833–1841.

Van Donk, P., Rickard, C., McGrail, M. & Doolan, G. (2009) Routine replacement versus clinical monitoring of peripheral intravenous catheters in a regional hospital in the home program: A randomized controlled trial. *Infection Control & Hospital Epidemiology*, 30(9), 915–917.

Verghese, S.T., Nath, A., Zenger, D., et al. (2002) The effects of the simulated Valsalva maneuver, liver compression, and/or Trendelenburg position on the cross-sectional area of the internal jugular vein in infants and young children. *Anesthesia & Analgesia*, 94(2), 250–254.

Vescia, S., Baumgartner, A.K., Jacobs, V.R., et al. (2008) Management of venous port systems in oncology: A review of current evidence. *Annals of Oncology*, 19(1), 9–15.

Vesely, T.M. (2002) Optimal positioning of CVC's. *Journal of Vascular Access Devices*, 7(3), 9–12.

Vesely, T.M. (2003) Central venous catheter tip position: A continuing controversy. *Journal of Vascular and Interventional Radiology*, 14(5), 527–534.

Vlahe, P.H. (2003) Complications associated with implantable vascular access devices in the patient with cancer. *Journal of Infusion Nursing*, 26(2), 97–102.

Volpicelli, G. (2011) Sonographic diagnosis of pneumothorax. *Intensive Care Medicine*, 37(2), 224–232.

Walker, E. (2009) Piloting a nurse-led ultrasound cannulation scheme. *British Journal of Nursing*, 18(14), 854–859.

Wall, C., Moore, J. & Thachil, J. (2016) Catheter-related thrombosis: A practical approach. *Journal of the Intensive Care Society*, 17(2), 160–167.

Wallach, S.G. (2004) Cannulation injury of the radial artery: Diagnosis and treatment algorithm. *American Journal of Critical Care*, 13(4), 315–319.

Wallis, M., McGrail, M., Webster, J., et al. (2014) Risk factors for peripheral intravenous catheter failure: A multivariate analysis of data from a randomized controlled trial. *Infection Control & Hospital Epidemiology*, 35(1), 63–68.

Warrington, W.G., Aragon Penoyer, D., Kamps, T.A., et al. (2012) Outcomes of using a modified Seldinger technique for long term intravenous therapy in hospitalized patients with difficult venous access. *Journal of the Association for Vascular Access*, 17(1), 24–30.

Washington, G.T. & Barrett, R. (2012) Peripheral phlebitis: A point-prevalence study. *Journal of Infusion Nursing*, 35(4), 252–258.

Webster, J., Clarke, S., Paterson, D., et al. (2008) Routine care of peripheral intravenous catheters versus clinically indicated replacement: Randomised controlled trial. *BMJ*, 337(7662), 157–160.

Weinstein, S. & Hagle, M.E. (2014) *Plumer's Principles & Practice of Infusion Therapy*, 9th edn. Philadelphia: Lippincott Williams & Wilkins.

Wells, S. (2008) Venous access in oncology and haematology patients: Part two. *Nursing Standard*, 23(1), 35–42.

Wendler, M.C. (2003) Effects of Tellington touch in healthy adults awaiting venipuncture. *Research in Nursing & Health*, 26 (1), 40–52.

White, M.L., Crawley, J., Rennie, E.A., et al. (2011) Examining the effectiveness of 2 solutions used to flush capped pediatric peripheral intravenous catheters. *Journal of Infusion Nursing*, 34(4), 260–270.

WHO (World Health Organization) (2009) *WHO Guidelines on Hand Hygiene in Health Care*. Available at: https://www.who.int/gpsc/5may/tools/9789241597906/en

Wigmore, T., Smythe, J., Hacking, M., et al. (2007) Effect of the implementation of NICE guidelines for ultrasound guidance on the complication rates associated with central venous catheter placement in patients presenting for routine surgery in a tertiary referral centre. *British Journal of Anaesthesia*, 99(5), 662–665.

Wilbeck, J. (2011) Evaluation methods for the assessment of acute care nurse practitioner inserted central lines: Evidence-based strategies for practice. *Journal of the Association for Vascular Access*, 16(4), 226–233.

Wilkes, G.M. (2011) Chemotherapy: Principles of administration. In: Yarbro, C.H., Wujcik, D. & Gobel, B.H. (eds) *Cancer Nursing: Principles and Practice*, 7th edn. Sudbury, MA: Jones & Bartlett, pp.390–457.

Williamson, E.E. & McKinney, J.M. (2001) Assessing the adequacy of peripherally inserted central catheters for power injection of intravenous contrast agents for CT. *Journal of Computer Assisted Tomography*, 25(6), 932–937.

Wise, M., Richardson, D. & Lum, P. (2001) Catheter tip position: A sign of things to come! *Journal of Vascular Access Devices*, 6(2), 18–27.

Witt, B. (2010) Vein selection. In: Phillips, S., Collins, M. & Dougherty, L. (eds) *Venepuncture and Cannulation*. Oxford: John Wiley & Sons, pp.91–107.

Wright, M.O., Tropp, J., Schora, D.M., et al. (2013) Continuous passive disinfection of catheter hubs prevents contamination and bloodstream infection. *American Journal of Infection Control*, 41, 33–38.

Yamada, R., Morita, T., Yashiro, E., et al. (2010) Patient-reported usefulness of peripherally inserted central venous catheters in terminally ill cancer patients. *Journal of Pain and Symptom Management*, 40(1), 60–66.

Yamamoto, A.J., Solomon, J.A., Soulen, M.C., et al. (2002) Sutureless securement device reduces complications of peripherally inserted central venous catheters. *Journal of Vascular and Interventional Radiology*, 13(1), 77–81.

Young, A., Begum, G., Billingham, L., et al. (2005) WARP-A multicentre prospective randomised controlled trial (RCT) of thrombosis prophylaxis with warfarin in cancer patients with central venous catheters (CVCs). *Journal of Clinical Oncology*, 23(16 Suppl.), LBA8004.

Yuan, R. & Cohen, M.J. (1985) Lateral antebrachial cutaneous nerve injury as a complication of phlebotomy. *Plastic and Reconstructive Surgery*, 76(2), 299–300.

Zhong, L., Wang, H., Xu, B., et al. (2017) Normal saline versus heparin for patency of central venous catheters in adult patients: A systematic review and meta-analysis. *Critical Care*, 21(1).

Zideman, D.A. & Morgan, M. (1981) Inadvertent intra-arterial injection of flucloxacillin. *Anaesthesia*, 36(3), 296–298.

Zinchenko, R., Prinsloo, N.J., Zarafov, A., et al. (2016) More needles less pain: The use of local anaesthesia during emergency arterial sampling. *Journal of Acute Disease*, 5(3), 244–247.

Chapter 18

Wound management

Jenni MacDonald with Kumal Rajpaul

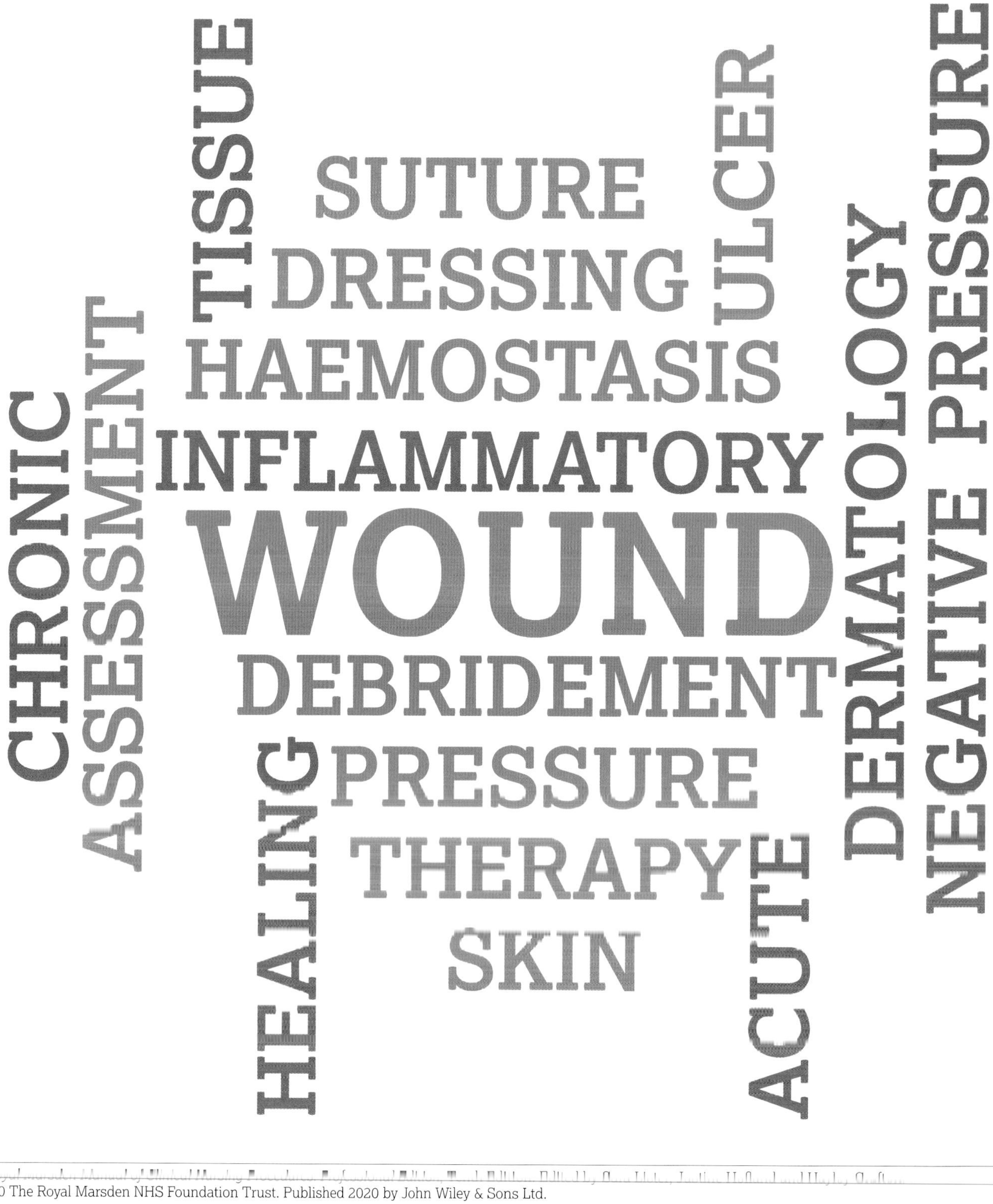

Procedure guidelines

Overview

This chapter provides a summary of the principles of wound care and current practice.

Wounds

Definition

A wound can be defined as a breach of the skin's epidermis, which may be attributable to an underlying, altered physiological state or a primary causation (HSE 2018). The causation of a wound may be intentional or accidental (Singh et al. 2017).

Wounds are a substantial burden for individuals and healthcare systems (Haesler et al. 2018). It has been estimated that 2.2 million wounds were managed, predominantly by nurses, in the NHS in the financial year 2012/13 (Guest et al. 2015).

Wounds can be divided into two categories: acute and chronic. There are no agreed definitions that enable differentiation between acute and chronic wounds (Kyaw et al. 2018). It is generally accepted that an acute wound is caused by a traumatic or surgical intervention (Doughty and Sparks 2016) and is expected to progress through the well-known phases of healing (Morton and Phillips 2016) in a predictable timeframe. In contrast, a chronic wound becomes 'stuck' in the inflammatory phase (Martin and Nunan 2015) and therefore does not heal as expected (Broderick 2009). Most chronic wounds occur on the lower limbs (Eming et al. 2014).

A holistic approach is essential for accurate assessment and planning of care (Eagle 2009). Both external and internal factors can contribute to the formation of a wound (Dhivya et al. 2015, Eagle 2009, Haesler et al. 2018):

- *External factors*: mechanical (friction, surgery or trauma), chemical, electrical, temperature extremes, radiation, micro-organisms, pressure and environment.
- *Internal factors*: circulatory system failure (venous, arterial or lymphatic), endocrine (diabetes), neuropathy, haematological causes (porphyria cutanea tarda or mycosis fungoides), nutritional status (smoking and alcohol history), malignancy, infection and age.

Anatomy and physiology

The skin is the largest organ in the body and makes up about 10% of an adult's total bodyweight (Hess 2012). The skin is important as it functions as an outer boundary for the body and helps to preserve the balance within (Tortora and Derrickson 2017). The skin needs to remain intact to perform vital functions (Tortora and Derrickson 2017); without it, humans would not survive insults from bacterial invasion, heat or water loss (Marieb and Hoehn 2018).

The skin varies in thickness from 1.5 to 4.0 mm depending upon which part of the body it is covering (Marieb and Hoehn 2018). The skin is made up of two main layers, the dermis and epidermis, which have six main functions: protection, sensation, thermoregulation, metabolism, excretion and non-verbal communication (Hess 2012).

The *epidermis* is the outermost layer and is avascular and thin. It regenerates every 4–6 weeks and functions as a protective barrier, preventing environmental damage and micro-organism invasion (Hess 2012). The thickness of the epidermis varies; it is thickest over the palms of the hands and soles of the feet (Marieb and Hoehn 2018) and thinnest on the eyelids (Jenkins and Tortora 2014).

The *dermis* provides support and transports nutrients to the epidermis. It contains blood and lymphatic vessels, sweat and oil glands, and hair follicles. The dermis is made up of collagen, fibroblasts, elastins and other extracellular proteins, which bind it together and keep it strong (Hess 2012). Its extracellular matrix contains fibroblasts, macrophages, and some mast cells and white blood cells (Marieb and Hoehn 2018). The connective tissue within the dermis is highly elastic and provides strength to maintain the skin's integrity and combat everyday stretching and wear and tear (Tortora and Derrickson 2011).

The subcutaneous layer just below the dermis is the deepest layer of skin and binds the skin to underlying tissues (Tortora and Derrickson 2011). This layer stores fat and is also known as the *hypodermis* or superficial fascia. It also assists the body as a protective layer and allows movement (Marieb and Hoehn 2018).

Wound healing: types and phases

Wound healing is a dynamic biological process of tissue regeneration (Dhivya et al. 2015) with the aim of full restoration of skin integrity (Harper et al. 2014).

Types of wound healing

There are three types of wound healing: primary, secondary and tertiary:

- Healing by *primary intention* involves the union of the edges of a wound under aseptic conditions, for example a traumatic laceration or surgical incision that is closed with sutures, skin adhesive, staples or clips (Flanagan 2013).
- Healing by *secondary intention* occurs when the wound's edges cannot be brought together. The wound is left open and allowed to heal by contraction and epithelialization. Epithelialization completes restoration of the skin's integrity (Giele and Cassell 2008). Wounds that heal by secondary intention heal at a slower rate due to the amount of tissue loss, are more susceptible to infection (Doughty and Sparks 2016) and often result in lesser cosmetic outcomes than other types of healing (Singh et al. 2017).
- Healing by *tertiary intention*, also known as 'delayed primary closure', occurs when a wound has been intentionally left open and is then closed, usually after a few days' delay, once swelling, infection or bleeding has decreased (Giele and Cassell 2008).

Phases of wound healing

The phases of wound healing are dynamic, depend upon each other and overlap (Eming et al. 2014). It is important to support a wound healing environment that encourages progression from one healing phase to the next without bacterial contamination.

The generally accepted phases of healing are:

1. haemostasis
2. inflammatory phase
3. proliferation or reconstructive phase
4. maturation or remodelling phase (Doughty and Sparks 2016).

Haemostasis (minutes)

Vasoconstriction occurs within a few seconds of tissue injury so blood flow from damaged blood vessels is reduced. When platelets come into contact with exposed collagen from damaged blood vessels, they release chemical messengers that stimulate a 'clotting cascade' (Timmons 2006). Platelets adhere to vessel walls, creating a fibrin clot that controls blood loss from compromised vessels (Doughty and Sparks 2016). Bleeding ceases when the blood vessels thrombose, usually within 5–10 minutes of injury (Hampton and Collins 2004) (Figure 18.1).

Inflammatory phase (1–5 days)

With the activation of clotting factors comes the release of histamine and associated vasodilation (Singh et al. 2017). The presence of histamine increases the permeability of the capillary walls, and plasma proteins, leucocytes, antibodies and electrolytes exude into the surrounding tissues. The wound becomes red, swollen and hot. These signs are accompanied by pain and tenderness at the wound site, last for 1–3 days and can be mistaken for wound infection (Hampton 2013) (Figure 18.2).

With haemostasis achieved, the focus then moves to preventing infection (Harper et al. 2014). Neutrophils, macrophages and then

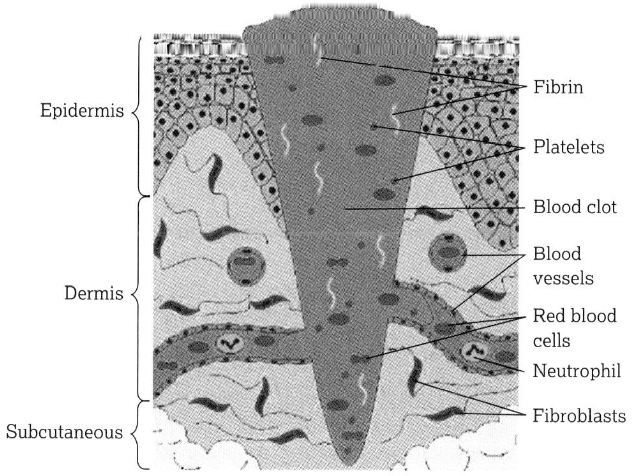

Figure 18.1 Haemostasis in a wound. *Source*: Reproduced with permission from Wayne Naylor.

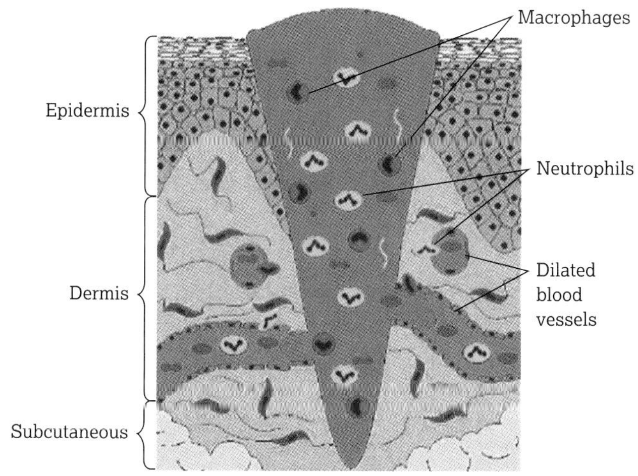

Figure 18.2 The inflammatory phase of wound healing. *Source*: Reproduced with permission from Wayne Naylor.

lymphocytes migrate to the wound within hours and these phagocytose debris and bacteria in the wound bed and secrete cytokines and growth factors (Stacey 2016). If the number and function of macrophages are reduced, as may occur in disease, for example diabetes (Snyder et al. 2016), healing processes are affected. Nutrients and oxygen are required to produce the aforementioned cellular activity and therefore malnourished patients and hypoxic wounds are more susceptible to infection (Singh et al. 2017). The breakdown of debris causes increased osmolarity within the area, resulting in further swelling. A chronic wound can become stuck in this phase of wound healing, resulting in prolonged healing, tendency to infection and higher levels of exudate (Martin and Nunan 2015). The phases that follow start the process of repair (Tortora and Derrickson 2017).

Proliferative phase (3–24 days)

The fibroblasts are activated to divide and produce collagen via processes initiated by the macrophages (Timmons 2006). Newly synthesized collagen creates a 'healing ridge' below an intact suture line, which gives an indication of how primary wound healing is progressing. The wound surface and the oxygen tension within encourage the macrophages to instigate the process of angiogenesis – the formation of new blood vessels (Singh et al. 2017). These vessels branch and join other vessels, forming loops. The fragile capillary loops are held within a framework of collagen. This complex is known as 'granulation tissue' (Gray et al. 2010). The combination of angiogenesis, granulation and collagen deposition encourages the wound edges to contract (Singh et al. 2017). Then, through mitosis and migration of epithelial cells, re-epithelialization occurs and covers the granulating wound bed, effectively restoring the bacterial barrier of the skin's surface (Doughty and Sparks 2016). Acute wounds start to granulate within 3 days, but the inflammatory and proliferative phases can overlap (Guo and DiPietro 2010) (Figure 18.3).

The mechanisms and processes within each phase of wound healing are dependent on an adequate oxygen supply at the wound bed and optimal nutrition, specifically iron, carbohydrates, protein, and vitamins A and C (Guo and DiPietro 2010, Singh et al. 2017).

Maturation phase (21 days onwards)

Maturation or remodelling of the healed wound begins at around 21 days following the initial injury and is the last phase of healing, which can last for up to 2 years (Harper et al. 2014) (Figure 18.4).

Collagen is reorganized and replaced, with the effect of emulating pre-wounded tissue. The new collagen provides increased tensile strength, though this will not achieve more than 80% of pre-wounded strength (Doughty and Sparks 2016).

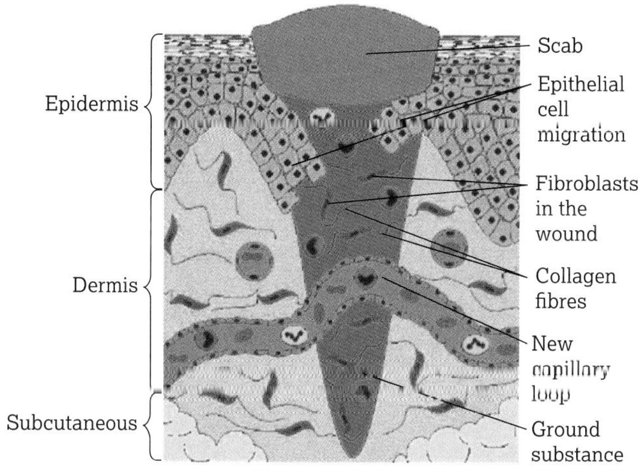

Figure 18.3 The proliferative phase of wound healing. *Source*: Reproduced with permission from Wayne Naylor.

1133

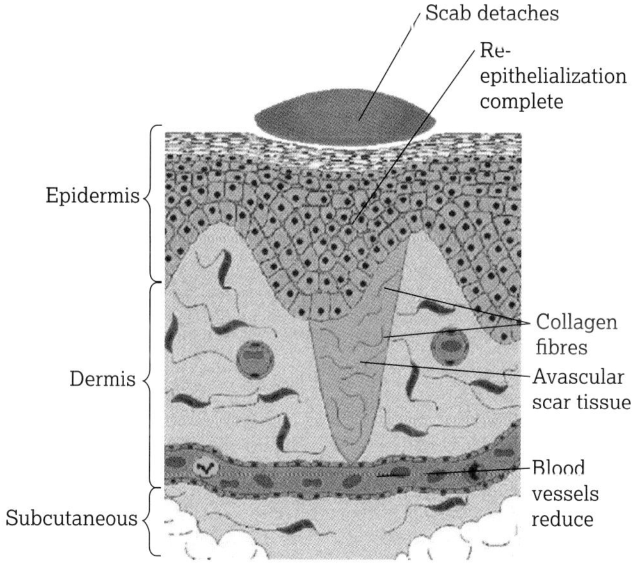

Figure 18.4 The maturation phase of wound healing. *Source*: Reproduced with permission from Wayne Naylor.

At the end of the maturation phase, the delicate granulation tissue of the wound will have been replaced by stronger avascular scar tissue. Rationalization of the blood vessels results in thinning and fading of the scar, although it is not fully known why this varies between people (Dealey 2005).

Related theory

Wound assessment

There are many frameworks available to aid a systematic approach to wound assessment (Flanagan 2013), though individually none are considered optimal (Greatrex-White and Moxey 2015).

The 'TIME' (tissue, infection/inflammation, moisture balance and edge of wound) acronym was developed in 2002 by an international group of wound care experts to provide a systematic approach to wound assessment and wound bed preparation (Dowsett and Ayello 2004, Leaper et al. 2012, Werdin et al. 2008) (Table 18.1).

Wound bed preparation (WBP) is a concept used to guide clinicians to focus on identifying and proactively addressing local barriers to wound healing in order to adequately 'prepare' the wound environment for healing (Kamolz and Wild 2013).

Goals of care should be determined early in the assessment process as full healing may not be the intention in fungating wounds or wounds at end of life. The underlying cause of the wound should be assessed, with a focus on details such as location, size and depth (Baranoski and Ayello 2015). The wound should be assessed each time a dressing is applied or if it gives cause for concern. The aim of assessing the wound is to determine the extent of healing and establish which treatment will best provide the ideal environment for healing. Regular wound photography provides a useful cumulative timeline of healing observation, but patient consent should always be gained (Baranoski and Ayello 2015). Figure 18.5 is an example of a wound assessment chart.

Factors that affect wound healing

The rate of wound healing varies depending on the general health, age and mobility of the individual; the location of the wound; the degree of tissue damage; and the treatment applied. It is necessary when assessing and treating a wound that all potential detrimental factors are addressed and minimized, where possible, in order to provide the optimum systemic, local and external conditions for healing.

Factors that may delay healing include disease, poor nutritional state, infection, body mass (Hess 2011) and medications such as chemotherapeutic drugs and steroids (Guo and DiPietro 2010) (Table 18.2). Lifestyle factors such as smoking, alcohol consumption and stress (Guo and DiPietro 2010, McDaniel and Browning 2014) can also affect wound healing. Other influences relate to the local microenvironment of the wound, including temperature, pH, humidity, air gas composition, oxygen tension, blood supply, inflammation and the presence of non-viable tissue (Hess 2011, Storch and Rice 2005). Whether this influence is positive or negative may depend on the stage of wound healing that has been reached. Other important considerations are external variables such as continuing trauma or the presence of foreign bodies.

Improving the blood flow to the wound bed will increase the availability of nutrients, oxygen, active cells and growth factors within the wound environment (Collier 2002). This may be achieved, if appropriate, through consideration of revascularization approaches or advanced therapies (Atkin et al. 2019).

Tissue (viable or non-viable)

Non-viable tissue in the wound bed will delay healing (Gray et al. 2010). Accurately identifying the different types of tissue in the wound bed by using the wound healing continuum (Figure 18.6) can guide the clinician to implement the correct actions and treatment plan to promote healing (Ousey and Cook 2012).

Debridement of devitalized tissue

Debridement is an essential component of wound bed preparation (Atkin 2014) and should be considered following a holistic patient assessment (Nazarko 2015). Debridement may not always be appropriate (McFarland and Smith 2014), for example in patients with clotting disorders, malignancy or ischaemic limbs, or in the palliative care environment (Wounds UK 2013).

Table 18.1 TIME principles for wound bed preparation

Clinical observations		Proposed pathophysiology	Wound bed preparation: clinical actions	Effect on wound bed of preparation actions	Clinical outcomes
Tissue (non-viable or viable)	**T**	Defective matrix and cell debris impair healing	Debridement (episodic or continuous)	Restoration of wound bed and functional extracellular matrix proteins	Viable wound bed
Infection or inflammation	**I**	High bacterial counts or prolonged inflammation ↑ Inflammatory cytokines ↑ Protease activity ↓ Growth factor activity	Remove infected foci with topical/systemic antimicrobials, anti-inflammatories or protease inhibition	Low bacteria counts or controlled inflammation ↓ Inflammatory cytokines ↓ Protease activity ↑ Growth factor activity	Bacterial balance and reduced inflammation
Moisture imbalance	**M**	Desiccation slows epithelial cell migration and causes maceration of wound margin	Identify root cause Apply moisture-balancing dressings, compression therapy or negative pressure wound therapy (NWPT)	Restored epithelial cell migration Desiccation avoided Oedema (excessive fluid) controlled Maceration avoided	Moisture balance
Edge of wound (non-advancing or undermined)	**E**	Non-migrating keratinocytes Non-responsive wound cells and abnormalities in extracellular matrix or abnormal protease activity	Reassess cause or consider corrective therapies Debridement Skin grafts Biological agents Adjunctive therapies	Migrating keratocytes and responsive wound cells Restoration of appropriate protease profile	Advancing edge of wound

Source: Royal Marsden NHS Foundation Trust (2013).

The ROYAL MARSDEN
NHS Foundation Trust

Wound Assessment Chart

Assessed by (Print name):	**Signature:**	**Role:**
Ward/Dept:	**Date:**	**Time:**
Patient Name:	**Hospital number:**	**Date of Birth:**

Factors affecting wound healing: (Please circle all that apply)

Diabetes Auto-Immune Conditions (rheumatoid arthritis, GVHD etc) Vascular Disease Neuropathy
Anaemia Radiotherapy Medication (cytotoxics, steroids, NSAIDs, Anticoagulants etc) Oedema
Reduced Mobility Malnutrition/Dehydration Pain Incontinence Smoking Infection
Non-Concordance Pressure Other (please specify):

Allergies/Sensitivities (please specify)

Impact of the wound on patient's life. *(body-image; pain; sleep, appetite; ability to eat/drink; socialization; sexuality; financial, etc)*

Patient's Treatment Goals and Information given:

Body Map: Please mark location of wounds with an x on diagram and number each wound

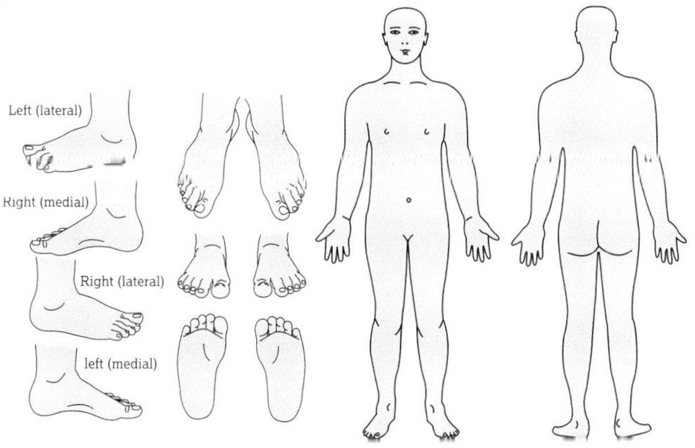

Pain Assessment: Please complete score in pain section overleaf

Visual Analogue Scale (VAS) for Patient's Rating of Pain

0 1 2 3 4 5 6 7 8 9 10

No Pain Mild Moderate Severe Worst Pain Imaginable

Wong-Baker FACES Pain Rating Scale

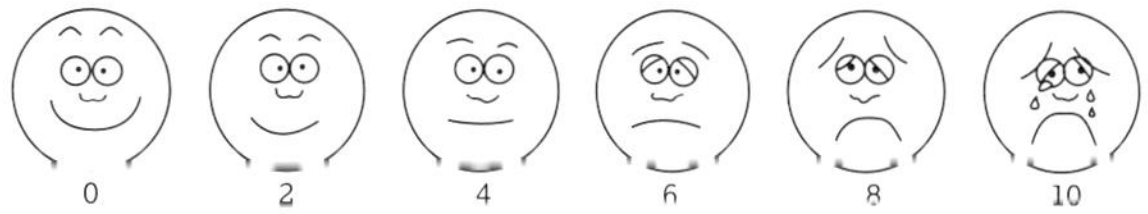

Key: Burn Diabetic Foot Ulcer Leg Ulcer - *Full Lower Limb assessment incl. Ankle-Brachial Pressure Index (ABPI)*
Malignant Fungating Wound Moisture Associated Skin Damage Pressure Ulcer *(specify category 1,2,3,4,U,SDTI)*
Surgical *(incision/drain site/skin graft/donor site)* Traumatic *(skin tear/abrasion/laceration/contusion, etc)* Other *(specify)*

Type	Number on body map	Date wound occurred/ duration	Referral (TVS, plastics, etc.)	Incident report number/date	Previous treatment/ ABPI	Investigations (bloods, imaging), comments

Figure 18.5 Wound assessment chart. *Source:* Reproduced with permission of The Royal Marsden NHS Foundation Trust.

The ROYAL MARSDEN
NHS Foundation Trust

Wound Assessment Complete/tick/select **bold** as appropriate							
Date of assessment:							
Wound Type and Body Map number:							
Measurements: (cm)							
Length (↕)							
Width (↔)							
Depth							
Undermining / **T**unnelling (clockwise)							
Photograph (**Y**es/ **N**o/ **D**eclined)							
TIMES framework:	Tissue Type Specify % of wound bed						
Epithelia (pink/white)							
Granulation (red)							
Hypergranulation (bright/dark red)							
Slough (yellow/green/brown)							
Necrotic (black)							
Haematoma							
Bone/tendon/fascia							
Infection/Inflammation Select **bold** as appropriate (1 or more signs may indicate infection)							
Increased or **P**urulent **E**xudate/**M**alodour/**P**ain							
Oedema/**E**rythema/**H**eat/**I**nduration							
Wound swab (**Y**/**N**)							
Moisture Balance: Please specify against each type **L**ow, **M**oderate or **H**igh							
Serous (straw/amber)							
Haemoserous (rose)							
Haematic (red)							
Purulent (green/brown/blue)							
Other							
Edges Tick as appropriate							
Healthy							
Dehisced							
Rolled							
Callused							
Raised							
Other							
Surrounding Skin Select **bold** as appropriate							
Healthy/**R**ash/**D**ry/**F**ragile/ **M**acerated/**E**xcoriated/**B**listers							
Pale/**D**usky/**R**ed/**N**ormal colour for the patient							
Oedema/**I**nduration/**B**oggy							
Hot/**C**old/**N**ormal temperature for the patient							
Other (skin nodules, ect)							
Pain Score (1–10)							
Continuous/**I**ntermittent/on **L**imb **M**obilisation/**D**ressing **C**hange							
Assessor Initials							

Figure 10.5 *Continued*

The ROYAL MARSDEN
NHS Foundation Trust

Wound Assessment Complete/tick/select **bold** as appropriate							
Date of assessment:							
Wound Type and Body Map number:							
Measurements: (cm)							
Length (↕)							
Width (↔)							
Depth							
Undermining / **T**unnelling (clockwise)							
Photograph (**Y**es/ **N**o/ **D**eclined)							
TIMES framework: Tissue Type Specify % of wound bed							
Epithelia (pink/white)							
Granulation (red)							
Hypergranulation (bright/dark red)							
Slough (yellow/green/brown)							
Necrotic (black)							
Haematoma							
Bone/tendon/fascia							
Infection/Inflammation Select **bold** as appropriate (1 or more signs may indicate infection)							
Increased or **P**urulent **E**xudate/**M**alodour/**P**ain							
Oedema/**E**rythema/**H**eat/**I**nduration							
Wound swab (**Y**/**N**)							
Moisture Balance: Please specify against each type **L**ow, **M**oderate or **H**igh							
Serous (straw/amber) Haemoserous (rose) Haematic (red)							
Purulent (green/brown/blue)							
Other							
Edges Tick as appropriate							
Healthy							
Dehisced							
Rolled							
Callused							
Raised							
Other							
Surrounding Skin Select **bold** as appropriate							
Healthy/**R**ash/**D**ry/**F**ragile/ **M**acerated/**E**xcoriated/**B**listers							
Pale/**D**usky/**R**ed/**N**ormal colour for the patient							
Oedema/**I**nduration/**B**oggy							
Hot/**C**old/**N**ormal temperature for the patient							
Other (skin nodules, ect)							
Pain Score (1–10)							
Continuous/**I**ntermittent/on **L**imb **E**levation/**D**ressing **C**hange							
Assessor Initials							

Figure 18.5 *Continued*

The ROYAL MARSDEN
NHS Foundation Trust

Date of assessment				
Wound Type and Body Map number:				
Wound healing process: Improving/ Static/ Deteriorating				
Treatment aim				
Cleansing agent				
Primary dressing				
Secondary dressing				
Planned frequency of dressing change				
Comments				
Assessor Print name and Initials				

Figure 10.5 *Continued*

Table 18.2 Factors that may delay wound healing

Factor	Action
Extrinsic factors	
Cold	Any drop in temperature delays healing by up to 4 hours
Excessive heat	Temperature over 30°C reduces tensile strength and causes vasoconstriction
Chronic excessive exudate	Wounds should not be too wet or too dry (see moisture imbalance in Table 18.1)
Poor dressing application and techniques	Delays may be caused by: • gaping of dressing material or multiple layers • tape/adhesive not being fastened securely, allowing slipping of wound exudates or dressing materials • bandaging too tight or loose
Poor surgical technique	Prolonged operating time, and inappropriate use of diathermy and drains can lead to haematomas and infection
Intrinsic factors	
Age	The elderly have a thinning of the dermis and underlying structural support for the wound (i.e. less moisture and subcutaneous fat); the metabolic process and circulation also slow with age
Medical and general health conditions	Diabetes, cardiopulmonary disease, hypovolaemic shock, rheumatoid arthritis, anaemia and obesity can delay healing
Malnutrition or protein–energy malnutrition	Malnutrition can cause generally poor healing, decreased tensile strength, and higher risk of wound dehiscence and infection; low serum albumin causes oedema
Psychosocial factors	Alcohol and smoking (carbon monoxide affects the blood vessels and circulation of oxygen), poor mobility, stress, isolation, anxiety and altered body image can delay healing
Drugs	Steroids, non-steroidal anti-inflammatories, anti-inflammatories, immunosuppressants and cytotoxic chemotherapy can delay wound healing

Source: Adapted from Bale and Jones (2006), ConvaTec (2004), Hampton and Collins (2004), Hess (2011).

Tissue colour	Description	Viable/non-viable	Treatment aim
Black/brown	Eschar/necrotic (dead) tissue	Non-viable	Debride
Yellow	Slough	Non-viable	Debride
Red	Granulation tissue	Viable	Promote healing – keep moist
Pink	Epithelial tissue	Viable	Protect

Figure 18.6 Wound healing continuum.

The aim of debridement is to:

- *remove* necrosis, slough, eschar, sources of inflammation or infection, exudate, serocrusts, hyperkeratosis, pus, haematomas, foreign bodies, debris and bone fragments
- *decrease* odour, excess moisture and risk of infection
- *stimulate* wound edges and epithelialization
- *improve* quality of life (Strohal et al. 2013).

Non-viable tissue and debris in a wound can:

- act as a physical barrier to healing
- impede normal extracellular matrix formation, angiogenesis, granulation and epidermal resurfacing
- reduce the effectiveness of topical preparations, such as antimicrobials
- mask or mimic signs of infection
- serve as a source of nutrients for bacteria
- contribute to overproduction of inflammatory cytokines, which can promote a septic response
- prevent the practitioner from gaining an accurate picture of tissue destruction and inhibit correct assessment of the wound
- lead to overproduction of exudate and odour (Wounds UK 2013).

Informed consent must be obtained before debridement. The healthcare professional must provide the patient with information regarding the methods of debridement available; this will include the predicted benefits and associated risks involved (Strohal et al. 2013).

There are many different approaches to wound debridement (Table 18.3). Various factors will inform the most appropriate method of debridement for a particular wound, such as suitability to the patient, type of wound, treatment aims, anatomical location and degree of debridement required (Madhok et al. 2013).

Inflammation and infection (or bacterial burden)

It is generally agreed that all chronic wounds harbour a variety of bacteria to some degree. As many chronic wounds fail to advance further than the inflammation phase of wound healing (Harries et al. 2016), their clinical presentation can often be mistaken for wound infection (Hampton 2013).

There are several stages in the continuum of wound infection: contamination, colonization, local infection, spreading infection and systemic infection (IWII 2016). The virulence of the infection involves a complex interaction between the individual and the condition of the wound (Butcher 2012). When a wound becomes infected, it displays the characteristic signs of heat, redness, swelling/inflammation, pain, increased exudate and malodour. The patient may also develop generalized pyrexia.

Table 18.3 Common debridement methods

Debridement method	Mechanisms of action	Advantages of this method	Disadvantages of this method	Who can implement this method?	How can this method be used?
Autolytic	A naturally occurring process in which the body's own enzymes and moisture rehydrate, soften and liquify hard eschar and slough	Least invasive method Can be used before or between other methods of debridement	Slow. Increasing the potential for infection and maceration	Any qualified nurse	Apply appropriate dressings (e.g. hydrogel or semi-occlusive) to achieve a moist wound healing environment
Mechanical	Physical disruption and removal of non-viable tissue from the wound bed	Can be used on devitalized tissues Quick and easy Can disturb biofilms Patients can self-administer under supervision	Not suitable for use on hard, dry eschar Not suitable for already painful wounds	Any qualified nurse	Employ single-use mechanical wound debridement product (e.g. monofilament pad or wipe) indicated in local wound dressings formulary
Bio-surgical (larvae)	Larvae quickly remove devitalized tissue from the wound; they are available loose or in a 'bagged' dressing	Highly selective and rapid	Costs higher than autolytic/ mechanical methods but treatment time is short Exercise caution with anticoagulants	Any qualified nurse with appropriate training or a specialist practitioner	Order and apply larvae as per local guidelines; seek specialist guidance if needed
Sharp	Removal of dead or devitalized tissue using a scalpel, curette, scissors and/ or forceps to just above the viable tissue level	Selective and quick Analgesia not normally required Works best on harder eschar that can be grasped with forceps Can be used at the bedside or in a clinic	Practitioners must be able to distinguish tissue types and understand anatomy as the procedure carries a risk of damage to blood vessels, nerves and tendons Not as effective on soft, adherent slough Does not result in total debridement of all non-viable tissue	Skilled practitioner (podiatrist or specialist nurse) with specialist training	Refer to specialist
Surgical	Excision or wider resection of non-viable tissue, including the removal of healthy tissue from the wound margins, until a bleeding wound bed is achieved	Selective and best used on large areas where rapid removal of devitalized tissue is required	Anaesthetic is usually required Higher costs related to theatre time	Must be performed by a surgeon, podiatrist or specialist nurse with appropriate training in the operating theatre	Refer to specialist

Source: Adapted from Vowden and Vowden (2011).

Clinicians must respond rapidly if a patient with a wound demonstrates signs of potentially fatal infection, including a systemic inflammatory response, sepsis, extensive tissue necrosis, gas gangrene or necrotizing fasciitis (Copeland-Halperin et al. 2016, IWII 2016). An essential role within wound management is therefore reducing bacterial burden, and many dressings are impregnated with antimicrobial compounds, such as silver, iodine or honey (Butcher 2012) (see Table 18.4). There is supporting evidence for the use of silver and other antimicrobials in reducing colonization and increasing healing rates (Leaper 2011). However, topical antimicrobials can be ineffective in the presence of biofilms (Percival 2017). Topical antibiotics are generally not advocated as they may increase bacterial resistance, and the use of antimicrobials prophylactically is controversial (Butcher 2012, Cutting 2011).

Immunosuppressed patients, diabetic patients and those on systemic steroid therapy may not present with the classic signs of infection. Instead, they may experience delayed healing, breakdown of the wound, presence of friable granulation tissue that bleeds easily, formation of an epithelial tissue bridge over the wound, increased production of exudate, malodour and increased pain.

There is currently no universally agreed-upon definition of wound infection that can be applied to all wounds (Cutting 2011). The clinical presentation of a wound should lead to the diagnosis of an infection. A wound swab should only be obtained if it is advocated by the clinical picture.

Wound swabs

There has been much debate and discussion as to which technique to use when obtaining a wound swab – the Z technique or the Levine technique (Myers 2011). The Z technique involves moving the swab in a zig-zag pattern across the wound while rotating the probe to achieve 10 points of contact without touching the edges of the wound. In the Levine technique, a swab is rotated over a 1 cm² area for 5 seconds with sufficient pressure to extract fluid (Copeland-Halperin et al. 2016).

The literature highlights that the Levine technique is more accurate when swabbing wounds than the Z technique because it takes

Table 18.4 Dressing groups (refer to the manufacturers' recommendations with regard to individual products)

Dressings	Description	Advantages	Disadvantages
Activated charcoal	Contains a layer of activated charcoal that traps and reduces odour-causing molecules	Easy to apply as either a primary or secondary dressing; can be combined with another dressing with absorbency	Need to obtain a good seal to prevent leakage of odour; some dressings lose effectiveness when wet*
Adhesive island	A low-adherent, absorbent pad located centrally on an adhesive backing	Quick and easy to apply; protects the suture line from contamination and absorbs exudate and blood	Only suitable for light exudate; some can cause skin damage (excoriation, blistering) if applied incorrectly
Alginates	A textile fibre dressing derived from seaweed; the soft woven fibres gel as they absorb exudate and promote autolytic debridement; available as a sheet, ribbon or packing	Suitable for moderate to heavy exudate; can be used on infected wounds; have haemostatic properties for bleeding wounds	Cannot be used on dry wounds or wounds with hard necrotic tissue (eschar); sometimes a mild burning or 'drawing' sensation is reported on application*
Antimicrobials (e.g. iodine, silver or honey)	Available as a primary or secondary layer and available topically (i.e. cream)	Suitable for chronic wounds with heavy exudate that need protection from bacterial contamination by providing a broad range of antimicrobial activities; can reduce or prevent infection	Sometimes sensitivity occurs with the use of silver and some skin staining can occur; instructions vary with products and dressings are expensive; evidence base for use is controversial and needs to be monitored*
Capillary wound dressings	Composed of 100% polyester filament outer layers and a 65% polyester and 35% cotton woven inner layer; the outer layer draws exudate, interstitial fluid and necrotic tissue into the inner layer via a capillary action	Suitable for light to heavy exudate; debride necrotic tissue; protect and insulate the wound; maintain a moist environment and prevent maceration; encourage development of granulation tissue; can be cut to any shape and are available in large rolls; can be used as a wick to drain sinus and cavity wounds	Can be hard to cut and have limited conformability to fit into wounds; cannot be used where there is the risk of bleeding due to the 'drawing' action and resultant increase in blood flow to the wound bed
Foams	Produced in a variety of forms, most being constructed of polyurethane foam; may have one or more layers	Suitable for use with open, exuding wounds; highly absorbent and non-adherent, and maintains a warm, moist wound bed; available for low to high exudates; available as non-adhesive and adhesive borders, which can negate the need for securing device	May be difficult to use in wounds with deep tracts and need a combined approach with an alginate or hydrofibre
Hydrocolloid	Usually consists of a base material containing gelatine, pectin and carboxymethylcellulose combined with adhesives and polymers; the base material may be bonded to either a semi-permeable film or a film plus polyurethane foam; some have a border	Suitable for acute and chronic wounds with low to no exudate; provides a moist wound environment; promotes wound debridement; provides thermal insulation; waterproof and provides a barrier to micro-organisms; easy to use; does not require secondary dressing	May release degradation products into the wound; strong odour produced as dressing interacts with exudate; not suitable for infected or dry wounds, or wounds with high exudate levels
Hydrofibre	Same consistency as hydrocolloid but in a soft woven sheet; has extra absorbency	Forms a soft, hydrophilic, gas-permeable gel on contact with the wound and manages exudate while preventing maceration of the wound edge; easy to remove without trauma to the wound bed	Does not have haemostatic property of alginates; not suitable for dry wounds*
Hydrogels	Contains 17.5–90% water, depending on the product; available as a gel or solid sheet; aids vertical exudate wicking	Suitable for light exudate wounds; donate fluid to dry necrotic tissue; can reduce pain and are cooling; low trauma at dressing changes; can be used as carriers for drugs	Cool the wound surface; use with caution in infected wounds; can cause peri-wound maceration due to leakage if too much gel is applied or the wound has moderate to heavy exudate*
Primary wound contact layer	Most are silicone based; applied directly to the wound bed	Conformable; non-adherent so can reduce trauma and pain on dressing change; some can reduce moisture loss; can be used with negative pressure wound therapy (NPWT)	Requires a secondary dressing

(continued)

Table 18.4 Dressing groups (refer to the manufacturers' recommendations with regard to individual products) *(continued)*

Dressings	Description	Advantages	Disadvantages
Semi-permeable films	Polyurethane film with a hypoallergenic acrylic adhesive; they have a variety of application methods, often consisting of a plastic or cardboard carrier	Only suitable for shallow, superficial wounds; suitable for prophylactic use against friction damage; useful as a retention dressing; allow passage of water vapour; allow monitoring of the wound	Not suitable for exuding wounds; possibility of adhesive trauma if removed incorrectly, can macerate, slip or leak
Skin barrier film	Alcohol-free liquid polymer that forms a protective film on the skin	Non-cytotoxic; does not sting if applied to raw areas of skin; high wash-off resistance; protects the skin from body fluids, friction and shear and the effects of adhesive products	Requires good manual dexterity to apply; may cause skin warming on application

* Requires a secondary dressing.
Source: Adapted from Skórkowska-Telichowska et al. (2013), Vowden and Vowden (2017).

samples from both the surface of the wound and the wound tissue due to the application of pressure to extract fluid (Angel et al. 2011). The Z technique has 63% sensitivity and 53% specificity while the Levine technique has 91% sensitivity and 57% specificity (Bonham 2009, Stotts 2012), which suggests that the Levine technique is more reliable in determining the organism in acute and chronic wounds when wound swabs are used to collect sample and cultures than the Z technique (Angel et al. 2011).

The procedure of obtaining a wound swab (see Chapter 13: Diagnostic tests) must always be explained to the patient and they must be informed that there may be some discomfort. The Levine technique involves cleansing the wound with normal saline. This will remove any debris on the wound bed. Avoid using antiseptics or antimicrobial agents prior to swabbing as this may influence the results (Reynolds 2013). Rotate the swab over a 1 cm^2 area of clean viable tissue with enough pressure to extract fluid from the inner part of the wound (Huang et al. 2016, IWII 2016).

Where possible, do not obtain sample from slough, pus or necrotic tissue as this will not provide an accurate profile of the microflora contained within the tissue (Cross 2014). Insert the wound swab into the culture container. Re-dress the wound after the procedure. Relevant clinical information about the patient and the wound should be provided with the sample, including the wound's aetiology, the anatomical location of the wound, current treatment, and presenting signs and symptoms (Cooper 2010).

Moisture balance

Wound exudate usually performs a useful function by aiding autolytic debridement and providing nutrients to the healing wound bed. It is required in the process of epithelialization, to allow the movement of cells across the surface of the wound (Jones 2013). However, in the presence of excess exudate, the process of wound healing can be adversely affected. This is especially so in chronic wounds, where there is increased proteolytic activity, leading to damage in the wound bed. Matrix metalloproteases are found in exudate, and, when present in chronic exudate, their beneficial properties, such as the provision of essential nutrients for cell metabolism, are hindered. This can be a significant factor in delayed healing (Hampton 2015).

The control of oedema or elevating the affected limb (e.g. in a lower leg wound) undoubtedly helps in the reduction of wound exudate. However, if the methods for achieving these goals are unsuccessful or contraindicated then exudate must be managed through the use of wound management products. These include absorbent wound dressings (e.g. alginates, hydrofibre or foams), non-adherent primary wound contact layers with a secondary absorbent pad, wound manager bags and negative pressure wound therapy (NPWT) (discussed later in this chapter). NPWT is highly effective in controlling excessive exudate (Probst and Huljev 2013). It is also vital to protect the skin surrounding the wound from maceration by excess exudate and excoriation from corrosive exudate. Useful products for skin protection include alcohol-free skin barrier films and thin hydrocolloid dressings, which can be cut and used to 'frame' the wound edges.

Edge non-advancement

Assessing and measuring the advancement of the wound edges towards wound contraction is an important indicator of wound progress (Harries et al. 2016). If wound edges fail to advance, the clinician should conduct a thorough reassessment using the TIME principles and interventions (Table 18.1).

Wound treatment planning

Clinicians must select appropriate dressings based on the tissue types in the wound bed, the treatment aims and the most suitable dressing properties. Based on the wound healing continuum, Figure 18.7 is an example dressing selection guide for wounds healing by secondary intention. It provides guidance on choice of products and their desired properties in relation to the tissue types in the wound bed, treatment aims and moisture levels. Where complete healing is the main aim, the clinician should use products that will create the optimal wound bed environment, ensuring the wound progresses through the wound healing continuum and subsequently completes the four phases of wound healing.

Caution must be exercised when considering hydrating wounds on the foot and/or at the end of life. Specialist referral may be required.

Principles of dressing a wound

With the exception of wounds where the main aim is to manage and improve symptoms, such as in malignant wounds or wounds at end of life, an ideal wound dressing must be capable of fulfilling the following functions:

- creates a moist, clean, warm environment
- provides hydration if the wound is dry or desiccated
- absorbs and adequately manages excess exudate
- provides protection to the peri-wound area
- allows for gaseous exchange
- is impermeable to micro-organisms
- is free of toxic or irritating particles
- does not shed particles or fibres
- can conform to the wound surface and anatomical location
- causes minimal pain and epidermal stripping during application and removal
- does not compromise the patient's religious or ethical beliefs
- is easy to use
- is cost-effective (Boyer 2013, Skórkowska-Telichowska et al. 2013, Sood et al. 2014).

Clinicians must be aware of the components of the wound care products used (Table 18.4). Dressings containing ingredients derived from animals, such as collagen and honey, may not be acceptable to patients from some faith, ethnic or ethical groups, such as Hindu, Islam, Sikhism or vegan (Eriksson et al. 2019, Sood et al. 2014).

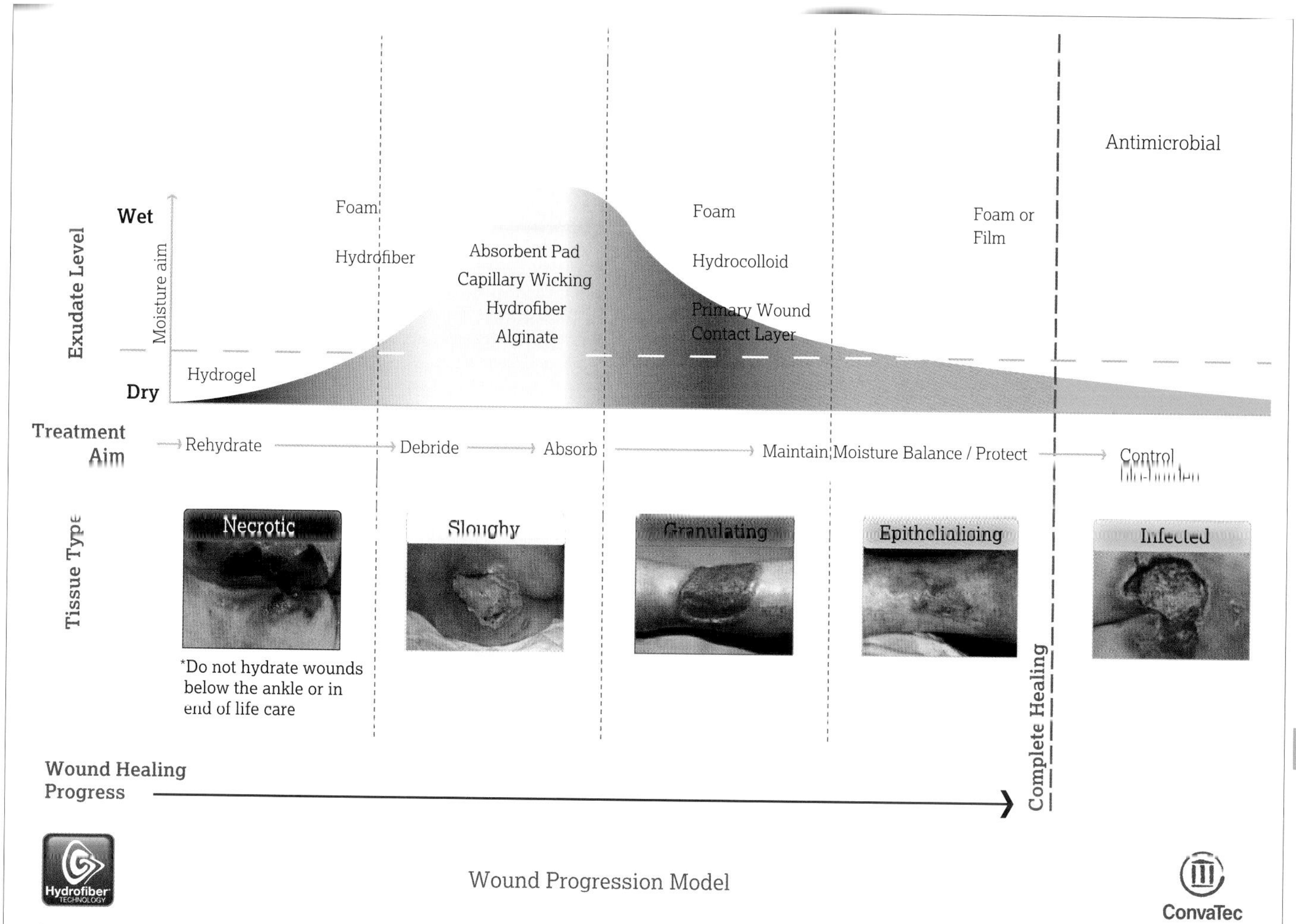

Figure 18.7 Treatment aims and dressing selection guide. *Source*: Reproduced from University College London Hospitals NHS Foundation Trust (2015) with permission of University College London.

Principles of cleansing a wound

The aim of wound cleansing is to help create the optimum local conditions for wound healing (Lloyd Jones 2012). Wound cleansing takes into consideration the wound bed, wound margins and peri-wound skin as all are central to successful healing (Kamolz and Wild 2013).

Wound cleansing can be considered ritualistic, non-evidence-based and often carried out unnecessarily (Lloyd Jones 2012). There is no robust evidence to suggest that routine cleansing of wounds expedites healing or reduces infection (Fernandez and Griffiths 2012). If a wound appears clean with little exudate, the clinician must consider the benefits and risks of cleansing the wound (McLain and Moore 2015).

When a wound bed is exposed to temperatures below core body temperature (36–38°C) or above 42°C, cellular activity is reduced, resulting in delayed wound healing (McGuiness et al. 2004). It can take 3 hours or longer for the wound to return to normal temperature (McKirdy 2001). Clinicians should consider warming cleansing solutions before use (HSE 2018).

Cleansing technique

Although swabbing wounds with soaked gauze swabs may be effective in removing foreign bodies from the surface of a wound, irrigation is the preferred technique as it is less damaging to new, fragile granulating tissue (Hall 2007, McLain and Moore 2015, Watret and Armitage 2002) and the potential of shedding gauze fibres into the wound is avoided (Wolcott and Fletcher 2014). Showering (at least 48 hours post-operatively) or immersing limbs may also be considered for those with chronic wounds located on the lower extremities (McLain and Moore 2015).

Cleansing solutions

Current evidence suggests that there is no significant difference in healing or infection rates between wounds cleansed with tap water (of drinkable quality) or 0.9% sodium chloride (Fernandez and Griffiths 2012, Hall 2007). NICE (2019) recommends using 0.9% sodium chloride for wound cleansing for 48 hours post-operatively. Wolcott and Fletcher (2014) repeat concerns that plumbing in healthcare facilities may be colonized with microbes, predominantly those of the genus *Pseudomonas*.

Where clinically indicated, there is evidence to support the use of modern, low-toxicity antimicrobial wound cleansing solutions such as polyhexamethylene biguanide (PHMB) or octenidine dihydrochloride in the reduction of wound microbial bio-burden (Andriessen and Eberlein 2008, Butcher 2012, Cutting and Westgate 2012).

Evidence-based approaches

Rationale

Indications

Indications for wound cleansing include the following:

- to remove debris and foreign bodies following a traumatic injury
- infected wounds, to remove excess exudate and manage malodour

- to remove superficial devitalized tissue or residual dressing material
- to provide patient comfort (Lloyd Jones 2012).

Pre-procedural considerations

Equipment

Dressings are grouped into categories under generic descriptions that reflect the products' properties and indications for use (see Table 18.4 for details of groups of dressings). The dressing that is applied directly to the wound bed (such as a primary wound contact layer) is the *primary* dressing. Not all primary dressings require a secondary dressing (e.g. a hydrocolloid does not).

A *secondary dressing* is applied on top of the primary dressing. An example is foam, although a foam can also be used alone as a primary dressing. Non-adhesive foams are helpful for patients with sensitivities to adhesives and will require securing with bandages (tubular or roll). Note that a dressing used to hold another in place in this way would be a secondary dressing.

Silicone-based products can be beneficial in protecting delicate wound beds and the peri-wound area due to their protective and atraumatic properties (Yarwood-Ross 2013). Dry dressings (such as gauze) do not fulfil the criteria for an ideal dressing and should not be used as a primary contact layer as they are likely to adhere, cause trauma and disturb healing (Sood et al. 2014).

It is important clinicians understand not only a dressing's properties but also how it behaves. For example, some dressings appear dry but 'gel' on contact with the wound, which maintains a moist environment, and are non-adhesive, thus becoming 'wet' (examples include hydrofibres, alginates and hydrocolloids). The wound itself has the ability to produce moisture. Wet dressings, such as hydrogels, can make a wound too wet and be responsible for maceration if used inappropriately (Hampton and Collins 2004).

Procedure guideline 18.1 Dressing a wound

Essential equipment

- Personal protective equipment
- Sterile dressing pack containing gallipots or an indented plastic tray, low-linting swabs, disposable forceps, sterile field and a disposable bag
- Fluids for cleaning and/or irrigation
- Appropriate dressings
- Disposable ruler
- Any other materials as determined by the nature of the dressing; special features of a dressing should be referred to in the patient's nursing care plan
- Detergent wipe
- Total traceability system for surgical instruments and patient record form

Optional equipment

- Sterile scissors
- Hypoallergenic tape

Action	Rationale
Pre-procedure	
1 Introduce yourself to the patient, explain and discuss the procedure with them, and gain their consent to proceed.	To ensure that the patient feels at ease, understands the procedure and gives their valid consent (NMC 2018, **C**).
2 Check analgesia requirements, allergy status, religious beliefs and ethical considerations that may affect wound dressing choice.	To reduce anxiety and discomfort during the procedure. Some dressings may not be suitable due to allergy, religion or ethical choices (Eriksson et al. 2013, **E**; Sood et al. 2014, **C**).
3 Wash hands with soap and water, and put on a disposable plastic apron.	Hands must be cleaned before and after every patient contact and before commencing the preparations for aseptic technique, to prevent cross-infection (Fraise and Bradley 2009, **E**).
4 Clean the trolley with a detergent wipe.	To provide a clean working surface (Fraise and Bradley 2009, **E**).
5 Place all the equipment required for the procedure on the bottom shelf of the clean dressing trolley. Check the integrity and use-by dates of all equipment (i.e. ensure that packs are undamaged, intact and dry).	To maintain the top shelf as a clean working surface. To ensure sterility of equipment prior to use. **E**
6 Close the treatment room door or screen the bed area. Position the patient comfortably so that the wound area is easily accessible without exposing the patient unduly.	To allow any airborne organisms to settle before the sterile field (and, in the case of a dressing, the wound) is exposed (Fraise and Bradley 2009, **E**). To maintain the patient's dignity and comfort. **E**
7 Take the trolley to the treatment room or patient's bedside, disturbing the screens as little as possible.	To minimize airborne contamination (Fraise and Bradley 2009, **E**).
Procedure	
8 Clean hands with an alcohol-based handrub.	To reduce the risk of wound infection and cross-contamination (Fraise and Bradley 2009, **E**).
9 Open the outer cover of the sterile dressing pack and slide the contents onto the top shelf of the trolley.	To ensure that only sterile products are used (Fraise and Bradley 2009, **E**).

10 Open the sterile field using only the corners of the paper. Open any other packs, tipping their contents gently onto the centre of the sterile field.	So that areas of potential contamination are kept to a minimum. **E**
11 Clean hands with an alcohol-based handrub.	Hands may become contaminated by handling outer packets, dressing and so on (Fraise and Bradley 2009, **E**).
12 Using the plastic bag in the pack as a sterile glove, arrange the sterile field. Pour cleaning solution into gallipots or an indented plastic tray.	The time the wound is exposed should be kept to a minimum to reduce the risk of contamination. To prevent contamination of the environment. To minimize the risk of contamination the cleaning solution. **E**
13 Attach the bag with the dressing to the side of the trolley below the top shelf on the side next to the patient.	To avoid taking soiled dressings across the sterile area. Contaminated material should be disposed of below the level of the sterile field. **E**
14 Apply non-sterile gloves and then loosen the adhesive of any existing dressing and remove it. Place the dressing in the disposal bag. Remove the gloves and dispose of them in the disposal bag.	To reduce the risk of cross-infection. To prevent contamination of the environment (Fraise and Bradley 2009, **E**).
15 Clean hands with an alcohol-based handrub and apply sterile gloves.	To reduce the risk of infection to the wound and contamination of the nurse. Gloves provide greater sensitivity than forceps and are less likely to traumatize the wound or the patient's skin. **E**
16 If necessary, gently irrigate the wound bed and peri-wound with 0.9% sodium chloride, unless another solution is indicated.	To reduce the possibility of physical and chemical trauma to granulation and epithelial tissue (Hess 2012, **E**).
17 Assess wound healing (see Figures 18.6 and 18.7). Obtain wound measurements and photography (with the consent of the patient) if required.	To assess healing and evaluate wound care (Hess 2012, **E**).
18 Apply the dressing that is most suitable for the wound using the criteria for dressings (see Table 18.4).	To promote healing and/or reduce symptoms. **E**
19 Ensure the patient is comfortable and the dressing is secure.	A dressing may slip or feel uncomfortable as the patient changes position. **E**
Post-procedure	
20 Dispose of waste in orange plastic clinical waste bags and sharps in a sharps bin. Remove gloves and apron and wash hands.	To prevent environmental contamination and sharps injury. Orange is the recognized colour for clinical waste (DH 2005, **C**).
21 Ensure the patient is comfortable and draw back the curtains (if applicable).	To promote wellbeing and maintain dignity and comfort. **E**
22 Clean hands with an alcohol-based handrub. Wipe trolley with detergent wipe and return to storage.	To prevent the risk of cross-contamination to the next episode of care (Fraise and Bradley 2009, **E**).
23 Record the assessment in the relevant documentation at the end of the procedure (see Figure 18.5 for an example).	To maintain an accurate record of wound healing progress (NMC 2018, **C**).

Post-procedural considerations

Ongoing care

Regular, accurate and in-depth wound assessment documentation is vital in monitoring wound healing and evaluating the effectiveness of a treatment plan (Baranoski and Ayello 2015). Regular wound measurements and photography can be helpful in communicating wound status to the multidisciplinary team and reducing unnecessary dressing changes.

Frequency of dressing changes should be carefully considered and based on the wound type, exudate level and dressing properties (NICE 2015b). High dressing change frequency should prompt a treatment plan reconsideration.

Pressure ulcers

Definition

Pressure ulcers are areas of localized tissue damage usually occurring over a bony prominence caused by excess pressure, shearing forces and medical devices (Haesler 2014).

Anatomy and physiology

A pressure ulcer usually results from compromised circulation secondary to unrelieved pressure on the tissues, compressed between a bone and an external surface (Hess 2012). During the period of unrelieved pressure, the local tissues are deprived of blood flow, oxygen and nutrients, resulting in ischaemia (House and Johnson 2014).

Pressure ulcers are categorized according to the degree of tissue damage using the International Pressure Ulcer Classification System developed by the National Pressure Ulcer Advisory Panel, the European Pressure Ulcer Advisory Panel and the Pan Pacific Pressure Injury Alliance (Haesler 2014), illustrated in Figure 18.8. Pressure ulcers are categorized into six stages. Stages I–IV are attributed according to wound depth. Depth is unknown in the 'unstageable' and 'suspected deep tissue injury' categories.

Evidence-based approaches

Pressure ulcers, although often preventable, remain a major healthcare issue and are debilitating for patients (NICE 2014). Pressure ulcers result in reduced quality of life, pain, infection, and prolonged hospital stay, and can be life threatening in the case of gangrene or sepsis (NICE 2015a).

INTERNATIONAL NPUAP/EPUAP PRESSURE ULCER CLASSIFICATION SYSTEM

A pressure ulcer is a localized injury to the skin and/or underlying tissue usually over a bony prominence, as a result of pressure, or pressure in combination with shear. A number of contributing or confounding factors are also associated with pressure ulcers; the significance of these factors is yet to be elucidated.

Category/Stage I: Nonblanchable Erythema

Intact skin with non-blanchable redness of a localized area usually over a bony prominence. Darkly pigmented skin may not have visible blanching; its color may differ from the surrounding area.

The area may be painful, firm, soft, warmer or cooler as compared to adjacent tissue. Category/Stage I may be difficult to detect in individuals with dark skin tones. May indicate 'at risk' individuals (a heralding sign of risk).

Category/Stage II: Partial Thickness Skin Loss

Partial thickness loss of dermis presenting as a shallow open ulcer with a red pink wound bed, without slough. May also present as an intact or open/ruptured serum-filled blister.

Presents as a shiny or dry shallow ulcer without slough or bruising.* This Category/Stage should not be used to describe skin tears, tape burns, perineal dermatitis, maceration or excoriation.

**Bruising indicates suspected deep tissue injury.*

Category/Stage III: Full Thickness Skin Loss

Full thickness tissue loss. Subcutaneous fat may be visible but bone, tendon or muscle are not exposed. Slough may be present but does not obscure the depth of tissue loss. May include undermining and tunneling.

The depth of a Category/Stage III pressure ulcer varies by anatomical location. The bridge of the nose, ear, occiput and malleolus do not have subcutaneous tissue and Category/Stage III ulcers can be shallow. In contrast, areas of significant adiposity can develop extremely deep Category/Stage III pressure ulcers. Bone/tendon is not visible or directly palpable.

Category/Stage IV: Full Thickness Tissue Loss

Full thickness tissue loss with exposed bone, tendon or muscle. Slough or eschar may be present on some parts of the wound bed. Often includes undermining and tunneling.

The depth of a Category/Stage IV pressure ulcer varies by anatomical location. The bridge of the nose, ear, occiput and malleolus do not have subcutaneous tissue and these ulcers can be shallow. Category/Stage IV ulcers can extend into muscle and/or supporting structures (e.g., fascia, tendon or joint capsule) making osteomyelitis possible. Exposed bone/tendon is visible or directly palpable.

Unstageable: Depth Unknown

Full thickness tissue loss in which the base of the ulcer is covered by slough (yellow, tan, gray, green or brown) and/or eschar (tan, brown or black) in the wound bed.

Until enough slough and/or eschar is removed to expose the base of the wound, the true depth, and therefore Category/Stage, cannot be determined. Stable (dry, adherent, intact without erythema or fluctuance) eschar on the heels serves as 'the body's natural (biological) cover' and should not be removed.

Suspected Deep Tissue Injury: Depth Unknown

Purple or maroon localized area of discolored intact skin or blood-filled blister due to damage of underlying soft tissue from pressure and/or shear. The area may be preceded by tissue that is painful, firm, mushy, boggy, warmer or cooler as compared to adjacent tissue.

Deep tissue injury may be difficult to detect in individuals with dark skin tones. Evolution may include a thin blister over a dark wound bed. The wound may further evolve and become covered by thin eschar. Evolution may be rapid exposing additional layers of tissue even with optimal treatment.

Figure 18.8 The International National Pressure Ulcer Advisory Panel/European Pressure Ulcer Advisory Panel Pressure Ulcer Classification System. *Source:* Reproduced from Haesler (2014).

It is important to use a structured approach that involves skin assessment and identification of risks (Haesler 2014). As part of an American initiative in 2004, the 'SKIN' acronym was developed to provide a structured approach to pressure ulcer prevention (Whitlock et al. 2011). This was introduced into the NHS in 2009 and was subsequently developed into 'SSKIN' in 2011 (by NHS Scotland) and 'ASSKING' (or aSSKINg) in 2018 (by NHS England). While it is recognized that the fundamentals of care required to prevent pressure ulcers are found in SSKIN, it is agreed that ASSKING (Assess risk, Skin inspection, Surface, Keep moving, Incontinence, Nutrition, Giving information) supports clinician actions. This structured approach is the foundation of all pressure ulcer prevention treatment plans and bedside care bundles (Figure 18.9).

Assessment of risk

The risk assessment (Figure 18.10) should be carried out within 6 hours (can vary locally) of admission and regularly thereafter (NICE

The ROYAL MARSDEN
NHS Foundation Trust

aSSKINg bundle assessment

Name			Date of birth
Hospital No.	NHS No.	Age	Weight

An aSSKINg (Assess risk, Skin inspection, Surface, Keep moving, Incontinence, Nutrition, Give information) bundle is a bedside tool to help staff and patients with skin concerns and proactively reduce the risks of developing a pressure ulcer. Documenting each aspect of the aSSKINg checklist can help to achieve this. Patients should be encouraged to inspect their own pressure areas and change position regularly and to document their findings on page 2. Please refer to the 'Preventing pressure ulcers' information leaflet

Complete daily if Waterlow ≥10 or if clinical judgement indicates

		Date (DD/MM/YY)					
		Time (HH:MM)					
Assess risk		Waterlow Score					
Nutrition and Hydration	Nutrition risk assessment completed in the last 7 days?	Y/N					
	Patient **E**ating/**N**il **B**y **M**outh/**P**arenteral **N**utrition/**E**nteral **N**utrition	E/NBM/PN/EN					
	Food record chart updated?	Y/N/NA					
	Patient **D**rinking/**I**ntra**V**enous **F**luids/**S**ips?	D/IVF/S					
	Fluid balance chart updated?	Y/N/NA					
	Snacks or supplements offered?	Y/N/NA/D					
	Meal assistance required?	Y/N/NA					
	If Nutrition Assessment ≥10+ or ANY category of pressure ulcer give date of referral to dietician	DD/MM/YY					
Surface	Date mattress and cushion ordered	DD/MM/YY					
	Mattress: **F**oam/**H**ybrid/**A**ir	F/H/A					
	Bed: **S**tandard/**L**ow/**P**lus size	S/L/P					
	Cushion: **A**ir/**S**pecialist (from OT/TVN)	A/S					
	Heels: **P**illows/**H**eel up boots	P/H					
	Giving information						
	Verbal **E**ducation provided and/or patient information **L**eaflet given and explained	VE/L					
		Staff initials					

STAFF

Figure 18.9 The Royal Marsden NHS Foundation Trust's ASSKING bundle.

2015a) by a registered nurse or healthcare professional who has undergone appropriate training in recognizing and reducing the risk factors that contribute to the development of pressure ulcers; this person should also understand how to initiate appropriate actions and maintain correct and suitable prevention measures (Waterlow 2007) (Figures 18.11 and 18.12). The use of risk assessment tools (e.g. Figure 18.10) should be undertaken in conjunction with clinical judgement and skin inspection (Haesler 2014).

Please note – if code V or D is entered, escalate to Nurse in Charge who must sign and date here. Please document on page 4.	
Signature	Date
Signature	Date

If patient has or develops any wound initiate the Wound Assessment booklet

Key: **1-4** – Grade **A** – Away from ward **B** – Blanching **C** – Changed dressing **D** – Declined **G** – Given analgesia **I** – Intact **IND** – Independent **MD** – Medical device **M** – Moisture lesion **N** – No **NA** – Not Applicable **R** – Reclined **S** – Suspected deep tissue injury **U** – Unstageable **UP** – Upright **V** – Variance **Y** – Yes

		Key / Date / Time																				
	Prescribed SSKIN frequency	eg 2/3/4 (hourly) or IND																				
Keep moving	Requires pain relief to turn/mobilise	Y/N/NA/G/D																				
	Laying on left side	✓																				
	Laying on right side	✓																				
	Laying flat on back	✓																				
	Chair – sitting Reclined/sitting fully Upright	R/UP																				
	Mobilised or repositioned >2 minutes	✓																				
	Appropriate manual handling equipment in use?	Y/N/NA																				
	Call bell is within easy reach of patient	Y/N																				
Incontinence	Skin clean and dry? If NO complete the following	Y/N																				
	Urinary/bowel/catheter functioning well?	Y/N/NA																				
	Have there been problems with Urine/Faeces/Sweat/Blood/Exudate/Other?	U/F/S/B/E/O																				
	Absorbent incontinence aids in use?	Y/N/NA																				
	Barrier cream/Spray applied	Y/N																				
Skin assessment – Staff to complete visual top to toe skin check at least twice in 24 hours	All skin checked?	Y/N																				
	If NO, state reason	eg splint/eating																				
	Head (specify)	I/B/M/1-4/S/U/D																				
	Shoulder L / R	I/B/M/1-4/S/U/D																				
	Elbow L / R	I/B/M/1-4/S/U/D																				
	Hip L / R	I/B/M/1-4/S/U/D																				
	Buttock L / R	I/B/M/1-4/S/U/D																				
	Heel L / R	I/B/M/1-4/S/U/D																				
	Ankles L / R	I/B/M/1-4/S/U/D																				
	Sacrum (tailbone)	I/B/M/1-4/S/U/D																				
	Other (specify)	I/B/M/1-4/S/U/D																				
	Skin under medical devices checked twice daily?	Y/N/NA																				
	Stockings/socks removed twice daily to check heels?	Y/N/NA																				
		Patient initials																				
		Staff initials																				

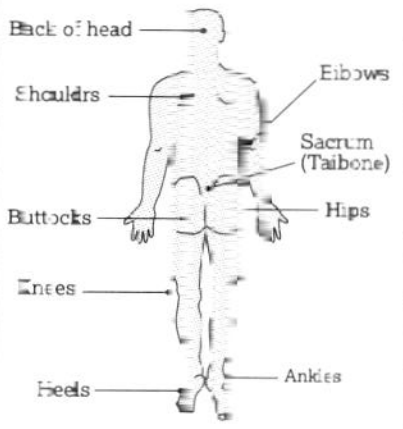

STAFF

STAFF

STAFF AND PATIENT/CARER

PATIENT

Figure 18.9 *Continued*

Body map

Indicate the location on the diagram with an X and number the wounds if more than one.

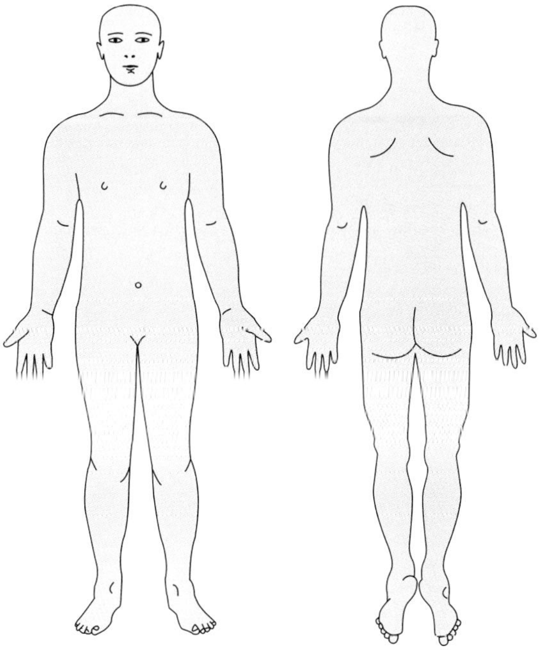

	Date						
	Time						
Wound chart updated	Y/N/NA						
If applicable, staff to refer to the Tissue Viability Nurse. (If no improvement after 72 hours, re-refer as appropriate.)	DD/MM/YY						
	Staff initials						

	Date	**DATIX number and description**
1.		
2.		
3.		
4.		

Date and time	**Variance** (if the code V is used on page 2 or 3 please provide details below)	**Print name and Signature**

Figure 18.9 *Continued*

The ROYAL MARSDEN
NHS Foundation Trust

Waterlow Pressure Ulcer Risk Assessment (within 4 hours of Admission and DAILY)

<10 Low Risk	10+ At Risk 15+ High Risk 20+ Very High Risk

Date (Day/Month/Year)		
Time (24-hour clock)		
GENDER	Male	1
	Female	2
AGE	14–49	1
	50–64	2
	65–74	3
	75–80	4
	81+	5
BUILD	Average	0
	Above average	1
	Obese	2
	Below average	3
APPETITE (select one option ONLY)	Average	0
	Poor	1
	NG tube/fluids only	2
	NBM/anorexic	3
VISUAL ASSESSMENT OF AT RISK SKINAREA (may select one or more options)	Healthy	0
	Thin and fragile and/or dry	1
	Oedematous	1
	Clammy (temp↑)	1
	Previous pressure ulcer or scarring	2
	Discoloured	2
	Broken	3
MOBILITY (select one option ONLY)	Fully	0
	Restless/fidgety	1
	Apathetic	2
	Restricted	3
	Bedbound	4
	Chairbound	5
CONTINENCE (select one option ONLY)	Continent/catheterised	0
	Incontinent of urine	1
	Incontinent of faeces	2
	Doubly incontinent	3
TISSUE MALNUTRITION (may select one or more options)	Smoking	2
	Anaemia	2
	Peripheral vascular disease	5
	Single organ failure	5
	Multiple organ failure	8
	Cachexia	8
NEUROLOGICAL DEFICIT (score depends on severity)	Diabetes, CVA, MS, motor/sensory paraplegia, epidural	4-6
MAJOR SURGERY TRAUMA (up to 48 hours post-surgery)	Above waist	2
	Orthopaedic, below waist, spinal >2 hours on theatre table	5
	> 6 hours on Theatre Table	8
MEDICATION	Cytotoxics, high dose steroids, anti inflammatory	4
		Total Score
Signature, print name and designation		

React to Risk

If total score is < 10	If total score is 10+ (or clinical judgement indicates): AT RISK
LOW RISK Re-assess daily OR if significant change in patient's condition	Initiate aSSKINg bundle in line with level of risk and clinical judgement **If patient has existing multiple grade 2 or a category 3, 4 or unstagable pressure ulcer** Complete SGA (safe-guarding) pressure ulcer protocol

Figure 18.10 The Waterlow Pressure Ulcer Risk Assessment Tool. *Source*: Reproduced with permission of The Royal Marsden NHS Foundation Trust.

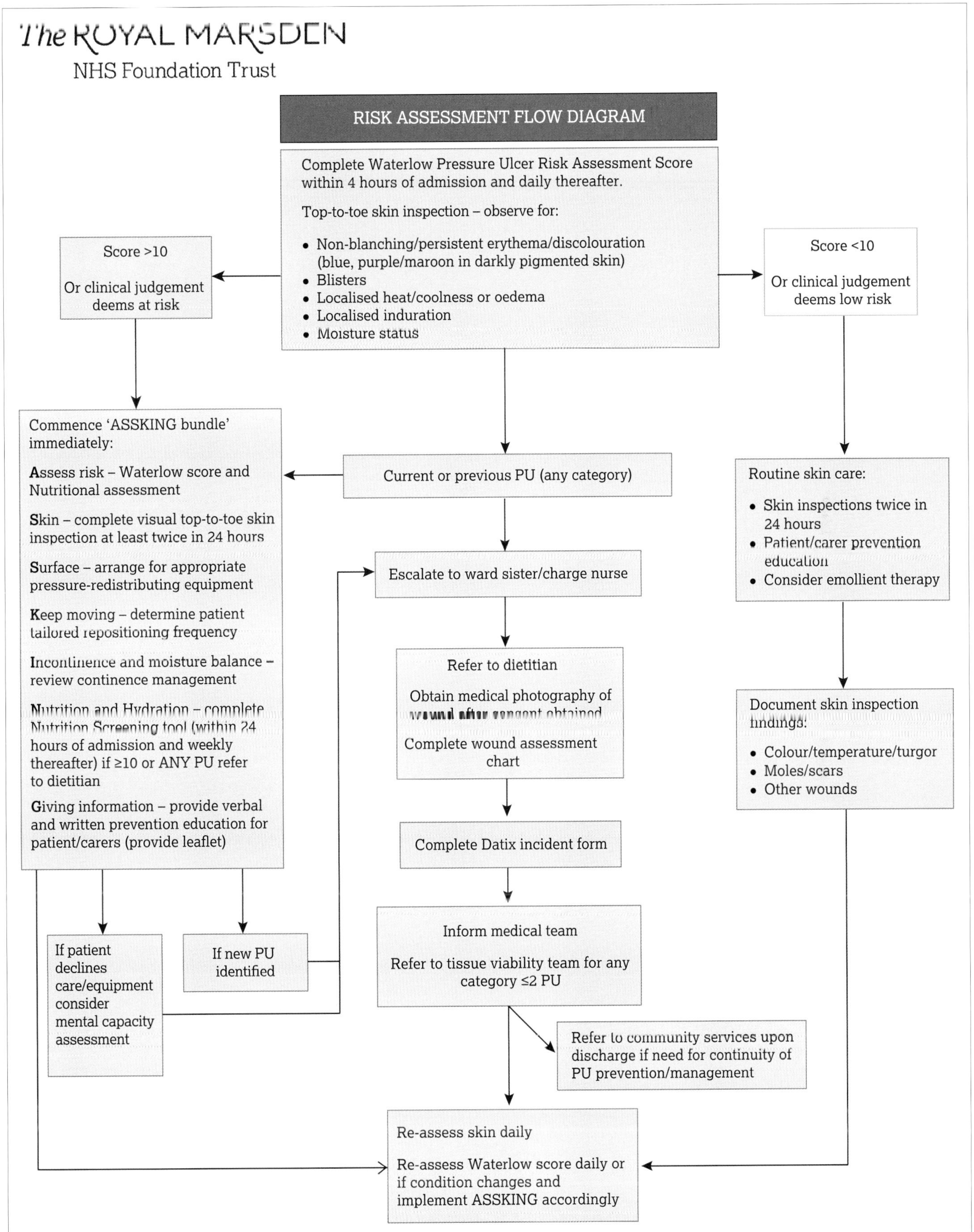
The ROYAL MARSDEN
NHS Foundation Trust
RISK ASSESSMENT FLOW DIAGRAM
Complete Waterlow Pressure Ulcer Risk Assessment Score within 4 hours of admission and daily thereafter.
Top-to-toe skin inspection – observe for:
• Non-blanching/persistent erythema/discolouration (blue, purple/maroon in darkly pigmented skin)
• Blisters
• Localised heat/coolness or oedema
• Localised induration
• Moisture status
Score >10
Or clinical judgement deems at risk
Score <10
Or clinical judgement deems low risk
Commence 'ASSKING bundle' immediately:
Assess risk – Waterlow score and Nutritional assessment
Skin – complete visual top-to-toe skin inspection at least twice in 24 hours
Surface – arrange for appropriate pressure-redistributing equipment
Keep moving – determine patient tailored repositioning frequency
Incontinence and moisture balance – review continence management
Nutrition and Hydration – complete Nutrition Screening tool (within 24 hours of admission and weekly thereafter) if ≥10 or ANY PU refer to dietitian
Giving information – provide verbal and written prevention education for patient/carers (provide leaflet)
Current or previous PU (any category)
Escalate to ward sister/charge nurse
Refer to dietitian
Obtain medical photography of wound after consent obtained
Complete wound assessment chart
Complete Datix incident form
Inform medical team
Refer to tissue viability team for any category ≤2 PU
Refer to community services upon discharge if need for continuity of PU prevention/management
Routine skin care:
• Skin inspections twice in 24 hours
• Patient/carer prevention education
• Consider emollient therapy
Document skin inspection findings:
• Colour/temperature/turgor
• Moles/scars
• Other wounds
If patient declines care/equipment consider mental capacity assessment
If new PU identified
Re-assess skin daily
Re-assess Waterlow score daily or if condition changes and implement ASSKING accordingly

Figure 18.11 Risk assessment flow diagram. PU, pressure ulcer. *Source*: Reproduced with permission of The Royal Marsden NHS Foundation Trust.

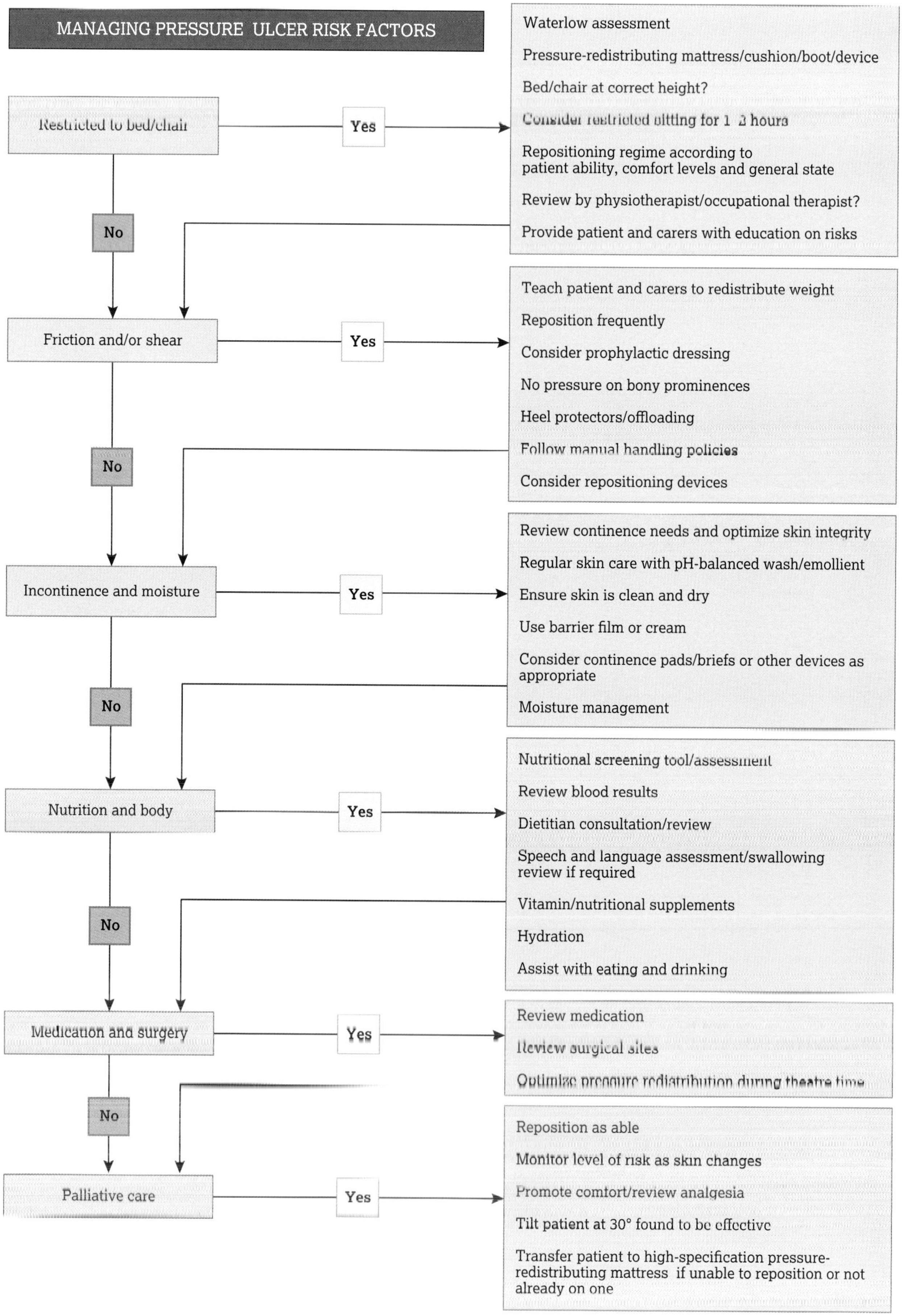

Figure 18.12 Managing pressure ulcer risk factors. *Source:* Reproduced with permission of The Royal Marsden NHS Foundation Trust.

An individual's potential for developing pressure ulcers may be influenced by the following intrinsic factors:

- reduced mobility or immobility
- acute illness
- level of consciousness
- extremes of age
- vascular disease
- severe, chronic or terminal illness
- previous history of pressure damage
- malnutrition and dehydration
- neurological compromise
- obesity
- poor posture.

The potential of an individual to develop pressure ulcers may be exacerbated by the following factors, which therefore should be considered when performing a risk assessment (Haesler 2014):

- Sedatives and hypnotics may make the patient excessively sleepy and thus reduce mobility.
- Analgesics may reduce normal stimulus to relieve pressure.
- Inotropes cause peripheral vasoconstriction and tissue hypoxia.
- Non-steroidal anti-inflammatory drugs impair inflammatory responses to pressure injury.
- Cytotoxics and high-dose steroids may induce immunosuppression, which impairs inflammatory responses to pressure injury and may lead to an increased risk of wound infection.
- Moisture to the skin (e.g. from incontinence, perspiration or wound exudate) can contribute to pressure ulcer formation.

Skin inspection

Systematic skin inspection should occur regularly, with increased or decreased frequencies determined in response to changes in the individual's condition. Individuals at risk should have their skin inspected (including under medical devices) at least twice per day (Haesler 2014) if an inpatient or at every visit in the community setting.

Skin inspection should be based on an assessment of the most vulnerable areas of risk for each patient (Figure 18.13), this should include daily removal of antiembolic stockings and/or non-slip socks. Areas for observation include heels, sacrum, ischial tuberosities, elbows, temporal region of skull, shoulders, backs of head and toes, and femoral trochanters, as well as parts of the body where pressure, friction and shear are exerted in the course of daily living activities, and parts of the body where external forces are exerted by equipment and clothing. Other areas should be inspected as necessitated by the patient's condition.

Individuals who are willing and able should be encouraged, following education, to inspect their own skin. Individuals who are wheelchair users should employ a mirror to inspect the areas that they cannot see easily or get others to inspect them.

Healthcare professionals should be aware of the following signs that may indicate incipient pressure ulcer development:

- persistent erythema
- non-blanching erythema
- blisters
- discoloration
- localized heat
- localized oedema
- localized induration
- purplish/bluish localized areas of skin
- localized heat that, if tissue becomes damaged, is replaced by coolness.

Skin observation and changes should be documented immediately using the aforementioned grading system (Haesler 2014) to classify the ulcer stage and extent of tissue damage (see Figure 18.6). Appropriate emollients should be prescribed and administered for dry skin conditions. Avoid excessive rubbing over bony prominences, as this does not prevent pressure damage and may cause additional damage.

Surface (equipment)

Support surfaces (i.e. mattresses and cushions) designed to redistribute pressure loading on the skin should be selected on an individual basis. While in hospital, a high-specification foam mattress and/or cushion should be provided to patients at risk as a minimum (NICE 2014).

An active support surface should be considered for patients:

- at high risk of pressure ulcer development
- who cannot be positioned off an existing pressure ulcer or who have pressure ulcers on opposing anatomical locations, limiting repositioning options
- who have existing pressure ulcers whose healing is stagnant or deteriorating (Haesler 2014).

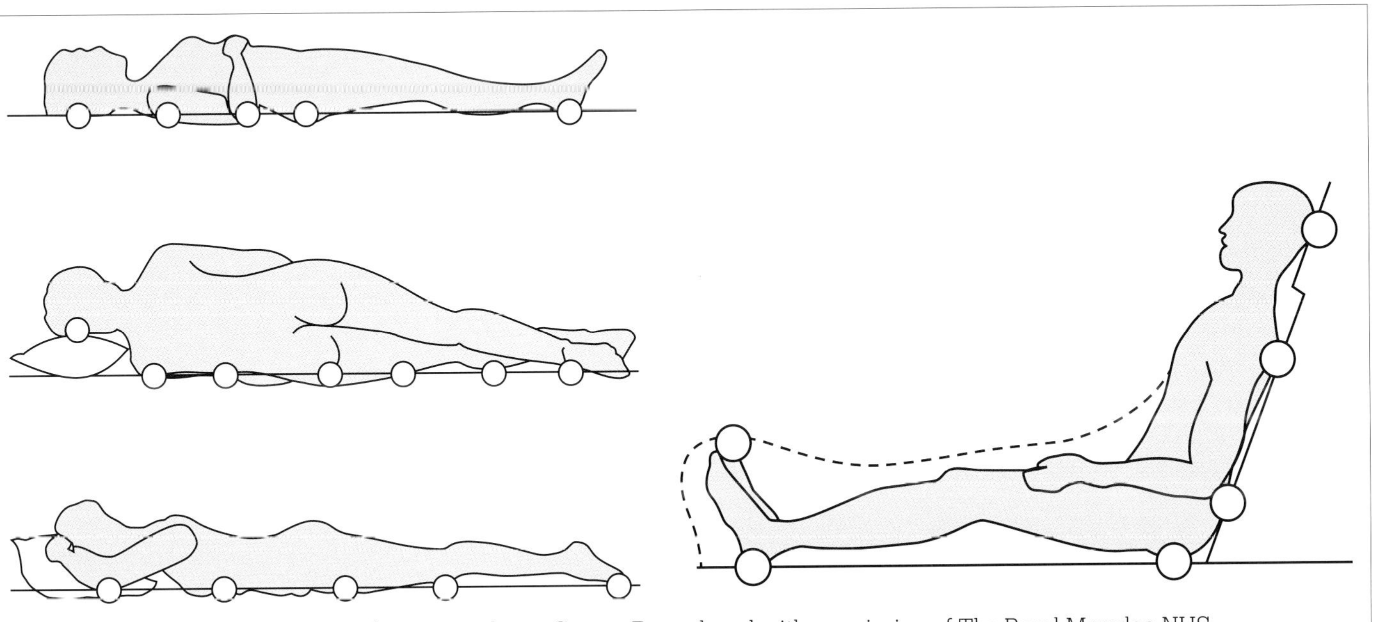

Figure 18.13 Common locations of pressure ulcers. *Source*: Reproduced with permission of The Royal Marsden NHS Foundation Trust.

Clinicians must be aware that the evidence to support the use of the various active support surfaces available is variable (McInnes et al. 2011, RCN 2005). A referral to an occupational therapist should be considered for complex equipment, seating and wheelchair needs.

Keep moving

The importance of 'keeping moving' should be discussed with each patient as appropriate. Mobility should be increased as quickly as tolerated (Haesler 2014) and a referral to physiotherapy should be considered.

Individuals who are willing and able should be taught how to redistribute their weight every 15 minutes via repositioning. Engage family and/or carers in how to assist patients to achieve this. Repositioning of patients who are unable do so independently aims to reduce prolonged pressure on bony prominences.

Individuals who are at risk of pressure ulcer development should be regularly repositioned and their heels elevated. The frequency of repositioning should be determined by the results of skin inspections and individual needs. A repositioning schedule, agreed with the individual, should be recorded and established for each person who is at risk, taking into consideration the following:

- Patients at high risk should be repositioned at least 4-hourly (NICE 2015a).
- Repositioning and factors affecting this should be documented after each intervention.
- Appropriate analgesia should be administered 20–30 minutes before repositioning patients who experience pain on movement (Haesler 2014).
- Individuals who are considered to be at risk of developing pressure ulcers should restrict chair sitting to less than 2 hours at a time until their general condition improves. Time sitting out can be increased incrementally.
- Avoid positioning individuals on an area of compromised skin integrity.
- Individuals with existing pressure ulcers anatomically located on or around the seating area should limit sitting out to 1 hour maximum for up to 3 times per day (Haesler 2014).
- Correct positioning of devices such as pillows and foam wedges should be used to keep bony prominences (e.g. knees, heels or ankles) out of direct contact with one another in accordance with a written plan. Care should be taken to ensure that these do not interfere with the action of any other pressure relieving support surfaces in use.
- Manual handling techniques and equipment should be used correctly in order to minimize shear and friction damage to the skin. After manoeuvring, slings, sleeves and other parts of the handling equipment should be removed from underneath individuals.
- In the community setting, patients and carers (both formal and informal) should be informed of the importance of repositioning (Royal Marsden NHS Foundation Trust 2013).

Incontinence and increased moisture

Excess moisture on the skin's surface causes softening and erosion of the epidermal layer, breaking the skin's barrier function. The link between excess skin moisture levels and pressure ulcers is widely acknowledged (Crook et al. 2014).

The source of excess moisture – whether incontinence, perspiration or wound drainage – should be eliminated where possible. When moisture cannot be controlled, interventions such as regular personal care using a pH-neutral cleanser and an application of barrier products is recommended (Haesler 2014).

Nutrition

Malnutrition is an independent risk factor in pressure ulcer development (NICE 2014) and can impede healing in established pressure ulcers (Taylor 2017). Malnutrition causes a reduction in fibroblast activity and collagen synthesis, and it delays angiogenesis in the proliferative and maturation phases of healing (Neloska et al. 2016).

Individuals must be assessed for the risk of malnutrition using a valid and reliable screening tool within 24 hours of hospital admission (Haesler 2014) and at least weekly thereafter. This assessment should include factors influencing poor food or fluid intake and unintended weight loss (Posthauer et al. 2015).

Individuals at risk of pressure ulcers should be offered high-caloric, high protein nutritional supplements in addition to their normal diet if their nutritional needs are not being met (ensure this is appropriate for the patient's renal function) (Haesler 2014). Individuals who have developed a pressure ulcer must be referred to a dietitian for assessment and intervention (Litchford et al. 2014). A referral to a speech and language therapist is advised in the case of actual or suspected chewing or swallowing difficulties (Posthauer et al. 2015).

Giving information

Healthcare professionals must provide tailored information and education about preventing pressure ulcers from developing for individuals at high risk and their family and/or carers, where appropriate (NICE 2015a). Patient and carer education leaflets should be made available and include information on the following:

- the risk factors associated with developing pressure ulcers
- the sites that are at the greatest risk of pressure damage
- how to inspect skin and recognize skin changes
- how to care for skin
- methods of pressure relief and reduction
- where patients can seek further advice and assistance should they need it
- the need for immediate visits to a healthcare professional should signs of damage be noticed (Royal Marsden NHS Foundation Trust 2013).

If a patient declines an aspect of recommended care, this should be documented; additionally, evaluations of whether the patient is improving or deteriorating should be recorded to keep their care plan up to date (Royal Marsden NHS Foundation Trust 2013). Nurses should consult additional guidance if they are unfamiliar with the patient or regimen (NMC 2018).

Surgical wounds

Definition

There are three main methods of wound closure for wounds healing by primary intention: sutures, skin adhesive and staples/clips (Flanagan 2013). Sutures are the most common.

Evidence-based approaches

Rationale

Suturing as a method of wound closure is appropriate in managing deep, large wounds. As there is a direct relationship between the time of wound closure and infection risk, suturing is usually best suited to primary closure in recently acquired, non-infected wounds (Jain 2013).

Indications

Suturing is used to promote primary healing, realign tissue layers and hold the skin edges together until enough healing has occurred for the wound to withstand stress without mechanical support (Wicker and O'Neill 2010).

Removal of sutures or clips

Evidence-based approaches

Rationale

Removal of sutures/clips is usually performed between days 4 and 14 after insertion, depending on the anatomical location of the wound (Trott 2012). Routinely, alternative sutures/clips are removed first, with the remainder removed if the incision stays securely closed. If the wound edges begin to separate during the procedure, the remaining sutures/clips should be left in place and reported to the responsible clinician (Cooper and Gosnell 2018).

Pre-procedural considerations

Assess the wound and surrounding skin for any areas of concern, such as infection. Surgical notes and instructions should be reviewed (NMC 2018). Analgesia may be offered depending on the patient and wound site.

Procedure guideline 18.2 Suture removal

Essential equipment

- Personal protective equipment
- Sterile dressing pack containing gallipots or an indented plastic tray, low-linting swabs and/or medical foam, disposable metal forceps, sterile field and disposable bag
- Fluids for cleaning and/or irrigation
- Appropriate dressing
- Any other materials as determined by the nature of the dressing; special features of a dressing should be referred to in the patient's nursing care plan
- Detergent wipe for cleaning trolley
- Total traceability system for surgical instruments and patient record form
- Any other equipment that may be needed during the procedure, for example sterile scissors, stitch cutter or sterile adhesive sutures

Action	Rationale
Pre-procedure	
1 Introduce yourself to the patient, explain and discuss the procedure with them, and gain their consent to proceed.	To ensure that the patient feels at ease, understands the procedure and gives their valid consent (NMC 2018, **C**).
2 Perform the procedure using aseptic technique (i.e. use of a trolley, clean hands, and apply apron and gloves).	To prevent infection (Fraise and Bradley 2009, **E**).
Procedure	
3 Clean the wound with an appropriate sterile solution, such as 0.9% sodium chloride, if required.	To remove crusts/dry skin to increase the visibility of the sutures to be removed (Perry et al. 2015, **E**).
4 Lift knot of suture with metal forceps.	Plastic forceps tend to slip against nylon sutures. **E**
5 Using a stitch cutter or scissors, snip the first stitch close to the skin. Pull the suture out gently. For intermittent sutures, alternate sutures should be removed first before the remaining sutures are removed.	To avoid previously exposed (potentially contaminated) aspects of the suture being pulled through underlying tissues (Trott 2012, **E**). To ensure wound closure and predict dehiscence (Cooper and Gosnell 2018, **E**).
6 Use the tips of the scissors slightly open or the side of the stitch cutter to gently press the skin when the suture is being drawn out. Continue until all appropriate sutures are removed as required.	To minimize pain by counteracting the adhesion between the suture and surrounding tissue. **E**
7 Apply a suitable dressing.	To protect the wound from further trauma or contamination and ensure optimum healing (Fraise and Bradley 2009, **E**).
Post-procedure	
8 Dispose of waste in orange plastic clinical waste bags and sharps in a sharps bin. Remove gloves and wash hands.	To prevent environmental contamination and sharps injury. Orange is the recognized colour for clinical waste (DH 2005, **C**).
9 Record the condition of the suture line and surrounding skin (amount of exudate, pus, inflammation, pain, etc.).	To document care and enable evaluation of the wound (Hess 2012, **E**; NMC 2018, **C**).

Procedure guideline 18.3 Clip removal

Essential equipment

- Personal protective equipment
- Sterile dressing pack containing gallipots or an indented plastic tray, low-linting swabs and/or medical foam, sterile field and disposable bag
- Fluids for cleaning and/or irrigation
- Appropriate dressing
- Any other materials as determined by the nature of the dressing; special features of a dressing should be referred to in the patient's nursing care plan
- Detergent wipe for cleaning trolley
- Total traceability system for surgical instruments and patient record form
- Clip remover

(continued)

Procedure guideline 18.3 Clip removal *(continued)*

Optional equipment

- Any extra equipment that may be needed during the procedure, for example sterile adhesive sutures

Action	Rationale
Pre-procedure	
1 Introduce yourself to the patient, explain and discuss the procedure with them, and gain their consent to proceed.	To ensure that the patient feels at ease, understands the procedure and gives their valid consent (NMC 2018, **C**).
2 Perform procedure using aseptic technique (i.e. use of a trolley, clean hands, apply apron and gloves).	To prevent infection (Fraise and Bradley 2009, **E**).
Procedure	
3 Clean the wound with an appropriate sterile solution, such as 0.9% sodium chloride, if required.	To remove crusts/dry skin to increase the visibility of the clips to be removed (Perry et al. 2015, **E**).
4 If the incision line is under tension, use free hand to gently support the skin either side of the surgical incision line.	To reduce the tension on the skin around the suture line and lessen pain on removal of the clip. **E**
5 Slide the lower bar of the clip remover with the V-shaped groove under the clip at an angle of 90°. Squeeze the handles of the clip remover together to open the clip.	To release the clip from the wound atraumatically. If the angle of the clip remover is not correct, the clip will not come out freely (Perry et al. 2015, **E**).
6 Repeat until all clips have been removed.	Clips should all be removed at the earliest possible point to avoid marks from the clips along the incision line (Widgerow 2013, **E**).
7 Apply a suitable dressing.	To protect the wound from further trauma or contamination and ensure optimum healing (Fraise and Bradley 2009, **E**).
Post-procedure	
8 Dispose of waste in orange plastic clinical waste bags and sharps in a sharps bin. Remove gloves and wash hands.	To prevent environmental contamination and sharps injury. Orange is the recognized colour for clinical waste (DH 2005, **C**).
9 Record the condition of the suture line and surrounding skin (amount of exudate, pus, inflammation, pain, etc.).	To document care and enable evaluation of the wound (Hess 2012, **E**; NMC 2018, **C**).

Post-procedural considerations

After removal of sutures or clips, patients should receive information on how to care for their wound, including dressing removal, cleansing the area without causing trauma, signs of infection, scar management and reducing exposure to direct sunlight (Perry et al. 2015).

Negative pressure wound therapy

Definition

Negative pressure wound therapy (NPWT), previously known as topical negative pressure (TNP), is the application of a controlled sub-atmospheric pressure across the wound bed via a suction unit attached to a dressing or wound filler (Sood et al. 2014).

Evidence-based approaches

Rationale

NPWT can expedite wound healing by creating a moist wound healing environment, removing bacteria, reducing oedema, increasing blood flow and oxygen to the wound bed, and stimulating angiogenesis and granulation (Bowers et al. 2016, Schreiber 2016). The benefits of NPWT include management of exudate, reduction of wound odour, reduction in the number of dressing changes required and improvement in quality of life (Janssen et al. 2016, Milne 2013, Ubbink et al. 2008). NPWT can be applied to open wounds (healing by secondary intention) or closed incisional wounds (healing by primary intention) (Anghel and Kim 2016).

The degree of negative pressure applied is dependent on the wound aetiology and patient tolerance (Henderson et al. 2010).

The suction unit (Figure 18.14) can be set on continuous or intermittent according to the therapy required (Apelqvist et al. 2017). Continuous therapy can be used:

- for highly exuding wounds
- over unstable structures to minimize movement and help to stabilize the wound bed, when used on flaps and grafts
- for patients with a high risk of bleeding (Smith & Nephew 2011).

Intermittent therapy stimulates the development of granulation tissue and can improve the rate of healing (Milne 2013). It has proven to be cost-efficient, safe and effective as a treatment modality for wound care (KCI 2014).

Indications

NPWT is indicated for:

- chronic wounds, such as venous leg ulcers and pressure ulcers
- diabetic and neuropathic ulcers
- post operative and dehisced surgical wounds
- partial thickness burns
- skin flaps and grafts
- traumatic wounds
- explored fistulae (Milne 2013, Smith & Nephew 2011).

Contraindications

NPWT is contraindicated in:

- clotting disorders (risk of bleeding) and acute mild to moderate bleeding in the wound after injury or debridement
- grossly contaminated wounds
- exposed organs, vessels, nerves and anastomotic sites, which might be altered or damaged by NPWT

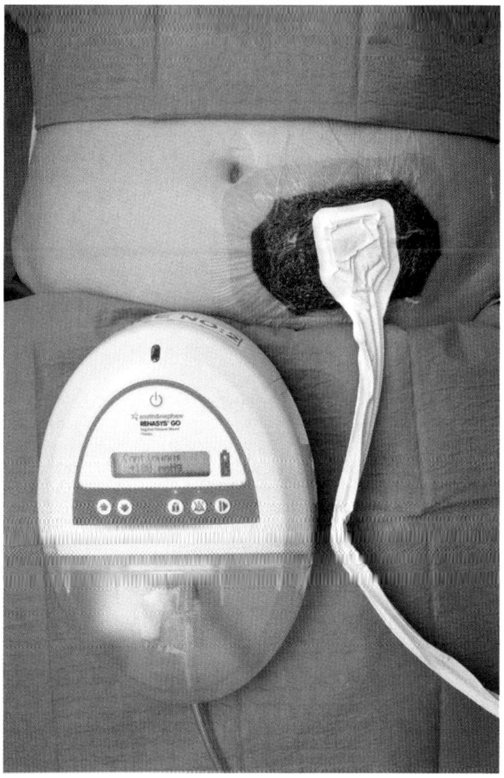

Figure 18.14 Negative pressure wound therapy dressing and unit (example of standard equipment and application).

- wounds with necrotic tissue, eschar or thick slough (these will require debridement prior to NPWT)
- malignant wounds due to the potential to stimulate proliferation of malignant cells (with the exception of palliative care to improve quality of life)
- untreated osteomyelitis
- non-enteric and unexplored fistulae (Apelqvist et al. 2017, Henderson et al. 2010, KCI 2014).

Precautions should be exercised:

- when there is active bleeding in the wound
- when there is difficult haemostasis

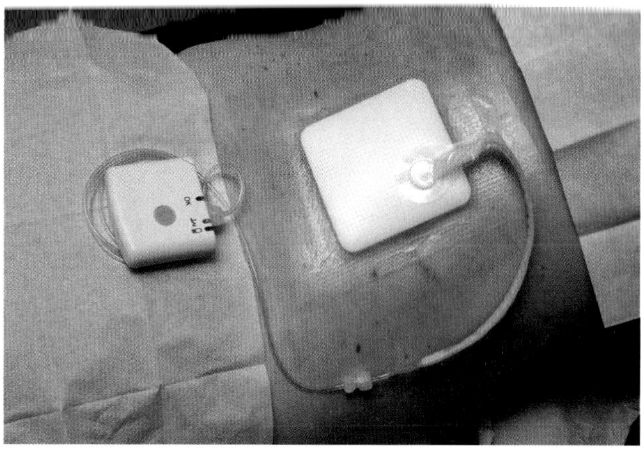

Figure 18.15 Single-use negative pressure wound therapy dressing and unit (example).

- when the patient is taking anticoagulants
- in cases of spinal cord injury
- in vascular anastomoses
- in wounds with sharp edges, such as bone fragments (Apelqvist et al. 2017, Henderson et al. 2010).

The wound site must be carefully assessed to ensure that NPWT is indeed the appropriate treatment modality. If signs of infection or complications develop, the therapy should be discontinued (KCI 2014). See Figures 18.14 and 18.15 for examples of NWPT devices.

Pre-procedural considerations

Consulting the appropriate manufacturer's representative for training is essential as application and approaches vary between different manufacturers. There are specific types of foams and gauze dressings that should be used in undermined wounds, tunnels and sinus tracts. If the patient is discharged into the community with NPWT, consideration should be given to the management of the dressings as well as the patient's mobility, risk of falls and psychological ability to cope with the therapy (Milne 2013).

Equipment

All equipment used should conform to the manufacturer's recommendations for the relevant system (KCI 2014).

Procedure guideline 18.4 Negative pressure wound therapy

Essential equipment

- Personal protective equipment
- NPWT unit
- NPWT dressing pack (foam or gauze)
- NPWT canister and tubing
- Forceps
- Sterile scissors
- Sterile gloves
- Dressing procedure pack
- Sterile 0.9% sodium chloride for irrigation (warmed to approx. 37°C in a jug of warm water)

Optional equipment

- Extra film dressings to seal any air leaks
- Non-adherent wound contact layer to prevent foam adhering to wound bed
- Alcohol-free skin barrier film to protect any fragile or macerated skin around the wound or thin hydrocolloid to protect the peri-wound area

(continued)

Procedure guideline 18.4 Negative pressure wound therapy *(continued)*

Action	Rationale
Pre-procedure	
1 Introduce yourself to the patient, explain and discuss the procedure with them, and gain their consent to proceed.	To ensure that the patient feels at ease, understands the procedure and gives their valid consent (NMC 2018, **C**).
2 Provide routine analgesia prior to the dressing procedure.	To prevent unnecessary procedural pain. **E**
3 Ensure there is adequate lighting and that the patient is comfortable and in a position where the wound can be accessed and viewed easily. Assemble all necessary equipment.	To allow access to the area for dressing change. Dressing application can be complicated and prolonged so the patient should be in a comfortable position for the procedure. **E**
Procedure	
4 Use aseptic technique and sterile equipment (as listed above).	To prevent infection (Fraise and Bradley 2009, **E**).
5 To remove the NPWT dressing, put on sterile gloves.	To reduce the risk of cross-infection (Pudner 2005, **E**).
6 Clamp the dressing tubing and disconnect it from the canister tubing. Allow any fluid in the canister tubing to be sucked into the canister. Switch off the pump and clamp the canister tubing.	To prevent spillage of body fluid waste from the tubing or canister. **E**
7 Remove and discard the canister (if full or at least weekly).	To prevent the pump alarm sounding and for infection control. **E**
8 Carefully remove the occlusive film drape by gently lifting one edge and then stretching the drape horizontally and slowly removing it from the skin.	To prevent damage to the peri-wound skin. **E**
9 Carefully remove the wound filler.	To prevent damage to newly formed tissue within the wound bed and prevent pain. **E**
10 Irrigate with sterile 0.9% sodium chloride if indicated.	To remove surface debris/necrotic tissue (Milne 2013, **E**).
11 Debride the wound if applicable and dry the peri-wound area.	To remove loose necrotic tissue, which may be a focus for infection (Vowden and Vowden 2011, **E**).
12 To apply the dressing, cut the NPWT foam/gauze filler to fit the size and shape of the wound. Appropriate foam or gauze should be used if tunnelling and undermined areas are present.	The foam should fit the wound exactly to ensure full benefit of the NPWT. **E**
13 Avoid cutting the foam over the wound bed.	To prevent loose particles of foam falling into the wound. **E**
14 Apply a skin barrier, drape or thin hydrocolloid to the peri-wound if required.	To prevent epidermal stripping on dressing removal. To protect vulnerable wound edges and to help achieve an air tight seal (Schreiber 2016, **E**).
15 Place the foam into the wound cavity.	The whole wound bed must be covered with foam. If multiple pieces of foam are used, they must all touch each other to ensure the negative pressure is transferred to each piece. **E**
16 A non-adherent wound contact layer should be used under the foam/gauze filler for protection in the case of a friable wound bed or exposed blood vessels, tendons, bone or muscle.	The extracellular matrix requires a trauma-free dressing removal (Ellis 2016, **E**).
17 Cut the occlusive film drape to size and apply it over the top of the foam. The film should extend 5 cm from the wound margin and not be stretched or applied under pressure. *Note*: do not compress the foam into the wound.	To obtain a good seal around the wound edges. **E**
18 Choose a location on the sealed occlusive film drape to apply the tubing where the tubing will not rub or cause pressure. Cut a hole through the film (size dependent on system being used), leaving the foam intact.	To reduce the risk of pressure injury to the skin. **E**
19 Align the opening of the port over the hole in the film. Apply gentle pressure to anchor the port to the film.	To ensure correct position and seal of the pad (Smith & Nephew 2011, **C**).
20 To commence the NPWT, insert the canister into the pump until it clicks into place. Do not clamp any part of the canister tubing.	The click indicates the canister is positioned correctly and is secure. **E** The pump will sound an alarm if the tubing is clamped or not connected. **E**
21 Connect the dressing tubing to the canister tubing.	To complete the circuit set-up. **E**
22 Press the power button and follow the on screen instructions to set the level and type of pressure required according to the instructions from the patient's NPWT prescriber	To ensure the therapy is set to the individual requirements of the patient (Milne 2013, **E**).

Action	Rationale
23 When therapy has commenced, the foam should collapse into the wound, be firm to touch and have a wrinkled appearance (Smith & Nephew 2011).	Any small air leak will prevent the foam dressing from contracting; reassessment will be required. **E**
Post-procedure	
24 Document the dressings and settings, frequency of changes, wound description and exudate in the patient's notes.	To provide a record of care in the patient's care plan (NMC 2018, **C**).

Post-procedural considerations

Ongoing care

It is imperative to carefully monitor the peri-wound area for signs of infection, skin breakdown or oedema, and to check the equipment while it is *in situ*, to ensure patient safety. Dressings should be changed every 48–72 hours and canisters changed as required and at least weekly (Anghel and Kim 2016). The NPWT unit should not be switched off for more than 2 hours without the dressing being replaced (KCI 2014).

Discontinuing NPWT should be considered when:

- a contraindication arises
- the exudate level is less than 20 mL per day
- the wound bed presents with 100% granulation tissue that is level with the wound edges (Milne 2013).

Single-use negative pressure wound therapy

Disposable NPWT systems provide a lightweight and portable alternative to the standard NPWT application. The same principles apply; however, disposable systems are typically applied to wounds with lesser exudate levels.

Websites

British Association of Dermatologists
www.bad.org.uk

British Lymphology Society
https://www.thebls.com

European Pressure Ulcer Advisory Panel (EPUAP)
www.epuap.org

European Wound Management Association
https://ewma.org

Healthcare Improvement Scotland: Tissue Viability
www.healthcareimprovementscotland.org/our_work/patient_safety/tissue_viability.aspx

International Skin Tear Advisory Panel (ISTAP)
www.skintears.org

International Wound Infection Institute
www.woundinfection-institute.com

Legs Matter
https://legsmatter.org

NHS Improvement: Stop the Pressure
http://nhs.stopthepressure.co.uk/index.html

NICE: *Negative Pressure Wound Therapy for the Open Abdomen* (2013)
https://www.nice.org.uk/guidance/ipg467

NICE: *Pressure Ulcers: Prevention and Management* (2014)
https://www.nice.org.uk/guidance/cg179

NICE: *Surgical Site Infections: Prevention and Treatment* (2017)
https://www.nice.org.uk/guidance/CG74/chapter/1-Guidance#postoperative-phase

Tissue Viability Society
https://tvs.org.uk

World Wide Wounds. Dressings Datacards
www.worldwidewounds.com/Common/ProductDatacards.html

Wounds UK.
https://www.wounds-uk.com

References

Andriessen, A.F. & Eberlein, T. (2008) Assessment of a wound cleansing solution in the treatment of problem wounds. *Wounds*, 20(6), 171–175.

Angel, D.E., Lloyd, P., Carville, K. & Santamaria, N. (2011) The clinical efficacy of two semi-quantitative wound-swabbing techniques in identifying the causative organism(s) in infected cutaneous wounds. *International Wound Journal*, 8(2), 176–185.

Anghel, E.L. & Kim, P.J. (2016) Negative-pressure wound therapy: A comprehensive review of the evidence. *Plastic and Reconstructive Surgery*, 138(3 Suppl.), 129S–137S.

Apelqvist, J., Willy, C., Fagerdahl, A.M., et al. (2017) EWMA document: Negative pressure wound therapy – Overview, challenges and perspectives. *Journal of Wound Care*, 26(Suppl. 3), S1–S154.

Atkin, L. (2014) Understanding methods of wound debridement. *British Journal of Nursing*, 23(Suppl. 12), S10–S15.

Atkin, L., Bućko, Z., Conde Montero, E., et al. (2019) Implementing TIMERS: The race against hard-to-heal wounds. *Journal of Wound Care*, 28(Suppl. 3a), S1–S49.

Bale, S. & Jones, V. (2006) *Wound Care Nursing: A Patient-Centred Approach*. Edinburgh: Mosby Elsevier.

Baranoski, S. & Ayello, E.A. (eds) (2015) *Wound Care Essentials: Practice Principles*, 4th edn. Philadelphia: Wolters Kluwer.

Bonham, P.A. (2009) Swab cultures for diagnosing wound infections: A literature review and clinical guideline. *Journal of Wound, Ostomy and Continence Nursing*, 36(4), 389–395.

Boyer, D. (2013) Cultural considerations in advanced wound care. *Advances in Skin & Wound Care*, 26(3), 110–111.

Broderick, N. (2009) Understanding chronic wound healing. *Nurse Practitioner*, 34(10), 16–22.

Butcher, M. (2012) PHMB: An effective antimicrobial in wound bioburden management. *British Journal of Nursing*, 21(Suppl. 12), S16–S21.

Collier, M. (2002) Wound-bed preparation. *Nursing Times*, 98(2), 55–57.

ConvaTec (2004) *ConvaTec Wound Care Reference Guide*. Uxbridge: ConvaTec.

Cooper, K. & Gosnell, K. (2018) *Foundations and Adult Health Nursing*, 8th edn. St Louis, MO: Elsevier.

Cooper, R.A. (2010) Ten top tips for taking a wound swab. *Wounds International*, 1(3), 19–20.

Copeland-Halperin, L.R., Kaminsky, A.J., Bluefeld, N. & Miraliakbari, R. (2016) Sample procurement for cultures of infected wounds: A systematic review. *Journal of Wound Care North American Supplement*, 25(4), S4–S10.

Crook, H., Evans, J., Pritchard, B., et al. (2014) *The All Wales Best Practice Statement on the Prevention and Management of Moisture Lesions.* Available at: www.welshwoundnetwork.org/files/5514/0326/4395/All_Wales-Moisture_Lesions_final_final.pdf

Cross, H.H. (2014) Obtaining a wound swab culture specimen. *Nursing,* 44(7), 68–69.

Cutting, K. (2011) Why use topical antiseptics? *Journal of Wound Care,* 20(Suppl. 2), 4–7.

Cutting, K.F. & Westgate, S.J. (2012) The use of wound cleansing solutions in chronic wounds. *Wounds UK,* 8(4), 130–133.

Dealey, C. (2005) *The Care of Wounds: A Guide for Nurses.* Oxford: Blackwell Science.

DH (Department of Health) (2005) *Saving Lives: A Delivery Programme to Reduce Health Associated Infection including MRSA.* London: Department of Health.

Dhivya, S., Padma, V.V. & Santhini, E. (2015) Wound dressings: A review. *BioMedicine,* 5(4), 22.

Doughty, D.B. & Sparks, B. (2016) Wound-healing physiology and factors that affect the repair process. In: Bryant, R.A. & Nix, D.P. (eds) *Acute and Chronic Wounds: Current Management Concepts,* 5th edn. St Louis, MO: Elsevier, pp.63–81.

Dowsett, C. & Ayello, E. (2004) TIME principles of chronic wound bed preparation and treatment. *British Journal of Nursing,* 13(15), S16–S23.

Eagle, M. (2009) Wound assessment: The patient and the wound. *Wound Essentials,* 4, 14–24.

Ellis, G. (2016) How to apply vacuum-assisted closure therapy. *Nursing Standard,* 30(27), 36–39.

Eming, S.A., Martin, P., & Tomic-Canic, M. (2014). Wound repair and regeneration: Mechanisms, signaling, and translation. *Science Translational Medicine,* 6(265), 265sr6.

Eriksson, A., Burcharth, J. & Rosenberg, J. (2013) Animal derived products may conflict with religious patients' beliefs. *BMC Medical Ethics,* 14(1), 48.

Fernandez, R. & Griffiths, R. (2012) Water for wound cleansing. *Cochrane Database of Systematic Reviews,* 2, CD003861.

Flanagan, M. (ed.) (2013) *Wound Healing and Skin Integrity: Principles and Practice.* Chichester: Wiley Blackwell.

Fraise, A.P. & Bradley, T. (eds) (2009) *Ayliffe's Control of Healthcare-Associated Infection: A Practical Handbook,* 5th edn. London: Hodder Arnold.

Giele, H. & Cassell, O. (2008) *Plastic and Reconstructive Surgery.* Oxford: Oxford University Press.

Gray, D., White, R., Cooper, P. & Kingsley, A. (2010) Applied wound management and using the wound healing continuum in practice. *Wound Essentials,* 5, 131–139.

Greatrex-White, S. & Moxey, H. (2015) Wound assessment tools and nurses' needs: An evaluation study. *International Wound Journal,* 12(3), 293–301.

Guest, J.F., Ayoub, N., McIlwraith, T., et al. (2015) Health economic burden that wounds impose on the National Health Service in the UK. *BMJ Open,* 5(12), e009283.

Guo, S.A. & DiPietro, L.A. (2010) Factors affecting wound healing. *Journal of Dental Research,* 89(3), 219–229.

Haesler, E. (ed) (2014) *Prevention and Treatment of Pressure Ulcers: Quick Reference Guide.* National Pressure Ulcer Advisory Panel, European Pressure Ulcer Advisory Panel and Pan Pacific Pressure Injury Alliance. Available at: www.epuap.org/wp-content/uploads/2016/10/NPUAP-EPUAP-PPPIA-Quick-Reference-Guide-2014-DIGITAL.pdf

Haesler, E., Frescos, N. & Rayner, R. (2018) The fundamental goal of wound prevention: Recent best evidence. *Wound Practice and Research,* 26(1), 14.

Hall, S. (2007) A review of the effect of tap water versus normal saline on infection rates in acute traumatic wounds. *Journal of Wound Care,* 16(1), 38–41.

Hampton, S. (2013) Exudate management. *Exudate Management,* 4–7.

Hampton, S. & Collins, F. (2004) *Tissue Viability: The Prevention, Treatment, and Management of Wounds.* London: Whurr.

Harper, D., Young, A., & McNaught, C.E. (2014). The physiology of wound healing. *Surgery,* 32(9), 445–450.

Harries, R.L., Bosanquet, D.C. & Harding, K.G. (2016) Wound bed preparation: TIME for an update. *International Wound Journal,* 13(Suppl. 3), 8–14.

Henderson, V., Timmins, J., Hurd, T., et al. (2010) NPWT in everyday practice made easy. *Wounds International,* 1(5), 1–6.

Hess, C.T. (2011) Checklist for factors affecting wound healing. *Advances in Skin & Wound Care,* 24(4), 192.

Hess, C.T. (2012) *Clinical Guide to Skin and Wound Care,* 7th edn. Lippincott Williams & Wilkins.

House, K.W. & Johnson, T.M. (2014) Prevention of pressure ulcers. In: Thomas, D.R. & Compton, G.A. (eds) *Pressure Ulcers in the Aging Population: A Guide for Clinicians.* New York: Humana Press, pp.27–46.

HSE (Health Service Executive) (2018) *HSE National Wound Management Guidelines 2018.* Available at: https://www.hse.ie/eng/services/publications/nursingmidwifery%20services/wound-management-guidelines-2018.pdf

Huang, Y., Cao, Y., Zou, M., et al. (2016) A comparison of tissue versus swab culturing of infected diabetic foot wounds. *International Journal of Endocrinology,* 2016, 1–6.

IWII (International Wound Infection Institute) (2016) *Wound Infection in Clinical Practice: Principles of Best Practice 2016.* Available at: www.woundinfection-institute.com/wp-content/uploads/2017/03/IWII-Wound-infection-in-clinical-practice.pdf

Jain, S. (2013) *Basic Surgical Skills and Techniques,* 2nd edn. London: Jaypee Brothers.

Janssen, A.H.J., Mommers, E.H.H., Notter, J., et al. (2016) Negative pressure wound therapy versus standard wound care on quality of life: A systematic review. *Journal of Wound Care,* 25(3), 154–159.

Jenkins, G. & Tortora, G.J. (2014) *Anatomy and Physiology: From Science to Life,* 3rd edn. Hoboken, NJ: Wiley.

Jones, J. (2013) Exploring the link between the clinical challenges of wound exudate and infection. *Exudate Management,* 8–12.

Kamolz, L.P. & Wild, T. (2013) Wound bed preparation: The impact of debridement and wound cleansing. *Wound Medicine,* 1, 44–50.

KCI (2014) *V.A.C. Therapy Clinical Guidelines: A Reference Source for Clinicians.* Available at: https://www.acelity.com/-/media/Project/Acelity/Acelity-Base-Sites/shared/PDF/2-b-128-ca-enb-clinical-guidelines---canada---en.pdf

Kyaw, B.M., Järbrink, K., Martinengo, L., et al. (2018). Need for improved definition of 'chronic wounds' in clinical studies. *Acta Dermato-Venereologica,* 98, 157–158.

Leaper, D. (2011) An overview of the evidence on the efficacy of silver dressings. *Journal of Wound Care,* 20(Suppl. 2), 8–14.

Leaper, D.J., Schultz, G., Carville, K., et al. (2012) Extending the TIME concept: What have we learned in the past 10 years? *International Wound Journal,* 9, 1–19.

Litchford, M.D., Dorner, B. & Posthauer, M.E. (2014) Malnutrition as a precursor of pressure ulcers. *Advances in Wound Care,* 3(1), 54–63.

Lloyd Jones, M. (2012) Wound cleansing: Is it necessary, or just a ritual? *Nursing & Residential Care,* 14(8), 396–399.

Madhok, B.M., Vowden, K. & Vowden, P. (2013) New techniques for wound debridement. *International Wound Journal,* 10, 247–251.

Marieb, E.N. & Hoehn, K. (2018) *Human Anatomy & Physiology,* 11th edn. Harlow: Pearson.

Martin, P. & Nunan, R. (2015) Cellular and molecular mechanisms of repair in acute and chronic wound healing. *British Journal of Dermatology,* 173, 370–378.

McDaniel, J.C. & Browning, K.K. (2014) Smoking, chronic wound healing, and implications for evidence-based practice. *Journal of Wound, Ostomy and Continence Nursing,* 41(5), E1–E2.

McFarland, A. & Smith, F. (2014) Wound debridement: A clinical update. *Nursing Standard,* 28(52), 51–58.

McGuiness, W., Vella, E. & Harrison, D. (2004) Influence of dressing changes on wound temperature. *Journal of Wound Care,* 13(9), 383–385.

McInnes, E., Jammali-Blasi, A., Bell-Syer, S., et al. (2011) Support surfaces for pressure ulcer prevention. *Cochrane Database of Systematic Reviews,* 4, CD001735.

McKirdy, L.W. (2001) Burn wound cleansing. *Journal of Community Nursing,* 15(5), 24–29.

McLain, N.E.M. & Moore, Z.E.H. (2015) Wound cleansing for treating venous leg ulcers. *Cochrane Database of Systematic Reviews,* 4, CD011675.

Milne, J. (2013) Effective use of negative pressure wound therapy. *Practice Nursing,* 24(1), 14–19.

Morton, L.M. & Phillips, T.J. (2016) Wound healing and treating wounds: Differential diagnosis and evaluation of chronic wounds. *Journal of the American Academy of Dermatology*, 74(4), 589–605.

Myers, B.A. (2011) *Wound Management: Principles and Practice*, 3rd edn. Harlow: Pearson.

Nazarko, L. (2015) Advances in wound debridement techniques. *British Journal of Community Nursing*, 20(Suppl. 6), S6–S8.

Neloska, L., Damevska, K., Nikolchev, A., et al. (2016) The association between malnutrition and pressure ulcers in elderly in long-term care facility. *Open Access Macedonian Journal of Medical Sciences*, 4(3), 423.

NICE (National Institute for Health and Care Excellence) (2014) *Pressure Ulcers: Prevention and Management* [CG179]. Available at: https://www.nice.org.uk/guidance/cg179

NICE (2015a) *Pressure Ulcers* [QS89]. Available at: https://www.nice.org.uk/guidance/qs89/resources/pressure-ulcers-pdf-2098916972485

NICE (2015b) *Wound Care Products*. Available at: https://www.nice.org.uk/advice/ktt14/chapter/evidence-context

NICE (2019) *Surgical Site Infections: Prevention and Treatment* [NG125]. Available at: https://www.nice.org.uk/guidance/ng125/chapter/Recommendations

NMC (Nursing and Midwifery Council) (2018) *The Code: Professional Standards of Practice and Behaviour for Nurses, Midwives and Nursing Associates*. Available at: https://www.nmc.org.uk/standards/code

Ousey, K. & Cook, L. (2012) Wound assessment made easy. *Wounds UK*, 8(2), 1–4.

Percival, S.L. (2017) Importance of biofilm formation in surgical infection. *British Journal of Surgery*, 104, e85–e94.

Perry, A.G., Potter, P.A. & Ostendorf, W. (2015) *Nursing Interventions and Clinical Skills*, 6th edn. St Louis, MO: Elsevier.

Posthauer, M.E., Banks, M., Dorner, B. & Schols, J.M. (2015) The role of nutrition for pressure ulcer management: National Pressure Ulcer Advisory Panel, European Pressure Ulcer Advisory Panel, and Pan Pacific Pressure Injury Alliance white paper. *Advances in Skin & Wound Care*, 28(4), 175–188.

Powers, J.G., Higham, C., Broussard, K. & Phillips, T.J. (2016) Wound healing and treating wounds: Chronic wound care and management. *Journal of the American Academy of Dermatology*, 74(4), 607–625.

Probst, S. & Huljev, D. (2013) The effective management of wounds with high levels of exudate. *British Journal of Nursing*, 22(6 Suppl.), S34.

Pudner, R. (2005) *Wound Healing in the Surgical Patient*. Edinburgh: Churchill Livingstone.

RCN (Royal College of Nursing) (2005) *The Management of Pressure Ulcers in Primary and Secondary Care: A Clinical Practice Guideline*. London: Royal College of Nursing.

Reynolds, V. (2013) Assessing and diagnosing wound infection (part one). *Nurse Prescribing*, 11(3), 114–121.

Royal Marsden NHS Foundation Trust (2013) *Pressure Ulcer Risk Assessment and Prevention*. London: Royal Marsden NHS Foundation Trust.

Schreiber, M.L. (2016) Negative pressure wound therapy. *MEDSURG Nursing*, 25(6), 425–428.

Singh, S., Young, A. & McNaught, C.E. (2017) The physiology of wound healing. *Surgery (Oxford)*, 35(9), 473–477.

Skórkowska-Telichowska, K., Czemplik, M., Kulma, A. & Szopa, J. (2013) The local treatment and available dressings designed for chronic wounds. *Journal of the American Academy of Dermatology*, 60(4), e117–e126.

Smith & Nephew (2011) *NPWT Clinical Guidelines*. Hull: Smith & Nephew.

Snyder, R.J., Lantis, J., Kirsner, R.S., et al. (2016) Macrophages: A review of their role in wound healing and their therapeutic use. *Wound Repair and Regeneration*, 24, 613–629.

Sood, A., Granick, M.S. & Tomaselli, N.L. (2014) Wound dressings and comparative effectiveness data. *Advances in Wound Care*, 3(8), 511–529.

Stacey, M. (2016) Why don't wounds heal? *Wounds International*, 7(1), 16–21.

Storch, J.E. & Rice, J. (2005) *Reconstructive Plastic Surgical Nursing: Clinical Management and Wound Care*. Oxford: Blackwell.

Stotts, N. (2012). Wound infection: Diagnosis and management. In: Bryant, R. & Nix, D. (eds) *Acute and Chronic Wounds: Current Management Concepts*. St Louis, MO: Elsevier Mosby, pp.270–278.

Strohal, R., Apelqvist, J., Dissemond, J., et al. (2013) EWMA document: Debridement. *Journal of Wound Care*, 22(Suppl. 1), S1–S52.

Taylor, C. (2017) Importance of nutrition in preventing and treating pressure ulcers. *Nursing Older People*, 29(6), 33–39.

Timmons, J. (2006) Skin function and wound healing physiology. *Wound Essentials*, 8–17.

Tortora, G.J. & Derrickson, B. (2011) *Principles of Anatomy & Physiology*, 13th edn. Hoboken, NJ: John Wiley & Sons.

Tortora, G.J. & Derrickson, B. (2017) *Principles of Anatomy & Physiology*, 15th edn. Hoboken, NJ: John Wiley & Sons.

Trott, A. (2012) *Wounds and Lacerations Emergency Care and Closure*, 4th edn. Philadelphia: Elsevier Saunders.

Ubbink, D., Westerbos, S., Evans, D., et al. (2008) Topical negative pressure for treating chronic wounds. *Cochrane Database of Systematic Reviews*, 3, CD001898.

University College London Hospitals NHS Foundation Trust (2015) *Wound Dressing Formulary*. London: University College London Hospitals.

Vowden, K. & Vowden, P. (2017) Wound dressings: Principles and practice. *Surgery (Oxford)*, 35(9), 489–494.

Vowden, P. & Vowden, K. (2011) Debridement made easy. *Wounds UK*, 7(4), 1–4.

Waterlow, J. (2007) *The Waterlow Assessment Tool*. Available at: www.judy-waterlow.co.uk/waterlow_score.htm

Watret, L. & Armitage, M. (2002) Making sense of wound cleansing. *Journal of Community Nursing*, 16(4), 27–34.

Werdin, F., Tenenhaus, M. & Rennekampff, H. (2008) Chronic wound care. *Lancet*, 372(9653), 1860–1862.

Whitlock, J., Rowlands, S., Ellis, G., et al. (2011) Using the SKIN Bundle to prevent pressure ulcers. *Nursing Times*, 107(35), 20–23.

Wicker, P. & O'Neill, J. (2010) *Caring for the Perioperative Patient*, 2nd edn. Oxford: Wiley Blackwell.

Widgerow, A. (2013) *Surgical Wounds*. Oxford: John Wiley & Sons.

Wolcott, R. & Fletcher, J. (2014) The role of wound cleansing in the management of wounds. *Wounds International*, 5(8), 25–30.

Wounds UK (2013) *Guidelines for Practice: Effective Debridement in a Changing NHS – A UK Consensus*. Available at: https://lohmann-rauscher.co.uk/downloads/clinical-evidence/Effective_debridemen.pdf

Yarwood-Ross, L. (2013) Silicone dressings are a good fit in the wound care jigsaw. *British Journal of Nursing*, 22(6 Suppl.), S22.

Part Five

Looking after ourselves so we can support patients

Chapter

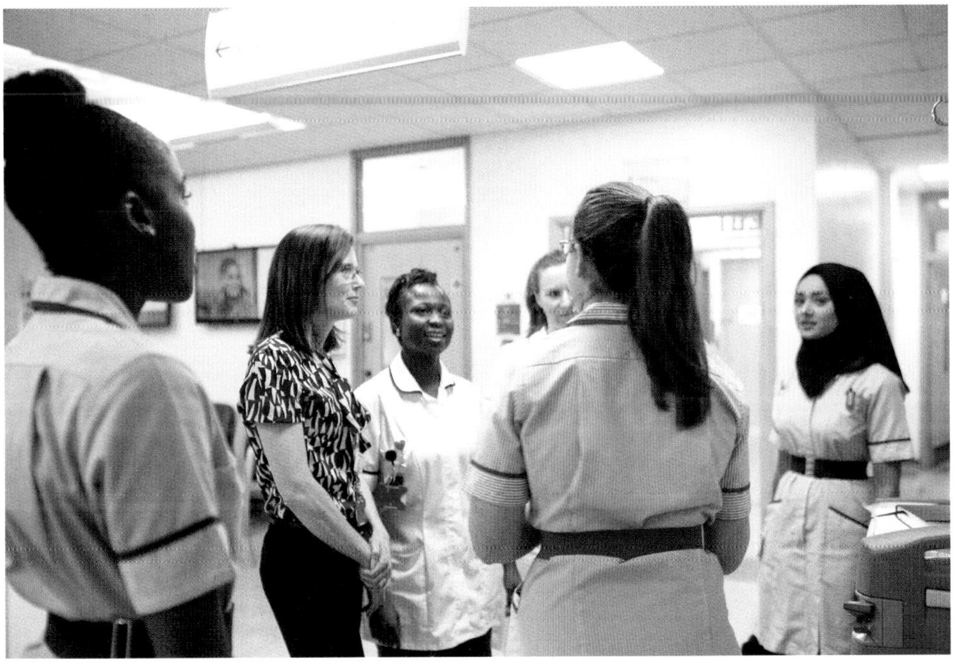

Chapter 19

Self-care and wellbeing

Sara Lister with Lorraine Bishop, Lucy Eldridge, Jayne Ellis, Tracey Shepherd and Sara Wright

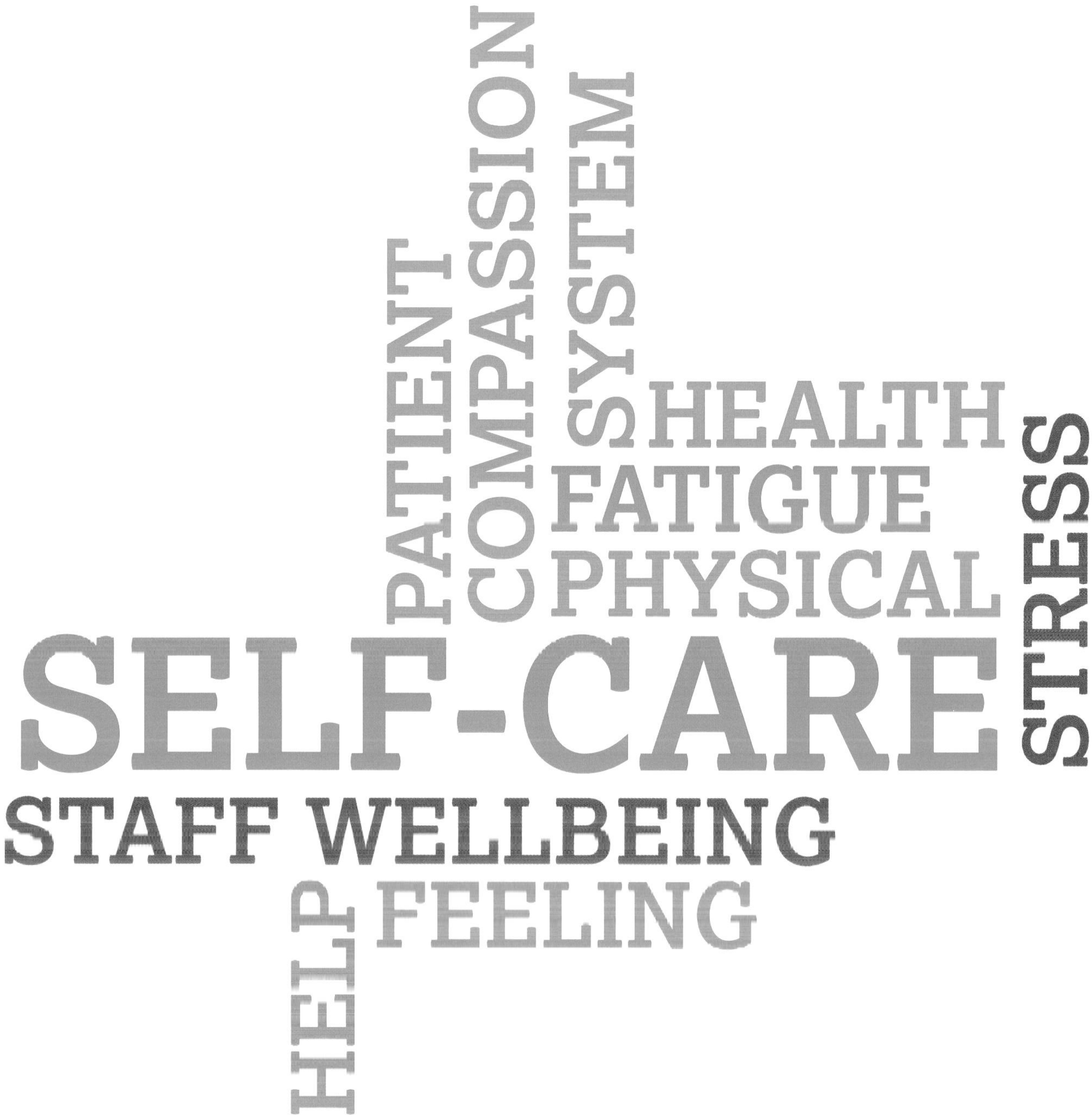

The Royal Marsden Manual of Clinical Nursing Procedures: Professional Edition, Tenth Edition. Edited by Sara Lister, Justine Hofland and Hayley Grafton.

Procedure guidelines

Being an accountable professional

At the point of registration, the nurse will:

1.5 Understand the demands of professional practice and demonstrate how to recognise signs of vulnerability in themselves or their colleagues and the action required to minimise risks to health

1.6 Understand the professional responsibility to adopt a healthy lifestyle to maintain the level of personal fitness and wellbeing required to meet people's needs for mental and physical care.

Future Nurse: Standards of Proficiency for Registered Nurses (NMC 2018)

Overview

This chapter considers why care of ourselves as nurses is important and explores specific strategies to maintain wellbeing in the following areas: self-care and wellbeing, mindfulness, eating and drinking, and physical wellbeing and musculoskeletal health.

Self-care and wellbeing

Definitions

Self-care

Self-care is 'the actions that individuals take for themselves, on behalf of and with others in order to develop, protect, maintain and improve their health, wellbeing or wellness' (Self Care Forum 2018).

Wellbeing

'Wellbeing is more than an avoidance of becoming physically sick. It represents a broader bio-psycho-social construct that includes physical, mental and social health. Well employees are physically and mentally able, willing to contribute in the workplace and likely to be more engaged at work' (CIPD 2016, p.2).

Related theory

Working in a caring role can be profoundly rewarding. Being alongside others when they are at their most vulnerable and scared is a privilege and incredibly fulfilling. Most choose the caring professions because they want to look after people and positively respond to human needs. Skovholt and Trotter-Mathison (2016) describe the joys, rewards and gifts of practice that this close connection to others in need can bring as 'having a ringside seat in the human drama and at times assist in making the drama turn out well' (p.12). In other words, we do it because we get a lot from giving and caring; specifically, Skovholt (1974) suggests four ways in which those in caring roles are rewarded:

- Caring roles provide a sense of identity and connection to others.
- Those in caring roles receive a type of love and status in the eyes of those they help (and of course money).
- Caring roles provide a unique opportunity to learn from those receiving care: this learning may encompass life and its deep, profound themes, such as how we cope with pain, what is important and what gives life meaning.
- Caring roles provide direct social reinforcement through affirmation, approval and positive feedback, which gives purpose and a sense of self-worth.

These ideas were first proposed as the 'helper therapy principle' by Riessman (1965).

When a person begins a career in care, they often have very high expectations of themselves and little thought is given to the effect of the work either physically or emotionally. Statistics show that caring work has an impact on the wellbeing of the carers. Drawing figures from the 2013 Absence Management Survey, carried out by the CIPD (2013), the Royal College of Physicians (RCP 2015) reported that 'NHS staff had 15.7 million days off sick in England alone in 2013–14' (p.2) and that 'sickness absence rates [in the NHS] are 27% higher than the UK public sector average, and 46% higher than the average for all sectors' (p.3).

Monthly absence figures reported by NHS Digital (2019) indicate that the number of days lost to sickness has not changed significantly in the past five years, with the highest rates in the following occupational groups: healthcare assistants, ambulance staff and nurses. NHS Employers (2018) suggests that the leading causes of absence in NHS staff are:

- *Mental ill health*: this is estimated to account for more than a quarter of staff sickness absence in the NHS. It was found that 38% of NHS staff in England reported having suffered work-related stress and/or being unwell as a result of work-related stress during 2013 (National NHS Staff Survey Co-ordination Centre 2013).
- *Musculoskeletal disorders*: with staff frequently engaging in physically demanding activities, musculoskeletal disorders are a major cause of illness and injury in the NHS workforce. They have been estimated to account for nearly half of all NHS staff absence (Boorman 2009).
- *Unhealthy lifestyles leading to problems such as obesity and overweight*: the government has estimated that around 300,000 NHS staff are obese, with a further 400,000 overweight (Cross-Government Obesity Unit 2009). Long hours of work, shift patterns and an environment that lacks facilities (e.g. a place to rest, exercise equipment, a café and a good working environment) contribute to the challenge of maintaining a healthy eating, sleeping and exercise routine (RCP 2015).

The national political response to these issues began with a review of health and wellbeing in the NHS, which was followed by the *Boorman Report* (Boorman 2009). These initiatives detailed the current health and wellbeing of the NHS workforce and highlighted the need for improvement so that absence rates would drop. It was anticipated that less absence would make a significant difference to the patient experience, outcomes and the quality of care, and would also have financial benefits.

It has taken some time for significant action to begin at a national level to drive and support a focus on staff wellbeing in the workplace, but such efforts are now forthcoming. For example, the Royal College of Physicians and other professional organizations have made the case that 'our healthcare system's greatest asset is the people who deliver it' and that 'for this system to provide safe, sustainable, patient-centred care, it is critically dependent on a healthy and engaged workforce with good mental and physical wellbeing' (RCP 2015, p.2). In 2018, NHS Employers published the NHS's *Workforce Health and Wellbeing Framework*, which gives equal recognition to organizational enablers (e.g. yoga classes and provision of healthy food) and specific health interventions (e.g. encouraging staff to take the required amount of exercise and eat healthy food) as necessary to improve the health and wellbeing of NHS staff (NHS Employers 2018).

Wellbeing

The ancient Greeks debated the concept of wellbeing: it was a core issue for philosophy and ethics. In recent years, as more research has been done on happiness, the term 'wellbeing' has gained more attention in economics and psychology, and has therefore been integrated into thinking and policy development (Fletcher 2015). Although a definition of wellbeing was offered at the beginning of this chapter, there is no agreement on a universal definition because it is dependent on why it is being defined.

The Department of Health report *Wellbeing: Why It Matters to Health Policy* (DH 2014a) proposed that wellbeing should be a core concept underpinning health policy and gave a number of reasons as to why it should matter (Box 19.1). The report defines

Box 19.1 Why wellbeing matters to health

- Adds years to life
- Improves recovery from illness
- Is associated with positive health behaviours in adults and children
- Is associated with broad positive outcomes
- Influences the wellbeing and mental health of those close to us
- Affects how staff and healthcare providers work
- Has implications for decisions for patient care practices and services
- Affects decisions about local services
- Has implications for treatment decisions and costs
- May ultimately reduce the healthcare burden

Source: Adapted from DH (2014a).

wellbeing in the context of health policy as 'feeling good and functioning well' and states that it 'comprises an individual's experience of their life; and a comparison of life circumstances with social norms and values' (DH 2014a, p.6). Wellbeing exists in two dimensions:

- *subjective wellbeing* (or personal wellbeing), which is how people think and feel about their own wellbeing, including their life satisfaction and whether their life is meaningful
- *objective wellbeing*, which is based on assumptions about basic human needs and rights, including aspects such as adequate food, physical health, education and safety.

Separately, the Office for National Statistics (2015) created the 'Well-Being Wheel', which illustrates the 41 statistical dimensions of national wellbeing (Figure 19.1).

Subjective wellbeing, it is proposed, increases life expectancy and improves not only health but also recovery from illness and injury. It is also associated with positive health behaviours in adults, such as eating a good diet, taking regular exercise, and less smoking and alcohol consumption (DH 2014a, pp.9–11). Significantly, if people are happy, this positively influences the subjective wellbeing of others they come into contact with, particularly their friends and neighbours (DH 2014a, p.13).

Thin (2012) describes people working in healthcare as 'happiness facilitators'. In a formal healthcare setting, nurses are generally in closest contact with patients compared to other healthcare professionals, which means that nurses' wellbeing is most likely to affect the quality of patients' experiences (Maben 2010).

Section 3a of the NHS Constitution states that 'the NHS commits to provide support and opportunities for staff to maintain their health, well-being and safety' (DH 2009, p.8). Therefore, the NHS encourages organizations to promote staff wellbeing, but it is also significant to note that staff wellbeing can improve the quality of patients' experiences and health outcomes (DH 2014b). Studies show that there is a connection between healthcare sector staff wellbeing (on the one hand) and how patients rate the care they receive and their health outcomes (on the other); NHS organizations that have more favourable indicators of staff wellbeing (e.g., in relation to bullying, harassment and stress) have better attendance, lower staff turnover, less agency spending, higher patient satisfaction and better outcome measures (Boorman 2009, Dawson 2009, Raleigh et al. 2009).

Stress

However, it is also recognized that work is not necessarily always good for wellbeing because, while employment can improve self-esteem, it can also be stressful (McManus and Perry 2012), so staff wellbeing initiatives need to involve the enhancement of positive psychological wellbeing as well as the reduction of negative pressure (e.g. stress) (DH 2014c). There is a great deal of disagreement both among academics and in popular opinion as to exactly what the definition of stress is, although all agree that it is very complex. In their study on workplace stress Sulsky and Smith (2005) define stress as 'any circumstance that places special physical and/or psychological demands on an organism leading to psychological, physiological and behavioural outcomes. If these demands persist over time, long term or chronic undesirable outcomes or strains may result' (p.6). This definition seems to

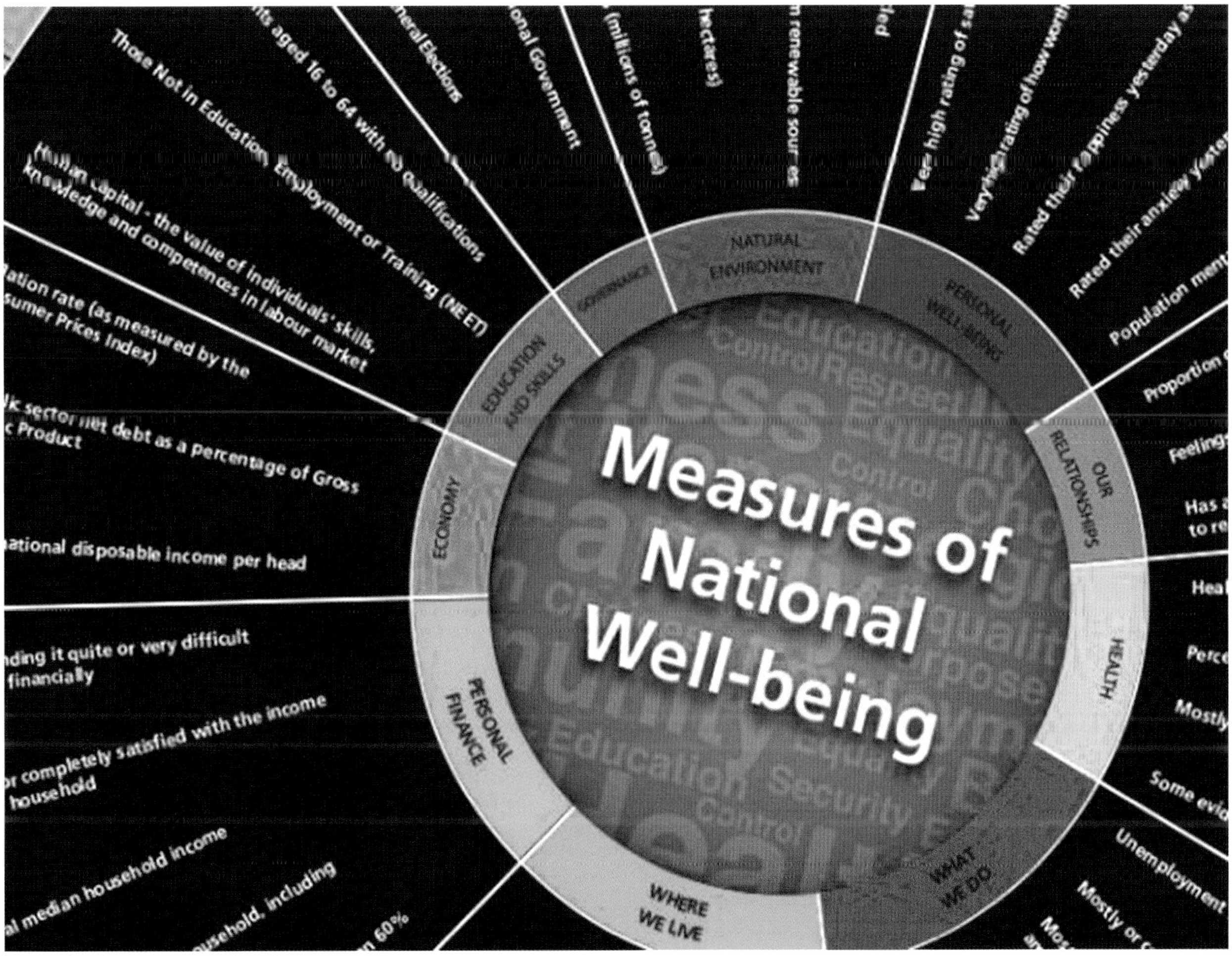

Figure 19.1 The 'Wheel of Wellbeing'. *Source:* Reproduced from Office for National Statistics (2015).

be in stark contrast to the World Health Organization's (2019) definition of occupational stress as 'the response people may have when presented with work demands and pressures that are not matched by their ability to cope'.

In the context of looking at how stress affects nurses, it seems to be most useful to define stress as a dynamic process, not just a reactive one. It is an ongoing process that affects the body and the mind, rather than an in-the-moment response to demands and pressure. This definition, which has been widely adopted in occupational stress literature, is called the 'transactional approach'. Mark and Smith (2012) use this definition to encompass both fields of thought on stress (i.e. that it is an ongoing process but also an in-the-moment response), stating that an environmental demand becomes a 'stressor' only when the individual perceives that it exceeds their available physical, emotional and psychological resources and threatens their wellbeing. This threat then triggers psychological, physiological and behavioural responses or 'strain' in an attempt to cope.

Anatomical and physiological factors

Recent studies in neuroscience have helped to develop a further understanding of the physiology of stress and its physical as well as emotional impacts. This knowledge has also assisted in the identification of evidence-based self-care strategies that can help individuals to cope more effectively with the demands of working in healthcare.

Physiologically, stress is the 'fight-or-flight response', in which the whole of a person becomes prepared to respond to a 'threat', either by recruiting all of their strength to physically defend themselves or by moving as quickly as they can to escape. This response can be switched on by an internal process – that is, by thoughts alone. As adrenaline and cortisol are released into the body, one of the immediate impacts is the redirection of blood to the muscles, lungs and heart, which prepares them to respond with as much strength and speed as they are able. This, however, means that other organs have less blood supply, with immediate – but survivable – consequences. Thus, blood is directed away from the prefrontal cortex and other parts of the brain, which affects our ability to make creative, logical and rational decisions in the moment and also our ability to remember the event afterwards. The gastrointestinal system also has less blood available, so digestion is impacted. In addition, many other micro-processes are interrupted, such as cell regeneration, which is important for processes including growing, learning and healing (Holroyd 2015). The cortisol also breaks down complex compounds in the body (such as sugars, fats and proteins) so they are available for energy to power the immediate fight or flight.

Physiologically, humans have evolved to survive brief periods of stress without any long-term damage (Cozolino 2017), but ongoing or chronic stress has physiological as well as psychological consequences. The continual release of cortisol and the continual breakdown of fats and proteins result in:

- inhibited inflammatory processes, which is a natural response to injury or a foreign agent in the body – this explains why cuts do not heal and we get mouth ulcers when we are stressed
- over the longer term, inhibition of white blood cell production, reducing immunity – this is why, after working for weeks in a busy, stressful environment, we may become ill as soon as we go on holiday
- damage to the hippocampus (the part of the brain that is essential for regulating emotions and memory)
- a decrease in plasticity and neural growth, inhibiting the ability to stop the fixed unhelpful and destructive thought patterns that can maintain the stress response (Cozolino 2017).

If we are experiencing stress for a considerable period of time, it can translate into our musculoskeletal system as well. It is experienced as tense muscles, rigid posture and a decrease in flexibility, which increases the risk of musculoskeletal injury. Additionally, when a person is stressed, awareness of body posture and position often decrease.

Psychological factors

What stresses an individual is very personal: what one individual views as stress, another will view as pressure and therefore their responses will be very different. A key driver that turns pressure into stress is what is known as 'rumination' (Waugh 2014). This is the mental process of thinking about the same thing over and over – either something that happened in the past or something that could happen in the future – and attaching a negative emotion to it.

The types of pressure that nurses experience are many and varied. Some are organizational (through targets and monitoring of performance) whereas others are political or managerial and are common to many professions. However, the unique pressures of healthcare are the expectations of patients and their families, which can often feel overwhelming. We add to this with the pressure we put on ourselves to fulfil our 'mission' to help, heal and show compassion.

Nursing requires a well-developed ability to empathize. Empathy allows nurses to connect with the people they are caring for and help them on a more than physical level. It is the empathetic connection to a patient that gives you the feeling that you have really been able to help them and that you have made a difference. Likewise, when a patient has experienced empathy from a nurse, they feel understood and valued as an individual.

Wiseman (1996) summarized the defining attributes of empathy in nursing as the ability to see the world as others see it, be non-judgemental, understand another's feelings and then communicate that understanding. Empathy is psychologically demanding; to be empathetic, you have to give up part of yourself and for a time connect with another person on a deeper level. Sometimes as a nurse this will be all you have to offer; you cannot 'fix' the problem for the person, just be with them in their distress and be the anchor for them to hold on to. However, sitting with those in distress can be psychologically or emotionally costly: Figley (2002) observes that 'the very act of being compassionate and empathic extracts a cost', that 'in our effort to view the world from the perspective of suffering, we suffer' and that 'the meaning of compassion is to bear suffering' (p.1434).

Empathy happens spontaneously and unconsciously and you may find yourself copying the facial expressions and body language of the person you are caring for. This is totally normal and the more naturally empathetic you are, the more this will happen. The empathetic response can be triggered by any part of the sensory nervous system: visual, auditory and touch are the most common. Empathy is not just a feeling and set of behaviours but also a physiological response to the distress of others; we all have mirror neurones, which can be described as chains of neurones inside us that communicate with those in others without any regard for the fact that we are distinct from each other (Ward 2010). Keyser (2011) uses the phrase 'a little bit of you becomes me, and a little bit of me becomes you' (p.221) to describe what happens when we see another in pain, and this assists humans in the ability to be empathetic. This can have a profound effect on our mental health; at the extreme this is 'burnout – a state of physical, emotional and mental exhaustion caused by long term involvement in emotionally demanding situations' (Pines and Aronson 1988, p.9) and there is often no return. As Victor Frankl (1959) said, 'what is to give light must endure burning' (cited in Gentry and Baranowsky 2013, p.16). This quote powerfully describes the inevitability that 'fixing the broken, healing the sick, comforting the lost and witnessing those who are dying' can be painful work (Gentry and Baranowsky 2013, p.16). To ensure that we don't burn out, we need to refuel – we need to learn self-care.

Compassion fatigue

'Compassion fatigue' is a term used to describe the occupational stressors unique to providers of healthcare (Sinclair et al. 2017). It has been suggested that the term was first used by a nurse (Carla Joinson) in 1992 to describe a unique form of burnout experienced by caregivers resulting in a 'loss of the ability to nurture' (Joinson 1992, p.119). However, the recognition of compassion fatigue as a concept is more commonly attributed to Dr Charles Figley, an American professor and expert in trauma, who in the 1980s observed that many of the care staff he worked with suffered from very similar symptoms to those they were caring for, even though the trauma was not happening directly to them (Coles 2017). Before this ground-breaking work, care staff affected by their work were labelled as suffering from stress or burnout, but Figley and his team identified that burnout can occur in situations where empathy and compassion have not been demanded, whereas compassion fatigue occurs where empathy and compassion are a key ask of the caregiver (Coles 2017). Compassion fatigue occurs when a carer feels overwhelmed by the amount they expect themselves to give. Burnout occurs when a carer feels they have nothing left to give.

Figley (1995) initially used the term 'secondary stress disorder' for what he was observing, but it is also referred to as 'vicarious trauma' and is increasingly referred to as 'compassion fatigue'. It is necessary to note that more recently there have been questions raised about the conceptual validity of compassion fatigue (Sinclair et al. 2017); however, naming it has significantly helped to develop interventions to address and prevent it among nurses and other healthcare professionals (Gentry and Baranowsky 2013).

Compassion fatigue is conceptualized as beginning with the *empathetic response* (explored in the previous section), which allows those in the caring profession to connect with a patient and feel how they are feeling, but also opens them up to absorbing and experiencing their trauma, suffering and pain, known as *vicarious traumatization*. This exposure stimulates our flight-or-fight response and its associated physiological responses (see above). However, the professional context in which we are working means these responses have to be suppressed. Continual suppression has consequences for both physical and mental health.

Compassion fatigue can be considered as an alarm system that alerts us that we need to take steps to care for ourselves before we experience burnout. It can be defined as 'the natural consequent behaviours and emotions resulting from knowing about a traumatizing event(s) experienced by another [and] resulting from helping or wanting to help a traumatized or suffering person' (Figley 1995, p.7). As Reman (1996) said, 'the expectation that we can be immersed in suffering and loss daily and not be touched by it, is as unrealistic as expecting to be able to walk through water without getting wet' (p.52).

Symptoms of compassion fatigue

The symptoms of compassion fatigue are caused by the body's empathetic response to vicarious trauma. It is vital that you recognize these feelings in yourself and see them as a call to action; if you ignore them, they will not go away and will only get worse.

Figley (1995) organized the symptoms into four phases: anxiety, irritability, withdrawal and robot.

Phase 1: anxiety

Physical symptoms

As the vicarious trauma stimulates your nervous system into flight or fight, you will experience the effects of adrenaline, which include raised heart and breathing rates, shaking and muscle tension. You will find it hard to think clearly and concentrate and may have trouble sleeping. You may find that you become hypervigilant, cannot relax and are very impulsive.

Internal narrative

You may find that you are telling yourself that you are the only one who can do the job properly: it's your mission and you are the first one in and the last one out from work every day. You know that your job is stressful, but you tell yourself that you are okay and coping, and you expect other people to do the same. Outside work you may find yourself volunteering for extra activities at clubs or societies or challenging yourself with sports or hobbies. You may have become accustomed to the feeling of anxiety and actively seek out the feeling. For example, when you are on holiday, you may find it impossible to relax and find that relaxing in itself causes you to feel stressed.

Grace's story

Grace had been working as a nurse for 20 years and had become a clinical nurse specialist. She had teenage children and a supportive partner. She had always been seen as extremely capable and the type of person who always got the job done; she went above and beyond what was expected of her. Away from work, Grace was the chair of her children's school's parent–teacher association, ran marathons for charity and worked as a St John Ambulance volunteer. She took a promotion with lots of extra responsibility and initially really enjoyed the work, but she began to notice that she was feeling different. She noticed that her memory was not as good as it had been and she was forgetting quite important things outside work, such as parents' evenings or family events. She began waking extremely early in the morning, feeling very fatigued and not enjoying her time off as much as she used to. One day in her car, on her way home from an important meeting, she suddenly felt as if she couldn't breathe and thought she was having a heart attack. She went to see her GP and was told that her blood pressure was very high and she was suffering from stress. She was completely devastated as she felt this meant she wasn't coping with her work. Although she felt guilty and initially said that she couldn't take time off, her GP insisted that she did. In the following weeks she hit rock bottom and at first she couldn't understand what was happening to her, but she began to realize the impact her job had been having on her mental and physical health and on her family and friends, who had been trying to tell her for a long time that things were not right.

Phase 2: irritability

Physical symptoms

These may include headaches, fatigue and multiple minor illnesses as the immune system is affected by the chronic stress. They might also include musculoskeletal problems, in particular chronic neck and back pain. You may also find that you are eating too much or too little, and eating things you know are not good for you.

Internal narrative

The people you are caring for are now starting to irritate you. You may feel that people at work and at home are putting unreasonable demands on you and you just can't deal with it all. You may feel very guilty about this but then start to worry about the guilt. You may tell yourself that there is nothing you can do to change the situation and that if you just ignore the way you are feeling it will go away. You may justify using alcohol or eating unhealthily to help you cope even though you know that this is not the right thing to do.

Phoebe's story

Phoebe had only ever wanted to work as a nurse. Her mother was a nurse and her father was a social worker, and lots of other family members also worked in health and social care. She trained in a big London hospital and then worked on busy wards gaining experience and promotions. She married a fellow nurse and had two young children. Her trust introduced an appraisal system that included feedback from both colleagues and patients. Staff were asked to write a reflective piece on how they saw themselves performing. Phoebe took the paperwork home to write the reflection on her day off. Having completed it, she left it out and having read it her daughter asked Phoebe who the document was describing; it said, 'this nurse is really great at her job, really funny and sweet and caring'. Phoebe thought her daughter was joking and laughed, saying that it was her. Her daughter looked at her strangely and said, 'but this person is nothing like you – you're irritable, short tempered, tired all the time and constantly complaining about everything!' Phoebe was horrified, and when she questioned her family and friends they all agreed. Phoebe began to realize that the job had taken over her life and that she had put her job first to the detriment of not only her mental health but also her home life.

Phase 3: withdrawal

Physical symptoms

You have chronic fatigue, and constant aches and pains. You neglect your physical and emotional health. You may need to take time off work but when you do, you don't feel any better on your return.

Internal narrative

You tell yourself that the only way you can carry on is to shut out the outside world after work. You may not feel like talking to anyone about how you feel as they will not understand, so you begin to withdraw from colleagues, family and friends. You may feel angry at the world and justified in complaining a lot about work and your colleagues. You may admit that you are feeling differently about work, and you may feel guilty that you are not as engaged as you once were and aware that you are protecting yourself emotionally. You won't admit it to them, but those who describe you as negative or pessimistic may have a point.

Steve's story

Steve had been working as an A&E nurse for just over a year. Following a very traumatic incident in the department, he started to feel very different at work and at home. His managers noticed that he was habitually late for shifts and training and was very disengaged from the rest of the team. They tried to talk to him about what was going on but he became very defensive. Steve was feeling anxious all the time, having problems sleeping and dreading going into work each day. He was having flashbacks and nightmares, and found that instead of going out with his mates after work or at the weekends, all he wanted to do was go home and shut the curtains and zone out.

Phase 4: Robot

Physical symptoms

The physical symptoms in this phase are very similar to those suffered by people with depression. They include headaches and generalized aches and pains, digestive problems, and a general feeling of low-level anxiety and very low mood.

Internal narrative

You tell yourself that just turning up and 'doing the job' is the best way to be. Nothing good is going to come from doing anything positive and nothing bad is going to come from being negative. Empathy and compassion for the people you care for are no longer required; the functional requirements are all that matter. You may admit that you are not coping and so feel resentful towards others who are. You are staying in your job because you're not able to do anything else.

Naheed's story

Naheed trained to be a nurse after becoming very disillusioned with the corporate job he'd had before. His first role was at a large dementia care home and he quickly became a dedicated and conscientious member of staff whom colleagues, clients and families universally loved. The workload was very heavy and Naheed soon found himself feeling that he was the only one who was doing the job properly. Over time, this turned into resentment and irritation with the rest of his team. He suffered from chronic back pain but never allowed himself to be off sick. Naheed felt less and less empathy towards the patients and their families; this upset him and he felt guilty. He felt compelled to continue as he had given up his other job for this one. Eventually his colleagues began to describe him as 'hard and unfeeling' and families no longer sought him out for support. A relative made a complaint and he was asked to explain his behaviour to the management team and forced to resign.

Evidence-based approaches

The NHS's *Workforce Health and Wellbeing Framework* (NHS Employers 2018) identified two ways in which staff wellbeing can be promoted: those that the organization can provide and facilitate, and self-care health interventions. The focus in this chapter is on self-care – that is, taking responsibility for our own physical health and wellbeing – because this has significant benefits, particularly empowerment, which is a sense of greater control of our own health, which in turn helps us to maintain our own emotional wellbeing (Self Care Forum 2018).

The general evidence underpinning strategies for self-care for nurses is no different from that for the general population. This general evidence base is vast and is readily accessible in many locations, such as https://www.nhs.uk/live-well, so the aspects of self-care that are more specific to nurses are the focus here. These include:

- preventing compassion fatigue
- physical wellbeing related to body posture and moving when working with patients
- eating and drinking well, particularly when on shifts.

These also reflect the three areas identified in the NHS's *Workforce Health and Wellbeing Framework* (NHS Employers 2018).

Preventing compassion fatigue

Studies conducted in the US show that specific skills can help to prevent compassion fatigue and also aid recovery from it when it occurs (Flarity et al. 2013, Gentry and Baranowsky 2013, Potter et al. 2013). Gentry and Baranowsky (2013) describe this as building up 'antibodies' or developing professional resilience skills to resist compassion fatigue. They name five skills – self-regulation, intentionality, self-compassion, connection and support, and self-care and revitalization – whose names have been adapted in the following sections.

Self-regulation

Self-regulation is the ability to recognize when the sympathetic nervous system is activated (the fight-or-flight response) because of a perceived threat in the workplace. Examples of threats include:

- a difficult relationship with colleagues, patients or relatives
- too much work to do and too little time to do it
- caring for critically ill or complex patients unsupported.

The bottom line is that in such situations, our body is telling us that we are in danger. Therefore, as described above, when the autonomic nervous system is activated, physical changes happen and cognitive functioning is affected, which is exhausting. Recognizing what is going on through using skills such as mindfulness (see below) can help us to consciously change our perceptions and thereby activate the parasympathetic nervous system.

It is known that one of the main factors that keeps our sympathetic nervous system activated is *perceived* threats. Our minds are very good at anticipating potential dangers around us and prompting a state of high alert. It is worth asking ourselves, however: how often, when we feel threatened on a shift or during a working day, is there any actual physical danger. For most people, the answer will be 'very infrequently', so we can learn to ask ourselves 'Am I in danger?' and tell ourselves 'No, I am not.'

However, this strategy will not automatically stop our minds perceiving threats in the workplace. These perceptions might be about the workplace, our managers or the organization as a whole.

Try this

This exercise lists *perceived* threats that you might recognize. If they are familiar to you, then read the possible alternative perceptions. Can you apply them in your work situation? If not, can you come up with any other alternatives that might help you to view the situation differently and therefore as less of a threat?

1. People are shouting and rushing around, and staff are looking anxious – there must be something critical happening.
   There might be, but it isn't dangerous, and you aren't dealing with it alone so there is no threat.
2. They just want more and more and I haven't got any more to give – I'm going to get in trouble, lose my job or get ill.
   The workplace is always going to demand more of you than you can give because the demand is always increasing and there are decreasing resources. This is not a dangerous situation, just a common one, so be kind to yourself and realize you are only employed to do a contracted number of hours.
3. You have made a mistake and you know you have a duty of candour, but you are afraid that if you own up you might lose your job.
   This can be a very frightening situation and you will be feeling very stressed because you have made a mistake and it could have real consequences for you and for your patient. As nurses, we are very hard on ourselves, and despite the pressure we are under and the emotional demands of the job we still expect that we will not make mistakes. But the consequences you are imagining may not be the reality. When you own up to the mistake as you know you should, the organization will probably take some kind of disciplinary action, there will be an investigation into what happened and why, and you may be offered additional training and supervision. One way of looking at this is that you should want this to happen as it will help you to avoid being in this situation again and also safeguard patients and potentially avoid other staff making a similar mistake. In addition, attending debriefing sessions, undertaking reflective practice or receiving clinical supervision can help us to talk about our perspective on a situation and to consider alternatives that might help us.

Intentionality

Intentionality is the ability to hold in mind our purpose and the values that are important to us at work.

Try this

Imagine that you are meeting a very wise person who is extremely kind and has your best interests at heart. As well as listening to you, they have the ability to see inside your mind and heart.

They want to know why you do your job, what is important to you in how you go about it each day, how you relate to your patients and their families, and how you interact with your colleagues. What would you tell them?

When we are stressed, we can unconsciously react impulsively in situations where we feel stressed in an attempt – without realizing it – to limit or get away from the 'threat' or difficult situation. This might take the form of an irritated request to a colleague or comforting ourselves during our break by eating more chocolate or cakes than we intend. The greater the stress or distress we experience, the greater the likelihood that our behaviour will be reactive.

Using processes such as mindfulness (see below) can help us to recognize when we are on automatic pilot and responding to others and ourselves in ways that are not intentional or reflective of our values.

Try this

During a shift, choose a time, perhaps using an alarm on your phone or choosing the beginning of a break or after you have finished an aspect of care for a patient. S.T.O.P. for no more than 30 seconds:

- S – STOP whatever you are doing and notice what is going on in your mind and body. Don't do anything about it, just notice.
- T – THINK: what were you actually doing just now? What were you thinking? Was it about the task or aspect of care you were doing? Was your mind focusing on the past, present or future? What was the mood of those thoughts? Were they anxious, angry, guilty or sad? If you don't know where your mind was, that is okay – maybe it was on automatic pilot. Notice whether any reactive ideas (i.e. automatic negative responses prompted by the situation) have crept in that don't match with your values.
- O – OPTIONS: if you find your mind was not where you wanted it to be, you can bring it to the 'here and now' using one of your five senses. For example, you can focus on:
  - The sounds around you – what can you hear?
  - The smells around you – what can you smell?
  - The sights around you – what colours can you see?
  - The touch sensations around you, such as your clothes against your body or your feet in your shoes – what can you feel?
  - The sensations in your body – are there any parts that need to stretch or need a rub? Do you need the toilet or a drink?
- P – PROCEED: go back to what you were doing, aware of your values and what is important to you in daily life.

Source: Adapted from Wax (2013).

Self-compassion

Self-compassion is described as:

> Being kind and understanding toward oneself in instances of pain or failure rather than being harshly self-critical; ... perceiving one's experiences as part of the larger human experience rather than seeing them as isolating; and ... holding painful thoughts and feelings in balanced awareness rather than over-identifying with them. (Neff 2011, p.85)

Working with distress in a stressful environment has an impact. Our immediate response can be that we aren't coping, we aren't good at time management, we aren't tough enough. If we become irritable or sad, or are getting to the point where we feel we can't face going into work, we need to recognize that this might be a sign that we have compassion fatigue and that these are normal responses to working with distress. It does not mean that you do not care or are emotionally unable to do your job. The combination of empathy and exposure to trauma *will* affect you and the key is to accept that it is normal and then respond to the symptoms.

Try this

- Take a selfie.
- Now say something *kind and positive* about the person you see in the picture.
- Don't be surprised if it is difficult.
- Are you a good listener?
- Are you a good organizer?
- Are you loyal?
- Are you fun?
- Are you ...?

We strive to take care of our patients in the way that we would like to be cared for if we were in their shoes. To achieve this, we must first take care of ourselves with kindness and compassion. As nurses, we take great pride in being kind and compassionate towards our patients but we are poor at showing ourselves the same compassion. We are very good at giving ourselves a hard time and very bad at forgiving ourselves for 'being human'. After a difficult day or incident, our tendency is to run over and over in our mind what we could have done differently, what we should have done but didn't, what we didn't know – the list can go on and on.

One important way you can begin to show yourself more compassion is to become very aware of how you talk to yourself when you are under pressure. Is your internal narrative helpful or unhelpful during times of stress? Are you actually making the situation worse by the way you are treating yourself? Think about the language you use under pressure and try to change it. As Lisa M. Hayes (2017), a famous relationship coach, said, 'Be careful what you say to yourself because you are listening.'

Try this

Find a notebook or use your phone and each day when you finish work write down three things that you did well. If this is difficult, write down a thank you or grateful comment from a patient or relative, or take a photo of a thank-you card.

When you are feeling really negative about yourself, read through what you have written to remind yourself that you are doing your best.

It can help to tell a close friend or family member that you have this list so they can remind you to look at it whenever they know you need a reminder to be kind to yourself.

Self-compassion is all about being warm and understanding towards yourself when you are suffering, failing or feeling inadequate rather than ignoring the pain or flagellating yourself with self-criticism. Self-compassionate people share some common traits (Neff 2011):

- They are kind to themselves when they fail or make mistakes.
- They recognize that failures are a shared human experience.
- They take a balanced approach to negative emotions when they stumble or fall short, allowing themselves to feel bad but not letting negative emotions take over.

Developing self-compassion has been shown to improve how we relate to others (Neff and Pommier 2012). It has also been shown to encourage willingness to learn from failure and try again without self-recrimination (Gustin and Wagner 2013).

Another aspect of our intentionality is how we define ourselves. Taking on a professional role like nursing can be very significant in our lives, giving us meaning and purpose (Skovholt and Trotter-Mathison 2016). However, it can become the dominant part of ourselves, and we may absorb society's ideas of what a nurse should be. This may mean we are unable to differentiate between our work and home lives, or between who we are and what we perceive a nurse should be.

Try this

If you asked a neighbour, a relative or a person serving behind the counter in your local coffee shop what the qualities of a nurse are, what do you think they would say? Write down a list of qualities that they might mention.

Look through your list and consider:

- Which qualities do you agree with, and how do they shape your values and why you do your job?
- Which ones are realistic and possible in the job you do?
- Has considering these qualities changed your values and how you see yourself?

Our perceptions of ourselves as nurses and particularly those 'put on us by others' make declining requests from those we work for feel like we are being less caring or committed. We can also develop an unrealistic sense of what doing a job is about as well as how we are meant to cope. It's okay to say 'no' to extra work or responsibilities, especially when you are feeling the effects of compassion fatigue – and, in fact, you must. You can only give so much and it's okay to need time away from work to refill your compassion and energy levels. If you keep saying 'yes' to everything, your body and mind will eventually say 'no' for you!

You 'work' as a nurse but you are so much more than this. You are a human being – someone's husband, wife, partner, parent, sister, brother, child, friend or colleague – the list is almost endless.

Connection and support

Feeling supported, heard and cared about by colleagues is crucial to maintaining our resilience (Tosone et al. 2010) and in helping to avoid compassion fatigue. As already explored, a component of compassion fatigue is exposure to the trauma, distress and suffering of others. One of the effective ways of overcoming the effects of this exposure is to share these difficult experiences with others in a relaxed, supportive and non-judgemental environment. Research shows that sharing these experiences helps us to process and make sense of what happened (Baranowsky et al. 2011). This is known as the 'universality of experience effect' and is a curative factor in groups (Yalom and Leszcz 2005). However, it is essential that the group is an environment in which everybody feels psychologically safe so they can talk openly and honestly.

In recent years, changes in shift patterns, establishments and training have led to increasing isolation rather than opportunities for professional connection. The individuals most immediately available to us for support are often therefore our family and friends. If they don't have a healthcare background, we may notice them withdrawing or changing the subject when we try to share difficult experiences, with the result that we internalize the experiences and don't talk about them. If we do, we can traumatize our friends and family because they are not trained to cope and do not have any opportunity to respond to the difficult situations we describe, so they are left feeling helpless. We therefore need to deliberately be aware of and nurture our professional support network.

Try this

Make a note of:

1. A professional colleague you can call in an 'emergency', when your thoughts and feelings about work have just got too much and you need to tell somebody. If you can identify somebody, it might be a good idea to check with them whether this is okay, and you can offer to be their emergency buddy in return.
2. The sources of support in your organization or other organizations that you know will listen – for example, occupational health, a staff counselling service, an employee assistance programme, a union hotline or a charity such as Cavell Nurses' Trust.
3. Are there any regular supervision or reflective practice groups for your area or role? Do you attend? If not, what do you need to do so you can? Who can support you with this?
4. As a team, what do you do to have fun together? Do you do this frequently enough? Who can help you make fun events happen regularly?

Self-care and revitalization

Our role as carers of those in distress is costly – we give of our emotional and physical energy to do it, so we need to have a plan to refuel or revitalize (Gentry and Baranowsky 2013). For each of us, how we do this will be different, but we have a professional responsibility to learn what it is that works for us and to regularly practise what will sustain our energy and hope.

Try this

This exercise focuses on things that nourish you and things that deplete you:

1. Make a list of things you do in a typical day when you work, from the time you get up until you go to bed. Make it as detailed as possible. For example:
   - Wake up and listen to the radio for 10 minutes.
   - Drink tea in bed.
   - Shower.
2. When you have finished, look at your list and put a letter beside each activity:
   - N – Nourishing: things that increase your energy, nourish you, and help you feel awake and alive.
   - D – Depleting: things that drain your energy, deplete you, and make you feel less awake and alive.
   - There may be some activities that could be either; if so, label them as both.
3. Have a look at the list:
   - What do you notice?
   - What is there more of?
   - Could some be either, depending on your attitude to them?
   - How easy is it to do the things that are nourishing and nurturing?
   - What are the proportions of each during your working hours?
   - If you did this exercise over a whole week, what would you notice? Would the proportions change?
4. Reflecting on this exercise with self-care in mind, do you need to make any changes? We don't have control over some depleting activities, but can you change them in any way to make them more nourishing? For example, you might find your commute very depleting if you spend a long time in slow-moving traffic. You may not be able to change your commute, but you could sign up for a talking book service and thereby come to love your time in the car listening to novels that you would otherwise not have time to enjoy.
5. Make a list of one or two things that you could add or change in your day so that the number of things you do to care for yourself increases.

Source: Adapted from Watt (2016).

Research shows that there are some core components of self-care that help prevent compassion fatigue (Gentry and Barnowsky 2013, Skovholt and Trotter-Mathison 2016):

- *Aerobic activity*: a minimum of 20 minutes will help to reduce stress levels by 'burning off' some of the adrenaline you have produced when in a threatening situation. This will reduce feelings of anxiety.
- *Deliberate, healthy sleep habits*: have a sleep routine no matter what time of the day you go to bed. Reduce the degree to which you are exposed to bright lights and screens at least 30 minutes

before you go to bed. Make the room dark and cool if at all possible, with no television. Avoid using your phone as an alarm clock; instead, leave it outside the room or at least in a bag or drawer.

- *Regular social connection with others outside work*: have a network of friends who are not connected with your work, and make a conscious effort to see them even when you are feeling emotionally or physically tired as they will give you a perspective beyond your world of work; this will give you emotional energy.
- *Opportunities to create, make, grow or collect*: we are by nature creative beings and many people gain great energy from things such as growing and tending plants, creating music or art, or spending time collecting objects they love and value. These activities give us joy and help to fill up our spiritual energy.
- *Time for solitude or spiritual practice*: time spent in prayer or meditation is valuable on many levels and gives you opportunities to reflect and think about what is important to you as well as allowing your brain time to just be 'in the moment'.
- *Eating well and maintaining fluid levels*: be aware that being hydrated and what we eat affect how we feel. This is even more essential when we are under pressure.

Recovery from compassion fatigue

It is recognized that, even if all preventive approaches are put into place, as individuals we can still experience compassion fatigue because of the intensity of distress we may witness and because events in our personal lives may reduce our resilience. So, what do we do if we experience the symptoms described above and our self-care strategies are not working? In such cases, it is vital to seek help. You have a number of options:

- your GP
- occupational health at your workplace
- a staff counselling service
- an employee assistance programme.

If you do not have a GP or occupational health advisor in your workplace, you are encouraged to contact your union, which will direct you to other sources of support for healthcare workers. More intense experiences of compassion fatigue are also known as 'secondary traumatic stress disorder', so therapeutic help similar to that given to individuals with post-traumatic stress disorder may be recommended (Coles 2017).

Mindfulness

Definition

Mindfulness means paying attention in the present moment, in a particular way, on purpose, without making any judgements or criticisms of self or others. It enables us to stop living life on automatic pilot and begin to live life more fully and responsively, rather than reactively. In this way, we increase the amount of choice we have over the things we do (Figure 19.2). For example, when we wash our hands, our minds are often thinking about what we are going to do next or later in the day, rather than noticing the temperature of the water, the sounds as the water pours from the tap or the scent of the soap.

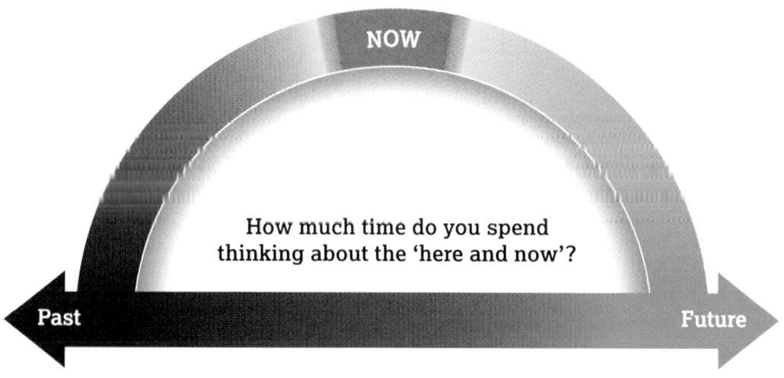

Figure 19.2 How much time do you spend thinking about the here and now?

Related theory

By keeping us in the present moment, mindfulness teaches us about 'anchors', such as focusing on the breath or attuning to the body. This helps us to manage any difficulties we might encounter. The ability to cultivate awareness in meditation enables us to observe patterns of thinking and responses to physical sensations, providing cues about ourselves and our behaviour that are transferable to everyday living. We observe and accept our thoughts, feelings and sensory reactions to experiences, and we allow fluctuations to pass by or simply tolerate them and remain with them, regardless of whether they are pleasurable, uncomfortable or neutral. We learn to tolerate and accept the desire we have for things to be different. The practice of mindfulness teaches us to manage everyday anxieties and stresses with kindness and compassion towards ourselves and others.

When practising mindfulness, there are no specific objectives or aims, unlike with other techniques such as relaxation (where the goal is to relax) or other forms of meditation (where the goal can be to eradicate all thinking from the mind). Nevertheless, people who participate in mindfulness often report feeling calm and tranquil after meditation, and research indicates that following sustained practice, EEG (electroencephalogram) patterns are associated with an altered resting pattern related to these responses. Investigators have also undertaken MRI scans of participants before and after they took part in mindfulness courses, and have found thickening in grey matter associated with attention, sensory processing and recognition of internal bodily sensations (e.g. taking time to drop your shoulders when you notice tension) (Lazar et al. 2005). Holzel et al. (2011) undertook similar MRI research, again comparing participants before and after a mindfulness course, and found increased grey-matter density in areas associated with learning and memory processing, emotion regulation, and the ability, psychologically speaking, to explore all aspects of ourselves and adopt a broad life view, such as when considering strategies for self-care and personal well-being (e.g. taking regular breaks to make refreshing drinks).

Evidence-based approaches

Evidence-based mindfulness-based interventions include Mindfulness-Based Stress Reduction (MBSR) (Williams and Penman 2011) and Mindfulness-Based Cognitive Therapy (MBCT) (Segal et al. 2013). Study outcomes show that those who satisfactorily complete an 8-week course of weekly sessions each lasting 2–3 hours are able to cultivate mindfulness and self-compassion. When mindfulness skills are developed, people also report improved mental health and resilience (Keng et al. 2011). Similarly, a systematic review demonstrated that nurses who undertook mindfulness based interventions and continued with practice showed significant changes in their health and wellbeing, self-compassion, empathy, stress and serenity compared to those who did not (Burton et al. 2017).

In workplaces, a range of mindfulness interventions are helpful (Burton et al. 2017), such as brief introductory courses to fit around working patterns, tailored one-off sessions for teams and 8-week courses. An 8-week mindfulness course adapted from MBSR and MBCT to be more accessible to employees in a healthcare setting has recently been piloted at The Royal Marsden Foundation NHS Trust. This showed significant benefits 3 months after completion for those who participated.

Rationale

Contraindications

Mindfulness is unsuitable for anyone diagnosed with post-traumatic stress disorder, any psychotic mental health disorder or anyone suffering with dissociative states

Pre-procedural considerations

Before taking part in any mindfulness practice, it is necessary to be able to sit physically for up to 20 minutes at a time and to have permission from a relevant manager, if attending during working hours. It is important that attendees declare any health conditions, so facilitators can respond appropriately to any symptoms that might be noticed or occur during sessions.

If attendees have any long-term or chronic health conditions or suffer with pain in any part of the body (this includes conditions that are invisible, such as epilepsy), it is essential for them to consult with their GP or medical consultant before taking part in any sessions.

Try this: 3-minute breathing space meditation

Deliberately adopt an erect and dignified posture, whether sitting or standing. If possible, close your eyes. Then bring your awareness to your inner experience and acknowledge it, asking: what is my experience right now?

- What thoughts are going through your mind? As best you can, acknowledge thoughts as mental events.
- What feelings are here? Turning towards any sense of discomfort or unpleasant feelings, acknowledge them without trying to make them different from how you find them.
- What body sensations are here right now? Perhaps quickly scan the body to pick up any sensations of tightness or bracing, acknowledging the sensations, but once again not trying to change them in any way.

Now, redirect the attention to a narrow spotlight on the physical sensations of the breath, moving in close to the physical sensations of the breath in the abdomen … Expanding as the breath comes in … and falling back as the breath goes out. Follow the breath all the way in and all the way out. Use each breath as an opportunity to anchor yourself into the present. And, if the mind wanders, gently escort the attention back to the breath.

Now, expand the field of awareness around the breathing so that it includes a sense of the body as a whole, your posture and facial expression, as if the whole body were breathing. If you become aware of any sensations of discomfort or tension, feel free to bring your focus of attention right in to the intensity by imagining that the breath could move into and around the sensations. In this, you are helping to explore the sensations, befriending them, rather than trying to change them in any way. If they stop pulling for your attention, return your focus to sitting, being aware of the whole body, moment by moment.

When you're ready, let go of this brief practice and open your eyes.

Source: Adapted from Williams and Penman (2011).

Try this: mindful hand washing

- Turn off your automatic pilot and soap up your hands as though you were doing it for the very first time. Slow down and be deliberate in your actions.
- Feeling each sensation: the warm water on your skin and the smell of the soap; take time to wash each finger, the backs of your hands, between your fingers and up to your wrists.
- Feel your feet anchored to the floor and the weight of your hands as they move over each other.
- Become aware of any sense of aliveness and vitality in your hands, noticing the simple pleasure of warm water on your skin and enjoying the feeling of clean hands.
- Picture all stress and worry spiralling down the drain with the water.
- As you dry your hands, continue being mindfully present, noticing all the sensations. No matter how many times you wash and dry your hands, each moment is refreshingly unique.

Source: Adapted from Sheridan (2016).

Problem solving

It is accepted that distractions will occur during mindfulness practice; these are expected and may include internal distractions (such as patterns of thinking, bodily feelings or sensations) and external distractions (such as noises). Such distractions offer an ideal opportunity to develop awareness of when the mind starts to wander, to observe where it has wandered to and then to practise, *gently and kindly*, bringing the focus of attention back to the meditation, *without self-criticism or judgement*.

Practising mindfulness can be experienced as challenging unless a habit has been established. Therefore, it can be helpful to set an alarm on your phone, laptop or PC and establish a preferred place and time to practise. Likewise, other supports (such as websites or mobile phone apps) can be useful resources. Often, finding time is not enough; it is important to *make* the time to practise. If you are practising at home, encourage family to join in with you, rather than being disturbed by them!

Eating and drinking

Related theory

It is not just patients whose nutritional needs should be considered; it is essential that all staff working in health establishments also have opportunities to eat and drink well. Food, water and rest are basic needs for all and if compromised significantly affect individuals' health. Evidence highlights that improved patient outcomes can be linked to good staff health and wellbeing; this effect is further enhanced by improved working environments and positive work experience (RCN 2018). A survey conducted by the Royal College of Nursing (RCN) in 2017 showed that almost 60% of staff did not take proper breaks (RCN 2017). This was further highlighted in a social media poll by the British Dietetic Association, which showed that one in ten of people who responded always skipped their breaks, and over half sometimes did (British Dietetic Association 2018). A House of Commons Health Committee (2018) report highlighted that retention is improved when staff can take breaks and refuel with food and drink.

Health and wellbeing within the workplace has increasingly become a priority. The NHS needs to be a beacon of good practice in supporting staff and visitors to make healthier choices when buying food and drink sold on NHS premises (British Dietetic Association 2017). There are various initiatives that have been brought in to support these plans, including a 'Healthier Food for NHS Staff and Visitors' commissioning strategy, and voluntary reduction targets to reduce the sale of sugar-sweetened beverages across the NHS (NHS England 2016). In 2015, the WIN project was set up; this is a healthy weight initiative for nurses (WIN) intended to help them achieve and maintain a healthy weight (RCN 2018).

Evidence-based approaches

The British Dietetic Association workplace initiative 'Work Ready' highlights that it is essential to the wellbeing of staff that they can take breaks to refuel and hydrate. What we eat can affect how we feel, our energy levels, our concentration, our decision making and how we deal with stressful situations. Most people feel better when they have had a healthy balanced meal. It is important to have adequate carbohydrates to eat.

The ability to concentrate and focus comes from the adequate supply of energy – from blood glucose – to the brain. The brain uses 20% of all energy needed by the body. Glucose is also vital to fuel muscles and maintain body temperature. Blood glucose comes from all the carbohydrates we eat, including fruit, vegetables, legumes, wholegrain cereals, bread, rice, and potatoes, sugars and low-fat dairy (Arens 2017) (see Boxes 19.2 and 19.3).

Box 19.2 Daily reference nutritional intakes for adults

- Total fat: less than 70 g
- Saturated fat: less than 20 g
- Carbohydrate: at least 260 g
- Total sugars: 90 g
- Protein: 50 g
- Salt: less than 6 g

Source: Adapted from NHS (2017).

Box 19.3 Ideas for healthy meals at work

- Wholemeal or seeded roll with lean meat, fish or egg, and a salad
- Wholemeal wrap with fish, avocado, humous and/or chicken
- Jacket potato with toppings such as beans, tomato ragu or tuna
- Sushi
- Fresh soup and a roll
- Salad with pasta, rice or cous cous

Eating from each of the four food groups

The British Nutrition Foundation (2019) recommends that everybody regularly eats from each of the four main food groups: starchy carbohydrates, fruit and vegetables, protein and low-fat dairy.

Starchy carbohydrates

Choose wholemeal options and aim for at least 260 g per day. Example foods include:

- bread: for a sandwich or with soup (approx. 12 g carbohydrate per slice)
- rice: 100 g cooked (approx. 28 g carbohydrate)
- pasta: 100 g cooked (approx. 31 g carbohydrate)
- potatoes: 100 g baked with skin on (approx. 22.6 g carbohydrate).

Fruit and vegetables

Aim for at least five different types per day. Example foods include:

- watermelon: 100 g (approx. 8 g carbohydrate)
- strawberries: 100 g (approx. 8 g carbohydrate)
- raspberries: 100 g (approx. 10 g carbohydrate)
- cucumber: 100 g (approx. 9g carbohydrate)
- broccoli: 100 g (approx. 7g carbohydrate)
- tomatoes: 100 g (approx. 3 g carbohydrate).

All fruits contain natural sugars and the water content in them supplements your daily recommended fluid intake as well.

Protein

Aim for 45–55 g per day (Public Health England 2016). Example foods include:

- chicken breast: 100 g grilled (approx. 32 g protein)
- lean beef steak: 100 g grilled (approx. 31 g protein)
- salmon: 100 g grilled (approx. 24 g protein)
- tuna: 100 g canned (approx. 24 g protein)
- eggs (chicken): 100 g (13 g protein)
- chickpeas: 100 g (approx. 8 g protein)
- kidney beans: 100 g (approx. 7 g protein)
- almonds: 100 g (approx. 21 g protein)
- walnuts: 100 g (approx. 14 g protein).

Low-fat dairy

Aim for two or three portions of low-fat dairy per day (Public Health England 2018). Example foods include:

- semi-skimmed milk: 100 g (approx. 3 g protein)
- low fat cheddar cheese: 100 g (approx. 26 g protein)
- yogurt (plain, low fat): 100 g (approx. 5 g protein).

Box 19.4 Ideas for snacks

- Fresh fruit
- Dried fruit mix with seeds and nuts
- Low-fat or 0% fat yogurts and fromage frais
- Cereal bars (wholegrain)
- Baked or popped crisps
- Chopped raw vegetables with dips such as humous

Source: Adapted from Hinton (2017).

Snacking

Many people snack, and these can be a useful energy source when working a long, busy day on the ward. Hignett (2017) suggests the following helpful hints relating to snacking:

- Snacks that are high in protein, fibre and wholegrains help to fill us up.
- Choose snacks that contain cereals, fruit and vegetables.
- Take care not to overindulge in snacks high in sugar.
- Choose low-fat snacks.
- Keep portions small.

Box 19.4 provides some ideas on snack choices, and the next section suggests snacking approaches that may help to sustain a positive mood.

Food and mood

When you work in an emotionally demanding job, being very mindful of what you are eating and drinking is essential, as food and hydration have a significant impact on how you feel. Eating well and staying hydrated will help you to cope better psychologically and physically, and will affect your concentration, energy levels, and ability to give compassionate and thoughtful care.

Food literally affects your mood. Under stress, the body craves rapidly acting carbohydrates to fuel the fight-or-flight response, which is why we favour sweet or starchy foods during times of stress. These foods temporarily give us an emotional lift but then add to our feelings of anxiety. This is because as they are quickly absorbed they cause a ‘crash’ in blood glucose, lowering mood and leading to further ‘sugar fix’ cravings. Fruit is good for you, but some is very high in natural sugar, so it is best to avoid eating it on an empty stomach and better to eat it with or after a meal. Controlling blood glucose levels during times of stress is therefore essential to avoid this swinging effect and subsequent mood changes.

To avoid this swinging, it is advised to choose foods with a low glycaemic index; they are harder for the body to absorb the glucose from. This means their glucose is released over a sustained period, preventing the rapid highs and lows that affect mood. As an example, choosing a wholegrain cereal, porridge, yogurt, smoothie or eggs for breakfast and avoiding white bread or very refined and sugary cereals will control your blood glucose better. Similarly, at lunch time, picking sandwiches made with brown bread over white, or choosing a jacket potato rather than chips, can make all the difference. After a long shift, it is essential to eat, but if a meal high in carbohydrates is eaten too close to bedtime, it may keep you awake. Therefore, it is better to choose smaller portion sizes that are high in protein if you are planning to go to sleep within 2 hours.

Snacks are important and can ‘keep you going’ until you are able to take a break, but avoid sugary sweets, chocolate and fizzy drinks as the glucose in these will be rapidly absorbed and have a negative effect on your mood. Nuts and seeds will give you energy without affecting your blood glucose, and both bananas and dark chocolate with a very high percentage of cocoa contain natural sources of serotonin, which can lift your mood. A good snack to make up at home and carry with you to work is the ‘good mood mix’ (Box 19.5).

Box 19.5 Good mood mix

Make up a mix of the following as a snack to lift your mood:
- mixed nuts
- dried banana chips
- dark chocolate chips.

You could also add other nuts, fruit and seeds that can help your mood, for example:
- Sunflower seeds are a natural source of norepinephrine, which can raise your mood.
- Pumpkin seeds contain magnesium, which is known to help alleviate anxiety.
- Dried cranberries can improve immunity.

Hydration

Water and good hydration are essential for life. Water has a number of roles within the body. For example, it:

- is a major constituent of the body
- transports nutrients and compounds in blood
- removes waste products, which are passed in the urine
- acts as a lubricant in joints
- regulates the body's temperature (Gandy 2017).

Dehydration affects concentration and cognitive function, and it also triggers fatigue. As a result, just like missing rest breaks, being inadequately hydrated is not just a wellbeing-at-work issue but an issue of patient and staff safety.

A study of the hydration levels of clinical staff at an NHS hospital found that 36% of participants were dehydrated before they started their shift. Using urine samples and short-term memory tests, the study also found that 45% of participants were dehydrated at the end of their shift, and that cognition was significantly impaired in dehydrated participants (El-Sharkawy 2016). Physical activity (such as being on a busy shift for 12 hours) and environmental temperatures can increase the need to keep hydrated. Nurses frequently complain of not being able to access drinking water while at work. In a survey of RCN members, 25% of respondents reported that they were not allowed to have water on the wards or at the nurses' station while at work (RCN 2017). Members who responded to this survey also reported that the pressure of work can lead to the inability to drink, go to the toilet or eat (RCN 2017).

Thirst is part of the way that the body regulates the body's hydration. However, it is important to note that people tend to stop drinking when their thirst subsides, but this normally occurs before true hydration. The colour of urine is the best indicator; if you are drinking enough fluid throughout the day, then your urine should be a straw or pale yellow colour (Figure 19.4). If it is dark, you must drink more. If you do not drink enough fluid, you may experience a variety of symptoms, such as tiredness, poor concentration, headache, and dizziness or light-headedness.

How much should I drink?

Men need a minimum of 2000 mL per day and women need a minimum of 1600 mL per day. The amount increases for women who are pregnant or lactating. It also increases in warm weather or in warm and dry environments, such as air-conditioned offices or wards. Additionally, centrally heated homes increase the need for water as they speed up the evaporation of sweat on the skin. The amount you need will also increase if you are busy with manual duties or engage in exercise (Figure 19.3).

What should I drink?

There are many options available. In the UK, drinking plain tap water is a good, cheap way to get enough to drink, and the water can be chilled or filtered depending on taste. Bottled water has the same hydrating abilities as tap water. Tea and coffee will also provide water. Fizzy and still drinks contain a lot of sugar and should only be drunk in small amounts; ideally choose sugar-free versions. Fruit juices provide water and other nutrients but contain sugar so only have one small serving per day. This counts towards your five servings a day of fruit and vegetables.

Caffeine

It is important to remember that caffeine is a stimulant, which means that although it will give you a quick burst of energy, it may then make you feel anxious and depressed, disturb your sleep (especially if you have it before bed) or give you withdrawal symptoms if you stop suddenly (Mind 2019). Caffeine-rich sources of liquid include tea, coffee, cola and other manufactured energy drinks. If you decide to drink less caffeine, you could try switching to decaffeinated versions of these drinks.

Physical wellbeing and musculoskeletal health

Related theory

An ergonomic work systems approach to preventing musculoskeletal disorders in the workplace has long been advocated and forms the basis of the Manual Handling Operations Regulations (1992). In order to ensure the health, safety, performance, comfort and wellbeing of all employees, it is essential for them to avoid hazardous physical tasks or for such tasks to be rigorously risk assessed if they cannot be avoided, so as to remove or reduce physical stresses and strains on the body. An ergonomic work systems approach takes into consideration all aspects of the work system, both in the assessment process and in the risk reduction process, to ensure that no hazard goes unnoticed and that all risks are identified and then removed or minimized. This includes:

- the nature of the task
- the characteristics of the individual staff member (weight, height, age, etc.) and their colleagues
- the nature of the load itself
- the environment
- any equipment available
- less tangible psychosocial hazards, such as time pressures and staff shortages.

It is a continuous and dynamic problem-solving approach, and is an essential component of a healthcare professional's clinical reasoning when caring for patients.

200 mL tea	**8:00** Morning handover
200 mL coffee	**10:00** Morning coffee
200 mL water	**12:00** Before serving lunches
200 mL decaffeinated tea	**14:00** During afternoon break
200 mL water	**17:00** Before serving supper
200 mL decaffeinated tea	**19:00** While writing up notes at the end of a shift

Figure 19.3 How many cups should I drink on a 12 hour shift?

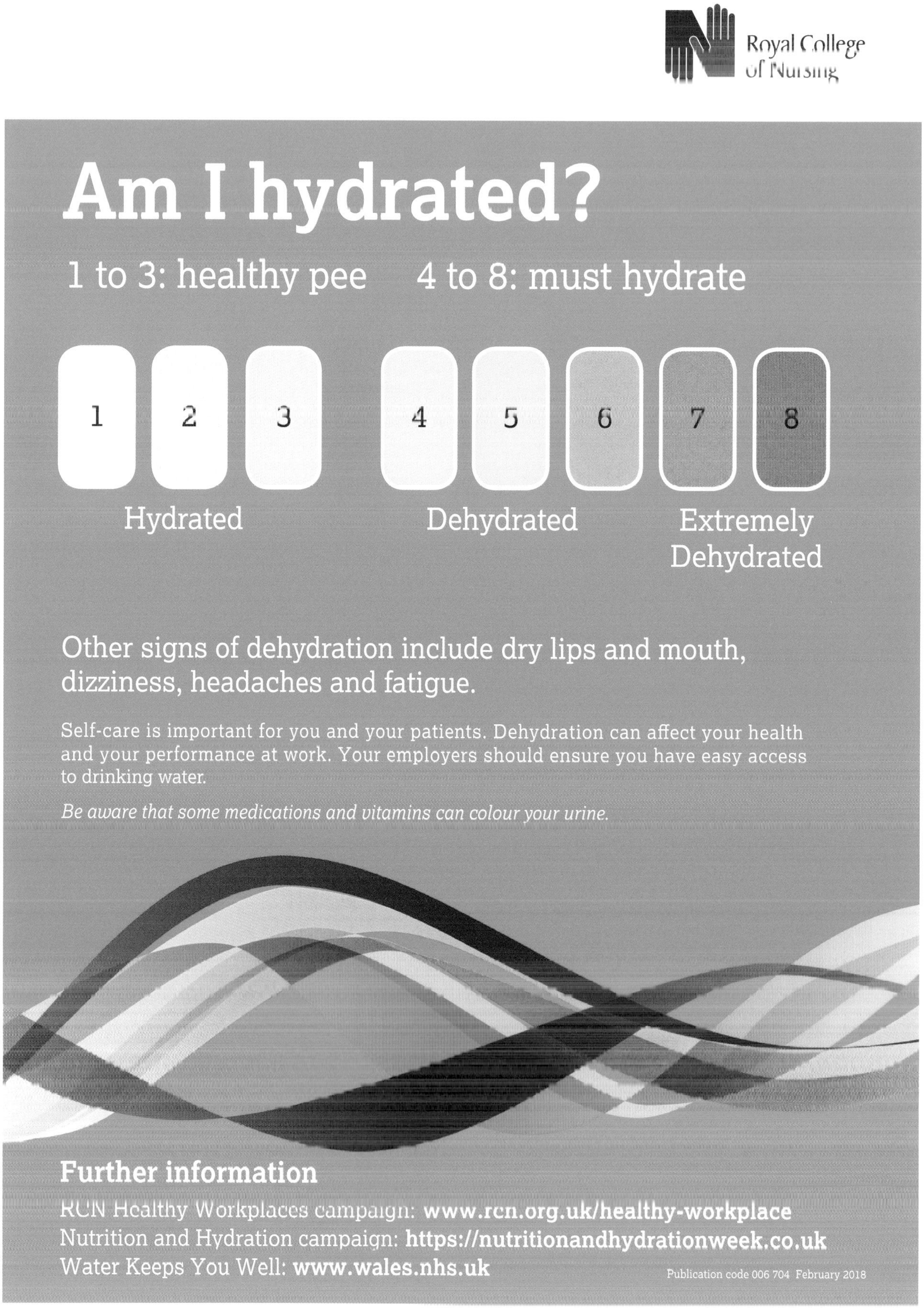
Royal College of Nursing
Am I hydrated?
1 to 3: healthy pee
4 to 8: must hydrate
1
2
3
4
5
6
7
8
Hydrated
Dehydrated
Extremely Dehydrated
Other signs of dehydration include dry lips and mouth, dizziness, headaches and fatigue.
Self-care is important for you and your patients. Dehydration can affect your health and your performance at work. Your employers should ensure you have easy access to drinking water.
Be aware that some medications and vitamins can colour your urine.
Further information
RCN Healthy Workplaces campaign: www.rcn.org.uk/healthy-workplace
Nutrition and Hydration campaign: https://nutritionandhydrationweek.co.uk
Water Keeps You Well: www.wales.nhs.uk
Publication code 006 704 February 2018

Figure 19.4 Am I hydrated? *Source*: Reproduced from RCN (2018) with permission of the Royal College of Nursing.

It is vital to ensure that staff are working within this safe system; for example, there should be:

- enough staff
- usable, adjustable and well-maintained equipment for which staff have received training
- good environmental workplace design
- training on the risk assessment and reduction process.

Once this system has been established, how healthcare professionals look after themselves and move their bodies when carrying out physical work tasks can further reduce the risk of injury.

Evidence-based approaches

Mandatory manual handling training educates staff about the biomechanical principles of safe moving and handling, for example:

- keeping the spine in line
- keeping the load close to the body
- bending the hips and knees rather than stooping and twisting
- keeping the feet in a wide, stable base.

The aim is to reduce physical stresses and strains on the lumbar spine but also the entire musculoskeletal system (HSE 2013). For tasks that involve handling patients, these principles can be adapted to include the following:

- keeping a walk-step stance (i.e. as if you are taking a step: legs apart, knees flexed, etc.)
- transferring bodyweight using the strong leg muscles
- avoiding overreaching by getting the patient to move closer or only handling the side of the patient closest to you
- raising the bed height or sinking down at the hips and knees (Smith 2011).

Where tasks are more static in nature and/or involve leaning or reaching forwards (e.g. assisting a patient to roll over in bed and supporting them in side-lying), a walk-step stance combined with attention to neck posture can reduce stresses and strains on the cervical, thoracic and lumbar spine regions.

For these tasks as well as those that involve prolonged sitting or standing (e.g. theatre tasks or computer use), the position of the head in relation to the trunk requires particular attention. If the head is directly above the trunk, it weighs approximately 5.5 kg. However, leaning the head forwards by just 5 cm increases its effective weight to approximately 15 kg; increasing this to 7.5 cm increases its effective weight to approximately 19 kg; and tilting the head down to a 60° angle increases its effective weight to approximately 27 kg (Figure 19.5). This forces the muscles of the neck and shoulders to work considerably harder; increases the loading and therefore the physical stresses and strains on the joints, soft tissues and nerves in the cervical spine; and heightens the risk of developing neck and upper limb musculoskeletal disorders over time (Kapandji 2019). This is a particular risk with computer use, where this issue may combine with poor seating and/or postures, lack of lumbar spine support, and overreaching to access the keyboard or mouse (Figure 19.6).

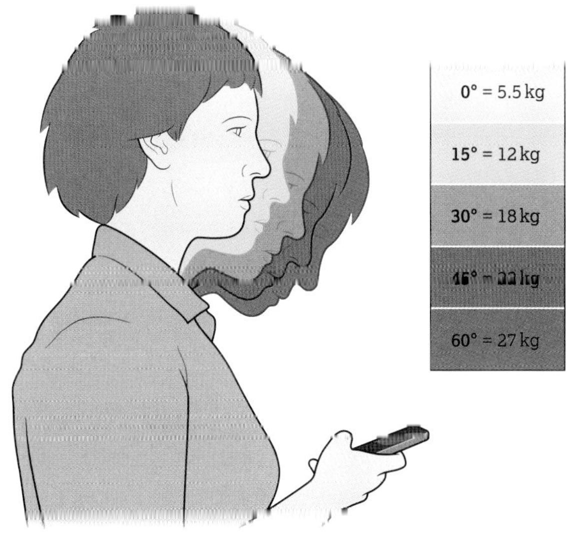

Figure 19.5 Illustration of weight burden on the spine as the head tips forward.

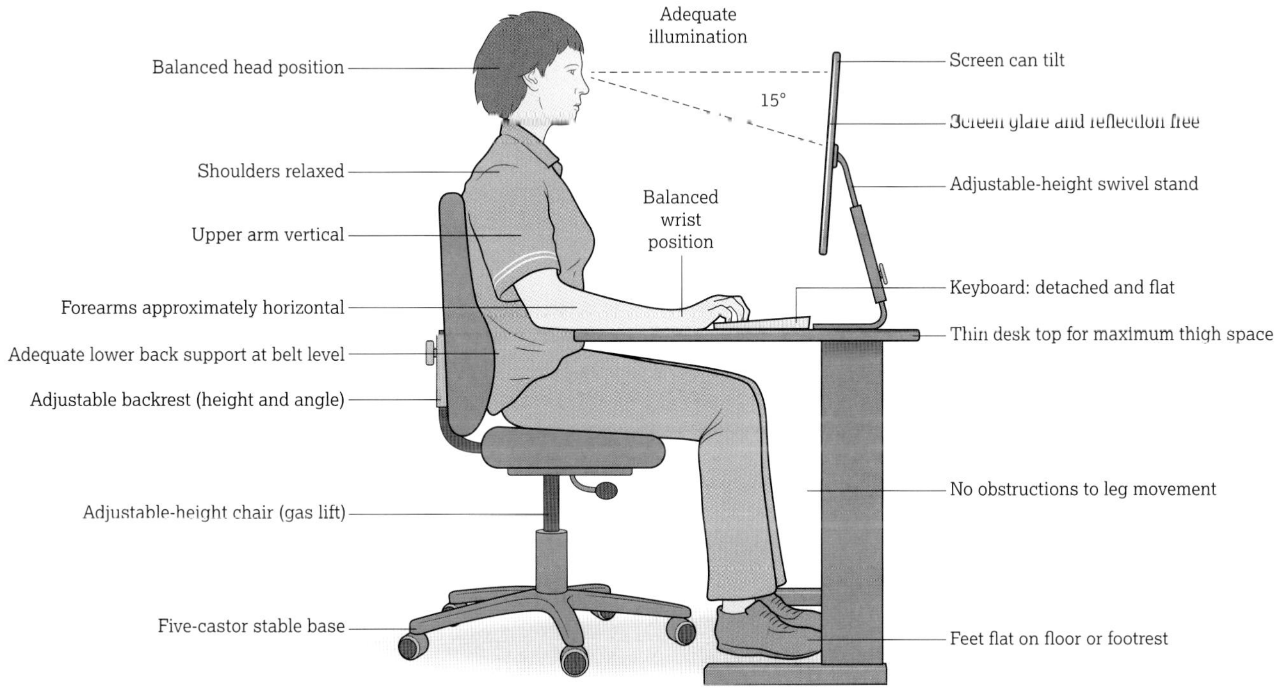

Figure 19.6 Workstation adjustment and efficient working posture.

It may seem inconsistent that bending and twisting the spine at a weekly yoga class is deemed beneficial whereas bending and twisting over a patient is high risk. The reason for this lies in repetition, as well as the potential for high forces. Risk factors for work-related musculoskeletal disorders are multifactorial and can be summarized as follows:

- poor postures (stooping and twisting)
- fixed or constrained body positions
- high forces (i.e. lifting, pulling and pushing)
- continual repetition of movements – doing these actions over and over again
- lack of recovery time
- psychosocial factors such as stress (HSE 2013).

Generally, none of these factors acts individually to cause injury; instead, injury occurs as a result of combinations of and interactions between these factors. Yoga may take your spine through the full range of movements a couple of times a week and improve your core strength, whereas a nurse may bend over a patient around 2000 times a day while also lifting, pushing and pulling at the same time (e.g. when lifting heavy legs into a bed, fitting hoist slings or repositioning patients in bed). Rather than improving flexibility and strengthening the core, adopting these compromised postures so excessively, especially when combined with high forces and psychosocial factors, may increase the risks of microtrauma and the development of cumulative musculoskeletal disorders over time (HSE 2013).

However, it is important to note that staff must not feel afraid to bend and twist; maintaining flexibility is very beneficial. The message is about reducing exposure to excessive bending and twisting during patient handling tasks, as well as reducing the accompanying high forces, for example by encouraging patient independence as much as possible, using equipment, adjusting working heights, using the strong leg muscles, and getting help to offload and share the physical stresses and strains. The Chartered Society of Physiotherapy (CSP) has published *Back Pain Myth Busters* (2016), which is an evidence-based guide to managing back pain and reducing fear; it also reinforces what the latest evidence says is best for the back when a person is experiencing discomfort. This includes not being afraid to bend and twist, keeping moving, and exercising regularly. Importantly, the CSP (2016) also suggests that pain does not always equal damage. The message is always about balance – to minimize excessive bending, twisting and heavy physical work and to adopt a balanced approach whereby staff consider the needs of patients and the goal of care, but where they do not forget to consider themselves in the process. This must all take place within a holistic, safe system of work that considers and addresses physical as well as psychosocial risk factors, which are the responsibility of both the employer and the employees (HSE 2013).

Healthcare professionals can further reduce the risk of developing musculoskeletal disorders by looking after their own health and fitness in terms of having a healthy lifestyle, maintaining a healthy weight and exercising regularly to ensure that they are fit for what can be quite physically demanding work. Shift patterns and constantly changing routines can make regular exercise a challenge, so the secret is to find something that is enjoyable so that it does not feel like another chore. Many hospital physiotherapy departments offer on-site staff yoga, Pilates or other exercise classes to make it easier for staff to get involved. Any exercise is better than none, even if it's simply parking your car further away from work and walking, or getting off the bus a couple of stops early.

In spite of this advice, those with pain or health concerns should always seek professional advice before embarking on a new exercise routine. Back care and musculoskeletal health require a 24-hour approach, and safe principles need to be incorporated into home and leisure activities as well as work tasks for maximum effect (Smith 2011).

Procedure guideline 19.1 Working at low or floor level

Essential equipment

- Low stool
- Kneeling pad
- Cushion for behind the knees

Action	Rationale
Pre-procedure	
1 Only work at floor level if there is no other option; always attempt to perform the task at a more functional height.	To minimize poor postures associated with working at or near floor level (HSE 2013, **C**).
2 Check there is sufficient space to kneel or sit on the floor close to the patient.	To reduce overreaching and stretching (Croshaw 2013, **C**).
Procedure	
3 Kneel in a comfortable position on a non-slip, wipeable kneeling pad or sit on a low stool if you are unable to kneel (**Action figure 3**). If kneeling, a cushion positioned behind the knees can improve comfort and posture.	To reduce the risk of prepatellar bursitis caused by kneeling on hard surfaces and to maintain a good spinal posture (Croshaw 2007, **E**). To help reduce the amount of flexion in the knees (Croshaw 2013, **E**).

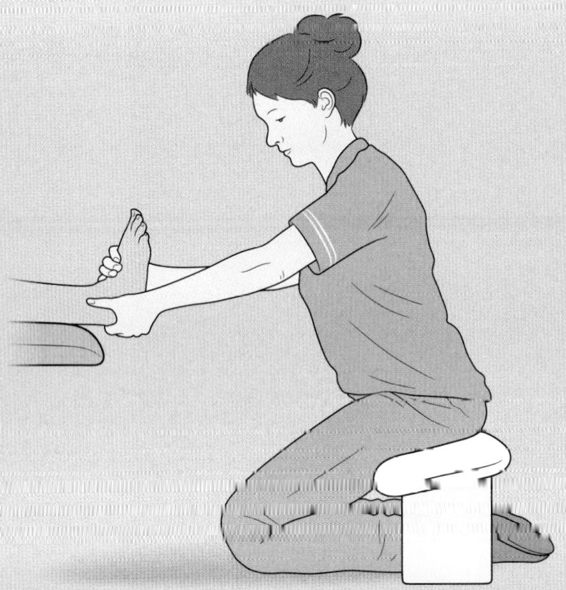

Action Figure 3a Combining a kneeling stool and a leg support to reduce strain on knees and keep the back upright. Some padding under the knees would make this position even more comfortable.

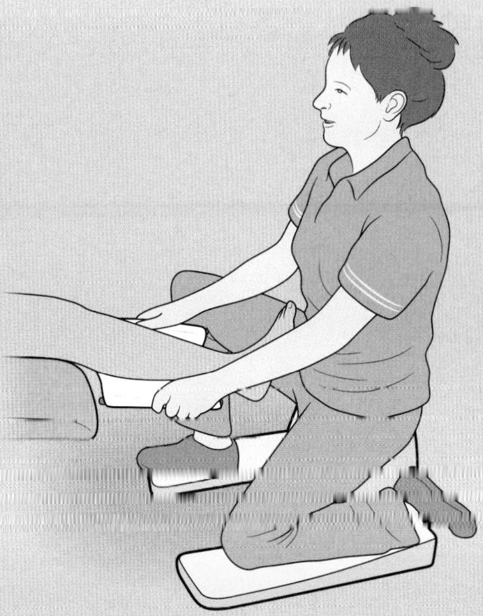

Action Figure 3b This stool can be used for sitting or kneeling on one or both knees. This allows for changes in posture while protecting the joints.

Procedure guideline 19.2 Working with a patient lying in a bed or on another raised supportive surface

Essential equipment

- Profiling hospital bed or other supine supportive surface (e.g. outpatient couch, theatre trolley or X-ray table)

Action	Rationale
Pre-procedure	
1 Familiarize yourself with the functions of the bed or supportive surface.	To ensure the bed or surface can be adjusted to the appropriate position (Smith 2011, **E**).
2 Ensure there is sufficient space around the bed or surface for all staff to move and position themselves freely.	To minimize poor posture for all staff involved (Smith 2011, **E**).
3 Ensure power cables are not interfering with the work area.	To minimize any trip hazards (HSE 2013, **C**).
Procedure	
4 Ensure that the bed is at the optimum height for the staff. If two members of staff are required, try to match staff heights as far as possible. Alternatively, raise the bed to the hip or waist height of the shortest team member.	To reduce the risk of cumulative strain and injury (Ruszala Alexander and Ruszala Alexander 2015, **E**).
5 Avoid reaching past the midline of the patient wherever it is reasonably practicable.	To minimize overreaching and stooping and to increase comfort. To reduce the risk of cumulative strain and injury (Ruszala Alexander and Ruszala Alexander 2015, **E**).
6 Adopt a walk stance with your feet close to the supportive surface.	To enable bodyweight transfer so as to facilitate techniques, and to maintain or improve posture (Smith 2011, **E**).

Procedure guideline 19.3 Carrying out clinical procedures in a seated posture (e.g. cannulation)

Essential equipment

- Adjustable wheeled chair or stool

Action	Rationale
Pre-procedure	
1 Familiarize yourself with the adjustable functions of the chair or stool.	To ensure the optimal seating position is achieved prior to undertaking the clinical procedure (Croshaw 2013, **C**).
2 Ensure the patient is in a comfortable position for the procedure and at the optimum height for your own posture.	To reduce the need to reposition the patient during the procedure and to improve staff posture. **P**
Procedure	
3 Sit up with your back in a neutral position with all three normal curves present. Where possible, your buttocks should touch the back of the chair. Adjust the back rest to support your spine in a neutral position.	To maintain a neutral spine and decrease physical stresses and strains on the spinal musculoskeletal system (HSE 2013, **C**).
4 Distribute your bodyweight evenly between both hips.	To minimize asymmetrical loading and physical stresses and strains on the musculoskeletal system (Smith 2011, **E**).
5 Flex your knees at a right angle. Keep your knees level with or slightly lower than the hips (use a footrest or stool if necessary).	To maintain a neutral lumbar spine and minimize drag and subsequent stresses and strains on the spinal musculoskeletal system (Smith 2011, **E**).
6 Do not cross your legs.	To reduce unnecessary twisting through the spine (Smith 2011, **E**).
7 Keep your feet flat on the floor	To ensure even weight distribution and muscle balance, and to minimize stresses and strains on the musculoskeletal system (Smith 2011, **E**).
8 Try to avoid sitting in the same position for more than 30 minutes.	To minimize physical stresses and strains on the musculoskeletal system and to ensure good blood flow and circulation (Smith 2011, **E**).

Procedure guideline 19.4 Working in a seated position: office work

Essential equipment

- Adjustable chair with a five-castor base

Action	Rationale
Procedure	
1 Adjust the chair so your lower back is properly supported. The chair should be adjustable so that the height, back position and tilt can all be changed easily.	A correctly adjusted chair will reduce the strain on your body (HSE 2013, **E**).
2 Adjust the chair height so that:	
• your buttocks are at the back of the chair and your lumbar spine is supported	To ensure a neutral spine is maintained (HSE 2013, **E**).
• your feet are placed flat on the floor or resting on a footrest if required	To ensure the lower limb joints are in a mid-range position (HSE 2013, **E**).
• your elbows are by the sides of your body so your arms form L shapes at the elbow joints with your wrists, and so your forearms are parallel to the floor and in neutral midline positions	To help reduce repetitive strain injuries (HSE 2013, **E**).
• the screen is positioned directly in front of you, approximately an arm's length away, with the top of the screen at eye level.	To reduce uncomfortable neck positions (HSE 2013, **E**).
3 Position and use the mouse as close to your body as possible. A mouse mat with a wrist pad may help to keep the wrist in a neutral position and avoid awkward bending.	To reduce unnecessary stresses and strains on the joints.

Post-procedural considerations

Continue to keep your and others' physical wellbeing and musculoskeletal health in mind. For example:

- Avoid remaining in any one position for a prolonged period of time.
- If you have adjusted the height of a bed or other raised supportive surface while working with a patient, lower the supporting surface after the procedure for patient safety.
- Avoid remaining in any one seated position for a prolonged period of time.
- Alter your posture as often as is practicable. Frequent short breaks are better for the back than fewer long ones.

Websites

British Dietetic Association: Food Facts
https://www.bda.uk.com/foodfacts/home

Collaborating for Health
https://www.c3health.org/our-programmes/health-professionals

Compendium of Factsheets: Wellbeing across the Lifecourse
https://www.bl.uk/collection-items/compendium-of-factsheets-wellbeing-across-the-lifecourse-what-works-to-improve-wellbeing

National Back Exchange
www.nationalbackexchange.org

NHS Live Well
https://www.nhs.uk/live-well

Sleepio (a sleep improvement program)
http://good-thinking.uk/sleepio

References

Arens, U. (2017) *Food and Mood*. British Dietetic Association. Available at: https://www.bda.uk.com/foodfacts/foodmood.pdf

Baranowsky, A.B., Gentry, J.E. & Schultz, F. (2011) *Trauma Practice: Tools for Stablisation and Recovery*, 2nd edn. Cambridge, MA: Hogrefe.

Boorman, S. (2009) *NHS Health and Well-being: Final Report, November 2009*. London: Department of Health.

British Dietetic Association (2016) *Protecting Your Lunch (or Meal) Breaks*. Available at: https://www.bda.uk.com/improvinghealth/awareness_raising/protecting_your_lunch_or_meal_breaks

British Dietetic Association (2017) *The Nutrition and Hydration Digest*, 2nd edn. Available at: https://www.bda.uk.com/regionsgroups/groups/foodservices/nutrition_hydration_digest

British Nutrition Foundation (2019) *Nutrients, Food and Ingredients*. Available at: https://www.nutrition.org.uk/nutritionscience/nutrients-food-and-ingredients

Burton, A., Burgess, C., Dean, S., et al. (2017) How effective are mindfulness-based interventions for reducing stress among healthcare professionals? A systematic review and meta-analysis. *Stress & Health*, 33(1), 3–13.

CIPD (Chartered Institute of Personnel and Development) (2013) *Absence Management: Annual Survey Report 2013*. London: CIPD.

CIPD (2016) *Growing the Health and Wellbeing Agenda: From First Steps to Full Potential*. Available at: https://www.cipd.co.uk/Images/health-well-being-agenda_2016-first-steps-full-potential_tcm18-10453.pdf

Coles, T.B. (2017) Compassion fatigue and burnout: History, definitions and assessment. *Veterinarian's Money Digest*, 27 October. Available at: https://www.vmdtoday.com/journals/vmd/2017/october2017/compassion-fatigue-and-burnout-history-definitions-and-assessment

Cozolino, L. (2017) *The Neuroscience of Psychotherapy*, 3rd edn. New York: W.W. Norton.

Croshaw, C. (2007) To kneel or not to kneel – that is the question. *Column: Journal of the National Back Exchange*, 19(3), 14–21.

Croshaw, C. (2013) *Working at or near Floor Level: A Survival Guide for Health and Social Care Staff*. Towcester, UK: National Back Exchange.

Cross-Government Obesity Unit (2009) *Healthy Weight, Healthy Lives: One Year On*. London: Department of Health.

CSP (Chartered Society of Physiotherapy) (2016) *Back Pain Myth Busters*. Available at: https://www.csp.org.uk/public-patient/back-pain-myth-busters

Dawson, D. (2009) *Does the Experience of Staff Working in the NHS Link to the Patient Experience of Care? An Analysis of the Link between the 2007 Acute Trust Inpatient and NHS Staff Surveys*. Institute for Health Services Effectiveness, Aston Business School. Available at: https://assets.publishing.service.gov.uk/government/uploads/system/uploads/attachment_data/file/215457/dh_129662.pdf

DH (Department of Health) (2009) *NHS Constitution: Interactive Version*. Available at: https://www.nhs.uk/NHSEngland/aboutnhs/Documents/NHS_Constitution_interactive_9Mar09.pdf

DH (2014a) *Wellbeing: Why It Matters to Health Policy*. Available at: https://assets.publishing.service.gov.uk/government/uploads/system/uploads/attachment_data/file/277566/Narrative__January 2014 .pdf

DH (2014b) *Healthcare Sector Staff Wellbeing, Service Delivery and Health Outcomes*. Available at: https://assets.publishing.service.gov.uk/government/uploads/system/uploads/attachment_data/file/277591/Staff_wellbeing__service_delivery_and_health_outcomes.pdf

DH (2014c) *Working Well: A Compendium of Factsheets – Wellbeing across the Lifecourse*. Available at: https://www.bl.uk/collection-items/compendium-of-factsheets-wellbeing-across-the-lifecourse-what-works-to-improve-wellbeing

El-Sharkawy, A.M. (2016) Hydration amongst nurses and doctors on-call (the HANDS on prospective cohort study). *Clinical Nutrition*, 35(4), 935–942.

Figley, C.R. (ed) (1995) *Compassion Fatigue: Coping with Secondary Traumatic Stress Disorder in Those Who Treat the Traumatized*. New York: Routledge.

Figley, C.R. (2002) Compassion fatigue: Psychotherapists' chronic lack of self care. *Journal of Clinical Psychology*, 58(11) 1433–1441.

Flarity, K., Gentry, J.E. & Mesnikoff, N. (2013) The effectiveness of an educational programme on preventing and treating compassion fatigue in emergency nurses. *Advanced Emergency Nursing Journal*, 35(3), 247–258.

Fletcher, G. (ed) (2015) *The Routledge Handbook of Philosophy of Wellbeing*. Routledge: New York.

Frankl, V. (1959) *Man's Search for Meaning*. New York: Pocket Books.

Gandy, J. (2017) *Fluid*. British Dietetic Association. Available at: https://www.bda.uk.com/foodfacts/fluid.pdf

Gentry, J.E. & Baranowsky, A.B. (2013) *Compassion Fatigue Resiliency: A New Attitude*. Available at: https://www.psychink.com/ti2012/wp-content/uploads/2013/10/Compassion-Resiliency-A-New-Attitude.pdf

Gustin, W. & Wagner, L. (2013) The butterfly effect of caring: Clinical nurse teachers' understanding of self compassion as a source of compassionate care. *Scandinavian Journal of Caring Sciences*, 27(1), 160–176.

Hayes, L. (2017) The power of self talk. *Lisa M. Hayes: Love Whisperer*, 11 October. Available at: https://www.lisamhayes.com/blog/post/the-power-of-self-talk

Hignett, J., ed. (2017) *Filling the Gap: Eating Well, Living Well*. Available at: www.eatingwellmag.co.uk

Hinton, F. (2017) *Healthy Snacks*. British Dietetic Association. Available at: https://www.bda.uk.com/foodfacts/healthysnacks.pdf

Holroyd, J. (2015) *Self-Leadership and Personal Resilience in Health and Social Care*. London: Sage.

Holzel, B.K., Carmody, J., Vangel, M., et al. (2011) Mindfulness practice leads to increases in regional brain gray matter density. *Psychiatry Research: Neuroimaging*, 191(1), 36–43.

House of Commons Health Committee (2018) *The Nursing Workforce: Second Report of Session 2017–19*. Available at: https://publications.parliament.uk/pa/cm201719/cmselect/cmhealth/353/353.pdf

HSE (Health and Safety Executive) (2013) *Ergonomics and Human Factors at Work: A Brief Guide*. Available at: www.hse.gov.uk/pubns/indg90.pdf

Joinson, C. (1992) Coping with compassion fatigue. *Nursing*, 22(116), 118–120.

Kapandji, A.I. (2019) *The Physiology of the Joints: Volume 3 – The Spinal Column, Pelvic Girdle and Head*, 7th edn. Pencaitland, UK: Handspring.

Keng, S.L., Smoski, M.J. & Robins, C.J. (2011) Effects of mindfulness on psychological health: A review of empirical studies. *Clinical Psychology Review*, 31(6), 1041–1056.

Keyser, C. (2011) *The Empathetic Brain: How the Discovery of Mirror Neurons Changes Our Understanding of Human Nature*. London: Social Brain Press.

Lazar, S.W., Kerr, C.E., Wasserman, R.H., et al. (2005) Meditation experience is associated with increased cortical thickness. *NeuroReport*, 16(17), 1893–1897.

Maben, J. (2010) The feel good factor. *Nursing Standard*, 24(30), 70–71.

Mark, G. & Smith, A.P. (2012) Effects of occupational stress, job characteristics, coping and attributional style on mental health and job satisfaction of university employees. *Anxiety, Stress & Coping*, 25, 63–78.

McManus, S. & Perry, J. (2012) *Work and Wellbeing* [British Social Attitudes Survey 29]. NatCen Social Research. Available at: www.bsa.natcen.ac.uk/latest-report/british-social-attitudes-29/work-and-wellbeing/introduction.aspx

MHOR (Manual Handling Operations Regulations) (1992) Available at: https://www.legislation.gov.uk/uksi/1992/2793/contents/made

Mind (2019) *Food and Mood*. Available at: https://www.mind.org.uk/information-support/tips-for-everyday-living/food-and-mood/#.XTwvy_7Fx0w

National NHS Staff Survey Co-ordination Centre (2013) *The 2013 NHS Staff Survey in England*. London: National NHS Staff Survey Co-ordination Centre.

Neff, K.D. (2003) Development and validation of a scale to measure self-compassion. *Self and Identity*, 2, 85–101.

Neff, K.D. (2011) *Self Compassion*. London: Hodder and Stoughton.

Neff, K.D. & Pommier, E. (2012) The relationship between self-compassion and other focused concern among college undergraduates, community adults, and practicing mediators. *Self and Identity*, 12(2), 160–176.

NHS (2017) *Reference Intakes Explained*. Available at: https://www.nhs.uk/live-well/eat-well/what-are-reference-intakes-on-food-labels

NHS Digital (2019) *NHS Sickness Absence Rates: November 2018 Provisional*. Available at: https://digital.nhs.uk/data-and-information/publications/statistical/nhs-sickness-absence-rates/november-2018-provisional-statistics

NHS Employers (2018) *Workforce Health and Wellbeing Framework*. Available at: https://www.nhsemployers.org/-/media/Employers/Publications/Health-and-wellbeing/NHS-Workforce-HWB-Framework_updated-July-18.pdf

NHS England (2016) *NHS Staff Health & Wellbeing: CQUIN Supplementary Guidance*. Available at: https://www.england.nhs.uk/wp-content/uploads/2016/03/HWB-CQUIN-Guidance.pdf.

Office for National Statistics (2015) *Measuring National Well-Being: Personal Well-Being in the UK, 2014 to 2015*. Available at: https://www.ons.gov.uk/peoplepopulationandcommunity/wellbeing/bulletins/measuringnationalwellbeing/2015-09-23

Pines, A.M. & Aronson, E. (1988) *Career Burnout Causes and Cures*. New York: Free Press.

Potter, P., Deshields, T., Allen Berger, J., et al. (2013) Evaluation of a compassion fatigue resiliency program for oncology nurses. *Oncology Nursing Forum*, 40(2), 180–187.

Public Health England (2016) *Government Dietary Recommendations: Government Recommendations for Energy and Nutrients for Males and Females Aged 1–18 Years and 19+ Years*. Available at: https://assets.publishing.service.gov.uk/government/uploads/system/uploads/attachment_data/file/618167/government_dietary_recommendations.pdf

Public Health England (2018) *Eatwell Guide*. Available at: https://assets.publishing.service.gov.uk/government/uploads/system/uploads/attachment_data/file/528193/Eatwell_guide_colour.pdf

Raleigh, V.S., Hussey, D., Seccombe, I. & Qi, R. (2009) Do associations between staff and inpatient feedback have the potential for improving patient experience? An analysis of surveys in NHS acute trusts in England. *Quality & Safety in Health Care*, 18(5), 347–354.

RCN (Royal College of Nursing) (2017) *Safe and Effective Staffing: Nursing against the Odds*. Available at: https://www.rcn.org.uk/professional-development/publications/pub-006415

RCN (2018) *Am I Hydrated?* London: Royal College of Nursing.

RCP (Royal College of Physicians) (2015) *Work and Wellbeing in the NHS: Why Staff Health Matters to Patient Care*. London: Royal College of Physicians.

Reman, R.N. (1996) *Kitchen Table Wisdom*. New York: Riverhead Books.

Riessman, F. (1965) The 'helper' therapy principle. *Social Work*, 10, 27–32.

Ruszala Alexander, S. & Ruszala Alexander, P. (2015) *Moving and Handling in Community and Residential Settings*. Towcester, UK: National Back Exchange.

Segal, Z., Williams, M. & Teasdale, J. (2013) *Mindfulness-Based Cognitive Therapy for Depression*, 2nd edn. London: Guilford Press.

Self Care Forum (2018) *What Do We Mean by Self Care and Why Is It Good For People?* Available at: www.selfcareforum.org/about-us/what-do-we-mean-by-self-care-and-why-is-good-for-people

Sheridan, C. (2016) *The Mindful Nurse: Using the Power of Mindfulness and Compassion to Help You Thrive in Your Work*. Galway, NY: Rivertime Press.

Sinclair, S., Raffin-Bouchal, S., Venturato, L., et al. (2017) Compassion fatigue: A meta-narrative review of healthcare literature. *International Journal of Nursing Studies*, 69, 9–24.

Skovholt, T.M. (1974) The client as helper: A means to promote personal growth. *Counselling Psychologist*, 4(3), 56–64.

Skovholt, T.M. & Trotter-Mathison, M. (2016) *The Resilient Practitioner: Burnout and Compassion Fatigue Prevention and Self-Care Strategies for the Helping Professionals*, 3rd edn. London: Routledge.

Smith, J. (2011) *Guide to the Handling of People: A Systems Approach*, 6th edn. Teddington, UK: Backcare.

Sulsky, L. & Smith, C.S. (2005) *Workplace Stress*. Belmont, CA: Thomas Wadsworth.

Thin, N. (2012) *Social Happiness: Theory into Policy and Practice*. Bristol: Policy Press.

Tosone, C., Bettmann, J.E., Minami, T. & Jasperson, R.A. (2010) New York City social workers after 9/11: Their attachment, resiliency and compassion fatigue. *International Journal of Emergency Mental Health*, 12(2), 103–116.

Ward, J. (2010) *The Student's Guide to Cognitive Neuroscience*, 2nd edn. Hove, UK: Psychology Press.

Watt, T. (2016) *Mindfulness: Your Step-by-Step Guide to a Happier Life*. London: Icon Books.

Waugh, C. (2014) The regulatory power of positive emotions in stress. In: Kent, M., Davis, M.C. & Reich, J.W. (eds) *The Resilience Handbook: Approaches to Stress and Trauma*. New York: Routledge, pp.73–85.

Wax, R. (2013) *Sane New World: Taming the Mind*. London: Hodder.

Williams, M. & Penman, D. (2011) *Mindfulness: A Practical Guide to Finding Peace in a Frantic World*. London: Piatkus.

Wiseman, T. (1996) A concept analysis of empathy. *Journal of Advanced Nursing*, 23(6), 1162–1167.

World Health Organization (2019) *Stress at the Workplace*. Available at: https://www.who.int/occupational_health/topics/stressatwp/en

Yalom, I.D. & Leszcz, M. (2005) *The Theory and Practice of Group Psychotherapy*, 5th edn. New York: Basic Books.

Appendix: Standards of Proficiency for Registered Nurses

Future Nurse: Standards of Proficiency for Registered Nurses (NMC 2018) mapped against the content of *The Royal Marsden Manual of Clinical Nursing Procedures*, 10th edition. Note that *Future Nurse* lists items 1.5 and 1.6 as outcomes rather than proficiencies, but they are included here because of their importance in nurses' practice.

Future Nurse proficiencies	Chapter in *The Royal Marsden Manual of Clinical Nursing Procedures*, 10th edition
Part 1: Procedures for assessing people's needs for person-centred care	
1. Use evidence-based, best practice approaches to take a history, observe, recognise and accurately assess people of all ages	
1.1 mental health and wellbeing status	Chapter 2: Admissions and assessment Chapter 5: Communication, psychological wellbeing and safeguarding
1.2 physical health and wellbeing	Chapter 2: Admissions and assessment
1.5 understand the demands of professional practice and demonstrate how to recognise signs of vulnerability in themselves or their colleagues and the action required to minimise risks to health	Chapter 19: Self-care and wellbeing
1.6 understand the professional responsibility to adopt a healthy lifestyle to maintain the level of personal fitness and wellbeing required to meet people's needs for mental and physical care	Chapter 19: Self-care and wellbeing
2. Use evidence-based, best practice approaches to undertake the following procedures	
2.1 take, record and interpret vital signs manually and via technological devices	Chapter 14: Observations
2.2 undertake venepuncture and cannulation and blood sampling, interpreting normal and common abnormal blood profiles and venous blood gases	Chapter 12: Respiratory care, CPR and blood transfusion Chapter 13: Diagnostic tests Chapter 17: Vascular access devices: insertion and management
2.3 set up and manage routine electrocardiogram (ECG) investigations and interpret normal and commonly encountered abnormal traces	Chapter 14: Observations
2.4 manage and monitor blood component transfusions	Chapter 12: Respiratory care, CPR and blood transfusion
2.5 manage and interpret cardiac monitors, infusion pumps, blood glucose monitors and other monitoring devices	Chapter 14: Observations
2.6 accurately measure weight and height, calculate body mass index and recognise healthy ranges and clinically significant low/high readings	Chapter 8: Nutrition and fluid balance
2.7 undertake a whole body systems assessment including respiratory, circulatory, neurological, musculoskeletal, cardiovascular and skin status	Chapter 2: Admissions and assessment Chapter 12: Respiratory care, CPR and blood transfusion Chapter 14: Observations
2.8 undertake chest auscultation and interpret findings	Chapter 2: Admissions and assessment

(continued)

The Royal Marsden Manual of Clinical Nursing Procedures: Professional Edition, Tenth Edition. Edited by Sara Lister, Justine Hofland and Hayley Grafton.

Future Nurse proficiencies	Chapter in *The Royal Marsden Manual of Clinical Nursing Procedures*, 10th edition
2.9 collect and observe sputum, urine, stool and vomit specimens, undertaking routine analysis and interpreting findings	Chapter 13: Diagnostic tests
2.10 measure and interpret blood glucose levels	Chapter 14: Observations
2.11 recognise and respond to signs of all forms of abuse	Chapter 5: Communication, psychological wellbeing and safeguarding
2.12 undertake, respond to and interpret neurological observations and assessments	Chapter 14: Observations
2.13 identify and respond to signs of deterioration and sepsis	Chapter 14: Observations
2.15 administer basic physical first aid	Chapter 12: Respiratory care, CPR and blood transfusion
2.16 recognise and manage seizures, choking and anaphylaxis, providing appropriate basic life support	Chapter 12: Respiratory care, CPR and blood transfusion
2.17 recognise and respond to challenging behaviour, providing appropriate safe holding and restraint.	Chapter 5: Communication, psychological wellbeing and safeguarding
Part 2: Procedures for the planning, provision and management of person-centred nursing care	
3. Use evidence-based, best practice approaches for meeting needs for care and support with rest, sleep, comfort and the maintenance of dignity, accurately assessing the person's capacity for independence and self-care and initiating appropriate interventions	Chapter 9: Patient comfort and supporting personal hygiene
4. Use evidence-based, best practice approaches for meeting the needs for care and support with hygiene and the maintenance of skin integrity, accurately assessing the person's capacity for independence and self-care and initiating appropriate interventions	Chapter 9: Patient comfort and supporting personal hygiene
5. Use evidence-based, best practice approaches for meeting needs for care and support with nutrition and hydration, accurately assessing the person's capacity for independence and self-care and initiating appropriate interventions	Chapter 8: Nutrition and fluid balance
6. Use evidence-based, best practice approaches for meeting needs for care and support with bladder and bowel health, accurately assessing the person's capacity for independence and self-care and initiating appropriate interventions	Chapter 6: Elimination
7. Use evidence-based, best practice approaches for meeting needs for care and support with mobility and safety, accurately assessing the person's capacity for independence and self-care and initiating appropriate interventions	Chapter 7: Moving and positioning
8. Use evidence-based, best practice approaches for meeting needs for respiratory care and support, accurately assessing the person's capacity for independence and self-care and initiating appropriate interventions	Chapter 12: Respiratory care, CPR and blood transfusion
9. Use evidence-based, best practice approaches for meeting needs for care and support with the prevention and management of infection, accurately assessing the person's capacity for independence and self-care and initiating appropriate interventions	Chapter 4: Infection prevention and control
10. Use evidence-based, best practice approaches for meeting needs for care and support at the end of life, accurately assessing the person's capacity for independence and self-care and initiating appropriate interventions	Chapter 11: Symptom control and care towards the end of life
11. Procedural competencies required for best practice, evidence-based medicines administration and optimisation	Chapter 15: Medicines optimization: ensuring quality and safety Chapter 17: Vascular access devices: insertion and management

Sources

Nursing and Midwifery Council (2018) Annexe B: Nursing procedures. In: *Future Nurse: Standards of Proficiency for Registered Nurses*. Available at: https://www.nmc.org.uk/globalassets/sitedocuments/education-standards/future-nurse-proficiencies.pdf

Nursing and Midwifery Council (2018) *The Code: Professional Standards of Practice and Behaviour for Nurses, Midwives and Nursing Associates*. Available at: https://www.nmc.org.uk/standards/code

List of abbreviations

AAC augmentative or alternative communication
AACCN American Association of Critical-Care Nurses
AAGBI Association of Anaesthetists of Great Britain and Ireland
ABCDE airway, breathing, circulation, disability, exposure
ABG arterial blood gas
ABHR alcohol-based handrub
ACBS Advisory Committee on Borderline Substances
ACPIN Association of Chartered Physiotherapists in Neurology
ACS acute coronary syndromes
ACT acceptance and commitment therapy
ACTH adrenocorticotropic hormone
AD autonomic dysreflexia
ADASS Association of Directors of Adult Social Services
ADCC antibody-dependent cell-mediated cytotoxic
ADH antidiuretic hormone
ADP adenosine diphosphate
ADR adverse drug reaction
ADRT Advance Decision to Refuse Treatment
A&E accident and emergency
AED automated external defibrillator
AfPP Association for Perioperative Practice
AIDS acquired immune deficiency syndrome
ALARP as low as reasonably practicable
ALS acute life support
ALT alanine aminotransferase
ANH acute normovolaemic haemodilution
ANS autonomic nervous system
ANTT aseptic non-touch technique
AORN Association of periOperative Registered Nurses
AP alkaline phosphatase/anteroposterior/alternating pressure
APTT activated partial thromboplastin time
ARDS acute respiratory distress syndrome
ART assisted reproductive technique
ASA American Society of Anesthesiologists
ASCN Association of Stoma Care Nurses
ASHP American Society of Hospital Pharmacists
ASIA American Spinal Injury Association
AST accelerated Seldinger technique/aspartate aminotransferase
AT anaerobic threshold
ATP adenosine triphosphate
AUC area under the curve
AV atrioventricular
AVPU Alert, Verbal, Pain, Unresponsive
BAL bronchoalveolar lavage
BAPEN British Association for Parenteral and Enteral Nutrition
BAUS British Association of Urological Surgeons
BCSP Bowel Cancer Screening Programme
BDA British Dietetic Association
BIA bioelectrical impedance analysis/bioimpedance analysis
BIPAP bilevel positive airway pressure
BLS basic life support
BMAS British Medical Acupuncture Society
BMF bone marrow failure
BMI body mass index
BNF British National Formulary
BP blood pressure
BPI Brief Pain Inventory
BPS Behavioural Pain Scale
BSA British Society of Audiology
BSACI British Society for Allergy and Clinical Immunology
BSE bovine spongiform encephalopathy
BSG British Society of Gastroenterology
BSH British Society for Haematology
BTS British Thoracic Society
BUN blood urea nitrogen
BVM bag valve mask
CAJ cavo-atrial junction
CAS Central Alerting System
CAUTI catheter-associated urinary tract infection
CBT cognitive–behavioural therapy
CCG Clinical Commissioning Group
CCU coronary care unit
CD controlled drug/curative dose
CDC complement-dependent cytotoxic
CDI *C. difficile* infection
CE Conformité Européenne (European Conformity)
CFT compassion-focused therapy
cfu colony-forming unit
CHB clinical handwash basin
CHG chlorhexidine gluconate
CISC clean intermittent self-catheterization
CJD Creutzfeldt–Jakob disease
CMC Coordinate My Care
CMV cytomegalovirus
CNS central nervous system
CO cardiac output
COMA Committee on Medical Aspects of Food Policy
COPD chronic obstructive pulmonary disease
COX-2 cyclo-oxygenase-2-selective inhibitor
CP cerebral palsy
CPAP continuous positive airway pressure
CPET cardiopulmonary exercise testing
CPNB continuous peripheral nerve block
CPOT Critical-Care Pain Observational Tool
CPR cardiopulmonary resuscitation
CQC Care Quality Commission
CRBSI catheter-related bloodstream infection
CRGSCI Clinical Reference Group for Spinal Cord Injury
CRP C-reactive protein
CSF cerebrospinal fluid
CSII continuous subcutaneous insulin infusion
CSNAT Carer Support Needs Assessment Tool
CSP Chartered Society of Physiotherapy
CSRDs closed system reconstitution devices
CSS central sterile services
CT computed tomography
CTZ chemoreceptor trigger zone
CVA cerebrovascular accident
CVAD central venous access device
CVC central venous catheter
CVP central venous pressure

The Royal Marsden Manual of Clinical Nursing Procedures: Professional Edition, Tenth Edition. Edited by Sara Lister, Justine Hofland and Hayley Grafton.

CXR	chest X-ray
DBEs	deep breathing exercises
DBT	dialectical behavioural therapy
DBWC	double-barrelled wet colostomy
DEFRA	Department for Environment, Food and Rural Affairs
DfE	Department for Education
DGSA	dangerous goods safety advisor
DH	Department of Health
DIC	disseminated intravascular coagulation
DIPC	director of infection prevention and control
DisDAT	Disability Distress Assessment Tool
DIVA	difficult intravenous access
DM	diabetes mellitus
DMSO	dimethylsulphoxide
DNA	did not attend
DNaCPR	do not attempt cardiopulmonary resuscitation
DNR	do not resuscitate
DoLS	Deprivation of Liberty Safeguards
DPG	diphosphoglycerate
DRE	digital rectal examination
DRF	digital removal of faeces
DRG	dorsal respiratory group (neurones)
DSU	day surgery unit
DVT	deep vein thrombosis
EASHW	European Agency for Health and Safety at Work
EAUN	European Association of Urology Nurses
EBN	evidence-based nursing
EBP	evidence-based practice
ECF	extracellular fluid
ECG	electrocardiogram/electrocardiography
ECHO	echocardiogram/echocardiography
ECOG	Eastern Cooperative Oncology Group
EDTA	ethylenediamine tetra-acetic acid
EEG	electroencephalogram
ELISA	enzyme-linked immunosorbent assay
EMLA	eutectic mixture of local anaesthetics
EMR	endoscopic mucosal resection
ENT	ear, nose and throat
EPaCCS	Electronic Palliative Care Co-ordination Systems
EPMA	electronic prescribing and medicines administration
EPR	electronic patient record
EPSG	Enteral Plastic Safety Group
EPUAP	European Pressure Ulcer Advisory Panel
ESD	endoscopic submucosal dissection
ESPAUR	English Surveillance Programme for Antimicrobial Utilisation and Resistance
ESR	erythrocyte sedimentation rate
ETT	endotracheal tube
EU	European Union
EWS	early warning scoring
FBC	full blood count
FEES	fibreoptic endoscopic evaluation of swallowing
FEV	forced expired volume
FFI	fatal familial insomnia
FFP	fresh frozen plasma
FGM	female genital mutilation
FPM	Faculty of Pain Management
FRC	functional residual capacity
FSA	Food Standards Authority
FVC	forced vital capacity
FWB	fully weight bearing
GABA	gamma-aminobutyric acid
GAD	generalized anxiety disorder
GAIN	Guidelines and Audit Implementation Network
GCS	Glasgow Coma Scale
GFR	glomerular filtration rate
GGT	gamma-glutamyl transpeptidase
GI	gastrointestinal
GMC	General Medical Council
GM-CSF	granulocyte-macrophage colony-stimulating factor
GTN	glyceryl trinitrate
GvHD	graft versus host disease
HAS	human albumin solution
HBN	Health Building Note
HBV	hepatitis B virus
HCAI	healthcare-associated infection
HCPC	Health and Care Professions Council
HCV	hepatitis C virus
HDFN	haemolytic disease of the foetus and newborn
HDU	high-dependency unit
HEE	Health Education England
HFEA	Human Fertilisation and Embryology Authority
HFN	high-flow nasal (oxygen)
HIT	heparin-induced thrombocytopenia
HIV	human immunodeficiency virus
HLA	human leucocyte antigen
HME	heat and moisture exchanger
HNA	Holistic Needs Assessment/human neutrophil antigen
HOCF	Home Oxygen Consent Form
HOOF	Home Oxygen Ordering Form
HPA	Health Protection Agency
HPN	home parenteral nutrition
HPV	human papillomavirus
HR	heart rate
HSCT	haemopoietic stem cell transplant
HSE	handling and storage errors/Health and Safety Executive
HTLV	human T cell leukaemia/lymphoma virus
HWR	Hazardous Waste Regulations
IAD	incontinence-associated dermatitis
IAPT	Improving Access to Psychological Therapies
IASP	International Association for the Study of Pain
IBCT	incorrect blood component transfused
ICD	implanted cardiac defibrillator
ICF	intracellular fluid
ICP	intracranial pressure
ICS	intraoperative cell salvage
ICSI	intracytoplasmic sperm injection
ICU	intensive care unit
IDDSI	International Dysphagia Diet Standardisation Initiative
IF	interstitial fluid/intestinal failure
IgA	immunoglobulin A
IgM	immunoglobulin M
IHORM	Initial Home Oxygen Risk Mitigation Form
IJV	internal jugular vein
ILS	intermediate life support
IMCA	Independent Mental Capacity Advocate
INR	international normalized ratio
INS	Infusion Nurses Society
IP	independent prescriber
IPC	intermittent pneumatic compression
IPCT	infection prevention and control team
IR(ME)R	Ionising Radiation (Medical Exposure) Regulations
ISC	intermittent self-catheterization
ITDD	intrathecal drug delivery
ITU	intensive therapy unit
IU	international unit
IV	intravenous
JVP	jugular venous pressure
KDIGO	Kidney Disease: Improving Global Outcomes
KVO	keep vein open
LA	local anaesthetic
LANSS	Leeds Assessment of Neuropathic Symptoms and Signs
LBC	liquid-based cytology
LCT	long-chain triglyceride
LMA	laryngeal mask airway
LMW(H)	low-molecular-weight (heparin)
LocSSIPs	Local Safety Standards for Invasive Procedures
LPA	lasting power of attorney
LSD	lysergic acid diethylamide

mAbs	monoclonal antibodies
MAE	medication administration error
MAGIC	Michigan Appropriateness Guide for Intravenous Catheters
MALDI-TOF MS	matrix-assisted laser desorption ionization time-of-flight mass spectrometry
MAOI	monoamine oxidase inhibitor
MAP	mean arterial pressure
MARSI	medical adhesive-related skin injury
MBCT	mindfulness-based cognitive therapy
MBSR	mindfulness-based stress reduction
MCCD	Medical Certificate of Cause of Death
MCT	medium-chain triglyceride
MDI	metered dose inhaler
MDT	multidisciplinary team
MESA	microepididymal sperm aspiration
MHOR	Manual Handling Operations Regulations
MHRA	Medicines and Healthcare products Regulatory Agency
MIC	minimum inhibitory concentration
MNA	Mini Nutrition Assessment
MND	motor neurone disease
MPQ	McGill Pain Questionnaire
MRA	magnetic resonance angiography
MRC	Medical Research Council
MRCP	magnetic resonance cholangiopancreatography
MRE	magnetic resonance enterography
MRI	magnetic resonance imaging
MRS	magnetic resonance spectroscopy
MRSA	meticillin-resistant *Staphylococcus aureus* (prefer to methicillin-resistant *Staphylococcus aureus*)
MS	multiple sclerosis
MSCC	metastatic spinal cord compression
MSD	musculoskeletal disorder
MST	Malnutrition Screening Tool/modified Seldinger technique
MSU	midstream urine
MUAC	mid upper arm circumference
MUST	Malnutrition Universal Screening Tool
MVTR	moisture vapour transmission rate
NAT	nucleic acid testing
NARI	noradrenaline reuptake inhibitor
NaSSA	noradrenergic and specific serotonergic antidepressant
NatSSIPs	National Safety Standards for Invasive Procedures
NBM	nil by mouth
NBTC	National Blood Transfusion Committee
NCA	National Comparative Audit
NCAA	National Cardiac Arrest Audit
NCCAC	National Collaborating Centre for Acute Care
NCEPOD	National Confidential Enquiry into Patient Outcome and Death
NDRUK	Nutrition and Diet Resources United Kingdom
NEWS	National Early Warning Score
NFD	nephrogenic fibrosing dermopathy
NG	nasogastric
NHS	National Health Service
NHSBSA	National Health Service Business Service Authority
NHSBT	National Health Service Blood and Transplant
NHSCSP	NHS cancer screening programmes
NHSI	NHS Improvement
NICE	National Institute for Health and Care Excellence
NIV	non-invasive ventilation
NIVAS	National Infusion and Vascular Access Society
NMC	Nursing and Midwifery Council
NMDA	N-methyl-D-aspartate
NNNG	National Nurses Nutrition Group
NOK	next of kin
NPC	National Prescribing Centre
NPQ	Neuropathic Pain Questionnaire
NPSA	National Patient Safety Agency
NPUAP	National Pressure Ulcer Advisory Panel
NPWT	negative pressure wound therapy
NRAT	Norgine Risk Assessment Tool
NREM	non-rapid eye movement
NRLS	National Reporting and Learning System
NRS	numerical rating scale
NSAID	non-steroidal anti-inflammatory drug
NSF	nephrogenic systemic fibrosis
NWB	non-weight bearing
OCD	obsessive compulsive disorder
ODP	operating department practitioner
OIH	opioid-induced hyperalgesia
OPA	oropharyngeal airway
OSA	obstructive sleep apnoea
OT	occupational therapist
OTFC	oral transmucosal fentanyl citrate
PaCO2	partial pressure of carbon dioxide
PACU	post-anaesthetic care unit
PAD	pre-operative autologous donation
PADS	Pain and Discomfort Scale
PaO2	partial pressure of oxygen
PCA	patient-controlled analgesia
PCEA	patient-controlled epidural analgesia
PCR	polymerase chain reaction
PCT	proximal convoluted tubule
PD	Parkinson's disease
PDT	percutaneous dilatational tracheostomy
PE	pulmonary embolus
PEA	pulseless electrical activity
PEEP	positive end-expiratory pressure
PEF	peak expiratory flow
PEG	percutaneous endoscopically placed gastrostomy
PENG	Parenteral and Enteral Nutrition Group
PESA	percutaneous epididymal sperm aspiration
PGD	patient group direction
PG-SGA	patient-generated subjective global assessment
PHE	Public Health England
PHMB	polyhexamethylene biguanide
PICC	peripherally inserted central cannula/catheter
PICD	paracentesis-induced circulatory dysfunction
PIVC	peripheral intravenous cannula
PJs	pyjamas
PLPH	post-lumbar puncture headache
PMR	progressive muscle relaxation
PN	parenteral nutrition
PNS	peripheral nervous system
POA	pre-operative assessment
PONV	post-operative nausea and vomiting
PPE	personal protective equipment
PPPIA	Pan Pacific Pressure Injury Alliance
PPSA	Pennsylvania Patient Safety Authority
PRO	patient-reported outcome
PT	prothrombin time
PTA	pure tone audiometry
PTFE	polytetrafluoroethylene
PTH	parathyroid hormone
PTHrP	parathormone-related polypeptide
PTP	post-transfusion purpura
PTSD	post-traumatic stress disorder
PTT	partial thromboplastin time
PU	pressure ulcer
PVC	polyvinyl chloride
PVS	persistent vegetative state
PWB	partially weight bearing
PWO	partial withdrawal occlusion

RAS	reticular activating system
RBC	red blood cell(s)
RCA	Royal College of Anaesthetists
RCCP	Registration Council for Clinical Physiologists
RCN	Royal College of Nursing
RCOG	Royal College of Obstetricians and Gynaecologists
RCOT	Royal College of Occupational Therapists
RCP	Royal College of Physicians
RCPsych	Royal College of Psychiatrists
RCR	Royal College of Radiologists
RCT	randomized controlled trial
REM	rapid eye movement
RFID	radiofrequency identification
RIG	radiologically inserted gastrostomy
RNI	reference nutrient intake
RNOH	Royal National Orthopaedic Hospital
RPECCAS	Rotherham Primary Ear Care Centre and Audiology Services
RPS	Royal Pharmaceutical Society
RR	relative risk/respiration rate
RSV	respiratory syncytial virus
RTO	resuscitation training officer
SA	sinoatrial
SABRE	Serious Adverse Blood Reactions and Events
SaBTO	Safety of Blood, Tissues and Organs
SAGM	saline, adenine, glucose and mannitol
SAM	self-administration of medicines
SAR	safeguarding adults review
SARS	severe acute respiratory syndrome
SBAR	Situation-Background-Assessment-Recommendation
SCC	spinal cord compression
SCI	spinal cord injury
SCST	Society for Cardiology Science and Technology
SDS	safety data sheet
SGA	subjective global assessment
SHOT	Serious Hazards of Transfusion
SIA	Spinal Injuries Association
SICP	standard infection control precaution
SIGN	Scottish Intercollegiate Guidelines Network
SLT	speech and language therapist
SNRI	serotonin–norepinephrine reuptake inhibitor
SNS	somatic nervous system
SP	supplementary prescriber
SPS	Specialist Pharmacy Service
SSI	surgical site infection
SSRI	selective serotonin reuptake inhibitor
STC	skin-tunnelled catheter
STEEP	Staying Steady Exercise and Education Programme
STI	sexually transmitted infection
SV	stroke volume
SVC	superior vena cava
SVR	surgical voice restoration/systemic vascular resistance
swg	standard wire gauge
TACO	transfusion-associated cardiac overload
TAD	transfusion-associated dyspnoea
TA-GVHD	transfusion-associated graft-versus-host disease
TB	tuberculosis
TBI	traumatic brain injury
TCA	tricyclic antidepressant
TCI	target controlled infusion
TED	thromboembolic deterrent
TENS	transcutaneous electrical nerve stimulation
TEP	tracheo-oesophageal puncture
TESE	testicular sperm extraction
TFT	thyroid function test
TIVA	total intravenous anaesthesia
TIVAD	totally implanted/implantable vascular access device
TO	total occlusion
TOE	transoesophageal echocardiogram
TPE	total pelvic exenteration
TPI	*Treponema pallidum* immobilization
TPN	total parenteral nutrition
TRALI	transfusion-related acute lung injury
TSE	transmissible spongiform encephalopathy
TSS	toxic shock syndrome
TTE	transthoracic echocardiogram
TTO	to take out
TTP	thrombotic thrombocytopenic purpura
TTS	transdermal therapeutic system
TURBT	transurethral resection of bladder tumour
TURP	transurethral resection of prostate
TVN	tissue viability nurse
UCLH	University College London Hospitals
UKOMiC	UK Oral Management in Cancer Care Group
UTI	urinary tract infection
VAD	vascular access device
VAP	ventilator-associated pneumonia
VAS	visual analogue scale
VAT	Venous Assessment Tool
VBG	venous blood gas
vCJD	variant Creutzfeldt–Jakob disease
VDRL	Venereal Disease Research Laboratory
VDS	verbal descriptor scale
VEGF	vascular endothelial growth factor
VF	ventricular fibrillation
VHP	vessel health preservation
VIP	visual infusion phlebitis (scoring system)
VPF	vascular permeability factor
V/Q	ventilation/perfusion
VRG	ventral respiratory group (neurones)
VT	ventricular tachycardia
VTE	venous thromboembolism
WBC	white blood cell(s)
WBIT	wrong blood in tube
WBP	wound bed preparation
WHO	World Health Organization
WR	Wassermann reaction

Index

Page numbers in *italics* refer to figures, and those in **bold** to tables or boxes.

The Royal Marsden Manual of Clinical Nursing Procedures: Professional Edition, Tenth Edition. Edited by Sara Lister, Justine Hofland and Hayley Grafton.